PARK'S TEXTBOOK OF PREVENTIVE AND SOCIAL MEDICINE

K. PARK
M.B.B.S., M.S.

TWENTY-SEVENTH EDITION

M/s BANARSIDAS BHANOT
PUBLISHERS

JABALPUR
1167, Prem Nagar,
Jabalpur - 482 001
Madhya Pradesh

PUNE
703, Konark Icon,
S.No. 134/1D/2, Hadapsar,
Magarpatta Road, Pune - 411 036

2023

M/s BANARSIDAS BHANOT
PUBLISHERS

JABALPUR
1167, Prem Nagar,
Jabalpur - 482 001 (M.P.)
Tel : +91-761 2424246, 94251 54030, 94251 52894
E-mail : banarsidasbhanot@gmail.com

PUNE
703, Konark Icon,
S.No. 134/1D/2, Hadapsar,
Magarpatta Road, Pune - 411 036
Tel : +91-20 48606788

ISBN No. 978-93-82219-19-4

1st	Edition	July,	1970
2nd	Edition	Nov,	1971
3rd	Edition	Sept,	1972
4th	Edition	April,	1974
5th	Edition	March,	1976
6th	Edition	July,	1977
7th	Edition	March,	1979
8th	Edition	Sept,	1980
9th	Edition	June,	1983
10th	Edition	Jan,	1985
11th	Edition	Nov,	1986
12th	Edition	Sept,	1989
13th	Edition	Dec,	1991
14th	Edition	Dec,	1994
15th	Edition	Sept,	1997
16th	Edition	Nov,	2000
17th	Edition	Nov,	2002
18th	Edition	Jan,	2005
19th	Edition	Feb,	2007
20th	Edition	Feb,	2009
21st	Edition	Feb,	2011
22nd	Edition	Feb,	2013
23rd	Edition	Jan,	2015
24th	Edition	Jan,	2017
25th	Edition	Feb,	2019
26th	Edition	Mar,	2021
27th	Edition	Feb,	2023

The twelfth edition was published under the title "Textbook of Preventive and Social Medicine"

PRICE Rs. 1700/-

NOTICE

The author and the publisher of this work have checked with sources believed to be reliable in their efforts to provide information that is complete and generally in accord with the standards accepted at the time of publication. However, in view of the possibility of human error or changes in medical sciences, neither the author nor the publisher warrants that the information contained herein is in every respect accurate or complete, and they disclaim all responsibility for any errors or omissions or for the results obtained from use of the information contained in this work. Readers are advised to confirm the information contained herein with other sources. In particular, readers are advised to check the product information sheet included in the package of each drug they plan to administer to be certain that the information contained in this work is accurate and that changes have not been made in the recommended dose or in the contraindications for administration.

The Book is dedicated to the revered memory of my husband

DR. JOHN EVERETT PARK

B.A., M.D., D.P.H., F.I.P.H.A., F.A.M.S.

the founder of this title

PREFACE

It is indeed gratifying that this book has seen twenty six successful editions and is now entering the twenty seventh edition – completing more than half century, with brand new look. The new edition is in keeping with the tradition of release of new editions at regular intervals with the objective to match the pace of everchanging subject matter.

The whole book has been updated thoroughly. The chapter of "Epidemiology of Communicable Diseases" have been updated, now it contains new treatment guidelines – particularly for COVID-19, tuberculosis, AIDS and new topic of Monkey Pox. Data from National Family Health Survey-5 has been incorporated as required. Every year, new schemes are being launched for the benefit of general public – like RMNCAH+N, SAANS, MAA programme, SUMAN, ANMOL etc. – have been added in the chapter of "Health Programmes in India". The chapter on "Preventive Medicine in Obstetrics, Paediatrics and Geriatrics" and chapter of "Demography and Family Planning" have been extensively updated.

The earlier chapter 24 – "Health Care of the Community" is now chapter 10 – it contains details of Indian Public Health Standards (2022) for all the levels of health care system – the new categorization of rural and urban Health and Wellness Centres – primary health centres and sub centres, citizen's charter, staff pattern and services available. Chapter of Essential Medicines (chapter 24) now contains the new (2022) recommendations.

In conclusion, I wish to express my gratitude to all those under graduate, post graduate students, and teachers whose comments and encouragement has helped me to keep the book up-to-date.

Lastly I extend my appreciation to Mr. Brij Mohan Bhanot for the care bestowed in publication of this book.

Jabalpur
February 2023

DR. MRS. KUMUD PARK

CONTENTS

1 Man and Medicine : Towards Health for All

"Those who fail to read history are destined to suffer the repetition of its mistakes"

From time immemorial man has been interested in trying to control disease. The medicine man, the priest, the herbalist and the magician, all undertook in various ways to cure man's disease and/or to bring relief to the sick. In an almost complete absence of scientific medical knowledge, it would not be fair to say that the early practitioners of medicine contributed nothing to the alleviation of man's suffering from disease. Medical knowledge in fact has been derived, to a very great degree, from the intuitive and observational propositions and cumulative experiences gleaned from others. A history of medicine thus contributes a review of accomplishments and errors, false theories and misinformation and mistaken interpretations. It is also a study of the evolution of man and of human knowledge down the ages; of the biographies of eminent individuals who developed medicine; of the discoveries and inventions in different historical periods; and of the ever-changing concepts, goals and objectives of medicine. In the course of its evolution, which proceeded by stages, with advances and halts, medicine has drawn richly from the traditional cultures of which it is a part, and later from biological and natural sciences and more recently from social and behavioural sciences. Medicine is thus built on the best of the past. In the crucible of time, medicine has evolved itself into a social system heavily bureaucratized and politicized. The "explosion" of knowledge during the 20th century has made medicine more complex, and treatment more costly, but the benefits of modern medicine have not yet penetrated the social periphery in many countries. The glaring contrasts in the state of health between the developed and developing countries, between the rural and urban areas, and between the rich and poor have attracted worldwide criticism as "social injustice". The commitment of all countries, under the banner of the World Health Organization, is to wipe out the inequalities in the distribution of health resources and services, and attain the Millenium Development Goals/ Sustainable Development Goals. The goal of modern medicine is no longer merely treatment of sickness. The other and more important goals which have emerged are prevention of disease, promotion of health and improvement of the quality of life of individuals and groups or communities. In other words, the scope of medicine has considerably broadened during recent years. It is also regarded as an essential component of socio-economic development.

I. MEDICINE IN ANTIQUITY

In ancient times, health and illness were interpreted in a cosmological and anthropological perspective. Medicine was dominated by magical and religious beliefs which were an integral part of ancient cultures and civilizations. Henry Siegerist, the medical historian has stated that every culture had developed a system of medicine, and medical history is but one aspect of the history of culture *(1)*. Dubos goes one step further and says that ancient medicine was the mother of sciences and played a large role in the integration of early cultures *(2)*. Since there is an organic relationship between medicine and human advancement, any account of medicine at a given period should be viewed against the civilization and human advancement at that time, i.e. philosophy, religion, economic conditions, form of government, education, science and aspirations of the people.

Primitive medicine

It has been truly said that medicine was conceived in sympathy and born out of necessity; and that the first doctor was the first man, and the first woman, the first nurse. The prehistoric man, motivated by feelings of sympathy and kindness, was always at the behest of his kindred, trying to provide relief, in times of sickness and suffering.

Since his knowledge was limited, the primitive man attributed disease, and in fact all human suffering and other calamities, to the wrath of gods, the invasion of body by "evil spirits" and the malevolent influence of stars and planets. The concept of disease in which the ancient man believed is known as the "supernatural theory of disease". As a logical sequence, the medicine he practised consisted in appeasing gods by prayers, rituals and sacrifices, driving out "evil spirits" from the human body by witchcraft and other crude means and using charms and amulets to protect himself against the influence of evil spirits. The administration of certain herbs or drugs whose effect is doubtful or nil, but hopefully harmless, may also be likened to a kind of magic ritual associated with the need to "do something". There is also evidence that prehistoric man improvised stone and flint instruments with which he performed circumcisions, amputations and trephining of skulls. It is thus obvious that medicine in the prehistoric times (about 5000 B.C.) was intermingled with superstition, religion, magic and witchcraft.

Primitive medicine is timeless. If we look around the world, we find that the rudiments of primitive medicine still persist in many parts of the world – in Asia, Africa, South America, Australia and the Pacific islands. The supernatural theory of disease in which the primitive man believed is as new as today. For example, in India, one may still hear the talk of curing snake bites by "mantras". Diseases such as leprosy are interpreted as being punishment for one's past sins in some cultures. Although primitive man may be extinct, his progeny – the so-called "traditional healers" are found everywhere. They live close to the people and their treatments are based on various combinations of religion, magic and empiricism.

Indian medicine *(3)*

The medical systems that are truly Indian in origin and development are the Ayurveda and the Siddha systems. Ayurveda is practised throughout India, but the Siddha system is practised in the Tamil-speaking areas of South India. These systems differ very little both in theory and practice *(4)*. Ayurveda by definition implies the "knowledge of life" or the knowledge by which life may be prolonged. Its origin is traced far back to the Vedic times, about 5000 B.C. During this period, medical history was associated with mythological figures, sages and seers. Dhanvantari, the Hindu god of medicine is said to have been born as a result of the churning of the oceans during a 'tug of war' between gods and demons. According to some authorities, the medical knowledge in the Atharvaveda (one of the four Vedas) gradually developed into the science of Ayurveda.

In ancient India, the celebrated authorities in Ayurvedic medicine were Atreya, Charaka, Sushruta and Vaghbhatt. Atreya (about 800 B.C.) is acknowledged as the first great Indian physician and teacher. He lived in the ancient university of Takshashila, about 20 miles west of modern Rawalpindi *(5)*. Ayurveda witnessed tremendous growth and development during the Buddhist times. King Ashoka (226 B.C.) and the other Buddhist kings patronized Ayurveda as State medicine and established schools of medicine and public hospitals. Charaka (200 A.D.), the most popular name in Ayurvedic medicine, was a court physician to the Buddhist king Kanishka. Based on the teachings of Atreya, Charaka compiled his famous treatise on medicine, the "Charaka Samhita". Charaka mentions some 500 drugs. The Indian snakeroot (rauwolfia) was employed for centuries by the Indian physicians, before *reserpine* was extracted from the root and found spectacularly effective in the treatment of hypertension.

Among the many distinguished names in Hindu medicine, that of Susruta, the "father of Indian surgery" stands out in prominence. He compiled the surgical knowledge of his time in his classic "Sushruta Samhita". It is believed that this classic was compiled between 800 B.C. and 400 A.D. Though this work is mainly devoted to surgery, it also includes medicine, pathology, anatomy, midwifery, ophthalmology, hygiene and bedside manners. The early Indians set fractures, performed amputations, excised tumours, repaired hernias and excelled in cataract operations and plastic surgery *(6)*. It is stated that the British physicians learned the art of rhinoplasty from Indian surgeons in the days of East India Company *(7)*. However, during Buddhist times, Indian surgery suffered a setback because of the doctrine of *ahimsa* (non-violence).

Of significance in Ayurveda is the "tridosha theory of disease". The *doshas* or humors are: *vata* (wind), pitta (gall) and kapha (mucus). Disease was explained as a disturbance in the equilibrium of the three humors; when these were in perfect balance and harmony, a person is said to be healthy *(8)*. This theory of disease is strikingly similar to the "theory of four humors" in Greek medicine. Medical historians admit that there was free exchange of thought and experience between the Hindu, Arab, Persian, Greek and Jewish scholars. The Samhitas of Charaka and Susruta were translated into Persian and Arabic in about 800 A.D.

Hygiene was given an important place in ancient Indian medicine. The laws of Manu were a code of personal hygiene. Archaeological excavations at Mohenjo-daro and Harappa in the Indus valley uncovered cities of over two thousand years old which revealed rather advanced knowledge of sanitation, water supply and engineering. The golden age of Indian medicine was between 800 B.C. and 600 A.D. During the Moghul period and subsequent years, Ayurveda declined due to lack of State support.

Medical historians admit that Indian medicine has played in Asia the same role as the Greek medicine in the west, for it has spread in Indochina, Indonesia, Tibet, Central Asia, and as far as Japan, exactly as the Greek medicine has done in Europe and Arab countries *(7)*.

Mention must be made of the other indigenous systems of medicine namely Unani-Tibb and Homoeopathy, which are not of Indian origin. The Unani-Tibb system of medicine, whose origin is traced to the ancient Greek medicine, was introduced into India by the Muslim rulers about the 10th century A.D. By the 13th century, the Unani system of medicine was firmly entrenched in certain towns and cities notably Delhi, Aligarh, Lucknow and Hyderabad *(5)*. It enjoyed State support under successive Muslim rulers in India, till the advent of the British in the 18th century. Homoeopathy, which was propounded by Samuel Hahnemann (1755–1843) of Germany gained foothold in India during 1810 and 1839 *(9)*. It is a system of pharmaco-dynamics based on "treatment of disease by the use of small amounts of a drug that, in healthy persons, produces symptoms similar to those of the disease being treated" *(10)*. Homoeopathy is practised in several countries, but India claims to have the largest number of practitioners of this system in the world *(9)*.

The Indian systems of medicine including Unani-Tibb and Homoeopathy are very much alive in India even today. In fact, they have become part of Indian culture, and they continue to be an important source of medical relief to the rural population.

Chinese medicine

Chinese medicine claims to be the world's first organized body of medical knowledge dating back to 2700 B.C. *(11)*. It is based on two principles – the yang and the yin. The yang is believed to be an active masculine principle and the yin a negative feminine principle. The balance of these two opposing forces meant good health. Hygiene, dietetics, hydrotherapy, massage, drugs were all used by the Chinese physicians.

The Chinese were early pioneers of immunization. They practised variolation to prevent smallpox. To a Chinese, "the great doctor is one who treats not someone who is already ill but someone not yet ill". The Chinese have great faith in their traditional medicine, which is fully integrated with modern medicine. The Chinese system of "barefoot doctors" and accupuncture have attracted worldwide attention in recent years *(12)*.

Egyptian medicine

Egypt had one of the oldest civilizations in about 2000 B.C. A lot is known about ancient Egypt because they invented picture writing and recorded their doings on papyrus. In Egyptian times, the art of medicine was mingled with religion. Egyptian physicians were co-equals of priests, trained in schools within the temples. They often helped priests care for the sick who were brought to the temples for treatment. There were no practical demonstrations in anatomy, for Egyptian religion enjoined strict preservation of the human body. Egyptian medicine reached its peak in the days of Imhotep (2800 B.C.) who was famous as a statesman, architect, builder of the step pyramid at Saqqarah and physician. The Egyptians worshipped many gods. Imhotep was considered both a doctor and divinity. Specialization prevailed in Egyptian times. There were eye doctors, head doctors and tooth doctors. All these doctors were officials paid by the State. Homer speaking of the doctors of the ancient world considered the Egyptians to be the "the best of all" *(13)*.

Egyptian medicine was far from primitive. They believed that disease was due to absorption from the intestine of harmful substances which gave rise to putrefaction of blood and formation of pus. They believed that the pulse was "the speech of the heart". Diseases were treated with cathartics, enema, blood-letting and a wide range of drugs. The best known medical manuscripts belonging to the Egyptian times are the Edwin Smith papyrus (3000–2500 B.C.), and the Ebers papyrus (1150 B.C.). The Edwin Smith papyrus, the oldest treatise on surgery, accurately describes partial paralysis following cerebral lesions in skull fractures. The Ebers papyrus which was found with a mummy on the banks of the Nile, is a unique record of some 800 prescriptions based on some 700 drugs. Castor oil, tannic acid, opium, turpentine, gentian, senna, minerals and root drugs were all used by the Egyptian physicians. A great number of diseases are reported in the papyri such as worms, eye diseases, diabetes, rheumatism, polio and schistosomiasis. Unfortunately, these ailments are still present in modern Egypt *(7)*.

In the realm of public health also, the Egyptians excelled. They built planned cities, public baths and underground drains which even the modern might envy. They had also some knowledge of inoculation against smallpox, the value of mosquito nets and the association of plague with rats. Their god of health was Horus. Egyptian medicine occupied a dominant place in the ancient world for about 2,500 years when it was replaced by Greek medicine.

Mesopotamian medicine

Contemporary with ancient Egyptian civilization, there existed another civilization in the land which lies between the Euphrates and Tigris rivers, Mesopotamia (now part of Iraq), often called the "Cradle of Civilization", as long as 6,000 years ago.

In ancient Mesopotamia, the basic concepts of medicine were religious, and taught and practised by herb doctors, knife doctors and spell doctors – a classification that roughly parallels our own internists, surgeons and psychiatrists. Mesopotamia was the cradle of magic and necromancy. Medical students were busy in classifying "demons", the causes of diseases. Geomancy, the interpretation of dreams, and hepatoscopic divination (the liver was considered the seat of life) are characteristic of their medical lore. Sumerians, Babylonians and Assyrians were the authors of a medical astrology which flourished in the whole of Eurasia. Prescriptions were written on tablets, in cuneiform writing. The oldest medical prescription comes to us from Mesopotamia, dating back to 2100 B.C.

Hammurabi, a great king of Babylon who lived around 2000 B.C. formulated a set of drastic laws known as the Code of Hammurabi that governed the conduct of physicians and provided for health practices *(14)*. Doctors whose proposed therapy proved wrong, ran the risk of being killed. Laws relating to medical practice, including fees payable to physicians for satisfactory services and penalties for harmful therapy are contained in the Babylonian Code of Hammurabi, the very first codification of medical practice. While the code of Hammurabi reflected a high degree of social organization, the medicine of his time was devoid of any scientific foundation.

Greek medicine

The classic period of Greek medicine was the year 460–136 B.C. The Greeks enjoyed the reputation – the civilizers of the ancient world. They taught men to think in terms of 'why' and 'how'. An early leader in Greek medicine was Aesculapius (1200 B.C.). Aesculapius bore two daughters – Hygiea and Panacea. The medical historian, Douglas Guthrie *(17)* has reminded us of the legend that Hygiea was worshipped as the goddess of health, and Panacea as the goddess of medicine. Panacea and Hygiea gave rise to dynasties of healers (curative medicine) and hygienists (preventive medicine) with different philosophies. Thus the dichotomy between curative medicine and preventive medicine began early and we know it remains true today. Hygiea (prevention) is at present fashionable among the intellectuals; but Panacea (cure) gets the cash. Aesculapius is still cherished in medical circles – his staff, entwined by a serpent, continues to be the symbol of medicine.

By far the greatest physician in Greek medicine was Hippocrates (460–370 B.C.) who is often called the "Father of Medicine". He was born on the little island of Cos, in the Aegean sea, about 460 B.C. He studied and classified diseases based on observation and reasoning. He challenged the tradition of magic in medicine, and initiated a radically new approach to medicine i.e., application of clinical methods in medicine. Hippocrate's lectures and writings, as compiled later by Alexandrian scholars into the "Corpus Hippocraticum", encompassed all branches of medicine. This 72 volume work contains the first scientific clinical case histories. Some of the sayings of Hippocrates later became favourites with physicians, such as "Life is short, the art (of medicine) long, opportunity fleeting, experience treacherous and judgement difficult", and "where there is love for mankind, there is love for the art of healing". His famous oath, the "Hippocratic oath" has become the keystone of medical ethics. It sets a high moral standard for the medical profession and demands absolute integrity of doctors. Hippocrates will always be regarded as one of the masters of the medical art.

Hippocrates was also an epidemiologist. Since he distinguished between diseases which were epidemic and those which were endemic, he was, in fact, the first true epidemiologist. He was constantly seeking the causes of disease. He studied such things as climate, water, clothing, diet, habits of eating and drinking and the effect they had in producing disease. His book "Airs, Water and Places" is considered a treatise on social medicine and hygiene. The Hippocratic concept of health and disease stressed the relation between man and his environment.

In short, the Greeks gave a new direction to medical thought. They rejected the supernatural theory of disease and looked upon disease as a natural process, not a visitation from a god of immolation. The Greeks believed that matter was made up of four elements – earth, air, fire and water. These elements had the corresponding qualities of being cold, dry, hot and moist and were represented in the body by the four humors – phlegm, yellow bile, blood and black bile – similar to the "tridosha theory" in Ayurveda. The Greeks postulated that health prevailed when the four humors were in equilibrium and when the balance was disturbed, disease was the result. The human body was assumed to have powers of restoration of humoral equilibrium, and it was the physician's primary role to assist in this healing process. While the humoral theory of Hippocrates was based on incorrect foundations, the concept of the innate capacity of the body of responding to disturbances in the equilibrium that constitutes health is highly relevant to modern medicine *(15)*.

Outstanding amongst post-Hippocratic medical centres was Alexandria's huge museum, the first University in the world which sheltered a library containing over 70,000 books. To this house of learning came eminent men. Between 300 B.C. and 30 B.C., thousands of pupils matriculated in the school of Alexandria, which replaced Athens as the world's centre of learning. In short, the Hippocratic school inspired in turn the Alexandria school, and the Arabo-Persian medicine. The Hippocratic school changed the destiny of medicine by separating it from magic and raising it to the status of a science. They had scientific method, although not scientific knowledge. The glorious Greek civilization fell into decay and was succeeded by the Roman civilization.

Roman medicine

By the first Century B.C., the centre of civilization shifted to Rome. The Romans borrowed their medicine largely from the Greeks whom they had conquered. While the politics of the world became Roman, medicine remained Greek. In the political philosophy of the Romans, the State and not the individual was supreme.

The Romans were a more practical-minded people than the Greeks. They had a keen sense of sanitation. Public health was born in Rome with the development of baths, sewers and aqueducts. The Romans made fine roads throughout their empire, brought pure water to all their cities through aqueducts, drained marshes to combat malaria, built sewerage systems and established hospitals for the sick.

An outstanding figure among Roman medical teachers was Galen (130–205 A.D.) who was born in the Greek city of Pergamon in Asia Minor (now Turkey). He was physician to the Roman emperor, Marcus Aurelius. His important contributions were in the field of comparative anatomy and experimental physiology. Galen was far ahead of his time in his views about health and disease. About health he stated: "Since both in importance and in time, health precedes disease, so we ought to consider first how health may be preserved, and then how one may best cure disease" *(16)*. About disease, Galen observed that disease is due to three factors – predisposing, exciting and environmental factors, a truly modern idea. The doctrines of Hippocrates and Galen were often in conflict since their approaches were so different – one is synthetic, the other analytic. The author of some 500 treatises on medical subjects, Galen was literally a "medical dictator" in his time, and also for a long time thereafter. His writings influenced European medicine. They were accepted as standard textbooks in medicine for 14 centuries, till his teachings and views were challenged by the anatomist, Vesalius in 1543, and the physiologist, William Harvey in 1628, almost 1500 years after his death.

Middle ages

The period between 500 and 1500 A.D. is generally known as "Middle Ages". With the fall of the Roman empire, the medical schools established in Roman times also disappeared. Europe was ravaged by disease and pestilence: plague, smallpox, leprosy and tuberculosis. The practice of medicine reverted back to primitive medicine dominated by superstition and dogma. Rejection of the body and glorification of the spirit became the accepted pattern of behaviour. It was regarded as immoral to see one's body; consequently, people seldom bathed. Dissection of the human body was prohibited. Consequently there was no progress of medicine. The medieval period is therefore called the "Dark Ages of Medicine" – a time of great strife, of socio-political change, of regression and progression *(7)*.

When Europe was passing through the Dark Ages, the Arabs stole a march over the rest of the civilization. They translated the Graeco-Roman medical literature into Arabic and helped preserve the ancient knowledge. Borrowing largely from the Greeks and Romans, they developed their own system of medicine known as the Unani system of medicine. They founded schools of medicine and hospitals in Baghdad, Damascus, Cairo and other Muslim capitals. The Arabs lit a brilliant torch from Greecian lamps, said Osler. Leaders in Arabic medicine were the Persians, Abu Becr (865–925) also known as Rhazes; and Ibn Sina (980–1037) known as Avicenna to the western world. Rhazes was a director of a large hospital in Baghdad and a court physician as well. Noted for keen observation and inventiveness, he was the first to observe pupillary reaction to light; to use mercurial purgatives; and to publish the first known book on Children's diseases *(7)*. However, the work most highly regarded today is his book on smallpox and measles which he distinguished clinically. Avicenna was an intellectual prodigy. He compiled a 21 volume encyclopaedia, the "Canon of Medicine", which was to leave its mark on medical theory and practice. He was responsible for elevating Islamic medicine to its zenith in the middle ages. The greatest contribution of Arabs, in general, was in the field of pharmacology. Seeking the "elixir of life", they developed pharmaceutical chemistry, introducing a large number of drugs, herbal and chemical. Pioneers in pharmacology, they invented the art of writing prescriptions, an art inherited by our modern pharmacists. They introduced a wide range of syrups, oils, poultices, plasters, pills, powders, alcoholates and aromatic waters. The words drug, alcohol, syrup and sugar are all Arabian *(17)*. The golden age of Arabic medicine was between 800–1300 A.D.

During the turbulent middle ages, Christianity exerted a wholesome influence. The spread of Christianity led to the establishment of hospitals. Early medieval hospitals rarely specialized in treatment of the sick. Usually the sick were received for the purpose of supplying their bodily wants and catering to their spiritual needs. The first hospital on record in England was built in York in 937 A.D. With the growth of medicine, a chain of hospitals sprang up from Persia to Spain– there were more than 60 in Baghdad and 33 in Cairo. Some hospitals, like Cairo's Al Mansur had separate departments for various diseases, wards for both sexes, fountains to cool fever patients, libraries, musicians and story tellers for the sleepless.

During the middle ages, religious institutions known as "monasteries" headed by monks, saints and abbotts also came up. These monasteries admitted men and women from all ranks including kings and queens. They not only helped preserve the ancient knowledge but also rendered active medical and nursing care to the sick.

II. DAWN OF SCIENTIFIC MEDICINE

The period following 1500 A.D. was marked by revolutions – political, industrial, religious and medical. Political revolutions took place in France and America, people claiming their just rights. The industrial revolution in the West brought great benefits leading to an improvement in the standard of living among people. With advancing degrees of civilization, medicine also evolved.

Revival of medicine

For many historians, the revival of medicine encompasses the period from 1453–1600 A.D. It was an age of individual scientific endeavour. The distinguished personalities during this period were: Paracelsus (1493–1541) who revived medicine. He was born at a time "when Europe stretched her limbs after a sleep of a thousand years in a bed of darkness". Labelled genius by some and quack by others, Swiss-born Paracelsus publicly burnt the works of Galen and Avicenna and attacked superstition and dogma and helped turn medicine towards rational research. Fracastorius (1483–1553), an Italian physician enunciated the "theory of contagion". He envisaged the transfer of infection *via* minute invisible particles and explained the cause of epidemics. Fracastorius recognized that syphilis was transmitted from person to person during sexual relations. He became the founder of epidemiology. Andreas Vasalius (1514–1564) of Brussels did lot of dissections on the human body and demonstrated some of Galen's errors. He raised the study of anatomy to a science, and has been called "the first man of modern science". Vesalius' great work Fabrica became a classic text in medical education. What Vesalius did for anatomy, Ambroise Pare (1510–1590), a French Army surgeon did for surgery and earned the title, "father of surgery". Pare advanced the art of surgery, but John Hunter (1728–1793) taught the science of it. In 1540, the United Company of Barber Surgeons was established in England, which later became the Royal College of Surgeons. Another great name in clinical medicine is that of Thomas Sydenham (1624–1689), the English Hippocrates who set the example of the true clinical method. He made a differential diagnosis of scarlet fever, malaria, dysentery and cholera. Sydenham is also regarded as the first distinguished epidemiologist.

The 17th and 18th centuries were full of even more exciting discoveries, e.g., Harvey's discovery of the circulation of blood (1628), Leeuwenhoek's microscope (1670) and Jenner's vaccination against smallpox (1796). However, the progress in medicine as well as surgery, during the 19th century would not have been possible but for Morgagni (1682–1771) who founded a new branch of medical science, pathologic anatomy.

Sanitary awakening

Another historic milestone in the evolution of medicine is the "great sanitary awakening" which took place in England in the mid-nineteenth century and gradually spread to other countries. It had a tremendous impact in modifying the behaviour of people and ushering an era of public health. The industrial revolution of the 18th century sparked off numerous problems – creation of slums, overcrowding with all its ill-effects, accumulation of filth in cities and towns, high sickness and death rates especially among women and children, infectious diseases like tuberculosis, industrial and social problems – which deteriorated the health of the people to the lowest ebb. The mean age at death in London was reported to be 44 years for the gentry and professionals, and 22 years for the working class, in 1842 *(14)*. Add to this, the frequent visitations of cholera compounded the misery of the people. The great cholera epidemic of 1832 led Edwin Chadwick (1800–1890), a lawyer in England to investigate the health of the inhabitants of the large towns with a view to improve the conditions under which they lived *(18)*. Chadwick's report on "The Sanitary Conditions of the Labouring Population in Great Britain", a landmark in the history of public health, set London and other cities slowly on the way to improve housing and working conditions. Chadwick's report focussed the attention of the people and government on the urgent need to improve public health. Filth was recognized as man's greatest enemy and with this began an anti-filth crusade, the "great sanitary awakening" which led to the enactment of the Public Health Act of 1848 in England. A new thinking began to take shape i.e., the State has a direct responsibility for the health of the people.

Rise of public health

The above events led to the birth of public health concept in England around 1840. Earlier, Johanna Peter Frank (1745–1821) a health philosopher of his time, conceived public health as good health laws enforced by the police and enunciated the principle that the State is responsible for the health of its people. The Public Health Act of 1848 was a fulfilment of his dream about the State's responsibility for the health of its people.

Cholera which is often called the "father of public health" appeared time and again in the western world during the 19th century. An English epidemiologist, John Snow, studied the epidemiology of cholera in London from 1848 to 1854 and established the role of polluted drinking water in the spread of cholera. In 1856, William Budd, another pioneer, by careful observations of an outbreak of typhoid fever in the rural north of England concluded that the spread was by drinking water, not by miasma and sewer gas. These two discoveries were all the more remarkable when one considers that the causative agents of cholera and typhoid fever were not identified. Then came the demand from people for clean water. At that time the Thames was both a source of drinking water and the depository for sewage. A comprehensive piece of legislation was brought into force in England, the Public Health Act of 1875 for the control of man's physical environment. The torch was already lit by Chadwick, but the man who was actually responsible more than any other for sanitary reforms was Sir John Simon (1816–1904), the first medical officer of health of London. He built up a system of public health in England which became the admiration of the rest of the world *(18)*. This early phase of public health (1880–1920) is often called the "disease control phase". Efforts were directed entirely towards general cleanliness, garbage and refuse disposal. Quarantine conventions were held to contain disease.

The development of the public health movement in Amercia follows closely the English pattern. In 1850, Lemuel Shattuck (1793–1859), a bookseller and publisher, published his report on the health conditions in Massachusetts. Like Chadwick's report it stirred the conscience of the American people to the improvement of public health. France, Spain, Australia, Germany, Italy, Belgium and the Scandinavian countries all developed their public health. By the beginning of the 20th century, the broad foundations of public health – clean water, clean surroundings, wholesome condition of houses, control of offensive trades, etc were laid in all the countries of the western world. After the First World War, there were three particular newcomers to the public health scene – Yugoslavia, Turkey and Russia *(19)*. These three countries in 1920 presented the typical picture of the underdeveloped world. Today they are quite advanced in public health.

While public health made rapid strides in the western world, its progress has been slow in the developing countries such as India where the main health problems continue to be those faced by the western world about 100 years ago. The establishment of the WHO providing a Health Charter for all people provided a great fillip to the public health movement in these countries.

Germ theory of disease

For long, man was groping in darkness about the causation of disease. Several theories were advanced from time to time to explain disease causation such as the supernatural theory of disease, the theory of humors by Greeks and Indians, the theory of contagion, the miasmatic theory which attributed disease to noxious air and vapours, the theory of spontaneous generation, etc. The breakthrough came in 1860, when the French bacteriologist Louis Pasteur (1822–1895) demonstrated the presence of bacteria in air. He disproved the theory of "spontaneous generation". In 1873, Pasteur advanced the "germ theory of disease". In 1877, Robert Koch (1843–1910) showed that anthrax was caused by a bacteria. The discoveries of Pasteur and Koch confirmed the germ theory of disease. It was the golden age of bacteriology. Microbe after microbe was discovered in quick succession – gonococcus in 1847; typhoid bacillus, pneumococcus in 1880; tubercle bacillus in 1882; cholera vibrio in 1883; diphtheria bacillus in 1884, and so on. These discoveries and a host of others at the turn of the century marked a turning point in our aetiological concepts. All attention was focussed on microbes and their role in disease causation. The germ theory of disease came to the forefront, supplanting the earlier theories of disease causation. Medicine finally shed the rags of dogma and superstition and put on the robes of scientific knowledge.

Birth of preventive medicine

Preventive medicine really dates back to the 18th century. It developed as a branch of medicine distinct from public health. Curiously, it came into existence even before the causative agents of disease were known. James Lind (1716–1794), a naval surgeon advocated the intake of fresh fruit and vegetables for the prevention of scurvy in 1753. Edward Jenner (1749–1823) of Great Britain, a pupil of John Hunter, discovered vaccination against smallpox in 1796. These two discoveries marked the beginning of a new era, the era of disease prevention by specific measures.

Preventive medicine got a firm foundation only after the discovery of causative agents of disease and the establishment of the germ theory of disease. The latter part of the 19th century was marked by such discoveries in preventive medicine as Pasteur's anti-rabies treatment (1883), cholera vaccine (1892), diphtheria antitoxin (1894), anti-typhoid vaccine (1898), antiseptics and disinfectants (1827–1912), etc. A further advance was the elucidation of the modes of disease transmission. For example, in 1896, Bruce, a British Army surgeon, demonstrated that the African sleeping sickness was transmitted by tsetse fly. In 1898, Ross demonstrated that malaria was transmitted by the Anopheles. In 1900, Walter Reed and his colleagues demonstrated that yellow fever was transmitted by the Aedes mosquito. With the knowledge derived from bacteriology, it became possible to control disease by specific measures such as blocking the channels of transmission, e.g., quarantine, water purification, pasteurization of milk, protection of foods, proper disposal of sewage, destruction of insects and disinfection. The development of laboratory methods for the early detection of disease was a further advance. In its early years, preventive medicine was equated with the control of infectious diseases. The modern concepts of primary, secondary and tertiary prevention were not known.

III. MODERN MEDICINE

The dichotomy of medicine into two major branches namely curative medicine, and public health/preventive medicine was evident at the close of the 19th century. After 1900, medicine moved faster towards specialization, and a rational, scientific approach to disease. The pattern of disease began to change. With the control of acute infectious diseases, the so-called modern diseases such as cancer, diabetes, cardiovascular disease, mental illness and accidents came into prominence and have become the leading causes of death in industrialized countries. These diseases could not be explained on the basis of the germ theory of disease, nor treated with "magic bullets". The realization began to dawn that there are other factors or causes in the aetiology of diseases, namely social, economic, genetic, environmental and psychological factors which are equally important. Most of these factors are linked to man's lifestyle and behaviour. The germ theory of disease gave place to a newer concept of disease – "multifactorial causation". In fact, it was Pettenkofer of Munich (1819–1901) who first mooted the concept of multifactorial causation of disease but his ideas were lost in the bacteriological era. The concept of multifactorial causation was revived by epidemiologists who have contributed significantly to our present-day understanding of multifactorial causation of disease and "risk-factors" in the aetiology of disease. The developments in modern medicine may be reviewed broadly under the following heads:

1. Curative medicine

Although curative medicine is thousands of years old, modern medicine, as we know today, is hardly 100 years old. Its primary objective is the removal of disease from the patient (rather than from the mass). It employs various modalities to accomplish this objective, e.g., diagnostic techniques, treatment. Over the years, the tools of diagnosis have become refined, sophisticated and numerous; the armamentarium for treatment more specific and potent. In the middle of the 20th century a profound revolution was brought in "allopathic medicine" which has been defined as "treatment of disease by the use of a drug which produces a reaction that itself neutralizes the disease" *(10)*, by the introduction of antibacterial and antibiotic agents. These discoveries, if they were to be recorded, would fill volumes. Suffice it to say that curative medicine, over the years, has accumulated a vast body of scientific knowledge, technical skills, medicaments and machinery – highly organized – not merely to treat disease but to preserve life itself as far as it could be possible.

In reviewing the history of medicine during the past 100 years, one cannot fail to note the tremendous growth of specialization that has taken place in response to advances in medical technology due to changes in the nature and distribution of health and disease pattern in the community, and to the changing emphasis placed by society upon age and sex groups. Some specialities have emerged, based on clearly defined skills such as surgery, radiology, and anaesthesia; some based on parts of the body such as ENT, ophthalmology, cardiology, gynaecology; and, some based on particular age or sex groups such as paediatrics, geriatrics and obstetrics. Again, within each speciality, there has been a growth of sub-specialities, as for example, neonatology, perinatology, paediatric cardiology, paediatric neurology and paediatric surgery – all in paediatrics. One wonders whether such microspecialization is needed.

Specialization has no doubt raised the standards of medical care, but it has escalated the cost of medical care and placed specialist medical care beyond the means of an average citizen, without outside aid or charity. It has infringed upon the basic tenets of socialism (i.e., the greatest good of the greatest number) and paved the way to varying degrees of social control over medicine. Specialization has also contributed to the decline of general practice and the isolation of medical practitioners at the periphery of the medical care system *(20)*.

2. Preventive medicine

Preventive medicine developed as a branch of medicine distinct from public health. By definition, preventive medicine is applied to "healthy" people, customarily by actions affecting large numbers or populations. Its primary objective is prevention of disease and promotion of health.

The early triumphs of preventive medicine were in the field of bacterial vaccines and antisera at the turn of the century which led to the conquest of a wide spectrum of specific diseases. Declines took place in the morbidity and mortality from diphtheria, tetanus, typhoid fever and others. Later, the introduction of tissue culture of viruses led to the development of anti-viral vaccines, e.g., polio vaccines (1955, 1960). The eradication of smallpox (the last case of smallpox occurred in Somalia in 1977) is one of the greatest triumphs of preventive medicine in recent times. The search for better and newer vaccines (e.g., against malaria, leprosy, syphilis and other parasitic diseases and even cancer) continues.

Preventive medicine did not confine itself to vaccination and quarantine. Discoveries in the field of nutrition have added a new dimension to preventive medicine. New strategies have been developed for combating specific deficiencies as for example, nutritional blindness and iodine deficiency disorders. The recognition of the role of vitamins, minerals, proteins and other nutrients, and more recently dietary fibre emphasize the nutrition component of preventive medicine.

Another glorious chapter in the history of preventive medicine is the discovery of synthetic insecticides such as DDT, HCH, malathion and others. They have brought about fundamental changes in the strategy in the control of vector-borne diseases (e.g., malaria, leishmaniasis, plague, rickettsial diseases) which have been among the most important world-wide health problems for many years. Despite insecticide resistance and environmental pollution mishaps (e.g., Bhopal tragedy in India in 1984), some of the chemical insecticides such as DDT still remain unchallenged in the control of disease.

The discovery of sulpha drugs, anti-malarials, antibiotics, anti-tubercular and anti-leprosy drugs have all enriched preventive medicine. Chemoprophylaxis and mass drug treatment have become important tools of preventive medicine. The pattern of disease in the community began to change with improved control of infectious diseases through both prevention and treatment, and people are now living for longer years, especially those in developing countries.

A new concept – concept of disease eradication – began to take shape. This concept found ready application in the eradication of smallpox. Eradication of certain other diseases (e.g., measles, tetanus, guineaworm and endemic goitre) are on the anvil.

Another notable development in the 20th century is the development of "screening" for the diagnosis of disease in its presymptomatic stage *(21)*. In the 1930s, the two most commonly used tests were the serologic blood test for syphilis, and the chest X-ray for tuberculosis. As the number of screening tests increased, the concept of screening for individual diseases entered the multiphasic epoch in early 1950s. In spite of the fact that the utility of screening has been increasingly debated in recent years, screening for disease among apparently healthy people has remained an important part of preventive medicine. An offshoot of the screening is screening for "risk-factors" of disease and identification of "high-risk groups". Since we do not have specific weapons against chronic diseases, screening and regular health checkups have acquired an important place in the early detection of cancer, diabetes, rheumatism and cardiovascular disease, the so-called "diseases of civilization".

Preventive medicine is currently faced with the problem of "population explosion" in developing countries where population overgrowth is causing social, economic, political and environmental problems. This is another kind of prevention – prevention of a problem that demands a mass attack, if its benefits are to accrue in the present and succeeding generations. Consequently, research in human fertility and contraceptive technology has gained momentum. Genetic counselling is another aspect of the population problem that is receiving attention.

Preventive medicine has become a growing point in medicine *(21)*. Advances in the field of treatment in no way has diminished the need for preventive care nor its usefulness. Preventive measures are already being applied not only to the chronic, degenerative and hereditary diseases but also to the special problems of old age. In fact, as medical science advances, it will become more and more preventive medical practice in nature. The emergence of preventive paediatrics, geriatrics and preventive cardiology reflect newer trends in the scope of preventive medicine.

Scientific advances, improved living standards and fuller education of the public have opened up a number of new avenues to prevention. Three levels of prevention are now recognized: primary, intended to prevent disease among healthy people; secondary, directed towards those in whom the disease has already developed; and tertiary, to reduce the prevalence of chronic disability consequent to disease. Preventive medicine ranges far beyond the medical field in the narrow sense of the word. Besides communicable diseases, it is concerned with the environmental, social, economic and more general aspects of prevention. Modern preventive medicine has been defined as "the art and science of health promotion, disease prevention, disability limitation and rehabilitation". It implies a more personal encounter between the individual and health professional than public health. In sum, preventive medicine is a kind of anticipatory medicine *(22)*.

3. Social medicine

Social medicine has been primarily a European speciality. The seeds that medicine is a social science were sown late in the 19th century by pioneers such as Neumann (1847) and Virchow (1848). But their ideas were far too ahead of their time. The germ theory of disease and discoveries in microbiology checked the development of these ideas.

In 1911, the concept of social medicine was revived by Alfred Grotjahn (1869–1931) of Berlin who stressed the importance of social factors in the aetiology of disease, which he called "social pathology". Others called it geographical pathology and population pathology. In 1912 Rene Sand had founded the Belgian Social Medicine Association. Developments in the field of social sciences (e.g., sociology, psychology, anthropology) rediscovered that man is not only a biological animal, but also a social being, and disease has social causes, social consequences and social therapy. The ideas of social medicine spread to other countries. John Ryle and his group in England were influenced by these ideas and visualized social medicine as an evolution of medicine. They promoted the concept of social medicine in England. A Chair of social medicine was set up at Oxford in 1942 followed by similar others in other Universities in England.

Social medicine has varying meanings attached to its label. By derivation, social medicine is the study of man as a social being in his total environment. Its focus is on the health of the community as a whole. Professor Crew *(23)* had ably stated that social medicine stands on two pillars – medicine and sociology. Others stated that the maiden sociology married public health and became social medicine *(24)*. McKeown *(25)* has this to say: "In contemporary usage social medicine has two meanings, one broad and ill-defined, the other more restricted and precise. In the broad sense, social medicine is an expression of the humanitarian tradition in medicine and people read into it any interpretation consistent with their own aspirations and interests. Thus it may be identified with care of patients, prevention of disease, administration of medical services; indeed with almost any subject in the extensive field of health and welfare. But in the more restricted sense, social medicine is concerned with a body of knowledge embodied in epidemiology and the study of the medical needs or medical care of society". In short, social medicine is not a new branch of medicine but rather a new orientation of medicine to the changing needs of man and society. It emphasizes the strong relationship between medicine and social sciences. The pre-eminent concern of social medicine has unquestionably been the development of epidemiological methods and their application to the investigation of disease. It has entered into a productive relationship with social sciences and statistics to be able to elucidate the role of social factors in disease aetiology *(26)*. These developments represent a forceful bid for the expanding concept of medicine. However, social medicine was criticized because it was virtually isolated from the service world and confined mostly to academic study of health services and chronic disease *(27)*.

Changing concepts in public health

In the history of public health, four distinct phases may be demarcated:

a. Disease control phase (1880–1920)

Public health during the 19th century was largely a matter of sanitary legislation and sanitary reforms aimed at the control of man's physical environment, e.g., water supply, sewage disposal, etc. Clearly these measures were not aimed at the control of any specific disease, for want of the needed technical knowledge. However, these measures vastly improved the health of the people due to disease and death control.

b. Health promotional phase (1920–1960)

At the beginning of the 20th century, a new concept, the concept of "health promotion" began to take shape. It was realized that public health had neglected the citizen as an individual, and that the State had a direct responsibility for the health of the individual. Consequently, in addition to disease control activities, one more goal was added to public health, that is, health promotion of individuals. It was initiated as personal health services such as mother and child health services, school health services, industrial health services, mental health and rehabilitation services. Public health nursing was a direct offshoot of this concept. Public health departments began expanding their programmes towards health promotional activities. C.E.A. Winslow, one of the leading figures in the history of public health, in 1920, defined public health as "the science and art of preventing disease, prolonging life and promoting health and efficiency through organized community effort". This definition summarizes the philosophy of public health, which remains largely true even today.

Since the State had assumed direct responsibility for the health of the individual, two great movements were initiated for human development during the first half of the present century, namely (a) provision of "basic health services" through the medium of primary health centres and subcentres for rural and urban areas. The evolution of health centres is an important development in the history of public health *(28)*. The concept of the health centre was first mooted in 1920 by Lord Dawson in England. In 1931, the League of Nations Health Organization called for the establishment of health centres. The Bhore Committee (1946) in India had also recommended the establishment of health centres for providing integrated curative and preventive services. Many developing countries have given the highest priority to the establishment of health centres for providing basic health services. (b) The second great movement was the Community Development Programme to promote village development through the active participation of the whole community and on the initiative of the community. This programme tried to do too much too quickly with inadequate resources. It was a great opportunity lost, because it failed to survive. However, the establishment of primary health centres and subcentres provided the much-needed infrastructure of health services, especially in the rural areas *(29)*.

c. Social engineering phase (1960–1980)

With the advances in preventive medicine and practice of public health, the pattern of disease began to change in the developed world. Many of the acute illness problems have been brought under control. However, as old problems were solved, new health problems in the form of chronic diseases began to emerge, e.g., cancer, diabetes, cardiovascular diseases, alcoholism and drug addiction etc. especially in the affluent societies. These problems could not be tackled by the traditional approaches to public health such as isolation, immunization and disinfection nor could these be explained on the basis of the germ theory of disease. A new concept, the concept of "risk factors" as determinants of these diseases came into existence. The consequences of these diseases, unlike the swift death brought by the acute infectious diseases, was to place a chronic burden on the society that created them. These problems brought new challenges to public health which needed reorientation more towards social objectives. Public health entered a new phase in the 1960s, described as the "social engineering" phase *(14)*. Social and behavioural aspects of disease and health were given a new priority. Public health moved into the preventive and rehabilitative aspects of chronic diseases and behavioural problems. In this process, the goals of public health and preventive medicine which had already considerable overlapping became identical, namely prevention of disease, promotion of health and prolongation of life. In short, although the term "public health" is still used, its original meaning has changed. In view of its changed meaning and scope, the term "community health" has been preferred by some leaders in public health. Community health incorporates services to the population at large as opposed to preventive or social medicine.

d. "Health for All" phase (1981–2000 A.D.)

As the centuries have unfolded, the glaring contrasts in the picture of health in the developed and developing countries came into a sharper focus, despite advances in medicine. Most people in the developed countries, and the elite of the developing countries, enjoy all the determinants of good health – adequate income, nutrition, education, sanitation, safe drinking water and comprehensive health care. In contrast, only 10 to 20 per cent of the population in developing countries enjoy ready access to health services of any kind *(30)*. Death claims 60–250 of every 1000 live births within the first year of life, and the life expectancy is 30 per cent lower than in the developed countries *(30)*. John Bryant in the introduction to his book: "Health and the Developing World" presented a gloomy picture and a challenge of inequalities in health by saying: "Large numbers of the world's people, perhaps more than half, have no access to health care at all, and for many of the rest, the care they receive does not answer the problems they have". The global conscience was stirred leading to a new awakening that the health gap between rich and poor within countries and between countries should be narrowed and ultimately eliminated. It was conceded that the neglected 80 per cent of the world's population too have an equal claim to health care, to protection from the killer diseases of childhood, to primary health care for mothers and children, to treatment for those ills that mankind has long ago learnt to control, if not to cure *(31)*. Against this background, in 1981, the members of the WHO pledged themselves to an ambitious target to provide "Health for All" by the year 2000, that is attainment of a level of health that will permit all people "to lead a socially and economically productive life" *(32)*. The public health, along with other medical sciences and other health-related sectors are engaged in this broad field of effort.

IV. MEDICAL REVOLUTION

State of the art

Medicine has moved from the organism to organ, and from the organ to the cell, and from the cell to molecular properties. The discovery of the biological role of nucleic acids, the uncovering of the genetic code and its role in regulating life processes are marvellous discoveries in recent years. Medicine has acquired a vast body of knowledge and has become highly technical. It has acquired new capabilities to modify and perhaps control the capacities and activities of men by direct intervention into and manipulation of their bodies and minds, viz. genetic counselling, genetic engineering, prenatal diagnosis of sex, prenatal diagnosis of genetic diseases, *in vitro* fertilization, the prospect of cloning (the asexual reproduction of unlimited number of genetically identical individuals from a single parent), organ transplantation, the use of artificial kidney machine, the development of an artificial heart, the practice of psychosurgery, etc. The data presented show that modern medicine has entered a new evolutionary stage with the promise of continued improvements in medical capabilities to preserve life, if not merely to solve problems of sickness.

Social control of medicine

When Virchow wrote in 1849 that "Medicine is a social science and politics is medicine on a large scale", he anticipated probably the social (political) control of medicine. Indeed, as medicine advanced, it became a highly personalized and institutionalized service. This generated a feeling that medicine was not rendering its full service to humanity. As the cost of medical care increased, two kinds of medical care came into existence – one for the rich and the other for the poor. The gap was bridged to a small extent by charitable and voluntary agencies providing free medical care to the poor. An attitude developed that charity was worthy of man and that the benefits of modern medicine should be available to all people. A solution was to be found – it was "socialization of medicine".

Social medicine should not be confused with state medicine or socialized medicine. State medicine implies provision of free medical service to the people at government expense. Socialized medicine envisages provision of medical service and professional education by the State as in state medicine, but the programme is operated and regulated by professional groups rather than by the government.

Germany led the way by instituting compulsory sickness insurance in 1883. Other countries followed suit – England in 1911, France in 1928 and so on. Great Britain nationalized its health services in 1946. A few other countries notably the socialist nations in Europe, New Zealand and Cuba took steps to socialize their health services. However, Russia was the first country to socialize medicine completely and to give its citizens a constitutional right to all health services. From a private ownership, medicine became a social institution, one more link in the chain of welfare institutions *(33)*.

Socialization is a noble idea. It eliminates the competition among physicians in search of clients. It ensures social equity, that is universal coverage by health services. Medical care becomes free for the patient, which is supported by the State. However, the varying degrees of social control over medicine, has resulted in a variety of health systems, each system having its own merits and demerits. It is now recognized that mere socialization was not sufficient to ensure utilization of health services. What is required is "community participation", which, as envisaged by WHO and UNICEF is "the process by which individuals and families assume responsibility for their own health and welfare and for those of the community, and develop the capacity to contribute to their and the community's development *(32)*. It also implies community participation in the planning, organization and management of their own health services. This is called simply "Health by the People" *(34)*. This is what Virchow had prophesied that medicine is nothing but politics on a large scale.

Family and community medicine

Way back in 1923, Dr. Francis Peabody, professor of medicine at Harvard, commented that specialization in medicine had already reached its apex and that modern medicine had fragmented the health care delivery system to too great a degree. He called for a rapid return of the general physician (family physician) who would give comprehensive and personalized care. In 1966, two reports (i.e., Millis Commission Report, Willard Committee Report) in United States made similar recommendations. In 1971, the American Academy of General Practice (which began in 1947) changed its name to "American Academy of Family Physicians" to place increased emphasis upon family-oriented health care and to gain academic acceptance for the new speciality.

The emergence of Family and Community Medicine represents a counterforce to the direction which medical science has taken lately. The field of specialization of family and community medicine is neither an organ system nor a disease syndrome, but rather in both instances, a designation of social categories namely family and community. Family and community medicine overlap and strengthen each other.

Family medicine

The emergence of family medicine has been hailed as a rediscovery of the human, social and cultural aspects of health and disease, and of the recognition of family as a focal point of health care and the right place for integrating preventive, promotive and curative services. Family medicine has been defined as "a field of specialization in medicine which is neither disease nor organ oriented. It is family oriented medicine or health care centred on the family as the unit – from first contact to the ongoing care of chronic problems (from prevention to rehabilitation). When family medicine is applied to the care of patients and their families, it becomes the speciality of *family* practice. Family practice is a horizontal speciality, which, like paediatrics and internal medicine, shares large areas of content with other clinical disciplines. The speciality of family practice is specially designed to deliver "primary care" *(35)*.

Community medicine

Like family medicine, community medicine is a newcomer. It is the successor of what was previously known as public health, community health, preventive and social medicine. All these share common ground, i.e., prevention of disease and promotion of health. The appearance of community medicine has caused confusion. The Faculty of Community Medicine of the Royal College of Physicians has defined community medicine as "that speciality which deals with populations...... and comprises those doctors who try to measure the needs of the population, both sick and well, who plan and administer services to meet those needs, and those who are engaged in research and teaching in the field" *(27)*. Besides this, there are at least four other definitions of community medicine *(36)*. To make matters worse, a WHO study group *(37)* stated that since health problems vary from country to country, each country should formulate its own definition of community medicine in the light of its traditions, geography and resources. There is still confusion and conflict about roles, tasks and professional identities in the service as well as the academic worlds of community medicine *(27)*.

V. HEALTH CARE REVOLUTION

Background

It was recognized that in both developed and developing countries, the standard of health services the public expected was not being provided *(38)*. The services do not cover the whole population. There is lack of services in some areas and unnecessary duplication in others. A very high proportion of the population in many developing countries, and especially in rural areas does not have ready access to health services. The health services favoured only the privileged few and urban dwellers. Although there was the recognition that health is a fundamental human right, there is a denial of this right to millions of people who are caught in the vicious circle of poverty and illhealth. There are marked differences in health status between people in different countries as well as between different groups in the same country; the cost of health care is rising without much improvement in their quality. In short, there has been a growing dissatisfaction with the existing health services and a clear demand for better health care.

Health for All

The spate of new ideas and concepts, e.g., increasing importance given to social justice and equity, recognition of the crucial role of community participation, changing ideas about the nature of health and development, the importance of political will called for new approaches to make medicine in the service of humanity more effective.

Against the above background, the 30th World Health Assembly resolved in May 1977, that "the main social target of governments and WHO in the coming decades should be the attainment by all citizens of the world by the year 2000 of a level of health that will permit them to lead a socially and economically productive life." This culminated in the international objective of HEALTH FOR ALL by the year 2000 as the social goal of all governments.

The goal of Health for All has two perspectives. Viewed in the long-term context, it simply means the realization of the WHO's objective of "attainment by all peoples of the highest possible level of health". But, what is of immediate relevance is the meaning that, as a minimum, all people in all countries should have at least such a level of health that they are capable of working productively and of participating actively in the social life of the community in which they live.

Health for All means that health is to be brought within the reach of every one in a given community. It implies the removal of obstacles to health – that is to say, the elimination of malnutrition, ignorance, disease, contaminated water supply, unhygienic housing, etc. It depends on continued progress in medicine and public health.

Health for All was a holistic concept calling for efforts in agriculture, industry, education, housing and communications, just as much as in medicine and public health. The attainment of Health for All by 2000 A.D. was the central issue and official target of WHO and its member countries. It symbolized the determination of the countries of the world to provide an acceptable level of health to all people. Health for All has been described as a revolutionary concept and a historic movement – a movement in terms of its own evolutionary process.

Primary health care *(39)*

With increasing recognition of the failure of existing health services to provide health care, alternative ideas and methods to provide health care have been considered and tried *(34,40)*. Discussing these issues at the Joint WHO–UNICEF international conference in 1978 at Alma-Ata (USSR), the governments of 134 countries and many voluntary agencies called for a **revolutionary approach** to health care. Declaring that "The existing gross inequality in the health status of people particularly between developed and developing countries as well as within countries is politically, socially and economically unacceptable", the Alma-Ata conference called for acceptance of the WHO goal of Health for All by 2000 A.D. and proclaimed primary health care as way to achieving "Health for All".

Primary health care is a new approach to health care, which integrates at the community level all the factors required for improving the health status of the population. It consists of at least eight elements (see page 37) described as "essential health care". This presupposes services that are both simple and efficient with regard to cost, techniques, and organization, that are readily accessible to those concerned, and that contribute to improving the living conditions of individuals, families and the community as a whole. Primary health care is available to all people at the first level of health care. It is based on principles of equity, wider coverage, individual and community involvement and intersectoral coordination. Viewed in these terms, primary health care is a radical departure from the conventional health care systems of the past. While it integrates promotive, preventive and curative services, it is also conceived as an integral part of the country's plan for socio-economic development.

The Alma-Ata Declaration called on all governments to formulate national policies, strategies and plans of action to launch and sustain primary health care as part of a national health system. It is left to each country to innovate, according to its own circumstances to provide primary health care. This was followed by the formulation and adoption of the **Global strategy** for Health for All by the 34th World Health Assembly in 1981. Primary health care got off to a good start in many countries with the theme "Health for All by 2000 A.D.". It presented a challenge so formidable that its implications boggle the bravest minds. The challenge brought us face-to-face with the Declaration of Alma-Ata.

Deprofessionalization of medicine

The practice of primary health care involves a good deal of "deprofessionalizaion" of medicine. Laymen have come to play a prominent role in the delivery of health care. While the physician still holds his unique position in the field of health care in general, the participation of a new cadre of health workers (e.g., community health workers, anganwadi workers, multipurpose workers, practitioners of indigenous medicine, social workers) with relatively little training and support have been considered and tried to provide health care. They now comprise part of the "health teams". The medical man can no longer restrict himself to his traditional role as diagnoser of ailments, prescriber of pills and potions, and exciser of lumps. He has acquired new roles – being an educator, case-finder, preventer, counsellor and an agent of social change.

The Millennium Development Goals

In September 2000, representatives from 189 countries met at the Millennium Summit in New York to adopt the United Nations Millennium Declaration. The leaders made specific commitments in seven areas : peace, security and disarmament; development and poverty eradication; protecting our common environment, human rights, democracy and good governance; protecting the vulnerable; meeting the special needs of Africa; and strengthening the United Nations. The Road Map established goals and targets to be reached by the year 2015 in each of seven areas. The goals in the area of development and poverty eradication are now widely referred to as *"Millennium Development Goals" (41, 42)*.

The Millennium Development Goals, place health at the heart of development and represent commitments by governments throughout the world to do more to reduce poverty and hunger, and to tackle ill-health, gender inequality, lack of education, access to clean water; and environmental degradation. Thus three of the eight goals are directly health related and all of other goals have important indirect effects on health; three of the 8 goals, 8 of the 18 targets required to achieve these goals, and 18 of the 48 indicators of progress, are health related.

Sustainable Development Goals

In September 2015, the United Nations General Assembly adopted the new development agenda : Transforming our world : the 2030 agenda for sustainable development. Comprising 17 Sustainable Development Goals (SDGs), the 2030 Agenda integrates all three dimensions of sustainable development (economic, social and environmental) around the themes of people, planet, prosperity, peace and partnership. The SDGs recognize that eradicating poverty and inequality, creating economic growth and preserving the planet are inextricably linked, not only to each other, but also to population health.

Health is centrally positioned within the 2030 Agenda, with one comprehensive goal – SDG 3 : "Ensure healthy lives and promote well-being for all at all ages"; and explicit links to many of the other goals. SDG 3 includes 13 targets covering all major health priorites, including four targets on the unfinished and expanded Millennium Development Goal agenda, four targets to address non-communicable diseases, mental health, injuries and environmental issues, and four "means of implementation" targets. The target for universal health coverage is key to the achievement of all other targets and the development of strong resilient health system. It will require an integrated approach to the provision of health services that minimize the fragmentation *(43)*.

Conclusion

Contemporary medicine is no longer solely an art and science for the diagnosis and treatment of diseases. It is also the science for the prevention of disease and the promotion of health. The scope of medicine has expanded during the last few decades to include not only health problems of individuals, but those of communities as well. This expansion of the scope of medicine has required a reformulation of its goals and objectives. Systems should integrate health promotion and disease prevention on the one hand, and treatment for acute illness and chronic care on the other. This should be done across all levels of the health care system, with the aim of delivering quality services equitably and efficiently to the whole population.

The real progress in health depends vitally on stronger health system based on primary health care.

It is left to the posterity to review our errors and accomplishments. This is how medicine has evolved down the centuries. Medicine will continue to evolve so long as man's quest for better health continues.

References

1. Siegerist Henry (1951). *A History of Medicine, Vol I* Oxford University Press, London.
2. Dubos, R.J. (1969). *Man, Medicine and Environment,* New American Library, New York.
3. Jaggi, O.P. (1973). *Indian System of Medicine,* Atma Ram and Sons.
4. Gokhale, B.V. (1960). *Swasth Hind,* 4, 165.
5. Banerjee, J.N. (1966). *Ind. J. Med. Edu.,* 5,79.
6. Bhatia, S.L. (1957). *Ind. J. Hist. Med.,* 2,70.
7. Parke-Davis (1961). *Great Moments in Medicine.* A History of Medicine in pictures, Parke-Davis & Co.
8. Kutumbiah, P. (1956). *Ind.J.Hist.Med.,* 2,6.
9. Kishore, Jugal (1974). *Swasth Hind,* 18,36.
10. WHO (1984). *World Health,* July 1984.
11. Smith, A.J. (1974). *Brit.Med.J.,* 2, 367.
12. Diamond, E.G. (1971). *JAMA* 218, 1558.
13. WHO (1970). *World Health,* May 1970.
14. Anderson, C.L. *et al* (1978). *Community Health,* C.V. Mosby.
15. Kark, S.L. (1974). *Epidemiology and Community Medicine,* Appleton Century Crofts.
16. Reiser, S.L. (1980). *World Health Forum,* 1, 103.
17. Guthrie Douglas (1947). *A History of Medicine,* Thomas Nelson & Sons, London.
18. Hobson, W. (1965). *World Health and History,* Oxford University Press, London.
19. Brockington, C.F. (1967). *World Health,* Churchill, London.
20. Noble, John (1976). *Primary Care and the Practice of Medicine,* Boston, Little, Brown & Co.
21. Norton Alan (1969). *The New Dimensions of Medicine,* 20th Century Studies, London, Hodder & Stoughton.
22. Clark Duncan, W and B. MacMahon (1981). *Preventive and Community Medicine,* 2nd ed. Boston, Little, Brown & Co.
23. Crew. F.A.E. (1960). *Med. Edu. Bull,* No.2, WHO, SEARO, New Delhi.
24. Stieglitz, Edward J. (1949). *In: Social Medicine, Its Derivatives and Objectives,* Ed.lago Galdstone, New York, The Commonwealth Fund.
25. Mckeown, T. and C.R. Lowe (1974). *An Introduction to Social Medicine,* 2nd ed., Blackwell, Oxford.
26. Martin, F.M. (1977). *Lancet,* 2, 1336.
27. Acheson, R.M. (1978). *Lancet,* 2, 1737.
28. Roemer, M.I. (1972). *Public Health Papers,* No.48 Geneva, WHO.
29. Fendall, R. (1984). *World Health Forum,* 5,300.
30. Morley, David, et al (1984). *Practising Health for All,* Oxford University Press.
31. Mahler, H. (1977). *World Health,* Nov.1977.
32. WHO-UNICEF (1978). *Health For All,* Sr.No.1.
33. Siegerist, (1947). *Medicine and Health in the Soviet Union,* Jaico Publishing House, Bombay.
34. Newell, K.W. *et al* (1975). *Health by the People,* WHO, Geneva.
35. Rakel, R.E. (1977). *Principles of Family Medicine,* Saunders.
36. Last, J.M. ed (1983) *A Dictionary of Epidemiology,* Oxford University Press.
37. WHO (1972). *Report on the Regional Seminar on Community Medicine of Medical teachers,* WHO/SEA/Med.Edu/187, 7 Sept.
38. WHO (1976). *WHO Chronicle,* 30 (1).8.
39. WHO (1978). *Health for All* Sr.No.1.
40. Djukanovic, V. and Mach, E.P. (1975). *Alternative approaches to meeting basic health needs in developing countries,* A joint UNICEF/WHO study, WHO, Geneva.
41. WHO (2003), *The World Health Report 2003,* Shaping the future.
42. UNDP, *Human Development Report 2003,* Millennium Development Goals : A compact among nations to end human poverty, Oxford University Press.
43. WHO (2016), *World Health Statistics 2016,* Monitoring Health for the SDGs.

2 Concept of Health and Disease

"*Health is NOT mainly an issue of doctors, social services and hospitals. It is an issue of social justice.*"

CONCEPT OF HEALTH

Health is a common theme in most cultures. In fact, all communities have their concepts of health, as part of their culture. Among definitions still used, probably the oldest is that health is the "absence of disease". In some cultures, health and harmony are considered equivalent, harmony being defined as "being at peace with the self, the community, god and cosmos". The ancient Indians and Greeks shared this concept and attributed disease to disturbances in bodily equilibrium of what they called "humors".

Modern medicine is often accused for its preoccupation with the study of disease, and neglect of the study of health. Consequently, our ignorance about health continues to be profound, as for example, the determinants of health are not yet clear; the current definitions of health are elusive; and there is no single yardstick for measuring health. There is thus a great scope for the study of the "epidemiology" of health.

However, during the past few decades, there has been a reawakening that health is a fundamental human right and a worldwide social goal; that it is essential to the satisfaction of basic human needs and to an improved quality of life; and, that it is to be attained by all people. In 1977, the 30th World Health Assembly decided that the main social target of governments and WHO in the coming decades should be "the attainment by all citizens of the world by the year 2000 of a level of health that will permit them to lead a socially and economically productive life", for brevity, called "Health for All" *(1)*. With the adoption of health as an integral part of socio-economic development by the United Nations in 1979 *(2)*, health, while being an end in itself, has also become a major instrument of overall socio-economic development and the creation of a new social order. In the year 2000, the Millennium Development Goals, and more recently in the year 2015, the Sustainable Development Goals kept health centrally positioned to ensure healthy lives and promote well-being for all at all ages.

CHANGING CONCEPTS

An understanding of health is the basis of all health care. Health is not perceived the same way by all members of a community including various professional groups (e.g., biomedical scientists, social science specialists, health administrators, ecologists, etc) giving rise to confusion about the concept of health. In a world of continuous change, new concepts are bound to emerge based on new patterns of thought. Health has evolved over the centuries as a concept from an individual concern to a worldwide social goal and encompasses the whole quality of life. A brief account of the changing concepts of health is given below:

1. Biomedical concept

Traditionally, health has been viewed as an "absence of disease", and if one was free from disease, then the person was considered healthy. This concept, known as the "biomedical concept" has the basis in the "germ theory of disease" which dominated medical thought at the turn of the 20th century. The medical profession viewed the human body as a machine, disease as a consequence of the breakdown of the machine and one of the doctor's task as repair of the machine *(3)*. Thus health, in this narrow view, became the ultimate goal of medicine.

The criticism that is levelled against the biomedical concept is that it has minimized the role of the environmental, social, psychological and cultural determinants of health. The biomedical model, for all its spectacular success in treating disease, was found inadequate to solve some of the major health problems of mankind (e.g., malnutrition, chronic diseases, accidents, drug abuse, mental illness, environmental pollution, population explosion) by elaborating the medical technologies. Developments in medical and social sciences led to the conclusion that the biomedical concept of health was inadequate.

2. Ecological concept

Deficiencies in the biomedical concept gave rise to other concepts. The ecologists put forward an attractive hypothesis which viewed health as a dynamic equilibrium between man and his environment, and disease a maladjustment of the human organism to environment. Dubos *(4)* defined health saying : "Health implies the relative absence of pain and discomfort and a continuous adaptation and adjustment to the environment to ensure optimal function". Human, ecological and cultural adaptations do determine not only the occurrence of disease but also the availability of food and the population explosion. The ecological concept raises two issues, viz. imperfect man and imperfect environment. History argues strongly that improvement in human adaptation to natural environments can lead to longer life expectancies and a better quality of life – even in the absence of modern health delivery services *(5)*.

3. Psychosocial concept

Contemporary developments in social sciences revealed that health is not only a biomedical phenomenon, but one which is influenced by social, psychological, cultural, economic and political factors of the people concerned *(5)*.

These factors must be taken into consideration in defining and measuring health. Thus health is both a biological and social phenomenon.

4. Holistic concept

The holistic model is a synthesis of all the above concepts. It recognizes the strength of social, economic, political and environmental influences on health. It has been variously described as a unified or multidimensional process involving the well-being of the whole person in the context of his environment. This view corresponds to the view held by the ancients that health implies a sound mind, in a sound body, in a sound family, in a sound environment. The holistic approach implies that all sectors of society have an effect on health, in particular, agriculture, animal husbandry, food, industry, education, housing, public works, communications and other sectors *(6)*. The emphasis is on the promotion and protection of health.

DEFINITION OF HEALTH

"Health" is one of those terms which most people find it difficult to define, although they are confident of its meaning. Therefore, many definitions of health have been offered from time to time.

WHO definition

The widely accepted definition of health is that given by the World Health Organization (1948) in the preamble to its constitution, which is as follows :

> *"Health is a state of complete physical, mental and social well-being and not merely an absence of disease or infirmity"*

In recent years, this statement has been amplified to include the ability to lead a "socially and economically productive life" *(6)*.

The WHO definition of health has been criticized as being too broad. Some argue that health cannot be defined as a "state" at all, but must be seen as a process of continuous adjustment to the changing demands of living and of the changing meanings we give to life. It is a dynamic concept. It helps people live well, work well and enjoy themselves.

Inspite of the above limitations, the concept of health as defined by WHO is broad and positive in its implications; it sets out the standard, the standard of "positive" health. It symbolizes the aspirations of people and represents an overall objective or goal towards which nations should strive.

Operational definition of health

The WHO definition of health is not an "operational" definition, i.e., it does not lend itself to direct measurement. Studies of epidemiology of health have been hampered because of our inability to measure health and well-being directly. In this connection an "operational definition" has been devised by a WHO study group *(7)*. In this definition, the concept of health is viewed as being of two orders. In a broad sense, health can be seen as "a condition or quality of the human organism expressing the adequate functioning of the organism in given conditions, genetic or environmental".

In a narrow sense – more useful for measuring purposes – health means: (a) there is no obvious evidence of disease, and that a person is functioning normally, i.e., conforming within normal limits of variation to the standards of health criteria generally accepted for one's age, sex, community, and geographic region; and (b) the several organs of the body are functioning adequately in themselves and in relation to one another, which implies a kind of equilibrium or homeostasis – a condition relatively stable but which may vary as human beings adapt to internal and external stimuli.

New philosophy of health

In recent years, we have acquired a new philosophy of health, which may be stated as below :

- health is a fundamental human right
- health is the essence of productive life, and not the result of ever increasing expenditure on medical care
- health is intersectoral
- health is an integral part of development
- health is central to the concept of quality of life
- health involves individuals, state and international responsibility
- health and its maintenance is a major social investment
- health is a worldwide social goal.

DIMENSIONS OF HEALTH

Health is multidimensional. The WHO definition envisages three specific dimensions – the physical, the mental and the social. Many more may be cited, viz. spiritual, emotional, vocational and political dimensions. As the knowledge base grows, the list may be expanding. Although these dimensions function and interact with one another, each has its own nature, and for descriptive purposes will be treated separately.

1. Physical dimension

The physical dimension of health is probably the easiest to understand. The state of physical health implies the notion of "perfect functioning" of the body. It conceptualizes health biologically as a state in which every cell and every organ is functioning at optimum capacity and in perfect harmony with the rest of the body. However, the term "optimum" is not definable.

The signs of physical health in an individual are: "a good complexion, a clean skin, bright eyes, lustrous hair with a body well clothed with firm flesh, not too fat, a sweet breath, a good appetite, sound sleep, regular activity of bowels and bladder and smooth, easy, coordinated bodily movements. All the organs of the body are of unexceptional size and function normally; all the special senses are intact; the resting pulse rate, blood pressure and exercise tolerance are all within the range of "normality" for the individual's age and sex. In the young and growing individual there is a steady gain in weight and in the future this weight remains more or less constant at a point about 5 lbs (2.3 kg) more or less than the individual's weight at the age of 25 years *(8)*. This state of normality has fairly wide limits. These limits are set by observation of a large number of "normal" people, who are free from evident disease.

Evaluation of physical health

Modern medicine has evolved tools and techniques which may be used in various combinations for the assessment of physical health. They include :

- self assessment of overall health
- inquiry into symptoms of ill-health and risk factors
- inquiry into medications

- inquiry into levels of activity (e.g., number of days of restricted activity within a specified time, degree of fitness)
- inquiry into use of medical services (e.g., the number of visits to a physician, number of hospitalizations) in the recent past
- standardized questionnaires for cardiovascular diseases
- standardized questionnaires for respiratory diseases
- clinical examination
- nutrition and dietary assessment, and
- biochemical and laboratory investigations.

At the community level, the state of health may be assessed by such indicators as death rate, infant mortality rate and expectation of life. Ideally, each piece of information should be individually useful and when combined should permit a more complete health profile of individuals and communities.

2. Mental dimension

Mental health is not mere absence of mental illness. Good mental health is the ability to respond to the many varied experiences of life with flexibility and a sense of purpose. In the recent past, mental health has been defined as "a state of balance between the individual and the surrounding world, a state of harmony between oneself and others, a coexistence between the realities of the self and that of other people and that of the environment" *(9)*.

Some decades ago, the mind and body were considered independent entities. However, researchers have discovered that psychological factors can induce all kinds of illness, not simply mental ones. They include conditions such as essential hypertension, peptic ulcer and bronchial asthma. Some major mental illnesses such as depression and schizophrenia have a biological component. The underlying inference is that there is a behavioural, psychological or biological dysfunction and that the disturbance in the mental equilibrium is not merely in the relationship between the individual and the society *(10)*.

Although mental health is an essential component of health, the scientific foundations of mental health are not yet clear. Therefore, we do not have precise tools to assess the state of mental health unlike physical health. Psychologists have mentioned the following characteristics as attributes of a mentally healthy person:

a. a mentally healthy person is free from internal conflicts; he is not at "war" with himself.
b. he is well-adjusted, i.e., he is able to get along well with others. He accepts criticism and is not easily upset.
c. he searches for identity.
d. he has a strong sense of self-esteem.
e. he knows himself: his needs, problems and goals (this is known as self-actualization).
f. he has good self-control-balances rationality and emotionality.
g. he faces problems and tries to solve them intelligently, i.e., coping with stress and anxiety.

Assessment of mental health at the population level may be made by administering mental status questionnaires by trained interviewers. The most commonly used questionnaires seek to determine the presence and extent of "organic disease" and of symptoms that could indicate psychiatric disorder; some personal assessment of mental well-being is also made. The most basic decision to be made in assessing mental health is whether to assess mental functioning, i.e., the extent to which cognitive or affective impairments impede role performance and subjective life quality, or psychiatric diagnosis *(10)*.

One of the keys to good health is a positive mental health. Unfortunately, our knowledge about mental health is far from complete.

3. Social dimension

Social well-being implies harmony and integration within the individual, between each individual and other members of society and between individuals and the world in which they live *(11)*. It has been defined as the "quantity and quality of an individual's interpersonal ties and the extent of involvement with the community" *(12)*.

The social dimension of health includes the levels of social skills one possesses, social functioning and the ability to see oneself as a member of a larger society. In general, social health takes into account that every individual is part of a family and of wider community and focuses on social and economic conditions and well-being of the "whole person" in the context of his social network. Social health is rooted in "positive material environment" (focussing on financial and residential matters), and "positive human environment" which is concerned with the social network of the individual *(10)*.

4. Spiritual dimension

Proponents of holistic health believe that the time has come to give serious consideration to the spiritual dimension and to the role this plays in health and disease. Spiritual health in this context, refers to that part of the individual which reaches out and strives for meaning and purpose in life. It is the intangible "something" that transcends physiology and psychology. As a relatively new concept, it seems to defy concrete definition. It includes integrity, principles and ethics, the purpose in life, commitment to some higher being and belief in concepts that are not subject to "state of the art" explanation *(13)*.

5. Emotional dimension

Historically the mental and emotional dimensions have been seen as one element or as two closely related elements. However, as more research becomes available a definite difference is emerging. Mental health can be seen as "knowing" or "cognition" while emotional health relates to "feeling". Experts in psychobiology have been relatively successful in isolating these two separate dimensions. With this new data, the mental and emotional aspects of humanness may have to be viewed as two separate dimensions of human health *(13)*.

6. Vocational dimension

The vocational aspect of life is a new dimension. It is part of human existence. When work is fully adapted to human goals, capacities and limitations, work often plays a role in promoting both physical and mental health. Physical work is usually associated with an improvement in physical capacity, while goal achievement and self-realization in work are a source of satisfaction and enhanced self-esteem *(14)*.

The importance of this dimension is exposed when individuals suddenly lose their jobs or are faced with mandatory retirement. For many individuals, the vocational dimension may be merely a source of income. To others, this dimension represents the culmination of the efforts of other dimensions as they function together to produce what the individual considers life "success" *(13)*.

7. Others

A few other dimensions have also been suggested such as *(15)*:

- philosophical dimension
- cultural dimension
- socio-economic dimension
- environmental dimension
- educational dimension
- nutritional dimension
- curative dimension
- preventive dimension.

A glance at the above dimensions shows that there are many "non-medical" dimensions of health, e.g., social, cultural, educational, etc. These symbolize a huge range of factors to which other sectors besides health must contribute if all people are indeed to attain a level of health that will permit them to lead a socially and economically productive life.

POSITIVE HEALTH

Health in the broad sense of the world does not merely mean the absence of disease or provision of diagnostic, curative and preventive services. It also includes as embodied in the WHO definition, a state of physical, mental and social well-being. The harmonious balance of this state of the human individual integrated into his environment, constitutes health, as defined by WHO.

The state of positive health implies the notion of "perfect functioning" of the body and mind. It conceptualizes health **biologically**, as a state in which every cell and every organ is functioning at optimum capacity and in perfect harmony with the rest of the body; **psychologically**, as a state in which the individual feels a sense of perfect well-being and of mastery over his environment, and **socially**, as a state in which the individual's capacities for participation in the social system are optimal *(16)*. These ideas were widely ventilated some years ago but now appear slightly ridiculous *(17)*.

Dubos *(4)* said, "The concept of perfect positive health cannot become a reality because man will never be so perfectly adapted to his environment that his life will not involve struggles, failures and sufferings". Positive health will, therefore, always remain a mirage, because everything in our life is subject to change. Health in this context has been described as a potentiality – the ability of an individual or a social group to modify himself or itself continually, in the face of changing conditions of life. In working for positive health the doctor and the community health expert are in the same position as the gardener or farmer faced with insects, moulds and weeds. Their work is never done *(18)*.

A broader concept of health has been emerging - that of improving the quality of life of which health is an essential component. This at once brings to focus that positive health depends not only on medical action, but on all the other economic, cultural and social factors operating in the community.

HEALTH – A RELATIVE CONCEPT

An alternative approach to positive health conceptualizes health not as an ideal state, but as a biologically "normal" state, based on statistical averages *(3)*. For example, a newborn baby in India weighs 2.8 kg on an average compared to 3.5 kg in the developed countries, and yet compares favourably in health. The height and weight standards vary from country to country, and also between socio-economic groups. Many normal people show heart murmurs, enlarged tonsils and X-ray shadows in the chest and yet do not show signs of ill-health. Thus health is a relative concept *(7)* and health standards vary among cultures, social classes and age-groups. This implies that health in any society should be defined in terms of prevailing ecological conditions. That is, instead of setting universal health standards, each country will decide on its own norms for a given set of prevailing conditions and then look into ways to achieve that level *(19)*.

CONCEPT OF WELL-BEING

Well-being is in general a term used to describe a condition of an individual or a group, with reference to social, economic, psychological, spiritual or medical attention.

Psychologists have pointed out that the "well-being" of an individual or group of individuals have objective and subjective components. The objective components relate to such concerns as are generally known by the term "standard of living" or "level of living". The subjective component of well-being (as expressed by each individual) is referred to as "quality of life" *(20)*. Let us consider these concepts separately.

1. Standard of living

The term "standard of living" refers to the usual scale of our expenditure, the goods we consume and the services we enjoy. It includes the level of education, employment status, food, dress, house, amusements and comforts of modern living *(20)*.

A similar definition, corresponding to the above, was proposed by WHO: "Income and occupation, standards of housing, sanitation and nutrition, the level of provision of health, educational, recreational and other services may all be used individually as measures of socio-economic status, and collectively as an index of the "standard of living" *(21)*.

There are vast inequalities in the standards of living of the people in different countries of the world. The extent of these differences are usually measured through the comparison of per capita GNP on which the standard of living primarily depends.

2. Level of living

The parallel term for standard of living used in United Nations documents is "level of living" *(22)*. It consists of nine components: health, food consumption, education, occupation and working conditions, housing, social security, clothing, recreation and leisure, and human rights. These objective characteristics are believed to influence human well-being. It is considered that health is the most important component of the level of living because its impairment always means impairment of the level of living.

3. Quality of life

Much has been said and written on the quality of life in recent years. It is the "subjective" component of well-being. "Quality of life" was defined by WHO *(23)* as: "the condition of life resulting from the combination of the effects of the complete range of factors such as those determining health, happiness (including comfort in the physical environment and a satisfying occupation), education, social and intellectual attainments, freedom of action, justice and freedom of expression".

A recent definition of quality of life by WHO is as follows: "the product of the interplay between social, health, economic, and environmental conditions which affect human and social development. It is a broad-ranging concept, incorporating a person's physical health, psychological state, level of independence, social relationships, personal belief and relationship to salient features in the environment" *(24)*.

Thus, a distinction is drawn between the concept of "level of living" consisting of objective criteria and of "quality of life" comprising the individual's own subjective evaluation of these. The quality of life can be evaluated by assessing a person's subjective feelings of happiness or unhappiness about the various life concerns.

People are now demanding a better quality of life. Therefore, governments all over the world are increasingly concerned about improving the quality of life of their people by reducing morbidity and mortality, providing primary health care and enhancing physical, mental and social well-being. It is conceded that a rise in the standard of living of the people is not enough to achieve satisfaction or happiness. Improvement of quality of life must also be added, and this means increased emphasis on social policy and on reformulation of societal goals to make life more liveable for all.

Physical quality of life index (PQLI)

As things stand at present, this important concept of quality of life is difficult to define and even more difficult to measure. Various attempts have been made to reach one composite index from a number of health indicators. The "Physical quality of life index" is one such index. It consolidates three indicators, viz. infant mortality, life expectancy at age one, and literacy. These three components measure the results rather than inputs. As such they lend themselves to international and national comparison.

For each component, the performance of individual countries is placed on a scale of 0 to 100, where 0 represents an absolutely defined "worst" performance, and 100 represents an absolutely defined "best" performance. The composite index is calculated by averaging the three indicators, giving equal weight to each of them. The resulting PQLI thus also is scaled 0 to 100.

It may be mentioned that PQLI has not taken per capita GNP into consideration, showing thereby that "money is not everything". For example, the oil-rich countries of Middle East with high per capita incomes have in fact not very high PQLIs. At the other extreme, Sri Lanka and Kerala state in India have low per capita incomes with high PQLIs. In short, PQLI does not measure economic growth; it measures the results of social, economic and political policies. It is intended to complement, not replace GNP *(25)*. The ultimate objective is to attain a PQLI of 100.

Human Development Index (HDI) *(26)*

Human development index (HDI) is defined as "a composite index focusing on three basic dimensions of human development : to lead a long and healthy life measured by life expectancy at birth; the ability to acquire knowledge, measured by mean years of schooling and expected years of schooling; and the ability to achieve a decent standard of living, measured by gross national income per capita in PPP US $. Fig. 1 summarizes how the human development index is constructed.

Thus the concept of HDI reflects achievements in the most basic human capabilities, viz, leading a long life, being knowledgeable and enjoying a decent standard of living. Hence, these three variables have been chosen to represent those dimensions. The HDI is a more comprehensive measure than per capita income. Income is only a means to human development, not an end. Nor is it a sum total of human lives. Thus by focussing on areas beyond income and treating income as a proxy for a decent standard of living, the HDI provides a more comprehensive picture of human life than income does.

The HDI values range between 0 to 1. The HDI value for a country shows the distance that it has already travelled towards maximum possible value to 1, and also allows comparisons with other countries.

STEPS TO ESTIMATE THE HUMAN DEVELOPMENT INDEX *(27)*

There are two steps to calculating the HDI.

Step 1. Creating the dimension indices

Minimum and maximum values (goalposts) are set in order to transform the indicators into indices between 0 and 1. The maximums are the highest observed values in the time series (1980–2011). The minimum values can be appropriately conceived of as subsistence values. The minimum values are set at 20 years for expectancy, at 0 years for both education variables and at $100 for per capita gross national income (GNI).

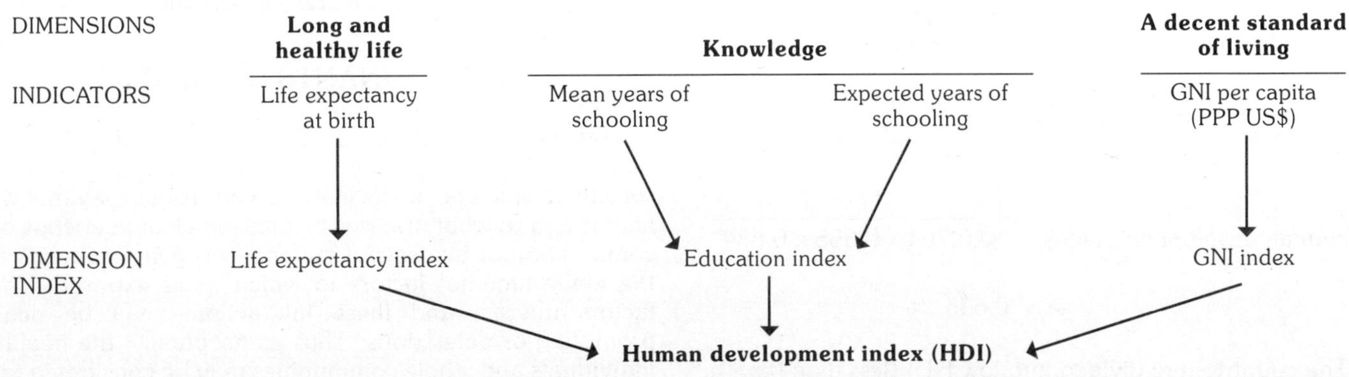

FIG. 1
Calculating the Human Development Index

Source : *(28)*

Goalposts for the Human Development Index

DIMENSION	OBSERVED MAXIMUM	MINIMUM
Life expectancy	85	20.0
Mean years of schooling	15	0
Expected years of schooling	18	0
Per capita income (PPP $)	75,000	100

Having defined the minimum and maximum values, the subindices are calculated as follows:

$$\text{Dimension index} = \frac{\text{Actual value} - \text{Minimum value}}{\text{Maximum value} - \text{Minimum value}} \qquad (1)$$

For education, equation 1 is applied to each of the two subcomponents, then a geometric mean of the resulting indices is created and finally, equation 1 is reapplied to the geometric mean of the indices using 0 as the minimum and the highest geometric mean of the resulting indices for the time period under consideration, as the maximum. This is equivalent to applying equation 1 directly to the geometric mean of the two subcomponents.

Step 2. Aggregating the subindices to produce the Human Development Index

The HDI is the geometric mean of the three dimension indices:

$$(I_{Life}^{1/3} \times I_{Education}^{1/3} \times I_{Income}^{1/3}) \qquad (2)$$

The construction of HDI methodology can be illustrated with the example of India for the year 2019.

Indicator	Value
Life expectancy at birth (years)	69.7
Mean years of schooling (years)	6.5
Expected years of schooling (years)	12.2
GNI per capita (PPP $)	6,681

$$\text{Life expectancy index} = \frac{69.7 - 20}{85 - 20} = \frac{49.7}{65} = 0.764$$

$$\text{Mean years of schooling index} = \frac{6.5 - 0}{15 - 0} = 0.433$$

$$\text{Expected years of schooling index} = \frac{12.2 - 0}{18.0 - 0} = 0.677$$

$$\text{Education index} = \frac{0.433 + 0.677}{2} = 0.555$$

$$\text{Income index} = \frac{\ln (6,681) - \ln (100)}{\ln (75,000) - \ln (100)} = 0.634$$

$$\text{Human development index} = \sqrt[3]{0.764 \times 0.555 \times 0.634}$$

$$= 0.645$$

The countries are divided into low HDI (less than 0.550), medium HDI (between 0.550 to 0.699), high HDI (between 0.700 to 0.799), and very high HDI for more than 0.800 values *(29)*.

For the year 2019, Norway, Ireland and Switzerland are at the top of HDI ranking, Niger and Central African Republic, are at the bottom. India comes in the medium human development category, ranking at number 131 *(29)*.

Disparities between regions can be significant with some regions having more ground to cover in making the shortfall than others. The link between the economic prosperity and human development is neither automatic nor obvious. Two countries with similar income per capita can have very different HDI values, and countries having similar HDI can have very different income levels.

SPECTRUM OF HEALTH

Health and disease lie along a continuum, and there is no single cut-off point. The lowest point on the health–disease spectrum is death and the highest point corresponds to the WHO definition of positive health (Fig. 2). It is thus obvious that health fluctuates within a range of optimum well-being to various levels of dysfunction, including the state of total dysfunction, namely the death. The transition from optimum health to ill-health is often gradual, and where one state ends and the other begins is a matter of judgment.

The spectral concept of health emphasizes that the health of an individual is not static; it is a dynamic phenomenon and a process of continuous change, subject to frequent subtle variations. What is considered maximum health today may be minimum tomorrow. That is, a person may function at maximum levels of health today, and diminished levels of health tomorrow. It implies that health is a state not to be attained once and for all, but ever to be renewed. There are degrees or "levels of health" as there are degrees or severity of illness. As long as we are alive there is some degree of health in us.

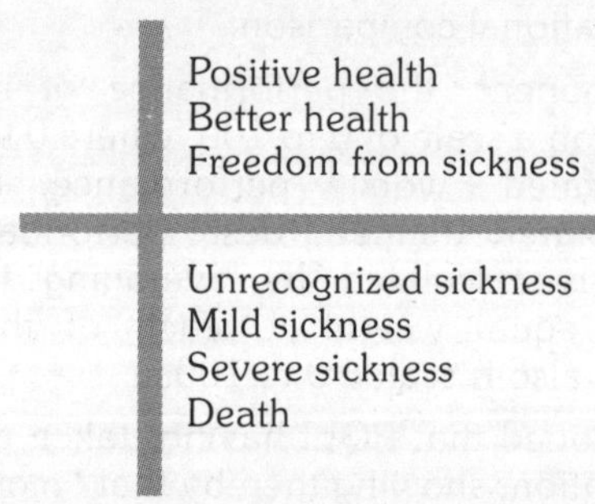

FIG. 2
The health sickness spectrum

DETERMINANTS OF HEALTH

Health is multifactorial. The factors which influence health lie both within the individual and externally in the society in which he or she lives. It is a truism to say that what man is and to what diseases he may fall victim depends on a combination of two sets of factors – his genetic factors and the environmental factors to which he is exposed. These factors interact and these interactions may be health-promoting or deleterious. Thus, conceptually, the health of individuals and whole communities may be considered to be the result of many interactions. Only a brief indication of the more important determinants or variables are shown in Fig. 3.

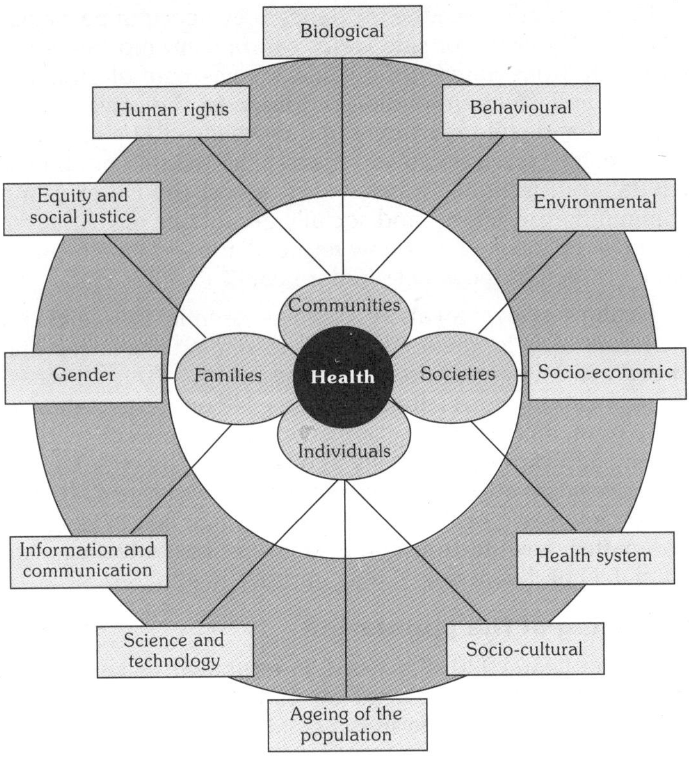

Source : *(30)*

FIG. 3
Determinants of health

1. Biological determinants

The physical and mental traits of every human being are to some extent determined by the nature of his genes at the moment of conception. The genetic make-up is unique in that it cannot be altered after conception. A number of diseases are now known to be of genetic origin, e.g., chromosomal anomalies, errors of metabolism, mental retardation, some types of diabetes, etc. The state of health, therefore depends partly on the genetic constitution of man. Nowadays, medical genetics offers hope for prevention and treatment of a wide spectrum of diseases, thus the prospect of better medicine and longer, healthier life. A vast field of knowledge has yet to be exploited. It plays a particularly important role in genetic screening and gene therapy.

Thus, from the genetic stand-point, health may be defined as that "state of the individual which is based upon the absence from the genetic constitution of such genes as correspond to characters that take the form of serious defect and derangement and to the absence of any aberration in respect of the total amount of chromosome material in the karyotype or stated in positive terms, from the presence in the genetic constitution of the genes that correspond to the normal characterization and to the presence of a normal karyotype" *(8)*.

The "positive health" advocated by WHO implies that a person should be able to express as completely as possible the potentialities of his genetic heritage. This is possible only when the person is allowed to live in healthy relationship with his environment – an environment that transforms genetic potentialities into phenotypic realities *(18)*.

2. Behavioural and socio-cultural conditions

The term "lifestyle" is rather a diffuse concept often used to denote "the way people live", reflecting a whole range of social values, attitudes and activities *(31)*. It is composed of cultural and behavioural patterns and lifelong personal habits (e.g., smoking, alcoholism) that have developed through processes of socialization. Lifestyles are learnt through social interaction with parents, peer groups, friends and siblings and through school and mass media.

Health requires the promotion of healthy lifestyle. A considerable body of evidence has accumulated which indicates that there is an association between health and lifestyle of individuals *(32)*. Many current-day health problems especially in the developed countries (e.g., coronary heart disease, obesity, lung cancer, drug addiction) are associated with lifestyle changes. In developing countries such as India where traditional lifestyles still persist, risks of illness and death are connected with lack of sanitation, poor nutrition, personal hygiene, elementary human habits, customs and cultural patterns.

It may be noted that not all lifestyle factors are harmful. There are many that can actually promote health. Examples include adequate nutrition, enough sleep, sufficient physical activity, etc. In short, the achievement of optimum health demands adoption of healthy lifestyles. Health is both a consequence of an individual's lifestyle and a factor in determining it *(31)*.

3. Environment

It was Hippocrates who first related disease to environment, e.g., climate, water, air, etc. Centuries later, Pettenkofer in Germany revived the concept of disease–environment association.

Environment is classified as "internal" and "external". The **internal** environment of man pertains to "each and every component part, every tissue, organ and organ–system and their harmonious functioning within the system". Internal environment is the domain of internal medicine. The **external** or macro-environment consists of those things to which man is exposed after conception. It is defined as "all that which is external to the individual human host" *(33)*. It can be divided into physical, biological and psychosocial components, any or all of which can affect the health of man and his susceptibility to illness. Some epidemiologists have used the term "micro-environment" (or domestic environment) to personal environment which includes the individual's way of living and lifestyle, e.g., eating habits, other personal habits (e.g., smoking or drinking), use of drugs, etc. It is also customary to speak about occupational environment, socio-economic environment and moral environment.

It is an established fact that environment has a direct impact on the physical, mental and social well-being of those living in it. The environmental factors range from housing, water supply, psychosocial stress and family structure through social and economic support systems, to the organization of health and social welfare services in the community.

The environmental components (physical, biological and psychological) are not water-tight compartments. They are so inextricably linked with one another that it is realistic and fruitful to view the human environment in toto when we consider the influence of environment on the health status of the population. If the environment is favourable to the individual, he can make full use of his physical and mental capabilities. Protection and promotion of family and environmental health is one of the major issues in the world today.

4. Socio-economic conditions

Socio-economic conditions have long been known to influence human health. For the majority of the world's people, health status is determined primarily by their level of socio-economic development, e.g., per capita GNP, education, nutrition, employment, housing, the political system of the country, etc. Those of major importance are :

(i) *Economic status* : The per capita GNP is the most widely accepted measure of general economic performance. There can be no doubt that in many developing countries, it is the economic progress that has been the major factor in reducing morbidity, increasing life expectancy and improving the quality of life (Table 7). The economic status determines the purchasing power, standard of living, quality of life, family size and the pattern of disease and deviant behaviour in the community. It is also an important factor in seeking health care. Ironically, affluence may also be a contributory cause of illness as exemplified by the high rates of coronary heart disease, diabetes and obesity in the upper socio-economic groups.

(ii) *Education* : A second major factor influencing health status is education (especially female education). The world map of illiteracy closely coincides with the maps of poverty, malnutrition, illhealth, high infant and child mortality rates. Studies indicate that education, to some extent, compensates the effects of poverty on health, irrespective of the availability of health facilities. The small state of Kerala in India is a striking example. Kerala has an estimated infant mortality rate of 6 compared to 28 for all-India in 2020. A major factor in the low infant mortality of Kerala is its high female literacy rate of 98.3 per cent as compared to 71.5 per cent for all-India for the year 2019–20 *(34)*.

(iii) *Occupation* : The very state of being employed in productive work promotes health, because the unemployed usually show a higher incidence of illhealth and death. For many, loss of work may mean loss of income and status. It can cause psychological and social damage.

(iv) *Political system* : Health is also related to the country's political system. Often the main obstacles to the implementation of health technologies are not technical, but rather political. Decisions concerning resource allocation, manpower policy, choice of technology and the degree to which health services are made available and accessible to different segments of the society are examples of the manner in which the political system can shape community health services *(35)*. The percentage of GNP spent on health is a quantitative indicator of political commitment. The WHO has set the target of at least 5 per cent expenditure of each country's GNP on health care. However India spends about 1 per cent of its GNP on health and family welfare *(36)*. What is needed is political commitment and leadership which is oriented towards social development, and not merely economic development. If poor health patterns are to be changed, then changes must be made in the entire socio-political system in any given community. Social, economic and political actions are required to eliminate health hazards in people's working and living environments.

5. Health services

The term health and family welfare services cover a wide spectrum of personal and community services for treatment of disease, prevention of illness and promotion of health. The purpose of health services is to improve the health status of the population. For example, immunization of children can influence the incidence/prevalence of particular diseases. Provision of safe water can prevent mortality and morbidity from water-borne diseases. The care of pregnant women and children would contribute to the reduction of maternal and child morbidity and mortality. To be effective, the health services must reach the social periphery, equitably distributed, accessible at a cost the country and community can afford, and socially acceptable *(6)*. All these are ingredients of what is now termed "primary health care", which is seen as the way to better health.

Health services can also be seen as essential for social and economic development. It is well to remind ourselves that "health care does not produce good health" *(37)*. Whereas, there is a strong correlation between GNP and expectation of life at birth, there is no significant correlation between medical density and expectation of life at birth *(38)*. The most we can expect from an effective health service is good care *(37)*. The epidemiological perspective emphasizes that health services, no matter how technically elegant or cost-effective, are ultimately pertinent only if they improve health *(39)*.

6. Ageing of the population

By the year 2020, the world is estimated to have more than 1.4 billion people aged 60 and over, and more than two-thirds of them living in developing countries. Although the elderly in many countries enjoy better health than hitherto, a major concern of rapid population ageing is the increased prevalence of chronic diseases and disabilities, both being conditions that tend to accompany the ageing process and deserve special attention.

7. Gender

The 1990s have witnessed an increased concentration on women's issues. In 1993, the Global Commission on Women's Health was established. The commission drew up an agenda for action on women's health covering nutrition, reproductive health, the health consequences of violence, ageing, lifestyle related conditions and the occupational environment. It has brought about an increased awareness among policy–makers of women's health issues and encourages their inclusion in all development plans as a priority.

8. Other factors

We are witnessing the transition from post industrial age to an information age and experiencing the early days of two interconnected revolutions, in information and in communication. The development of these technologies offers tremendous opportunities in providing an easy and instant access to medical information once difficult to retrieve. It contributes to dissemination of information worldwide, serving the needs of many physicians, health professionals, biomedical scientists and researchers, the mass media and the public.

Other contributions to the health of population derive from systems outside the formal health care system, i.e., health related systems (e.g., food and agriculture, education, industry, social welfare, rural development), as well as adoption of policies in the economic and social fields that would assist in raising the standard of living. This would include employment opportunities, increased wages, prepaid medical programmes and family support systems.

In short, medicine is not the sole contributor to the health and well-being of population. The potential of intersectoral contributions to the health of communities is increasingly recognized.

ECOLOGY OF HEALTH

Ecology is a key word in present–day health philosophy. It comes from the Greek "Oikos" meaning a house. Ecology is defined as the science of mutual relationship between living organisms and their environments. Human ecology is a subset of more general science of ecology. It is defined as the study of human groups as influenced by environmental factors, including social and behavioural factors. A macro-level, holistic approach to the study of human organization *(40)*.

A full understanding of health requires that humanity be seen as part of an ecosystem. The human ecosystem includes in addition to the natural environment, all the dimensions of the man-made environment – physical, chemical, biological, psychological: in short, our culture and all its products *(41)*. Disease is embedded in the ecosystem of man. Health, according to ecological concepts, is visualized as a state of dynamic equilibrium between man and his environment.

By constantly altering his environment or ecosystem by such activities as urbanization, industrialization, deforestation, land reclamation, construction of irrigation canals and dams, man has created for himself new health problems. For example, the greatest threat to human health in India today is the ever–increasing, unplanned urbanization, growth of slums and deterioration of environment. As a result, diseases at one time thought to be primarily "rural" have acquired serious urban dimensions. The agents of a number of diseases, for example, dengue and chikungunya fever, which were effectively controlled have shown a recrudescence. The reasons for this must be sought in changes in the human ecology. Man's intrusion into ecological cycles of disease has resulted in zoonotic diseases such as kyasanur forest disease, rabies, yellow fever, monkeypox, lassa fever, etc. The Bhopal gas tragedy in 1984 highlights the danger of locating industries in urban areas. The nuclear disaster in Soviet Russia in April 1986 is another grim reminder of environmental pollution. Construction of irrigation systems and artificial lakes has created ecological niches favouring the breeding of mosquitoes and snails. In fact, ecological factors are at the root of the geographic distribution of disease. Therefore it has been said that good public health is basically good ecology.

Some have equated ecology with epidemiology. The main distinction between epidemiology and ecology is that while epidemiology is the study of the relationship between variations in man's environment and his state of health (or disease), ecology embraces the interrelationship of all living things. In this regard, epidemiology constitutes a special application of human ecology or that part of ecology relating to the state of human health *(42)*.

It is now being increasingly recognized that environmental factors and ecological considerations must be built into the total planning process to prevent degradation of ecosystems. Prevention of disease through ecological or environmental manipulations or interventions is much safer, cheaper and a more effective rational approach than all the other means of control. It is through environmental manipulations that diseases such as cholera and other diarrhoeal diseases, typhoid, malaria and other vector borne diseases, and hookworm disease could be brought under control or eliminated. The greatest improvement in human health thus may be expected from an understanding and modification of the factors that favour disease occurrence in the human ecosystem. Professor Rene Dubos believes that man's capacity to adapt himself to ecological changes is not unlimited. Man can adapt himself only in so far as the mechanisms of adaptations are potentially present in his genetic code *(18)*.

RIGHT TO HEALTH

With the establishment of WHO, for the first time the right to health was recognized internationally. The WHO constitution affirms that "the enjoyment of the highest attainable standard of health is one of the fundamental right of every human being, without distinction of race, religion, political belief, economic or social condition". Over the time this recognition was reiterated in a wide array of formulation in several international and regional human rights *(43)*.

The International Covenant on Economic, Social and Cultural Rights, widely considered as the central instrument of protection for the right to health recognizes "the right to health of everyone to the enjoyment of the highest attainable standard of physical and mental health". It is important to note that the covenant gives both physical health and mental health equal consideration *(44)*. The steps to be taken to achieve the full realization of the right to health include those necessary for *(45)* :

(a) The provision for the reduction of stillbirth rate and infant mortality, and for the healthy development of the child;

(b) The improvement of all aspects of environmental and industrial hygiene;

(c) The prevention, treatment and control of epidemic, endemic, occupational and other diseases; and

(d) The creation of conditions which would assure to all medical service and medical attention in the event of sickness.

To operationalize the above provisions, the UN Committee on Economic, Social and Cultural Rights adopted a General Comment on "Right to Health" in the year 2000, and set out that the right to health extends not only to timely and appropriate health care but also to the underlying determinants of health, such as access to safe and potable water, adequate sanitation, an adequate supply of safe food, nutrition and housing, healthy occupational and environmental conditions and access to health-related education and information, including on sexual and reproductive health *(45)*. According to General Comment, the right to health also has a "core content" referring to the minimum essential level of the right with above mentioned key elements in addition to the supply of essential drugs.

The human right to health care means that hospitals, clinics, medicines and doctor's services must be accessible, available, acceptable (non-discrimination, physical accessibility, affordability and information accessibility), and of good quality for everyone, on an equitable basis, where and when needed. The key principles are : (a) Universality; (b) Equity; (c) Accountability; (d) Transparency; and (e) Participation.

At the international level, the Universal Declaration of Human Rights (Art. 25) established in 1948 acknowledges the relationship between health and well-being, and its link with other rights. The other international human rights treaties recognizing the right to health are as follows:

1. The 1965 International Convention on the Elimination of all forms of Racial Discrimination (Art. 5);
2. The 1966 International Covenant on Economic, Social and Cultural Rights (Art. 12);

3. The 1979 Convention on the Elimination of all forms of Discrimination against Women (Art. 11, 12 and 14);
4. The 1989 Convention on the Rights of the Child (Art. 24);
5. The 1990 International Convention on the Protection of the Rights of All Migrant Workers and Members of their Families (Art. 28, 43 and 45);
6. The 2006 Convention on the Rights of Persons with Disabilities (Art. 25).

Numerous conferences and declarations, such as declaration of Alma-Ata on Primary Health Care and WHO designed plan "Health for all by the year 2000", which consists of a series of goals and programmes, to achieve minimum level of health for all. Later on, "Promoting Health", one of the fundamental aspect of primary health care, has been addressed independently by four successive conferences – Ottawa, Canada in 1986; Jakarta, Indonesia in 1997; Cairo in 1994 and Conference on Women in Beijing, 1995. The United Nation's Millennium Development Goals, Declaration of Commitment on HIV/AIDs and more recently Sustainable Development Goals, 2015 : the 2030 Agenda for Sustainable Development has health centrally positioned. The right to health or the right to health care is recognized in at least 115 countries constitution.

RESPONSIBILITY FOR HEALTH

Health is on one hand a highly personal responsibility and on the other hand a major public concern. It thus involves the joint efforts of the whole social fabric, viz. the individual, the community and the state to protect and promote health.

1. Individual responsibility

Although health is now recognized a fundamental human right, it is essentially an individual responsibility. It is not a commodity that one individual can bestow on another. No community or state programme of health services can give health. In large measure, it has to be earned and maintained by the individual himself, who must accept a broad spectrum of responsibilities, now known as "self care".

Self care in health

Presently the trend in health care is self care. It is defined as "health activities, including promotion, maintenance, treatment care and health related decision making, carried out by individuals and families" *(24)*. It refers to those activities individuals undertake in promoting their own health, preventing their own disease, limiting their own illness, and restoring their own health. These activities are undertaken without professional assistance, although individuals are informed by technical knowledge and skills. The generic attribute of self care is its non-professional, non-bureaucratic, non-industrial character; its natural place in social life *(46)*.

Self care activities comprise observance of simple rules of behaviour relating to diet, sleep, exercise, weight, alcohol, smoking and drugs. Others include attention to personal hygiene, cultivation of healthful habits and lifestyle, submitting oneself to selective medical examinations and screening; accepting immunization and carrying out other specific disease–prevention measures, reporting early when sick and accepting treatment, undertaking measures for the prevention of a relapse or of the spread of the disease to others. To these must be added family planning which is essentially an individual responsibility.

The shift in disease patterns from acute to chronic disease makes self care both a logical necessity and an appropriate strategy. For example, by teaching patients self care (e.g., recording one's own blood pressure and blood sugar level, the burden on the official health services would be considerably reduced. In other words, health must begin with the individual.

2. Community responsibility

Health can never be adequately protected by health services without the active understanding and involvement of communities whose health is at stake. Until quite recently, throughout the world, people were neglected as a health resource; they were merely looked upon as sources of pathology or victims of pathology and consequently as a "target" for preventive and therapeutic services. This negative view of people's role in health has changed because of the realization that there are many things which the individual cannot do for himself except through united community effort. The individual and community responsibility are complementary, not antithetical. The current trend is to "demedicalize" health and involve the communities in a meaningful way. This implies a more active involvement of families and communities in health matters, viz. planning, implementation, utilization, operation and evaluation of health services. In other words, the emphasis has shifted from **health care for the people to health care by the people.** The concept of primary health care centres round people's participation in their own activities. The Village Health Guides' scheme in India, launched in 1977 and ASHA under National Health Mission are examples of community participation.

There are three ways in which a community can participate *(47)*: (i) the community can provide in the shape of facilities, manpower, logistic support, and possibly funds (ii) it also means the community can be actively involved in planning, management, and evaluation, and (iii) an equally important contribution that people can make is by joining in and using the health services. This is particularly true of preventive and protective measures. Further, no standard pattern of community participation can be recommended since there is a wide range of economic and social problems, as well as political and cultural traits among and within the communities. What is essential is flexibility of approach.

However, community involvement is not easy to obtain as extensive experience has indicated *(48)*. The traditional Indian society is cut across on rigid religion and caste lines, and appropriate role for each caste group has been a serious obstacle in securing complete community participation *(49)*. And in the health sector, the greatest resistance to health guide's involvement in primary health care came from the medical profession than the lay public *(50)*. Community participation has become an aphorism that is still awaiting genuine realization in many countries of the world.

Long ago, Henry Sigerist, the medical historian stated that "The people's health ought to be the concern of the people themselves. They must struggle for it and plan for it. The war against disease and for health cannot be fought by physicians alone. It is a people's war in which the entire population must be mobilized permanently" *(51)*.

3. State responsibility

The responsibility for health does not end with the individual and community effort. In all civilized societies, the

State assumes responsibility for the health and welfare of its citizens. The Constitution of India provides that health is a State responsibility. The relevant portions are to be found in the Directive Principles of State Policy, which are as below :

The State shall, in particular, direct the policy towards securing–

....that the health and strength of workers, men and women and the tender age of children are not abused and that citizens are not forced by economic necessity to enter avocations unsuited to their age or strength.

....that childhood and youth are protected against exploitation and against moral and material abandonment.

The State shall, within the limits of its economic capacity and development, make effective provision for securing the right to work, to education and to public assistance in cases of unemployment, old age, sickness and disablement, and in other cases of undeserved want.

The State shall make provision for securing just and humane conditions of work and maternity relief.

The State shall regard the raising of the level of nutrition and standard of living of its people and the improvement of public health as among its primary duties.

– The Constitution of India; Part IV

India is a signatory to the Alma-Ata Declaration of 1978 and the Millennium Development Goals of 2000. The National Health Policy, approved by Parliament in 1983 and later on in 2002 have resulted in a greater degree of state involvement in the management of health services, and the establishment of nation-wide systems of health services with emphasis on primary health care approach.

4. International responsibility

The health of mankind requires the cooperation of governments, the people, national and international organizations both within and outside the United Nations system in achieving our health goals. This cooperation covers such subjects as exchange of experts, provision of drugs and supplies, border meetings with regard to control of communicable diseases. The TCDC (Technical Cooperation in Developing Countries), ASEAN (Association of South–East Asian Nations) and SAARC (South Asia Association for Regional Cooperation) are important regional mechanisms for such cooperation.

The eradication of smallpox and polio, the pursuit of "Health for All", Millennium Development Goals, Sustainable Development Goals, and The Global Strategy for Women's, Children's and Adolescent's Health (2016–2030); and the campaign against smoking and AIDS are a few recent examples of international responsibility for the control of disease and promotion of health. Today, more than ever before, there is a wider international understanding on matters relating to health and "social injustices" in the distribution of health services. The WHO is a major factor in fostering international cooperation in health. In keeping with its constitutional mandate, WHO acts as a directing and coordinating authority on international health work.

HEALTH AND DEVELOPMENT

"Health is essential to socio-economic development" has gained increasing recognition. It was commonly thought in the 1960s that socio-economic progress was not essential for improving the health status of people in developing countries, and that substantial and rapid progress could be made through introduction of modern public health measures alone. According to this way of thinking, the role of human beings in the developing process was grossly underestimated.

The period 1973–1977 witnessed considerable rethinking on this subject *(49)*. There was profound modification of the economic theory. It became increasingly clear that economic development alone cannot solve the major problems of poverty, hunger, malnutrition and disease. In its place, "non-economic" issues (e.g., education, productive employment, housing, equity, freedom and dignity, human welfare) have emerged as major objectives in development strategies.

The experiences of a few developing countries (e.g., Sri Lanka, Costa Rica, and the state of Kerala in India) illustrate dramatically the way in which health forms part of development. This was because the efforts in the health field were simultaneously reinforced by developments in other sectors such as education, social welfare and land reforms *(52)*. The link between health and development has been clearly established, the one being the starting point for the other and vice versa.

Since health is an integral part of development, all sectors of society have an effect on health. In other words, health services are no longer considered merely as a complex of solely medical measures but a "subsystem" of an overall socio-economic system. In the final analysis, human health and well-being are the ultimate goal of development.

Lessons from Kerala State

Kerala is the southern-most state of India. With a population of 3.56 crore, and an estimated population density of 926 per sq.km, the state of Kerala is extremely crowded. Its annual *per capita* income of Rs. 2,36,093 (2021–22) was more than the national average of Rs. 1,28,829. Kerala has surpassed all the Indian states in certain important measures of health and social development, as shown in Table 1.

TABLE 1

Comparison of Kerala and all–India Health Statistics

	Kerala	All India
Death rate/1000 (2020)	7.0	6.0
Rural birth rate (2020)	13.1	21.1
Infant mortality rate (2020)	6.0	28
Under-five mortality rate (2019)	9.0	35
Maternal mortality ratio (2017–19)	30	103
Annual growth rate, per cent (2020)	0.62	1.35
Life expectancy at birth (2014–17)	75.2	69.6
Literacy rate, per cent (2021)	96.2	77.7
Female literacy rate (2019–20)	98.3	71.5
Mean age at marriage, females (2019)	23.2	22.3
Per capita income (2021–22)	Rs. 2,36,093	Rs. 1,28,829

Kerala has demonstrated that, in a democratic system with a strong political commitment to equitable socio-economic development, high levels of health can be achieved even on modest levels of income. Kerala can therefore be considered a **yardstick** for judging health status in the country.

Studies have shown that the efforts in the health field

were simultaneously reinforced by developments in other sectors. Literacy (especially female literacy) has played a key role in improving the health situation. This was probably responsible for the high rate of utilization of health facilities. Long-standing programmes directed at social welfare raised not only educational levels of the population but also developed a social infrastructure, including a transport network which provided easy access to services. An effective programme of land reform had given poor people access to land resources for food production at the household level. Kerala has demonstrated that good health at low cost is attainable by poor countries, but requires major political and social commitment.

HEALTH DEVELOPMENT

Health development is defined as "the process of continuous progressive improvement of the health status of a population" *(53)*. Its product is rising level of human well-being, marked not only by reduction in the burden of disease, but also by the attainment of positive physical and mental health related to satisfactory economic functioning and social integration *(54)*.

The concept of **health development** as distinct from the provision of medical care is a product of recent policy thinking. It is based on the fundamental principle that governments have a responsibility for the health of their people and at the same time people should have the right as well as the duty, individually and collectively to participate in the development of their own health.

Health development contributes to and results from social and economic development. Therefore, health development has been given increasing emphasis in the policies and programmes of the United Nations system. One example is that of World Bank which is providing funds for the health component of economic development programmes. The UNDP has also shown a growing interest in health development, as has the World Bank.

INDICATORS OF HEALTH

A question that is often raised is: How healthy is a given community ? Indicators are required not only to measure the health status of a community, but also to compare the health status of one country with that of another; for assessment of health care needs; for allocation of scarce resources; and for monitoring and evaluation of health services, activities, and programmes. Indicators help to measure the extent to which the objectives and targets of a programme are being attained.

As the name suggests, indicators are only an indication of a given situation or a reflection of that situation. In WHO's guidelines for health programme evaluation *(55)* they are defined as **variables** which help to measure changes. Often they are used particularly when these changes cannot be measured directly, as for example health or nutritional status *(54)*. If measured sequentially over time, they can indicate direction and speed of change and serve to compare different areas or groups of people at the same moment in time *(55)*.

There has been some confusion over terminology: **health indicator** as compared to **health index** (plural: indices or indexes). It has been suggested that in relation to health trends, the term **indicator** is to be preferred to **index**, whereas **health index** is generally considered to be an amalgamation of health indicators *(56)*.

Characteristics of indicators

Indicators have been given scientific respectability; for example **ideal** indicators

a. should be **valid**, i.e., they should actually measure what they are supposed to measure;
b. should be **reliable** and objective, i.e., the answers should be the same if measured by different people in similar circumstances;
c. should be **sensitive**, i.e., they should be sensitive to changes in the situation concerned,
d. should be **specific**, i.e., they should reflect changes only in the situation concerned,
e. should be **feasible**, i.e., they should have the ability to obtain data needed, and;
f. should be **relevant**, i.e., they should contribute to the understanding of the phenomenon of interest.

But in real life there are few indicators that comply with all these criteria. Measurement of health is far from simple. No existing definition (including the WHO definition) contains criteria for measuring health. This is because health, like happiness, cannot be defined in exact measurable terms. Its presence or absence is so largely a matter of subjective judgement. Since we have problems in defining health, we also have problems in measuring health and the question is largely unresolved. Therefore, measurements of health have been framed in terms of illness (or lack of health), the consequences of ill-health (e.g., morbidity, disability) and economic, occupational and domestic factors that promote ill-health – all the antitheses of health.

Further, health is multidimensional, and each dimension is influenced by numerous factors, some known and many unknown. This means we must measure health multidimensionally. Thus the subject of health measurement is a complicated one even for professionals. Our understanding of health, therefore, cannot be in terms of a single indicator; it must be conceived in terms of a profile, employing many indicators, which may be classified as:

1. Mortality indicators
2. Morbidity indicators
3. Disability rates
4. Nutritional status indicators
5. Health care delivery indicators
6. Utilization rates
7. Indicators of social and mental health
8. Environmental indicators
9. Socio-economic indicators
10. Health policy indicators
11. Indicators of quality of life, and
12. Other indicators.

1. Mortality indicators

(a) *Crude death rate:* This is considered a fair indicator of the comparative health of the people. It is defined as the number of deaths per 1000 population per year in a given community. It indicates the rate at which people are dying. Strictly speaking, health should not be measured by the number of deaths that occur in a community. But in many countries, the crude death rate is the only available indicator of health. When used for international comparison, the usefulness of the crude death rate is restricted because it is influenced by the age–sex composition of the population. Although not a perfect measure of health status, a decrease in death rate provides a good tool for assessing the overall health improvement in a population. Reducing the number of deaths in the population is an obvious goal of medicine and health care, and success or failure to do so is a measure of a nation's commitment to better health.

(b) *Expectation of life :* Life expectancy at birth is "the average number of years that will be lived by those born alive into a population if the current age-specific mortality rates persist". Life expectancy at birth is highly influenced by the infant mortality rate where that is high. Life expectancy at the age of 1 excludes the influence of infant mortality, and life expectancy at the age of 5 excludes the influence of child mortality. Life expectancy at birth is used most frequently *(57)*. It is estimated for both sexes separately. An increase in the expectation of life is regarded, inferentially, as an improvement in health status.

Life expectancy is a good indicator of socio-economic development in general. As an indicator of long-term survival, it can be considered as a positive health indicator. It has been adopted as a global health indicator.

(c) *Age-specific death rates :* Death rates can be expressed for specific age groups in a population which are defined by age. An age-specific death rate is defined as total number of deaths occurring in a specific age group of the population (e.g. 20–24 years) in a defined area during a specific period per 1000 estimated total population of the same age group of the population in the same area during the same period.

(d) *Infant mortality rate :* Infant mortality rate is the ratio of deaths under 1 year of age in a given year to the total number of live births in the same year; usually expressed as a rate per 1000 live births. It is one of the most universally accepted indicators of health status not only of infants, but also of whole population and of the socio-economic conditions under which they live. In addition, the infant mortality rate is a sensitive indicator of the availability, utilization and effectiveness of health care, particularly perinatal care.

(e) *Child death rate :* Another indicator related to the overall health status is the early childhood (1–4 years) mortality rate. It is defined as the number of deaths at ages 1–4 years in a given year, per 1000 children in that age group at the mid-point of the year concerned. It thus excludes infant mortality.

Apart from its correlation with inadequate MCH services, it is also related to insufficient nutrition, low coverage by immunization and adverse environmental exposure and other exogenous agents. Whereas the IMR may be more than 10 times higher in the least developed countries than in the developed countries, the child mortality rate may be as much as 25 times higher. This indicates the magnitude of the gap and the room for improvement.

(f) *Under–5 proportionate mortality rate :* It is the proportion of total deaths occurring in the under–5 age group. This rate can be used to reflect both infant and child mortality rates. In communities with poor hygiene, the proportion may exceed 60 per 1000 live births. In some European countries, the proportion is less than 2 per 1000 live births. High rate reflects high birth rates, high child mortality rates and shorter life expectancy *(28)*.

(g) *Adult mortality rate :* The adult mortality rate is defined as the probability of dying between the age of 15 and 60 years per 1000 population. The adult mortality rate offers a way to analyze health gaps between countries in the main working groups. The probability of dying in adulthood is greater for men than for women in almost all countries, but the variations between countries is very large. In Japan, less than 1 in 10 men (and 1 in 20 women) die in these productive age group, compared to almost 2–3 in 10 men (and 1–2 women) in Angola *(58)*.

(h) *Maternal (puerperal) mortality rate :* Maternal (puerperal) mortality accounts for the greatest proportion of deaths among women of reproductive age in most of the developing world. There are enormous variations in maternal mortality rate according to country's level of socio-economic status.

(i) *Disease-specific mortality rate :* Mortality rates can be computed for specific diseases. As countries begin to extricate themselves from the burden of communicable diseases, a number of other indicators such as deaths from cancer, cardiovascular diseases, accidents, diabetes, etc have emerged as measures of specific disease problems.

(j) *Proportional mortality rate :* The simplest measure of estimating the burden of a disease in the community is proportional mortality rate, i.e., the proportion of all deaths currently attributed to it. For example, coronary heart disease is the cause of 25 to 30 per cent of all deaths in most western countries. The proportional mortality rate from communicable diseases has been suggested as a useful health status indicator; it indicates the magnitude of preventable mortality.

(k) *Case fatality rate :* Case fatality rate measures the risk of persons dying from a certain disease within a given time period. Case fatality rate is calculated as number of deaths from a specific disease during a specific time period divided by number of cases of the disease during the same time period, usually expressed as per 100. The case fatality rate is used to link mortality to morbidity. One function of the case fatality rate is to measure various aspects or properties of a disease such as its pathogenicity, severity or virulence *(59)*. It can also be used in poisonings, chemical exposures or other short-term non-disease cause of death.

(l) *Years of potential life lost (YPLL) :* Years of potential life lost is based on the years of life lost through premature death. It is defined as one that occurs before the age to which a dying person could have expected to survive (before an arbitrary determined age, usually taken age 75 years). A 30 year old who dies in a road accident could theoretically have lived to an average life expectancy of 75 years of age; thus 45 years of life are lost.

Mortality indicators represent the traditional measures of health status. Even today they are probably the most often used indirect indicators of health. As infectious diseases have been brought under control, mortality rates have declined to very low levels in many countries. Consequently mortality indicators are losing their sensitivity as health indicators in developed countries. However, mortality indicators continue to be used as the starting point in health status evaluation.

2. Morbidity indicators

To describe health in terms of mortality rates only is misleading. This is because, mortality indicators do not reveal the burden of ill-health in a community, as for example mental illness and rheumatoid arthritis. Therefore, morbidity indicators are used to supplement mortality data to describe the health status of a population. Morbidity statistics have also their own drawback; they tend to overlook a large number of conditions which are subclinical or inapparent, that is, the hidden part of the iceberg of disease.

The following morbidity rates are used for assessing ill-health in the community *(60)*.

a. incidence and prevalence
b. notification rates
c. attendance rates at out-patient departments, health centres, etc.
d. admission, readmission and discharge rates
e. duration of stay in hospital, and
f. spells of sickness or absence from work or school.

3. Disability rates

Since death rates have not changed markedly in recent years, despite massive health expenditures, disability rates related to illness and injury have come into use to supplement mortality and morbidity indicators. The disability rates are based on the premise or notion that health implies a full range of daily activities. The commonly used disability rates fall into two groups: (a) Event–type indicators and (b) person–type indicators *(10, 61)*.

(a) *Event–type indicators*

i) Number of days of restricted activity
ii) Bed disability days
iii) Work-loss days (or school-loss days) within a specified period

(b) *Person–type indicators*

i) *Limitation of mobility*: For example, confined to bed, confined to the house, special aid in getting around either inside or outside the house.
ii) *Limitation of activity*: For example, limitation to perform the basic activities of daily living (ADL)– e.g., eating, washing, dressing, going to toilet, moving about, etc; limitation in major activity, e.g., ability to work at a job, ability to housework, etc.

HALE (Health-Adjusted Life Expectancy) : The name of the indicator used to measure healthy life expectancy has been changed from disability–adjusted life expectancy (DALE) to health–adjusted life expectancy (HALE). HALE is based on life expectancy at birth but includes an adjustment for *time spent in poor health*. It is most easily understood as the equivalent number of years in full health that a newborn can expect to live based on current rates of ill-health and mortality.

Quality-adjusted life years (QALY) : QALY is a measure of disease burden including both the quality and quantity of life lived. It is used in assessing the value for money of a medical intervention. The QALY is based on the number of years of life that would be added by intervention. Each year in perfect health is assigned a value of 1.0 down to a value of 0.0 for death, i.e. 1 QALY (1 year of life × 1 utility value = 1 QALY) is a year of life lived in perfect health. Half a year lived in perfect health is equivalent to 0.5 QALY (1 year × 0.5 utility value).

Disability-free life expectancy (Syn : active life expectancy) : Disability-free life expectancy (DFLE) is the average number of years an individual is expected to live free of disability if current pattern of mortality and disability continue to apply *(62)*.

Disability-adjusted life years (DALY) : DALY is a measure of overall disease burden, expressed as a number of years lost due to ill-health, disability or early death. Originally developed by Harvard University for the World Bank in 1990, the WHO subsequently adopted the method in the year 2000. The DALY is becoming increasingly common in the field of public health and health impact assessment. The Global Burden of Disease project combines the impact of premature mortality with that of disability. It captures the population impact of important fatal and non-fatal disabling conditions through a single measure. The major measure used is disability–adjusted life years (DALYs) which combines *(58)* :

– years of lost life (YLL) – calculated from the number of deaths at each age multiplied by the expected remaining years of life according to a global standard life expectancy
– years lost to disability (YLD) where the number of incident cases due to injury and illness is multiplied by the average duration of the disease and a weighting factor reflecting the severity of the disease on a scale from 0 (perfect health) to 1 (dead).

It is calculated by formula : DALY = YLL + YLD

The DALY relies on an acceptance that the most appropriate measure of the effects of the chronic illness is time. One DALY, therefore, is equal to one year of healthy life lost. Japanese life expectancy statistics are used as a standard for measuring premature death, as Japanese have the longest life expectancy.

DALY can reveal surprising things about a population's health. For example, the 1990 WHO report indicated that 5 out of 10 leading causes of disability were psychiatric conditions. Psychiatric and neurological conditions account for about 28 per cent of years lived with disability, but accounts for only 1.4 per cent of all deaths and 1.1 per cent of years of life lost. Thus they have a huge impact on population. A crucial distinction among DALY studies is the use of "social weighting", in which the value of each year of life depends on age. Commonly, years lived as a young adult are valued more highly than years spent as a young child or older adults. This weighting system reflects societie's interest in productivity and receiving a return on its investment in upbringing of the children. The effects of the interplay between life expectancy and years lost, discounting, and social weighting are complex, depending on the severity and duration of illness.

4. Nutritional status indicators

Nutritional status is a positive health indicator. Three nutritional status indicators are considered important as indicators of health status. They are *(57)* :

a. anthropometric measurements of preschool children, e.g., weight and height, mid-arm circumference;
b. heights (and sometimes weights) of children at school entry; and
c. prevalence of low birth weight (less than 2.5 kg).

5. Health care delivery indicators

The frequently used indicators of health care delivery are:

a. Doctor–population ratio
b. Doctor–nurse ratio
c. Population–bed ratio
d. Population per health/subcentre, and
e. Population per trained birth attendant.

These indicators reflect the equity of distribution of health resources in different parts of the country, and of the provision of health care.

6. Utilization rates

In order to obtain additional information on health status, the extent of use of health services is often investigated. Utilization of services – or actual coverage – is expressed as the proportion of people in need of a service who actually receive it in a given period, usually a year *(57)*. It is argued that utilization rates give some indication of the care needed by a population, and therefore, the health status of the population. In other words, a relationship exists between utilization of health care services and health needs and status. Health care utilization is also affected by factors such as availability and accessibility of health services and the attitude of an individual towards his health and the health care system. A few examples of utilization rates are cited below:

a. proportion of infants who are "fully immunized" against the 9 EPI diseases.
b. proportion of pregnant women who receive antenatal care, or have their deliveries supervised by a trained birth attendant.
c. percentage of the population using the various methods of family planning.
d. bed–occupancy rate (i.e., average daily in-patient census/average number of beds).
e. average length of stay (i.e., days of care rendered/discharges), and
f. bed turnover ratio (i.e., discharges/average beds).

The above list is neither exhaustive nor all–inclusive. The list can be expanded depending upon the services provided. These indicators direct attention away from the biological aspects of disease in a population towards the discharge of social responsibility for the organization in delivery of health care services.

7. Indicators of social and mental health

As long as valid positive indicators of social and mental health are scarce, it is necessary to use indirect measures, viz. *indicators of social and mental pathology.* These include suicide, homicide, other acts of violence and other crime; road traffic accidents, juvenile delinquency; alcohol and drug abuse; smoking; consumption of tranquillizers; obesity, etc *(57)*. To these may be added family violence, battered–baby and battered–wife syndromes and neglected and abandoned youth in the neighbourhood. These social indicators provide a guide to social action for improving the health of the people.

8. Environmental indicators

Environmental indicators reflect the quality of physical and biological environment in which diseases occur and in which the people live. They include indicators relating to pollution of air and water, radiation, solid wastes, noise, exposure to toxic substances in food or drink. Among these, the most useful indicators are those measuring the proportion of population having access to safe water and sanitation facilities, as for example, percentage of households with safe water in the home or within 15 minutes' walking distance from a water standpoint or protected well; adequate sanitary facilities in the home or immediate vicinity *(57)*.

9. Socio-economic indicators

These indicators do not directly measure health. Nevertheless, they are of great importance in the interpretation of the indicators of health care. These include :

a. rate of population increase
b. per capita GNP
c. level of unemployment
d. dependency ratio
e. literacy rates, especially female literacy rates
f. family size
g. housing: the number of persons per room, and
h. per capita "calorie" availability.

10. Health policy indicators

The single most important indicator of political commitment is "allocation of adequate resources". The relevant indicators are: (i) proportion of GNP spent on health services (ii) proportion of GNP spent on health-related activities (including water supply and sanitation, housing and nutrition, community development), and (iii) proportion of total health resources devoted to primary health care.

11. Indicators of quality of life

Increasingly, mortality and morbidity data have been questioned as to whether they fully reflect the health status of a population. The previous emphasis on using increased life expectancy as an indicator of health is no longer considered adequate, especially in developed countries, and attention has shifted more towards concern about the quality of life enjoyed by individuals and communities. Quality of life is difficult to define and even more difficult to measure (see page 16). Various attempts have been made to reach one composite index from a number of health indicators. The physical quality of life index is one such index (see page 17). It consolidates three indicators, viz. infant mortality, life expectancy at age one, and literacy. Obviously more work is needed to develop indicators of quality of life.

12. Social indicators

Social indicators, as defined by the United Nations

Statistical Office, have been divided into 12 categories:– population; family formation, families and households; learning and educational services; earning activities; distribution of income, consumption, and accumulation; social security and welfare services; health services and nutrition; housing and its environment; public order and safety; time use; leisure and culture; social stratification and mobility *(63)*.

13. Basic needs indicators

Basic needs indicators are used by ILO. Those mentioned in "Basic needs performance" *(64)* include calorie consumption; access to water; life expectancy; deaths due to disease; illiteracy, doctors and nurses per population; rooms per person; GNP per capita.

SPECIAL INDICATORS SERIES

1. "Health for All" indicators

For monitoring progress towards the goal of Health for All by 2000 AD, the WHO has listed the following four categories of indicators (Table 2).

TABLE 2

Indicators selected for monitoring progress towards "Health for All"

(1) Health policy indicators: – political commitment to "Health for All" – resource allocation – the degree of equity of distribution of health services – community involvement – organizational framework and managerial process
(2) Social and economic indicators related to health: – rate of population increase – GNP or GDP – income distribution – work conditions – adult literacy rate – housing – food availability
(3) Indicators for the provision of health care: – availability – accessibility – utilization – quality of care
(4) Health status indicators: – low birth weight (percentage) – nutritional status and psychosocial development of children – infant mortality rate – child mortality rate – life expectancy at birth – maternal mortality rate – disease specific mortality – morbidity – incidence and prevalence – disability prevalence

Source : *(57)*

2. Millennium Development Goals – Indicators

The Millennium Development Goals adopted by the United Nations in the year 2000 provide an opportunity for concerted action to improve global health. The health related goals and their indicators of progress are listed in Table 3.

TABLE 3

Health-related Millennium Development Goals, and Indicators

Goal: 1. Eradicate extreme poverty and hunger		
Indicator :	4.	Prevalence of underweight children under five years of age
	5.	Proportion of population below minimum level of dietary energy consumption
Goal: 4. Reduce child mortality		
Indicator :	13.	Under-five mortality rate
	14.	Infant mortality rate
	15.	Proportion of 1-year-old children immunized against measles
Goal: 5. Improve maternal health		
Indicator :	16.	Maternal mortality ratio
	17.	Proportion of births attended by skilled health personnel
Goal: 6. Combat HIV/AIDS, malaria and other diseases		
Indicator :	18.	HIV prevalence among young people aged 15 to 24 years
	19.	Condom use rate of the contraceptive prevalence rate
	20.	Number of children orphaned by HIV/AIDS
	21.	Prevalence and death rates associated with malaria
	22.	Proportion of population in malaria-risk areas using effective malaria prevention and treatment measures
	23.	Prevalence and death rates associated with tuberculosis
	24.	Proportion of tuberculosis cases detected and cured under Directly Observed Treatment, Short-course (DOTS)
Goal: 7. Ensure environmental sustainability		
Indicator :	29.	Proportion of population using solid fuel
Indicator :	30.	Proportion of population with sustainable access to an improved water source, urban and rural
Indicator :	31.	Proportion of urban population with access to improved sanitation
Goal: 8. Develop a global partnership for development		
Indicator :	46.	Proportion of population with access to affordable essential drugs on a sustainable basis

Source : *(65)*

3. Sustainable Development Goals

On 25th September 2015, the United Nations General Assembly adopted the new development agenda "Transforming our world : the 2030 agenda for sustainable development". The post-2015 framework goes beyond the MDGs. It has 17 goals and 169 targets, including one specific (3rd goal) for health with 13 targets as shown in Table 4.

TABLE 4
Health Targets in Sustainable Development Goal 3

Goal	Target
3.1	By 2030, reduce the global maternal mortality ratio to less than 70 per 100,000 live births.
3.2	By 2030, end preventable deaths of newborns and children under five years of age, with all countries aiming to reduce neonatal mortality to at least as low as 12 per 1000 live births, and under-five mortality to at least as low as 25 per 1000 live births.
3.3	By 2030, end the epidemics of AIDS, tuberculosis, malaria and neglected tropical diseases and combat hepatitis, water-borne diseases and other communicable diseases.
3.4	By 2030, reduce by one-third premature mortality from non-communicable diseases through prevention and treatment, and promote mental health and well-being.
3.5	Strengthen the prevention and treatment of substance abuse, including narcotic drug abuse and harmful use of alcohol.
3.6	By 2020, halve the number of global deaths and injuries from road traffic accidents.
3.7	By 2030, ensure universal access to sexual and reproductive health-care services, including for family planning, information and education, and the integration of reproductive health into national strategies and programmes.
3.8	Achieve universal health coverage, including financial risk protection, access to quality essential health-care services and access to safe, effective, quality and affordable essential medicines and vaccines for all.
3.9	By 2030, substantially reduce the number of deaths and illnesses from hazardous chemicals and air, water and soil pollution and contamination.
3.a	Strengthen the implementation of the World Health Organization Framework Convention on Tobacco Control in all countries, as appropriate.
3.b	Support the research and development of vaccines and medicines for the communicable and non-communicable diseases that primarily affect developing countries, provide access to affordable essential medicines and vaccines, in accordance with the Doha Declaration on the TRIPS Agreement and Public Health, which affirms the right of developing countries to use to the full the provisions in the Agreement on Trade-Related Aspects of Intellectual Property Rights regarding flexibilities to protect public health, and, in particular, provide access to medicines for all.
3.c	Substantially increase health financing and the recruitment, development, training and retention of the health work-force in developing countries, especially in least-developed countries and small island developing states.
3.d	Strengthen the capacity of all countries, in particular developing countries, for early warning, risk reduction and management of national and global health risks.

Source : *(66)*

4. Global Reference list of Core Health Indicators (2018)

"The Global Reference List", is a standard set of 100 core indicators prioritized by the global community to provide concise information on the health situation and trends, including responses at national and global levels.

The 2018 revision of the Global Reference List builds on the previous 2015 version. The 2018 list of indicators contains modifications and additions that were made in 2017 to reflect the recommended health and health related indicators of Sustainable Development Goals (SDG), including universal health coverage, non-communicable diseases and other key health-related environmental, social, economic and behavioural risk factors *(67)*.

The list includes a selection of priority indicators relating to 4 domains that include health status, risk factors, service coverage and health systems. They are as follows *(67)*:

1. Health status indicators

Mortality by age and sex

- Life expectancy at birth
- Adolescent mortality rate
- Adult mortality rate between 15 and 60 years of age
- Under-five mortality rate (SDG 3.2.1)
- Infant mortality rate
- Neonatal mortality rate (SDG 3.2.2)
- Stillbirth rate

Mortality by cause

- Maternal mortality ratio (SDG 3.1.1)
- TB mortality rate
- AIDS-related mortality rate
- Malaria mortality rate
- Premature non-communicable disease (NCD) mortality (SDG 3.4.1)
- Mortality from household and ambient air pollution (SDG 3.9.1)
- Mortality from unsafe water, unsafe sanitation and lack of hygiene (SDG 3.9.2)
- Mortality from unintentional poisoning (SDG 3.9.3)
- Suicide rate (SDG 3.4.2)
- Death rate due to road traffic injuries (SDG 3.6.1)
- Number of deaths, missing persons and persons affected by disaster per 100,000 people (SDG 1.5.1, 11.5.1, 13.1.1)
- Mortality rate due to homicide (SDG 16.1.1)

Fertility

- Adolescent birth rate (SDG 3.7.2)
- Total fertility rate

Morbidity

- New cases of vaccine-preventable diseases
- New cases of IHR-notifiable diseases and other notifiable diseases
- HIV prevalence rate
- HIV incidence rate (SDG 3.3.1)
- Hepatitis B surface antigen prevalence
- Hepatitis B incidence (SDG 3.3.4)
- Sexually transmitted infections (STIs) incidence rate
- Congenital syphilis rate
- TB incidence rate (SDG 3.3.2)
- TB notification rate
- Malaria parasite prevalence among children aged 6–59 months
- Malaria incidence rate (SDG 3.3.3)
- Cancer incidence, by type of cancer

2. Risk factor indicators

Nutrition

- Exclusive breast-feeding rate 0–5 months of age
- Early initiation of breast-feeding
- Incidence of low birth weight among newborns
- Children under 5 years who are stunted (SDG 2.2.1)
- Children under 5 years who are wasted (SDG 2.2.2)

- Children under 5 years who are overweight (SDG 2.2.2)
- Anaemia prevalence in children
- Anaemia prevalence in women of reproductive age (also: severe anaemia)

Infections

- Prevention of HIV in key populations

Environmental risk factors

- Population using safely managed drinking-water services (SDG 6.1.1)
- Population using safely managed sanitation services (SDG 6.2.1a/6.2.1b) (also: population with handwashing facility with soap and water)
- Population with primary reliance on clean fuels and technologies (SDG 7.1.2)
- Air pollution level in cities (SDG 11.6.2)

Non-communicable diseases

- Total alcohol per capita (age 15+ years) consumption (SDG 3.5.2)
- Tobacco use among persons aged 15+ years (SDG 3.a.1) (also adolescents)
- Raised blood pressure among adults
- Overweight and obesity in adults (also: School-age children and adolescents)
- Raised blood glucose/diabetes among adults
- Salt intake
- Insufficient physical activity in adults (also: adolescents)

Injuries/harmful traditional practices

- Intimate partner violence prevalence (SDG 5.2.1)
- Non-partner sexual violence prevalence (SDG 5.2.2)
- Prevalence of female genital mutilation/cutting (SDG 5.3.2)
- Sexual violence against children (SDG 16.2.3)
- Early marriage (SDG 5.3.1)
- Frequency rates of occupational injuries (SDG 8.8.1)

3. Service coverage indicators

Reproductive, maternal, newborn, child and adolescent

- Demand for family planning satisfied with modern methods (SDG 3.7.1)
- Contraceptive prevalence rate
- Antenatal care coverage
- Births attended by skilled health personnel (SDG 3.1.2) (also: institutional delivery – overall and in "baby-friendly" institutions)
- Postpartum care coverage – women
- Postnatal care coverage – newborn
- Care-seeking for symptoms of pneumonia
- Coverage of diarrhoea treatment
- Vitamin A supplementation coverage

Immunization

- Immunization coverage rate by vaccine for each vaccine in the national schedule (SDG 3.b.1)

HIV

- People living with HIV who know their status
- Prevention of mother-to-child transmission
- Antiretroviral therapy (ART) coverage
- HIV viral load suppression

HIV/TB

- Coverage of treatment for latent TB infection (LTBI)
- HIV test results for TB patients
- HIV-positive new and relapse TB patients on ART during TB treatment

Tuberculosis

- Drug susceptibility testing coverage for TB patients
- TB treatment coverage
- Treatment coverage for drug-resistant TB

Malaria

- Intermittent preventive therapy for malaria during pregnancy (IPTp)
- Use of insecticide treated nets (ITNs)
- Treatment of confirmed malaria cases
- Indoor residual spraying (IRS) coverage

Neglected tropical diseases

- Number of people requiring interventions against neglected tropical diseases (SDG 3.3.5)
- Coverage of preventive chemotherapy for selected neglected tropical diseases

Screening and preventive care

- Cervical cancer screening

Mental Health

- Coverage of services for severe mental health disorders

Substance abuse

- Treatment coverage for alcohol and drug dependence (SDG 3.5.1)

Essential health services

- Coverage of essential health services (SDG 3.8.1)

4. Health system indicators

Quality and safety of care

- Perioperative mortality rate
- Obstetric and gynaecological admissions owing to abortion
- Institutional maternal mortality ratio
- Maternal death reviews
- ART retention rate
- TB treatment success rate
- Service-specific availability and readiness

Access

- Out-patient service utilization (also: in-patient admissions and surgical volume)
- Health facility density and distribution (also: access to emergency surgery)
- Hospital bed density
- Access to a core set of relevant essential medicines (SDG 3.b.3)

Health work-force

- Health worker density and distribution (SDG 3.c.1)
- Output training institutions

Health information

- Birth registration (SDG 16.9.1)
- Death registration (SDG 17.19.2)
- Completeness of reporting by facilities (also: completeness and timeliness for notifiable diseases)

Health financing

- Total current expenditure on health as % of gross domestic product (also: total capital expenditure on health as % of current + capital expenditure on health)

- Public domestic sources of current spending on health as % of current health expenditure (also: private)
- External source of current spending on health (% of current expenditure on health)
- Proportion of the population with impoverishing health expenditure
- Proportion of the population with large household expenditure on health as a share of total household consumption or income (SDG 3.8.2)
- Total net official development assistance to medical research and basic health sectors (SDG 3.b.2)

Health security

- International Health Regulations (IHR) core capacity index (SDG 3.d.1)

Governance

- Existence of national health sector policy/strategy/plan

The list also presents the indicators according to level of the results of chain framework (input, output, outcome and impact).

100 CORE HEALTH INDICATORS (PLUS HEALTH-RELATED SDGs) BY RESULTS CHAIN

Inputs and processes → **Output** → **Outcome** → **Impact**

Inputs and processes

Health financing
- Total current expenditure on health as % of gross domestic product (Also: total capital expenditure on health as % of current + capital expenditure on health)
- Public domestic sources of current spending on health as % of current health expenditure (Also: private)
- External source of current spending on health (% of current expenditure on health)
- Total net official development assistance to medical research and basic health sectors (SDG 3.b.2)

Health work-force
- Health worker density and distribution (SDG 3.c.1)
- Output training institutions

Health infrastructure
- Health facility density and distribution (Also: access to emergency surgery)
- Hospital bed density

Health information
- Birth registration (SDG 16.9.1)
- Death registration (SDG 17.19.2)
- Completeness of reporting by facilities (Also: completeness and timeliness for notifiable diseases)
- Existence of national health sector policy/strategy/plan

Output

Service access and availability
- Out-patient service utilization (Also: in-patient admissions and surgical volume)
- Service-specific availability and readiness
- Access to a core set of relevant essential medicines (SDG 3.b.3)

Service quality and safety
- Perioperative mortality rate
- Obstetric and gynaecological admissions owing to abortion
- Institutional maternal mortality ratio
- Maternal death reviews
- ART retention rate
- HIV test results for TB patients
- TB notification rate
- TB treatment success rate

Health security
- International Health Regulations (IHR) core capacity index (SDG 3.d.1)

Outcome

Coverage of interventions
- Demand for family planning satisfied with modern methods (SDG 3.7.1)
- Contraceptive prevalence rate
- Antenatal care coverage
- Births attended by skilled health personnel (SDG 3.1.2) (Also: institutional delivery – overall and in "baby-friendly" institutions)
- Postpartum care coverage – women
- Postnatal care coverage – newborn
- Care-seeking for symptoms of pneumonia
- Coverage of diarrhoea treatment
- Vitamin A supplementation coverage
- Immunization coverage rate by vaccine for each vaccine in the national schedule (SDG 3.b.1)
- People living with HIV who know their status
- Prevention of mother-to-child transmission
- Antiretroviral therapy (ART) coverage
- HIV viral load suppression
- Coverage of treatment for latent TB infection (LTBI)
- HIV-positive new and relapse TB patients on ART during TB treatment
- Drug susceptibility testing coverage for TB patients
- TB treatment coverage
- Treatment coverage for drug-resistant TB
- Intermittent preventive therapy for malaria during pregnancy (IPTp)
- Use of insecticide treated nets (ITNs)
- Treatment of confirmed malaria cases
- Indoor residual spraying (IRS) coverage
- Number of people requiring interventions against neglected tropical diseases (SDG 3.3.5)
- Coverage of preventive chemotherapy for selected neglected tropical diseases
- Cervical cancer screening
- Coverage of services for severe mental health disorders
- Treatment coverage for alcohol and drug dependence (SDG 3.5.1)
- Coverage of essential health services (SDG 3.8.1)

Risk factors and behaviours
- Exclusive breast-feeding rate 0–5 months of age
- Early initiation of breast-feeding
- Incidence of low birth weight among newborns
- Children under 5 years who are stunted (SDG 2.2.1)
- Children under 5 years who are wasted (SDG 2.2.2)
- Children aged under 5 years who are overweight (SDG 2.2.2)
- Anaemia prevalence in children
- Anaemia prevalence in women of reproductive age (Also: severe anaemia)
- Prevention of HIV in key populations
- Population using safely managed drinking-water services (SDG 6.1.1)
- Population using safely managed sanitation services (SDG 6.2.1a/6.2.1b (forthcoming)) (Also population with handwashing facility with soap and water)
- Population with primary reliance on clean fuels and technologies (SDG 7.1.2)
- Air pollution level in cities (SDG 11.6.2)
- Total alcohol per capita (age 15+ years) consumption (SDG 3.5.2)
- Tobacco use among persons aged 15+ years (SDG 3.a.1) (Also adolescents)
- Raised blood pressure among adults
- Overweight and obesity in adults (Also: School-age children and adolescents)
- Raised blood glucose/diabetes among adults
- Salt intake
- Insufficient physical activity in adults (Also: adolescents)
- Intimate partner violence prevalence (SDG 5.2.1)
- Non-partner sexual violence prevalence (SDG 5.2.2)
- Prevalence of female genital mutilation/cutting (SDG 5.3.2)
- Sexual violence against children (SDG 16.2.3)
- Early marriage (SDG 5.3.1)
- Frequency rates of occupational injuries (SDG 8.8.1)

Impact

Health status
- Life expectancy at birth
- Adolescent mortality rate
- Adult mortality rate between 15 and 60 years of age
- Under-five mortality rate (SDG 3.2.1)
- Infant mortality rate
- Neonatal mortality rate (SDG 3.2.2)
- Stillbirth rate
- Maternal mortality ratio (SDG 3.1.1)
- TB mortality rate
- AIDS-related mortality rate
- Malaria mortality rate
- Premature non-communicable disease (NCD) mortality (SDG 3.4.1)
- Mortality from household and ambient air pollution (SDG 3.9.1)
- Mortality from unsafe water, unsafe sanitation and lack of hygiene (SDG 3.9.2)
- Mortality from unintentional poisoning (SDG 3.9.3)
- Suicide rate (SDG 3.4.2)
- Death rate due to road traffic injuries (SDG 3.6.1)
- Number of deaths, missing persons and persons affected by disaster per 100,000 people (SDG 1.5.1, 11.5.1, 13.1.1)
- Mortality rate due to homicide (SDG 16.1.1)
- Adolescent birth rate (SDG 3.7.2)
- Total fertility rate
- New cases of vaccine-preventable diseases
- New cases of IHR-notifiable diseases and other notifiable diseases
- HIV prevalence rate
- HIV incidence rate (SDG 3.3.1)
- Hepatitis B surface antigen prevalence
- Hepatitis B incidence (SDG 3.3.4)
- Sexually transmitted infections (STIs) incidence rate
- Congenital syphilis rate
- TB incidence rate (SDG 3.3.2)
- Malaria parasite prevalence among children aged 6–59 months
- Malaria incidence rate (SDG 3.3.3)
- Cancer incidence, by type of cancer

Financial risk protection
- Proportion of the population with impoverishing health expenditure
- Proportion of the population with large household expenditure on health as a share of total household consumption or income (SDG 3.8.2)

5. Health Index of India (Niti Aayog) *(68)*

Niti Aayog of India recently ranked all states and UTs in an attempt to measure the nations health performance. The states and UTs are grouped in three categories to ensure comparisons among similar entities namely 21 larger states, 8 smaller states and 7 Union Territories as shown in Table 5.

TABLE 5
Categorization of states and UTs

Category	Number of States and UTs	States and UTs
Larger states	21	Andhra Pradesh, Assam, Bihar, Chhattisgarh, Gujarat, Haryana, Himachal Pradesh, Jammu & Kashmir, Jharkhand, Karnataka, Kerala, Madhya Pradesh, Maharashtra, Odisha, Punjab, Rajasthan, Tamil Nadu, Telangana, Uttar Pradesh, Uttarakhand, West Bengal
Smaller states	8	Arunachal Pradesh, Goa, Manipur, Meghalaya, Mizoram, Nagaland, Sikkim, Tripura
Union Territories	7	Andaman & Nicobar, Chandigarh, Dadra & Nagar Haveli, Daman & Diu, Delhi, Lakshadweep, Puducherry

The health index is a weighted composite index, which is based on indicators in three domains : (a) Health outcomes (70 per cent); (b) Governance and information (12 per cent); and (c) Key inputs and processes (18 per cent). Each domain is assigned a weight based on its importance. Within a domain or sub-domain, the weight has been equally distributed among the indicators. Table 6 provides the detailed health index with indicators, their definitions, the data sources and specifics of base year (BY) and reference year (RY) *(68)*.

DEVELOPED AND DEVELOPING REGIONS

The world today is divided into developed and developing regions on the basis of some common features shared by them. The former is represented by countries such as USA and UK, and the latter by countries such as India. If one defined development as the organization of society to provide adequate housing, food, health services, education and employment for the majority of people, then many developing countries are wide of the mark. Social medicine is concerned with disparities that exist among countries. This is because socio-economic factors and health problems are interlinked. An account of these disparities is given below:

1. Social and economic characteristics

Most people in the developing countries live in rural areas

TABLE 6
Health Index : Indicators, definitions, base and reference years

S.No.	Indicator	Definition	Base Year (BY) & Reference Year (RY)
		DOMAIN 1 - HEALTH OUTCOMES *Sub-domain 1.1 - Key outcomes (Weight : larger states - 500, smaller states & UTs-100)*	
1.1.1	Neonatal mortality rate (NMR)	Number of infant deaths of less than 29 days per thousand live births during a specific year.	BY : 2015 RY : 2016
1.1.2	Under-five mortality rate (U5MR)	Number of child deaths of less than 5 years per thousand live births during a specific year.	BY : 2015 RY : 2016
1.1.3	Total fertility rate (TFR)	Average number of children that would be born to a woman if she experiences the current fertility pattern throughout her reproductive span (15-49 years), during a specific year.	BY : 2015 RY : 2016
1.1.4	Proportion of low birth weight (LBW) among newborns	Proportion of low birth weight (≤ 2.5 kg) newborns out of the total number of newborns weighed during a specific year born in a public health facility.	BY : 2015–16 RY : 2017–18
1.1.5	Sex ratio at birth (SRB)	The number of girls born for every 1,000 boys born during a specific year.	BY : 2012–15 RY : 2014–16
		Sub-domain 1.2 - Intermediate outcomes (Weight : larger & smaller states - 300, UTs-250)	
1.2.1	Full immunization coverage	Proportion of infants 9–11 months old who have received BCG, 3 doses of DPT, 3 doses of OPV and one dose of measles against estimated number of infants during a specific year.	BY : 2015–18 RY : 2017–18
1.2.2	Proportion of institutional deliveries	Proportion of deliveries conducted in public and private health facilities against the number of estimated deliveries during a specific year.	BY : 2015–16 RY : 2017–18
1.2.3	Total case notification rate of tuberculosis (TB)	Number of new and relapsed TB cases notified (public + private) per 100,000 population during a specific year.	By : 2016 RY : 2017
1.2.4	Treatment success rate of new microbiologically confirmed TB cases	Proportion of new cured and their treatment completed against the total number of new microbiologically confirmed TB cases registered during a specific year.	BY : 2015 RY : 2016
1.2.5	Proportion of people living with HIV (PLHIV) on antiretroviral therapy (ART)	Proportion of PLHIVs receiving ART treatment against the number of estimated PLHIVs who needed ART treatment for the specific year.	BY : 2015–16 RY : 2017–18

S.No.	Indicator	Definition	Base Year (BY) & Reference Year (RY)
		DOMAIN 2 - GOVERNANCE AND INFORMATION *Sub-domain 2.1 - health monitoring and data integrity (Weight : 70)*	
2.1.1	Data Integrity Measure : a. Institutional deliveries b. ANC registered within first trimester	Percentage deviation of reported data from standard survey data to assess the quality/integrity of reported data for a specific period.	BY & RY 2015–16 (NFHS) BY & RY : 2011–12 to 2015–2016 (HMIS)
		Sub-domain 2.2 - Governance (Weight -60)	
2.2.1	Average occupancy of an officer (in months), combined for following three posts at state level for last three years 1. Principal Secretary 2. Mission Director (NHM) 3. Director (Health Services)	Average occupancy of an officer (in months), combined for following posts in last three years : 1. Principal Secretary 2. Mission Director (NHM) 3. Director (Health Services)	BY : April 1, 2013– March 31, 2016 RY : April 1, 2015– March 31, 2018
2.2.2	Average occupancy of a full-time officer (in months) for all the districts in last three years - District Chief Medical Officers (CMOs) or equivalent post (heading District Health Services)	Average occupancy of a CMO (in months) for all the districts in last three years.	BY : April 1, 2013– March 31, 2016 RY : April 1, 2015– March 31, 2018
		DOMAIN 3 - KEY INPUTS/PROCESSES *Sub-domain 3.1 - health systems/service delivery (Weight - 200)*	
3.1.1	Proportion of vacant health-care provider positions (regular + contractual) in public health facilities	Vacant health-care provider positions in public health facilities against total sanctioned health-care provider positions for following cadres (separately for each cadre) during a specific year : a. Auxiliary nurse mid-wife (ANM) at sub-centers (SCs) b. Staff nurse (SN) at Primary Health Centers (PHCs) and Community Health Centers (CHCs) c. Medical officers (MOs) at PHCs d. Specialists at District Hospitals (Medicine, Surgery, Obstetrics and Gynaecology, Paediatrics, Anaesthesia, Ophthalmology, Radiology, Pathology, Ear-Nose-Throat (ENT), Dental, Psychiatry)	BY : As on March 31, 2016 RY : As on March 31, 2018
3.1.2	Proportion of total staff (regular + contractual) for whom an e-payslip can be generated in the IT-enabled Human Resources Management System (HRMIS).	Availability of a functional IT-enabled HRMIS measured by the proportion of staff (regular + contractual) for whom an e-payslip can be generated in the IT- enabled HRMIS against total number of staff (regular + contractual) during a specific year.	BY : As on March 31, 2016 RY : As on March 31, 2018
3.1.3	a. Proportion of specified type of facilities functioning as First Referral Units (FRUs)	Proportion of public sector facilities conducting specified number of C-sections* per year (FRUs) against the norm of one FRU per 500,000 population during a specific year.	BY : 2015–16 RY : 2017–18
	b. Proportion of functional 24x7 PHCs	Proportion of PHCs providing all stipulated health-care services** round the clock against the norm of one 24x7 PHC per 100,000 population during a specific year.	BY : 2015–16 RY : 2017–18
3.1.4	Proportion of districts with functional Cardiac Care Units (CCUs)	Proportion of districts with functional CCUs [with desired equipment (ventilator, monitor, defibrillator, CCU beds, portable ECG machine, pulse oxymeter etc.), drugs, diagnostics and desired staff as per programme guidelines] against total number of districts.	BY : As on March 31, 2016 RY : As on March 31, 2018
3.1.5	Proportion of ANC registered within first trimester against total registrations	Proportion of pregnant women registered for ANC within 12 weeks of pregnancy during a specific year.	BY : 2015–16 RY : 2017–18

S.No.	Indicator	Definition	Base Year (BY) & Reference Year (RY)
3.1.6	Level of registration of births	Proportion of births registered under Civil Registration System (CRS) against the estimated number of births during a specific year.	BY : 2014 RY : 2016
3.1.7	Completeness of IDSP reporting of P and L forms	Proportion of Reporting Units (RUs) reporting in stipulated time period against total RUs, for P and L forms during a specific year.	BY : 2015 RY : 2017
3.1.8	Proportion of CHCs with grading above 3 points	Proportion of CHCs that are graded above 3 points against total number of CHCs during a specific year.	BY : 2015–16 RY : 2017–18
3.1.9	Proportion of public health facilities with accreditation certificates by a standard quality assurance program (NQAS/NABH/ISO/AHPI)	Proportion of specified type of public health facilities with accreditation certificates by a standard quality assurance program against the total number following specified type of facilities during a specific year. 1. District hospital (DH)/Sub-district hospital (SDH) 2. CHC/Block PHC	BY : As on March 31, 2016 RY : As on March 31, 2018
3.1.10	Average number of days for transfer of Central NHM fund from State Treasury to implementation agency (Department/Society) based on all tranches of the last financial year	Average time taken (in number of days) by the State Treasury to transfer funds to implementation agencies during a specific year.	BY : 2015–16 RY : 2017–18

* Criteria for fully operational FRUs: SDHs/CHCs - conducting minimum 60 C-sections per year (36 C-sections per year for Hilly and North-Eastern States except for Assam); DHs - conducting minimum 120 C-sections per year (72 C-sections per year for Hilly and North-Eastern States except Assam).

** Criteria for functional 24x7 PHCs: 10 deliveries per month (5 deliveries per month for Hilly and North-Eastern States except Assam)

\# Centre NHM Finance data includes the RCH flexi-pool and NHM-Health System Strengthening flexi-pool data (representing a substantial portion of the NHM funds) for calculating delay in transfer of funds.

and urban slums. There is a rigid hierarchy and class structure moulded by tradition and long-standing customs. The family, often a joint family, is a strong binding force. People depend mainly on agriculture and there is a lack of alternative employment opportunities. The GNP *per capita* ranges from US $ 2000 to 6000 in most developing countries. The production and consumption per capita are low. They have an economic potential which is not fully realized; this refers to unemployed labour, natural resources and fertility of the soil. Science and technology are not fully applied. The level of literacy is low – it averages only 63 per cent in the least developed countries. The quality of life is poor because of the scarcity of essential goods, facilities and money. There is isolation caused by distance, poor communication and transport facilities. The environment is unfavourable predisposing to communicable diseases and malnutrition. The vast majority of people are not able to pay for medical services. There is a long tradition of free medical services provided by the State.

In the developed countries, most people (8 out of 10) are urban residents. Urban life differs from that in the villages by being more impersonal. Women are economically employed. Agriculture is second to industry. Great use is made of scientific disciplines. The standard of living and quality of life are high. The GNP per capita ranges from US $ 5000 to 40,600 in most developed countries. The adult literacy is almost universal.

2. Demographic characteristics

Demographic trends fundamentally influence country's economic, social and health conditions. Population growth, changes in fertility rates and population structure, all have a profound influence, as do migration (which is increasingly a cross-border issue) and growing urbanization which may spur economic growth but also put strain on food and water resources.

Fertility rates are falling globally and as a consequence, population growth is slowing down almost everywhere except Africa. The fertility rate is now at or below replacement level in 44 per cent of countries in the world. High fertility has multiple consequences for health and health related issues. Continued rapid population growth in low and lower-middle-income countries, along with higher fertility rates in poorest segments of the population makes it harder to eradicate poverty, combat hunger and malnutrition, invest in health and education, improve access to basic services, plan and develop cities, protect local ecosystems and promote peaceful societies *(66)*.

In mid-2017, the World Population reached 7.4 billion, of which 60 per cent live in Asia. The population in developing countries is a "young" population; the proportion of persons under 15 years of age in the year 2016 was about 41 per cent in the least developed countries and 24 in other developing countries, as compared to about 16 per cent in the developed countries. The proportion of people over 65 years of age in developing countries is about 5 per cent, compared to 18 per cent in the developed countries *(69)*. The social and economic backlashes of this age distribution are being felt in both the developing and developed countries – the former having to bear the heavy burden of providing for a population which is mainly young; and the latter having to deal with the problems of ageing.

3. Contrasts in health (Health gap)

While accurate statistical data are difficult to obtain, even perfunctory glance at available data (Table 7) are sufficient to illustrate the wide health gap between population in the developed and developing countries.

Table 7 shows that the present gap in life expectancy at birth between developed and developing countries is 15–20 years. Developed countries are characterized by longer life expectancy and lower infant and child mortality rates, and the opposite is true of developing countries.

TABLE 7

Selected health and socio-economic indicators

Indicator	Least developed countries	Developing countries	High HDI countries
1. Life expectancy at birth (2019)	65.3	71.1	79.5
2. IMR (per 1000 live births) (2019)	45	33.0	3
3. Under 5 mortality per 1000 live births (2019)	63	40	4
4. Maternal mortality per 100,000 live births (2017)	412	224	14
5. Doctor–population ratio per 10,000 (2010–18)	2.5	11.5	30.4
6. Nurse–population ratio per 10,000 (2007–13)	9	33	114
7. GNI, per capita (US $ PPP) (2019)			
Male	3,846	14,136	55,720
Female	2,083	6,923	33,668
8. Public health expenditure (as % of GDP) US $ (2019)	4.9	5.8	12.5
9. Projected expected years of schooling (2020)			
Male	10.4	12.3	16.0
Female	9.4	12.2	16.6
10. Access to safe water % population (2017)	61	92	95
11. Access to adequate sanitation % population (2017)	34	69	98
12. Universal service coverage (2019)	46	61	79

Source : *(29)*

The burden of disease pattern of developed, developing high mortality, and developing low mortality countries in the world differ substantially. This phenomenon reflects what is known as the "epidemiological transition". As life expectancy increases, the major causes of death and disability in general shift from communicable, maternal and perinatal causes to chronic, non-communicable ones.

To sum up, the world health situation leaves much to be desired. Millions of people in the developing countries have incomes too low to ensure basic nutrition and have little access to essential health services. In a number of industrialized countries, rapid increases in health cost have called into question the relationship between health care and health indicators. A search for alternative approaches has led to the view that primary health care is the most important means, whereby, the health sector, with intersectoral coordination, can close the health gap and improve the health status of the population.

THE URBAN-RURAL DIVIDE IN HEALTH AND DEVELOPMENT

A majority of world's population live in urban areas, a milestone that was reached only within the last decade. The world continues to become more urban, yet in Africa and Asia, the majority of the population is still rural. The average annual rate of change of percentage to urban is 1.1 per cent in Africa and 1.5 per cent in Asia. Despite the rise of an unprecedented number of large cities, most urban residents in developing countries live in places with a populatin of less than half a million.

There is no universal definition of "Urban". Countries differ in their definitions of urban, although it is fairly common for the urban population to consist of those living in towns and cities of a few thousand or more. How countries define urban can affect our ability to compare "urban" across countries. For example, in India the term "urban" refers to towns (places with a municipal corporation, municipal area committee, town committee, notified area committee, or cantonment board); or, all places having 5,000 or more inhabitants, a density of not less than 1,000 persons per square mile or 400 per square kilometer, pronounced urban characteristics, and at least three fourths of the adult male population employed in pursuits other than agriculture. In contrast, Peru defines "urban" simply as populated centers with 100 or more dwellings *(70)*.

During the year 2020, the total urban population in the world was 56 per cent. In more developed countries, 81 per cent population was urban, compared to 68 per cent in less developed countries and 43 per cent in least develped countries.

Across indicators, those living in urban areas usually fare better than their rural counter-parts. Young people are more likely to stay in school longer; women marry later and have small families; fewer infants die in their first year of life. Rate of modern contraceptive use in urban and rural areas are steadly increasing in most developing countries, although urban areas have consistently shown high use. Nevertheless, progress can vary significantly by country, even in the same region. Country level data, however, can mask further disparities within urban areas, where the gaps between poor and rich can be striking. The urban poor frequently remain marginalized and may fare no better than rural dwellers. In many developing countries where urbanization is occurring rapidly, infrastructure and services including health care; water and sanitation cannot keep pace leaving the urban poor unable to find or afford services. Often, the poorest urban children are at least twice as likely to die before they reach their fifth birthday.

In Delhi, India, only 19 per cent of the poorest women have a skilled attendant at birth compared to 99 per cent amont wealthiest women, yet data at the national level in India show skilled attendance at delivery in urban and rural areas at 74 per cent and 43 per cent respectively *(70)*.

The indicators used in urban-rural divide are as follows : The year of the Indian data is given in bracket with each indicator.

	Urban	Rural
Demography		
Population % Urban (2021)	35.39	
Total Fertility Rate (2019–21)	1.6	2.1
Women Ages 15-19 who have begun childbearing (%) (2019–21)	3.8	7.9
Socio-economic		
Population below National Poverty Line (%) (2011–12)	13.7	25.7
Employment in agriculture (% of total employment) 2004/2013		47
Women who are literate (%) (2019–21)	83	69.3

	Urban	Rural
Maternal and Child Health		
Antenatal Care (at least 4 visits) (%) (2019–21)	68.1	54.2
Skilled attendance at delivery (%) (2019–21)	94	81.8
Infant Mortality Rate (2020)	19	31
Children under age 5 who are underweight (%) (2019–21)	27.3	33.8
Children who are stunted (2019–21)	30.1	37.3
Children who are overweight (2019–21)	4.2	3.2
Family Planning		
Married women ages 15–49 using modern contraception (%) (2019–21)	58.6	55.5
Unmet need for family planning (%) (2019–21)	8.4	9.9
Drinking water and sanitation		
Population with access to improved drinking water source (%) (2019–21)	98.7	94.6
Population with access to improved sanitation facility (%) (2019–21)	81.5	64.9

Source : *(34)*

HEALTH SERVICE PHILOSOPHIES

Health care

Health care is an expression of concern for fellow human beings. It is defined as a "multitude of services rendered to individuals, families or communities by the agents of the health services or professions, for the purpose of promoting, maintaining, monitoring or restoring health" *(33)*. Such services might be staffed, organized, administered and financed in every imaginable way, but they all have one thing in common: people are being "served", that is, diagnosed, helped, cured, educated and rehabilitated by health personnel *(21)*. In many countries, health care is completely or largely a government function.

Health care includes "medical care". Many people mistakenly believe that both are synonymous. Medical care is a subset of a health care system. The term "medical care (which ranges from domiciliary care to resident hospital care) refers chiefly to those personal services that are provided directly by physicians or rendered as a result of the physician's instructions" *(71)*.

Health care has many characteristics; they include:

i. **appropriateness** (relevance), i.e., whether the service is needed at all in relation to essential human needs, priorities and policies;
ii. **comprehensiveness** i.e., whether there is an optimum mix of preventive, curative and promotional services;
iii. **adequacy**, i.e., if the service is proportionate to requirement;
iv. **availability**, i.e., ratio between the population of an administrative unit and the health facility (e.g., population per centre; doctor–population ratio);
v. **accessibility**, i.e., this may be geographic accessibility, economic accessibility or cultural accessibility;
vi. **affordability**, i.e., the cost of health care should be within the means of the individual and the state; and
vii. **feasibility**, i.e., operational efficiency of certain procedures, logistic support, manpower and material resources.

Health system

The "health system" is intended to deliver health services. It can be defined as "the human and material resources that a nation or community deploys to preserve, protect, and restore health and to minimize suffering caused by disease and injury, and the corresponding administrative and organizational arrangements" *(40)*.

The components of the health system include: **concepts** (e.g., health and disease); **ideas** (e.g., equity, coverage, effectiveness, efficiency, impact); **objects** (e.g., hospitals, health centres, health programmes) and **persons** (e.g., providers and consumers). Together, these form a whole in which all the components interact to support or control one another *(72)*. The aim of a health system is **health development** – a process of continuous and progressive improvement of the health status of a population.

Levels of health care

Health services are usually organized at three levels, each level supported by a higher level to which the patient is referred. These levels are:

(a) **Primary health care** : This is the first level of contact between the individual and the health system where "essential" health care (primary health care) is provided. A majority of prevailing health complaints and problems can be satisfactorily dealt with at this level. This level of care is closest to the people. In the Indian context, this care is provided by the primary health centres and their subcentres, with community participation.

(b) **Secondary health care** : At this level, more complex problems are dealt with. This care comprises essentially curative services and is provided by the district hospitals and community health centres. This level serves as the first referral level in the health system.

(c) **Tertiary health care** : This level offers super-specialist care. This care is provided by the regional/central level institutions. These institutions provide not only highly specialized care, but also planning and managerial skills and teaching for specialized staff. In addition, the tertiary level supports and complements the actions carried out at the primary level.

Health team concept

It is recognized that the physician of today is overworked professionally. It is also recognized that many of the functions of the physician can be performed by auxiliaries, given suitable training. An auxiliary worker has been defined as one "who has less than full professional qualifications in a particular field and is supervised by a professional worker". The WHO no longer uses the term "paramedical" for the various health professions allied with medicine *(53)*.

The practice of modern medicine has become a joint effort of many groups of workers, both medical and non-medical, viz. physicians, nurses, social workers, health assistants, ASHA and a host of others. The composition of the team varies. The hospital team is different from the team that works in the community. Whether it is a hospital team or community health work team, it is important for each team member to have a specific and recognized function in the team and to have freedom to exercise his or her particular skills. In this context, a **health team** has been defined as "a group of persons who share a common health goal and common objectives, determined by community needs and towards the achievement of which each member of the team contributes in accordance with her/his competence and skills, and respecting the functions of the other" *(73)*. The auxiliary is an essential member of the team. The team must have a leader. The leader should be able to evaluate the team adequately and should know the motivations of each member in order to stimulate and enhance their potentialities. The health team concept has taken a firm root in the delivery of health services both in the developed and developing countries. The health team approach aims to produce the right "mix" of health personnel for providing full health coverage of the entire population. The mere presence of a variety of health professionals is not sufficient to establish teamwork; it is the proper division and combination of their operations from which the benefits of divided labour will be derived *(74)*.

Health for All

After three decades of trial and error and dissatisfaction in meeting people's basic health needs, the World Health Assembly, in May 1977, decided that the main social goal of governments and WHO in the coming years should be the "attainment by all the people of the world by the year 2000 A.D. of a level of health that will permit them to lead a socially and economically productive life". This goal has come to be popularly known as "Health for All by the year 2000" (HFA). The background to this "new" philosophy was the growing concern about the unacceptably low levels of health status of the majority of the world's population especially the rural poor and the gross disparities in health between the rich and poor, urban and rural population, both between and within countries. The essential principle of "HFA" is the concept of "equity in health", that is, all people should have an opportunity to enjoy good health.

Primary health care

The concept of primary health care came into lime-light in 1978 following an international conference in Alma-Ata, USSR. It has been defined as:

> *"Essential health care based on practical, scientifically sound and socially acceptable methods and technology made universally accessible to individuals and families in the community through their full participation and at a cost that the community and the country can afford to maintain at every stage of their development in the spirit of self–determination"*

The primary health care approach is based on principles of social equity, nation-wide coverage, self-reliance, intersectoral coordination, and people's involvement in the planning and implementation of health programmes in pursuit of common health goals. This approach has been described as "Health by the people" and "placing people's health in people's hands". Primary health care was accepted by the member countries of WHO as the key to achieving the goal of HFA by the year 2000 A.D.

The **Declaration of Alma-Ata** *(6)* stated that primary health care includes at least:

- education about prevailing health problems and methods of preventing and controlling them;
- promotion of food supply and proper nutrition;
- an adequate supply of safe water and basic sanitation;
- maternal and child health care, including family planning;
- immunization against infectious diseases;
- prevention and control of endemic diseases;
- appropriate treatment of common diseases and injuries; and
- provision of essential drugs.

The concept of primary health care involves a concerted effort to provide the rural population of developing countries with at least the bare minimum of health services. The list can be modified to fit local circumstances. For example, some countries have specifically included mental health, physical handicaps, and the health and social care of the elderly. The primary health care approach integrates at the community level all the factors required for improving the health status of the population. As a signatory to the Alma-Ata Declaration, the Government of India, has pledged itself to provide primary health care. Obstacles to the implementation of primary health care in India include shortage of health manpower, entrenchment of a curative culture within the existing health system, and a high concentration of health services and health personnel in urban areas *(49)*.

Health promotion *(75)*

The first international conference on health promotion was held in Ottawa in November 1986, primarily in response to growing expectation for a new public health movement around the world. It was built on progress made through Declaration on Primary Health Care at Alma-Ata, and the debate at the World Health Assembly on intersectoral action for health. The conference resulted in proclamation of the **Ottawa Charter for Health Promotion**, which has been a source of guidance and inspiration for health promotion since that time.

Health is a basic human right and is essential for social and economic development. Increasingly health promotion is being recognized as an essential element of health development. Health promotion, through investment and action, has a marked impact on the determinants of health so as to create the greatest health gain for people, to contribute significantly to the reduction of inequities of health, and to further human rights. The ultimate goal is to increase health expectancy.

The **Jakarta Declaration on Health Promotion** (the fourth conference held in July 1997) offered a vision and focus for health promotion into the 21st century. The determinants of health; new challenges in the 21st century; and the fundamental conditions and resources for health are peace, shelter, education, social security, social relations, food, income, the empowerment of women, a stable ecosystem, sustainable resource use, social justice, respect for human rights, and equity. Above all, poverty is the greatest threat to health.

Demographic trends such as urbanization, an increase in the number of older people and the high prevalence of chronic diseases pose new problems in all countries. Other social, behavioural and biological changes such as increased sedentary behaviour, resistance to antibiotics and other commonly available drugs, increased drug abuse, and civil and domestic violence threaten the health and well-being of hundreds of millions of people. New and re-emerging infectious diseases, and the greater recognition of mental health problems, require an urgent response. It is vital that approaches to health promotion evolve to meet changes in the determinants of health. To address emerging threats to health, new forms of action are needed. The challenges for the coming years will be to unlock the potential for health promotion inherent in many sectors of society, among local communities, and within families.

The Ottawa charter incorporates five key action areas in health promotion. They are :

a. build healthy public policy,
b. create supportive environment for health,
c. strenghthen community action for health,
d. develop personal skills, and
e. re-orient health services

A Logo was created for Ottawa conference. Since then, WHO kept this symbol as the **Health Promotion Logo,** as it stands for the approaches to health promotion as outlined in Ottawa Charter. The Logo represents a circle with 3 wings. It incorporates five key action areas in health promotion and three basic health promotion strategies.

Health promotion strategies and programmes should be adapted to the local needs and possibilities of individual countries and regions to take into account differing social, cultural and economic systems.

Millennium Development Goals (MDGs)

In the Millennium Declaration of September 2000, Member States of the United Nations made a most passionate committment to address the crippling poverty and multiplying misery that grip many areas of the world. Governments had set a date of 2015 by which they would meet the Millennium Development Goals: eradicate extreme poverty and hunger, achieve universal primary education, promote gender equality and empower women, reduce child mortality, improve maternal health, combat HIV/AIDS, malaria and other diseases, ensure environmental sustainability and develop a global partnership for development.

Sustainable Development Goals *(66)*

The 2030 Sustainable Development Agenda is of unprecedented scope and ambition, applicable to all countries, and goes well beyond the MDGs. While poverty eradication, health, education, and food security and nutrition remain priorities, the Sustainable Development Goals (SDGs) comprise a broad range of economic, social and environmental objectives, and offer the prospect of more peaceful and inclusive societies.

Paragraph 26 of the 2030 agenda for sustainable development addresses health as follows:

> *To promote physical and mental health and well-being, and to extend life expectancy for all, we must achieve universal health coverage and access to quality health care. No one must be left behind. We commit to accelerating the progress made to date in reducing newborn, child and maternal mortality by ending all such preventable deaths before 2030. We are committed to ensuring universal access to sexual and reproductive health-care services, including for family planning, information and education. We will equally accelerate the pace of progress made in fighting malaria, HIV/AIDS, tuberculosis, hepatitis, Ebola and other communicable diseases and epidemics, including by addressing growing anti-microbial resistance and the problem of unattended diseases affecting developing countries. We are committed to the prevention and treatment of non-communicable diseases, including behavioural, developmental and neurological disorders, which constitute a major challenge for sustainable development.*

Out of the 17 goals, 3rd goal is devoted specifically to health, and is framed in deliberately broad terms that are relevant to all countries and all populations. "Ensure healthy lives and promote well-being for all at all ages". The health goal is associated with 13 targets, including four means of implementation targets labelled 3.a to 3.d. Overall, the SDGs have 169 targets. (See chapter 9 for details).

Health policy

Policies are general statements based on human aspirations, set of values, commitments, assessment of current situation and an image of a desired future situation *(53)*. A national health policy is an expression of goals for improving the health situation, the priorities among these goals, and the main directions for attaining them *(76)*. Health policy is often defined at the national level.

Each country will have to develop a health policy of its own aimed at defined goals, for improving the people's health, in the light of its own problems, particular circumstances, social and economic structures, and political and administrative mechanisms. Among the crucial factors affecting realization of these goals are: a political commitment; financial implications; administrative reforms; community participation and basic legislation *(77)*.

A landmark in the development of health policy was the worldwide adoption of the goal of HFA by 2000 A.D. A further landmark was the Alma-Ata Declaration (1978) calling on all governments to develop and implement primary health care strategies to attain the target of "HFA" by 2000 A.D. and more recently, Millennium Development Goals, and Sustainable Development Goals.

Health services research

Health research has several ramifications. It may include (a) **Biomedical research**, to elucidate outstanding health problems and develop new or better ways of dealing with them; (b) **Intersectoral research**, for which relationships would have to be established with the institutions concerned with the other sectors, and (c) **Health services research** or health practice research (now called "health systems research").

The concept of health services research (HSR) was developed during 1981–1982. It has been defined as "the systematic study of the means by which biomedical and other relevant knowledge is brought to bear on the health of individuals and communities under a given set of conditions" *(78)*. HSR is wide in scope. It deals with all aspects of management of health services, viz. prioritization of health problems, planning, management, logistics and delivery of health care services. It deals with such topics as manpower, organization, the utilization of facilities, the quality of health care, cost-benefit and cost-effectiveness *(79)*.

Thousands of people suffer morbidity, mortality and disability not because of deficiencies in biomedical knowledge but as a result of the failure to apply this knowledge effectively. Health services research aims to correct this failure *(80)*.

The concept of HSR is holistic and multidisciplinary. The prime purpose of HSR is to improve the health of the people through improvement not only of conventional health services but also of other services that have a bearing on health. HSR is essential for the continuous evolution and refinement of health services *(78)*.

CONCEPT OF DISEASE

There have been many attempts to define disease. Webster defines disease as "a condition in which body health is impaired, a departure from a state of health, an alteration of the human body interrupting the performance of vital functions". The Oxford English Dictionary defines disease as "a condition of the body or some part or organ of the body in which its functions are disrupted or deranged". From an **ecological** point of view, disease is defined as "a maladjustment of the human organism to the environment" *(81)*. From a **sociological** point of view, disease is considered a social phenomenon, occurring in all societies *(82)* and defined and fought in terms of the particular cultural forces prevalent in the society. The simplest definition is, of course, that disease is just the opposite of health – i.e., any deviation from normal functioning or state of complete physical or mental well-being – since health and disease are mutually exclusive. These definitions are considered inadequate because they do not give a criterion by which to decide when a disease state begins, nor do they lend themselves to measurement of disease.

The WHO has defined health but not disease. This is because disease has many shades ("spectrum of disease") ranging from inapparent (subclinical) cases to severe manifest illness. Some diseases commence acutely (e.g., food poisoning), and some insidiously (e.g., mental illness, rheumatoid arthritis). In some diseases, a "carrier" state occurs in which the individual remains outwardly healthy, and is able to infect others (e.g., typhoid fever). In some instances, the same organism may cause more than one clinical manifestation (e.g., streptococcus). In some cases, the same disease may be caused by more than one organism (e.g., diarrhoea). Some diseases have a short course, and some a prolonged course. It is easy to determine illness when the signs and symptoms are manifest, but in many diseases the border line between normal and abnormal is indistinct as in the case of diabetes, hypertension and mental illness. The end-point or final outcome of disease is variable – recovery, disability or death of the host.

Distinction is also made between the words disease, illness and sickness which are not wholly synonymous. The term "disease" literally means "without ease" (uneasiness) – disease, the opposite of ease – when something is wrong with bodily function. "Illness" refers not only to the presence of a specific disease, but also to the individual's perceptions and behaviour in response to the disease, as well as the impact of that disease on the psychosocial environment *(83)*. "Sickness" refers to a state of social dysfunction. Susser *(84)* has suggested the following usage:

> Disease is a physiological/psychological dysfunction;
>
> Illness is a subjective state of the person who feels aware of not being well;
>
> Sickness is a state of social dysfunction, i.e., a role that the individual assumes when ill ("sickness role").

The clinician sees people who are ill rather than the diseases which he must diagnose and treat *(85)*. However, it is possible to be victim of disease without feeling ill, and to be ill without signs of physical impairment. In short, an adequate definition of disease is yet to be found – a definition that is satisfactory or acceptable to the epidemiologist, clinician, sociologist and the statistician.

CONCEPT OF CAUSATION

Upto the time of Louis Pasteur (1822–1895), various concepts of disease causation were in vogue, e.g., the supernatural theory of disease, the theory of humors, the concept of contagion, miasmatic theory of disease, the theory of spontaneous generation, etc. Discoveries in microbiology marked a turning point in our aetiological concepts .

Germ theory of disease

Mention has already been made about the germ theory of disease in chapter 1. This concept gained momentum during the 19th and the early part of 20th century. The emphasis had shifted from empirical causes (e.g., bad air) to microbes as the sole cause of disease. The concept of cause embodied in the germ theory of disease is generally referred to as a **one-to-one** relationship between causal agent and disease. The disease model accordingly is :

Disease agent → Man → Disease

The germ theory of disease, though it was a revolutionary concept, led many epidemiologists to take one–sided view of disease causation. That is, they could not think beyond the germ theory of disease. It is now recognized that a disease is rarely caused by a single agent alone, but rather depends upon a number of factors which contribute to its occurrence. Therefore, modern medicine has moved away from the strict adherence to the germ theory of disease.

Epidemiological triad

The germ theory of disease has many limitations. For example, it is well-known, that not everyone exposed to tuberculosis develops tuberculosis. The same exposure, however, in an undernourished or otherwise susceptible person may result in clinical disease. Similarly, not everyone exposed to beta-haemolytic streptococci develops acute rheumatic fever. There are other factors relating to the host and environment which are equally important to determine whether or not disease will occur in the exposed host. This demanded a broader concept of disease causation that synthesized the basic factors of agent, host and environment (Fig. 4).

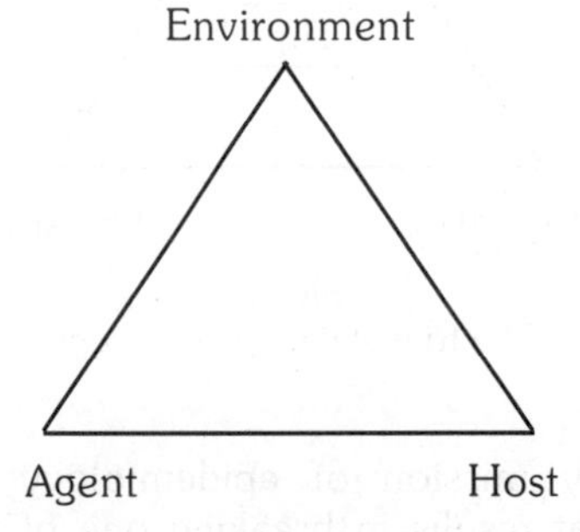

FIG. 4
Epidemiological triad

The above model – agent, host and environment – has been in use for many years. It helped epidemiologists to focus on different classes of factors, especially with regard to infectious diseases *(86)*.

The triangle of epidemiology *(59)*

The traditional triangle of epidemiology is shown in Figure 5. This triangle is based on the communicable disease model and is useful in showing the interaction and interdependence of agent, host, environment, and time as used in the investigation of diseases and epidemics. The agent is the cause of disease; the host is an organism, usually a human or an animal, that harbours the disease, the environment is those surroundings and conditions external to the human or animal that cause or allow disease transmission; and time accounts for incubation periods, life expectancy of the host or the pathogen, and duration of the course of illness or condition.

Agents of infectious diseases include bacteria, viruses, parasites, fungi, and molds. With regard to non-infectious disease, disability, injury, or death, agents can include chemicals from dietary foods, tobacco smoke, solvents, radiation or heat, nutritional deficiencies, or other substances, such as poison. One or several agents may contribute to an illness.

A host offers subsistence and lodging for a pathogen and may or may not develop the disease. The level of immunity, genetic makeup, level of exposure, state of health, and overall fitness of the host can determine the effect a disease organism will have on it. The makeup of the host and the ability of the pathogen to accept the new environment can also be a determining factor because some pathogens thrive only under limited ideal conditions. For example, many infectious disease agents can exist only in a limited temperature range.

Environmental factors can include the biological aspects as well as social, cultural, and physical aspects of the environment. The surroundings in which a pathogen lives and the effect the surroundings have on it are a part of the environment. Environment can be within a host or external to it in the community. Finally, time includes severity of illness in relation to how long a person is infected or until the condition causes death or passes the threshold of danger towards recovery. Delays in time from infection to when symptoms develop, duration of illness, and threshold of an epidemic in a population are time elements with which the epidemiologist is concerned.

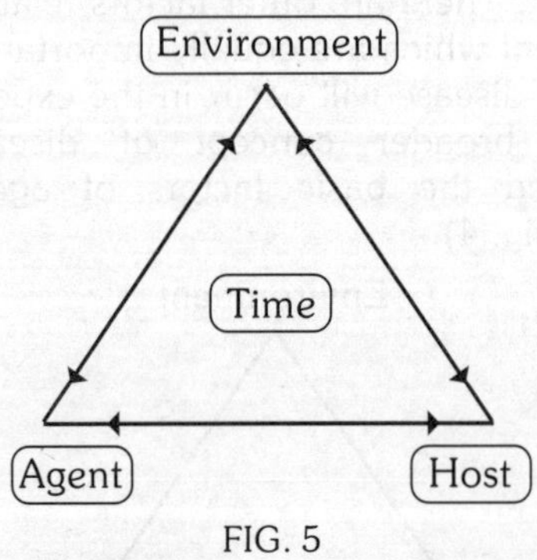

FIG. 5
The triangle of epidemiology

Source : *(59)*

The primary mission of epidemiology is to provide information that results in breaking one of the legs of the triangle, thereby disrupting the connection among environment, host, and agent, and stopping the outbreak.

Multifactorial causation

The concept that disease is due to multiple factors is not a new one. Pettenkofer of Munich (1819–1901) was an early proponent of this concept. But the "germ theory of disease" or "single cause idea" in the late 19th century overshadowed the multiple cause theory.

As a result of advances in public health, chemotherapy, antibiotics and vector control communicable diseases began to decline – only to be replaced by new types of diseases, the so-called "modern" diseases of civilization, e.g., lung cancer, coronary heart disease, chronic bronchitis, mental illness, etc. These diseases could not be explained on the basis of the germ theory of disease nor could they be prevented by the traditional methods of isolation, immunization or improvements in sanitation. The realization began to dawn that the "single cause idea" was an oversimplification and that there are other factors in the aetiology of diseases – social, economic, cultural, genetic and psychological which are equally important. As already mentioned, tuberculosis is not merely due to tubercle bacilli; factors such as poverty, overcrowding and malnutrition contribute to its occurrence. The doctrine of one-to-one relationship between cause and disease has been shown to be untenable, even for microbial diseases, e.g., tuberculosis, leprosy.

It is now known that diseases such as coronary heart disease and cancer are due to multiple factors. For example, excess of fat intake, smoking, lack of physical exercise and obesity are all involved in the pathogenesis of coronary heart disease. Most of these factors are linked to lifestyle and human behaviour. Epidemiology has contributed significantly to our present day understanding of multifactorial causation of disease. Medical men are looking "beyond the "germ theory" of disease into the total life situation of the patient and the community in search of multiple (or risk) factors of disease. Fig. 6 presents an adapted and ***advanced model of the triangle of epidemiology***. This new model includes all facets of the communicable disease model, and to make it more relevant and useful with regard to today's diseases, conditions, disorders, defects, injuries, and deaths; it also reflects the causes of current illnesses and conditions. Behaviour, lifestyle factors, environmental causes, ecologic elements, physical factors, and chronic diseases must also be taken into account. The term ***agent*** is replaced by ***causative factors***, which implies the need to identify multiple causes or a aetiologic factors of disease, disability, injury and death *(59)*.

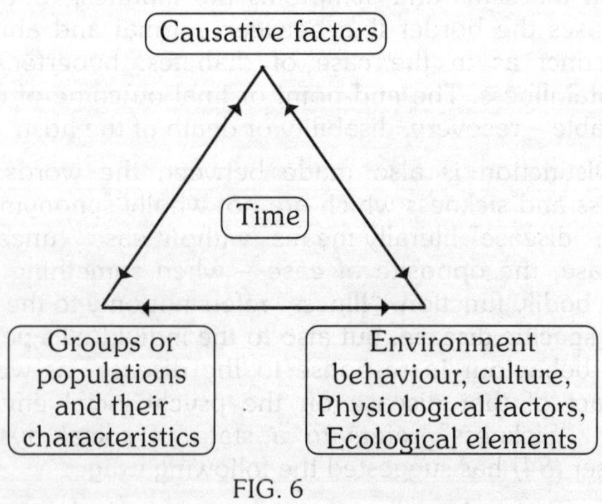

FIG. 6
Advanced model of the triangle of epidemiology

Source : *(59)*

The purpose of knowing the multiple factors of disease is to quantify and arrange them in priority sequence (prioritization) for modification or amelioration to prevent or control disease. The multifactorial concept offers multiple approaches for the prevention/control of disease.

Web of causation

This model of disease causation was suggested by MacMahon and Pugh in their book: "Epidemiologic Principles and Methods" *(87)*. This model is ideally suited in the study of chronic disease, where the disease agent is often not known, but is the outcome of interaction of multiple factors.

The "web of causation" considers all the predisposing factors of any type and their complex interrelationship with each other. Fig. 7 illustrates the complexities of a causal web of myocardial infarction (which is by no means complete). The basic tenet of epidemiology is to study the clusters of causes and combinations of effects and how they relate to each other *(88)*. It can be visualized that the causal web (Fig. 7) provides a model which shows a variety of possible interventions that could be taken which might reduce the occurrence of myocardial infarction.

The web of causation does not imply that the disease cannot be controlled unless all the multiple causes or chains of causation or at least a number of them are appropriately controlled or removed. This is not the case. Sometimes removal or elimination of just only one link or chain may be sufficient to control disease, provided that link is sufficiently important in the pathogenetic process. In a multifactorial event, therefore, individual factors are by no means all of equal weight. The relative importance of these factors may be expressed in terms of "relative risk" (see page 81).

NATURAL HISTORY OF DISEASE

Disease results from a complex interaction between man, an agent (or cause of disease) and the environment. The term ***natural history of disease*** is a key concept in epidemiology. It signifies the way in which a disease evolves over time from the earliest stage of its prepathogenesis phase to its termination as recovery, disability or death, in the absence of treatment or prevention. Each disease has its own unique natural history, which is not necessarily the same in all individuals, so much so, any general formulation of the natural history of disease is necessarily arbitrary.

The natural history of disease is best established by cohort studies (see page 83). As these studies are costly and laborious, our understanding of the natural history of disease is largely based on other epidemiological studies, such as cross-sectional and retrospective studies, undertaken in different population settings, both national and international. What the physician sees in the hospital is just an "episode" in the natural history of disease. The epidemiologist, by studying the natural history of disease in the community setting, is in a unique position to fill the gaps in our knowledge about the natural history of disease.

A schematic diagram of the natural history of disease is shown in Fig. 8. It is a necessary framework to understand the pathogenetic chain of events for a particular disease, and for the application of preventive measures. It is customary to describe the natural history of disease as consisting of two phases: prepathogenesis (i.e., the process in the environment) and pathogenesis (i.e., the process in man). Let us consider the events that take place in the natural history of disease, using infectious disease as a principal model *(89)*.

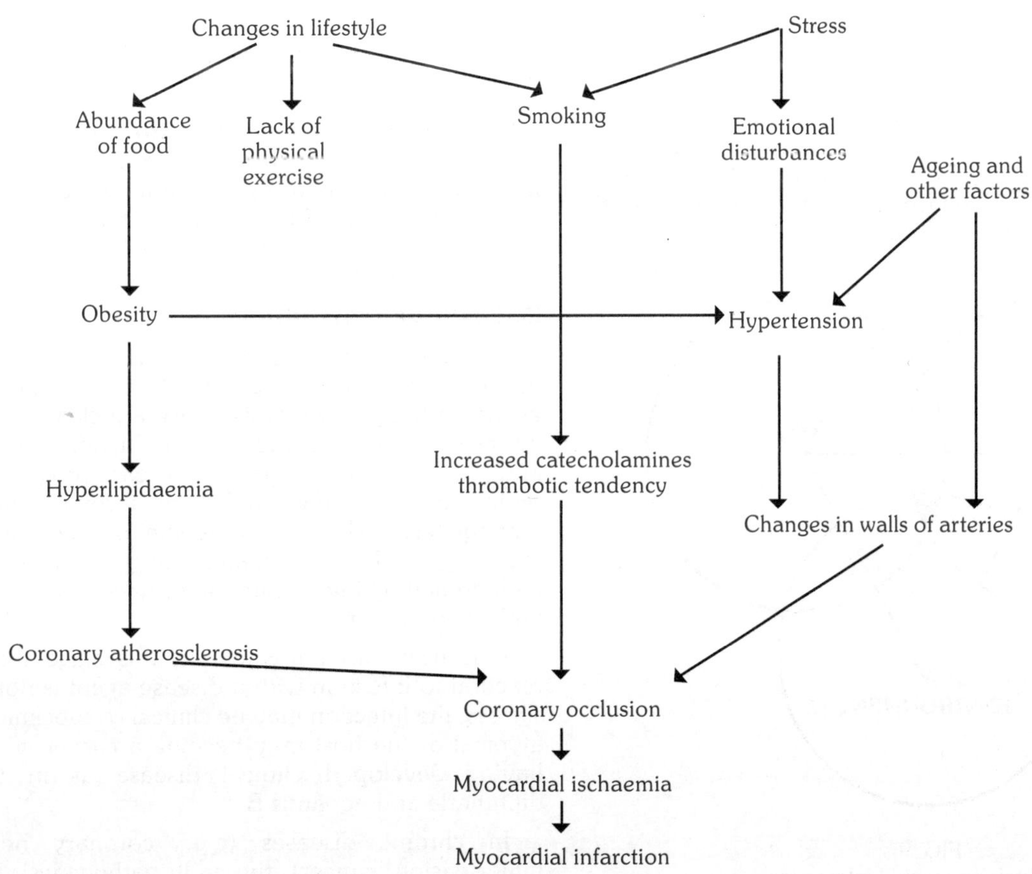

FIG. 7
Web of casuation for myocardial infarction

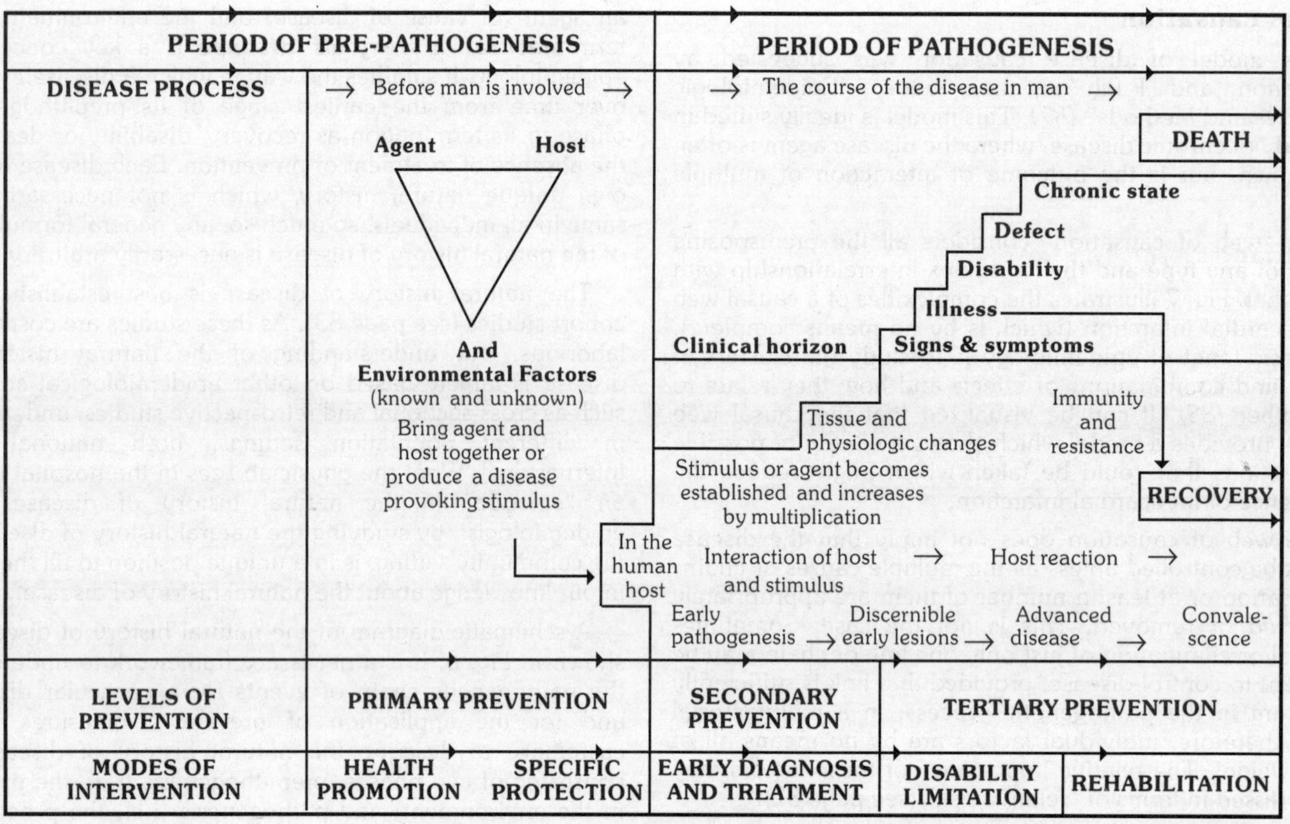

FIG. 8
Natural history of disease
(From Preventive Medicine for the Doctor in His Community, by Leavell & Clark with permission of McGraw-Hill Book Co.)

1. Prepathogenesis phase

This refers to the period preliminary to the onset of disease in man. The disease agent has not yet entered man, but the factors which favour its interaction with the human host are already existing in the environment. This situation is frequently referred to as "man in the midst of disease" or "man exposed to the risk of disease". Potentially we are all in the prepathogenesis phase of many diseases, both communicable and non-communicable.

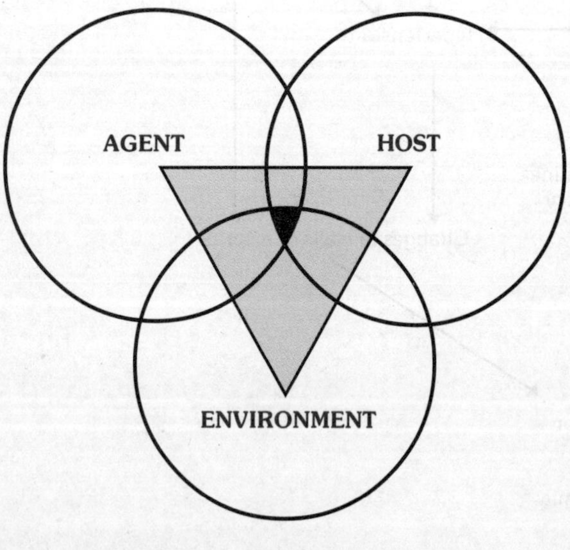

FIG. 9
Epidemiologic concept of interactions of
Agent, Host and Environment
(Adapted from Health Services Reports, Vol. 87, page 672)

The causative factors of disease may be classified as AGENT, HOST and ENVIRONMENT. These three factors are referred to as **epidemiological triad**. The mere presence of agent, host and favourable environmental factors in the prepathogenesis period is not sufficient to start the disease in man. What is required is an **interaction** of these three factors to initiate the disease process in man. The agent, host and environment operating in combination determine not only the onset of disease which may range from a single case to epidemics (as depicted in Fig. 9's black area) but also the distribution of disease in the community.

2. Pathogenesis phase

The pathogenesis phase begins with the entry of the disease "agent" in the susceptible human host. The further events in the pathogenesis phase are clear-cut in infectious diseases, i.e., the disease agent multiplies and induces tissue and physiological changes, the disease progresses through a period of incubation and later through early and late pathogenesis. The final outcome of the disease may be recovery, disability or death. The pathogenesis phase may be modified by intervention measures such as immunization and chemotherapy.

It is useful to remember at this stage that the host's reaction to infection with a disease agent is not predictable. That is, the infection may be clinical or subclinical; typical or atypical or the host may become a carrier with or without having developed clinical disease as in the case of diphtheria and hepatitis B.

In chronic diseases (e.g., coronary heart disease, hypertension, cancer), the early pathogenesis phase is less dramatic. This phase in chronic diseases is referred to as presymptomatic phase. During the presymptomatic stage, there is no manifest disease. The pathological changes are essentially below the level of the "clinical horizon". The clinical stage begins when recognizable signs or symptoms appear. By the time signs and symptoms appear, the disease phase is already well advanced into the late pathogenesis phase. In many chronic diseases, the agent-host-environmental interactions are not yet well understood.

Agent factors

The first link in the chain of disease transmission is a disease agent. The disease "agent" is defined as a substance, living or non-living, or a force, tangible or intangible, the excessive presence or relative lack of which may initiate or perpetuate a disease process. A disease may have a single agent, a number of independent alternative agents or a complex of two or more factors whose combined presence is essential for the development of the disease *(33)*.

Disease agents may be classified broadly into the following groups :

1. Biological agents

These are living agents of disease, viz, viruses, rickettsiae, fungi, bacteria, protozoa and metazoa. These agents exhibit certain "host–related" biological properties such as: (i) **infectivity**: this is the ability of an infectious agent to invade and multiply (produce infection) in a host; (ii) **pathogenicity**: this is the ability to induce clinically apparent illness, and (iii) **virulence**: this is defined as the proportion of clinical cases resulting in severe clinical manifestations (including sequelae). The case fatality rate is one way of measuring virulence *(86)*.

2. Nutrient agents

These are proteins, fats, carbohydrates, vitamins, minerals and water. Any excess or deficiency of the intake of nutritive elements may result in nutritional disorders. Protein energy malnutrition (PEM), anaemia, goitre, obesity and vitamin deficiencies are some of the current nutritional problems in many countries.

3. Physical agents

Exposure to excessive heat, cold, humidity, pressure, radiation, electricity, sound, etc may result in illness.

4. Chemical agents

(i) Endogenous: Some of the chemicals may be produced in the body as a result of derangement of function, e.g., urea (uraemia), serum bilirubin (jaundice), ketones (ketosis), uric acid (gout), calcium carbonate (kidney stones), etc.

(ii) Exogenous: Agents arising outside of human host, e.g., allergens, metals, fumes, dust, gases, insecticides, etc. These may be acquired by inhalation, ingestion or inoculation.

5. Mechanical agents

Exposure to chronic friction and other mechanical forces may result in crushing, tearing, sprains, dislocations and even death.

6. Absence or insufficiency or excess of a factor necessary to health

These may be (i) Chemical factors: e.g., hormones (insulin, oestrogens, enzymes) (ii) Nutrient factors: given under no. 2 above (iii) Lack of structure: e.g., thymus (iv) Lack of part of structure, e.g., cardiac defects (v) Chromosomal factors, e.g., mongolism, turner's syndrome, and (vi) Immunological factors, e.g., agammaglobulinemia.

7. Social agents

It is also necessary to consider social agents of disease. These are poverty, smoking, abuse of drugs and alcohol, unhealthy lifestyles, social isolation, maternal deprivation, etc.

Thus the modern concept of disease "agent" is a very broad one; it includes both living and non-living agents.

Host factors (intrinsic)

In epidemiological terminology, the human host is referred to as "soil" and the disease agent as "seed". In some situations, host factors play a major role in determining the outcome of an individual's exposure to infection (e.g., tuberculosis).

The host factors may be classified as (i) Demographic characteristics such as age, sex, ethnicity; (ii) Biological characteristics such as genetic factors; biochemical levels of the blood (e.g., cholesterol); blood groups and enzymes; cellular constituents of the blood; immunological factors; and physiological function of different organ systems of the body (e.g., blood pressure, forced expiratory ventilation). etc. (iii) Social and economic characteristics such as socio-economic status, education, occupation, stress, marital status, housing, etc. and (iv) Lifestyle factors such as personality traits, living habits, nutrition, physical exercise, use of alcohol, drugs and smoking, behavioural patterns, etc. The association of a particular disease with a specific set of host factors frequently provides an insight into the cause of disease. The host factors of importance are further discussed in chapter 3.

Environmental factors (extrinsic)

The study of disease is really the study of man and his environment. Hundreds of millions of people are affected by preventable diseases originating in the environment in which they live. For human beings the environment is not limited, as it normally is for plants and animals, to a set of climatic factors. For example, for man, social and economic conditions are more important than the mean annual temperature. Thus the concept of environment is complex and all-embracing. The external or **macro-environment** is defined as "all that which is external to the individual human host, living and non-living, and with which he is in constant interaction". This includes all of man's external surroundings such as air, water, food, housing, etc.

For descriptive purposes, the environment of man has been divided into three components – physical, biological and psychosocial. It should be emphasized that this separation is artificial. They are closely related to each other and with host factors.

a. Physical environment

The term "physical environment" is applied to non-living things and physical factors (e.g., air, water, soil, housing, climate, geography, heat, light, noise, debris, radiation, etc) with which man is in constant interaction. Man's victory over his physical environment has been responsible for most of the improvement in health during the past century. In most developing countries, defective environment (e.g., lack of sanitation) continues to be the main health problem. Man has altered practically everything in his physical environment to his advantage. In doing so, he has created for himself a host of new health problems such as air pollution, water pollution, noise pollution, urbanization, radiation hazards, etc. The increasing use of electrical and electronic devices, including the rapid growth of telecommunication system (e.g., satellite systems), radio-broadcasting, television transmitters and radar installations have increased the possibility of human exposure to electromagnetic energy.

Man is living today in a highly complicated environment which is getting more complicated as man is becoming more ingenious. If these trends continue, it is feared that the very "quality of life" we cherish may soon be in danger.

b. Biological environment

The biological environment is the universe of living things which surrounds man, including man himself. The living things are the viruses and other microbial agents, insects, rodents, animals and plants. These are constantly working for their survival, and in this process, some of them act as disease–producing agents, reservoirs of infection, intermediate hosts and vectors of disease. Between the members of the ecological system (which includes man) there is constant adjustment and readjustment. For the most part, the parties manage to effect a harmonious inter-relationship, to achieve a state of peaceful co-existence, even though this may not be always enduring. When for any reason, this harmonious relationship is disturbed, ill-health results. In the area of biological environment also, preventive medicine has been highly successful in protecting the health of the individual and of the community.

c. Psychosocial environment

It is difficult to define "psychosocial environment" against the background of the highly varied social, economic and cultural contexts of different countries and their social standards and value systems. It includes a complex of psychosocial factors which are defined as "those factors affecting personal health, health care and community well-being that stem from the psychosocial make-up of individuals and the structure and functions of social groups" *(60)*. They include cultural values, customs, habits, beliefs, attitudes, morals, religion, education, lifestyles, community life, health services, social and political organization.

In addition to this broad aspect of psychosocial environment, man is in constant interaction with that part of the social environment known as "people". He is a member of a social group, the member of a family, of a caste, of a community and of a nation. Between the individual and other members of the group, there can be harmony or disharmony, interests and points of view that are shared or that are in conflict. The behaviour of one individual can affect others more or less directly; conflict and tension between the individual and the group as a whole or between the individual and other members of the group can yield great distress. The law of the land, customs, attitudes, beliefs, traditions, all regulate the interactions among groups of individuals and families.

The impact of social environment has both positive and negative aspects on the health of individuals and communities. A favourable social environment can improve health, provide opportunities for man to achieve a sense of fulfilment, and add to the quality of life. Therefore, customs and traditions favouring health must be preserved. Beneficial social behaviour (e.g., community participation) should be restored where it has disappeared due to social changes.

Psychosocial factors can also affect negatively man's health and well-being. For example, poverty, urbanization, migration and exposure to stressful situations such as bereavement, desertion, loss of employment, birth of a handicapped child may produce feelings of anxiety, depression, anger, frustration, and so forth; and these feelings may be accompanied by physical symptoms such as headache, palpitation and sweating. But these emotional states also produce changes in the endocrine, autonomic and motor systems, which, if prolonged and in interaction with genetic and personality factors, may lead to structural changes in various bodily organs. The resulting psychosomatic disorders include conditions such as duodenal ulcer, bronchial asthma, hypertension, coronary heart disease, mental disorders and socially deviant behaviour (e.g., suicide, crime, violence, drug abuse). Of primary concern is coronary heart disease which may be related to lifestyle and psychosocial stress. In many countries, road accidents are now the principal cause of death in young people. It is related to psychosocial states such as boredom, anxiety, frustration and other pre-occupations that can impair attention.

Man today is viewed as an "agent" of his own diseases; his state of health is determined more by what he does to himself than what some outside germ or infectious agent does to him. For example, the medical cause of lung cancer may be a chemical substance in cigarettes, but the psychosocial cause is behaviour – smoking. From a psychosocial point of view, disease may be viewed as a maladjustment of the human organism to his psychosocial environment resulting from misperception, misinterpretation and misbehaviour *(90)*. The epidemiologists today are as much concerned with psychosocial environment, as with physical or biological environment, in search for aetiological causes of disease.

Because of the fact that man exists concurrently in so many environmental contexts, it has become customary to speak of man in his "total environment". The social environment is so inextricably linked with the physical and biological environments that it is realistic and necessary to view the human environment in toto to promote health. A stable and harmonious equilibrium between man and his environment is needed to reduce man's vulnerability to disease and to permit him to lead a more productive and satisfying life.

Risk factors

For many diseases, the disease "agent" is still unidentified, e.g. coronary heart disease, cancer, peptic ulcer, mental illness, etc. Where the disease agent is not firmly established, the aetiology is generally discussed in terms of "risk factors".

The term "risk factor" is used by different authors with at least two meanings *(33)*:

a. an attribute or exposure that is significantly associated with the development of a disease *(91)*;
b. a determinant that can be modified by intervention, thereby reducing the possibility of occurrence of disease or other specified outcomes *(33)*;

Risk factors are often suggestive, but absolute proof of cause and effect between a risk factor and disease is usually lacking. That is, the presence of a risk factor does not imply that the disease will occur, and in its absence, the disease will not occur. The important thing about risk factors is that they are observable or identifiable prior to the event they predict. It is also recognized that combination of risk factors in the same individual may be purely additive or synergistic (multiplicative). For example, smoking and occupational exposure (shoe, leather, rubber, dye and chemical industries) were found to have an additive effect as risk factors for bladder cancer *(87)*. On the other hand, smoking was found to be synergistic with other risk factors such as hypertension and high blood cholesterol *(92)*. That is, the effects are more than additive.

Risk factors may be truly causative (e.g., smoking for lung cancer); they may be merely contributory to the undesired outcome (e.g., lack of physical exercise is a risk factor for coronary heart disease), or they may be predictive only in a statistical sense (e.g., illiteracy for perinatal mortality).

Some risk factors can be modified; others cannot be modified. The modifiable factors include smoking, hypertension, elevated serum cholesterol, physical activity, obesity, etc. They are amenable to intervention and are useful in the care of the individual. The unmodifiable or immutable risk factors such as age, sex, race, family history and genetic factors are not subject to change. They act more as signals in alerting health professionals and other personnel to the possible outcome *(93)*.

Risk factors may characterize the individual, the family, the group, the community or the environment. For example, some of the individual risk factors include age, sex, smoking, hypertension, etc. But there are also collective community risks – for example, from the presence of malaria, from air pollution, from substandard housing, or a poor water supply or poor health care services. The degree of risk in these cases is indirectly an expression of **need**. Therefore, it is stated that a risk factor is a proxy for need – indicating the need for promotive and preventive health services.

Epidemiological methods (e.g., case control and cohort studies) are needed to identify risk factors and estimate the degree of risk. These studies are carried out in population groups among whom certain diseases occur much more frequently than other groups. By such comparative studies, epidemiologists have been able to identify smoking as a risk for lung cancer; high serum cholesterol and high blood pressure as risk factors for coronary heart disease. The contribution of epidemiology in the identification of risk factors has been highly significant. Risk factors associated with some major disease groups are as shown in Table 8.

TABLE 8
Prominent risk factors

Disease	Risk factors
Heart disease	Smoking, high blood pressure, elevated serum cholesterol, diabetes, obesity, lack of exercise, type A personality
Cancer	Smoking, alcohol, solar radiation, ionizing radiation, work–site hazards, environmental pollution, medications, infectious agents, dietary factors
Stroke	High blood pressure, elevated cholesterol, smoking
Motor vehicle accidents	Alcohol, non-use of seat belts, speed, automobile design, roadway design
Diabetes	Obesity, diet
Cirrhosis of liver	Alcohol

Source : *(94)*

The detection of risk factors should be considered a prelude to prevention or intervention. For each risk factor ascertained, the question has to be asked whether it can be reduced in a cost-effective way and whether its reduction will prevent or delay the unwanted outcome *(95)*. Since the detection procedure usually involves whole population, it bears some similarity to presymptomatic screening for disease *(93)*.

Risk groups

Another approach developed and promoted by WHO is to identify precisely the "risk groups" or "target groups" (e.g., at-risk mothers, at-risk infants, at-risk families, chronically ill, handicapped, elderly) in the population by certain defined criteria and direct appropriate action to them first. This is known as the "risk approach". It has been summed up as "something for all, but more for those in need – in proportion to the need" *(53)*. In essence, the risk approach is a managerial device for increasing the efficiency of health care services within the limits of existing resources *(96)*. WHO has been using the risk approach in MCH services since a long time (Table 9).

TABLE 9
Guidelines for defining "at-risk" groups

a. *Biological situation:*
- age group, e.g., infants (low birth weight), toddlers, elderly
- sex, e.g., females in the reproductive age period
- physiological state, e.g., pregnancy, cholesterol level, high blood pressure
- genetic factors, e.g. family history of genetic disorders
- other health conditions (disease, physical functioning, unhealthy behaviour)

b. *Physical situation:*
- rural, urban slums
- living conditions, overcrowding
- environment: water supply, proximity to industries

c. *Sociocultural and cultural situation:*
- social class
- ethnic and cultural group
- family disruption, education, housing
- customs, habits and behaviour (e.g., smoking, lack of exercise, over-eating, drug addicts)
- access to health services
- lifestyles and attitudes

Source : *(97)*

Modern epidemiology is concerned with the identification of risk factors and high-risk groups in the population. Since resources are scarce, identification of those at risk is imperative. It helps to define priorities and points to those most in need of attention. The knowledge of risk factors and risk groups can be used to prevent disease in so far as we are able to remove or minimize the risk.

Spectrum of disease

The term "spectrum of disease" is a graphic representation of variations in the manifestations of disease. It is akin to the spectrum of light where the colours vary from one end to the other, but difficult to determine where one colour ends and the other begins. At one end of the disease spectrum are subclinical infections which are not ordinarily identified, and at the other end are fatal illnesses. In the middle of the spectrum lie illnesses ranging in severity from mild to severe. These different manifestations are simply reflections of individuals' different states of immunity and receptivity. Leprosy is an excellent example of the spectral concept of disease. For almost every disease there exists a spectrum of severity, with few exceptions such as rabies. In infectious diseases, the spectrum of disease is also referred to as the "gradient of infection".

The sequence of events in the spectrum of disease can be interrupted by early diagnosis and treatment or by preventive measures which if introduced at a particular point will prevent or retard the further development of the disease. The concept of spectrum of disease provides for inclusion of all cases, both subclinical and clinical, in the study of disease.

Iceberg of disease

A concept closely related to the spectrum of disease is the concept of the iceberg phenomenon of disease. According to this concept, disease in a community may be compared with an iceberg (Fig. 10). The floating tip of the iceberg represents what the physician sees in the community, i.e., clinical cases. The vast submerged portion of the iceberg represents the hidden mass of disease, i.e., latent, inapparent, presymptomatic and undiagnosed cases and carriers in the community. The "waterline" represents the demarcation between apparent and inapparent disease.

In some diseases (e.g., hypertension, diabetes, anaemia, malnutrition, mental illness) the unknown morbidity (i.e., the submerged portion of the iceberg) far exceeds the known morbidity. The hidden part of the iceberg thus constitutes an important, undiagnosed reservoir of infection or disease in the community, and its detection and control is a challenge to modern techniques in preventive medicine. One of the major deterrents in the study of chronic diseases of unknown aetiology is the absence of methods to detect the subclinical state – the bottom of the iceberg *(98)*.

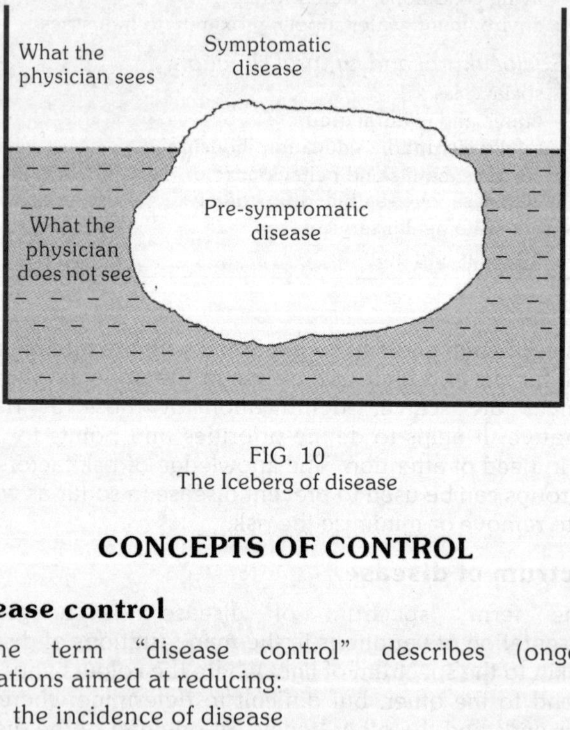

FIG. 10
The Iceberg of disease

CONCEPTS OF CONTROL

Disease control

The term "disease control" describes (ongoing) operations aimed at reducing:

i. the incidence of disease
ii. the duration of disease, and consequently the risk of transmission
iii. the effects of infection, including both the physical and psychosocial complications; and
iv. the financial burden to the community.

Control activities may focus on primary prevention or secondary prevention, most control programmes combine the two. The concept of tertiary prevention is comparatively less relevant to control efforts.

In disease control, the disease "agent" is permitted to persist in the community at a level where it ceases to be a public health problem according to the tolerance of the local population. A state of equilibrium becomes established between the disease agent, host and environment components of the disease process. An excellent embodiment of this concept is malaria control, which is distinct from malaria eradication.

Disease elimination

Between control and eradication, an intermediate goal has been described, called "regional elimination" *(99)*. The term "elimination" is used to describe interruption of transmission of disease, as for example, elimination of measles, polio and diphtheria from large geographic regions or areas *(33)*. Regional elimination is now seen as an important precursor of eradication *(99)*.

Disease eradication

Eradication literally means to "tear out by roots". Eradication of disease implies termination of all transmission of infection by extermination of the infectious agent *(33)*. As the name implies, eradication is an absolute process, and not a relative goal. It is "all or none phenomenon". The word eradication is reserved to cessation of infection and disease from the whole world *(99)*.

Today, smallpox is the only disease that has been eradicated globally. Every disease like every human being is unique with its own epidemiological characteristics and specific strategies for control.

During recent years, three diseases have been seriously advanced as candidates for global eradication within the foreseeable future: polio, measles and dracunculiasis. The feasibility of eradicating polio appears to be greater than that of others and the goal is in sight as Afghanistan and Pakistan are the only two countries endemic for poliomyelitis at present.

Experience gained from eradication programmes (e.g., malaria, yaws) has shown that once the morbidity of a disease reaches a very low level, a "residual" infection usually persists in the population leading to a state of equilibrium between the agent, host and environmental components of the disease process. In this situation, there are always hidden foci of infection, unrecognized methods of transmission, resistance of the vector or organism, all of which may again flare up when the agent–host–environment equilibrium is disturbed *(100)*. Failure to understand this led to disappointment in the eradication programmes mounted against malaria, yaws, plague, kala-azar and yellow fever.

Monitoring and surveillance

According to standard dictionaries, the words monitoring and surveillance are almost synonymous. But in public health practice they have taken on rather specific and somewhat different meanings *(101)*:

i) Monitoring

Monitoring is "the performance and analysis of routine measurements aimed at detecting changes in the environment or health status of population" *(33)*. Thus we have monitoring of air pollution, water quality, growth and nutritional status, etc. It also refers to on-going measurement of performance of a health service or a health professional, or of the extent to which patients comply with or adhere to advice from health professionals.

In management, monitoring refers to "the episodic oversight of the implementation of an activity, seeking to ensure that input deliveries, work schedules, targeted outputs, and other required actions are proceeding according to plan" *(102)*. It keeps track of achievements, staff movements and utilization, supplies and equipment, and the money spent in relation to the resources available so that if anything goes wrong, immediate corrective measures can be taken.

ii) Surveillance

Surveillance is defined in many ways *(40)* :

1. Continuous analysis, interpretation, and feedback of systematically collected data, generally using methods distinguished by their practicality, uniformity, and rapidity rather than by accuracy or completeness. By observing trends in time, place, and persons, changes can be observed or anticipated and appropriate action, including investigative or control measures, can be taken. Sources of data may relate directly to disease or to factors influencing disease. Thus they may include mortality and morbidity reports based on death certificates, hospital records, general practice sentinels, or notifications; laboratory diagnosis; outbreak reports; vaccine uptake and side effects; sickness absence records; changes in disease agents, vectors, or reservoirs; serological surveillance through serum banks. The latter can also be seen as an example of biological monitoring.
2. Systematic and continuous collection, analysis, and interpretation of data, closely integrated with the timely and coherent dissemination of the results and assessment to those who have the right to know so that action can be taken. It is an essential feature of epidemiological and public health practice. The final phase in the surveillance chain is the application of information to health promotion and to disease prevention and control. A surveillance system includes a functional capacity for data collection, analysis, and dissemination linked to public health programmes. It is often distinguished from monitoring by the notion that surveillance is continuous and ongoing, whereas monitoring tends to be more intermittent or episodic.

Surveillance programmes can assume any character and dimension – thus we have epidemiological surveillance, demographic surveillance, nutritional surveillance, etc.

According to the above definitions, monitoring becomes one specific and essential part of the broader concept embraced by surveillance. Monitoring requires careful planning and the use of standardized procedures and methods of data collection, and can then be carried out over extended periods of time by technicians and automated instrumentation. Surveillance, in contrast, requires professional analysis and sophisticated judgement of data leading to recommendations for control activities.

Sentinel surveillance

No routine notification system can identify all cases of infection or disease. A method for identifying the missing cases and thereby supplementing the notified cases is required. This is known as "sentinel surveillance." The sentinel data is extrapolated to the entire population to estimate the disease prevalence in the total population. The advantages of such a system are that the reporting biases are minimized, and feed-back of information to the providers is simplified.

Sentinel surveillance agencies could be interested and competent physicians (or institutions) in selected areas to report the cases of disease in their areas. This system would provide more valuable and detailed information than could be obtained from the traditional notification system *(103)*. Finally, these sentinel sites could be developed into a notification system for providing more detailed information, which, in some settings, may be less costly than developing and maintaining an ongoing notification system.

Evaluation of control

Evaluation is the process by which results are compared with the intended objectives, or more simply the assessment of how well a programme is performing. Evaluation should always be considered during the planning and implementation stages of a programme or activity. Evaluation may be crucial in identifying the health benefits derived (impact on morbidity, mortality, sequelae, patient satisfaction). Evaluation can be useful in identifying performance difficulties. Evaluation studies may also be carried out to generate information for other purposes, e.g., to attract attention to a problem, extension of control activities, training and patient management, etc. The principles of evaluation are discussed in chapter 23.

CONCEPTS OF PREVENTION

The goals of medicine are to promote health, to preserve health, to restore health when it is impaired, and to minimize suffering and distress. These goals are embodied in the word "prevention" *(33)*. Successful prevention depends upon a knowledge of causation, dynamics of transmission, identification of risk factors and risk groups, availability of prophylactic or early detection and treatment measures, an organization for applying these measures to appropriate persons or groups, and continuous evaluation of and development of procedures applied *(104)*.

It is not necessary (although desirable) to know everything about the natural history of a disease to initiate preventive measures. Often times, removal or elimination of a single known essential cause may be sufficient to prevent a disease. The objective of preventive medicine is to intercept or oppose the "cause" and thereby the disease process. This epidemiological concept permits the inclusion of treatment as one of the modes of intervention *(89)*.

Levels of prevention

In modern day, the concept of prevention has become broad-based. It has become customary to define prevention in terms of four level:

1. primordial prevention
2. primary prevention
3. secondary prevention
4. tertiary prevention

These levels of prevention are shown in Fig.10 in relation to the natural history of disease. Authorities on preventive medicine do not agree on the precise boundaries between these levels, but that does not minimize their importance. For example, the supply of food supplements to a family could be primary prevention for some members, and secondary prevention (curative) for others. These differences of opinion are more semantic than substantive *(33)*. A general discussion of these concepts is given below:

1. Primordial prevention

Primordial prevention, a new concept, is receiving special attention in the prevention of chronic diseases. This is primary prevention in its purest sense, that is, prevention of the emergence or development of risk factors in countries or population groups in which they have not yet appeared. For example, many adult health problems (e.g., obesity, hypertension) have their early origins in childhood, because this is the time when lifestyles are formed (for example, smoking, eating patterns, physical exercise). In primordial prevention, efforts are directed towards discouraging children from adopting harmful lifestyles. The main intervention in primordial prevention is through individual and mass education.

2. Primary prevention

Primary prevention can be defined as "action taken prior to the onset of disease, which removes the possibility that a disease will ever occur". It signifies intervention in the pre-pathogenesis phase of a disease or health problem (e.g., low birth weight) or other departure from health. Primary prevention may be accomplished by measures designed to promote general health and well-being, and quality of life of people or by specific protective measures. These are discussed in detail elsewhere under "Mode of Intervention".

Primary prevention is far more than averting the occurrence of a disease and prolonging life. It includes the concept of "positive health", a concept that encourages achievement and maintenance of "an acceptable level of health that will enable every individual to lead a socially and economically productive life". It concerns an individual's attitude towards life and health and the initiative he takes about positive and responsible measures for himself, his family and his community.

The concept of primary prevention is now being applied to the prevention of chronic diseases such as coronary heart disease, hypertension and cancer based on elimination or modification of "risk-factors" of disease. The WHO has recommended the following approaches for the primary prevention of chronic diseases where the risk factors are established *(105)* :

a. population (mass) strategy
b. high-risk strategy

a. Population (mass) strategy

Another preventive approach is "population strategy" which is directed at the whole population irrespective of individual risk levels. For example, studies have shown that even a small reduction in the average blood pressure or serum cholesterol of a population would produce a large reduction in the incidence of cardiovascular disease *(106)*. The population approach is directed towards socio-economic, behavioural and lifestyle changes *(106)*.

b. High-risk strategy

The high-risk strategy aims to bring preventive care to individuals at special risk. This requires detection of individuals at high risk by the optimum use of clinical methods.

Primary prevention is a desirable goal. It is worthwhile to recall the fact that the industrialized countries succeeded in eliminating a number of communicable diseases like cholera, typhoid and dysentery and controlling several others like plague, leprosy and tuberculosis, not by medical interventions but mainly by raising the standard of living (primary prevention). And much of this success came even before immunization became universal routine. The application of primary prevention to the prevention of chronic disease is a recent development. To have an impact on the population, all the above three approaches (primordial prevention, population strategy and high-risk strategy) should be implemented as they are usually complementary.

In summary, primary prevention is a "holistic" approach. It relies on measures designed to promote health or to protect against specific disease "agents" and hazards in the environment. It utilizes knowledge of the prepathogenesis phase of disease, embracing the agent, host and environment. Fundamental public health measures and activities such as sanitation; infection control; immunization; protection of food, milk, and water supplies; environmental protection; and protection against occupational hazards and accidents are all basic to primary prevention. Basic personal hygiene and public health measures, have had a major impact on halting communicable disease epidemics. Immunization, infection control (eg, hand washing), refrigeration of foods, garbage collection, solid and liquid waste management, water supply protection and treatment, and general sanitation have reduced infectious disease threats to populations. The safety and low cost of primary prevention justifies its wider application. Primary prevention has become increasingly identified with "health education" and the concept of individual and community responsibility for health *(107)*.

3. Secondary prevention

Secondary prevention can be defined as "action which halts the progress of a disease at its incipient stage and prevents complications". The specific interventions are early diagnosis (e.g., screening tests, case finding programmes) and adequate treatment. By early diagnosis and adequate treatment, secondary prevention attempts to arrest the disease process; restore health by seeking out unrecognized disease and treating it before irreversible pathological changes have taken place; and reverse communicability of infectious diseases. It may also protect others in the community from acquiring the infection and thus provide, at once, secondary prevention for the infected individuals and primary prevention for their potential contacts *(86)*.

Secondary prevention is largely the domain of clinical medicine. The health programmes initiated by governments are usually at the level of secondary prevention. The drawback of secondary prevention is that the patient has already been subject to mental anguish, physical pain; and the community to loss of productivity. These situations are not encountered in primary prevention.

Secondary prevention is an imperfect tool in the control of transmission of disease. It is often more expensive and less effective than primary prevention. In the long run, human health, happiness and useful longevity will be achieved at far less expense with less suffering through primary prevention than through secondary prevention *(108)*.

4. Tertiary prevention

When the disease process has advanced beyond its early stages, it is still possible to accomplish prevention by what might be called "tertiary prevention" *(89)*. It signifies intervention in the late pathogenesis phase. Tertiary prevention can be defined as "all measures available to reduce or limit impairments and disabilities, minimize suffering caused by existing departures from good health and to promote the patient's adjustment to irremediable conditions" *(33)*. For example, treatment, even if undertaken late in the natural history of disease may prevent sequelae and limit disability. When defect and disability are more or less stabilized, rehabilitation may play a preventable role. Modern rehabilitation includes psychosocial, vocational, and medical components based on team work from a variety of professions. Tertiary prevention extends the concept of prevention into fields of rehabilitation.

Table 10 summarizes the levels of prevention.

MODES OF INTERVENTION

"Intervention" can be defined as any attempt to intervene or interrupt the usual sequence in the development of disease in man. This may be by the provision of treatment, education, help or social support. Five modes of intervention have been described which form a continuum corresponding to the natural history of any disease. These levels are related to agent, host and environment and are shown in Fig. 9. They are:

1. Health promotion
2. Specific protection
3. Early diagnosis and treatment
4. Disability limitation
5. Rehabilitation

1. Health promotion

Health promotion is "the process of enabling people to increase control over, and to improve health " *(109)*. It is not directed against any particular disease, but is intended to strengthen the host through a variety of approaches (interventions). The well–known interventions in this area are:

i. health education
ii. environmental modifications
iii. nutritional interventions
iv. lifestyle and behavioural changes

(i) **Health education**: This is one of the most cost–effective interventions. A large number of diseases could be prevented with little or no medical intervention if people were adequately informed about them and if they were encouraged to take necessary precautions in time. Recognizing this truth, the WHO's constitution states that "the extension to all people of the benefits of medical, psychological and related knowledge is essential to the fullest attainment of health". The targets for educational efforts may include the general public, patients, priority groups, health providers, community leaders and decision–makers.

(ii) **Environmental modifications**: A comprehensive approach to health promotion requires environmental modifications, such as provision of safe water; installation of sanitary latrines; control of insects and rodents; improvement of housing, etc. The history of medicine has shown that many infectious diseases have been successfully controlled in western countries through environmental modifications, even prior to the development of specific vaccines or chemotherapeutic drugs. Environmental interventions are non-clinical and do not involve the physician.

(iii) **Nutritional interventions**: These comprise food distribution and nutrition improvement of vulnerable groups; child feeding programmes; food fortification; nutrition education, etc.

(iv) **Lifestyle and behavioural changes**: The conventional public health measures or interventions have not been successful in making inroads into lifestyle reforms. The action of prevention in this case, is one of individual and community responsibility for health (see page 22), the physician and in fact each health worker acting as an educator than a therapist. Health education is a basic element of all health activity. It is of paramount importance in changing the views, behaviour and habits of people.

TABLE 10

Levels of prevention

Level	Phase of disease	Aim	Actions	Target
Primordial	Underlying economic, social, and environmental conditions leading to causation	Establish and maintain conditions that minimize hazards to health	Measures that inhibit the emergence of environmental, economic, social and behavioural conditions.	Total population or selected groups; achieved through public health policy and health promotion.
Primary	Specific causal factors	Reduce the incidence of disease	Protection of health by personal and community efforts, such as enhancing nutritional status, providing immunizations, and eliminating environmental risks.	Total population, selected groups and individuals at high-risk; achieved through public health programmes
Secondary	Early stage of disease	Reduce the prevalence of disease by shortening its duration	Measures available to individuals and communities for early detection and prompt intervention to control disease and minimize disability (e.g. through screening programmes).	Individuals with established disease; achieved through early diagnosis and treatment.
Tertiary	Late stage of disease (treatment, rehabilitation)	Reduce the number and/or impact of complications	Measures aimed at softening the impact of long-term disease and disability; minimizing suffering; maximizing potential years of useful life.	Patients; achieved through rehabilitation.

Source : *(58)*

Since health promotion comprises a broad spectrum of activities, a well-conceived health promotion programme would first attempt to identify the "target groups" or at-risk individuals in a population and then direct more appropriate message to them *(110)*. Goals must be defined. Means and alternative means of accomplishing them must be explored. It involves "organizational, political, social and economic interventions designed to facilitate environmental and behavioural adaptations that will improve or protect health" *(111)*.

2. Specific protection

To avoid disease altogether is the ideal but this is possible only in a limited number of cases. The following are some of the currently available interventions aimed at specific protection: (a) immunization (b) use of specific nutrients (c) chemoprophylaxis (d) protection against occupational hazards (e) protection against accidents (f) protection from carcinogens (g) avoidance of allergens (h) the control of specific hazards in the general environment, e.g. air pollution, noise control (i) control of consumer product quality and safety of foods, drugs, cosmetics, etc.

Health protection

The term "health protection" which is quite often used, is not synonymous with specific protection. Health protection is defined as "The provision of conditions for normal mental and physical functioning of the human being individually and in the group. It includes the promotion of health, the prevention of sickness and curative and restorative medicine in all its aspects" *(58)*. In fact, health protection is conceived as an integral part of an overall community development programme, associated with activities such as literacy campaigns, education and food production *(112)*. Thus health protection covers a much wider field of health activities than specific protection.

3. Early diagnosis and treatment

A WHO Expert Committee *(113)* defined early detection of health impairment as "the detection of disturbances of homoeostatic and compensatory mechanism while biochemical, morphological, and functional changes are still reversible." Thus, in order to prevent overt disease or disablement, the criteria of diagnosis should, if possible, be based on early biochemical, morphological and functional changes that precede the occurrence of manifest signs and symptoms. This is of particular importance in chronic diseases.

Early detection and treatment are the main interventions of disease control. The earlier a disease is diagnosed and treated the better it is from the point of view of prognosis and preventing the occurrence of further cases (secondary cases) or any long-term disability. It is like stamping out the "spark" rather than calling the fire brigade to put out the fire.

Strictly speaking, early diagnosis and treatment cannot be called prevention because the disease has already commenced in the host. However, since early diagnosis and treatment intercepts the disease process, it has been included in the schema of prevention, in as much as the goal of prevention is "to oppose or intercept a cause to prevent or dissipate its effect." *(89)*.

Early diagnosis and treatment though not as effective and economical as "primary prevention" may be critically important in reducing the high morbidity and mortality in certain diseases such as essential hypertension, cancer cervix and breast cancer. For many others such as tuberculosis, leprosy and STD, early diagnosis and treatment are the only effective mode of intervention. Early effective therapy has made it possible to shorten considerably the period of communicability and reduce the mortality from acute communicable diseases.

Mass treatment: A mass treatment approach is used in the control of certain diseases, viz. yaws, pinta, bejel, trachoma and filaria, The rationale for a mass treatment programme is the existence of at least 4–5 cases of latent infection for each clinical case of active disease in the community. Patients with a latent (incubating) infection may develop disease at any time. In such cases, mass treatment is a critical factor in the interruption of disease transmission. There are many variants of mass treatment – total mass treatment, juvenile mass treatment, selective mass treatment, depending upon the nature and prevalence of disease in the community *(103)*.

4. Disability limitation

When a patient reports late in the pathogenesis phase, the mode of intervention is disability limitation. The objective of this intervention is to prevent or halt the transition of the disease process from impairment to handicap.

Concept of disability

The sequence of events leading to disability and handicap have been stated as follows *(114)*:

Disease ⟶ impairment ⟶ disability ⟶ handicap

The WHO *(115)* has defined these terms as follows:

(i) **Impairment** : An impairment is defined as "any loss or abnormality of psychological, physiological or anatomical structure or function", e.g., loss of foot, defective vision or mental retardation. An impairment may be visible or invisible, temporary or permanent, progressive or regressive. Further, one impairment may lead to the development of "secondary" impairments as in the case of leprosy where damage to nerves (primary impairment) may lead to plantar ulcers (secondary impairment).

(ii) **Disability** : Because of an impairment, the affected person may be unable to carry out certain activities considered normal for his age, sex, etc. This inability to carry out certain activities is termed "disability". A disability has been defined as "any restriction or lack of ability to perform an activity in the manner or within the range considered normal for a human being".

(iii) **Handicap** : As a result of disability, the person experiences certain disadvantages in life and is not able to discharge the obligations required of him and play the role expected of him in the society. This is termed "handicap", and is defined as "a disadvantage for a given individual, resulting from an impairment or a disability, that limits or prevents the fulfilment of a role that is normal (depending on age, sex, and social and cultural factors) for that individual".

Taking accidents as an example, the above terms can be explained further as follows *(95)*:

Accident.............	Disease (or disorder)
Loss of foot	Impairment (extrinsic or intrinsic)
Cannot walk	Disability (objectified)
Unemployed	Handicap (socialized)

FIG. 11
Concept of disability

The intervention in disability will often be social or environmental as well as medical. While impairment which is the earliest stage has a large medical component, disability and handicap which are later stages have large social and environmental components in terms of dependence and social cost *(95)*.

Disability prevention

Another concept is "disability prevention". It relates to all the levels of prevention: (a) reducing the occurrence of impairment, viz. immunization against polio (primary prevention); (b) disability limitation by appropriate treatment (secondary prevention); and, (c) preventing the transition of disability into handicap (tertiary prevention) *(115)*.

The major causes of disabling impairments in the developing countries are communicable diseases, malnutrition, low quality of perinatal care and accidents. These are responsible for about 70 per cent of cases of disability in developing countries. Primary prevention is the most effective way of dealing with the disability problem in developing countries *(115)*.

5. Rehabilitation

Rehabilitation has been defined as "the combined and coordinated use of medical, social, educational and vocational measures for training and retraining the individual to the highest possible level of functional ability" *(116)*. It includes all measures aimed at reducing the impact of disabling and handicapping conditions and at enabling the disabled and handicapped to achieve social integration *(115)*. Social integration has been defined as the active participation of disabled and handicapped people in the mainstream of community life *(117)*.

It involves Rehabilitation medicine or Physical medicine or Physiatry has emerged in recent years as a medical speciality. It aims to enhance and restore functional ability and quality of life to those with physical impairments or disabilities. A physiatrist specializes in restoring optional function to people with injuries to the muscles, bones, ligaments or nervous system. Six formal sub-specialization are recognized are: neuromuscular medicine, pain medicine, paediatric rehabilitation medicine, spinal cord injury medicine, sports medicine and brain medicine. Paramedical and non-medical persons are involved in the discipline. They are physical medicine or physiotherapy, occupational therapy, speech therapy, audiology, psychology, education, social work, vocational guidance and placement services. The following areas of concern in rehabilitation have been identified:

(a) Medical rehabilitation – restoration of function.
(b) Vocational rehabilitation – restoration of the capacity to earn a livelihood.
(c) Social rehabilitation – restoration of family and social relationships.
(d) Psychological rehabilitation – restoration of personal dignity and confidence.

Rehabilitation is no longer looked upon as an extra-curricular activity of the physician. The current view is that the responsibility of the doctor does not end when the "temperature touches normal and stitches are removed". The patient must be restored and retrained "to live and work within the limits of his disability but to the hilt of his capacity". As such medical rehabilitation should start very early in the process of medical treatment.

Examples of rehabilitation are: establishing schools for the blind, provision of aids for the crippled, reconstructive surgery in leprosy, muscle re-education and graded exercises in neurological disorders, change of profession for a more suitable one and modification of life in general in the case of tuberculosis, cardiac patients and others. The purpose of rehabilitation is to make productive people out of non-productive people.

It is now recognized that rehabilitation is a difficult and demanding task that seldom gives totally satisfactory results; but needs enthusiastic cooperation from different segments of society as well as expertise, equipment and funds not readily available for this purpose even in affluent societies. It is further recognized that interventions at earlier stages are more feasible, will yield results, and are less demanding of scarce resources.

CHANGING PATTERN OF DISEASE

Although diseases have not changed significantly through human history, their patterns have. It is said that every decade produces its own pattern of disease. The truth of this will be obvious when one compares the leading causes of death globally for the year 2000 and 2019, as shown in Fig. 11 *(118)*.

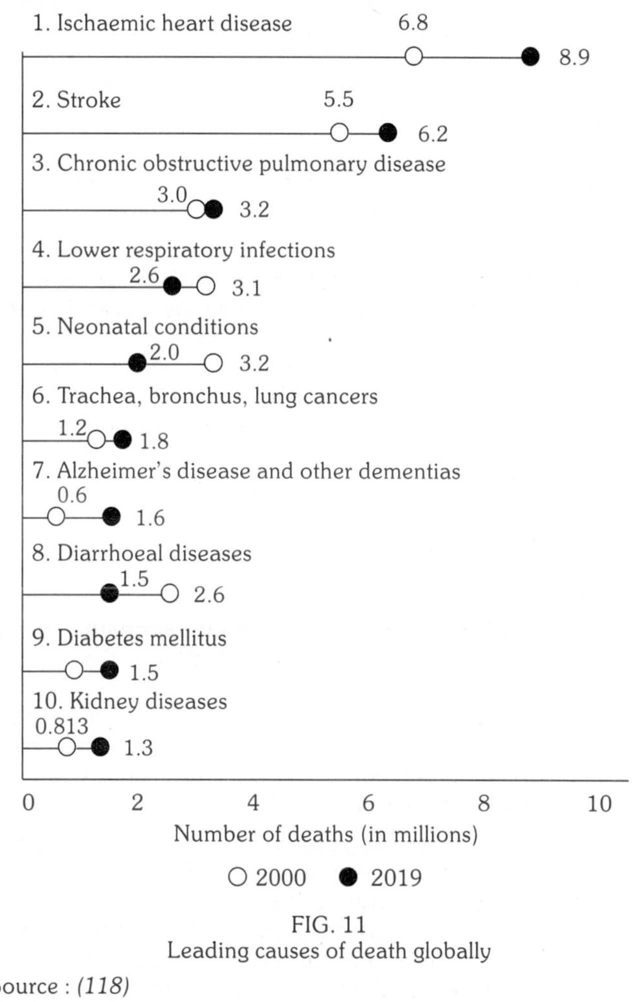

FIG. 11
Leading causes of death globally

Source : *(118)*

In the year 2019, the top 10 causes of death accounted for 55 per cent of the 55.4 million deaths worldwide. The top global causes of death, in order of total number of lives lost, are associated with three broad topics : cardiovascular (ischaemic heart disease, stroke), respiratory (chronic obstructive pulmonary disease, lower respiratory infections) and neonatal conditions, which include birth asphyxia and birth trauma, neonatal sepsis and infections, and preterm birth complications. In the year 2019, globally, 7 of the 10 leading causes of deaths were noncommunicable diseases. These seven causes accounted for 80 per cent of the top 10 deaths.

The world's biggest killer is ischaemic heart disease, responsible for 16.59 per cent of the total deaths. Since year 2000, the largest increase in deaths has been for this disease. Stroke and chronic obstructive pulmonary disease are the 2nd and 3rd leading causes of death responsible for approximately 10.16 and 5.34 per cent of total deaths respectively. Lower respiratory infection ranked as the 4th leading cause of death. However, the number of deaths has gone down substantially : in 2020 it claimed 2.55 million lives, 460,000 fewer than in year 2000 *(118)*.

Neonatal conditions are ranked 5th in the list. However, deaths from neonatal conditions are one of the categories for which the global decrease in deaths in absolute numbers over the past two decades has been the greatest : these conditions killed 2 million newborns and young children in 2019, 1.2 million fewer than in 2000 *(118)*.

Deaths from trachea, bronchus and lung cancers have risen from 1.2 million to 1.8 million and are now ranked 6th among the leading cause of death. In 2019, Alzheimer's disease and other forms of dementia ranked as 7th leading cause. Women are disproportionately affected. Globally, 65 per cent of deaths from Alzheimer's disease and dementia are in women *(118)*.

One of the largest decline in the number of deaths is from diarrhoeal diseases with global deaths falling from 2.6 million in year 2000 to 1.5 million in year 2019.

Diabetes has entered the top 10 causes list following a significant increase of 70 per cent since 2000. Diabetes is also responsible for the largest rise in male deaths among the top 10 diseases. Other diseases which were among the top 10 causes of death in 2000 are no longer on the list, HIV/AIDS is one of them. Deaths from HIV/AIDS have fallen by 51 per cent during the last 20 years, moving from the world's 8th leading cause of death in 2000 to the 19th position in the year 2019. Kidney diseases have risen from the world's 13th position to the 10th position in the list, mortality has increased from 813,000 in year 2000 to 1.3 million in year 2019 *(118)*. Tuberculosis is no longer in the global top 10, falling from 7th place in 2000 to 13th in 2019, with a 30 per cent reduction in global deaths. Yet, it remains among the top 10 causes of deaths in the African and South-East Asian regions, where it is the 8th and 5th leading cause respectively. The new estimates show that 6 of the top 10 causes of death in the low-income countries are still due to communicable diseases. This includes malaria (6th), tuberculosis (8th) and HIV/AIDS (9th position).

In 2019, people are living longer (73 years) than in 2000 (67 years). Likewise, disability is also on the rise. To a large extent, the diseases and health conditions that are causing the most deaths are those that are responsible for the greatest number of healthy life-years lost. Heart disease, diabetes, stroke, lung cancer and chronic obstructive pulmonary disease were collectively responsible for nearly 100 million additional healthy life-years lost in 2019 compared to 2000. Injuries are also major cause of disability and death. There has been significant rise in road traffic injuries in the African region since 2000, with an almost 50 per cent increase in both death and DALYs. Globally, 75 per cent deaths from road traffic injuries are male. The region of Americas is the only one for which drug use disorder is in top 10 contributors to life-years lost due to premature deaths and disability *(119)*.

Top 10 global causes of disability-adjusted life years (DALYs) in 2019 are as follows *(120)* :

1. Neonatal conditions
2. Ischaemic heart disease
3. Stroke
4. Lower respiratory infections
5. Diarrhoeal diseases
6. Road injury
7. Chronic obstructive pulmonary disease
8. Diabetes mellitus
9. Tuberculosis
10. Congenital anomalies

However, these data do not include COVID-19 as death statistics available actually releate to 2019. However, the WHO estimated COVID-19 to have caused more than 1.5 million deaths worldwide in 2020. This would have tied it with diarrhoeal diseases and diabetes, which were 8th on the list of top causes of deaths worldwide, assuming these figures stay more or less the same *(121)*.

INDIA

TABLE 11

Top 10 causes of death in rural & urban areas: 2015–2017

Rank	Cause of Death	Percentage Proportion of death		
		Male	Female	Person
	Rural Area			
1.	Cardiovascular diseases	27.0	24.0	25.8
2.	Respiratory diseases	7.2	8.0	7.5
3.	Malignant and other neoplasms	5.6	7.0	6.2
4.	Fever of unknown origin	4.4	6.4	5.2
5.	Digestive diseases	5.8	3.8	4.9
6.	Perinatal conditions	6.0	2.6	4.6
7.	Unintentional injuries : other than motor vehicle accidents	4.5	4.4	4.5
8.	Unintentional injuries : motor vehicle accidents	5.4	1.6	3.9
9.	Diarrhoeal diseases	2.8	4.1	3.3
10.	Ill-defined/All other symptoms, signs and abnormal clinical and laboratory findings	11.8	18.7	14.7
	All other remaining causes	19.4	19.3	19.4
	Urban Area			
1.	Cardiovascular diseases	33.7	28.3	31.5
2.	Malignant and other neoplasms	6.0	8.1	6.8
3.	Respiratory diseases	5.7	6.6	6.1
4.	Digestive diseases	6.7	4.1	5.6
5.	Fever of unknown origin	3.8	5.5	4.5
6.	Unintentional injuries : motor vehicle accidents	5.9	1.9	4.3
7.	Diabetes mellitus	3.7	4.1	3.8
8.	Perinatal conditions	4.6	1.9	3.5
9.	Unintentional injuries: other than motor vehicle accidents	3.4	3.6	3.5
10.	Ill-defined/All other symptoms, signs and abnormal clinical and laboratory findings	10.5	17.9	13.5
	All other remaining causes	16.2	18.2	17.0

Note : Symptoms, signs and abnormal clinical and laboratory findings not elsewhere classified (NEC) (R00-R99) was not properly diagnosed, so it may not be considered as second leading cause group.

Source : *(122)*

Table 11 shows the top causes of death in rural and urban area for period of year 2015–2017. The top 10 causes of deaths in the rural and urban areas are common except for deaths due to diarrhoeal diseases in rural area and diabetes mellitus in urban area. However, their relative order varies. Cardiovascular diseases which is leading cause of death both the areas accounts for 31.5 per cent of deaths in urban vis-a-vis 25.8 per cent in rural area. The difference in proportion of male deaths due to perinatal condition is higher than female deaths both in rural and urban areas. Higher proportion of deaths of female due to respiratory diseases and malignant & other neoplasm is noted *(122)*.

The factors which play a role in the changing patterns of disease are multiple. They include changing lifestyles and living standards, demographic factors, urbanization and industrialization, medical interventions, maintenance of people with transmissible genetic defects, and the widespread effects of technology on ecology.

The changing pattern of disease in both developed and developing countries and the emergence of new problems emphasize the need for forward-looking approaches in health planning and management.

POPULATION MEDICINE

Knowledge about human health and disease is sum of the contributions of a large number of disciplines, classified as (a) basic sciences (b) clinical sciences, and (c) population medicine. The basic sciences (e.g., biochemistry, physiology, microbiology) are primarily sited in laboratories; clinical activities are carried out in hospitals, and population medicine in the community. Tuberculosis provides a good illustration of the three different approaches to the same disease. The basic sciences are concerned with tubercle bacilli; the clinical sciences with the treatment of tuberculosis in the individual, and population medicine with prevention and control of tuberculosis in the community *(86)*. All these approaches are highly interrelated.

In different settings, **population medicine** is referred to as hygiene, public health, preventive medicine, social medicine or community medicine. All these share common ground in their concern for promotion of health and prevention of disease. Each has originated at a different time, and each has introduced a new direction or emphasis. So there should be little expectation that definitions can be other than arbitrary and imprecise *(123)*. It has been truly said that every definition is dangerous.

Hygiene

The world "hygiene" is derived from **Hygeia**, the goddess of health in Greek mythology. She is represented as a beautiful woman holding in her hand a bowl from which a serpent is drinking. In Greek mythology, the serpent testifies the art of healing which symbol is retained even today. Hygiene is defined as "the science of health and embraces all factors which contribute to healthful living".

Public health

The term "public health" came into general use around 1840. It arose from the need to protect "the public" from the spread of communicable diseases. Later, it appeared in 1848 in the name of a law, the Public Health Act in England to crystallize the efforts organized by society to protect, promote, and restore the people's health.

In 1920, C.E.A. Winslow, a former professor of public health at Yale University, gave the oft-quoted definition of public health. The WHO Expert Committee on Public Health Administration, adapting Winslow's earlier definition, has defined it as *(124)*:

> *"the science and art of preventing disease, prolonging life, and promoting health and efficiency through organized community efforts for the sanitation of the environment, the control of communicable infections, the education of the individual in personal hygiene, the organization of medical and nursing services for early diagnosis and preventive treatment of disease, and the development of social machinery to ensure for every individual a standard of living adequate for the maintenance of health, so organizing these benefits as to enable every citizen to realize his birthright of health and longevity".*

Whereas in developing countries, public health has not made much headway in terms of sanitary reforms and control of communicable diseases, it has made tremendous strides in the industrialized western countries resulting in longer expectation of life and significant decline in death rates. As a result of improvements in public health during the past 50 or 60 years, public health in the developed countries has moved from sanitation and control of communicable diseases (which have been largely controlled) to preventive, therapeutic and rehabilitative aspects of chronic diseases and behavioural disorders.

A EURO symposium in 1966 *(56)* suggested that the definition of public health should be expanded to include the organization of medical care services. This was endorsed by another Expert Committee of WHO in 1973 *(125)*. Thus modern public health also includes organization of medical care, as a means of protecting and improving the health of people *(126)*. Since the organization of public health tends to be determined by cultural, political and administrative patterns of the countries, there is a wide mosaic of organizational arrangements.

Public health, in its present form, is a combination of scientific disciplines (e.g., epidemiology, biostatistics, laboratory sciences, social sciences, demography) and skills and strategies (e.g., epidemiological investigations, planning and management, interventions, surveillance, evaluation) that are directed to the maintenance and improvement of the health of the people *(126)*.

With the adoption of the goal of "Health for All", a new public health was evident worldwide, which may be defined as:

> *"the organized application of local, state, national and international resources to achieve "Health for All", i.e., attainment by all people of the world by the year 2000 of a level of health that will permit them to lead a socially and economically productive life".*

Although the term "public health" has lost its original meaning, the term is still widely used. Terms like preventive medicine, social medicine and community medicine are used as synonyms for public health. Public health is not only a discipline but has become a "social institution" *(33)* created and maintained by society to do something about the death rate and sanitary conditions and many other matters relating to life and death *(127)*. In this sense public health is both a body of knowledge and also a means to apply that knowledge.

Preventive medicine

Preventive medicine developed as a branch of medicine distinct from public health, based on aetiology. It is, by definition, applied to "healthy" people. It scored several successes in the prevention of communicable diseases based on immunization, so much so, in its early years, preventive medicine was equated with the control of infectious diseases. A brief account of the advances made in preventive medicine is given in chapter 1.

As concepts of the aetiology of disease changed through time, so too have the techniques and activities of preventive medicine. Preventive medicine is no longer concerned, as it used to be, with immunization, important though it may be. The concept of preventive medicine has broadened to include health promotion, treatment, and prevention of disability as well as specific protection *(90)*. Preventive medicine has thus come to include both specific medical measures (e.g., immunization), as well as general health promotional measures (e.g., health education). Within this change in the definition and scope of preventive medicine, it has become clear that promoting health and preventing illness involve responsibilities and decisions at many levels – individual, public and private; and that these efforts are applied to whole population or to segments. In this, preventive medicine has become akin to public health.

Preventive medicine has become a growing point in medicine *(128)*. It has branched into newer areas such as screening for disease, population control, environmental control, genetic counselling and prevention of chronic diseases. Community prevention and primordial prevention (see page 47) are relatively new concepts which are being applied in the community control of coronary heart disease, hypertension and cancer with palpable success *(106)*. The emergence of preventive paediatrics, preventive geriatrics and preventive cardiology are relatively new dimensions of prevention.

Since preventive medicine has increasingly tended to be applied to the organized health activities of the community *(56)*, the term "preventive medicine" is regarded as synonymous with public health. Both terms often appear in combination (e.g., Maxcy–Rosenau Textbook of "Public Health and Preventive Medicine").

Associated with the concept of public health, preventive medicine has been defined as meaning "not only the organized activities of the community to prevent occurrence as well as progression of disease and disability, mental and physical, but also the timely application of all means to promote the health of individuals, and of the community as a whole, including prophylaxis, health education and similar work done by a good doctor in looking after individuals and families" *(56)*. In this the goals of preventive medicine and public health have become identical, i.e., Health for All. In line with this extension of the scope of preventive medicine, it is now customary to speak of primary, secondary and tertiary levels of prevention *(56)*. The cornerstone of preventive medicine is, however, "primary prevention".

Community health

The term "community health" has replaced in some countries, the terms public health, preventive medicine and social medicine. A EURO symposium in 1966 *(56)* defined community health as including "all the personal health and environmental services in any human community, irrespective of whether such services were public or private ones". In some instances, community health is used as a synonym for "environmental health". It is also used to refer to "community health care". Therefore, a WHO Expert Committee in 1973 *(125)* observed that without further qualification, the term "community health" is ambiguous, and suggested caution in the use of the term.

Social medicine

The term "social medicine" was first introduced by Jules Guerin, a French physician in 1848. In 1911, the concept of social medicine was revived by Alfred Grotjahn of Berlin who stressed the importance of social factors as determinants of health and disease. These ideas of social medicine spread throughout Europe and England after the First World War (see page 8).

By derivation, social medicine is "the study of man as a social being in his total environment". It is concerned with all the factors affecting the distribution of health and illhealth in population, including the use of health services *(129)*. Social medicine is not a new branch of medicine, but rather an extension of the public health idea reflecting the strong relationship between medicine and social sciences.

Professor Crew of Edinburgh defined social medicine as follows: "Social medicine stands upon two pillars, medicine and sociology. Social medicine, by derivation is concerned with the health of groups of individuals and individuals within these groups with a view to create, promote, preserve, and maintain optimum health. The laboratory to practice social medicine is the whole community; the tools for diagnosing community ills are epidemiology and biostatistics; and social therapy does not consist in administration of drugs, but social and political action for the betterment of conditions of life of man. Social medicine is one more link in the chain of social organizations of a civilized community". Terms such as social anatomy, social physiology, social pathology and social therapy came into vogue to describe the various aspects of social medicine.

Although the term "social medicine" was introduced more than 150 years ago, the characteristic aspect was its repeated advent and disappearance. It never came to be generally accepted. There was no unanimity in its objectives or subject matter. This is reflected in more than 50 definitions given to social medicine.

Social medicine had achieved academic respectability in England when John Ryle was appointed as professor of social medicine at Oxford, and Crew at Edinburgh. The post–war period (1945–1967) saw considerable expansion of social medicine as an academic discipline *(129)*.

With the development of epidemiology as a new discipline and a practical tool in the planning, provision and evaluation of health services, interest in social medicine began to wane. In 1968, the Report of the Royal Commission on Medical Education (Todd Report) for the first time referred to "community medicine" instead of social medicine, and defined it in terms which embraced social medicine, but went beyond it, by giving greater emphasis to the organizational and administrative aspects than had academic social medicine in the past *(129)*. This gave a blow to the further development of social medicine which had tended in many countries to be displaced by the newer term "community medicine" *(56)*.

Community medicine

The term "community medicine" is a newcomer. It is the successor of what has been previously known as public health, preventive medicine, social medicine and community health. Since community medicine is a recent introduction, it has borrowed heavily from the concepts, approaches and methods of public health, preventive medicine and social medicine.

The history of community medicine in England is

interesting. It was instituted by Ordinance and by Act of Parliament *(130)*. The Todd Commission (1968) forcibly recommended that every medical school in England should have a department of community medicine. The Royal College of Physicians of Edinburgh and London and the Royal College of Physicians and Surgeons of Glasgow established the Faculty of community medicine, which came into being in March 1972 as the central body with a responsibility of setting standards and overseeing the quality of postgraduate education and training in the field *(131)*. On the night of 31st March 1974, the traditional medical officer of health passed into the pages of the history book, and was thereafter designated as the "community physician".

The term community medicine means different things in different countries *(56)*. For example, in most European countries various aspects of community medicine are taught at medical universities, though under different names, such as general practice, family medicine, community medicine or social medicine *(132)*. Even in the same country and region, the variation in the amount and range of teaching remains remarkable *(131)*. These variations are reflected in the definitions quoted below *(56)*.

(a) The field concerned with the study of health and disease in the population of a defined community or group. Its goal is to identify the health problems and needs of defined population (community diagnosis) and to plan, implement and evaluate the extent to which health measures effectively meet these needs.

(b) The practice of medicine concerned with groups or population rather than with individual patients. This includes the elements listed in definition (a), together with the organization and provision of health care at a community or group level.

(c) The term is also used to describe the practice of medicine in the community, e.g., by a family physician. Some writers equate the terms "family medicine" and "community medicine"; others confine its use to public health practice.

(d) Community oriented primary health care is an integration of community medicine with the primary health care of individuals in the community. In this form of practice, the community practitioner or community health team has responsibility for health care at a community or at an individual level.

It will be seen that a common thread runs through all the above definitions. Diagnosis of the state of health of a community is an important foundation of community medicine. As used in the present context, community medicine is a practice which focuses on the health needs of the community as a whole. The combination of community medicine with "primary health care" extends the functioning of both elements to a health care system which aims to change the state of health of the community by intervention both at the individual and group level. The foundations of community medicine are in no way different from those of modern public health and social medicine, viz. epidemiology, biostatistics, social sciences and organization of health care which includes planning, implementation and evaluation *(133)*.

It is anomalous that in England and United States where the term community medicine is freely used, their standard textbooks on the subject are still titled **Public Health** (e.g., Oxford "Textbook of Public Health;" Maxcy-Rosenau: "Public Health and Preventive Medicine").

HOSPITALS AND COMMUNITY

The hospital is a unique institution of man. A WHO Expert Committee in 1963 *(134)* proposed the following working definition of a hospital: "A hospital is a residential establishment which provides short-term and long-term medical care consisting of observational, diagnostic, therapeutic and rehabilitative services for persons suffering or suspected to be suffering from a disease or injury and for parturients. It may or may not also provide services for ambulatory patients on an out-patient basis".

The criticism levelled against the hospital is that it exists in splendid isolation in the community, acquiring the euphemism "an ivory tower of disease"; it absorbs vast proportion (50 to 80 per cent) of health budget; it is not people-oriented; its procedures and styles are inflexible; it overlooks the cultural aspects of illness (treating the disease without treating the patient); the treatment is expensive; it is intrinsically resistant to change, and so on. The relative isolation of hospitals from the broader health problems of the community which has its roots in the historical development of health services has contributed to the dominance of hospital model of health care.

In 1957, an Expert Committee of WHO *(135)* emphasized that the general hospital cannot work in isolation; it must be a part of a social and medical system that provides complete health care for the population. Subsequent years witnessed the efforts of WHO, UNICEF and non-governmental agencies to involve hospitals in providing basic and referral services. The establishment of primary health centres was a step forward to integrate preventive and curative services.

The community hospital should be a flexible institution, capable of adapting its resources to the total health care needs of the community. This adaptation requires hospital administration that is both a science and art. Dr. Rene Sand has said that the right patient should receive the right care at the right time in the right place at the right cost *(136)*. This ideal, seemingly simple, is perhaps never achieved, like all other ideals because of a complex set of interacting and often conflicting social forces operating both within and outside the hospital system.

With the acceptance of the goal of "Health for All", there is involvement of hospitals in primary health care activities. Member countries of WHO have enunciated in their national policies to reorient and restructure their health care systems on the basis of primary health care. Primary health care cannot work unless there is effective hospital support to deal with referred patients, and to refer patients who do not require hospital attention to one of the other primary health care services. Without hospital support primary health care could not achieve its full potential. The trend is now set to redefine the role of the hospital as a community health oriented institution, which means that it is not only disease oriented but has responsibilities in the field of preventive medicine and health promotion *(137)*.

Functions of a physician

The object of medical education is to prepare a doctor (physician) for the tasks he is likely to be given. In view of the fact that there is no internationally accepted definition of the word "physician", the WHO has adopted the following definition *(138)*.

"A physician is a person who, having been regularly admitted to a medical school, duly recognized in the

country in which it is located, has successfully completed the prescribed courses of studies in medicine and has acquired the requisite qualification to be legally licensed to practise medicine (comprising prevention, diagnosis, treatment and rehabilitation) using independent judgement to promote community and individual health".

In India, at present, a doctor soon after graduation, has often to take charge of a health centre (population 30,000) which is usually in a rural area. He is called upon to provide promotive, preventive, curative, rehabilitative and emergency care services appropriate to meet the main health problems in the community, with special attention to vulnerable groups. The functions of the health centre are discussed elsewhere. The functions of a doctor (physician) may be summarized as follows:

(a) *The care of the individual*: A physician must be able to assess the state of health of the individual. This would include a clinical diagnosis, a simple laboratory diagnosis as well as an assessment of the individual's state of nutrition, level of development, social and emotional state and the health needs. He must then be able to take any further measures necessary for treatment, prevention and referral to higher levels of health care. He must be particularly expert in common conditions, in first-aid and in the management of acute emergencies. Because of the large numbers involved, he must know how to delegate work to his auxiliaries.

(b) *The care of community*: The care of the community centres round the eight essential elements of primary health care as stated in the Alma-Ata Declaration (see page 37). The physician is the leader of the "health team". He provides primary health care through the health team at the grass-root level. He should be familiar with community diagnosis, prioritization of health problems and community treatment.

(c) *The physician as a teacher*: The term "doctor" by derivation means to teach. Therefore the physician has a major responsibility as a teacher and educator. In his practice, in his professional associations and in his community activities, the physician has wide educational opportunities. But unfortunately, the physician's role as a teacher is a neglected one. Many physicians are reluctant to capitalize on their role as educators. As a teacher, the physician can play an effective role in community health education so that individuals, families and communities assume greater responsibility for their own health and welfare, including self-care. He can also generate and mobilize community participation in health programmes through effective propagation of relevant information.

Community diagnosis

The diagnosis of disease in an individual patient is a fundamental idea in medicine. It is based on signs and symptoms and the making of inferences from them. When this is applied to a community, it is known as community diagnosis. The community diagnosis may be defined as the pattern of disease in a community described in terms of the important factors which influence this pattern *(139)*.

The community diagnosis is based on collection and interpretation of the relevant data such as (a) the age and sex distribution of a population; the distribution of population by social groups; (b) vital statistical rates such as the birth rate, and the death rate; (c) the incidence and prevalence of the important diseases of the area. In addition, a doctor must be able to find information on a wide variety of social and economic factors that may assist him in making a community diagnosis. The focus is on the identification of the basic health needs and health problems of the community. The needs **as felt** by the community (some of which may have no connection at all with health) should be next investigated and listed according to priority for community treatment.

Community treatment

Community treatment or community health action is the sum of steps decided upon to meet the health needs of the community taking into account the resources available and the wishes of the people, as revealed by community diagnosis. Improvement of water supplies, immunization, health education, control of specific diseases, health legislation are examples of community health action or interventions. Action may be taken at three levels: at the level of the individual, at the level of the family and at the level of the community *(139)*.

A programme of community action must have the following characteristics: (a) it must effectively utilize all the available resources, (b) it must coordinate the efforts of all other agencies in the community, now termed as "intersectoral coordination", and (c) it must encourage the full participation of the community in the programme. These are the principles on which primary health care, as defined in the Alma-Ata Declaration, is based. This approach is a significant departure from the earlier basic services approach.

DISEASE CLASSIFICATION

There is a wide variation among countries in the criteria and standards adopted for diagnosis of diseases and their notification, making it difficult to compare national statistics. A system of classification was needed whereby diseases could be grouped according to certain common characteristics, that would facilitate the statistical study of disease phenomena. Over the years, many approaches were tried to classify diseases. John Graunt in the 17th century in his study of Bills of Mortality, arranged diseases in an alphabetical order. Later, a more scientific approach was adopted in classifying diseases according to certain characteristics of the disease or injuries such as (a) the part of the body affected (b) the aetiologic agent (c) the kind of morbid change produced by the disease, and (d) the kind of disturbance of function produced by the disease or injury. Thus there are many axes of classification, and the particular axis selected will depend on the interest of the investigator *(140)*.

International classification of diseases

All the above criteria formed the basis of the International classification of diseases (ICD) produced by WHO and accepted in the year 1940 for national and international use. Since its inception, ICD has been revised about once every 10 years; the 10th revision, came into effect on January 1, 1993. Earlier, the scope of ICD was expanded in the sixth revision in 1948 to cover morbidity from illness and injury. The ICD also provides a basis that can be adapted for use in other fields.

ICD is the foundation for the identification of health trends and statistics globally and is the international standard for reporting diseases and health conditions. It is a diagnostic classification standard for all clinical and research purposes. ICD defines the universe of diseases, disorders, injuries and other related health conditions, listed in a comprehensive, hierarchical fashion that allows for : easy storage, retrieval and analysis of health information for evidence-based decision-making; sharing and comparing health information between hospitals, regions, settings and countries; and data comparison in the same location across different time period.

ICD-11 *(141)*

The ICD-11 has been updated for the 21st century to reflect the significant progress in science and medicine over the past 30 years and has been designed for the use with digital health applications and application systems. The digital platform for ICD-11 can be accessed online or downloaded remotely free of charge and in multiple languages via the online browser. It comprises over 55,000 entities.

Besides diseases, ICD includes disorders, injuries, external causes, signs and symptoms, substances, medicaments, anatomy, devices, histopathology, severity and much more and 120,000 clinical terms (and can code millions of terms), with thousands of new categories and updated classification schemes, and is intended to supersede the 10th Revision, which was more than 28 years old and clinically outdated.

New to ICD-11 is a chapter on sexual health, which brings together several conditions that were previously classified differently. Gender incongruence is included in this new chapter, reflecting an understanding that it is not a mental health condition. Re-classification should help to reduce the stigma attached to gender-defined states. Another new chapter focuses on traditional medicine, commonly used across many countries. In a landmark decision, stroke is now listed as a neurological disorder and not as a disorder of the circulatory system. This important change was long overdue and it brings stroke out of the shadow of heart disease.

The new classification of HIV recognizes advances in HIV therapy, which should be seen as a chronic condition. Allergy is coded under diseases of the immune system. Attention deficit hyperactivity disorder's updated description states that the symptoms no longer have to occur within fixed age range to lead to diagnosis. The updates also enable better reporting of antimicrobial resistance, with codes that are more in line with the Global Antimicrobial Resistance Surveillance System.

In this iteration of the ICD, special attention has been dedicated to mental health. Simpler diagnostic descriptions will make mental health diagnosis more accessible to health-care professionals globally. For instance, the ICD-11 list of post-traumatic stress disorder criteria have been reduced to facilitate easier diagnosis and improve access to treatment. Addictive conditions, such as gaming and hoarding disorders, have been added. Compulsive sexual behaviour was included as an impulse control disorder.

The International Classification of Diseases 11th Revision has been adopted by the World Health Assembly in 2019 and it will come into effect from 1st January 2022.

The ICD-11 contains following chapters :

1. Certain infectious and parasitic diseases.
2. Neoplasms.
3. Diseases of blood and blood forming organs.
4. Disorders of the immune system.
5. Endocrine, nutritional and metabolic diseases.
6. Mental, behavioural or neurodevelopmental disorders.
7. Sleep-wake disorders.
8. Disease of the visual system.
9. Diseases of the nervous system.
10. Diseases of the ear and mastoid process.
11. Diseases of the circulatory system.
12. Diseases of the respiratory system.
13. Diseases of the digestive system.
14. Diseases of the skin.
15. Diseases of the musculoskeletal system and connective tissue.
16. Diseases of the genitourinary system.
17. Conditions related to sexual health.
18. Pregnancy, childbirth and the puerperium.
19. Certain conditions originating in the perinatal and neonatal period.
20. Developmental anomalies.
21. Symptoms, signs or clinical findings, not elsewhere classified.
22. Injury, poisoning or certain other consequences of external causes.
23. External causes of morbidity and mortality.
24. Factors influencing health status or contact with health services.
25. Codes for special purposes.
26. Supplementary chapter, Traditional Medicine Conditions – Module I.

V. Supplementary section for functioning assessment.

X. Extension codes.

Linkages with other classifications and terminologies *(139)*

The ICD-11 incorporates on links with the following classifications and terminologies through the ICD-11 foundation :

a. International Classification of Disease for Oncology – ICD-O
b. International Classification of External Causes of Injury – ICECI
c. International Classification of Functioning, Disability and Health – ICF
d. International Classification of Primary Care – ICPC
e. Other terminologies such as OrphaNet and SNOMED-CT

The International Classification of Functioning, Disability and Health (ICF) *(142)*

The ICF is a framework for organizing and documenting information on functioning and disability (WHO 2001). It conceptualizes functioning as a "dynamic interaction between a person's health condition, environmental factors and personal factors".

ICF provides a standard language and conceptual basis for the definition and measurement of disability, and it provides classification and codes. It integrates the major models of disability – the medical model and the social model – as a bio-psycho-social synthesis. It recognizes the role of environmental factors in the creation of disability, as well as the health conditions.

Functioning and disability are understood as umbrella terms denoting the positive and negative aspects of functioning from a biological, individual and social perspective. ICF, therefore provides definitions and categories in neutral language, wherever possible. ICF is aetiology – neutral, i.e., disability is not differentiated by aetiology. The ICF covers the entire life span. ICF organizes information in two parts. Part 1 deals with functioning and disability while part 2 covers contextual factors. Each part has two components :

a. Functioning and disability :
   - Body function and body structures.
   - Activities and participation.
b. Contextual factors :
   - Environment factors
   - Personal factors

ICF can be used to structure a holistic approach to management of any patient with any health condition, ensuring person – centred care. As ICF does not belong to any single discipline, it is ideal tool to link and integrate information to different health professionals. This can result in better patient experience; a bio-psycho-social-spiritual approach to patient care; improved health outcomes; the strengthening of health systems; improved inter-professional education, collaboration and practice, task sharing and task shifting.

References

1. WHO (1979). *Health for All*, Sr.No.2.
2. WHO (1980). *WHO Chr.*, 34 (2) 80.
3. Ahmed, and Coelho, (1979). *Toward a New Definition of Health*, Pleum, N. Y.
4. Dubos, R. (1965). *Man Adapting*, New Haven, Yale Uni.Press.
5. WHO (1986). *Concepts of Health Behaviour Research*, Reg. Health Paper No.13, SEARO, New Delhi.
6. WHO (1978). *Health for All*, Sr.No.1.
7. WHO (1957). *Techn.Rep.Ser.*,No.137.
8. Crew, F.A.E. (1965). *Health its Nature and Conservation*, Pergamon Press, London.
9. Sartorius, N. (1983). *Bull WHO*, 61 (1) 5.
10. Fillenbaum, G.G. (1984) *The Wellbeing of the Elderly*, WHO Offset Publ.No.84.
11. Cmich, D.E. (1984) *Jr.School Health*, 54 (1) 30–32.
12. Donald, C.A. et al (1978). *Social Health. In : Conceptualization and measurement of health for adults in the health insurance study*, Santa Monica, CA, Rand Corporation, Vol 4.
13. Eberst, R.M. (1984). *Jr.School Health*, 54 (3) 99–104.
14. WHO (1985). *Techn.Rep.Ser.*,No.714.
15. Indian Council of Social Science Research and ICMR (1981). *Health for All*, an alternative strategy, Voluntary Health Asso. of India, New Delhi.
16. Twaddle, A.C. and Hassler, R.M. (1977). *A Sociology of Health*, St. Louis, Mosby.
17. Charles, Sir John (1970). *WHO Chr.*, 24 (9) 391.
18. Dubos, R. (1969). *WHO Chro.*, 23:499.
19. Carlos, M. (1978). *Bull PAHO*, 12:7.
20. Nagpal, R. and Sell, H. (1985). *Subjective Wellbeing*, Reg. Health Papers No.7, SEARO, WHO New Delhi.
21. WHO (1975). *Promoting Health in the Human Environment*, Geneva.
22. United Nations (1961). *International Definition and Measurement of Levels of Living*–an interim guide, UN Publ. 61, IV F.
23. WHO (1976). *WHO Chr*, 30 (8) 312.
24. WHO (2004), *A Glossary of Terms for Community Health Care and Services for Older Persons, Vol. 5*. Ageing and Health Technical Report.
25. Morris, D.M. and Michelle, B.M. (1982). *Measuring the condition of India's poor–PQLI*, Promilla & Co., New Delhi–1.
26. UNDP, *Human Development Report* 2015, Oxford University Press.
27. India Study Channel (2011), *Difference between old and new calculation methods of HDI*.
28. UNDP (2011), *Human Development Report* 2011, Oxford University Press.
29. UNDP (2020), *Human Development Report 2020*.
30. WHO (1998), *International Digest of Health Legislation*, Vol. 49, No. 1, 1998.
31. WHO (1986). *Techn.Rep.Ser.*,No.731.
32. Wingard, D.L. (1982). *Am.J.Epid*, 116 (5) 765.
33. Last, J.M. (1983). *A Dictionary of Epidemiology*, Oxford University Press.
34. Govt. of India (2021), *National Family Health Survey (NFHS-5), 2019–20*, Ministry of Health and Family Welfare, New Delhi.
35. Banerji, (1985). *Health & Family Planning Services in India*, Lok Paksh, N. D.
36. UNICEF (2018), *The State of World's Children 2018*.
37. WHO (1986). *WHO Chr.*, 32 (7) 295.
38. WHO (1978). *WHO Chr.*, 32 (9) 356.
39. Noble, John, (1976). *Primary Care & Practice of Med.*, Little Brown, Boston.
40. Miquel Porta, *A Dictionary of Epidemiology*, Sixth Edition, Oxford University Press.
41. Editorial (1982). *Canad. J. Pub. Hlth*, 73 (3) 153.
42. Susser, M.W. (1973). *Causal thinking in the health sciences*, Ox.U.P.
43. Circle of Rights, Economic, Social and Cultural Rights Activisms : A Training Resource, *Module 14, The Right to Health*.
44. WHO, *Fact Sheet No. 31*, The Right to Health.
45. WHO (2007), *Joint - Fact Sheet WHO/OHCHR/323*.
46. Levin, L.S. and E.L. Idler (1983). *Ann.Rev.Pub.Health*, 4: 181–201.
47. Djukanovic, V. and Mach, E.P. (1975). *Alternative approaches to meeting basic health needs in developing countries*, A Joint UNICEF/ WHO Study.
48. WHO (1987). *Techn.Rep.Ser.*, No.744.
49. WHO (1986). *Seventh Report World Health Situation*, Vol.4 Evaluation of the strategy for health for all, WHO, SEARO.
50. WHO (1984). *Strengthening Ministries of Health for Primary Health Care*, WHO Offset Publ.No.82.
51. Sigerist, H.E. (1941). *Medicine and Human Welfare*, New Haven, Yale University Press.
52. WHO (1984). *Intersectoral Linkages and Health Development*, WHO Offset Publ.No.83.
53. WHO (1984). *Health for All*, Ser.No.9.
54. WHO (1984). *Health Planning and Management Glossary. Reg.Health Paper 2*, SEARO, New Delhi.
55. WHO (1981). *Health for All*, Sr.No.6.
56. Hogarth, J. (1978). *Glossary for Health Care Terminology*, Public Health in Europe–4.
57. WHO (1981). *Health for All*, Sr.No.4.
58. WHO (2006). *Basic Epidemiology*, Second Ed., R. Bonita, R. Beaglehole, T. Kjellstrom.
59. Ray M. Merrill, Thomas C. Timmreck, *Introduction to Epidemiology*, 4th Ed., Jones and Bartlett Publishers.
60. WHO (1976). *Techn. Rep.Ser.*, No.587.
61. Wilson, R.W. and T.F. Drury (1984). *Ann Rev. Pub.Health*. 5:83–106.
62. Last, John M., *A Dictionary of Epidemiology*, Fourth Ed. (2001), Ox.U.P.
63. UN Dept. of Economic and Social Affairs (1978). *Social Indicators*, Statistical Paper Series M.No.63.
64. Sheehan, and Hopkins, (1979). *Basic needs performance*, ILO, Geneva.
65. WHO (2003), *World Health Report 2003*, Shaping the future.
66. WHO (2015), *Health in 2015, from MDGs (Millennium Development Goals) to SDGs (Sustainable Development Goals)*.
67. WHO (2018), *Global Reference List of 100 Core Health Indicators, 2018*.
68. Govt. of India (2019), *Healthy States, Progressive India*, Report of the Niti Aayog on the Ranks of States and Union Territories.
69. UNFPA (2017), *State of World's Population 2017*, Worlds Apart, Reproductive health and rights in an age of inequality.
70. Population Reference Bureau (2015), *The Urban-Rural Divide in Health and Development*.
71. Lee P.R. and P.E. Franks (1977). *Preventive Medicine*, 6, 209: 226.

72. WHO (1980). *Information systems for health services,* Public Health in Europe–13, Regional Office for Europe.
73. WHO (1987). *Techn.Rep.Ser.*,No.746.
74. Kohn,R. (1983). *The health centre concept in primary health care,* Public health in Europe-22, Regional Office for Europe.
75. WHO (1986). *Health promotion, Ottawa Charter,* First International Conference, 21st Nov. 1986.
76. WHO (1981). *Health for All,* Sr.No.5.
77. WHO (1980). *Sixth Report* , World Health Situation.
78. WHO (1983). *The concept of Health Services Research,* SEARO Techn.Publ.1, New Delhi.
79. Grundy, F.and W.A. Reinke (1973). *Health Practice Research and Formalized Management Methods,* WHO, Geneva.
80. WHO (1979). *WHO Chr.,* 33 (2) 49.
81. Gregg Alan (1956). *Amer. J. Public Health,* 46: 1384.
82. Suchman, E.A. (1963). *Sociology and the field of Public Health,* Russel Sage Foundation, New York.
83. Ouslander, J.G. and J.C. Beck (1982). *Ann.Rev.Public Health,* 3:58.
84. Susser, M.W. and Waston, W. (1971). *Sociology in Medicine,* 2nd ed. London, Oxford University Press.
85. Le Riche, W.H. and Jean Milner (1971). *Epidemiology as Medical Ecology,* Churchill Livingstone, Edinburgh.
86. Mausner, J.S. and Kramer, S. (1985). *Mausner and Bahn: Epidemiology*–An Introductory Text, Saunders.
87. MacMahon, B.and Pugh, T.F. (1970). *Epidemiology: Principles and Methods,* Boston: Little, Brown.
88. Stallones, R.A. (1971). *Environmental Ecology and Epidemiology,* PAHO Scientific Publ. No. 231.
89. Leavell, H.R. and Clark, E.G. (1965). *Preventive Medicine for the Doctor in his Community,* McGraw Hill, New York.
90. Suchman, E.A. (1970). *Arch.Env. Health,* 20:105.
91. WHO (1980). *WHO Chr.,* 34 (5) 189.
92. WHO (1979). *Techn.Rep.Ser.*,No.636.
93. Backett, E.M. et al (1984). *The risk approach to health care,* Public health papers No.76.
94. Fielding, J.E. (1984). *Ann.Rev.Public Health,* 5:239.
95. WHO (1984). *Techn.Rep.Ser.,* No.706.
96. WHO (1977). *WHO Chr.,* 31:150.
97. WHO (1976). *Tech.Rep.Ser.*No.593.
98. Lilienfeld, A.M. and Lilienfeld, D. (1979). *Foundations of Epidemiology,* New York, Oxford University Press.
99. Stuart–Harris, Charles (1981). *World Health Forum,* 2 (2) 305.
100. Soper, F.L. (1962). *Am.J.Public Health,* 52:724–745.
101. WHO (1972). *Health Hazards of the Human Environment,* WHO Geneva.
102. John M. Last (2001), *A Dictionary of Epidemiology,* 4th Ed.
103. WHO (1986). *Techn.Rep.Ser.*,No.736.
104. WHO (1979). *WHO Chr.*,33 (2) 50.
105. WHO (1982). *Techn.Rep.Ser.*,No.678.
106. WHO (1986). *Techn. Rep.Ser.,* No.732.
107. Dept, of Health and Social Security (1976). *Prevention and Health Everybody's Business,* London, HMSO.
108. Suchman, L.M. (1970). *Public Health Reports,* 85:1.
109. WHO (1987). *World Health,* May 1987.
110. Lauzon, R.R. J. (1977). *Canad. J.Pub.Health,* 68:311.
111. WHO (1984). *Techn.Rep.Ser.*,No.713.
112. WHO (1976). *WHO Chr.*,30 (1) 16.
113. WHO (1973). *Tech.Rep.Ser.,* No.535.
114. WHO (1980). *International classification of impairments*, disabilities, handicaps. WHO, Geneva.
115. WHO (1981). *Techn.Rep.Ser.,* No.668.
116. WHO (1969). *Techn.Rep.Ser.,* No.419.
117. WHO (1984). *World Health,* May 1984.
118. WHO (2020). *The top 10 causes of death,* 9th Dec. 2020.
119. WHO (2020). *WHO reveals leading causes of death and disability world-wide 2000–2019,* 9th Dec. 2020.
120. WHO (2020). *Global Health Observatory, Global health estimates life expectancy and leading causes of death and disability,* 2020.
121. WHO (2020). *World's leading causes of death statistics,* 11th Dec. 2020.
122. Govt. of India (2022), *Causes of death statistics 2015–17,* Office of the Registrar General and Census Commissioner, India, New Delhi, Ministry of Home Affairs, March 2022.
123. Clark, Duncan and B. MacMohan (1981). *Preventive and Community Medicine,* 2nd ed., Boston: Little, Brown & Co.
124. WHO (1952). *Techn.Rep.Ser.,* No.55.
125. WHO (1973). *Techn.Rep.Ser.,* No.533.
126. Roger Detels and Lester Breslow (1984). In: *Oxford Textbook of Public Health.* Vol *1. W.W. Holland,* et al (eds) Oxford University Press.
127. Brockington, F. (1958). *World Health,* A pelican book.
128. Norton, Alan (1969). *The New Dimensions of Medicine,* 20th century studies, Hodder and Stoughton, London.
129. Chave, S.P.W. (1984). In: *Oxford Textbook of Public Health,* Vol 1, Oxford University Press.
130. Stewart, G.T. (1974). *Int.J.Epid,* 3 (3) 275.
131. Warren, M.D. and Roy M.Acheson (1973). *Int.J.Epi.,* 2 (4) 371–378.
132. WHO (1985). *Primary prevention coronary heart disease,* EURO Reports and Studies 98.
133. Kark, S.L. et al (1973). *Int J. Epid,* 2 (4) 419.
134. WHO (1963) *Techn.Rep.Ser.*,No. 261.
135. WHO (1957). *Techn.Rep.Ser.,* No. 122.
136. Rene Sand (1952). *The Advance to Social Medicine,* Lon. Staples Press.
137. WHO (1987). *Techn.Rep.Ser.,* No.744.
138. WHO (1972). *WHO Chr.,* 26 (4) 181.
139. King Maurice ed (1982). *Medical Care in Developing Countries,* Ox.U.P.
140. Kupka, K. (1978). *WHO Chr.,* 32:219–225.
141. WHO (2019), *ICD 11, Implementation or Transition Guide,* 2019, Revision.
142. WHO (2013), *How to use the ICF, A practical manual for using the International Classification of Functioning, Disability and Health,* Oct. 2013.

3 Principles of Epidemiology and Epidemiologic Methods

"I keep six honest serving men; they taught me all I know.
Their names are what, why, when, how, where and who."

Epidemiology is the basic science of preventive and social medicine. Although of ancient lineage, it made only slow progress upto the start of 20th century. Epidemiology has evolved rapidly during the past few decades. Its ramifications cover not only study of disease distribution and causation (and thereby prevention), but also health and health-related events occurring in human population. Modern epidemiology has entered the most exciting phase of its evolution. By identifying risk factors of chronic disease, evaluating treatment modalities and health services, it has provided new opportunities for prevention, treatment, planning and improving the effectiveness and efficiency of health services. The current interest of medical sciences in epidemiology has given rise to newer off-shoots such as infectious disease epidemiology, chronic disease epidemiology, clinical epidemiology, serological epidemiology, cancer epidemiology, malaria epidemiology, neuro epidemiology, genetic epidemiology, occupational epidemiology, psychosocial epidemiology, and so on. This trend is bound to increase in view of the increasing importance given to the pursuit of epidemiological studies. That these studies have added substantially to the advancement of medical knowledge is indisputable. This Chapter studies the basic concepts and principles of epidemiology as an introduction to the subject.

History

Epidemiology began with Adam and Eve, both trying to investigate the qualities of the "forbidden fruit". Epidemiology is derived from the word epidemic (epi=among; demos=people; logos=study), which is a very old word dating back to the 3rd century B.C. The foundation of epidemiology was laid in the 19th century, when a few classic studies made a major contribution to the saving of life. Mention is made of an Epidemiological Society in London in 1850s under the presidency of the Earl of Shaftesbury *(1)*. The Society's main concern was the investigation of infectious diseases. The sudden growth of bacteriology had smothered the development of epidemiology in the Universities.

In the United States, Winslow and Sedgwick both lectured in epidemiology in the early 1920s, although the subject was not given departmental status. In 1927, W.H. Frost became the first professor of epidemiology in US. Later Major Greenwood became the first professor of epidemiology and medical statistics in the University of London *(1)*. Epidemiology has grown rapidly during the past few decades. It has now become firmly established in medical education.

There appears to be almost as many definitions of epidemiology as there are authors who have written on the subject, ranging from Hippocrates to those of the present day. A short list is given below *(2, 3)* :

1. That branch of medical science which treats epidemics (Parkin, 1873).
2. The science of the mass phenomena of infectious diseases (Frost, 1927).
3. The study of disease, any disease, as a mass phenomenon (Greenwood, 1934), and
4. The study of the distribution and determinants of disease frequency in man (MacMahon, 1960).

Definition

Epidemiology has been defined as *(4)* :–

> *"The study of the occurrence and distribution of health-related events, states, and processes in specified populations, including the study of the determinants influencing such processes, and the application of this knowledge to control relevant health problems."*

Study includes surveillance, observation, screening, hypothesis testing, analytic research, experiments, and prediction. Distribution refers to analysis by time, place (or space), and population (i.e. classes or subgroups of persons affected in an organization, population or society, or at regional and global scales). Determinants are the geophysical, biological, behavioural, social, cultural, economic, and political factors that influence health. Health-related events, states and processes include outbreaks, diseases, disorders, causes of death, behaviours, environmental and socio-economic processes, effects of preventive programmes, and use of health and social services. Specified populations are those with common contexts and identifiable characteristics. Application to control ... makes explicit the aim of epidemiology – to promote, protect, and restore health, and to advance scientific knowledge *(4)*.

The wide variety of meanings attached to epidemiology is the expression of the wide ranging subject–matter. The diseases included in the subject–matter have increased from those which occur in epidemics to include those infectious diseases which are endemic in nature, and more recently chronic diseases, accidents and mental health. Modern epidemiology has also taken within its scope the study of health-related states, events and "facts of life" occurring in human population. This includes study of the health services used by the population, and to measure their impact. Epidemiology, like public health itself, is often more concerned with the well-being of society as a whole, than with the well-being of individuals.

Although there is no single definition to which all epidemiologists subscribe, three components are common to most of them. First, studies of disease frequency; second, studies of the distribution; and third, studies of the determinants. Each of these components confers an important message.

1. Disease frequency

Inherent in the definition of epidemiology is measurement of frequency of disease, disability or death, and summarizing this information in the form of rates and ratios (e.g., prevalence rate, incidence rate, death rate, etc). Thus the basic measure of disease frequency is a rate or ratio. These rates are essential for comparing disease frequency in different populations or subgroups of the same population in relation to suspected causal factors. Such comparisons may yield important clues to disease aetiology. This is a vital step in the development of strategies for prevention or control of health problems.

Equally, epidemiology is also concerned with the measurement of health-related events and states in the community (e.g., health needs, demands, activities, tasks, health care utilization) and variables such as blood pressure, serum cholesterol, height, weight, etc. In this respect, epidemiology has the features of a quantitative science. Much of the subject matter of measurement of disease and health-related events falls in the domain of biostatistics, which is a basic tool of epidemiology.

2. Distribution of disease

It is well-known that disease, or for that matter health, is not uniformly distributed in human populations. The basic tenet of epidemiology is that the distribution of disease occurs in *patterns* in a community *(3)* and that the patterns may lead to the generation of hypotheses about causative (or risk) factors. An important function of epidemiology is to study these distribution patterns in the various subgroups of the population by time, place and person. That is, the epidemiologist examines whether there has been an increase or decrease of disease over time span; whether there is a higher concentration of disease in one geographic area than in others; whether the disease occurs more often in men or in a particular age-group, and whether most characteristics or behaviour of those affected are different from those not affected *(5)*. Epidemiology addresses itself to a study of these variations or patterns, which may suggest or lead to measures to control or prevent the disease. An important outcome of this study is formulation of aetiological hypothesis. This aspect of epidemiology is known as "descriptive epidemiology".

3. Determinants of disease

A unique feature of epidemiology is to test aetiological hypotheses and identify the underlying causes (or risk factors) of disease. This requires the use of epidemiological principles and methods. This is the real substance of epidemiology. This aspect of epidemiology is known as "analytical epidemiology". Analytical strategies help in developing scientifically sound health programmes, interventions and policies. In recent years, analytical studies have contributed vastly to our understanding of the determinants of chronic diseases, e.g., lung cancer and cardiovascular diseases.

Aims of epidemiology

According to the International Epidemiological Association (IEA), epidemiology has three main aims *(6)*:

a. to describe the distribution and magnitude of health and disease problems in human populations
b. to identify aetiological factors (risk factors) in the pathogenesis of disease; and
c. to provide the data essential to the planning, implementation and evaluation of services for the prevention, control and treatment of disease and to the setting up of priorities among those services.

In order to fulfil these aims, three rather different classes of epidemiological studies may be mentioned: descriptive studies, analytical studies, and experimental or intervention studies *(7)*. These studies are described in the following pages.

The ultimate aim of epidemiology is to lead to effective action :

a. to eliminate or reduce the health problem or its consequences; and
b. to promote the health and well-being of society as a whole.

Epidemiology and clinical medicine

The basic difference between epidemiology and clinical medicine is that in epidemiology, the unit of study is a "defined population" or "population at-risk"; in clinical medicine, the unit of study is a "case" or "cases". In clinical medicine, the physician is concerned with disease in the individual patient, whereas the epidemiologist is concerned with disease patterns in the entire population. Epidemiology is thus concerned with both the sick and healthy. It has been stated that clinicians are interested in cases with the disease, the statistician with the population from which the cases are derived, and the epidemiologist is interested in the relationship between cases and the population in the form of a rate *(8)*.

In clinical medicine, the physician seeks a diagnosis from which he derives a prognosis and prescribes specific treatment. In epidemiology, an analogous situation exists. The epidemiologist is confronted with relevant data derived from a particular epidemiological study. He seeks to identify a particular source of infection, a mode of spread or an aetiological factor in order to determine a future trend and recommend specific control measures *(9)*. The epidemiologist also evaluates the outcome of preventive and therapeutic measures instituted which provides the necessary guidance and feed-back to the health care administrator for effective management of public health programmes.

In clinical medicine, the patient comes to the doctor; in epidemiology, the investigator goes out into the community to find persons who have the disease or experience of the suspected causal factor in question. Clinical medicine is based on biomedical concepts with an ever-increasing concern for refining the technique of diagnosis and treatment at the individual level. The subject matter of clinical medicine is easily "perceived" by such techniques as clinical and laboratory examinations including postmortem reports. In contrast, the subject matter of epidemiology is "conceptual" and can only be symbolized in the form of tables and graphs *(10)*.

Finally, it may be stated that clinical medicine and epidemiology are not antagonistic. Both are closely related, co-existent and mutually helpful. Most epidemiological enquiries could never be established without appropriate clinical consideration as to how the disease in question can be identified among individuals comprising the group under scrutiny. Likewise, a knowledge of prevalence, aetiology and prognosis derived from epidemiological research is important to the clinician for the diagnosis and management of individual patients and their families *(10)*.

Epidemiological approach

The epidemiological approach to problems of health and disease is based on two major foundations:

a. Asking questions
b. Making comparisons.

a. *Asking questions*

Epidemiology has been defined as "a means of learning or asking questions....and getting answers that lead to further questions" *(11)*. For example, the following questions could be asked *(12)* :

RELATED TO HEALTH EVENTS

a. What is the event ? (the problem)
b. What is its magnitude?
c. Where did it happen?
d. When did it happen?
e. Who are affected?
f. Why did it happen?

RELATED TO HEALTH ACTION

a. What can be done to reduce this problem and its consequences ?
b. How can it be prevented in the future ?
c. What action should be taken by the community ? By the health services? By other sectors ? Where and for whom these activities be carried out ?
d. What resources are required ? How are the activities to be organized ?
e. What difficulties may arise, and how might they be overcome ?

Answer to the above questions may provide clues to disease aetiology, and help the epidemiologist to guide planning and evaluation.

b. *Making comparisons*

The basic approach in epidemiology is to make comparisons and draw inferences. This may be comparison of two (or more groups) – one group having the disease (or exposed to risk factor) and the other group(s) not having the disease (or not exposed to risk factor), or comparison between individuals. By making comparisons, the epidemiologist tries to find out the crucial differences in the host and environmental factors between those affected and not affected. In short the epidemiologist weighs, balances and contrasts. Clues to aetiology come from such comparisons.

One of the first considerations before making comparisons is to ensure what is known as "comparability" between the study and control groups. In other words, both the groups should be similar so that "like can be compared with like". For facts to be comparable, they must be accurate, and they must be gathered in a uniform way. For example, the study and control groups should be similar with regard to their age and sex composition, and similar other pertinent variables. The best method of ensuring comparability, in such cases, is by randomization or random allocation (see page 90). Where random allocation is not possible (as in case control and cohort studies) what is known as "matching" is done for selected characteristics that might confound the interpretation of results. Another alternative is standardization which usually has a limited application to a few characteristics such as age, sex and parity. These biostatistical concepts are elaborated in the following pages. It may be mentioned that international comparisons may be difficult because of differences in terminology. It requires standardization of definitions, classifications, criteria and nomenclature.

BASIC MEASUREMENTS IN EPIDEMIOLOGY

Epidemiology focuses, among other things, on measurement of mortality and morbidity in human populations. The first requirement is therefore definition of what is to be measured and establishment of criteria or standards by which it can be measured. This is not only a prerequisite of epidemiological studies, but also one of its goals *(13)*. The clinician may not require a precise definition of disease (e.g., migraine) for immediate patient care, but the epidemiologist needs a definition (a) that is acceptable and applicable to its use in large populations; and (b) that is precise and valid, to enable him to identify those who have the disease from those who do not *(10)*. Clear definitions help to minimize errors in classification of data. Standardized methods of observation and recording are therefore essential before commencing any epidemiological study.

Measurements in Epidemiology

The scope of measurements in epidemiology is very broad and unlimited and includes the following : *(14)*

a. Measurement of mortality
b. Measurement of morbidity
c. Measurement of disability
d. Measurement of natality
e. Measurement of the presence, absence or distribution of the characteristic or attributes of the disease
f. Measurement of medical needs, health care facilities, utilization of health services and other health-related events
g. Measurement of the presence, absence or distribution of the environmental and other factors suspected of causing the disease, and
h. Measurement of demographic variables.

Inspite of a wide range of presently available measurements, there are many areas which are not fully covered. As for example, measurement of the psycho-social aspects of health and disease. The components of well-being need to be better identified.

The basic requirements of measurements are validity, reliability, accuracy, sensitivity and specificity. These are discussed in the next chapter. Finally, measurement errors are unavoidable, no matter where and by whom measurements are taken. The purpose of quality control in measurement is, therefore, not to eliminate errors, but to reduce them as much as possible or at least to an acceptable level.

In the above connection, the following terminology needs explanation: (a) *Variate*: Any piece of information referring to the patient or his disease is called a variate. A variate can be discrete, that is it can be present or absent, e.g., cancer lung, broken leg, or rash in measles or it can be *continuously distributed,* e.g., blood pressure, serum cholesterol, height, etc. (b) *Circumstance*: Any factor in the environment that might be suspected of causing a disease, e.g., air pollution, polluted water, etc *(10)*.

The frequency of a discrete variable or circumstance can be expressed as a rate in relation to population. The frequency of continuously distributed variables or circumstances is expressed in the form of a *frequency distribution* using the summarizing indices of mean, centiles, standard deviations, etc.

Tools of measurement

The epidemiologist usually expresses disease magnitude as a rate, ratio or proportion. A clear understanding of the term is required for proper interpretation of epidemiological data. The basic tools of measurement in epidemiology are :

1. Rates
2. Ratios, and
3. Proportions

1. RATE

When we say there were 500 deaths from motor vehicle accidents in City A during 2010, it is just nothing more than counting deaths in that city during that particular year. Such a statement might be sufficient for the municipal administrator to provide necessary health services. But it conveys no meaning to an epidemiologist who is interested in comparing the frequency of accidents in City A with that in City B. To allow such comparisons, the frequency must be expressed as a rate.

A rate measures the occurrence of some particular event (development of disease or the occurrence of death) in a defined population during a given time period. It is a statement of the risk of developing a condition. It indicates the change in some event that takes place in a population over a period of time. An example of a typical rate is the death rate. It is written as below:

$$\text{Death rate} = \frac{\text{Number of deaths in one year}}{\text{Mid-year population}} \times 1000$$

A rate comprises the following elements – numerator, denominator, time specification and multiplier. The time dimension is usually a calendar year. The rate is expressed per 1000 or some other round figure (10,000; 100,000) selected according to the convenience or convention to avoid fractions.

The various categories of rates are :

(1) Crude rates: These are the actual observed rates such as the birth and death rates. Crude rates are also known as unstandardized rates.

(2) Specific rates: These are the actual observed rates due to specific causes (e.g., tuberculosis); or occurring in specific groups (e.g., age-sex groups) or during specific time periods (e.g., annual, monthly or weekly rates).

(3) Standardized rates: These are obtained by direct or indirect method of standardization or adjustment, e.g., age and sex standardized rates (see page 66, 67).

2. RATIO

Another measure of disease frequency is a ratio. It expresses a relation in size between two random quantities. The numerator is not a component of the denominator. The numerator and denominator may involve an interval of time or may be instantaneous in time. Broadly, ratio is the result of dividing one quantity by another. It is expressed in the form of:

$$x : y \quad \text{or} \quad \frac{x}{y}$$

Example 1:

The ratio of white blood cells relative to red cells is 1:600 or 1/600, meaning that for each white cell, there are 600 red cells.

Example 2:

$$\frac{\text{The number of children with scabies at a certain time}}{\text{The number of children with malnutrition at a certain time}}$$

Other examples include: sex–ratio, doctor–population ratio, child–woman ratio, etc.

3. PROPORTION

A proportion is a ratio which indicates the relation in magnitude of a part of the whole. The numerator is always included in the denominator. A proportion is usually expressed as a percentage.

$$\text{Example : } \frac{\text{The number of childern with scabies at a certain time}}{\text{The total number of children in the village at the same time}} \times 100$$

CONCEPT OF NUMERATOR AND DENOMINATOR

1. Numerator

Numerator refers to the number of times an event (e.g., sickness, birth, death, episodes of sickness) has occurred in a population, during a specified time–period. The numerator is a component of the denominator in calculating a rate, but not in a ratio.

2. Denominator

The lower portion of a ratio. Numerator has little meaning unless it is related to the denominator, The epidemiologist has to choose an appropriate denominator while calculating a rate. It may be (a) related to the population, or (b) related to the total events.

a. Related to the population

The denominators related to the population comprise the following: (i) *MID-YEAR POPULATION:* Because the population size changes daily due to births, deaths and migration, the mid-year population is commonly chosen as a denominator. The mid-point refers to the population estimated as on the first of July of an year. (ii) *POPULATION AT-RISK:* This is an important concept in epidemiology because it focuses on groups at risk of disease rather than on individuals. The term is applied to all those to whom an event could have happened whether it did or not. For example, if we are determining the rate of accidents for a town, the population at risk is all the people in the town. But sometimes, it may be necessary to exclude people because they are not at risk, as for example, in food poisoning, only those who ate the food are at risk of becoming ill. Similarly in calculating "general fertility rate", the denominator is restricted to women of child-bearing age (i.e., 15–49 years); older women and little girls are excluded because they are not "at risk" of becoming pregnant. In short, "population at risk" is restricted solely to those who are capable of having or acquiring the disease or condition in question. (iii) *PERSON–TIME:* In some epidemiological studies (e.g., cohort studies), persons may enter the study at different times. Consequently, they are under observation for varying time periods. In such cases, the denominator is a combination of persons and time. The most frequently used person–time is person–years. Sometimes, this may be person–months, person–weeks or man-hours. For example, if 10 persons remain in the study for 10 years, there are said to be 100 person–years of observation. The same figure would be derived if 100 persons were under observation for one year. These denominators have the advantage of summarizing the experience of persons with different durations of observation or exposure. (iv) *PERSON–DISTANCE:* A variant of person–time is person–distance, as for example passenger–miles. (v) *SUB-GROUPS OF THE POPULATION:* The denominator may be subgroups of a population, e.g., age, sex, occupation, social class, etc.

b. Related to total events

In some instances, the denominator may be related to total events instead of the total population, as in the case of infant mortality rate and case fatality rate. In the case of accidents, the number of accidents "per 1000 vehicles" or "per million vehicle–miles" will be a more useful denominator than the total population, many of them may not be using vehicles.

MEASUREMENT OF MORTALITY

Traditionally and universally, most epidemiological studies begin with mortality data. Mortality data are relatively easy to obtain, and, in many countries, reasonably accurate. Many countries have routine systems for collecting mortality data. Each year, information on deaths is analyzed and the resulting tabulations are made available by each government. Mortality data provide the starting point for many epidemiological studies. In fact, they are the major resource for the epidemiologist.

Death Certificate (Certificate of cause of death)

The basis of mortality data is the Death Certificate. For ensuring national and international comparability, it is very necessary to have a uniform and standardized system of recording and classifying deaths. The death certificate recommended by WHO for international use is given in Fig. 1 *(4)*.

In India, Death Certificate is a vital record signed by a licensed physician or another designated health worker, that includes cause of death, decedant's name, sex, birth date, adhar number, place of residence and of death, and whether the deceased had been medically attended before death. Occupation, birth place, and other information may be included.

It will be seen from Fig. 1 that the international certificate of cause of death is in two parts. Part I deals with the immediate cause of death and the underlying cause.

"Causes of death : The causes of death to be entered on the medical certificate of cause of death are all those diseases, morbid conditions, or injuries that either resulted in or contributed to death and circumstances of the accident or violence which produced any such injuries.

Underlying cause of death : The underlying cause of death is (1) the disease or injury that initiated the train of events leading to death or (2) the circumstances of the accident or violence that produced the fatal injury."

In Part II is recorded any significant associated disease that contributed to the death but did not directly lead to it.

Death Certificate used in India

In order to improve the quality of maternal mortality and infant mortality data and to provide alternative method of collecting data on deaths during pregnancy and infancy, a set of questions are added to the basic structure of international death certificate for use in India.

Limitations of mortality data

Mortality data are not without limitations. Problems are posed by (a) *Incomplete reporting of deaths.* This is not a problem in developed countries, but in India and other developing countries, this may be considerable. (b) *Lack of accuracy:* That is inaccuracies in the recording of age and cause of death. The practice of medical certification of death is not widespread. If it does exist, the cause of death is often inaccurate or incomplete due to such difficulties as lack of diagnostic evidence, inexperience on the part of the certifying doctor and absence of postmortem which may be important in deciding the cause of death. (c) *Lack of uniformity:* There is no uniform and standardized method of collection of data. This hampers national and international comparability (d) *Choosing a single cause of death:* Most countries tabulate mortality data only according to the underlying cause of

CAUSE OF DEATH	**Approximate interval between onset and death**
I	
*Disease or condition directly leading to death** (a) Bronchopneumonia	....
due to (or as a consequence of)	
Antecedent causes (b)	....
Morbid conditions, if any, giving rise to the above cause, stating the underlying condition last — due to (or as a consequence of)	
(c) Strangulated Hernia	....
due to (or as a consequence of)	
(d)	....
II	
Other significant conditions contributing to the death, but not related to the disease or condition causing it — Diabetes	....
***This does not mean the mode of dying, e.g., heart failure, respiratory failure. It means the disease, injury, or complication that caused death**	

FIG. 1

Death Certificate. The International Standard Form (ICD-10)

Source : *(4)*

death. Other diseases (or risk factors) and conditions which contribute to the patient's death are not tabulated, and valuable information is thereby lost. (e) *Changing:* Changing coding systems and changing fashions in diagnosis may affect the validity. We also need uniform definitions and nomenclature. (f) *Diseases with low fatality:* Lastly, mortality statistics are virtually useless, if the disease is associated with low fatality (e.g., mental diseases, arthritis).

Uses of mortality data

Statistics on causes of death are important and widely used for a number of purposes. They may be employed in explaining trends and differentials in overall mortality, indicating priorities for health action and the allocation of resources, in designing intervention programmes, and in the assessment and monitoring of public health problems and programmes – moreover, they give important clues for epidemiological research.

MORTALITY RATES AND RATIOS

The commonly used measures are described below :

1. Crude death rate

The simplest measure of mortality is the 'crude death rate'. It is defined as "the number of deaths (from all causes) per 1000 estimated mid-year population in one year, in a given place". It measures the rate at which deaths are occurring from various causes in a given population, during a specified period. The crude death rate is calculated from the formula:

$$\frac{\text{Number of deaths during the year}}{\text{Mid-year population}} \times 1000$$

It is important to recognize that the crude death rate summarizes the effect of two factors:

a. population composition
b. age-specific death rates (which reflect the probability of dying)

Table 1 shows the crude death rates of two populations, A and B. The crude death rate for population A is 15.2 per 1000. The crude death rate for population B is 9.9 per 1000. Apparently, population B appears healthier, than population A.

The limitation of the crude death rate is exposed, when we compare the age-specific rates between the two populations as shown in Table 1. It can be seen that population B has higher age-specific rates in all age groups. This seeming contradiction is due to differences in the age-composition of the population. The higher crude death rate in population A is due to its older population compared with population B which has a relatively younger population. Currently, this is the prevailing situation in most developing countries with low crude death rates, but high age-specific death rates.

TABLE 1
Crude and age-specific death rates

Popula -tion	Crude death rate	Age-specific death rates per 1000 population					
		0–1	1–4	5–7	8–44	45–64	65+
A	15.2	13.5	0.6	0.4	1.5	10.7	59.7
B	9.9	22.6	1.0	0.5	3.6	18.8	61.1

In summary, the crude death rates have a major disadvantage, that is, they lack comparability for communities with populations that differ by age, sex, race, etc. However, they should always be examined first, and later the age-specific death rates which are the most useful single measures of mortality. By moving away from the crude death rate to the more detailed age-specific rates, an attractive feature of the crude death rate, that is, its ability to portray an impression in a single figure is lost.

2. Specific death rates

When analysis is planned to throw light on aetiology, it is essential to use specific death rates. The specific death rates may be – (a) cause or disease specific – e.g., tuberculosis, cancer, accident; (b) related to specific groups – e.g., age-specific, sex-specific, age and sex specific, etc. Rates can also be made specific for many other variables such as income, religion, race, housing, etc. Specific death rates can help us to identify particular groups or groups "at-risk", for preventive action. They permit comparisons between different causes within the same population. Specific death rates are obtained mainly in countries in which a satisfactory civil registration system operates and in which a high proportion of deaths is certified medically.

Table 2 illustrates how some specific death rates in common use are computed :

TABLE 2
Specific death rates

1.	Specific death rate due to tuberculosis	=	$\frac{\text{Number of deaths from tuberculosis during a calendar year}}{\text{Mid-year population}} \times 1{,}000$
2.	Specific death rate for males	=	$\frac{\text{Number of deaths among males during a calendar year}}{\text{Mid-year population of males}} \times 1{,}000$
3.	Specific death rate in age group 15-20 years	=	$\frac{\text{Number of deaths of persons aged 15–20 during a calendar year}}{\text{Mid-year population of persons aged 15–20}} \times 1{,}000$
4.	Death rate for January (Note: The deaths are multiplied by 12 in order to make the monthly death rate comparable with the annual death rate)	=	$\frac{\text{Deaths in January} \times 12}{\text{Mid-year population}} \times 1{,}000$
5.	Weekly death rate	=	$\frac{\text{Deaths in the week} \times 52}{\text{Mid-year population}} \times 1{,}000$

3. Case fatality rate (Ratio)

$$= \frac{\text{Total number of deaths due to a particular disease}}{\text{Total number of cases due to the same disease}} \times 100$$

Case fatality rate represents the killing power of a disease. It is simply the ratio of deaths to cases. The time interval is not specified. Case fatality rate is typically used in acute infectious diseases (e.g., food poisoning, cholera, measles). Its usefulness for chronic diseases is limited, because the period from onset to death is long and variable. The case fatality rate for the same disease may vary in different epidemics because of changes in the agent, host and environmental factors. Case fatality is closely related to virulence.

4. Proportional mortality rate (Ratio)

It is sometimes useful to know what proportion of total deaths are due to a particular cause (e.g., cancer) or what proportion of deaths are occurring in a particular age group (e.g., above the age of 50 years). Proportional mortality rate expresses the "number of deaths due to a particular cause (or in a specific age group) per 100 (or 1000) total deaths". Thus we have:

(a) *Proportional mortality from a specific disease*

$$= \frac{\text{Number of deaths from the specific disease in a year}}{\text{Total deaths from all causes in that year}} \times 100$$

(b) *Under-5 proportionate mortality rate*

$$= \frac{\text{Number of deaths under 5 years of age in the given year}}{\text{Total number of deaths during the same period}} \times 100$$

(c) *Proportional mortality rate for aged 50 years and above*

$$= \frac{\text{Number of deaths of persons aged 50 years and above}}{\text{Total deaths of all age groups in that year}} \times 100$$

Proportional mortality rate is computed usually for a broad disease group (such as communicable diseases as a whole) and for a specific disease of major public health importance, such as cancer or coronary heart disease in industrialized countries *(15)*.

Proportional rates are used when population data are not available. Since proportional mortality rate depends upon two variables, both of which may differ, it is of limited value in making comparison between population groups or different time periods. However, proportional rates are useful indicators within any population group of the relative importance of the specific disease or disease group, as a cause of death. Mortality from communicable diseases is especially important as it relates mostly to preventable conditions. Since the prevailing causes of death vary according to age and sex, it is desirable to compute proportionate mortality separately for each age and sex group in order to determine measures directed to particular age–sex groups for the reduction of preventable mortality *(15)*. Proportional mortality rate does not indicate the risk of members of the population contracting or dying from the disease.

5. Survival rate

It is the proportion of survivors in a group, (e.g., of patients) studied and followed over a period (e.g., a 5–year period). It is a method of describing prognosis in certain disease conditions. Survival experience can be used as a yardstick for the assessment of standards of therapy. The survival period is usually reckoned from the date of diagnosis or start of the treatment. Survival rates have received special attention in cancer studies.

$$\text{Survival rate} = \frac{\text{Total number of patients alive after 5 years}}{\text{Total number of patients diagnosed or treated}} \times 100$$

6. Adjusted or standardized rates

If we want to compare the death rates of two populations with different age–composition, the crude death rate is not the right yardstick. This is because, rates are only comparable if the populations upon which they are based are comparable. And it is cumbersome to use a series of age specific death rates. The answer is "age adjustment" or "age standardization", which removes the confounding effect of different age structures and yields a single standardized or adjusted rate, by which the mortality experience can be compared directly. The adjustment can be made not only for age but also sex, race, parity, etc. Thus one can generate age–sex, and race-adjusted rates.

Standardization is carried out by one of two methods – direct or indirect standardization. Both the methods begin by choosing a "standard population", not the age–structures of the populations.

DIRECT STANDARDIZATION

Two examples of direct standardization are given. In the first, a "standard population" is selected. A standard population is defined as one for which the numbers in each age and sex group are known. A frequently used standard age-composition *(15)* is shown in Table 3. The standard population may also be "created" by combining 2 populations; this is shown in the second example.

The next step is to apply to the standard population, the age-specific rates of the population whose crude death rate is to be adjusted or standardized. As a result, for each age group, an "expected" number of deaths (or events) in the standard population is obtained; these are added together for all the age groups, to give the total expected deaths. The final operation is to divide the "expected" total number of deaths by the total of the standard population, which yields the standardized or age-adjusted rate.

Example 1

Example 1 shows: (a) the computation of age-specific death rates per 1000 population for city X (Table 3); and (b) application of these rates to a standard population to obtain the "expected deaths" and the standardized or age-adjusted death rate (Table 4).

TABLE 3

Calculation of age-specific death rates for City "X"

Age	Mid-year population	Deaths in the year	Age-specific death rates
0	4,000	60	15.0
1–4	4,500	20	4.4
5–14	4,000	12	3.0
15–19	5,000	15	3.0
20–24	4,000	16	4.0
25–34	8,000	25	3.1
35–44	9,000	48	5.3
45–54	8,000	100	12.5
55–64	7,000	150	21.4
	53,500	446	
Crude death rate per 1000 = **8.3**			

TABLE 4

Calculation of the standardized death rate for City "X"

Age	Standard population	Age-specific death rates per 1000	Expected deaths
0	2,400	15.0	36
1–4	9,600	4.4	42.24
5–14	19,000	3.0	57
15–19	9,000	3.0	27
20–24	8,000	4.0	32
25–34	14,000	3.1	43.4
35–44	12,000	5.3	63.6
45–54	11,000	12.5	137.5
55–64	8,000	21.4	171.2
	93,000		609.94

Standardized death rate per 1000 = $\frac{609.94}{93,000} \times 1000 = \mathbf{6.56}$

It can be seen from Tables 3 and 4 that standardizing for age distribution has reduced the crude death rate from 8.3 to 6.56. The choice of the standard population is, to some extent, arbitrary. Clearly, use of a different standard population will give rise to a different value for the standardized death rate, but it must be remembered that these standardized rates have been calculated so that they can be compared between themselves – they have no intrinsic meaning other than for this purpose *(16)*.

It is usual to use the national population as standard when inter–regional comparisons between cities within a range are made. In order that comparisons can be made over a period of years, a 'standard population' can be maintained for that period *(16)*. The standard population used in Table 4 is given by WHO in its publication "Health for All" Series No. 4, on page 77 *(15)*.

Example 2

Table 5 shows that in a study of lung cancer and smoking, 42 per cent of cases and 18 per cent of controls were heavy smokers.

TABLE 5

Proportion of heavy smokers in cases and controls (lung cancer)

Age	Total subjects	CASES No.	CASES Heavy smokers	CASES %	CONTROLS No.	CONTROLS Heavy smokers	CONTROLS %
40–49	500	400	200	50	100	50	50
50–59	500	100	10	10	400	40	10
Total	1,000	500	210	42	500	90	18

Source : *(6)*

Age adjustments were carried out (a) first, by combining the number of subjects in both the age groups (500+500=1,000) to create a standard population, and (b) applying the observed age-specific proportions of heavy smokers (i.e., 50% and 10% in both cases and controls) to the same standard population. The results (or "expected" values) are shown in Table 6, which shows that the age adjusted proportions of heavy smokers are identical (30%) for cases and controls. The previously observed difference is explained entirely by the difference in age composition.

TABLE 6

Age-adjusted proportions

Age	Subjects	Expected number of heavy smokers: CASES	Expected number of heavy smokers: CONTROLS
40–49	500	$\frac{500 \times 50}{100} = 250$	$\frac{500 \times 50}{100} = 250$
50–59	500	$\frac{500 \times 10}{100} = 50$	$\frac{500 \times 10}{100} = 50$
Total	1000	300	300
Standardized rates		$\frac{300}{1000} \times 100 = 30$	$\frac{300}{1000} \times 100 = 30$

The direct method of standardization is feasible only if the actual specific rates in subgroups of the observed population are available, along with the number of individuals in each subgroup.

INDIRECT AGE STANDARDIZATION

1. Standardized mortality ratio (SMR)

The simplest and most useful form of indirect standardization is the Standardized Mortality Ratio (SMR). In England, it is the basis for the allocation of government money to the health regions of the country. The concept is that the regions with higher mortality also have the higher morbidity, and should therefore receive proportionately higher funding to combat ill-health *(16)*.

Standard mortality ratio is a ratio (usually expressed as a percentage) of the total number of deaths that occur in the study group to the number of deaths that would have been expected to occur if that study group had experienced the death rates of a standard population (or other reference population). In other words. SMR compares the mortality in a study group (e.g., an occupational group) with the mortality that the occupational group would have had if they had experienced national mortality rates. In this method, the more stable rates of the larger population are applied to the smaller study group. It gives a measure of the likely excess risk of mortality due to the occupation.

$$*SMR = \frac{\text{Observed deaths}}{\text{Expected deaths}} \times 100$$

If the ratio had value greater than 100, then the occupation would appear to carry a greater mortality risk than that of the whole population. If the ratio had value less than 100, then the occupation risks of mortality would seem to be proportionately less than that for the whole population.

Table 7 shows that the mortality experience of coal workers was 129 per cent, which meant that their mortality was 29 per cent more than that experienced by the national population. Values over 100 per cent represent an unfavourable mortality experience and those below 100 per cent relatively favourable mortality experience. Table 7 displays the calculations.

TABLE 7

Calculation of the SMR for coal workers

Age	National population death rates per 1000	Coal workers population	Observed deaths	Expected deaths
25–34	3.0	300	*	0.9
35–44	5.0	400	*	2.0
45–54	8.0	200	*	1.6
55–64	25.0	100	*	2.5
		1,000	9	7.0

SMR = 9/7 × 100=129

* It is not necessary to know these values; only the total for the whole age–range is required

The SMR has the advantage over the direct method of age adjustment in that it permits adjustment for age and other factors where age-specific rates are not available or are unstable because of small numbers. One needs to know only the number of persons in each age group in the study population and the age-specific rates of the national population (or other reference population). It is possible to use SMR if the event of interest is occurrence of disease rather than death.

2. Other standardization techniques

(a) A more complicated method of indirect adjustment which yields absolute age adjusted rate, involves the calculation of an index death rate and a standardizing factor for each population of interest. The reader is referred to A.B. Hill's "Principles of Medical Statistics". (b) *Life* table is an age-adjusted summary of current all-causes mortality. (c) *Regression techniques:* These are an efficient means of standardization. (d) *Multivariate analysis:* A computer, using regression or similar methods, can standardize for many variables simultaneously *(17)*.

MEASUREMENT OF MORBIDITY

Morbidity has been defined as "any departure, subjective or objective, from a state of physiological well-being" *(18, 19)*. The term is used equivalent to such terms as sickness, illness, disability etc. The WHO Expert Committee on Health Statistics noted in its 6th Report *(18)* that morbidity could be measured in terms of 3 units – (a) persons who were ill; (b) the illnesses (periods or spells of illness) that these persons experienced; and (c) the duration (days, weeks, etc) of these illnesses.

Three aspects of morbidity are commonly measured by *morbidity rates* or *morbidity ratios,* namely frequency, duration and severity. Disease frequency is measured by *incidence* and prevalence rates. The average duration per case or the disability rate, which is the average number of days of *disability* per person, may serve as a measure of the duration of illnesses. The case fatality rate may be used as an index of severity *(20)*. This section focuses on incidence and prevalence rates, which are widely used to describe disease occurrence in a community.

The value of morbidity data may be summarized as follows:

a. they describe the extent and nature of the disease load in the community, and thus assist in the establishment of priorities.
b. they usually provide more comprehensive and more accurate and clinically relevant information on patient characteristics, than can be obtained from mortality data, and are therefore essential for basic research.
c. they serve as starting point for aetiological studies, and thus play a crucial role in disease prevention.
d. they are needed for monitoring and evaluation of disease control activities.

INCIDENCE

Incidence rate is defined as "the number of NEW cases occurring in a defined population during a specified period of time". It is given by the formula :

$$\text{Incidence} = \frac{\text{Number of new cases of specific disease during a given time period}}{\text{Population at-risk during that period}} \times 1000$$

For example, if there had been 500 new cases of an illness in a population of 30,000 in a year, the incidence rate would be:

$$= 500/30{,}000 \times 1000$$
$$= 16.7 \text{ per 1000 per year}$$

Note: Incidence rate must include the unit of time used in the final expression. If you write 16.7 per 1000, this would be inadequate. The correct expression is 16.7 per 1,000 per year *(21)*.

It will be seen from the above definition that incidence rate refers

a. only to new cases
b. during a given period (usually one year)
c. in a specified population or "population at risk", unless other denominators are chosen.
d. it can also refer to new spells or episodes of disease arising in a given period of time, per 1000 population. For example, a person may suffer from common cold more than once a year. If he had suffered twice, he would contribute 2 spells of sickness in that year. The formula in this case would be:

$$\text{Incidence rate (spells)} = \frac{\text{Number of spells of sickness starting in a defined period}}{\text{Mean number of persons exposed to risk in that period}} \times 1000$$

Incidence measures the rate at which new cases are occurring in a population. It is not influenced by the duration of the disease. The use of incidence is generally restricted to acute conditions.

Special incidence rates

Examples include: Attack rate (case rate), Secondary attack rate, Hospital admission rate, etc.

a. *Attack rate*

An attack rate is an incidence rate (usually expressed as a per cent), used only when the population is exposed to risk for a limited period of time such as during an epidemic. It relates the number of cases in the population at risk and reflects the extent of the epidemic. Attack rate is given by the formula:

$$\text{Attack rate} = \frac{\text{Number of new cases of a specified disease during a specified time interval}}{\text{Total population at risk during the same interval}} \times 100$$

b. *Secondary attack rate*

It is defined as the number of exposed persons developing the disease within the range of the incubation period following exposure to a primary case. (see page 103).

USES OF INCIDENCE RATE

The incidence rate, as a health status indicator, is useful for taking action (a) to control disease, and (b) for research into aetiology and pathogenesis, distribution of diseases, and efficacy of preventive and therapeutic measures *(15)*.

For instance, if the incidence rate is increasing, it might indicate failure or ineffectiveness of the current control programmes. Rising incidence rates might suggest the need for a new disease control or preventive programme, or that reporting practices had improved. A change or fluctuation in the incidence of disease may also mean a change in the aetiology of disease, e.g., change in the agent, host and environmental characteristics. Analysis of differences in incidence rates reported from various socio-economic groups and geographical areas may provide useful insights into the effectiveness of the health services provided *(15)*.

PREVALENCE

The term "disease prevalence" refers specifically to all current cases (old and new) existing at a given point in time, or over a period of time in a given population. A broader definition of prevalence is as follows: "the total number of all individuals who have an attribute or disease at a particular time (or during a particular period) divided by the population at risk of having the attribute or disease at this point in time or midway through the period *(2)*". Although referred to as a rate, prevalence rate is really a ratio.

Prevalence is of two types :

(a) Point prevalence

(b) Period prevalence

(a) Point prevalence

Point prevalence of a disease is defined as the number of all current cases (old and new) of a disease at one point of time, in relation to a defined population. The "point" in point prevalence, may for all practical purposes consist of a day, several days, or even a few weeks, depending upon the time it takes to examine the population sample *(21)*.

Point prevalence is given by the formula:

$$= \frac{\text{Number of all current cases (old and new) of a specified disease existing at a given point in time}}{\text{Estimated population at the same point in time}} \times 100$$

When the term "prevalence rate" is used, without any further qualification, it is taken to mean "point prevalence" *(18)*.

Point prevalence can be made specific for age, sex and other relevant factors or attributes.

(b) Period prevalence

A less commonly used measure of prevalence is period prevalence. It measures the frequency of all current cases (old and new) existing during a defined period of time (e.g., annual prevalence) expressed in relation to a defined population. It includes cases arising before but extending into or through to the year as well as those cases arising during the year (Fig. 2). Period prevalence is given by the formula:

$$= \frac{\text{Number of existing cases (old and new) of a specified disease during a given period of time interval}}{\text{Estimated mid-interval population at-risk}} \times 100$$

The terms incidence and prevalence are illustrated in Fig. 2

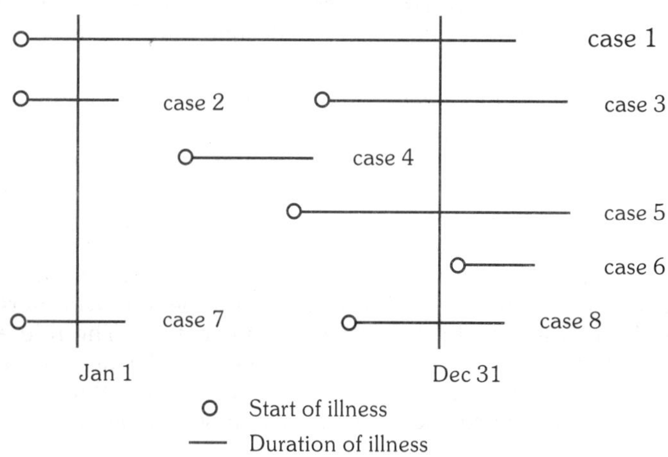

Incidence would include cases – 3,4,5, and 8
Point prevalence (Jan 1) cases – 1,2, and 7
Point prevalence (Dec.31) cases – 1,3,5 and 8
Period prevalence (Jan–Dec) cases – 1,2,3,4,5,7, and 8

FIG. 2
Number of cases of a disease beginning, developing and ending during a period of time

Relationship between prevalence and incidence

Prevalence depends upon 2 factors, the incidence and duration of illness. Given the assumption that the population is stable, and incidence and duration are unchanging, the relationship between incidence and prevalence can be expressed as :

$P = I \times D$

$= \text{incidence} \times \text{mean duration}$

Example (for a stable condition)
Incidence = 10 cases per 1000 population per year
Mean duration of disease = 5 years
Prevalence = $10 \times 5 = 50$ per 1000 population

Conversely, it is possible to derive incidence and duration as follows:

Incidence = P/D

Duration = P/I

The above equation ($P = I \times D$) shows that the longer the duration of the disease, the greater its prevalence. For example, tuberculosis has a high prevalence rate relative to incidence. This is because new cases of tuberculosis keep cropping up throughout the year, while the old ones may persist for months or years. On the other hand, if the disease is acute and of short duration either because of rapid recovery or death, the prevalence rate will be relatively low compared with the incidence rate. In some diseases (e.g., food poisoning), the disease is so short–lived, there are no "old" cases. The same is true of conditions which are rapidly fatal, such as homicides. Strictly speaking, these events have no prevalence. In other words, decrease in prevalence may take place not only from a decrease in incidence, but also from a decrease of the duration of illness through either more rapid recovery or more rapid death.

When we see a change in prevalence from one time period to another, this can result from changes in incidence, changes in duration of disease or both. For example, improvements in treatment may decrease the duration of illness and thereby decrease prevalence of a disease. But if the treatment is such that by preventing death, and at the same time not producing recovery, may give rise to the apparently paradoxical effect of an increase in prevalence. Further, if duration is decreased sufficiently, a decrease in prevalence could take place despite an increase in incidence.

Prevalence has been compared with a photograph, an instantaneous record; and incidence with a film, a continuous record. Both the terms may perhaps be better understood by taking into consideration a coffee house. After the coffee house opens in the morning, people keep entering and leaving, each one remaining inside the coffee house for a short while. At any point of time, say 10 AM, we could go into the coffee house and count people over there. This corresponds to estimating the *prevalence*. The rate at which people enter the coffee house, say 10 people per hour, is equivalent to the incidence. The relationship between incidence and prevalence is shown in Fig. 3 *(22)*.

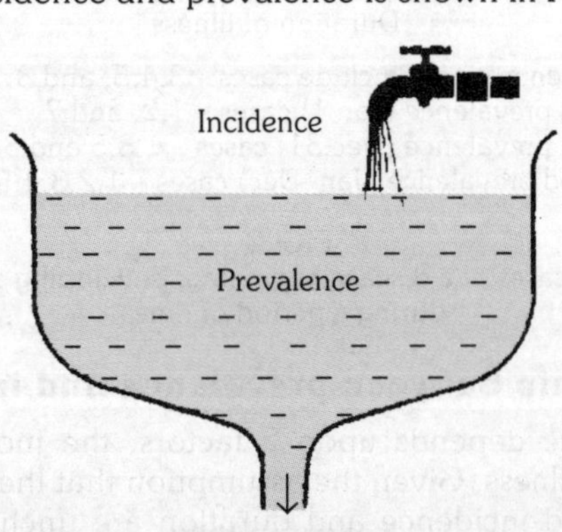

FIG. 3
Relationship between incidence and prevalence

It is important to note the limitations of prevalence rate. It is not the ideal measure for studying disease aetiology or causation. We have seen that two factors determine prevalence, namely incidence and duration. Incidence is related to the occurrence of disease and duration to factors which affect the course of the disease. In other words, the element of *duration* reflects the prognostic factors, and incidence reflects the causal factors. Therefore, incidence rates should be optimally used in the formulation and testing of aetiological hypotheses. When incidence rates are not available, prevalence rates (which are readily obtainable) may have to be used, but the contribution of duration element always has to be assessed.

Uses of prevalence

(a) Prevalence helps to estimate the magnitude of health/disease problems in the community, and identify potential high-risk populations (b) Prevalence rates are especially useful for administrative and planning purposes, e.g., hospital beds, manpower needs, rehabilitation facilities, etc.

EPIDEMIOLOGIC METHODS

The primary concern of the epidemiologist is to study disease occurrence in people, who during the course of their lives are exposed to numerous factors and circumstances, some of which may have a role in disease aetiology. Unlike the clinician or the laboratory investigator, who is able to study disease conditions more precisely, the epidemiologist employs carefully designed research strategies to explore disease aetiology.

Epidemiological studies can be classified as observational studies and experimental studies with further subdivisions :

1. *Observational studies*

a. Descriptive studies

b. Analytical studies

(i) Ecological	or	Correlational,	with populations as unit of study
(ii) Cross-sectional	or	Prevalence,	with individuals as unit of study
(iii) Case-control	or	Case-reference,	with individuals as unit of study
(iv) Cohort	or	Follow-up,	with individuals as unit of study

2. Experimental studies Intervention studies

a. Randomized controlled trials	or	Clinical trials	with patients as unit of study
b. Field trials			with healthy people as unit of study
c. Community trials	or	Community intervention studies	with communities as unit of study

These studies or methods cannot be regarded as watertight compartments; they complement one another. Observational studies allow nature to take its own course; the investigator measures but does not intervene. Descriptive study is limited to a description of the occurrence of a disease in a population. An analytical study goes further by analyzing relationship between health status and other variables. Experimental or intervention studies involve an active attempt to change a disease determinant or the progress of a disease, and are similar in design to experiments in other sciences. However, they are subject to extra constraints, since the health of the people in the study group may be at stake. The major experimental design is the randomized controlled trial using patients as subjects. Field trials and community trials are other experimental studies in which the participants are healthy people and community respectively *(23)*.

In all epidemiological studies, it is essential to have a clear definition of a case of the disease being investigated and of an exposed person. In absence of clear definitions of disease and exposure, great difficulties are likely to be experienced in interpreting the data.

DESCRIPTIVE EPIDEMIOLOGY

The best study of mankind is man. This statement emphasizes the importance of making the best use of observations on individuals or populations exposed to suspected factors of disease. Meticulous observations made in Africa by Burkitt led to the eventual incrimination of Epstein-Barr virus (EBV) as the aetiological factor (possibly conditioned by other factors such as malarial infection) of the type of cancer known as Burkitt's lymphoma. It was the epidemiological study in New Guinea of "Kuru", a hereditary neurological disorder, that led to the discovery of slow virus infections as the cause of chronic degenerative neurological disorders in human beings. The list is endless.

Descriptive studies are usually the first phase of an epidemiological investigation. These studies are concerned with observing the distribution of disease or health-related characteristics in human populations and identifying the characteristics with which the disease in question seems to be associated. Such studies basically ask the questions.

a. When is the disease occurring ? – time distribution

b. Where is it occurring ? – place distribution

c. Who is getting the disease? – person distribution

The various procedures involved in descriptive studies may be outlined as below (Table 8).

TABLE 8

Procedures in descriptive studies

1. Defining the population to be studied
2. Defining the disease under study
3. Describing the disease by
   a. time
   b. place
   c. person
4. Measurement of disease
5. Comparing with known indices
6. Formulation of an aetiological hypothesis

1. Defining the population

Descriptive studies are investigations of populations, not individuals. The first step is, therefore, to define the "population base" not only in terms of the total number, but also its composition in terms of age, sex, occupation, cultural characters and similar information needed for the study.

The "defined population" can be the whole population in a geographic area, or more often a representative sample taken from it. The defined population can also be a specially selected group such as age and sex groups, occupational groups, hospital patients, school children, small communities as well as wider groupings – in fact, wherever a group of people can be fairly accurately counted.

The defined population needs to be large enough so that age, sex and other specific rates are meaningful. The community chosen should be stable, without migration into or out of the area. It should be clear who does and who does not belong to the population, as for example, visitors and relations. Perhaps the most essential ingredient is community participation, which must be forthcoming. Furthermore, the population should not be overtly different from other communities in the region. Finally, a health facility should be close enough to provide relatively easy access for patients requiring medical services. In the famous Framingham Heart Study in US, all the above criteria were taken into consideration in choosing the study population.

The concept of 'defined population' (or population at risk) is crucial in epidemiological studies. It provides the denominator for calculating rates which are essential to measure the frequency of disease and study its distribution and determinants. Epidemiologists therefore have been labelled as men in search of a denominator *(24)*.

2. Defining the disease under study

Once the population to be studied is defined or specified, one must then define the disease or condition being investigated. Here the needs of the clinician and epidemiologist may diverge. The clinician may not need a precise definition of disease (e.g., migraine) for immediate patient care. If the diagnosis is wrong, he can revise it subsequently. But the epidemiologist, whose main concern is to obtain an accurate estimate of disease in a population, needs a definition that is both precise and valid to enable him (or observers working in field conditions) to identify those who have the disease from those who do not *(10)*. The diagnostic methods for use in epidemiological studies must be acceptable to the population to be studied, and applicable to their use in large populations.

In other words, the epidemiologist looks out for an "operational definition", i.e., a definition by which the disease or condition can be identified and measured in the defined population with a degree of accuracy. For example, tonsillitis might be defined clinically as an inflammation of the tonsils caused by infection, usually with *streptococcus pyogenes*. This definition, like many other clinical definitions (and the WHO definition of 'health') serves to convey particular information, but cannot be used to measure disease in the community. On the other hand, an "operational definition" spells out clearly the criteria by which the disease can be measured. Such criteria in the case of tonsillitis would include the presence of enlarged, red tonsils with white exudate, which on throat swab culture grow predominantly *S. pyogenes*. If the definition is not valid, it would be a powerful source of error in the presentation and comparability of measurements from different sources. With regard to certain diseases (e.g., neurological diseases) which often do not have pathognomonic signs and symptoms, disease definition is a crucial concern for the epidemiologist. In such cases, the epidemiologist frames his own definition keeping the objectives of his study in view and aiming at the same time a degree of accuracy sufficient for his purpose. Once established, the case definition must be adhered to throughout the study.

3. Describing the disease

The primary objective of descriptive epidemiology is to describe the occurrence and distribution of disease (or health-related events or characteristics within populations) by time, place and person, and identifying those characteristics associated with presence or absence of disease in individuals. This involves systematic collection and analysis of data. Some of the characteristics most frequently examined by epidemiologists in descriptive studies are given in Table 9. It is only an initial separation or grouping of variables according to time, place and person and NOT a classification of causal factors.

TABLE 9
Characteristics frequently examined in descriptive studies

Time	Place	Person	
Year, season	Climatic zones	Age	Birth order
Month, week	Country, region	Sex	Family size
Day, hour of onset,	Urban/rural Local community	Marital state	Height Weight
Duration	Towns Cities Institutions	Occupation Social status Education	Blood pressure Blood cholesterol Personal habits

TIME DISTRIBUTION

The pattern of disease may be described by the time of its occurrence, i.e., by week, month, year, the day of the week, hour of onset, etc. It raises questions whether the disease is seasonal in occurrence; whether it shows periodic increase or decrease; or whether it follows a consistent time trend. Such studies may yield important clues about the source or aetiology of the disease, thereby suggesting potential preventive measures. Epidemiologists have identified three kinds of time trends or fluctuations in disease occurrence.

I. Short-term fluctuations
II. Periodic fluctuations, and
III. Long-term or secular trends

I. Short-term fluctuations

The best known short-term fluctuation in the occurrence of a disease is an epidemic. According to modern concepts an epidemic is defined as "the occurrence in a community or region of cases of an illness or other health-related events clearly in excess of normal expectancy". The community or region, and the time period in which the cases occur, are specified precisely. Epidemicity is thus relative to usual frequency of the disease in the same area, among the specified population, at the same season of the year *(2)*. The data in Table 10 illustrates this point.

Types of epidemics

Three major types of epidemics may be distinguished.

A. Common-source epidemics
  (a) Single exposure or "point-source" epidemics.
  (b) Continuous or multiple exposure epidemics
B. Propagated epidemics
  (a) Person-to-person
  (b) Arthropod vector
  (c) Animal reservoir
C. Slow (modern) epidemics.

A graph of the time distribution of epidemic cases is called the "epidemic curve" (Fig. 4). The epidemic curve may suggest : (1) a time relationship with exposure to a suspected source, (2) a cyclical or seasonal pattern suggestive of a particular infection, and common source or propagated spread of the disease.

A. *Common-source epidemics*

(a) Common-source, single exposure epidemics

These are also known as "point-source" epidemics. The exposure to the disease agent is brief and essentially simultaneous, the resultant cases all develop within one incubation period of the disease (e.g., an epidemic of food poisoning). Fig. 4 illustrates a common-source, single exposure epidemic. The curve has usually one peak. One point of interest is the "median incubation period", it is the time required for 50 per cent of the cases to occur following exposure.

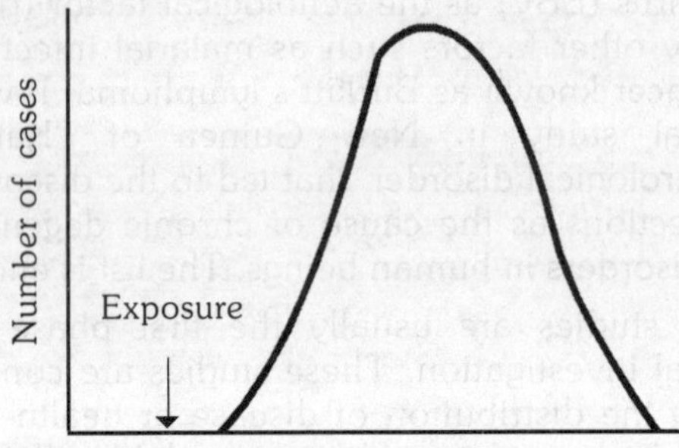

FIG. 4
Epidemic curve

Source : *(3)*

The main features of a "point-source" epidemic are : (i) the epidemic curve rises and falls rapidly, with no secondary waves (ii) the epidemic tends to be explosive, there is clustering of cases within a narrow interval of time, and (iii) more importantly, all the cases develop within one incubation period of disease.

Common-source epidemics are frequently, but not always, due to exposure to an infectious agent. They can result from contamination of the environment (air, water, food, soil) by industrial chemicals or pollutants, e.g., Bhopal gas tragedy in India and Minamata disease in Japan resulting from consumption of fish containing high concentration of methyl mercury.

If the epidemic continues over more than one incubation period, there is either a continuous or multiple exposure to a common source, or a propagated spread.

(b) Common-source, continuous or repeated exposure

Sometimes the exposure from the same source may be prolonged – continuous, repeated or intermittent – not necessarily at the same time or place. A prostitute may be a common source in a gonorrhoea outbreak, but since she will infect her clients over a period of time there may be no explosive rise in the number of cases. A well of contaminated water, or a nationally distributed brand of vaccine (e.g. polio vaccine), or food, could result in similar outbreaks. In these instances, the resulting epidemics tend to be more extended or irregular. The outbreak of respiratory illness, the Legionnaire's disease, in the summer of 1976 in Philadelphia (USA) was a common-source, continuous or repeated exposure outbreak. This outbreak, as in other outbreaks of this type, continued beyond the range of one incubation period. There was no evidence of secondary cases among persons who had contact with ill persons *(25)*.

A variation to the above model is that an epidemic may

be initiated from a common source and then continue as a propagated epidemic. Water-borne cholera is a familiar example, the epidemic reaches a sharp peak, but tails off gradually over a longer period of time.

B. *Propagated epidemics*

A propagated epidemic is most often of infectious origin and results from person-to-person transmission of an infectious agent (e.g., epidemics of hepatitis A and polio). The epidemic usually shows a gradual rise and tails off over a much longer period of time. Transmission continues until the number of susceptibles is depleted or susceptible individuals are no longer exposed to infected persons or intermediary vectors. The speed of spread depends upon herd immunity, opportunities for contact and secondary attack rate. Propagated epidemics are more likely to occur where large number of susceptibles are aggregated, or where there is a regular supply of new susceptible individuals (e.g., birth, immigrants) lowering herd immunity. Fig. 5 illustrates the course of a typical propagated epidemic in which the agent is transmitted by contact between individuals.

II. Periodic fluctuations

(i) *Seasonal trend* : Seasonal variation is a well-known characteristic of many communicable diseases, e.g., measles, varicella, cerebro-spinal meningitis, upper respiratory infections, malaria, etc. For example, measles is usually at its height in early spring and so is varicella. Upper respiratory infections frequently show a seasonal rise during winter months. Bacterial gastrointestinal infections are prominent in summer months because of warm weather and rapid multiplication of flies. The seasonal variations of disease occurrence may be related to environmental conditions (e.g., temperature, humidity, rainfall, overcrowding, life cycle of vectors, etc.) which directly or indirectly favour disease transmission. However, in many infectious diseases (e.g., polio), the basis for seasonal variation is unknown. Non-infectious diseases and conditions may sometimes exhibit seasonal variation, e.g., sunstroke, hay fever, snakebite. Some epidemiologists would regard seasonal trend as a form of cyclic trend. Table 10 shows a typical pattern of seasonal trend, – the outbreaks of dengue/DF starting by month of July and peaking in September, October and November, coinciding with late summer and rain.

TABLE 10

Seasonal trend of dengue/DHF in India 2005–2007

Month	2005	2006	2007
January	151	281	83
February	80	193	64
March	59	178	46
April	68	166	50
May	172	181	127
June	130	269	175
July	742	478	487
August	946	577	487
September	4,852	1,275	974
October	2,482	5,880	1,507
November	1,507	1,934	802
December	801	905	221
Total	11,990	12,317	5,023

Source : *(26)*

(ii) *Cyclic trend* : Some diseases occur in cycles spread over short periods of time which may be days, weeks, months or years. For example, measles in the pre-vaccination era appeared in cycles with major peaks every 2–3 years and rubella every 6–9 years. This was due to naturally occurring variations in herd immunity. A build-up of susceptibles is again required in the "herd" before there can be another attack. Influenza pandemics are known to occur at intervals of 7–10 years, due to antigenic variations. Non-infectious conditions may also show periodic fluctuations, e.g., automobile accidents in US are more frequent on week-ends, especially Saturdays. A knowledge of cyclicity of disease is useful in that it may enable communities to defend themselves.

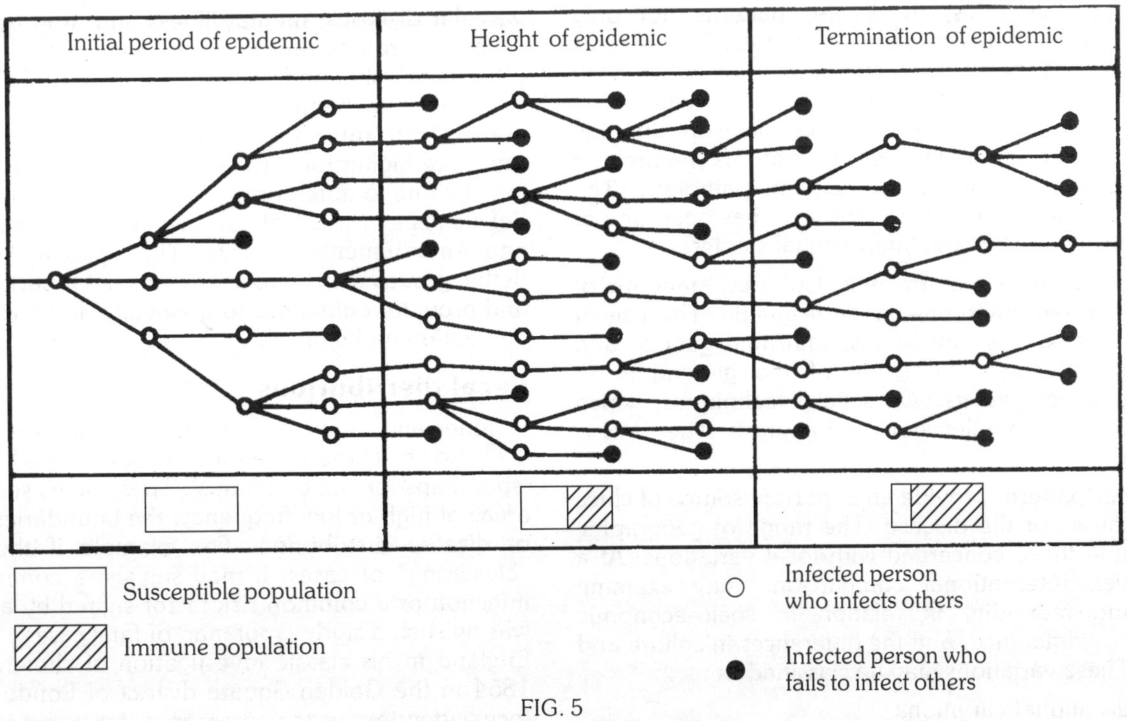

FIG. 5
Course of typical propagated epidemic

Source : *(5)*

III. Long-term or secular trends

The term "secular trend" implies changes in the occurrence of disease (i.e., a progressive increase or decrease) over a long period of time, generally several years or decades. Although it may have short-term fluctuations imposed on it, a secular trend implies a consistent tendency to change in a particular direction or a definite movement in one direction. Examples include coronary heart disease, lung cancer and diabetes which have shown a consistent upward trend in the developed countries during the past 50 years or so, followed by a decline of such diseases as tuberculosis, typhoid fever, diphtheria and polio.

Interpretation of time-trends

By surveillance or monitoring of time-trends, the epidemiologist seeks which diseases are increasing, which decreasing, and which are the emerging health problems and of the effectiveness of measures to control old ones *(17)*. He tries to formulate aetiological hypotheses, and seeks explanations whether these changes were due to changes in the aetiological agent or variations in diagnosis, reporting, case fatality or changes in age distribution, or some other determinants, specific and non-specific (e.g., changes in quality of life, socio-economic status and personal habits). For example the "time-clustering" of cases of adenocarcinoma of vagina in young women led to the incrimination of its cause, viz. *in utero* exposure to diethylstilbestrol *(27)*. Even changes taking place over several years or decades can be productive of hypotheses, as in the cases of lung cancer. By studying time trends, the epidemiologist seeks to provide guidelines to the health administrator in matters of prevention or control of disease.

PLACE DISTRIBUTION

(Geographical comparisons)

Studies of the geography of disease (or geographical pathology) is one of the important dimensions of descriptive epidemiology. By studying the distribution of disease in different populations we gain perspective on the fascinating differences (or variations) in disease patterns not only between countries, but also within countries. The relative importance of genes versus environment; changes with migration; and the possible roles of diet and other aetiological factors. In short geographical studies have profoundly influenced our understanding of disease, its nature, its detriments and its relation to subsequent pathology. The geographic variation in disease occurrence has been one of the stimulants to national and international studies.

The world is not a uniform unit. Cultures, standard of living and external environments vary greatly. The use of migrant studies is one way of distinguishing genetic and environmental factors. The study of the geography of diseases has developed its own special techniques, which sometimes involve complex statistical analysis. The SMR is one of them.

Geographic patterns provide an important source of clues about the causes of the disease. The range of geographic studies include those concerned with local variations. At a broader level, international comparisons may examine mortality and morbidity in relation to socio-economic factors, dietary differences and the differences in culture and behaviour. These variations may be classified as :

a. International variations
b. National variations
c. Rural–urban variations
d. Local distributions

International variations

Descriptive studies by place have shown that the pattern of disease is not the same everywhere. For example, we know that cancer exists all over the world. There is, however, a marked difference between the incidence of each cancer in different parts of the world. Thus cancer of the stomach is very common in Japan, but unusual in US. Cancers of the oral cavity and uterine cervix are exceedingly common in India as compared to industrialized countries. An international study of breast cancer showed that rates differ widely from country to country with the lowest prevalence in Japan and the highest in the western countries. Similarly, there are marked international differences in the occurrence of cardiovascular diseases. These variations have stimulated epidemiologists to search for cause–effect relationships between the environmental factors and disease. The aim is to identify factors which are crucial in the cause and prevention of disease.

National variations

It is obvious that variations in disease occurrence must also exist within countries or national boundaries. For example the distribution of endemic goitre, lathyrism, fluorosis, leprosy, malaria, nutritional deficiency diseases have all shown variations in their distribution in India, with some parts of the country more affected and others less affected or not affected at all. Such situations exist in every country. One of the functions of descriptive epidemiology is to provide data regarding the type of disease problems and their magnitude in terms of incidence, prevalence and mortality rates. Such information is needed to demarcate the affected areas and for providing appropriate health care services.

Rural-urban variations

Rural/urban variations in disease distribution are well known. Chronic bronchitis, accidents, lung cancer, cardiovascular diseases, mental illness and drug dependance are usually more frequent in urban than in rural areas. On the other hand, skin and zoonotic diseases and soil-transmitted helminths may be more frequent in rural areas than in urban areas. Death rates, especially infant and maternal mortality rates, are higher for rural than urban areas. These variations may be due to differences in population density, social class, deficiencies in medical care, levels of sanitation, education and environmental factors. The epidemiologist seeks to define groups which are at higher risk for particular diseases, and provides guidelines to the health administrator for their prevention and control.

Local distributions

Inner and outer city variations in disease frequency are well known. These variations are best studied with the aid of 'spot maps' or 'shaded maps'. These maps show at a glance areas of high or low frequency, the boundaries and patterns of disease distribution. For example if the map shows "clustering" of cases, it may suggest a common source of infection or a common risk factor shared by all the cases. It was by such a study (spot map of fatal cases), John Snow of England in his classic investigation of cholera epidemic in 1854 in the Golden Square district of London was able to focus attention on the common water pump in Broad street as the source of infection (Fig. 6). Based on his descriptive

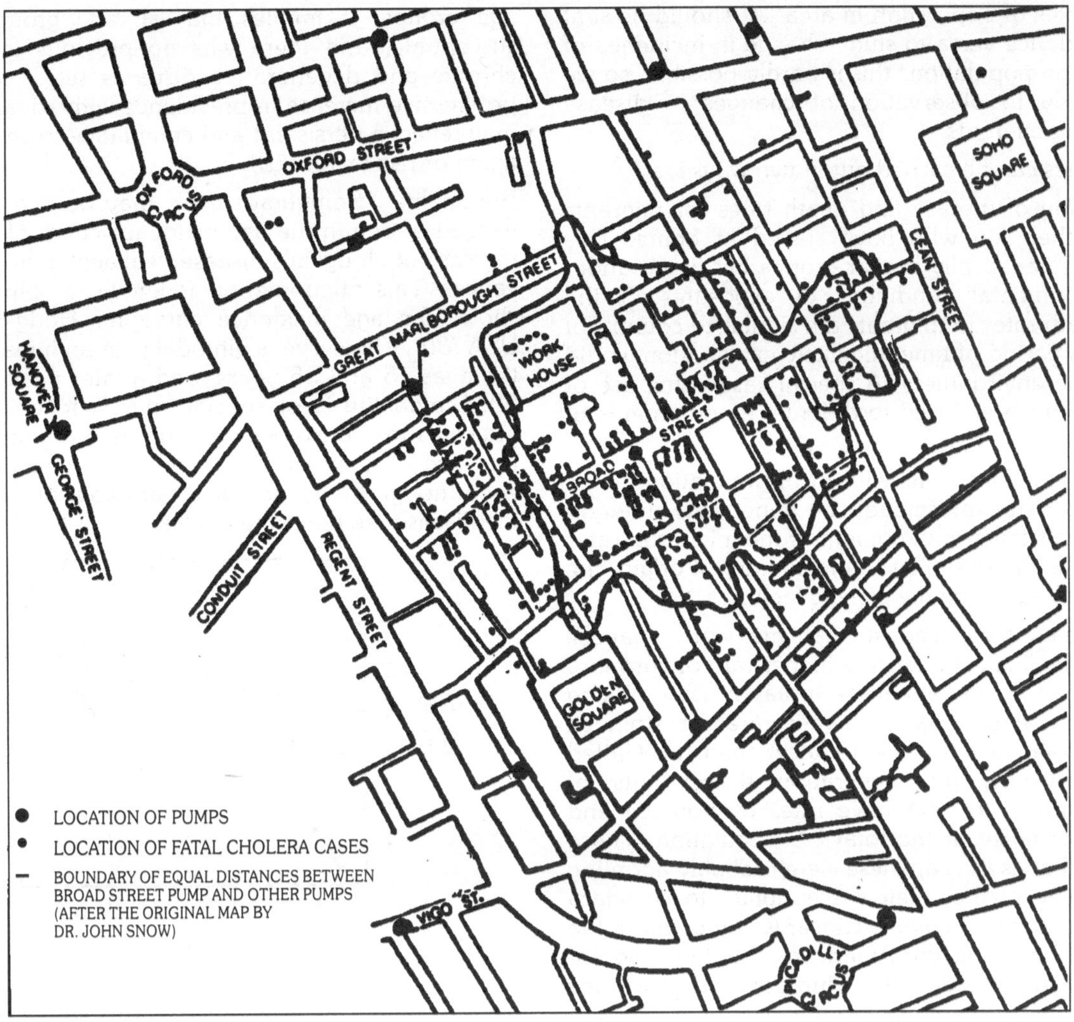

FIG. 6
Spot map of Asiatic cholera in London

findings, Snow was able to hypothesize that cholera was a water-borne disease, long before the birth of bacteriology. It was by a spot map by "place of employment" Maxcy hypothesized a rodent reservoir for typhus fever in 1920s which led to the discovery that typhus fever was not a single disease entity, as it was earlier thought. Also, the evidence of case clustering based on sexual contact or blood product use provided the clue that AIDS (Acquired Immune Deficiency Syndrome) was an infectious disease.

In short the geographic differences in disease occurrence is an important dimension of a descriptive study. These differences are determined by the agent, host and environmental factors. The classic example of place-related diseases include yellow fever, schistosomiasis, sleeping sickness and endemic goitre. There have also been studies on asthma, cancer, cardiovascular diseases, blood groups and abnormal haemoglobins by geographic location. In short, all diseases whether acute or chronic, communicable or non-communicable, show definite patterns of geographic distribution.

The epidemiologist is interested in geographic variations in disease occurrence. Geographic distribution may provide evidence of the source of disease and its mode of spread. By relating these variations to agent, host and environmental factors, he tries to derive clues to the source of disease and its mode of spread to formulate and test aetiological hypotheses. The clinician is also benefited from knowledge that a patient comes to him from a certain geographic area which is endemic for certain infrequent diseases such as yaws or leishmaniasis, as it helps him to focus attention on these diseases to which the patient may have been exposed.

The geographic distribution of disease may change, if changes occur in the agent, host and environmental factors. The empires of malaria, plague and many other diseases have shrunk due to changes in the epidemiological triad. On the other hand, since 1961 cholera has shown an increasing geographic distribution due to changes in the disease agent. Since the mode of living and environmental factors vary from country to country, one would expect to find differences in the geographic distribution and frequency of disease.

Migration studies

Large scale migration of human populations from one country to another provides a unique opportunity to evaluate the role of the possible genetic and environmental factors in the occurrence of disease in a population. Supposing there are marked geographic differences in the occurrence of a disease in two areas, area "A" and area "B". Let us assume that the environments in these two places are very different. The question arises whether the environmental differences in the two areas account for the variations in the occurrence of the disease in question.

Ideally, samples of population in area "A" should be sent to area "B", and vice versa to study change in incidence of disease. In human populations this is hardly possible, so we restrict our study to observation of changes in disease frequency among migrants.

Migrant studies can be carried out in two ways :

(a) comparison of disease and death rates for migrants with those of their kin who have stayed at home. This permits study of genetically similar groups but living under different environmental conditions or exposures. If the disease and death rates in migrants are similar to country of adoption over a period of time, the likely explanation would be change in the environment. A special case is the use of twins who have been exposed to different environments of migration.

(b) comparison of migrants with local population of the host country provides information on genetically different groups living in a similar environment. If the migration rates of disease and death are similar to the country of origin, the likely explanation would be the genetic factors.

Migrant studies have shown that men of Japanese ancestry living in USA experience a higher rate of coronary heart disease than do the Japanese in Japan *(28)*. Taking another example, Japan has a higher rate for stomach cancer and a lower rate for colon cancer than the United States has. However, third-generation descendants of Japanese immigrants to USA have rates of stomach and colon cancer like those of the total US population. These studies suggest that as the Japanese were probably adopting the American way of life, their susceptibility to coronary heart disease, gastric and colonic cancer was moving in the direction of that found in the Americans. Further, migrant studies may also indicate the duration of residence necessary to acquire susceptibility to the disease in question by comparing groups that left home at different ages. Studies of this kind provide a basis for further studies of specific environmental factors to which the migrants may have been exposed or of changes in their habits of life that may be of aetiological importance.

Migrant studies suffer from the usual defects of observational studies, deriving from lack of random assignment to the groups under observation. Migrants may be self-selected in that fit, vigorous and perhaps the temperamentally unstable are more likely to migrate *(29)*. The environmental factors may only act at a certain critical point or at a certain specific age. If the incubation period of the disease is very long, migrants may not show any increased incidence or mortality from the disease for many years.

PERSON DISTRIBUTION

In descriptive studies, the disease is further characterized by defining the persons who develop the disease by age, sex, occupation, martial status, habits, social class and other host factors. These factors do not necessarily represent aetiological factors, but they contribute a good deal to our understanding of the natural history of disease. Some of the host factors basic to epidemiological studies (Table 9) are discussed below.

(a) *Age* : Age is strongly related to disease than any other single host factor. Certain diseases are more frequent in certain age groups than in others, e.g., measles in childhood, cancer in middle age and atherosclerosis in old age. If the attack rate of a communicable disease is uniform in all the age groups, it implies that all age groups are equally susceptible, and there was no previous immunity. Many chronic and degenerative diseases (e.g., cancer) show a progressive increase in prevalence with advancing age. This may reflect a persistent and cumulative exposure to a causal agent or risk factor *(13)*.

Bimodality : Sometimes there may be two separate peaks instead of one in the age incidence curve of a disease as in the case of Hodgkin's disease, leukaemia, and female breast cancer. This phenomenon is known as bimodality. Fig. 7 shows the age incidence curve for Hodgkin's disease in USA *(30)*. The curve is bimodal with an initial peak between the ages 15 and 35 years, and a later peak starting at age 50. Bimodality is of special interest to epidemiologists. It indicates that the study material is not homogeneous, and that two distinct sets of causal factors might be operative, even though the clinical and pathological manifestations of the disease are the same at all ages.

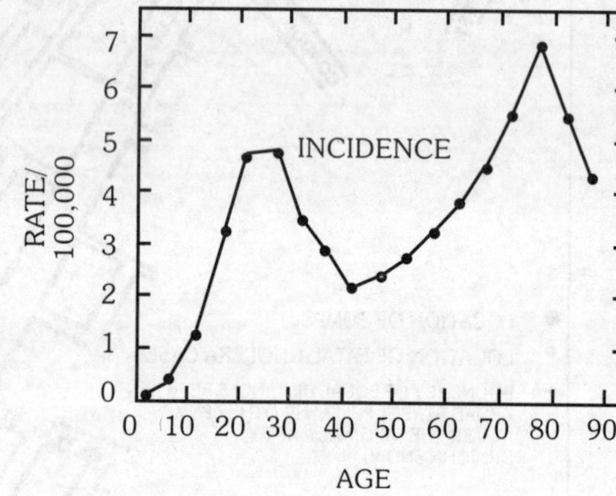

FIG. 7
Bimodality in Hodgkin's disease

However, there are two points relating to bimodality which make their interpretation difficult : (a) small numbers of observations are a frequent source of bimodality; (b) the absence of bimodality does not signify that data have come from a homogeneous source.

(b) *Sex* : Sex is another host characteristic which is often studied in relation to disease, using such indices as sex–ratio, sex–specific morbidity and mortality rates. It has been found that certain chronic diseases such as diabetes, hyperthyroidism and obesity are strikingly more common in women than in men, and diseases such as lung cancer and coronary heart disease are less frequent in women.

Variations in disease frequency between sexes have been ascribed to (a) basic biological differences between the sexes, including sex–linked genetic inheritance, and (b) cultural and behavioural differences between the sexes (e.g., smoking, automobile use, alcoholism) due to different roles in social setting. In fact, it is the 4:1 male to female ratio in lung cancer that has helped to identify cigarette smoking as a causal factor. Even larger differences exist in, for example, duodenal ulcer and coronary heart disease, that are as yet unexplained *(31)*.

(c) *Ethnicity* : Differences in disease occurrence have been noted between population subgroups of different racial and ethnic origin. These include tuberculosis, essential hypertension, coronary heart disease, cancer, and sickle cell anaemia. These differences, whether they are related to genetic or environmental factors, have been a stimulus to further studies.

(d) *Marital status* : In countries where studies on mortality in relation to marital status have been conducted, it was found that mortality rates were always lower for married males and females than for the unmarried, of the same age and sex. According to demographers and sociologists, the reason for this phenomenon may be found in the fact that marriages are selective with respect to the health status of persons, for those who are healthy are more likely to get married, with the result that the risk of dying is also less. Besides, married persons are generally more secure and protected and they usually lead a more sober life than those who are unmarried. All these factors are thought to contribute to lower mortality rates among married persons.

Marital status can be a risk factor for some diseases and conditions. The observation that cancer cervix is rare in nuns led to the hypothesis regarding marital status and cancer cervix. Further studies led to the suggestion that cancer cervix may be associated with multiple sexual contacts and promiscuity. This in turn raised the possibility of a possible infectious agent transmitted venereally. Although the viral aetiology of cancer cervix is not yet proved, this chain of thinking serves to illustrate how an observation can be a starting point of an epidemiological enquiry.

(e) *Occupation* : It is now well recognized that man's occupation from which he earns his livelihood has an important bearing on his health status. Occupation may alter the habit pattern of employees e.g., sleep, alcohol, smoking, drug addiction, night shifts etc. It is obvious that persons working in particular occupations are exposed to particular types of risks. For instance, while workers in coal mines are more likely to suffer from silicosis, those in sedentary occupations face the risk of heart disease.

(f) *Social class* : Epidemiological studies have shown that health and diseases are not equally distributed in social classes. Individuals in the upper social classes have a longer life expectancy and better health and nutritional status than those in the lower social classes. Certain diseases (e.g., coronary heart disease, hypertension, diabetes) have shown a higher prevalence in upper classes than in the lower classes. Social class differences have also been observed in mental illness and utilization of medical and health care services.

However, there is one snag. Social classification varies from country to country. It has different meanings for different persons. Therefore associations of disease with social class vary according to one's concept of social class. Consequently, it is difficult to compare the results of studies in which social class has been used differently by different investigators *(31)*.

(g) *Behaviour* : Human behaviour is increasingly looked upon as a risk factor in modern–day diseases such as coronary heart disease, cancer, obesity and accidents. The behavioural factors which have attracted the greatest attention are cigarette smoking, sedentary life, over-eating and drug abuse. To this must be added the mass movement of people, such as occurs in pilgrimages, which lends themselves to the transmission of infectious diseases such as cholera and diarrhoeal diseases, insect–borne and sexually transmitted diseases.

(h) *Stress* : Stress has been shown to affect a variety of variables related to patients response, e.g., susceptibility to disease, exacerbation of symptoms, compliance with medical regimen, etc.

(i) *Migration* : In India diseases like leprosy, filaria and malaria are considered to be rural problems. However, because of the movement of people from rural to urban areas these diseases have created a serious problem in urban areas also.

Human movement may be classified (i) as short-term, long-term, and permanent (ii) according to age, sex, education, occupation, (iii) internal or external (iv) urban versus rural, etc. Migration has presented challenge to control/prevention of disease.

To sum up, a study of the host factors in relation to disease occurrence is an important dimension of descriptive epidemiology. Variations in the distribution of disease in age, sex, occupation and other subgroups of the population can be the starting point for an epidemiological enquiry leading to formulation of an aetiological hypothesis for further study. Knowledge of the frequency of disease in subgroups of the population has also generated the concept of "high risk groups".

4. Measurement of disease

It is mandatory to have a clear picture of the amount of disease ("disease load") in the population. This information should be available in terms of mortality, morbidity, disability and so on, and should preferably be available for different subgroups of the population. Measurement of mortality is straightforward. Morbidity has two aspects – incidence and prevalence (see page 68, 69). Incidence can be obtained from "longitudinal" studies, and prevalence from "cross-sectional" studies. Descriptive epidemiology may use a cross-sectional or longitudinal design to obtain estimates of magnitude of health and disease problems in human populations.

Cross-sectional studies

Cross-sectional study is the simplest form of an observational study. It is based on a single examination of a cross-section of population at one point in time – the results of which can be projected on the whole population provided the sampling has been done correctly. Cross-sectional study is also known as "prevalence study".

Cross-sectional studies are more useful for chronic than short-lived diseases. For example, in a study of hypertension, we can also collect data during the survey about age, sex, physical exercise, body weight, salt intake and other variables of interest. Then we can determine how prevention of hypertension is related to certain variables simultaneously measured. Such a study tells us about the distribution of a disease in population rather than its aetiology.

The most common reason that epidemiologist examines the inter-relationships between a disease, or one of its precursors, and other variables is to attempt to establish a causal chain and so give lead to possible ways of preventing that disease. A point which must be stressed is that the time sequence which is essential to the concept of causativity cannot be deduced from cross-sectional data. However, frequently there is evidence that permits ranking of events to form such a sequence. That is, the distribution patterns may suggest causal hypothesis which can be tested by analytical studies. Although a cross-sectional study provides information about disease prevalence, it provides very little information about the natural history of disease or about the rate of occurrence of new cases (incidence).

Longitudinal studies

There is an increasing emphasis on the value of longitudinal studies in which observations are repeated in the same population over a prolonged period of time by means of follow-up examinations. Cross-sectional studies have been likened to a photograph, and longitudinal studies to a cine film. Longitudinal studies are useful (i) to study the natural history of disease and its future outcome (ii) for identifying risk factors of disease, and (iii) for finding out incidence rate or rate of occurrence of new cases of disease in the community. Longitudinal studies provide valuable information which the cross-sectional studies may not provide, but longitudinal studies are difficult to organize and more time-consuming than cross-sectional studies.

Measurement can also be extended to health states and events. For example, the study of blood pressure levels in a population will reveal the normal values, rather than abnormal ones related to disease.

5. Comparing with known indices

The essence of epidemiology is to make comparisons and ask questions. By making comparisons between different populations, and subgroups of the same population, it is possible to arrive at clues to disease aetiology. We can also identify or define groups which are at increased risk for certain diseases.

6. Formulation of a hypothesis

By studying the distribution of disease, and utilizing the techniques of descriptive epidemiology, it is often possible to formulate hypotheses relating to disease aetiology. A hypothesis is a supposition, arrived at from observation or reflection. It can be accepted or rejected, using the techniques of analytical epidemiology. An epidemiological hypothesis should specify the following *(13)* :

a. the population – the characteristics of the persons to whom the hypothesis applies
b. the specific cause being considered
c. the expected outcome – the disease
d. the dose–response relationship – the amount of the cause needed to lead to a stated incidence of the effect
e. the time–response relationship – the time period that will elapse between exposure to the cause and observation of the effect.

In other words, a hypothesis should be formulated in a manner that it can be tested taking into consideration the above elements. In practice, the components of a hypothesis are often less well–defined.

For example :

"Cigarette smoking causes lung cancer" – is an incomplete hypothesis.

An improved formulation

"The smoking of 30–40 cigarettes per day causes lung cancer in 10 per cent of smokers after 20 years of exposure"

The improved formulation suggests data needed to test the hypothesis, i.e., the number of cigarettes smoking per day, years of exposure, and so on. The success or failure of a research project frequently depends upon the soundness of the hypothesis *(13)*.

Uses of descriptive epidemiology

Descriptive studies : (a) provide data regarding the magnitude of the disease load and types of disease problems in the community in terms of morbidity and mortality rates and ratios (b) provide clues to disease aetiology, and help in the formulation of an aetiological hypothesis. That is, the existence of a possible causal association between a factor and a disease is usually recognized in descriptive studies. Thus, if the disease is observed to be more frequent in a particular group than in others, hypotheses are formulated to explain the increased frequency (c) provide background data for planning, organizing and evaluating preventive and curative services, and (d) they contribute to research by describing variations in disease occurrence by time, place and person.

ANALYTICAL EPIDEMIOLOGY

Analytical studies are the second major type of epidemiological studies. In contrast to descriptive studies that look at entire populations, in analytical studies, the subject of interest is the individual within the population. The object is not to formulate, but to test hypotheses. Nevertheless, although individuals are evaluated in analytical studies, the inference is not to individuals, but to the population from which they are selected.

Analytical studies comprise two distinct types of observational studies :

a. case control study
b. cohort study.

From each of these study designs, one can determine :

a. whether or not a statistical association exists between a disease and a suspected factor; and
b. if one exists, the strength of the Association.

A schematic design of case control and cohort studies is shown in Fig. 8.

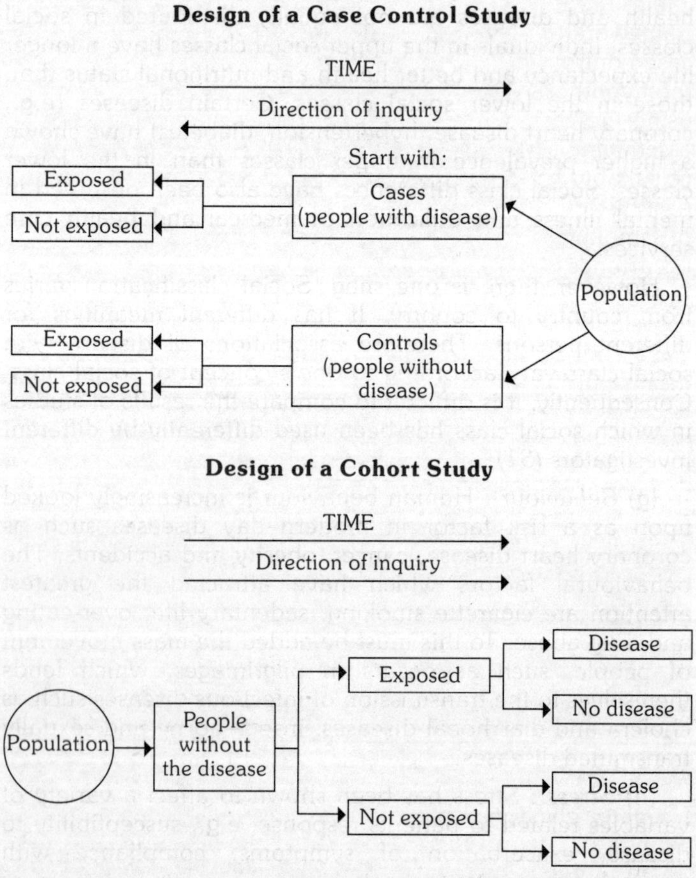

FIG. 8
Schematic diagram of the design of case control and cohort studies
Source : *(32)*

CASE CONTROL STUDY

Case control studies, often called "retrospective studies" are a common first approach to test causal hypothesis. In recent years, the case control approach has emerged as a permanent method of epidemiological investigation. The case control method has three distinct features :

a. both exposure and outcome (disease) have occurred before the start of the study
b. the study proceeds backwards from effect to cause; and
c. it uses a control or comparison group to support or refute an inference.

By definition, a case control study involves two populations – cases and controls. In case control studies, the unit is the individual rather than the group. The focus is on a disease or some other health problem that has already developed.

Case control studies are basically comparison studies. Cases and controls must be comparable with respect to known "confounding factors" such as age, sex, occupation, social status, etc. The questions asked relate to personal characteristics and antecedent exposures which may be responsible for the condition studied. For example, one can use as "cases" the immunized children and use as "controls" un-immunized children, and look for factors of interest in their past histories. Case control studies have been used effectively for studies of many cancers, and other serious conditions such as cirrhosis of the liver, lupus erythematosis, and congestive heart failure.

The basic design of a case control study is shown in Table 11. It is a 2×2 table which provides a very useful framework to discuss the various elements which make up a case control study. To illustrate, if it is our intention to test the hypothesis that "cigarette smoking causes lung cancer", using the case control method, the investigation begins by assembling a group of lung cancer cases (a+c), and a group of suitably matched controls (b+d). One then explores the past history of these two groups for the presence or absence of smoking, which is suspected to be related to the occurrence of cancer lung. If the frequency of smoking, a/(a+c) is higher in cases than in controls b/(b+d), an association is said to exist between smoking and lung cancer. Case control studies have their major use in the chronic disease problem when the causal pathway may span many decades.

TABLE 11

Framework of a case control study
(The 2 × 2 contingency table)

Suspected or risk factors	Cases (Disease present)	Control (Disease absent)
Present	a	b
Absent	c	d
	a+c	b+d

Basic steps

There are four basic steps in conducting a case control study :

1. Selection of cases and controls
2. Matching
3. Measurement of exposure, and
4. Analysis and interpretation.

1. Selection of cases and controls

The first step is to identify a suitable group of cases and a group of controls. While identification of cases is relatively easy, selection of suitable controls may present difficulties. In this connection, definite guidelines have been laid down such as the following *(5, 10, 13)*.

(1) SELECTION OF CASES

(a) *Definition of a case* : The prior definition of what constitutes a "case" is crucial to the case control study. It involves two specifications : (i) DIAGNOSTIC CRITERIA : The diagnostic criteria of the disease and the stage of disease, if any (e.g., breast cancer Stage I) to be included in the study must be specified before the study is undertaken. Supposing we are investigating cases of cancer, we should be quite clear that we have, for our cases, a group histologically the same. Once the diagnostic criteria are established, they should not be altered or changed till the study is over. (ii) ELIGIBILITY CRITERIA : The second criterion is that of eligibility. A criterion customarily employed is the requirement that only newly diagnosed ***(incident)*** cases within a specified period of time are eligible than old cases or cases in advanced stages of the disease ***(prevalent cases)***.

(b) *Sources of cases* : The cases may be drawn from (i) hospitals, or (ii) general population. (i) HOSPITALS : It is often convenient to select cases from hospitals. The cases may be drawn from a single hospital or a network of hospitals, admitted during a specified period of time. The entire case series or a random sample of it is selected for study. (ii) GENERAL POPULATION : In a population–based case control study, all cases of the study disease occurring within a defined geographic area during a specified period of time are ascertained, often through a survey, a disease registry or hospital network. The entire case series or a random sample of it is selected for study. The cases should be fairly representative of all cases in the community.

(2) SELECTION OF CONTROLS

The controls must be free from the disease under study. They must be as similar to the cases as possible, except for the absence of the disease under study. As a rule, a comparison group is identified before a study is done, comprising of persons who have not been exposed to the disease or some other factor whose influence is being studied. Difficulties may arise in the selection of controls if the disease under investigation occurs in subclinical forms whose diagnosis is difficult. Selection of an appropriate control group is therefore an important prerequisite, for it is against this, we make comparisons, draw inferences and make judgements about the outcome of the investigation *(10)*.

Sources of controls : The possible sources from which controls may be selected include hospitals, relatives, neighbours and general population. (i) HOSPITAL CONTROLS: The controls may be selected from the same hospital as the cases, but with different illneses other than the study disease. For example, if we are going to study cancer cervix patients, the control group may comprise patients with cancer breast, cancer of the digestive tract, or patients with non-cancerous lesions and other patients. Usually it is unwise to choose a control group from a group of patients with one disease. This is because hospital controls are often a source of "selection bias". Many hospital patients may have diseases which are also influenced by the factor under study. For example, if one was studying the relationship of smoking and myocardial infarction and chooses bladder cancer cases as controls, the relationship between smoking and myocardial infarction may not have been demonstrated. Therefore, great care must be taken when using other patients as comparison subjects, for they differ in many ways from a normal healthy population. Ideally the controls should have undergone the same diagnostic work-up as cases, but have been found to be negative. But this may not be acceptable to most controls (ii) RELATIVES : The controls may also be taken up from relatives (spouses and siblings). Sibling controls are unsuitable where genetic conditions are under study. (iii) NEIGHBOURHOOD CONTROLS : The controls may be drawn from persons living in the same locality as cases, persons working in the same factory or children attending the same school. (iv) GENERAL POPULATION : Population controls can be obtained from defined geographic areas, by taking a random sample of individuals free of the study disease. We must use great care in the selection of controls to be certain that they accurately reflect the population that is free of the disease of interest.

How many controls are needed ? If many cases are available, and large study is contemplated, and if the cost to collect case and control is about equal, then one tends to use one control for each case. If the study group is small (say under 50) as many as 2,3, or even 4 controls can be selected for each study subject.

To sum up, selection of proper cases and controls is crucial to the interpretation of the results of case control studies. Some investigators select cases from one source and controls from more than one source to avoid the influence of "selection bias". Such studies are recommended by epidemiologists. It is also desired to conduct more than one case control study, preferably in different geographic areas. If the findings are consistent, it serves to increase the validity (i.e., accuracy) of the inferences. Failure to select comparable controls can introduce "bias" into results of case control studies and decrease the confidence one can place in the findings.

2. Matching

The controls may differ from the cases in a number of factors such as age, sex, occupation, social status, etc. An important consideration is to ensure *comparability* between cases and controls. This involves what is known as "matching". Matching is defined as the process by which we select controls in such a way that they are similar to cases with regard to certain pertinent selected variables (e.g., age) which are known to influence the outcome of disease and which, if not adequately matched for comparability, could distort or confound the results. A "confounding factor" is defined as one which is associated both with exposure and disease, and is distributed unequally in study and control groups. More specifically a "confounding factor" is one that, although associated with "exposure" under investigation, is itself, independently of any such association, a "risk factor" for the disease. Two examples are cited to explain confounding.

(a) In the study of the role of alcohol in the aetiology of oesophageal cancer, smoking is a confounding factor because (i) it is associated with the consumption of alcohol and (ii) it is an independent risk factor for oesophageal cancer. In these conditions, the effects of alcohol consumption can be determined only if the influence of smoking is neutralized by matching *(33)*.

(b) Age could be a confounding variable. Supposing, we are investigating the relationship between steroid contraceptive and breast cancer. If the women taking these contraceptives were younger than those in the comparison group, they would necessarily be at lower risk of breast cancer since this disease becomes increasingly common with increasing age. This "confounding" effect of age can be neutralized by matching so that both the groups have an equal proportion of each age group. In other words, matching protects against an unexpected strong association between the matching factor (e.g., age) and the disease (e.g., breast cancer). In a similar fashion other confounding variables will have to be matched.

While matching it should be borne in mind that the suspected aetiological factor or the variable we wish to measure should not be matched, because by matching, its aetiological role is eliminated in that study. The cases and controls will then become automatically alike with respect to that factor. In the above example, it would be useless to match cases and controls on steroid contraceptive use; by doing so, the aetiological role of steroid contraceptive cannot be investigated.

There are several kinds of matching procedures. One is group matching. This may be done by assigning cases to sub-categories (strata) based on their characteristics (e.g., age, occupation, social class) and then establishing appropriate controls. The frequency distribution of the matched variable must be similar in study and comparison groups. Matching is also done by *pairs*. For example, for each case, a control is chosen which can be matched quite closely. Thus, if we have a 50 year old mason with a particular disease, we will search for 50 year old mason without the disease as a control. Thus one can obtain pairs of patients and controls of the same sex, age, duration and severity of illness, etc. But there may be great difficulties in obtaining cases and controls matched on all characteristics, and it may be necessary to wait a considerable period of time before obtaining a sufficient number of matched pairs. Therefore, some leeway is necessary in matching for variables *(34, 35)*. It should be noted that if matching is overdone, it may be difficult to find controls. Further with excess zeal in matching, there may be a tendency to reduce the odds ratio.

3. Measurement of exposure

Definitions and criteria about exposure (or variables which may be of aetiological importance) are just as important as those used to define cases and controls. Information about exposure should be obtained in precisely the same manner both for cases and controls. This may be obtained by interviews, by questionnaires or by studying past records of cases such as hospital records, employment records, etc. It is important to recognize that when case control studies are being used to test associations, the most important factor to be considered, even more important than the *P. values* obtained, is the question of "bias" or systematic error which must be ruled out (see page 81).

4. Analysis

The final step is analysis, to find out

(a) Exposure rates among cases and controls to suspected factor

(b) Estimation of disease risk associated with exposure (Odds ratio)

(a) EXPOSURE RATES

A case control study provides a direct estimation of the exposure rates (frequency of exposure) to a suspected factor in disease and non-disease groups. Table 12 shows how exposure rates may be calculated from a case control study.

TABLE 12

A case control study of smoking and lung cancer

	Cases (with lung cancer)	Controls (without lung cancer)	Total
Smokers (less than 5 cigarettes a day)	33 (a)	55 (b)	88 (a+b)
Non-smokers	2 (c)	27 (d)	29 (c+d)
Total	35 (a+c)	82 (b+d)	n = a+b +c+d

Source : *(36)*

Exposure rates

a. Cases = a/(a+c) = 33/35 = 94.2 per cent
b. Controls = b/(b+d) = 55/82 = 67.0 per cent
$P < 0.001$

Table 12 shows that the frequency rate of lung cancer was definitely higher among smokers than among non-smokers. The next step will be to ascertain whether there is a *statistical association* between exposure status and occurrence of lung cancer. This question can be resolved by calculating the *P. value,* which in this case is less than 0.001.

The particular test of significance will depend upon the variables under investigation. If we are dealing with discrete variables, as in the present case (smoking and lung cancer; exposure and disease) the results are usually presented as rates or proportions of those present or absent in the study and in the control group. The test of significance usually adopted is the standard error of difference between two proportions or the Chi–square test. On the other hand, if we are dealing with *continuous variables* (e.g., age, blood pressure), the data will have to be grouped and the test of significance used is likely to be the standard error of difference between two means, or test.

According to convention, if *P* is less than or equal to 0.05, it is regarded as "statistically significant". The smaller the *P.* value, the greater the statistical significance or probability that the association is not due to chance alone. However, statistical association (*P.* value) does not imply causation. Statement of *P.* value is thus an inadequate, although common end-point of case control studies.

(b) ESTIMATION OF RISK

The second analytical step is estimation of disease risk associated with exposure. It should be noted (Table 12) that if the exposure rate was 94.2 per cent in the study group, it does not mean that 94.2 per cent of those smoked would develop lung cancer. The estimation of disease risk associated with exposure is obtained by an index known as "Relative Risk" (RR) or "risk ratio", which is defined as the ratio between the incidence of disease among exposed persons and incidence among non-exposed. It is given by the formula:

$$\text{Relative risk} = \frac{\text{Incidence among exposed}}{\text{Incidence among non-exposed}}$$

$$= \frac{a}{(a+b)} \div \frac{c}{(c+d)}$$

A typical case control study does not provide incidence rates from which relative risk can be calculated directly, because there is no appropriate denominator or population at risk, to calculate these rates. In general, the relative risk can be exactly determined only from a cohort study.

Odds Ratio (Cross-product ratio)

From a case control study, we can derive what is known as Odds Ratio (OR) which is a measure of the strength of the association between risk factor and outcome. Odds ratio is closely related to relative risk. The derivation of odds ratio is based on three assumptions : (a) the disease being investigated must be relatively rare; (b) the cases must be representative of those with the disease, and (c) the controls must be representative of those without the disease. The odds ratio is the cross product of the entries in Table 11 which is reproduced below :

	Diseases	
	Yes	*No*
Exposed	a	b
Not exposed	c	d

Odds ratio = ad/bc

Using the data in Table 12, the odds ratio would be estimated as follows :

$$\text{Odds ratio} = \left(\frac{a}{b}\right)/\left(\frac{c}{d}\right) = \frac{ad}{bc}$$

$$= \frac{33 \times 27}{55 \times 2} = 8.1$$

In the above example, smokers of less than 5 cigarettes per day showed a risk of having lung cancer 8.1 times that of non-smokers. Odds ratio is a key parameter in the analysis of case control studies.

Bias in case control studies

Bias is any systematic error in the determination of the association between the exposure and disease. The relative risk estimate may increase or decrease as a result of the bias; it reflects some type of non-comparability between the study and control groups. The possibility of bias must be considered when evaluating a possible cause and effect relationship.

Many varieties of bias may arise in epidemiological studies. Some of these are : (a) *Bias due to confounding* : Mention has already been made about confounding as an important source of bias. This bias can be removed by matching in case control studies. (b) *Memory or recall bias* : When cases and controls are asked questions about their past history, it may be more likely for the cases to recall the existence of certain events or factors, than the controls who are healthy persons. For example, those who have had a myocardial infarction might be more likely to remember and recall certain habits or events than those who have not. Thus cases may have a different recall of past events than controls. (c) *Selection bias* : The cases and controls may not be representative of cases and controls in the general population. There may be systematic differences in characteristics between cases and controls. The selection bias can be best controlled by its prevention (d) *Berkesonian bias* : A special example of bias is Berkesonian bias, termed after Dr. Joseph Berkeson who recognized this problem. The bias arises because of the different rates of admission to hospitals for people with different diseases (i.e., hospital cases and controls). (e) *Interviewer's bias* : Bias may also occur when the interviewer knows the hypothesis and also knows who the cases are. This prior information may lead him to question the cases more thoroughly than controls regarding a positive history of the suspected causal factor. A useful check on this kind of bias can be made by noting the length of time taken to interview the average case and the average control. This type of bias can be eliminated by double-blinding (see page 91).

Advantages and disadvantages

Table 13 summarizes the advantages and disadvantages of case control studies.

TABLE 13

Advantages and disadvantages of case control studies

ADVANTAGES

1. Relatively easy to carry out.
2. Rapid and inexpensive (compared with cohort studies).
3. Require comparatively few subjects.
4. Particularly suitable to investigate rare diseases or diseases about which little is known. But a disease which is rare in the general population (e.g., leukaemia in adolescents) may not be rare in special exposure group (e.g. prenatal X-rays).
5. No risk to subjects.
6. Allows the study of several different aetiological factors (e.g., smoking, physical activity and personality characteristics in myocardial infarction).
7. Risk factors can be identified. Rational prevention and control programmes can be established.
8. No attrition problems, because case control studies do not require follow-up of individuals into the future.
9. Ethical problems minimal.

DISADVANTAGES

1. Problems of bias relies on memory or past records, the accuracy of which may be uncertain; validation of information obtained is difficult or sometimes impossible.
2. Selection of an appropriate control group may be difficult.
3. We cannot measure incidence, and can only estimate the relative risk.
4. Do not distinguish between causes and associated factors.
5. Not suited to the evaluation of therapy or prophylaxis of disease.
6. Another major concern is the representativeness of cases and controls.

Source : *(37, 38)*

Examples of case control studies

Case control studies have provided much of the current base of knowledge in epidemiology. Some of the early case control studies centred round cigarette smoking and lung cancer *(36, 39, 40)*. Other studies include: maternal smoking and congenital malformations *(41)*, radiation and leukaemia *(42)*, oral contraceptive use and hepatocellular adenoma *(43)*, herpes simplex and Bell palsy *(44)*, induced abortion and spontaneous abortion *(45)*, physical activity and coronary death *(46)*, artificial sweeteners and bladder cancer *(47)*, etc.

A few studies are cited in detail :

Example 1: *Adenocarcinoma of vagina (27).*

An excellent example of a case control study is adenocarcinoma of the vagina in young women. It is not only a rare disease, but also the usual victim is over 50 years of age. There was an unusual occurrence of this tumor in 7 young women (15 to 22 years) born in one Boston hospital between 1966 and 1969. The apparent "time clustering" of cases – 7 occurring within 4 years at a single hospital – led to this enquiry. An eighth case occurred in 1969 in a 20 year old patient who was treated at another Boston hospital in USA.

The cause of this tumor was investigated by a case control study in 1971 to find out the factors that might be associated with this tumor. As this was a rare disease, for each case, four matched controls were put up. The controls were identified from the birth records of the hospital in which each case was born. Female births occurring closest in time to each patient were selected as controls. Information was collected by personal interviews regarding (a) maternal age (b) maternal smoking (c) antenatal radiology, and (d) diethyl-stilbestrol (DES) exposure in foetal life. The results of the study are shown in Table 14 which shows that cases differed significantly from the controls in their past history. Seven of the eight cases had been exposed to DES in foetal life. This drug had been given to their mothers during the first trimester of pregnancy to prevent possible miscarriage. But none of the mothers in the control group had received DES. Since this study, more cases have been reported and the association with DES has been confirmed. The case control method played a critical role in revealing exposure to DES *in utero* as the cause of vaginal adenocarcinoma in the exposed child 10–20 years later.

TABLE 14

Association between maternal DES therapy and adenocarcinoma of vagina amongst female offspring

Information acquired retrospectively	Cases (8)	Controls (32)	Significance level
Maternal age	26.1	29.3	n.s.
Maternal smoking	7	21	n.s.
Antenatal radiology	1	4	n.s.
Oestrogen exposure	7	–	P<0.00001

Source : *(27)*

Example 2: *Oral contraceptives and thromboembolic disease (48, 49).*

By August 1965, the British Committee on Safety of Drugs had received 249 reports of adverse reactions and 16 reports of death in women taking oral contraceptives. It became apparent that epidemiological studies were needed to determine whether women who took oral contraceptives were at greater risk of developing thromboembolic disease.

In 1968 and 1969, Vassey and Doll reported the findings of their case control studies in which they interviewed women who had been admitted to hospitals with venous thrombosis or pulmonary embolism without medical cause and compared the history with that obtained from other women who had been admitted to the same hospital with other diseases and who were matched for age, marital status and parity.

It was found that out of 84, 42 (50%) of those with venous thrombosis and pulmonary embolism had been using oral contraceptives, compared with 14% of controls (Table 15). The studies confirmed that taking the pill and having pulmonary embolism co-existed more frequently than would be expected by chance. The relative risk of users to non-users was 6.3:1. That is, the investigators found that users of oral contraceptives were about 6 times as likely as non-users to develop thromboembolic disease.

TABLE 15
Case control studies on the safety of oral contraceptives

	No.	Per cent who used oral contraceptives
Cases (venous thrombosis and pulmonary embolism)	84	50
Controls	168	14

Source : *(48, 49)*

Example 3 : Thalidomide tragedy (50).

Thalidomide was first marketed as a safe, non-barbiturate hypnotic in Britain in 1958. In 1961, at a congress of Gynaecologists, attention was drawn to the birth of a large number of babies with congenital abnormalities, which was previously rare. In the same year, it was suggested that thalidomide might be responsible for it.

A retrospective study of 46 mothers delivered of deformed babies showed that 41 were found to have thalidomide during their early pregnancy. This was compared with a control of 300 mothers who had delivered normal babies; none of these had taken thalidomide. Laboratory experiments confirmed that thalidomide was teratogenic in experimental studies *(50)*.

COHORT STUDY

Cohort study is another type of analytical (observational) study which is usually undertaken to obtain additional evidence to refute or support the existence of an association between suspected cause and disease. Cohort study is known by a variety of names : prospective study, longitudinal study, incidence study, and forward–looking study. The most widely used term, however, is "cohort study" *(5)*.

The distinguishing features of cohort studies are :

a. the cohorts are identified prior to the appearance of the disease under investigation
b. the study groups, so defined, are observed over a period of time to determine the frequency of disease among them
c. the study proceeds forward from cause to effect.

Concept of cohort

In epidemiology, the term "cohort" is defined as a group of people who share a common characteristic or experience within a defined time period (e.g., age, occupation, exposure to a drug or vaccine, pregnancy, insured persons, etc). Thus a group of people born on the same day or in the same period of time (usually a year) form a "birth cohort". All those born in 2010 form the birth cohort of 2010. Persons exposed to a common drug, vaccine or infection within a defined period constitute an "exposure cohort". A group of males or females married on the same day or in the same period of time form a "marriage cohort". A cohort might be all those who survived a myocardial infarction in one particular year.

The comparison group may be the general population from which the cohort is drawn, or it may be another cohort of persons thought to have had little or no exposure to the substance in question, but otherwise similar.

Indications for cohort studies

Cohort studies are indicated : (a) when there is good evidence of an association between exposure and disease, as derived from clinical observations and supported by descriptive and case control studies (b) when exposure is rare, but the incidence of disease high among exposed, e.g., special exposure groups like those in industries, exposure to X-rays, etc (c) when attrition of study population can be minimized, e.g., follow-up is easy, cohort is stable, co-operative and easily accessible, and (d) when ample funds are available.

Framework of a cohort study

In contrast to case control studies which proceed from "effect to cause", the basic approach in cohort studies is to work from "cause to effect" (Fig. 8). That is, in a case control study, exposure and disease have already occurred when the study is initiated. In a cohort study, the exposure has occurred, but the disease has not.

The basic design of a simple cohort study is shown in Table 16. We begin with a group or cohort (a+b) exposed to a particular factor thought to be related to disease occurrence, and a group (c+d) not exposed to that particular factor. The former is known as "study cohort", and the latter "control cohort".

TABLE 16
Framework of a cohort study

	Disease		
Cohort	yes	no	Total
Exposed to putative aetiologic factor	a	b	a + b
Not exposed to putative aetiologic factor	c	d	c + d

In assembling cohorts, the following general considerations are taken into account :

a. The cohorts must be free from the disease under study. Thus, if the disease under study is coronary heart disease, the cohort members are first examined and those who already have evidence of the disease under investigation are excluded.
b. Insofar as the knowledge of the disease permits, both the groups (i.e., study and control cohorts) should be equally susceptible to the disease under study, or efficiently reflect any difference in disease occurrence (for example, males over 35 years would be appropriate for studies on lung cancer).
c. Both the groups should be comparable in respect of all the possible variables, which may influence the frequency of the disease; and
d. The diagnostic and eligibility criteria of the disease must be defined beforehand; this will depend upon the availability of reliable methods for recognizing the disease when it develops.

The groups are then followed, under the same identical conditions, over a period of time to determine the outcome of exposure (e.g., onset of disease, disability or death) in both the groups. In chronic diseases such as cancer the time required for the follow-up may be very long.

Table 16 shows (a+b) persons were exposed to the factor under study, 'a' of which developed the disease during the follow-up period; (c+d) persons were not exposed, 'c' of which became cases (it is assumed for simplicity of presentation that there were no intermittent deaths or losses during the follow-up period). After the end of the follow-up, the incidence rate of the disease in both the groups is determined. If it is found that the incidence of the disease in the exposed group, a/(a+b) is significantly higher than in the non-exposed group, c/(c+d), it would suggest that the disease and suspected cause are associated. Since the approach is prospective, that is, studies are planned to observe events that have not yet occurred, cohort studies are frequently referred to as "prospective" studies.

A well-designed cohort study is considered the most reliable means of showing an association between a suspected risk factor and subsequent disease because it eliminates many of the problems of the case control study and approximates the experimental model of the physical sciences.

Types of cohort studies

Three types of cohort studies have been distinguished on the basis of the time of occurrence of disease in relation to the time at which the investigation is initiated and continued :

1. Prospective cohort studies
2. Retrospective cohort studies, and
3. A combination of retrospective and prospective cohort studies.

1. Prospective cohort studies

A prospective cohort study (or "current" cohort study) is one in which the outcome (e.g., disease) has not yet occurred at the time the investigation begins. Most prospective studies begin in the present and continue into future. For example, the long-term effects of exposure to uranium was evaluated by identifying a group of uranium miners and a comparison group of individuals not exposed to uranium mining and by assessing subsequent development of lung cancer in both the groups. The principal finding was that the uranium miners had an excess frequency of lung cancer compared to non-miners. Since the disease had not yet occurred when the study was undertaken, this was a prospective cohort design. The US Public Health Service's Framingham Heart Study *(51)*, Doll and Hills *(52)* prospective study on smoking and lung cancer, and study of oral contraceptives and health by the Royal College of General Practitioners *(53)* are examples of this type of study.

2. Retrospective cohort studies

A retrospective cohort study (or "historical" cohort study) is one in which the outcomes have all occurred before the start of the investigation. The investigator goes back in time, sometimes 10 to 30 years, to select his study groups from existing records of past employment, medical or other records and traces them forward through time, from a past date fixed on the records, usually up to the present. This type of study is known by a variety of names : retrospective cohort study, "historical" cohort study, prospective study in retrospect and non-concurrent prospective study.

The successful application of this approach is illustrated in one study undertaken in 1978 – a cohort of 17,080 babies born between January 1, 1969 and December 31, 1975 at a Boston hospital were investigated of the effects of electronic foetal monitoring during labour. The outcome measured was neonatal death. The study showed that the neonatal death rate was 1.7 times higher in unmonitored infants *(54)*. The most notable retrospective cohort studies to date are those of occupational exposures, because the recorded information is easily available, e.g., study of the role of arsenic in human carcinogenesis, study of lung cancer in uranium miners, study of the mortality experience of groups of physicians in relation to their probable exposure to radiation *(55,56,57)*. More recently, angiosarcoma of the liver, a very rare disease, has been reported in excess frequency in relation to poly-vinyl chloride *(58)*. This association was picked up only because of the retrospective cohort design. Retrospective cohort studies are generally more economical and produce results more quickly than prospective cohort studies.

3. Combination of retrospective and prospective cohort studies

In this type of study, both the retrospective and prospective elements are combined. The cohort is identified from past records, and is assessed of date for the outcome. The same cohort is followed up prospectively into future for further assessment of outcome.

Court–Brown and Doll (1957) applied this approach to study the effects of radiation. They assembled a cohort in 1955 consisting of 13,352 patients who had received large doses of radiation therapy for ankylosing spondylitis between 1934 and 1954. The outcome evaluated was death from leukaemia or aplastic anaemia between 1935 and 1954. They found that the death rate from leukaemia or aplastic anaemia was substantially higher in their cohort than that of the general population. A prospective component was added to the study and the cohort was followed, as established in 1955, to identify deaths occurring in subsequent years *(59)*.

ELEMENTS OF A COHORT STUDY

The elements of a cohort study are :

1. Selection of study subjects
2. Obtaining data on exposure
3. Selection of comparison groups
4. Follow-up, and
5. Analysis.

1. Selection of study subjects

The subjects of a cohort study are usually assembled in one of two ways – either from general population or select groups of the population that can be readily studied (e.g., persons with different degrees of exposure to the suspected causal factor).

(a) *General population* : When the exposure or cause of death is fairly frequent in the population, cohorts may be assembled from the general population, residing in well-defined geographical, political and administrative areas (e.g., Framingham Heart Study). If the population is very large, an appropriate sample is taken, so that the results can be generalized to the population sampled. The exposed and unexposed segments of the population to be studied should be representative of the corresponding segments of the general population.

(b) *Special groups* : These may be special groups or exposure groups that can readily be studied : (i) *Select groups* : These may be professional groups (e.g., doctors, nurses, lawyers, teachers, civil servants), insured persons, obstetric population, college alumni, government employees, volunteers, etc. These groups are usually a homogeneous population. Doll's prospective study on smoking and lung cancer was carried out on British doctors listed in the Medical Register of the UK in 1951 *(60)*. The study by Dorn on smoking and mortality in 293,658 veterans (i.e., former military service) in United States having life insurance policies is another example of a study based on special groups *(61)*. These groups are not only homogeneous, but they also offer advantages of accessibility and easy follow-up for a protracted period (ii) *Exposure groups* : If the exposure is rare, a more economical procedure is to select a cohort of persons known to have experienced the exposure. In other words, cohorts may be selected because of special exposure to physical, chemical and other disease agents. A readily accessible source of these groups is workers in industries and those employed in high-risk situations (e.g., radiologists exposed to X-rays).

When cohorts have been selected because of special exposure, it facilitates classification of cohort members according to the degree or duration of exposure to the suspected factor for subsequent analytical study.

2. Obtaining data on exposure

Information about exposure may be obtained directly from the (a) *Cohort members :* through personal interviews or mailed questionnaires. Since cohort studies involve large numbers of population, mailed questionnaires offer a simple and economic way of obtaining information. For example, Doll and Hill *(62)* used mailed questionnaires to collect smoking histories from British doctors. (b) *Review of records :* Certain kinds of information (e.g., dose of radiation, kinds of surgery, or details of medical treatment) can be obtained only from medical records. (c) *Medical examination or special tests :* Some types of information can be obtained only by medical examination or special tests, e.g., blood pressure, serum cholesterol, ECG. (d) *Environmental surveys :* This is the best source for obtaining information on exposure levels of the suspected factor in the environment where the cohort lived or worked. In fact, information may be needed from more than one or all of the above sources.

Information about exposure (or any other factor related to the development of the disease being investigated) should be collected in a manner that will allow classification of cohort members :

(a) according to whether or not they have been exposed to the suspected factor, and
(b) according to the level or degree of exposure, at least in broad classes, in the case of special exposure groups (Table 17).

In addition to the above, basic information about demographic variables which might affect the frequency of disease under investigation, should also be collected. Such information will be required for subsequent analysis.

3. Selection of comparison groups

There are many ways of assembling comparison groups :

(a) Internal comparisons

In some cohort studies, no outside comparison group is required. The comparison groups are in-built. That is, single cohort enters the study, and its members may, on the basis of information obtained, be classified into several comparison groups according to the degrees or levels of exposure to risk (e.g., smoking, blood pressure, serum cholesterol) before the development of the disease in question. The groups, so defined, are compared in terms of their subsequent morbidity and mortality rates. Table 17 illustrates this point. It shows that mortality from lung cancer increases with increasing number of cigarettes smoked reinforcing the conclusion that there is valid association between smoking and lung cancer.

TABLE 17

Age standardized death rates per 100,000 men per year by amount of current smoking

Classification of exposure (cigarettes)	No. of deaths	Death rate
1/2 pack	24	95.2
1/2–1 pack	84	107.8
1–2 packs	90	229.2
2 packs +	97	264.2

Source : *(6)*

(b) External comparisons

When information on degree of exposure is not available, it is necessary to put up an external control, to evaluate the experience of the exposed group, e.g., smokers and non-smokers, a cohort of radiologists compared with a cohort of ophthalmologists, etc. The study and control cohorts should be similar in demographic and possibly important variables other than those under study.

(c) Comparison with general population rates

If none is available, the mortality experience of the exposed group is compared with the mortality experience of the general population in the same geographic area as the exposed people, e.g., comparison of frequency of lung cancer among uranium mine workers with lung cancer mortality in the general population where the miners resided *(56)*; comparison of frequency of cancer among asbestos workers with the rate in general population in the same geographic area *(63)*.

Rates for disease occurrence in sub-groups of the control cohort by age, sex, and other variables considered important may be applied to the corresponding sub-groups of the study cohort (exposed cohort) to determine the "expected" values in the absence of exposure. The ratio of "observed" and "expected" values provides a measure of the effect of the factor under study.

The limiting factors in using general population rates for comparison are : (i) non-availability of population rates for the outcome required; and (ii) the difficulties of selecting the study and comparison groups which are representative of the exposed and non-exposed segments of the general population.

4. Follow-up

One of the problems in cohort studies is the regular follow-up of all the participants. Therefore, at the start of the study, methods should be devised depending upon the outcome to be determined (morbidity or death), to obtain data for assessing the outcome. The procedures required comprise :

(a) periodic medical examination of each member of the cohort
(b) reviewing physician and hospital records
(c) routine surveillance of death records, and
(d) mailed questionnaires, telephone calls, periodic home visits – preferably all three on an annual basis.

Of the above, periodic examination of each member of the cohort, yields greater amount of information on the individuals examined, than would the use of any other procedure.

However, inspite of best efforts, a certain percentage of losses to follow-up are inevitable due to death, change of residence, migration or withdrawal of occupation. These losses may bias the results. It is, therefore, necessary to build into the study design a system for obtaining basic information on outcome for those who cannot be followed up in detail for the full duration of the study *(14)*. The safest course recommended is to achieve as close to a 95 per cent follow-up as possible *(13)*.

5. Analysis

The data are analyzed in terms of :

(a) Incidence rates of outcome among exposed and non-exposed,

(b) Estimation of risk.

(a) Incidence rates

In a cohort study, we can determine incidence rates directly in those exposed and those not exposed. A hypothetical example is given in Table 18 showing how incidence rates may be calculated :

TABLE 18

Contingency table applied to hypothetical cigarette smoking and lung cancer example

Cigarette smoking	Developed lung cancer	Did not develop lung cancer	Total
Yes	70 (a)	6930 (b)	7000 (a + b)
No	3 (c)	2997 (d)	3000 (c + d)

Incidence rates

(a) among smokers = 70/7000 = 10 per 1000

(b) among non-smokers = 3/3000 = 1 per 1000

Statistical significance : $P < 0.001$

(b) Estimation of risk

Having calculated the incidence rates, the next step is to estimate the risk of outcome (e.g., disease or death) in the exposed and non-exposed cohorts. This is done in terms of two well-known indices: (a) relative risk, (b) attributable risk.

RELATIVE RISK

Relative risk (RR) is the ratio of the incidence of the disease (or death) among exposed and the incidence among non-exposed. Some authors use the term "risk ratio" to refer to relative risk.

$$RR = \frac{\text{Incidence of disease (or death) among exposed}}{\text{Incidence of disease (or death) among non-exposed}}$$

In our hypothetical example (Table 18)

$$\text{RR of lung cancer} = \frac{10}{1} = 10$$

Estimation of relative risk (RR) is important in aetiological enquiries. It is a direct measure (or index) of the "strength" of the association between suspected cause and effect. A relative risk of one indicates no association; relative risk greater than one suggests "positive" association between exposure and the disease under study. A relative risk of 2 indicates that the incidence rate of disease is 2 times higher in the exposed group as compared with the unexposed. Equivalently, this represents a 100 per cent increase in risk. A relative risk of 0.25 indicates a 75% reduction in the incidence rate in exposed individuals as compared with the unexposed *(37)*. It is often useful to consider the 95 per cent confidence interval of a relative risk since it provides an indication of the likely and maximum levels of risk.

In our hypothetical example (Table 18), the relative risk is 10. It implies that smokers are 10 times at greater risk of developing lung cancer than non-smokers. The larger the RR, the greater the "strength" of the association between the suspected factor and disease. It may be noted that risk does not necessarily imply causal association.

ATTRIBUTABLE RISK

Attributable risk (AR) is the difference in incidence rates of disease (or death) between an exposed group and non-exposed group. Some authors use the term "risk difference" to attributable risk.

Attributable risk is often expressed as a per cent. This is given by the formula :

$$= \frac{\text{Incidence of disease rate among exposed} - \text{incidence of disease rate among non-exposed}}{\text{Incidence rate among exposed}} \times 100$$

Attributable risk in our example (Table 18) would be :

$$\frac{10-1}{10} \times 100 = 90 \text{ per cent}$$

Attributable risk indicates to what extent the disease under study can be attributed to the exposure. The figure in our example indicates that the association between smoking and lung cancer is causal, 90 per cent of the lung cancer among smokers was due to their smoking. This suggests the amount of disease that might be eliminated if the factor under study could be controlled or eliminated.

POPULATION–ATTRIBUTABLE RISK

Another concept is "population–attributable risk". It is the incidence of the disease (or death) in the total population minus the incidence of disease (or death) among those who were not exposed to the suspected causal factor (Table 19).

TABLE 19

Lung cancer death rates among smokers and non-smokers : UK physicians

Deaths per 100,000 person-years		
Heavy smokers	224	Exposed to suspected factor (a)
Non-smokers	10	Non-exposed to suspected causal factor (b)
Deaths in total population	74 (c)	
Individual RR	a/b = $\frac{224}{10}$ = 22.40	
Population AR	(c–b)/c = 86 per cent	

Source : *(60)*

The concept of population attributable risk is useful in that it provides an estimate of the amount by which the disease could be reduced in that population if the suspected factor was eliminated or modified. In our example (Table 19) one might expect that 86 per cent of deaths from lung cancer could be avoided if the risk factor of cigarettes were eliminated.

Relative risk versus attributable risk

Relative risk is important in aetiological enquiries. Its size is a better index than is attributable risk for assessing the aetiological role of a factor in disease. The larger the relative risk, the stronger the association between cause and effect. But relative risk does not reflect the potential public health importance as does the attributable risk. That is, attributable risk gives a better idea than does relative risk of the impact of successful preventive or public health programme might have in reducing the problem.

Two examples are cited (Tables 20 and 21) to show the practical importance of distinguishing relative and absolute risk. In the first example, (Table 20) the RR of a cardiovascular complication in users of oral contraceptives is independent of age, whereas the AR is more than 5 times higher in the older age groups. This epidemiological observation has been the basis for not recommending oral contraceptive in those aged 35 years and over.

TABLE 20

The relative and attributable risks of cardiovascular complications in women taking oral contraceptives

Cardiovascular risk 100,000 patient years	Age	
	30–39	40–44
Relative risk	2.8	2.8
Attributable risk	3.5	20.0

Source : *(64)*

The second example (Table 21) shows that smoking is attributable to 92 per cent of lung cancer, and 13.3 per cent of CHD. In CHD, both RR and AR are not very high suggesting not much of the disease could be prevented as compared to lung cancer.

TABLE 21

Risk assessment, smokers *vs* non-smokers

Cause of death	Death rate/1000		RR	AR (%)
	Smokers	Non-smokers		
Lung cancer	0.90	0.07	12.86	92.2
CHD	4.87	4.22	1.15	13.3

Source : *(65)*

Advantages and disadvantages of cohort studies

Advantages

(a) Incidence can be calculated. (b) Several possible outcomes related to exposure can be studied simultaneously – that is, we can study the association of the suspected factor with many other diseases in addition to the one under study. For example, cohort studies designed to study the association between smoking and lung cancer also showed association of smoking with coronary heart disease, peptic ulcer, cancer oesophagus and several others. (c) Cohort studies provide a direct estimate of relative risk. (d) Dose–response ratios can also be calculated, and (e) Since comparison groups are formed before disease develops, certain forms of bias can be minimized like mis-classification of individuals into exposed and unexposed groups.

Disadvantages

Cohort studies also present a number of problems : (a) Cohort studies involve a large number of people. They are generally unsuitable for investigating uncommon diseases or diseases with low incidence in the population. (b) It takes a long time to complete the study and obtain results (20–30 years or more in cancer studies) by which time the investigators may have died or the participants may have changed their classification. Even in very common chronic diseases like coronary heart disease, cohort studies are difficult to carry out. It is difficult to keep a large number of individuals under medical surveillance indefinitely. (c) Certain administrative problems such as loss of experienced staff, loss of funding and extensive record keeping are inevitable. (d) It is not unusual to lose a substantial proportion of the original cohort – they may migrate, lose interest in the study or simply refuse to provide any required information. (e) Selection of comparison groups which are representative of the exposed and unexposed segments of the population is a limiting factor. Those who volunteer for the study may not be representative of all individuals with the characteristic of interest. (f) There may be changes in the standard methods or diagnostic criteria of the disease over prolonged follow-up. Once we have established the study protocol, it is difficult to introduce new knowledge or new tests later. (g) Cohort studies are expensive. (h) The study itself may alter people's behaviour. If we are examining the role of smoking in lung cancer, an increased concern in the study cohort may be created. This may induce the study subjects to stop or decrease smoking. (i) With any cohort study we are faced with ethical problems of varying importance. As evidence accumulates about the implicating factor in the aetiology of disease, we are obliged to intervene and if possible reduce or eliminate this factor, and (j) Finally, in a cohort study, practical considerations dictate that we must concentrate on a limited number or factors possibly related to disease outcome.

The main differences between case control and cohort studies are summarized in Table 22.

TABLE 22

Main differences between case control and cohort studies

Case control study	Cohort study
1. Proceeds from "effect to cause".	Proceeds from "cause to effect".
2. Starts with the disease.	Starts with people exposed to risk factor or suspected cause.
3. Tests whether the suspected cause occurs more frequently in those with the disease than among those without the disease.	Tests whether disease occurs more frequently in those exposed, than in those not similarly exposed.
4. Usually the first approach to the testing of a hypothesis, but also useful for exploratory studies.	Reserved for testing of precisely formulated hypothesis.
5. Involves fewer number of subjects.	Involves larger number of subjects.
6. Yields relatively quick results.	Long follow-up period often needed, involving delayed results.
7. Suitable for the study of rare diseases.	Inappropriate when the disease or exposure under investigation is rare.
8. Generally yields only estimate of RR (odds ratio).	Yields incidence rates, RR as well as AR.
9. Cannot yield information about diseases other than that selected for study.	Can yield information about more than one disease outcome.
10. Relatively inexpensive.	Expensive.

Examples of cohort studies

Example 1 : Smoking and lung cancer.

At least eight prospective studies on the relation of smoking to lung cancer had been done. Doll and Hill *(52, 62, 66)*, Hammond and Horn *(67, 68)* and Dorn *(61)* were the first to report their findings.

In October 1951, Doll and Hill sent a questionnaire to 59,600 British doctors listed in the Medical Register of the UK enquiring about their smoking habits. This enabled them to form two cohorts (smokers and non-smokers) who were similar in all other respects like age, education and social class. They received usable replies from 40,701 physicians - 34,494 men and 6,207 women. These were followed for 4 years and 5 months by obtaining notifications of physicians' deaths from the Registrar General, the General Medical Council and the British Medical Association. For every death certified as due to lung cancer, confirmation was obtained by writing to the physician certifying the death and also, when necessary to the hospital or consultant to whom the patient had been referred. The results of the study are shown in Table 19.

Example 2 : The Framingham heart study (51).

The Framingham heart study was initiated in 1948 by the United States Public Health Service to study the relationship of a number of (risk) factors (e.g., serum cholesterol, blood pressure, weight, smoking) to the subsequent development of cardiovascular disease. The town of Framingham (Massachusetts) had a population of 28,000 in 1948. The study was planned for 20 years in view of the slow development of heart disease.

The lower and upper limits of the study population was set at 30 and 59 years. Out of 10,000 people in this age group a sample of 6,507 persons of both sexes were invited to participate in the study, out of which 5,209 participated. The initial examination revealed that 82 subjects had clinically evident CHD. These were excluded from the sample leaving a total of 5,127.

4,469 (69 per cent) of the 6,507 in the initial sample actually underwent the first examination. After the first examination, the study population was examined every 2 years for a 20 year period. Information was obtained with regard to serum cholesterol, blood pressure, weight and cigarette smoking. Although biennial examinations were the main source of follow up information, other means were also adopted to detect CHD (e.g., Death certificate records).

Among other things, the study showed increasing risk of CHD with increasing serum cholesterol levels in the 45–54 age group. The study also showed that the association between smoking and CHD varied with manifestations of the disease. Thus, smoking was more strongly associated with sudden death from CHD than with less fatal forms of the disease. Risk factors have been found to include male sex, advancing age, high serum lipid concentration, high blood pressure, cigarette smoking, diabetes mellitus, obesity, low vital capacity and certain ECG abnormalities. The predictive value of serum lipids, blood pressure and cigarette smoking have been repeatedly demonstrated. The Framingham heart study became a prototype of similar studies in US and other countries.

Example 3 : Oral contraceptives and health (53).

Another example is the cohort study of oral contraceptives and health conducted by the Royal College of General Practitioners in England (1974). It was initiated in 1968, after 2 years of planning. 23,000 users of the pill aged 15–49 years together with a similar number of controls using other methods or no method of contraception were brought under observation of 1400 general practitioners. During follow-up doctors recorded the diagnoses of episodes of illness, and information about pregnancies and deaths.

The study brought out the risks and benefits of oral contraceptive use. For example, the study showed that the risk of hypertension increases, and the risk of benign breast disease decreases with the dose of norethisterone acetate (progestogen) in the combined pill which is an important finding. The study found an increased mortality from diseases of cardiovascular system in pill users confirming the results of retrospective case control studies *(69)*.

EXPERIMENTAL EPIDEMIOLOGY

In the 1920s, "experimental epidemiology" meant the study of epidemics among colonies of experimental animals such as rats and mice. In modern usage, experimental epidemiology is often equated with RANDOMIZED CONTROLLED TRIALS *(2)*.

Experimental or intervention studies are similar in approach to cohort studies excepting that the conditions in which study is carried out are under the direct control of the investigator. Thus experimental studies involve some action, intervention or manipulation such as deliberate application or withdrawal of the suspected cause or changing one variable in the causative chain in the experimental group while making no change in the control group, and observing and comparing the outcome of the experiment in both the groups. This contrasts sharply with observational studies (e.g., descriptive, case control and cohort studies), where the epidemiologist takes no action but only observes the natural course of events or outcome.

The aims of experimental studies may be stated as follows : (a) to provide "scientific proof" of aetiological (or risk) factors which may permit the modification or control of those diseases : and (b) to provide a method of measuring the effectiveness and efficiency of health services for the prevention, control and treatment of disease and improve the health of the community.

Experimental studies have all the advantages and disadvantages of the usual prospective cohort studies plus three additional problems namely cost, ethics and feasibility. Experimental studies have become a major area of epidemiological studies. They may be conducted in animals or human beings.

Animal studies

Throughout history animals have played an important role in men's quest for knowledge about himself and his environment. Animal studies have contributed to our knowledge of anatomy, physiology, pathology, microbiology, immunology, genetics, chemotherapy and so many others. At the beginning of this century, Webster in United States and Topley, Wilson and Greenwood in England had carried out classical animal experiments. Their studies centred round inducing epidemics in animals and in studies of herd immunity under laboratory conditions.

More important application of animal experiments have been in (a) experimental reproduction of human disease in animals to confirm aetiological hypothesis and to study the pathogenetic phenomena or mechanisms (b) testing the efficacy of preventive and therapeutic measures such as vaccines and drugs, and (c) completing the natural history of disease. For example, naturally occurring leprosy has been found in armadillos. Data obtained from studying these animals indicate that lepra bacilli might exist outside of humans.

Animal experiments have their own advantages and limitations. The **advantages** are that the experimental animals can be bred in laboratories and manipulated easily according to the wishes of the investigator. A more important point is that they multiply rapidly and enable the investigators to carry out certain experiments (e.g., genetic experiments) which in human population would take several years and involve many generations. The **limitations** of animal experiments are that not all human diseases can be reproduced in animals. Secondly, all the conclusions derived from animal experiments may not be strictly applicable to human beings. An excellent example to illustrate this point is the WHO trial of typhoid vaccine in Yugoslavia in the mid-1950s. Laboratory tests in animals showed the alcohol-killed and preserved vaccine to be more effective than the traditional heat-killed phenol-preserved vaccine. But randomized controlled trials in human beings demonstrated that, contrary to laboratory evidence, the alcohol-preserved vaccine was found to be less than half as effective in preventing typhoid fever as the traditional phenol-preserved vaccine introduced by Almorth Wright. This highlights the difficulties encountered in extrapolating findings from animal experiments in man.

Human experiments

Human experiments will always be needed to investigate disease aetiology and to evaluate the preventive and therapeutic measures. These studies are even more essential in the investigation of diseases that cannot be reproduced in animals.

Historically, in 1747, James Lind performed a human experiment (clinical trial) in which he added different substances to diet of 12 soldiers who were suffering from scurvy. He divided his patients into 6 pairs and supplemented the diets of each pair with cider, elixir vitriol, vinegar, sea water; a mixture of nutmeg, garlic, mustard and tamarind in barley water; and two oranges and one lemon daily. All the subjects were studied for 6 days. At the end of 6 days the LIMEYS recovered from scurvy and were found fit for duty. Then came Edward Jenner's experiment with cowpox in 1796. Other classical experiments are Finlay and Reed's experiments (1881–1900) to elucidate the mosquito–borne nature of yellow fever and Goldberger's classical experiments in 1915 inducing pellagra by diets deficient in nicotinic acid, thereby proving pellagra to be a nutritional deficiency disease, not an infectious disease as was then supposed. Since then, human beings have participated in studies of malaria, syphilis, hepatitis, measles, polio and others. These experiments have played decisive roles in investigating disease aetiology and in testing preventive and therapeutic measures.

Although the experimental method is unquestionably the most incisive approach to scientific problem, ethical and logistic considerations often prevent its application to the study of disease in humans. Therefore, before launching human experiments, the benefits of the experiment have to be weighed against risks involved. The volunteers should be made fully aware of all possible consequences of the experiment. Thus when an illness is fatal (e.g., excessive haemorrhage) and the benefit of treatment (e.g., blood transfusion) is self-evident, it would be ethically unacceptable to prove or disprove the therapeutic value of blood transfusion. However, such instances represent only a small part of the total research effort. On the other hand, in the present era of scientific medicine, many unscientific or scientifically unsound procedures are still being carried out. For instance, in the study of prescription drugs, a panel of experts in USA found that only 23 per cent of some 16,000 drugs could be classified unequivocally as "effective" *(38)*. It is now conceded that it is equally unethical if a drug or procedure is brought into general use without establishing its effectiveness by controlled trials. The thalidomide disaster and the occurrence of carcinoma of the vagina in the offspring of pregnant women treated with diethylstilbestrol highlight the unfortunate consequence of therapy on the basis of uncontrolled observations. The WHO in 1980 has laid down a strict code of practice in connection with human trials *(70)*.

Experimental studies are of two types :

a. Randomized controlled trials (i.e., those involving a process of random allocation); and
b. Non-randomized or "non-experimental" trials (i.e., those departing from strict randomization for practical purposes, but in such a manner that non-randomization does not seriously affect the theoretical basis of conclusions).

RANDOMIZED CONTROLLED TRIALS

Too often physicians are guided in their daily work by clinical impressions of their own or their teachers. These impressions, particularly when they are incorporated in textbooks and repeatedly quoted by reputed teachers and their students acquire authority, just as if they were proved facts. Similarly many public health measures are introduced on the basis of assumed benefits without subjecting them to rigorous testing. The history of medicine amply illustrates this. For instance, it took centuries before therapeutic blood letting and drastic purging were abandoned by the medical profession.

It is mainly in the last 35 to 40 years, determined efforts have been made to use scientific techniques to evaluate methods of treatment and prevention. An important advance in this field has been the development of an assessment method, known as Randomized Controlled Trial (RCT). It is really an epidemiologic experiment. Since its introduction, the RCT has questioned the validity of such widely used treatments as oral hypoglycaemic agents, varicose vein stripping, tonsillectomy, hospitalization of all patients with myocardial infarction, multiphasic screening, and toxicity and applicability of many preventive and therapeutic procedures.

The design of a randomized controlled trial is given in Fig. 9. For new programmes or new therapies, the RCT is the No.1 method of evaluation. The basic steps in conducting a RCT include the following :

1. Drawing up a protocol.
2. Selecting reference and experimental populations.
3. Randomization.
4. Manipulation or intervention.
5. Follow-up.
6. Assessment of outcome.

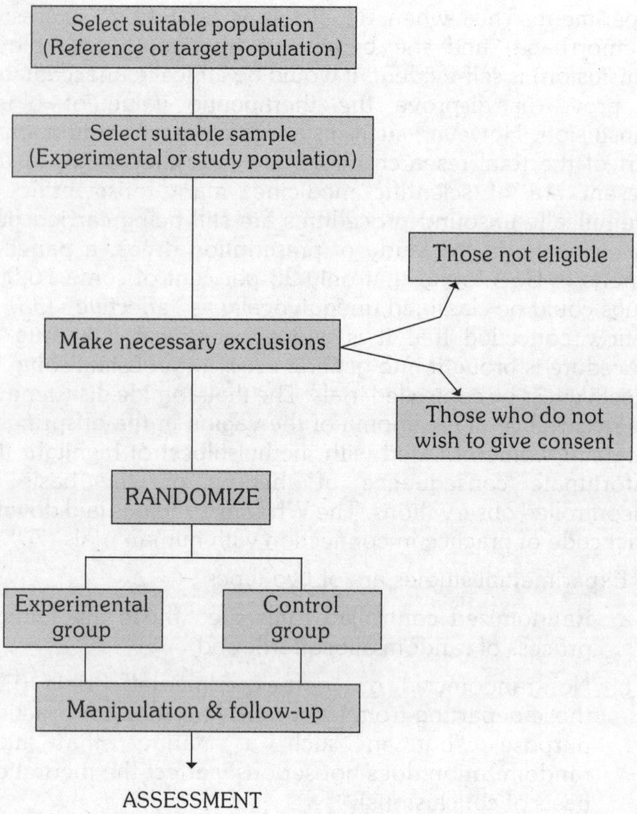

FIG.9
Design of a randomized controlled trial

1. The protocol

One of the essential features of a randomized controlled trial is that the study is conducted under a strict protocol. The protocol specifies the aims and objectives of the study, questions to be answered, criteria for the selection of study and control groups, size of the sample, the procedures for allocation of subjects into study and control groups, treatments to be applied – when and where and how to what kind of patients, standardization of working procedures and schedules as well as responsibilities of the parties involved in the trial, upto the stage of evaluation of outcome of the study. A protocol is essential especially when a number of centres are participating in the trial. Once a protocol has been evolved, it should be strictly adhered to throughout the study. The protocol aims at preventing bias and to reduce the sources of error in the study.

Preliminary test runs : Sometimes, before a protocol is completed, preliminary (pilot) studies have to be made to find out the feasibility or operational efficiency of certain procedures, or unknown effects, or on the acceptability of certain policies. Sometimes it is useful to have a short test run of the protocol to see whether it contains any flaws. It is important that the final version of the protocol should be agreed upon by all concerned before the trial begins.

2. Selecting reference and experimental populations

(a) *Reference or target population* : It is the population to which the findings of the trial, if found successful, are expected to be applicable (e.g., a drug, vaccine or other procedure). A reference population may be as broad as mankind or it may be geographically limited or limited to persons in specifiç age, sex, occupational or social groups. Thus the reference population may comprise the population of a whole city, or a population of school children, industrial workers, obstetric population and so on according to the nature of the study.

(b) *Experimental or study population* : The study population is derived from the reference population. It is the actual population that participates in the experimental study. Ideally, it should be randomly chosen from the reference population, so that it has the same characteristics as the reference population. If the study population differs from the reference population, it may not be possible to generalize the findings of the study to the reference population.

When an experimental population has been defined, its members are invited to participate in the study. It is important to choose a stable population whose cooperation is assured to avoid losses to follow-up. The participants or volunteers must fulfil the following three criteria :

a. they must give "informed consent", that is they must agree to participate in the trial after having been fully informed about the purpose, procedures and possible dangers of the trial;

b. they should be representative of the population to which they belong (i.e., reference population); and

c. they should be qualified or eligible for the trial. That is, let us suppose, we are testing the effectiveness of a new drug for the treatment of anaemia. If the volunteers are not anaemic, we will then say, they are not eligible or qualified for the trial. Similarly, let us suppose; we are going to test the effectiveness of a new vaccine against whooping cough. If the volunteers are already immune to the disease in question, we will then say, they are not qualified for the trial. In other words, the participants must be fully susceptible to the disease under study.

It must be recognized that persons who agree to participate in a study are likely to differ from those who do not, in many ways that may affect the outcome under investigation.

3. Randomization

Randomization is a statistical procedure by which the participants are allocated into groups usually called "study" and "control" groups, to receive or not to receive an experimental preventive or therapeutic procedure, manoeuvre or intervention. Randomization is an attempt to eliminate "bias" and allow for *comparability.* Theoretically it is possible to assure comparability by matching. But when one matches, one can only match those factors which are known to be important. There may be other factors which are important but whose effect is not recognized or cannot be determined. By a process of randomization, hopefully, these factors will be distributed equally between the two groups.

Randomization is the "heart" of a control trial. It will give the greatest confidence that the groups are comparable so that "like can be compared with like". It ensures that the investigator has no control over allocation of participants to either study or control group, thus eliminating what is known as "selection bias". In other words, by random allocation, every individual gets an equal chance of being allocated into either group or any of the trial groups.

It is crucial that both the groups should be alike with regard to certain variables or characteristics that might affect the outcome of the experiment (e.g., age, sex), the entire study population can be stratified into sub-groups according to the variable, and individuals within each sub-group can then be randomly allocated into study and control groups. It is always desirable to check that the groups formed initially are basically similar in composition. Randomization is done only after the participant has entered the study, that is after having been qualified for the trial and has given his informed consent to participate in the study. Randomization is best done by using a table of random numbers (see chapter 20).

The essential difference between a randomized controlled trial and an analytical study is that in the latter, there is no randomization because a differentiation into diseased and non–diseased (exposed or non–exposed) groups has already taken place. The only option left to ensure comparability in analytical studies is by matching.

4. Manipulation

Having formed the study and control groups, the next step is to intervene or manipulate the study (experimental) group by the deliberate application or withdrawal or reduction of the suspected causal factor (e.g., this may be a drug, vaccine, dietary component, a habit, etc) as laid down in the protocol.

This manipulation creates an *independent* variable (e.g., drug, vaccine, a new procedure) whose effect is then determined by measurement of the final outcome, which constitutes the *dependent* variable (e.g., incidence of disease, survival time, recovery period).

5. Follow-up

This implies examination of the experimental and control group subjects at defined intervals of time, in a standard manner, with equal intensity, under the same given circumstances, in the same time frame till final assessment of outcome. The duration of the trial is usually based on the expectation that a significant difference (e.g., mortality) will be demonstrable at a given point in time after the start of the trial. Thus the follow-up may be short or may require many years depending upon the study undertaken.

It may be mentioned that some losses to follow-up are inevitable due to factors, such as death, migration and loss of interest. This is known as attrition. If the attrition is substantial, it may be difficult to generalise the results of the study to the reference population. Every effort, therefore, should be made to minimize the losses to follow-up.

6. Assessment

The final step is assessment of the outcome of the trial in terms of : (a) *Positive results* : that is, benefits of the experimental measure such as reduced incidence or severity of the disease, cost to the health service or other appropriate outcome in the study and control groups. (b) *Negative results* : that is, severity and frequency of side-effects and complications, if any, including death. Adverse effects may be missed if they are not sought.

The incidence of positive/negative results is rigorously compared in both the groups, and the differences, if any, are tested for statistical significance. Techniques are available for the analysis of data as they are collected (sequential analysis), but it is more useful to analyze the results at the end of the trial.

Bias may arise from errors of assessment of the outcome due to human element. These may be from three sources : *First,* there may be bias on the part of the participants, who may subjectively feel better or report improvement if they knew they were receiving a new form of treatment. This is known as "subject variation". *Secondly* there may be observer bias, that is the investigator measuring the outcome of a therapeutic trial may be influenced if he knows beforehand the particular procedure or therapy to which the patient has been subjected. This is known as "observer bias." *Thirdly*, there may be bias in evaluation – that is, the investigator may subconsciously give a favourable report of the outcome of the trial. Randomization cannot guard against these sorts of bias, nor the size of the sample. In order to reduce these problems, a technique known as "blinding" is adopted, which will ensure that the outcome is assessed objectively.

Blinding : Blinding can be done in three ways – (a) *SINGLE BLIND TRIAL* : The trial is so planned that the participant is not aware whether he belongs to the study group or control group. (B) *DOUBLE BLIND TRIAL* : The trial is so planned that neither the doctor nor the participant is aware of the group allocation and the treatment received. (C) *TRIPLE BLIND TRIAL* : This goes one step further. The participant, the investigator and the person analyzing the data are all "blind". Ideally, of course, triple blinding should be used; but the double blinding is the most frequently used method when a blind trial is conducted *(5)*. When an outcome such as death is being measured, blinding is not so essential.

SOME STUDY DESIGNS

It is useful to consider here some of the study designs of controlled trials :

1. Concurrent parallel study designs

In this situation (Fig. 10–a), comparisons are made between two randomly assigned groups, one group exposed to specific treatment, and the other group not exposed. Patients remain in the study group or the control group for the duration of the investigation.

2. Cross-over type of study designs

This is illustrated in Fig. 10–b. With this type of study design, each patient serves as his own control. As before, the patients are randomly assigned to a study group and control group. The study group receives the treatment under consideration. The control group receives some alternate form of active treatment or placebo. The two groups are observed over time. Then the patients in each group are taken off their medication or placebo to allow for the elimination of the medication from the body and for the possibility of any "carry over" effects, as shown in Fig. 10–b by the diagonal lines. After this period of medication (the length of this interval is determined by the pharmacologic properties of the drug being tested), the two groups are switched. Those who received the treatment under study are changed to the control group therapy or placebo, and vice versa.

Cross-over studies offer a number of advantages. With such a design, all patients can be assured that sometime during the course of investigation, they will receive the new therapy. Such studies generally economize on the total number of patients required at the expense of the time necessary to complete the study. This method of study is not suitable if the drug of interest cures the disease, if the drug is effective only during a certain stage of the disease or if the disease changes radically during the period of time required for the study.

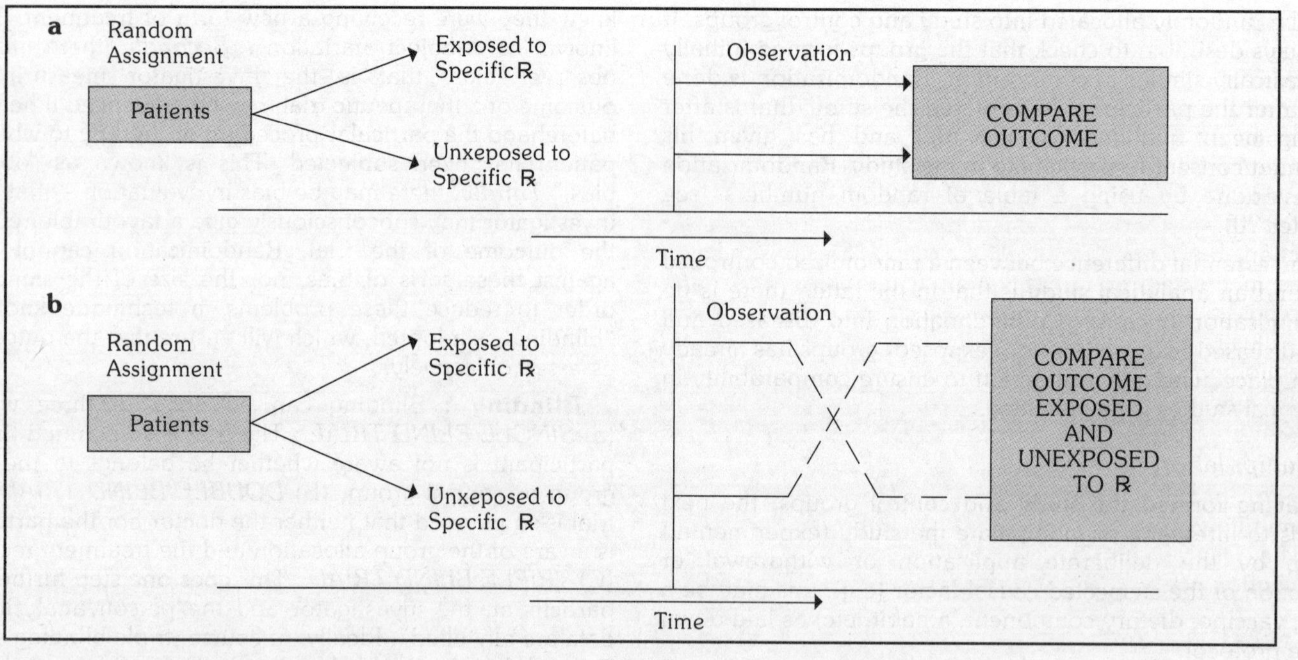

FIG. 10
Schematic diagram of the design of concurrent parallel and cross-over controlled therapeutic trials *(73)*.

TYPES OF RANDOMIZED CONTROLLED TRIALS

1. Clinical trials

For the most part, "clinical trials" have been concerned with evaluating therapeutic agents, mainly drugs. The last decades have seen clearly the utility of clinical trials. Some of the recent examples include – evaluation of beta-blockers in reducing cardiovascular mortality in patient surviving the acute phase of myocardial infarction *(71)*; trials of folate treatment/supplementation before conception to prevent recurrence of neural tube defects *(72)*; trials of aspirin on cardiovascular mortality and beta-carotene on cancer incidence; efficacy of tonsillectomy for recurrent throat infection *(73)*; randomized controlled trial of coronary bypass surgery for the prevention of myocardial infarction *(74)*, etc. The list is endless.

Unfortunately, not all clinical trials are susceptible to being blinded. For example, there is no way to perform a clinical trial of tonsillectomy and adenoidectomy without its being obvious who received surgery and who did not, a reason why the value of these procedures continues to be uncertain. Many ethical, administrative and technical problems are involved in the conduct of clinical trials. Nevertheless, they are a powerful tool and should be carried out before any new therapy, procedure or service is introduced.

2. Preventive trials

In general usage, prevention is synonymous with primary prevention, and the term "preventive trials" implies trials of primary preventive measures. These trials are purported to prevent or eliminate disease on an experimental basis. The most frequently occurring type of preventive trials are the trials of vaccines and chemoprophylactic drugs. The basic principles of experimental design are also applicable to these trials. It may be necessary to apply the trial to groups of subjects instead of to individual subjects. For example, in 1946, the Medical Research Council of UK conducted an extensive trial *(76)* to test whooping cough vaccine from three manufacturers in ten separate field trials. Those children between 6–18 months who were entered into the trial were randomly allocated in study and control groups. The vaccine was given in three, monthly injections, and the children were followed up at monthly intervals to detect the occurrence of whooping cough. The study group comprised of 3,801 children who were vaccinated, and 149 developed whooping cough. The control group consisted of 3,757 unvaccinated children, and 687 of them developed the infection. This gave an attack rate of 1.45 per 1000 child months in the vaccinated group and 6.72 per 1000 child months in the control group. The difference was significant.

Analysis of a preventive trial must result in a clear statement about (a) the benefit the community will derive from the measure (b) the risks involved, and (c) the costs to the health service in terms of money, men and material resources *(22)*. Since preventive trials involve larger number of subjects and sometimes a longer time span to obtain results, there may be greater number of practical problems in their organisation and execution.

3. Risk factor trials

A type of preventive trial is the trial of risk factors in which the investigator intervenes to interrupt the usual sequence in the development of disease for those individuals who have "risk factor" for developing the disease; often this involves risk factor modification. The concept of "risk factor" gave a new dimension to epidemiological research.

For example, the major risk factors of coronary heart disease are elevated blood cholesterol, smoking, hypertension and sedentary habits. Accordingly, the four main possibilities of intervention in coronary heart disease are : reduction of blood cholesterol, the cessation of smoking, control of hypertension and promotion of regular physical activity. Risk factor trials can be "single-factor" or "multi-factor" trials. Both the approaches are complementary, and both are needed.

The WHO *(77)* promoted a trial on primary prevention of coronary heart disease using clofibrate to lower serum cholesterol, which was accepted as a significant risk factor for CHD. This study is the largest preventive trial yet conducted, comprising more than 15,000 men of whom one-third received clofibrate and two-third received olive oil as a control treatment. The study was conducted in 3 centres in Europe (Edinburgh, Prague, and Budapest). The design was double-blind and randomization was successfully achieved. The mean observation was 9.6 years. The trial showed a significant reduction in non-fatal cardiac infarction, but unfortunately, there were 25 per cent more deaths in the clofibrate-treated group than in the control group possibly due to long-term toxic effect of the drug. The trial illustrates the kind of contribution that an epidemiological approach can make to protect the public health against possible adverse effects of long-term medication with potent drugs *(77)*.

The other widely reported risk-factor intervention trials in coronary heart disease are : (a) The Stanford Three Community Study (b) The North Karelia Project in Finland (c) The Oslo Study, and (d) The Multiple Risk Factor Intervention Trial (MRFIT) in USA.

4. Cessation experiments

Another type of preventive trial is the cessation experiment. In this type of study, an attempt is made to evaluate the termination of a habit (or removal of suspected agent) which is considered to be causally related to a disease. If such action is followed by a significant reduction in the disease, the hypothesis of cause is greatly strengthened. The familiar example is cigarette smoking and lung cancer. If in a randomized controlled trial, one group of cigarette smokers continue to smoke and the other group has given up, the demonstration of a decrease in the incidence of lung cancer in the study group greatly strengthens the hypothesis of a causal relationship. A large randomized controlled trial has been mounted to study the role of smoking cessation in the primary prevention of coronary heart disease *(78)*.

5. Trial of aetiological agents

One of the aims of experimental epidemiology is to confirm or refute an aetiological hypothesis. The best known example of trial of an aetiological agent relates to retrolental fibroplasia (RLF). Retrolental fibroplasia, as a cause of blindness, was non-existent prior to 1938. It was originally observed and reported by T.L.Terry, a Boston ophthalmologist in 1942 *(79)*, and later in many other countries outside the USA.

RLF was recognized as a leading cause of blindness by descriptive studies which showed that beginning in about 1940–1941, the incidence of the disease increased at an alarming rate (Fig. 11), and that this previously unknown disease was occurring only in premature babies. Analytical studies demonstrated its close association with administration of oxygen to premature babies. A large randomized controlled trial was mounted involving 18 hospitals in United States by Kinsey and Hemphill *(80, 81)* in which premature babies with birth weight of 1500 gram or less were allocated into experimental and control groups. In the experimental group, all the babies received 50 per cent oxygen therapy for 28 days, while in the control group ("curtailed oxygen group") oxygen was used only for clinical emergency. It was later found that all of the babies in the "curtailed oxygen group" who developed RLF had received some oxygen. There were no cases among those who received none, confirming the aetiological hypothesis.

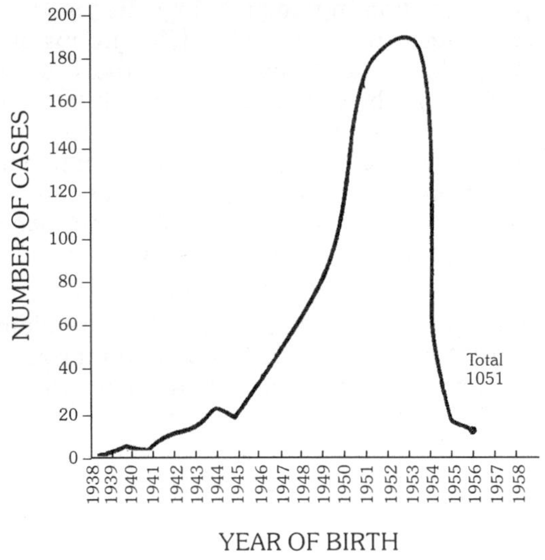

FIG. 11
Incidence of retrolental fibroplasia in New York, 1938–1956

The dramatic rise and fall in frequency of RLF can be seen in Fig. 11. It will be noted that RLF reached its peak during the years 1952–53. The sharp drop in the graph after 1953 highlights the results of the decreased use of oxygen. RLF illustrates one of the problems often introduced by technological or scientific advances.

Since most diseases are fatal, disabling or unpleasant, human experiments to confirm an aetiological hypothesis are rarely possible.

6. Evaluation of health services

Randomized controlled trials have been extended to assess the effectiveness and efficiency of health services. Often, choices have to be made between alternative policies of health care delivery. The necessity of choice arises from the fact that resources are limited, and priorities must be set for the implementation of a large number of activities which could contribute to the welfare of the society. An excellent example of such an evaluation is the controlled trials in the chemotherapy of tuberculosis in India, which demonstrated that "domiciliary treatment" of pulmonary tuberculosis was as effective as the more costlier "hospital or sanatorium" treatment. The results of the study have gained international acceptance and ushered in a new era – the era of domiciliary treatment, in the treatment of tuberculosis.

More recently, multiphasic screening which has achieved great popularity in some countries, was evaluated by a randomized controlled trial in South-East London. The study led to the withholding of vast outlay of resources required to mount a national programme of multiphasic screening in UK *(82, 83)*. Another example is that related to studies which have shown that many of the health care delivery tasks traditionally performed by physicians can be performed by nurses and other paramedical workers, thus saving physician time *(84)*. These studies are also labelled as "health services research" studies.

NON-RANDOMIZED TRIALS

Although the experimental method is almost always to be preferred, it is not always possible for ethical, administrative and other reasons to resort to a randomized controlled trial in human beings. For example, smoking and lung cancer and induction of cancer by viruses have not lent themselves to direct experimentation in human beings. Secondly, some preventive measures can be applied only to groups or on a community-wide basis (e.g., community trials of water fluoridation). Thirdly, when disease frequency is low and the natural history long (e.g., cancer cervix) randomized controlled trials require follow-up of thousands of people for a decade or more. The cost and logistics are often prohibitive. These trials are rare. In such situations, we must depend upon other study designs – these are referred to as non-randomized (or non-experimental) trials.

Where the approach is sophisticated in randomized controlled trials, it is rather crude in non-randomized trials. As there is no randomization in non-experimental trials, the degree of comparability will be low and the chances of a spurious result higher than where randomization had taken place. In other words, the validity of causal inference remains largely a matter of extra-statistical judgement. Nevertheless, vital decisions affecting public health and preventive medicine have been made by non-experimental studies. A few examples of non-randomized trials are discussed below :

1. Uncontrolled trials

There is room for uncontrolled trials (i.e., trials with no comparison group). For example, there were no randomized controlled studies of the benefits of the Pap test (cervical cancer) when it was introduced in 1920s. Today, there is indirect epidemiological evidence from well over a dozen uncontrolled studies of cervical cancer screening that the Pap test is effective in reducing mortality from this disease. Initially uncontrolled trials may be useful in evaluating whether a specific therapy appears to have any value in a particular disease, to determine an appropriate dose, to investigate adverse reactions, etc. However, even in these uncontrolled trials, one is using implied "historical controls", i.e., the experience of earlier untreated patients affected by the same disease.

Since most therapeutic trials deal with drugs which do not produce such remarkably beneficial results, it is becoming increasingly common to employ the procedures of a double-blind controlled clinical trial in which the effects of a new drug are compared to some concurrent experience (either placebo or a currently utilized therapy).

2. Natural experiments

Where experimental studies are not possible in human populations, the epidemiologist seeks to identify "natural circumstances" that mimic an experiment. For example, in respect of cigarette smoking, people have separated themselves "naturally" into two groups, smokers and non-smokers. Epidemiologists have taken advantage of this separation and tested hypothesis regarding lung cancer and cigarette smoking. Other populations involved in natural experiments comprise the following groups : (a) migrants (b) religious or social groups (c) atomic bombing of Japan (d) famines (e) earthquakes, etc. A major earthquake in Athens in 1981 provided a "natural experiment" to epidemiologists who studied the effects of acute stress on cardiovascular mortality. They showed an excess of deaths from cardiac and external causes on the days after the major earthquake, but no excess deaths from other causes *(85)*.

John Snow's discovery that cholera is a water-borne disease was the outcome of a natural experiment. Snow in his "grand experiment" identified two randomly mixed populations, alike in other important respects, except the source of water supply in their households. The results of the experiment are given in Table 23.

TABLE 23

Deaths from cholera per 10,000 houses and sources of water supply of these houses, London 1853

Sources of water supply	Number of houses	Deaths from cholera	Deaths in each 10,000 houses
Southwark & Vauxhall Co.	40,046	1263	315
Lambeth Co.	26,107	98	37

It will be seen from Table 23 that deaths were fewer in houses supplied by Lambeth company compared to houses supplied by Southwark and Vauxhall company. The inference was obvious – the Lambeth company water came from an intake on the River Thames well above London, whereas the Southwark and Vauxhall company water was derived from the sewage polluted water basin. The great difference in the occurrence of cholera among these two populations gave clear demonstration that cholera is a water-borne disease. This was demonstrated long before the advent of the bacteriological era; it also led to the institution of public health measures to control cholera.

3. Before and after comparison studies

These are community trials which fall into two distinct groups:

A. Before and after comparison studies without control, and

B. Before and after comparison studies with control.

*A. Before and after comparison studies **without** control*

These studies centre round comparing the incidence of disease before and after introduction of a preventive measure. The events which took place prior to the use of the new treatment or preventive procedure are used as a standard for comparison. In other words, the experiment serves as its own control; this eliminates virtually all group differences. The classic examples of "before and after comparison studies" were the prevention of scurvy among sailors by James Lind in 1750 by providing fresh fruit; studies on the transmission of cholera by John Snow in 1854; and later, prevention of polio by Salk and Sabin vaccines.

In order to establish evidence in before and after comparison studies, the following are needed; (a) data regarding the incidence of disease, before and after introduction of a preventive measure must be available (b) there should be introduction or manipulation of only one factor or change relevant to the situation, other factors remaining the same, as for example, addition of fluorine to drinking water to prevent dental caries (c) diagnostic criteria of the disease should remain the same (d) adoption of preventive measures should be over a wide area (e) reduction in the incidence must be large following the introduction of the preventive measure, because there is no control, and (f) several trials may be needed before the evaluation is considered conclusive.

Table 24 gives an example of a "before and after comparison study" in Victoria (Australia) following introduction of seat-belt legislation for prevention of deaths and injuries caused by motor vehicle accidents.

TABLE 24

Effect of adoption of compulsory seat-belt legislation in Victoria, Australia–1971

	1970	1971	% change
Deaths	564	464	- 17.7
Injuries	14620	12454	- 14.8

Table 24 shows a definite fall in the numbers of deaths and injuries in occupants of cars, following the introduction of compulsory seat-belts in one state of Australia.

*B. Before and after comparison studies **with** control*

In the absence of a control group, comparison between observations before and after the use of a new treatment or procedure may be misleading. In such situations, the epidemiologist tries to utilize a "natural" control group i.e., the one provided by nature or natural circumstances. If preventive programme is to be applied to an entire community, he would select another community as similar as possible, particularly with respect to frequency and characteristics of the disease to be prevented. One of them is arbitrarily chosen to provide the study group and the other a control group. In the example cited (e.g., seat-belt legislation in Victoria, Australia), a natural "control" was sought by comparing the results in Victoria with other states in Australia where similar legislation was not introduced. The findings are given in Table 25.

TABLE 25

Effect of adoption of compulsory seat-belt legislation in Victoria, 1971 compared with other states where similar legislation was not introduced

	1970	1971	% change
Deaths			
Victoria	564	464	- 17.7
Other states	1,426	1,429	0.2
Injuries			
Victoria	14,620	12,454	- 14.8
Other states	39,980	40,396	1.0

In the example cited above, the existence of a control with which the results in Victoria could be compared strengthens the conclusion that there was definite fall in the number of deaths and injuries in occupants of cars after the introduction of compulsory seat-belt legislation.

In the evaluation of preventive measures, three questions are generally considered : (a) How much will it benefit the community ? This will depend upon the effectiveness of the preventive measure and the acceptance of the measure by the community. The combined outcome of effectiveness and acceptability is measured by the difference in the incidence rate among the experimental and control groups. (b) What are the risks to the recipients? These include the immediate and long-term risks. (c) Cost in money and man power? This is done to find out whether the preventive measure is economical and practical in terms of money spent. It is now conceded that no health measure should be introduced on a large scale without proper evaluation.

Recent problems that have engaged the attention of epidemiologists are studies of medical care and health services; planning and evaluation of health measures, services and research.

ASSOCIATION AND CAUSATION

Descriptive studies help in the identification of the disease problem in the community; and by relating disease to host, agent and environmental factors, it endeavours to suggest an aetiological hypothesis. Analytical and experimental studies test the hypotheses derived from descriptive studies and confirm or refute the observed association between suspected causes and disease. When the disease is multifactorial (e.g., coronary heart disease) numerous factors or variables become implicated in the web of causation, and the notion of "cause" becomes confused. The more associations, the more investigations to disentangle the web of causation. The epidemiologist whose primary interest is to establish a "cause and effect" relationship has to sift the husk from the grain. He proceeds from demonstration of statistical association to demonstration that the association is causal.

The terms "association" and "relationship" are often used interchangeably. Association may be defined as the concurrence of two variables more often than would be expected by chance. In other words, events are said to be associated when they occur more frequently together than one would expect by chance *(2)*. Association does not necessarily imply a causal relationship.

It will be useful to consider here the concept of correlation. Correlation indicates the *degree* of association between two characteristics. The correlation coefficients range from –1.0 to +1.0. A correlation coefficient of 1.0 means that the two variables exhibit a perfect linear relationship. However, correlation cannot be used to invoke causation, because the sequence of exposure preceding disease (temporal association) cannot be assumed to have occurred. Secondly, correlation does not measure risk. It may be said that causation implies correlation, but correlation does not imply causation.

Association can be broadly grouped under three headings :

a. Spurious association
b. Indirect association
c. Direct (causal) association
   (i) one-to-one causal association
   (ii) multifactorial causation.

a. Spurious association

Sometimes an observed association between a disease and suspected factor may not be real. For example, a study in UK of 5174 births at home and 11,156 births in hospitals showed perinatal mortality rates of 5.4 per 1000 in the home births, and 27.8 per 1000 in the hospital births *(86)*. Apparently, the perinatal mortality was higher in hospital births than in the home births. It might be concluded that homes are a safer place for delivery of births than hospitals. Such a conclusion is spurious or artifactual, because in general, hospitals attract women at high risk for delivery because of their special equipment and expertise, whereas this is not the case with home deliveries. The high perinatal mortality rate in hospitals might be due to this fact alone, and not because the quality of care was inferior. There might be other factors also such as differences in age, parity, prenatal care, home circumstances, general health and disease state between the study and control groups. This type of bias where "like" is not compared with "like" (selection bias) is very important in epidemiological studies. It may lead to a spurious association or an association when none actually existed.

b. Indirect association

Many associations which at first appeared to be causal have been found on further study to be due to indirect association. The indirect association is a statistical association between a characteristic (or variable) of interest and a disease due to the presence of another factor, known or unknown, that is common to both the characteristic and the disease. This third factor (i.e., the common factor) is also known as the "confounding" variable. Since it is related both to the disease and to the variable, it might explain the statistical association between disease and a characteristic wholly or in part. Such confounding variables (e.g., age, sex, social class) are potentially and probably present in all data and represent a formidable obstacle to overcome in trying to assess the causal nature of the relationship. Two examples of an indirect association are given below.

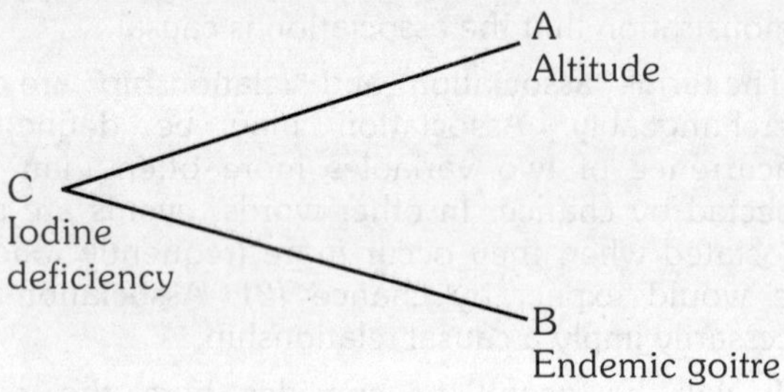

FIG. 12
Model of an indirect association

(a) Altitude and endemic goitre

Endemic goitre is generally found in high altitudes, showing thereby an association between altitude and endemic goitre (Fig. 12). We know, that endemic goitre is not due to altitude but due to environmental deficiency of iodine. Fig. 12 illustrates how a common factor (i.e., iodine deficiency) can result in an apparent association between two variables, when no association exists. This amplifies the earlier statement that statistical association does not necessarily mean causation.

(b) Sucrose and CHD

Yudkin and Roddy *(87)* found a higher intake of sugar by patients with myocardial infarction. Their study was based on an enquiry by questionnaire method into dietary habits of cases and controls. They put forward an attractive hypothesis that people who consume lot of sugar are far more likely to have a heart attack than those who take little.

Further studies were undertaken to test whether sugar intake was associated with other variables such as cigarette smoking, which might be causally related to CHD. Bennet and others *(88)* found that heavy cigarette smoking was positively associated with an increase in the number of cups of hot drinks consumed daily and the amount of sugar consumed. They concluded that it was cigarette smoking and not sugar consumption which was implicated in the aetiology of CHD. In their study, they did not find any evidence of increasing trend of CHD with increasing consumption of sugar. Finally, proof came from experimental studies that high sucrose feeding did not induce arteriosclerotic disease in animals.

Sometimes knowledge of indirect associations can be applied towards reducing disease risk. Before the discovery of the cholera vibrio, elimination of certain water supplies achieved a marked decrease in new cases of the disease. Such indirect associations must be pursued, for it is likely that they may provide aetiological clues.

c. Direct (causal) association

(i) One-to-one causal relationship

Two variables are stated to be causally related **(AB)** if a change in A is followed by a change in B. If it does not, then their relationship cannot be causal. This is known as "one-to-one" causal relationship. This model suggests that when the factor **A** is present, the disease **B** must result. Conversely, when the disease is present, the factor must also be present. Measles may be one disease in which such a relation exists *(3)*.

Epidemiologists are interested in identifying the "cause". The most satisfactory procedure to demonstrate this would be by direct experiment. But this procedure is scarcely available to the epidemiologist. And, in some cases, the "cause" is not amenable to manipulation.

The above concept of one-to-one causal relationship was the essence of Koch's postulates. The proponents of the germ theory of disease insisted that the cause must be :

a. necessary, and
b. sufficient for the occurrence of disease

before it can qualify as cause of disease. In other words, whenever the disease occurs, the factor or cause must be present.

Although Koch's postulates are theoretically sound, the "necessary and sufficient" concept does not fit well for many diseases. Taking for example tuberculosis, tubercle bacilli cannot be found in all cases of the disease but this does not rule out the statement that tubercle bacilli are the cause of tuberculosis *(5)*. That the cause must be "sufficient" is also not always supported by evidence. In tuberculosis, it is well–known that besides tubercle bacilli, there are additional factors such as host susceptibility which are required to produce the disease.

The concept of one-to-one causal relationship is further complicated by the fact that sometimes, a single cause or factor may lead to more than one outcome, as shown in Fig. 13. In short, one-to-one causal relationship, although ideal in disease aetiology, does not explain every situation.

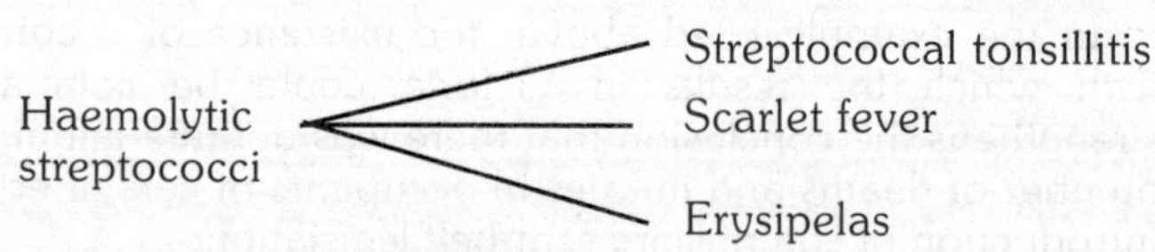

FIG. 13
Model in which one factor is shown to lead to more than one disease

(ii) Multifactorial causation

The causal thinking is different when we consider a non-communicable disease or condition (e.g., CHD) where the aetiology is multifactorial. Two models are presented in Figures 14 and 15 to explain the complex situation. In one model (Fig. 14), there are alternative causal factors (Factors 1, 2 and 3) each acting independently. This situation is exemplified in lung cancer where more than one aetiological factor (e.g., smoking, air pollution, exposure to asbestos) can produce the disease independently. It is possible as our knowledge of cancer increases, we may discover a common biochemical event at the cellular level that can be produced by each of the factors. The cellular or molecular factor will then be considered necessary as a causal factor *(5)*.

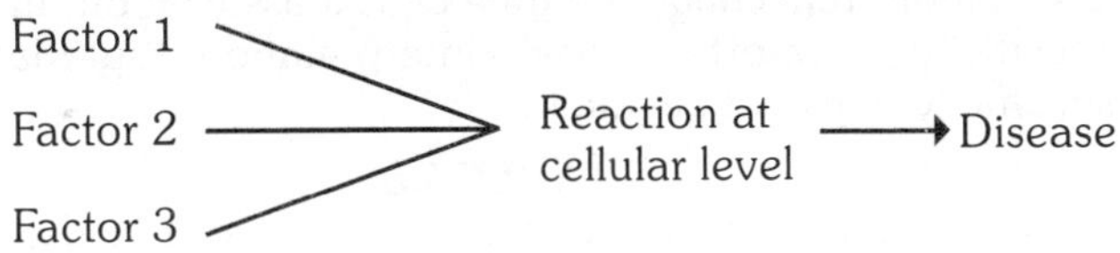

FIG. 14
A model of multifactorial causation *(4)*.

In the second model (Fig. 15) the causal factors act cumulatively to produce disease. This is probably the correct model for many diseases. It is possible that each of the several factors act independently, but when an individual is exposed to 2 or more factors, there may be a synergistic effect.

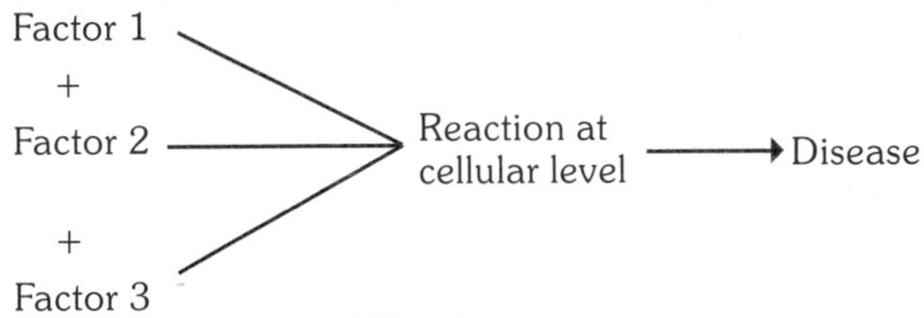

FIG. 15
A model of multifactorial causation showing synergism *(4)*

From the above discussion, it is reasonable to conclude that "one-to-one" relationship in causation is an oversimplification. In biological phenomena, the requirement that "cause" is both "necessary" and "sufficient" condition is not easily reached, because of the existence of multiple factors in disease aetiology. This has created a serious problem to the epidemiologist, who is in search of causes of disease.

ADDITIONAL CRITERIA FOR JUDGING CAUSALITY

In the absence of controlled experimental evidence to incriminate the "cause", certain additional criteria have been evolved for deciding when an association may be considered a causal association. An elegant elucidation of these criteria appears in "Smoking and Health" the Report of the Advisory Committee to the Surgeon General of the Public Health Service in US *(89)*. Bradford Hill *(90, 91)* and others *(92)* have pointed out that the likelihood of a causal relationship is increased by the presence of the following criteria.

1. Temporal association
2. Strength of association
3. Specificity of the association
4. Consistency of the association
5. Biological plausibility
6. Coherence of the association

The Surgeon–General's Report (1964) states that the causal significance of an association is a matter of judgement which goes beyond any statement of statistical probability. To judge or evaluate the causal significance of an association, all the above criteria must be utilized, no one of which by itself is self-sufficient or *sine qua-non* for drawing causal inferences from statistical associations, but each adds to the quantum of evidence, and all put together contribute to a probability of the association being causal.

ASSOCIATION BETWEEN CIGARETTE SMOKING AND LUNG CANCER

Cigarette smoking and lung cancer hypothesis provides an excellent example to illustrate the epidemiological criteria for establishing whether or not an observed association plays a causal role in the aetiology of a disease. The data fulfilling the criteria were covered adequately in *Smoking* and *Health*, the initial report of the Advisory Committee to the Surgeon General of the Public Health Service in 1964 *(89)*. The later reports of US Public Health Service from 1964–1973, and similar other reports (e.g., Report of the Royal College of Physicians, London : *Smoking or Health*, 1977) summarized newer data supporting the validity of the hypothesis. Let us examine the cigarette smoking and lung cancer hypothesis in the light of the above criteria.

1. Temporal association

This criterion centres round the question: Does the suspected cause precede the observed effect ? A causal association requires that exposure to a putative cause must precede temporarily the onset of a disease which it is purported to produce to allow for any necessary period of induction and latency. This requirement is basic to the causal concept.

In certain acute diseases such as water and food-borne outbreaks, discovery of temporal sequence of two variables (e.g., drinking contaminated water and diarrhoea) is not often a serious problem. However, in many chronic diseases, because of insidious onset and ignorance of precise induction periods, it becomes hard to establish a temporal sequence as to which came first – the suspected agent or the disease, because one is dealing with a continuous evolving process.

Lung cancer occurs in smokers of long-standing; this satisfies the temporal requirement. Further, the increase in consumption of cigarettes preceded by about 30 years the increase in death rates from lung cancer. These observations are compatible with the long latent period characteristic of carcinogenesis.

2. Strength of association

The strength of association is based on answers to two questions:

a. Relative risk – is it large ?
b. Is there a dose–response, duration–response relationship ?

In general, the larger the relative risk, the greater the likelihood of a causal association. Furthermore, the likelihood of a causal relationship is strengthened if there is a biological gradient or dose–response relationship – i.e., with increasing levels of exposure to the risk factor, an increasing rise in incidence of the disease is found. If there is no dose–response or duration–response relationship, that would be an argument against the relationship being causal.

In the absence of experimental data on humans, the causal relationship of cigarette smoking and lung cancer has been based on three points : (a) relative risk (b) dose–response relationship, and (c) the decrease in risk on cessation of smoking. Table 26 presents data showing relative risk and dose–response relationship. Such high relative risks are rarely seen in epidemiological studies. It has been stated that the relationship between lung cancer and smoking is one of the most impressive demonstrations of a dose–response relationship that can be found in epidemiology *(3)*. The dose–response relationship has, in fact, played a major role in acceptance of relationship as causal *(13)*. If there has been no dose–response relationship, that would have been a strong argument against the causal hypothesis. Another factor that has added to the weight of evidence is the fact that lung cancer death rates among moderate smokers were intermediate between those among light smokers and heavy smokers.

TABLE 26

Death rate and relative risk for smokers and non-smokers

Daily average cigarettes smoked	Death rate per 1000		Relative risk
	Smokers	Non-smokers	
1–14	0.47	0.07	6.7
15–24	0.86	0.07	12.3
25+	1.66	0.07	23.7

Source : *(62)*

Cessation experiment

Another piece of evidence is provided by the cessation experiment. Table 27 shows the mortality ratios in ex-cigarette smokers by number of years stopped smoking among British doctors. The results confirmed that the mortality ratios were reduced in a way that would be expected if smoking were the cause of the disease. This is a strong point in the evidence favouring the hypothesis.

TABLE 27

Lung cancer mortality ratios in ex-cigarette-smokers, by number of years stopped smoking, British physicians

Years stopped smoking	Mortality ratio
Still smoking	15.8
1–4	16.0
5–9	5.9
10–14	5.3
15 +	2.0
Non-smokers	1.0

Source : *(60)*

3. Specificity of the association

The concept of specificity implies a "one-to-one" relationship between the cause and effect. In the past, much of the controversy over cigarette smoking and lung cancer centred round lack of specificity of the association. That is, cigarette smoking is linked with not only lung cancer but several others such as coronary heart disease, bronchitis, emphysema, cancer cervix, etc. This was used, for several years, as an argument against the acceptance of the association as causal. It is true that cigarette smoking is associated with so many diseases reflecting an apparent lack of specificity, but that cannot be a strong argument, so as to dismiss the causal hypothesis. This is because the requirement of specificity is a most difficult criterion to establish not only in chronic disease but also in acute diseases and conditions. The reasons are : first, a single cause or factor can give rise to more than one disease. Secondly, most diseases are due to multiple factors with no possibility of demonstrating one-to-one relationship.

The lack of specificity can be further explained by the fact that tobacco smoke is a complex of substances containing several harmful ingredients or factors such as nicotine, carbon monoxide, benzpyrene, particulate matter and many other ingredients with possible additive and synergistic action. The different components of tobacco smoke could as well be responsible for different states. In spite of this, it can be seen from Table 28 that the association of lung cancer with cigarette smoking is far more striking than any other association, reflecting a definite causal association. In short, specificity supports causal interpretation but lack of specificity does not negate it.

TABLE 28

Expected and observed deaths for smokers of cigarettes compared to non-smokers; Seven prospective studies combined, for selected causes of death

Underlying cause of death	Expected deaths (E)	Observed deaths (O)	Mortality ratio (O/E)
Cancer of lung	170.3	1,833	10.8
Bronchitis and emphysema	89.5	546	6.1
Cancer of larynx	14.0	75	5.4
Cancer oesophagus	37.0	152	4.1
Peptic ulcer	105.1	294	2.8
Cancer bladder	111.6	216	1.9
CHD	6,430.7	11,177	1.7
Cancer rectum	207.8	213	1.0
All causes of death	15,653.9	23,223	1.7

Source : *(38)*

The concept of specificity cannot be entirely dissociated from the concept of association. It has been estimated that about 80–90 per cent of lung cancer can be attributed to cigarette smoking. To say this, it is assumed that the association between smoking and lung cancer is causal. Under the heading of specificity, two more observations require comment : (a) not everyone who smokes develops cancer, and (b) not everyone who develops lung cancer has smoked. The first apparent paradox is related to the multifactorial nature of lung cancer. It may well be that there are other factors as yet unidentified which must be present in conjunction with smoking for lung cancer to develop. As for lung cancer in non-smokers, it is known that there are factors other than smoking which increase the risk of lung cancer such as occupational exposure to chromates, asbestos, nickel, uranium and exposure to air pollution. Deviations from one-to-one relationship between cigarette smoking and lung cancer therefore, cannot be said to rule out a causal relationship.

4. Consistency of the association

The association is consistent if the results are replicated when studied in different settings and by different methods. That is, evidence from a single study is seldom sufficient to establish "causal" association. If there is no consistency, it will weaken a causal interpretation.

A consistent association has been found between cigarette smoking and lung cancer. More than 50 retrospective studies and at least nine prospective studies in different countries had shown a consistent association between cigarette smoking and subsequent development of lung cancer, lending support to a causal association.

5. Biological plausibility

Causal association is supported if there is biological credibility to the association, that is, the association agrees with current understanding of the response of cells, tissues, organs, and systems to stimuli. For example, the notion that food intake and cancer are interrelated is an old one. The positive association of intestine, rectum and breast cancers is biologically logical, whereas the positive association of food and skin cancer makes no biological sense suggesting that strength of association by itself does not imply causality.

This is one of the pitfalls of correlation studies. Further, the criterion of biological plausibility should not be applied rigidly. That is, even if a biological mechanism cannot be postulated, it does not rule out the possibility of a cause and effect relationship, for it may be merely due to the limits of current knowledge.

The cigarette smoking and lung cancer hypothesis is biologically plausible. It is not hard to visualize the inhalation of hot smoke into the lungs and deposition of a chemical carcinogen over a period of time probably building itself up to a threshold level and initiating neoplastic changes in the lungs. Experimental studies in animals have strengthened the evidence for the aetiological role of cigarette smoking, although one cannot directly translate the results of such studies in humans. Many such studies have shown that lung cancer can be produced by tracheobronchial implantation of tobacco extracts or by inhalation of cigarette smoke or of aerosols of its constituents. Carcinogenic substances have been isolated from cigarette smoke, although the precise carcinogens responsible for lung cancer in man are unknown. The biological credibility, in fact, provides a convincing evidence in favour of a causal association.

6. Coherence of the association

A final criterion for the appraisal of causal significance of an association is its coherence with known facts that are thought to be relevant. For example, the historical evidence of the rising consumption of tobacco in the form of cigarettes and the rising incidence of lung cancer are coherent. Male and female differences in trends of lung cancer death rates are also coherent with the more recent adoption of cigarette smoking by women. Death rates rose first in males and are now increasing relatively more rapidly in females. The fall in the relative risk of lung cancer when cigarette smoking is stopped, and the occurrence of lung cancer from occupational exposure to other carcinogens such as asbestos and uranium and the demonstrated increase in lung cancer risk when workers exposed to these substances also smoked, enhance the significance of a causal association.

In conclusion, it may be stated that the association between cigarette smoking and lung cancer can never be proved by a direct experiment on humans. It is an illusory and virtually unattainable goal. It is well known that epidemiology depends heavily on inferences drawn from observations rather than on the ultimate experiment. The nearest approach to "scientific proof", therefore is the vast body of convincing evidence we have accumulated during the past few years meeting all the criteria proposed for judging the causality of such associations.

USES OF EPIDEMIOLOGY

While the study of disease distribution and causation remains central to epidemiology; the techniques of epidemiology have a wider application covering many more important areas relating not only to disease but also health and health services. In more utilitarian terms, epidemiology has been defined as "a means of learning, or asking questions....and getting answers that lead to further questions". In this context, Morris *(11)* has identified seven distinct uses of epidemiology, five of which extend epidemiology beyond the search for causes of disease and bring it closer to day-to-day concerns of modern medicine.These are :

1. To study historically the rise and fall of disease in the population

Winston Churchill said : "The farther back you look, the farther forward you can see". The first use of epidemiology relates to this aspect, that is, study of the history of disease in human population. It is well known that the health and disease pattern in a community is never constant. There are fluctuations both over short and long periods of time. For example, the first contribution of epidemiology to the study of coronary heart disease was that it was an "epidemic". Later many others such as accidents, cancer and diabetes were found to be "epidemic". As old diseases (e.g., smallpox) are conquered, new ones (e.g., Legionnaires' disease, Lassa fever, AIDS) have been identified, in which epidemiology has played a major role. Epidemiology provides a means to study disease profiles and time trends in human population. By a study of these trends, we can make useful projections into the future and identify emerging health problems and their correlates.

2. Community diagnosis

One of the uses of epidemiology is community diagnosis. Community diagnosis generally refers to the identification and quantification of health problems in a community in terms of mortality and morbidity rates and ratios, and identification of their correlates for the purpose of defining those individuals or groups at risk or those in need of health care. By quantification of health problems, we lay down priorities in disease control and prevention. Secondly, quantification of morbidity and mortality can serve as a benchmark for the evaluation of health services at a later date. Thirdly, the quantification of health problems can be a source of new knowledge about disease distribution, causation and prevention. Community diagnosis has also been effectively extended beyond population distributions and profiles of illness to include an understanding of the social, cultural and environmental characteristics of the community *(93)*. Epidemiology, therefore, has been described as a "diagnostic tool" of community medicine.

3. Planning and evaluation

Planning is essential for a rational allocation of the limited resources. For example, in developing countries, too many hospitals have been built and equipped without knowledge of the particular disease problems in the community. Epidemiologic information about the distribution of health problems over time and place provides the fundamental basis for planning and developing the needed health services and for assessing the impact of these services on the people's problems. The application of epidemiological principles to problems of health care constitutes the "new epidemiology" *(94)*. Examples of planning include planning facilities for medical care (e.g., number of hospital beds required for patients with specific diseases, health manpower planning); planning facilities for preventive services (e.g., screening programmes, immunization campaigns; provision of sanitary services); and planning for research.

Evaluation is an equally important concern of epidemiology. Any measures taken to control or prevent a disease must be followed by an evaluation to find out whether the measures undertaken are effective in reducing the frequency of the disease. Evaluation of a control method such as hepatitis vaccine requires more than the demonstration of its effectiveness in reducing disease frequency. We have to measure the cost of its large-scale application in terms of the cost of the vaccine, trained personnel, storage, transport and other factors. The value of one method in relation to others is assessed by cost-effectiveness studies. It is now being recognized that not only vaccines, but in time all health services will have to submit to evaluation *(95)*. The development of randomized controlled trial has made it possible to evaluate treatment modalities on a firm scientific basis. Such trials have raised doubts about the utility of multiphasic screening, certain operative procedures (e.g., tonsillectomy, varicose vein, stripping), prolonged hospitalization of patients with myocardial infarction, etc. Clearly it is not enough to know that a programme provides some benefit; we need to know how much benefit and at what risk and cost *(95)*.

4. Evaluation of individual's risks and chances

One of the important tasks of epidemiologists is to make a statement about the degree of risk in a population. Besides the incidence rate and specific rates which are measures of absolute risk, the epidemiologists calculate relative risk and attributable risk for a factor related to or believed to be a cause of the disease. The risk of bearing a mongol child and of some hereditary disorders are classic examples of evaluating individual's risks and chances. The risk assessment for smokers and non-smokers, for selected causes of death (e.g., cancer CHD) is another well-known example.

5. Syndrome identification

Medical syndromes are identified by observing frequently associated findings in individual patients. It is worth recalling that, although approximately 3000 so-called syndromes are described in the contemporary paediatric literature, a primary defect is known only in about 20 per cent of these *(96)*. Epidemiological investigations can be used to define and refine syndromes. By observation of groups, such studies have been able to correct misconceptions concerning many disease syndromes. For example, there was less appreciation of the two main types of peptic ulcer (gastric and duodenal) till 1920. But the "poverty" gradient in the certification of the gastric ulcer and its absence in duodenal ulcer led to differentiation of gastric and duodenal ulcers. Another example is that of Patterson-Kelly syndrome of association between dysphagia and iron-deficiency anaemia, but when the association was tested by epidemiological methods, it was not found *(11)*. Clinical studies using plasma renin levels have suggested that aetiologically, prognostically and therapeutically distinct syndromes of essential hypertension may exist. It has been the subject of hot debate *(97, 98)*.

6. Completing the natural history of disease

Epidemiology is concerned with the entire spectrum of disease in a population. The picture of disease constructed on the basis of hospital patients is quite different from that found in the community. The epidemiologist by studying disease patterns in the community in relation to agent, host and environmental factors is in a better position to fill up the gaps in the natural history of disease than the clinician. For example an outstanding contribution by epidemiology to the natural history of atherosclerosis is the recognition that one-third to two-thirds of all deaths due to ischaemic heart disease are sudden, i.e., occur in less than one hour. Hospital studies could never have come to this conclusion, for most victims do not reach the hospital. This gave tremendous impetus to the development of intensive coronary care units *(99)*. Epidemiological investigations have yielded a large amount of data on risk factors in relation to chronic disease. The impact of these findings on our knowledge of the natural history of chronic disease remains to be elucidated. Since the epidemiologist is concerned with all cases in the defined population, regardless of severity or source of medical care, his perspective of disease is consequently the broadest.

7. Searching for causes and risk factors

Epidemiology, by relating disease to interpopulation differences and other attributes of the population or cohorts examined, tries to identify the causes of disease. The contributions of epidemiology have been many in this regard. Numerous examples can be cited : epidemiological studies have incriminated that rubella is the cause of congenital defects in the newborn, that thalidomide is a teratogenic agent, cigarette smoking is a cause of lung cancer, exposure of premature babies to oxygen is the cause of retrolental fibroplasia, etc. in the case of chronic disease, hopes of finding a single cause remains unfulfilled, but an important conceptual change has occurred – that is, search for risk factors. The concept of "risk factors" gave renewed impetus to epidemiological research. The search for causes and risk factors will be a ceaseless effort, as our ignorance about disease aetiology, particularly chronic disease, is profound, not to speak of the "new" diseases which are appearing.

INFECTIOUS DISEASE EPIDEMIOLOGY

Infectious disease epidemiology is a fundamental part of the whole of epidemiology. In fact, the subject of epidemiology originally developed from the study of epidemics of infectious diseases. There is a renaissance in the study of communicable diseases, stimulated by (a) changes in the pattern of communicable diseases, (b) by the discovery of "new" infections, and (c) by the possibility that some chronic diseases have an infective origin. The development of vaccines and antibiotics was not followed, as predicted, by the virtual disappearance of infectious disease. Its prevention and control needs epidemiological knowledge and experience *(100)*. This section focuses on infectious disease epidemiology.

Selected definitions

Definitions are essential for any kind of epidemiological activity, e.g., disease reporting, measurement of mortality and morbidity, etc. Clear-cut definitions of the terms such as "infection", "epidemic" and "surveillance" are needed in the study of infectious diseases. A few selected definitions pertaining to infectious disease epidemiology are given below :

INFECTION

The entry and development or multiplication of an infectious agent in an organism, including the body of man or animals *(4)*. It also implies that the body responds in some way to defend itself against the invader, either in the form of an immune response (evidence of this may not be readily available) or disease. An infection does not always cause illness.

There are several levels of infection : *colonization* (e.g., *S. aureus* in skin and normal nasopharynx); subclinical or *inapparent infection* (e.g., polio); latent infection (e.g., virus of herpes simplex); and manifest or *clinical infection*.

CONTAMINATION

The presence of an infectious agent on a body surface; also on or in clothes, beddings, toys, surgical instruments or dressings, or other inanimate articles or substances including water, milk and food. *Pollution* is distinct from contamination and implies the presence of offensive, but not necessarily infectious matter in the environment. Contamination on a body surface does not imply a carrier state *(100)*.

INFESTATION

For persons or animals the lodgement, development and reproduction of arthropods on the surface of the body or in the clothing, e.g., lice, itch mite *(100)*. Some authorities use the term also to describe invasion of the gut by parasitic worms, e.g., ascariasis *(100)*.

Infested articles or premises are those which harbour or give shelter to animal forms, especially arthropods and rodents *(100)*.

HOST

A person or other living animal, including birds and arthropods, that affords subsistence or lodgement to an infectious agent under natural (as opposed to experimental) conditions. An *obligate* host means the only host, e.g., man in measles and typhoid fever. Hosts in which the parasite attains maturity or passes its sexual stage are primary or *definitive* hosts; those in which the parasite is in a larval or asexual state are secondary or *intermediate* hosts. A *transport* host is a carrier in which the organism remains alive but does not undergo development *(100)*.

INFECTIOUS DISEASE

A disease due to an infectious agent. While some infectious diseases are contagious, others are non-contagious. All infectious diseases and infestations are communicable diseases *(4)*.

CONTAGIOUS DISEASE

A disease that is transmitted through contact *(100)*. Examples include scabies, trachoma, STD and leprosy.

COMMUNICABLE DISEASE

An illness due to a specific infectious agent or its toxic products that arises through transmission of that agent or its products from an infected person, animal, or reservoir to a susceptible host, either directly or indirectly through an intermediate plant or animal host, vector, or the inanimate environment *(100)*.

EPIDEMIC

[*Epi* (upon), *demos* (people)]. The occurrence in a community or region of cases of an illness, specific health-related behaviour, or other health-related events clearly in excess of normal expectancy. The community or region and the period in which the cases occur must be specified precisely. The number of cases indicating the presence of an epidemic varies according to the agent, size, and type of population exposed; previous experience or lack of exposure to the disease; and time and place of occurrence. Epidemicity is thus relative to usual frequency of the disease in the same area, among the specified population, at the same season of the year.

A single case of a communicable disease long absent from a population or first invasion by a disease not previously recognized in that area requires immediate reporting and full field investigation; two cases of such disease associated in time and place may be sufficient evidence to be considered an epidemic. The purpose of surveillance systems is to identify epidemics as early as possible, so that effective control measure can be put in place. This remains the most important task for epidemiology *(4)*.

ENDEMIC

(En=in; demos=people). It refers to the constant presence of a disease or infectious agent within a given geographic area or population group, without importation from outside; may also refer to the "usual" or expected frequency of the disease within such area or population group. For instance, common cold is endemic because somebody always has one.

The term "hyperendemic" expresses that the disease is constantly present at a high incidence and/or prevalence rate and affects all age groups equally; and the term "holoendemic" a high level of infection beginning early in life and affecting most of the child population, leading to a state of equilibrium such that the adult population shows evidence of the disease much less commonly than do the children, as in the case of malaria *(100)*.

An endemic disease when conditions are favourable may burst into an epidemic (e.g., hepatitis A, typhoid fever). As new control or preventive measures are applied, the endemic status of a disease may change.

SPORADIC

The word sporadic means scattered about. The cases occur irregularly, haphazardly from time to time, and generally infrequently *(100)*. The cases are so few and separated widely in space and time that they show little or no connection with each other, nor a recognizable common source of infection, e.g., tetanus, herpes-zoster and meningococcal meningitis. A sporadic disease may be the starting point of an epidemic when conditions are favourable for its spread. Many zoonotic diseases are characterised by sporadic transmission to man.

PANDEMIC

An epidemic occurring over a very wide area, crossing international boundaries, and usually affecting a large number of people. Only some pandemics cause severe disease in some individuals or at a population level. Characteristics of an infectious agent influencing the causation of a pandemic include : the agent must be able to infect humans, to cause disease in humans and to spread easily from human to human *(4)*. Examples are influenza pandemics and cholera pandemics.

EXOTIC

Diseases which are imported into a country in which they do not otherwise occur.

ZOONOSES

An infection or infectious disease transmissible under natural conditions from vertebrate animals to man. May be enzootic or epizootic – e.g., rabies, plague, bovine tuberculosis, anthrax, brucellosis, salmonellosis, endemic typhus, hydatidosis, kyasanur forest disease, monkeypox, lassa fever, etc.

The term zoonoses has been further amplified as follows : (a) *anthropozoonoses* : that is, infections transmitted to man from vertebrate animals, e.g., rabies, plague, hydatid disease, anthrax and trichinosis; (b) *zooanthroponoses* : that is, infections transmitted from man to vertebrate animals, e.g., human tuberculosis in cattle; and (c) *amphixenoses* : that is infections maintained in both man and lower vertebrate animals that may be transmitted in either direction, e.g., *T.cruzi,* and *S.japonicum (100).*

EPIZOOTIC

An outbreak (epidemic) of disease in an animal population (often with the implication that it may also affect human populations) *(100).* Only a few zoonotic agents cause major epidemics. Notable among these are the agents of anthrax, brucellosis, rabies, influenza, Rift valley fever, Q fever, Japanese encephalitis and equine encephalitis. The study of epizootic diseases is given the name of epizootiology.

EPORNITHIC

An outbreak (epidemic) of disease in a bird population *(100).*

ENZOOTIC

An endemic occurring in animals e.g., anthrax, rabies, brucellosis, bovine tuberculosis, endemic typhus and tick typhus.

NOSOCOMIAL INFECTION

Nosocomial (hospital acquired) infection is an infection originating in a patient while in a hospital or other health care facility. It denotes a new disorder (unrelated to the patient's primary condition) associated with being in a hospital *(100).* That is, it was not present or incubating at the time of admission or the residual of an infection acquired during a previous admission. It includes infections acquired in the hospital but appearing after discharge, and also such infections among the staff of the facility *(100).* Examples include infection of surgical wounds, hepatitis B and urinary tract infections.

OPPORTUNISTIC INFECTION

Infection with organism(s) that are normally innocuous (e.g. commensals in the human) but become pathogenic when the body's immunological defenses are compromised, as in AIDS *(4).*

IATROGENIC DISEASE

Literally, "doctor-generated"; often, broadly used to refer to adverse effects of preventive, diagnostic, therapeutic, surgical, and other medical, biotechnical, cosmetic, sanitary, and public health products, services, procedures, interventions, or policies. The process through which a professional activity generates an adverse health effect. There is a natural plurality of views on what constitutes iatrogenesis and its scope. Medicine and public health are obviously not the only professions that cause adverse health effects *(4).*

The disease may be serious enough to prolong the hospital stay, require special treatment or actually threaten life. Most of the episodes are related to drug therapy, immunization or diagnostic procedures, e.g., reactions to penicillin and immunizing agents, aplastic anaemia following the use of chloramphenicol, childhood leukaemia due to prenatal X-rays, hepatitis B following blood transfusion, etc. These are all preventable. In short, iatrogenic disease is a hazard of health care.

SURVEILLANCE

Continuous analysis, interpretation, and feedback of systematically collected data, generally using methods distinguished by their practicality, uniformity, and rapidity rather than by accuracy or completeness. By observing trends in time, place, and persons, changes can be observed or anticipated and appropriate action, including investigative or control measures, can be taken. Sources of data may relate directly to disease or to factors influencing disease. Thus they may include mortality and morbidity reports based on death certificates, hospital records, general practice sentinels, or notifications; laboratory diagnosis; outbreak reports; vaccine uptake and side effects; sickness absence records; changes in disease agents, vectors, or reservoirs; serological surveillance through serum banks *(4).*

ERADICATION

Termination of all transmission of infection by extermination of the infectious agent through surveillance and containment *(4, 100).* Eradication is an absolute process, an "all or none" phenomenon, restricted to termination of an infection from the whole world. It implies that disease will no longer occur in a population. To-date, only one disease has been eradicated, that is smallpox.

The term *elimination* is sometimes used to describe "eradication" of disease (e.g., measles) from a large geographic region or political jurisdiction *(100).* In the state of our present knowledge, diseases which are amenable to eradication are measles, diphtheria, polio and guinea worm.

DYNAMICS OF DISEASE TRANSMISSION

Communicable diseases are transmitted from the reservoir/source of infection to susceptible host. Fig.16 illustrates the medical model of an infectious disease. Basically there are three links in the chain of transmission, viz, the reservoir, modes of transmission and the susceptible host.

Sources and reservoir

The starting point for the occurrence of a communicable disease is the existence of a reservoir or source of infection. The **source** of infection is defined as "the person, animal, object or substance from which an infectious agent passes or is disseminated to the host" *(100).* A **reservoir** is defined as "any person, animal, arthropod, plant, soil or substance (or combination of these) in which an infectious agent lives and multiplies, on which it depends primarily for survival, and where it reproduces itself in such manner that it can be transmitted to a susceptible host" *(100).* In short, the reservoir is the natural habitat in which the organism metabolizes and replicates.

The terms reservoir and source are not always synonymous. For example, in hookworm infection, the reservoir is man, but the source of infection is the soil contaminated with infective larvae. In tetanus, the reservoir and source are the same, that is soil. In typhoid fever, the reservoir of infection may be a case or carrier, but the source of infection may be faeces or urine of patients or contaminated food, milk or water. Thus the term "source"

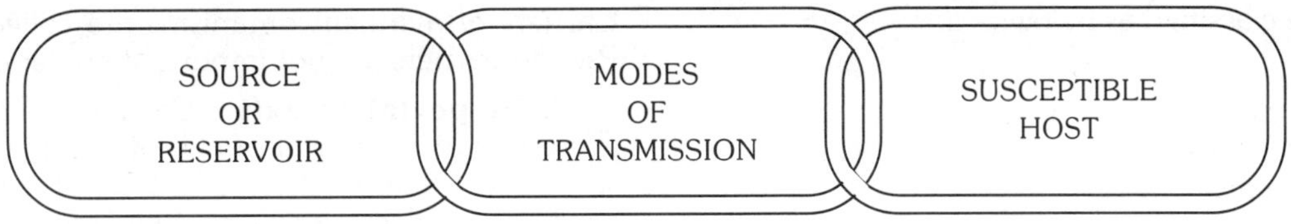

FIG. 16
Chain of Infection

refers to the immediate source of infection and may or may not be a part of reservoir.

The term *homologous reservoir* is applied when another member of the same species is the victim, as for example man is the principal reservoir for some enteric pathogens, e.g., *vibrio cholerae*. The term heterologous is applied when the infection is derived from a reservoir other than man, as for example animals and birds infected with salmonella.

The reservoir may be of three types :

1. Human reservoir
2. Animal reservoir, and
3. Reservoir in non-living things.

1. Human reservoir

By far the most important source or reservoir of infection for humans is man himself. He may be a case or carrier. Man is often described as his own enemy because most of the communicable diseases of which man is heir to are contracted from human sources.

a. CASES

A case is defined as "a person in the population or study group identified as having the particular disease, health disorder or condition under investigation" *(100)*. A variety of criteria (e.g., clinical, biochemical, laboratory registries and notifications, abstracts of clinical records, surveys of the general population, population screening and reporting of defects etc.) may be used to identify cases. Broadly, the presence of infection in a host may be clinical, subclinical or latent. These variations in the manifestations of disease are referred to as "spectrum of disease" or "gradient of infection" (see page 45).

(1) The *clinical* illness may be mild or moderate, typical or atypical, severe or fatal depending upon the gradient of involvement. Epidemiologically, mild cases may be more important sources of infection than severe cases because they are ambulant and spread the infection wherever they go, whereas severe cases are usually confined to bed.

(2) The *subclinical cases* are variously referred to as inapparent, covert, missed or abortive cases. They are equally important as sources of infection. The disease agent may multiply in the host but does not manifest itself by signs and symptoms. The disease agent is, eliminated and contaminates the environment in the same way as clinical cases. Persons who are thus sick (unbeknown to themselves and others) contribute more than symptomatic patients to the transmission of infection to others and what is more, they do not appear in any of the statistics. Subclinical cases play a dominant role in maintaining the chain of infection (endemicity) in the community.

Subclinical infection can be detected only by laboratory tests, e.g., recovery of the organism, antibody response, biochemical and skin sensitivity tests.

Barring a few (e.g., measles), subclinical infection occurs in most infectious diseases. In some diseases (e.g., rubella, mumps, polio, hepatitis A and B, Japanese encephalitis, influenza, diphtheria), a great deal of subclinical infection occurs. Since subclinical infections occur frequently during a person's life time, they are responsible for the immunity shown by adult humans to a variety of disease–producing microbes.

(3) The term *latent infection* must be distinguished from subclinical infection. In latent infection, the host does not shed the infectious agent which lies dormant within the host without symptoms (and often without demonstrable presence in blood, tissues or bodily secretions of the host). For example, latent infection occurs in herpes simplex, Brill–Zinser disease, infections due to slow viruses, ancylostomiasis, etc. The role of latent infection in the perpetuation of certain infectious agents appears to be great.

In epidemiological terminology, the term **primary case** refers to the first case of a communicable disease introduced into the population unit being studied. The term **index case** refers to the first case to come to the attention of the investigator; it is not always the primary case. **Secondary cases** are those developing from contact with primary case. A **suspect** case is an individual (or a group of individuals) who has all of the signs and symptoms of a disease or condition, yet has not been diagnosed as having the disease or had the cause of the symptoms connected to the suspected pathogen.

Whatever may be the "gradient of infection", all infected persons, whether clinical or subclinical, are potential sources of infection, because the disease agent is leaving the body through frequent stools, vomiting, coughing, sneezing or other means and is potentially available for transfer to a new host.

b. CARRIERS

In some diseases, either due to inadequate treatment or immune response, the disease agent is not completely eliminated, leading to a carrier state. A carrier is defined as "an infected person or animal that harbours a specific infectious agent in the absence of discernible clinical disease and serves as a potential source of infection for others" *(100)*. As a rule carriers are less infectious than cases, but epidemiologically, they are more dangerous than cases because they escape recognition, and continuing as they do to live a normal life among the population or community, they readily infect the susceptible individuals over a wider area and longer period of time, under favourable conditions. The "Typhoid Mary" is a classic example of a carrier.

The elements in a carrier state are : (a) the presence in the body of the disease agent (b) the absence of recognizable symptoms and signs of disease, and (c) the shedding of the disease agent in the discharges or excretions, thus acting as a source of infection for other persons.

Carriers may be classified as below :

A. Type
- (a) Incubatory
- (b) Convalescent
- (c) Healthy

B. Duration
- (a) Temporary
- (b) Chronic

C. Portal of exit
- (a) Urinary
- (b) Intestinal
- (c) Respiratory
- (d) Others

A. **By type** : (a) INCUBATORY CARRIERS : Incubatory carriers are those who shed the infectious agent during the incubation period of disease. That is, they are capable of infecting others before the onset of illness. This usually occurs during the last few days of the incubation period, e.g., measles, mumps, polio, pertussis, influenza, diphtheria and hepatitis B. (b) CONVALESCENT CARRIERS : That is, those who continue to shed the disease agent during the period of convalescence, e.g., typhoid fever, dysentery (bacillary and amoebic), cholera, diphtheria and whooping cough. In these diseases, clinical recovery does not coincide with bacteriological recovery. A convalescent carrier can pose a serious threat to the unprotected household members and those in the immediate environment, as in the case of a typhoid fever patient who may excrete the bacilli for 6–8 weeks. This highlights the importance of bacteriological surveillance of carriers, after clinical recovery. (c) HEALTHY CARRIERS : Healthy carriers emerge from subclinical cases. They are victims of subclinical infection who have developed carrier state without suffering from overt disease, but are nevertheless shedding the disease agent, e.g., poliomyelitis, cholera, meningococcal meningitis, salmonellosis, and diphtheria. It is well to remember that a person whose infection remains subclinical may or may not be a carrier. For example, in polio the infection may remain subclinical and the person may act as a temporary carrier by virtue of shedding the organism. On the other hand, in tuberculosis, most persons with positive tuberculin test do not actively disseminate tubercle bacilli and therefore are not labelled as carrier *(38)*.

B. **By duration** : (a) TEMPORARY CARRIERS : Temporary carriers are those who shed the infectious agent for short periods of time. In this category may be included the incubatory, convalescent and healthy carriers. (b) CHRONIC CARRIERS : A chronic carrier is one who excretes the infectious agent for indefinite periods. Chronic carrier state occurs in a number of diseases, e.g., typhoid fever, hepatitis B, dysentery, cerebro-spinal meningitis, malaria, gonorrhoea, etc. Chronic carriers are far more important sources of infection than cases. The longer the carrier state, the greater the risk to the community. Some carriers excrete the infectious agent only intermittently and some continuously. The duration of the carrier state varies with the disease. In typhoid fever and hepatitis B, the chronic carrier state may last for several years; in chronic dysentery, it may last for a year or longer. In diphtheria, the carrier state is associated with infected tonsils; in typhoid fever with gall bladder disease. Chronic carriers are known to reintroduce disease into areas which are otherwise free of infection (e.g., malaria). Therefore their early detection and treatment are essential to limit the spread of infection. Carriers of avirulent organisms are called *pseudo-carriers*. Pseudo-carriers are not important epidemiologically.

C. **By portal of exit** : Carriers may also be classified according to the portal of exit of the infectious agent. Thus we have urinary carriers, intestinal carriers, respiratory carriers, nasal carriers, etc. Skin eruptions, open wounds and blood are also portals of exit. In typhoid fever, the urinary carrier is more dangerous than an intestinal carrier. A typhoid carrier working in a food establishment or water works is more dangerous than a typhoid carrier working in an office establishment. Thus the portal of exit and the occupational status of the carrier are important epidemiological considerations.

2. Animal reservoir

The source of infection may sometimes be animals and birds. These, like the human sources of infection, may be cases or carriers. The diseases and infections which are transmissible to man from vertebrates are called zoonoses. There are over 100 zoonotic diseases which may be conveyed to man from animals and birds. The best known examples are rabies, yellow fever and influenza. The role of pigs and ducks in the spread of epidemic and pandemic influenza both as reservoirs, carriers and "amplifying hosts" is now well established. Pigeons in cities can lead to infection with chlamydia; dust mites from them can cause allergy in man. Ornithosis and arboviruses can be transmitted to man from various birds. Wild birds, in particular, are important hosts in the transmission cycles of most of the mosquito-borne encephalitis and several mosquito-borne undifferentiated febrile diseases *(101)*. Histoplasmosis is carried all over the world by birds. As birds migrate from one locality to another they may carry ticks infected with viruses and rickettsiae that may cause disease in humans. In short, the migrations and movements of animals and birds may carry serious epizootiological and epidemiological risks. There is evidence that genetic recombination between animal and human viruses might produce "new" strains of viruses (e.g., influenza viruses).

3. Reservoir in non-living things

Soil and inanimate matter can also act as reservoirs of infection. For example, soil may harbour agents that cause tetanus, anthrax, coccidioidomycosis and mycetoma.

MODES OF TRANSMISSION

Communicable diseases may be transmitted from the reservoir or source of infection to a susceptible individual in many different ways, depending upon the infectious agent, portal of entry and the local ecological conditions. As a rule, an infectious disease is transmitted by only one route, e.g., typhoid fever by vehicle transmission and common cold by direct contact. But there are others which may be transmitted by several routes e.g., AIDS, salmonellosis, hepatitis B, brucellosis, Q fever, tularemia etc. The multiple transmission routes enhance the survival of the infectious agent. The mode of transmission of infectious diseases may be classified as below *(2, 99)*.

A DIRECT TRANSMISSION
1. Direct contact
2. Droplet infection
3. Contact with soil
4. Inoculation into skin or mucosa
5. Transplacental (vertical)

B INDIRECT TRANSMISSION
1. Vehicle-borne
2. Vector-borne
   a. Mechanical
   b. Biological
3. Air-borne
   a. Droplet nuclei
   b. Dust
4. Fomite-borne
5. Unclean hands and fingers

A. Direct transmission

(1) *Direct contact* : Infection may be transmitted by direct contact from skin to skin, mucosa to mucosa, or mucosa to skin of the same or another person. This implies direct and essentially immediate transfer of infectious agents from the reservoir or source to a susceptible individual, without an intermediate agency, e.g., skin–to–skin contact as by touching, kissing or sexual intercourse or continued close contact. Direct contact not only reduces the period for which the organism will have to survive outside the human host but also ensures a larger dose of infection. Diseases transmitted by direct contact include STD and AIDS, leprosy, leptospirosis, skin and eye infections. (2) *Droplet infection* : This is direct projection of a spray of droplets of saliva and nasopharyngeal secretions during coughing, sneezing, (Fig. 17) or speaking and spitting, talking into the surrounding atmosphere. The expelled droplets may impinge directly upon the conjunctiva, oro-respiratory mucosa or skin of a close contact. Particles of 10 mmm or greater in diameter are filtered off by nose. Those 5 mmm or less can penetrate deeply and reach the alveoli. The droplet spread is usually, limited to a distance of 30–60 cm between source and host *(102)*. In infectious diseases, these droplets, which may contain millions of bacteria and viruses can be a source of infection to others. When a healthy susceptible person comes within the range of these infected droplets he is likely to inhale some of them and acquire infection. Diseases transmitted by droplet spread include many respiratory infections, eruptive fevers, many infections of the nervous system, common cold, diphtheria, whooping cough, tuberculosis, COVID-19, meningococcal meningitis, etc. The potential for droplet spread is increased in conditions of close proximity, overcrowding and lack of ventilation. (3) *Contact with soil* : The disease agent may be acquired by direct exposure of susceptible tissue to the disease agent in soil, compost or decaying vegetable matter in which it normally leads a saprophytic existence e.g., hookworm larvae, tetanus, mycosis etc. (4) *Inoculation into skin or mucosa* : The disease agent may be inoculated directly into the skin or mucosa e.g., rabies virus by dog bite, hepatitis B virus through contaminated needles and syringes etc., and (5) *Transplacental (or vertical) transmission* : Disease agents can be transmitted transplacentally *(103, 104)*. This is another form of direct transmission. Examples include the so-called TORCH agents (Toxoplasma gondii, rubella virus, cytomegalovirus and herpes virus), varicella virus, syphilis, hepatitis B, Coxsackie B and AIDS. Some of the non-living agents (e.g., thalidomide, diethylstilbestrol) can also be transmitted vertically. In these cases, the disease agent produces malformations of the embryo by disturbing its development.

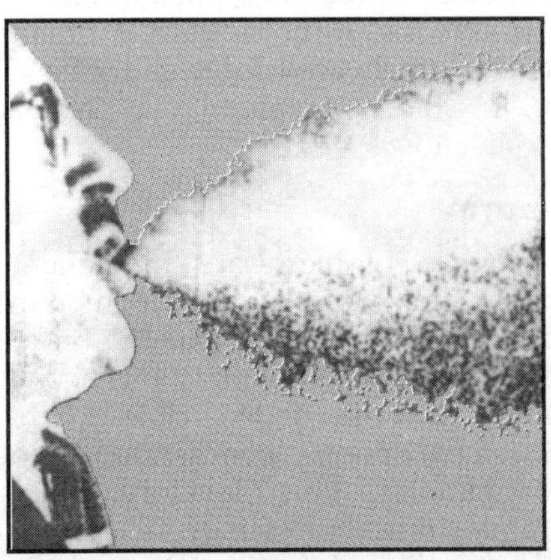

FIG. 17
Droplets sprayed into the air from a sneeze
(From : The Medical Clinics of North America, 1944 . p. 1301)

B. Indirect transmission

This embraces a variety of mechanisms including the traditional 5 F's – "flies, fingers, fomites, food and fluid". An essential requirement for indirect transmission is that the infectious agent must be capable of surviving outside the human host in the external environment and retain its basic properties of pathogenesis and virulence till it finds a new host. This depends upon the characteristics of the agent, the inanimate object and the influence of environmental factors such as temperature and humidity. If the disease agent acquires drug resistance, it will further facilitate its spread. Indirect transmission can occur in a variety of settings :

1. Vehicle-borne

Vehicle-borne transmission implies transmission of the infectious agent through the agency of water, food (including raw vegetables, fruits, milk and milk products), ice, blood, serum, plasma or other biological products such as tissues and organs. Of these water and food are the most frequent vehicles of transmission, because they are used by everyone. The infectious agent may have multiplied or developed in the vehicle (e.g., *S.aureus* in food) before being transmitted; or only passively transmitted in the vehicle (e.g., hepatitis A virus in water). Diseases transmitted by water and food include chiefly infections of the alimentary tract, e.g., acute diarrhoeas, typhoid fever, cholera, polio, hepatitis A, food poisoning and intestinal parasites. Those transmitted by blood include hepatitis B, malaria, syphilis, brucellosis, trypanasomes (Chaga's disease), infectious mononucleosis and cytomegalovirus infection *(105)*. Organ transplantation may result in the introduction of the disease agent such as cytomegalovirus in association with kidney transplants.

The epidemiological features of vehicle transmission are : (a) if the dose of contamination is heavy, the outbreak may be explosive as in the case of cholera and hepatitis A epidemics (b) cases are initially confined to those who are exposed to the contaminated vehicle, in some infections (c) when secondary cases occur, the primary case may be obscured (d) the distance travelled by the infectious agent may be great, e.g., outbreaks of food poisoning (e) it is not always possible to isolate the infectious agent in the incriminated vehicle, e.g., typhoid bacilli in contaminated water (f) when the vehicle is controlled or withdrawn, the epidemic subsides, e.g., epidemics of cholera, and (g) the common source of infection is often traceable.

2. Vector-borne

In infectious disease epidemiology, vector is defined as an arthropod or any living carrier (e.g., snail) that transports an infectious agent to a susceptible individual. Transmission by a vector may be mechanical or biological. In the latter case, the disease agent passes through a developmental cycle or multiplication in the vector.

Epidemiological classification of vector-borne diseases

I. By vector

a) Invertebrate type : Arthropod vectors fall into seven orders largely
   (1) Diptera – flies and mosquitoes
   (2) Siphonaptera – fleas
   (3) Orthoptera – cockroaches
   (4) Anoplura – sucking lice
   (5) Hemiptera – bugs, including kissing bugs
   (6) Acarina – ticks and mites
   (7) Copepoda – cyclops

b) Vertebrate type – Mice, rodents, bats.

II. By transmission chain

Vector-borne diseases are classified under heterogeneous infection chain and involve three principal patterns :

a) Man and a non–vertebrate host
   1) Man–arthropod–man (malaria)
   2) Man–snail–man (schistosomiasis).

b) Man, another vertebrate host, and a non–vertebrate host
   1) Mammal–arthropod–man (plague)
   2) Bird–arthropod–man (encephalitis).

c) Man and 2 intermediate hosts
   1) Man–cyclops-fish–man (fish tape worm)
   2) Man–snail–fish–man (Clonorchis sinensis)
   3) Man–snail–crab–man (Paragonimiasis).

III. By methods in which vectors transmit agent

a) Biting
b) Regurgitation
c) Scratching-in of infective faeces
d) Contamination of host with body fluids of vectors.

IV. By methods in which vectors are involved in the transmission and propagation of parasites

(a) *Mechanical transmission* : The infectious agent is mechanically transported by a crawling or flying arthropod through soiling of its feet or proboscis; or by passage of organisms through its gastrointestinal tract and passively excreted. There is no development or multiplication of the infectious agent on or within the vector.

(b) *Biological transmission* : The infectious agent undergoing replication or development or both, in vector and requires an incubation period before vector can transmit. Biological transmission is of three types : (i) *Propagative* : The agent merely multiplies in vector, but no change in form, e.g., plague bacilli in rat fleas. (ii) *Cyclo-propagative* : The agent changes in form and number, e.g., malaria parasites in mosquito. (iii) *Cyclo-developmental* : The disease agent undergoes only development but no multiplication, e.g., microfilaria in mosquito.

When the infectious agent is transmitted vertically from the infected female to her progeny in the vector, it is known as *transovarial transmission*. Transmission of the disease agent from one stage of the life cycle to another as for example nymph to adult is known as *transstadial transmission.*

The factors which influence the ability of vectors to transmit disease are : (a) host feeding preferences (b) infectivity, that is ability to transmit the disease agent (c) susceptibility, that is ability to become infected (d) survival rate of vectors in the environment (e) domesticity, that is degree of association with man, and (f) suitable environmental factors. Seasonal occurrence of some diseases (e.g., malaria) may be related to intense breeding and thereby greater density of the insect vector during certain periods of the year.

3. Airborne

(1) *Droplet nuclei* : "Droplet nuclei" are a type of particles implicated in the spread of airborne infection. They are tiny particles (1–10 microns range) that represent the dried residue of droplets *(100)*. They may be formed by (a) evaporation of droplets coughed or sneezed into the air or (b) generated purposefully by a variety of atomizing devices (aerosols). They may also be formed accidentally in microbiological laboratories, in abattoirs, rendering plants or autopsy rooms *(106)*. The droplet nuclei may remain airborne for long periods of time, some retaining and others losing infectivity or virulence. They not only keep floating in the air but may be disseminated by air currents from the point of their origin. Particles in the 1–5 micron range are liable to be easily drawn into the alveoli of the lungs and may be retained there. Diseases spread by droplet nuclei include tuberculosis, influenza, chickenpox, measles, Q fever, COVID-19, and many respiratory infections. (Not considered airborne are droplets and other large particles which promptly settle out). Mention must also be made of the role of airborne spread of toxic air pollutants including "smog" resulting in air pollution epidemics.

(2) *Dust* : Some of the larger droplets which are expelled during talking, coughing or sneezing, settle down by their sheer weight on the floor, carpets, furniture, clothes, bedding, linen and other objects in the immediate environment and become part of the dust. A variety of infectious agents (e.g., streptococci, other pathogenic bacteria, viruses and fungal spores) and skin squamae have been found in the dust of hospital wards and living rooms. Some of them (e.g., tubercle bacilli) may survive in the dust for considerable periods under optimum conditions of temperature and moisture. During the act of sweeping, dusting and bed–making, the dust is released into the air and becomes once again airborne. Dust particles may also be blown from the soil by wind; this may include fungal spores. Coccidioidomycosis is an example of a disease spread through airborne transmission of fungal spores *(38)*. Other diseases carried by infected dust include streptococcal and staphylococcal infection, pneumonia, tuberculosis, Q fever and psittacosis. Airborne dust is primarily inhaled, but may settle on uncovered food and milk. This type of transmission is most common in hospital–acquired (nosocomial) infection.

4. Fomite-borne

Fomites (singular; fomes) are inanimate articles or substances other than water or food contaminated by the infectious discharges from a patient and capable of harbouring and transferring the infectious agent to a healthy person. Fomites include soiled clothes, towels, linen, handkerchiefs, cups, spoons, pencils, books, toys, drinking glasses, door handles, taps, lavatory chains, syringes, instruments and surgical dressings. The fomites play an important role in indirect infection. Diseases transmitted by fomites include diphtheria, typhoid fever, bacillary dysentery, hepatitis A, eye and skin infections.

5. Unclean hands and fingers

Hands are the most common medium by which pathogenic agents are transferred to food from the skin, nose, bowel, etc as well as from other foods. The transmission takes place both directly (hand-to-mouth) and indirectly. Examples include staphylococcal and streptococcal infections, typhoid fever, dysentery, hepatitis A and intestinal parasites. Unclean hands and fingers imply lack of personal hygiene. Lack of personal hygiene coupled with poor sanitation favour person-to-person transmission of infection, an example is the 1984 dysentery epidemic in India.

SUSCEPTIBLE HOST

Successful parasitism

Four stages have been described in successful parasitism : (a) First, the infectious agent must find a PORTAL OF ENTRY by which it may enter the host. There are many portals of entry, e.g., respiratory tract, alimentary tract, genitourinary tract, skin, etc. Some organisms may have more than one portal of entry, e.g., hepatitis B, Q fever, brucellosis. (b) On gaining entry into the host, the organisms must reach the appropriate tissue or "SITE OF ELECTION" in the body of the host where it may find optimum conditions for its multiplication and survival. (c) Thirdly, the disease agent must find a way out of the body (PORTAL OF EXIT) in order that it may reach a new host and propagate its species. If there is no portal of exit, the infection becomes a dead-end infection as in rabies, bubonic plague, tetanus and trichinosis. (d) After leaving the human body, the organism must survive in the external environment for sufficient period till a new host is found. In addition, a successful disease agent should not cause the death of the host but produce only a low-grade immunity so that the host is vulnerable again and again to the same infection. The best example is common cold virus.

Incubation period

An infection becomes apparent only after a certain incubation period, which is defined as "the time interval between invasion by an infectious agent and appearance of the first sign or symptom of the disease in question" *(2)*. During the incubation period, the infectious agent undergoes multiplication in the host. When a sufficient density of the disease agent is built up in the host, the health equilibrium is disturbed and the disease becomes overt. Also of interest to the epidemiologist is the **median incubation period,** defined as the time required for 50 per cent of the cases to occur following exposure. These concepts are explained in Fig. 18. The factors which determine the incubation period include the generation time of the particular pathogen, infective dose, portal of entry and individual susceptibility. As a rule, infectious diseases are not communicable during the incubation period, but there are exceptions, as for example, measles, chickenpox, whooping cough and hepatitis A are communicable during the later part of the incubation period.

The length of the incubation period is characteristic of each disease. There is a minimum incubation period for every disease before which no illness can occur. That is, incubation period varies for different infectious diseases, and also from one person to another with the same disease. In some, the incubation period is very short ranging from a few hours to 2–3 days, e.g., staphylococcal food poisoning, cholera, bacillary dysentery and influenza. In some, the incubation period is of median length ranging from 10 days to 3 weeks; in this category, there are many examples : typhoid infections, virus diseases such as chickenpox, measles, COVID-19, and mumps. Then there are infections with longer incubation periods (ranging from weeks to months or years) and whose incubation time is difficult to measure precisely, e.g., hepatitis A and B, rabies, leprosy and slow virus diseases.

Non-infectious diseases such as cancer, heart disease and mental illness also have incubation periods, which may be months or years. The term **latent period** is used in non-infectious diseases as the equivalent of incubation period in infectious diseases *(36)*. Latent period has been defined as "the period from disease initiation to disease detection" *(2)*. In chronic disease, the agent–host interactions leading to a sequence of cellular changes are not well understood.

Incubation period is of fundamental importance in epidemiological studies : (a) *Tracing the source of infection and contacts* : In the case of a disease with a short incubation period ranging from a few hours to a few days, it is relatively simple to trace the source of infection and "follow the trail" of the spread of infection as in the case of food poisoning, bacillary dysentery or typhoid fever. The position is quite different with diseases whose incubation period is of medium length (10 days to 3 weeks) or longer. So many things will have happened and such varied contacts taken place that the cause–effect relationship becomes "diluted". We will have a whole gamut of possible causes from among which we have to single out the main cause. Once the source of infection is traced, then only it will be possible to institute appropriate control measures. (b) *Period of surveillance* : Incubation period is useful in determining the period of surveillance (or quarantine) which may be advised (A in Fig. 18). This period is usually equal to the maximum incubation period of

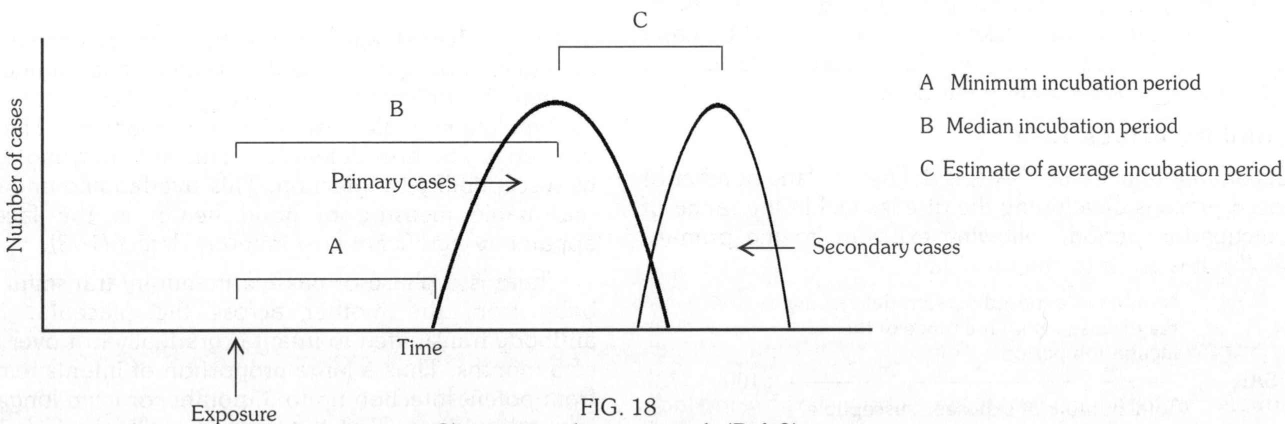

FIG. 18
Showing incubation periods (Ref. 3)

the disease. (c) *Immunization* : Prophylactically, a knowledge of incubation period helps us to prevent clinical illness by human immunoglobulins and antisera. (d) *Identification of point source or propagated epidemics* : In a point source epidemic, all the cases occur within one incubation period of the disease; in a propagated epidemic, cases occur later than the known length of the incubation period; and (e) *Prognosis* : Incubation period can also be used in estimating the prognosis of a disease. In some diseases (e.g., tetanus, rabies), the shorter the incubation period, the worse the prognosis of the disease. Thus prognosis is related to the incubation period of the disease *(14)*.

Serial interval

In actual practice we seldom know precisely the incubation period of a disease. But we know, when an outbreak of disease occurs, say in a family which is the smallest group and also a closed group, there is an initial primary case. The primary case is followed by 2 or 3 secondary cases within a short time. The gap in time between the onset of the primary case and the secondary case is called the "serial interval". By collecting information about a whole series of such onsets, we get a distribution of secondary cases from which we can guess the incubation period of disease.

Generation time

Another concept in infectious disease epidemiology is "generation time". It is defined as "the interval of time between receipt of infection by a host and maximal infectivity of that host" *(2)*. In general, generation time is roughly equal to the incubation period. However, these two terms are not the same. The time of maximum communicability may precede or follow the incubation period. For example, in mumps, communicability appears to reach its height about 48 hours before the onset of swelling of the salivary glands *(38)*. With person-to-person transmission of infection, the interval between cases is determined by the generation time *(2)*. A further difference is that the term "incubation period" can only be applied to infections that result in manifest disease, whereas "generation time" refers to transmissions of infection, whether clinical or subclinical *(38)*.

Communicable period

The communicable period is defined as "the time during which an infectious agent may be transferred directly or indirectly from an infected person to another person, from an infected animal to man, or from an infected person to an animal, including arthropods" *(2)*. Communicability varies in different diseases. Some diseases are more communicable during the incubation period than during actual illness. Communicability of some diseases can be reduced by early diagnosis and treatment. An important measure of communicability is Secondary attack rate.

Secondary attack rate

Secondary attack rate (SAR) is defined as "the number of exposed persons developing the disease within the range of the incubation period, following exposure to the primary case" *(5)*. It is given by the formula :

$$\text{SAR} = \frac{\text{Number of exposed persons developing the disease within the range of the incubation period}}{\text{Total number of exposed/"susceptible" contacts}} \times 100$$

The denominator consists of all persons who are exposed to the case. More specifically, the denominator may be restricted only to "susceptible" contacts, if means are available to distinguish the susceptible persons from the immune *(5)*. The primary case is excluded from both the numerator and denominator.

Supposing there is a family of 6 consisting of 2 parents (already immune) and 4 children who are susceptible to a specific disease, say measles. There occurs a primary case and within a short time 2 secondary cases among the remaining children. The secondary attack rate is 2/3 or 66.6 per cent. The primary case is excluded from both numerator and denominator.

Secondary attack rate is limited in its application to infectious diseases in which the primary case is infective for only a short period of time measured in days (e.g., measles and chickenpox). When the primary case is infective over a long period of time (e.g., tuberculosis), duration of exposure is an important factor in determining the extent of spread *(14)*. It is indicated by the formula :

$$\text{SAR} = \frac{\text{Number of contacts developing tuberculosis}}{\text{Number of person–weeks (months or years) of exposure}} \times 100$$

Another limitation of secondary attack rate is to identify "susceptibles". It is feasible only in diseases such as measles and chickenpox where history can be used as a basis for identification; but in many others, susceptibles cannot be readily identified (e.g., influenza). In such cases, secondary attack rate is based on all exposed family members and still remains a useful tool *(14)*. Where there are numerous subclinical cases, secondary attack rate has a limited meaning. Further spread cannot be measured without laboratory investigations *(107)*.

An additional advantage of the secondary attack rate is that vaccinees and non-vaccinees from several families can be added to determine the overall attack rates in the vaccinated and unvaccinated populations, provided the same definitions for cases and immunization status are used.

Secondary attack rate was initially developed to measure the spread of an infection within a family, household or any closed aggregate of persons who have had contact with a case of disease. It is also useful to determine whether a disease of unknown aetiology (e.g., Hodgkin's disease) is communicable or not; and in evaluating the effectiveness of control measures such as isolation and immunization.

HOST DEFENCES

Host defences against infection are at once local and systemic, non-specific and specific, and humoral and cellular. It is difficult to identify any infectious agent that fails to stimulate multiple host defence mechanisms. The concept of overlapping host defences is crucial to our understanding of susceptibility to infection. This overlapping underlies the reasonable measure of good health in the face of an apparently significant host immune defect *(108)*.

There is a phase of passive immunity transmitted to the baby from the mother across the placenta. Maternal antibody transmitted to infant is gradually lost over a period of 6 months. Thus a large proportion of infants remain free from potent infection up to 3 months, or even longer. There is good evidence that this protective "biological shield" is due to the presence of high levels of immunoglobulins IgM and especially IgG in the cord blood and plasma of infants born of immune mothers. It has been postulated that some other factors (breast milk, presence of fetal haemoglobulin), are also responsible for the transient protection of infants.

SPECIFIC DEFENCES

Specific defences come into play, once microorganisms have breached local defence mechanisms. By virtue of these defences, the host is able to recognize, destroy and eliminate antigenic material (e.g., bacteria, viruses, proteins, etc.) foreign to his own. A person is said to be immune when he possesses "specific protective antibodies or cellular immunity as a result of previous infection or immunization, or is so conditioned by such previous experience as to respond adequately to prevent infection and/or clinical illness following exposure to a specific infectious agent" *(106)*.

The specific defences may be discussed for convenience under the following heads :

1. Active immunity
    (1) Humoral immunity
    (2) Cellular immunity
    (3) Combination of the above.
2. Passive immunity
    (1) Normal human Ig
    (2) Specific human Ig
    (3) Animal antitoxins or antisera.

1. Active immunity

It is the immunity which an individual develops as a result of infection or by specific immunization and is usually associated with presence of antibodies or cells having a specific action on the microorganism concerned with a particular infectious disease or on its toxin *(106)*. In other words, active immunity depends upon the humoral and cellular responses of the host. The immunity produced is specific for a particular disease, i.e., the individual in most cases is immune to further infection with the same organism or antigenically related organism for varying periods depending upon the particular disease.

Active immunity may be acquired in 3 ways :

(a) following clinical infection, e.g., chickenpox, rubella and measles.

(b) following subclinical or inapparent infection, e.g., polio and diphtheria.

(c) following immunization with an antigen which may be a killed vaccine, a live attenuated vaccine or toxoid.

The immune response

(a) PRIMARY RESPONSE : When an antigen is administered for the first time to an animal or human who has never been exposed to it, there is a latent period of induction of 3 to 10 days before antibodies appear in the blood (Fig. 19). The antibody that is elicited first is entirely of the IgM type. The IgM antibody titre rises steadily during the next 2–3 days or more, reaches a peak level and then declines almost as fast as it developed. Meanwhile, if the antigenic stimulus was sufficient, IgG antibody appears in a few days. IgG reaches a peak in 7–10 days and then gradually falls over a period of weeks or months (Fig. 19).

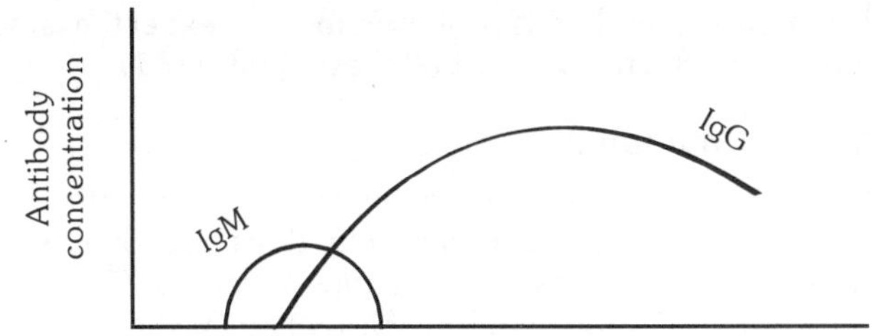

FIG. 19
The primary response

The nature and extent of primary response to an antigen is determined by a number of factors, e.g., dose of antigen, nature of antigen, route of administration, adjuvants, presence of maternal antibody, nutritional status of the host, genetic and co-existing diseases etc *(109)*. For example, with small doses of antigen, only IgM type of response may be induced, and successive small doses of antigen at suitable intervals may also induce IgM antibody. The antigenic dose required for the induction of IgG is about 50 times that which is required to induce IgM antibody.

An important outcome of primary antigenic challenge is education of the reticuloendothelial system of the body. There is production of what are known as "memory cells" or "primed cells" by both B and T lymphocytes. These cells are responsible for the "immunological memory" which becomes established after immunization. In fact, the purpose of immunization is to develop immunological memory.

(b) SECONDARY (BOOSTER) RESPONSE: The response to a booster dose differs in a number of ways from the primary response : (1) shorter latent period. (2) production of antibody more rapid. (3) antibody more abundant. (4) antibody response maintained at higher levels for a longer period of time, and (5) the antibody elicited tends to have a greater avidity or capacity to bind to the antigen.

The secondary response also involves the production of IgM and IgG antibody. Collaboration between B and T cells is necessary to initiate a secondary response. There is a brief production of IgM antibody and much larger and more prolonged production of IgG antibody. This accelerated response is attributed to immunological memory. The immune response (primary and secondary) and immunological memory are the basis of vaccination and revaccination.

(1) Humoral immunity

Humoral immunity comes from the B-cells (bone-marrow derived lymphocytes) which proliferate and manufacture specific antibodies after antigen presentation by macrophages. The antibodies are localized in the immunoglobulin fraction of the serum. Immunoglobulins are divided into 5 main classes – IgG, IgM, IgA, IgD and IgE (and sub-classes within them) – each class representing a different functional group. These antibodies circulate in the body and act directly by neutralizing the microbe, or its toxin or rendering the microbe susceptible to attack by the polymorphonuclear leucocyte and the monocyte. The complement system, together with antibodies is necessary for efficient phagocytosis of bacteria *(110)*.

The antibodies are specific, i.e., they react with the same antigen which provoked their production, or a closely related one. As a result of this specificity, host response mediated by antibodies is somewhat limited in that it will not provide protection against more than one antigen *(111)*. This specificity has been a formidable problem in the production of vaccines. For example, there are numerous antigenic types of rhinoviruses, and it is not possible to expect a single vaccine to be effective against all these types *(111)*.

(2) Cellular immunity

Although antibodies are quite effective in combating most infectious diseases, humoral immunity does not cover all the situation that one finds in infectious diseases *(111)*. For example, some pathogens (e.g., *M. leprae, M. tuberculosis, S. typhi, Candida albicans* and many viruses) escape the bactericidal action of leukocyte. They can even multiply in the mononuclear leukocyte (macrophage). However, these macrophages can be stimulated by substances (lymphokines) secreted by specific stimulated T–lymphocytes (thymus – derived lymphocytes). The activated macrophages perform a much more efficient phagocytic function than non-activated macrophages *(108)*.

It is now well-recognized that cellular immunity plays a fundamental role in resistance to infection. It is mediated by the T–cells which differentiate into sub-populations able to help B–lymphocytes. The T–cells do not secrete antibody, but are responsible for recognition of antigen. On contact with antigen, the T–cells initiate a chain of responses e.g., activation of macrophages, release of cytotoxic factors, mononuclear inflammatory reactions, delayed hypersensitivity reactions, secretion of immunological mediators (e.g., immune interferon), etc. There is growing evidence that cellular immunity is responsible for immunity against many diseases including tuberculosis, brucellosis and also for the body's rejection of foreign material, such as skin grafts. The importance of cell–mediated immunity can be appreciated from the fact that a child born with a defect in humoral antibody production may survive for as long as 6 years without replacement therapy, but a severe defect in cell–mediated immunity will result in death within the first six months of life *(112)*.

(3) Combination of the above

In addition to the B and T lymphoid cells which are responsible for recognizing self and non–self, very often, they cooperate with one another and with certain accessory cells such as macrophages and human K (killer) cells, and their joint functions constitute the complex events of immunity. For instance, one subset of T–cells (helper T–cells) are required for the optimal production of antibody to most antigens. Another set of T–cells (suppressor T–cells) inhibit immunoglobulin synthesis. Antibody-dependant cell-mediated (K) cytotoxic cells recognize membrane viral antigens through specific antibody, whereas natural killer (NK) cells destroy non-specifically virus-infected target cells. It is now increasingly recognized that vaccines to be effective must elicit both humoral and cell-mediated responses *(113)*.

Active immunity takes time to develop. It is superior to passive immunity because (a) the duration of protection, like that of the natural infection is frequently long–lasting (b) with few exceptions, severe reactions are rare (c) the protective efficacy of active immunization exceeds that of passive immunization, and in some instances, approaches 100 per cent, and (d) active immunization is less expensive than passive immunization. Vaccines are cheaper to produce than are antisera.

It is important to realize at this stage that an individual is immunized only against small doses of pathogenic agents or toxins. There exists a "threshold" at which resistance fails. Beyond a certain dosage, which here again varies with the individual, his physiological state and the micro-organism, the immune systems are overwhelmed and the disease develops. Many examples of this can be seen among individuals who, though immunized, nevertheless contact a typhoid or paratyphoid infection, diphtheria, or some other disease.

Moreover, many factors are involved in the maintenance of immunity. Fatigue, strange surroundings, change of diet, ingestion of drugs, and emotional shock are examples of these factors that can produce a fall in immunity or a lowering of the threshold at which resistance to infection fails *(114)*.

2. Passive immunity

When antibodies produced in one body (human or animal) are transferred to another to induce protection against disease, it is known as passive immunity. In other words, the body does not produce its own antibodies but depends upon ready-made antibodies. Passive immunity may be induced :

(a) by administration of an antibody–containing preparation (immune globulin or antiserum)

(b) by transfer of maternal antibodies across the placenta. Human milk also contains protective antibodies, (IgA).

(c) by transfer of lymphocytes, to induce passive cellular immunity – this procedure is still experimental.

Passive immunity differs from active immunity in the following respects : (a) immunity is rapidly established (b) immunity produced is only temporary (days to months) till the antibody is eliminated from the body, and (c) there is no education of the reticuloendothelial system.

Passive immunization is useful for individual who cannot form antibodies, or for the normal host who takes time to develop antibodies following active immunization.

Herd immunity

Herd immunity (or community immunity) describes a type of immunity that occurs when the vaccination of a portion of population (or herd) provides protection to unprotected individuals. Herd immunity theory proposes that in diseases passed from individual to individual, it is difficult to maintain a chain of infection when large numbers of a population are immune. The higher the number of immune individuals, the lower the likelihood that a susceptible person will come in contact with an infectious agent *(115)*.

Herd immunity provides an immunological barrier to the spread of disease in the human herd. For example, when an infectious disease is introduced into a "virgin" population, that is, population with a very low or no immunity, the attack and case fatality rates tend to be very high involving practically all susceptibles as it had happened in the very severe measles epidemic in the Faroe islands, in 1854, where the population had no previous experience of measles. The epidemic wave declined with a build-up of herd immunity following natural infection.

Elements which contribute to herd immunity are (a) occurrence of clinical and subclinical infection in the herd, (b) immunization of the herd, and (c) herd structure. Herd structure is never constant. It is subject to constant variation because of new births, deaths and population mobility. An on-going immunization programme will keep up the herd immunity at a very high level.

The herd structure includes not only the hosts (population) belonging to the herd species but also the presence and distribution of alternative animal hosts and possible insect vectors as well as those environmental and social factors that favour or inhibit the spread of infection from host to host. The herd structure thus plays a decisive role in the immunity status of the herd.

If the herd immunity is sufficiently high, the occurrence of an epidemic is regarded as highly unlikely. If that high level of immunity is maintained and stepped up, by an on-going immunization programme, to the point where the susceptible persons are reduced to a small proportion of the population, it may lead (but not necessarily) to elimination of the disease in due course. This has been achieved in such diseases as diphtheria and poliomyelitis. In the case of smallpox, however, it may be mentioned that it was not herd immunity (although important as it was) that played a crucial role in its eradication, but elimination of the source of infection, by surveillance and containment measures. With the abolition of vaccination against smallpox, the herd immunity in the case of smallpox will naturally tend to decline with the passage of time. In the case of tetanus, however, herd immunity does not protect the individual.

Studies have shown that it is neither possible nor necessary to achieve 100 per cent herd immunity in a population to halt an epidemic or control disease, as for example, eradication of smallpox and poliomyelitis. Just how much less than 100 per cent is required above which the disease may no longer exist, is a crucial question.

The proportion of immune individuals in a population, above which a disease may no longer persist, is *herd immunity threshold*. It's value varies with the virulence of the disease, the efficacy of the vaccine and the contact parameter for the population.

Herd immunity may be determined by serological surveys (serological epidemiology).

IMMUNIZING AGENTS

The immunizing agents may be classified as vaccines, immunoglobulins and antisera.

Vaccines

Over the last century, vaccination has been the most effective medical strategy to control infectious diseases. Smallpox has been eradicated world-wide and poliomyelitis has been almost eradicated. Most viral and bacterial diseases traditionally affecting children world-wide are now preventable by vaccines. Vaccination is estimated to save at least 2–3 million lives every year. The vaccines currently used are as shown in Table 29.

Vaccine is an immuno-biological substance designed to produce specific protection against a given disease. It stimulates the production of protective antibody and other immune mechanisms. Vaccines may be prepared from live modified organisms, inactivated or killed organisms, extracted cellular fractions, toxoids or combination of these.

a. Live vaccines

Live vaccines (e.g., BCG, measles, oral polio) are prepared from live or wild (generally attenuated) organisms. These organisms have been passed repeatedly in the laboratory in tissue culture or chick embryos and have lost their capacity to induce full–blown disease but retain their immunogenicity. In general, live vaccines are more potent immunizing agents than killed vaccines, the reasons being : (i) live organisms multiply in the host and the resulting antigenic dose is larger than what is injected, (ii) live vaccines have all the major and minor antigenic components, (iii) live vaccines engage certain tissues of the body, as for example, intestinal mucosa by the oral polio vaccine, and (iv) there may be other mechanisms such as the persistence of latent virus.

Live vaccines should not be administered to persons with immune deficiency diseases or to persons whose immune response may be suppressed because of leukaemia, lymphoma or malignancy or because of therapy with corticosteroids, alkylating agents, antimetabolic agents, or radiation *(117, 118)*. Pregnancy is another contraindication unless the risk of infection exceeds the risk of harm to the foetus of some live vaccines.

When two live vaccines are required they should be given either simultaneously at different sites or with an interval of atleast 3 weeks. In the case of live vaccines, protection is generally achieved with a single dose of vaccine. An additional dose is given to ensure seroconversion, e.g., 95 to 98 per cent of recipient will respond to single dose of measles vaccine. The second dose is given to ensure that 100 per cent of persons are immune. The other exception is polio vaccine which needs three or more doses to be given at spaced intervals to produce effective immunity. Live vaccines usually produce a durable immunity, but not always as long as that of the natural infection.

Live vaccines must be properly stored to retain effectiveness. Serious failures of measles and polio

TABLE 29
Vaccines currently in use

Live attenuated	Killed whole organism	Toxoid/Protein	Polysaccharide	Glycoconjugate	Recombinant
Tuberculosis (BCG)	Typhoid	Diphtheria	Pneumococcus	Hib	HBV
Yellow fever	Cholera	Tetanus	Meningococcus	Pneumococcus	Lyme disease
Polio (OPV)	Plague	Acellular Pertussis	Hib	MenACWY	Cholera toxin B
Measles	Pertussis	Anthrax	Typhoid (Vi)		HPV
Mumps	Influenza	Influenza subunit			COVID-19
Rubella	Typhus				
Typhoid	Polio (IPV)				
Varicella	Rabies				
Rotavirus	JE				
Cholera	TBE				
Cold-adapted influenza	HAV				
Rotavirus reassortants	COVID-19				
Zoster					

BCG – Bacille Calmette-Guerin; HAV – hepatitis A virus; HBV – hepatitis B virus; Hib – Haemophilus influenzae type b; IPV – inactivated polio vaccine; JE – Japanese encephalitis; Men – meningococcus, OPV – oral polio vaccine; TBE – tick-borne encephalitis.

Source : *(116)*

immunization have resulted from inadequate refrigeration prior to use.

b. Inactivated or killed vaccines

Inactivated vaccines are produced by growing virus or bacteria in culture media and then inactivating them with heat or chemicals (usually formalin), when injected into the body they stimulate active immunity. They are usually safe but generally, less efficacious than live vaccines. For example, cholera vaccine offers only 50 per cent protection. The efficacy of 3 doses of pertussis vaccine is about 80 per cent in the first three years, and almost "nil" 12 years after immunization. Killed vaccines usually require a primary series of 2 or 3 doses of vaccine to produce an adequate antibody response, and in most cases "booster" injections are required. The duration of immunity following the use of inactivated vaccines varies from months to many years. Inactivated polio vaccine has been quite an effective vaccine, the widespread use of which in certain countries has led to the elimination of the disease. Killed vaccines are usually administered by subcutaneous or intramuscular route.

Because the vaccine is inactivated, the infective agent cannot grow in the vaccinated individual and therefore, can not cause the disease, even in an immunodeficient person.

The only absolute contraindication to their administration is a severe local or general reaction to a previous dose. Unlike live antigens, inactivited antigens are not affected by circulating antibody. They are often more stable than live attenuated vaccines.

Some features of attenuated vaccines versus inactivated (killed) vaccines are listed in Table 30 and some of the very important developments in the field of vaccines are listed in Table 31.

TABLE 30

Comparison of characteristics of killed and live vaccines

Characteristic	Killed vaccine	Live vaccine
Number of doses	Mutiple	Single
Need for adjuvant	Yes	No
Duration of immunity	Shorter	Longer
Effectiveness of protection (more closely mimics natural infection)	Lower	Greater
Immunoglobulins produced	IgG	IgA and IgG
Mucosal immunity produced	Poor	Yes
Cell-mediated immunity produced	Poor	Yes
Residual virulent virus in vaccine	Possible	No
Reversion to virulence	No	Possible
Excretion of vaccine virus and transmission to non-immune contacts	No	Possible
Interference by other viruses in host	No	Possible
Stability at room temperature	High	Low

Source : *(119)*

TABLE 31

Milestones in vaccination

Year	Milestone
1798	Smallpox vaccine
1885	Rabies vaccine
1897	Plague vaccine
1917	Cholera vaccine
1917	Typhoid vaccine (parenteral)
1923	Diphtheria toxoid
1926	Pertussis vaccine
1927	Tuberculosis (BCG)
1927	Tetanus toxoid
1935	Yellow fever vaccine
1940s	DTP
1945	The first influenza vaccines
1955	Inactivated polio vaccine (IPV).
1955	Tetanus and diphtheria toxoids adsorbed (adult use, Td)
1961	Monovalent oral polio vaccine
1963	Trivalent oral polio vaccine (OPV).
1963	The first measles vaccine
1967	Mumps vaccine
1969	Rubella vaccine
1970	Anthrax vaccine
1971	Measles, Mumps, Rubella (MMR) vaccine licensed.
1978	Fluzone, the current flu vaccine.
1980	Smallpox declared eradicated from the world.
1981	Meningococcal polysaccharide vaccine, groups A, C, Y, W135 combined (Menomune)
1982	Hepatitis B vaccine
1983	Pneumococcal vaccine, 23 valent
1988	Worldwide Polio Eradication Initiative launched; supported by Rotary International, CDC and others.
1990	The Vaccine Adverse Reporting System (VAERS), a national programme monitoring the safety of vaccines established.
1990	Haemophilus influenzae type B (Hib) polysaccharide conjugate vaccine licensed for infants.
1990	Typhoid vaccine (oral)
1991	Hepatitis B vaccine recommended for all infants.
1991	Acellular pertussis vaccine (DTaP) licensed for use in older children aged 15 months to six years old.
1993	Japanese encephalitis vaccine.
1995	Varicella vaccine licensed.
1995	Hepatitis A vaccine licensed.
1996	Acellular pertussis vaccine (DTaP) licensed for use in young infants.
2000	Pneumococcal conjugate vaccine (Prevnar) recommended for all young children.
2003	First live attenuated influenza vaccine licensed (FluMist) for use in 5 to 49 year old persons.
2003	First Adult Immunization Schedule introduced.
2004	Inactivated influenza vaccine recommended for all children 6 to 23 months of age.
2004	Pediarix, a vaccine that combines the DTaP, IPV, and Hep B vaccines, into one shot, is approved.
2005	Boostrix and Adacel, Tdap vaccines, are approved for teens.
2005	Menatra, a new menigococcal vaccine is approved for people between the age of 11 to 55 years.
2006	Rota Teq is a new rotavirus vaccine from Merck. ProQuad is a new vaccine that combines the MMR and Varivax vaccines for measles, mumps, rubella, and chicken pox into a single shot.
2006	Gardasil, the first HPV vaccine is approved.
2007	A booster dose of Varivax, the chickenpox vaccine, is recommended for all children.
2007	The recommended age for Flumist, the nasal spray flu vaccine, was lowered to two years.
2008	Rotarix, a two dose rotavirus vaccine is approved.
2009	Influenza-A (H_1N_1) vaccine approved.
2011	FDA approved the first vaccine (Menactra) to prevent meningococcal disease in infants and toddlers. FDA approved Boostrix Tdap (Glaxo Smith Klin) to prevent tetanus, diphtheria and pertussis in older people. HPV vaccine for adolescent boys.
2012	Approved quadrivalent formulation of fluarix.
2013	Inactivated and intranasal influenza vaccine-quadrivalent
2020	COVID-19

Source : *(120)*

c. Subunit vaccines (116)

A vaccine can be made of single or multiple antigenic components of a microorganism that are capable of stimulating a specific immune response sufficient to protect from the relevant pathogen infection or from the clinical manifestation of the disease. Depending on the molecular composition of the purified antigen used to prepare the vaccine, and on the techniques applied to obtain the final material used as a vaccine, different types of subunit vaccines can be defined.

1. Toxoids

Certain organisms produce exotoxins, e.g., diphtheria and tetanus bacilli. The toxins produced by these organisms are detoxicated and used in the preparation of vaccines. The antibodies produced neutralize the toxic moiety produced during infection, rather than act upon the organisms. In general, toxoid preparations are highly efficacious and safe immunizing agents.

2. Protein vaccines

In case, immunization with a single protein or a combination of proteins from a pathogen is sufficient to stimulate a protective immune response against that particular microorganism, the approach of a protein-based vaccine is appropriate. Proteins can be purified from *in-vitro* cultures of a pathogenic microorganism. The resulting vaccine preparations contain different amounts of contaminants depending on the efficiency of the purification process. Licensed acellular pertussis vaccines currently available contain from two to four different proteins purified from *B. pertussis* and are able to confer protection against whooping cough comparable to that obtained with the whole cell vaccine. One of the most widely used subunit protein vaccines is the influenza vaccine composed of haemagglutinin (HA) and neuraminidase (NA) purified from the inactivated influenza virus.

3. Recombinant protein vaccines

Development of the recombinant deoxyribonucleic acid (DNA) technology has made possible the expression of protective protein antigens in heterologous expression systems such as *E. coli*, yeast, mammalian cells, or baculovirus. This technology avoids the problems related to growing and manipulating large amounts of a pathogen from which the antigen is purified. Moreover, recombinant proteins are generally better purified from cultured microorganisms resulting in cleaner vaccine preparations with a better safety profile. A drawback of a clean vaccine preparation containing pure recombinant protein(s) is their reduced immunogenicity that may require the addition of an adjuvant to achieve enhanced efficacy. For example, the hepatitis B vaccine is made by inserting a segment of the hepatitis B virus gene into a yeast cell. The modified yeast cell produces large amounts of hepatitis B surface antigen, which is purified and harvested and used to produce the vaccine. The recombinant hepatitis B vaccine is identical to the natural hepatitis B surface antigen, but does not contain virus DNA and is unable to produce infection.

4. Polysaccharide-based vaccines

The surface of many pathogenic bacteria is covered by a capsular shell that is mainly assembled from polymeric glycans. This extensive polysaccharide coat entirely shields the bacteria outer membrane, preventing other surface bacterial components from becoming a target of the host immune response. Nevertheless, antibodies to bacterial surface polysaccharides can clear the bacteria from the host by different mechanisms, such as complement-mediated killing and opsonophagocytosis. Hence, stimulation of an antibody response against the surface polysaccharide of pathogenic bacteria is a strategy for the development of vaccines against capsulated bacteria. The chemical structure or capsular polysaccharides varies not only between bacteria of different species but also between different strains within a single species, which are usually differentiated and typed based on their capsular polysaccharides. As a consequence, a limitation of polysaccharide-based vaccine is that the immune responses they elicit are often serotype specific. In addition to *S. pneumoniae*, for which a vaccine against 23 serotypes is available, polysaccharide-based vaccines have been developed for MenACWY, Hib, and *Salmonella typhimurium (116)*.

5. Conjugated vaccines

Children under two years of age do not respond well to antigens, such as polysaccharides, which produce antibodies via a T-cell independent mechanism. If these polysaccharide antigens are chemically linked (conjugated) to a protein that T-cells recognize, then these conjugate vaccines can elicit strong immune responses and immune memory in young children. Similar to the polysaccharide-based vaccines, the conjugate vaccines are also sero-type specific, and, therefore, multivalent formulations are required to achieve protection against multiple serotypes. Examples are *S. pneumococcal* and *meningococcal* vaccines *(115)*.

d. Combinations

If more than one kind of immunizing agent is included in the vaccine, it is called a mixed or combined vaccine. The aim of combined vaccines is to simplify administration, reduce costs, minimize the number of contacts of the patient with the health system, reducing the storage cost, improving timelines of vaccination, and facilitating the addition of new vaccine into immunization programme. No evidence exists that the administration of several antigens in combined vaccines increases the burden on the immune system which is capable of responding to millions of antigens at a time. Combining antigens usually does not increase the risk of adverse reactions and can infact lead to an overall reduction in adverse reactions *(115)*. The following are some of the well-known combinations :

- DPT (Diphtheria–pertussis–tetanus)
- DT (Diphtheria–tetanus)
- DP (Diphtheria–pertussis)
- DPT and typhoid vaccine
- MMR (Measles, mumps and rubella)
- DPTP (DPT plus inactivated polio)
- Hepatitis A, and B
- Hepatitis A, and typhoid.
- DTwP (Diphtheria, tetanus, whole-cell pertussis)
- DPT–Hep B–Hib (Diphtheria, pertussis, tetanus, hepatitis B and haemophilus influenzae type B).

The term “polyvalent” is applied to vaccines (e.g., polio, influenza vaccines) which are prepared from two or more strains of the same species. The term “auto” or “autogenous” vaccine is applied when the organism in the vaccine is obtained from the same patient.

OTHER COMPONENTS IN VACCINES (EXCIPIENTS)

Adjuvant

Sometimes a substance is added to a vaccine to enhance the immune response by degree and/or duration, making it possible to reduce the amount of immunogen per dose or the total number of doses needed to achieve immunity. The commonly used adjuvant are aluminium salts (aluminium hydroxide, aluminium phosphate or potassium aluminium sulfate) which primarily enhance the immune response to proteins. They have been shown to be safe over several decades of use. Rarely, they may cause injection site reactions, including subcutaneous nodules, sterile abscess, granulomatous inflammation or contact hypersensitivity *(115)*.

Table 32 shows the approved human vaccine adjuvants in use, their class, components and the vaccines in which they are used *(116)*.

Antibiotics

Antibiotics are used during the manufacturing phase to prevent bacterial contamination of the tissue culture cells in which the viruses are grown. For example, MMR vaccine and IPV each contains less than 25 micrograms of neomycin per dose (less than 0.000025g). Persons who are known to be allergic to neomycin should be closely observed after vaccination so that any allergic reaction can be treated at once *(115)*.

Preservatives

These are chemicals (e.g. thiomersal, formaldehyde) added to killed or subunit vaccines in order to inactivate viruses, detoxify bacterial toxins, and to prevent serious secondary infections as a result of bacterial or fungal contamination *(115)*.

Stabilizers

To confirm product quality or stability, compounds may be added to vaccines for a variety of manufacture-related issues: controlling acidity (pH); stabilizing antigens through necessary steps in the manufacturing process, such as freeze drying; and preventing antigens from adhering to the sides of glass vials with a resultant loss in immunogenicity. Examples of such additives include potassium or sodium salts, lactose, human serum albumin and a variety of animal proteins, such as gelatine and bovine serum albumin *(115)*.

Different types of vaccine presentations *(116A)*

1. Single–dose vials (SDVs)

   A single–dose vial (SDV) contains one dose and is used one time for one patient. Never combined leftover vaccine from one SDV with another to obtain a dose.

2. Manufacturer–filled syringes

   A manufacturer–filled syringe (MFS) is prepared with a single dose of vaccine and sealed under sterile conditions by the manufacturer. An MFS does not contain a preservative to help prevent the growth of microorganisms. An MFS is intended for one patient and one injection. Once the sterile seal has been broken, the vaccine should be used or discarded by the end of the workday.

3. Multidose vials

   A multidose vial (MDV) contains more than one dose of vaccine. MDVs canbe punctured more than once (using sterile technique) because they typically contain a preservative to help prevent the growth of microorganisms. Only the number of doses indicated in the manufacturer's package insert should be withdrawn from the vial.

Routes of administration

The routes of administration of vaccine varies to maximise effectiveness of the vaccine. The routes of administration of vaccine are as follows :

1. *Intramuscular (IM) injection* administers the vaccine into the muscle mass. Vaccine containing adjuvants should be injected IM to reduce adverse local effects.

2. *Subcutaneous (SC) injection* administers the vaccine into the subcutaneous layer above the muscle and below the skin.

3. *Intradermal (ID) injection* administers the vaccine in the topmost layer of the skin. BCG is the only vaccine with this route of administration. Intradermal injection of BCG vaccine reduces the risk of neurovascular injury.

4. *Oral administration* of vaccine makes immunization easier by eliminating the need for a needle and syringe.

5. *Intranasal spray application* of a vaccine offers a needle free approach through the nasal mucosa of the vaccine.

The manufacturer's usually recommend the route of administration that limits best the adverse reactions of the respective vaccine. The recommended routes of different vaccines are as shown on Fig. 20. The correct angle of the needle while giving injection is shown in Fig. 21.

TABLE 32
Human vaccine adjuvants

Name	Class	Components	Vaccine
Alum	Mineral salts	Aluminium phosphate, aluminium hydroxide	Diphtheria, tetanus, pneumococcus, HAV, HBV, anthrax, tick-borne encephalitis, MenC, HPV
MF59	Oil-in-water emulsion	Squalene, Tween 80, Span 85	Seasonal and pandemic influenza
AS03	Oil-in-water emulsion	Squalene, Tween 80, α-tocopherol	Pandemic influenza
AF03	Oil-in-water emulsion	Squalene, Montane 80, Eumulgin B1PH	Pandemic influenza
Virosomes	Liposomes	Phospholipids, cholesterol, HA	Seasonal influenza, HAV
AS04	Alum-adsorbed TLR4 agonist	Aluminium hydroxide, MPL	HBV, HPV
RC-529	Alum-adsorbed TLR4 agonist	Aluminium hydroxide, synthetic MPL	HBV

HAV – hepatitis A virus; HBV – hepatitis B virus; HPV – human papillomavirus; Men – meningococcus, MPL – monophosphoryl lipid A; TLR – toll-like receptor

Source : *(116)*

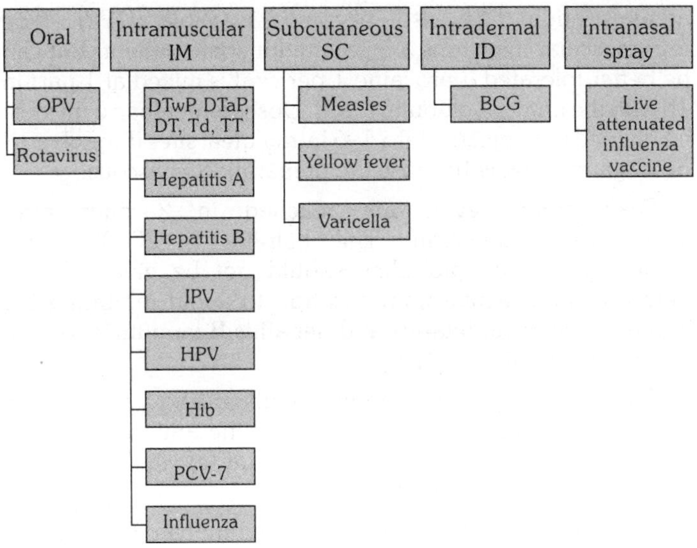

FIG. 20
Recommended route of administration of vaccines
Source : *(116A)*

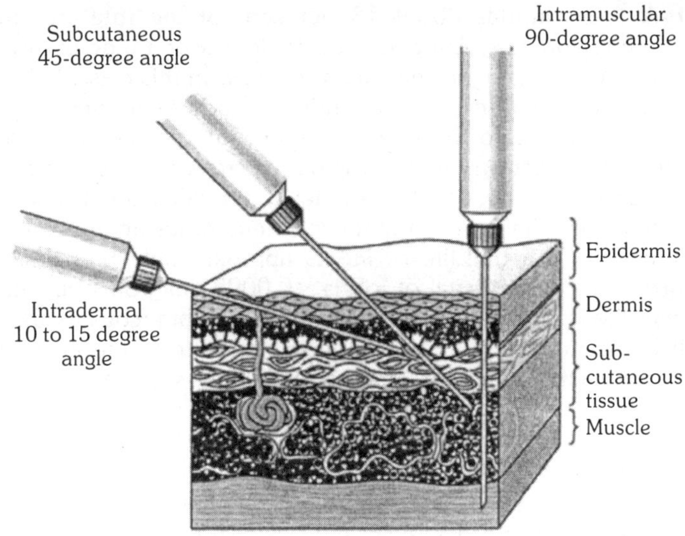

FIG. 21
Technique of giving vaccine injection
Source : *(116A)*

Order of injections *(116A)*

Frequently children and adults receive 2 or more injections at an immunization encounter. Some vaccines are associated with more pain than others. Because procedure pain can increase with each injection, the order of the vaccines administered may effect the overall pain response. Some vaccines cause a painful or stinging sensation; examples include measles, mumps and rubella (MMR) and human papillomavirus (HPV) vaccines. Injecting the most painful vaccine (e.g. MMR, PCV13 or HPV) last when multiple injections are being administered can decrease the pain associated with the injections.

FUTURE PROSPECTS *(119)*

Molecular biology and modern technologies are combining to devise novel approaches to vaccine development. Many of these approaches avoid the incorporation of viral nucleic acid in the final product, improving vaccine safety. Examples of what is ongoing in this field can be listed as follows. The ultimate success of these new approaches remains to be determined.

(1) Use of recombinant DNA techniques to insert the gene coding for the protein of interest into the genome of an avirulent virus that can be administered as the vaccine (such as vaccinia virus).

(2) Including in the vaccine only those subviral components needed to stimulate protective antibody, thus minimizing the occurrence of adverse reactions to the vaccine.

(3) Use of purified proteins isolated from purified virus or synthesized from cloned genes (a recombinant hepatitis B virus vaccine contains viral proteins synthesized in yeast cells). Expression of cloned gene(s) sometimes results in formation of empty virus–like particles (VLPs).

(4) Use of synthetic peptides that correspond to antigenic determinants on a viral protein, thus avoiding any possibility of reversion to virulence since no viral nucleic acid would be present–although the immune response induced by synthetic peptides is considerably weaker than that induced by intact protein.

(5) Development of edible vaccines whereby transgenic plants synthesizing antigens from pathogenic viruses may provide new cost-effective ways of delivering vaccines.

(6) Use of naked DNA vaccines–potentially simple, cheap, and safe–in which recombinant plasmids carrying the gene for the protein of interest are injected into hosts and the DNA produces the immunizing protein.

(7) Administration of vaccine locally to stimulate antibody at the portal of entry (such as aerosol vaccines for respiratory disease viruses).

Immunoglobulins

The human immunoglobulin system is composed of 5 major classes (IgG, IgM, IgA, IgD and IgE) and sub-classes within them. The various classes and sub-classes of immunoglobulins represent different functional groups that are required to meet different types of antigenic challenges. All antibodies are immunoglobulins, but it is still an open question whether all immunoglobulins are antibodies *(108)*. The WHO recommends that the term "gamma globulin" should not be used as a synonym for "immunoglobulin" *(121)*.

IgG : IgG is the major immunoglobulin of serum, comprising about 80 per cent of the total serum immunoglobulins. Because of its relatively smaller molecular weight (150,000), IgG can diffuse into the interstitial fluid. In other words, IgG is largely extravascular. IgG is the only class of IgGs which is transported across the placenta. Antibodies to gram-positive pyogenic bacteria, anti-viral and anti-toxic antibodies are found exclusively among IgG globulins. Its half life is about 21 days. **IgM** : It accounts for about 6 per cent of normal serum immunoglobulins. It represents antibody that is promptly formed with exposure to antigen (Fig. 19). Its presence may be indicative of recent infection. IgM antibody has high agglutinating and complement–fixing ability. Its half life is about 7 days. It can be produced by a foetus undergoing an infection.

IgA : Constitutes about 13 per cent of the total serum immunoglobulins. Antibody activity to a wide range of viral and bacterial antigens has been reported in this class. IgA is found relatively in large quantities in body secretions, e.g., saliva, milk, colostrum, tears, bronchial secretions, nasal mucosa, prostatic fluid, vaginal secretions and mucus secretions of the small intestine; it provides the primary defence mechanism at the mucos membranes against local infection. The half-life of IgA is approximately 6–8 days. **IgE** : The serum level of IgE is <0.0005 miligrams per ml. Half-life is 2 days. IgE is concentrated in submucous tissues. It is the major antibody responsible for immediate allergic anaphylactic reactions. In persons with such antibody–mediated allergic hypersensitivity, IgE concentration is greatly increased, and IgE may appear in external secretions. Serum IgE is also typically increased during helminth infestations. **IgD :** IgD acts as an antigen receptor when present on the surface of certain B lymphocytes. In serum it is present only in trace amount (<0.003 mg per ml). Its half-life is 2 days.

Immunoglobulin preparations

Two types of immunoglobulin preparations are available for passive immunization. These are (a) Normal human immunoglobulin and (b) Specific (hyper-immune) human immunoglobulin. These are used in the prophylaxis of viral and bacterial infections, and in replacement of antibodies in immunodeficient patients.

a. Normal human Ig

Normal human Ig is an antibody-rich fraction (Cohn fraction II), obtained from a pool of at least 1000 donors. The WHO has laid down definite standards for its preparation. For example, the preparation should contain at least 90 per cent intact IgG; it should be as free as possible from IgG aggregates; all IgG sub-classes should be present; there should be a low IgA concentration; the level of antibody against at least two bacterial species and two viruses should be ascertained etc. *(122)*.

Normal human Ig is used to prevent measles in highly susceptible individuals and to provide temporary protection (upto 12 weeks) against hepatitis A infection for travellers to endemic areas and to control institutional & household outbreaks of hepatitis A infection.

Live vaccines should not normally be given for 12 weeks after an injection of normal human Ig, and if a live vaccine has already been given. NHIg injection should be deferred for 2 weeks.

b. Specific human Ig

The specific (hyperimmune) human Ig should contain at least 5 times the antibody potential of the standard preparation per unit volume. These preparations are made from the plasma of patients who have recently recovered from an infection or are obtained from individuals who have been immunized against a specific infection. They therefore have a high antibody content against an individual infection and provide immediate protection e.g., specific human Igs are used for chickenpox prophylaxis of highly susceptible individuals and for post-exposure prophylaxis of hepatitis B, and rabies and for tetanus prophylaxis in the wounded.

Immunoglobulin is administered by intramuscular injection. Immunoglobulin suitable for intravenous administration has also become available *(122)*. The intramuscular injections are painful for some patients but can be better tolerated if procaine 1 per cent is mixed at 1 part in 10 with the immunoglobulin *(123)*. Doses larger than 5 ml must be divided and injected into 4–6 intragluteal sites through a 18 or 20 gauge needle because the preparation is viscous.

Peak blood levels are reached in 2 days after intramuscular injection. The half-life is 20–35 days. Generally, immunoglobulins should not be given shortly before or after active immunization to avoid inhibiting the immune response; tetanus and hepatitis B immunization are exceptions to this rule *(122)*.

The advantages of immunoglobulins are : (a) freedom from hepatitis B, (b) concentration of the antibodies into a small volume for intramuscular use, and (c) stable antibody content, if properly stored.

Adverse reactions to immunoglobulin can be local or systemic. Local reactions (e.g., pain, sterile abscesses) are relatively common when large volumes are injected intramuscularly. Systemic reactions can be rapid or late. Rapid reactions occur during or within minutes of administration, and are anaphylactic in type (flushing, flank pain, rigor, dyspnoea, and signs of shock). Late reactions may occur within hours or days, are usually less severe, and may include urticaria, arthralgia, pyrexia or diarrhoea. Systemic reactions are less common occurring once in every 500–1000 injections. They are more common with intravenous administration. Systemic reactions can be prevented by giving hydrocortisone before the injection *(122)*.

The uses of human immunoglobulin are listed in Table 33. Use is recommended only where the efficacy has been proved; where efficacy has not been established conclusively, use is listed as optional. The target populations listed in the table have been well-defined in controlled studies, and use should be limited to these individuals *(122)*.

Antisera or antitoxins

The term *antiserum* is applied to materials prepared in animals. Originally passive immunization was achieved by the administration of antisera or antitoxins prepared from non-human sources such as horses. Since human immunoglobulin preparations exist only for a small number of diseases, antitoxins prepared from non-human sources (against tetanus, diphtheria, botulism, gas gangrene and snake bite) are still the mainstay of passive immunization. Administration of antisera may occasionally give rise to serum sickness and anaphylactic shock due to abnormal sensitivity of the recipient. The current trend is in favour of using immunoglobulins wherever possible. The uses of antisera are listed in Table 34.

THE COLD CHAIN

The "cold chain" is a system of storage and transport of vaccines at low temperature from the manufacturer to the actual vaccination site. The cold chain system is necessary because vaccine failure may occur due to failure to store and transport under strict temperature controls. This is of concern in view of the fairly frequent reports of vaccine–preventable disease occurrence in populations thought to have been well immunized. In other words – the success of

TABLE 33

Appropriate uses of human immunoglobulin in the prevention and treatment of disease

Agent/ Condition	Target population	Preparation[ab]	Dose[c]	Status
Hepatitis A	Family contacts Institutional outbreaks	IG	(0.02 ml/kg of body weight) (3.2mg/kg of body weight)	Recommended for prevention
	Travellers exposed to unhygienic conditions in tropical or developing countries	IG	0.02-0.05 ml/kg of body weight (3.2-8.0 mg/kg of body weight) every 4 months	
Hepatitis C	Percutaneous or mucosal exposure	IG	0.05 ml/kg of body weight (8 mg/kg of body weight)	Optional for prevention
Hepatitis B	Percutaneous or mucosal exposure	HBIG	0.05-0.07 ml/kg of body weight (8-11 mg/kg of body weight) Repeat in one month	Recommended for prevention
	Newborns of mothers with HBsAg	HBIG	0.05ml (8 mg) at birth, 3, and 6 months	Recommended for prevention
	Sexual contacts of acute hepatitis B patients	HBIG	0.05 ml/kg of body weight (8 mg/kg of body weight) Repeat after one month	Optional for prevention
Rubella	Women exposed during early pregnancy	IG	20 ml	Optional for prevention
Varicella-zoster	Immuno-suppressed contacts of acute cases or newborn contacts	VZIG[d]	15-25 units/kg body weight; minimum 125 units	Recommended for prevention
Measles (rubeola)	Infants less than 1 year old or immuno-suppressed contacts of acute cases exposed less than 6 days previously	IG	0.25 ml/kg of body weight or 0.5 ml/kg of body weight if immuno-suppressed	Recommended for prevention
Rabies	Subjects exposed to rabid animals	RIG	20 IU/kg of body weight	Recommended for prevention
Tetanus	Following significant exposure of unimmunized or incompletely immunized person or immediately on diagnosis of disease	TIG	250 units for prophylaxis 3000-6000 units for therapy	Recommended for prevention or treatment
Rh isoimmunization	Rh (D)-negative mother on delivery of Rh-positive infant, or after uncompleted pregnancy with Rh-positive father, or after transfusion of Rh-positive blood to Rh-negative mother	RhIG	1 vial (200-300 μg) per 15 ml of Rh (+) blood exposure	Recommended for prevention

a IG = immune globulin (human); HBIG = hepatitis B immune globulin; VZIG = varicella-zoster immune globulin; RIG = rabies immune globulin; TIG = tetanus immune globulin; RhIG = rhesus factor immune globulin.

b Hyperimmune immunoglobulins have also been used in prophylaxis of mumps and prophylaxis and treatment of pertussis and diphtheria; there are no conclusive data available, and no recommendations can be given.

c Dose based on intramuscular administration of 16.5% solution

d Of limited availability at the present time.

TABLE 34

Passive immunization procedures with antisera

Disease	Passive immunization (ANTISERA)
1. Diphtheria	A dose of 500-1,000 of IU of diphtheria antitoxin is given intramuscularly to susceptible contacts immediately after exposure. Protection does not last more than 2-3 weeks.
2. Tetanus	The usual prophylactic dose is 1,500 units of horse A.T.S. given subcutaneously or intramuscularly, soon after injury.
3. Gas gangrene	A polyvalent antitoxin is used. A patient who has sustained a wound possibly contaminated with spores of gas gangrene should receive a dose of 10,000 IU of *Cl. perfringens. (Cl. welchii)* antitoxin, 5,000 units of *Cl. septicum* antitoxin and 10,000 units of *Cl. oedematiens* antitoxin, intramuscularly, or in urgent cases intravenously.
4. Rabies	Antirabies serum in a dose of 40 IU per kg. of body weight should be given intramuscularly within 72 hours and preferably within 24 hours of exposure. A part of the antiserum is applied locally to the wound.
5. Botulism	When botulism is suspected, 10,000 units of polyvalent antitoxin is recommended every 3 to 4 hours.

national immunization programme is highly dependant on supply chain system for delivery of vaccines and equipment, with a functional system that meets 6 rights of supply chain – The right vaccine in the right quantity at the right place at the right time in the right condition (no temperature breaks in cold chain) and at the right cost *(124)*.

Temperature requirements for vaccines *(125)*

Vaccines are sensitive biological products. Some vaccines are sensitive to freezing, some to heat and others to light. Vaccine potency, meaning its ability to adequately protect the vaccinated patient, can diminish when the vaccine is exposed to inappropriate temperatures. Once lost, vaccine potency cannot be regained. To maintain quality, vaccines must be protected from temperature extremes. Vaccine quality is maintained using a cold chain that meets specific temperature requirements. It is essential that all those who handle vaccines and diluents know the temperature sensitivities and the recommended storage temperature for all the vaccines in the national schedule.

Sensitivity to heat and freezing

Fig. 22 shows the relative heat sensitivity of vaccines. These vaccines are grouped into six categories. Within each of these six categories, the vaccines are arranged in alphabetical order, not in order of sensitivity to heat, within the group. The most heat sensitive vaccines are in group A and the least heat sensitive vaccines are in group F.

The heat stability information shown for freeze-dried vaccines applies only to unopened vials; most freeze-dried vaccines rapidly lose potency after reconstitution. In addition, it is important to keep opened multi-dose vaccine vials that do not contain preservative – whether lyophilized or liquid – cooled at temperature between +2°C and +8°C during the immunization session, or used within 4 hours after opening, whichever comes first.

Vaccines that are sensitive to freezing and should be protected from sub-zero temperature are *(125)* :

- Cholera
- DTaP-hepatitis B-Hib-IPV (hexavalent)
- DTwP or DTwP-hepatitis B-Hib (pentavalent)
- Hepatitis B (Hep B)
- Hib (liquid)
- Human papillomavirus (HPV)
- Inactivated poliovirus (IPV)
- Influenza
- Pneumococcal
- Tetanus, DT, Td
- Rotavirus (liquid and freeze-dried)

Sensitivity to light *(125)*

Some vaccines are very sensitive to light and lose potency when exposed to it. Such vaccines should always be protected against sunlight and strong artificial light. Vaccines sensitive to light are BCG, measles, measles-rubella, measles-mumps-rubella and rubella. These vaccine are supplied in dark glass vials that give them some protection; but they should be kept in their secondary packaging for as long as possible during storage and transportation.

At the health facility level (usually health centres and health posts), health workers can adequately protect vaccines by doing the following : (a) Keep vaccines in appropriate vaccine refrigeration equipments; (b) Use a temperature monitoring device to ensure temperatures remain between +2°C and +8°C; (c) Transport vaccines to immunization sessions in a vaccine carrier, correctly packed, using coolant packs that have been properly prepared; and (d) During immunization sessions, fit a foam pad (if available) at the top of the vaccine carrier.

At the health facility, one person must have overall responsibility for managing the vaccine cold chain. A second person can fill in when the primary person is absent. Their responsibilities should include : (a) checking and recording vaccine temperatures twice daily; typically in the morning and at the end of the session or day; (b) properly storing vaccines, diluents and water packs; and (c) handling preventive maintenance of the cold chain equipment.

All health workers in a facility should know how to monitor the cold chain and what to do if temperature is out of range.

Most sensitive to heat ——————————▶ Least sensitive to heat

Group A	Group B	Group C	Group D	Group E	Group F
Oral poliovirus (OPV)	Influenza	Inactivated poliovirus (IPV) Japanese encephalitis (freeze-dried) Measles or measles-rubella or measles-mumps-rubella (freeze-dried)	Cholera DTaP-hepatitis B-Hib-IPV (hexavalent) DTwP or DTwP-hepatitis B-Hib (pentavalent) Hib (liquid) Measles (freeze-dried) Rotavirus (liquid and freeze-dried) Rubella (freeze-dried) Yellow fever (freeze-dried)	Bacillus Calmette Guerin (BCG) Human papillomavirus (HPV) Japanese encephalitis (JE) Tetanus, TD, Td	Hepatitis B Hib (freeze-dried) Meningoccal A Pneumococcal

FIG. 22
Vaccine heat sensitivity

Source : *(125)*

Cold chain equipment *(126)*

The cold chain equipment used in Universal Immunization Programme are classified as follows :

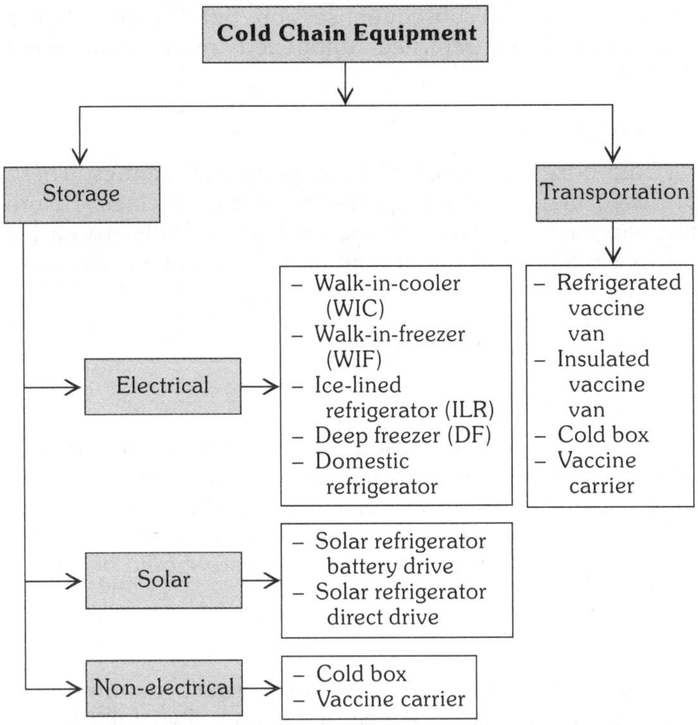

Electrical Cold Chain Equipment

There are equipments of different capacity for storage of vaccines at different levels, which are dependant on electric supply to maintain the recommended temperature.

1. Walk-in-freezers (WIF)

The Walk-in-freezer is a pre-fabricated modular polyurethane foam (PUF) insulated panel assembled cold room with two identical refrigeration units and a standby generator set to provide uninterruprted power supply. The generator set starts automatically as soon as the power cuts off. It maintains a temperature between – 15°C to – 25°C. WIF are usually installed at national, state and regional vaccine stores. It is used for bulk storage of OPV vaccine and for preparation of frozen ice packs for vaccine transportation.

2. Walk-in-coolers (WIC)

The Walk-in-cooler is a pre-fabricated modular polyurethane (PUF) insulated panel assembled cold room. They maintain a temperature of +2°C to +8°C. In India, under UIP usually WIC with capacity of 16.5, 32 and 40 Cubic meter are in use.

These are used for storage of large quantities of all UIP vaccines like BCG, hepatitis B, DPT, pentavalent, IPV, measles and TT. They have two identical cooling units and a standby generator with automatic start and stop function.

These Walk-in-coolers are installed at government medical store depots, state and regional vaccine stores. The WICs have been installed in some district vaccine stores based on the target beneficiary and requirement.

WIC and WIF come with continuous temperature recorder and alarm system. Once the temperature of WIC/WIF exceeds the recommended storage temperature the alarm system gives alarm loudly.

3. Deep freezer (DF)

The Deep freezer is an equipment, which operates on a vapour compression system similar to any conventional type of refrigerator operating on 220 volts A.C. mains supply. However DF has top opening lid to prevent loss of cold air during door opening.

The cabinet temperature is maintained between –15° to –25°C. This is used for storing of OPV vaccine for 3 months (district level and above only) and also for freezing of ice packs (at sub-district level only). Unlike the ice-lined refrigerator (ILR), the DF has got little or limited hold-over time which is dependent on the number of frozen ice packs in it and the frequency of opening. These are available in different sizes.

The DF which is used for storing vaccines should not be used for preparation of icepacks, as it may increase the cabinet temperature and can be potentially harmful to the vaccines (OPV). However adequate frozen icepacks can be kept permanently inside the vaccine storing DF for increasing the hold-over time.

4. Ice lined refrigerator (ILR)

One of the most important link in the cold chain is ice lined refrigerator (ILR). This is an equipment which operates on a vapour compression system similar to any conventional type of refrigerator operating on 220 volts A.C. mains supply. ILRs are to maintain a cabinet temperature between +2°C to + 8°C and are used to store vaccines at district and sub-district level. These type of refrigerators are top opening because they can hold the cold air inside better than a refrigerator with a front opening. It can keep vaccine safe with minimum 8 hours continuous electricity supply in a 24-hour period. The ILRs are categorized on the basis of vaccine storage capacity. These are available in different sizes. Usually the larger ILR is supplied to district headquarters and smaller ILR to PHC headquarters, based on the size and population.

Inside the ILR there is a lining of water containers (ice packs or tubes) fitted all around the walls and held in place by a frame.

When the refrigerator is functioning the water in the containers freezes and cools the cabinet. When the electricity supply fails, then the ice lining maintains the inside temperature of the refrigerator at a safe level for vaccines. Therefore, the temperature is maintained in ILR for much longer duration than in the deep freezers and domestic refrigerator. Thus ILR is an ideal option for safe storage of vaccines.

Based on the temperature zone, inside of the ILR can be divided into 2 parts, upper part and lower part. In most of the ILR models, the lower part is cooler compared to the upper part, as the cooler air is heavier and settles down at the bottom of ILR. Hence upper part is preferred location for storing the freeze sensitive vaccines.

All the vaccines should be kept in the basket provided with the ILR. Vaccines like OPV, BCG, measles, and JE (in the sub-district stores, OPV is kept in ILR, unlike higher level vaccine stores, where it is kept in DF) can be kept at bottom of the basket while DPT, TT, hep B, IPV and pentavalent vaccines and diluents are kept in upper part of the basket. These vaccines should never be kept directly on the floor of the refrigerator as they can freeze and get damaged. In case basket is not available, two layers of empty ice-packs can be laid flat on the bottom of the ILR.

Hold-over time of the equipment *(126)*

In the event of power failure, hold-over time is defined as the "time taken by the equipment to raise the inside cabinet temperature from its temperature at the time of power cut, to maximum temperature limit of its recommended range." For example, in case of ILR if the cabinet temperature is +4°C at the time of power-cut, then the time taken to reach +8°C from +4°C will be hold-over time for that ILR.

Hold-over time depends on the following factors : (a) Ambient temperature: More the ambient temperature less will be the hold-over time; (b) Frequency of opening of lid and use of basket; (c) Quantity of vaccines kept inside with adequate space between the containers (Equipment empty/ loaded); and (d) Condition of ice-pack lining (Frozen/ partially frozen/melted).

5. Domestic refrigerator (front load refrigerator)

Domestic refrigerators can also maintain the cabinet temperature between +2°C to +8°C, but the hold-over time and capacity to store vaccines/freeze icepacks is limited. They can be used for storage of vaccine at private clinics and nursing homes, provided continuous power supply is ensured.

Load a domestic refrigerator as following : (a) Freeze and store ice-packs in the freezer compartment, they should be kept vertically to avoid leaking with a space of at least 2 mm. Ice-packs should be taken out from the left; (b) All the vaccines and diluents are stored in the refrigerator compartment. Arrange the boxes of vaccine in stacks so air can pass between them. Placement of vaccines in the refrigerator with freezer on top is as follows: measles, BCG, rota virus vaccine and OPV on the top shelf. DPT, pentavalent vaccine, TT, IPV, hepatitis B, and JE vaccine on the middle shelf and diluents next to vaccine with which they are supplied; (c) Keep ice-packs filled with water on the bottom shelf and in the door of the refrigerator. They help to maintain temperature in case of power-cut; and (d) Closer expiry date vaccines should be kept in front.

A dial thermometer should be kept in the ILR and temperature recorded twice a day. At the time of defrosting the vaccines are shifted to the cold boxes containing required number of frozen ice packs. In case of equipment failure or electric supply failure, vaccines should be transferred to ice boxes and then to alternate vaccine storage.

There are some DOs and DONTs for the use of ILR/ freezer. **DOs:** keep the equipment in cool room away from direct sunlight and at least 10 cms away from the wall; keep the equipment levelled; fix the equipment through voltage stabilizer; keep vaccines neatly with space between the stacks for circulation of air; keep the equipment locked and open only when necessary; defrost periodically, supervise the temperature record; and if vaccines are kept in cartons, make holes on the sides of the cartons for cold air circulation. **DONTs :** do not keep any object on these equipments; do not store any other drug; do not keep drinking water or food in them; do not keep more than one months requirements at PHC level; and do not keep date expired vaccines. Reconstituted BCG, Rota virus vaccine and measles vaccines can be kept at +2°C to +8°C for maximum of 4 hours and JE vaccine for 2 hours. To be on safe side, write the time of reconstitution on the label of these vaccine vials and discard them after 4 hours (2 hours for JE vaccine). ***Do not*** keep any used vials in the cold chain. Return the unused vaccine vials from session site to the PHC on the same day in the cold chain through alternative vaccine delivery. Keep the box labeled ***"returned unused"*** in the ILR for all unused vaccines that can be used in the subsequent session, but discard vaccines that have been returned unopened more than three times *(127)*.

6. Cold boxes

Cold boxes are supplied to all peripheral centres. These are used mainly for transportation of the vaccines. Before the vaccines are placed in the cold boxes, fully frozen ice packs are placed at the bottom and sides. The vaccines are first kept in cartons or polythene bags. The vials of DPT, DT, TT, vaccines and diluents should not be placed in direct contact with the frozen ice packs.

7. Vaccine carriers

Vaccine carriers are used to carry small quantities of vaccines (16–20 vials) for the out of reach sessions. 4 fully frozen ice-packs are used for lining the sides, and vials of DPT, DT, TT and diluents should not be placed in direct contact with frozen ice-packs. The carriers should be closed tightly.

8. Day carriers

Day carriers are used to carry small quantities of vaccines (6–8 vials) to a nearby session. Two fully frozen packs are to be used. It is used only for few hours period.

9. Ice packs

The ice packs contain water and no salt should be added to it. The water should be filled upto the level marked on the side. If there is any leakage such ice-packs should be discarded.

The risk of cold chain failure is greatest at sub-centre and village level. For this reason, vaccines are not stored at the sub-centre level and must be supplied on the day of use.

Solar cold chain equipment *(126)*

Solar systems used in UIP are mainly of two types.

1. Solar refrigerators battery drive.
2. Solar refrigerators direct drive.

1. Solar refrigerator battery drive

A solar refrigerator operates on the same principle as normal compression refrigerator but incorporates low voltage (12 or 24V) DC compressors in place of mains AC voltage operated compressors. The battery is charged by solar energy. A solar refrigerator has good PUF insulation around the storage compartments to maximize energy efficiency. Battery, charge controller and solar panels are the major additional components associated with solar refrigerator.

Vaccine refrigerator/freezer :

It is a refrigerator cum freezer having basket for storing of vaccine and freezing of ice-packs. It has two separate compartments :

1. Vaccine storage compartment maintains temperature range of +2°C to + 8°C.
2. Freezer compartment is for storing frozen ice-pack maintaining temperature upto –7°C.

For each refrigerator and freezer compartment, it has separate DC compressor. The refrigerator is designed for continuous operation, therefore an ON/OFF switch is not provided, as it is not necessary. The freezer however, does have an ON/OFF switch to allow for defrosting.

2. Solar refrigerator direct drive

The "direct drive" technology uses the sun's energy to freeze water or other phase change material and then uses the cooling from that "ice bank" to keep the refrigerator cold during night and cloudy days. These refrigerators are wired directly to the photovolatic generators.

OPEN VIAL POLICY (2015)

Implementation of open vial policy allows reuse of partially used multidose vials of applicable vaccines under UIP in subsequent session (both fixed and outreach) upto four weeks (28 days) subject to meeting certain conditions and thus reduce vaccine wastage. The guidelines on open vial policy 2015 are summarized in Fig. 23.

Open Vial Policy

ENSURE SAFETY
PRESERVE LIFE

✓ Open Vial policy applies only for DPT, TT, Hepatitis B, Oral Polio Vaccine (OPV), Liquid Pentavalent, PCV and injectable IPV.

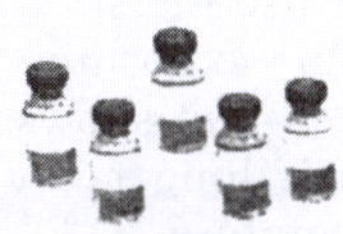

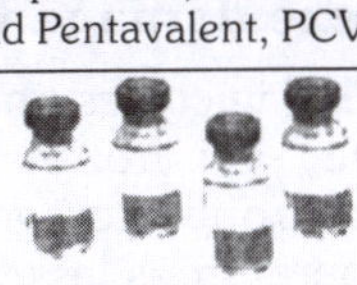

× Does not apply to Measles/MR, BCG, Japanese Encephalitis (JE) vaccines, Rota virus

✓ Vaccine vials opened in session-site can be used in more than one immunization session upto four weeks provided:-

- Expiry date has not passed.
- Vaccines are stored strictly under appropriate temperature range both during transportation & storage at cold chain point.
- Vaccine vial septum has not submerged in water or contaminated in any way.
- Aseptic technique has been used to withdraw all doses.
- Vaccine vial monitor (VVM), has not reached discard point.

× Open vials should never be submerged in water (e.g. Water accumulated in vaccine carrier) as it increases the risk of contamination of the vial septum.

✓ Ensure all open vials have recorded date and time of opening.

- At the end of the session, all open vials should be returned to Cold Chain Point.
- At Cold Chain Point, open vials should be segregated into :
  - Re-usable DPT, TT, Hep B and Pentavalent vaccine vials fulfilling the above mentioned criteria.
  - Non-reusable open vials of Measles/MR, BCG & JE.
- All open vials of BCG, Measles and JE should be destroyed after 48 hours or before next session, whichever is earlier.
- In case of any AEFI reported, all open vials (usable & non-usable) should not be discarded or used. All open vials should be stored under proper cold chain till investigation is complete.

✓ All vials (open or unopened) should be transported in a zipper bag in the vaccine carrier and recorded in the stock register.

✓ Well-sealed conditioned ice-packs should be used in vaccine carriers and water should not be allowed to accumulate where vaccine vials and diluents are stored.

FIG. 23
Open Vial Policy 2015

Source : *(126)*

Monitoring heat exposure using vaccine vial monitors

Vaccine vial monitors (VVMs) are the only temperature monitoring devices that routinely accompany vaccines throughout the entire supply chain. A VVM is a chemical indicator label attached to the vaccine container (vial, ampoule or dropper) by the vaccine manufacturer. As the container moves through the supply chain, the VVM records its cumulative heat exposure through a gradual change in colour. If the colour of the inner square is the same colour or darker than the outer circle, the vaccine has been exposed to too much heat and should be discarded. Fig. 24 shows the colour change sequence.

There are currently four types of VVM, chosen to match the heat sensitivity of the vaccine. These four types are VVM2, VVM7, VVM14 and VVM30. The VVM number is the time in days that it takes for the inner square to reach the colour indicating a discard point, if the vial is exposed to a constant temperature of 37°C.

The main purpose of VVMs is to ensure that heat-damaged vaccines are not administered. The VVM status is also used to decide which vaccines can safely be kept after a cold chain break occurs thus minimizing unnecessary vaccine wastage. In addition, VVM status helps the user to decide which vaccine should be used first – a batch of vaccine showing significant heat exposure should be distributed and used before a batch that shows lower heat exposure, even if its expiry date is longer. VVMs do not measure exposure to freezing temperature.

There are two different locations for VVMs (Fig. 25) and each is associated with specific guidance for handling opened multi-dose vials of vaccine :

1. WHO-prequalified vaccines, where the VVM, if attached, is on the label of the vaccine. The vaccine vial, once opened, can be kept for subsequent immunization sessions up to 28 days, regardless of the formulation of the product (liquid or freeze-dried).
2. WHO-prequalified vaccines where the VVM is attached in a location other than on the label (e.g., cap or neck of ampoule). In this instance, the vaccine vial, once opened, must be discarded at the end of the immunization session or within six hours of opening, whichever comes first. This is regardless of the formulation of the product (liquid or freeze-dried).

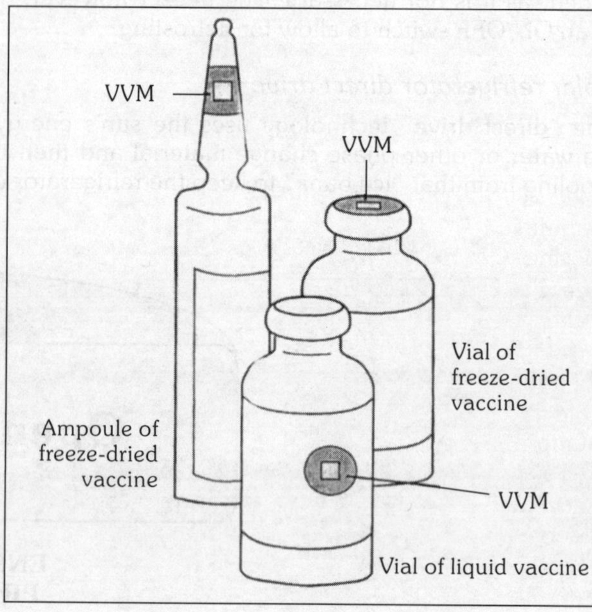

FIG. 25
Location of VVMs on ampoules and vials

Source : *(125)*

Freeze damage to the vaccine

The vaccines that are freeze sensitive will get spoiled if they get frozen. The causes of vaccine freezing are : (a) Improper storage in ILR; (b) Cold climates and if ambient temperature is less than 0°C; (c) Storage and transport with non-conditioned frozen ice-packs; (d) Defective ILR; (e) Incorrect thermostat adjustment; and (f) Untrained or improperly trained staff handling vaccine/cold chain.

The "Shake Test" is used to check whether freeze sensitive vaccines have been damaged by exposure to temperature below 0°C. After it has thawed, a vial of vaccine that has been frozen no longer has the apperance of a cloudy liquid, but tends to form flakes that settle down at the bottom of the vial.

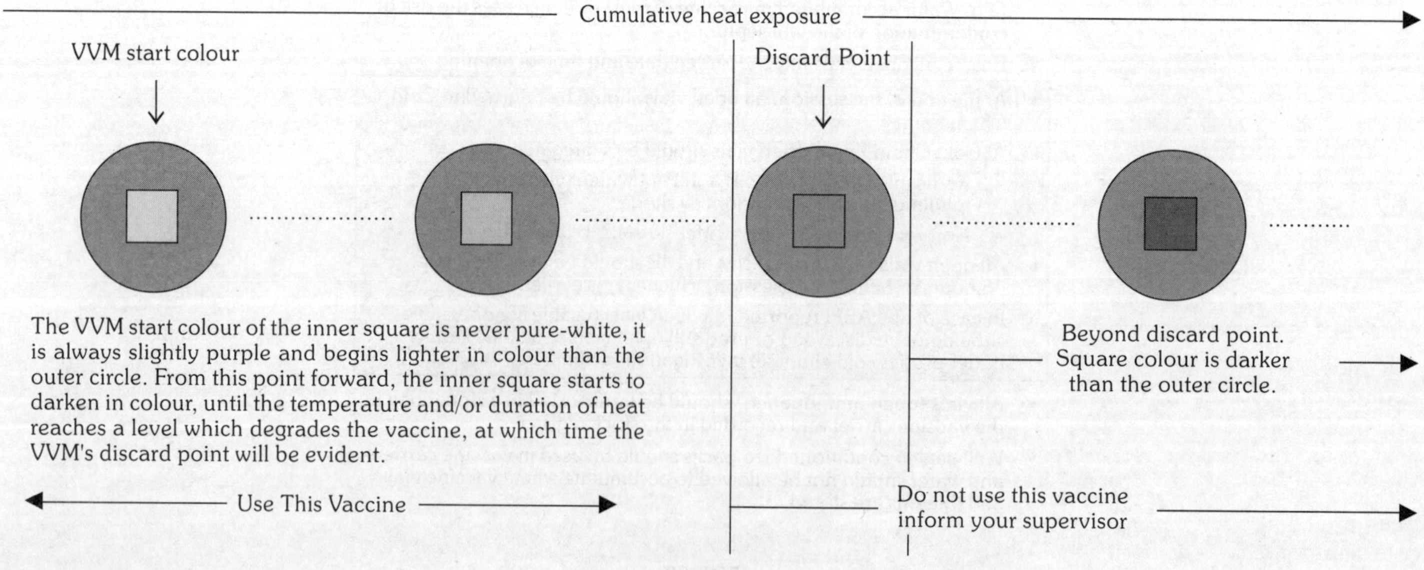

FIG. 24
VVM showing colour change sequence and interpretation.

Source : *(128)*

Shake Test *(125, 126)*

There is only one way to conduct a Shake Test. The protocol must not be altered. The procedure is as follows :

Test Vial

- Take a vaccine vial you suspect that may have been frozen – This is "TEST" vial.

Frozen control vial

- Take a vaccine vial of the same antigen, same manufacturer, and same batch number as the suspect vaccine vial you want to test.
- Freeze solid this vial at – 20°C overnight in the DF. This is the "frozen control" vial, and label it accordingly to avoid its usage.
- Let it thaw. Do NOT heat it.
- Hold the Control and the Test vials together between thumb and forefinger, and vigorously shake the vials for 10-15 seconds.
- Place both vials to rest on a flat surface, side-by-side observe them for 30 minutes.
- Compare for rate of sedimentation as shown in Fig. 26.
- If the sedimentation in the "Test vial" is slower than in the "Frozen control vial", the vaccine has not been damaged, it passes the shake test. Use the vaccine batch – it is not damaged.
- If the sedimentation is similar in both vials or if sedimentation is faster in the "Test" vial than in the "Frozen" vial, the vaccine is damaged, it failed in shake test. Do NOT use. Notify your supervisor.

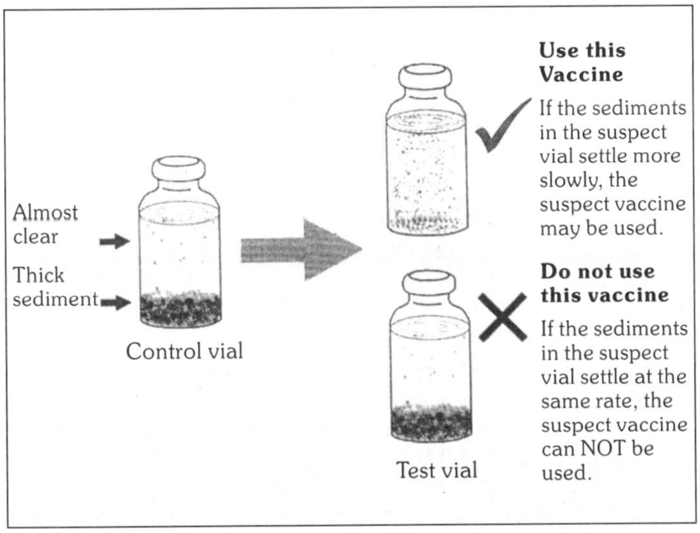

FIG. 26
Comparison of deliberately frozen vial next to the suspect test vial.
Source : *(125)*

Correct Storage and Use of Diluents *(124, 127)*

Only use the diluents supplied and packaged by the manufacturer with the vaccine, since the diluent is specifically designed for the needs of that vaccine, with respect to volume, pH level and chemical properties.

Store the diluents, between +2° to + 8° C in the ILR. If there are constraints of space, then store diluents outside the cold chain. However, remember to cool diluents for at least 24 hours before use to ensure that vaccines and diluents are at the same temperature (+2° to +8°C) when being reconstituted. Otherwise, it can lead to thermal shock i.e. the death of some or all the essential live organisms in the vaccine. Store the diluents and droppers with the vaccines in the vaccine carrier during transportation. Diluents should not come in direct contact with the ice-pack.

ADVERSE EVENTS FOLLOWING IMMUNIZATION

Vaccines used in national immunization programmes are extremely safe and effective. However, no immune response is entirely free from the risk of adverse reactions or remote sequelae.

An AEFI is any untoward medical occurrence which follows immunization and which does not necessarily have a causal relationship with the usage of the vaccine. The adverse event may be any unfavourable or unintended sign, abnormal laboratory finding, symptom or disease. Reported adverse events can either be true adverse events, i.e. really a result of the vaccine or immunization process, or coincidental events that are not due to the vaccine or immunization process but are temporally associated with immunization.

In 2012, the Council for International Organizations of Medical Sciences (CIOMS) and WHO revised the existing classification relevant to cause-specific categorization of AEFIs and a new categorization has been introduced which is as follows :

1. Vaccine product-related reaction

   An AEFI that is caused or precipitated by a vaccine due to one or more of the inherent properties of the vaccine product.

   Example : Extensive limb swelling following DTP vaccination.

2. Vaccine quality defect-related reaction

   An AEFI that is caused or precipitated by a vaccine that is due to one or more quality defects of the vaccine product, including its administration device as provided by the manufacturer.

   Example : Failure by the manufacturer to completely inactivate a lot of inactivated polio vaccine leads to cases of paralytic polio.

3. Immunization error-related reaction

   An AEFI that is caused by inappropriate vaccine handling, prescribing or administration and thus by its nature is preventable.

   Example : Transmission of infection by contaminated multidose vial.

4. Immunization anxiety-related reaction

   An AEFI arising from anxiety about the immunization.

   Example : Vasovagal syncope in an adolescent during/ following vaccination.

5. Coincidental event

   An AEFI that is caused by something other than the vaccine product, immunization error or immunization anxiety.

   Example : A fever occurs at the time of the vaccination (temporal association) but is in fact caused by malaria.

   Coincidental events reflect the natural occurrence of health problems in the community with common problems being frequently reported.

Source : *(128A)*

1. Vaccine reactions *(115, 128, 130)*

The new cause-specific categorization is important for decision-making on a vaccine-product, since it clearly differentiates the two types of possible vaccine reactions. The first, **vaccine product-related reaction**, is a reaction in an individual's response to the inherent properties of the vaccine, even when the vaccine has been prepared, handled and administered correctly. The second, **vaccine quality defect-related reaction**, is the defect in a vaccine that occurred during manufacturing process. Such a defect may have an impact on an individual's response and thus increase the risk of adverse vaccine reactions. In early years of immunization programmes, a few major incidences of vaccine quality defect-related reactions were reported (e.g. Cutter case study). However, due to introduction of improved Good Manufacturing Practices (GMP), such defects are now very rare.

Vaccine reactions may be classified into common, minor reactions or rare, more serious reactions. Most vaccine reactions are minor and settle on their own. More serious reactions are very rare and, in general, do not result in long-term problems.

COMMON, MINOR VACCINE REACTIONS

The purpose of a vaccine is to induce immunity by causing the recipient's immune system to react to the vaccine. Local reaction, fever and systemic symptoms can result as part of the immune response. In addition, some of the vaccine's components (e.g. aluminium adjuvant, stabilizers or preservatives) can lead to reactions. A successful vaccine reduces these reactions to a minimum while producing the best possible immunity.

The local reactions include pain, swelling and/or redness at the injection site and can be expected in about 10% of vaccinees, except for those injected with DTP (whole cell), or tetanus boosters, where up to half can be affected. BCG causes a specific local reaction that starts as a papule (lump) two or more weeks after immunization, that then becomes ulcerated and heals after several months, leaving a scar. Keloid (thickened scar tissue) from the BCG lesion is more common among asian and african populations.

The systemic reactions include fever and occur in about 10% or less of vaccinees, except for DTP where it is again about half. Other common systemic reactions (e.g., irritability, malaise, 'off-colour', loss of appetite) can also occur after DTP. For measles/MMR and OPV the sytemic reactions arise from vaccine virus infection. Measles vaccine causes fever, rash and/or conjunctivitis, and affects 5–15% of vaccinees. It is very mild compared to 'wild' measles, but for severely immunocompromised individuals, it can be severe, even fatal. Vaccine reactions for mumps (swollen parotid gland) and rubella (joint pains and swollen lymph nodes) affect less than 1% of children. Rubella vaccine causes symptoms more often in adults, with 15% suffering from joint pains. Systemic reactions from OPV affect less than 1% of vaccinees with diarrhoea, headache and/or muscle pain.

The common minor vaccine reactions and their expected frequency are as shown in Table 35.

TABLE 35

Summary of common minor vaccine reactions

Vaccine	Possible minor adverse reaction	Expected frequency
BCG	Local reaction (pain, swelling, redness)	Common
Cholera	Oral presentation–none	
DTP	Local reaction (pain, swelling, redness) Fever	Upto 50% [a] Upto 50%
Hepatitis A	Local reaction (pain, swelling, redness)	Upto 50%
Hepatitis B	Local reaction (pain, swelling, redness) Fever	Adults up to 30%, Children upto 5% 1-6%
Hib	Local reaction (pain, swelling, redness) Fever	5-15% 2-10%
Japanese encephalitis	Local reaction, low-grade fever, myalgia, gastrointestinal upset	Upto 20%
Measles/ MMR	Local reaction (pain, swelling, redness) Irritability, malaise and non-specific symptoms, fever	Upto 10% Upto 5%
Pneumococcal	Local reaction (pain, swelling, redness)	30-50%
Poliomyelitis (OPV)	None	
Poliomyelitis (IPV)	None	
Rabies	Local and/or general reaction depending on type of vaccine (see product information)	15-25%
Meningococcal disease	Mild local reactions	Upto 71%
Tetanus/Td	Local reaction (pain, swelling, redness)[b] Malaise and non-specific symptoms	Upto 10% Upto 25%
Tick-borne encephalitis	Local reaction (pain, swelling, redness)	Upto 10%
Typhoid fever	Depends on type of vaccine use (see product information)	–
Yellow fever	Headache Influenza-like symptoms Local reaction (pain, swelling, redness)	10% 22% 5%

[a] With whole-cell pertussis vaccine. Rates for acellular pertussis vaccine are lower.

[b] Rate of local reactions likely to increase with booster doses, up to 50-85%.

Source : *(129)*

RARE, MORE SERIOUS VACCINE REACTIONS *(115)*

'Serious' and 'severe' are often used as interchangeable terms but they are not. An AEFI will be considered **serious**, if it results in death, is life-threatening, requires in-patient hospitalization or prolongation of existing hospitalization, results in persistent or significant disability/incapacity, is a congenital anomaly/birth defect, or required intervention to prevent permanent impairment or damage. **Severe** is used to describe the intensity of a specification event (as in mild, moderate or severe). The event itself, however, may be of relatively minor medical significance. (For example, fever is a common relatively minor medical event, but according to its severity it can be graded as mild fever or moderate fever. Anaphylaxis is always a serious event and life-threatening.) Table 36 details the rare vaccine reactions; the onset interval, the rate per doses and the case definitions. Most of the rare and more serious vaccine reactions (e.g. seizures, thrombocytopenia, HHEs, persistent inconsolable screaming) do not lead to long-term problems. Anaphylaxis, while potentially fatal, is treatable without leaving any long-term effects. Although encephalopthy is included as a rare reaction to measles or DTP vaccine, it is not certain that these vaccines in fact cause encephalopathy.

TABLE 36

Rare vaccine reactions, onset interval and rate per doses

Vaccine	Reaction	Onset interval	Rate/doses
BCG	Suppurative lymphadenitis BCG osteitis Disseminated BCG infection	2–6 months 1–12 months 1–12 months	$1–10/10^4$ $1–700/10^6$ $0.19–1.56/10^6$
Hib	None		
Hepatitis B	Anaphylaxis	0–1 hour	$1.1/10^6$
Influenza (inactivated)	Anaphylaxis Guillain-Barre syndrome (GBS) Oculo-respiratory syndrome		$0.7/10^6$ $1–2/10^6$ $76/10^6$
Influenza (live-attenuated)	Anaphylaxis Wheezing (children 6-11 months age)		$2/10^6$ 14/100
Japanese encephalitis (inactivated)	Neurologic events (encephalitis, encephalopathy $, peripheral neuropathy)		$1–2.3/10^6$
Measles/MMR/MR *	Febrile seizures Thrombocytopenia Anaphylaxis Encephalopathy $	6–12 days 15–35 days 0–1 hour 6–12 days	$3/10^3$ $3/10^4$ $\sim 1/10^6$ $<1/10^6$
Oral poliomyelitis	VAPP	4–30 days	$2\text{-}4/10^{6\dagger}$
Pertussis (DTwP)	Persistent (>3 hours) inconsolable screaming Seizures †† Hypotonic, hypo responsive episode (HHE) Anaphylaxis Encephalopathy $	0–24 hours 0–3 days 0–48 hours 0–1 hour 0–2 days	<1/100 <1/100 $1–2/10^3$ $20/10^6$ $0–1/10^6$
Pneumococcal	None proven ±		
Rotavirus	None known **		
Tetanus toxoid, DT	Brachial neuritis Anaphylaxis	2–28 days 0–1 hour	$5–10/10^6$ $1–6/10^6$
Yellow fever	Vaccine-associated viscerotropic disease ***		$1/10^6$
Varicella	Febrile seizures		$4\text{-}9/10^{4\dagger\dagger}$

Notes:

* Reactions (except anaphylaxis) do not occur if already immune (~90% of those receiving a second dose are immune): children over six years unlikely to have febrile seizures.

† VAPP Risk is higher following the first dose (1 in 750,000 compared to 1 in 5.1 million for subsequent doses), and for adults and immunocompromised.

± No proven risk of severe febrile or anaphylactic reactions or neurological disorders (e.g. Guillain-Barre syndrome)

** Post-marketing surveillance of currently available rotavirus vaccines has detected a small increased risk of intussusception (~1-2 cases per 100,000 infants vaccinated) in some settings shortly after the first dose of rotavirus vaccine.

*** Very rare in children

†† Seizures are mostly febrile and the risk depends on age, with much lower risk in infants under the age of four months.

$ Although encephalopathy is included as a rare possible reaction to measles, JE or DTP vaccines, it is not certain that these vaccines in fact cause encephalopathy. Hence, further scientific evaluation is necessary.

Although other serious events have been reported following immunization, it is likely that these events are coincidental, not true reactions.

The case definitions and treatments of adverse events following immunization are as follows *(115, 130)* :

Adverse event	Case definition	Treatment	Vaccines
Acute flaccid paralysis (vaccine associated paralytic poliomyelitis)	Acute onset of flaccid paralysis within 4 to 30 days of receipt of oral poliovirus (OPV), or within 4 to 75 days after contact with a vaccine recipient with isolation of vaccine virus and absence of wild polio virus in the stool, and neurological deficits remaining 60 days after onset, or death.	No specific treatment available; supportive care.	OPV
Anaphylactoid reaction (acute hypersensitivity reaction)	Exaggerated acute allergic reaction, occurring within 2 hours after immunization, characterized by one or more of the following: • wheezing and shortness of breath due to bronchospasm • laryngospasm/laryngeal oedema • one or more skin manifestations, e.g. hives, facial oedema, or generalized oedema. Less severe allergic reactions do not need to be reported.	Self-limiting; anti-histamines may be helpful.	All
Anaphylaxis	Severe immediate (within 1 hour) allergic reaction leading to circulatory failure with or without bronchospasm and/or laryngospasm/laryngeal oedema	Adrenaline injection	All
Arthralgia	Joint pain usually including the small peripheral joints. Persistent, if lasting longer than 10 days, transient; if lasting up to 10 days.	Self-limiting; analgesics	Rubella, MMR
Brachial neuritis	Dysfunction of nerves supplying the arm/shoulder without other involvement of nervous system. A deep steady, often severe aching pain in the shoulder and upper arm followed in days or weeks by weakness and wasting in arm/shoulder muscles. Sensory loss may be present, but is less prominent. May present on the same or the opposite side to the injection and sometimes affects both arms.	Symptomatic only; analgesics.	Tetanus
Disseminated BCG infections	Widespread infection occurring within 1 to 12 months after BCG vaccination and confirmed by isolation of *Mycobacterium bovis* BCG strain. Usually in immunocompromised individuals.	Should be treated with anti-tuberculous regimens including isoniazid and rifampicin.	BCG
Encephalopathy	Acute onset of major illness characterized by any two of the following three conditions: • seizures • severe alteration in level of consciousness lasting for one day or more • distinct change in behaviour lasting one day or more. Needs to occur within 48 hours of DTP vaccine or from 7 to 12 days after measles or MMR vaccine, to be related to immunization.	No specific treatment available; supportive care.	Measles, Pertussis
Fever	The fever can be classified (based on rectal temperature) as mild (38 to 38.9°C), high (39 to 40.4°C) and extreme (40.5°C or higher). Fever on its own does not need to be reported.	Symptomatic; paracetamol.	All
Hypotonic, hyporesponsive episode (HHE or shock-collapse)	Event of sudden onset occurring within 48 (usually less than 12) hours of vaccination and lasting from one minute to several hours, in children younger than 10 years of age. All of the following must be present : • limpness (hypotonic) • reduced responsiveness (hyporesponsive) • pallor or cyanosis – or failure to observed/recall.	The episode is transient and self-limiting, and does not require specific treatment. It is not a contraindication to further doses of the vaccine.	Mainly DTP, rarely others

Adverse event	Case definition	Treatment	Vaccines
Injection site abscess	Fluctuant or draining fluid-filled lesion at the site of injection. Bacterial if evidence of infection (e.g. purulent, inflammatory signs, fever, culture), sterile abscess if not.	Incise and drain; antibiotics if bacterial.	All
Lymphadenitis (includes suppurative lymphadenitis)	Either at least one lymph nodes enlarged to >1.5 cm in size (one adult finger width), or a draining sinus over a lymph node. Almost exclusively caused by BCG and then occurring within 2 to 6 months after receipt of BCG vaccine, on the same side as inoculation (mostly axilliary).	Heals spontaneously (over months) and best not to treat unless lesion is sticking to skin. If so,or already draining, surgical drainage and local instillation of anti-tuberculous drug. Systemic treatment with anti-tuberculous drugs is ineffective.	BCG
Osteitis/ Osteomyelitis	Inflammation of the bone with isolation of *Mycobacterium bovis* BCG strain.	Should be treated with anti-tuberculous regimens including isoniazid and rifampicin.	BCG
Persistent inconsolable screaming	Inconsolable continuous crying lasting 3 hours or longer accompanied by high-pitched screaming.	Settles within a day or so; analgesics may help	DTP, Pertussis
Seizures	Occurrence of generalized convulsions that are not accompanied by focal neurological signs or symptoms. Febrile seizures: if temperature elevated >38°C (rectal) Afebrile seizures : if temperature normal.	Self-limiting supportive care; paracetamol and cooling if febrile; rarely anticonvulsants.	All, especially Pertussis, Measles
Sepsis	Acute onset of severe generalized illness due to bacterial infection and confirmed (if possible) by positive blood culture. Needs to be reported as possible indicator of programme error.	Critical to recognize and treat early. Urgent transfer to hospital for parenteral antibiotics and fluids	All
Severe local reaction	Redness and/or swelling centred at the site of injection and one or more of the following: • swelling beyond the nearest joint • pain, redness, and swelling of more than 3 days duration • requires hospitalization. Local reactions of lesser intensity occur commonly and are trivial and do not need to be reported.	Settles spontaneously within a few days to a week. Symptomatic treatment with analgesics. Antibiotics are inappropriate.	All
Thrombocytopenia	Serum platelet count of less than 50,000/ml leading to bruising and/or bleeding.	Usually mild and self-limiting; occasionally may need steroid or platelets.	MMR
Toxic shock syndrome (TSS)	Abrupt onset of fever, vomiting and watery diarrhoea within a few hours of immunization. Often leading to death within 24 to 48 hours. Needs to be reported as possible indicator of programme error.	Critical to recognize and treat early. Urgent transfer to hospital for parenteral antibiotics and fluids.	All

RECOGNITION OF ANAPHYLAXIS *(115, 130)*

Administration of antisera may occasionally give rise to anaphylactic shock and serum sickness. Many viral vaccines contain traces of various antibiotics used in their preparation and some individuals may be sensitive to the antibiotic which it contains.

Anaphylaxis is a severe reaction of rapid onset, characterized by circulatory collapse. The early signs of anaphylaxis are generalized erythema and urticaria with upper and/or lower respiratory tract obstruction. In more severe cases, limpness, pallor, loss of consciousness and hypotension may also become evident. Vaccinators should be able to recognize the following signs and symptoms of anaphylaxis:

Diagnostic features of anaphylaxis	
Respiratory	*Airway* • Throat and tongue swelling (pharyngeal/laryngeal oedema) – the patient has difficulty in breathing and swallowing and feels that the throat is closing up. • Hoarse voice. • Stridor *Breathing* • Bronchospasm • Respiratory distress :– 2 or more of the following: – Tachypnoea – Increased use of accessory respiratory muscles – Recession – Cyanosis • Grunting • Respiratory arrest
Cardiovascular	• Hypotension • Clinical diagnosis of uncompensated shock, indicated by the combination of at least three of the following: – Tachycardia – Capillary refill time >3 seconds – Reduced central pulse volume – Decreased level of consciousness or loss of consciousness • Cardiac arrest • Bradycardia (a slow pulse) is usually a late feature, often preceding cardiac arrest
CNS	• Confusion/Agitation • Headache • Loss of consciousness
Dermatologic or mucosal	• Tingling of lips • Generalized urticaria or generalized erythema • Angioedema, localized or generalized (angioedema is similar to urticaria but involves swelling of deeper tissues, most commonly in the eyelids and lips, and sometimes in the mouth and throat) • Generalized itching of skin especially hands, forehead and eyes in children Note : Skin changes alone without life threatening cardio-respiratory signs do not signify an anaphylactic reaction
Gastrointestinal	• Diarrhoea • Colic abdominal pain • Vomiting • Incontinence

In general, the more severe the reaction, the more rapid the onset. Most life-threatening reactions begin within 10 minutes of immunization. It is advisable to keep the recipient under observation for at least 20 minutes after the injection. Symptoms limited to only one system can occur, leading to delay in diagnosis. Biphasic reactions where symptoms recur 8 to 12 hours after onset of the original attack and prolonged attacks lasting up to 48 hours have been described.

Time Scale	Signs and symptoms of anaphylaxis	Severity
Early warning signs	Dizziness, perineal burning, warmth, pruritus	Mild
↓	Flushing, urticaria, nasal congestion, sneezing, lacrimation, angioedema	Mild to moderate
	Hoarseness, nausea, vomiting, sub-sternal pressure	Moderate
	Laryngeal oedema, dyspnoea, abdominal pain	Moderate to severe
Late, life-threatening symptoms	Bronchospasm, stridor, collapse, hypotension, dysrhythmias	Severe

2. Immunization error-related reactions *(115, 130)*

"Immunization" means the usage of a vaccine for the purpose of immunizing individuals. "Usage" includes all processes that occur after a vaccine product has left the manufacturing/packaging site, i.e. handling, prescribing and administration of the vaccine.

An immunization error-related reaction may lead to a cluster of events associated with immunization. These clusters are usually associated with a particular provider, or health facility, or even a single vial of vaccine that has been inappropriately prepared or contaminated. Immunization errors-related reactions can also affect many vials. For example, freezing vaccine during transport may lead to an increase in local reactions.

Table 37 shows the immunization error-related reactions *(115)*.

TABLE 37
Immunization error-related reactions

Immunization error		Related reaction
Error in vaccine handling	Exposure to excess heat or cold as a result of inappropriate transport, storage or handling of the vaccine (and its diluent) where applicable.	Systemic or local reactions due to changes in the physical nature of the vaccine such as agglutination of aluminium-based excipients in freeze-sensitive vaccines.
	Use of a product after the expiry date.	Failure to vaccinate as a result of loss of potency or non-viability of an attenuated product.
Error in vaccine prescribing or non-adherence to recommendations for use	Failure to adhere to a contraindication.	Anaphylaxis, disseminated infection with an attenuated live, VAPP.
	Failure to adhere to vaccine indications or prescription (dose or schedule).	Systemic and/or local reactions, neurologic, muscular, vascular or bony injury due to incorrect injection site, equipment or technique.
Error in administration	Use of an incorrect diluent or injection of a product other than the intended vaccine.	Failure to vaccinate due to incorrect diluent. Reaction due to the inherent properties of whatever was administered other than the intended vaccine or diluent.
	Incorrect sterile technique or inappropriate procedure with a multidose vial.	Infection at the site of injection/beyond the site of injection.

In the past, the most common immunization error was an infection (including bloodborne virus) as a result of non-sterile-injection. The infection could manifest as a local reaction (e.g. suppuration, abscess), systemic effect (e.g. sepsis or toxic shock syndrome), or blood-borne virus infection (e.g. HIV, hepatitis B or hepatitis C). However, with the introduction of auto disabled (AD) syringes, infection occurrence has reduced significantly. Still, infection can occur in cases of mass vaccination or disaster stituations, particularly if there is any shortage or problems with logistics and supplies. This can be avoided by proper planning and preparedness of programme managers.

The symptoms arising from an immunization error may help to identify the likely cause. For example, children immunized with contaminated vaccine (usually the *bacterium Staphylococcus aureus*) become sick within a few hours; local tenderness and tissue infiltration, vomiting, diarrhoea, cyanosis and a high temperature are the most frequent symptoms. Bacteriological examination of the vial, if still available, can confirm the source of the infection.

3. Immunization stress–related–response *(115, 115A)*

Previously it was known as immunization anxiety-related reaction. Individuals and groups can react in anticipation to and as a result of an injection of any kind. This reaction is unrelated to content of the vaccine. Fainting is relatively common. During fainting, the individual suddenly becomes pale, loses consciousness and collapses to the ground. Fainting is sometimes accompanied by brief clonic seizure activity (i.e. rhythmic jerking of the limbs), but this requires no specific treatment or investigation. Fainting is relatively common after immunization of adults and adolescents, but very rare in young children. It is managed by simply placing the patient in a recumbent position. Recovery of consciousness occurs within a minute or two, but patients may take some more time to recover fully. Table 38 shows the difference between fainting attack and anaphylaxis.

An anxiety spell can lead to pale, fearful appearance and symptoms of hyperventilation (light-headedness, dizziness, tingling in the hands and around the mouth). Breath-holding occurs in young children and will lead to facial flushing and cyanosis. It can end in unconsciousness, during which breathing resumes. Anaphylaxis develops over several minutes upto a few hours and usually involves multiple body systems. Unconsciousness is rarely the sole manifestation of anaphylaxis – it only occurs as a late event in severe cases. A strong central pulse (e.g. carotid) is maintained during a faint, but not in anaphylaxis.

4. Coincidental events

Occasionally following immunization there may occur a disease totally unconnected with the immunizing agent. Vaccines are normally scheduled early in life, when infections and other illnesses are common, including manifestations of an underlying congenital or neurological condition. The mechanism seems to be that the individual is harbouring the infectious agent and the administration of the vaccine shortens the incubation period and produces the disease or what may have been otherwise only a latent infection is converted into a clinical attack.

PRECAUTIONS TO BE TAKEN

Before administration of the antiserum or antitoxin, it is necessary to test for sensitivity reaction. This can be done in 2 ways: (a) instilling a drop of the preparation into the conjunctival sac. A sensitized person will develop pricking of the conjunctiva. (b) a more reliable way of testing is by intradermal injection of 0.2 ml of antiserum diluted 1 : 10 with saline. A sensitized patient will develop a wheal and flare within 10 minutes at the site of injection. It should be borne in mind that these tests are not infallible.

Adrenaline (1:1000 solution) should be kept ready when giving foreign serum. In the event of anaphylaxis, for an adult, 0.5 ml of adrenaline solution should be injected intramuscularly immediately, followed by 0.5 ml every 20 minutes if the systolic blood pressure is below 100 mm of mercury. An injection of antihistaminic drug should also be given, e.g., 10–20 mg of chlorpheniramine maleate by the intramuscular route, to minimize the after-effects such as urticaria or oedema. The patient should be observed for 30 minutes after any serum injection.

The risk of adverse reactions can be reduced by proper sterilization of syringes and needles, by proper selection of the subject and the product, and if due care is exercised in carrying out the procedure. Measles and BCG vaccines should be reconstituted only with the diluent supplied by the manufacturer. Reconstituted vaccine should be discarded at the end of each immunization session and NEVER retained for use in subsequent sessions. In the refrigerator of the immunization centre, no other drug and substances should be stored beside vaccines. Training of immunization worker and their close supervision to ensure that proper procedures are being followed are essential to prevent complications and deaths following immunization. Careful epidemiological investigation should be carried out when an adverse event following immunization occurs to pinpoint the cause of the incident and to correct immunization practices *(131, 115)*.

TABLE 38
Difference between a fainting attack and anaphylaxis

Clinical features	Fainting	Anaphylaxis
Timing	Before, during or few minutes after injection	A short time, upto a few hours
Skin	Generalized pallor, cold clammy skin	Itching, generalized erythema, urticaria, swelling of lips, face, tingling around lips
Respiratory system	Normal breathing Shallow breathing	Tachypnoea, difficulty in breathing, wheezing, stridor, hoarseness, cyanosis, recession of intercostal spaces
Cardiovascular	Bradycardia, weak pulse, carotid pulse felt, hypotension may occur-reversed by supine position	Tachycardia, weak pulse, carotid pulse may be weak, hypotension – not reversed by supine position
GIT	Vomiting	Vomiting, diarrhoea, abdominal cramps
CNS	Faintishness, light-headedness relieved by supine posture	Anxiety and distress, loss of consciousness not relieved by supine posture
Panic attack – no hypotension, pallor, wheeze, or urticarial rash or swelling. May have flushing or blotchy skin.		

Investigating adverse events following immunization *(115)*

The suggested reportable events believed by the public or health workers to be caused by immunization are listed below and could be considered for inclusion in the AEFI surveillance system. There is no point in reporting common minor reactions such as local reactions, fever and self-limiting systemic symptoms.

Events that should be reported after immunization

Occurring within 24–48 hours of immunization	• Anaphylactoid reaction (acute hypersensitivity reaction) • Anaphylaxis • Persistent (more than 3 hours) inconsolable screaming • Hypotonic hyporesponsive episode (HHE) • Toxic shock syndrome (TSS)
Occurring within 7 days of immunization	• Severe local reaction • Sepsis • Injection site abscess (bacterial/sterile)
Occurring within 14 days of immunization	• Seizures, including febrile seizures (6–12 days for measles/MMR; 0–2 days for DTP) • Encephalopathy (6–12 days for measles/MMR; 0–2 days for DTP)
Occurring within 3 months of immunization	• Acute flaccid paralysis (4–30 days for OPV recipient; 4–75 days for contact) • Brachial neuritis (2–28 days after tetanus containing vaccine) • Thrombocytopenia (15–35 days after measles/MMR) • Intussusception commonly after rotavirus
Occurring between 1 and 12 months after BCG immunization	• Lymphadenitis • Disseminated BCG infection • Osteitis/Osteomyelitis
No time limit	Any death, hospitalization, disability or other severe and unusual events that are thought by health workers or the public to be related to immunization

Once the report has been received, an assessment should be made to determine whether or not an investigation is needed. The urgency of the investigation depends on the situation.

Investigating AEFI clusters

A cluster of AEFI is defined as two or more cases of the same adverse event related in time, place or vaccine administration. Cluster investigation begins by establishing the case definition and identifying all cases that meet the case definition.

A cluster of similar adverse events is likely to arise from programme errors. If the event also occured in unimmunized people, it may be coincidental. If all cases received the same vaccine or lot, and there are no similar cases in the community, a problem with the vaccine is likely. If the event is a known vaccine reaction but occurring at an increased rate, a programme error or a vaccine problem are likely causes (Fig. 27).

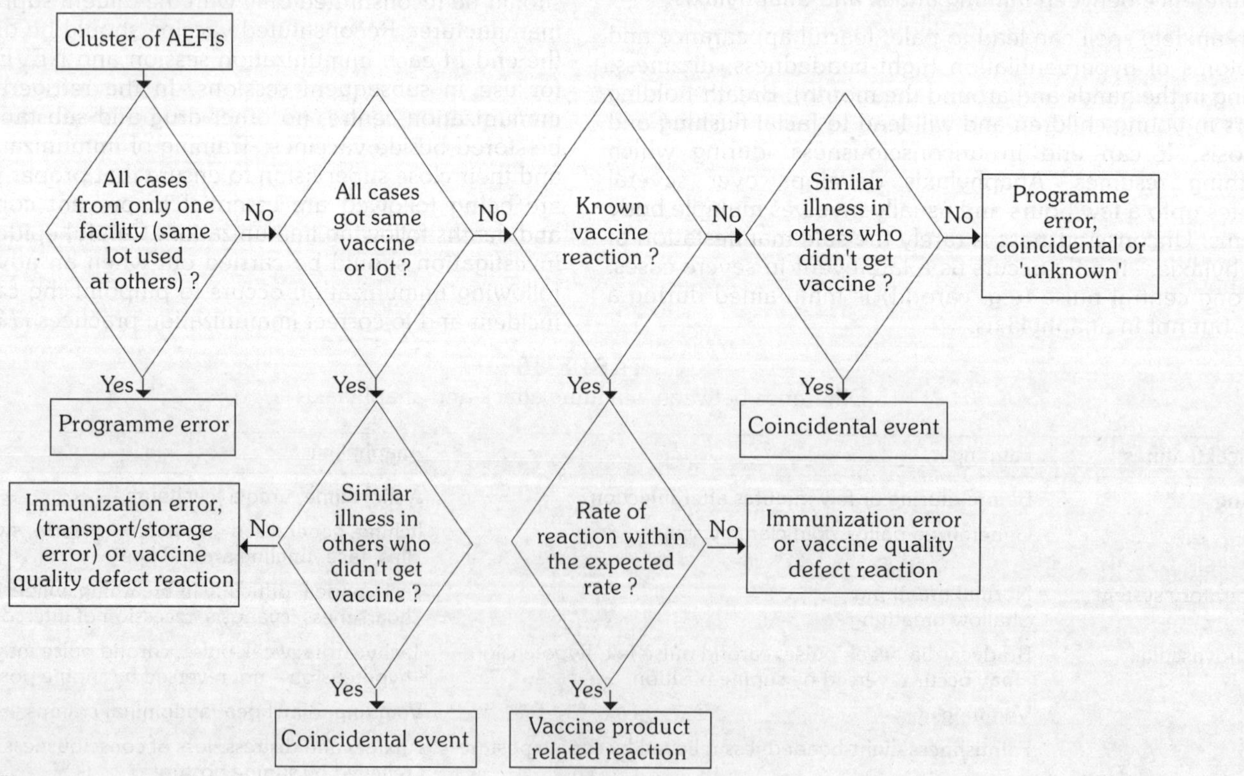

Source : *(115)*

FIG. 27
Identifying cause of AEFI cluster

Investigation of an AEFI *(115)*

AN AEFI investigation follows standard epidemiological investigation principles. In addition, investigation of the vaccine(s), immunization techniques and procedures, and service in action needs to be conducted.

STEPS IN AN AEFI INVESTIGATION

Step	Actions
1. Confirm information in report	• Obtain patient's medical file (or other clinical record). • Check details about patient and event from medical file and document information. • Identify any other cases that need to be included in the investigation.
2. Investigate and collect data: About the patient:	• Immunization history. • Previous medical history, including prior history of similar reaction or other allergies. • Family history of similar events.
About the event:	• History, clinical description, any relevant laboratory results about the AEFI and diagnosis of the event. • Treatment, whether hospitalized, and outcome.
About the suspected vaccine(s):	• Conditions under which the vaccine was shipped, its present storage condition, state of vaccine vial monitor, and temperature record of refrigerator. • Storage of vaccine before it arrived at health facility, where it has come from higher up the cold chain, vaccine monitor card.
About other people:	• Whether others received the same vaccine and developed illness. • Whether others had similar illness (may need case definition); if so exposure of cases of suspect vaccine(s). • Investigate the local immunization service.
3. Assess the service by: asking about:	• Vaccine storage (including open vials), distribution, and disposal. • Diluent storage and distribution. • Reconstitution (process and time kept). • Use and sterilization of syringes and needles. • Details of training in immunization practice, supervision and vaccinator(s). • Number of immunizations greater than normal ?
Observing the service in action:	• Refrigerator – what else is stored (note if similar containers stored next to vaccine vials which could be confused); which vaccines/diluents stored with other drugs; whether any vials have lost their label. • Immunization procedures (reconstitution, drawing up vaccine, injection technique, safety of needles and syringes; disposal of opened vials). • Do any open vials look contaminated ?
4. Formulate a working hypothesis:	• On the likely/possible cause(s) of the event.
5. Test working hypothesis	• Does case distribution match working hypothesis ? • Occasionally, laboratory tests may help.
6. Conclude investigation	• Reach a conclusion on the cause. • Complete AEFI Investigation Form. • *Take corrective action, and recommend further action*

A series of cases without comparison of disease and exposure among controls is not likely to reveal the cause of the AEFI, except in the case of programme errors. Clear case definitions, from the guidelines on reporting or defined during the investigation, are essential. The investigation needs to identify all cases in the community and find out the outcomes for all those who received the suspect vaccine. A working hypothesis should be established as soon as there is sufficient information. Laboratory testing may sometimes confirm or rule out the suspected cause. The vaccine may be tested for sterility and adjuvant (e.g. aluminium content); the diluent for sterility and chemical composition; and the needles and syringe for sterility. Testing should be requested on a *clear suspicion* and not as a routine, and *never* before the working hypothesis has been formulated.

Contraindications to vaccination

Vaccines are very rarely contraindicated. However, it is important to check for contraindications to avoid serious reactions. For example, vaccines are contraindicated if there is serious allergy to the vaccine or its components. Live vaccines should not be given to immune-deficient children.

The main contraindication to the administration of vaccines are summarized in Table 39.

DISEASE PREVENTION AND CONTROL

Every disease has certain weak points susceptible to attack. The basic approach in controlling disease is to identify these weak points and break the weakest links in the chain of transmission (Fig. 16). This requires sound epidemiological knowledge of the disease – that is its magnitude, distribution in time, place and person, multifactorial causation, sources of infection and dynamics of transmission.

Frequently it may be necessary to institute more than one method of control simultaneously. The choice of methods will depend upon factors such as availability of proper tools and techniques, relative cost effectiveness, efficiency and acceptability. Although effective control of a disease requires knowledge of its multifactorial causation, removal or elimination of a single known essential link or the weakest link may be sufficient to control a disease, even if complete knowledge about the aetiology of the disease in question is lacking. The classic example is that of John Snow controlling the cholera epidemic in London, by removing the handle of the incriminated water pump.

Disease control involves all the measures designed to prevent or reduce as much as possible the incidence, prevalence and consequences of disease *(132)*. This includes community participation, political support and intersectoral coordination *(133)*. Control measures should not be delayed because of incomplete or lack of accurate knowledge of the aetiological agent.

TABLE 39
Contraindications to vaccines

Vaccine	Contraindications
All	An anaphylactic reaction[a] following a previous dose of a particular vaccine is a true contraindication to further immunization with the antigen concerned and a subsequent dose should not be given, OR, Current serious illness.
Live vaccines (MMR, BCG, yellow fever)	Pregnancy. Radiation therapy (i.e. total-body radiation).
Yellow fever	Egg allergy. Immunodeficiency (from medication, disease or symptomatic HIV infection[b]).
BCG	Symptomatic HIV infection.
Influenza, yellow fever	History of anaphylactic reactions[a] following egg ingestion. No vaccines prepared in hen's egg tissues (i.e. yellow fever and influenza vaccines) should be given. (Vaccine viruses propagated in chicken fibroblast cells, e.g. measles or MMR vaccines, can however usually be given.)
Pertussis-containing	Anaphylactic reaction to a previous dose. Evolving neurological disease (e.g. uncontrolled epilepsy or progressive encephalopathy). Vaccines containing the whole-cell pertussis component should not be given to children with this problem. Acellular vaccine is less reactogenic and is used in many industrialized countries instead of whole-cell pertussis vaccine.

[a] Generalized urticaria, difficulty in breathing, swelling of the mouth and throat, hypotension or shock.
[b] In many industrialized countries yellow fever vaccine is administered to individuals with symptomatic HIV infection or who are suffering from other immunodeficiency diseases, provided that their CD_4 count is at least 400 cells/mm^3 and if they plan to visit areas where epidemic or endemic yellow fever actually occurs.

Source : *(129)*

Broadly these are measures, pending results of epidemiologic investigation.

1. The reservoir or source of infection
2. The route(s) of transmission
3. The susceptible host (people at risk).

The activities of disease prevention and control are now included in primary health care – it requires community participation (involvement), political support and inter-sectoral coordination *(133)*.

1. Controlling the reservoir

If the first link in the chain of causation (i.e., the disease agent) is deemed to be the weakest link, logically, the most desirable control measure would be to eliminate the reservoir or source, if that could be possible. Elimination of the reservoir may be pretty easy with the animal reservoir (e.g., bovine tuberculosis, brucellosis), but is not possible in humans in whom the general measures of reservoir control comprise : early diagnosis, notification, isolation, treatment, quarantine, surveillance and disinfection – all directed to reduce the quantity of the agent available for dissemination.

(1) EARLY DIAGNOSIS

The first step in the control of a communicable disease is its rapid identification. It is the cornerstone on which the edifice of disease control is built. It has been aptly said that prompt detection of cases (and carriers) and their treatment is like stamping out the "spark" rather than calling the fire brigade to put out the fire caused by the spark. Frequently, laboratory procedures may be required to confirm the diagnosis.

Early diagnosis is needed for (a) the treatment of patients (b) for epidemiological investigations, e.g., to trace the source of infection from the known or index case to the unknown or the primary source of infection (c) to study the time, place and person distribution (descriptive epidemiology) and (d) for the institution of prevention and control measures.

(2) NOTIFICATION

Once an infectious disease has been detected (or even suspected), it should be notified to the local health authority, whose responsibility is to put into operation control measures, including the provision of medical care to patients, perhaps in a hospital.

Certain diseases are statutorily notifiable. The diseases to be notified vary from country to country; and even within the same country. Usually, diseases which are considered to be serious menaces to public health are included in the list of notifiable diseases. Notifiable diseases may also include non-communicable diseases and conditions such as cancer, congenital defects, accidents, etc.

Notification is an important source of epidemiological information. It enables early detection of disease outbreaks, which permits immediate action to be taken by the health authority to control their spread. The other uses of notification are discussed elsewhere.

Notification of infectious diseases is often made by the attending physician or the head of the family, but any one, including the lay people (e.g., religious, political and administrative leaders, teachers and others) can report, even on suspicion. In all cases, the diagnosis is verified by the local health authority.

Under the **International Health Regulations (IHR)**, certain prescribed diseases are notified by the national health authority to WHO. These can be divided into :

(a) Those diseases subject to International Health Regulations (1969), Third Annotated Edition, 1983 – cholera, plague and yellow fever.
(b) Diseases under surveillance by WHO – louse-borne typhus fever, relapsing fever, paralytic polio, malaria, viral influenza–A, SARS, smallpox etc.

Health administrations are required to notify to WHO Geneva for any notification of communicable diseases under international surveillance and International Health Regulations.

(3) EPIDEMIOLOGICAL INVESTIGATIONS

An epidemiological investigation is called for whenever there is a disease outbreak, the methodology for which is given elsewhere (see page 147). Broadly, the investigation covers the identification of the source of infection and of the factors influencing its spread in the community. These may include geographical situation, climatic condition, social, cultural and behavioural patterns, and more importantly the character of the agent, reservoir, the vectors and vehicles, and the susceptible host populations.

(4) ISOLATION

Isolation is the oldest communicable disease control measure. It is defined as "separation, for the period of communicability of infected persons or animals from others in such places and under such conditions, as to prevent or limit the direct or indirect transmission of the infectious agent from those infected to those who are susceptible, or who may spread the agent to others" *(106)*. In general, infections from human/animal sources can be controlled by physical isolation of the case or carrier, and if necessary, treatment until free from infection, provided cases and carriers can be easily identified and carrier rates are low.

The *purpose* of isolation is to protect the community by preventing transfer of infection from the reservoir to the possible susceptible hosts. The *type* of isolation varies with the mode of spread and severity of the disease. There are several types of isolation – standard isolation, strict isolation, protective isolation, high security isolation *(134)*. For each patient, the relative risks to the patient and to others should be assessed and the appropriate type of isolation determined. Hospital isolation, wherever possible, is better than home isolation. Isolation is particularly difficult in rural areas. In some situations (e.g., cholera outbreaks) the entire village or rural community may have to be isolated. Isolation may also be achieved in some diseases by "ring immunization", that is encircling the infected persons with a barrier of immune persons through whom the infection is unable to spread. This method when applied worldwide in the 1960s and 1970s eradicated smallpox. In North America, ring immunization is being applied in measles control and eradication. The duration of isolation is determined by the duration of communicability of the disease and the effect of chemotherapy on infectivity (Table 40).

Isolation has a distinctive value in the control of some infectious diseases, e.g., diphtheria, cholera, streptococcal respiratory disease, pneumonic plague, etc. In some diseases where there is a large component of subclinical infection and carrier state (polio, hepatitis A, and typhoid fever), even the most rigid isolation will not prevent the spread of the disease. It is also futile to impose isolation if the disease is highly infectious before it is diagnosed as in the case of mumps. Isolation has failed in the control of diseases such as leprosy, tuberculosis and STD. In the control of these diseases, the concept of physical isolation has been replaced by chemical isolation, i.e., rapid treatment of cases in their own homes and rendering them non-infectious as quickly as possible. Lastly, cases are usually reported after the disease has spread widely. Taking all these limitations into consideration, it may be stated that isolation which is a "barrier approach" to the prevention and control of infectious disease is not as successful as one would imagine and may well give rise to a false sense of security *(135)*. In modern–day disease control, isolation is more judiciously applied and in most cases replaced by surveillance because of improvements in epidemiological and disease control technologies. Today, isolation is recommended only when the risk of transmission of the infection is exceptionally serious.

TABLE 40
Periods of isolation recommended

Disease	Duration of isolation
Chickenpox	Until all lesions crusted; usually about 6 days after onset of rash.
Measles	From the onset of catarrhal stage through 3rd day of rash.
German measles	None, except that women in the first trimester or sexually active, non immune women in child-bearing years not using contraceptive measures should not be exposed.
Cholera, Diphtheria	3 days after tetracyclines started, until 48 hours of antibiotics (or negative cultures after treatment).
Shigellosis, Salmonellosis	Until 3 consecutive negative stool cultures.
Hepatitis A	3 weeks.
Influenza	3 days after onset.
Polio	2 weeks adult, 6 weeks paediatric.
Tuberculosis (sputum +)	Until 3 weeks of effective chemotherapy.
Herpes zoster	6 days after onset of rash.
Mumps	Until swelling subsides.
Pertussis	4 weeks or until paroxysms cease.
Meningococcal meningitis, Streptococcal pharyngitis	Until the first 6 hours of effective antibiotic therapy are completed.

Source : *(136, 137)*

(5) TREATMENT

Many communicable diseases have been tamed by effective drugs. The object of treatment is to kill the infectious agent when it is still in the reservoir, i.e., before it is disseminated. Treatment reduces the communicability of disease, cuts short the duration of illness and prevents development of secondary cases. In some diseases (e.g., syphilis, tuberculosis, and leprosy), early diagnosis and treatment is of primary importance in interrupting transmission. Treatment is also extended to carriers.

Treatment can take the form of individual treatment or mass treatment. In the latter category, all the people in the community are administered the drugs whether they have the disease or not (e.g., trachoma). If the treatment is inadequate or inappropriate, it may induce drug resistance in the infectious agent and may frustrate attempts to control the disease by chemotherapy. It is well to remember that no disease has ever been conquered through attempting to treat every affected individual *(138)*. Yaws is a shining example.

(6) QUARANTINE

Quarantine has been defined as "the limitation of freedom of movement of such well persons or domestic animals exposed to communicable disease for a period of time not longer than the longest usual incubation period of the disease, in such manner as to prevent effective contact with those not so exposed" *(139)*. Quarantine measures are also "applied by a health authority to a ship, an aircraft, a train, road vehicle, other means of transport or container, to prevent the spread of disease, reservoirs of disease or vectors of disease" *(140)*.

Quarantine may comprise (a) *absolute quarantine*, as defined above; (b) *modified quarantine,* e.g., a selective partial limitation of freedom of movement, such as exclusion of children from school; and (c) *segregation* which has been defined as "the separation for special consideration, control of observation of some part of a group of persons (or domestic animals) from the others to facilitate control of a communicable disease, e.g., removal of susceptible children to homes of immune persons" *(2)*.

In contrast to isolation, quarantine applies to restrictions on the healthy contacts of an infectious disease. Quarantine which was once a popular method of disease control has now declined in popularity *(135)*. With better techniques of early diagnosis and treatment, quarantine, as a method of disease control, has become outdated. It has been replaced by active surveillance.

2. Interruption of transmission

A major aspect of communicable disease control relates to "breaking the chain of transmission" or interruption of transmission (Fig. 16). This may mean changing some components of man's environment to prevent the infective agent from a patient or carrier from entering the body of susceptible person. For example, water can be a medium for the transmission of many diseases such as typhoid, dysentery, hepatitis A, cholera and gastroenteritis. Water treatment will eliminate these diseases. Depending upon the level of pollution, this may vary from simple chlorination to complex treatment. However, control of the source of contamination is an important long-term measure. Food-borne disease is particularly prevalent in areas having low standards of sanitation. Clean practices such as hand-washing, adequate cooking, prompt refrigeration of prepared foods and withdrawal of contaminated foods will prevent most food–borne illnesses *(141)*. When the disease is vector–borne, control measures should be directed primarily at the vector and its breeding places. Vector control also includes destruction of stray dogs, control of cattle, pets and other animals to minimize spread of infection among them, and from them to man. On the other hand, episodes of infection either by droplets or droplet nuclei are not usually controlled effectively by attempting to interrupt their mode of spread; reliance is placed on early diagnosis and treatment of patients, personal hygiene and proper handling of secretions and excretions. In short, blocking the routes of transmission imply an attack on environmental factors, that is, to bring about an adjusted equilibrium between host and environment through encouraging some ecological influences and inhibiting others *(138)*.

3. The susceptible host

The third link in the chain of transmission is the susceptible host or people at risk. They may be protected by one or more of the following strategies.

(1) ACTIVE IMMUNIZATION

One effective way of controlling the spread of infection is to strengthen the host defences. Under certain circumstances this may be accomplished by active immunization, which is one of the most powerful and cost-effective weapons of modern medicine. There are some infectious diseases whose control is solely based on active immunization, e.g., polio, tetanus, diphtheria and measles. Vaccination against these diseases is given as a routine during infancy and early childhood (Table 42), with periodic boosters to maintain adequate levels of immunity. Then there are immunizations against certain diseases (Table 41) which are offered to high-risk groups or restricted to definite geographic areas where the disease is endemic or a public health problem (e.g., yellow fever). Unfortunately we do not have vaccines for every infectious disease (e.g., malaria, diarrhoeal diseases). Diseases for which improved or less costly vaccines are needed include tuberculosis, pertussis, meningococcal meningitis, hepatitis B, rabies, Japanese encephalitis, etc. *(142)*.

Immunization is a mass means of protecting the greatest number of people. By reducing the number of susceptibles in the community, it augments "herd immunity" making the infection more difficult to spread. It also reduces the risk for those individuals who have escaped vaccination or those who have not developed satisfactory protection. It is well to bear in mind that immunizations are not all 100 per cent effective, particularly when an individual is exposed to a large dose of pathogenic organisms.

Immunization has to be planned according to the needs of the situation. Every country has its own immunization schedule, so does each medical society and each paediatric society, adding to confusion. Thus there is an infinite number of immunization schedules, each having its merits and demerits. If each vaccine were to be given separately, a minimum of at least 14 visits would be needed to the

TABLE 41
Active Immunization recommended under special circumstances

	Disease	Immunization
1.	Cholera	Two types of safe and effective oral cholera vaccines currently available. Given orally in two doses between seven days and six weeks apart.
2.	Plague	Given subcutaneously or intramuscularly in 2 doses at an interval of 7 to 14 days. Immunity starts 5 to 7 days after inoculation and lasts for about 6 months.
3.	Typhoid fever	Two vaccines are available for prevention of typhoid. Typhoid polysaccharide vaccine is injectable given subcutaneously or intramuscularly. One dose is required. Confers protection after 7 days. The other is oral Ty21a vaccine, administered on 1, 3 and 5th day. Protective immunity achieved 7 days after 3rd dose.
4.	Influenza	Inactivated vaccines are widely used. Two adequately spaced doses (1.0 ml each) of an aqueous or saline vaccine are recommended for primary immunization, although one dose may be given when an epidemic is threatened. The immunity lasts for about 3 to 6 months. Oil-adjuvanted vaccines give immunity of longer duration, but they tend to produce unpleasant local reaction.
5.	Yellow fever	The dose of the vaccine (17 D vaccine) is 0.5 ml given subcutaneously. Immunity begins 10-12 days after vaccination, and extends upto 10 years.

immunization clinic. The current trend is to combine immunizing agents into small packages and thus reduce the number of injections an individual must receive.

A well thought-out immunization schedule must be (a) *epidemiologically relevant*, that is, vaccinations should be included only against diseases which are public health problems and against which an effective vaccine exists (b) *immunologically effective :* children must be vaccinated at an age when they can benefit from it, i.e., when they are capable of forming defences and when they have lost the antibodies transmitted by the mother. Above all, children must be vaccinated at the right time, that is before they are exposed to possible infection. An immunization may not be effective if given within too short an interval between subsequent doses (c) *operationally feasible :* this includes cost and ability to achieve a high percentage of coverage which is a key factor in an effective immunization programme. The schedule must minimize the number of visits, by simultaneous administration of vaccines, and (d) *socially acceptable :* the schedule must take into account the local customs, beliefs and practices, seasonal and climatic factors and daily work pattern of the community. One important factor is to reduce long waiting time for patients whose sole purpose in visiting the clinic was to be immunized.

Universal Immunization Programme (UIP)

In May 1974, the WHO officially launched a global immunization programme, known as Expanded Programme on Immunization (EPI) to protect all children of the world against six vaccine–preventable diseases, namely – diphtheria, whooping cough, tetanus, polio, tuberculosis and measles by the year 2000. EPI was launched in India in January 1978 *(143)*.

The Programme is now called *Universal Child Immunization*, 1990–that's the name given to a declaration sponsored by UNICEF as part of the United Nations' 40th anniversary in October 1985. It is aimed at adding impetus to the global programme of EPI.

The Indian version, the *Universal Immunization Programme,* was launched on November 19, 1985 and was dedicated to the memory of Smt. Indira Gandhi. The National Health Policy was aimed at achieving universal immunization coverage of the eligible population by 1990.

IMMUNIZATION SCHEDULES

1. National Immunization Schedule

The National Immunization Schedule is given in Table 43. The first visit may be made when the infant is 6 weeks old; the second and third visits, at intervals of 1–2 months. Oral polio vaccine may be given concurrently with pentavalent vaccine. BCG can be given with any of the three doses but the site for the injection should be different. The schedule also covers immunization of women during pregnancy against tetanus.

The Indian Academy of Paediatrics recommends inclusion of more vaccines in the immunization schedule. These vaccines are not included in the UIP because of financial constraints. The immunization schedule approved by the IAP is as follows :

BCG	–	Birth – 2 weeks
OPV	–	Birth; 6 weeks, 10 weeks and 14 weeks; 16–18 months, 5 years
DPT	–	6 weeks, 10 weeks and 14 weeks; 16–18 months and 5 years
Hepatitis B	–	Birth, 6 weeks and 14 weeks *or* 6 weeks, 10 weeks and 14 weeks
Hib Conjugate	–	6 weeks, 10 weeks and 14 weeks
Measles	–	9 months, 16–24 months
MMR	–	15 months
Typhoid	–	2 years, 5 years, 8 years, 12 years
TT/Td	–	10 years, 16 years
TT	–	2 doses one month apart for pregnant women, or booster dose if previously immunized.
Pneumococcal conjugate vaccine	–	6 weeks, 14 weeks and booster dose at 9–12 months.

Pentavalent vaccine has replaced DPT, Hepatitis B and Hib conjugate vaccine in NIS, therefore DPT, Hepatitis and Hib conjugate vaccine should not be given at 6, 10, and 14 weeks if pentavalent vaccine is being used.

Vaccines that can be given after discussion with parents

Varicella	–	15 months (or after 1 year)
Hepatitis A	–	high-risk selected infants, 18 months, and 6 months later
Influenza vaccine	–	6 months of age to high risk selected infants annually

2. WHO EPI Schedule

Table 44 summarizes the WHO recommendations for routine vaccination for children. The purpose is to assist health planners to develop an appropriate country specific immunization schedule based on local conditions. The health care workers should refer to their national immunization schedules.

The WHO EPI Global Advisory Committee has strongly recommended BCG and Polio vaccine to be given at birth or at first contact, in countries where tuberculosis and polio have not been controlled. In all countries routine immunization with DPT and oral polio vaccine can be safely and effectively initiated at 6 weeks of age. New vaccines are being added for the vaccination schedule e.g., hepatitis B, rubella, Rota virus vaccine Hib, pneumococcal and Japanese encephalitis vaccines are now included in several country's programmes.

The immunization schedule may be altered to suit the local needs of individuals and groups. Interruption of the schedule with a delay between doses does not interfere with the final immunity achieved. There is no basis for the mistaken belief that if a second (or third) dose in an immunization is delayed, the immunization schedule must be started all over again *(109)*. The ages shown in Table 43 for the various immunizations are considered the best. However, if there is any delay in starting the first dose the site for the injection should be different, the periods may be adjusted accordingly.

Immunization is frequently postponed if children are ill or malnourished. This is not acceptable in the light of present knowledge. In fact, it is particularly important to immunize children with malnutrition. Low grade fever, mild respiratory infections or diarrhoea and other minor illnesses should not be considered as contraindications to immunization. These are the very children who are most in need of immunization. They are most likely to die should they acquire a vaccine–preventable disease *(145)*.

TABLE 42
National Immunization Schedule (NIS) for infants, children and pregnant women (vaccine-wise), India (2020)

Vaccine	When to give	Dose	Route	Site
For Pregnant Women				
Tetanus Toxoid (TT)/ Tetanus & adult Diphtheria (Td)-1	Early in pregnancy	0.5 ml	Intra-muscular	Upper Arm
TT/Td-2	4 weeks after TT-1	0.5 ml	Intra-muscular	Upper Arm
TT/Td-Booster	If received 2 TT doses in a pregnancy within the last 3 years*	0.5 ml	Intra-muscular	Upper Arm
For Infants				
Bacillus Calmette Guerin (BCG)	At birth or as early as possible till one year of age	0.1ml (0.05ml until 1 month age)	Intra-dermal	Left Upper Arm
Hepatitis B - Birth dose	At birth or as early as possible within 24 hours	0.5 ml	Intra-muscular	Antero-lateral side of mid-thigh
Oral Polio Vaccine (OPV)-0	At birth or as early as possible within the first 15 days	2 drops	Oral	Oral
OPV 1, 2 & 3	At 6 weeks, 10 weeks & 14 weeks (OPV can be given till 5 years of age)	2 drops	Oral	Oral
Pentavalent 1, 2 & 3	At 6 weeks, 10 weeks & 14 weeks (can be given till one year of age)	0.5 ml	Intra-muscular	Antero-lateral side of mid-thigh
Pneumococcal Conjugate Vaccine (PCV)	Two primary doses at 6 and 14 weeks followed by booster dose at 9-12 months	0.5 ml	Intra-muscular	Antero-lateral side of mid-thigh
Rotavirus (RVV)[#]	At 6 weeks, 10 weeks & 14 weeks 5 drops Rotavac (liquid vaccine) or 2.5 ml Rotasill (lyophilized vaccine) (can be given till one year of age)	–	Oral	Oral
Inactivated Polio Vaccine (IPV)	Two fractional dose at 6 and 14 weeks of age	0.1 ml ID	Intra dermal, two fractional dose	Right Upper Arm
Measles Rubella (MR) 1st dose	9 completed months-12 months. (Measles can be given till 5 years of age)	0.5 ml	Sub-cutaneous	Right Upper Arm
Japanese Encephelitis (JE) - 1**	9 completed months-12 months.	0.5 ml	Sub-cutaneous	Left Upper Arm
Vitamin A (1st dose)	At 9 completed months with Measles-Rubella	1 ml (1 lakh IU)	Oral	Oral
For Children				
Diphtheria, Pertussis & Tetanus (DPT) booster-1	16-24 months	0.5 ml	Intra-muscular	Antero-lateral side of mid-thigh
MR 2nd dose	16-24 months	0.5 ml	Sub-cutaneous	Right Upper Arm
OPV Booster	16-24 months	2 drops	Oral	Oral
JE-2	16-24 months	0.5 ml	Sub-cutaneous	Left Upper Arm
Vitamin A*** (2nd to 9th dose)	16-18 months. Then one dose every 6 months upto the age of 5 years	2 ml (2 lakh IU)	Oral	Oral
DPT Booster-2	5-6 years	0.5 ml.	Intra-muscular	Upper Arm
TT/Td	10 years & 16 years	0.5 ml	Intra-muscular	Upper Arm

* One dose if previously vaccinated within 3 years
** JE Vaccine is introduced in select endemic districts after the campaign.
*** 2nd to 9th doses of Vitamin A can be administered to children 1-5 years old during bi-annual rounds, in collaboration with ICDS.
[#] Rotavirus vaccine : lyophilized vaccine in all states/UT (D&N Haveli, Daman & Diu, Goa, Gujarat, Jharkhand, Karnataka, Kerala, Maharashtra, Puducherry, Telangana, West Bengal), Liquid vaccine in remaining 25 states/UT.

Source : *(143A)*

TABLE 43

WHO Recommendations for Routine Immunizations for Children (updated April 2018)

Antigen		Age at 1st Dose	Doses in Primary Series	Interval Between Doses 1st to 2nd	2nd to 3rd	3rd to 4th	Booster Dose
Recommendations for all children							
BCG		As soon as possible after birth	1				
Hepatitis B	Option 1	As soon as possible after birth (<24h)	3	4 weeks (min) with DTPCV1	4 weeks (min) with DTPCV2		
	Option 2	As soon as possible after birth (<24h)	4	4 weeks (min) with DTPCV1	4 weeks (min) with DTPCV2	4 weeks (min) with DTPCV3	
Polio	bOPV + IPV	6 weeks	4 (IPV dose to be given with bOPV dose from 14 weeks)	4 weeks (min) with DTPCV2	4 weeks (min) with DTPCV3		
	IPV/bOPV Sequential	8 weeks (IPV 1st)	1–2 IPV 2 bOPV	4–8 weeks	4–8 weeks	4–8 weeks	
	IPV	8 weeks	3	4–8 weeks	4–8 weeks		
DTP-containing vaccine		6 weeks (min)	3	4 weeks (min) – 8 weeks	4 weeks (min) – 8 weeks		3 Boosters 12–23 months (DTP-containing vaccince) 4–7 years (Td); and 9–15 years (Td)
Haemophilus influenzae type b	Option 1	6 weeks (min) 59 months (max.)	3	4 weeks (min) with DTPCV2	4 weeks (min) with DTPCV3		
	Option 2		2–3	8 weeks (min) if only 2 doses, 4 weeks (min) if 3 doses	4 weeks (min) if 3 doses		At least 6 months (min) after last dose
Pneumococcal (Conjugate)	Option 1	6 weeks (min)	3	4 weeks (min)	4 weeks		
	Option 2	6 weeks (min)	2	8 weeks (min)			9–15 months
Rotavirus	Rotarix	6 weeks (min) with DTP1	2	4 weeks (min) with DTPCV2			
	Rota Teq	6 weeks (min) with DTP1	3	4 weeks (min)– 10 weeks with DTPCV2	4 weeks (min) with DTPCV3		
Measles		9 or 12 months (6 months min)	2	4 weeks (min)			
Rubella		9 or 12 months with measles containing vaccine	1				
HPV		As soon as possible from 9 years of age (females only)	2	6 months (min 5 months)			
Recommendations for children residing in certain regions							
Japanese Encephalitis	Inactivated Vero cell-derived	6 months	2 generally	4 weeks (generally)			
	Live attentuated	8 months	1				
	Live recombinant	9 months	1				
Yellow Fever		9–12 months with measles containing vaccine	1				
Tick-borne Encephalitis		≥ 1 yr FSME-Immune and Encepur ≥ 3 yrs TBE-Moscow and EnceVir	3	1–3 months FSME-Immun and Encepur 1–7 months TBE-Moscow and EnceVir	5–12 months FSME-Immun and Encepur 12 months TBE-Moscow and EnceVir		At least 1 Every 3 years
Recommendations for children in some high-risk populations							
Typhoid	TCV (Typbar)	> 6 months	1				
	Vi PS	2 years (min)	1				Every 3 years
	Ty21a	Capsules 5 years (min)	3 or 4	1 day	1 day	1 day	Every 3–7 years
Cholera	Dukoral (WC-rBS)	2 years (min)	3 (2–5 years) 2 (≥ 6 years)	≥ 7 days (min) < 6 weeks (max.)	≥ 7 days (min) < 6 weeks (max)		Every 6 months Every 2 years
	Shanchol, Euvchol and mORCVAX	1 year (min)	2	14 days			After 2 years
Meningococcal	MenA conjugate	9–18 months (5 µg)	1				
	MenC conjugate	2–11 months	2	8 weeks			After 1 year
		≥ 12 months	1				
	Quadrivalent conjugate	9–23 months	2	12 weeks			
		≥ 2 years	1				
Hepatitis A		1 year	At least 1				
Rabies		As required	2	7 days			
Dengue (CYD-TDV)		9 years (min)	3	6 months	6 months		
Recommendations for children receiving vaccinations from immunization programmes with certain characteristics							
Mumps		12–18 months with measles containing vaccine	2	1 month (min) to school entry			
Seasonal Influenza (inactivated tri- and quadri-valent)		6 months (min)	2 (< 9 years) 1 (≥ 9 years)	4 weeks			Revaccinate annually 1 dose only
Varicella		12-18 months	1-2	4 weeks to 3 months per manufacturer recommendations			

Source : *(144)*

Since the success of EPI is now being seen to have important long-term effects on the traditional epidemiological patterns of major infectious diseases, often raising the average age of incidence, the adolescent age group of 10–19 years represent an important additional target group for immunization. In the pre-immunization era, large proportion of adults had disease induced immunity to common infections, now majority of individuals have *vaccine induced* immunity, which may or may not have the same long-term stability. Questions therefore arise as to policy and strategy implications for post-infancy immunization programmes.

The WHO Scientific Advisory Group of Experts to EPI has indicated the need to expand immunization activities beyond infancy, either as part of routine immunization services or as part of disease elimination or eradication measure.

Adolescence presents certain challenges for immunization in relation to lifestyle and other social issues, while also offering special opportunities, such as a vaccine delivery in the setting of educational institutions. The vaccines of interest are MR and MMR as part of measles outbreak prevention or elimination campaign, Td as booster dose for neonatal tetanus elimination, hepatitis B, influenza, varicella and HPV vaccines etc.

Immunization of health care workers : The information in Table 44 is provided by WHO to assist countries to develop policies for the vaccination of health care workers, as per the national vaccination schedule in use in their countries.

TABLE 44

Immunization of health care workers

Antigen	***Vaccination of Health Care Workers recommended***
BCG	BCG vaccination is recommended for unvaccinated TST- or IGRA-negative persons at risk of occupational exposure in low and high TB incidence areas (e.g. health-care workers, laboratory workers, medical students, prison workers, other individuals with occupational exposure)
Hepatitis B	Immunization is suggested for groups at risk of acquiring infection who have not been vaccinated previously (for example HCWs who may be exposed to blood and blood products at work).
Polio	All HCWs should have completed a full course of primary vaccination against polio.
Diphtheria	HCWs who may have occupational exposure to *C. diphtheriae*. All health-care workers should be upto date with immunization as recommended in their national immunization schedules.
Measles	All HCWs should be immune to measles and proof/documentation of immunity or immunization should be required as a condition of enrollment into training and employment.
Rubella	If rubella vaccine has been introduced into the national programme, all HCWs should be immune to rubella and proof/ documentation of immunity or immunization should be required as a condition of enrollment into training and employment.
Meningococcal	One booster dose 3–5 years after the primary dose may be given to persons considered to be at continued risk of exposure, including HCWs.
Influenza	HCWs are an important group for influenza vaccination. Annual immunization with a single dose is recommended.
Varicella	Countries should consider vaccination of potentially susceptible health-care workers (i.e. unvaccinated and with no history of varicella) with 2 doses of varicella vaccine
Pertussis	HWCs should be prioritized as a group to receive pertussis vaccine.
Antigen	***No current recommendation for vaccination of Health Care Workers***
Tetanus	There is currently no recommendation regarding HCWs.
Haemophilus influenzae type b	The main burden of disease lies in infants under 5 years of age. Work in a health care setting is not indicated as a factor for increased risk. There is currently no recommendation regarding HCWs.
Pneumococcal	The main burden of disease lies in infants under 5 years of age. Immunocompetent adults are not at an increased risk for serious pneumococcal disease. HCWs are not indicated as a group at increased risk of pneumococcal disease.
Rotavirus	Children are the target group for rotavirus vaccination as they have the greatest burden of disease. Adults including HCWs are not at increased risk of severe disease.
HPV	HCWs are not at increased risk of HPV. The primary target group for vaccination is girls aged 9–14.
Japanese Encephalitis	Health-care workers are generally not at special risk of contracting JE. Workers at high-risk in endemic areas, such as those involved in vector control, should be vaccinated.
Yellow Fever	Individuals in endemic countries and travellers to these countries should receive a single dose of yellow fever vaccine. Work in a health care setting is not indicated as a factor for increased risk. There is currently no recommendation regarding HCWs.
Tick-borne Encepalitis	Health-care workers are generally not at special risk of contracting JE. Workers at high-risk in endemic areas, such as those involved in vector control, should be vaccinated.
Typhoid	Typhoid vaccines should be employed as part of comprehensive control strategies in areas where the disease is endemic. Work in a health care setting is not indicated as a factor for increased risk. There is currently no recommendation regarding HCWs.
Cholera	Cholera vaccines may be employed as part of comprehensive control strategies in areas where the disease is endemic as well as to prevent and respond to cholera outbreaks. There is currently no recommendation regarding HCWs.
Hepatitis A	Hepatitis A is transmitted through contaminated food and water or direct contact with an infectious person. HCWs are not indicated as a group at increased risk of hepatitis A infection.
Rabies	PrEP may be considered for medical professionals who regularly provide care to persons with rabies.
Mumps	Routine mumps vaccination is recommended in countries with a well-established, effective childhood vaccination programme and the capacity to maintain high level vaccination coverage with measles and rubella vaccination. HCWs are not indicated as a group at increased risk.
Dengue (CYD-TDV)	HCWs are not at increased risk of dengue

Source : *(144A)*

(2) PASSIVE IMMUNIZATION

Three types of preparations are available for passive immunity – (a) Normal human immunoglobulin, (b) Specific (hyperimmune) human immunoglobulin, and (c) antisera or anti-toxins.

Passive immunization is a short-term expedient useful only when exposure to infection has just occurred or is imminent within the next few days. The duration of immunity induced is short and variable (1–6 weeks). Undesirable reactions may occur, especially if antiserum is of non-human origin.

Passive immunization has a limited value in the mass control of disease. It is recommended for non-immune persons under special circumstances. The commonly employed passive immunization procedures are listed in Table 33 and 34.

(3) COMBINED PASSIVE AND ACTIVE IMMUNIZATION

In some diseases (e.g., tetanus, diphtheria, rabies) passive immunization is often undertaken in conjunction with inactivated vaccine products, to provide both immediate (but temporary) passive immunity and slowly developing active immunity. If the injections are given at separate sites, the immune response to the active agent, may or may not be impaired by immunoglobulin *(108)*.

But, according to current recommendations immunoglobulin should not be given within 3 weeks before, or until 2 weeks after administration of a live attenuated vaccine *(146)*. For example, the antibody response to live attenuated measles vaccine is diminished in persons who receive immunoglobulin concurrently *(147)*. However, there are exceptions to this rule, as for example, the simultaneous administration of hepatitis B vaccine and hepatitis B immunoglobulin *(122)*.

(4) CHEMOPROPHYLAXIS

Chemoprophylaxis implies the protection from, or prevention of, disease. This may be achieved by causal prophylaxis, or by clinical prophylaxis :

(i) Causal prophylaxis implies the complete prevention of infection by the early elimination of the invading or migrating causal agent. For example, there is causal prophylaxis available against malaria.

(ii) Clinical prophylaxis implies the prevention of clinical symptoms; it does not necessarily mean elimination of infection.

The indications for chemoprophylaxis are given as in Table 45.

TABLE 45
Indications for chemoprophylaxis

Disease	Chemoprophylaxis
Cholera	Tetracycline or furazolidone for house-hold contacts
Conjunctivitis, bacterial	Erythromycin ophthalmic ointment (no effect on viral conjunctivitis)
Diphtheria	Erythromycin (and first dose of vaccine)
Influenza	Oseltamivir (effective only for type A) for contacts suffering from chronic diseases
Malaria	See Chapter 5
Meningitis, meningococcal	Ciprofloxacin and minocycline, for household and close community contacts; immunization should be initiated in all cases (against serogroups A and C).
Plague	Tetracycline for contacts of pneumonic plague.

(5) NON-SPECIFIC MEASURES

Most of the non-specific measures to interrupt pathways of transmission are of general applicability. Improvements in the quality of life (e.g., better housing, water supply, sanitation, nutrition, education) fall into this category. Non-specific measures will also include "legislative measures", wherever needed, to formulate integrated programme and permit effective programme implementation. In fact, these non-specific factors have played a dominant role in the decline of tuberculosis, cholera, leprosy and child mortality in the industrialized world, long before the introduction of specific control measures. Another important non-specific measure is community involvement in disease surveillance, disease control and other public health activities. If community involvement is not an integral part of public health programmes, they are unlikely to succeed. Laws, regulations and policy measures alone will not bring the desired results *(101)*.

It is well worth considering some obstacles and new developments in the control of infectious diseases in developing countries. First and foremost is the scarcity of funds, lack of an effective health infrastructure, public health laboratory facilities, equipment, supplies, trained personnel (e.g., epidemiologists) and public awareness needed for the investigation and control of communicable diseases. This handicap is shared by all developing countries. A development which has been supported by WHO is integration of communicable disease control into *primary health care*. This integration has been successfully carried out. Some authorities emphasize the need for maintaining intensive vertical programmes for the control of the highly prevalent and controllable diseases such as malaria, tuberculosis and leprosy until their frequency has been reduced to low levels. The failure of the malaria eradication programmes emphasize this point.

Finally a major obstacle to disease control is human behaviour. Medical technology is often ineffective in changing behaviour. In this regard, health education remains the only approach to enlist public co-operation and to induce relevant changes in the behaviour and life-styles of people. Such changes could, in themselves, be powerful methods of disease control.

Surveillance

Surveillance must follow control measures. It has been defined as "the continuous scrutiny of all aspects of occurrence and spread of disease that are pertinent to effective control" *(106)*. Surveillance goes beyond the passive reporting of cases. It includes laboratory confirmation of presumptive diagnosis; finding out the source of infection, routes of transmission, identification of all cases and susceptible contacts; and still others who are at risk in order finally to prevent the further spread of the disease. Serological surveillance identifies patterns of current and past infection. Included in surveillance are systematic collection of pertinent morbidity and mortality data, the orderly consolidation of these data, special field investigations and rapid dissemination of this information to those responsible for control or prevention. Once control measures have been instituted, their effectiveness should be *evaluated*. If they have not been successful, the reason(s) for failure should be identified, the existing measures modified and evaluation continued *(102)*. The ultimate objective of surveillance is prevention.

Surveillance may comprise : (a) *Individual surveillance* : This is surveillance of infected persons until they are no longer a significant risk to other individuals, (b) *Local population surveillance* : e.g., surveillance of malaria, (c) *National population surveillance :* e.g., surveillance of smallpox after the disease has been eradicated, and (d) *International surveillance :* At the international level, the WHO maintains surveillance of important diseases (e.g., influenza, malaria, polio, etc.) and gives timely warning to all national governments. Surveillance, if properly pursued, can provide the health agencies with an overall intelligence and disease–accounting capability. Surveillance is an essential pre-requisite to the rational design and evaluation of any disease control programme.

HEALTH ADVICE TO TRAVELLERS

Emporiatrics is the term coined to describe the science of the health of travellers *(148)*. Travellers face special health risks. In the age of jet travel, international travellers are subject to various forms of stress that may reduce their resistance to disease, e.g., crowding, long hours of waiting, disruption of eating habit, change in the climate and time zone. These factors may in themselves provoke nausea, indigestion, extreme fatigue and insomnia.

Secondly, in developing countries, they are exposed to diseases which are not covered by International Health Regulations (IHR), e.g., malaria, giardiasis, dengue, influenza, filariasis, STD and AIDS, intestinal parasites, typhoid and paratyphoid fever, viral hepatitis, etc. Many of these may not manifest themselves immediately but occur during a varying period after the traveller returns to his normal way of life. Poor hygiene by food handler, poor water quality and improper disposal of wastes are other important causes of disease transfer *(149)*. International travellers have a personal responsibility to recognize these risks of travel, which can be minimized by immunization and chemoprophylaxis or chemotherapy. Thirdly, travellers are separated from familiar and accessible sources of medical care.

Some of the recommendations pertain to the following : (1) Avoid bathing with polluted water as this may result in ear, eye and skin infections. Excessive heat and humidity or over–exertion in these conditions may lead to exhaustion from loss of water and salt. (2) The measures for prevention of insect bites. (3) *Diarrhoeal Diseases :* "Be careful what you eat" is common advice to travellers, but very few truely understand its implications. Diarrhoea affects an estimated 20–50 per cent of all travellers. Contaminated food drinks are the most common source of these infections. Careful selection and preparation of food and drink offer the best protection. Unfortunately appearance of food is no guide as to its safety. The main personal protection is to consider unpasteurized milk, non–bottled drinks, uncooked food (apart from the fruits and vegetables that can be peeled or shelled), as likely to be contaminated and therefore unsafe. The food should be thoroughly and freshly cooked. Use boiled water or bottled mineral water (now available everywhere). Travellers should be aware of the importance of oral rehydration fluids containing salt and glucose for countering dehydration. (4) *Malaria :* There is a high risk of acquiring malaria in endemic areas. Travellers are advised to protect themselves by chemoprophylaxis. Drug prophylaxis should begin at the latest on the day of arrival in the malarious areas and continued for 4–6 weeks after leaving the malarious areas. (5) *Hepatitis A :* Normal human immunoglobulin in a dose of 0.02–0.05 mg/kg of body weight has been recommended every 4 months. Ideally immunoglobulin should not be given within 3 weeks before, or until 2 weeks after administration of a live vaccine. A highly safe, inactivated HAV vaccine is available in several European countries. (6) *Hepatitis E :* There is no vaccine against hepatitis E and immunoglobulin prepared in Europe and USA does not give much of protection. Avoidance of contaminated food and water is the only effective protective measure. (7) *Hepatitis B :* Hepatitis B vaccines are available and are safe. Three doses of vaccine constitute the complete course. The first two doses are given one month apart and the third dose about 6 months later. (8) *STD and HIV :* Measures for preventing STD are the same whether the individual is travelling abroad or not, i.e., avoidance of sex altogether or limit it to a single faithful, uninfected partner. Use of condom is an important preventive measure. To reduce the risk of acquiring HIV and hepatitis B from syringes and needles, travellers should avoid injectable drugs and if an injection is essential they should make sure that the needle and syringe come from sterile pack. (9) *Yellow fever:* Vaccination certificate for yellow fever is the only certificate required for international travel. Yellow fever vaccine is recommended for travellers to countries designated as yellow fever endemic zone. (10) *Tetanus :* It is a wise precaution for the traveller to have a booster dose of tetanus toxoid if 10 years or more have elapsed since the last injection of a complete course or booster.

Medical kit for travellers should contain a disinfectant and dressing that can be applied easily. Sun cream, mosquito repellent, oral rehydration salts and first-aid articles are basic necessities. Patients with chronic diseases like diabetes, cardiac problems etc. should carry enough medicines to avoid the risk of break in medication *(150)*. It is advisable to carry a card with noting of their blood group, drug sensitivity if any and name of any chronic disease he or she is suffering from.

For the benefit of travellers, the WHO publishes every year a booklet, now entitled "International Travel and Health, Vaccination requirements and Health advice ". It provides guidance on some of the main health risks to which travellers may be exposed in different parts of the world and advice on precautions that may be taken against them.

DISINFECTION

Semmelweis (1818–1865) demonstrated the value of handwashing with antiseptic solutions, when he obtained considerable reduction in the death rate from puerperal fever. Lister (1827–1912) was also successful in reducing the number of wound infections by prophylactic application of an antiseptic (carbolic acid) to wounds. The importance of antiseptics and disinfectants has not diminished in this "golden age of antibiotics". Their uses range from control of communicable diseases to sterilization of sophisticated instruments, and treatment of fungal and bacterial infections of the skin and mucous membrane.

Definitions

Disinfectant : Usually a chemical agent (but sometimes a physical agent) that destroys disease causing pathogens or other harmful microorganisms, but might not kill bacterial spores. It refers to substances applied to inanimate objects.

Disinfection : Thermal or chemical destruction of pathogen and other types of microorganisms. Disinfection is less lethal than sterilization because it destroys most recognized pathogenic microorganisms but not necessarily all microbial forms (e.g., bacterial spores).

Sterilization : Validated process used to render a product free of all forms of viable microorganisms including bacterial spores. Sterilizer is the apparatus used to sterilize medical devices, equipment or supplies by direct exposure to the sterilizing agent.

Antiseptic : Substance that prevents or arrests the growth or action of micro-organisms by inhibiting their activity or by destroying them. The term is used especially for preparations applied topically to living tissue.

Asepsis : Prevention of contact with micro-organism.

Sanitizer : Agent that reduces the number of bacterial contaminants to safe levels as judged by public health requirements. Commonly used with substances applied to inanimate objects.

Sterile : State of being free from all living micro-organisms.

Hospital disinfectant : Disinfectant registered for use in hospitals, clinics, dental offices or any other medical-related facility. Efficacy is demonstrated against *Salmonella choleraesuis, Staphylococcus aureus,* and *Pseudomonas aeruginosa*.

Germicide : Agent that destroys micro-organisms, especially pathogenic organisms.

Detergent : Surface cleaning agent that makes no antimicrobial claims on the label. They comprise a hydrophilic component and a lipohilic component. It acts by lowering surface tension e.g. soap which removes bacteria along with dirt.

Cleaning : Removal, usually with detergent and water or enzyme cleaner and water, of adherent visible soil, blood, protein substances, micro-organisms and other debris from the surfaces, crevices, serrations, joints, and lumens of instruments, devices and equipment by a manual or mechanical process that prepares the items for safe handling and/or further decontamination.

Deodorant : Deodarant is a substance which suppresses or neutralizes bad odours, e.g., lime and bleaching powder.

Properties of an ideal disinfectant *(151)*

An ideal disinfectant fulfils the following criteria :

1. Broad spectrum: should have a wide antimicrobial spectrum.
2. Fast acting: should produce a rapid kill.
3. Not affected by environmental factors: should be active in the presence of organic matter (e.g., blood, sputum, faeces) and compatible with soaps, detergents, and other chemicals encountered in use.
4. Nontoxic: should not be harmful to the user or patient.
5. Surface compatibility: should not corrode instruments and metallic surfaces, and should not cause the deterioration of cloth, rubber, plastics, and other materials.
6. Residual effect on treated surfaces: should leave an antimicrobial film on the treated surface.
7. Easy to use with clear label directions.
8. Odourless: should have a pleasant odour or no odour to facilitate its routine use.
9. Economical: should not be prohibitively high in cost.
10. Solubility: should be soluble in water.
11. Stability: should be stable in concentrate and use-dilution.
12. Cleaner: should have good cleaning properties.
13. Environmentally friendly: should not damage the environment on disposal.

Types of disinfection

(a) **Concurrent disinfection** : It is the application of disinfective measures as soon as possible after the discharge of infectious material from the body of an infected person, or after the soiling of articles with such infectious discharges *(2)*. In other words, the disease agent is destroyed as soon as it is released from the body, and in this way further spread of the agent is stopped. Concurrent disinfection consists of usually disinfection of urine, faeces, vomit, contaminated linen, clothes, hands, dressings, aprons, gloves, etc throughout the course of an illness. (b) **Terminal disinfection** : It is the application of disinfective measures after the patient has been removed by death or to a hospital or has ceased to be a source of infection or after other hospital isolation practices have been discontinued *(10, 106)*. Terminal disinfection is now scarcely practised; terminal cleaning is considered adequate, along with airing and sunning of rooms, furniture and bedding *(10, 106)*. (c) **Precurrent (prophylactic) disinfection** : Disinfection of water by chlorine, pasteurization of milk and handwashing may be cited as examples of precurrent disinfection.

Natural agents

(1) *Sunlight* : Direct and continuous exposure to sunlight is destructive to many disease producing organisms. The ultraviolet rays of sunlight (these do not penetrate through glass) are particularly lethal to bacteria and some viruses. Articles such as linen, bedding, and furniture may be disinfected by exposure to direct sunlight for several hours (2) *Air* : Exposure to open air (airing) acts by drying or evaporation of moisture which is lethal to most bacteria. In general, natural agents such as sunlight and air, because of their vagaries, cannot be totally depended upon for disinfection.

Physical agents

(1) *Burning* : Burning or incineration is an excellent method of disinfection. Inexpensive articles such as contaminated dressings, rags and swabs can be disposed off by burning. Addition of sawdust, paper, kerosene or other combustible material aid in burning. Faeces can be disposed off by burning. Burning should not be done in open air; it is best done in an incinerator. (2) *Hot air* : Hot air is very useful for sterilizing articles such as glassware, syringes, swabs, dressings, french chalk, oils, vaseline and sharp instruments. The drawback of hot air is that it has no penetrating power, and is therefore not suitable for disinfection of bulky articles such as mattresses. Hot air sterilization is usually done in a hot air oven. The temperature of the air in the oven should be maintained at 160–180 deg C for at least one hour to kill spores. Unfortunately, such elevated temperatures destroy plastic, rubber and other delicate substances. (3) *Boiling* : Boiling is an effective method of disinfection. It provides an atmosphere of boiling and steam. Boiling for 5–10 minutes

(rolling boil) will kill bacteria, but not spores or viruses. Boilers provide temperature well above 90 deg C in an atmosphere of steam, which is exposed to open air. To ensure destruction of spores, temperatures above 100 deg C would be required which cannot be achieved in boilers. Boiling is suitable for disinfection of small instruments, tools which are not used for subcutaneous insertion, linen and rubber goods such as gloves. Linen stained with faeces, pus or blood should be first washed in cold water (preferably with a disinfectant such as $2^1/_2$ per cent cresol) and then subjected to boiling, with frequent stirring because linen and clothes are poor conductors of heat. Addition of 1 per cent soap and 0.3 per cent of washing soda enhances the effect of boiling. Boiling for about 30 minutes is adequate to disinfect linen, utensils and bedpans. The drawbacks of boiling are that it is a slow process, unsuitable for thick beddings and woollen materials as they shrink, and it fixes albuminous stains. (4) *Autoclaving :* Sterilizers which operate at high temperatures (in excess of 100 deg C) and pressure are called autoclaves. They generate steam under pressure (saturated steam) which is the most effective sterilizing agent. Autoclaves fall into two categories – gravity displacement autoclaves and the high–speed prevaccum sterilizers. Basically, the autoclave works on the same principle as the domestic pressure cooker. Autoclaving is widely used in hospital and laboratory practice. It destroys all forms of life, including spores. Steam attains a higher temperature under pressure, and has greater powers of penetration than ordinary steam. For example, it attains a temperature of 122 deg C under 15 lbs/sq. inch (1 kg/sq. cm.) pressure. It acts by giving off its latent heat. Absolute sterility can be obtained only by raising the temperature of articles to over 135 deg C. Autoclaving is the most effective method for sterilization of linen, dressings, gloves, syringes, certain instruments and culture media. It is not suitable for sterilization of plastics and sharp instruments. (5) *Radiation :* Ionizing radiation is being increasingly used for sterilization of bandages, dressings, catgut and surgical instruments. The objects to be sterilized are placed in plastic bags before radiation, and they will remain sterile until opened. Ionizing radiation has great penetrating powers with little or no heating effect. This method is most effective, but very costly. Commercial methods of sterilization are normally carried out by gamma radiation (atomic). This technique requires special packing and equipment. It is now one of the most viable, safe and economic methods used today.

Chemical agents

Articles which cannot be sterilized by boiling or autoclaving may be immersed in chemical disinfectants. Chemical agents may also be used for the disinfection of faeces, urine and other contaminated material. There are a wide range of chemical disinfectants, each with its advantages and disadvantages. These are discussed below :

1. Phenol and related compounds

(1) *Phenol :* Pure phenol or carbolic acid is the best known member of this group. On exposure to air, the colourless crystals of phenol become pinkish, and on longer exposure, the colour deepens to dark red. Pure phenol is not an effective disinfectant. It is used as a standard to compare the germicidal activity of disinfectants. (2) *Crude phenol :* The phenol that is commonly used for disinfection is "crude phenol", which is a mixture of phenol and cresol. It is a dark oily liquid. It is effective against gram-positive and gram-negative bacteria, but only slowly effective against spores and acid–fast bacteria. It is also effective against certain viruses. Phenol disinfectants are not readily inactivated by organic matter. Its effect is greatly weakened by dilution. Therefore, it should not be used in less than 10 per cent strength for disinfection of faeces. In 5 per cent strength, it may be used for mopping floors and cleaning drains. Aqueous solutions of 0.2 to 1 per cent are bacteriostatic. (3) *Cresol :* Cresol is an excellent coal-tar disinfectant. It is 3 to 10 times as powerful as phenol, yet no more toxic. Cresol is best used in 5 to 10 per cent strength for disinfection of faeces and urine. A 5 per cent solution may be prepared by adding 8 ounces of cresol to one gallon of water (or 50 ml to one litre of water). Cresol is an all-purpose general disinfectant. (4) *Cresol emulsions :* Cresol emulsified with soap is known as "saponified cresol". Lysol, izal and cyllin are cresol emulsions. Lysol contains 50–60 per cent cresol. They are very powerful disinfectants. A 2 per cent solution of lysol may be used for disinfection of faeces. (5) *Chlorhexidine (hibitane) :* This is one of the most useful skin antiseptics. Highly active against vegetative gram-positive organisms, and moderately active against gram-positive microbes. It is soluble in water and alcohol. It is inactivated by soaps and detergents. 0.5 per cent alcoholic or aqueous solutions can be used as effective handlotions. Creams and lotions containing 1 per cent chlorhexidine are recommended for burns and hand disinfection. (6) *Hexachlorphane :* This antiseptic is highly active against gram-positive organisms, but less active against gram-negative organisms. It is slow in action, but shows a cumulative effect on the skin and is compatible with soaps. Thus it may be incorporated in soap preparations without loss of activity. (7) *Dettol :* Dettol (chloroxylenol) is a relatively non-toxic antiseptic and can be used safely in high concentrations. It is more easily inactivated by organic matter than many other phenolic disinfectants. It is active against streptococci, but worthless against some gram-negative bacteria. Dettol (5%) is suitable for disinfection of instruments and plastic equipment; a contact of at least 15 minutes will be required for disinfection.

2. Quaternary ammonia compounds

(1) *Cetrimide :* It is manufactured under the trade name "cetavlon". It is actively bactericidal against vegetative gram-positive organisms, but much less so against gram-negative organisms. Cetavlon is soluble in water; it has a soapy feel. It may be used in 1–2 per cent strength. (2) *Savlon :* Savlon is a combination of cetavlon and hibitane. Plastic appliances may be disinfected by keeping them in normal strength savlon for 20 minutes. Savlon 1 in 6 in spirit is more effective than savlon 1 in 20 aqueous solution. Clinical thermometers may be best disinfected in savlon 1 in 6 in spirit in just under 3 minutes.

3. Halogens and their compounds

a. *Chlorine and chlorine compounds :* They are potent bactericidal, fungicidal, sporicidal, tuberculocidal and virucidal. Since long time chlorine has been used as disinfectant in water treatment.

(1) *Bleaching powder :* Bleaching powder or chlorinated lime ($CaOCl_2$) is a white amorphous powder with a pungent smell of chlorine. A good sample of bleaching powder contains about 33 per cent of "available chlorine". It kills most of the organisms when used in the strength of 1 to 3 per cent. Bleaching powder is widely used in public health

practice in India for disinfection of water, faeces and urine; and as a deodorant. The chief drawback of bleaching powder is that it is an unstable compound and loses its chlorine content on storage. Its action is rapid but brief. A 5 per cent solution (3 to 4 rounded tablespoons to 1 litre of water) is suitable for disinfection of faeces and urine allowing a period of one hour for disinfection. (2) *Hypochlorites* : Hypochlorites are the most widely used chlorine disinfectant, available as liquid (e.g. sodium hypochlorite) or solid (e.g. calcium hypochlorite). The most prevalent chlorine products are aqueous solutions of 5.25–6.15 per cent of sodium hypochlorite, usually called household bleach. They have a broad spectrum of antimicrobial activity, do not leave toxic residues, are unaffected by water hardness, are inexpensive and fast acting, remove dried or fixed organisms and biofilms from surfaces *(151)*. (3) *Chlorine tablets* : Under various trade names (viz., halazone tablets) they are available in the market. They are quite good in disinfecting small quantities of water. (4) Alternative compounds that release chlorine and are used in the health-care setting include demand-release chlorine dioxide, sodium dichloroisocyanurate, and chloramine–T. The advantage of these compounds over hypochlorites is that they retain chlorine longer and so exert a more prolonged bactericidal effect. (5) The microbicidal activity of a new disinfectant, "superoxidized water" has been examined. The concept of electrolyzing saline to create a disinfectant or antiseptic is appealing because the basic materials of saline and electricity are inexpensive and the end product (i.e., water) does not damage the environment. The main products of this water are hypochlorous acid (e.g., at a concentration of about 144 mg/L) and chlorine.

b. *Iodine* : (1) Iodine solutions or tinctures have been used by health professionals primarily as antiseptic on skin (e.g.to prepare incision site prior to surgery) or tissue since long time. Iodine is bactericidal, fungicidal, virucidal and lethal to spore-bearing organisms. Iodine is cheap, readily available and quick in action. (2) *Iodophores* : An iodophore is a combination of iodine and a solubilizing agent or carrier; the resulting complex provides a sustained-release reservoir of iodine and releases small amounts of free iodine in aqueous solution. The best known and most widely used iodophore is povidone-iodine (Betadine). They are non-irritant and do not stain the skin. Besides their use as an antiseptic, iodophores have been used for disinfecting blood culture bottles and medical equipment.

4. Alcohols

Ethyl and isopropyl alcohols are commonly used as antiseptics and disinfectants. Ethyl alcohol in the form of industrial methylated spirit is the alcohol most commonly used for skin disinfection and hand washing. Pure alcohol has no powers of disinfection but when diluted with water to 60–90 per cent vol/vol, it is potent bactericidal, fungicidal, virucidal and tuberculocidal, but does not destroy bacterial spores *(151)*. Its activity decreases rapidly below 50 per cent concentration. 70 per cent alcohol is lethal in a period of seconds to all types of non-sporing bacteria, but when applied to the skin and other surfaces, its activity disappears as the alcohol dries off. Because of expense and flammability, its use is limited to small article disinfection. Available evidence suggests that the most effective skin antiseptics are alcoholic solutions of chlorhexidine and iodine. Alcohols are inflammable and consequently must be stored in cool areas. They also evaporate rapidly, making extended exposure time difficult to achieve unless the items are immersed *(151)*.

5. Formaldehyde

More commonly known in solution as formalin, formaldehyde is a highly toxic and irritant gas which precipitates and destroys protein. It is effective against vegetative bacteria, fungi and many viruses but only slowly effective against bacterial spores (e.g., tetanus spores) and acid-fast bacteria. It does not injure fabrics and metals. It may be used as a 2–3 per cent solution (20–30 ml of 40 per cent formalin in one litre of water) for spraying rooms, walls and furniture.

Formaldehyde gas is most commonly used for disinfection of rooms. The gas is most effective at a high temperature and a relative humidity of 80–90 per cent. The gas may also be used for disinfection of blankets, beds, books and other valuable articles which cannot be boiled.

6. Oxidizing agents

a. *Potassium permanganate* : It is a purplish black crystelline powder that colours everything it touches through strong oxidizing action, which limits its use. It is used to disinfect aquariums and is also widely used in community swimming pools to disinfect ones feet before entering the pool. It is also used to disinfect fruits and vegetables.

b. *Hydrogen peroxide* : Hydrogen peroxide is bactericidal, virucidal, sporicidal and fungicidal. It is used in hospital setting to disinfect surfaces. It is used as solution alone or in combination with other chemicals as a high level disinfectant. A 0.5 per cent accelerated hydrogen peroxide demonstrated bactericidal and virucidal activity in 1 minute and mycobactericidal and fungicidal activity in 5 minutes. A 3 per cent solution is also used as an antiseptic and for cleaning wounds and discharging ulcers.

c. *Paracetic acid* : It is a disinfectant produced by reacting hydrogen peroxide with acetic acid. It is broadly effective against microorganisms and is not deactivated by catalase and peroxidase, the enzymes that break down hydrogen peroxide. It inactivates gram-positive and gram-negative bacteria, fungi and yeast in less than 5 minutes at less than 100 ppm. In the presence of organic matter, 200–250 ppm is required. For viruses, the dose range is wide (12–2250 ppm). It breaks down to environment friendly residue (acetic acid and hydrogen peroxide) and therefore can be used in non–rinse applications.

7. Metals as microbicides

Anti-infective activity of some heavy metals has been known since antiquity. Heavy metals such as silver have been used for prophylaxis of conjunctivitis of the new-born, topical therapy for burn wounds, and bonding to indwelling catheters. Inactivation of bacteria on stainless steel surfaces by zeolite ceramic coating containing silver and zinc ions has also been demonstrated. Metals such as silver, iron, and copper could be used for environmental control, disinfection of water or reusable medical devices, or incorporated into medical devices.

8. Lime

Lime is the cheapest of all disinfectants. It is used in the form of fresh quick lime or 10–20 per cent aqueous suspension known as "milk of lime". Faeces and urine can be disinfected by mixing 10–20 per cent aqueous suspension of lime and allowing the disinfectant to act for 2 hours. As lime wash, it is used for treating walls. As a deodorant, lime is sprinkled in cattle sheds and stables and in public places where urinals and latrines are located.

9. Ethylene oxide

Heat-sensitive articles may be sterilized at 55–60 deg.C by ethylene oxide which kills bacteria, spores (e.g., tetanus spores) and also viruses. Ethylene oxide is explosive, therefore, it is mixed with carbon dioxide (12 per cent). Water vapour is also often added to the mixture (relative humidity 33 per cent) since it increases the efficiency of the gas. Ethylene oxide has been effectively used to sterilize fabrics, plastic equipment, cardiac catheters, books, etc; but the process is difficult to control. Therefore ethylene oxide disinfection is discouraged when alternatives are available.

10. Miscellaneous inactivating agents

a. *Pasteurization :* Pasteurization is not a sterilization process; its purpose is to destroy all pathogenic microorganisms. However, pasteurization does not destroy bacterial spores. The time-temperature relation for hot-water pasteurization is generally 70°C (158°F) for 30 minutes.

b. *Microwave :* Microwaves are used in medicine for disinfection of soft contact lenses, dental instruments, dentures, milk, and urinary catheters for intermittent self-catheterization. However, microwaves must only be used with products that are compatible (e.g., do not melt). Microwaves are radio-frequency waves, which are usually used at a frequency of 2450 MHz. The microwaves produce friction of water molecules in an alternating electrical field. The intermolecular friction derived from the vibrations generates heat. The microwaves produced by a "home-type" microwave oven (2.45 GHz) completely inactivate bacterial cultures, mycobacteria viruses, and *G. stearothermophilus* spores within 60 seconds to 5 minutes depending on the challenge organism.

c. *Flushing and Washer Disinfectors :* Flushing and washer-disinfectors are automated and closed equipment that clean and disinfect objects from bedpans, urinals and washbowls to surgical instruments and anesthesia tubes. They have a short cycle of a few minutes. They clean by flushing with warm water, possibly with a detergent, and then disinfect by flushing the items with hot water or with steam. Because this machine empties, cleans, and disinfects, manual cleaning is eliminated, fewer disposable items are needed, and fewer chemical gemicides are used.

d. *Ultraviolet radiation :* The wavelength of UV radiation ranges from 328 nm to 210 nm. Its maximum bactericidal effect occurs at 240–280 nm. Mercury vapour lamps emit more than 90 per cent of their radiation at 253.7 nm, which is near the maximum microbicidal activity *(155)*. UV radiation has been employed in the disinfection of drinking water, air, titanium implants and contact lenses. Bacteria and viruses are more easily killed by UV light than the bacterial spores.

e. Ozone : Ozone has been used for years as a drinking water disinfectant. Ozone is produced when O_2 is energized and split into two monatomic (O_1) molecules. The monatomic oxygen molecules then collide with O_2 molecules to form ozone, which is O_3. Ozone is a powerful oxidant that destroys microorganisms but it is highly unstable (i.e. half-life of 22 minutes of room temperature).

Factors affecting the efficacy of sterilization *(151)*

Following factors should be kept in mind while sterilizing the medical equipment :

Factors	**Effect**
1. Cleaning	Failure to adequately clean instruments results in higher bioburden, protein load, and salt concentration. These will decrease sterilization efficacy.
2. Pathogen type	Spore-forming organisms are most resistant to sterilization. However, the contaminating microflora on surgical instruments consists mainly of vegetative bacteria.
3. Biofilm accumulation	Biofilm accumulation reduces efficacy of sterilization by impairing exposure of the sterilant to the microbial cell.
4. Luman length and luman diameter	Increasing lumen length and decreasing lumen diameter impairs sterilant penetration. May require forced flow through lumen to achieve sterilization.
5. Restricted flow	Sterilant must come into contact with microorganisms. Device designs that prevent or inhibit this contact (e.g. sharp bends, blind lumens) will decrease sterilization efficacy.
6. Device design and construction	Materials used in construction may affect compatibility with different sterilization processes.

Recommended disinfection procedures

1. Faeces and urine

Faeces and urine should be collected in impervious vessels and disinfected by adding an equal volume of one of the disinfectants listed in Table 46 and allowed to stand for 1–2 hours. Faeces should be broken up with a stick to allow proper disinfection. If the disinfectants listed in Table 47 are not available, an equal amount of quicklime or freshly prepared milk of lime (1 of lime to 4 of water) may be added, mixed and left for 2 hours. If none is available, a bucket of boiling water may be added to the faeces which is then covered and allowed to stand until cool. After disinfection, the excretal matter may be emptied into water closet or buried in ground. Bedpans and urinals should ideally be steam disinfected. Alternatively, they may be disinfected with $2^1/_2$ per cent cresol for an hour after cleaning.

TABLE 46

Agents suitable for disinfection of faeces and urine

Disinfectant	Amount per litre	Per cent
1. Bleaching powder	50 g	5
2. Crude phenol	100 ml	10
3. Cresol	50 ml	5
4. Formalin	100 ml	10

2. Sputum

This is best received in gauze or paper handkerchiefs and destroyed by burning. If the amount is considerable (as in TB hospitals), it may be disinfected by boiling or autoclaving for 20 minutes at 20 lbs pressure. Alternatively, the patient may be asked to spit in a sputum cup half filled with 5 per cent cresol. When the cup is full, it is allowed to stand for an hour and the contents may be emptied and disposed off. 5 per cent phenol or 4.8 per cent chloroxylenol is also used for safe disposal of sputum.

3. Room

Usually thorough cleaning, airing and exposure to direct sunlight, when possible, for several hours will be sufficient. If necessary, floors and hard surfaces in the room should be prohibited for 48 hours *(152)*. For chemical disinfection, floors and hard surfaces should be sprayed or mopped with one of the following disinfectants : chlorine preparations such as chlorinated lime in concentrations that leave 25 ppm or more of free chlorine; formaldehyde solution at a concentration of 1 per cent or more; phenolic disinfectants such as $2^1/_2$ per cent cresol. The solution should remain in contact with the surface for at least 4 hours before final washing *(152)*.

On rare occasions, when fumigation is required, the gas most commonly used is formaldehyde. It may be generated by boiling commercial formalin in 2 volumes of water (500 ml of formalin plus 1 litre of water per 30 cu. metres of space) in a stainless steel vessel, over an electric hot plate or by adding potassium permanganate to commercial formalin in large jars (170–200 gram to 500 ml of formalin plus 1 litre of water per 30 cu. metres) *(152)*. There is vigorous boiling and liberation of formaldehyde gas. The room is kept closed for 6–12 hours to allow disinfection. Formaldehyde disinfection is most effective at a high temperature and a relative humidity of 80–90 per cent.

Special Disinfection Procedures (In COVID-19 context)

Sanitization tunnel

It is a tunnel or gateway for the sanitization and decontamination of items and people when combined with appropriately atomized biocides and/or virucide spray. These sanitary and decontamination tunnels and gates represent a safe protection and entry for everyone, in particular for those who work in close contact with groups and are therefore at higher risk. It can be installed at the entrance of public offices, pharmacies, supermarkets, airports, hospitals, ports, stations and for companies who need to sanitize the workforce, goods, vehicles and materials.

The tunnel creates an obligatory passage and is equipped with internal arc-shaped atomizing nozzles that saturate the environment. The nebulization system is connected to control system capable of automatically mixing and sanitizing products at percentage indicated by the manufacturer. The liquid is sprayed in the form of mist for 6–8 seconds on the person walking through the tunnel. Access to the tunnel is regulated by a traffic light with motion detection. By placing a barrier floor inside the sanitary gate, it is possible to sanitize the surface in contact with the ground.

The chemical used is : (a) hydrogen peroxide and isopropyl alcohol with distilled water; (b) sodium hypochlorite for material sanitization; (c) sodium hypochlorite for humans under PPE protection; and (d) concentrated chemical free and alcohol free ayurvedic solution with enriched 100 per cent silver nano particles.

Presently, WHO advises against the use of tunnel for human use, as it can cause skin irritation and respiratory tract allergy; and it does not give protection from the infective agent in the respiratory tract.

Guidelines on disinfection of common public places including offices *(156)*

It provides interim guidance about the environmental cleaning/decontamiation of common public places including offices in areas reporting COVID-19.

1. Indoor areas including office spaces

Office spaces, including conference rooms should be cleaned every evening after office hours or early in the morning before the rooms are occupied. If contact surface is visibly dirty, it should be cleaned with soap and water prior to disinfection. Prior to cleaning, the worker should wear disposable rubber boots, gloves (heavy duty), and a triple layer mask.

- Start cleaning from cleaner areas and proceed towards dirtier areas.
- All indoor areas such as entrance lobbies, corridors and staircases, escalators, elevators, security guard booths, office rooms, meeting rooms, cafeteria should be mopped with a disinfectent with 1% sodium hypochlorite or phenolic disinfectants.
- High contact surfaces such as elevator buttons, handrails/handles and call buttons, escalator handrails, public counters, intercom systems, equipment like telephone, printers/scanners, and other office machines should be cleaned twice daily by mopping with a linen/ absorbable cloth soaked in 1% sodium hypochloride. Frequently touched areas like table tops, chair handles, pens, diary files, keyboards, mouse, mouse pad, tea/ coffee dispensing machines etc. should specially be cleaned.
- For metallic surfaces like door handles, security locks, keys etc., 70% alcohol can be used to wipe down surfaces where the use of bleach is not suitable.
- Hand sanitizing stations should be installed in office premises (specially at the entry) and near high contact surfaces.
- In a meeting/conference/office room, if someone is coughing, without following respiratory etiquettes or mask, the areas around his/her seat should be vacated and cleaned with 1% sodium hypochlorite.
- Carefully clean the equipment used in cleaning at the end of the cleaning process.
- Remove PPE, discard in a yellow disposable bag and wash hands with soap and water.

In addition, all employees should consider cleaning the work area in front of them with a disinfecting wipe prior to use and sit one seat further away from others, if possible.

2. Outdoor areas

Outdoor areas have less risk then indoor areas due to air currents and exposure to sunlight. These include bus stops, railway platforms, park, roads, etc. Cleaning and disinfection efforts should be targeted to frequently touched/ contaminated surfaces as already detailed above.

3. Public toilets

Sanitary workers must use separate set of cleaning equipment for toilets (mops, nylon scrubber) and seperate set for sink and commode). They should always wear disposable protective gloves while cleaning a toilet.

Areas	Agents / Toilet cleaner	Procedure
Toilet pot/ commode	Sodium hypochlorite 1%/detergent Soap powder/long handle angular brush	• Inside of toilet pot/commode: Scrub with the recommended agents and the long handle angular brush. • Outside: clean with recommended agents; use a scrubber.
Lid/ commode	Nylon scrubber and soap powder/detergent 1% Sodium Hypochlorite	• Wet and scrub with soap powder and the nylon scrubber inside and outside. • Wipe with 1% Sodium Hypochlorite.
Toilet floor	Soap powder / detergent and scrubbing brush/ nylon broom 1% Sodium Hypochlorite	• Scrub floor with soap powder and the scrubbing brush • Wash with water • Use sodium hypochlorite 1% dilution.
Sink	Soap powder / detergent and nylon scrubber 1% Sodium Hypochlorite	• Scrub with the nylon scrubber. • Wipe with 1% sodium hypochlorite.
Showers area / Taps and fittings	Warm water Detergent powder Nylon Scrubber 1% Sodium Hypochlorite/ 70% alcohol	• Thoroughly scrub the floors/ tiles with warm water and detergent. • Wipe over taps and fittings with a damp cloth and detergent. • Care should be taken to clean the underside of taps and fittings. • Wipe with 1% sodium hypochlorite/ 70% alcohol.
Soap dispensers	Detergent and water	• Should be cleaned daily with detergent and water and dried.

- 70% Alcohol can be used to wipe down surfaces where the use of bleach is not suitable, e.g. metal. Chloroxylenol (4.5–5.5%)/ Benzalkonium Chloride or any other disinfectants found to be effective against coronavirus may be used as per manufacturer's instructions.
- Always use freshly prepared 1% sodium hypochlorite.

- Do not use disinfectants spray on potentially highly contaminated areas (such as toilet bowl or surrounding surfaces) as it may create splashes which can further spread the virus.
- To prevent cross contamination, discard cleaning material made of cloth (mop and wiping cloth) in appropriate bags after cleaning and disinfecting. Wear new pair of glove and fasten the bag.
- Disinfect all cleaning equipment after use and before using in other areas.
- Disinfect buckets by soaking in bleach solution or rinse in hot water.

Guidelines for preparation of 1% sodium hypochlorite solution

Product	Available chlorine	1per cent solution
Sodium hypochlorite – liquid bleach	3.5%	1 part bleach to 2.5 parts water
Sodium hypochlorite – liquid	5%	1 part bleach to 4 parts water
NaDCC (sodium dichloro-isocyanurate) powder	60%	17 grams to 1 litre water
NaDCC (1.5 g/ tablet) – tablets	60%	11 tablets to 1 litre water
Chloramine – powder	25%	80 g to 1 litre water
Bleaching powder	70%	7 g to 1 litre water
Any other	As per manufacturer's Instructions	

4. Personal Protective Equipment (PPE)

Wear appropriate PPE which would include the following while carrying out cleaning and disinfection work.

- Wear disposable rubber boots, gloves (heavy duty), and a triple layer mask
- Gloves should be removed and discarded/damaged, and a new pair worn.
- All disposable PPE should be removed and discarded after cleaning activities are completed.
- Hands should be washed with soap and water immediately after each piece of PPE is removed, following completion of cleaning.

Masks are effective if worn according to instructions and properly fitted. Masks should be discarded and changed if they become physically damaged or soaked.

Hand washing technique

Fig. 28 shows steps of hand washing technique with soap and water *(156)*.

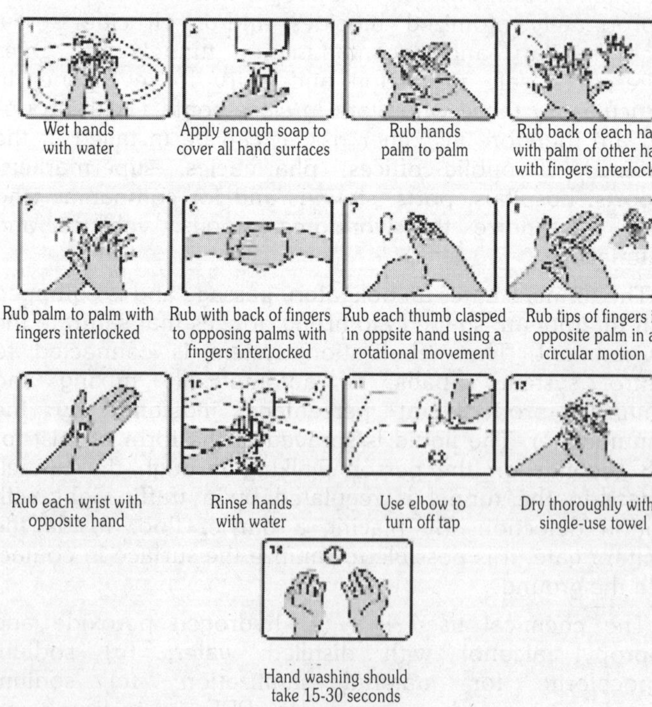

FIG. 28
Hand washing technique with soap and water

Guidelines for use of mask *(156)*

The correct procedure of wearing triple layer surgical mask is as follows :

1. Perform hand hygiene
2. Unfold the pleats; make sure that they are facing down.
3. Place over nose, mouth and chin.
4. Fit flexible nose piece over nose bridge.
5. Secure with tie strings (upper string to be tied on top of head above the ears – lower string at the back of the neck.)
6. Ensure there are no gaps on either side of the mask, adjust to fit.
7. Do not let the mask hanging from the neck.
8. Change the mask after six hours or as soon as they become wet.
9. Disposable masks are never to be reused and should be disposed off.
10. While removing the mask great care must be taken not to touch the potentialy infected outer surface of the mask.
11. To remove mask first untie the string below and then the string above and handle the mask using the upper strings.
12. Disposal of used masks: Used mask should be considered as potentially infected medical waste. Discard the mask in a closed bin immediately after use.

INVESTIGATION OF AN EPIDEMIC

The occurrence of an epidemic always signals some significant shift in the existing balance between the agent, host and environment. It calls for a prompt and thorough investigation of the cases to uncover the factor(s) responsible and to guide in advocating control measures to prevent further spread. Emergencies caused by epidemics remain one of the most important challenges to national health administrations. Epidemiology has an important role to play in the investigation of epidemics. The objectives of an epidemic investigation are *(3, 22, 153)*.

a. to define the magnitude of the epidemic outbreak or involvement in terms of time, place and person.
b. to determine the particular conditions and factors responsible for the occurrence of the epidemic.
c. to identify the cause, source(s) of infection, and modes of transmission to determine measures necessary to control the epidemic; and
d. to make recommendations to prevent recurrence.

An epidemic investigation calls for inference as well as description. Frequently, epidemic investigations are called for after the peak of the epidemic has occurred; in such cases, the investigation is mainly retrospective. No step by step approach applicable in all situations can be described like a "cook–book" *(153)*. However, in investigating an epidemic, it is desired to have an orderly procedure or practical guidelines as outlined below which are applicable for almost any epidemic study. Some of the steps can be done concurrently.

1. Verification of diagnosis

Verification of diagnosis is the first step in an epidemic investigation, as it may happen sometimes that the report may be spurious, and arise from misinterpretation of signs and symptoms by the lay public. It is therefore necessary to have the verification of diagnosis on the spot, as quickly as possible. It is not necessary to examine all the cases to arrive at a diagnosis. A clinical examination of a sample of cases may well suffice. Laboratory investigations wherever applicable, are most useful to confirm the diagnosis but the epidemiological investigations should not be delayed until the laboratory results are available.

2. Confirmation of the existence of an epidemic

The next step is to confirm if epidemic exists. This is done by comparing the disease frequencies during the same period of previous years. An epidemic is said to exist when the number of cases (observed frequency) is in excess of the expected frequency for that population, based on past experience. An arbitrary limit of two standard errors from the endemic occurrence is used to define the epidemic threshold for common diseases such as influenza *(3)*. Often the existence of an epidemic is obvious needing no such comparison, as in the case of common-source epidemics of cholera, food poisoning and hepatitis A. These epidemics are easily recognized. In contrast the existence of modern epidemics (e.g., cancer, cardiovascular diseases) is not easily recognized unless comparison is made with previous experience.

3. Defining the population at-risk

(a) Obtaining a map of the area : Before beginning the investigation, it is necessary to have a detailed and current map of the area. If this is not available, it may be necessary to prepare such a map. It should contain information concerning natural landmarks, roads and the location of all dwelling units along each road or in isolated areas. The area may be divided into segments, using natural landmarks as boundaries. This may again be divided into smaller sections. Within each section, the dwelling units (houses) may be designated by numbers.

(b) Counting the population : The denominator may be related to the entire population or sub-groups of a population. It may also be related to total events (see page 45 for more details). For example, if the denominator is the entire population a complete census of the population by age and sex should be carried out in the defined area by house–to–house visits. For this purpose lay health workers in sufficient numbers may be employed. Using this technique it is possible to establish the size of the population. The population census will help in computing the much–needed attack rates in various groups and subgroups of the population later on. Without an appropriate denominator of "population at risk" attack rates cannot be calculated.

4. Rapid search for all cases and their characteristics

(a) *Medical survey* : Concurrently, a medical survey should be carried out in the defined area to identify all cases including those who have not sought medical care, and those possibly exposed to risk. Ideally, the complete survey (screening each member of the population for the presence of the disease in question) will pick up all affected individuals with symptoms or signs of the disorder. Lay health workers may be trained to administer the "epidemiological case sheet" or questionnaire to collect relevant data.

(b) Epidemiological case sheet : The epidemiologist should be armed with an "epidemiological case sheet" for collecting data from cases and from persons apparently exposed but unaffected. The epidemiological case sheet or "case interview form" should be carefully designed (based on the findings of a rapid preliminary inquiry) to collect relevant information. This includes : name, age, sex, occupation, social class, travel, history of previous exposure, time of onset of disease, signs and symptoms of illness, personal contacts at home, work, school and other places; special events such as parties attended, foods eaten and exposure to common vehicles such as water, food and milk; visits out of the community, history of receiving injections or blood products, attendance at large gathering, etc. The information collected should be relevant to the disease under study. For example, if the disease is food-borne, detailed food histories are necessary. A case review form will ensure completeness and consistency of data collection.

If the outbreak is large, it may not be possible to interview all the cases (e.g., influenza). In such cases, a random sample should be examined and data collected.

(c) Searching for more cases : The patient may be asked if he knew of other cases in the home, family, neighbourhood, school, work place having an onset within the incubation of the index case. Cases admitted to the local hospitals should also be taken into consideration. This may reveal not only additional cases but also person-to-person spread. The search for new cases (secondary cases) should be carried out everyday, till the area is declared free of epidemic. This period is usually taken as twice the incubation period of the disease since the occurrence of last case.

5. Data analysis

The data collected should be analyzed on ongoing basis, using the classical epidemiological parameters – time, place and person. If the disease agent is known, the characteristics of time, place and person may be rearranged into Agent–Host–Environment model *(3)*.

a. Time : Prepare a chronological distribution of dates of onset and construct an "epidemic curve". Look for time clustering of cases. An epidemic curve may suggest : (a) a time relationship with exposure to a suspected source (Fig. 4), (b) whether it is a common-source or propagated epidemic, and (c) whether it is a seasonal or cyclic pattern suggestive of a particular infection.

b. Place : Prepare a "spot map" (geographic distribution) of cases, and if possible, their relation to possible sources of infection, e.g., water supply, air pollution, foods eaten, occupation, etc. Clustering of cases may indicate a common source of infection. Analysis of geographic distribution may provide evidence of the source of disease and its mode of spread. This was demonstrated by John Snow in the cholera outbreak in the Golden Square district, London (Figure 6).

c. Person : Analyze the data by age, sex, occupation and other possible risk factors. Determine the attack rates/case fatality rates, for those exposed and those not exposed and according to host factors. For example, in most food-borne outbreaks, food-specific attack rates must be calculated for each food eaten to determine the source of infection.

The purpose of data analysis is to identify common event or experience, and to delineate the group involved in the common experience.

6. Formulation of hypothesis

On the basis of time, place and person distribution or the Agent–Host–Environment model, formulate hypothesis to explain the epidemic in terms of (a) possible source (b) causative agent (c) possible modes of spread, and (d) the environmental factors which enabled it to occur. These hypothesis should be placed in order of relative likelihood. Formulation of a tentative hypothesis should guide further investigation.

7. Testing of hypothesis

All reasonable hypothesis need to be considered and weighed by comparing the attack rates in various groups for those exposed and those not exposed to each suspected factor. This will enable the epidemiologist to ascertain which hypothesis is consistent with all the known facts. When divergent theories are presented, it is not easy to distinguish immediately between those which are sound and those which are merely plausible. Therefore it is instructive to turn back to arguments which have been tested by the subsequent course of events *(154)*.

8. Evaluation of ecological factors

An investigation of the circumstances involved should be carried out to undertake appropriate measures to prevent further transmission of the disease. Ecological factors which have made the epidemic possible should be investigated such as sanitary status of eating establishments, water and milk supply; breakdown in the water supply system; movements of the human population, atmospheric changes such as temperature, humidity and air pollution, population dynamics of insects and animal reservoirs. The outbreak can be studied in a case control fashion. One of the primary concerns of the epidemiologist is to relate the disease to environmental factors to know the source(s) of infection, reservoirs and modes of transmission.

9. Further investigation of population at risk

A study of the population at risk or a sample of it may be needed to obtain additional information. This may involve medical examination, screening tests, examination of suspected food, faeces or blood samples, biochemical studies, assessment of immunity status, etc. The approach may be retrospective or prospective. For example, serological study may reveal clinically inapparent cases and throw light on the pathogenesis of the condition. Healthy individuals (those who are not ill) from the same universe may be studied in a case control fashion. This will permit classification of all members as to :

a. exposure to specific potential vehicles.

b. whether ill or not.

10. Writing the report

The report should be complete and convincing. Information to be included in the final report on an epidemic is given in Table 47 *(155)*.

TABLE 47

Information to be included in the final report on an epidemic

Section	Contents
1. Background	Geographical location Climatic conditions Demographic status (population pyramid) Socio-economic situation Organization of health services Surveillance and early warning systems Normal disease prevalence.
2. Historical data	Previous occurrence of epidemics – of the same disease, – locally or elsewhere Occurrence of related diseases, if any – in the same area – in other areas Discovery of the first cases of the present outbreak.
3. Methodology of investigations	Case definition Questionnaire used in epidemiological investigation Survey teams Household survey Retrospective survey Prospective surveillance Collection of laboratory specimens Laboratory techniques.
4. Analysis of data	Clinical data : – frequency of signs and symptoms – course of disease – differential diagnosis – death or sequelae rates Epidemiological data : – mode of occurrence – in time – by place – by population groups Modes of transmission : – source(s) of infection – route(s) of excretion and portal(s) of entry – factors influencing transmission Laboratory data : – isolation of agent(s) – serological confirmation – significance of results Interpretation of data : – comprehensive picture of the outbreak – hypotheses as to cause(s) – formulation and testing of hypotheses by statistical analysis.
5. Control measures	Definition of strategies and methodology of implementation – constraints – results Evaluation : – significance of results – cost/effectiveness Preventive measures.

It may be necessary to implement temporary control measures at the commencement of an epidemic on the basis of known facts of the disease. These measures may be modified or replaced in the light of new knowledge acquired by the epidemic investigation. As Frost *(154)* observed, an epidemiological investigation is more than the collection of established facts. It includes their orderly arrangement into chains of inference, which extend more or less beyond the bounds of direct observation.

References

1. Acheson, R.M. (1978). *Brit. Med. J.*, 2 : 1737.
2. Last, John M.ed. (1983). *A Dictionary of Epidemiology*, A Handbook sponsored by the IEA, Oxford Univ. Press.
3. Roht, L.H. et al (1982). *Principles of Epidemiology*, A self–teaching guide, London, Academic Press.
4. IEA (2014), *A Dictionary of Epidemiology*, 6th ed., Edited by Miquel Porta, Oxford University Press.
5. Lilienfeld, A.M. and Lilienfeld, D.E. (1980) *Foundations of Epidemiology*, 2nd ed., Oxford University Press.
6. Lowe, C.R. and J. Kostrzewski (1973). *Epidemiology*, A guide to teaching methods, Churchill Livingstone.
7. Alderson, M. (1983). *An Introduction to Epidemiology*, 2nd ed., London, Macmillan.
8. Lilienfeld, A.M. (1973). *Am. J. Epi.*, 97 : 135.
9. Langmuir, A.D. (1975). *Int. J. Epi.*, 4 (4) 253.
10. Roberts, C.J. (1977) *Epidemiology for Clinicians*, London, Pitam Medical.
11. Morris, J.N. (1975). *Uses of Epidemiology*, 3rd ed., London, Churchill Livingstone.
12. WHO (1982). *The Place of Epidemiology in Local Health Work*, Offset Pub. No. 70, Geneva, WHO.
13. Macmahon, B. and T.F. Pugh (1970). *Epidemiology : Principles and Methods*, Boston, Little, Brown.
14. Fox, J.P. et al (1970). *Epidemiology : Man and Disease*, New York, Macmillan.
15. WHO (1981). *Health for All*, Sr. No. 4.
16. Hall, David J. (1984). *The Islamic World Med.J.*, April 84 p. 22.
17. Rose, G and D.J.P. Barker (1979). *Epidemiology for the Uninitiated*, British Medical Association, London.
18. WHO (1959). *Techn. Rep. Ser.*, No.164.
19. WHO (1968). *Techn. Rep. Ser.*, No. 389.
20. Hogarth, J. (1978). *Glossary of Health Care Terminology*, Geneva, WHO.
21. Lowe, C.R. and S.K. Lwanga (1978). *Health Statistics*, A manual for teachers of medical students, IEA/WHO handbook, Oxford Medical Publications.
22. Barker, D.J.P. and G. Rose (1976). *Epidemiology in Medical Practice*, Churchill Livingstone.
23. WHO (1993), *Basic Epidemiology* by R. Beaglehole R. Bonita, T.Kjelistrom.
24. Austin, D.F. and Werner, S.B. (1970). *Epidemiology for the Health Sciences*, Illionis, C.C. Thomas.
25. Fraser, D.W. et al (1977). *N. Eng. Med. J.*, 299 : 1189.
26. WHO (2008). *Health Situation in South East Asia Region*, 2001-2007.
27. Herbst, A.L. et al (1971). *N. Eng. J. Med.*, 284 : 878.
28. Marmot, M.G. (1979). *Bull WHO*, 57 (3) 332.
29. WHO (1967). *Techn. Rep. Ser.*, No. 365.
30. Austin–Seymour, Mary M et al (1984). *Ann. Int. Med.*, 100 : 17.
31. MacMahon, B. (1981). In : *Preventive and Community Medicine*, 2nd ed., Duncan Clark (ed) Boston, Little, Brown & Co.
32. WHO (2006). *Basic Epidemiology*, 2nd Ed., R. Bonita, R. Beaglehole and T. Kjellstrom.
33. WHO (1972). *Techn. Rep. Ser.*, No. 510, P. 20.
34. Thompson, D.W. et al (1982). *Am. J. Epid.*, 116 (5) 840.
35. Karon, J.M. and Kupper, L.L. (1982). *Am. J. Epi.*, 116 (5) 852.
36. Doll, R. and Hill, A.B. (1950). *Brit. Med. J.*, 2 : 739.
37. Schlesselman, J.J. (1982). *Case Control Studies*, New York, Oxford University Press.
38. Mausner, J.S. and Bahn, A.K. (1974). *Epidemiology : An Introductory Text*, Philadelphia, Saunders.
39. Wynder, E.L. and Graham, E.A. (1950). *JAMA*, 143 : 329.
40. Levin, M.I. et al (1950). *JAMA* 143 : 336–338.
41. Kelsey, J.K. et al (1978). *J. Epi. and Comm. Hlth.* 32 : 102–107.
42. Linos, A. et al (1980). *N. Eng. J. Med.*, 302 : 1101.
43. Rooks, J.B. et al (1979). *JAMA*, *242* : 644–648.
44. Adour, K.K. et al (1975). *JAMA*. 233 : 527–539.
45. Kline, J. et al (1978). *Am. J. Epi.*, 107 : 290–298.
46. Hennekens, C.H. et al (1977). *Int. J. Epi.*, 6 : 243–246.
47. Hoover, R.N. and P.H. Strasser (1980). *Lancet*, 1 : 837–840.
48. Vassey, M.P. and R.Doll (1968). *Brit. Med. J.*, 2 : 199.
49. Vassey, M.P. and R.Doll (1969). *Brit. Med. J.*, 2 : 651.
50. Speirs, A.L. (1962). *Lancet*, 1 : 303.
51. Dawber, T.R. et al (1951). *Am. J. Pub. Hlth*, 41 : 249.
52. Doll, R. and A.B.Hill (1964). Brit. Med. J. 1 : 1399-1410;1460-1467.
53. Royal College of General Practitioners (1974). *Oral Contraceptives and Health*, London, Pitman Medical.
54. Neutra, R.R. et al (1978). *N. Eng. J. Med.*, 299 : 324–326.
55. Lee, A.M. et al (1969). *J. Natl. Cancer Inst.*, 42 : 1045.
56. Wagoner, J.K. et al (1965). *N. Eng. J. Med.*, 273 : 181–188.
57. Selter, R. and P.E. Sartwell (1965). *Am. J. Epi.*, 81 : 2–22.
58. Makka, L. et al (1974). *JAMA*, 230 : 64.

59. Court–Brown, W.M. and R. Doll (1957). *Leukaemia and Aplastic anaemia in patients irradiated for ankylosing spondylitis,* MRC Spl Res.Ser.No.295, London, HMSO.
60. Doll, R. and Peto (1976). *Brit. Med.* J., 2 : 1525.
61. Dorn, H.F. (1959). *Pub. Health Rep.,* 74 : 581–593, Washington DC, Govt. Printing Press.
62. Doll, R. and A.B. Hill (1956). *Brit.Med.J.,* 2 : 1071–1081.
63. Selikoff, I.J. et al (1968). *JAMA,* 204 : 106–112.
64. Mann, J.I. (1977). In : *Proceedings of an International Symposium on CHD in young women,* Edinburgh, 30 June–2 July 1977, Edinburgh, Churchill Livingstone.
65. Doll, R. and A.B. Hill (1956). *Brit. Med.* J., 2 : 1071.
66. Doll, R. and A.B. Hill (1954). *Brit. Med.* J., 1 : 1451–1455.
67. Hammond, E.C. and D.Horn (1954). *JAMA,* 155 : 1316–1328.
68. Hammond, E.C. et al (1958). *JAMA,* 116 : 1159–1172; 1294–1308.
69. Editorial (1977). *Lancet,* 2 : 747.
70. WHO (1980). *Medical Experimentation and the protection of Human Rights.*
71. Weser, J.K. et al (1984). *N. Eng. J. Med.,* 310:830.
72. Smithells, R.W. et al (1983). *Lancet,* 1 : 1027–31.
73. Paradise, J.L. et al (1984). *N. Eng. J. Med.,* 310:674.
74. Coronary Artery Surgery Study Randomized Trial (1984). *N. Eng. J. Med.,* 310 : 750.
75. Schoenberg, B.S. (1982). *Neuroepidemiology,* 1 : 85–101.
76. Medical Research Council (1951), *Brit. Med. J.,* 2:1463–71.
77. WHO cooperative Trial on Primary Prevention of IHD (1980) *Lancet,* 2:379.
78. Rose, G. and P.J.S. Hamilton (1978). *J. Epi and Community Health,* 32 : 275–81.
79. Terry, T.L. (1942). *Am. J. Ophthalmology,* 25:203–204; 1409–1423
80. Kinsey, V.E. and F.M. Hemphill (1955). *Am. J. Oph,* 56:481.
81. Kinsey, V.E. (1956). *Archives of Oph,* 56, 481–543.
82. South–East London Screening Study Group (1977). *Inj. J. Epi.,* 6 (4) 357–63.
83. Bennet, A.E. (1978). *Recent Advances in Community Medicine,* Churchill Livingstone.
84. Sackett, D.L. et al (1974). *Ann. Int. Med.,* 80 : 137.
85. Trichopoulos, D. et al (1983). *Lancet,* 1:441–443.
86. Moses, L.E. et al (1984). *Annual Rev. P. H.,* 5:267–92.
87. Yudkin, J.Roddy, J. (1964). *Lancet,* 2:6.
88. Bennet, A.E. et al (1970). *Lancet,* 1:1012.
89. US Public Health Service (1964). *Smoking and Health,* P.H. Service Pub; No.1103 Washington, US Govt. Printing Press.
90. Hill, A.B. (1965). *Proc. Roy. Soc. Med.,* 58:295–300.
91. Hill, A.B. (1971). *Principles of Medical Statistics,* 9th ed., Oxford University Press.
92. Susser, M.W. (1977). *Am. J. Epi.,* 105:1–15
93. Noble, John (1976). *Primary Care and the Practice of Medicine,* Boston, Little Brown.
94. White, K.L. (1978). In : *Basic Health Care in Developing Countries,* An Epidemiological perspective, Basil S. Hetzel (ed). IEA/WHO Handbook, Oxford Med. Publications.
95. Mckeown, T and C.R. Lowe (1974). *An Introduction to Social Medicine,* 2nd ed., Blackwell.
96. WHO (1980). *Early Detection of Handicap in Children,* EURO Rep and Studies, 30 Reg.Office WHO, Copenhagen.
97. Melby. J.C. (1975). *JAMA,* 231 : 399.
98. Finnerty, F.A. (1975). *JAMA,* 231 : 402.
99. WHO (1972). *WHO Chr.,* 26 (1) 7–11.
100. IEA (2001), *A Dictionary of Epidemiology,* 4th ed., Edited by John M. Last.
101. WHO (1982). *Techn. Rep. Ser.,* No.682.
102. Brachman, P.S. (1984). In : *Oxford Textbook of Public Health,* Vol II.
103. Waterson, A.P. (1979). *Brit. Med.* J., 2:564.
104. Dudgeon, J.A. (1976). *Brit. Med. Bull,* 32:77–85.
105. WHO (1978). *Techn. Rep. Ser.,* No.626.
106. Benenson, A.S. ed (1981). *Control of Communicable Diseases in Man,* 13th ed. American P.H. Association, New York.
107. Last, J.M. (1980). *Maxcy–Rosenau Public Health and Preventive Medicine,* 11th ed., Appleton Century Crofts.
108. Fudenberg, H.H. et al (1976). *Basic and Clinical Immunology,* Los Altos, Ca, Lange
109. Gell, P.G.H. et al (1975). *Clinical Aspects of Immunology,* 3rd ed., Blackwell, Oxford.
110. Mims, C.A. (1977). *The Pathogenesis of Infectious Disease,* London, Academic Press.
111. Youmans, G.P. et al (1980). *The Biological and Clinical Basis of Infectious Diseases,* 2nd ed., Saunders.
112. Turk, J.L. (1975). In : *Clinical Aspects of Immunology,* P.G.H. Cell et al (eds), 3rd ed., Blackwell, Oxford.
113. McConnel, I. et al (1981). *The Immune System,* a Course on the moleculer and cellular basis of immunity, 2nd ed. Oxford, Blackwell.
114. WHO (1976). *Public Health Papers,* No.62.
115. WHO (2013), *Immunization Safety Surveillance,* Guidelines for managers of immunization programmes on reporting and investigating adverse events following immunization, 2nd ed.
115A. WHO (2019). *Weekly Epidemiological Record,* No.22/23, 2019.
116. William E. Paul (2013), *Fundamental Immunology,* Seventh ed.
116A. Centre for Disease Control and Prevention(2020), *Epidemiology and prevention of vaccine - preventable diseases.*
117. Galazka, A.M. et al (1984). *World Health Forum,* 5 (3).
118. Galazka, A.M. et al (1984). *Bull WHO,* 62:357
119. Jawetz, Melnick and Adelberg's *Medical Microbiology,* 24th edition (2007), A Lange medical book.
120. Internet.
121. WHO (1983). *Bull WHO,* 61 (1) Directions to Contributors to Bulletin.
122. WHO (1982). *Bull WHO,* 60 (1) 43–47.
123. WHO (1978) *Techn. Rep. Ser.* No. 630.
124. Govt. of India (2011), *Immunization Handbook for Health Workers,* Ministry of Health and Family Welfare, New Delhi.
125. WHO (2015), *Vaccine Cold Chain Module 2,* 2015.
126. Govt. of India (2016), *Hand book for vaccine and Cold Chain handlers,* 2nd edition, Ministry of Health and Family Welfare, New Delhi.
127. Govt. of India (2008), *Immunization Handbook for Medical Officers,* Ministry of Health and Family Welfare, New Delhi.
128. Govt. of India (2015), *AEFI – Adverse Events Following Immunization, Surveillance and Response Operational Guidelines,* 2015, Ministry of Health and Family Welfare, New Delhi.
128A. WHO (2020), *Module 3, Adverse events following immunization.*
129. WHO (2006), *International travel and Health 2006.*
130. Govt. of India (2017), *Immunization Handbook for Medical Officers,* Ministry of Health and Family Welfare, New Delhi.
131. WHO (1996), *Weekly Epidemiological Record* No. 32, 9 August 1996.
132. WHO (1984). *Health for All,* Sr.No.9.
133. WHO (1978). *Health for All,* Sr.No.1, pp 24–25.
134. Bagshawe, K.D. et al (1978). *Brit.Med.J.,* 2:879–881.
135. WHO (1978). *WHO Chronicle,* 32:439–447.
136. Clark Duncan, W and B. MacMahon (1981). *Preventive and Community Medicine,* 2nd ed., Boston, Little Brown & Co.
137. American Academy of Paediatrics (1977). *Report of Committee on infectious Diseases* (Red Book, 18th ed).
138. Le Riche and J. Milner (1971). *Epidemiology as Medical Ecology,* Churchill, Livingstone.
139. Council for International Organizations of Medical Sciences (1973). *Communicable Diseases,* Provisional International Nomenclature, CIOMS/WHO, Geneva.
140. WHO (1983). *International Health Regulations,* 1969. 3rd Annotated edition, WHO, Geneva.
141. Salvato, J.A. (1976). *Guide to Sanitation in Tourist Establishments,* WHO Geneva.
142. WHO (1984). *The Work of WHO,* 1982–83.
143. WHO (1978). *Expanded Programme on Immunization,* Report and Working Papers, 31st Session of the WHO Reg. Committee, Mongolia, 21–28 Aug, 1978, SEARO.
143A. Govt. of India (2022), *Annual Report 2021–2022,* Ministry of Health and Family Welfare, New Delhi.
144. WHO (2016), WHO recommendations for routine immunizations, Immunization, Vaccines and Biologicals.
144A. WHO (2020), *Immunization, Vaccines and Biologicals,* WHO recommendations for immunization, summary tables.
145. Galazka, A.M. et al (1984). *Bull WHO,* 62 (3) 357.
146. Centre for Disease Control (1982). *Health Information for International Travel,* Washington DC. Govt. Printing Office (H.H.S. Publication (CDC) 82–8280), p.64.
147. Krugman, S. et al (1963). *Pediatrics,* 31:919–928.
148. Editorial (1982). *Brit.Med.J.,* 285:582.
149. WHO (1983). *WHO Chronicle,* 37 (6) 210.
150. WHO (1996), *International Travel and Health,* Vaccination Requirements and Health Advice.
151. William A. Rutala, David J. Weber and Health Care Infection Control Advisory Committee (2008), *Guidelines for Disinfection and Sterilization in Healthcare Facilities,* CDC.
152. WHO (1972). *Techn.Rep.Ser.,* No.493, p. 58.
153. Friedman, G.D. (1974). *Primer of Epidemiology,* McGraw Hill.
154. Frost, W.H. (1936). In : *Snow on Cholera,* New York, Commonwealth Fund, p.ix.
155. Bres, P. (1986). *Public Health action in Emergencies caused by Epidemics,* WHO, Geneva.
156. COVID-19 : *Guidelines on disinfection of common public places including offices,* 2020.

4 Screening for Disease

> *"Health should mean a lot more than escape from death or, for that matter, escape from disease."*

Iceberg phenomenon of disease

Epidemiologist and others who study disease find that the pattern of disease in hospitals is quite different from that in a community. That is, a far larger proportion of disease (e.g., diabetes, hypertension) is hidden from view in the community than is evident to physicians or to the general public. The analogy of an **iceberg**, only the tip of which is seen, is widely used to describe disease in the community.

The concept of the "iceberg phenomenon of disease" (Page 46) gives a better idea of the progress of a disease from its sub-clinical stages to overt or apparent disease than the familiar **spectrum of disease**. The submerged portion of the iceberg represents the hidden mass of disease (e.g., sub-clinical cases, carriers, undiagnosed cases). The floating tip represents what the physician sees in his practice. The hidden part of the iceberg thus constitutes the mass of unrecognized disease in the community, and its detection and control is a challenge to modern techniques in preventive medicine.

Concept of screening

The active search for disease among apparently healthy people is a fundamental aspect of prevention. This is embodied in screening, which has been defined as "the search for unrecognized disease or defect by means of rapidly applied tests, examinations or other procedures in apparently healthy individuals."

Historically, the annual health examinations were meant for the early detection of "hidden" disease. To bring such examinations within the reach of large masses of people with minimal expenditures of time and money, a number of alternative approaches have come into use. They are based primarily on conserving the physician–time for diagnosis and treatment and having technicians to administer simple, inexpensive laboratory tests and operate other measuring devices. This is the genesis of screening programmes. The original screening programmes were for individual diseases such as tuberculosis, syphilis or selected groups such as antenatal mothers, school children and occupational groups. Over the years, the screening tests have steadily grown in number (Table 8). Screening is considered a preventive care function, and some consider it a logical extension of health care.

Screening differs from **periodic health examinations** in the following respects *(1)*:

1) capable of wide application
2) relatively inexpensive, and
3) requires little physician–time. In fact the physician is not required to administer the test, but only to interpret it.

Screening and diagnostic tests

A screening test is not intended to be a diagnostic test. It is only an initial examination. Those who are found to have positive test results are referred to a physician for further diagnostic work-up and treatment. Screening and diagnostic tests may be contrasted as in Table 1.

TABLE 1
Screening and diagnostic tests contrasted

	Screening test	Diagnostic test
1	Done on apparently healthy	Done on those with indications or sick.
2	Applied to groups	Applied to single patients, all diseases are considered.
3	Test results are arbitrary and final	Diagnosis is not final but modified in light of new evidence, diagnosis is the sum of all evidence.
4	Based on one criterion or cut-off point	Based on evaluation of a number of symptoms, signs (e.g., diabetes) and laboratory findings.
5	Less accurate	More accurate.
6	Less expensive	More expensive.
7	Not a basis for treatment	Used as a basis for treatment.
8	The initiative comes from the investigator or agency providing care.	The initiative comes from a patient with a complaint.

Source : *(2)*

However, the criteria in Table 1 are not hard and fast. There are some tests which are used both for screening and diagnosis, e.g., test for anaemia and glucose tolerance test. Screening and diagnosis are not competing, and different criteria apply to each.

Concept of "lead time"

Fig. 1 shows the possible outcomes for a given disease process. There is nothing to be gained in screening for diseases whose onset is quite obvious. Detection programmes should be restricted to those conditions in which there is considerable **time lag** between disease onset and the usual time of diagnosis. In this period, there are usually a number of critical points which determine both the severity of the disease and the success of any treatment in reversing the disease process. There is clearly little value in detecting disease in advance of the usual time of diagnosis unless such detection precedes the final critical point beyond which treatment would be unsuccessful and/or permanent damage would be done. Detection programmes should, therefore, concentrate on those conditions where the time lag between the disease's onset and its final critical point is sufficiently long to be suitable for population screening *(3)*.

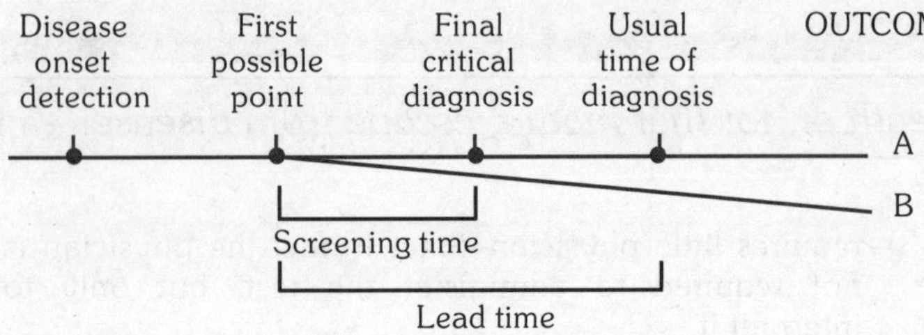

FIG.1
Model for early detection programmes

"Lead time" is the advantage gained by screening, i.e., the period between diagnosis by early detection and diagnosis by other means. In Fig.1, **A** is the usual outcome of the disease, and **B** is the outcome to be expected when the disease is detected at the earliest possible moment. The benefits of the programme are therefore **B–A**. The benefits of the programme must be seen in terms of its outcomes. It is also necessary for the complexities and costs of any detection programme to be viewed against the benefits accruing therefrom *(3)*.

Aims and objectives

The basic purpose of screening is to sort out from a large group of apparently healthy persons those likely to have the disease or at increased risk of the disease under study, to bring those who are "apparently abnormal" under medical supervision and treatment (Fig.2). Screening is carried out in the hope that earlier diagnosis and subsequent treatment favourably alters the natural history of the disease in a significant proportion of those who are identified as "positive" *(4)*.

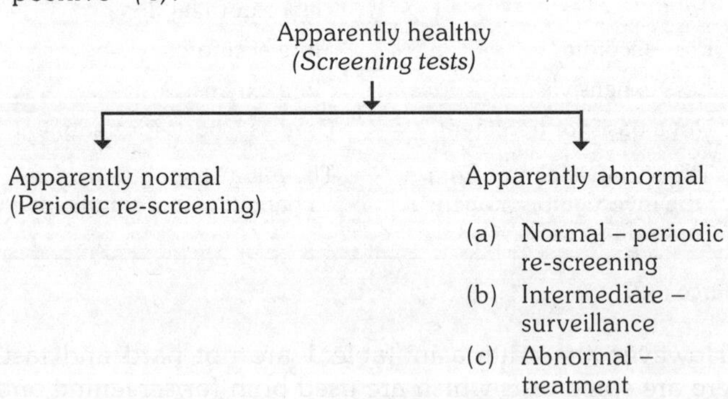

FIG.2
Possible outcomes of screening

Explanation of terms

a. Screening

Strictly speaking, screening is testing for infection or disease in populations or in individuals *who are not seeking health* care; for example, serological testing for AIDS virus in blood donors, neonatal screening, premarital screening for syphilis.

b. Case-finding

This is use of clinical and/or laboratory tests to detect disease in individuals *seeking health care* for other reasons; for example, the use of VDRL test to detect syphilis in pregnant women. Other diseases include pulmonary tuberculosis in chest symptomatics, hypertension, cervical cancer, breast cancer, diabetes mellitus, etc.

c. Diagnostic tests

Use of clinical and/or laboratory procedures to *confirm* or refute the existence of disease or true abnormality in patients with signs and symptoms presumed to be caused by the disease; for example, VDRL testing of patients with lesions suggestive of secondary syphilis; endocervical culture for *N. gonorrhoea.*

The distinction between screening, case-finding or diagnosis should be clear-cut. Often, however, it is blurred by the multiplicity of tests used and the haphazard nature of diagnostic decision-making. Thus the same test may be used in different contexts for both screening and diagnosis. Each step may involve multiple tests as in the case of syphilis. In evaluating a test, then, one must consider whether it is for screening or diagnosis, alone or in conjunction with other tests *(19)*.

Uses of screening

Four main uses have been described:

a. Case detection

This is also known as "prescriptive screening". It is defined as the presumptive identification of unrecognized disease, which does not arise from a patient's request, e.g., neonatal screening. In other words, people are screened primarily for their own benefit. Specific diseases sought by this method have included bacteriuria in pregnancy, breast cancer, cervical cancer, deafness in children, diabetes mellitus, iron deficiency anaemia, PKU, pulmonary tuberculosis, haemolytic disease of the newborn, etc. *(5)*. Since disease detection is initiated by medical and public health personnel, they are under special obligation to make sure that appropriate treatment is started early.

b. Control of disease

This is also known as "prospective screening". People are examined for the benefit of others, e.g., screening of immigrants from infectious diseases such as tuberculosis and syphilis to protect the home population; and screening for streptococcal infection to prevent rheumatic fever. The screening programme may, by leading to early diagnosis permit more effective treatment and reduce the spread of infectious disease and/or mortality from the disease.

c. Research purposes

Screening may sometimes be performed for research purposes. For example, there are many chronic diseases whose natural history is not fully known (e.g., cancer, hypertension). Screening may aid in obtaining more basic knowledge about the natural history of such diseases, as for example, initial screening provides a prevalence estimate and subsequent screening, an incidence figure. Where screening is done for research purposes, the investigator should inform the study participants that no follow-up therapy will be available.

d. Educational opportunities

Apart from possible benefits to the individual and the acquisition of information of public health relevance, screening programmes (as for example, screening for diabetes) provide opportunities for creating public awareness and for educating health professionals.

Types of screening

Three types of screening have been described:

a. Mass screening
b. High-risk or selective screening
c. Multiphasic screening.

a. Mass screening

Mass screening simply means the screening of a whole population *(6)* or a sub-group, as for example, all adults *(7)*. It is offered to all, irrespective of the particular risk individual may run of contracting the disease in question (e.g., tuberculosis).

Mass screening for disease received enthusiastic support in the past. However, when a number of mass screening procedures were subjected to critical review, there appeared to be little justification for their use in many instances *(8)*. Indiscriminate mass screening, therefore, is not a useful preventive measure unless it is backed up by suitable treatment that will reduce the duration of illness or alter its final outcome.

b. High-risk or selective screening

Screening will be most productive if applied selectively to high-risk groups, the groups defined on the basis of epidemiological research *(7)*. For example, since cancer cervix tends to occur relatively less often in the upper social groups, screening for cancer cervix in the lower social groups could increase the yield of new cases. One population sub-group where certain diseases (e.g., diabetes, hypertension, breast cancer) tend to be aggregated in the family. By screening the other members of the family (and close relatives), the physician can detect additional cases.

Epidemiologists have extended the concept of screening for disease to screening for "risk factors", as these factors apparently antedate the development of actual disease. For example, elevated serum cholesterol is associated with a high risk of developing coronary heart disease. Risk factors, particularly those of a patho-physiological nature such as serum cholesterol and blood pressure are amenable to effective interventions. In this way, preventive measures can be applied before the disease occurs. Besides effectiveness, economical use of resources will also occur if the screening tests are selectively applied to individuals in high-risk group.

c. Multiphasic screening

It has been defined as the application of two or more screening tests in combination to a large number of people at one time than to carry out separate screening tests for single diseases. The procedure may also include a health questionnaire, clinical examination and a range of measurements and investigations (e.g., chemical and haematological tests on blood and urine specimens, lung function assessment, audiometry and measurement of visual acuity) – all of which can be performed rapidly with the appropriate staffing organization and equipment *(7)*.

Multiphasic screening has enjoyed considerable popularity, and evidence from randomized controlled studies in UK and USA suggested that multiphasic screening has not shown any benefit accruing to the population in terms of mortality and morbidity reduction *(9)*. On the other hand, it has increased the cost of health services without any observable benefit. Furthermore, in multiphasic screening, as currently practised, most of the tests have not been validated. These observations have cast doubts on the utility of multiphasic screening *(10, 11)*.

CRITERIA FOR SCREENING

Before a screening programme is initiated, a decision must be made whether it is worthwhile, which requires ethical, scientific, and, if possible financial justification *(4)*. The criteria for screening are based on two considerations: the DISEASE to be screened, and the TEST to be applied *(12,13,14,15)*.

Disease

The disease to be screened should fulfil the following criteria before it is considered suitable for screening:

1. the condition sought should be an important health problem (in general, prevalence should be high);
2. there should be a recognizable latent or early asymptomatic stage;
3. the natural history of the condition, including development from latent to declared disease, should be adequately understood (so that we can know at what stage the process ceases to be reversible);
4. there is a test that can detect the disease prior to the onset of signs and symptoms;
5. facilities should be available for confirmation of the diagnosis;
6. there is an effective treatment;
7. there should be an agreed–on policy concerning whom to treat as patients (e.g., lower ranges of blood pressure; border-line diabetes);
8. there is good evidence that early detection and treatment reduces morbidity and mortality;
9. the expected benefits (e.g., the number of lives saved) of early detection exceed the risks and costs.

When the above criteria are satisfied, then only, it would be appropriate to consider a suitable screening test.

Screening test

The test must satisfy the criteria of acceptability, repeatability and validity, besides others such as yield, simplicity, safety, rapidity, ease of administration and cost. Tests most likely to fulfil one condition may however, be least likely to fulfil another – for example, tests with greater accuracy may be more expensive and time consuming. The choice of the test must therefore often be based on compromise.

1. Acceptability

Since a high rate of cooperation is necessary, it is important that the test should be acceptable to the people at whom it is aimed. In general, tests that are painful, discomforting or embarrassing (e.g., rectal or vaginal examinations) are not likely to be acceptable to the population in mass campaigns.

2. Repeatability

An attribute of an ideal screening test or any measurement (e.g., height, weight) is its repeatability (sometimes called reliability, precision or reproducibility). That is, the test must give consistent results when repeated more than once on the same individual or material, under the same conditions. The repeatability of the test depends upon three major factors, namely observer variation, biological (or subject) variation and errors relating to technical methods. For example, the measurement of blood pressure is poorly reproducible because it is subjected to all these three major factors.

A. Observer variation

All observations are subjected to variation (or error). These may be of two types:

a. Intra-observer variation

If a single observer takes two measurements (e.g., blood pressure, chest expansion) in the same subject, at the same time and each time, he obtained a different result, this is termed as **intra-observer** or **within-observer** variation. This is variation between repeated observations by the same observer on the same subject or material at the same time. Intra-observer variation may often be minimized by taking the average of several replicate measurements at the same time.

b. Inter-observer variation

This is variation between different observers on the same subject or material, also known as **between-observer** variation. Inter-observer variation has occurred if one observer examines a blood-smear and finds malaria parasite, while a second observer examines the same slide and finds it normal.

Table 2 shows the results when 14,867 chest X-ray films were each read independently by the same eight radiologists.

TABLE 2

Showing observer variation among radiologists

"Positive" readings	No.of films	Per cent
0/8	13,560	91.21
1/8	877	5.90
2/8	168	1.13
3/8	66	.44
4/8	42	.28
5/8	28	.19
6/8	23	.16
7/8	39	.26
8/8	64	.43
	14,867	100.00

Source : *(16)*

The results shown in Table 2 are sobering and instructive. There was concurrence of all 8 readers that 91.21 per cent of the films had one or more positive readings.

Observational errors are common in the interpretation of X-rays, ECG tracings, readings of blood pressure and studies of histopathological specimens. Observer errors can be minimized by (a) standardization of procedures for obtaining measurements and classifications (b) intensive training of all the observers (c) making use of two or more observers for independent assessment, etc. It is probable that these errors can never be eliminated absolutely.

B. Biological (subject) variation

There is a biological variability associated with many physiological variables such as blood pressure, blood sugar, serum cholesterol, etc. The fluctuation in the variate measured in the same individual may be due to: (a) *Changes in the parameters observed*: This is a frequent phenomena in clinical presentation. For example, cervical smears taken from the same woman may be normal one day, and abnormal on another day. Myocardial infarction may occur without pain. Subject variation of blood pressure is a common phenomenon. (b) *Variations in the way patients perceive their symptoms and answer*: This is a common subject variation. There may be errors in recollection of past events when a questionnaire is administered. When the subject is aware that he is being probed, he may not give correct replies. In short, subject variation can be a potential source of error in epidemiological studies. (c) *Regression to the mean*: An important example of biological variability is regression to the mean. There is a tendency for values at the extremes of a distribution, either very high or low, to regress towards the mean or average on repeat measurements. Many features of disease states vary considerably over time, for example, the pain of rheumatoid arthritis, stool frequency in ulcerative colitis, blood pressure in hypertension or the blood glucose in diabetes. This concept is particularly important to remember in evaluating the effects of a specific therapy on a variable such as the use of a specific drug to reduce blood pressure or serum cholesterol.

Whereas observer variation may be checked by repeat measurements at the *same time,* biological variation is tested by repeat measurements *over time.* This is due to the fact that measurement is done only on a tiny sample of the normal distribution of the physiological variable.

C. Errors relating to technical methods

Lastly, repeatability may be affected by variations inherent in the method, e.g., defective instruments, erroneous calibration, faulty reagents; or the test itself might be inappropriate or unreliable. Where these errors are large, repeatability will be reduced, and a single test result may be unreliable.

3. Validity (accuracy)

The term **validity** refers to what extent the test accurately measures which it purports to measure. In other words, validity expresses the ability of a test to separate or distinguish those who have the disease from those who do not. For example, glycosuria is a useful screening test for diabetes, but a more valid or accurate test is the glucose tolerance test. Accuracy refers to the closeness with which measured values agree with "true" values.

Validity has two components – sensitivity and specificity. When assessing the accuracy of a diagnostic test, one must consider both these components. Both measurements are expressed as percentages. Sensitivity and specificity are usually determined by applying the test to one group of persons having the disease, and to a reference group not having the disease (Table 3). Sensitivity and specificity, together with "predictive accuracy" are inherent properties of a screening test. These are discussed below.

TABLE 3–A

Screening test result by diagnosis

Screening test results	Diagnosis		Total
	Diseased	Not diseased	
Positive	a (True-positive)	b (False-positive)	a+b
Negative	c (False-negative)	d (True-negative)	c + d
Total	a + c	b + d	a + b + c + d

The letter "a" (Table 3–A) denotes those individuals found positive on the test who have the condition or disorder being studied (i.e., true-positives). The group labelled "b" includes those who have a positive test result but who do not have the disease (i.e., false-positives). Group "c" includes those with negative test results but who have the disease (i.e., false-negatives). Finally, those with negative results who do not have the disease are included in group "d" (i.e., true-negatives).

Evaluation of a screening test

The following measures are used to evaluate a screening test:

(a) Sensitivity = a/ (a + c) × 100

(b) Specificity = d/(b + d) × 100

(c) Predictive value of a positive test = a/(a + b) × 100

(d) Predictive value of a negative test = d/(c + d) × 100

(e) Percentage of false-negatives = c/(a + c) × 100

(f) Percentage of false-positive = b/(b + d) × 100

Let us rewrite Table 3–A substituting hypothetical figures (Table 3–B) and calculate the above measures:

TABLE 3–B

Screening test result by diagnosis

Screening test results	Diagnosis		Total
	Diseased	Not diseased	
Positive	40 (a)	20 (b)	60 (a+b)
Negative	100 (c)	9,840 (d)	9,940 (c + d)
	140 (a + c)	9,860 (b + d)	10,000 (a + b + c + d)

(a) Sensitivity (true-positive) = (40/140) × 100 = 28.57%

(b) Specificity (true-negative) = (9840/9860) × 100 = 99.79%

(c) False-negative = (100/140) × 100 = 71.4%

(d) False-positive = (20/9860) × 100 = 0.20%

(e) Predictive value of a positive test = (40/60) × 100 = 66.66%

(f) Predictive value of a negative test = (9840/9940) × 100 = 98.9%

Sensitivity

The term **sensitivity** was introduced by Yerushalmy *(17)* in 1940s as a statistical index of diagnostic accuracy. It has been defined as the ability of a test to identify correctly all those who have the disease, that is "true-positive". A 90 per cent sensitivity means that 90 per cent of the diseased people screened by the test will give a "true-positive" result and the remaining 10 per cent a "false-negative" result.

Specificity

It is defined as the ability of a test to identify correctly those who do not have the disease, that is, "true-negatives". A 90 per cent specificity means that 90 per cent of the non-diseased persons will give "true-negative" result, 10 per cent of non-diseased people screened by the test will be wrongly classified as "diseased" when they are not.

To illustrate, let us compare the sensitivity and specificity of EEG and CAT screening for diagnosis of brain tumours (Tables 4 and 5).

It can be seen from Tables 4 and 5, the CAT screening test is both more sensitive and more specific than EEG in the diagnosis of brain tumours.

In dealing with diagnostic tests that yield a quantitative result (e.g., blood sugar, blood pressure) the situation is different. There will be overlapping of the distributions of an attribute for diseased and non-diseased persons (Fig. 3). False positives and false negatives comprise the area of the overlap. When the distributions overlap, it is not possible to correctly assign individuals with these values to either the normal or the diseased group on the basis of screening alone.

For example, if we decide to use the 2–hour post-prandial blood glucose level of 180 mg/100 ml as an index of the presence of diabetes mellitus, the sensitivity and specificity are 50 and 99.8 per cent respectively (Table 6). In other words, sensitivity is low, but specificity very high. Further it will be seen from Table 6 that sensitivity and specificity are inversely related. That is, sensitivity may be increased only at the expense of specificity and vice versa. An ideal screening test should be 100 per cent sensitive and 100 per cent specific. In practice, this seldom occurs.

TABLE 4

Diagnosis of brain tumours by EEG

EEG results	Brain tumour	
	Present	Absent
Positive	36	54,000
Negative	4	306,000
	40	360,000

Sensitivity = 36/40 × 100 = 90 per cent
Specificity = 306,000/360,000 × 100 = 85 per cent

TABLE 5

Diagnosis of brain tumours by computer assisted axial tomography

CAT results	Brain tumour	
	Present	Absent
Positive	39	18,000
Negative	1	342,000
	40	360,000

Sensitivity = 39/40 × 100 = 97.5 per cent

Specificity = 342,000/360,000 × 100 = 95 per cent

TABLE 6

Sensitivity and specificity of a 2–hour postprandial blood test for glucose for 70 true diabetics and 510 true non-diabetics at different levels of blood glucose

Blood glucose level (mg/100 ml)	Sensitivity	Specificity
80	100.0	1.2
90	98.6	7.3
100	97.1	25.3
110	92.9	48.4
120	88.6	68.2
130	81.4	82.4
140	74.3	91.2
150	64.3	96.1
160	55.7	98.6
170	52.9	99.6
180	50.0	99.8
190	44.3	99.8
200	37.1	100.0

Source : *(18)*

Predictive accuracy

In addition to sensitivity and specificity, the performance of a screening test is measured by its "predictive value" which reflects the diagnostic power of the test. The predictive accuracy depends upon sensitivity, specificity and disease prevalence. The "predictive value of a positive test" indicates the probability that a patient with a positive test result has, in fact, the disease in question. The more prevalent a disease is in a given population, the more accurate will be the predictive value of a positive screening test. The predictive value of a positive result falls as disease prevalence declines.

Table 7 shows the predictive value of positive Gram's stained cervical smear test to detect gonorrhoea at prevalences of 5,15 and 25 per cent. In this example, the predictive value of a positive test was calculated to be 21, 47 and 63 per cent respectively. Thus in female populations in which the gonorrhoea is low (5 per cent prevalence), only 21 per cent of patients with positive results really have gonorrhoea; the remaining 79 per cent have false-positive results. Furthermore, as the sensitivity of this test is only 50 per cent, half of the cases are not detected, which greatly reduces the impact of the detection programme on disease transmission.

False negatives and positives

Whereas the epidemiologist thinks in terms of sensitivity and specificity, the clinician thinks in terms of false negatives and false positives.

False-negatives: The term "false-negative" means that patients who actually have the disease are told that they do not have the disease. It amounts to giving them a "false reassurance". The patient with a "false-negative" test result might ignore the development of signs and symptoms and may postpone the treatment. This could be detrimental if the disease in question is a serious one and the screening test is unlikely to be repeated within a short period of time. A screening test which is very sensitive has few "false negatives". The lower the sensitivity, the larger will be the number of false negatives.

False-positives: The term "false-positive" means that patients who do not have the disease are told that they have the disease. In this case, normal healthy people may be subjected to further diagnostic tests, at some inconvenience, discomfort, anxiety and expense – until their freedom from disease is established. A screening test with a high specificity will have few false positives. False-positives not only burden the diagnostic facilities, but they also bring discredit to screening programmes.

In fact, no screening test is perfect, i.e., 100 per cent sensitive and 100 per cent specific.

Yield

"Yield" is the amount of previously unrecognized disease that is diagnosed as a result of the screening effort. It depends upon many factors, viz. sensitivity and specificity of the test, prevalence of the disease, the participation of the individuals in the detection programme. For example, by limiting a diabetes screening programme to persons over 40 years, we can increase the yield of the screening test. High-risk populations are usually selected for screening, thus increasing yield.

Combination of tests

Two or more tests can be used in combination to enhance the specificity or sensitivity of screening. For example, syphilis screening affords an example whereby all screenees are first evaluated by an RPR test. This test has high sensitivity, yet will yield false positives. However, all those positive to RPR are then submitted to FTA–ABS, which is a more specific test, and the resultant positives now truly have syphilis.

TABLE 7

Predictive value of a positive gram-stained cervical smear test (with constant sensitivity of 50% and specificity of 90%) at three levels of prevalence

Prevalence 5%

		Culture +	Culture –	Total
Smear	+	25	95	120
	–	25	855	880
Total		50	950	1000

Positive predictive value $\frac{25}{120} \times \frac{100}{1} = 21\%$

Prevalence 15%

		Culture +	Culture –	Total
Smear	+	75	85	160
	–	75	765	840
Total		150	850	1000

Positive predictive value $\frac{75}{160} \times \frac{100}{1} = 47\%$

Prevalence 25%

		Culture +	Culture –	Total
Smear	+	125	75	200
	–	125	675	800
Total		250	750	1000

Positive predictive value $\frac{125}{200} \times \frac{100}{1} = 63\%$

The problem of the borderline *(20)*

The question arises which of the two qualities (sensitivity or specificity) is more important in screening? No categorical answer can be given. Figure 3 illustrates graphically the concepts of sensitivity and specificity.

Figure 3–a is a bimodal distribution of a variable in the "normal" and "diseased" populations. Note that the two curves overlap. If the disease is bimodal, as may be expected in certain genetically transmitted characteristics such as phenylketonuria, the shaded area or the "borderline" group will comprise a mixture of persons with the disease and persons without the disease (i.e., a mixture of false positives and false negatives). The point at which the distributions intersect (i.e., at level E) is frequently used as the **cut-off** point between the "normal" and "diseased" persons, because it will generally minimize the false positives and false negatives.

Figure 3–b is a unimodal distribution. Many physiological variables such as blood pressure, blood sugar and serum cholesterol show this type of distribution. Their values are continuously distributed around the mean, confirming to a normal or skewed distribution. In these observations, there is no sharp dividing line between the "normal" and "diseased". The "borderline" group (C–D) will comprise a homogeneous sample of persons. The question arises whether the cut-off point between "disease" and "normality" should be set at C or D as in Figure 3-b. If the **cut-off** point is set at the level of A or C, it will render the test highly sensitive, missing few cases but yielding many false positives. If the **cut-off** point is set at B or D, it will increase specificity of the test. Furthermore, in the unimodal distribution, once a cut-off point level has been adopted, all persons above that level (i.e., above level C or D in Figure 3-b) would be regarded as "diseased".

Taking diabetes as our example, if the cut-off point for

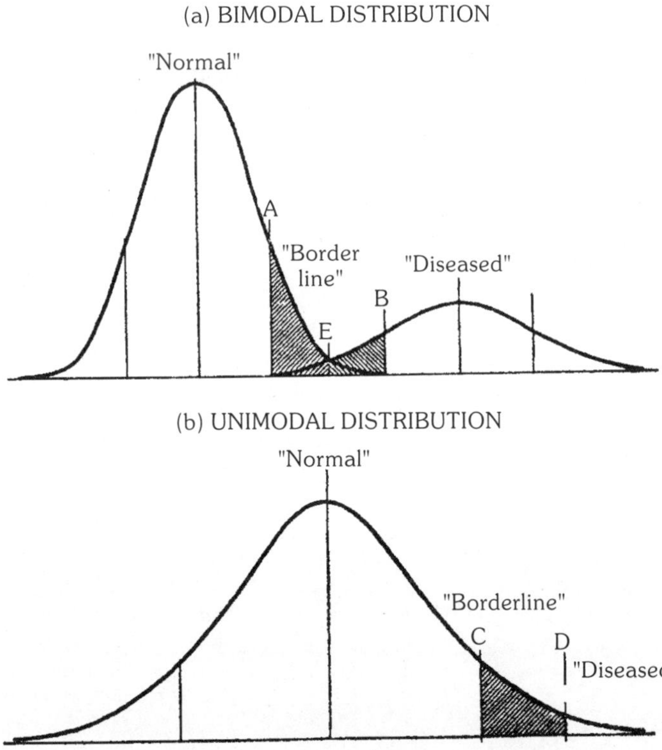

FIG. 3
Distribution of a variable in a population

blood glucose is lowered to detect diabetes (say less than 120 mg per cent), the sensitivity of the test is increased at the cost of specificity. If the cut-off point is raised (say to 180 mg per cent), the sensitivity is decreased (Table 6). In other words, there is no blood sugar level which will ensure the separation of all those with the disease from those without the disease.

In screening for disease, a prior decision is made about the cut-off point, on the basis of which individuals are classified as "normal" or "diseased". In making this decision, the following factors are taken into consideration: (a) *Disease prevalence*: When the prevalence is high in the community, the screening level is set at a lower level, which will increase sensitivity. (b) *The disease*: If the disease is very lethal (e.g., cervical cancer, breast cancer) and early detection markedly improves prognosis, a greater degree of sensitivity, even at the expense of specificity, is desired. In these cases, subsequent diagnostic work-up can be relied on to rule out the disease in the false-positives. That is, a proportion of false-positives is tolerable but not false-negatives. On the other hand, in a prevalent disease like diabetes for which treatment does not markedly alter outcome, specificity must be high and early cases may be missed, but false-positives should be limited; otherwise the health system will be overburdened with diagnostic demands on the positives, both true and false. That is, high specificity is necessary when false-positive errors must be avoided. A useful index in making this decision is the predictive value of a positive test. This index measures the percentage of positive results that are true positives; it is a function of the sensitivity and specificity as well as the frequency of the disease.

There are various other points which must also be taken into account in screening. First, people who participate in the screening programme may not be those who have most to gain from it, as for example, those at greatest risk of cancer of the cervix uteri are least likely to attend for cervical cytology. Therefore screening must be applied selectively to those people most likely to benefit. Selection might be based on a person's age, sex, medical history, occupation, family history or other factors. Secondly, tests with greater accuracy may be more expensive and time-consuming, and the choice of the test therefore often be based on compromise. Thirdly, screening should not be developed in isolation; it should be integrated into the existing health services. Lastly, the risks as well as the expected benefits must be explained to the people to be screened. These risks include any possible complications of the examination procedures, and the possibility of false-positive and false-negative test results.

Regardless of the approach taken to screening tests, regular patient follow-up visits are important (not to leave the patients high and dry) if effective health and medical care are to result from the effort. Garfield *(21)* has stressed the need to meet demands for medical care by separating screenees into well, asymptomatic-sick, and sick groups. This separation makes possible the optimal use of health care services.

Evaluation of screening programmes

Many screening tests (Table 8) were introduced in the past without subjecting them to rigid scrutiny. They were introduced because it was thought a good thing to detect and treat cases before they should reach an advanced stage. The modern view is that new screening programmes should be introduced only after proper evaluation.

TABLE 8
Some screening tests

Pregnancy	Infancy
Anaemia	LCB
Hypertension Toxaemia	Congenital dislocation of hip
Rh status	Congenital heart disease
Syphilis (VDRL Test)	Spina bifida
Diabetes	Cerebral palsy
Cardiovascular disease	Hearing defects
Neural tube defects	Visual defects
Down's syndrome	Hypothyroidism
HIV	Developmental screening tests
	Haemoglobinopathies
Middle-aged men and women	Sickle cell anaemia
Hypertension	Undescended testis
Cancer	**Elderly**
Diabetes mellitus	Nutritional disorders
Serum cholesterol	Cancer
Obesity	Tuberculosis
	Chronic bronchitis
	Glaucoma
	Cataract

(1) *Randomized controlled trials*: Ideally evaluation should be done by a randomized controlled trial in which one group (randomly selected) receives the screening test, and a control which receives no such test. Ideally RCT should be performed in the setting where the screening programme will be implemented, and should employ the same type of personnel, equipment and procedures that will be used in that programme. If the disease has a low frequency in the population, and a long incubation period (e.g., cancer) RCT may require following tens of thousands of people for 10–20 years with virtually perfect record keeping. The cost and logistics are often prohibitive.

(2) *Uncontrolled trials*: Sometimes, uncontrolled trials are used to see if people with disease detected through screening appear to live longer after diagnosis and treatment than patients who were not screened. One such example is uncontrolled studies of cervical cancer screening which indicated that deaths from that disease could be very much reduced if every woman was examined periodically.

(3) *Other methods*: There are also other methods of evaluation such as case control studies and comparison in trends between areas with different degrees of screening coverage. Thus it can be determined whether intervention by screening is any better than the conventional method of managing the disease.

To conclude, the screening concept, filled with potential has been overburdened with problems, many of which remain unsolved. The construction of accurate tests that are both sensitive and specific is a key obstacle to the wide application of screening. Scientific and technical puzzles abound.

References

1. Reiser, S.J. (1980). *World Health Forum*, 1 (1 and 2) 99–103.
2. Blumberg, M.S. (1966). In: *Chronic Diseases and Public Health*, A.M. Lilienfeld, et al (eds). Johns Hopkins.
3. WHO (1980). *Early detection of handicap in children*, EURO Reports and Studies No.30.
4. Cochrane, A.L. and Holland, W.w. (1971). *Br.Med.Bull*, 27:3.
5. McKeown, T. et al (1968). *Screening in Medical Care*, Reviewing the evidence for Nuffield Provincial Hospital Trust, London and Oxford.
6. Last, J.M. ed (1980). *A Dictionary of Epidemiology*, Oxford University Press.
7. Whitby, L.G. (1974), *Lancet*, 2:819–821.
8. Rakel, R.E. (1977). *Principles of Family Medicine*, Saunders.
9. WHO (1981). *World Health Forum*, 2:294.
10. South-East London Screening Study Group (1977). *Int.J.Epidemiology*, 6:357.
11. Collen, M. (1978). *Multiphasic health testing services*, New York, Wiley.
12. Wilson, J.M.G. and Jungner, G. (1968). *Principles and Practice for Screening for Disease*, Pub.Hlth.Paper No.34, Geneva, WHO.
13. WHO (1971). *Mass Health Examinations*, P.H. Paper No.45.
14. Roberts, C.J. (1977). *Epidemiology for Clinicians*, Pitman Medical.
15. WHO (1980). *World Health Forum*, 1:105.
16. Yerushalmy, J. (1956). *Bull Int.Union Tuberculosis*, 26:110–124.
17. Yerushalmy, J. (1947). *Pub.Hlth.Rep.*,62:1432.
18. Lilienfeld, A.M. and D.Lilienfeld (1979). *Foundations of Epidemiology*, 2nd ed. New York, Oxford Publications.
19. Grant, A and Mohide, P. (1982). In: *Effectiveness and Satisfaction in Antenatal Care*, M. Ekin and I. Chalmers (eds). Heinemann, London.
20. Le Riche, W.H. and Jean Milner (1971). *Epidemiology as Medical Ecology*, Churchill Livingstone.
21. Garfield, S.R. (1970). *N. Eng. J. Med.*, 283: 1087.

5 Epidemiology of Communicable Diseases

"Infectious diseases will last as long as humanity itself"

I. RESPIRATORY INFECTIONS

SMALLPOX
(VARIOLA)

An acute infectious disease caused by *variola virus*, and clinically characterized by a sudden onset of fever, headache, backache, vomiting and sometimes convulsions, especially in children. On the third day of fever, a typical rash appears which is centrifugal in distribution and passes through successive stages of macule, papule, vesicle, pustule, and scab with subsequent scarring.

Previously, it was one of the greatest killer disease. In 1967, WHO began an intensified worldwide campaign to eradicate smallpox, based on the technique of surveillance and containment. The last known case of smallpox in India occurred on 24th May 1975. India was declared smallpox free on 5th July 1975. The eradication of smallpox was confirmed in April 1977 by an international commission. The World Health Assembly confirmed the global eradication of smallpox in May 1980. All countries have discontinued routine vaccination against smallpox. However, WHO maintains a reserve stock of smallpox vaccine and vaccination needles – sufficient to protect more than 200 million people, should an emergency arise *(1)*.

Case definition for notification of smallpox under the International Health Regulations, 2005 *(2)*

Member states to the IHR (2005) are required to notify to WHO immediately of any confirmed case of smallpox. The case definition for a confirmed smallpox case includes the following :

Confirmed case of smallpox

An individual of any age presenting with acute onset of fever (≥38.3°C/101°F), malaise, and severe prostration with headache and backache occurring 2–4 days before onset of rash

AND

Subsequent development of a maculopapular rash starting on the face and forearms then spreading to the trunk and legs, and evolving within 48 hours to deep-seated, firm or hard and round well-circumscribed vesicles, and later pustules, which may become umbilicated or confluent

AND

Lesions that appear at the same stage of development (i.e. all are vesicles or all are pustules) on any given part of the body (e.g. the face or arm)

AND

No alternative diagnosis explaining the illness

AND

Laboratory confirmation.

Smallpox eradication surveillance

Despite the absence of smallpox, surveillance of "rumours" continues in order to sustain public confidence in the eradication of the disease. However, the final chapter of the smallpox story remains to be written, as the smallpox virus has not been completely destroyed. Stocks are still held at government research centres in the Russian Federation and at the United States.

References

1. WHO (1980), *The Global Eradication of Smallpox*, Final Report, Geneva.
2. WHO (2009), *Weekly Epidemiological Record*, No. 7, Feb 13, 2009.

HUMAN MONKEYPOX

Monkeypox is a viral zoonosis (a virus transmitted to humans from animals) with symptoms similar to those seen in the past in smallpox patients, although it is clinically less severe. With the eradication of smallpox in 1980 and subsequent cessation of smallpox vaccination, monkeypox has emerged as the most important orthopoxvirus for public health. Monkeypox primarily occurs in central and west Africa, often in proximity to tropical rainforests, and has been increasingly appearing in urban areas. Animal hosts include a range of rodents and non-human primates *(1)*.

Problem statement

Monkeypox is a disease of global public health importance as it not only affects countries in west and central Africa, but also the rest of the world. In 2003, the first monkeypox outbreak outside of Africa was in the United States of America and was linked to contact with infected pet prairie dogs. This outbreak led to over 70 cases of monkeypox in the U.S. Monkeypox has also been reported in travelers from Nigeria to Israel in September 2018, to the United Kingdom in September 2018, December 2019, May 2021 and May 2022, to Singapore in May 2019, and to the

United States of America in July and November 2021. In May 2022, multiple cases of monkeypox were identified in several non-endemic countries. Studies are currently underway to further understand the epidemiology, sources of infection, and transmission patterns.

Agent factor

Monkeypox virus is an enveloped double-stranded DNA virus that belongs to the *Orthopoxvirus* genus of the *Poxviridae* family. There are two distinct genetic clades of the monkeypox virus : the central African (Congo Basin) clade and the west African clade. The Congo Basin clade has historically caused more severe disease and was thought to be more transmissible. The geographical division between the two clades has so far been in Cameroon, the only country where both virus clades have been found.

Natural host

Various animal species have been identified as susceptible to monkeypox virus. This includes rope squirrels, tree squirrels, Gambian pouched rats, dormice, non-human primates and other species. Uncertainty remains on the natural history of monkeypox virus and further studies are needed to identify the exact reservoir(s) and how virus circulation is maintained in nature.

Transmission of disease *(1, 2)*

Animal-to-human (zoonotic) transmission can occur from direct contact with the blood, bodily fluids, or cutaneous or mucosal lesions of infected animals. Eating inadequately cooked meat and other animal products of infected animals is a possible risk factor. People living in or near forested areas may have indirect or low-level exposure to infected animals.

Human-to-human transmission can result from close contact with respiratory secretions, skin lesions of an infected person, or recently contaminated objects. Transmission via droplet respiratory particles usually requires prolonged face-to-face contact, which puts health workers, household members and other close contacts of active cases at greater risk. However, the longest documented chain of transmission in a community has risen in recent years from 6 to 9 successive person-to-person infections. This may reflect declining immunity in all communities due to cessation of smallpox vaccination. Transmission can also occur via the placenta from mother to fetus (which can lead to congenital monkeypox) or during close contact during and after birth. While close physical contact is a well-known risk factor for transmission, studies are needed to better understand this risk, if monkeypox can be transmitted specifically through sexual transmission routes *(1, 2)*.

Incubation period

The incubation period of monkeypox is usually from 6 to 13 days, but can range from 5 to 21 days.

Clinical picture

The infection can be divided into two periods :

- the invasion period (lasts between 0–5 days) characterized by fever, intense headache, lymphadenopathy, back pain, myalgia and intense asthenia. Lymphadenopathy is a distinctive feature of monkeypox compared to other diseases that may initially appear similar (chickenpox, measles, smallpox).
- the skin eruption usually begins within 1–3 days of appearance of fever. The rash tends to be more concentrated on the face and extremities rather than on the trunk. It affects the face (in 95 per cent of cases), and palms of the hands and soles of the feet (in 75 per cent of cases). Also affected are oral mucous membranes (in 70 per cent of cases), genitalia (30 per cent), and conjunctivae (20 per cent), as well as the cornea. The rash evolves sequentially from macules (lesions with a flat base) to papules (slightly raised firm lesions), vesicles (lesions filled with clear fluid), pustules (lesions filled with yellowish fluid), and crusts which dry up and fall off. The number of lesions varies from a few to several thousand. In severe cases, lesions can coalesce until large sections of skin slough off.

Monkeypox is usually a self-limited disease with the symptoms lasting from 2 to 4 weeks. Severe cases occur more commonly among children and are related to the extent of virus exposure, patient health status and nature of complications. Underlying immune deficiencies may lead to worse outcomes. Although vaccination against smallpox was protective in the past, today persons younger than 40 to 50 years of age (depending on the country) may be more susceptible to monkeypox due to cessation of smallpox vaccination campaigns globally after eradication of the disease. Complications of monkeypox can include secondary infections, bronchopneumonia, sepsis, encephalitis, and infection of the cornea with ensuing loss of vision. The extent to which asymptomatic infection may occur is unknown. The case fatality ratio has been around 3–6 per cent *(1)*.

Diagnosis

Polymerase chain reaction (PCR) is the preferred laboratory test given its accuracy and sensitivity. For this, optimal diagnostic samples for monkeypox are from skin lesions - the roof or fluid from vesicles and pustules, and dry crusts. Where feasible, biopsy is an option.

Treatment

Clinical care for monkeypox should be fully optimized to alleviate symptoms, manage complications and prevent long-term sequelae. Patients should be offered fluids and food to maintain adequate nutritional status. Secondary bacterial infections should be treated as indicated. An antiviral agent known as tecovirimat that was developed for smallpox was licensed by the European Medical Association (EMA) for monkeypox in 2022 based on data in animal and human studies. It is not yet widely available.

Vaccination

Vaccination against smallpox was demonstrated through several observational studies to be about 85 per cent effective in preventing monkeypox. Prior smallpox vaccination may result in milder illness. A still newer vaccine based on a modified attenuated vaccinia virus (Ankara strain) was approved for the prevention of monkeypox in 2019 *(1)*. This is a two-dose vaccine for which availability is limited.

Prevention *(1)*

Raising awareness of risk factors and educating people about the measures they can take to reduce exposure to the virus is the main prevention strategy for monkeypox. Scientific studies are now underway to assess the feasibility and appropriateness of vaccination for the prevention and control of monkeypox. Some countries have, or are developing, policies to offer vaccine to persons who may be at risk such as laboratory personnel, rapid response teams and health workers.

Reducing the risk of human-to-human transmission *(1)*

Surveillance and rapid identification of new cases is critical for outbreak containment. During human monkeypox outbreaks, close contact with infected persons is the most significant risk factor for monkeypox virus infection. Health workers and household members are at a greater risk of infection. Health workers caring for patients with suspected or confirmed monkeypox virus infection, or handling specimens from them, should implement standard infection control precautions. If possible, persons previously vaccinated against smallpox should be selected to care for the patient.

References

1. WHO (2022), *Fact sheet on Monkeypox*, 19th May 2022.
2. CDC (2022), *Monkeypox, How it spreads.*

CHICKENPOX (VARICELLA)

Chickenpox or varicella is an acute, highly infectious disease caused by *varicella-zoster* (V–Z) virus. It is characterized by vesicular rash that may be accompanied by fever and malaise. It is worldwide in distribution and occurs in both epidemic and endemic forms. Chickenpox and herpes zoster are now regarded as different host responses to the same aetiological agent. Inoculation of zoster vesicle fluid into children produces chickenpox, and children who have recovered from zoster virus related infection are resistant to varicella *(1)*.

Problem Statement

Based on conservative estimates, the global annual chickenpox disease burden includes 4.2 million severe complications leading to hospitalization and 4,200 deaths. In the pre-vaccine era in high-income developed countries, case fatality rate was about 3 per lac cases compared to 1–3 per 1000 cases for measles. Factors which influence the severity of disease and outcome in populations include the proportion of cases among infants, pregnant women and other adults, the prevalence of immunocompromising conditions including HIV infections and the extent of access to care and appropriate treatment. In otherwise healthy children, the disease is usually self-limiting *(2)*.

The incidence and severity of herpes-zoster disease increases with age, with marked increase after 50 years of age, which correlates with ageing related decline in cell-mediated immunity. Among adults who reach 85 years of age, it is estimated that approximately half will have suffered atleast one episode of herpes zoster *(2)*.

In India, during the year 2020, about 29,481 cases of chickenpox were reported with 15 deaths. The case fatality rate was about 0.050 per cent. Kerala reported the highest number of cases (17,086) and West Bengal reported the maximum number of deaths (8) due to chickenpox *(3)*.

Epidemiological determinants

Agent factors

(a) AGENT : The causative agent of chickenpox, V–Z virus is also called "Human (alpha) herpes virus 3". Primary infection causes chickenpox. Recovery from primary infection is commonly followed by the establishment of latent infection in the cranial nerves, sensory, ganglia, and spinal dorsal root ganglia, often for decades, without clinical manifestations. When the cell-mediated immunity wanes with age or following immuno-suppressive therapy, the virus may reactivate, resulting in herpes zoster in about 10–30 per cent of persons *(4)*. It is, a painful, vesicular, pustular eruption in the distribution of one or more sensory nerve roots. The virus can be grown in tissue culture. (b) SOURCE OF INFECTION: Usually a case of chickenpox. The virus occurs in the oropharyngeal secretions and lesions of skin and mucosa. Rarely the source of infection may be a patient with herpes zoster. The virus can be readily isolated from the vesicular fluid during the first 3 days of illness. The scabs however are not infective *(5)*. (c) INFECTIVITY: The period of communicability of patients with varicella is estimated to range from 1 to 2 days before the appearance of rash, and 4 to 5 days thereafter *(5)*. The virus tends to die out before the pustular stage *(6)*. The patient ceases to be infectious once the lesions have crusted. (d) SECONDARY ATTACK RATE: Varicella is a highly contagious disease with secondary attack ratio of approximately 85 per cent (range between 61 per cent to 100 per cent) in susceptible household contacts. Herpes zoster is approximately 20 per cent as infectious as chickenpox; in susceptible people, contact with herpes zoster rash causes varicella, not herpes zoster *(9)*.

Host factors

(a) AGE : Chickenpox occurs primarily among children under 10 years of age. Few persons escape infection until adulthood. The disease can be severe in normal adults. (b) IMMUNITY : One attack gives durable immunity; second attacks are rare. The acquisition of maternal antibody protects the infant during the first few months of life. No age, however, is exempt in the absence of immunity. The IgG antibodies persist for life and their presence is correlated with protection against varicella. The cell-mediated immunity appears to be important in recovery from V–Z infections and in protection against the reactivation of latent V–Z virus *(8)*. (c) PREGNANCY : Infection during pregnancy presents a risk for the foetus leading to congenital varicella syndrome. It occurs in 0.4–2.0 per cent of children born to mothers who become infected with VZV during the first 20 weeks of gestation. Infants, whose mothers had chickenpox during pregnancy, have a higher risk of developing herpes zoster in the first years of life *(2)*.

Environmental factors

Chickenpox shows a seasonal trend in temperate settings and in most tropical settings, with peak incidence during winter and spring, or in coolest, driest months in the tropics. Periodic large outbreaks occur with an inter-epidemic cycle of 2–5 years *(2)*.

VZV is heat labile. Outside host cell, the virus survives in the external environment for only a few hours, occasionally for a day or two, and it is readily inactivated by lipid solvents, detergents, and proteases *(2)*.

Transmission

Chickenpox is transmitted from person to person by droplet infection and by droplet nuclei. Most patients are infected by "face-to-face" (personal) contact. The portal of entry of the virus is the upper respiratory tract or the conjunctiva. Since the virus is extremely labile, it is unlikely that fomites play a significant role in its transmission. Contact infection undoubtedly plays a role when an individual with herpes zoster is an index case. The virus can cross the placental barrier and infect the foetus, a condition known as congenital varicella.

Incubation period

Usually 14 to 16 days, although extremes as wide as 10 to 21 days have been reported.

Clinical features

The clinical spectrum of chickenpox may vary from a mild illness with only a few scattered lesions to a severe febrile illness with widespread rash. Inapparent infection is estimated to occur in no more than 5 per cent of susceptible children *(7)*. In the majority of cases, the disease tends to be mild and typical *(6)*. The clinical course of chickenpox may be divided into two stages :

(A) PRE-ERUPTIVE STAGE : Onset is sudden with mild or moderate fever, pain in the back, shivering and malaise. This stage is very brief, lasting about 24 hours. In adults, the prodromal illness is usually more severe and may last for 2–3 days before the rash comes out *(6)*.

(B) ERUPTIVE STAGE : In children the rash is often the first sign. It comes on the day the fever starts. The distinctive features of the rash are :

(a) *Distribution :* The rash is symmetrical. It first appears on the trunk where it is abundant, and then comes on the face, arms and legs where it is less abundant. Mucosal surfaces (e.g., buccal, pharyngeal) are generally involved. Axilla may be affected, but palms and soles are not usually affected. The density of the eruption diminishes centrifugally.

(b) *Rapid evolution :* The rash advances quickly through the stages of macule, papule, vesicle and scab. In fact, the first to attract attention are often the vesicles filled with clear fluid and looking like "dew-drops" on the skin. They are superficial in site, with easily ruptured walls and surrounded by an area of inflammation. Usually they are not umbilicated. The vesicles may form crusts without going through the pustular stage. Many of the lesions may abort. Scabbing begins 4 to 7 days after the rash appears.

(c) *Pleomorphism :* A characteristic feature of the rash in chickenpox is its pleomorphism, that is, all stages of the rash (papules, vesicles and crusts) may be seen simultaneously at one time, in the same area. This is due to the rash appearing in successive crops for 4 to 5 days in the same area.

(d) *Fever :* The fever does not run high but shows exacerbations with each fresh crop of eruption.

The main points of difference between chickenpox and smallpox are given in Table 1.

TABLE 1
Differences between smallpox and chickenpox

	Smallpox	Chickenpox
1.	*Incubation :* About 12 days (range: 7–17 days).	About 15 days (range 7–21 days).
2.	*Prodromal symptoms:* Severe.	Usually mild.
3.	*Distribution of rash :*	
	(a) centrifugal	(a) centripetal
	(b) palms and soles frequently involved	(b) seldom affected
	(c) axilla usually free	(c) axilla affected
	(d) rash predominant on extensor surfaces and bony prominences.	(d) rash mostly on flexor surfaces.
4.	*Characteristics of the rash:*	
	(a) deep-seated	(a) superficial
	(b) vesicles multilocular and umbilicated	(b) unilocular; dew-drop like appearance
	(c) only one stage of rash may be seen at one time	(c) rash pleomorphic, i.e., different stages of the rash evident at one given time, because rash appears in successive crops
	(d) No area of inflammation is seen around the vesicles.	(d) an area of inflammation is seen around the vesicles.
5.	*Evolution of rash :*	
	(a) evolution of rash is slow, deliberate and majestic, passing through definite stages of macule, papule, vesicle and pustule.	(a) evolution of rash very rapid
	(b) scabs begin to form 10–14 days after the rash appears	(b) scabs begin to form 4–7 days after the rash appears
6.	*Fever :* Fever subsides with the appearance of rash, but may rise again in the pustular stage (secondary rise of fever).	Temperature rises with each fresh crop of rash.

Complications

In most cases, chickenpox is a mild, self–limiting disease. The mortality is less than 1 per cent in uncomplicated cases.

However, varicella may be accompanied by severe complications particularly in immunosuppressed patients and may also occur in normal children and adults. These include haemorrhages (varicella haemorrhagical), pneumonia, encephalitis, acute cerebellar ataxia and Reye's syndrome (acute encephalopathy associated with fatty degeneration of the viscera especially liver) *(10)*. Varicella pneumonia is rare in healthy children but is the most common complication in neonates, adults and immuno-compromised patients. It is related to many varicella-related deaths. Maternal varicella during pregnancy may cause foetal wastage and birth defects such as cutaneous scars, atrophied limbs, microcephaly and low birth weight, cataract, microphthalmia, chorioretinitis, deafness and cerebro-cortical atrophy. If varicella develops in a mother within 5 days after delivery, the newborn is at risk of disseminated disease and should receive varicella-zoster immunoglobulin *(4)*. The virus has a potential for oncogenicity.

Varicella-zoster virus is the major virus associated with acute retinal necrosis and progressive outer retinal necrosis, both of which occur with increased frequency among AIDS patients *(4)*.

Secondary bacterial infections, particularly with group A β-haemolytic streptococci and *staphylococcus aureus* are common. Cellulitis, erysipelas, epiglottitis, osteomyelitis, scarlet fever and rarely meningitis are observed. Pitted scars are frequent sequelae.

Immunocompromised patients are at increased risk of complications of varicella, including those with malignancies, organ transplants or HIV infection and those receiving high doses of corticosteroids. Disseminated intravascular coagulation may occur which is rapidly fatal. Children with leukaemia are especially prone to develop severe disseminated varicella-zoster virus disease *(1)*.

Laboratory diagnosis

During the smallpox post-eradication era the diagnosis of chickenpox is of great importance because of its resemblance to mild smallpox. Laboratory diagnosis is rarely required as clinical signs are usually clear-cut.

Laboratory confirmation of varicella or herpes zoster (HZ) is by detecting VZV DNA using polymerase chain reaction (PCR) or isolating VZV in cell culture from vesicular fluid, crusts, saliva, cerebrospinal fluid or other specimens. Direct immunofluorescence can also be used for rapid testing though this method has lower sensitivity than PCR. Detection of VZV-specific serum IgM antibody is considerably less sensitive than PCR and is not the method of choice for confirming varicella. Detection of serum IgM and PCR are of limited value for the confirmation of HZ. Serologic screening of serum for IgG antibodies is used to assess immunity or susceptibility to varicella in unvaccinated persons, e.g. in health-care workers *(2)*.

Control

The usual control measures are notifications, isolation of cases for about 6 days after onset of rash and disinfection of articles soiled by nose and throat discharges *(11)*.

Several antiviral compounds provide effective therapy for varicella including acyclovir, valaciclovir, famiciclovir and foscarnet. Acyclovir can prevent the development of systemic disease in varicella-infected immunosuppressed patients and can halt the progression of zoster in adults. Acyclovir does not appear to prevent post herpic neuralgia *(1)*.

Prevention

1. VARICELLA-ZOSTER IMMUNOGLOBULIN (VZIG)

Varicella-Zoster Immunoglobulin *(VZIG)* given within 72 hours of exposure has been recommended for prevention of chickenpox in exposed susceptible individuals particularly in immunosuppressed persons. These include (a) susceptible persons receiving immunosuppressive therapy; (b) persons with congenital cellular immunodeficiency; (c) persons with acquired immunodeficiency including HIV/AIDS; (d) susceptible and exposed persons, in particular pregnant women; (e) newborns; and (f) premature infants of low birth weight. It has no therapeutic value in established disease. *VZIG* is given by intramuscular injection in a dose of 12.5 units/kg body weight up to a maximum of 625 units, with a repeat dose in 3 weeks, if a high-risk patient remains exposed. Because *VZIG* appears to bind the varicella vaccine, the two should not be given concomitantly *(4)*.

2. VACCINE

A live attenuated varicella virus vaccine is safe and currently recommended for children between 12–18 months of age who have not had chickenpox.

Recommendations on dosage and interval between doses vary by manufacturer. Monovalent vaccine can be administered following one or two dose schedule (0.5 ml each by subcutaneous injection. A 2 dose schedule is recommended for all persons aged ≥13 years. When 2 doses are administered, the minimum interval between doses is from 4 weeks to 3 months for children (12 months to 12 years of age inclusive), and 4 or 6 weeks for adolescents and adults (13 years of age and older).

Combination vaccines (MMRV) can be administered to children from 9 months to 12 years. If 2 doses of MMRV are used, the minimum interval between doses should be 4 weeks. It is preferred that the 2nd dose be administered from 6 weeks to 3 months after the first dose or at 4–6 years of age *(2)*.

The duration of immunity is not known but is probably 10 years. Although the vaccine is very effective in preventing disease, breakthrough infections do occur – but are much milder than in unvaccinated individuals (usually less than 50 lesions, with milder systemic symptoms). Although the vaccine is very safe, adverse reactions can occur as late as 4–6 weeks after vaccination. Tenderness and erythema at the injection site are seen in 25%, fever in 10–15%, and a localized maculopapular or vesicular rash in 5%; a smaller percentage develops a diffuse rash, usually with five or fewer vesicular lesions.

Spread of virus from vaccinees to susceptible individuals is possible, but the risk of such transmission even to immuno-compromised patients is small, and disease, when it develops, is mild and treatable with acyclovir. Nonetheless, the vaccine, being a live attenuated virus, should not be given to immunocompromised individuals. The use of varicella vaccine may be considered in clinically stable HIV-infected children or adults with CD4+ T-cell levels ≥ 15 per cent including those receiving highly active antiretroviral therapy. HIV testing is not a prerequisite for varicella vaccination *(2)*. It is contraindicated in persons allergic to neomycin. For theoretic reasons, it is recommended that following vaccination, salicylates should be avoided for 6 weeks (to prevent Reye's syndrome).

Varicella vaccination is contraindicated during pregnancy and pregnancy should be delayed for 4 weeks after vaccination. Termination of pregnancy is not indicated if vaccination was carried out inadvertently during pregnancy *(9)*.

POST-EXPOSURE PROPHYLAXIS

Vaccine: Varicella vaccine is recommended for post exposure administration to un-vaccinated healthy people aged ≥12 months and without other evidence of immunity, to prevent or modify the disease. The vaccine should be administered as soon as possible within 5 days after exposure to rash, if there is no contraindication to use. Among children, protective efficacy was reported as ≥90 per cent when vaccination occurred within 3 days of exposure. However, administration of a second dose is recommended for exposed people to bring them up-to-date on vaccination and for best protection against future exposure *(9)*.

Several unresolved issues remain, including the need for booster doses, whether universal childhood vaccination will shift the incidence of disease to adolescence or adulthood with the possibility of more severe disease, and whether vaccination might prevent development of herpes zoster.

References

1. Jawetz, Melnick and Adelberg's *Medical Microbiology,* (2007), 24th Ed., A Lange Publication.
2. WHO (2014), *Weekly Epidemiological Record,* No. 25, June 20, 2014.
3. Govt. of India (2021), *National Health Profile of India 2021,* Ministry of Health and Family Welfare, New Delhi.
4. Lawrence, M., Tierney, Jr. (2008), *Current Medical Diagnosis and Treatment,* (2008), 47th Ed., A Lange Publication.
5. Weller, Thomas H. (1977). in *Viral Infections of Humans: Epidemiology and Control,* Evans Alfred, S. et al (eds), 2nd ed., Plenum Medical, New York.
6. Christie, A.B. (1980). *Infectious Diseases:* Epidemiology and Clinical Practice, 3rd ed., Churchil Livingstone.
7. Stephen, R Preblud and A.R. Hinman (1980), *Maxcy–Rosenau : Public* Health and Preventive Medicine, Last, J.M. (ed), 11th ed, Appleton – Century – Crofts.
8. WHO (1985) *Bull WHO* 63 : 433.
9. CDC Pink Book (2019), *Epidemiology and Prevention of Vaccine-Preventable Diseases.*
10. WHO (1985) *Techn. Rep. Ser.*, No.725.
11. Bres, P. (1986) *Public Health Action in Emergencies* caused by Epidemics. Geneva, WHO.

MEASLES
(RUBEOLA)

An acute highly infectious disease of childhood caused by a specific virus of the group myxoviruses. It is clinically characterized by fever and catarrhal symptoms of the upper respiratory tract (coryza, cough), followed by a typical rash. Measles is associated with high morbidity and mortality in developing countries. Measles occurs only in humans. There is no animal reservoir of infection.

Problem statement

Measles is endemic virtually in all parts of the world. It tends to occur in epidemics when the proportion of susceptible children reaches about 40 per cent *(1)*. When the disease is introduced into a virgin community more than 90 per cent of that community will be infected *(2)*. While measles is now rare in industrialized countries, it remains a common illness in many developing countries. The primary reason for continuing high childhood measles mortality and morbidity is the failure to deliver at least one dose of measles vaccine to all infants *(3)*.

The challenges for measles elimination include : (1) weak immunization systems; (2) high infectious nature of measles; (3) populations that are inaccessible due to conflict; (4) the increasing refusal of immunization by some populations; (5) the changing epidemiology of measles which has led to increased transmission among adolescents and adults; (6) the gaps in human and financial resources at the country, regional and global levels *(6)*.

In 1980, before widespread use of measles vaccine, an estimated 2.6 million measles deaths occurred worldwide. Recognizing this burden, WHO and UNICEF developed an accelerated measles mortality reduction strategy of delivering 2 doses of measles containing vaccine (MCV) to all children through routine services and supplementary immunizing activities (SIAs), and improving disease surveillance. Implementation of this strategy began in 2001. At the 2010 World Health Assembly, member states endorsed the following targets to be met by 2015 as milestones towards eventual global measles eradication : (1) raise routine coverage with the first dose of MCV (MCV_1) to ≥90 per cent nationally, and ≥80 per cent in every district or equivalent administrative unit; (2) reduce and maintain annual measles incidence to <5 cases per million; and (3) reduce measles mortality by ≥95 per cent in comparison with the estimated level in the year 2000 *(5)*.

The Global Measles and Rubella Strategic Plan 2012–20 period saw a significant reduction in the measles and rubella disease burden, a steep increase in the introduction of a second dose of measles-containing (MCV_2) and rubella vaccines, and improvements in surveillance. An increase in measles cases in January and February 2022 is a worrying sign of a heightened risk for the spread of vaccine-preventable diseases and could trigger large outbreaks. Pandemic-related disruptions, increasing inequalities in access to vaccines and the diversion of resources from routine immunization are leaving too many children without protection against measles. In addition, with millions of people being displaced due to conflicts and crises, disruptions of routine immunization and COVID-19 vaccine services, lack of clean water, sanitation and overcrowding increase the risk of disease outbreak. Almost 17,338 measles cases were reported globally in January and February 2022, compared to 9,665 during the first two months of 2021. As measles is very contageous, cases tend to show up quickly when vaccination level declines (In 2020, 23 million children missed out on basic childhood vaccines through health services).

Based on updated annual data, the estimated number of measles cases decreased 79 per cent, from 3,67,63,000 in year 2000 to 75,49,000 in 2020; and estimated annual measles deaths decreased 94 per cent from 10,72,800 to 60,700 in year 2020. During 2000–2020, measles vaccination prevented an estimated 31.7 million deaths globally compared with no measles vaccination *(6)*.

In India, measles is a significant cause of childhood morbidity. Prior to the immunization programme, cyclical increase in the incidence of measles were recorded every third year. With the increase in immunization coverage levels, the intervals between cyclical peaks has increased and the intensity of the peak minimized. However, several outbreaks are reported in tribal and remote areas. The retrospective data indicate a declining trend of measles in the country. During 1987 about 2.47 lakh cases were reported, whereas, after implementation of UIP, the number of cases has come down to 12,081 with 1 death during the year 2020.

The states majorly affected were West Bengal (4,863 cases and 1 death), Odisha (3,151 cases, no deaths), Uttar Pradesh (1,372 cases without any death), Assam (931 cases, no deaths), Andhra Pradesh (373 cases, no deaths), and Gujarat (254 cases and no deaths) *(7)*. The country is making significant progress towards the goal of measles elimination and rubella/congenital rubella syndrome control. The strategies for measles and rubella elimination include : (1) 95 per cent coverage with measles and rubella vaccination; (2) Case-based measles-rubella surveillance with adequate laboratory support; (3) Linkage with other child health interventions; and (4) Increased public confidence and demand for immunization *(8)*.

Epidemiological determinants

Agent factors

(a) AGENT : Measles is caused by an RNA paramyxovirus. So far as is known, there is only one serotype. The virus cannot survive outside the human body for any length of time, but retains infectivity when stored at sub-zero temperature. The virus has been grown in cell cultures. (b) SOURCE OF INFECTION : The only source of infection is a case of measles. Carriers are not known to occur. There is some evidence to suggest that subclinical measles occurs more often than previously thought. (c) INFECTIVE MATERIAL : Secretions of the nose, throat and respiratory tract of a case of measles during the prodromal period and the early stages of the rash. (d) COMMUNICABILITY : Measles is highly infectious during the prodromal period and at the time of eruption. Communicability declines rapidly after the appearance of the rash. The period of communicability is approximately 4 days before and 4 days after the appearance of the rash. Isolation of the patient for a week from the onset of rash more than covers the period of communicability *(9)*. (e) SECOND ATTACK RATE : There is only one antigenic type of measles virus. Infection confers life long immunity. Most so-called second attacks represent errors in diagnosis either in initial or second illness *(10)*.

Host factors

(a) AGE : Affects virtually everyone in infancy or childhood – between 6 months and 3 years of age in developing countries where environmental conditions are generally poor, and older children usually over 5 years in developed countries *(11)*. Following the use of measles vaccine, the disease is now seen in somewhat older age-groups *(12)*. This highlights the importance of periodic serological checking of the immunity status of the susceptible population. (b) SEX : Incidence equal. (c) IMMUNITY : No age is immune if there was no previous immunity. One attack of measles generally confers life-long immunity. Second attacks are rare. Infants are protected by maternal antibodies up to 6 months of age; in some, maternal immunity may persist beyond 9 months. Immunity after vaccination is quite solid and long-lasting. (d) NUTRITION : Measles tends to be very severe in the malnourished child, carrying a mortality upto 400 times higher than in well-nourished children having measles *(13)*. This may possibly be related to poor cell-mediated immunity response, secondary to malnutrition *(14)*. Additionally, severely malnourished children have been shown to excrete measles virus for longer periods than better nourished children indicating prolonged risk to themselves, and of intensity of spread to others *(15)*. Even in a healthy child, an attack of severe measles may be followed by weight loss, precipitating the child into malnutrition.

Environmental factors

Given a chance, the virus can spread in any season *(10)*. In tropical zones, most cases of measles occur during the dry season. In temperate climates, measles is a winter disease, probably because people crowd together indoors. Epidemics of measles are common in India during winter and early spring (January to April). Population density and movement do affect epidemicity *(16)*. In general, the less favourable the prevailing socio-economic conditions, the lower the average age at which children are attacked.

Transmission

Transmission occurs directly from person to person mainly by droplet infection and droplet nuclei, from 4 days before onset of rash until 4 days thereafter. The portal of entry is the respiratory tract. Infection through conjunctiva is also considered likely as the virus instilled into the conjunctiva can cause infection. Recipients of measles vaccine are not contagious to others *(17)*.

Incubation period

Incubation period is commonly 10 days from exposure to onset of fever, and 14 days to appearance of rash. When measles infection is artificially induced bypassing the respiratory tract (as with injection of live measles vaccine), the incubation period is somewhat shortened, averaging 7 days.

Clinical features

There are three stages in the natural history of measles, viz. the prodromal or pre-eruptive stage, eruptive stage and post-measles stage.

1. PRODROMAL STAGE

It begins 10 days after infection, and lasts until day 14. It is characterized by fever, coryza with sneezing and nasal discharge, cough, redness of the eyes, lacrimation and often photophobia. There may be vomiting or diarrhoea. A day or two before the appearance of the rash Koplik's spots like table salt crystals appear on the buccal mucosa opposite the first and second lower molars. They are small, bluish–white spots on a red base, smaller than the head of a pin *(10)*. Their presence is pathognomonic of measles.

2. ERUPTIVE PHASE

This phase is characterized by a typical, dusky–red, macular or maculo-papular rash which begins behind the ears and spreads rapidly in a few hours over the face and neck, and extends down the body taking 2 to 3 days to progress to the lower extremities. The rash may remain discrete, but often it becomes confluent and blotchy. In the absence of complications, the lesions and fever disappear in another 3 or 4 days signalling the end of the disease. The rash fades in the same order of appearance leaving a brownish discoloration which may persist for 2 months or more.

During the prodromal phase (2–4 days) and the first 2–5 days of rash, virus is present in tears, nasal and throat secretions, urine and blood. Just as the maculo-papular rash appears, the circulating antibodies become detectable, the viraemia disappears and the fever falls. The rash develops as a result of interaction of immune T cells with virus-infected cells in the small blood vessels. In patients with defective cell-mediated immunity, no rash develops *(10)*.

Diagnosis of measles is based on the typical rash and Koplik's spots seen in oral mucosa. The diagnosis would normally be incorrect in any febrile exanthem in which red eyes and cough are absent. In developed countries, where measles is uncommon, specific IgM antibodies by ELISA, or the detection of measles virus RNA by RT-PCR (reverse transcriptase polymerase chain reaction) in throat swabs, oral fluid or nasopharyngeal mucus; or urine are being used for diagnosis *(18)*.

3. POST–MEASLES STAGE

The child will have lost weight and will remain weak for a number of days. There may be failure to recover and a gradual deterioration into chronic illness – due to increased susceptibility to other bacterial and viral infections, nutritional and metabolic effects and the tissue destructive effects of the virus. There may be growth retardation and diarrhoea, cancrum oris, pyogenic infections, candidosis, reactivation of pulmonary tuberculosis etc.

Complications *(18)*

The severity of measles varies widely, depending on several host and environmental factors. The risk of developing severe or fatal measles increases for children aged <5 years, and persons living in overcrowded conditions, those who are malnourished especially with vitamin A deficiency, and those with immunological disorders, such as AIDS. Complications occur in approximately 30% of reported cases depending on age and predisposing conditions. Relatively common complications of measles include otitis media, laryngotracheo-bronchitis (croup), diarrhoea and pneumonia. In children in developed countries, otitis media occurs in 7–9% of cases, diarrhoea in 8% of cases, and pneumonia in 1–6%. Post-infectious measles encephalitis occurs in about 1–4 per 1000–2000 cases, and sub-acute sclerosing panencephalitis (SSPE) develops several years after the infection in about 1 per 10,000–100,000 cases. Particularly severe complications of measles which occur in immunocompromised individuals are an acute progressive encephalitis (measles inclusion-body encephalitis), and a characteristic giant cell pneumonia. In developing countries, persistent diarrhoea with protein-losing enteropathy may ensue, particularly in infants. In these countries, where malnutrition, particularly vitamin A deficiency, and exposure to other infectious diseases are common, the case-fatality rate for measles is usually 3–6%, but can be as high as 30% particularly among displaced or isolated, immunologically naive populations. In developed countries death due to measles is rare and the case-fatality rate is usually 0.01–0.1%. The greatest risk of death is in children younger than 1 year and in adults older than 30 years. In HIV-infected children, the case-fatality rate has been reported to be as high as 50% *(18)*.

Measles during pregnancy is not known to cause congenital abnormalities of the foetus. However, it is associated with spontaneous abortion and premature delivery. Measles in the offspring of mothers with measles ranges from mild to severe; therefore, it is recommended that infants born to such mothers be passively immunized with immunoglobulin at birth *(19)*.

Treatment *(18)*

There is no specific treatment for measles. Case management of measles focuses on supportive care as well as the prevention and treatment of measles complications and secondary infections. Supportive care should be provided, including relieving common symptoms such as fever, cough, nasal congestion or rhinorrhea, conjunctivitis, and sore mouth. Nutritional support is recommended to reduce the risk of malnutrition due to diarrhoea, vomiting and poor appetite associated with measles. Breast-feeding should be encouraged where appropriate. Oral rehydration salts should be used as needed to prevent dehydration.

Since measles is highly contagious, patient isolation is an important intervention to prevent further spread of the virus. However, increasing population immunity through vaccination is the most effective way to prevent outbreaks.

All cases of severe measles, and all cases of measles in areas with high case–fatality rates should be treated with vitamin A, as many children develop acute deficiency of vitamin A, which may lead to keratomalacia and blindness from corneal scarring. A high dose of vitamin A is given immediately on diagnosis and repeated the next day. The recommended age-specific daily doses are 50,000 IU for infants aged <6 months, 100,000 IU for infants aged 6–11 months, and 200,000 IU for children aged ≥ 12 months. If the child has clinical signs of vitamin A deficiency (such as Bitot's spots) a third dose should be given 4–6 weeks later *(20)*.

Measles and chickenpox

It has been noted that sometimes measles and chickenpox may occur together and one most remarkable finding in these cases of double infection is that the first infection may diminish the severity of the rash of the second infection *(21)*.

Prevention of measles

The following guidelines are important in combating measles:

a. achieving an immunization rate of over 95 per cent, and
b. on-going immunization against measles through successive generations of children.

1. Measles vaccination

Measles is best prevented by active immunization.

VACCINE : Only live attenuated vaccines are recommended for use; they are both safe and effective, and may be used interchangeably within immunization programmes. Person to person transmission of measles vaccine strains has never been documented. The vaccine is presented as a freeze-dried product. Before use, the lyophilized vaccine is reconstituted with sterile diluent. Each dose of 0.5 ml contains ≥1000 viral infective units of the vaccine strain; this is also true when it is presented as an MCV combination. Measles vaccine may also contain sorbitol and hydrolysed gelatin as stabilizers, as well as a small amount of neomycin, but it does not contain thiomersal. In general, it is recommended that freeze-dried vaccine be stored in a refrigerated condition *(20)*. The diluent must not be frozen but should be cooled before reconstitution. Reconstituted measles vaccine loses about 50 per cent of its potency after 1 hour at 20°C; it loses almost all potency after 1 hour at 37°C. The vaccine is also sensitive to sunlight, hence it is kept in coloured glass vials. After reconstitution, the vaccine must be stored in the dark at 2–8°C and used within 4 hours.

Measles vaccine is available in monovalent (measles only) form and in combination : measles-rubella (MR), measles-mumps-rubella (MMR) vaccine, and measles-mumps-rubella-varicella (MMRV) vaccine.

Reaching all children with 2 doses of measles containing vaccine (MCV) should be the standard for all national immunization programmes. In countries with ongoing transmission in which the risk of measles mortality remains high, MCV_1 should be given at age 9 months. MCV_2 should be given between 15–18 months, as providing MCV_2 in the 2nd year of life reduces the rate of accumulation of susceptible children and the risk of an outbreak. The minimum interval between MCV_1 and MCV_2 is 4 weeks. Every opportunity (e.g. when children come into contact with health services) should be taken to vaccinate all children that missed one or both MCV routine doses, particularly those under 15 years of age. Policies which prohibit use of vaccine in children >1 year of age, older children and teenagers should be changed to allow these individuals to be vaccinated.

In countries with low levels of measles transmission (i.e. those that are near elimination or verified as having eliminated endemic measles virus transmission), and therefore the risk of measles virus infection among infants is low, MCV_1 may be administered at 12 months of age to take advantage of the higher sero-conversion rates achieved at this age. In these countries, the optimal age for delivering MCV_2 is based on programmatic considerations to achieve the highest coverage of MCV_2 and, hence, the highest population immunity. Administration of MCV_2 at 15–18 months of age ensures early protection of the individual, slows accumulation of susceptible young children, and may correspond to the schedule for other routine immunizations (for example, a DTP-containing booster, PCV, or meningococcal vaccines). This measure also supports the establishment of a policy on immunization and other health interventions in the second year of life. If MCV_1 coverage is high (>90%) and school enrolment is high (>95%), administration of routine MCV_2 at school entry may prove an effective strategy for achieving high coverage and preventing outbreaks in schools *(22)*.

MCV administered before 9 months of age should be considered a supplementary dose and recorded on the child's vaccination record as "MCV_0". Children who receive MCV_0 should also receive MCV_1 and MCV_2 at the recommended ages according to the national schedule. A supplementary dose of MCV should be given to infants from 6 months of age : (1) during a measles outbreak as part of intensified service delivery; (2) during campaigns in settings where the risk of measles among infants < 9 months of age remains high (e.g. in endemic countries experiencing regular outbreaks); (3) for internally displaced populations and refugees, and populations in conflict zones; (4) for individual infants at high risk of contracting measles (e.g. contacts of known measles cases or in settings with increased risk of exposure during outbreaks such as day-care facilities); (5) for infants travelling to countries experiencing measles outbreaks; (6) for infants known to be HIV-infected or exposed (i.e. born to an HIV-infected woman) *(22)*.

Given the severe course of measles in patients with AIDS, measles vaccination should be routinely administered to potentially susceptible, asymptomatic HIV infected children and adults. Vaccination may even be considered for those with symptomatic HIV infection if they are not severely immuno-suppressed according to conventional definitions. In areas where there is a high incidence of both HIV infection and measles, an initial dose of MCV may be offered as early as age 6 months (recorded as MCV_0). The 2 routine doses of MCV (MCV_1 and MCV_2) should then be administered to these children according to the national immunization schedule *(22)*.

CONTRAINDICATIONS TO VACCINATION *(23)* : MMR and other measles-containing vaccines are not recommended for HIV-infected persons with evidence of severe immunosuppression. MMRV is not approved for and should not be administered to a person known to be infected with HIV.

Persons with moderate or severe acute illness should not be vaccinated until the patient has improved. This precaution is intended to prevent complicating the management of an ill patient with a potential vaccine adverse reaction, such as fever. Minor illness (e.g., otitis media, mild upper respiratory infections), concurrent antibiotic therapy, and exposure to or recovery from other illness are not contraindications to measles vaccination.

Receipt of antibody-containing blood products (e.g., immune globulin, whole blood or packed red blood cells, intravenous immune globulin) may interfere with sero-conversion after measles vaccine. The length of time that such passively acquired antibody persists depends on the concentration and quantity of blood product received. For instance, it is recommended that vaccination be delayed for 3 months following receipt of immune globulin for prophylaxis of hepatitis A; a 7 to 11 months delay is recommended following administration of intravenous immune globulin, depending on the dose.

Replication of vaccine viruses can be prolonged in persons who are immunosuppressed or immunodeficient. Severe immunosuppression can be due to a variety of conditions, including congenital immunodeficiency, HIV infection, leukaemia, lymphoma, generalized malignancy, or therapy with alkylating agents, antimetabolites, radiation, or large doses of corticosteroids. For this reason, persons who are severely immunocompromised for any reason should not be given measles containing vaccine.

Women known to be pregnant should not receive measles vaccine. Pregnancy should be avoided for 4 weeks following MMR vaccine. Close contact with a pregnant woman is not a contraindication to MMR vaccination of the contact. Breastfeeding is not a contraindication to vaccination of either the woman or a breastfeeding child.

Do tuberculin skin testing (TST) at the same visit as MMR vaccination, or delay TST at least 4 weeks if MMR is given first. The least favoured option is to do TST first and administer MMR when TST is read as it delays the vaccination. TST has no effect on the response to MMR vaccination. However, measles containing vaccines may transiently suppress the response to TST in a person infected with *M. tuberculosis (23)*.

ADMINISTRATION : The reconstituted vaccine is generally injected subcutaneously, but it is also effective when administered intramuscularly.

REACTIONS : When injected into the body, the attenuated virus multiplies and induces a mild "measles" illness (fever and rash) 5 to 10 days after immunization, but in reduced frequency and severity. This may occur in 15 to 20 per cent of vaccinees. The fever may last for 1–2 days and the rash for 1–3 days. There is no cause for alarm. The vaccines now given rarely cause severe reaction *(10)*. There is no spread of the virus from the vaccinees to contacts.

IMMUNITY : The vaccine has convincingly demonstrated to provide immunity to even severely malnourished children. Immunity develops 11 to 12 days after vaccination and appears to be of long duration, probably for life. One dose of the vaccine given at 11–12 months of age appears to give 95 per cent protection and with two doses 98 per cent protection. Infants vaccinated at the age of 9 months show sero-conversion of about 90 per cent *(20)*.

CONTACTS : Susceptible contacts over the age of 9–12 months may be protected against measles with measles vaccine, provided that this is given within 3 days of exposure. This is because, the incubation period of measles induced by the vaccine is about 7 days, compared with 10 days for the naturally acquired measles.

ADVERSE EFFECTS OF VACCINE : Toxic shock syndrome (TSS) occurs when measles vaccine is contaminated or the same vial is used for more than one session on the same day or next day. The vaccine should not be used after 4 hours of opening the vial. TSS is totally preventable and reflects poor quality of immunization services. The symptoms of TSS are typical. Severe watery diarrhoea, vomiting and high fever are reported within few hours of measles vaccination. There are usually a cluster of cases as all infants vaccinated from contaminated vial will be affected. This may cause death within 48 hours. Case fatality rates are high *(20)*.

2. Immunoglobulin

Measles may be prevented by administration of immunoglobulin (human) early in the incubation period.

The dose recommended by WHO is 0.25 ml per kg of body weight (see Table 33 on page 116). It should be given within 3–4 days of exposure. The person passively immunized should be given live measles vaccine 8–12 weeks later. The need for immunoglobulin is now much reduced because of the availability of an effective live attenuated vaccine.

Global measles and rubella strategic framework 2021–2030 (MRSF) *(24)*

The measles and rubella strategic framework 2021–2030 aims to provide a high-level framework that will guide the regional and national strategies and operational plans, within the umbrella of the Immunization Agenda 2030 structure. It aims to establish convergence with other key agency strategy documents. It envisions "A world free from measles and rubella". The goal for the 2021–2030 period is to "achieve and sustain the regional measles and rubella elimination goals".

The core strategies identified in the 2012–20 MRSP will remain relevant in the post 2020 period. The strategic priorities are as follows :

1. Incorporate all measles and rubella activities, including surveillance and case management, as key components of effective PHC system in support of universal health coverage.
2. Improve ownership and accountability of measles and rubella goals and targets at all levels and improve community demand for uptake of measles and rubella containing vaccines.
3. Identify and close immunity gaps to measles and rubella by effectively utilizing all relevant contacts between individuals and the health system, establishing or strengthening new contact points where required, and using targeted approaches to reach under-served populations.
4. Leverage the life-course approach for delivery of the second routine dose of measles and rubella containing vaccines and for catch-up vaccination; and integrate measles and rubella activities with other health and non-health activities.
5. Ensure outbreak preparedness for timely detection and effective response to limit the spread of measles and rubella and reduce related morbidity and mortality.
6. Ensure continued, timely and quality supply of measles and rubella containing vaccines, vaccination supplies and laboratory reagents and that measles and rubella activities, including surveillance, are sustainably financed.
7. Foster research and innovation to overcome barriers to achieve high measles and rubella population immunity and to generate and use high quality disease and programme data.

Outbreak control measures

The following control measures have been recommended : (a) isolation for 7 days after onset of rash, (b) immunization of contacts within 2 days of exposure (if vaccine is contraindicated, immunoglobulin should be given within 3–4 days of exposure), and (c) prompt immunization at the beginning of an epidemic is essential to limit the spread.

Eradication of measles

It is believed that measles, like smallpox, is amenable to eradication. Measles immunization has in its favour the fact that only two doses are needed, and that a measles vaccine has now been developed which is more heat stable. It requires (a) achieving an immunization coverage of at least 96 per cent of children under one year of age, and that (b) the cumulation in the immunity gap be prevented.

References

1. Coovidia H. (1988). *Med. Int.* 53 : 2177.
2. Morley David (1975). *Trans.Roy.Soc.trop.Med.Hyg.*, 69:22.
3. WHO (2006), *Fact Sheet No. 286*, WHO Website.
4. WHO (2011), *Weekly Epidemiological Record,* No. 1–2, 2011.
5. WHO (2018), *Fact sheet on measles,* March 2018.
6. UNICEF and WHO (2022), *UNICEF and WHO warn of perfect storm of conditions for measles outbreak affecting children,* 27th April, 2022.
7. Govt. of India 2021, *National Health Profile of India-2021,* Central Bureau of Health Intelligence, Ministry of Health and Family Welfare, New Delhi.
8. WHO 2014, *World Health Statistics 2014*.
9. Govt. of India (2020), *Annual Report 2019–20,* Ministry of Health and Family Welfare, New Delhi.
10. Jawetz, Melnick, and Adelberg's *Medical Microbiology,* 24th ed. (2007), A Lange publication.
11. WHO (1978), *Tech.Rep.Ser.,* 629.
12. Pan American Health Organization (1978). *Bull PAHO,* 12 (2): 162.
13. Morley David (1973). *Paediatric Priorities in the Developing World,* Butterworths.
14. Katz, M and Stiehm, E.R. (1977). *Pediatrics,* 59 : 490.
15. Dossetor, J et al (1977) *B M J 1* : 1633 – 35.
16. Last, John M. (1980). *Maxcy–Rosenau : Public Health and Preventive Medicine,* 11th ed., Appleton–Century–Crofts, New York.
17. Gershon, A.A. (1979). In *Principles and Practice of Infectious Diseases,* Mandell, G.L. et al (eds), Wiley.
18. WHO (2017), *Weekly Epidemiological Record,* No. 17, 2017.
19. Lawrence, M. et al. *Current Medical Diagnosis and Treatment,* 47th Ed. (2008), A Lange Medical Publication.
20. WHO 2009, *Weekly Epidemiological Record,* No. 35, 28 Aug. 2009.
21. Alter Milton (1976). *Lancet,* 1: 456.
22. WHO (2020), *Summary of WHO position papers - Recommended Routine Immunization for Children.*
23. CDC (2019), *Epidemiology and Prevention of Vaccine Preventable Diseases,* Yellow Book.
24. Measles and Rubella Initiative (2020), *Measles and Rubella Strategic Framework, 2021–2030.*

RUBELLA
(GERMAN MEASLES)

Rubella or german measles is an acute childhood infection, usually mild, of short duration (approximately 3 days) and accompanied by low–grade fever, lymphadenopathy and a maculopapular rash. Infection in early pregnancy may result in serious congenital defects, including death of the foetus. The disease is worldwide in distribution and tends to occur in epidemics. In pre- vaccination era epidemics occurred every 5 to 9 years. However, extent and periodicity of rubella are highly variable in industrialized and developing countries. Worldwide over 100,000 babies are born with congenital rubella syndrome every year *(1, 2)*.

History

Rubella was considered a mild and benign disease until 1941 when Norman Gregg, an ophthalmologist reported an epidemic of congenital cataracts associated with other congenital defects in children born to mothers who had rubella during their pregnancies *(3)*. This discovery changed the concept that rubella is not merely a benign disease of childhood but also one with teratogenic potential. In 1962, the virus was isolated; in 1967, an attenuated vaccine was developed.

Epidemiological determinants

Agent factors

(a) AGENT : Rubella is caused by an RNA virus of the togavirus family. Only one antigenic type of the virus seems to exist. The virus has been recovered from the nasopharynx, throat, blood, CSF and urine. It can be propagated in cell culture. (b) SOURCE OF INFECTION : Clinical or subclinical cases of rubella. A large number of rubella infections are, in fact, subclinical. This represents one of the major differences between measles and rubella. There is no known carrier state for postnatally acquired rubella. Infants born with congenital rubella may shed the virus for many months. The vaccine virus is not communicable. (c) PERIOD OF COMMUNICABILITY: Rubella is much less communicable than measles, probably because of the absence of coughing in rubella. It is difficult to state the exact period of infectivity. It probably extends from a week before symptoms to about a week after rash appears. Infectivity is greatest 1–5 days after the appearance of rash *(1)*.

Host factors

(a) AGE: Mainly a disease of childhood particularly in the age group 3 to 10 years. Persons older than 15 years now account for over 70 per cent cases in developed countries – this is similar to the changing epidemiological pattern with measles, following widespread immunization campaigns against the disease. (b) IMMUNITY : One attack results in life-long immunity; second attacks are rare. Infants of immune mothers are protected for 4 to 6 months. It is estimated that 10 to 40 per cent of the population could reach adulthood without experiencing rubella infection in the absence of immunization.

Environmental factors

Disease usually occurs in a seasonal pattern i.e. in temperate zones during the late winter and spring, with epidemics every 4–9 years.

Transmission

The virus is transmitted directly from person to person by droplets from nose and throat, and droplet nuclei (aerosols), from one week before onset of rash to one week after it has faded. The portal of entry is *via* the respiratory route. The virus is maintained in human population by chain transmission. The virus can cross the placenta (vertical transmission) and infect the foetus *in utero*, leading to congenital rubella in the newborn.

Incubation period

2 to 3 weeks; average 18 days.

Clinical features

A large percentage of infections (20–50 per cent) are asymptomatic *(2)*. In a typical case, the clinical features comprise the following: (a) PRODROMAL : The prodromal symptoms (coryza, sore throat, low–grade fever) herald the onset of viraemia. They are generally mild and insignificant, and less frequent in children. (b) LYMPHADENOPATHY : In susceptible individuals, the enlargement of the post–auricular, occipital and posterior cervical lymph nodes appears as early as 5–10 days before the appearance of the rash. This, however, is not pathognomonic since cases of clinical rubella without enlargement of lymph nodes have been documented *(2)*. The glands may be found enlarged for 10 to 14 days after the rash. (c) RASH: The rash is often the first indication of the disease in children. It appears first on the face, usually within 24 hours of the onset of prodromal symptoms. It is a minute, discrete, pinkish, macular rash and not confluent as the rash of measles and it may be pruritic. Conjunctivitis may occur. The rash spreads rapidly to the trunk and extremities, by which time it is often no longer apparent on the face. The rash spreads much faster and clears more rapidly than the rash of measles. It disappears altogether by the third day. The rash is an inconstant feature of the disease; it is absent in subclinical cases. The incidence of rubella infection without rash may be upto 25 per cent *(4)*. (d) COMPLICATIONS : In rare instances arthralgia may occur in several joints in adults, especially young women. Encephalitis is very rare. Thrombocytopenic purpura has also been observed as a complication. Mention has been made already about the congenital malformations.

Diagnosis

Because of its mildness and variability of symptoms, the disease can go unrecognized unless it is an epidemic. A definitive diagnosis of rubella is possible only through virus isolation and serology. Throat swabs should be cultured for virus isolation; it takes longer than serological diagnosis. The haemagglutination inhibition (HI) test is a standard serological test for rubella. However, serum must be pretreated to remove non-specific inhibitors before testing. ELISA tests are preferred because serum pretreatment is not required and they can be adapted to detect specific IgM. Detection of IgG is evidence of immunity because there is only one serotype of rubella virus. To accurately confirm a recent rubella infection, either a rise in antibody titer must be demonstrated between two serum samples taken at least 10 days apart or rubella-specific IgM must be detected in a single specimen. It is critically important in a pregnant woman *(6)*.

CONGENITAL RUBELLA SYNDROME (CRS)

Congenital rubella syndrome (CRS) refers to infants born with defects secondary to intrauterine infection or who manifest symptoms or signs of intrauterine infection sometime after birth *(5)*. Congenital infection is considered to have occurred if the infant has IgM rubella antibodies shortly after birth (as IgM antibodies do not cross the placenta, their presence indicate that they must have been synthesized by the infant *in utero*) or if IgG antibodies persist for more than 6 months, by which time maternally derived antibodies would have disappeared. Intrauterine infection with rubella is associated with chronic persistence of the virus in the newborn. At birth, virus is easily detectable in pharyngeal secretions, multiple organs, cerebrospinal fluid, urine, and rectal swabs. Viral excretion may last for 12–18 months after birth, but the level of shedding gradually decreases with age *(6)*.

Rubella infection inhibits cell division, and this is probably the reason for congenital malformations and low birth weight *(7)*. The classic triad of congenital defects are deafness, cardiac malformations and cataracts.

Rubella infection in a woman who becomes infected (i.e. with asymptomatic or symptomatic disease) just before conception and upto the first 8–10 weeks of gestation causes multiple congenital abnormalities in upto 90% of infections, and may result in miscarriage or stillbirth. Congenital anomalies associated with maternal rubella infection are rare after the 16th week of pregnancy, although sensorineural hearing deficits may occur after exposure upto week 20 of gestation. The defects associated with CRS include ophthalmic (e.g. cataracts, microphthalmia, glaucoma, pigmentary retinopathy, chorioretinitis), auditory (e.g. sensorineural deafness), cardiac (e.g. peripheral pulmonary artery stenosis, patent ductus arteriosus or ventricular septal defects) and craniofacial (e.g. microcephaly) anomalies. CRS can also present with other manifestations, such as meningoencephalitis, hepatosplenomegaly, hepatitis, thrombocytopenia, interstitial pneumonitis and radio-lucency in the long bones (a characteristic radiological pattern of CRS). Infants who survive the neonatal period may have serious developmental disabilities (such as autism, visual and hearing impairment), and developmental delay. Viral shedding can continue in CRS cases beyond 1 year of age, which may result in virus transmission *(2)*.

Prevention

The currently used rubella vaccines are based on the live attenuated RA 27/3 strain. Most rubella vaccines are available in combination with other vaccine antigens such as measles, mumps and varicella (MR, MMR, MMRV, respectively) and also in a monovalent formulation. Each dose of an RCV contains a minimum number of infectious units (≥1000 plaque-forming units or 50% cell culture infectious dose). When stored at 4°C, most RCVs have a shelf-life of 2–3 years. Monovalent rubella, MR and MMR vaccines should be stored at 2–8°C, protected from light. Diluent vials may be stored at ambient temperatures but must never be frozen. The standard volume of a single dose of RCV is 0.5 ml, and the vaccine is usually injected subcutaneously. The preferred site of injection is the anterolateral thigh or outer aspect of upper arm, depending on the age of the individual *(2)*.

Because rubella is not as highly infectious as measles and because the effectiveness of 1 dose of an RCV is >95%, even at 9 months of age, only 1 dose of rubella vaccine is required to achieve rubella elimination if high coverage is achieved. However, when combined with measles vaccination, it may be easier to implement a second dose of RCV's using the same combined MR vaccine or MMR vaccine for both doses. RCV's can be administered concurrently with inactivated vaccines. As a general rule, live vaccines should be given either simultaneously with RCV's, or at least 4 weeks apart. An exception to this is oral polio vaccine, which can be given at any time before or after RCV's without interfering in the response to either vaccine. Interference may occur between MMR and yellow fever vaccines if they are simultaneously administered to children <2 years of age *(8)*.

The vaccine induced immunity persists for life time. In order to provide direct protection against rubella, all non-pregnant women of reproductive age who are not already vaccinated or who are sero-negative for rubella receive one dose of RCV *(2)*.

Precautions and contraindications

RCVs should not be given to anyone who has experienced a severe allergic reaction after a previous vaccine dose or vaccine component. It is recommended not to provide the vaccine to those with active TB or severe immunodeficiency (including individuals with symptomatic HIV infection, AIDS, congenital immune disorders, malignancies or aggressive immunosuppressive therapy).

Rubella vaccination should be avoided in pregnancy because of a theoretical (but never demonstrated) risk of teratogenic outcomes. Women planning a pregnancy are advised to avoid pregnancy for 1 month after rubella vaccination. Inadvertent vaccination with RCV during pregnancy is not an indication for terminating the pregnancy. People who receive blood products wait at least 3 months before vaccination with RCV, and, if possible, avoid administration of blood products for 2 weeks after vaccination *(2)*.

Global measles and rubella strategic framework (2021–2030)

Refer to page 168 for the details.

References

1. WHO (2016), *Rubella Fact sheet*, March 2016.
2. WHO (2020), *Weekly Epidemiological Record*, No. 27, 3rd July 2020.
3. Fovbes, J.A. (1969). *American J. Dis.Child.*, 118 :5.
4. Valman, H.B. (1981), *Brit.Med.J.* 283 : 1038.
5. Walter, A.O. et al (1984). *JAMA* 251 : 1988.
6. Jewetz, Melnick and Adelberg's *Medical Microbiology*, 28th ed., 2019.
7. Dudgeon, J.A. (1969). *Am.J.Dis.Child*, 118 : 35.
8. WHO (2020), *Summary of WHO Position Papers - Recommended Routine Immunization for Children.*

MUMPS

An acute infectious disease caused by an RNA virus classified as genus *Rubulavirus* of the family paramyxoviridae which has a predilection for glandular and nervous tissues. Clinically, the disease is recognized by non-suppurative enlargement and tenderness of one or both the parotid glands. Other organs may also be involved. Constitutional symptoms vary, or may be inapparent. The disease occurs throughout the world. Although morbidity rate tends to be high, mortality rate is negligible.

In most parts of the world, the annual incidence of mumps in the absence of immunization is in the range of 100–1000 cases/100,000 population with epidemic peak every 2–5 years. Natural infection with this virus is thought to confer lifelong protection *(1)*.

Agent factors

(a) AGENT : The causative agent, *Myxovirus parotiditis* is a RNA virus of the myxovirus family. The virus can be grown readily in chick embryo or tissue culture. There is only one serotype. (b) SOURCE OF INFECTION : Both clinical and subclinical cases. Subclinical cases which account for 30–40 per cent of all cases *(2)* appear to be responsible for maintaining the cycle of infection. The virus can be isolated from the saliva or from swabs taken from the surface of Stenson's duct. Virus has also been found in the blood, urine, human milk and on occasion in the CSF. (c) PERIOD OF COMMUNICABILITY : Usually 4–6 days before the onset of symptoms and a week or more thereafter. The period of maximum infectivity is just before and at the onset of parotitis. Once the swelling of the glands has subsided, the case may be regarded as no longer infectious. (d) SECONDARY ATTACK RATE : Estimated to be about 86 per cent.

Host factors

(a) AGE AND SEX : Mumps is the most frequent cause of parotitis in children in the age group 5–9 years. The average

age of incidence of mumps is higher than with measles, chickenpox or whooping cough. However, no age is exempt if there is no previous immunity. The disease tends to be more severe in adults than in children. (b) IMMUNITY : One attack, clinical or subclinical, is assumed to induce lifelong immunity. There is only one antigenic type of mumps virus, and it does not exhibit significant antigenic variation *(3)*. Most infants below the age of 6 months are immune because of maternal antibodies.

Environmental factors

Mumps is largely an endemic disease. Cases occur throughout the year, but the peak incidence is in winter and spring. Epidemics are often associated with overcrowding.

Mode of transmission

The disease is spread mainly by droplet infection and after direct contact with an infected person.

Incubation period

Varies from 2 to 4 weeks, usually 14–18 days.

Clinical features

Mumps is a generalized virus infection. In 30–40 per cent of cases mumps infection is clinically non-apparent. In clinically apparent cases, it is characterized by pain and swelling in either one or both the parotid glands but may also involve the sublingual and submandibular glands. Often the child complains of "ear ache" on the affected side prior to the onset of swelling. There may be pain and stiffness on opening the mouth before the swelling of the gland is evident. Mumps may also affect the testes, pancreas, CNS, ovaries, prostate, etc. In severe cases, there may be fever, headache and other constitutional symptoms which may last from 3–5 days. The swelling subsides slowly over 1–2 weeks.

COMPLICATIONS : Though frequent, are not serious. These include orchitis, ovaritis, pancreatitis, meningo-encephalitis, thyroiditis, neuritis, hepatitis and myocarditis. Testicular swelling and tenderness denote orchitis, which is the most common extrasalivary gland manifestation of mumps in adults. It is unilateral in about 75 per cent of cases. High fever usually accompanies orchitis, which develops typically 7–10 days after the onset of parotitis in about 25–40 per cent of post-pubertal men *(4)*. Bilateral orchitis is rare and the assumption that mumps orchitis may lead to sterility is ill-founded *(5)*. Upper abdominal pain, nausea and vomiting suggest pancreatitis. Mumps is a leading cause of pancreatitis in children. It occurs in about 4 per cent of patients *(6)*. Lower abdominal pain and ovarian enlargement suggest oophoritis which occurs in 5 per cent of post pubertal women, usually unilateral *(4)*. While some instances of diabetes have occurred in children following mumps infection, a causal relationship has yet to be demonstrated *(5)*. Rarer complications include nerve deafness, polyarthritis, hydrocephalus, encephalitis, cerebellar ataxia, facial palsy and transverse myelitis. Encephalitis is associated with cerebral oedema, serious neurologic manifestations and sometimes death *(4)*. Upto 15% of mumps patients may develop meningitis, and a much smaller proportion (0.02–0.03%) may develop encephalitis. Mumps is one of the main infectious causes of sensorineural deafness, which affects approximately 5 per 100,000 mumps cases *(6)*.

Mumps infection in the first trimester of pregnancy is associated with a 25% incidence of spontaneous abortion, although congenital malformations following mumps infection in pregnancy have not been reported *(6)*.

Prevention

VACCINATION : Highly effective live attenuated vaccine is now available for the prevention of mumps. Widely-used live attenuated mumps vaccine strains include the Jeryl-Lynn, RIT 4385, Leningrad-3, L-Zagreb and Urabe strains. Live attenuated mumps vaccine strains used only on a limited scale include the Hoshino, Torii and NKM-46 strains. The WHO recommends that the Rubini mumps vaccine strain should not be used in national immunization programmes because of its demonstrated low effectiveness *(6)*.

A single dose (0.5 ml) intramuscularly produces detectable antibodies in 95 per cent of vaccinees. The duration of long-term immunity is not known. It is recommended for routine immunization for children over 1 year of age, either alone or in combination with other virus vaccines, eg. in MMR vaccine or as a quadrivalent vaccine with varicella. A second dose is recommended for children at 4–6 years of age i.e., before starting the school. The current mumps strain (Jeryl Lynm) has the lowest associated incidence of post vaccine aseptic meningitis (from 1 in 150,000 to 1 in 1.8 million). There are no known cases of long-term sequelae associated with mumps vaccination *(4)*.

Countries including mumps vaccines in their national immunization programme are advised by WHO to set disease control targets (control or elimination) and to design their mumps immunization strategy accordingly. Strategies to achieve mumps elimination include very high coverage with the first dose of mumps vaccine, ensuring a second opportunity for vaccination and conducting catch-up immunization of susceptible cohorts *(6)*.

As with most other live virus vaccines, mumps vaccine should not be administered to pregnant women, patients receiving immunosuppressive therapy or those who are severely ill. For further details, please refer to page 164.

Mumps surveillance *(6)*

Case definitions : WHO recommends the following case definitions for mumps surveillance :

a. *Clinical mumps* : acute onset of unilateral or bilateral tender, self-limited swelling of the parotid or other salivary gland, lasting 2 or more days and without other apparent cause.

b. *Laboratory confirmed mumps* : a patient with clinical mumps and laboratory confirmation by positive-mumps IgM antibody (without mumps immunization in the previous 6 weeks) or; sero-conversion with 4–fold or greater rise in mumps IgG titre; or isolation of mumps virus from saliva, urine or cerebrospinal fluid.

c. *Epidemiologically–confirmed mumps* : a patient with clinical mumps who is epidemiologically linked to a laboratory–confirmed mumps case.

Control

The control of mumps is difficult because the disease is infectious before a diagnosis can be made. The long and variable incubation period, and the occurrence of subclinical cases make the control of spread difficult. However, cases should be isolated till the clinical manifestations subside. Steps should be taken to disinfect the articles used by the patient. Contacts should be kept under surveillance.

References

1. WHO (2007), *Weekly Epidemiological Record*, 16th Feb, No. 7, 2007.
2. Christie, A.B. (1980). *Infectious Disease : Epidemiology and Clinical Practice*, 3rd ed., Churchill Livingstone.
3. Jawetz, E. et al (2007), *Medical Microbiology*, 24th ed., Lange Medical Book.
4. Stephen, J. McPhee et al (2008), *Current Medical Diagnosis and Treatment*, 47th ed., A Lange Medical Book.
5. Feldman, Harry A (1977) in *Viral Infections of Humans: Epidemiology and Control*, Evans Alfred, S. et al (eds), 2nd ed., Plenum Medical, New York and London.
6. WHO (2005), *Weekly Epidemiological Record*, No. 48, 2nd Dec. 2005.

INFLUENZA

Influenza is an acute respiratory tract infection caused by influenza virus, of which there are 4 types – A, B, C and D. All known epidemics are caused by influenza A and B strains. The disease is characterized by sudden onset of chills, malaise, fever, muscular pains and cough.

Problem statement

Influenza is truly an international disease. It occurs in all countries and affects millions of people every year. Its behaviour is unpredictable. It may occur in several forms. It may smoulder in a community without clinical recognition, being manifest only by serological surveys. It may occur in pandemics every 10–40 years due to major antigenic changes, as occurred in 1918 (Spanish influenza), 1957 (Asian influenza) and 1968 (Hong Kong influenza) *(1)*. More recently, influenza A (H_1N_1) virus of swine origin emerged in Mexico during the spring of 2009 and was given name – pandemic influenza A (H_1N_1) 2009 virus. It spreads with travellers worldwide, resulting in the first influenza pandemic of this century. In between pandemics, epidemics tend to occur at intervals of 2–3 years in case of influenza A and 3–6 years in the case of influenza B – but the periodicity is not regular as in the case of measles or whooping cough because several strains of the virus may be in simultaneous circulation, which means that there may be outbreaks of influenza practically every year, and sometimes even twice a year *(2)*.

Once an epidemic begins, the picture is quite characteristic. Preceded by a few early cases, there is a sudden outburst of the disease. This may be indicated by reports of increased febrile respiratory illness in children, followed by the same in adults. The next event is increased hospitalization of cases and sickness–absenteeism in schools and places of work. Attack rates tend to be high, varying from 5 to 10 per cent in adults and 20–30 per cent in children. The peak of the epidemic is reached in 3–4 weeks, before tending to decline. The time scale is compressed for smaller geographic areas *(1)*. The unique features of influenza epidemics are the suddenness with which they arise, and the speed and ease with which they spread. The short incubation period, large number of subclinical cases, high proportion of susceptible population, short duration of immunity, and absence of cross-immunity, all contribute to its rapid spread. Worldwide, the annual epidemics are estimated to result in about 3–5 million cases of severe illness and about 290,000 to 650,000 deaths *(3)*. The fate of the virus during inter-epidemic periods is not known. Possible explanations include transmission of virus to extra-human reservoirs (pigs, horses, birds), latent infection in humans or continuous transfer from one human to another. This explains the occurrence of sporadic cases.

At present three types of influenza virus are circulating in the world: A(H_1N_1), A(H_3N_2) and B viruses. Influenza A predominated in most countries accounting for 59 per cent of all influenza viruses detected.

SEASONAL INFLUENZA

Epidemiological determinants

Agent factors

(a) AGENT : Influenza viruses are classified within the family Orthomyxoviridae. There are four viral subtypes, namely influenza type A, type B, type C and type D. These four viruses are antigenically distinct. There is no cross immunity between them. Of importance are the influenza A and B viruses which are responsible for epidemics of disease throughout the world *(4)*. Influenza A virus has 2 distinct surface antigens – the haemagglutinin (H) and the neuraminidase (N) antigens. The H antigen initiates infection following attachment of the virus to susceptible cells. The N antigen is responsible for the release of the virus from the infected cell. The currently identified subtypes are 18 HA and 11 NA. Humans are generally infected by viruses of the subtype H1, H2 or H3, and N1 or N2. Type B virus does not exhibit antigenic shifts and is not divided into subtypes.

The influenza A virus is unique among the viruses because it is frequently subject to antigenic variation, both major and minor. When there is a sudden complete or major change, it is called a **shift,** and when the antigenic change is gradual over a period of time, it is called a **drift**. Antigenic shift appears to result from genetic recombination of human with animal or avian virus, providing a major antigenic change. This can cause a major epidemic or pandemic involving most or all age groups. Antigenic drift involves "point mutation" in the gene owing to selection pressure by immunity in the host population. Antigenic changes occur to a lesser degree in the B group influenza viruses. Influenza C appears to be antigenically stable.

Since the isolation of the virus A in 1933, major antigenic changes have occurred twice – once in 1957 (H_2N_2) and again in 1968 (H_3N_2). Strains occurring between 1946 and 1957 have been called (H_1N_1) strains. The shift in 1968 involved only the H antigen.

(b) RESERVOIR OF INFECTION : It has become increasingly evident that a major reservoir of influenza virus exists in animals and birds. Many influenza viruses have been isolated from a wide variety of animals and birds (e.g., swine, horses, dogs, cats, domestic poultry, wild birds, etc). Some of these include the major H and N antigens related to human strains. It is hypothesized. There is an increasing evidence that the animal reservoirs provide new strains of influenza virus by recombination between the influenza viruses of man, animals and birds.

(c) SOURCE OF INFECTION : Usually a case or subclinical case. During epidemics, a large number of mild and asymptomatic infections occur, which play an important role in the spread of infection. The secretions of the respiratory tract are infective.

(d) PERIOD OF INFECTIVITY : Virus is present in the nasopharynx from 1 to 2 days before and 1 to 2 days after onset of symptoms.

Host factors

(a) AGE AND SEX : Influenza affects all ages and both

sexes. In general, the attack rate is lower among adults. Children constitute an important link in the transmission chain. The highest mortality rate during an epidemic occurs among certain high-risk groups in the population such as old people (generally over 65 years of age), children under 18 months, and persons with diabetes or chronic heart disease, kidney and respiratory ailments *(5)*. (b) HUMAN MOBILITY : This is an important factor in the spread of infection. (c) IMMUNITY : Immunity to influenza is subtype-specific. Antibodies against HA and NA are important in immunity to influenza. Resistance to initiation of infection is related to antibody against HA, which neutralizes the virus, whereas decreased severity of disease and decreased ability to transmit virus to contacts are related to antibody directed against the NA. Antibodies against ribonucleoprotein are type-specific and are useful in typing viral isolates as in influenza A and B. Protection correlates with both serum antibodies and secretory IgA antibodies in nasal secretions. The local secretory antibody is probably important in preventing infection. Serum antibodies persist for many months, whereas secretory antibodies are shorter-lived (usually only few months). Antibody also modifies the course of illness. A person with low titres of antibody may be infected but will experience a mild form of illness. Immunity can be incomplete as reinfection with the same virus can occur. The three types of influenza viruses are antigenically unrelated and therefore induce no cross-protection. When a viral type undergoes antigenic drift, a person with pre-existing antibody to the original strain may suffer only mild infection with the new strain *(6)*. Antibodies appear in about 7 days after the attack and reach a maximum level in about 2 weeks. After 8 to 12 months, the antibody level drops to pre-infection level.

Environmental factors

(a) Season : The seasonal incidence is striking, epidemics usually occurring in winter months in the Northern Hemisphere and in the winter or rainy season in the Southern Hemisphere *(4)*. In tropical countries, influenza virus circulates throughout the year with one or two peaks during rainy season. *(b) Overcrowding* : Enhances transmission. The attack rates are high in close population groups, e.g., schools, institutions, ships, etc.

Mode of transmission

Influenza is spread mainly from person to person by droplet infection or droplet nuclei created by sneezing, coughing or talking. The portal of entry of the virus is the respiratory tract.

Incubation period

1–4 days.

Pathogenesis and clinical features

The virus enters the respiratory tract and causes inflammation and necrosis of superficial epithelium of the tracheal and bronchial mucosa, followed by secondary bacterial invasion. There is no viraemia. Both the viruses cause much the same symptoms – fever, chills, aches and pains, coughing and generalized weakness. Fever lasts from 1–5 days, averaging 3 days in adults. Frequent complications are acute sinusitis, otitis media, purulent bronchitis and pneumonia. The most dreaded complication is pneumonia, which should be suspected if fever persists beyond 4 or 5 days or recurs abruptly after convalescence *(1)*.

Reye syndrome (fatty liver with encephalopathy) is a rare and severe complication of influenza, usually A and B type, particularly in young children between 2 and 16 years of age. It consists of rapidly progressive hepatic failure and encephalopathy, and there is about 10–40 per cent mortality rate. The pathogenesis is unknown, but the syndrome is associated with aspirin use in a variety of viral infections *(7)*.

AVIAN INFLUENZA *(8)*
(BIRD FLU)

Avian influenza refers to a large group of different influenza viruses that primarily affect birds. On rare occasions, these bird viruses can infect other species, including pigs and humans. The vast majority of avian influenza viruses do not infect humans. However, avian H_5N_1 is a strain with pandemic potential, since it might ultimately adapt into a strain that is contagious among humans. Once this adaptation occurs, it will no longer be a bird virus – it will be a human influenza virus. Influenza pandemics are caused by new influenza viruses that have adapted to humans. Health experts have been monitoring a new and extremely severe influenza virus – the H_5N_1 strain – for almost 15 years. Fortunately, the virus does not jump easily from birds to humans or spread readily and sustainably among humans. Once a fully contagious virus emerges, its global spread is considered inevitable.

Transmission

Human infections with avian influenza viruses, though rare, have been reported sporadically. Human infections are primarily acquired through direct contact with infected live or dead poultry birds or contaminated environments, such as live bird markets.

Incubation period

2–5 days.

Diagnosis

Diagnosis is confirmed by RT-PCR. Rapid influenza diagnostic tests (RDTs) are available, but they have lower sensitivity compared to RT-PCR.

Treatment

Some antiviral drugs, notably oseltamivir and zanamivir can reduce the duration of viral replication and improve prospects of survival.

Prevention

Public health management includes personal protective measures like regular hand washing and proper drying; good respiratory hygiene (covering mouth and nose when coughing or sneezing); early self-isolation; avoid close contact with sick people; and avoid touching eyes, mouth and nose.

Vaccine

In the year 2007, a vaccine for bird flu was licensed, this vaccine is for people 18 years through 64 years of age. It is an inactivated influenza vaccine given in two doses, 28 days apart. The recipient can have pain and tenderness at the injection site, headache, muscle pain and general ill feeling.

Some other vaccines were approved, but at the time of pandemic, (as the H_5N_1 continually mutates), the current sample of H_5N_1 cannot be depended upon to work.

PANDEMIC INFLUENZA A (H_1N_1) 2009 (SWINE FLU)

The pandemic influenza A (H_1N_1) 2009 virus differs in its pathogenicity from seasonal influenza in two key aspects. First, as the majority of human population has little or no pre-existing immunity to the virus, the impact of the infection has been in a wider age range, in particular among children and young adults. Secondly, the virus can infect the lower respiratory tract and can cause rapidly progressive pneumonia, especially in children and young to middle-aged adults.

Following its emergence in March 2009, pandemic A (H_1N_1) 2009 virus spread rapidly throughout the world, leading to the declaration of an inlfuenza pandemic by WHO on 11th June 2009 *(9)*. The world is now in post-pandemic period. In India it causes local outbreaks. During 2020, India reported 2,752 cases and 44 deaths, a case fatality rate of 1.6 per cent *(10)*.

Based on knowledge about past pandemics, the (H_1N_1) 2009 virus is expected to continue to circulate as a seasonal virus for some years to come. While level of concern is now greatly diminished, vigilance on the part of national health authorities remains important, when the behaviour of H_1N_1 virus as a seasonal virus cannot be reliably predicted *(11)*. On 26th September 2011 WHO has adapted a new nomenclature as Influenza A (H_1N_1) pdm09 *(12)*.

Incubation period

The incubation period appears to be approximately 1–4 days, but could range upto 7 days.

Case definitions *(13)*

Suspected case : A suspected case of influenza A (H_1N_1) 2009 is defined as a person with acute febrile respiratory illness (fever ≥ 38°C) with onset (a) within 7 days of close contact with a person who is a confirmed case of influenza A (H_1N_1) 2009 virus infection, or; (b) within 7 days of travel to areas where there are one or more confirmed cases, or (c) resides in a community where there are one or more confirmed influenza A (H_1N_1) 2009 cases.

Probable case : A probable case of influenza A (H_1N_1) 2009 virus infection is defined as a person with an acute febrile respiratory illness who : (1) is positive for influenza A, but unsubtypable for H_1 and H_3 by influenza RT–PCR or reagents used to detect seasonal influenza virus infection, or; (2) is positive for influenza A by an influenza rapid test or an influenza immunofluoresence assay (IFA) and meets criteria for a suspected case, or; (3) individual with a clinically compatible illness who died of an unexplained acute respiratory illness who is considered to be epidemiollogically linked to a probable or confirmed case.

Confirmed case : A confirmed case of pandemic influenza A (H_1N_1) 2009 virus infection is defined as a person with an acute febrile respiratory illness with laboratory confirmed influenza A (H_1N_1) 2009 virus infection at WHO approved laboratory by one or more of the following tests :

a. Real Time PCR
b. Viral culture
c. Four–fold rise in influenza A (H_1N_1) virus specific neutralizing antibodies.

Clinical features *(14)*

A wide clinical spectrum of disease ranging from non-febrile mild upper respiratory illness, febrile influenza like illness (ILI), to severe or even fatal complications including rapidly progressive pneumonia has been described. The case fatality rate is smilar to seasonal influenza i.e. about 0.5 per cent; however this could change *(15)*. The clinical features are as described below :

(a) *Uncomplicated influenza*

(1) ILI symptoms include : fever, cough, sore throat, rhinorrhoea, headache, muscle pain, and malaise, but no shortness of breath and no dyspnoea. Patients may present with some or all of these symptoms.
(2) Gastrointestinal illness may also be present, such as diarrhoea and/or vomiting, especially in children, but without evidence of dehydration.

(b) *Complicated or severe influenza*

(1) Presenting clinical (e.g. shortness of breath/ dyspnoea, tachypnea, hypoxia) and/or radiological signs of lower respiratory tract disease (e.g. pneumonia), central nervous system (CNS) involvement (e.g. encephalopathy, encephalitis), severe dehydration, or presenting secondary complications, such as renal failure, multiorgan failure, and septic shock. Other complications can include rhabdomyolysis and myocarditis.
(2) Exacerbation of underlying chronic disease, including asthma, COPD, chronic hepatic or renal failure, diabetes, or other cardiovascular conditions.
(3) Any other condition or clinical presentation requiring hospital admission for clinical management.
(4) Any of the signs of progressive disease.

As COVID-19 and influenza, both are respiratory illnesses, they share many similarities. It is very important to differentiate these both diseases so as to take timely appropriate action to manage the disease. The differentiating points are as follows *(16)* :

	COVID-19	INFLUENZA
Incubation period	2–14 days	1–4 days
Common symptoms	– Fever – Cough – Fatigue – Shortness of breath – Loss of smell – Loss of taste	– Fever – Chills – Cough – Fatigue – Body aches and pains – Headache – Runny or stuffy nose – Sore throat
Less common symptoms	– Body aches and pains – Headache – Runny or stuffy nose – Sore throat – Nausea or diarrhoea	– Nausea or diarrhoea
Symptom onset	– Gradual	– Rapid
Vaccine and medications	– Vaccines are available	– Seasonal and swine flu vaccine and antiviral medication available.

Signs and symptoms of progressive disease

Patients who present initially with uncomplicated influenza may progress to more severe disease. Progression can be rapid (i.e. within 24 hours). The following are some of the indicators of progression, which would necessitate an urgent review of patient management.

(a) Symptoms and signs suggesting oxygen impairment or cardiopulmonary insufficiency :
   - Shortness of breath (with activity or at rest), difficulty in breathing, turning blue, bloody or coloured sputum, chest pain, and low blood pressure;
   - In children, fast or laboured breathing; and
   - Hypoxia, as indicated by pulse oximetry.

(b) Symptoms and signs suggesting CNS complications:
   - Altered mental status, unconsciousness, drowsiness, or difficult to awaken and recurring or persistent convulsions (seizures), confusion, severe weakness, or paralysis.

(c) Evidence of sustained virus replication or invasive secondary bacterial infection based on laboratory testing or clinical signs (e.g. persistent high fever and other symptoms beyond 3 days).

(d) Severe dehydration, manifested as decreased activity, dizziness, decreased urine output, and lethargy.

Risk factors for severe disease *(14)*

Risk factors for severe disease from pandemic influenza A (H_1N_1) 2009 virus infection reported to date are considered similar to those risk factors identified for complications from seasonal influenza. These include the following groups :

(1) Infants and young children, in particular <2 years

(2) Pregnant women

(3) Persons of any age with chronic pulmonary disease (e.g. asthma, COPD)

(4) Persons of any age with chronic cardiac disease (e.g. congestive cardiac failure)

(5) Persons with metabolic disorders (e.g. diabetes)

(6) Persons with chronic renal disease, chronic hepatic disease, certain neurological conditions (including neuromuscular, neurocognitive, and seizure disorders), haemoglobinopathies, or immunosuppression, whether due to primary immunosuppressive conditions, such as HIV infection, or secondary conditions, such as immunosuppressive medication or malignancy

(7) Children receiving chronic aspirin therapy

(8) Persons aged 65 years and older.

A higher risk of severe complications from pandemic influenza A (H_1N_1) 2009 virus infection has also been reported in individuals who are obese particularly in those who are morbidly obese.

Laboratory diagnosis *(14)*

Laboratory diagnosis of pandemic influenza A (H_1N_1) 2009 virus, especially at the beginning of a new community outbreak or for unusual cases, has important implications for case managment, such as infection control procedures, consideration of antiviral treatment options and avoiding the inappropriate use of antibiotics. Currently, the diagnostic tests can be done by specialized laboratories in many countries. Reverse transcriptase polymerase chain reaction (RT–PCR) will provide the most timely and sensitive detection of the infection.

Clinical specimens to be collected for laboratory diagnosis are respiratory samples. Samples from the upper respiratory tract, including a combination of nasal or nasopharyngeal samples, and a throat swab are advised. Recent evidence supports viral replication and recovery of pandemic A (H_1N_1) 2009 virus from lower respiratory tract samples (tracheal and bronchial aspirates) in patients presenting lower respiratory tract symptoms and in these patients, such samples have higher diagnostic yields than samples from the upper respiratory tract.

When influenza viruses are known to be circulating in a community, patients presenting with features of uncomplicated influenza can be diagnosed on clinical and epidemiological grounds. All patients should be instructed to return for follow-up, should they develop any signs or symptoms of progressive disease or fail to improve within 72 hours of the onset of symptoms.

Diagnostic testing, when available, should be prioritized for patients in whom confirmation of influenza virus infection may affect clinical management, including patients considered at-risk and/or those with complicated, severe, or progressive respiratory illness. In addition, results of diagnostic testing may also be valuable in guiding infection control practices and management of a patient's close contacts. Under no circumstances should influenza diagnostic testing delay initiation of infection control practices or antiviral treatment, if pandemic influenza A (H_1N_1) 2009 disease is suspected clinically and epidemiologically *(14)*.

Several rapid influenza diagnostic tests including (so-called *point-of-care* diagnostic tests) are commercially available. However, studies indicate that rapid diagnostic tests miss many infections with pandemic (H_1N_1) 2009 virus and, therefore, negative results cannot rule out disease, and should not be used as grounds to withhold therapy or lift infection control measures.

Infection control

Evidence to date suggests that pandemic (H_1N_1) 2009 virus is transmitted similarly as seasonal influenza A and B viruses. Appropriate infection control measures (standard plus droplet precautions) should be adhered to at all times, which includes strict adherence to hand hygiene with soap and water or an alcohol based hand sanitizer, and to cover mouth and nose with tissue or handkerchief when coughing or sneezing. If ill persons must go into the community e.g. to seek medical care, they should wear a face mask to reduce the risk of spreading the virus in the community.

Whenever performing high-risk aerosol-generating procedures (for example, bronchoscopy or any procedure involving aspiration of the respiratory tract) use a particulate respirator (N95, FFP2 or equivalent), eye protection, gown, and gloves, and carry out the procedure in an adequately ventilated room, either naturally or mechanically.

The duration of isolation precautions for hospitalized patients with influenza symptoms should be continued for 7 days after onset of illness or 24 hours after the resolution of fever and respiratory symptoms, whichever is longer, while a patient is in a health-care facility. For prolonged illness with complications (i.e. pneumonia), control measures should be used during the duration of acute illness (i.e. until the patient has improved clinically). Special attention is needed in caring for immunosuppressed patients who may shed virus for a longer time period and are also at increased risk for development of antiviral resistant virus.

Influenza vaccine

Currently, there are three different influenza technologies in use, to produce influenza vaccines. These include egg-based, cell-cultured, and recombinant technologies. Egg-based inactivated influenza vaccines (IIVs) are prepared from inactivated and detergent-solubilized virion particles containing HA and NA proteins prepared in embryonated chicken eggs. The live attenuated vaccine (LAIV) is prepared from attenuated, less virulent virus strains. Cell-cultured vaccines are produced by growing the influenza virus in animal cells, allowing for a faster manufacturing process. Although hen's eggs are not used, trace amounts of egg protein may be found in these vaccines. The recombinant flu vaccine is an alternative method that isolates the HA gene and proteins in order to obtain an immunogenic response without the use of chicken eggs. This vaccine is produced in insect cell cultures and contains three times the amount of HA compared with the standard-dose preparation. It is currently the only available influenza vaccine that is completely egg-free *(17)*.

Two types of influenza viruses are included in the influenza vaccine: human influenza A virus and influenza B virus. Vaccine composition is reviewed annually and updated as needed based on the circulating viruses, extent to which those viruses are spreading, and how good the response was to the previous year's vaccine. The World Health Organization makes recommendations about the specific viruses to be included.

Inactivated influenza vaccine (IIVs)

IIVs are available since 1940. Trivalent IIVs contain three inactivated viruses: type A (H_1N_1), type A (H_3N_2), and type B. Quadrivalent influenza vaccines were introduced in the year 2013–2014 season. They contain the same antigens as trivalent vaccines, with addition of another B strain virus, increasing the likelihood for adequate protection. IIV is administered by intramuscular or intradermal route. The vaccine is available in both paediatric (0.25 ml) and adult (0.5 ml) dose formulation. One dose of IIV may be administered annually for persons 9 years of age and older. Children 6 months through 8 years of age receiving influenza vaccine for the first time should receive two doses administered at least 28 days apart. Annual immunization is recommended *(18)*.

The vaccine is about 60 per cent effective among healthy persons younger than 65 years of age. On vaccination, the vaccine becomes effective after 14 days. Those infected shortly before (1–3 days) or shortly after immunization can still get the disease *(18)*. Vaccinated individuals can also get infected with other strain of influenza virus for which the vaccine dose not provide protection *(18)*. The immunity lasts from 6–12 months. The vaccine is 50–60 per cent effective in preventing hospitalization and 80 per cent effective in preventing death among elderly persons *(18)*.

The vaccine should be stored at temperature of 2–8°C. It should not be frozen.

For those persons aged 65 years and older, there are currently two influenza vaccines designed to overcome the waning immune response found in this patient population high-dose IIV (HD-IIV) and adjuvanted IIV (aIIV). Both formulations are available only as a trivalent vaccine. The HD-IIV contains four times the HA-antigen compared with standard influenza vaccines, providing a better immune response and reducing clinical outcomes associated with influenza infection in this patient population. When compared with patients who received standard-dose trivalent influenza vaccines, HD-IIV was shown to be 24% more effective in preventing laboratory confirmed influenza *(17)*.

SIDE EFFECTS

Inactivated vaccines, administered by injection, commonly cause local reactions such as soreness, swelling and redness at the injection site, and less often can cause fever, muscle or joint-aches or headache. These symptoms are generally mild and do not need medical attention, and last for 1–2 days. Fever, aches and headaches can occur more frequently in children compared to elderly people. Rarely, these inlfuenza vaccines can cause allergic reactions such as hives, rapid swelling of deeper skin layers and tissues, asthma or a severe multisystem allergic reaction due to hypersensitivity to certain components.

CONTRAINDICATIONS

As a general rule, inactivated vaccines should not be administered to *(19)* :

(1) People who have a severe allergy to chicken eggs;
(2) People with a history of anaphylactic reactions or other life–threatening allergic reactions to any of the constituents or trace residue of the vaccine;
(3) People with history of a severe reaction to influenza vaccination;
(4) People who developed Guillain-Barre syndrome (GBS) within 6 weeks of getting an influenza vaccine;
(5) Children less than 6 months of age (inactivated influenza vaccine is not approved for this age group); and
(6) People who have a moderate-to-severe illness with a fever (they should wait till they recover to get vaccinated).

Live attenuated influenza vaccine

Live attenuated influenza vaccine (LAIV) was approved for use in 2003. It contains the same influenza viruses as IIV. The viruses are cold-adapted, and replicate effectively in the mucosa of the nasopharynx. The vaccine viruses are grown in chicken eggs, and the final product contains residual egg protein. The vaccine is provided in a single-dose sprayer unit; half of the dose is sprayed into each nostril. LAIV dose not contain thimerosal or any other preservative. LAIV is approved for use only in healthy, non-pregnant persons 2 to 49 years of age. Vaccinated children can shed vaccine virus in nasopharyngeal secretions for up to 3 weeks.

LAIV is 87 per cent effective against culture confirmed influenza in children 60–84 months old; results in 27 per cent reduction in febrile otitis media; 28 per cent reduction in otitis media with accompanying antibiotic use.

SIDE EFFECTS

Live attenuated vaccines are given *via* a nasal spray, and can commonly cause runny nose, nasal congestion, cough and can less frequently cause sore throat, low grade fever, irritability and muscle-aches and headache. Wheezing and vomiting episodes have been described in children receiving live influenza vaccines *(19)*.

CONTRAINDICATIONS

Persons who should not receive LAIV include children younger than 2 years of age; persons 50 years of age and older; persons with chronic medical conditions, including asthma, a recent wheezing episode, reactive airways disease or other chronic pulmonary or cardiovascular conditions, metabolic disease such as diabetes, renal disease, or hemoglobinopathy, such as sickle cell disease; and children or adolescents receiving long-term therapy with aspirin or aspirin-containing therapy, because of the association of Reye syndrome with wild-type influenza infection. Persons in these groups should receive inactivated influenza vaccine.

As with other live-virus vaccines, LAIV should not be given to persons who are immuno-suppressed because of disease, including HIV, or who are receiving immuno-suppressive therapy. Pregnant women should not receive LAIV. Immuno-suppressed persons and pregnant women should receive inactivated influenza vaccine. Since LAIV contains residual egg protein, it should not be administered to persons with a history of severe allergy to egg or any other vaccine component. A history of Guillain-Barre syndrome (GBS) within 6 weeks following a previous dose of influenza vaccine is a precaution for LAIV.

Since the spread of the epidemics of influenza virus is unstoppable and there is limitation of vaccine availability, WHO recommends that all the countries should immunize their health care workers as the first priority to protect the essential health infrastructure, and to prevent initiation of nosocomial spread of disease to vulnerable patients. WHO recommends the following groups of persons be vaccinated according to their order of priority : (a) pregnant women; (b) individuals aged more than 6 months with one of the several chronic medical conditions; (c) healthy young adults between age 15–49 years, (d) healthy children; (e) healthy adults between age 49–65 years; and (f) healthy adults aged more than 65 years.

The time difference between a dose of COVID-19 vaccine and influenza vaccine should be atleast 7 days.

Treatment

Key principles for clinical management include basic symptomatic care, early use of antiviral drugs if available, for high risk populations, antimicrobials for co-infections, and proactive observation for progression of illness.

Hospital care requires early supplemental oxygen therapy to correct hypoxaemia, with saturation monitoring at triage and during hospitalization, if possible, careful fluid replacement, antimicrobials, and other supportive care. It is important to provide appropriate antimicrobials for other infections which also present with severe respiratory distress. A number of severely ill patients with pandemic (H_1N_1) 2009 disease develop respiratory distress requiring mechanical ventilation and intensive care support.

Antiviral therapy *(14)*

Pandemic influenza A (H_1N_1) 2009 virus is currently susceptible to the neuraminidase inhibitors (NAIs) oseltamivir and zanamivir, but resistant to the M2 inhibitors amantadine or rimantadine.

The following is a summary of treatment recommendations.

(1) Patients who have severe or progressive clinical illness should be treated with oseltamivir. Treatment should be initiated as soon as possible.

   (a) This recommendation applies to all patient groups, including pregnant women, and young children <2 years, including neonates.

   (b) In patients with severe or progressive illness not responding to normal treatment regimens, higher doses of oseltamivir and longer duration of treatment may be appropriate. In adults, a dose of 150 mg twice daily is being used in some situations.

   (c) Where oseltamivir is not available or not possible to use, or if the virus is resistant to oseltamivir, patients who have severe or progressive clinical illness should be treated with zanamivir.

(2) Patients at higher risk of developing severe or complicated illness, but presenting with uncomplicated illness due to influenza virus infection, should be treated with oseltamivir or zanamvir. Treatment should be initiated as soon as possible following onset of illness.

(3) Patients not considered to be at higher risk of developing severe or complicated illness and who have uncomplicated illness due to confirmed or strongly suspected influenza virus infection need not be treated with antivirals.

If used, antiviral treatment should ideally be started early following the onset of symptoms, but it may also be used at any stage of active disease when ongoing viral replication is anticipated or documented. Recent experience strongly indicates that earlier treatment is associated with better outcomes. Therefore, antiviral treatment should be initiated immediately and without waiting for laboratory confirmation of diagnosis.

In patients who have persistent severe illness despite oseltamivir treatment, there are few licensed alternative antiviral treatments. In these situations, clinicians have considered intravenous administration of alternative antiviral drugs such as zanamivir, peramivir, and ribavirin. The use of such treatments should be done only in the context of prospective clinical and virological data collection and with regard to the following cautions:

- ribavirin should not be administered as monotherapy;
- ribavirin should not be administered to pregnant women; and
- zanamivir formulated as a powder for inhalation should not be delivered *via* nebulization due to the presence of lactose, which may compromise ventilator function.

Standard antiviral treatment regimens *(14)*

Oseltamivir

Oseltamivir is indicated for treatment of influenza. For adults the recommended oral dose is 75 mg oseltamivir twice daily for 5 days.

For infants less than 1 year of age recommended oral doses are as follows:

>3 months to 12 months	3 mg/kg, twice daily for 5 days
>1 month to 3 months	2.5 mg/kg, twice daily for 5 days
0 to 1 month *	2 mg/kg, twice daily for 5 days
* There are no data available regarding the adminstration of oseltamivir to infants less than one month of age.	

For children older than 1 year up to 12 years of age, the recommended oral doses according to body weight are as follows:

15 kg or less	30 mg twice a day for 5 days
15-23 kg	45 mg twice a day for 5 days
24-40 kg	60 mg twice a day for 5 days
>40 kg	75 mg twice a day for 5 days

Zanamivir

Zanamivir is indicated for treatment of influenza in adults and children (>5 years). The recommended dose for treatment of adults and children from the age of 5 years is two inhalations (2 x 5 mg) twice daily for 5 days.

Chemoprophylaxis *(13)*

Oseltamivir is the drug of choice for chemoprophylaxis to health care personnels and close contacts of suspected, probable or confirmed case of pandemic influenza A (H_1N_1) 2009. It should be given till 10 days after last exposure. The dose by body weight is a follows :

Weight less than 15 kg	–	30 mg OD
15–23 kg	–	45 mg OD
24–40 kg	–	60 mg OD
> 40 kg	–	75 mg OD
For infants		
< 3 months	–	not recommended unless situation is critical
3–5 months	–	20 mg OD
6–11 months	–	25 mg OD

Influenza surveillance

Influenza surveillance is intended to monitor the prevalence of the circulating strains and to detect new strains necessary for vaccine information; to estimate influenza related impact on morbidity, mortality and economic loss; rapidly detect outbreaks; and disease control through rapid action.

References

1. WHO (2012), *Weekly Epidemiological Record No. 47,* 23 Nov. 2012.
2. Maxine A. Papadakis, Stephen J. McPhee, *Current Medical Diagnosis and Treatment,* 53rd Ed. 2014, Lange Publication.
3. WHO 2018, Fact Sheet, March 14, 2018.
4. WHO (1980). *Techn.Rep.Ser.,* No.642.
5. WHO (1985) *Bull. WHO* 63 (1) 51.
6. Jawetz, et al (2001) *Medical Microbiology, 22nd ed., A Lange Med. Publication.*
7. Jawetz, et.al. (2019), *Medical Microbiology,* 28th ed, A Lange Medical Publication.
8. WHO (2005). *Weekly Epidemiological Record,* No.49/50, Oct 14, 2005.
9. WHO (2009), *Weekly Epidemiological Record,* No. 41, 9th Oct, 2009.
10. Govt. of India (2021), *National Health Profile 2021,* Central Bureau of Health Intelligence, Ministry of Health and Family Welfare, New Delhi.
11. WHO (2010), *WHO Recommendations for the post-pandemic,* Pandemic (H_1N_1) 2009 briefing note 23.
12. WHO (2011), *Weekly Epidemiological Record,* No. 43, 21st Oct, 2011.
13. Govt. of India (2010), *Guidelines for Swineflu (Influenza A H_1N_1),* Ministry of Health and Family Welfare, New Delhi.
14. WHO (2009), *Clinical Management of human infection with pandemic,* (H_1N_1) 2009 : revised guidance, November, 2009.
15. Stephen J. Mcphee et al (2010), *Current Medical Diagnosis and Treatment,* 49th Ed., A Lange & Med. Publication.
16. *Flu Vaccine Medically reviewed by Alan Carter,* 8th Sept. 2020.
17. Austin D. Yung etc. (2019), *U.S. Pharmacist,* The pharmacist resource for clinical excellence, 12th Nov. 2019 US pharm. 2019 : 44 (11) 18–22.
18. CDC (2019), *Epidemiology and Prevention of Vaccine Preventable Diseases,* 15th April 2019.
19. WHO (2010), *Safety of pandemic (H_1N_1) 2009 vaccines,* 30th Oct, 2009.

DIPHTHERIA

Diphtheria is an acute bacterial infectious disease caused by toxigenic strains of *Corynebacterium diphtheriae.* Three major clinical types have been described : anterior nasal, faucial and laryngeal; however, the skin, conjunctiva, vulva and other parts of the body may be affected. The bacilli multiply locally, usually in the throat, and elaborate a powerful exotoxin which is responsible for :

(a) the formation of a greyish or yellowish membrane ("false membrane") commonly over the tonsils, pharynx or larynx (or at the site of implantation), with well–defined edges and the membrane cannot be wiped away;
(b) marked congestion, oedema or local tissue destruction;
(c) enlargement of the regional lymph nodes; and
(d) signs and symptoms of toxaemia.

Fatality rate on the average is about 5–10 per cent which has changed little in the past decades in untreated cases, and in children under 5 years of age, and adults over 40 years of age, one out of 5 persons who get diphtheria dies *(1).*

Problem statement

WORLD : Diphtheria is a rare disease in most developed countries owing to routine children vaccination. In countries where satisfactory vaccination schemes have been instituted the disease has so declined that it is no longer regarded as a public health problem. However the disease is seen occasionally among non-immunized children in developed countries.

Improved socio-economic conditions are changing the epidemiology of diphtheria. Changes in lifestyle allow far less opportunity to maintain natural immunity, such as through frequent skin infection with *C.diphtheriae (2).* These epidemics are largely due to decreasing immunization coverage among infants and children, waning immunity to diphtheria in adults, movement of large groups of population in the last few years, and an irregular supply of vaccine *(3).* These outbreaks highlight the need for booster vaccinations. Recent diphtheria outbreaks in a number of countries have demonstrated a shift in the age distribution of cases to older children and adults *(4).* In developing countries, the disease continues to be endemic due to lack of adequate widespread immunization. The true numbers of diphtheria cases and deaths are unknown because of incomplete reporting from most countries where the disease occurs. During the year 2021, about 8,639 diphtheria cases were reported globally *(5).*

INDIA : Diphtheria is an endemic disease. The available retrospective data indicate a declining trend of diphtheria in the country. It is due to increasing coverage of child population by immunization. During the year 2020, about 1,991 cases of diptheria were reported in India with about 28 deaths. Most of the cases reported were from West Bengal (950 cases, 1 death), Telangana (254 cases and no deaths), Andhra Pradesh (202 cases no deaths), Rajasthan (148 cases and 8 deaths) and Delhi (136 cases and 15 deaths) *(6).*

Epidemiological determinants

Agent factors

(a) AGENT : The causative agent, *C.diphtheriae* is a gram–positive, non–motile organism. It has no invasive power, but produces a powerful exotoxin. Four types of diphtheria bacilli are differentiated – *gravis, mitis, belfanti* and *intermedius,* all pathogenic to man. In general, *gravis* infections tend to be more severe than *mitis* infections. Not all the strains of the organism are toxigenic. There is evidence that a non–toxigenic strain may become toxigenic when exposed to a particular bacteriophage – the beta phage – carrying the gene for toxin production *(7)*. The toxin can affect the heart leading to myocarditis or the nerves leading to paralysis. Diphtheria bacilli are sensitive to penicillin and are readily killed by heat and chemical agents. They may survive for short periods in dust and fomites. (b) SOURCE OF INFECTION : The source of infection may be a case or carrier: *(i) CASE* : Cases range from subclinical to frank clinical cases. Mild or silent infections may exhibit no more than a mere running nose or sore throat; these cases play a more important role than frank cases in spreading the infection. *(ii) CARRIER* : Carriers are common sources of infection *(8)*. Carriers may be temporary or chronic; nasal or throat carriers. The nasal carriers are particularly dangerous as source of infection because of frequent shedding of the organism into the environment, than do throat carriers. The temporary carrier state may last for about a month, but the chronic carrier state may persist for a year or so, unless the patient is treated. Immunization does not prevent the carrier state. (c) INFECTIVE MATERIAL : Nasopharyngeal secretions, discharges from skin lesions, contaminated fomites and possibly infected dust. (d) PERIOD OF INFECTIVITY : Unless treated, the period of infectivity may vary from 14 to 28 days from the onset of the disease, but carriers may remain infective for much longer periods. A case or carrier may be considered non-communicable, when at least two cultures properly obtained from nose and throat, 24 hours apart, are negative for diphtheria bacilli.

Host factors

(a) AGE : Diphtheria particularly affects children aged 1 to 5. In countries where widespread immunization is practised, a shift in age incidence has been observed from preschool to school age. (b) SEX : Both sexes are affected. (c) IMMUNITY : Infants born of immune mothers are relatively immune during the first few weeks or months of life. Before artificial immunization, large proportion of population in developing countries were acquiring active immunity through inapparent infection which resulted in widespread production of antitoxin in the population. Thus most members of the population except children were immune. By age 6–8 years, approximately 75 per cent of children in developing countries where skin infection with *C. diphtheriae* are common have protective serum antitoxin levels *(9)*.

Since diphtheria is principally the result of action of the toxin formed by the organism rather than invasion by the organism, resistance to the disease depends largely on the availability of specific neutralizing antitoxin in the bloodstream and tissues. It is generally true that diphtheria occurs only in persons who possess no antitoxin (or less than 0.01 Lf unit/ml.). Assessment of immunity to diphtheria toxin for individual patients can best be made by review of documented diphtheria toxoid immunizations and primary or booster immunization if needed *(9)*.

Environmental factors

Cases of diphtheria occur in all seasons, although winter months favour its spread.

Mode of transmission

The disease is spread mainly by droplet infection. It can also be transmitted directly to susceptible persons from infected cutaneous lesions. Transmission by objects (e.g., cups, thermometers, toys, pencils), contaminated by the nasopharyngeal secretions of the patient is possible, but for only short periods.

Portal of entry

(a) RESPIRATORY ROUTE : Commonly the portal of entry is the respiratory tract. *(b) NON–RESPIRATORY ROUTES* : The portal of entry sometimes may be the skin where cuts, wounds and ulcers not properly attended to, may get infected with diphtheria bacilli, and so is the umbilicus in the newborn. Occasionally, the site of implantation may be the eye, genitalia or middle ear. The non–respiratory routes of infection are less common in developed countries where spread by droplet infection is more common.

Incubation period

2 to 6 days, occasionally longer.

Clinical features

Respiratory tract forms of diphtheria consist of pharyngotonsillar, laryngotracheal, nasal, and combinations thereof. Patients with pharyngotonsillar diphtheria usually have a sore throat, difficulty in swallowing, and low grade fever at presentation. Examination of the throat may show only mild erythema, localized exudate, or a pseudo-membrane. The membrane may be localized or a patch of the posterior pharynx or tonsil, may cover the entire tonsil, or, less frequently, may spread to cover the soft and hard palates and the posterior portion of the pharynx. In the early stage the pseudo-membrane may be whitish and may wipe off easily. The membrane may extend to become thick, blue–white to grey–black, and adherent. Attempts to remove the membrane result in bleeding. A minimal area of mucosal erythema surrounds the membrane. Patients with severe disease may have marked oedema of the submandibular area and the anterior portion of the neck, along with lymphadenopathy, giving a characteristic "bull-necked" appearance *(1)*.

Laryngotracheal diphtheria most often is preceded by pharyngotonsillar disease, usually is associated with fever, hoarseness and croupy cough at presentation, and, if the infection extends into bronchial tree, it is the most severe form of disease. Initially it may be clinically indistinguishable from viral croup or epiglottitis. Prostration and dyspnoea soon follow because of the obstruction caused by the membrane. This obstruction may even cause suffocation if not promptly relieved by intubation or tracheostomy.

The diphtheria bacilli within the membrane continue to produce toxin actively. This is absorbed and results in distant toxic damage, particularly parenchymatous degeneration, fatty infiltration and necrosis in heart muscle, liver, kidneys, and adrenals, sometimes accompanied by gross haemorrhage. Irregularities of cardiac rhythm indicate damage to the heart. Later, there may be difficulties with vision, speech, swallowing, or movement of the arms or legs. The toxin also produces nerve damage, resulting often in paralysis of the soft palate, eye muscles, or extremities *(9)*. Patients who survive complications recover completely.

Nasal diphtheria, the mildest form of respiratory diphtheria, usually is localized to the septum or turbinates of one side of the nose. Occasionally a membrane may extend into the pharynx.

Non-respiratory mucosal surface i.e., the conjunctiva and genitals may also be sites of infection.

Cutaneous diphtheria is common in tropical areas. It often appears as a secondary infection of a previous skin abrasion or infection. The presenting lesion, often an ulcer, may be surrounded by erythema and covered with a membrane. Patients generally seek treatment because of the chronicity of the skin lesion.

CONTROL OF DIPHTHERIA

1. CASES AND CARRIERS

(a) ***Early detection :*** An active search for cases and carriers should start immediately amongst family and school contacts. Carriers can be detected only by culture method. Swabs should be taken from both the nose and throat and examined by culture methods for diphtheria bacilli. Tests should be made for the virulence of the organism. (b) ***Isolation :*** All cases, suspected cases and carriers should be promptly isolated, preferably in a hospital, for at least 14 days or until proved free of infection. At least 2 consecutive nose and throat swabs, taken 24 hours apart, should be negative before terminating isolation. (c) ***Treatment :*** (i) CASES : When diphtheria is suspected, diphtheria antitoxin should be given without delay, IM or IV, in doses ranging from 20,000 to 100,000 units or more, depending upon the severity of the case, after a preliminary test dose of 0.2 ml subcutaneously to detect sensitization to horse serum. For mild early pharyngeal or laryngeal disease the dose is 20,000–40,000 units; for moderate nasopharyngeal disease, 40,000–60,000 units; for severe, extensive or late (3 days or more) disease, 80,000–100,000 units *(10)*. In addition to antitoxin, every case should be treated with penicillin or erythromycin for 5 to 6 days to clear the throat of *C.diptheriae* and thereby decrease toxin production, (ii) CARRIERS : The carriers should be treated with 10 days course of oral erythromycin, which is the most effective drug for the treatment of carriers. The immunity status should be upgraded as discussed below.

2. CONTACTS

Contacts merit special attention. They should be throat swabbed and their immunity status determined. Different situations pose different options : (a) where primary immunization or booster dose was received within the previous 5 years, no further action would be needed (b) where primary course or booster dose of diphtheria toxoid was received more than 5 years before, only a booster dose of diphtheria toxoid need be given (c) non-immunized close contact should receive prophylactic penicillin or erythromycin. They should be given 1000–2000 units of diphtheria antitoxin and actively immunized against diphtheria. Contacts should be placed under medical surveillance and examined daily for evidence of diphtheria for at least a week after exposure. The bacteriological surveillance of close contacts should be continued for several weeks by repeated swabbing.

3. COMMUNITY

The only effective control is by active immunization with diphtheria toxoid of all infants as early in life as possible, as scheduled, with subsequent booster doses every 10 years thereafter. The aim should be to immunize before the infant loses his maternally derived immunity so that there will be continuous protection from birth without any gap in immunity to natural disease. The vaccine being a toxoid is not directed against organisms. Therefore immunization does not prevent the carrier state; consequently, the non-immune individuals are not protected by a high level of population immunity *(11)*. This implies that immunization rate must be maintained at a high level.

DIPHTHERIA IMMUNIZATION

Current prophylactics

These may be grouped as below :

a. Combined or mixed vaccines

- DPT (diphtheria–pertussis–tetanus vaccine)
- DTPw (diphtheria, tetanus, whole–cell pertussis)
- DTPa (diphtheria, tetanus, acellular pertussis)
- DT (diphtheria–tetanus toxoid)
- dT (diphtheria–tetanus, adult type)
- Pentavalent (diphtheria, tetanus, pertussis, hepatitis B and Hib).

b. Single vaccines

- FT (formal–toxoid)
- APT (alum–precipitated toxoid)
- PTAP (purified toxoid aluminium phosphate)
- PTAH (purified toxoid aluminium hydroxide)
- TAF (toxoid–antitoxin flocculus)

c. Antisera

- Diphtheria antitoxin.

a. COMBINED VACCINES

1. DPT vaccine

For immunizing infants, the preparation of choice is DPT. Firstly because, the infant can be immunized simultaneously against three diseases, viz., diphtheria, pertussis and tetanus which is a great gain administratively. Secondly the pertussis component in DPT vaccine enhances the potency of the diphtheria toxoid.

There are two types of DPT vaccines – plain and adsorbed. Adsorption is usually carried out on a mineral carrier like aluminium phosphate or hydroxide. Studies have shown that adsorption increases the immunological effectiveness of the vaccine. The WHO recommends that only adjuvant DPT preparations be utilized in immunization programmes *(12)*.

STORAGE : DPT/DT vaccines should not be frozen. They should be stored in a refrigerator between 2 to 8 deg. C.

(a) *Optimum age :* It has been found that young infants respond well to immunization with potent vaccines and toxoids even in the presence of low to moderate levels of maternal antibodies. Accordingly, the Global Advisory Group of the Expanded Programme on Immunization (EPI), has recommended that DPT vaccine can be safely and effectively administered as early as 6 weeks after birth.

(b) *Number of doses :* Three doses of DPT each of which is usually 0.5 ml, should be considered optimal for primary immunization. It is associated with higher and more sustained levels of diphtheria and tetanus antitoxin and acceptable level of pertussis protection i.e., vaccine efficiency 95 per cent *(13)*.

(c) *Interval between doses :* The current recommendation is to allow an interval of 4 weeks between the 3 doses, with a booster injection at 16–24 months, followed by another booster at the age of 5 to 6 years.

(d) *Mode of administration :* DPT should be administered intramuscularly in antero (lateral aspect) of the thigh.

(e) *Reactions :* Fever and mild local reactions following DPT immunization are common. It is estimated that 2 to 6 per cent of vaccinees develop fever of 39 deg. C or higher, and that 5 to 10 per cent experience swelling and induration or pain lasting more than 48 hours.

The most severe complications following DPT immunization are neurological (encephalitis/ encephalopathy, prolonged convulsions, infantile spasms and Reye's syndrome) and are thought to be due primarily to the pertussis component of the vaccine – the estimated risk is 1:170,000 doses administered.

(f) *Contraindications* : Minor illnesses such as cough, cold, mild fever are not considered contraindications to vaccination, only such children who are seriously ill or need hospitalization are not vaccinated. DPT should not be repeated if a severe reaction occurred after a previous dose. Such reactions include collapse or shock–like state, persistent screaming episodes, temperature above 40 deg.C, convulsions, other neurological symptoms and anaphylactic reactions. In the case of DPT, subsequent immunization with DT only is recommended, without the pertussis component. Local reactions at the site of injection or mild fever do not by themselves preclude the further use of DPT.

Since the severity of pertussis infection decreases with age, the pertussis component in DPT vaccine is not usually recommended after the age of 6 years *(1)*. Therefore, children over the age of 5 years who have not received DPT, need only 2 doses of DT vaccine, 4 weeks apart, with a booster dose 6 months to 1 year later. Those children who received the primary course of DPT earlier, should receive only DT as booster at 5–6 years or at school entry.

For immunizing children over 12 years of age and adults, the preparation of choice is dT, which is an adult–type of diphtheria tetanus vaccine *(13)*. This preparation contains no more than 2 Lf of diphtheria toxoid per dose, compared with 25 Lf in the ordinary (paediatric) DPT/DT vaccines. Administration of dT vaccine to adults is carried out in 2 doses at an interval of 4 to 6 weeks, followed by a booster 6 to 12 months after the second dose *(13)*. This vaccine (DT) is not followed by the high incidence of reactions associated with the use of DPT or DT. Alternatively, for primary immunization of adults, FT or TAF may be used and they cause fewer reactions than APT or PTAP.

2. Pentavalent vaccine

Pentavalent vaccine provides protection to a child from 5 life threatening diseases – diphtheria, pertussis, tetanus, hepatitis B and haemophilus influenzae type b (Hib). Giving pentavalent vaccine reduces the number of pricks to a child. When used, it replaces Hepatitis B and DPT primary vaccination schedule at 6, 10 and 14 weeks in the immunization programme, except that the birth dose of hepatitis B and booster doses of DPT are continued.

The UIP pentavalent vaccine comes in liquid form in a vial. Each dose (0.5 ml) is given by intramuscular injection in anterolateral aspect of the mid-thigh, using auto-disabled syringe. Pentavalent vaccine is a freeze sensitive vaccine and should be stored and transported at 2–8°C temperature.

Pentavalent vaccine is very safe. As with all medicines, a few side effects are possible. Pain, redness and swelling at the site of injection, fever, vomiting, loss of appetite, abnormal crying, irritability are the common side effects. The rare side effects are high fever (more than 39.5°C) and fits or seizures, and very rarely severe allergic reaction can occur.

b. SINGLE VACCINES

Single vaccines (e.g., FT, PTAP, APT, PTAH) are less frequently used. They are all good immunizing agents. APT is hardly used because it is prone to give rise to serious reactions. Each dose of these antigens generally contains 25 Loeffler *(Lf)* units of diphtheria toxoid.

c. ANTISERA

Diphtheria antitoxin prepared in horse serum is still the mainstay of passive prophylaxis and also for treatment of diphtheria.

It has been shown, protection against diphtheria toxin is a quantitative phenomenon, so that a serum antitoxin titre that protects against a small dose of toxin may not protect against a large dose: for this reason, failures of diphtheria immunization may take place *(14)*.

References

1. WHO (2017), *Weekly Epidemiological Record,* No. 31, 4th Aug. 2017.
2. WHO (1999), *Health Situation in the South East Asia Region* 1994–1997, Regional office for SEAR, New Delhi.
3. WHO (1996), *World Health Report,* Fighting disease Fostering development.
4. WHO (1995), *World Health Report,* Bridging the gaps.
5. WHO (2021), *Diphtheria – Reported cases by WHO region.*
6. Govt. of India (2021), *National Health Profile 2021,* DGHS, Ministry of Health and Family Welfare, New Delhi.
7. Youmans, G.P. et al (1980). *The Biological and Clinical Basis of Infectious Diseases,* 2nd ed., Saunders.
8. CDC *Fact sheet for parents,* reviewed in Feb. 2013.
9. Jawetz, et al, *Medical Microbiology,* 2013, 26th ed., A Lange Medical Book.
10. Lawrence, M. et al, *Current Medical Diagnosis and Treatment,* 2008, 47th ed., A Lange Medical Book.
11. Downham, M.A.P.S. (1976). *Brit.Med.J.,* 1 : 1063.
12. WHO (1985), *Bull WHO* 63 (6) 1151–1169.
13. CDC (2019), *Epidemiology and Prevention of Vaccine Preventable Diseases.*
14. Edsall, G (1975) *Clinical Aspect of Immunology* (Eds) P.G.H. Gell et al Blackwell, Oxford.

WHOOPING COUGH *(PERTUSSIS)*

An acute infectious disease, usually of young children, caused by *B. pertussis.* It is clinically characterized by an insidious onset with mild fever and an irritating cough, gradually becoming paroxysmal with the characteristic "whoop" (loud crowing inspiration) often with cyanosis and vomiting. The spectrum of disease varies from severe illness to atypical and mild illness without whoop. The Chinese call it a "Hundred Day Cough" *(1)*.

Problem statement

Pertussis is an important cause of death in infants worldwide, and continues to be a public health concern even in countries with high vaccination coverage. During 2020, about 69,414 cases were reported to WHO globally *(2)* and the DPT_3 immunization rate was 83 per cent.

It is one of the most lethal diseases of the infants and young children who have not been immunized, particularly those with underlying malnutrition and other respiratory infections *(3)*. Pertussis is increasingly reported in older children, adolescents and adults. A serological study from the United States showed that 21 per cent of adults with prolonged cough (lasting more than 2 weeks) had pertussis *(4)*.

In India, there is marked decline of the disease after launch of universal immunization programme. During the year 1987; the reported incidence was about 1.63 lakh cases, whereas during 2020 only 11,985 cases with 50 deaths were reported showing a decline of about 92.648 per cent *(5)*.

Epidemiological determinants

Agent factors

(a) AGENT : The causative agent in a large proportion of cases is *B. pertussis.* In a small percentage of cases (less than 5 per cent), *B. parapertussis* is probably responsible. Certain viruses (e.g., adenoviruses, parainfluenza viruses) are also implicated in the whooping cough syndrome, but their presence in cases of whooping cough is probably coincidental and not causal *(6)*. *B. pertussis* occurs in smooth and rough phases, capsulated and non-capsulated forms, and elaborates an exotoxin and endotoxin. Clinical disease is associated with encapsulated, phase 1 strains. *B. pertussis* is antigenically highly complex. It carries 3 major agglutinogens – 1, 2 and 3 and several minor ones. The nature of the protective antigen is not known *(6)*. The bacterium survives only for very short periods outside the human body. (b) SOURCE OF INFECTION : *B.pertussis* infects only man. The source of infection is a case of pertussis. More often, the source may be mild, missed and unrecognized cases. There is no evidence that infection is ever subclinical *(6)*. A chronic carrier state does not exist. (c) INFECTIVE MATERIAL : The bacilli occurs abundantly in the nasopharyngeal and bronchial secretions, which are infective. Objects freshly contaminated by such discharges are also infective. (d) INFECTIVE PERIOD : Whooping cough is most infectious during catarrhal stage. The infective period may be considered to extend from a week after exposure to about 3 weeks after the onset of the paroxysmal stage although communicability diminishes rapidly after the catarrhal stage. Asymptomatic chronic carriers of *B. pertussis* are uncommon *(7)*. (e) SECOND ATTACK RATE : Averages 90 per cent in unimmunized household contacts *(7)*.

Host factors

(a) AGE : Whooping cough is primarily a disease of infants and pre-school children. The highest incidence is found below the age of 5 years. The median age of infection, i.e., the age when half the children are likely to develop whooping cough is between 20–30 months in developing countries as compared to 50 months in developed countries *(1)*. Infants below 6 months have the highest mortality. In older children, adolescents and adults, pertussis is often unrecognized because of its atypical course. However, older age groups represent an important source of infection for susceptible infants *(7)*. (b) SEX : Incidence and fatality are observed to be more among female than male children *(6)*. (c) IMMUNITY : Recovery from whooping cough or adequate immunization is followed by immunity. Second attacks may occur in persons with declining immunity, but these are usually mild. It is possible that the first defence against pertussis infection is the antibody that prevents attachment of the bacteria to the cilia of the respiratory epithelium *(8)*. Infants are susceptible to infection from birth because maternal antibody does not appear to give them protection. There is no cross immunity with *B. parapertussis.*

Environmental factors

Pertussis occurs throughout the year, but the disease shows a seasonal trend with more cases occurring during winter and spring months, due to overcrowding. Socio-economic conditions and ways of life also play a role in the epidemiology of the disease. Thus, the risk of exposure is greater in the lower social classes living in overcrowded conditions than in well-to-do groups.

Mode of transmission

Whooping cough is spread mainly by droplet infection and direct contact. Each time the patient coughs, sneezes or talks, the bacilli are sprayed into the air. Most children contract infection from their playmates who are in the early stages of the disease. The role of fomites in the spread of infection appears to be very small, unless they are freshly contaminated.

Incubation period

Usually 7 to 14 days, but not more than 3 weeks.

Clinical course

B. pertussis produces a local infection; the organism is not invasive. It multiplies on the surface epithelium of the respiratory tract and causes inflammation and necrosis of the mucosa leading to secondary bacterial invasion. Three stages are described in the clinical course of the disease: (a) catarrhal stage, lasting for about 10 days. It is characterized by its insidious onset, lacrimation, sneezing and coryza, anorexia and malaise, and a hacking night cough that becomes diurnal. (b) paroxysmal stage, lasting for 2–4 weeks. It is characterized by bursts of rapid, consecutive coughs followed by a deep, high-pitched inspiration (whoop). It is usually followed by vomiting. In young infants it may cause cyanosis and apnoea. In adults and adolescents, uncharacteristic, persistent cough may be the only manifestation of the disease, and (c) convalescent stage, lasting for 1–2 weeks. The illness generally lasts 6 to 8 weeks.

Complications occur in 5–6 per cent of cases, most frequently in infants aged less than 6 months. The chief complications of pertussis are bronchitis; bronchopneumonia and bronchiectasis. The violence of the paroxysms may precipitate subconjunctival haemorrhages, epistaxis, haemoptysis and punctate cerebral haemorrhages which may cause convulsions and coma.

Bronchopneumonia occurs in about 5.2 per cent of cases. It is the most prominent problem, with relatively high mortality. The incidence of pertussis-associated encephalopathy is 0.9 per cent 100,000. In industrialized countries, lethality of pertussis is very low (<1/1000), whereas in developing countries the average mortality is estimated at 3.9 per cent in infants and 1 per cent in children aged 1–4 years *(7)*.

Control of Whooping Cough

1. CASES AND CONTACTS

(i) Cases : Early diagnosis, isolation and treatment of cases, and disinfection of discharges from nose and throat are the general principles of control of whooping cough. Early diagnosis is possible only by bacteriological examination of nose and throat secretions which may be obtained by naso-pharyngeal swabs. The chances of isolating the organism are < 60 per cent if the material is obtained within 10–14 days from the onset of illness. The value of fluorescent antibody technique has been emphasized in facilitating the rapid diagnosis of pertussis. The patient should be isolated until considered to be non-infectious. Although several antibiotics are effective against *B. pertussis*, erythromycin is probably the drug of choice. A dose of 30–50 mg/kg of body weight in 4 divided doses for 10 days has been recommended. Possible alternatives are Azithromycin,

Clarithromycin. Antibiotics may prevent or moderate clinical pertussis when given during incubation period or in early catarrhal stage. During paroxysmal phase of disease, antimicrobial drugs will not change the clinical course but may eliminate the bacterium from the nasopharynx and thus reduce transmission of disease *(7)*. They are useful in controlling secondary bacterial infections.

(ii) Contacts : Infants and young children should be kept away from cases. Those known to have been in contact with whooping cough may be given prophylactic antibiotic (erythromycin or azithromycin) treatment for 10 days to prevent the infecting bacteria to become established. The best protection that can be given to an infant is to administer a booster dose of DPT/DT to his siblings before he is born *(6)*.

2. ACTIVE IMMUNIZATION

The vaccine is usually administered in the national childhood immunization programme as combined DPT, DTWP or DTaP vaccine. In India, the national policy is to immunize against diphtheria, whooping cough and tetanus simultaneously, by administering 3 doses (each dose about 0.5 ml) of DPT vaccine intramuscularly, at one month interval, starting at the age of 6 weeks. A booster dose is given at 18–24 months. Children whose vaccination series has been interrupted should have their series resumed, without repeating previous doses. In some countries, an additional vaccine dose is now offered to health-care workers and young parents. Only acellular pertussis vaccines are used for vaccination of older children and adults *(7)*.

Despite major differences in the content, mode of preparation and efficacy among both whole-cell pertussis vaccines and acellular pertussis vaccines; comprehensive clinical trials have demonstrated that the most efficacious vaccines of either category will protect 85 per cent of the recipients from clinical disease. The duration of protection following the primary 3-dose course in infants and 1 booster dose atleast 1 year later is believed to be on an average 6–12 years for both whole-cell and acellular pertussis vaccines. This is similar to, or somewhat shorter than, immunity following natural infection *(7)*. Some studies suggest that pertussis vaccination affects pharyngeal colonization of *B. pertussis*, resulting in some reduction of bacterial transmission in the community *(7)*. All infants, including HIV-positive individuals should be immunized against pertussis.

In principle, the same type of acellular vaccine should be given throughout the primary course of vaccination. However, if the previous type of vaccine is unknown, any type of acellular vaccine may be used *(7)*.

Commercially available vaccines containing acelluar pertussis include combination with some or all of the following components : diphtheria toxoid, tetanus toxoid, Hib, HepB and IPV.

UNTOWARD REACTIONS : With some vaccines available in the early 1960s, persistent screaming and collapse were reported, but these reactions are rarely observed with the vaccines now available. Pertussis vaccines may give rise to local reactions at the site of injection, mild fever and irritability. The rare vaccine reactions are persistent (more than 3 hours) inconsolable screaming, seizures, hypotonic hypo-responsive episodes, anaphylactic reaction and very rarely encephalopathy. For details kindly refer to Table 36 of chapter 3 page 125.

CONTRAINDICATIONS : The contraindications to pertussis vaccination are anaphylactic reaction, encephalopathy, a personal or strong family history of epilepsy, convulsions or similar CNS disorders: any febrile upset until fully recovered: or a reaction to one of the previously given triple vaccine injections *(10)*.

3. PASSIVE IMMUNIZATION

The merit of hyperimmune globulin in pertussis prophylaxis has yet to be established. So far, there is no evidence of its efficacy in well-controlled trials *(9)*.

The control of pertussis by immunization is still an unsolved problem. Even if the level of immunization reaches 100 per cent, it is possible that the disease would not be entirely eliminated because whooping cough vaccines have never been claimed to be more than 90 per cent effective.

References

1. Morley, David (1973). *Paediatric Priorities in the Developing World,* Butterworths.
2. WHO (2022), *Global Health Observatory Data.*
3. WHO (1996), *The World Health Report 1996,* Fighting disease Fostering development.
4. WHO (2010), *Weekly Epidemiological Record,* No. 40, 1st Oct, 2010.
5. Govt. of India (2021), *National Health Profile 2021,* DGHS, Ministry of Health and Family Welfare, New Delhi.
6. Christie, A.B. (1980). *Infectious Diseases : Epidemiology and Clinical Practice,* 3rd ed., Churchill Livingstone.
7. WHO (2005), *Weekly Epidemiological Record,* No. 4, Jan. 28, 2005.
8. Jawetz, et al, *Medical Microbiology,* 24th ed. 2007, A Lange Medical Book.
9. Manclark, C.R. (1981). *Bull WHO,* 59: 9–15.
10. Gray, James A (1981). *Medicine International,* 3, 112.

MENINGOCOCCAL MENINGITIS

Meningococcal meningitis or cerebrospinal fever is an acute communicable disease caused by *N.meningitidis*. It usually begins with intense headache, vomiting and stiff neck and progresses to coma within a few hours. The meningitis is part of a septicaemic process. The fatality of typical untreated cases is about 50 per cent. With early diagnosis and treatment, case fatality rates have declined to less than 8–15 per cent.

Problem statement

Distribution worldwide, occurring sporadically and in small outbreaks in most parts of the world. In some regions this endemic situation may alternate with devastating, unpredictable epidemics. This is the case in the African meningitis belt, which is the region in sub–Saharan Africa stretching from Senegal in the west to Ethiopia in the east. This region is inhabited by around 400 million people. In the African meningitis belt, the WHO definition of a meningococcal epidemic is >100 cases per 100,000 population per year. In the endemic countries, the incidence of >10 cases, 2–10 cases and <2 cases per 100,000 population per year characterize high, moderate and low endemicity respectivety. An outbreak outside the meningitis belt may be defined as a substantial increase in invasive meningococcal disease in a defined population above that which is expected by place and time *(1)*.

During recent years, several serious outbreaks affecting numerous countries have occurred in tropical and temperate zones of other continents, viz, Americas, Asia and Europe. In Europe, the incidence of disease ranges from 0.2 to 14 cases per 100,000 population and majority cases are caused by serogroup B strains. In Americas, the incidence of disease is in the range of 0.3 to 4 cases per 100,000 population. In United States, the majority cases are caused by serogroups B, C and Y. In Asia, most meningococcal disease is caused by meningococci belonging to serogroup A or C *(1)*.

Meingococcal disease is endemic in India. Cases of meningococcal meningitis are reported sporadically or in small clusters. During 2020, about 2,266 cases of meningococcal meningitis were reported in India with about 27 deaths. Majority of the cases were reported from only few states as shown in Table 1.

TABLE 1

Reported cases and deaths due to meningococcal meningitis in some states in India – 2020

State	Cases	Deaths
Andhra Pradesh	364	5
Telangana	814	0
Uttar Pradesh	16	1
Rajasthan	293	0
West Bengal	218	13
Uttarakhand	3	1
Karnataka	31	0
Maharashtra	45	0
Bihar	33	0
Delhi	37	0
Odisha	5	0
Haryana	218	0
Chhattisgarh	11	2
India	2,266	27

Source : *(2)*

Epidemiological features

(a) AGENT : The causative agent, *N. meningitidis* is a gram-negative diplococci. 12 serotypes have been identified, viz. Groups A, B, C, 29E, H, I, K, L, W135, X, Y, Z based on the structure of the polysaccharide capsule. The majority of invasive meningococcal infections are caused by organisms of serogroups A, B, C, X, W135 and Y. Meningococci of these serogroups have the potential to cause both endemic disease and outbreaks. In African meningitis belt, subgroup A has been the most important cause of disease *(1)*. *N. meningitidis* is a delicate organism; it dies rapidly on exposure to heat and cold. (b) SOURCE OF INFECTION : The organism is found in the nasopharynx of cases and carriers. Clinical cases present only a negligible source of infection. More often the infection causes mild or even unnoticeable symptoms of naso-pharyngitis. 4 to 35 per cent of the normal population may harbour the organism in the nasopharynx during inter-epidemic periods. Carriers are the most important source of infection. The mean duration of temporary carriers is about 10 months *(3)*. During epidemics, the carrier rate may go up to 70–80 per cent. (c) PERIOD OF COMMUNICABILITY : Until meningococci are no longer present in discharges from nose and throat. Cases rapidly lose their infectiousness within 24 hours of specific treatment. (d) AGE AND SEX : This is predominantly a disease of children and young adults of both sexes with highest attack rate in infants aged 3–12 months. (e) IMMUNITY : All ages are susceptible. Younger age groups are more susceptible than older groups as their antibodies are lower. Immunity is acquired by subclinical infection (mostly), clinical disease or vaccination. Infants derive passive immunity from the mother. (f) ENVIRONMENTAL FACTORS : The seasonal variation of the disease is well established; outbreaks occur more frequently in the dry and cold months of the year from December to June. Overcrowding, as occurs in schools, barracks, refugee and other camps, is an important predisposing factor. The incidence is also greater in the low socio-economic groups living under poor housing conditions, with exposure to tobacco smoke, asplenia, HIV infection and travel to endemic areas.

Mode of transmission

The disease spreads mainly by droplet infection. The portal of entry is the nasopharynx.

Incubation period

Usually 3 to 4 days, but may vary from 2 to 10 days.

Clinical course

Most infections do not cause clinical disease. Many infected people become asymptomatic carriers of the bacteria and serve as a reservoir and source of infection for others. In general, susceptibility to meningococcal disease decreases with age. Meningococcal meningitis has a sudden onset of intense headache, fever, nausea, vomiting, photophobia, stiff neck and various neurological signs. The disease is fatal within 24–48 hours in 5–10 per cent of cases even with prompt antimicrobial treatment in good health care facility. Among individuals who survive, upto 15–20 per cent have permanent neurological sequelae. Meningococcal septicaemia, in which there is rapid dissemination of bacteria in the bloodstream, is a less common form of meningococcal disease, characterized by circulatory collapse, haemorrhagic skin rash and high fatality rate *(4)*.

Prevention and control

(a) CASES : Treatment with antibiotics can save the lives of 95 per cent of patients provided that it is started during the first 2 days of illness. Penicillin is the drug of choice. In penicillin–allergic patients, ceftriaxone and other third-generation cephalosporin should be substituted. A single dose of long–acting chloramphenicol or cetriaxone is used for treatment of epidemic meningococcal meningitis in sub–Saharan Africa. Septicaemic shock and raised intracranial pressure in meningitis are particular problems in the management of meningococcal disease. Treatment of cases has practically no effect on the epidemiological pattern of the disease because it only reduces the fatality rate of the disease according to the treatment efficiency *(3)*. Isolation of cases is of limited usefulness in controlling epidemics because the carriers outnumber cases.

(b) CARRIERS : Treatment with penicillin does not eradicate the carrier state; more powerful antibiotics such as rifampicin are needed to eradicate the carrier state *(5)*.

(c) CONTACTS : Close contacts of persons with confirmed meningococcal disease are at an increased risk of developing meningococcal illness. Antibiotics are effective in preventing additional cases through eradicating carriage of the invasive strain. Most secondary case occur within the first 72 hours after presentation of the index case; risk of secondary disease decreases to near baseline by 10–14 days. Close contacts include household, child care, and preschool contacts. In outbreaks involving limited populations, those with direct, prolonged contact with a case of meningococcal disease may also be offered clearance treatment. Ideally, where indicated, treatment should be started within 24 hours of identification of the index case. Antibiotics effective for this purpose include rifampicin, ciprofloxacin, ceftriaxone or azithromycin.

(d) MASS CHEMOPROPHYLAXIS : This is in fact mass medication of the total population some of which are not infected. It is recommended that mass chemoprophylaxis be restricted to closed and medically supervised communities. Mass treatment causes an immediate drop in the incidence rate of meningitis and in the proportion of carriers. The efficacy of this preventive measure depends to a large extent on the population coverage *(3)*. The drugs of choice are ciprofloxacin, minocycline, spiramycin and ceftriaxone.

(e) VACCINE *(1, 4)* : Currently available meningococcal vaccines include polysaccharide vaccines and polysaccharide–protein conjugate vaccines. The conjugate vaccines are more immunogenic and also induce immunogenic memory. Both vaccines are available against meningococci of serogroup A, C, W135 and Y.

Polysaccharide vaccines : Internationally marketed meningococcal polysaccharide vaccines are available in bivalent (A, C), trivalent (A,C, W 135), and quadrivalent (A, C, W135, Y) formulations. The vaccines contain 50 µg of each of the individual polysaccharides. Meningococcal polysaccharide vaccines are administered as a single dose to persons ≥2 years old; most of these vaccines are given subcutaneously.

Adverse reactions to polysaccharide meningococcal vaccines are usually mild; the most frequent reaction is 1–2 days of pain and redness at the site of injection, which occur in 4%–56% of vaccine recipients. Transient fever is reported in <5% of recipients.

Conjugate vaccines : Licensed meningococcal conjugate vaccines are monovalent (A or C) or quadrivalent (A, C, W135, Y), and also include a combination vaccine based on *Haemophilus influenzae type b* and *Neisseria meningitidis* serogroup C vaccines (Hib/MenC).

Conjugate vaccine should be given as intramuscular injection, preferably in the deltoid muscle (or in the anterolateral aspect of the upper thigh in children <12 months of age).

Monovalent Men A conjugate vaccine should be given as a single dose to individuals 1–29 years of age. For monovalent Men C conjugate vaccine, one single intramuscular dose is recommended for children aged ≥12 months, teenagers and adults. Children 2–11 months of age require 2 dose administration at an interval of at least 2 months and a booster about 1 year thereafter. Quadrivalent vaccines are administered as a single dose to individuals aged ≥ 2 years.

Meningococcal vaccines should be stored at 2–8°C. Conjugate vaccines are preferred over polysaccharide vaccines due to their potential for herd protection and their increased immunogenicity, particularly in children < 2 years of age. Both vaccines are safe when used during pregnancy *(1)*. WHO recommends that countries with high or medium endemic rates of invasive meningococcal disease and countries with frequent epidemics should introduce appropriate large-scale meningococcal vaccination programmes *(1)*.

References

1. WHO (2011), *Weekly Epidemiological Record*, No. 47, 18th Nov. 2011.
2. Govt. of India (2021), *National Health Profile 2021*, DGHS, Ministry of Health and Family Welfare, New Delhi.
3. Cvjetanovic, B. et al (1978). *Bull WHO*, 56 (Supplement No.1): 81.
4. WHO (2012), *International travel and Health*, 2012.
5. Jawetz, et al, (2007), *Medical Microbiology*, 24th ed., A Lange Medical Book.

ACUTE RESPIRATORY INFECTIONS

Infections of the respiratory tract are perhaps the most common human ailment. While they are a source of discomfort, disability and loss of time for most adults, they are a substantial cause of morbidity and mortality in young children and the elderly. Many of these infections run their natural course in older children and in adults without specific treatment and without complications. However, in young infants, small children and in the elderly, or in persons with impaired respiratory tract reserves, it increases the morbidity and mortality rates.

Acute respiratory infections (ARI) may cause inflammation of the respiratory tract anywhere from nose to alveoli, with a wide range of combination of symptoms and signs. ARI is often classified by clinical syndromes depending on the site of infection and is referred to as ARI of upper (AURI) or lower (ALRI) respiratory tract. The upper respiratory tract infections include common cold, pharyngitis and otitis media. The lower respiratory tract infections include epiglottitis, laryngitis, laryngotracheitis, bronchitis, bronchiolitis and pneumonia.

The clinical features include running nose, cough, sore throat, difficult breathing and ear problem. Fever is also common in acute respiratory infections. Most children with these infections have only mild infection, such as cold or cough. However, some children may have pneumonia which is a major cause of death. In less developed countries, measles and whooping cough are important causes of severe respiratory tract infection.

Problem statement

Pneumonia continues to kill more children under five worldwide than any other single infectious disease, claiming an estimated 0.80 million children's life in 2018. Young children are at particularly high risk of developing severe pneumonia disease and death. More than 80 per cent of deaths associated with pneumonia occur in children during the first 2 years of life. It is more prevalent in the developing countries in South Asia and sub-Saharan Africa *(1)*. Before widespread introduction of PCV into national immunization programmes since 2006, the reported mean annual incidence of invasive pneumococcal disease (IPD) in children less than 2 years of age was 44.4 per lakh population per year in Europe and United States of America, 60 per 100,000 population in South Africa and somewhere in between in Asia and Latin America *(2)*.

It is difficult to determine the proportion of *Straptococcus pneumoniae* to pneumonia cases. In a compilation data, it was found to be responsible for 78 per cent of the lobar pneumonia cases and 13 per cent of bronchopneumonia cases.

The other common causes of pneumonia are *Haemophilus influenzae* type b (the second most common cause of pneumonia), respiratory syncytial virus is the most common viral cause of pneumonia, and in HIV infected infants *pneumocystis jirovecii* is the most common cause of pneumonia responsible for at least one quarter of all pneumonia deaths in HIV-infected infants *(3)*.

Continuous spread of infection from nasopharynx can cause otitis media or sinusitis. Pneumonia is often caused by aspiration of pneumococci from nanopharynx and may also be caused by blood-borne spread. When associated with bacteraemia, pneumonia is classified as IPD. Case fatality rates from IPD in children can be high, ranging up-to 20 per cent for septicaemia and 50 per cent for meningitis in low middle income countries. Long-term neurological sequelae such as hearing loss, mental retardation, motor abnormalities and seizures have been observed in 24.7 per cent of survivors of pneumococcal meningitis.

The risk of pneumococcal disease decreases after early childhood and increases again in old age, suggesting acquisition of natural immunity and loss of immunity in older adults due to immunosenescence and increased susceptibility due to other diseases. The mechanism of natural immunity are not fully understood *(2)*.

H. influenzae colonizes the upper respiratory tract of humans and is transmitted person–to–person by inhalation of respiratory droplets or by direct contact with respiratory tract secretions. Neonates can acquire infection by aspiration of amniotic fluid or contact with genital tract secretions during delivery. The contagious potential of invasive hib disease is considered to be limited. However, certain circumstances particularly close contact with a case (patient e.g. household, child care, institutional settings) can lead to outbreaks of direct secondary transmission of the disease *(4)*.

The exposure factors include household crowding, small household size, child care attendance, low socio-economic status, low parental educational levels and school-age siblings, chronic diseases, HIV infection, immunoglobulin deficiency, chemotherapy or stem cell transplant *(4)*.

In India, in the states and districts with high infant and child mortality rates, ARI is one of the major causes of death. ARI is also one of the major reasons for which children are brought to the hospitals and health facilities. Hospital records from states with high infant mortality rates show that upto 13% of inpatient deaths in paediatric wards are due to ARI. The proportion of death due to ARI in the community is much higher as many children die at home. The reason for high case fatality may be that children are either not brought to the hospitals or brought too late.

In India during 2020, about 2,36,71,178 cases of ARI were reported with 5,160 deaths. Same year 4,22,250 cases of pneumonia were reported with 4,624 deaths *(5)*.

Epidemiological determinants

Agent factors

The microbial agents that cause acute respiratory infections are numerous and include bacteria and viruses. Even within species they can show a wide diversity of antigenic type. The agents are those most frequently encountered in a normal population. The bacteria involved can all be isolated with varying frequency from carriers, and cause illness in only minority of infected persons. The viruses that have been found in association with acute respiratory disease are numerous. They are the primary cause of the great majority of respiratory illnesses. However, the severity of the illness is often determined by whether or not secondary bacterial infection occurs, particularly in the case of lower respiratory tract infections. The agents considered to be capable of acute respiratory diseases, the age group most frequently affected, and the characteristic clinical features are as shown in Table 1.

TABLE 1

The agents causing ARI, age group affected and clinical features

Agent	Age group (s) most frequently affected	Characteristic clinical features
Bacteria		
Bordetella pertussis	Infants and young children	Paroxysmal cough
Corynebacterium diphtheriae	Children	Nasal/tonsillar/pharyngeal membranous exudate ± severe toxaemia
Haemophilus influenzae	Adults	Acute exacerbations of chronic bronchitis pneumonia
	Children	Acute epiglottitis (*H.influenzae* type B)
Klebsiella pneumoniae	Adults	Lobar pneumonia ± lung abscess
Legionella pneumophila	Adults	Pneumonia
Staphylococcus pyogenes	All ages	Lobar and broncho-pneumonia (esp. secondary to influenza) ± lung abscess
Streptococcus pneumoniae	All ages	Pneumonia (lobar or multilobular) Acute exacerbations of chronic bronchitis
Streptococcus pyogenes	All ages	Acute pharyngitis and tonsillitis
Virus		
Adenoviruses – endemic types (1,2,5)	Young children	Lower respiratory
– epidemic types (3,4,7)	Older children and young adults	Febrile pharyngitis and influenza-like illness
Enteroviruses (ECHO and Coxsackie)	All ages	Variable respiratory
Influenza A	All ages	Fever, aching, malaise, variable respiratory
B	School children	Occasional primary pneumonia Secondary bacterial pneumonia in elderly
C	Rare	Mild upper respiratory
Measles	Young children	Variable respiratory with characteristic rash
Parainfluenza 1, 2	Young children	Croup — re-infection in later life : mild upper respiratory
3	Infants	Bronchiolitis and pneumonia
Respiratory syncytial virus	Infants and young children	Severe bronchiolitis and pneumonia
Rhinoviruses (multiple serotypes) Coronavirus	All ages	Common cold
Other agents		
Chlamydia type B (Psittacosis)	Adults exposed to infected birds	Influenza-like illness and atypical pneumonia
Coxiella burnetti (Q fever)	Adults exposed to sheep and cattle	Atypical pneumonia
Mycoplasma pneumoniae	School children and young adults	Febrile bronchitis and atypical pneumonia

Source : *(6)*

Host factors

Small children can succumb to the disease within a matter of days. Case fatality rates are higher in young infants and malnourished children. Age-specific mortality rates show wide differences between countries. In general, rates tend to be high in infants and young children, and in the elderly in all countries, although the age group with the highest rates can differ. In developing countries where malnutrition and low birth weight is often a major problem, the rates in children tend to be the highest. By contrast, in developed countries respiratory infections are only exceptionally fatal in infants but are commonly terminal in the elderly.

Upper respiratory tract infections, e.g., common cold and pharyngitis are several times higher in children than in adults. Rates for pharyngitis and otitis media increase from infancy to a peak at the age of 5 years. Illness rates are highest in young children and decrease with the increasing age, except in the third decade of life when young adults are exposed to infection by their own young children. Adult women experience more illness than men. The greater exposure of women to small children may be responsible for this. Under 3 years of age boys are affected more often and more severely.

Risk factors

Many risk factors for respiratory tract infections have been identified. They include not only the climatic conditions but also the housing, level of industrialization and socio-economic development. In developing countries, overcrowded dwellings, poor nutrition, low birth weight and intense indoor smoke pollution underline the high rates. Local mortality rates are particularly affected by the extent of influenza epidemics. Studies in developed countries have shown that higher rate of infection is common in younger sibling of school going children who introduce infection into the household. Maternal cigarette smoking has also been linked to increased occurrence of respiratory tract infections during the first year of life. Children from low socio-economic status tend to have more respiratory infections. The infection is more common in preschool children attending day-care centres. The infections tend to be more common in urban communities than in rural communities.

Mode of transmission

All the causative organisms are normally transmitted by the airborne route. As most viruses do not survive for long outside the respiratory tract, the chain of transmission is maintained by direct person–to–person contact.

CONTROL OF ACUTE RESPIRATORY INFECTIONS

Improving the primary medical care services and developing better methods for early detection, treatment and where possible, prevention of acute respiratory infections is the best strategy to control ARI. Effective reduction of mortality due to pneumonia is possible if children suffering from pneumonia are treated correctly. Education of mother is also crucial since compliance with treatment and seeking care promptly when signs of pneumonia are observed, are among the key factors which determine the outcome of the disease. The recommendations by WHO for the management of acute respiratory infections in children and the practical guidelines for out-patient care are discussed below *(7)*. The same guidelines are followed in India.

Clinical assessment

History taking and clinical assessment is very important in the management of the acute respiratory infections. Note the age of the child, for how long the child is coughing, whether the child is able to drink (if the child is aged 2 months upto 5 years), has the young infant stopped feeding well (child less than 2 months), has there been any antecedent illness such as measles, does the child have fever, is the child excessively drowsy or difficult to wake (if yes, for how long), did the child have convulsions, is there irregular breathing, short periods of not breathing or the child turning blue, any history of treatment during the illness.

Physical examination

Look and listen for the following :

(1) COUNT THE BREATHS IN ONE MINUTE : As the children get older, their breathing rate slows down. Therefore, the cut-off point used to determine if a child has fast breathing will depend on the age of the child. Count the respiratory rate for full one minute using the second's hand of the watch looking at the abdominal movement or lower chest when the child is calm. The chest and abdomen must be exposed for counting. Increased respiratory rate is of significance only if it persists.

Fast breathing is present when the respiratory rate is :

- 60 breaths per minute or more in a child less than 2 months of age
- 50 breaths per minute or more in a child aged 2 months upto 12 months
- 40 breaths per minute or more in a child aged 12 months upto 5 years.

However, repeat the count for a young infant (age less than 2 months) if the count is 60 breaths per minute or more. This is important because the breathing rate of young infant is often erratic. Occasionally young infants stop breathing for a few seconds, and then breath very rapidly for a short period.

(2) LOOK FOR CHEST INDRAWING : Look for chest indrawing when the child breaths IN. The child has indrawing *if the lower chest wall goes in when the child breaths in.* Chest indrawing occurs when the effort required to breath in, is much greater than normal.

(3) LOOK AND LISTEN FOR STRIDOR : A child with stridor makes a harsh noise when breathing IN. Stridor occurs when there is narrowing of the larynx, trachea or epiglottis which interferes with air entering the lungs. These conditions are often called *croup.*

(4) LOOK FOR WHEEZE : A child with wheezing makes a soft whistling noise or shows signs that breathing *OUT* is difficult, wheezing is caused by narrowing of the air passage in the lungs. The breathing–out phase takes longer than normal and requires effort.

If the child is wheezing, ask the mother if her child has had a previous episode of wheezing within the past year. If so, the child should be classified as having recurrent wheeze.

(5) See if the child is abnormally sleepy or difficult to wake. An abnormally sleepy child is drowsy most of the time when he or she should be awake and alert.

(6) Feel for fever or low body temperature.

(7) CHECK FOR SEVERE MALNUTRITION : Malnutrition when present is a high risk factor and case fatality rates are higher in such children. In severely malnourished children with pneumonia, fast breathing and chest indrawing may not be as evident as in other children. A severely malnourished child may have an impaired or absent response to hypoxia and

a weak or absent cough reflex. These children need careful evaluation for pneumonia as well as careful management.

(8) Cyanosis is a sign of hypoxia. Cyanosis must be checked in good light.

CLASSIFICATION OF ILLNESS AND TREATMENT

In the early 1980s, the global burden of childhood mortality due to pneumonia led the World Health Organization to develop a pneumonia control strategy suitable for countries with limited resources and constrained health systems. Management of pneumonia cases formed the cornerstone of this strategy. Simple signs were identified to classify varying severities of pneumonia in settings with little or no access to diagnostic technology; the classifications determined the appropriate case management actions. These pneumonia classification and management guidelines were based on evidence generated in the 1970s and early 1980s, and were incorporated into the original version of Integrated Management of Childhood Illness (IMCI). In the intervening time, new evidence has emerged which prompted the development of revised guidelines *(7)*.

The revisions include changing the recommendation for the first-line antibiotic and re-defining the classification of pneumonia severity. The data shows that oral amoxicillin is preferable to oral cotrimoxazole for the treatment of "fast breathing pneumonia" and is equivalent to injectable penicillin/ampicillin in cases of "chest indrawing pneumonia". Hence, in a programmatic context, the distinction between previously defined "pneumonia" (fast breathing) and "severe pneumonia" (chest indrawing) loses its significance. The new classification is therefore simplified to include only two categories of pneumonia; "pneumonia" with fast breathing and/or chest indrawing, which requires home therapy with oral amoxicillin, and "severe pneumonia", pneumonia with any general danger sign, which requires referral and injectable therapy. Fig. 1 shows the difference between previous and revised classification and the treatment recommended.

A. Child aged 2 months upto 5 years

The revised recommendations for children aged 2 months to 59 months are as follows *(7)* :

1. Children with fast breathing pneumonia with no chest indrawing or general danger sign should be treated with oral amoxicillin : at least 40 mg/kg/dose twice daily (80 mg/kg/day) for five days. In areas with low HIV prevalence, give amoxicillin for three days.
   Children with fast-breathing pneumonia who fail on first-line treatment with amoxicillin should have the option of referral to a facility where there is appropriate second-line treatment.
2. Children age 2–59 months with chest indrawing pneumonia should be treated with oral amoxicillin : at least 40 mg/kg/dose twice daily for five days.
3. Children aged 2–59 months with severe pneumonia should be treated with parenteral ampicillin (or penicillin) and gentamicin as a first-line treatment.
   – Ampicillin : 50 mg/kg, or benzyl penicillin: 50,000 units per kg IM/IV every 6 hours for at least five days
   – Gentamicin : 7.5 mg/kg IM/IV once a day for at least five days

   Ceftriaxone should be used as a second-line treatment in children with severe pneumonia having failed on the first-line treatment.
4. Ampicillin (or penicillin when ampicillin is not available) plus gentamicin or ceftriaxone are recommended as a first-line antibiotic regimen for HIV-infected and HIV-exposed infants and for children under 5 years of age with chest indrawing pneumonia or severe pneumonia.
   For HIV-infected and HIV-exposed infants and for children with chest indrawing pneumonia or severe pneumonia, who do not respond to treatment with ampicillin or penicillin plus gentamicin, ceftriaxone alone is recommended for use as second-line treatment.
5. Empiric cotrimoxazole treatment for suspected *Pneumocystis jirovecii* (previously *Pneumocystis carinii*)

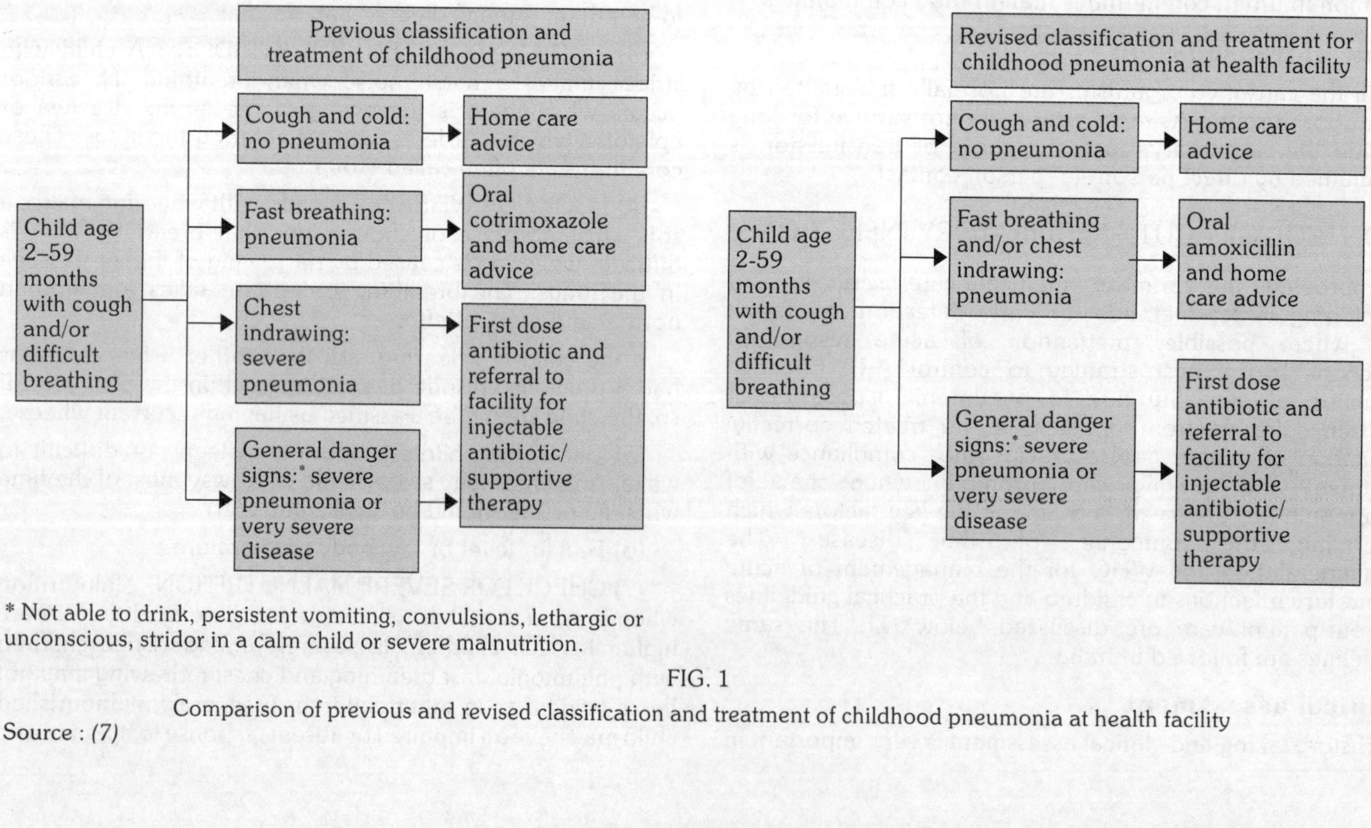

* Not able to drink, persistent vomiting, convulsions, lethargic or unconscious, stridor in a calm child or severe malnutrition.

FIG. 1

Comparison of previous and revised classification and treatment of childhood pneumonia at health facility

Source : *(7)*

pneumonia (PCP) is recommended as an additional treatment for HIV-infected and HIV-exposed infants aged from 2 months up to 1 year with chest indrawing or severe pneumonia.

Empirical cotrimoxazole treatment for *Pneumocystis jirovecii* pneumonia (PCP) is not recommended for HIV-infected and HIV-exposed children over 1 year of age with chest indrawing or severe pneumonia.

Dosages of amoxicillin for pneumonia treatment at health facilities have been revised to reflect three age bands as shown in Table 2 : 2 months up to 12 months (4–<10 kg); 12 months up to 3 years (10–<14 kg); 3 years up to 5 years (14–19 kg). Dosages and age bands for treatment of fast breathing pneumonia by community health workers (CHWs) have not changed.

The revised recommendations present a number of advantages such as :

- Oral amoxicillin can be used to treat both fast breathing pneumonia and chest indrawing pneumonia;
- Pneumonia classification and management are simplified to two categories instead of three;
- Access to antibiotic treatment closer to home is increased;
- The need for referrals to higher level facilities is decreased;
- The probability of hospitalization and thus the risk of nosocomial and injection borne diseases is reduced;
- The probability of antimicrobial resistance is diminished, due to better adherence to the simplified treatment; and
- Training of health workers is simplified.

B. Pneumonia in Young Infants under 2 Months of Age

The treatment in these conditions is, basically the same. The child must be hospitalized. Treatment may be started by the health worker before referring the child. If pneumonia is suspected the child should be treated with intramuscular injections of benzyl penicillin or injection ampicillin, along with injection gentamycin. Chloramphenicol is not recommended as the first line of treatment in young infants. The treatment plan is as shown in Table 3.

TABLE 3
Treatment of pneumonia in children aged less than 2 months

ANTIBIOTIC	DOSE	FREQUENCY	
		Age < 7 days	Age 7 days to 2 months
Inj. Benzyl Penicillin	50,000 IU/kg/dose	12 hourly	6 hourly
OR			
Inj Ampicillin	50 mg/kg/dose	12 hourly	8 hourly
AND			
Inj. Gentamycin	2.5 mg/kg/dose	12 hourly	8 hourly

Besides antibiotics, therapy for the associated conditions, if any, must be instituted immediately. The child should be kept warm and dry. Breast-feeding must be promoted strongly as the child who is not breast-fed is at a much higher risk of diarrhoea.

MANAGEMENT OF AURI (NO PNEUMONIA)

Many children with presenting symptoms of cough, cold and fever do not have pneumonia (no fast breathing or chest indrawing) and DO NOT require treatment with antibiotics.

Antibiotics are not recommended for coughs and colds because majority of cases are caused by viruses and antibiotics are not effective, they increase resistant strains and cause side-effects while providing no clinical benefit, and are wasteful expenditure. Symptomatic treatment and care at home is generally enough for such cases. The mothers must be advised on how to take care of the child at home.

Prevention of Acute Respiratory Infections

Present understanding of risk factors of respiratory tract infection in childhood indicates several approaches for primary prevention. In developing countries, improved living conditions, better nutrition and reduction of smoke pollution indoors will reduce the burden of mortality and morbidity associated with ARI. Other preventive measures include better MCH care. Immunization is an important measure to reduce cases of pneumonia which occur as a complication of vaccine preventable disease, especially measles. It is obvious that community support is essential to reduce the disease burden. Families with young children must be helped to recognize pneumonia. Health promotional activities are specially important in vulnerable areas *(8)*.

Immunization

Vaccines hold promise of saving millions of children from dying of pneumonia. Three vaccines have potential of reducing deaths from pneumonia. These vaccines work to reduce the incidence of bacterial pneumonia.

1. MEASLES VACCINE

Pneumonia is a serious complication of measles and the most common cause of death associated with measles worldwide. Thus, reducing the incidence of measles in young children through vaccination would also help to reduce deaths from pneumonia. A safe and effective vaccine against measles is available for past 40 years. Please refer to page 166 for details.

2. HIB VACCINE

Haemophilus influenzae type B (Hib), is an important cause of pneumonia and meningitis among children in developing countries. Hib vaccine has been available for more than a decade. It reduces dramatically the incidence of Hib meningitis and pneumonia in infants and nasopharyngeal colonization by Hib bacteria. It's high cost has posed obstacle to its introduction in developing countries.

TABLE 2
Doses of amoxicillin for children 2–59 months of age with pneumonia

Tools	Category of pneumonia	Age/weight of child	Dosage of Amoxicillin dispersible tablets (250 mg)
ICCM tool for community health workers : no change	Fast breathing pneumonia	2 months up to 12 months (4–<10 kg)	1 tab twice a day × 5 days (10 tabs)
		12 months up to 5 years (10–19 kg)	2 tabs twice a day × 5 days (20 tabs)
IMCI tool for professional health workers at health facilities : revised	Fast breathing and chest indrawing pneumonia	2 months up to 12 months (4–<10 kg)	1 tab twice a day × 5 days (10 tabs)
		12 months up to 3 years (10–<14 kg)	2 tabs twice a day × 5 days (20 tabs)
		3 years up to 5 years (14–19 kg)	3 tabs twice a day × 5 days (30 tabs)

The vaccine is often given as a combined preparation with DPT and poliomyelitis vaccine. Three or four doses are given depending on the manufacturers and type of vaccine used, and is given intramuscularly. The vaccine schedule is at 6, 10, and 14 weeks of age or according to national immunization schedule. In many industrialized countries a booster dose is given between 12–18 months which provides additional benefit to limit burden of Hib disease among children *(9)*. For children more than 12 months of age, who have not received their primary immunization series a single dose is sufficient for protection. The vaccine is not generally offered to children aged more than 24 months *(9)*.

No serious side-effects have been recorded, and no contraindications are known, except for hyper-sensitivity to previous dose of vaccine. All conjugate vaccine have an excellent safety record, and where tested, do not interfere substantially with immunogenecity of other vaccines given simultaneously *(10)*.

3. PNEUMOCOCCAL PNEUMONIA VACCINE

a. *PPV23* : For years, the polysaccharide non-conjugate vaccine containing capsular antigens of 23 serotypes against this infection have been available for adults and children over 2 years of age. Children under 2 years of age and immunocompromised individuals do not respond well to the vaccine. It is recommended for selected groups, e.g., those who have undergone splenectomy or have sickle-cell disease, chronic diseases of heart, lung, liver or kidney; diabetes mellitus, alcoholism, generalized malignancies, organ transplants etc. In some industrialized countries like USA it is routinely advised for everyone aged above 65 years *(10)*.

A dose of 0.5 ml of PPV23 contains 25 micrograms of purified capsular polysaccharide from each 23 serotypes. For primary immunization, PPV23 is administered as a single intra-muscular dose preferably in the deltoid muscle or as subcutaneous dose. The vaccine should not be mixed in the same syringe with other vaccines, for e.g. with influenza vaccine, but may be administered at the same time by separate injection in the other arm. Simultaneous administration does not increase adverse events or decrease the antibody response to either vaccine. Protective capsular type-specific antibody levels generally develop by the third week following vaccination *(11)*.

Minor adverse reactions, such as transient redness and pain at the site of injection occur in 30–50 per cent of those who have been vaccinated, more commonly following subcutaneous administration. Local reactions are more frequent in recipients of the 2nd dose of the vaccine *(11)*.

b. *PCV* : Two conjugate vaccines are available since 2009, PCV_{10} and PCV_{13}. The PCV_7 conjugate vaccine is gradually being removed from the market *(1)*. Both PCV_{10} and PCV_{13} are preservative free and their recommended storage temperature is 2–8°C. The vaccine must not be frozen. The shake test is applicable to PCV vaccine.

For PCV administration to infants, WHO recommends 3 primary doses (the 3p+0 schedule) or, as an alternative, 2 primary doses plus one booster (the 2p+1 schedule). In 3p+0 schedule, vaccination can be initiated as early as 6 weeks of age with an interval betweeen doses of 4–8 weeks, with doses given at 6, 10 and 14 weeks or 2, 4, and 6 months, depending on programme convenience *(2)*.

If 2p+1 schedule is selected, the 2 primary doses are given during infancy as early as 6 weeks of age at an interval preferably of 8 weeks or more for young infant, and 4–8 weeks or more between primary doses for infants ≥7 months of age. One booster dose should be given between 9–15 months of age *(2)*.

The National Immunization Schedule of India recommends PCV for infants up to 1 year of age in three doses (2 primary doses and 1 booster dose) at 6 weeks, 14 weeks and 9 months. 0.5 ml is given using auto-disable syringe as intramuscular injection in the anterolateral aspect of the right mid thigh *(1)*.

PCV efficacy is more than 80 per cent for serotypes present in the vaccine. It can be co-administered with other UIP vaccines. If two injections are being given in the same limb, then they should be administered at least one inch apart *(1)*.

PCV is a safe vaccine. Severe reactions are extremely rare. The most common side effects are irritability, crying, swelling and tenderness at injection site, and transient fever >39°C (102°F). PCV should not be administered to children with severe allergic reaction to a prior dose, or to vaccines containing diphtheria toxoid, such as pentavalent vaccine *(1)*. It should not be given to a child with severe illness. It is not intended to be used for treatment of active infection.

HIV positive and preterm babies who have received their 3 primary doses of vaccine before reaching 12 months of age may benefit from a booster dose in the second year of life. Interrupted schedules should be resumed without repeating the previous doses *(2)*.

When primary immunization is initiated with one of these vaccines, it is recommended that remaining doses are administered with the same product. Interchangeability between PCV_{10} and PCV_{13} has yet not been documented. WHO recommends inclusion of PCVs in childhood immunization programme worldwide, particularly in countries with high under-five mortalities *(2)*.

The Integrated Global Action Plan for the Prevention and Control of Pneumonia and Diarrhoea *(12)*

The Integrated Global Action Plan for the Prevention and Control of Pneumonia and Diarrhoea (GAPPD) proposes a cohesive approach to ending preventable pneumonia and diarrhoea deaths. It brings together critical services and interventions to create healthy environments, promotes practices known to protect children from disease, and ensures that every child has access to proven and appropriate preventive and treatment measures.

The specific goals for 2025 are to:

- reduce mortality from pneumonia in children less than 5 years of age to fewer than 3 per 1000 live births;
- reduce mortality from diarrhoea in children less than 5 years of age to fewer than 1 per 1000 live births;
- reduce the incidence of severe pneumonia by 75% in children less than 5 years of age as compared to 2010 levels;
- reduce the incidence of severe diarrhoea by 75% in children less than 5 years of age as compared to 2010 levels;
- reduce by 40% the global number of children less than 5 years of age who are stunted as compared to 2010 levels.

Theses goals are ambitious and will require significant political will and mobilization of additional resources if they are to be reached.

Coverage targets to be maintained or reached have also been set to define efforts needed to attain the above goals. These are:

- By the end of 2025:
  - 90% full-dose coverage of each relevant vaccine (with 80% coverage in every district);

  - 90% access to appropriate pneumonia and diarrhoea case management (with 80% coverage in every district);
  - at least 50% coverage of exclusive breast-feeding during the first 6 months of life;
  - virtual elimination of paediatric HIV.
- By the end of 2030:
  - universal access to basic drinking-water in health care facilities and homes;
  - universal access to adequate sanitation in health care facilities by 2030 and in homes by 2040;
  - universal access to handwashing facilities (water and soap) in health care facilities and homes;
  - universal access to clean and safe energy technologies in health care facilities and homes.

References

1. Govt. of India (2021), *National operational guidelines, Introduction of Pneumococcal Conjugate Vaccine (PCV),* Immunization Division, Ministry of Health and Family Welfare, New Delhi, January 2021.
2. WHO (2019), *Weekly Epidemiological Record,* No. 8, 22nd Feb. 2019.
3. WHO (2019), *Fact Sheet Pneumonia*, 2019.
4. CDC (2020), *Pink Book,* Epidemiology and Prevention of Vaccine Preventable Diseases.
5. Govt. of India (2021), *National Health Profile 2021,* DGHS, Ministry of Health and Family Welfare, New Delhi.
6. *Epidemiology of Diseases,* Edited by Miller, D.L. and Farmer, R.D., Blackwell Scientific Publications.
7. WHO (2014), *Revised WHO classification and treatment of childhood pneumonia at health facilities,* Evidence summaries.
8. Govt of India (1994), *National Child Survival and Safe Motherhood Programme,* Programme Interventions, MCH Division, Ministry of Health and Family Welfare, New Delhi.
9. WHO (2006), *Weekly Epidemiological Record,* No. 47, 24th Nov. 2006.
10. WHO (2006), *International Travel and Health*.
11. WHO (2008), *Weekly Epidemiological Record,* No. 42, 17th Oct, 2008.
12. WHO, UNICEF (2013), *Ending Preventable Child Deaths from Pneumonia and Diarrhoea by 2025.* The Integrated Global Action Plan for Pneumonia and Diarrhoea.

SEVERE ACUTE RESPIRATORY SYNDROME (SARS)

Severe acute respiratory syndrome (SARS) is a communicable viral disease, caused by a new strain of coronavirus, which differs considerably in genetic structure from previously recognized coronavirus.

The most common symptoms in patient progressing to SARS include fever, malaise, chills, headache myalgia, dizziness, cough, sore throat and running nose. In some cases there is rapid deterioration with low oxygen saturation and acute respiratory distress requiring ventilatory support. It is capable of causing death in as many as 10 per cent cases *(1)*.

Chest X-ray findings typically begin with a small, unilateral patchy shadowing, and progress over 1–2 days to become bilateral and generalized, with interstitial/confluent infiltration. Adult respiratory distress syndrome has been observed in a number of patients in the end stages.

Problem statement

The earliest case was traced to a health care worker in China, in late 2002, with rapid spread to Hong Kong, Singapore, Vietnam, Taiwan and Toranto. As of early August 2003, about 8,422 cases were reported to the WHO from 30 countries with 916 fatalities *(2)*.

Incubation period

The incubation period has been estimated to be 2 to 7 days, commonly 3 to 5 days *(1)*.

Mode of transmission

The primary mode of transmission appears to be through direct or indirect contact of mucous membranes of eyes, nose, or mouth with respiratory droplets or fomites. The use of aerosol–generating procedures (endotracheal intubation, bronchoscopy, nebulization treatments) in hospitals may amplify the transmission of the SARS coronavirus. The virus is shed in stools but the role of faecal–oral transmission is unknown. The natural reservoir appears to be the horseshoe bat (which eats and drops fruits ingested by civets, the earlier presumed reservoir and a likely amplifying host).

The SARS virus can survive for hours on common surfaces outside the human body, and up to four days in human waste. The virus can survive at least for 24 hours on a plastic surface at room temperature, and can live for extended periods in the cold.

Case definition *(4)*

The case definition is based on current understanding of the clinical features of SARS, and available epidemiological data. It may be revised as new information accumulates.

Case definition for notification of SARS under the International Health Regulation (2005)

In the period following an outbreak of SARS, a notifiable case of SARS is defined as an individual with laboratory confirmation of infection with SARS coronavirus (SARS-CoV) who either fulfils the clinical case definition of SARS or has worked in a laboratory handling live SARS-CoV or storing clinical specimens infected with SARS-CoV.

Clinical case definition of SARS

1. A history of fever, or documented fever

   AND
2. One or more symptoms of lower respiratory tract illness (cough, difficulty in breathing, shortness of breath)

   AND
3. Radiographic evidence of lung infiltrates consistent with pneumonia or acute respiratory distress syndrome (ARDS) or autopsy findings consistent with the pathology of pneumonia or ARDS without an identifiable cause

   AND
4. No alternative diagnosis fully explaining the illness.

Diagnostic tests required for laboratory confirmation of SARS

(a) Conventional reverse transcriptase PCR (RT-PCR) and real-time reverse transcriptase PCR (real-time RT-PCR) assay detecting viral RNA present in:

1. At least 2 different clinical specimens (e.g. nasopharyngeal and stool specimens)

   OR
2. The same clinical specimen collected on 2 or more occasions during the course of the illness (e.g. sequential nasopharyngeal aspirates)

   OR
3. A new extract from the original clinical sample tested positive by 2 different assays or repeat RT-PCR or real-time RT-PCR on each occasion of testing

   OR
4. Virus culture from any clinical specimen.

(b) Enzyme-linked immunosorbent assay (ELISA) and immunofluorescent assay (IFA)
   1. Negative antibody test on serum collected during the acute phase of illness, followed by positive antibody test on convalescent-phase serum, tested simultaneously OR
   2. A 4-fold or greater rise in antibody titre against SARS-CoV between an acute-phase serum specimen and a convalescent-phase serum specimen (paired sera), tested simultaneously.

In the absence of known SARS-CoV transmission to humans, the positive predictive value of a SARS-CoV diagnostic test is extremely low; therefore, the diagnosis should be independently verified in one or more WHO international SARS reference and verification network laboratories. Every single case of SARS must be reported to WHO.

Epidemiological aspect

Health care workers, especially those involved in procedures generating aerosols, accounted for 21 per cent of all cases. Maximum virus excretion from the respiratory tract occurs on about day 10 of illness and then declines. The efficiency of transmission appears to be greatest following exposure to severely ill patients or those experiencing rapid clinical deterioration, usually during the second week of illness. When symptomatic cases were isolated within 5 days of the onset of illness, few cases of secondary transmission occurred. There was no evidence that patient transmits infection 10 days after fever has resolved.

Children are rarely affected by SARS. To date, there have been two reported cases of transmission from children to adults and no report of transmission from child to child. Three separate epidemiological investigations have not found any evidence of SARS transmission in schools. Furthermore, no evidence of SARS has been found in infants of mothers who were infected during pregnancy.

International flights have been associated with the transmission of SARS from symptomatic probable cases to passengers or crew. WHO recommends exit screening and other measures to reduce opportunities for further international spread associated with air travel during the epidemic period.

Complications

As with any viral pneumonia, pulmonary decompensation is the most feared problem. ARDS occurs in about 16% patients, and about 20–30% of patients require intubation and mechanical ventilation. Sequelae of intensive care include infection with nosocomial pathogens, tension pneumothorax from ventilation at high peak pressures, and non-cardiogenic pulmonary edema.

Treatment

Severe cases require intensive support. Although a number of different agents including ribavirin (400–600 mg/d and 4 g/d), lopinavir/ritonavir (400 mg/100 mg), interferon type 1, intravenous immunoglobulin, and systemic corticosteroids were used to treat SARS patients during the 2003 epidemic, the treatment efficacy of these therapeutic agents remains inconclusive and further research is needed. Subsequent studies with ribavirin show no activity against the virus in vitro, and a retrospective analysis of the epidemic in Toronto suggests worse outcomes in patients who receive the drug *(5)*.

Prognosis

The overall mortality rate of identified cases is about 14%. Mortality is age-related, ranging from less than 1% in persons under 24 years of age to greater than 50% in persons over 65 years of age. Poor prognostic factors include advanced age, chronic hepatitis B infection treated with lamivudine, high initial or high peak lactate dehydrogenase concentration, high neutrophil count on presentation, diabetes mellitus, acute kidney disease, and low counts of CD4 and CD8 on presentation. Many subclinical cases probably go undiagnosed. Seasonality, as with influenza, is not established *(5)*.

Prevention

As there is no vaccine against SARS, the preventive measures for SARS control are appropriate detection and protective measures which include :

1. Prompt identification of persons with SARS, their movements and contacts;
2. Effective isolation of SARS patients in hospitals;
3. Appropriate protection of medical staff treating these patients;
4. Comprehensive identification and isolation of suspected SARS cases;
5. Simple hygienic measures such as hand-washing after touching patients, use of appropriate and well-fitted masks, and introduction of infection control measures;
6. Exit screening of international travellers;
7. Timely and accurate reporting and sharing of information with other authorities and/or governments.

References

1. WHO (2003), *Weekly Epidemiological Record No. 12,* 21 March 2003.
2. WHO (2003), *World Health Report 2003,* Shaping the future.
3. WHO (2003), *Weekly Epidemiological Record No. 43,* 24th Oct. 2003.
4. WHO (2009), *Weekly Epidemiological Record No. 7,* 13th Feb. 2009.
5. Stephen J. Mcphee et al, (2010), *Current Medical Diagnosis and Treatment,* 49th Ed. A Lange Medical Publication.

CORONAVIRUS DISEASE-19

Coronavirus disease-2019 (COVID-19) is caused by SARS-CoV-2, a newly emergent coronavirus, that was first recognized in Wuhan, China, in December 2019. Genetic sequencing of the virus suggests that it is a betacoronavirus closely linked to SARS virus. It is from the family of single-stranded RNA virus (+ss RNA) with a crown like appearance under an electronic microscope, of approximately 60–140 nm diameter, contains large widely spread club or petal shaped spikes. Although high temperature decreases the replication of the virus, it can resist the cold temperature. It is sensitive to ultraviolet rays, and is effectively inactivated by lipid solvents including ether (75 per cent), ethnol, chlorine-containing disinfectants, peroxyacetic acid and chloroform except for chlorhexidine *(1)*.

The dynamics of SARS-CoV-2 are currently unknown, but it is speculated that it has an animal origin.

Global scenario

In late December 2019, investigation of a cluster of pneumonia cases of unknown origin in Wuhan, China, resulted in identification of a novel coronavirus. The virus is distinct from both Severe Acute Respiratory Syndrome (SARS) coronavirus and Middle East Respiratory Syndrome (MERS) coronavirus, although closely related. Early epidemiological findings suggest that the virus is more contagious than its predecessors. Severe Acute Respiratory Syndrome Coronavirus-2 (SARS-CoV-2) is a newly identified pathogen and it is assumed that there is no existing human immunity to the virus. Every one is susceptible, although there may be risk factors that increase an individuals illness severity.

The disease since its first detection in China, has now spread to over 220 countries/territories. COVID-19 was declared a Pandemic by WHO on 11th March 2020, resulting in shift of focus from China to Europe and North America and later on to the world. As such WHO advised countries to take a whole-of-government, whole-of-society approach, built around a comprehensive strategy to prevent disease, save lives and minimize the effect. Countries closed their borders against travel related activities (by air, road, railway or sea), and lockdown was imposed to minimize the public movements.

The pandemic has taught the world that "global problem requires global solution". International co-operation is the requirement of the day. Whether in detection of virus or development of vaccines or action on economic and social fronts. COVID-19 has imposed many restrictions on our daily behaviour whether it is social distancing or wearing masks. We have also discovered that work-from-home-study-from-home, and shop-from-home, no visit to malls and markets are workable concepts. E commerce portals witnessed record traffic, which may become a permanent feature *(2)*.

The global scenario of COVID-19 and the trend of disease in top 5 countries affected are as shown in Table 1.

When compared globally, India's cases per million population were amongst the lowest in the world. Like-wise the number of deaths per million was also one of the lowest. USA reported the highest number of cases and deaths.

SARS-CoV-2 variants

Viruses constantly change through mutation and sometimes these mutations result in a new variant of the virus. Some variants emerge and disappear while others persist. Most changes have little or no impact on the virus properties. However, some changes may affect the virus's properties, such as how easily it spreads, the associated disease severity, or the performance of vaccines, therapeutic medicines, diagnostic tools or public health and social measures *(4)*.

Scientists monitor all variants but may classify certain ones as variants being monitored, variants of interest, variants of concern and variants of high consequence. Some variants spread more easily and quickly than other variants, which may lead to more cases of COVID-19. Even if a variant causes less severe disease in general, an increase in the overall number of cases could cause an increase in hospitalizations, put more strain on healthcare resources and potentially lead to more deaths.

Variants of concern

Following is the variant of concern :

Omicron - B.1.1.529, BA.1, BA.1.1, BA.2, BA.3, BA.4 and BA.5.

First identified in South Africa. Spreads more easily than other variants. Data suggest that Omicron is less severe in general. However, a surge in cases may lead to significant increase in hospitalization and death. Breakthrough infection in people who are vaccinated are expected but being up to date on recommended vaccine, is effective at preventing severe illness, hospitalization and death.

Variants being monitored (VBM)

Variants designated as VBM include those where data indicates there is a potential or clear impact on approved or authorized medical countermeasures, or that have been associated with more severe disease or increased transmission but are no longer detected, or are circulating at very low levels. These variants do not pose a significant and imminent risk to public health.

The variants being monitored are as follows *(5)* :

WHO Label	Pango Lineage
Alpha	B.1.1.7 and Q lineages
Beta	B.1.351 and descendent lineages
Gamma	P.1and descendent lineages
Delta	B.1.617.2 and AY lineages
Epsilon	B.1.427 B.1.429
Eta	B.1.525
Iota	B.1.526
Kappa	B.1.617.1
N/A	B.1.617.3
Zeta	P.2

INDIA

In India, the first case of COVID-19 was reported on 30th January 2020 in Kerala. India currently has the largest number of confirmed cases in Asia. The outbreak of the disease was declared an epidemic and Epidemic Disease Act, 1897 was invoked leading to temporary closure of educational, religious, entertainment and commercial establishments. It was followed by gradual un-lockdown spread in 6 phases (one month each) upto 30th November 2020.

A three-tier arrangement of health facilities was created for appropriate management of COVID-19 cases. [(i) COVID Care Centre with isolation beds for mild or pre-symptomatic cases; (ii) Dedicated COVID Health Centre (DCHC) with oxygen supported isolation beds for moderate cases; and (iii) Dedicated COVID Hospital (DCH) with ICU beds for severe cases] has been implemented. Tertiary care hospitals

TABLE 1

The global scenario and the trend of disease in top 5 countries affected by COVID-19 (20.09.2022)

Trend	Global	USA	India	France	Brazil	Germany
Total cases	61,81,41,427	9,75,94,686	4,45,47,599	3,49,73,419	3,46,44,407	3,27,97,308
Total deaths	65,33,467	10,79,206	5,28,403	1,54,824	6,85,569	1,49,169
Total recovered cases	59,80,84,372	9,41,52,770	4,39,72,980	3,43,74,410	3,37,50,459	3,20,38,000
Active cases	1,35,23,588	23,62,710	46,216	4,44,218	2,08,379	6,10,139
Serious critical cases	40,191	3,260	698	869	8,318	1,406
Total cases/million population	79,302	2,91,311	31,593	5,33,186	1,60,461	3,88,699
Deaths/million population	838.2	3,221	375	2,360	2,360	1,768
Tests/million population	–	33,17,878	6,32,877	41,38,995	2,95,390	14,49,830
Population	7,97,58,74,244	33,50,19,427	1,41,07,41,415	6,55,93,263	21,59,05,241	8,43,77,058

Source : *(3)*

under ESIC, Defence, Railways, paramilitary forces, Steel Ministry etc. have been leveraged for case management.

The top five states contributing to over 80 per cent active cases are Kerala, Maharashtra, Tamil Nadu, West Bengal and Karnataka. In India, about 92 per cent of the reported cases were having mild disease, 5.8 per cent cases required oxygen therapy and about 1.7 per cent cases required intensive care *(6)*.

Aarogya Setu App : Aarogya Setu App was launched by the Government of India on the 2nd April 2020, and is available in 11 languages including Hindi and English. It is one of the many location-based surveillance app. to let the users check whether they have been in contact with infected people by using location and bluetooth data from smartphones. The app. is available on both Android and iOS devices. It asks a set of questions to the user to identify whether they are at the risk of the coronavirus infection.

Mode of transmission *(7)*

Transmission of SARS-CoV-2 can occur through direct, indirect or close contact with infected people through secretions such as saliva and respiratory secretions or their respiratory droplets, which are expelled when infected person coughs, sneezes or talks. Respiratory droplets are >5–10 μm in diameter whereas droplets ≤5 μm in diameter are droplet nuclei or aerosols. Respiratory droplet transmission can occur when person is in close contact (within 1 metre) with an infected person who has respiratory symptoms or who is talking. In these circumstances, respiratory droplets that include virus can reach the mouth, nose or eyes of a susceptible person and can result in infection.

Airborne transmission is defined as spread of an infectious agent caused by transmission of droplet nuclei (aerosols) that remain infectious when suspended in air over long distances and time. Airborne transmission of SARS-CoV-2 can occur during medical procedures that generate aerosols or it may also spread in indoor settings with poor ventilation. High variability is suggested between individuals in terms of particle emission rate speech, with increased rates correlate with increased amplitude of vocalization *(7)*.

Fomite transmission is possible. Respiratory secretions or droplets expelled by infected persons can contaminate surfaces and objects, creating fomites. Viable SARS-CoV-2 virus and or RNA detected by RT-PCR can be found on those surfaces for periods ranging from hours to days, depending on the ambient environment (including temperature and humidity) and the type of surface. Therefore, transmission may also occur indirectly through touching surfaces in the immediate environment or objects contaminated with virus from an infected person, followed by touching mouth, eyes or nose.

SARS-CoV-2 has also been detected in other biological samples, including urine and faeces of some patients. However, there have been no published reports of transmission of SARS-CoV-2 through faeces or urine.

Period of communicability

Knowing when an infected person can spread COVID-19 is important. Evidence suggests that COVID-19 can be detected in people 1–3 days before their symptoms appear, with the highest viral loads as measured by RT-PCR, observed around the day of symptom onset, followed by a gradual decline over time. The duration of RT-PCR positivity generally appears to be 1–2 weeks for asymptomatic persons, and up to 3 weeks or more for patients with mild to moderate disease. In patients with severe COVID-19 disease, it can be longer *(8)*.

A study of the first patients in the Republic of Korea showed that 9–13 secondary cases occurred among household contacts.

Incubation period

2–14 days.

Clinical spectrum of SARS-CoV-2 infection

Most patients with COVID-19 predominantly have a respiratory tract infection. However, in a small proportion of cases, they can progress to a more severe and systemic disease characterized by the Acute Respiratory Distress Syndrome (ARDS), sepsis and septic shock, multiorgan failure, including acute kidney injury and cardiac injury *(8, 9)*. The definition of a case, a contact, and clinical presentation and risk factors are as shown in Table 2. Table 3 shows the progress of mild disease to a severe disease.

TABLE 2

Symptoms and risk factors associated with COVID-19

Clinical presentation	Presenting signs and symptoms of COVID-19 vary Most persons experience fever (83–99%), cough (59–82%), fatigue (44–70%), anorexia (40–84%), shortness of breath (31–40%), myalgias (11–35%). Other non-specific symptoms, such as sore throat, nasal congestion, headache, diarrhoea, nausea and vomiting, have also been reported. Loss of smell (anosmia) or loss of taste (ageusia) preceding the onset of respiratory symptoms has also been reported. Older people and immunosuppressed patients in particular may present with atypical symptoms such as fatigue, reduced alertness, reduced mobility, diarrhoea, loss of appetite, delirium, and absence of fever. Symptoms such as dyspnoea, fever, gastrointestinal (GI) symptoms or fatigue due to physiologic adaptations in pregnant women, adverse pregnancy events, or other diseases such as malaria, may overlap with symptoms of COVID-19. Children might not have reported fever or cough as frequently as adults.
Risk factors for severe disease	Age more than 60 years (increasing with age). Underlying non-communicable diseases (NCDs): diabetes, hypertension, cardiac disease, chronic lung disease, cerebrovascular disease, chronic kidney disease, immunosuppression and cancer have been associated with higher mortality. Smoking.

Source : *(8, 9)*

TABLE 3

COVID-19 disease severity

Mild disease		Symptomatic patients (Table 1) meeting the case definition for COVID-19 without evidence of viral pneumonia or hypoxia.
Moderate disease	Pneumonia	Adolescent or adult with clinical signs of pneumonia (fever, cough, dyspnoea, fast breathing) but no signs of severe pneumonia, including $SpO_2 \geq 90\%$ on room air. Child with clinical signs of non-severe pneumonia (cough or difficulty breathing + fast breathing and/or chest indrawing) and no signs of severe pneumonia. Fast breathing (in breaths/min) : < 2 months : ≥ 60; 2–11 months : ≥ 50; 1–5 years : ≥ 40. While the diagnosis can be made on clinical grounds; chest imaging (radiograph, CT scan, ultrasound) may assist in diagnosis and identify or exclude pulmonary complications.
Severe disease	Severe pneumonia	Adolescent or adult with clinical signs of pneumonia (fever, cough, dyspnoea, fast breathing) plus one of the following: respiratory rate > 30 breaths/min; severe respiratory distress; or $SpO_2 < 90\%$ on room air. Child with clinical signs of pneumonia (cough or difficulty in breathing) + at least one of the following: – Central cyanosis or $SpO_2 < 90\%$; severe respiratory distress (e.g. fast breathing, grunting, very severe chest indrawing); general danger sign: inability to breastfeed or drink, lethargy or unconsciousness, or convulsions. – Fast breathing (in breaths/min) : < 2 months : ≥ 60; 2–11 months : ≥ 50; 1–5 years : ≥ 40. While the diagnosis can be made on clinical grounds; chest imaging (radiograph, CT scan, ultrasound) may assist in diagnosis and identify or exclude pulmonary complications.
Critical disease	Acute respiratory distress syndrome (ARDS)	Onset : within 1 week of a known clinical insult (i.e. pneumonia) or new or worsening respiratory symptoms. Chest imaging : (radiograph, CT scan, or lung ultrasound): bilateral opacities, not fully explained by volume overload, lobar or lung collapse, or nodules. Origin of pulmonary infiltrates : respiratory failure not fully explained by cardiac failure or fluid overload. Need objective assessment (e.g. echocardiography) to exclude hydrostatic cause of infiltrates/oedema if no risk factor present. Oxygenation impairment in adults : – Mild ARDS : 200 mmHg < PaO_2/FiO_2[a] ≤ 300 mmHg (with PEEP or CPAP ≥ 5 cmH_2O).[b] – Moderate ARDS : 100 mmHg < PaO_2/FiO_2 ≤ 200 mmHg (with PEEP ≥ 5 cmH_2O).[b] – Severe ARDS : PaO_2/FiO_2 ≤ 100 mmHg (with PEEP ≥ 5 cmH_2O).[b] Oxygenation impairment in children : note OI and OSI.[c] Use OI when available. If PaO_2 not available, wean FiO_2 to maintain $SpO_2 \leq 97\%$ to calculate OSI or SpO_2/FiO_2 ratio : – Bilevel (NIV or CPAP) ≥ 5 cmH_2O via full face mask : PaO_2/FiO_2 ≤ 300 mmHg or SpO_2/FiO_2 ≤ 264. – Mild ARDS (invasively ventilated) : 4 ≤ OI < 8 or 5 ≤ OSI < 7.5. – Moderate ARDS (invasively ventilated) : 8 ≤ OI < 16 or 7.5 ≤ OSI < 12.3. – Severe ARDS (invasively ventilated) : OI ≥ 16 or OSI ≥ 12.3.
Critical disease	Sepsis	Adults : acute life-threatening organ dysfunction caused by a dysregulated host response to suspected or proven infection. Signs of organ dysfunction include: altered mental status, difficult or fast breathing, low oxygen saturation, reduced urine output, fast heart rate, weak pulse, cold extremities or low blood pressure, skin mottling, laboratory evidence of coagulopathy, thrombocytopenia, acidosis, high lactate, or hyperbilirubinaemia. Children : suspected or proven infection and ≥ 2 age-based systemic inflammatory response syndrome (SIRS) criteria,[e] of which one must be abnormal temperature or white blood cell count.
	Septic shock	Adults : persistent hypotension despite volume resuscitation, requiring vasopressors to maintain MAP ≥ 65mmHg and serum lactate level > 2 mmol/L. Children : any hypotension (SBP < 5th centile or > 2 SD below normal for age) or two or three of the following: altered mental status; bradycardia or tachycardia (HR < 90 bpm or > 160 bpm in infants and heart rate < 70 bpm or > 150 bpm in children); prolonged capillary refill (> 2 sec) or weak pulse; fast breathing; mottled or cool skin or petechial or purpuric rash; high lactate; reduced urine output; hyperthermia or hypothermia.

Other complications that have been described in COVID-19 patients include acute, life-threatening conditions such as : acute pulmonary embolism, acute coronary syndrome, acute stroke and delirium. Clinical suspicion for these complications should be heightened when caring for COVID-19 patients, and appropriate diagnostic and treatment protocols available.

a If altitude is higher than 1000 m, then the correction factor should be calculated as follows: $PaO_2/FiO_2 \times$ barometric pressure/760.

b When PaO_2 is not available, $SpO_2/FiO_2 \leq 315$ suggests ARDS (including in non-ventilated patients).

c Oxygenation Index (OI) is an invasive measurement of the severity of hypoxaemic respiratory failure and may be used to predict outcomes in paediatric patients. It is calculated as follows: percentage of fraction of inhaled oxygen multiplied by the mean airway pressure (in mmHg), divided by the partial pressure of arterial oxygen (in mmHg). Oxygen saturation index (OSI) is a non-invasive measurement and has been shown to be a reliable surrogate marker of OI in children and adults with respiratory failure. OSI replaces PaO_2 with oxygen saturation as measured by pulse oximetry (SpO_2) in the OI equation.

d The SOFA score ranges from 0 to 24 and includes points related to six organ systems: respiratory (hypoxaemia defined by low PaO_2/FiO_2); coagulation (low platelets); liver (high bilirubin); cardiovascular (hypotension); central nervous system (low level of consciousness defined by Glasgow Coma Scale); and renal (low urine output or high creatinine). Sepsis is defined by an increase in the sepsis-related SOFA score of ≥ 2 points. Assume the baseline score is 0 if data are not available.

e SIRS criteria : abnormal temperature (> 38.5°C or < 36°C); tachycardia for age or bradycardia for age if < 1 year; tachypnoea for age or need for mechanical ventilation; abnormal white blood cell count for age or > 10% bands.

ABBREVIATIONS : BP blood pressure; bpm beats per minute; CPAP continuous positive airway pressure; CT computed tomography; FiO_2 fraction of inspired oxygen; MAP mean arterial pressure; NIV non-invasive ventilation; OI Oxygenation Index; OSI Oxygenation Index using SpO_2; PaO_2 partial pressure arterial oxygen; PEEP positive end-expiratory pressure; SBP systolic blood pressure; SD standard deviation; SIRS systemic inflammatory response syndrome; SOFA sequential organ failure assessment; SpO_2 oxygen saturation.

Source : *(8, 9)*

Case definitions

1. Suspect case *(10)*

A patient with acute respiratory illness (fever and at least one sign/symptom of respiratory disease (e.g., cough, shortness of breath), AND a history of travel to or residence in a country/area or territory reporting local transmission of COVID-19 disease during the 14 days prior to symptom onset;

OR

A patient/health care worker with any acute respiratory illness AND having been in contact with a confirmed COVID-19 case in the last 14 days prior to onset of symptoms;

OR

A patient with severe acute respiratory infection (fever and at least one sign/symptom of respiratory disease (e.g., cough, shortness of breath) and requiring hospitalization and with no other etiology that fully explains the clinical presentation;

OR

A case for whom testing for COVID-19 is inconclusive.

2. Laboratory confirmed case *(10)*

A person with laboratory confirmation of COVID-19 infection, irrespective of clinical signs and symptoms.

Definition of contact

A contact is a person that is involved in any of the following:

- Providing direct care without proper personal protective equipment (PPE) for COVID-19 patients
- Staying in the same close environment of a COVID-19 patient (including workplace, classroom, household, gatherings).
- Travelling together in close proximity (1 m) with a symptomatic person who later tested positive for COVID-19.

High risk contact

- Touched body fluids of the patient (Respiratory tract secretions, blood, vomit, saliva, urine, faeces)
- Had direct physical contact with the body of the patient including physical examination without PPE.
- Touched or cleaned the linens, clothes, or dishes of the patient.
- Lives in the same household as the patient.
- Anyone in close proximity (within 3 ft) of the confirmed case without precautions.
- Passenger in close proximity (within 3 ft) of a conveyance with a symptomatic person who later tested positive for COVID-19 for more than 6 hours.

Low risk contact

- Shared the same space (Same class for school/worked in same room/similar and not having a high risk exposure to confirmed or suspect case of COVID-19).
- Travelled in same environment (bus/train/flight/any mode of transit) but not having a high-risk exposure.

Long COVID or Post-COVID conditions *(11)*

Post-COVID conditions are a wide range of new, returning, or ongoing health problems that people experience after first being infected with the virus that causes COVID-19. Most people with COVID-19 get better within a few days to a few weeks after infection, so at least four weeks after infection is the start of time when post-COVID conditions could first be identified.

Post-COVID conditions can include a wide range of ongoing health problems; these conditions can last weeks, months, or years. The conditions are found more often in people who had severe COVID-19 illness, but anyone can experience post-COVID conditions, even people who had mild illness or no symptoms from COVID-19. People who are not vaccinated against COVID-19 and become infected are at higher risk of developing post-COVID conditions compared to people who were vaccinated and had breakthrough infections. There is no single test for post-COVID conditions. While most people with post-COVID conditions have evidence of infection or COVID-19 illness, in some cases, a person with post-COVID conditions may not have tested positive for the virus or known they were infected.

Symptoms of post-COVID conditions *(11)*

People with post-COVID conditions may experience many symptoms. The most common symptoms are as follows :

1. *General symptoms :* (a) Tiredness or fatigue that interferes with daily life; (b) Symptoms that get worse after physical or mental effort (also known as "post-exertional malaise"); and (c) Fever.
2. *Respiratory and heart symptoms :* (a) Difficulty in breathing or shortness of breath; (b) Cough; (c) Chest pain; and (d) Fast-beating or pounding heart (also known as heart palpitations).
3. *Neurological symptoms :* (a) Difficulty in thinking or concentrating (sometimes referred to as "brain fog"); (b) Headache; (c) Sleep problems; (d) Dizziness when you stand up (lightheadedness); (e) Pins-and-needles feelings; (f) Change in smell or taste; and (g) Depression or anxiety.
4. *Digestive symptoms :* Diarrhoea and stomach pain.
5. *Other symptoms :* Joint or muscle pain, rash, and changes in menstrual cycles.

Some people, especially those who had severe COVID-19, experience multiorgan effects or autoimmune conditions with symptoms lasting weeks or months after COVID-19 illness. Multiorgan effects can involve many body systems, including the heart, lung, kidney, skin, and brain. As a result of these effects, people who have had COVID-19 may be more likely to develop new health conditions such as diabetes, heart conditions, or neurological conditions compared with people who have not had COVID-19 *(11)*.

Living with post-COVID conditions can be hard, especially when there are no immediate answers or solutions. The best way to prevent post-COVID conditions is to protect yourself from becoming infected. Getting vaccinated is the best way to avoid the disease or getting serious illness. However, people experiencing post-COVID conditions can seek personal medical management plan that can help improve their symptoms and quality of life.

Black Fungus Infection

Mucormycosis or Black Fungus is a rare fungal infection caused by a group of fungi called 'mucormycetes'. They commonly exist in the environment, especially in animal dung, compost, soil, leaves, and rotting produce. These fungi can enter the body through exposed wounds in the skin, inhaling, and breathing. Once they enter the body, these fungi have the potential to affect the brain, skin, lungs, and sinuses.

The risk factors are uncontrolled pre-existing diabetes; rampant overuse of steroids in management of COVID-19; new onset of diabetes due to steroid overuse or severe cases of COVID-19; prolonged ICU stay and irrational use of broad spectrum antibiotics; pre-existing co-morbidities such as haematological malignancies, use of immunosuppressants, solid organ transplant etc.; and contamination through the pipes and prongs used for the mechanical supply of oxygen to patients.

Signs and symptoms : 1. Facial pain, pain over sinuses, pain in teeth and gums; 2. Decreased sensation over half of face; 3. Blackish discoloration of skin over nasolabial groove/alae nasi; 4. Nasal crusting and nasal discharge which could be blackish or blood tinged; 5. Conjunctival redness; 6. Periorbital swelling; 7. Blurring of vision or diplopia; 8. Loosening of teeth/discoloration of palate/ gangrenous inferior turbinates; and 9. Worsening of respiratory symptoms, haemoptysis, chest pain, alteration of consciousness, headache *(12)*.

Diagnosis

1. KOH staining and microscopy, histopathology of debrided tissue and culture.
2. Imaging techniques : CT scan of paranasal sinuses brain and lungs.
3. Molecular assays.

Treatment

Liposomal Amphotericin B in initial dose of 5mg/kg body weight (10 mg/kg body wt in case of CNS involvement) is the treatment of choice. Each vial contains 50 mg. It should be diluted in 5% or 10% dextrose, it is incompatible with normal saline/Ringer Lactate. It has to be continued till a favourable response is achieved and disease is stabilized which may take several weeks following which step down to oral Posaconazole (300 mg delayed release tablets twice a day for 1 day followed by 300 mg daily) or Isavuconazole (200 mg 1 tablet 3 times daily for 2 days followed by 200 mg daily). Conventional Amphotericin B (deoxy cholate) in the dose 1–1.5 mg/kg may be used if liposomal form is not available and renal functions and serum electrolytes are within normal limits.

In severe cases, surgery is required to remove dead or infected tissues. Surgery can lead to permanent damage, both mentally and physically, as it involves removing parts of the nose or eyes. India reported more than 11,000 cases of black fungus in COVID cases *(6)*.

Diagnosis of COVID-19

Testing strategies for Covid-19 diagnosis : There are two types of testings for SARS-CoV-2. (1) *Diagnostic testing :* It is intended to identify current infection at the individual level and is performed when a person has signs and symptoms consistent with COVID-19, or when a person is asymptomatic but has recent known or suspected exposure, and (2) *Screening testing :* It is intended to identify infected persons who are asymptomatic and without known or suspected exposure to SARS-CoV-2. Screening testing is performed to identify persons who may be contagious so that measures can be taken to prevent further transmission of the disease.

MOLECULAR TEST

Respiratory sample collection method (8)

A. Lower respiratory tract
   - Bronchoalveolar lavage, tracheal aspirate, sputum
   - Collect 2–3 mL into a sterile, leak-proof, screw-cap sputum collection cup or sterile dry container.

B. Upper respiratory tract
   - Nasopharyngeal swab and oropharyngeal swab

Oropharyngeal swab (e.g. throat swab) : Tilt patient's head back 70 degrees. Rub swab over both tonsillar pillars and posterior oropharynx and avoid touching the tongue, teeth, and gums. Use only synthetic fiber swabs with plastic shafts. Do not use calcium alginate swabs or swabs with wooden shafts. Place swabs immediately into sterile tubes containing 2–3 ml of viral transport media.

Combined nasal & throat swab : Tilt patient's head back 70 degrees. While gently rotating the swab, insert swab less than one inch into nostril (until resistance is met at turbinates). Rotate the swab several times against nasal wall and repeat in other nostril using the same swab. Place tip of the swab into sterile viral transport media tube and cut off the applicator stick. For throat swab, take a second dry polyester swab, insert into mouth, and swab the posterior pharynx and tonsillar areas (avoid the tongue). Place tip of swab into the same tube and cut off the applicator tip.

Nasopharyngeal swab : Tilt patient's head back 70 degrees. Insert flexible swab through the nares parallel to the palate (not upwards) until resistance is encountered or the distance is equivalent to that from the ear to the nostril of the patient. Gently, rub and roll the swab. Leave the swab in place for several seconds to absorb secretions before removing.

Clinicians may also collect lower respiratory tract samples when these are readily available (for example, in mechanically ventilated patients). In hospitalized patients in Dedicated Covid Hospitals (severe cases with confirmed COVID-19 infection), repeat upper respiratory tract samples should be collected to demonstrate viral clearance.

Nucleic acid amplification testing (NAAT) for SARS-CoV-2

Reverse transcriptase polymerase chain reaction (RT-PCR)-based diagnostic tests (which detect viral nucleic acids) are considered the gold standard for detecting current SARS-CoV-2 infection.

The CT score or value in the RT-PCR report is an important part of the result and stands for 'Cycle Threshold'. The RT-PCR test involves converting the RNA collected from the patient's sample into DNA and then amplifying it. The CT value or score in the RT-PCR test refers to the number of cycles it took for the fluorescence to be detected over the background signal. In simpler words, the CT score in RT-PCR is the number of cycles it took to detect the viral load. If the virus is not detected in a few cycles, the CT score of the RT-PCR test will keep increasing. A higher number of cycles means that the virus was undetectable in lower cycles. So, the CT value in RT-PCR report helps determine the viral load and transmission potential of the virus. If the CT value is low, it means it took a lesser number of cycles to detect the virus, implying a higher viral load and higher transmissibility. A higher CT value on the other hand means a lower viral load as well as transmissibility.

The CT Range in RT-PCR

The ICMR has defined a basic CT range for RT-PCR tests to help diagnose the COVID-19 infection:

- *More than 35* : If the CT value in the report is 35 or more, it is considered to be a negative report. Additionally, it could also mean that the virus is in its initial stages and replication in the body has just started. It can also indicate later phases of the infection when the person is recovering. Clinical interpretation is necessary here.
- *25–35* : Moderate viral load and transmissibility. Whether the person is having symptoms or is asymptomatic, there is need for isolation and to begin treatment as soon as possible.
- *Less than 25* : High viral load and transmissibility. Immediate isolation and medical consultation.

More recently, NAATs have included a variety of additional platforms (e.g., real-time loop mediated isothermal amplification). Clinically, there may be a window period of up to 5 days after exposure before viral nucleic acids can be detected. However, false negative NAAT results can also occur outside of this 5-day window. Therefore, a single negative test result does not completely exclude SARS-CoV-2 infection in people with a high likelihood of infection based on their exposure history and/or their clinical presentation, and repeat testing using a NAAT should be considered.

SARS-CoV-2 poses several diagnostic challenges, including potentially discordant shedding of virus from the upper versus the lower respiratory tract. Due to the high specificity of NAAT, there is no need to obtain a lower respiratory tract sample to diagnose COVID-19 when a patient with recent onset of COVID-19-compatible symptoms has a positive NAAT on an upper respiratory sample.

Antigen testing for SARS-CoV-2

When compared with RT-PCR-based tests, antigen-based diagnostic tests (which detect viral antigens in nasal or nasopharyngeal swabs, also called RDT) are less sensitive but have a similarly high specificity. Antigen tests perform best early in the course of symptomatic SARS-CoV-2 infection, when the viral load is thought to be highest. When a person who is strongly suspected of having SARS-CoV-2 infection receives a negative result on an initial antigen test, repeat testing using a NAAT should be considered. Advantages of antigen-based tests are their low cost and rapid turnaround. The availability of immediate results makes antigen-based tests an attractive option for point-of-care testing in high-risk congregate settings where preventing transmission is critical. Antigen-based tests also allow for repeat testing to quickly identify persons with SARS-CoV-2 infection. Currently, there are limited data to guide the use of rapid antigen tests to detect or exclude SARS-CoV-2 infection in asymptomatic persons or to determine whether a person who was previously confirmed to have SARS-CoV-2 infection is still infectious.

Serologic or antibody testing for diagnosis of SARS-CoV-2

Unlike NAATs and antigen tests for SARS-CoV-2 that detect the presence of the virus, serologic or antibody tests are intended to identify persons with recent or prior SARS-CoV-2 infection. Because it may take 21 days or longer after symptom onset for seroconversion or detection of immunoglobulin IgM and/or IgG antibodies to SARS-CoV-2. The use of serologic testing as the sole basis for diagnosing acute SARS-CoV-2 infection is not recommended. Given that NAATs and antigen tests for SARS-CoV-2 occasionally yield false negative results, serologic tests have been used in some settings as an additional diagnostic test for patients who are strongly suspected to have SARS-CoV-2 infection. Using serology in combination with a NAAT to detect IgG or total antibodies 3 to 4 weeks after onset of symptoms maximizes the sensitivity and specificity to detect past infection *(10)*.

CHEST IMAGING

Chest X-ray examination

Since the disease manifests itself as pneumonia, radiological imaging has a fundamental role in the diagnostic process, management, and follow-up. Standard radiographic examination (X-ray) of the chest has a low sensitivity in identifying early lung changes in the initial stages of the disease. At this stage, it can be completely negative. In the more advanced stages of infection, the chest X-ray examination generally shows bilateral multifocal alveolar opacities, which tend to confluence up to the complete opacity of the lung. Pleural effusion can be associated.

Chest computed tomography

Given the high sensitivity of the method, chest computed tomography (CT), in particular high-resolution CT (HRCT), is the method of choice in the study of COVID-19 pneumonia, even in the initial stages. Several non-specific HRCT findings and patterns can be found. The most common findings are multifocal bilateral "ground glass" (GG) areas associated with consolidation areas with patchy distribution, mainly peripheral/subpleural and with greater involvement of the posterior regions and lower lobes. Other findings are the "reversed halo sign" which is a focal area of GG delimited by a peripheral ring with consolidation, and the findings of cavitations, calcifications, lymphadenopathies and pleural effusion *(10)*.

Lung ultrasound

Ultrasound can allow evaluating the evolution of the disease, from a focal interstitial pattern up to "white lung" with evidence often of subpleural consolidations. It should be performed within the first 24 hours in the suspect and every 24/48 hours and can be useful for patient follow-up, choice of the setting of mechanical ventilation, and for the indication of prone positioning.

Laboratory examinations (10)

- In the early stage of the disease, a normal or decreased total white blood cell count (WBC) and a decreased lymphocyte count can be demonstrated. Interestingly, lymphopenia appears to be a negative prognostic factor.
- Increased values of liver enzymes, lactate dehydrogenase (LDH), muscle enzymes, and C-reactive protein can be detected.
- Unless a bacterial overlap, a normal procalcitonin value is found.

- The elevated neutrophil-to-lymphocyte ratio (NLR), derived NLR ratio (d-NLR) (neutrophil count divided by the result of WBC count minus neutrophil count), and platelet-to-lymphocyte ratio, can be the expression of the inflammatory storm. The correction of these indices is an expression of a favourable trend.
- Increased D-dimer.
- In critical patients, D-dimer value is increased, blood lymphocytes decrease persistently, and laboratory alterations of multiorgan imbalance (high amylase, coagulation disorders etc.) are found.

For COVID-19 patients with severe disease, collect blood for blood culture, ideally prior to initiation of antimicrobial therapy. Dual infection with other respiratory infections (viral, bacterial and fungal) have been found in COVID-19 patients. Depending on local epidemiology and clinical symptoms, test for other potential aetiologies, e.g., influenza, other respiratory viruses, malaria, dengue fever, typhoid fever as appropriate *(8)*.

Management of COVID-19

In the containment phase, to break the chain of transmission of COVID-19, patients with suspected or confirmed disease are isolated. Cases can be managed at Covid Care Centre, First Referral Units, Community Health Centres (CHC), Sub-district Hospitals, District Hospitals, and Medical Colleges.

Detailed clinical history is taken including that of co-morbidities. The patient is followed up daily for temperature, vitals and oxygen saturation (SpO_2). Patients should be monitored for signs and symptoms of complications that should prompt urgent referral. Patients with risk factors for severe illness should be monitored closely, given the possible risk of deterioration. If they develop any worsening symptoms (such as mental confusion, difficulty breathing, persistent pain or pressure in the chest, bluish coloration of face/lips, dehydration, decreased urine output etc.), they should be immediately admitted to a Dedicated Covid Health Centre or Dedicated Covid Hospital. Children with mild COVID-19 should be monitored for signs and symptoms of clinical deterioration requiring urgent re-evaluation. These include difficulty in breathing/fast or shallow breathing (for infants: grunting, inability to breast-feed), blue lips or face, chest pain or pressure, new confusion, inability to awaken/not interacting when awake, inability to drink or keep down any liquids.

An algorithm for clinical guidance for management of COVID-19 suspect/confirmed case is as shown in Fig. 1 and 2.

The mainstay of treatment is supplemental oxygen and other supporting therapy. No specific antivirals have been proven effective. However, drugs like Ivermectin, Hydroxychloroquine, inhalational Budesonide, Dexamethasone, Methylprednisolne and Low Molecular Weight Heparin have been recommended. In addition, provisions for Investigational Therapies have also been made using Remdesivir, and Tocilizumab for defined sub-group of patients under medical supervision *(6)*.

Prevention of complications

Implementation of the following interventions can prevent complications associated with critical illness.

Prevention of complications

Anticipated outcome	Interventions
Reduce days of invasive mechanical ventilation	• Use weaning protocols that include daily assessment for readiness to breathe spontaneously • Minimize continuous or intermittent sedation, targeting specific titration endpoints (light sedation unless contraindicated) or with daily interruption of continuous sedative infusions • Early mobilization • Implementation of the above as a bundle of care (may also reduce delirium); such as the Awakening and Breathing Coordination, Delirium assessment/management, and Early mobility (ABCDE)
Reduce incidence of ventilator-associated pneumonia	• Oral intubation is preferable to nasal intubation in adolescents and adults • Keep patient in semi-recumbent position (head of bed elevation 30–45°) • Use a closed suctioning system; periodically drain and discard condensate in tubing • Use a new ventilator circuit for each patient; once patient is ventilated, change circuit if it is soiled or damaged, but not routinely • Change heat moisture exchanger when it malfunctions, when soiled, or every 5–7 days
Reduce incidence of catheter-related bloodstream infection	• Use a checklist with completion verified by a real-time observer as a reminder of each step needed for sterile insertion and as a daily reminder to remove catheter if no longer needed
Reduce incidence of pressure ulcers	• Turn patient every 2 hours
Reduce incidence of stress ulcers and GI bleeding	• Give early enteral nutrition (within 24–48 hours of admission) • Administer histamine-2 receptor blockers or proton-pump inhibitors in patients with risk factors for GI bleeding. Risk factors for GI bleeding include mechanical ventilation for ≥ 48 hours, coagulopathy, renal replacement therapy, liver disease, multiple comorbidities, and higher organ failure score
Reduce the development of antimicrobial resistance	• Utilize de-escalation protocols as soon as patient is clinically stable and there is no evidence of bacterial infection
Reduce the development of adverse drug effects	• Expose patient to empiric antimicrobial therapy for the shortest time possible, to prevent nephrotoxicity, cardiac and other side-effects from unnecessary antimicrobial use
Promote appropriate antimicrobial prescribing and use during the COVID-19 pandemic	• Do not prescribe antibiotics to suspected or confirmed COVID-19 patients with low suspicion of a bacterial infection, to avoid more short-term side-effects of antibiotics in patients and negative long-term consequences of increased antimicrobial resistance

Source : *(8)*

Adult patient diagnosed with COVID-19

Mild disease

Upper respiratory tract symptoms and/or fever WITHOUT shortness of breath or hypoxia

Home Isolation & Care (Refer to relevant guideline)

MUST DOs

- Physical distancing, indoor mask use, strict hand hygiene
- Symptomatic management (hydration, anti-pyretics, anti-tussive)
- Stay in contact with treating physician
- Monitor temperature and oxygen saturation (by applying a SpO_2 probe to fingers)

Seek immediate medical attention if :

- Difficulty in breathing or SpO_2 <93%
- High grade fever/severe cough, particularly if lasting for >5 days
- A low threshold to be kept for those with any of the high-risk features*

MAY DOs

Therapies based on low certainty of evidence especially for those with high-risk of progression*

Inhalational Budesonide (given via Metered dose inhaler/Dry powder inhaler) at a dose of 800 mcg BD for 5 days) to be given if symptoms (fever and/or cough) are persistent beyond 5 days of disease onset

*High-risk for severe disease or mortality

- Age > 60 years
- Cardiovascular disease, hypertension, and CAD
- Diabetes mellitus and other immunocompromised states (such as HIV)
- Active tuberculosis
- Chronic lung/kidney/liver disease
- Cerebrovascular disease
- Obesity

If cough persists for more than 2–3 weeks, investigate for tuberculosis and other conditions

Moderate disease

Any one of :

1. Respiratory rate ≥ 24/min, breathlessness
2. SpO_2 : 90% to ≤ 93% on room air

ADMIT IN WARD

Oxygen Support :

- Target SpO_2 : 92-96% (88-92% in patients with COPD)
- Preferred devices for oxygenation : non-rebreathing face mask
- Awake proning encouraged in all patients requiring supplemental oxygen therapy (sequential position changes every 2 hours)

Anti-inflammatory or immunomodulatory therapy :

- Inj. Methylprednisolone 0.5 to 1 mg/kg in 2 divided doses (or an equivalent dose of dexamethasone) usually for a duration of 5 to 10 days
- Patients may be initiated or switched to oral route if stable and/or improving
- There is no evidence for benefit for injectable steroids in those NOT requiring oxygen supplementation, or on continuation after discharge
- Anti-inflammatory or immunomodulatory therapy (such as steroids) can have risk of secondary infection such as invasive mucormycosis when used too early, at higher dose or for longer than required

Anticoagulation :

- Conventional dose prophylactic unfractionated heparin or Low Molecular Weight Heparin (weight based e.g., enoxaparin 0.5mg/kg per day SC). There should be no contraindication or high risk of bleeding

Monitoring :

- Clinical Monitoring : breathing rate, Hemodynamic instability, Change in oxygen requirement
- Serial CXR; HRCT chest to be done ONLY if there is worsening
- Lab monitoring : CRP, D-dimer, blood sugar 48 to 72 hrly; CBC, KFT, LFT 24 to 48 hrly

Severe disease

Any one of :

1. Respiratory rate > 30/min, breathlessness
2. SpO_2 < 90% on room air

ADMIT IN HDU/ICU

Respiratory support :

- Consider use of NIV (Helmet or face mask interface depending on availability) in patients with increasing oxygen requirement, if work of breathing is LOW
- Consider use of HFNC in patients with increasing oxygen requirement
- Intubation should be prioritized in patients with high work of breathing/if NIV is not tolerated
- Use institutional protocol for ventilator management when required

Anti-inflammatory or immunomodulatory therapy :

- Inj Methylprednisolone 1 to 2 mg/kg IV in 2 divided doses (or an equivalent dose of dexamethasone) usually for a duration 5 to 10 days
- Anti-inflammatory or immunomodulatory therapy (such as steroids) can have risk of secondary infection such as invasive mucormycosis when used too early, at higher dose or for longer than required

Supportive measures :

- Maintain euvolemia (if available, use dynamic measures for assessing fluid responsiveness)
- If sepsis/septic shock : manage as per existing protocol and local antibiogram

Monitoring :

- Clinical Monitoring : work of breathing, Hemodynamic instability, Change in oxygen requirement
- Serial CXR; HRCT chest to be done ONLY if there is worsening
- Lab monitoring : CRP, D-dimer, blood sugar 48 to 72 hrly; CBC, KFT, LFT 24 to 48 hrly

After clinical improvement, discharge as per revised discharge criteria

EUA/Off label use (based on limited available evidence and only in specific circumstances) :

Remdesivir (EUA) may be considered ONLY in patients with

- 10 days of onset of symptoms, in those having moderate to severe disease (requiring supplemental oxygen), but who are NOT on IMV or ECMO
- Consider remdesivir for 5 days to treat hospitalized patients with COVID-19 (No evidence of benefit for treatment more than 5 days)
- NOT to be used in patients who are NOT on oxygen support or in home setting
- Monitor for RFT and LFT (remdesivir not recommended if eGFR <30 ml/min/m2; AST/ALT >5 times UNL) (not an absolute contraindication)
- Recommended dose : 200 mg IV on day 1 followed by 100 mg IV OD for next 4 days

Tocilizumab may be considered when ALL OF THE BELOW CRITERIA ARE MET

- Rapidly progressing COVID-19 needing oxygen supplementation or IMV and not responding adequately to steroids (preferably with in 24–48 hours of onset of severe disease/ICU admission)
- Preferably to be given with steroids
- No active TB, fungal, systemic bacterial infection
- Long term follow up for secondary infections (such as reactivation of TB, flaring of Herpes etc.)
- Significantly raised inflammatory markers (CRP and/or IL-6)
- Recommended single dose : 4 to 6 mg/kg (400 mg in 60 kg adult) in 100 ml NS over 1 hour

FIG. 1

Clinical guidance for management of adult COVID-19 patients (Revised on 14.01.2022)

Source : *(13)*

Asymptomatic

- Suspected contact [RAT or RTPCR negative or not available]
- Incidentally detected [RAT or RTPCR positive]

Home isolation (tele consultation SOS)

Mainstay of Treatment

- Infants and younger children to stay under immediate care of parents/guardians
- No specific medication required for COVID-19 infection
- Continue medications for other conditions, if any
- Promote COVID appropriate behaviour (mask, strict hand hygiene, physical distancing; please see guide for using mask)
- Fluids and feeds : ensure oral fluids to maintain hydration and give a nutritious diet
- Advise older children and family to stay connected and engage in positive talks through phone, video-calls, etc.
- Parent/caregivers to contact the doctor in case of appearance of symptoms

Investigations

- No investigations needed

Mild

- Sore throat, rhinorrhoea
- Cough without breathing difficulty
- $SpO_2 \geq 94\%$ on room air

Home isolation (tele consultation SOS) or COVID Care Centre (⇄ Admit in DCHC or COVID-19 Hospital)

Mainstay of Treatment

- For fever, give paracetamol 10–15mg/kg/dose; may repeat every 4–6 hours
- For cough, give throat soothing agents and warm saline gargles in older children and adolescents
- Fluids and feeds: ensure oral fluids to maintain hydration and give a nutritious diet
- No other COVID-19 specific medication needed
- Antimicrobials are not indicated
- Maintain monitoring chart including counting of respiratory rate 2–3 times a day, look for chest indrawing, cold extremities, urine output, oxygen saturation, fluid intake, activity level, especially for young children
- Promote COVID appropriate behaviour (mask, strict hand hygiene, physical distancing)
- Advise older children and family to stay connected and engage in positive talks through phone, video-calls, etc.
- Parent/caregivers to contact the doctor in case of deterioration of symptoms

Investigations

- No investigations needed

Moderate

- In addition to symptoms in mild cases, check for pneumonia which may not be apparent
- Rapid respiration (age-based) : <2 months RR ≥ 60/min; 2–12 months, RR ≥ 50/min; 1–5 years, RR ≥ 40/min; >5 years, RR ≥ 30/min; AND/OR SpO_2 90–93% on room air

Admit in DCHC or COVID-19 Hospital (⇄ Admit in HDU/ICU of COVID-19 Hospital)

Mainstay of Treatment

- Initiate oxygen if SpO_2 is <94% and maintain between 94–96%
- Maintain fluid and electrolyte balance
  - Encourage oral fluids (breast feeds in infants)
  - Initiate intravenous fluid therapy if oral intake is poor
- Corticosteroids are not required in all children with moderate illness; they may be administered in rapidly progressive disease
- Fever with temperature >38°C (or 100.4°F) : Paracetamol 10–15mg/kg/dose; may repeat every 4–6 hours
- Anti-microbials to be administered if there is evidence/strong suspicion of superadded bacterial infection
- Supportive care for comorbid conditions, if any

Investigations

- Baseline : CBC including ESR, blood glucose
- Chest X-Ray

Severe

- SpO_2<90% on room air
- Any of the following - signs of severe pneumonia, acute respiratory distress syndrome, septic shock, multi-organ dysfunction syndrome, or pneumonia with cyanosis, grunting, severe retraction of chest, lethargy, somnolence, seizure

Admit in HDU/ICU of COVID-19 Hospital

Mainstay of Treatment

- Initiate immediate oxygen therapy and maintain target SpO_2 94–96%
- Maintain fluid and electrolyte balance
- Corticosteroids therapy to be initiated
- Anticoagulants may also be indicated; see anticoagulants guide
- Exercise caution - see use of corticosteroids and anticoagulants guide
- In case Acute Respiratory Distress Syndrome (ARDS) or shock develops, initiate necessary management
- Antimicrobials to be administered if there is evidence/strong suspicion of superadded bacterial infection
- May need organ support in case of organ dysfunction e.g. renal replacement therapy

Investigations

- Baseline : CBC including ESR, blood glucose, CRP, LFT, KFT, serum ferritin, D-Dimer
- Chest X-Ray

As of now, in absence of safety and efficacy data, the use of antivirals such as Remdesivir, Favipiravir, Molnupiravir, Fluvoxamine, and monoclonal antibodies such as Sotrovimab, Casirivimab+Imdevimab, are NOT recommended for children less than 18 years of age irrespective of severity of illness

Children with comorbidities should continue to receive appropriate management for their underlying disease

CT chest is not indicated in diagnosis or management of COVID-19 infection in children

Consider CT chest only if no improvement in respiratory status

FIG. 2

Comprehensive guidelines for management of COVID-19 in children and adolescents (below 18 years) (Revised on 17.01.2022)

Source : *(14)*

Home care for COVID-19 patients

To ensure both safety and quality of health care of the patient, isolation and monitoring is preferable in a hospital setting. However, for several reasons, in situations when inpatient care is not available or in case of informed refusal for hospitalization, patients with mild symptoms and without chronic lung, heart or renal diseases may be cared for in the home environment. The same principle of care applies to symptomatic patients no longer requiring hospitalization. The patient and family should be provided with ongoing support, education and monitoring. They should adhere to the following recommendations *(15)* :

1. Place the patient in a well-ventilated single room.
2. Limit the number of caretakers of the patient, ideally assign one person who is in a good health without risk conditions. No visitors.
3. Household members should stay in a different room or, if that is not possible, maintain a distance of at least 1 m from the ill person (e.g. sleep in a separate bed).
4. Limit the movement of the patient and minimize shared space. Ensure that shared spaces (e.g. kitchen, bathroom) are well ventilated (e.g. keep windows open).
5. The caregiver should wear a medical mask fitted tightly to the face when in the same room with the ill person. Masks should not be touched or handled during use. If the mask gets wet or dirty with secretions, it must be changed immediately. Discard the mask after use and perform hand hygiene after removal of the mask.
6. Perform hand hygiene following all contacts with the ill persons. Refer to page 145 for details. Dry hands with towel.
7. Respiratory hygiene should be practiced by all, especially ill person.
8. Discard the material used to cover the mouth and nose or clean them appropriately.
9. Avoid direct contact with body fluid, particularly oral and nasal secretions.
10. Clean and disinfect frequently touched surfaces such as bedside tables, bedframes, and other bedroom furniture daily with household disinfectant containing diluted bleach.
11. Clean bathroom and toilet surfaces once daily.
12. Clean clothes and bed clothes, bath and hand towels etc.
13. Persons with symptoms should remain at home until their symptoms are resolved based on either clinical and/or laboratory findings (two negative RT-PCR tests at least 24 hours apart).
14. All household members should be considered contacts and their health should be monitored for respiratory infection, fever, cough, sore throat, difficult breathing.
15. Use of pulse oximeter to monitor oxygen saturation.

Pulse oximeter : It is a compact portable device, measures arterial blood oxygen saturation (SpO_2), heart rate and signal strength. Measuring range : SpO_2 30 to 100 per cent (minimum graduation 1 per cent), heart rate – 20 to 250 beats per minute (minimum graduation 1 beat per minute).

Revised discharge policy for hospitalized patients

The recommendation of Government of India on the discharge policy is summarized and is as shown in the algorithm in Fig. 3.

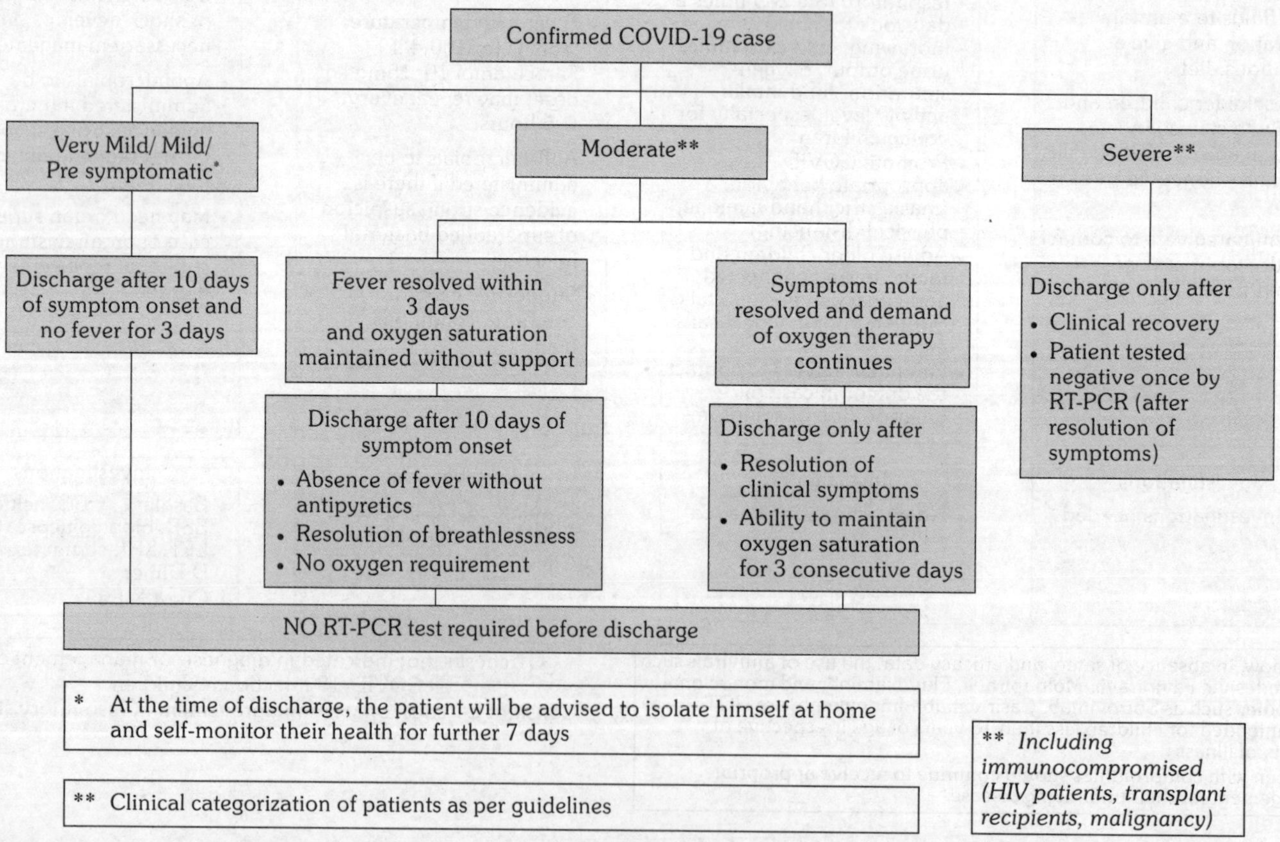

FIG. 3
Revised discharge policy for COVID-19

Source : *(16)*

Post COVID-19 management protocol *(17)*

After acute COVID-19 illness, recovered patients may continue to report wide variety of signs and symptoms including fatigue, body ache, cough, sore throat, difficulty in breathing etc. For details please refer to page 196. A holistic approach is required for follow-up care and well-being of all post-COVID-19 recovering patients. The recovery period is likely to be longer for patients who suffered more severe form of the disease and those with pre-existing illness.

POST-COVID FOLLOW-UP PROTOCOL

1. At individual level

- Continue COVID appropriate behaviour (use of mask, hand and respiratory hygiene, physical distancing).
- Drink adequate amount of warm water (if not contra-indicated).
- Take immunity promoting AYUSH medicine, to be practiced and prescribed by a qualified practitioner of AYUSH.
- If health permits, regular household work to be done. Professional work to be resumed in graded manner.
- Mild/ moderate exercise
  - Daily practice of yogasana, pranayama and meditation, as much as health permits or as prescribed.
  - Breathing exercises as prescribed by treating physician.
  - Daily morning or evening walk at a comfortable pace as tolerated.
- Balanced nutritious diet, preferably easy to digest freshly cooked soft diet.
- Have adequate sleep and rest.
- Avoid smoking and consumption of alcohol.
- Take regular medications as advised for COVID and also for managing comorbidities, if any. Doctor to be always informed about all medicines that the individual is taking (allopathic/AYUSH) so as to avoid prescription interaction.
- Self-health monitoring at home-temperature, blood pressure, blood sugar (especially, if diabetic), pulse oximetry etc. (if medically advised)
- If there is persistent dry cough / sore throat, do saline gargles and take steam inhalation. The addition of herbs/ spices for gargling/steam inhalation can help. Cough medications, should be taken on advice of medical doctor or qualified practitioner of Ayush.
- Look for early warning signs like high grade fever, breathlessness, $SpO_2 < 95\%$, unexplained chest pain, new onset of confusion, focal weakness.

2. At the level of community

- Recovered individuals to share their positive experiences with their friends and relatives using social media, community leaders, opinion leaders, religious leaders for creating awareness, dispelling myths and stigma.
- Take support of community based self-help groups, civil society organizations, and qualified professionals for recovery and rehabilitation process (medical, social, occupational, livelihood).
- Seek psycho-social support from peers, community health workers, counsellor. If required seek mental health support service.
- Participate in group sessions of Yoga, Meditation etc. while taking all due precautions like physical distancing.

3. In health-care facility setting

- The first follow-up visit (physical/telephonic) should be within 7 days after discharge, preferably at the hospital where he/she underwent treatment.
- Subsequent treatment/follow-up visits may be with the nearest qualified allopathic/AYUSH practitioner/medical facility of other systems of medicine. Poly-therapy is to be avoided due to potential for unknown drug-drug interaction, which may lead to Serious Adverse Events (SAE) or Adverse Effects (AE).
- The patients who had undergone home isolation, if they complain of persisting symptoms, will visit the nearest health facility.
- Severe cases requiring critical care support will require more stringent follow-up.

Public health surveillance for COVID-19 *(18)*

The aim of national surveillance for COVID-19 is to enable public health authorities to reduce transmission of SARS-CoV-2, thereby limiting associated morbidity and mortality.

The objectives of COVID-19 surveillance are to :

- Enable rapid detection, isolation, testing, and management of cases
- Detect and contain clusters and outbreaks, especially among vulnerable populations
- Identify, follow-up and quarantine contacts
- Guide the implementation and adjustment of targetted control measures, while enabling safe resumption of economic and social activities
- Evaluate the impact of the pandemic on health care systems and society
- Monitor longer term epidemiologic trends and evolution of SARS-CoV-2 virus and monitor trends in COVID-19 deaths
- Contribute to the understanding of the co-circulation of SARS-CoV-2 virus, influenza and other respiratory viruses, and other pathogens.

Surveillance approaches

Most countries need significantly strengthened surveillance capacities to rapidly identify and care for cases of COVID-19, trace and quarantine their contacts and monitor disease trends over time. Comprehensive national surveillance for COVID-19 will require the adaptation and reinforcement of existing national systems, where appropriate, and the scale-up of additional surveillance capacities, as needed. Digital technologies for rapid reporting, contact tracing and data management and analysis may support these capacities.

Robust comprehensive surveillance, once in place, should be maintained even in areas where transmission has been suppressed or controlled, even if there are few or no cases. It is critical that new cases and clusters of SARS-CoV-2 infection be detected rapidly before outbreaks or widespread transmission occurs. Ongoing surveillance for COVID-19 is also important to understand longer-term epidemiological trends, such as incidence and mortality among different age groups, which population groups are at higher risk for severe disease and death, and potential epidemiological changes over time.

Key actions for comprehensive COVID-19 surveillance include:

- Use, adaptation and strengthening of existing surveillance systems

- Strengthen laboratory and testing capacities
- Use, adaptation and enhancement of public health workforce to carry out case finding, contact tracing and testing
- Include COVID-19 as a mandatory notifiable disease
- Implement immediate reporting
- Establish systems to monitor contact tracing activity.

It is important to maintain routine syndromic surveillance for other infectious diseases, especially those caused by respiratory pathogens, such as influenza and respiratory syncytial virus, through surveillance for influenza-like-illness (ILI), severe acute respiratory infection (SARI), atypical pneumonia and unexplained fever, with sampling and laboratory testing of all or a subset of cases. This is critical for understanding trends in other diseases with similar presentations to guide appropriate public health preparedness and clinical management.

Essential surveillance for COVID-19

Surveillance systems should be geographically comprehensive, and surveillance for vulnerable or high-risk populations should be enhanced. This will require a combination of surveillance systems including contact tracing for all levels of the health care system, at the community level, in closed residential settings and in other vulnerable groups. Table 4 shows how surveillance systems can be combined across different sites.

Global surveillance

The objectives of the global surveillance are as follows:

- Monitor trends in COVID-19 at national and global levels
- Monitor mortality caused by, and indirectly associated with, COVID-19
- Estimate morbidity and mortality for health care workers
- Assess the impact of control measures.

Weekly aggregated reporting

The aim of ongoing weekly aggregate reporting is to obtain further information on global COVID-19 trends for enhanced analysis. The variables are as follows *(19)* :

- Number of confirmed cases
- Number of probable cases
- Number of confirmed deaths
- Number of probable deaths
- Number of individuals hospitalized (confirmed and probable)
- Number discharged (confirmed and probable)
- Number of health care workers infected (confirmed + probable) as a subset of total cases count
- Number of health care workers who died due to COVID-19 (confirmed + probable) as a subset of total death count
- Number of persons tested
- Number of persons tested by PCR
- Confirmed + probable cases by age group and sex
- Confirmed + probable deaths by age group and sex

Categories for transmission pattern *(19)*

WHO recommends using the following categories to describe transmission patterns at national and sub-national levels to guide decisions for preparedness, readiness and response activities. The definitions of categories are as shown in Table 5.

Prevention of the disease

"Do gaj ki doori, mask hai jaroori" is the slogan of the day. Although the vaccine is now available in India, it is critical that people should continue to follow all the "COVID Appropriate Behaviour". They should use mask, maintain a physical distance of at least 6 feet when in public place, not touch nose, eyes and mouth, cover mouth and nose while coughing and sneezing and avoid spitting in open, prompt testing on observing symptoms, and isolation if having the disease or for contacts quarantine for 14 days.

While UK and USA have emerged as the first two countries in the world to launch the COVID vaccine, India has also launched one of the world's largest COVID vaccination drive. This is the first time that a vaccine for COVID-19 has been developed and launched in the country.

Dry run for the vaccine : The dry run is a mock drill to test the laid out mechanisms for COVID-19 vaccination roll out in the health system and to assess the operational feasibility of using Co-Win application in field environment for planning, implementation and reporting at the block, district and state levels *(20, 21)*.

TABLE 4
Surveillance systems across different sites/contexts

Site/Context \ System	Immediate case notification	Contact tracing	Virologic surveillance	Cluster investigations	Mortality surveillance	Serologic surveillance
Community	×	×		×	×	×
Primary Care Sites (non-sentinel ILI/ARI)	×		×	×		
Hospitals (non-sentinel ILI/SARI)	×		×	×	×	×
Sentinel ILI/ARI/ SARI sites	×		×			
Closed settings*	×	×		×	×	×
Health care-associated SARS-CoV-2 infection	×	×		×	×	×
Travellers at points of entry	×	×		×		

*Including but not limited to long-term living facilities, prisons and dormitories.

Source : *(19)*

TABLE 5

Definition of the categories for transmission pattern

Category name	Definition
No (active) cases	No new cases detected for at least 28 days (two times the maximum incubation period), in the presence of a robust surveillance system. This implies a near-zero risk of infection for the general population.
Imported / Sporadic cases	Cases detected in the past 14 days are all imported, sporadic (e.g. laboratory acquired or zoonotic) or are all linked to imported/sporadic cases, and there are no clear signals of further locally acquired transmission. This implies minimal risk of infection for the general population.
Clusters of cases	Cases detected in the past 14 days are predominantly limited to well-defined clusters that are not directly linked to imported cases, but which are all linked by time, geographic location and common exposures. It is assumed that there are a number of unidentified cases in the area. This implies a low risk of infection to others in the wider community if exposure to these clusters is avoided.
Community transmission – level 1 (CT1)	Low incidence of locally acquired widely dispersed cases detected in the past 14 days not linked to specific clusters; transmission may be focussed in certain population sub-groups. Low risk of infection for the general population.
Community transmission – level 2 (CT2)	Moderate incidence of locally acquired widely dispersed cases detected in the past 14 days; transmission less focussed in certain population sub-groups. Moderate risk of infection for the general population.
Community transmission – level 3 (CT3)	High incidence of locally acquired widely dispersed cases in the past 14 days; transmission not focussed in certain population sub-groups. High risk of infection for the general population.
Community transmission – level 4 (CT4)	Very high incidence of locally acquired widely dispersed cases in the past 14 days. Very high risk of infection for the general population.

Source : *(19)*

Vaccination for COVID-19 is voluntary. However, it is advisable to receive the complete schedule of COVID-19 vaccine for protecting one-self against this disease and also to limit the spread of this disease to the close contacts. It is advisable to receive complete schedule of COVID vaccine irrespective of past history of infection with COVID-19. This will help in developing a strong immune response against the disease. Person with confirmed or suspected COVID-19 infection may increase the risk of spreading the same to others at vaccination site. For this reason, infected individuals should defer vaccination for 14 days after symptoms resolution.

Based on the potential availability of vaccines the Government of India selected the priority groups which are at higher risk. The first group includes healthcare workers because they are at high risk of contracting the infection and protecting them helps to sustain essential health services. The vaccination of frontline workers (police, home-guard, municipal worker, armed forces etc.) will help in reducing the societal and economic impact by reducing COVID-19 mortalities. The next group to receive COVID-19 vaccine was persons over 50 years of age and persons under 50 years with comorbid conditions because there is high mortality in this category. The reason for including more than 50 years of age group for vaccination was that it will be able to cover 78% of persons having co-morbidities and thereby reduce mortality on account of COVID-19. More than 50 years of age group was divided into two sub-groups. One sub-group was 60 years and above, they were vaccinated first. Second sub-group was between 50 to 60 years age group, they were vaccinated after the first sub group is covered. In subsequent phases the vaccine was given to the remaining persons above 18 years of age. COVID-19 vaccination for children in the age group 15–18 years started from 3rd January 2022. Covaxin is the only option for them *(22)*. Only 100 persons were vaccinated at each designated vaccination site per day.

The vaccination may not be sequential. It can go in parallel for all beneficiaries depending on the availability of the vaccine. Photo ID is a must for both registration and verification of beneficiary at session site to ensure that the intended person is vaccinated.

Any of the following mentioned ID with Photo may be produced at the time of registration : Aadhar Card, Driving License, Health Insurance Smart Card issued under the scheme of Ministry of Labour, MGNREGA Job Card, official identity cards issued to MPs/MLAs/MLCs, PAN Card, passbooks issued by bank/post Office, passport, pension document, service identity card with photograph issued to employees by Central/ State Govt./PSUs/Public Limited Companies, Voter ID and Smart card issued by RGI under NPR.

Following online registration, beneficiary will receive SMS on their registered mobile number for the due date, place, and time of vaccination. On getting due dose of COVID-19 vaccine, the beneficiary will receive SMS on their registered mobile number. After all doses of vaccine are administered, a QR code based certificate will also be sent to the registered mobile number of the beneficiary.

It must be ensured that the entire schedule of vaccination is completed by only one type of vaccine, as different COVID-19 vaccines are not interchangeable.

COVID-19 Vaccines

In the light of urgent need due to COVID pandemic in the country, Central Drugs Standard Control Organization (CDSCO) has granted permissions to following six COVID-19 vaccines for restricted use in emergency situation :

1. ChAdOx1 nCoV-19 Corona Virus Vaccine (Recombinant) (Covishield) manufactured by M/s Serum Institute of India Pvt., Ltd., Pune.
2. Whole Virion Inactivated Corona Virus Vaccine (Covaxin) manufactured by M/s Bharat Biotech International Limited, Hyderabad.
3. Gam-COVID-Vac Combined vector vaccine (SPUTNIK-V) imported by M/s Dr. Reddy's Laboratories Ltd, Hyderabad OR manufactured by M/s Ra (biologicals) Panacea Biotec Ltd., New Delhi.

4. mRNA-1273 COVID-19 vaccine (Moderna) imported by M/s Cipla Limited, Mumbai
5. Janssen/Ad 26. CoV2-S – Adenovirus vector platform based Vaccine manufactured by M/s Johnson & Johnson.
6. ZyCoV-D, a DNA based COVID-19 vaccine manufactured by M/s Zydus Cadilla Ltd.

Currently, three COVID-19 vaccines are being used under the vaccination program namely Covishield manufactured by M/s Serum Institute of India, Covaxin manufactured by M/s Bharat Biotech International Limited and Sputnik V vaccine developed by Gamaleya Research Institute, Russia (imported by Dr Reddy's Lab and is being administered in few private hospitals, presently).

Persons who are temporarily not eligible to get the vaccine are *(23)* :

(a) Persons showing active symptoms of SARS-CoV-2 infection;
(b) COVID-19 patients who have been given anti-SARS-CoV-2 monoclonal antibodies or convalescent plasma;
(c) The vaccine should be given with caution to persons with a history of any bleeding or coagulation disorder platelet disorder, clotting factor deficiency or coagulopathy; and
(d) Actually unwell and hospitalized patients (with or without intensive care) due to any illness.

Persons with a past history of COVID-19 infection can be administered the vaccine. Persons with a history of chronic disease and comorbidities (cardiac, neurological, pulmonary, and metabolic) are eligible for the vaccine although efficiency of the vaccine may be less in these patients. Administration of vaccine to pregnant women should only be considered when the potential benefits out weigh any potential risks for the mother and foetus. According to recent guidelines a pregnant women who opts for vaccination could be vaccinated at any time of pregnancy. It is unknown whether the vaccine is secreted in human milk. However the current guidelines of the Indian Government recommends COVID-19 vaccination for all lactating mothers. The vaccines are not interchangeable.

Covishield vaccine *(23)*

Covishield vaccine is a recombinant chimpanzee adenovirus vector vaccine, administered intramuscularly in deltoid muscle. Given in two doses, 12–16 weeks apart. The protective level of antibodies are generally developed two weeks after the 2nd dose of the vaccine. The vaccine has been approved for individuals 18 years of age and above. To be stored at 2–8°C.

Side effects

The common side effects with Covishield vaccine are : injection site pain and tenderness, headache, fatigue, myalgia, discomfort, pyrexia, chills and nausea. Very rare events of demyelination disorder have been reported following vaccine "without the causal relationship establishment".

Contraindications

1. Vaccine should not be given if there is severe allergic reaction after the previous dose of this vaccine;
2. Had a severe allergic reaction to any ingredient of this vaccine.

Covaxin vaccine *(23)*

The Bharat Biotech's vaccine, developed in collaboration with ICMR and NIV Pune, is a whole virion inactivated coronavirus vaccine. It is given intramuscularly in deltoid muscle in two doses 28 days apart, to persons above 18 years of age and recently approved for 15–18 year age group *(22)*. The vaccine should be stored at 2–8°C.

Side effects

The common side effects following Covaxin are : injection site pain, fatigue, fever, headache, bodyache, nausea, abdominal pain, dizziness, sweating, and cold and cough.

Contraindications

1. Those below 18 years of age;
2. Those with allergic reaction to any componant of Covaxin vaccine, plasma centrical products and notable food allergies;
3. Anyone who has had adverse reaction to COVID-19 vaccine earlier; and
4. Currently having an acute infection or fever.

Individuals with HIV infection or other immunocompromising conditions, or who take immunosuppressive medications might be at increased risk of severe COVID-19. However, data is not currently available to establish vaccine safety and efficacy in these groups. Individuals may not generate a full immune response to COVID-19. As Covaxin is not a live virus vaccine, it is not likely to pose a safety risk.

Sputnik V Vaccine

Sputnik V Vaccine (Gam-COVID-Vac) is manufactured by Gamaleya Research Institute, Russia. It is a non-replicating viral vector vaccine administered by intramuscular injection in two doses to people 18 years and above. The second dose is taken 21 days after the 1st dose. For both the Jabs, two different vectors are used (Adenovirus 26 and Adenovirus 5). The use of two varying serotypes is unique that provides long-lasting immunity. Vaccine can be stored at 2 to 8°C.

Some people reported mild side effects such as pain, redness or swelling at the site of injection, Asthenia, fatigue, body and muscle pain, cough and sore throat, runny nose, fever and chills, nausea and vomiting, diarrhoea and headache *(24)*.

In India vaccination is not mandatory. But if you choose to get vaccinated, you cannot choose which vaccine you will get. You will be vaccinated by the vaccine that is available at the site. 16th January, 2021 is the historical day when India launched the vaccination drive.

Pfizer-BioNtech COVID-19 Vaccine *(25)*

It is a messenger RNA vaccine with 95 per cent efficacy. People 16 years and older are eligible for the vaccine, administered in two doses intramuscularly, 3 weeks apart. It is authorized for emergency use. It is not interchangeable. Storage is at –70°C.

Contraindications : (a) history of severe allergic reaction after the previous dose of this vaccine; (b) had a severe reaction to any ingredient of this vaccine.

Before taking the vaccine the provider must know the medical history of the person : any allergy, fever, bleeding disorder if any, or taking blood thinner, if the person is immunocompromised or on a medicine that affects immune system, pregnancy and breast-feeding, and have received another COVID-19 vaccine.

Side effects : Injection site pain, tiredness, headache, muscle pain, chills, joint pain, fever, injection site swelling and redness, nausea, feeling unwell, swollen lymph nodes. There are remote chances of severe allergic reaction (within a few minutes to one hour after getting the dose).

Moderna COVID-19 Vaccine *(26)*

It is a messenger RNA vaccine, with efficacy of about 94.1 per cent, meant for people 18 years of age and above, two doses given intramuscularly 1 month apart. It should be stored between –25°C and –15°C temperature.

The vaccine provider must know about the history of allergies, fever, bleeding disorders or history of taking blood thinner, pregnancy and breast-feeding in mothers, history of taking another COVID-19 vaccine and if the recipient is immunocompromised.

Side effects : Side effects reported are : (a) injection site reactions are pain, redness, swelling, tenderness; (b) general side effects are fatigue, headache, muscle pain, joint pain, vomiting, and fever. Severe side effects are difficulty in breathing, swelling of face and throat, fast heart beat, bad rash all over the body, dizziness and weakness.

COVID-19 dead body management

All staff identified to handle dead bodies in the isolation area, mortuary, ambulance and those workers in the crematorium/burial ground should be trained in the infection prevention control practices. The health worker attending to the dead body should perform hand hygiene, ensure proper use of PPE. Plug oral, nasal orifices of the dead body to prevent leakage of body fluids. Place the body in leak-proof plastic body bag. The exterior of the body bag be decontaminated with 1 per cent hypochlorite.The body bag can be wrapped with a mortuary sheet or sheet provided by the family members. Embalming of the dead body should not be allowed. Autopsies should be avoided. The crematorium/ burial ground staff should be sensitized that COVID-19 does not pose additional risk to them. Viewing of the dead body by unzipping the face, for the relatives to see the body for one last time is allowed. Bathing, kissing, hugging, etc. of the dead body should not be allowed. Religious rituals such as reading from religious scripts, sprinkling holy water and any other last rites that does not require touching of the body can be allowed. Large gathering at the crematorium/burial ground should be avoided. The funeral staff and family members should perform hand hygiene after cremation/burial *(27)*.

References

1. NCBI Book Shelf (2020), *Features, evaluation and treatment of corona virus,* last updated 4th Oct. 2020.
2. WHO (2020), *Weekly update of global corona virus impact and implications.*
3. Worldometer.info, *COVID-19 Corona virus pandemic,* 20th Sept. 2022.
4. WHO (2022), *Tracking SARS-CoV-2 variants,* May 2022.
5. *Centers for Disease Control and Prevention,* 26th April 2022.
6. Govt. of India (2022), *Annual Report 2021-22,* Ministry of Health and Family Welfare, New Delhi.
7. WHO (2020), *Transmission of SARS-CoV-2, implications of infection prevention, precautions.*
8. Govt. of India (2020), *Clinical Management Protocol : COVID-19,* 5th version, 3rd July 2020.
9. WHO (2020), *Clinical Management of COVID-19,* 27th May 2020.
10. Govt. of India (2020), *National Centre for Disease Control, updated case definition and contact categories,* Director General of Health Services.
11. CDC (2022), *Long COVID or Post COVID conditions.*
12. Govt. of India, *Guidelines for management of mucormycosis in COVID-19 patients.*
13. AIIMS/ICMR/COVID-19 Task Force/Monitoring Group (2022), *Clinical guidance for management of adult COVID-19 patients,* Ministry of Health and Family Welfare, New Delhi, 14th Jan. 2022.
14. Govt. of India (2022), *Comprehensive guidelines for management of COVID-19 in children and adolescents (below 18 years),* DGHS, Ministry of Health and Family Welfare, New Delhi.
15. WHO, *Home care for patients with suspected noval corona infection presenting with mild symptoms and management of contacts,* 20th Jan. 2021.
16. Govt. of India (2020), *Final guidance on management of COVID cases.*
17. Govt. of India (2020), *Post COVID management protocol,* 13th Sept. 2020.
18. WHO (2020), *Public health guidelines for COVID-19 : Interim guidance,* 16th Dec. 2020.
19. WHO (2020), *Public Health Surveillance,* 16th Dec. 2020.
20. Govt. of India (2020), *COVID-19 vaccine strategy communication strategy, help us help you.*
21. Govt. of India (2020), *Frequently asked questions on COVID-19 vaccine,* target group : general public.
22. Govt. of India, *Guidelines for COVID-19 vaccination of children between 15–18 years and precaution dose to health care workers, frontline workers and 60+ population with comorbidities,* 3rd Jan. 2022.
23. Govt. of India, *Press release.*
24. *Sputnik V Vaccine, efficacy, doses, side effects and price,* Pace Hospital.
25. Pfizer-BioNtech COVID-19 Vaccine - *fact sheet for recipient and provider of the vaccine.*
26. Moderna COVID-19 Vaccine - *fact sheet for recipient and provider of the vaccine.*
27. Govt. of India (2020), *COVID-19 : Guidelines on dead body management,* 15th March 2020.

TUBERCULOSIS

Tuberculosis is a specific infectious disease caused by *M. tuberculosis.* The disease primarily affects lungs and causes pulmonary tuberculosis. It can also affect intestine, meninges, bones and joints, lymph glands, skin and other tissues of the body. The disease is usually chronic with varying clinical manifestations. The disease also affects animals like cattle; this is known as "bovine tuberculosis", which may sometimes be communicated to man. Pulmonary tuberculosis, the most important form of tuberculosis which affects man, will be considered here.

Problem statement

WORLD

Tuberculosis remains a worldwide public health problem despite the fact that the causative organism was discovered more than 100 years ago and highly effective drugs and vaccine are available making tuberculosis a preventable and curable disease. Technologically advanced countries have achieved spectacular results in the control of tuberculosis. This decline started long before the advent of BCG or chemotherapy and has been attributed to changes in the "non-specific" determinants of the disease such as improvements in the standard of living and the quality of life of the people coupled with the application of available technical knowledge and health resources.

It is estimated that about one-third of the current global population is infected asymptomatically with tuberculosis, of whom 5–10 per cent will develop clinical disease during their lifetime *(1)*. Most new cases and deaths occur in developing countries where infection is often acquired in childhood. The annual risk of tuberculosis infection in high burden countries is estimated to be 0.5–2 per cent *(2)*. Patients with infectious pulmonary tuberculosis disease can infect 10–15 persons in a year.

Globally, the COVID-19 pandemic has reversed years of progress in providing essential TB services and reducing TB disease burden. The most obvious impact is a large global drop in the number of people newly diagnosed with TB and reported. The fall is from 7.1 million cases in 2019 to 5.8 million in 2020, an 18 per cent decline back to the level of 2012 and far short of the estimated 10 million people who developed TB in 2020. 16 countries accounted for 93 per cent of this reduction, with India, Indonesia and the Philippines the worst affected *(3)*.

Reduced access to TB diagnosis and treatment has resulted in an increase in TB deaths. The estimates for year 2020 are 1.3 million TB deaths among HIV-negative people and an additional 2,14,000 among HIV-positive people, with the combined total back to the level of 2017. People who are infected with HIV are 18 times more likely to develop active TB.

In the year 2020, out of estimated 10 million cases, 5.6 million were men, 3.3 million women and 1.1 million children. The severity of national TB epidemics, in terms of the number of incident TB cases per 1,00,000 population per year, varies widely among countries, from less than five to more than 500 new and relapse cases per 1,00,000 population per year. In 2020, 57 countries had a low incidence of TB (<10 cases/1,00,000 population), mostly in the WHO region of the Americas and European region. There were 150–400 cases/1,00,000 population in most of the 30 high TB burden countries *(3)*.

Drug-resistant TB continues to be a public health threat. Resistance to isoniazid and rifampicin - the two most effective first-line drugs - is of greatest concern. Globally, the burden of MDR-TB or RR-TB is stable. For more than 10 years, the best estimate of the proportion of people diagnosed with MDR/RR-TB has remained at about 3–4 per cent and the best estimate for MDR-TB in those previously treated for TB has remained at about 18–21 per cent *(3)*.

In year 2020, the success rate among patients treated for DR-TB remained at 59 per cent as large proportion of patients were lost due to discontinuation of treatment or death *(4)*.

The preventive treatment for TB is expanding, especially in the priority risk groups of people living with HIV and children under 5 years of age. However, most people eligible for TB preventive treatment are not accepting it *(5)*.

The actual burden of paediatric TB is not known due to diagnostic difficulties. It is assumed that about 10 per cent of total TB load is found in children. Globally, about 1 million cases of paediatric TB are estimated to occur every year, with more than 100,000 deaths *(6)*. Childhood deaths from TB are usually caused by meningitis or disseminated disease *(2)*. Though MDR-TB and XDR-TB is documented among paediatric age groups, there are no estimates of overall burden because of diagnostic difficulties and exclusion of children in most of the drug resistant surveys *(6)*.

In many developing countries, acquired drug resistance remains high, because national tuberculosis control programmes in these countries have not been able to achieve a high cure rate over a very long period of time, even after the introduction of short–course chemotherapy. Poverty, economic recession, malnutrition, overcrowding, indoor air pollution, tobacco, alcohol abuse and diabetes make populations more vulnerable to tuberculosis. Increase in human migration has rapidly mixed infected with uninfected communities. To make global situation worse, tuberculosis has formed a lethal combination with HIV.

The WHO has set *International Standards for Tuberculosis Care.* These standards are intended to facilitate the effective engagement of all care-providers in delivering high-quality care for patients of all ages, including those with smear-positive, smear-negative, extrapulmonary tuberculosis, drug-resistant tuberculosis, and tuberculosis combined with HIV infection. The basic principles of care for people with, or suspected of having tuberculosis are the same worldwide. The standards are intended to be complementary to local and national tuberculosis control policies that are consistent with WHO recommendations. They are not intended to replace local guidelines. There are 6 standards for diagnosis, 9 standards for treatment and 2 standards for public health responsibilities. Please refer to WHO publication : Weekly Epidemiological Record, No. 5, dated 3rd Feb. 2006 for further details.

For the past two decades, national and international efforts in TB prevention, diagnosis and treatment have been guided by the DOTS strategy (mid–1990 until 2005) and subsequently the Stop TB Strategy (2006–2015). The Stop TB strategy was designed to achieve global TB targets set for 2015 within the context of the Millennium Development Goals *(7)*. It focused on five indicators to measure the implementation and impact of TB control. They are; case detection, treatment success, incidence, prevalence and death. The core of the strategy was DOTS. The WHO End TB strategy, adopted by the World Health Assembly in May 2014, is a blueprint for countries to end the TB epidemic by driving down TB deaths, incidence and eliminating catastrophic costs. It outlines global impact targets to reduce TB deaths by 90 per cent and to cut new cases by 80 per cent between 2015 and 2030, and to ensure that no family is burdened with the costs due to TB. Ending the TB epidemic by 2030 is among the health targets of the newly adopted Sustainable Development Goals. WHO has gone one step further and set a 2035 target of 95 per cent reduction in deaths and a 90 per cent decline in TB incidence – similar to current levels in low TB incidence countries today *(8)*. For further details, please refer to page 237.

In September 2018, the UN General Assembly held its first-ever high level meeting on TB. The outcome was a political declaration in which commitments to SDGs and End TB Strategy were reaffirmed and new ones added. Global targets for funding to be mobilized for TB prevention, care and research, and for the number of people to be treated for TB infection and disease, were set for the first time. The targets are as follows *(1)* :

1. 40 million people treated for TB from 2018 to 2022, including :
   - 3.5 million children
   - 1.5 million people with drug-resistant TB, including 115,000 children.
2. At least 30 million people provided with TB preventive treatment from 2018 to 2022, including
   - 6 million people living with HIV
   - 4 million children under 5 years of age and 20 million people in other age groups, who are household contacts of people affected by TB.
3. Funding of at least US$ 13 billion per year for universal access to TB prevention, diagnosis, treatment and care by 2022.
4. Funding of at least US$ 2 billion per year for TB research from 2018 to 2022.

INDIA

India is the highest TB burden country in the world in terms of absolute number of incident cases that occur each year. It accounts for 26 per cent of the estimated global incident TB cases in 2020. Table 1 shows the burden of tuberculosis in India, the estimated and reported cases for the year 2020.

TABLE 1

Burden of tuberculosis in India (2020)
(Population : 1,380 million)

	Number (thousands)	Rate (per 100,000 population)
Estimates of TB burden, 2020*		
Total TB incidence	2590 (1780–3550)	188 (129–257)
HIV positive TB incidence	53 (36–72)	3.8 (2.6–5.2)
HIV negative TB mortality	493 (453–536)	36 (33–39)
HIV positive TB mortality	11 (9.8–12)	0.78 (0.71–0.84)
*Universal health coverage and social protection**		
TB treatment coverage (notified/estimated incidence), 2020		63% (46–92)
TB case fatality ratio (estimated mortality/estimated incidence), 2020		20% (14–27)
TB case notifications, 2020		
Total new and relapse		1,629,301
– % tested with rapid diagnostics at time of diagnosis		18%
– % with known HIV status		92%
– % pulmonary		71%
– % bacteriologically confirmed^		54%
– % children aged 0–14 years		6%
– % women (aged ≥ 15 years)		36%
– % men (aged ≥ 15 years)		58%
Total cases notified		1,812,643
TB/HIV care in new and relapse TB patients, 2020		
	Number	(%)
Patients with known HIV-status who are HIV-positive	30,496	2%
– on antiretroviral therapy	28,931	95%
*Drug-resistant TB care**, 2020*		
% of bacteriologically confirmed TB cases tested for rifampicin resistance - New cases^		98%
% of bacteriologically confirmed TB cases tested for rifampicin resistance - Previously treated cases^		96%
Laboratory-confirmed cases : MDR/RR-TB^^		49,679
Patients started on treatment : MDR/RR-TB^^^		42,505
Laboratory-confirmed cases : pre-XDR-TB or XDR-TB^^		8,982
Patients started on treatment : pre-XDR-TB or XDR-TB^^^		8,256
MDR/RR-TB cases tested for resistance to any fluoroquinolone		16,354
Treatment success rate and cohort size		
	Success	Cohort
New and relapse cases registered in 2019	84%	2,152,563
Previously treated cases, excluding relapse, registered in 2019	77%	147,159
HIV-positive TB cases registered in 2019	71%	40,031
MDR/RR-TB cases started on second-line treatment in 2018	56%	47,284
XDR-TB cases started on second-line treatment in 2018	48%	2,661
TB preventive treatment, 2020		
% of HIV-positive people (newly enrolled in care) on preventive treatment		39%
% of children (aged<5) household contacts of bacteriologically-confirmed TB cases on preventive treatment		42% (39–46)

* Estimates of TB burden are produced by WHO in consultation with countries. Ranges represent uncertainty intervals.

** RR is TB resistant to rifampicin (R); MDR is TB resistant to R + isoniazid; pre-XDR is TB resistant to R + any fluoroquinolone.

^ Calculated for pulmonary cases only.

^^ Includes cases with unknown previous TB treatment history.

^^^ Includes patients diagnosed before 2020 and patients who were not laboratory-confirmed.

Source : *(9)*

AGE DISTRIBUTION : Overall the age distribution of TB diagnosed incident cases shows a predominance in adolescent and young adult age groups between 15 to 30 years of age, indicating ongoing disease transmission as shown in Fig. 1. However, there is a wide variation in the age distribution pattern among the states. In southern states of Kerala, Karnataka, Tamil Nadu, Andhra Pradesh and UTs of Puducherry, Lakshadweep there is a general elderly prevalence of TB towards the age 50+ year ranges. In other states the incidence is similar to that of the country.

THE ECONOMIC AND SOCIAL BURDEN OF DISEASE : Besides the disease burden, TB also causes an enormous socio-economic burden to India. TB primarily affects people in their most productive years of life. While two-thirds of the cases are male, TB takes disproportionately larger toll among young females, with more than 50 per cent of female cases occurring before the age of 34 years *(11)*.

Tuberculosis kills more women in reproductive age group than all causes of maternal mortality combined, and it may create more orphans than any other infectious disease. Nearly one-third of female infertility in India, is caused by tuberculosis. The indirect impact of tuberculosis on children is considerable, as nearly 3 lacs children of tuberculosis patients, either leave the school or take up employment to help support their families *(8)*. A patient of tuberculosis takes an average of three to four months to recuperate, losing that much income. The loss is disastrous for those struggling against poverty. They are most likely to be defaulters of treatment. The vast majority (more than 90 per cent) of the economic burden of TB in India is caused by the loss of life rather than morbidity.

In India, tuberculosis is mainly a disease of the poor. The majority of its victims are migrant labourers, slum dwellers, residents of backward areas and tribal pockets. Poor living conditions, malnutrition, shanty housing and overcrowding are the main reasons for the spread of the disease *(12)*.

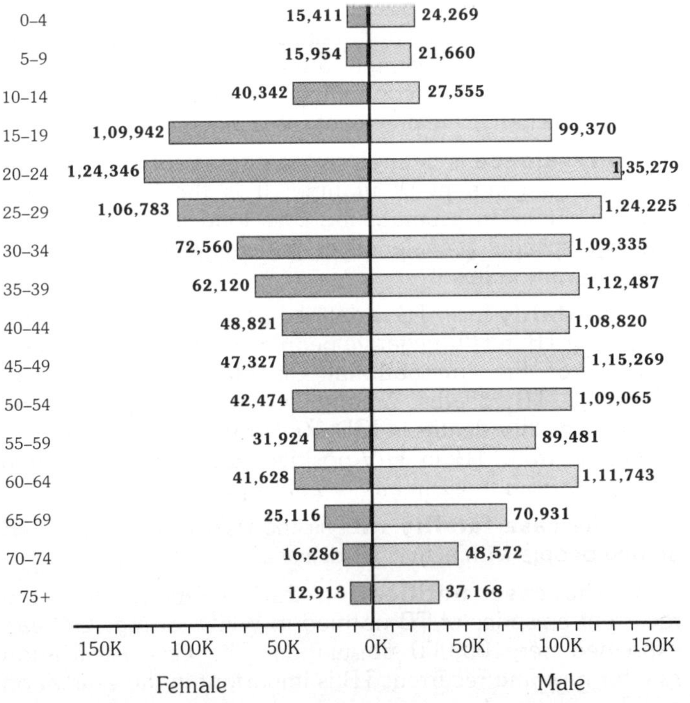

FIG. 1

Age distribution of TB cases, India (2019)

Source : *(10)*

HIV increases a person's susceptibility to tuberculosis infection, and tuberculosis is one of the earliest opportunistic disease to develop amongst persons infected with HIV. It increases morbidity and mortality in HIV infected persons. HIV is the most potent risk factor for progression of TB infection to disease.

Since death rate is declining and the disease is showing a decline in younger age groups, epidemiologists are beginning to think that perhaps we may have crossed the peak of the secular epidemic curve and are somewhere at the beginning of the declining limb.

Despite a comprehensive national TB control programme guiding states for implementation of TB diagnosis and treatment, there is still a long way to go. The vision of RNTCP is that the people suffering from TB receive the highest standards of care and support from healthcare providers of their choice. It is spelt out in the National strategic plan 2012–17 to extend the umbrella of quality TB care and control to include those provided by the private sector. Thus Standards of TB care relevant in Indian context and acceptable to medical fraternity were developed. These standards represent what is expected from Indian health care system *(13)*.

Epidemiological indices *(14)*

Indices or parameters are needed to measure the tuberculosis problem in a community as well as for planning and evaluation of control measures. Indices are also required for international comparison. The following epidemiological indices are generally used in tuberculosis problem measurement and programme strategy :

1. **Incidence** is defined as the number of new and recurrent (relapse) episodes of TB (all forms) occurring in a given year. Recurrent episodes are defined as a new episode of TB in people who have had TB in the past and for whom there was bacteriological confirmation of cure and/or documentation that treatment was completed. Relapse cases are referred to as recurrent cases because the term is more useful when explaining the estimation of TB incidence. Recurrent cases may be true relapses or a new episode of TB caused by reinfection. In current case definitions, both relapse cases and patients who require a change in treatment are called 'retreatment cases'. However, people with a continuing episode of TB that requires a treatment change are prevalent cases, not incident cases.

2. **Prevalence** is defined as the number of TB cases (all forms) at a given point in time. It is the best available practical index to estimate the case load in a community. The age-specific prevalence of patients is considered the most relevant index.

3. **Mortality** from TB is defined as the number of deaths caused by TB in HIV-negative people, according to the latest revision of the International Classification of Diseases (ICD-10). TB deaths among HIV-positive people are classified as HIV deaths in ICD-10. For this reason, estimates of deaths from TB in HIV-positive people are presented separately from those in HIV-negative people.

4. The **case fatality rate** is the risk of death from TB among people with active TB disease.

5. The **case notification rate** refers to new and recurrent episodes of TB notified to WHO for a given year, expressed per 100,000 population. The case notification rate for new and recurrent TB is important in the estimation of TB incidence. In some countries, however, information on treatment history may be missing for some cases. When data on treatment history are not available, recurrent cases cannot be distinguished from cases whose treatment was changed, since both are registered and reported in the category "retreatment". Patients reported in the "unknown history" category are considered incident TB episodes (new or relapse). This is a change from previous years in view of past difficulties to estimate with NTPs the proportion of true new, or relapse TB episodes in this category of patients.

6. **Case detection rate** : The case detection rate is calculated as the number of notification of new and relapse cases in a year divided by the estimated incidence of such cases in the same year.

7. **Prevalence of drug-resistant cases** : It is the prevalence of patient excreting tubercle bacilli resistant to anti-tuberculosis drugs. This index is directly related to chemotherapy.

(a) *Prevalence of infection* : It is the percentage of individuals who show a positive reaction to the standard tuberculin test. When the test is done in defined age-groups, it yields age-specific prevalence which is a far superior indicator than the mere percentage of positive reactors in the total population *(15)*. Prevalence represents a cumulative experience of a population to recent and remote infection with *M. tuberculosis*. It may be mentioned that the interpretation of tuberculin test has become complicated in countries with a high coverage of BCG vaccination at birth, since most of the vaccinees become positive reactors to tuberculin test. This presents a problem in identifying true prevalence of infection. Further, cross-sensitivity to atypical mycobacteriae, where it occurred, has also caused the prevalence to be over-estimated. Despite these limitations, tuberculin-testing is widely used for estimating the prevalence of tuberculous infection in a population.

(b) *Incidence of infection* : (Annual Infection Rate) : It is the percentage of population under study who will be newly infected by Mycobacterium tuberculosis among the non-infected of the preceding survey during the course of one year. It reflects the annual risk of being infected (or reinfected) in a given community. In other words, it expresses the attacking force of tuberculosis in a community *(16)*. In developing countries, every 1% of annual risk of infection is said to correspond to 50 new cases of smear–positive pulmonary tuberculosis, per year for 100,000 general population *(17)*. Also known as "tuberculin conversion" index, this parameter is considered one of the best indicators for evaluating the tuberculosis problem and its trend. The higher the rate, the greater the problem *(16, 18)*. It may be mentioned that a good treatment programme, lowers the risk of tuberculosis infection in the community.

Definitions of tuberculosis cases and treatment *(19)*

WHO has issued updated guidance on definitions of cases and treatment outcomes and associated reporting framework. These updates were necessary to accomodate diagnosis using Xpert MTB/RIF and other WHO-endorsed molecular tests, as well as offering an opportunity to improve aspects of the existing (2006) framework, such as inclusion of more comprehensive reporting of TB cases among children. The updated definitions are used from 2014 in global data collection *(14)*.

Presumptive case: Presumptive TB refers to a patient who presents with symptoms or signs suggestive of TB (previously known as a TB suspect).

A. CASE DEFINITIONS

a. *A bacteriologically confirmed TB case* is one from whom a biological specimen is positive by smear microscopy, culture or WRD (such as Xpert MTB/RIF). All such cases should be notified, regardless of whether TB treatment has started.

b. *A clinically diagnosed TB case* is one who does not fulfil the criteria for bacteriological confirmation but has been diagnosed with active TB by a clinician or other medical practitioner who has decided to give the patient a full course of TB treatment. This definition includes cases diagnosed on the basis of X-ray abnormalities or suggestive histology and extrapulmonary cases without laboratory confirmation. Clinically diagnosed cases subsequently found to be bacteriologically positive (before or after starting treatment) should be reclassified as bacteriologically confirmed.

Bacteriologically confirmed or clinically diagnosed cases of TB are also classified according to:

1. anatomical site of disease;
2. history of previous treatment;
3. drug resistance;
4. HIV status.

1. Classification based on anatomical site of disease

a. *Pulmonary tuberculosis (PTB)* refers to any bacteriologically confirmed or clinically diagnosed case of TB involving the lung parenchyma or the tracheobronchial tree. Miliary TB is classified as PTB because there are lesions in the lungs. Tuberculous intra-thoracic lymphadenopathy (mediastinal and/or hilar) or tuberculous pleural effusion, without radiographic abnormalities in the lungs, constitutes a case of extrapulmonary TB. A patient with both pulmonary and extrapulmonary TB should be classified as a case of PTB.

b. *Extrapulmonary tuberculosis (EPTB)* refers to any bacteriologically confirmed or clinically diagnosed case of TB involving organs other than the lungs, e.g. pleura, lymph nodes, abdomen, genitourinary tract, skin, joints and bones, meninges.

2. Classification based on history of previous TB treatment (patient registration group)

Classifications based on history of previous TB treatment are slightly different from those previously defined. They focus only on history of previous treatment and are independent of bacteriological confirmation or site of disease.

New patients: Patients who have never been treated for TB or have taken anti-TB drugs for less than 1 month.

Previously treated patients: Patients who received 1 month or more of anti-TB drugs in the past. They are further classified by the outcome of their most recent course of treatment as follows:

a. *Relapse patients* have previously been treated for TB, were declared cured or treatment completed at the end of their most recent course of treatment, and are now diagnosed with a recurrent episode of TB (either a true relapse or a new episode of TB caused by reinfection).

b. *Treatment after failure patients* are those who have previously been treated for TB and whose treatment failed at the end of their most recent course of treatment.

c. *Treatment after loss to follow-up patients* have previously been treated for TB and were declared lost to follow-up at the end of their most recent course of treatment. (These were previously known as treatment after default patients.)

d. *Other previously treated patients* are those who have previously been treated for TB but whose outcome after their most recent course of treatment is unknown or undocumented.

e. *Patients with unknown previous TB treatment history* do not fit into any of the categories listed above. New and relapse cases of TB are incident TB cases.

3. Classification based on drug resistance

Cases are classified in categories based on drug susceptibility testing (DST) of clinical isolates confirmed to be *M. tuberculosis* :

a. *Monoresistance:* resistance to one first-line anti-TB drug only.

b. *Polydrug resistance:* resistance to more than one first-line anti-TB drug (other than both isoniazid and rifampicin).

c. *Multidrug resistance:* resistance to at least both isoniazid and rifampicin.

d. *Extensive drug resistance:* resistance to any fluoroquinolone and at least one of three second-line injectable drugs (capreomycin, kanamycin and amikacin), in addition to multidrug resistance.

e. *Rifampicin resistance:* resistance to rifampicin detected using phenotypic or genotypic methods, with or without resistance to other anti-TB drugs. It includes any resistance to rifampicin, whether monoresistance, multidrug resistance, polydrug resistance or extensive drug resistance.

These categories are not all mutually exclusive. When enumerating rifampicin-resistant TB (RR-TB), for instance, multidrug-resistant TB (MDR-TB) and extensively drug-resistant TB (XDR-TB) are also included. While it has been the practice until now to limit the definitions of monoresistance and polydrug resistance to first-line drugs only, future drug regimens may make it important to classify patients by their strain resistance patterns to fluoroquinolones, second-line injectable agents and any other anti-TB drug for which reliable DST becomes available.

4. Classification based on HIV status

a. *HIV-positive TB patient* refers to any bacteriologically confirmed or clinically diagnosed case of TB who has a positive result from HIV testing conducted at the time of TB diagnosis or other documented evidence of enrolment in HIV care, such as enrolment in the pre-ART register or in the ART register once ART has been started.

b. *HIV-negative TB patient* refers to any bacteriologically confirmed or clinically diagnosed case of TB who has a negative result from HIV testing conducted at the time of TB diagnosis. Any HIV-negative TB patient subsequently found to be HIV-positive should be reclassified accordingly.

c. *HIV status unknown TB patient* refers to any bacteriologically confirmed or clinically diagnosed case of TB who has no result of HIV testing and no other documented evidence of enrolment in HIV care. If the patient's HIV status is subsequently determined, he or she should be reclassified accordingly.

B. TREATMENT OUTCOME DEFINITIONS

The new treatment outcome definitions make a clear distinction between two types of patients:

- patients treated for drug-susceptible TB;
- patients treated for drug-resistant TB using second-line treatment (defined as combination chemotherapy for drug-resistant tuberculosis which includes drugs other than the first-line drugs (see page 218).

The two groups are mutually exclusive. Any patient found to have drug-resistant TB and placed on second-line treatment is removed from the drug-suscepitible TB outcome cohort. This means that management of the standard TB register and of the second-line TB treatment register needs to be coordinated to ensure proper accounting of the outcomes of treatment.

1. Treatment outcomes for TB patients (excluding patients treated for RR-TB or MDR-TB)

All bacteriologically confirmed and clinically diagnosed TB cases should be assigned an outcome from this list except those with RR-TB or MDR-TB, who are placed on a second-line drug regimen.

Outcome	Definition
Cured	A pulmonary TB patient with bacteriologically confirmed TB at the beginning of treatment who was smear or culture-negative in the last month of treatment and on at least one previous occasion.
Treatment completed	A TB patient who completed treatment without evidence of failure BUT with no record to show that sputum smear or culture results in the last month of treatment and on at least one previous occasion were negative, either because tests were not done or because results are unavailable.
Treatment failed	A TB patient whose sputum smear or culture is positive at month 5 or later during treatment.
Died	A TB patient who dies for any reason before starting or during the course of treatment.
Lost to follow-up	A TB patient who did not start treatment or whose treatment was interrupted for 2 consecutive months or more.
Not evaluated	A TB patient for whom no treatment outcome is assigned. This includes cases "transferred out" to another treatment unit as well as cases for whom the treatment outcome is unknown to the reporting unit.
Treatment success	The sum of cured and treatment completed.
Cohort	A group of patients in whom TB has been diagnosed, and who were registered for treatment during a specified time period (e.g. the cohort of new smear-positive cases registered in the calendar year 2011). This group forms the denominator for calculating treatment outcomes. The sum of the treatment outcomes, plus any case for which no outcome is recorded (eg. still on treatment) should equal the number of cases registered *(5)*.

Patients found to have an RR-TB or MDR-TB strain at any point in time should be started on an adequate second-line drug regimen. These cases are excluded from the main TB cohort when calculating treatment outcomes and included only in the second-line TB treatment cohort analysis. If treatment with a second-line drug regimen is not possible, the patient is kept in the main TB cohort and assigned an outcome from above table.

2. Outcomes for RR-TB/MDR-TB/XDR-TB patients treated using second-line treatment

Outcome	Definition
Cured	Treatment completed as recommended by the national policy without evidence of failure AND three or more consecutive cultures taken at least 30 days apart are negative after the intensive phase.[a]
Treatment completed	Treatment completed as recommended by the national policy without evidence of failure BUT no record that three or more consecutive cultures taken at least 30 days apart are negative after the intensive phase.[a]
Treatment failed	Treatment terminated or need for permanent regimen change of at least two anti-TB drugs because of: – lack of conversion[b] by the end of the intensive phase,[a] or – bacteriological reversion[b] in the continuation phase after conversion[b] to negative, or – evidence of additional acquired resistance to fluoroquinolones or second-line injectable drugs, or – adverse drug reactions (ADRs).
Died	A patient who dies for any reason during the course of treatment.
Lost to follow-up	A patient whose treatment was interrupted for 2 consecutive months or more.
Not evaluated	A patient for whom no treatment outcome is assigned. (This includes cases "transferred out" to another treatment unit and whose treatment outcome is unknown)
Treatment success	The sum of cured and treatment completed
Cohort	A group of patients where RR-TB has been diagnosed (including MDR-TB and XDR-TB), and who were started on a full course of a second-line MDR-TB drug regimen during a specified time period (e.g. the cohort of MDR-TB cases registered in the calendar year 2010). This group forms the denominator for calculating treatment outcomes. With the revised definitions, any patient found to have drug-resistant TB and placed on second-line treatment is removed from the drug-susceptible TB outcome cohort. This means that management of the basic management unit TB register and of the second-line TB treatment register needs to be coordinated to ensure proper accounting of the outcomes of treatment *(14)*.

[a] For *Treatment failed*, lack of conversion by the end of the intensive phase implies that the patient does not convert within the maximum duration of intensive phase applied by the programme. If no maximum duration is defined, an 8-month cut-off is proposed. For regimens without a clear distinction between intensive and continuation phases, a cut-off 8 months after the start of treatment is suggested to determine when the criteria for Cured, Treatment completed and Treatment failed start to apply.

[b] The terms "conversion" and "reversion" of culture as used here are defined as follows:

Conversion (to negative) : culture is considered to have converted to negative when two consecutive cultures, taken at least 30 days apart, are found to be negative. In such a case, the specimen collection date of the first negative culture is used as the date of conversion.

Reversion (to positive) : culture is considered to have reverted to positive when, after an initial conversion, two consecutive cultures, taken at least 30 days apart, are found to be positive. For the purpose of defining treatment failed, reversion is considered only when it occurs in the continuation phase.

NATURAL HISTORY OF TUBERCULOSIS

Agent factors

(a) AGENT : *M. tuberculosis* is a facultative intracellular parasite, i.e., it is readily ingested by phagocytes and is resistant to intracellular killing *(20)*. Of importance to man are the human and bovine strains. The human strain is responsible for the vast majority of cases. The bovine strain affects mainly cattle and other animals. Regarding virulence, the Indian tubercle bacillus is said to be less virulent than the European bacillus. In recent years, a number of "atypical" mycobacteria have been isolated from man *(21)*. These have been classified into four groups – (i) photochromogens (e.g., *M. Kansasii*); (ii) scotochromogens (e.g., *M. scrofulaceum*); (iii) non–photochromogens (e.g., *M. intercellulare*)) and, (iv) rapid growers (e.g., *M. fortuitum*). All these are mainly saprophytic. Diseases attributed to them have resembled pulmonary tuberculosis and chronic cervical lymphadenitis.

(b) SOURCE OF INFECTION : There are two sources of infection – human and bovine. (i) *Human source :* The most common source of infection is the human case whose sputum is positive for tubercle bacilli and who has either received no treatment or has not been treated fully. An estimated annual average of 10–15 persons contract the infection from one case of infectious pulmonary TB. Such sources can discharge the bacilli in their sputum for years. The tubercle bacilli in a human case are usually a mixed group – some multiply very rapidly and some slowly. The more rapidly a bacillary strain multiplies the more susceptible it is to the bactericidal action of chemotherapeutic drugs. The slow multipliers are the source of persister or dormant bacilli; they can remain alive for years without causing harm to the host, but when conditions are favourable they may start multiplying again and cause active disease. That is, they are the seeds of a future relapse *(22)*. (ii) *Bovine source:* The bovine source of infection is usually infected milk. There is no definite evidence that bovine tuberculosis is a problem in this country because of the practice of boiling milk before consumption.

(c) COMMUNICABILITY : Patients are infective as long as they remain untreated. Effective anti–microbial treatment reduces infectivity by 90 per cent within 48 hours *(23)*.

Host factors

(a) AGE : Tuberculosis affects all ages. Developing countries show a sharp rise in infection rates from childhood to adolescence. In India, from an average of 2 per cent in the "0–14 years age group", the infection rate climbs to about 20 per cent at age 15–24 years age group. In the developed countries, the disease is now more common in the elderly. (b) SEX : More prevalent in males than in females. (c) HEREDITY : Tuberculosis is not a hereditary disease. However, twin studies *(24)* indicate that inherited susceptibility is an important risk factor. (d) NUTRITION : Malnutrition is widely believed to predispose to tuberculosis. As malnutrition is widely prevalent in developing world, it will continue to affect the development of active disease, out- come of treatment and spread of the disease. (e) IMMUNITY : Man has no inherited immunity against tuberculosis. It is acquired as a result of natural infection or BCG vaccination. Past infection with atypical mycobacteria is also credited with certain amount of naturally acquired immunity. It is now known that both delayed hypersensitivity and acquired resistance to tuberculosis are cell–mediated responses. In most cases, the cellular immunity proves adequate to limit further multiplication and spread of bacilli.

Social factors

Tuberculosis is a social disease with medical aspects. It has also been described as a barometer of social welfare. The social factors include many non-medical factors such as poor quality of life, poor housing, and overcrowding, population explosion, undernutrition, smoking, alcohol abuse, lack of education, large families, early marriages, lack of awareness of causes of illness, etc. All these factors are interrelated and contribute to the occurrence and spread of tuberculosis. In fact, tuberculosis began to decline in the western world long before the advent of chemotherapeutic drugs. This has been attributed to improvements in the quality of life.

Mode of transmission

Tuberculosis is transmitted mainly by droplet infection and droplet nuclei generated by sputum-positive patients with pulmonary tuberculosis. To transmit infection, the particles must be fresh enough to carry a viable organism. Coughing generates the largest number of droplets of all sizes. The frequency and vigour of cough and the ventilation of the environment influence transmission of infection. Tuberculosis is not transmitted by fomites, such as dishes and other articles used by the patients. Sterilization of these articles is therefore of little or no value. Patients with extrapulmonary tuberculosis or smear-negative tuberculosis constitute a minimal hazard for transmission of infection.

Incubation period

The time from receipt of infection to the development of a positive tuberculin test ranges from 3 to 6 weeks, and thereafter, the development of disease depends upon the closeness of contact, extent of the disease and sputum positivity of the source case (dose of infection) and host–parasite relationship. Thus the incubation period may be weeks, months or years.

THE CONTROL OF TUBERCULOSIS

Tuberculosis control means reduction in the prevalence and incidence of disease in the community.

Since tuberculosis is an infectious disease, the basic principles of prevention and control are the same as for any other infectious disease. The control measures consist of a **curative** component – namely case finding and treatment; and a **preventive** component – namely BCG vaccination. These are the two fundamental components of a national tuberculosis programme. The most powerful weapon, however, is the combination of case-finding and treatment.

Case-finding in public sector *(25)*

The first step in a tuberculosis control programme is early detection of sputum-positive cases. This should be an intensive, on-going programme. The evolution of strategies for improving case findings are as shown below :

Evolution of strategies for improving case findings

Passive Case Finding (1962–)	Intensified Case Finding (2001–)	Active Case Finding (2017–)	Population based screening (2020–)
Based on footfall in Health Facility	Co-morbid conditions - HIV, DM	Systematic screening of vulnerable population (migrant, slums, prisons, contact of DR TB, Paediatrics)	Vulnerability mapping Periodic screening of vulnerable

STRATEGIES ADOPTED FOR CASE FINDING

a. *Passive case finding :* An overwhelming majority of patients of pulmonary tuberculosis have one or more of the symptoms referable to chest, such as persistent cough and fever, and many of them (over 60 per cent) seek medical advice on their own initiative. The chest symptoms often develop early, that is before the disease has gone on to an advanced stage. This is the most fertile group for case-finding.
b. *Intensified case finding :* Screening patients attending health facilities with comorbidities, for TB (HIV care settings, diabetes clinic, tobacco cessation clinic, nutritional rehabilitation centre) and OPDs (Gynaecology, orthopaedics etc.). This is a provider-initiated screening of outpatient clinic/hospital attendees for symptoms of TB.
c. *Active case finding :* Actively searching for TB patients among vulnerable population in the community (Slum, tribal, prison etc.). This activity adopted by the programme enables early detection of TB patients.
d. Vulnerability mapping is done followed by periodic screening of vulnerable population. Leveraging outreach of other Health Programmes in Health and wellness centres.

Screening strategies

1. Community screening can be done by :

Inviting people to attend screening at a mobile facility or a fixed facility. Invitations may target specifically people within a given vulnerable group, those

- who have had recent close contact with someone who has TB and people with symptoms of TB.
- Going door-to-door to screen households.

2. Institutional screening

- In health care facilities : Systematically perform active screening of vulnerable individuals attending hospitals and other health care institution.
- In congregate settings : Systematically perform active screening of vulnerable individuals in shelters, old age homes, refugee camps, correctional facilities and other specific locations such as workplaces.

Recommendations on at risk or vulnerable groups to be screened

A vulnerable group is any group of people in which the prevalence or incidence of TB is significantly higher than in the general population. The recommended vulnerable groups to be considered for intensified case finding are discussed in detail on page 239.

d. CASE-FINDING TOOLS

Tools for microbiological confirmation of TB are *(26)* :

1. Sputum Smear Microscopy (for AFB) :
   - Zeihl-Neelsen staining
   - Fluorescence staining
2. Culture :
   - Solid (Lowenstein Jensen) media
   - Automated Liquid culture systems e.g. BACTEC MGIT 960, BacT Alert or Versatrek etc.
3. Drug Sensitivity Testing:
   - Modified proportionate sensitivity testing (PST) for MGIT 960 system
   - Economic variant of proportion sensitivity testing (1%) using LJ medium
4. Rapid molecular diagnostic tests:
   - Line probe assay (LPA) for MTB complex and detection of RIF & INH resistance (FL LPA), and FQ and SLI resistance (SL LPA)
   - Nucleic acid amplification test (NAAT) (CBNAAT/ truenat)

Supportive tools for the clinical diagnosis of TB

- Chest X-ray and other radiological tests.
- Tuberculin skin test (TST), Interferon gamma release assay (IGRA) and other blood tests, histopathology and other tissue-based tests.

Smear microscopy being the most commonly used method for microbiological diagnosis of TB for the last several decades, has had enormous value in TB diagnosis but with limited sensitivity, more so in children and PLHIV. Under the programme, two methods of microscopy are currently being used – ZN stain-based microscopy using conventional microscope and light emitting.

Diode based fluorescent microscopy (LED FM) : Culture though highly sensitive and specific method for TB diagnosis, requires 2–8 weeks to yield results and hence does not help in early diagnosis. However, culture is used for follow-up of patients on drug resistant TB treatment to detect early recurrence. In addition, it is also used for long term follow-up for DS TB patients, to ensure relapse free cure.

Liquid culture system : Mycobacteria growth indicator tube system (MGIT-B) is an automated culture system that detects the growth of mycobacteria. The culture results are usually available upto 42 days. DST results are available 14–26 days after the cultures turn positive.

Molecular assays : Polymerase-chain-reaction (PCR) based technologies using various modifications are used for detecting the presence of putative resistance genes (rpoB for rifampicin, katG and inhA for Isoniazid etc.).

Sputum examination : Sputum smear examination by direct microscopy is now considered the method of choice. The reliability, cheapness and ease of direct microscopic examination has made it number one case-finding method all over the world. It enables us to discover the epidemiologically most important cases of pulmonary tuberculosis, i.e., those excreting tubercle bacilli in their sputum. This is the group which contributes most of the new cases to the "pool of infection" every year.

Collection of sputum samples

A pulmonary tuberculosis suspect should submit two sputum samples for microscopy. The chances of finding TB bacilli are greater with two samples than with one sample. Secretions build up in the airways overnight. So an early morning sputum sample is more likely to contain TB bacilli than one taken later in the day. It may be difficult for an out-patient to provide two early morning sputum samples. Therefore in practice an out-patient usually provides sputum samples as follows:

day 1	sample 1	Patient provides an "on-the-spot" sample under supervision when presenting to the health facility. Give the patient a sputum container to take home for an early morning sample the following morning.
day 2	sample 2	Patient brings an early morning sample.

If the patient is coming from a long distance or there is likelihood that the patient may default to give a second sample, 2 spot specimens are collected with a gap of one hour *(27)*.

Ziehl-Neelsen acid-fast stain

This simple stain detects acid fast bacilli. The procedure is as follows:

1. Fix the smear on the slide by passing the slide with the smear up about three times slowly through a flame. It can also be done by covering the smear with alcohol and letting this evaporate.
2. Cover with carbol fuchsin, steam gently for 5 minutes over direct flame (or for 20 minutes over a water bath). Do not permit slide to boil or dry out.
3. Wash with deionized water.
4. Decolourize in 3.0 per cent acid–alcohol (95 per cent ethanol and 3.0 per cent hydrochloric acid) until only a faint pink colour remains.
5. Wash with water.
6. Counter stain for 1 minute with Loeffler's methylene blue.
7. Wash with deionized water and let it dry.

Slide reporting *(28)*

The number of bacilli seen in a smear reflects disease severity and patient infectivity. Therefore, it is important to record the number of bacilli seen on each smear. The table below shows the standard method of reporting using 1000 X magnification.

Number of bacilli			Result reported
No	AFB	per 100 oil immersion fields	0
1-9	AFB	per 100 oil immersion fields	scanty (or number AFB seen)
10-99	AFB	per 100 oil immersion fields	+ (1+)
1-10	AFB	per oil immersion field	++ (2+)
> 10	AFB	per oil immersion field	+++ (3+)

Laboratory technicians should examine both the sputum samples from each TB suspect. They must record the result of each sputum sample with the laboratory reference number in the laboratory register and on the sputum request form. Results as indicated above are made available to the clinician who can then categorize the patient. It is advised that the smear examined by one microscopist should not exceed 20 per day as visual fatigue leads to a deterioration of reading quality *(29)*. One positive specimen out of the two is enough to declare a patient as smear positive TB.

Sputum smear microscopy for tubercle bacilli is positive when there are at least 10,000 organisms present per ml of sputum. The sputum smear positivity rate in TB/HIV patient depends on the degree of immunocompromise. If the degree of immunocompromise is mild, the likelihood of positive sputum smear is similar to HIV negative patient. If immunocompromise is severe, the likelihood of positive sputum smear is decreased because of decreased inflammation in lungs *(28)*.

False-positive results of sputum smear microscopy

A false-positive result means that the sputum smear result is positive even though the patient does not really have sputum smear-positive PTB. This may arise because of the following: red stain retained by scratches on the slide; accidental transfer of AFBs from a positive slide to a negative one; contamination of the slide or smear by environmental mycobacteria; presence of various particles that are acid-fast (e.g. food particles, precipitates, other microorganisms).

False-negative results of sputum smear microscopy

A false-negative result means that the sputum smear result is negative even though the patient really does have sputum smear-positive PTB. This may arise because of problems in collecting (patient provides inadequate sample, inappropriate sputum container used or sputum stored too long before smear microscopy), processing (faulty sampling of sputum for smear or faulty smear preparation and staining), or interpreting sputum smears (inadequate time spent examining smear or inadequate attention to smear examination), or because of administrative errors (misidentification of patient, incorrect labelling of sample or mistakes in documentation).

Fluorescence microscopy

Fluorescence microscopy is mainly used in industralized countries. It is performed with auramine stain. The advantage of FA microscopy is from the speed of examination. The field of view is 5–10 times bigger. Scanning of one length of smear will require only 1–2 minutes.

Light-emitting diode fluorescence microscopy (LEDs)

LEDs provide a much less expensive light source for fluorescence microscopy. In a recent WHO evaluation, the diagnostic accuracy of LED microscopy was found to be comparable to that of conventional fluorescence microscopy and superior to that of conventional Ziehl-Neelsen microscopy. It is therefore recommended that LED microscopy be phased in as an alternative to conventional Z–N light microscopy in both high and low-volume laboratories *(29)*.

Rapid diagnostic tools include

The CB-NAAT system detects DNA sequences, specific for Mycobacterium tuberculosis complex and rifampicin resistance by polymerase chain reaction. It concentrates mycobacterium tuberculosis bacilli from sputum samples, isolates genomic material from the captured bacteria by sonication and subsequently amplifies the genomic DNA by PCR. The process identifies clinically relevant, rifampicin resistance inducing mutations in the RNA polymerase beta (rpoB) gene in the Mycobacterium tuberculosis genome in a real time format using fluorescent probes called molecular beacons. Results are obtained from unprocessed sputum samples in 90 minutes.

Line Probe Assay (LPA) :

Line Probe Assays detect DNA sequences specific for Mycobacterium tuberculosis complex as well as mutations conferring resistance. Sputum samples are decontaminated and the concentrated deposit subjected to smear microscopy. DNA is extracted from all smear positive samples and subjected to PCR; while all smear negative samples are inoculated in liquid culture and LPA performed using the culture isolate obtained upon growth of Mycobacteria. The PCR amplified products are reverse hybridized on nitrocellulose strips containing probes specific for detection of *M. tuberculosis* and mutations associated with drug resistance. First line LPA detects resistance to Rifampicin (rpoB) and Isoniazid (katG, inhA), while second line LPA detects fluoroquinolone class resistance (gyrA, gyrB) and second line injectable class resistance (rrs, eis).

Nucleic Acid Amplification Test (NAAT) provides accurate and rapid diagnosis of TB by detecting Mycobacterium tuberculosis (*M. tuberculosis*) and Rifampicin (Rif) resistance conferring mutations, in sputum specimen as well as specimen from extra-pulmonary sites. Under the programme, its use is recommended for diagnosis of DR-TB, in presumptive DR-TB patients and TB preferentially in key population such as children, PLHIV, Extra-pulmonary TB and in smear negative TB as per the diagnostic algorithm.

Radiography

Chest X-rays are useful for the diagnosis of smear negative pulmonary TB and TB in children. It is not routinely indicated in smear-postive cases. X-rays are valuable tools for the diagnosis of pleural and pericardial effusion, especially in early stages of the disease when clinical signs are minimal. It is essential in the diagnosis of miliary TB. The other indications are frequent or severe haemoptysis to exclude bronchiectasis or aspergilloma and in patients needing specific treatment for pneumothorax.

TUBERCULIN TEST

The tuberculin test was discovered by Von Pirquet in 1907. A positive reaction to the test is generally accepted as evidence of past or present infection by *M. tuberculosis*. The tuberculin test is the only means of estimating the prevalence of infection in a population.

Tuberculin : Only two tuberculins have been accepted as standard tuberculin by WHO, i.e., purified protein derivative–S (PPD–S) and PPD–RT 23. PPD is standardized in terms of its biological reactivity as tuberculin units (TU). A standard 5 tuberculin unit (5 TU) dose of PPD-S is defined as delayed skin activity contained in a 0.1 μg/0.1 ml dose of PPD–S. 1 TU of PPD–RT 23 is equivalent to 5 TU of PPD–S. In India PPD–RT 23 with Tween 80 is used. Tween 80 is a detergent added to tuberculin to prevent their adsorption on glass or plastic surface. Use of tuberculin strength of 1 TU is recommended for standard Mantoux test in India.

MANTOUX TEST : The Mantoux test is carried out by injecting 1 TU of PPD in 0.1 ml intradermally on the flexor surface of the left forearm, mid-way between elbow and wrist. The injection should be made with a tuberculin syringe, with the needle bevel facing upward. When placed correctly, injection should produce a pale wheal of the skin, 6 to 10 mm in diameter. The result of the test is read after 48–96 hours but 72 hours (3rd day) is the ideal.

Tuberculin reaction consists of erythema and induration. Since erythema is sometimes difficult to measure, induration alone is measured (horizontal transverse diameter of induration in millimetres, using a transparent plastic ruler or callipers). Reactions exceeding 10 mm are considered "positive". Those less than 6 mm are considered "negative". Those between 6 and 9 mm are considered "doubtful", i.e., the reaction may be due to *M. tuberculosis* or atypical mycobacteria. If there is no induration, the result should be recorded as '0'.

It has been further observed that strong reactors (i.e., those showing 20 mm or more induration) have greater chances of developing tuberculosis than those showing 10 mm induration. Those with less than 5 mm induration have more risk of developing tuberculosis than those with 6–9 mm induration. Studies indicate that 92 per cent of new cases occur in persons who are already tuberculin reactors *(30)*. These findings illustrate the prognostic significance of the test.

Classification of positive tuberculin skin test reaction *(31)*

A tuberculin skin test reaction is considered positive if the transverse diameter of the indurated area reaches the size required for the specific group. All other reactions are considered negative. The classification is as follows :

Induration size	Group
≥ 5 mm	1. HIV-positive persons. 2. Recent contacts of individuals with active tuberculosis. 3. Persons with fibrotic changes on chest films suggestive of prior tuberculosis. 4. Patients with organ transplants and other immunosuppressed patients (receiving the equivalent of >15 mg/d of prednisone for 1 month or more).
≥ 10 mm	1. Recent immigrants (<5 years) from countries with a high prevalence of tuberculosis (eg, Asia, Africa, Latin America). 2. HIV-negative injection drug users. 3. Mycobacteriology laboratory personnel. 4. Residents of and employees in the following high-risk congregate settings: correctional institutions; nursing homes and other long-term facilities for the elderly; hospitals and other health care facilities; residential facilities for AIDS patients; and homeless shelters. 5. Persons with the following medical conditions that increase the risk of tuberculosis: gastrectomy, ≥ 10% below ideal body weight, jejunoileal bypass, diabetes mellitus, silicosis, advanced chronic kidney disease, some hematologic disorders, (eg. leukemias, lymphomas) and other specific malignancies (eg, carcinoma of the head or neck and lung). 6. Children <4 years of age or infants, children and adolescents exposed to adults at high risk.
≥ 15 mm	1. Persons with no risk factors for tuberculosis.

A negative tuberculin test must also be interpreted with caution. For many years, it has been assumed that a negative test constituted strong evidence against the presence of active tuberculous disease in the majority of cases. It has been shown that in the majority of patients with tuberculosis, the cellular immune response may be depressed. It means a negative tuberculin test cannot be relied upon to exclude tuberculosis. The dermal hypersensitivity to tuberculin can also be lost in various states of immune suppression, e.g., malignancy, Hodgkin's disease, HIV infection, malnutrition, severe bacterial infection (including TB itself), viral infections (e.g. measles, chickenpox, glandular fever), recent live-virus vaccination (e.g. measles), immunosuppresive drugs (e.g. steroids) and incorrect injection of PPD. Therefore, too great a diagnostic significance should not be placed on a negative tuberculin test *(20)*.

Two-step testing

Some people who were previously infected with TB may have a negative reaction when tested years after infection, as the immune system response may gradually wane. This initial skin test, though negative, may stimulate (boost) the body's ability to react to tuberculin in future tests. Thus, a positive reaction to a subsequent test may be misinterpreted as a new infection, when in fact it is the result of the boosted reaction to an old infection. Giving a second TST after an initial negative TST reaction is called a two-step testing. Use of two-step testing is recommended for initial skin testing of adults who will be retested periodically (e.g, health care workers).

- The first test is read 48–72 hours after injection.
  - If the first test is positive, consider the person infected.
  - If the first test is negative, give a second test one to three weeks after the first injection.
- The second test is read 48–72 hours after injection.
  - If the second test is positive, consider the person previously infected.
  - If the second test is negative, consider the person uninfected.

The validity of tuberculin test, like all medical tests, is subject to variability. It is limited by lack of specificity. Apart from errors associated with the mode of administration, reading of results and the test material used, there are other factors such as cross-reactions due to sensitization by other mycobacteria, which should be taken into account. In countries with a high coverage of BCG, which also produces tuberculin hypersensitivity, tuberculin test has lost its sensitivity as an indicator of the "true" prevalence of infection. The true prevalence rates of infection may be exaggerated by infection with atypical mycobacteria as well as the "boosting effect" of a second dose of tuberculin producing a larger reaction than the first *(32)*.

It is often assumed that delayed hypersensitivity as measured by tuberculin testing is a correlate of the protective immune response. But evidence indicates that this hypersensitivity is irrelevant to the ability of the host to combat the disease. Despite these limitations, the tuberculin test continues to be the only tool for measuring the prevalence of tuberculous infection in a community. It has been aptly said that tuberculin test "must be approached with respect, administered with care, read with deliberation and interpreted with sentient discrimination".

TB Interferon gamma release assays (IGRAs)

The Interferon Gamma Release Assays (IGRAs) are a new type of more accurate test for TB. IGRAs are blood tests that measure a person's immune response to the bacteria that cause TB. The immune system produces some special molecules called cytokines. These TB tests work by detecting a cytokine called the interferon gamma cytokine. In practice you carry out one of these TB tests by taking a blood sample and mixing it with special substances to identify if the cytokine is present. Two IGRAs that have been approved and are commercially available, are the QuantiFERON® TB Gold test, and the T-SPOT® TB test. The advantages of an IGRA TB test includes the fact that it only requires a single patient visit to carry out the TB test. Results can be available within 24 hours, and prior BCG vaccination does not cause a false positive result. Disadvantages include the fact that the blood sample must be processed fairly quickly, laboratory facilities are required, and the test is only for latent TB. It is also thought that the IGRAs may not be as accurate in people who have HIV. In low prevalence resource rich settings, IGRAs are beginning to be used in place of the TB skin test *(33)*.

Case-finding should not be an end in itself. It is of little value as a control measure unless followed by chemotherapy. Resources and efforts should be directed towards primary health care, rather than irrational case finding.

Please refer to page 220 for the flow chart for diagnosis of tuberculosis in adults, as followed by NTEP.

Chemotherapy

The development of effective treatment for tuberculosis has been one of the most significant advances during this century. With the evolution of controlled trials (see page 92), the chemotherapy of tuberculosis is now more rationally based, than in the treatment of other infectious diseases.

Chemotherapy is indicated in every case of active tuberculosis. The objective of treatment is cure – that is, the elimination of both the fast and slowly multiplying bacilli (including the persisters) from the patient's body. The effects of chemotherapy are judged not by the anatomic healing of lesions, but mainly by the elimination of bacilli from the patient's sputum. Chemotherapy should be easily available, free of charge to every patient detected. It should be adequate, appropriate and applied to the entire pool of infectors in the community. Patient compliance is critically important; the patient must take the correct drugs at the correct dosage for the correct length of time. Incomplete treatment puts the patient at risk of relapse and the development of bacterial resistance and, importantly, the community at risk of infection with resistant organisms.

Anti-tuberculosis drugs

There are now twelve or thirteen drugs active against ***M. tuberculosis,*** of which, six are considered to be essential. An antitubercular drug should satisfy the following criteria : (a) highly effective (b) free from side-effects (c) easy to administer, and (d) reasonably cheap. The currently used drugs may be classified into two groups : bactericidal and bacteriostatic. The bactericidal drugs kill the bacilli *in vivo*. The bacteriostatic drugs inhibit the multiplication of the bacilli and lead to their destruction by the immune mechanism of the host. A brief review of these drugs is given below.

THE FIRST–LINE DRUGS

BACTERICIDAL DRUGS

Rifampicin (RMP)

RMP is a powerful bactericidal drug. It is a better sterilizing agent than INH. It permeates all tissue membranes including the blood–brain and placental barriers. It is equally effective against intracellular as well as extracellular bacilli. It is the only bactericidal drug active against the "persisters" or dormant bacilli which are found in the solid caseous lesions, all other drugs being inactive *(34)*. In this regard, it has a distinct advantage over INH. Rifampicin is of special value when the bacilli resists other drugs. In combination with INH, it can cure even extensive tuberculosis, in about 9 months.

RMP is used only as oral drug. It is so well absorbed that there is little need for parenteral administration. The dose should be taken at least one hour before or 2 hours after food because absorption is reduced by food. It is never used alone for the treatment of tuberculosis, but always used in combination with INH or another drug.

Many patients develop nausea at the start of treatment, but this passes off. The toxic effects include hepatotoxicity, gastritis, influenza–like illness, purpura, thrombocytopenia and nephrotoxicity. The patient should be told that the drug will turn the urine red; this can be used as test of compliance.

PAS delays its absorption; hence concurrent administration with PAS should be avoided. If RMP is stopped for some reason, it should not be restarted within 3 weeks to avoid hypersensitivity.

INH

INH ranks among the most powerful drugs in the treatment of tuberculosis. It can easily penetrate the cell membrane, and is thus active against intracellular and extracellular bacilli. Its action is most marked on rapidly multiplying bacilli. It is less active against slow multipliers. INH gets widely distributed in the body including CSF. Its ease of administration, freedom from toxicity and low cost makes it an ideal component for any drug regimen.

INH should be given as a single dose. INH reaches its peak level in blood 1 to 2 hours after the dose. It has been found that its peak level in serum is more important than sustained inhibitory level. It is for this reason, INH should not be given in divided doses *(35)*.

Patient may experience gastrointestinal irritation, peripheral neuropathy, blood dyscrasias, hyperglycaemia and liver damage. Those patients who are slow inactivators experience a higher incidence of toxicity. The addition of pyridoxine (10–20 mg daily) helps prevent the occurrence of peripheral neuropathy.

Streptomycin

Streptomycin is bactericidal. It acts entirely on rapidly multiplying bacilli. It has been shown that when bacilli are multiplying rapidly, they come out of the phagocytes and are mostly extracellular and are, therefore, susceptible to streptomycin. Streptomycin is less active against slow multipliers. It has no action on persisters. It does not permeate cell walls or normal biological membranes such as meninges or pleura.

The daily dose of streptomycin is 0.75 g in a single injection. This is a disadvantage because of the organizational problem involved in the long term treatment. It can cause side-effects which include vestibular damage and nystagmus rather than deafness. Renal damage may also occur.

Pyrazinamide

This drug is bactericidal and is particularly active against the slow-multiplying intracellular bacilli which are unaffected by other drugs. It has been found to increase the sterilizing ability of rifampicin. Therefore, pyrazinamide has been incorporated in short-course chemotherapy regimens.

Complications include hepatotoxicity and hyperuricaemia. Pyrazinamide achieves high levels in CSF and is, therefore, recommended in tuberculous meningitis.

BACTERIOSTATIC DRUGS

Ethambutol

Ethambutol is bacteriostatic and is used in combination to prevent the emergence of resistance to other drugs. It is given orally. Its major side-effect is retrobulbar neuritis; this however does not occur at the usual dosage. Ethambutol has replaced para–aminosalicylic acid (PAS) almost entirely among adults.

THE SECOND–LINE DRUGS

Fluoroquinolones

Ciprofloxacin, ofloxacin, levofloxacin, moxifloxacin and gatifloxacin are active against *M. tuberculosis*, even those resistant to other drugs. They are given orally or IV. They are useful in treating infections resistant to standard drugs and in cases with relapse.

Ethionamide

Ethionamide is structurally related to INH and acts by inhibiting the mycolic acid synthesis. It is effective against bacilli resistant to other drugs and has proved effective in infections due to atypical mycobacteria. It is effective against intracellular as well as extracellular organisms.

Capreomycin

It is bactericidal. Its mechanism of action, pharmacokinetics and adverse reactions are similar to those of streptomycin. It should be administered with caution in presence of renal impairment.

Kanamycin and amikacin

They are bactericidal and are active against bacilli resistant to streptomycin, INH and cycloserine.

Cycloserine

The drug is mainly bacteriostatic. It is effective against bacilli resistant to INH or streptomycin and against atypical mycobacteria, although antitubercular activity is less than that of these two drugs. It acts by inhibiting the synthesis of the bacterial cell wall.

Thioacetazone

It is a bacteriostatic drug. It rapidly diffuses into various body tissues and also crosses the placenta barrier. It is also secreted in milk. It should never be used in HIV patients as it can cause severe and fatal skin reactions. Side-effects include gastrointestinal disturbances, blurring of vision, haemolytic anaemia and urticaria. The incidence of these side-effects seem to differ in different ethnic groups.

Macrolides

Newer macrolides azithromycin and clarithromycin also have action against tubercular bacilli. They are used to treat atypical mycobacterial infection and cases with relapse.

Bedaquiline (BDQ)

Bedaquiline (BDQ) is a new class of drug diarylquinoline, that specifically targets mycobacterial ATP synthase, an enzyme essential to supply of energy to *mycobacterium*. It is a bactericidal drug with high volume of tissue distribution, highly bound to plasma proteins and hepatically metabolized. The drug has extended half-life, which means that it is still present in the plasma up to 5.5 months post stopping BDQ. The drug has shown significant benefits in improving the time to culture convertion in MDR–TB patients. The basic criteria for patient selection is : (1) age of the patient should be ≥ 18 years having MDR–TB; (2) Pregnancy is a contraindication for BDQ therapy and the patient should be using non-hormonal based birth control measure throughout the treatment period or have been post-menopausal for past 2 years; and (3) Cardiac arrythmia is a contraindication for BDQ treatment *(36)*.

The following group of patients are eligible for BDQ therapy :

1. MDR/RR TB with resistance to any/all fluoroquinolones (FQ) or to any/all second-line injectable agents (SLI)
2. XDR–TB
3. Mixed pattern resistant TB (XDR–TB + additional first line / second line resistant TB)
4. Treatment failure of MDR–TB + FQ/SLI resistance or XDR–TB

Delamanid (DLM)

Delamanid is a recently approved drug for the treatment of TB conditional use under programmatic setting only. The phase III clinical trial results for safety and effectiveness of the drug is yet to be published. The Drug Controller General of India has issued permission to use Delamanid (50 mg) as part of an appropriate combination regimen for pulmonary MDR-TB in adult patients when an effective treatment regimen cannot otherwise be composed for reasons of resistance or tolerability *(37)*.

For dosage of different second-line drugs, kindly refer to page 224.

Most TB patients complete their treatment without any significant drug side-effects. However, a few patients do develop major reactions and it is important to monitor clinically all the patients. A patient who develops one of the following reactions must never receive that drug again *(34)* :

Reaction	Drug responsible
a. Severe rash, agranulocytosis	Thioacetazone
b. Hearing loss or disturbed balance	Streptomycin
c. Visual disturbance (poor vision and colour perception)	Ethambutol
d. Renal failure, shock or thrombocytopenia	Rifampicin
e. Hepatitis	Pyrazinamide

Two-phase chemotherapy

It is well recognized that there are two phases in the effective treatment of tuberculosis : (i) the first is a short, aggressive or intense phase, early in the course of treatment, lasting 1–3 months. During this intensive phase, three or more drugs are combined to kill off as many bacilli as possible. The more rapidly the bacilli are killed initially, the less likely are "persisters" to emerge. The risk of relapse is also lessened. (ii) the second or "continuation" phase is aimed at sterilizing the smaller number of dormant or persisting bacilli. In the standard anti-tuberculous therapy, the duration of treatment was not less than 18 months to achieve complete sterilization of the bacilli. With the introduction of rifampicin and pyrazinamide, this period is now successfully reduced to 6–9 months.

DOMICILIARY TREATMENT

The self-administration of drugs (generally oral drugs) by the patients themselves without recourse to hospitalization is called domiciliary or ambulatory treatment. The classical controlled clinical trials *(38)* carried out at the Tuberculosis Chemotherapy Centre, Chennai showed that the incidence of tuberculosis was no greater in the contacts of patients treated at home than in the contacts of patients treated in sanatoria. It is now universally accepted that with good chemotherapy, hospital treatment has no advantage over domiciliary treatment, and domiciliary treatment is to be preferred because in the long run, it is so much cheaper than hospital treatment, and that it can be managed by the primary health care system and the general health services of the country. It may be mentioned that it was this study, the classical Chennai Study, that prompted a radical departure from the traditional sanatorium to ambulatory or domiciliary treatment.

SHORT-COURSE CHEMOTHERAPY

For a long time, the standard duration of tuberculosis chemotherapy was 18 months. In 1972, Wallace Fox and his colleagues from the British Medical Research Council showed that the addition of rifampicin or of pyrazinamide to regimens containing INH made it possible to reduce the duration of treatment.

There are a number of advantages of short–course chemotherapy, viz. rapid bacteriological conversion, lower failure rates and a reduction in the frequency of emergence of drug–resistant bacilli. Patient compliance is improved, they become non-infectious earlier. The disadvantage is that the high cost of short-term chemotherapy militates against its wider use in developing countries.

There are now a number of short–course regimens of 6 months duration that are highly effective, of low toxicity, and well–tolerated. These potent regimens are based on an initial intensive phase with 4 drugs (INH, rifampicin and pyrazinamide, supplemented by either streptomycin or ethambutol) for a period of 2 months, followed by 2 drugs in the continuation phase, (INH plus rifampicin or thioacetazone) given daily or intermittently. The treatment must be fully supervised and monitored mainly by bacteriological examination.

DIRECTLY OBSERVED TREATMENT, SHORT COURSE (DOTS) CHEMOTHERAPY

DOTS is a strategy to ensure cure by providing the most effective medicine and confirming that it is taken. It is the only strategy which has been documented to be effective worldwide on a programme basis. In DOTS, during the intensive phase of treatment a health worker or other trained person watches as the patient swallows the drug in his presence. During continuation phase, the patient is issued medicine for one week in a multiblister combipack, of which the first dose is swallowed by the patient in the presence of health worker or trained person. The consumption of medicine in the continuation phase is also checked by return of empty multiblister combipack, when the patient comes to collect medicine for the next week. The drugs are provided in patient–wise boxes with sufficient shelf-life.

INTRODUCTION OF DAILY DOSE REGIMEN IN NTEP

The technical and operational guidelines–2016 for TB control in India, define major groups of TB patients who are offered standard treatment regimen. Patient's classification is based on drug susceptibility result as drug-sensitive TB; and mono, poly, RR, multi and extensively drug resistant TB. For drug-sensitive TB patients, the thrice weekly intermittent TB regimen used since inception of the programme has been switched to a daily fixed dose combination regimen *(37)*.

1. MANAGEMENT OF DRUG SENSITIVE TUBERCULOSIS (2019)

Early identification of people with a high probability of having active TB (presumptive TB) is the most important activity of the case finding strategy. Screening and diagnosing patients with appropriate tests and strategies will largely determine the response to appropriate treatment. Passive case finding alone can lead to missed cases or delayed diagnosis.

All presumptive TB will undergo sputum smear examination (ZN/LEDFM). Two specimens are collected (spot–early morning or spot–spot). If the first smear is positive and the patient is not at the risk of drug resistant TB, he will be categorized as microscopically confirmed TB (sensitivity status not known). If the first smear is negative, CXR may be considered and if reported as suggestive of TB, the 2nd sample will be subjected to smear and CBNAAT simultaneously. Based on CBNAAT results, patient will be categorized as microbiologically confirmed drug sensitive TB.

For NTEP endorsed TB diagnostics, Fig. 2 shows the diagnostic algorithm for pulmonary tuberculosis.

Pre-treatment counselling and evaluation

The patient and his/her family members should be counselled about the type of disease, mode of spread, the treatment duration and dosage schedule, common drug side-effects and methods to prevent them, importance of regular treatment and consequences of irregular treatment, screening of co-morbidities like diabetes, liver or renal diseases and neurological disorder etc. It is also important to look for substance abuse especially tobacco (in any form) and alcohol. Socio-economic status of the patient may be assessed to link him/her with appropriate treatment support schemes. HIV testing should be done in all the cases of TB. This is important to ensure that all HIV positive cases of TB receive anti-retroviral therapy and co-trimoxazole preventive therapy *(36)*.

Since the drugs used in the treatment of tuberculosis are known to produce adverse effects, a proper pre-treatment evaluation is essential to identify patients who are at increased risk of developing such adverse effects. The pre-treatment evaluation includes the following :

1. Detailed history (including mental illness, seizure, drug and alcohol abuse etc).
2. Weight and height.
3. Complete blood count.
4. Blood sugar to screen for diabetes mellitus.
5. Liver function test.
6. Blood urea and creatinine to assess kidney function.
7. Urine examine – routine and microscopic.
8. Chest X-ray
9. Pregnancy test (for all women in child bearing age group).

Most TB patients on first line drugs complete their treatment without any serious drug side effects. Trivial side effects may lead to reduced compliance with the treatment, hence asymptom-based approach to the management of the common adverse effect should be adopted.

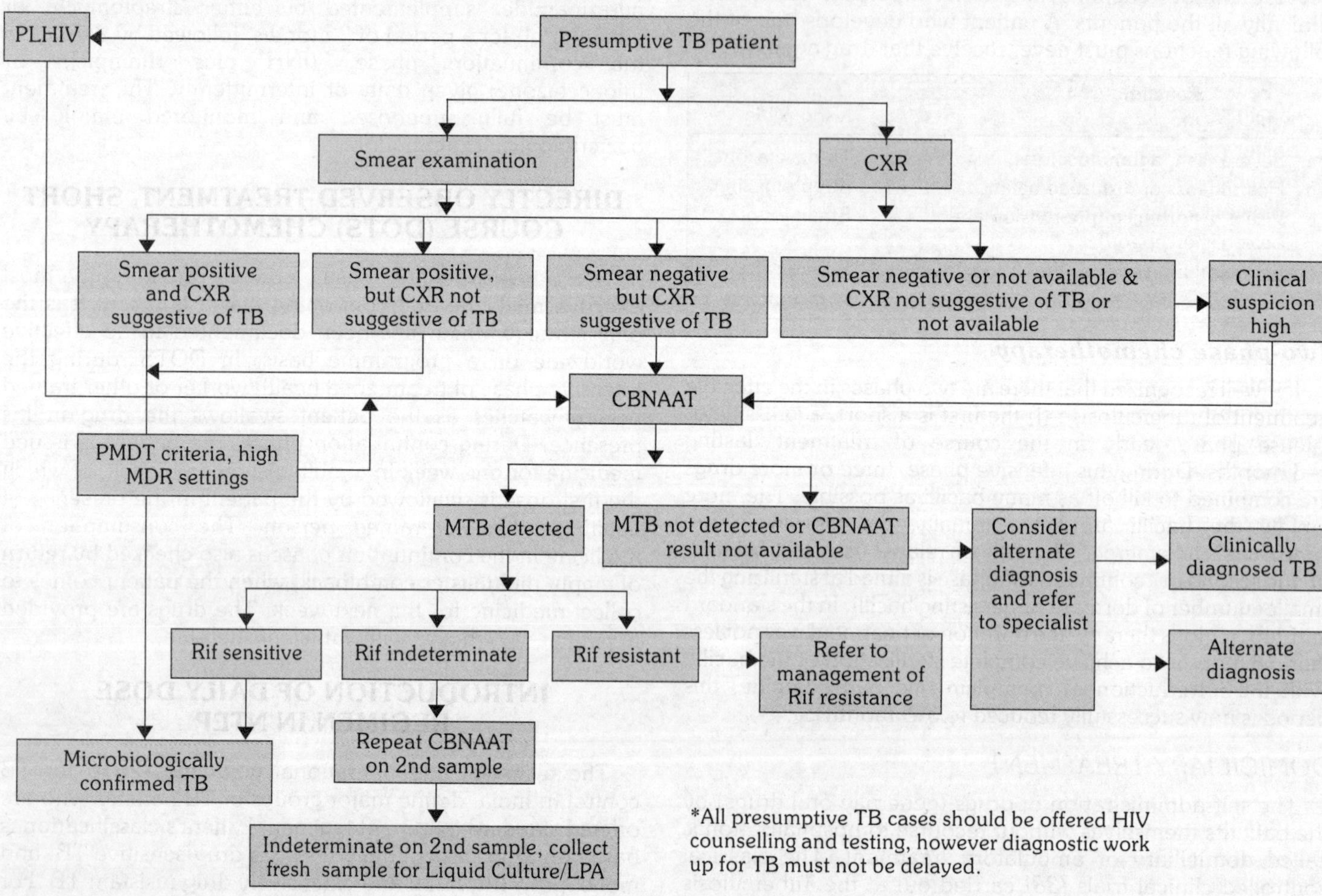

*All presumptive TB cases should be offered HIV counselling and testing, however diagnostic work up for TB must not be delayed.

FIG. 2
Diagnostic algorithm for pulmonary TB

Source : *(39)*

Pharmacovigilance in TB control programme : Pharmacovigilance is defined by the WHO as the "science and activities relating to the detection, assessment, understanding and prevention of adverse effects or any other drug-related problem". It is fundamental activity to inform the management of patient safety measurement in health care. It is a public health surveillance activity. Priority is given to establish pharmacovigilance at drug resistance TB centres.

Recommended daily dose regimen for drug sensitive TB (2019)

The principle of treatment for tuberculosis (other than confirmed drug resistant forms of TB) with daily regimen is to administer daily fixed dose combinations of first-line anti-tuberculosis drugs in appropriate weight bands.

Fixed dose combinations (FDCs)

Fixed dose combinations (FDCs) refer to products containing two or more active ingredients in fixed doses, used for a particular indication(s).

In NTEP, for Adults – 4-FDC (given in IP) consists of HRZE and 3-FDC (given in CP) consists of HRE. For paediatric patients – dispersible 3 FDC consists of HRZ and dispersible 2 FDC consists of HR.

Advantages of FDCs

- Simplicity of treatment
- Increased patient acceptance
  - Fewer tablets to swallow
  - Prevents 'concealed' irregularity
- Increased health worker compliance
  - Fewer tablets to handle, hence quicker supervision of DOT
- Easier drug management
- Reduced use of monotherapy
  - Lower risk of misuse of single drugs
- Lower risk of emergence of drug resistance
- Easier to adjust dosages by body weight

Treatment is given in two phases (26):

- Intensive phase (IP) consists of 8 weeks (56 doses) of isoniazid (H), rifampicin (R), pyrazinamide (Z) and ethambutol (E) given under direct observation in daily dosages as per weight band categories.
- Continuation phase (CP), consists of 16 weeks (112 doses) of isoniazid, rifampicin and ethambutol in daily dosages. Only pyrazinamide will be stopped in the continuation phase. The CP may be extended by 12–24 weeks in certain forms of TB like CNS TB, skeletal TB, disseminated TB etc. based on clinical decision of the treating physician on case to case basis. Extension beyond 12 weeks should only be on recommendation of specialists.

Type of TB case	Treatment regimen in IP	Treatment regimen in CP
New and previously treated cases (H and R sensitive / unknown)	2 HRZE	4 HRE

Prefix to the drugs stands for number of months.

Loose drugs could be used as substitutions in case of adverse drug reaction or with comorbid conditions.

Steroids as an adjunctive therapy is useful in patients with TB pericarditis and meningeal TB, with an initial high dose tapered downwards gradually over 6–8 weeks.

Drug dosages for first line anti-TB drugs

Drugs	Adults	Children	Maximum in children
Isoniazid	10 mg/kg daily (7–15 mg/kg)	5 mg/kg daily (4 to 6 mg/kg)	300 mg
Rifampicin	15 mg/kg daily (10–20 mg/kg)	10 mg/kg daily (8–12 mg/kg)	600 mg
Pyrazinamide	35 mg/kg daily (30–40 mg/kg)	25 mg/kg daily (20–30 mg/kg)	2000 mg
Ethambutol**	20 mg/kg daily (15–25 mg/kg)	15 mg/kg daily (12–15 mg/kg)	1500 mg
Streptomycin*	20 mg/kg daily (15–20 mg/kg)	15 mg/kg daily (15–20 mg/kg)	1000 mg

* Streptomycin is administered only in certain situations, like TB meningitis or if any first line drug need to be replaced due to ADR as per weight of the patient

** Ethambutol is given separately for children to monitor ophthalmic ADR.

Daily dose schedule for adults (as per weight bands) *(26)*

Weight category	Number of tablets (FDCs)	
	Intensive phase HRZE	Continuation phase HRE
	75/ 150/ 400/275	75/150/275
25–34 kg	2	2
35–49 kg	3	3
50–64 kg	4	4
65–75 kg	5	5
≥ 75 kg	6	6

During treatment if the weight of the patient increases by more than 5 kg and crosses to the next weight band category then patient should be given the next higher weight band FDC drugs.

Treatment of paediatric TB

Paediatric cases are to be treated under NTEP in daily dosages as per 6 weight band categories. All adolescents upto 18 years of age and weighing less than 39 kg, are to be treated using paediatric weight bands and children weighing more than 39 kg with adult weight bands.

Key product information (for paediatric)

1. Dispersible FDC, flavoured
   Rifampicin 75 mg + Isoniazid 50 mg + Pyrazinamide 150 mg
   Rifampicin 75 mg + Isoniazid 50 mg
2. Dispersible Loose drugs
   Ethambutol 100 mg
   Isoniazid 100 mg

Drug dosage for paediatric TB *(26)*

Weight category	Number of tablets (dispersible FDCs)			
	Intensive phase		Continuation phase	
	HRZ	E	HR	E
	50/75/ 150	100	50/75	100
4–7 kg	1	1	1	1
8–11 kg	2	2	2	2
12–15 kg	3	3	3	3
16–24 kg	4	4	4	4
25–29 kg	3 + 1A*	3	3 + 1A*	3
30–39 kg	2 + 2A*	2	2 + 2A*	2

* A=Adult FDC (HRZE = 75/150/400/275; HRE = 75/150/275). It is added in higher weight band categories i.e. > 25 kg as these children may be able to swallow tablets.

Change in weight bands to be effective upon crossing of weight bands irrespective of the quantum of weight gain/loss.

Pyridoxine may be given at a dosage of 10 mg per day to all children receiving INH containing therapy irrespective of age group.

Nikshay entry : Once the treatment regimen is finalized, all patients should be initiated on treatment after opening the treatment card and entries are done in Nikshay. MO-PHI should ensure that the treatment details are entered in Nikshay by the PHI staff. Nikshay entry should not be a separate activity. All events starting from notification to treatment outcome are from Nikshay as it is integrated part of documentation *(26)*.

Follow-up of the treatment

There are two components of the follow-up :

a. *Clinical follow up :* It should be done at monthly interval. Improvement in chest symptoms, increase in weight etc, may indicate good prognosis.

b. *Laboratory investigations* : Sputum smear microscopy should be done at the end of intensive phase and end of treatment. A negative sputum smear at the end of IP indicate good prognosis. However, in the presence of clinical deterioration, the medical officer may consider repeating sputum smear microscopy even during continuation phase. This will provide the patient an early opportunity to undergo drug susceptibility testing. At completion of the treatment, a sputum smear and/or culture should be done for every patient, as culture is more specific and sensitive compared to smear microscopy to detect the presence of *M. tuberculosis* in biological specimens.

Long term follow-up at the end of 6, 12, 18, and 24 months should be done. In presence of any clinical symptoms and /or cough, sputum microscopy and/or culture should be considered *(36)*.

2. MANAGEMENT OF DRUG-RESISTANT TB

Providing treatment to diagnosed DR-TB patients is extremely important. To begin with, only MDR-TB patients were offered treatment with a standard second-line regimen. Later, treatment with standard regimen was offered to extensively drug resistant (XDR) TB patients and MDR-TB with additional resistance to fluoroquinolones or second-line injectable. Procurement and supply chain management of second-line drugs is complex, since no standardized patient-wise boxes are manufactured and drugs do need temperature regulated storage and repacking.

Since 2016, new drugs like Bedaquiline (Bdq) are made accessible to DR-TB patients through expanded access under NTEP. In 2016, with the release of the Revised Technical and Operational Guidelines, regimens to treat other forms of drug resistance, such as mono and poly resistance to first and second-line drugs were also included.

The new guidelines of 2019 and later on 2020, has substaintially changed the approach to the treatment of MDR/XDR-TB. It recommends as follows *(26)* :

- policy recommendations on treatment regimens for isoniazid resistant TB and multidrug and rifampicin resistant TB (MDR/RR-TB), including longer and shorter regimens;
- culture monitoring of patients on treatment;
- the timing of antiretroviral therapy in MDR/RR-TB patients infected with HIV;
- the use of surgery for patients receiving MDR-TB treatment;
- optimal models of patient support and care; and
- fully oral regimens should have priority and should become option for most patients.

It needs to be emphasized that treatment for drug resistant TB should only be provided under the supervision of an experienced doctor. This includes the choice of a shorter or longer regimen, and also whether injectable drugs are used.

Accordingly, India has made some changes in its PMDT guidelines. The revised integrated DR-TB diagnostic algorithm recommends testing of all TB patients for rifampicin and isoniazid resistance and all RR-TB patients for fluoroquinolone and second line injectable. Fig. 3 on page 223 shows the integrated drug resistant TB algorithm.

The medicines recommended for longer MDR-TB regimens are classified into three groups (A, B and C) based on efficacy, experience of use and drug class and aligned with revised classification as per WHO consolidated guidelines for treatment of drug resistant TB. The groups are as listed below :

Grouping of medicines recommended for use in longer MDR-TB regimens

Groups & steps	Medicine	
Group A: Include all three medicines	levofloxacin OR moxifloxacin	Lfx Mfx
	bedaquiline	Bdq
	linezolid	Lzd
Group B: Add one or both medicines	clofazimine	Cfz
	cycloserine OR terizidone	Cs Trd
Group C: Add to complete the regimen and when medicines from Groups A and B cannot be used	ethambutol	E
	delamanid	Dlm
	pyrazinamide	Z
	imipenem–cilastatin OR meropenem	Ipm–Cln Mpm
	amikacin (OR streptomycin)	Am (S)
	ethionamide OR prothionamide	Eto Pto
	p-aminosalicylic acid	PAS

Source : *(40, 26)*

Inclusion criteria for newer drugs (Bdq/Dlm)

- Patient aged >6 years having MDR/RR TB. (Bdq/Dlm can be provided to the patient ≥18 yrs) for children & adolescents between 6 to 17 years, Dlm can be provided. Use of Bdq for 6 to 17 yrs and Dlm for 3 to 6 yrs may be considered only after approval of DCGI; and
- patients with controlled stable arrhythmia can be considered after obtaining cardiac consultation.

Exclusion criteria for newer drugs (Bdq/Dlm)

- Pregnancy & lactating mother
- currently having uncontrolled cardiac arrhythmia that requires medication;
- having any of the following QTcF interval characteristics at screening:
- QTcF ≥500 at baseline & normal electrolytes, ECG to be repeated after 6 hours and if both ECGs show QTcF>500 then the patient should not be challenged with cardiotoxic drugs.
- history of additional risk factors for Torsade de Pointes, e.g. heart failure, hypokalaemia, family history of long QT syndrome.

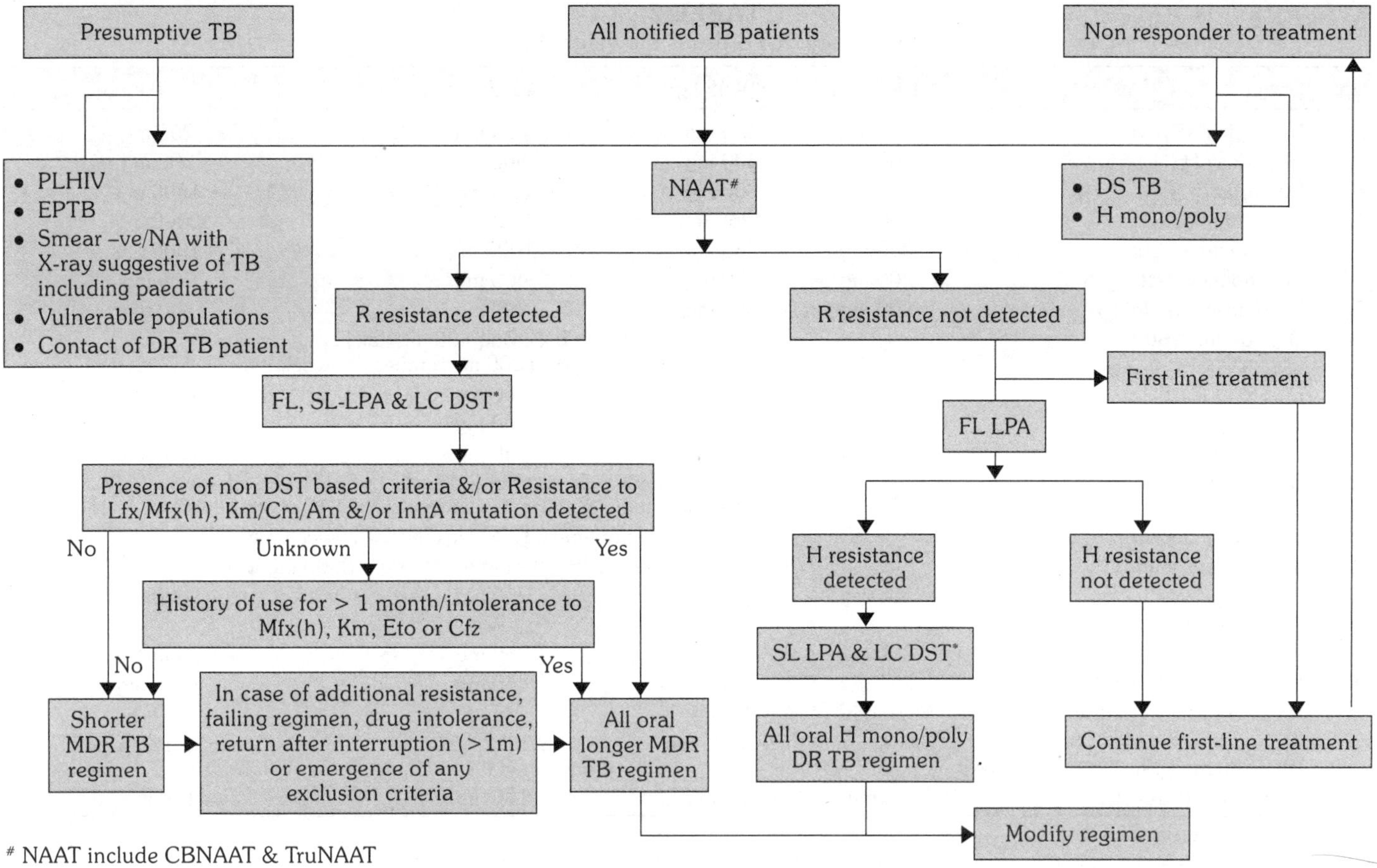

NAAT include CBNAAT & TruNAAT

* LC DST will be done as per the diagnostic algorithm

FIG. 3
Integrated drug resistant TB algorithm (2019)

Source : *(26)*

Bedaquiline (26)

Week 0–2 : Bdq 400 mg (4 tablets of 100 mg) daily (7 days per week) + other drugs; Week 3–24 : Bdq 200 mg (2 tablets of 100 mg) 3 times per week (with at least 48 hours between doses) for a total dose of 600 mg per week + other drugs; and Week 25 (start of month 7) to end of treatment : Continue other second-line anti-TB drugs only as per NTEP recommendations.

If taking a light meal with Bdq and other anti-TB drugs, patients should not consume milk-containing products at the same time, as the calcium in these can decrease the absorption of FQs. Also, large fatty meals should be avoided, as these can impair absorption of some of the other anti-TB drugs (Cs, H, etc.).

The following medications are disallowed during the 24-week administration of Bdq and upto one month after the last dose of Bdq because of potential drug–drug interactions :

- systemic use of moderate and strong CYP3A4 inhibitors, e.g. azole antifungals: ketoconazole, voriconazole, itraconazole, fluconazole; ketolides such as telithromycin and macrolide antibiotics other than azithromycin for more than 2 consecutive weeks;
- systemic use of strong CYP3A4 inducers, e.g. phenytoin, carbamazepine, phenobarbital, St. John's wort and rifamycins (rifampin, rifabutin, rifapentine); and
- cholesterol lowering medications of the "statin" class.

Delamanid (26)

All patients >12 yrs of age will receive Tab. Delamanid 100 mg (two tablets of 50 mg) orally twice a day for 24 weeks in combination with other drugs in the regimen while patients belonging to 6 to 11 yrs of age group will receive Tab. Delamanid 50 mg (one tablet of 50 mg) twice a day for 24 weeks. Remaining drugs in regimen will be continued beyond the 24 weeks of Dlm administration for the NTEP recommended duration of treatment. It is important that Dlm be taken daily preferably after a standard meal to improve bioavailability.

Patients should not consume milk-containing products at the same time, as calcium can decrease the absorption of FQs. Also, large fatty meals should be avoided as these can impair absorption of some of the other anti-TB drugs (Cs, H, etc).

Dosage of DR TB drugs

The dosage for drugs used in various DR TB regimens by weight bands for adults are enumerated in Table 2. These are in accordance to the WHO recommended doses of anti-TB drugs for adults and paediatric patients.

Pretreatment evaluation for drug-resistant patients

Since the drugs used for the treatment of DR-TB have significant adverse effects, a pretreatment evaluation is essential to identify patients at increased risk of developing

TABLE 2
Dosage of DR TB drugs by weight bands

S.No.	Drugs	16–29 kg	30–45 kg	46–70 kg	>70 kg
1	Rifampicin (R)[1]	300 mg	450 mg	600 mg	750 mg
2	High dose H (H^h)	300 mg	600 mg	900 mg	900 mg
3	Ethambutol (E)	400 mg	800 mg	1200 mg	1600 mg
4	Pyrazinamide (Z)	750 mg	1250 mg	1750 mg	2000 mg
5	Levofloxacin (Lfx)	250 mg	750 mg	1000 mg	1000 mg
6	Moxifloxacin (Mfx)	200 mg	400 mg	400 mg	400 mg
7	High dose Mfx (Mfx^h)	400 mg	600 mg	800 mg	800 mg
8	Bedaquiline (Bdq)	Week 0–2: Bdq 400 mg daily Week 3–24: Bdq 200 mg 3 times per week			
9	Linezolid (Lzd)	300 mg	600 mg	600 mg	600 mg
10	Clofazimine (Cfz)	50 mg	100 mg	100 mg	200 mg
11	Cycloserine (Cs)[4]	250 mg	500 mg	750 mg	1000 mg
12	Delamanid (Dlm)	50 mg twice daily (100 mg) for 24 weeks in 6–11 years of age 100 mg twice daily (200 mg) for 24 weeks for >11 years of age			
13	Imipenem/cilastatin (Ipm/Cls)[4]	1000 mg imipenem/1000 mg cilastatin twice daily			
14	Meropenem (Mpm)[4]	1000 mg three times daily (alternative dosing is 2000 mg twice daily)			
15	Amikacin (Am)[2]	500 mg	750 mg	750 mg	1000 mg
16	Capreomycin (Am)[2]	-	-	-	-
17	Kanamycin (Km)[2]	500 mg	750 mg	750 mg	1000 mg
18	Ethionamide (Eto)[4]	375 mg	500 mg	750 mg	1000 mg
19	Na-PAS (60% weight/vol)[3,4]	10 gm	14 gm	16 gm	22 gm
20	Amoxyclav (Amx/Clv) (In child: WHO 80 mg/kg in 2 divided doses)	875/125 mg BD	875/125 mg BD	875/125 mg (2 morning + 1 evening)	875/125 mg (2 morning + 1 evening)
21	Pyridoxine (Pdx)	50 mg	100 mg	100 mg	100 mg

[1] For H mono/poly resistant TB;
[2] For adult more than 60 years of age, dose of SLI should be reduced to 10mg/kg (max upto 750 mg)
[3] In patient of PAS with 80% weight/volume the dose will be changed to 7.5gm (16–29kg); 10gm (30–45 kg); 12 gm (46–70 kg) and 16 gm (>70 kg)
[4] Drugs can be given in divided doses in a day in the event of intolerance

Source : *(26)*

such adverse effects. This pretreatment evaluation is as follows :

Pretreatment evaluations

1 Detailed history (including screening for mental illness, seizure disorder, drug/alcohol abuse, etc.)
2 Previous history of ATT taken especially SLI/FQ
3 Weight & height
4 Thorough clinical examination
5 Complete blood count with haemoglobin & platelets count
6 Blood sugar to screen for Diabetes Mellitus
7 Blood urea and S. Creatinine to assess renal function
8 Urine examination – routine and microscopic
9 UPT (for all women in the child-bearing age)
10 Chest X-ray
11 HIV counselling and testing*
12 Audiogram
13 Liver function tests#
14 TSH levels to assess the thyroid function
15 Mental health evaluation
16 Surgical evaluation
17 ECG (if Mfx^h, Dlm, Bdq, Cfz used)
18 Serum electrolytes – potassium, magnesium, calcium
19 Serum proteins, lipase, amylase
20 Ophthalmologist opinion to rule out chorioretinitis/uveitis

* All DR-TB patients will be offered referral for HIV counselling and testing at the nearest centre if the HIV status is not known or HIV test result is negative with results more than 6 months old. If patient is HIV positive, refer to ART centre (if not on ART)
\# including HBsAg at baseline

Source : *(26)*

Pretreatment evaluation and treatment initiation must be done at the DR-TBC (Drug-Resistant TB centre) i.e., DDR-TBC (District DR-TBC) and NDR-TBC (Nodal DR-TBC). The concerned DR-TBC committee provides counselling, initiates activities related to active drug safety monitoring (aDSM) like, assessing the baseline history of known adverse/serious adverse events, biochemical investigations, ECG etc., and initiates him/her on an appropriate treatment regimen. Care must be taken to correct any electrolyte imbalance before treatment initiation.

Newer treatment regimen

NTEP provides simplified regimen for various types of DR-TB including shorter oral Bedaquiline-containing MDR/RR-TB regimen and longer oral M/XDR-TB regimen based on DST/DRT results with scope in difficult patients to extend Bdq beyond 6 months, combined use of Bdq and Dlm and Bdq use in pregnancy. As the fully oral regimens get scaled up nationwide, the current shorter MDR-TB regimen with injectable SLDs will be phased out. Injectable SLDs will be available for use under PMDT to substitute oral SLDs based on DST and ADR. Guidance is also provided for using Bdq for children above 5 years and Dlm for children above 6 years. Use of BPaL regimen consisting of Bdq, pretomanid (Pa) & linezolid (Lzd) are ongoing in select group of patients on a research mode. H mono/poly DR-TB treatment to be initiated at HF level. To further improve the quality of care offered by the DR-TB centres, difficult-to-treat TB clinics (DT3C) are established at state and national levels.

1. Shorter oral Bedaquiline-containing MDR/RR-TB regimen *(41, 42)*

Following the recommendations of WHO to implement short oral Bedaquiline-containing MDR/RR-TB regimen, Govt. of India decided on transitioning from the current shorter injectable containing MDR/RR-TB regimen to the shorter oral Bedaquiline-containing MDR/RR-TB regimen in patients >5 years of age weighing 15 kg or more in a phased manner starting with selected states to gain programmatic experience to guide future expansion within 2021.

Eligibility criteria *(41)*

Shorter oral Bedaquiline-containing MDR/RR-TB regimen is recommended for those MDR/RR-TB patients in whom resistance to the component drugs has been excluded or those who have not been previously treated for more than one month with second-line drugs used in shorter oral Bedaquiline-containing MDR/RR-TB regimen and have no other exclusion criteria. The criteria to include or exclude the patients from offering shorter oral Bedaquiline-containing MDR/RR-TB regimen are given below.

Inclusion criteria

1. DST based inclusion criteria
   - Rifampicin resistance detected/inferred;
   - MDR/RR-TB with H resistance detected/inferred based on InhA mutation only or based on KatG mutation only (not both); and
   - MDR/RR-TB with FQ resistance not detected.
2. Other inclusion criteria
   - Children, aged 5 years to less than 18 years of age and weighing at least 15 kg, given their special needs, in consultation with the pediatrician;
   - No history of exposure to previous treatment with second-line medicines in the regimen (Bdq, Lfx, Eto or Cfz) for more than 1 month (unless susceptibility to these medicines is confirmed);
   - No extensive TB disease;
   - No severe extra-pulmonary TB; and
   - Women who are not pregnant or lactating.

Exclusion criteria

1. DST based exclusion criteria
   - MDR/RR-TB patients with H resistance detected with both KatG and InhA mutation; and
   - MDR/RR-TB patients with FQ resistance detected.
2. Other exclusion criteria
   - If result for FL-LPA, SL-LPA and DST to Z, BDQ & Cfz is not available after pre-treatment evaluation is completed and it is a time to initiate the first dose of the regimen, then, exclude those with history of exposure for > 1 month to Bdq, Lfx, Eto or Cfz;
   - Intolerance to any drug or risk of toxicity from a drug in shorter oral Bedaquiline-containing MDR/RR-TB regimen (e.g. drug-drug interactions);
   - Extensive TB disease found in presence of bilateral cavitary disease or extensive parenchymal damage on chest radiography. In children aged under 15 years, presence of cavities or bilateral disease on chest radiography;
   - Severe EP-TB disease where there is a presence of miliary TB or TB meningitis or central nervous system (CNS) TB. In children aged under 15 years, extrapulmonary forms of disease other than lymphadenopathy (peripheral nodes or isolated mediastinal mass without compression);
   - Pregnant and lactating women; and
   - Children below 5 years.

The regimen consists of an initial phase of 4 months that may be extended up to 6 months and a continuation phase of 5 months, giving a total duration of 9–11 months. Bdq is used for a duration of 6 months.

(4–6) Bdq $_{(6\ m)}$, Lfx, Cfz, Z, E, H^h, Eto (5) Lfx, Cfz, Z, E

The composition or the duration of the initial or continuation phase cannot be changed :

1. From start to end of 4th month – Bdq, Lfx, Cfz, Z, E, H^h, Eto;
2. From start of 5th month to end of 6 th month – (If IP not extended) – Bdq, Lfx, Cfz, Z, E;
3. From start of 7th month to end of 9th month – Lfx, Cfz, Z, E; and
4. If the IP is extended up to 6 months then all 3 drugs Bdq, H^h and Eto are stopped together.

Treatment extension

- Total duration of shorter oral Bedaquiline-containing MDR/RR-TB regimen is for 9–11 months, depending on IP duration.
- IP should be given for at least 4 months. After 4th month of treatment, if the result of sputum microscopy is negative then CP should be initiated with Bdq continued for another 2 months.
- If sputum smear microscopy does not become negative by the 4th month of treatment, subject the patient to FL-LPA and SL-LPA and culture & DST and the IP should be extended. IP can be extended to 5th or 6th month based on smear results at the end of 4th and 5th month of treatment. This will be done for a maximum of 2 months (i.e., total duration of IP is not more than 6 months). If any additional resistant to Z/Cfz on C&DST of the baseline sample is detected or to FQ/InhA & KatG mutation of the 4th month sample is detected, the patient needs to be reassessed at N/DDR-TBC for stopping shorter oral Bedaquiline-containing MDR/RR-TB regimen and initiation of longer oral M/XDR-TB regimen, immediately on receiving the report.
- Duration of CP is fixed for 5 months.

Additional considerations for the use of Bdq

- Bdq can be provided to adults and children aged 5 years to less than 18 years of age and weighing at least 15 kg, given their special needs, in consultation with pediatrician;
- Patients with controlled stable arrhythmia can be considered after obtaining cardiac consultation; and
- Pregnancy & lactating women.

The drug dose administration is as shown in Table 2.

Shorter injectable containing regimen *(41)*

Till the complete geographical coverage by shorter oral Bedaquiline-containing MDR/RR-TB regimen, the states will continue to use shorter injectable containing regimen for MDR/RR-TB. The regimen composition and duration is as follows :

(4–6) Mfx^h, Km/Am, Eto, Cfz, Z, H^h, E/ (5) Mfx^h, Cfz, Z, E

- If the intensive phase is prolonged, the injectable agent is only given three times a week in the extended intensive phase;

- Neither replacement of drug (except the use of Am instead of Km) nor extension of treatment duration (beyond 11 months) is permitted; and
- Pyridoxine is to be given as per weight band.

The drug dose administration is as shown in Table 2.

Follow-up evaluation of Shorter oral Bedaquiline-containing MDR/RR-TB regimen

Duration	9–11 months (4–6m IP, 5m CP)
Clinical + Wt.	Monthly in IP or extended IP if previous month S+ve, quarterly in CP
Smear Microscopy	Monthly from 3rd month onwards till end of IP Monthly in extended IP only if previous month S+ve Conduct SM within 7 days, if the smear at 6 months is positive to rapidly ascertain bacteriological conversion/reversion
Culture	At the end of month 3, end of month 6 and/or end of treatment If the culture results of month 6 is positive, collect one repeat sample immediately to rapidly ascertain the bacteriological conversion/reversion If the repeat sample is culture negative, then do end of treatment specimen collection
DST	FL-SL LPA (Lfx, Mfx, Eto) and LC&DST (Z, Bdq*, Cfz*, Mfx, Lzd, Dlm*) if any – culture +ve (end of month 3 or later and end of treatment) or – smear +ve at end of IP, end of extended IP and end of treatment
UPT	As and when clinically indicated
CBC	As and when clinically indicated
TSH & LFT#	At end of IP, then as and when clinically indicated
CXR	At end of IP, then as and when clinically indicated, end of treatment
ECG$	At 2 weeks, then monthly in first 6 months, then as and when clinically indicated
S. Electrolytes (Na, K, Mg, Ca)	As and when indicated and in case of any QTcF prolongation
Specialist consultation	As and when clinically indicated
Color vision test	Once in two months (in children)

\# HBsAG and other viral markers (Hepatitis A, C & E) to be done in case of Jaundice.

$ In case of baseline ECG abnormality or QTcF ≥ 450ms with shorter oral Bedaquiline-containing MDR/RR-TB regimen that contains Bdq & Cfz, ECG must be done on daily basis for initial 3 days or as suggested by cardiologist. Repeat ECG with long II lead after an hour to reconfirm abnormal ECG

* DST whenever available

Source : *(41)*

2. H mono/poly DR-TB regimen *(41)*

H mono/poly DR-TB regimen (R resistance not detected and H resistance detected) under NTEP is as follows :

(6 or 9) Lfx R E Z

Total duration of H mono/poly DR-TB regimen is 6 months. It can be extended directly to 9 months in certain conditions. In patients with extensive disease; uncontrolled comorbidity; extra-pulmonary TB; if smear at the end of month 4 is found positive and when regimen is modified, the treatment may be directly extended to 9 months. There would be no monthly extensions in this regimen. In patients who remain sputum smear positive at the end of month 5 or later, the treatment outcome will be declared as 'treatment failed' and the patient will be re-evaluated as per the diagnostic algorithm as a non-responder.

Follow-up evaluation schedule of H mono/poly DR-TB patients

Duration	6 or 9 months (no separate IP/CP)
Clinical + Wt.	Monthly till the end of treatment
Smear microscopy	Monthly from month 3 onwards till the end of treatment Conduct SM within 7 days, if the smear at month 4 or later is positive to rapidly ascertain bacteriological conversion/reversion
Culture	At end of month 3, end of treatment (month 6 and/or 9 if applicable) If the culture results of month 3 are positive, collect one repeat specimen for culture to rapidly ascertain bacteriological conversion/ reversion. If the repeat specimen is culture negative, then ensure specimen collection at the end of treatment
DST	NAAT, FL LPA, SL LPA (R, Eto, Lfx, Mfx) and LC DST (Mfx, Z, Lzd & Cfz) if smear/ culture +ve at month 3, end of treatment (month 6 and/or 9 if applicable)

3. Longer oral M/XDR-TB treatment regimen *(41)*

The longer oral M/XDR-TB regimen is as follows :

(18–20) Lfx Bdq $_{(6\ \text{month or longer})}$ Lzd#Cfz Cs

\# dose of Lzd will be tapered to 300 mg after the initial 6–8 months of treatment

Bdq will be given for 6 months & extended beyond 6 months as an exception

Pyridoxine to be given to all DR-TB patients as per weight band

For Pre-XDR-TB and XDR-TB patients the duration of longer oral XDR-TB regimen would be for 20 months with appropriate modifications.

Once a patient is placed on a longer oral M/XDR-TB regimen for at least 4 weeks, normally that patient can no longer be switched to the shorter oral Bedaquiline-containing MDR/RR-TB regimen because this 4-weeks treatment would represent an exposure to second-line medicines.

Treatment extension (41)

Total duration of longer oral M/XDR-TB regimen is 18–20 months.

a. After month 6 of treatment, the patient must be reviewed based on month 5 culture results. If month 5 culture result is not available at the end of month 6, decision to taper the dose of Lzd to 300 mg will be based on month 4 culture result. If the month 5 or 4 culture result (whichever applicable) remains positive, the dose of Lzd (600 mg) and the regimen is extended by 1 month to month 7 and for a maximum till month 8 based on monthly culture results of month 6 and 7 respectively and clinical/radiographic response. If the month 8 culture is also positive, subject the culture isolate to FL-LPA, SL-LPA and C&DST. If any additional resistant to Group A, B or C drugs in use is detected, the patient needs to be reassessed at N/DDR-TBC for modification of longer oral M/XDR-TB regimen immediately on receiving the report.

b. The duration of Bedaquiline is limited to 6 months. Extension beyond 6 months is to be considered in patients in whom an effective regimen cannot otherwise be designed if only 2 of 5 drugs are available from Groups A & B and adequate number of Group C drugs are not available due to high background resistance, non-availability or unreliability of DST.

c. Maximum duration of treatment is not more than 20 months. A treatment duration of 15–17 months after culture conversion is suggested for most patients. The duration may be modified according to the patient's response to treatment.

The drug dose administration is as shown in Table 2.

Follow up evaluation schedule of longer oral M/XDR-TB regimen during treatment is as follows

Duration	18–20 months (no separate IP/CP)
Clinical + Wt.	Monthly up to month 6 or 7 or 8 if previous month S+ve Quarterly in from month 7 or 9 onwards
Smear microscopy	With culture at C&DST lab Conduct SM within 7 days, if any smear at 6 month or later is positive to rapidly ascertain bacteriological conversion/reversion C&DST lab to update the result on Nikshay and inform the concerned field staff of collection center on same day
Culture	Monthly from month 3 onwards to end of 6 months or 7 or 8 if the previous month's culture is +ve Quarterly month 6 or 7 or 8 onwards based on previous month's culture results If the culture results of month 6 or any of the quarterly culture is positive, collect one repeat specimen immediately and send it for culture to rapidly ascertain bacteriological conversion/ reversion and if the repeat specimen is culture negative, then the subsequent quarterly or end of treatment specimen collection.
DST	FL & SL-LPA (Lfx, Mfx, Am, Eto) and LC&DST (Mfx, Lzd, Cfz*, Bdq*, Dlm*, Z) if culture +ve at the end of 6 months or any time beyond
UPT	As and when clinically indicated
CBC/platelets^	Day 15, monthly in first 6 months, 6 or 7 or 8 if previous month S+ve, then as and when clinically indicated
TSH & LFT#	LFT quarterly, then as and when clinically indicated. TSH every 6 months
CXR	At the end of month 6, end of treatment and as and when clinically indicated
ECG$	At 2 weeks, monthly in first 6 months and till Bdq/Mfx/Cfz/Dlm is extended, then as and when clinically indicated.
S. electrolytes (K, Mg, Ca)	As and when indicated and in case of any QTcF prolongation

^ If Lzd is part of the regimen to rule out bone marrow suppression

HBsAG and other viral markers (Hepatitis A, C & E) to be done in case of jaundice

$ In case of baseline ECG abnormality or QTcF ≥ 450ms with longer oral M/XDR-TB regimen that contains Bdq, Mfx, Cfz or Dlm, ECG must be done on daily basis for initial 3 days or as suggested by cardiologist. Repeat ECG with long II lead after an hour to reconfirm abnormal ECG.

* DST whenever available.

The most important evidence of response to DR-TB treatment is conversion of sputum smear and culture to negative. Good quality sputum specimen is therefore essential to get reliable results that form the basis of monitoring bacteriological response to treatment.

Treatment Interruptions & DRTB

Management of DR TB patients with treatment interruptions and lost to follow-up

All efforts must be made to ensure that DR TB patients do not interrupt treatment or are lost to follow-up. Action should be taken to promptly retrieve patients who fail to come for their daily dose by the treatment supporter. The following strategies are applicable for patients who interrupt treatment :

Patients who miss doses : In shorter MDR TB regimen, all missed doses during IP must be completed prior to switching the patient to CP. Similarly, all missed doses during CP must be administered prior to ending treatment. In longer MDR TB regimen, all missed doses during treatment must be administered prior to ending treatment.

Patients who interrupt treatment for less than one month : When the patient returns to resume treatment, the treatment will be continued. However, the duration of treatment will be extended to complete the regimen. The follow-up cultures will be done as per the schedule.

Patients who are "lost to follow-up" (interrupt treatment continuously for one month or more) and return back for treatment: Such patients will be given an outcome of "lost to follow-up". The patient would be subjected to repeat NAAT & FL/SL LPA and LC DST as per the diagnostic algorithm to restart with appropriate treatment. If there are signs of impending treatment failure for any MDR/RR TB patient with or without additional resistance to second line drugs, the patient should be switched to an all oral longer DR TB regimen and evaluated further to modify appropriately based on DST results if required. If a patient has received the shorter MDR TB regimen for more than one month and returns for treatment after an interruption of one month or more, the patient is not restarted on a shorter MDR TB regimen.

MDR/RR TB patients on Bdq/Dlm containing regimen who interrupt treatment or are "lost to follow-up" or recurrent DR TB :

Patients who interrupt Bedaquiline treatment during the first two weeks of Bdq course and return to resume the treatment :

- if interruption is upto 7 days, Bdq containing regimen will be continued to complete the doses and the duration of treatment will be extended to complete IP. Follow-up cultures will be done as per the revised schedule; and
- if interruption is more than 7 consecutive days, Bdq course will be reloaded (started afresh) and a fresh specimen collected for culture. The culture isolate must be stored for Bdq DST in future.

Patients who interrupt Bedaquiline treatment during 3–24 weeks of Bdq course and return to resume treatment *(26)* :

- if interruption is upto one month, Bdq containing regimen will be continued to complete the doses and duration of treatment will be extended to complete full course of Bdq. Follow-up cultures will be done as per revised schedule; and
- if interruption is more than one month, Bdq will be permanently discontinued. Such patients will be given an outcome of "Lost to follow-up" (LTFU), registered afresh and initiate all oral longer MDR TB regimen with appropriate modification. A sputum specimen will be collected for culture. The culture isolate must be stored for Bdq DST in future.

Delamanid : If the patient misses one or more doses of Dlm during treatment upto a maximum of one month, one should continue the treatment and complete the Dlm for rest of the period which may prolong the Dlm containing phase beyond 24 weeks from initiation of treatment to make the adjustment of missed dosage.

Patients who initiated on Bdq/Dlm containing regimen and return after treatment interruption of one month or more will be declared as "lost to follow-up". Such patients would not be considered eligible for administration of same drug (Bdq/Dlm) anymore.

Where further treatment is concerned, if the patient has any indication of a treatment failure or recurrence, the NDR TBC Committee will be contacted to discuss whether s/he should be retreated. The decision will be made on a case-to-case basis, using all available bacteriological and clinical data.

Providing health education and counselling to patient and family members (36) :

All MDR-TB cases are offered referral for counselling and HIV testing at the nearest centre. Patients should receive counselling on the nature and duration of treatment, need for regular treatment and possible side effects of these drugs and the consequences of irregular treatment or pre-mature cessation of treatment and cough etiquette. It is advisable to involve close family members during the counselling, since family support is an essential component in the management. Patients should be advised to report any side-effects experienced by them. Female patients should receive special counselling on family planning.

While the MDR-TB case is undergoing pre-treatment evaluation, the DTO should ensure an initial home visit to verify the address and meet the family members. The medical officer needs to open a treatment card for the patient at the time of initiating the treatment. Each patient must be given TB Identity Card. A DOT provider (who can either be a health care worker or a community volunteer), should be identified in consultation with the patient. The DOT centre can be either at the sub-centre of the health system or in the community. The DOT provider should be given training for drug administration, identification of adverse effects during treatment and the frequency of follow-up.

Monthly patient-wise box for DR-TB patients *(41)*

The district drug store will supply the monthly patient-wise boxes as per standard regimens. The shorter oral MDR/RR TB regimen will have two types of boxes – type A for intensive phase and type B for continuation phase. The longer oral M/XDR-TB regimen and H mono/poly DR-TB regimen will standard patient-wise box as there is no separate intensive and continuation phase. The DR-TB patients on longer/shorter injectable containing regimen will be supplied drugs continuously till the state/districts fully transitions to all oral regimen.

CHILDHOOD TUBERCULOSIS

Cases of tuberculosis in children usually represent between 6–8 per cent of all reported tuberculosis in the age group of under 15 years, although the estimates are about 11 per cent cases are in children *(43)*. The source of infection to a child is usually an adult, often a family member with sputum smear-positive tuberculosis. The frequency of childhood TB in a given population depends on : (a) the number of infectious cases; (b) closeness of contact with an infectious case; (c) the age of child when exposed to TB; and the age structure of the population.

Children rarely have sputum smear-positive TB and it is unlikely that they are a powerful source of transmission of TB. Tuberculosis in children is mainly due to failure of TB control in adults. The risk of infection to a child depends on extent of exposure to infectious droplet nuclei. An infant whose mother has sputum smear-positive PTB has a high chance of becoming infected. The chance of developing disease is greatest shortly after infection, and steadily decreases as the time goes by. Because of less-developed immune system, children under 5 years of age are more prone to develop (upto 20 per cent) the disease mostly within 2 years following infection *(28)*. The commonest age of childhood TB disease is 1 to 4 years. Young age is a risk factor for spread of disease to other parts of the body, i.e. dissemination.

In order to simplify the management of paediatric TB, RNTCP in association with Indian Academy of Paediatrics (IAP) has described criteria for suspecting TB among children, has separate algorithms for diagnosing pulmonary TB and peripheral TB lymphadenitis and a strategy for treatment and monitoring patients who are on treatment. In brief, TB diagnosis is based on clinical features, smear examination of sputum where this is available, positive family history, tuberculin skin testing, chest radiography and histo-pathological examination as appropriate. The treatment strategy comprises of components. First, as in adults, children with TB are classified, categorized, registered and treated with daily dose short-course chemotherapy from treatment initiation to completion, given under direct observation of a treatment provider (DOT provider) and the disease status is monitored during the course of treatment. Based on their pre-treatment weight, children are assigned to one of the pre-treatment weight bands and are treated with good quality anti-TB drugs through "ready-to-use" fixed dose combination tablets in patient-wise boxes containing the patients' complete course of anti-TB drugs, made available to every registered TB patient according to programme guidelines. India is the first country to introduce paediatric patient-wise boxes *(6)*.

Diagnosis of Paediatric TB

In children with presumptive paediatric TB, every attempt must be made to microbiologically prove diagnosis through examination of appropriate respiratory/non-respiratory specimens with quality assured diagnostic tests. Diagnosis of tuberculosis should not be made only on clinical features, and further investigations are always necessary to establish the diagnosis.

In case of suspicion of pulmonary TB, sputum examination should be carried out among children who are able to give good quality specimens. CBNAAT is the preferred investigation of choice. If CBNAAT is not readily available or testing is not possible even by referral, smear microscopy should be performed. If *M. tuberculosis* is detected, by either of methods patient is diagnosed as microbiologically confirmed pulmonary TB. In situations where *M. tubeculosis* is not detected or specimen is not available, chest X-ray and Tuberculin skin test (TST) by Mantoux technique using 2 TU of PPD RT 23 should be done. For interpretation and further course of action, refer to the diagnostic algorithm for childhood pulmonary TB (Fig. 4).

While following the flow chart, it is important to note the following points :

1. This algorithm is for children who are likely to have drug sensitive disease i.e. have not received ATT previously

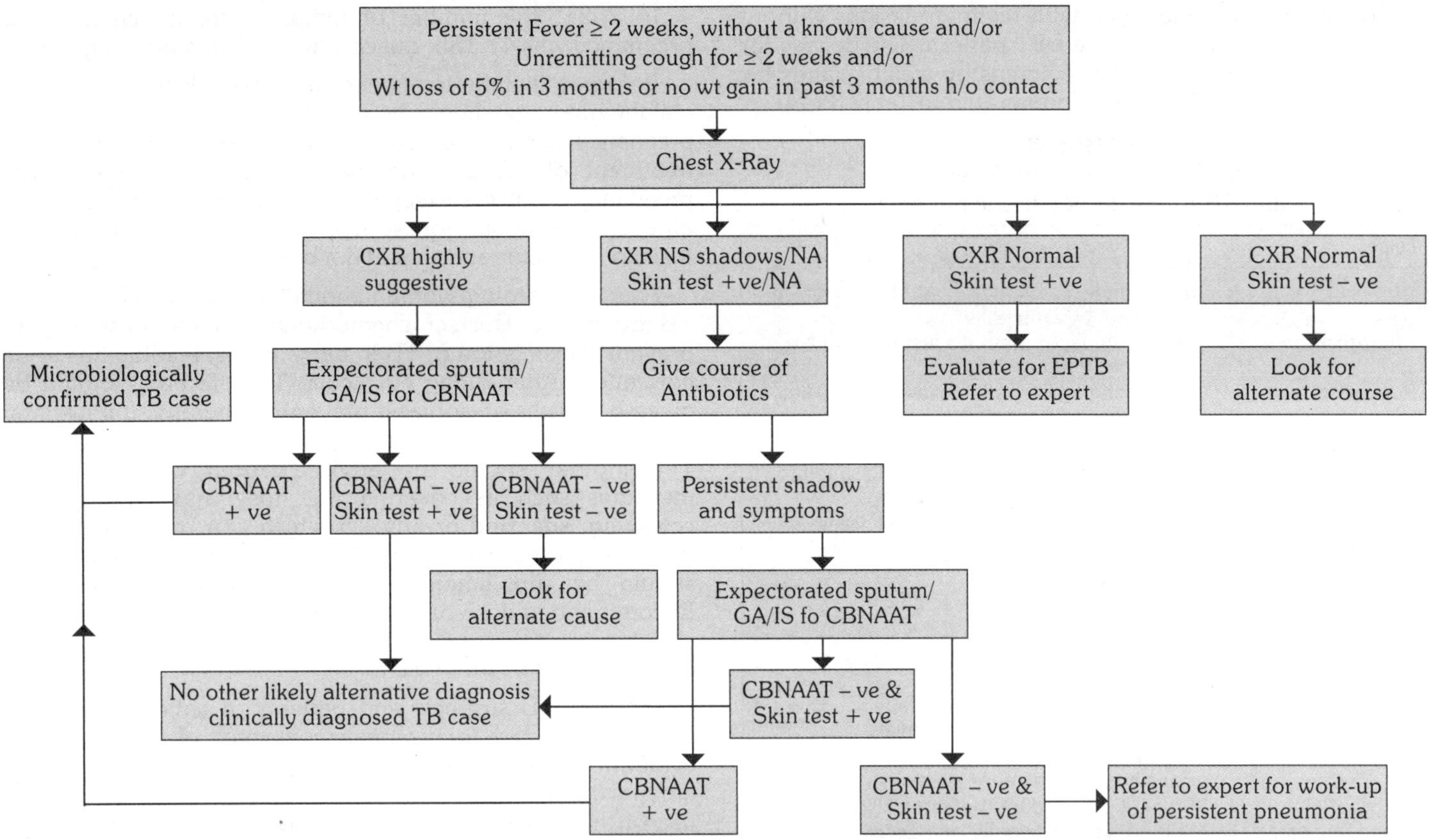

FIG. 4
Diagnostic algorithm for paediatric pulmonary tuberculosis

Source : *(39)*

ever and are not presumptive drug resistant TB cases (lost to follow-up, recurrent, treatment failure, HIV).

2. Proper characterization of symptoms is very important starting point. Weight loss or not gaining weight should always be documented with appropriate and proper weighing.
3. Where CBNAAT is doable, smear examination may not be done. Whenever smear is used for diagnosis at least 2 samples should be sent while a single sample is subjected to CBNAAT. If a specimen is positive by any of these methods, the disease is labelled as microbiologically confirmed TB.
4. Highly suggestive chest X-ray refers to skiagrams showing either miliary or lymphadenopathy (hilar or mediastinal) or chronic fibro-cavitatory shadows. If the radiological picture is highly suggestive of TB, then proceed to do further investigations irrespective of the TST result as the sensitivity of the test is not 100%.
5. Non specific chest X-ray : Refer to patterns other than highly suggestive like consolidations in homogenous shadows or bronchopneumonia, etc.
6. Whenever indicated, alternative specimens (gastric aspirate/induced sputum/bronchoalveolar lavage) should be collected by a skilled health care provider, depending upon available infrastructure and sample should be subjected to CBNAAT.
7. Antibiotics like linezolid or any quinolone or Amoxicillin-clavulanic acid should not be used as they have anti-TB action.
8. Children with persistent symptoms, non specific shadows and negative smears and negative other samples (GA/IS) by CBNAAT should be referred to experts for further work-up of persistent pneumonia.
9. All TB cases diagnosed must be offered testing for HIV.
10. Whenever Rif resistant result is reported on CBNAAT further management should be carried out as per the guidelines on drug resistant TB.

TB preventive therapy :

The dose of INH for chemoprophylaxis is 10 mg/kg (instead of earlier recommended dosage of 5 mg/kg) administered daily for 6 months. TB preventive therapy should be provided to:

a. All asymptomatic contacts (under 6 years of age) of a smear positive case, after ruling out active disease and irrespective of their BCG or nutritional status.
b. Chemoprophylaxis is also recommended for all HIV infected children who either had a known exposure to an infectious TB case or are tuberculin skin test (TST) positive (≥5 mm induration) but have no active TB disease.
c. All TST positive children who are receiving immunosuppressive therapy (e.g. children with nephrotic syndrome, acute leukemia, etc).
d. A child born to mother, who was diagnosed to have TB in pregnancy, should receive prophylaxis for 6 months, provided congenital TB has been ruled out followed by BCG vaccination.

Drug-resistant TB in children:

The principles of treatment of drug-resistant TB in children are : (1) Always treat the child in consultation with an expert; (2) Include at least 4–6 bactericidal medication to which the strain is known to or likely to be susceptible; (3) Do not add a single drug to a failing regimen; (4) Ensure treatment is given for at least 12 months after *M. tuberculosis* culture has converted to negative; and extend treatment to 24 months in case of HIV infection or cavitatory lesions.

The children are managed with regimen designs without newer drugs, depending on the DST pattern. The dosage for drugs used in various DR-TB regimens by weight bands for paediatric DR-TB patients are enumerated in Table 3 *(44)*.

TABLE 3
WHO recommended doses of anti TB drugs for paediatric patients

Drugs	Daily Dose (Paediatric)
Isoniazid [1]	7–15 mg/kg for patients less than 30 kg; max dose 300 mg daily
Rifampicin	10–20 mg/kg for patients less than 30 kg; max dose 600 mg daily
Pyrazinamide	30–40 mg/kg for patients less than 30 kg; max dose 2000 mg daily
Ethambutol	15–25 mg/kg once daily
Levofloxacin	5 years and under : 15–20 mg/kg split into two doses (morning and evening) Over 5 years: 10–15 mg/kg once daily
Moxifloxacin	7.5–10 mg/kg
Ethionamide/ Protionamide	15–20 mg/kg
Cycloserine	10–20 mg/kg
p-aminosalicylic acid	200–300 mg/kg for patients less than 30 kg
Linezolid	10 mg/kg given three times daily (pyridoxine should also be given)
Clofazimine	Limited data, but 1 mg/kg once daily has been given
Amoxicillin clavulanic acid 7/1	80 mg/kg (based on the amoxicillin component) in two divided doses
Kanamycin	15–30 mg/kg once daily (Max 1000 mg)
Amikacin	15–30 mg/kg once daily (Max 1000 mg)
Capreomycin	15–30 mg/kg once daily (Max 1000 mg)
Imipenem cilastatin	Meropenem is preferred in children
Meropenem	20–40 mg/kg intravenous every eight hours
Bedaquiline	Refer to page 223
Delamanid	Refer to page 223

[1] Children at risk for peripheral neuropathy (e.g. malnutrition or HIV co-infection) should also receive pyridoxine 5–10 mg/day as therapeutic dose.

Source : *(44)*

TB IN PREGNANCY AND LACTATING WOMEN *(36)*

While the burden of TB is higher in men in India, the impact of TB in women is far-reaching, especially for women in the reproductive age group (15–49 years). Due to common non-specific symptoms in both TB and pregnancy, diagnosing TB disease in pregnant women is complex. TB in pregnancy has a wide spectrum of short and long-term implications and could have sequential effects : repeated reproductive failure, foetal ill-health, preterm delivery, and TB of the new-borns and infants, leading to high maternal and perinatal morbidity and mortality. For example, there is a six-fold increase in perinatal deaths and a two-fold risk of premature birth and low birth weight in mothers with active TB disease.

The NTEP and the Maternal Health (MH) division have developed a collaborative framework for management of TB in pregnant women to reduce morbidity and mortality due to TB in pregnant women and new-borns through prevention, screening for early detection, and prompt management of TB in pregnant women and achieve optimum maternal and perinatal outcomes. This screening for TB will be made an essential component of ANC services. The National-level sensitization workshop for all the state nodal officers of both the programmes has been conducted, and the training will be cascaded *(43)*.

In 2021, the number of female patients screened for pregnancy was 47,185, out of which 4,048 were pregnant.

Before initiating treatment for tuberculosis, women of childbearing age should be asked about current or planned pregnancy and counselled appropriately. A successful treatment of TB is important for successful outcome of pregnancy. With the exception of streptomycin, the first line anti-TB drugs are safe for use in pregnancy. Streptomycin is oto-toxic to the foetus and should not be used during pregnancy.

A breast feeding woman should receive a full course of TB treatment. Correct chemotherapy is the best way to prevent transmission of TB to baby. Breast feeding has to be continued. After ruling out active TB, the baby should be given 6 months of isoniazid preventive therapy, followed by BCG vaccination. Breast-feeding should not be discouraged. The mother should be advised about cough hygiene measures such as covering the nose and mouth while coughing, sneezing or any act which can produce sputum droplets. Mothers receiving INH and their breastfed infants should be supplemented with vitamin B6 (pyridoxine). Recommended dose of Pyridoxine in infants is 5 mg/day.

Pregnancy with MDR-TB

All MDR-TB suspects and patients of child-bearing age should be tested for pregnancy as part of pre-treatment evaluation and while on treatment, if there is a history of amenorrhoea of any duration. They should be advised to use birth control measures because of the potential risk to both mother and foetus. Oral contraceptives should be avoided. Use of barrier methods (condoms/diaphragms), IUDs are recommended, based on individual preference and eligibility. The management of MDR-TB patients with pregnancy is summarized in Fig. 5.

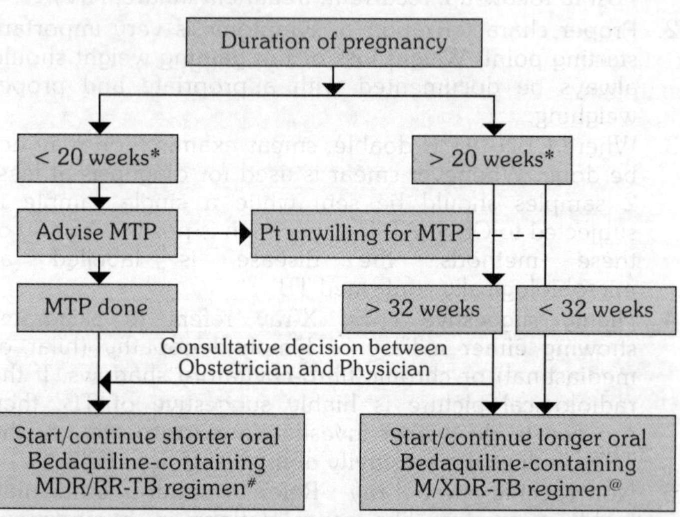

* 24 weeks will apply wherever the bill is passed.

\# Regimen : 4–6 Bdq (6m) Lfx, Cfz, Eto, Hh, Z, E / 5 Lfx, Cfz, Z, E. No modifications allowed.

@ Regimen :18–20 Lfx, Bdq (6m or longer) Lzd#, Cfz, Cs. Lzd dose to be tapered to half after 6–8 months based on bacteriological response. Modify regimen if one or more drug cannot be used due to reasons of resistance, tolerability, contraindication, availability etc.
- in the order of Z E PAS.
- Eto may be considered after 32 weeks' gestation.
- Am may be considered in post-partum period only. Am will not be started in the final 12 months of treatment.

FIG. 5
Management of MDR-TB patients during pregnancy

Source : *(41)*

Pregnant DR-TB patients need to be monitored carefully, both in relation to the treatment and progress of the pregnancy. This approach should lead to good results, since the patient should be smear-negative at the time of parturition and mother and infant do not need to be separated. Breast-feeding should be encouraged as long as the patient is sputum negative.

In the end it may be stated that the main problem of chemotherapy today is not the need to introduce new regimens or more potent drugs, but to apply the existing ones successfully. The cornerstone of successful chemotherapy is adequate and regular drug intake. Patient compliance is critically important throughout the prescribed period of treatment. All other considerations are secondary.

BCG VACCINATION

Ever since Koch discovered *M. tuberculosis,* attempts have been made to prepare a prophylactic vaccine against tuberculosis using either attenuated or killed tubercle bacilli. Initially BCG was given orally during 1921 to 1925. The first human was vaccinated by the intradermal technique in 1927. Recognition of the value of BCG came in 1948 when it was accepted by tuberculosis workers from all over the world as a safe preventive measure.

(1) AIM : The aim of BCG vaccination is to induce a benign, artificial primary infection which will stimulate an acquired resistance to possible subsequent infection with virulent tubercle bacilli, and thus reduce the morbidity and mortality from primary tuberculosis among those most at risk.

(2) VACCINE : BCG is the only widely used live bacterial vaccine. It consists of living bacteria derived from an attenuated *bovine* strain of tubercle bacilli. The bacilli used for vaccine production are descendants of the original Calmette strain of BCG. Due to different methods of maintenance in various vaccine–production laboratories, many substrains have evolved during the past few decades. The WHO has recommended the "Danish 1331" strain for the production of BCG vaccine. Since January 1967, the BCG Laboratory at Guindy, Chennai, has been using the "Danish 1331" strain for the production of BCG vaccine *(45)*. Emphasis has been laid on regular checking of the quality of vaccines at the International Reference Centre for BCG quality control at Copenhagen.

(3) TYPES OF VACCINE : There are two types of BCG vaccine – the liquid (fresh) vaccine and the freeze-dried vaccine. Freeze-dried vaccine is a more stable preparation than liquid vaccine with vastly superior keeping qualities. Present–day vaccines are distributed in the freeze-dried form.

BCG vaccine is stable for several weeks at ambient temperature in a tropical climate, and for up to 1 year if kept away from direct light and stored in a cool environment preferably refrigerated at a temperature below 10 deg C *(46)*.

The vaccine must be protected from exposure to light during storage (wrapped up in a double layer of red or black cloth) and in the field. Normal saline is recommended as a diluent for reconstituting the vaccine, as distilled water may cause irritation. The reconstituted vaccine may be used up within 3 hours, and the left–over vaccine should be discarded.

(4) DOSAGE : For vaccination, the usual strength is 0.1 mg in 0.1 ml volume *(47)*. The dose to newborn aged below 4 weeks is 0.05 ml. This is because the skin of newborn is rather thin and an intradermal injection with full dose (0.1 ml) in some of them might penetrate into deeper tissue and give rise to local abscess formation and enlarged regional (axillary) lymph nodes.

(5) ADMINISTRATION : The standard procedure recommended by WHO is to inject the vaccine intradermally using a "Tuberculin" syringe (Omega microstat syringe fitted with a 1 cm steel 26 gauge intradermal needle). The syringe and needle technique remains the most precise way of administering the desired dose. All other techniques (e.g., bifurcated needle, dermo–jet) are reported to be less accurate, and do not permit the desired dose to be injected *(48)*. If the vaccine is injected subcutaneously an abscess is more likely to develop *(49)*. The site of injection should be just above the insertion of the left deltoid muscle. If it is injected too high, too forward or too backward, the adjacent lymph nodes may become involved and tender. A satisfactory injection should produce a wheal of 5 mm in diameter.

The vaccine must not be contaminated with an antiseptic or detergent. If alcohol is used to swab the skin, it must be allowed to evaporate before the vaccine is given.

(6) AGE : The national vaccination policies differ from country to country *(47)*. In countries where tuberculosis is prevalent and the risk of childhood infection is high (as in India), the national policy is to administer BCG very early in infancy either at birth (for institutional deliveries) or at 6 weeks of age simultaneously with other immunizing agents such as DPT and polio. BCG administered early in life provides a high level of protection, particularly against the severe forms of childhood tuberculosis and tuberculous meningitis.

In countries with a low prevalence of tuberculosis, perhaps there is a diminishing need for widespread BCG vaccination. In this situation, it would seem reasonable to restrict BCG vaccination to high risk groups, for example, hospital personnel and tuberculin-negative contacts of known cases of tuberculosis particularly multi-drug resistant TB (MDR-TB) *(46, 50)*.

(7) PHENOMENA AFTER VACCINATION : Two to three weeks after a correct intradermal injection of a potent vaccine, a papule develops at the site of vaccination. It increases slowly in size and reaches a diameter of about 4 to 8 mm in about 5 weeks. It then subsides or breaks into a shallow ulcer, rarely open, but usually seen covered with a crust. Healing occurs spontaneously within 6 to 12 weeks leaving a permanent, tiny, round scar, typically 4–8 mm in diameter. This is a normal reaction *(51)*. However, with overdosage, the local lesion and the later scar may be considerably larger and of irregular size. Normally the individual becomes Mantoux–positive after a period of 8 weeks has elapsed, but sometimes about 14 weeks are needed.

(8) COMPLICATIONS : BCG has been associated with adverse reactions which include : prolonged severe ulceration at the site of vaccination, suppurative lymphadenitis, osteomyelitis, disseminated BCG infection and death. Ulceration and lymphadenitis occurs in 1–10 per cent of vaccinations, and disseminated infection occurs in less than one per million vaccinations. The disseminated infection is usually associated with severe abnormalities of cellular immunity. The risk of adverse reactions is related to the BCG strain used by different manufacturers, the dose, the age of the child, the method of immunization and the skill of the vaccinator *(52)*.

If there is a local abscess formation, it should be treated by aspiration, in case it does not clear spontaneously. If this is not successful, it should be incised and treated with local applications daily with PAS or INH powder. There is no need for systemic treatment with INH. The patient should be assured of the harmless nature of the lesion *(53)*. In order to avoid these complications, the vaccination should be strictly intradermal and no other injection should be given for at least 6 months into the arm which received BCG vaccine *(54)*.

(9) PROTECTIVE VALUE : The duration of protection is from 15 to 20 years. The local BCG infection generates an immunity response, which is associated with the development of tuberculin hypersensitivity and with it, possibly, some immunity. The first prospective control trial of BCG showed it to be 80 per cent effective over an observation period of 20 years *(55)*. Since then several well–planned, controlled trials have been conducted in various parts of the world, including the "Tuberculosis Prevention Trial" in South India *(56, 57)*.

Studies have shown that the range of protection offered by BCG varied from 0 to 80 per cent in different parts of the world. The full explanation for the varying degrees of protection has yet to be found *(58, 59)*. One suggestion for which there is an increasing epidemiological support, is that prior exposure to some non-tuberculous environmental mycobacteria (e.g., *M. vaccae, M. non–chromogenicum*) may have conferred partial immunity on the population and thus masked the potential benefit of BCG vaccination *(60)*. There is also evidence that exposure to other species (e.g., *M. kansasii, M. scrofulaceus*) have an antagonistic action against BCG *(55)*. This may be one reason why BCG was not found to be protective in the South Indian trial *(51)*. However, infants and young children, BCG–vaccinated before they had contact with environmental mycobacteria, derived protection.

There is a large body of evidence which supports the conclusion that BCG gives an appreciable degree of protection against childhood tuberculosis *(61)*. The WHO, on the basis of an extended review of BCG including the South Indian trial *(62)* holds that it would seem unreasonable to stop current BCG vaccination programmes *(59)* and recommends that the use of BCG should be continued as an antituberculosis measure *(62)*.

(10) REVACCINATION : The duration of protection conferred by BCG is a matter of dispute. Even 90 years after the development of the vaccine, it is not known whether booster doses are indicated or advisable. In fact, BCG revaccination has not been included in the official immunization schedule in India under the expanded programme on immunization.

(11) CONTRAINDICATIONS : Unless specifically indicated, BCG should not be given to patients suffering from generalized eczema, infective dermatosis, hypogammaglobulinaemia, to those with a history of deficient immunity (symptomatic HIV infection, known or suspected congenital immunodeficiency, leukaemia, lymphoma or generalized malignant diseases), patients under immunosuppressive treatment (corticosteroids, alkylating agents, antimetabolites, radiation), and in pregnancy. The effect of BCG may be exaggerated in these patients.

(12) DIRECT BCG VACCINATION : Direct BCG vaccination, i.e., vaccination without a prior tuberculin test, has been adopted as a national policy in many developing countries, including India. It permits a more rapid and complete coverage of the eligible population, while reducing the cost. No adverse effects have been reported even if BCG is given to tuberculin–positive reactors *(51)*. However, it is sound practice to administer BCG during infancy before the child has had contact with environmental mycobacteria, than to resort to direct BCG at a later date, when the benefits of BCG are doubtful as shown by the South Indian trial *(63)*.

(13) IMPACT : BCG vaccination is less effective in controlling tuberculosis as compared to active case-finding and chemotherapy, as BCG offers only partial protection. In 1982, a WHO Expert Committee *(64)* concluded that although BCG vaccination of uninfected individuals (usually children) can prevent tuberculosis in them, it can have only a relatively small epidemiological effect in that it will not contribute significantly to the reduction in the overall risk of infection in the community as a whole.

(14) BCG VACCINATION AND HIV INFECTION : Following a review of relevant data, the Global Advisory Committee on Vaccine Safety (GACVS) has revised its previous recommendations concerning BCG vaccination of children infected with HIV.

WHO had previously recommended that in countries with a high burden of TB, a single dose of BCG vaccine should be given to all healthy infants as soon as possible after birth unless the child presented with symptomatic HIV infection. However, evidence shows that children who were HIV-infected, when vaccinated with BCG at birth, and who later developed AIDS, were at an increased risk of developing disseminated BCG disease. Among these children, the benefits of potentially preventing severe TB are out weighted by the risks associated with the use of BCG vaccine. GACVS, therefore, advised WHO to change its recommendation such that *children who are known to be HIV-infected, even if asymptomatic, should no longer be immunized with BCG vaccine (65)*. However, population with high prevalence of HIV also have the greatest burden of TB, and in such populations, uninfected children will benefit from the use of BCG vaccine. Furthermore, with the increasing range and coverage of interventions to prevent vertical transmission from mother to child – including early diagnosis of maternal HIV infections; management of sexually transmitted infections; safe delivery practices; maternal and infant preventive antiretroviral medicines or maternal antiretroviral therapy; and safe infant feeding – the majority of infants born to HIV-infected mothers are not infected and would also be expected to benefit from BCG vaccination *(65)*.

Unfortunately, accurate diagnosis of HIV infection in the first year of life relies upon direct demonstration of the HIV virus, as maternal HIV antibody is passively transferred to the infant *in utero*. Currently available assays that can be used to diagnose HIV in the first year of life are expensive and technically demanding in many countries with generalized HIV epidemics. WHO recommends that these tests are first performed at or around 6 weeks age, yet this is often after BCG vaccination has already been given *(66)*.

(15) COMBINED VACCINATION : BCG may be given at the same time as oral polio vaccine. DPT vaccine may also be given at the same time as BCG, but in different arm without reducing the immune responses or increasing the rate of complications *(56)*. Mixed vaccines containing BCG have not yet been introduced.

An increasing number of industrialized countries are likely to reconsider their BCG vaccination policy during the coming years. To change from general to selective BCG vaccination, an efficient notification system must be in place in addition to the following "low endemicity" criteria : (a) an average annual notification rate of smear-positive pulmonary TB cases below 5 per 100,000; or (b) an average annual notification rate of tubercular meningitis in children aged under five years, below 1 per 10 million population during the previous five years; or (c) an average annual risk of tuberculosis infection below 0.1 per cent *(66)*.

To sum up, BCG vaccination is a fundamental component of a national tuberculosis programme. Despite the contradictory evidence of controlled trials, there is evidence that BCG plays a valuable role in preventing severe forms of childhood tuberculosis, viz. meningitis and miliary tuberculosis. Today, BCG vaccination is part of WHO Expanded Programme on Immunization. The greatest need for BCG vaccination today is undoubtedly in the developing countries of the world where tuberculosis is still a major health problem.

LATENT TB INFECTION

Persons with latent tuberculosis infection are infected with *M. tuberculosis*, but do not have TB disease. The only sign of TB infection is a positive reaction to the tuberculin skin test or IGRA TB blood test. They are not infectious and cannot spread TB infection to others. Overall, without treatment, about 5–10 per cent of infected persons will develop TB disease at some time in their lives. About half of those people who develop TB will do so within the first two years of infection. For persons whose immune systems are weak, especially those with HIV infection, the risk of developing TB disease is considerably higher than for persons with normal immune systems. Of special concern are persons infected by someone with extensively drug-resistant TB (XDR TB) who later develop TB disease, these persons will have XDR TB, not regular TB disease.

A person with latent TB infection has a skin test or blood test result indicating TB infection; has a normal chest X-ray and a negative sputum test; has TB bacteria in the body that are alive, but inactive; does not feel sick, cannot spread TB bacteria to others; needs treatment for latent TB infection to prevent TB disease. However, if infected by a person with MDR TB or XDR TB, preventive treatment may not be an option *(67)*.

Health care interventions

Currently, three major categories of health care interventions are available for TB prevention :

1. TB preventive treatment;
2. prevention of transmission of TB infection through infection prevention and control; and
3. vaccination of children with BCG vaccine.

Latent tuberculosis treatment (68)

It is not recommended that everyone with latent TB infection (LTBI) should have TB treatment. Rather it is recommended that certain "target" groups should receive treatment. The main "target" groups considered to be most at risk for progressing from latent to active TB include people in low TB burden countries :

- who have had recent contact with an infectious patient;
- with silicosis;
- infected with both TB and HIV;
- who have been or who are in prison;
- who are immigrants to a low burden country from a high burden country;
- who are homeless;
- who are an illicit drug user;
- who have certain clinical conditions, or conditions which compromise their immune system, such as people with diabetes, and people with chronic renal failure.

In high TB burden countries the populations that are most strongly recommended for the treatment of latent TB infection are people living with HIV, and children under-five, who are household contacts of pulmonary TB cases.

Recommended regimens (68)

Currently the following three regimens are recommended:

- Isoniazid daily or twice weekly for nine months
- Isoniazid plus rifapentine once weekly for 12 weeks
- Rifampicin (or rifabutin) daily for 4 months (with this regimen dots must be used)

The WHO also recommends two other regimens of 3 or 4 months of isoniazid plus rifampicin daily, and six months of isoniazid daily. In 2019 the results were reported of 2 clinical trials looking specifically at side effects. An important problem limiting the treatment of latent TB infection is the occurrence of adverse events with isoniazid. Therefore, it was recommended that in patients without contraindications, rifampicin is likely to be the safest TB infection treatment option.

Rehabilitation

In recent years, there has been a good deal of fresh thinking on the subject of rehabilitation, because of the success achieved in treating patients on domiciliary lines without interfering with their normal work and life. The proportion of patients who need rehabilitation and work under sheltered conditions is becoming less and less. The groups that need rehabilitation are those who are chronically ill and are still excreting tubercle bacilli. Some of those who had lung resection may require rehabilitation to suit their physical and mental abilities.

Surveillance

Surveillance is an integral part of any effective tuberculosis programme. It should be concerned with two distinct aspects : (a) surveillance of the tuberculosis situation, for example, by measuring the "annual infection rates" which will guide the epidemiologist and health administrator by indicating whether the TB problem is static, increasing or decreasing; (b) surveillance of control measures applied such as BCG vaccination and chemotherapy.

Role of hospitals

Inspite of effective domiciliary treatment services, there will always be some patients who will be needing hospitalization. The main indications for hospitalization are : (a) emergencies such as massive haemoptysis and spontaneous pneumothorax (b) surgical treatment (c) management of serious types of tuberculosis such as meningeal tuberculosis, and (d) certain social indications, such as when there is no one to look after the patient at home.

DRUG RESISTANCE

All drugs used in the treatment of tuberculosis tend to produce resistant strains. The resistance may be of two types : (a) *PRIMARY OR PRE–TREATMENT RESISTANCE :* It is the resistance shown by the bacteria in a patient, who has not received the drug in question before. That this is not always due to infection of the individual with drug–resistant bacilli, is well known. It is an accepted fact that when the bacilli are rapidly multiplying, resistant mutants appear irrespective of the administration of any particular drug. According to one hypothesis, drug resistance is induced by transference through what are called "episomes". Episomes are non–chromosomal heritable genes which can pass from one bacterial cell to another. If there is a direct contact between the cell containing episomes, the episomes leave the resistant cell and invade susceptible cells *(69)*. (b) *SECONDARY OR ACQUIRED RESISTANCE :* Here the bacteria were sensitive to the drug at the start of the treatment but became resistant to the particular drug during the course of treatment with it.

Drug resistance means that certain strains of tuberculosis bacilli are not killed by the anti–tuberculosis drugs given during the treatment. Some strains can be resistant to one or more drugs.

Definitions

Please refer to page 210 for classification of cases based on drug resistance.

Causes of drug-resistant tuberculosis *(27)*

Drug-resistant TB has microbial, clinical and programmatic causes. From a microbiological perspective, the resistance is caused by a genetic mutation that makes a drug ineffective against the mutant bacilli. An inadequate or poorly administered treatment regimen allows drug-resistant mutants to become the dominant strain in a patient infected with TB. Table 4 summarizes the common causes of inadequate treatment. However it should be stressed that MDR-TB is man-made phenomenon – poor treatment, poor drugs and poor adherence lead to the development of MDR-TB.

In all countries and especially those where the number of cases of tuberculosis is rising rapidly because of the association with HIV, the development of resistant strains of tuberculosis is a serious concern. In 2016, about 0.60 million people worldwide, are estimated to be infected with strains of drug resistant tuberculosis. An accurate picture of drug resistance is not available because few countries have a reliable drug resistance surveillance system *(5)*.

It is estimated that primary MDR-TB in India is around 2.8 per cent. The drug resistance in re-treatment cases is 12 (10–13) per cent. Although the level of MDR-TB in the country is low in relation to percentage and proportion, it translates into large absolute numbers *(70)*.

XDR-TB has been reported in India by isolated studies with non-representative and highly selected clinical samples. The magnitude of the problem remains to be determined due to the absence of laboratories capable of conducting quality assured second line drug susceptibility test *(12)*.

It has been observed that resistance to isoniazid alone does not affect the results of treatment so much, if proper regimens for treatment or retreatment are prescribed, but simultaneous resistance to isoniazid and rifampicin limits severely the results of the treatment.

The most serious danger of MDR Tuberculosis is that it is much more difficult to treat, even where second line drugs are available. Treatment of MDR tuberculosis can take at least two years and the results are poor. Second line drugs cost 30 times as much as drugs used in SCC treatment of non–resistant tuberculosis patients. Patients with MDR tuberculosis may need to be hospitalised and isolated which adds to the cost of treatment, to prevent transmission of primary resistant strains to others. Careful precautions are necessary to prevent transmission, especially to health workers caring for MDR tuberculosis patients *(71)*.

The emergence of XDR-TB and high case fatality rate in patients with HIV infection was the subject of an emergency consultations held in Johannesburg on 7–8 September, 2006. The issues included strengthening treatment adherence to achieve high levels of completion (≥ 85 per cent) for all TB patients ensuring that second line drugs used to treat MDR-TB and XDR-TB are strictly controlled and properly used according to WHO guidelines. The steps required to limit the impact of MDR-TB and XDR-TB were identified and incorporated into a 7-point plan of action *(72)*.

In the short term, countries should:

1. develop national emergency response plans for MDR-TB and XDR-TB and ensure that basic TB control measures meet international standards for TB care and are fully implemented;
2. conduct rapid surveys of MDR-TB and XDR-TB using a standardized protocol to assess the geographical and temporal distribution of XDR-TB in vulnerable populations;
3. strengthen and expand national TB laboratory capacity by addressing all aspects of laboratory procedures and managment;
4. implement infection control precautions in health-care facilities according to WHO guidelines, with special emphasis on those facilities providing care for people living with HIV/AIDS.

In the long term, countries should:

5. establish capacity for clinical and public health managers to respond effectively to MDR-TB and XDR-TB;
6. promote universal access to antiretroviral therapy for all TB patients through close collaboration with treatment and care programmes for people living with HIV/AIDS;
7. support and increase funding for research into the development of new anti-tuberculosis drugs and rapid diagnostic tests for MDR-TB and XDR-TB.

Prevention of Drug Resistance : Since incomplete, inadequate and irregular treatment is the main cause of drug resistance, this can be prevented by (a) treatment with two or more drugs in combination (b) using drugs to which the bacteria are sensitive, and (c) ensuring that the treatment is complete, adequate and regular.

Please refer to page 222 for details of guidelines about management of MDR and XDR-TB.

Tuberculosis and comorbidities

Several medical conditions are risk factors for TB and poor TB treatment outcomes. Similarly TB can complicate

TABLE 4

Causes of inadequate treatment

Providers/programmes : inadequate regimens	Drugs: inadequate supply/quality	Patients: inadequate drug intake
– Absence of guidelines or inappropriate guidelines – Non-compliance with guidelines – Inadequate training of health staff – No monitoring of treatment – Poorly organized or funded TB control programmes	– Non-availability of certain drugs (stock-outs or delivery disruptions) – Poor quality – Poor storage conditions – Wrong dosages or combination	– Poor adherence (or poor DOT) – Lack of information – Non-availability of free drugs – Social and economic barriers – Malabsorption – Substance abuse disorders

course of some diseases. It is therefore important to identify these comorbidities in people diagnosed with TB in order to ensure early detection and improved outcome.

TUBERCULOSIS AND HIV

Worldwide the number of people infected with both HIV and tuberculosis is rising. The HIV virus damages the body's natural defences – the immune system – and accelerates the speed at which tuberculosis progresses from a harmless infection to life–threatening condition. The estimated 10 per cent activation of dormant tuberculosis infection over the life span of an infected person, is increased to 10 per cent activation in one year, if HIV infection is superimposed. Tuberculosis is already the opportunistic infection that most frequently kills HIV–positive people.

Even in HIV positive cases, tuberculosis can be cured if diagnosed in time and treated properly. Good TB control programme is the best thing that can be done to cure and extend the lives of HIV positive individuals. With correct TB treatment, the HIV positive person having tuberculosis can gain, on an average two additional years of life *(73)*.

Epidemiological impact

HIV and tuberculosis interact in several ways *(71)* :

1. *Reactivation of latent infection :* People who are infected with both tuberculosis and HIV, are 25–30 times more likely to develop tuberculosis disease, than people infected only with tuberculosis. This is because HIV stops the immune system working effectively and tuberculosis bacilli are able to multiply rapidly. In developing countries HIV associated tubercular disease is very common.

2. *Primary infection :* People with HIV are at risk of being newly infected, if they are exposed to tuberculosis because their weakened immune system makes them more vulnerable. New tubercular infection in people with HIV can progress to active disease very quickly.

3. *Recurring infection :* People with HIV who have been cured of tuberculosis infection may be more at risk of developing tuberculosis again. However, it is not clear whether this is because of reinfection or relapse.

4. *In the community :* There are more new cases of active tuberculosis because more people infected with tuberculosis develop active disease, and those newly infected become ill faster. This means that there are more people in the community who are infectious to others. Larger number of people with active disease mean more people will die from tuberculosis unless they are treated. The association of tuberculosis with HIV means that people suffer additional discrimination. Community education is needed to increase awareness that tuberculosis is curable and, most important, that people are no longer infectious after the first few weeks of treatment.

Diagnosis of tuberculosis in people with HIV

The salient features are as follows *(36)* :

1. Emphasis on integrated TB and HIV services, eg., HIV screening at RNTCP designated microscopy centre.
2. Focus on early detection and early care.
   a. Early detection of TB in PLHIV (persons living with HIV/AIDS) : Early suspicion of TB-symptoms of any duration among PLHIV; use of an expanded clinical algorithm for TB screening that relies on presence of four clinical symptoms (current cough, weight loss, fever or night sweats) instead of only cough, to identify patients with presumptive TB; strengthen intensified case finding at ART, Link ART centre and targeted intervention projects for high risk group specially injection drug users; female sex workers and men having sex with men etc. and offering upfront CBNAAT among presumptive TB cases among PLHIV.
   b. Early detection and care of HIV infected drug-resistant TB patients by strengthening HIV testing in presumptive DR-TB cases; ensure access to culture and drug susceptibility test for HIV infected TB patients, prompt linkage of HIV infected DR-TB cases to ART centres, and prompt initiation of ART in HIV infected DR-TB cases.
   c. Strengthen HIV/TB activities among children and pregnant women.

In most people in the early stages of HIV infection, symptoms of tuberculosis are similar as in people without HIV infection. In areas where many people have HIV infection, tuberculosis programmes should continue to focus on identifying infectious sputum–smear–positive cases through microscopy. However, diagnosis of tuberculosis in individual patients using the standard diagnostic tools can be more difficult if they have advanced HIV infection because :

(a) HIV positive people with pulmonary tuberculosis may have a higher frequency of negative sputum smears. Confirming the diagnosis may require sputum culture.

(b) The tuberculin skin test often fails to work in people who are HIV positive because it relies on measuring the response of a person's immune system. If the immune system has been damaged by HIV, it may not respond even though the person is infected with tuberculosis. HIV positive people with tuberculosis, therefore, have a higher frequency of false negative tuberculin skin test results.

(c) Chest radiography may be less useful in people with HIV because they have less cavitation. Cavities usually develop because the immune response to the tubercular bacilli leads to some destruction of lung tissue. In people with HIV, who do not have a fully functioning immune system, there is less tissue destruction and hence less lung cavitation.

(d) Cases of extra-pulmonary tuberculosis seem to be more common in people who are co–infected.

In short-screen for tuberculosis using sputum smear microscopy, if the result is positive, start treatment; if the result is negative, but it is suspected that the patient has tuberculosis, sputum culture should be carried out where feasible to confirm the diagnosis and give treatment to those with positive culture results.

Treatment for HIV infected TB patients

Based on the clinical history and investigation reports ART medical officer will categorize patients as rifampicin sensitive/ rifampicin sensitivity status not known/clinically diagnosed TB case, prior history of taking anti-TB drugs (Cat I/Cat II), and initiate daily anti TB treatment in Fixed Dosage Combination as per RNTCP guidelines at ART centre itself. The treatment of HIV positive individual with MDR-TB is same as for HIV negative patients. However, treament is more difficult and adverse events more common, hence rigorous monitoring in this particular group of patients is required in order to ensure adherence to treatment, early detection and treatment of adverse events reduce "lost to follow-up" *(36)*.

ART must be offered to all patients with HIV and TB and HIV and MDR-TB, irrespective of CD_4 cell count. Start anti-tuberculosis treatment first and then start ART as soon as TB treatment is tolerated (between 2 weeks and 2 months). In the absence of ART, TB treatment alone does not significantly increase the CD_4 cell count, nor does it significantly decrease the HIV viral load. The use of Highly Active Anti-Retroviral Therapy (HAART) in patients with TB can lead to a sustained reduction in the HIV viral load. It can also facilitate immunological reconstitution, and decrease AIDS – defining illness and mortality. This benefit is seen across different range of CD_4 counts.

In addition to TB treatment, all HIV-infected TB patients must be provided access to care and support for HIV disease, including co-trimoxazole preventive therapy to reduce mortality among PLHIV by preventing opportunistic infections.

Immune reconstitution inflammatory syndrome (IRIS) :

Occasionally, patients with HIV-related TB may experience a temporary exacerbation of symptoms, signs of radiographic manifestations of TB after beginning TB treatment. This paradoxical reaction occurs in HIV-infected patients with active TB and is thought to be a result of immune restitution due to the simultaneous administration of antiretroviral and tuberculosis medication. Symptoms and signs may include high fever, lymphadenopathy, expanding intra-thoracic lesions and worsening of chest radiographic findings. The diagnosis of paradoxical reaction should be made only after a thorough evaluation has excluded other aetiologies, particularly TB treatment failure. For severe paradoxical reactions prednisone (1–2 mg/kg for 1–2 weeks, then gradually decreasing doses) may be used *(36)*.

Isoniazid preventive therapy for PLHIVs

Isoniazid preventive therapy (IPT) is one of the 3–I's globally recommended for prevention of incident TB among HIV infected individuals. It is the most effective bactericidal, anti TB drug available currently. While it protects against progression of latent TB infection to active disease i.e reactivation, it also prevents TB reinfection in persons who are exposed to open TB cases.

All children living with HIV who have completed treatment for TB successfully should receive INH for an additional six months. These children who do not have poor weight gain, fever or cough currently, are unlikely to have active TB. Those who have above symptoms may have TB and should be evaluated for TB and other conditions. If evaluation shows no TB, such children should be offered IPT regardless of their age. Children living with HIV who are more than 12 months of age and who are unlikely to have active TB on symptom-based screening, and have no contact with a TB case should receive six months of IPT (10 mg/kg/day) as part of a comprehensive package of HIV prevention and care services.

Providing IPT to people living with HIV does not increase risk of developing INH resistant TB later. Therefore, concern regarding development on INH resistance should not be a barrier to providing IPT *(36)*.

For details regarding HIV and TB co-activities please refer to chapter 7 also.

TUBERCULOSIS AND DIABETES

Diabetes has been shown to be an independent risk factor for tuberculosis in community based study from south India and multiple studies globally. It is suggested that diabetes accounts for 20 per cent of all tuberculosis and 10 per cent of smear positive TB *(36)*. People with weak immune system as in diabetes are at higher risk of progressing from latent to active tuberculosis. The risk is 2–3 times higher than people without diabetes. A large proportion of people with diabetes and TB are diagnosed very late.

It is suggested that all people with TB should be screened for diabetes and screening for TB in diabetes should be considered, particularly in setting with high TB prevalence. People with diabetes and TB have a high risk of death during TB treatment and of TB relapse after treatment. As diabetes is complicated by presence of other infectious diseases also, it is important to take proper care of diabetes in patients suffering from diabetes/TB *(74)*.

National framework for joint TB-diabetes collaborative activities are as follows *(36)* :

a. Activities to improve diagnosis and management of diabetes among TB patients :
   - screening of all registered TB patients for diabetes mellitus.
   - ensuring diabetes mellitus management among TB patients.
b. Activities to improve diagnosis and management of TB among diabetic patients :
   - Intensified detection of active TB disease among diabetic patients.
   - Ensuring TB infection control measures in health care settings where diabetes mellitus is managed.
   - Ensuring TB treatment and management in comorbid patients.
c. Joint monitoring and evaluation.
d. TB patients diagnosed with diabetes should receive the same duration of TB treatment with daily regimen as non-diabetic patients.

TB AND TOBACCO *(36)*

Tobacco smoke contains toxic chemicals which cause disturbances in the bronchial surface of the lung. It also weakens the immunity of the patient to fight with TB bacteria. The following evidence emerges from several studies conducted to look at the association of TB and tobacco in India :

- Almost 38% of TB deaths are associated with the use of tobacco.
- Prevalence of TB is 3 times as high among ever-smokers as compared to that of among never-smokers.
- Mortality from TB is 3 to 4 times as high among ever-smokers as compared to that among never-smokers.
- Smoking contributes to half the male deaths in 25–69 age groups from TB in India.

Exposure to tobacco smoke has also been found to affect TB in the following ways :

- Increase the risk of tuberculous infection and the risk of developing TB.
- Affect clinical manifestations and increase risk of relapse among TB patients.
- Affect microbiological conversion (sputum smear or culture) and outcome of treatment in TB patients.
- Increase tuberculosis mortality and drug resistance to anti-tubercular drugs.

When a patient gets registered as a TB case, the status of tobacco use is recorded in the TB treatment card. He/she is advised to quit tobacco use with 5 R's : Relevance of quitting; Risk of continuing; Reward of quitting; Roadblock to quitting; and Repeat at each visit.

TUBERCULOSIS AND COVID-19 *(1)*

Since the beginning of 2020, the COVID-19 pandemic has caused enormous health, social and economic impacts, which are likely to continue. Even after some of these impacts have been mitigated or contained, there will be medium- and longer-term consequences, including for the tuberculosis (TB) epidemic and response. The pandemic threatens to reverse the progress made towards global TB targets. Although physical distancing policies may help to reduce TB transmission, this effect could be offset by longer durations of infectiousness, increased household exposure to TB infection, worsening treatment outcomes and higher levels of poverty. In the absence of effective mitigation strategies, such as social protection and health insurance, severe economic contractions and loss of income (particularly among the most vulnerable populations) are likely to worsen some of the factors that determine TB epidemics, especially the prevalence of undernutrition.

The newer scientific evidence available on TB and COVID-19 suggests that TB is a comorbidity for COVID-19 and impacts its progression and severity and vice versa. Hence as an effort to ensure early detection and timely and effective management of TB and COVID-19, the following recommendations have been approved and are under process of being shared with the states in the form of a guidance document on "TB & COVID-19 screening and follow up."

- Screening patients with a history of TB in the past two years for COVID-19 at a six-monthly interval as post-treatment follow-up for two years. For COVID testing, modalities like home-based kits/ Rapid Antigen test/ RT-PCR may be utilized.
- Screening for TB among post COVID-19 patients at six-monthly intervals for two years.
  - COVID-19 patients with active TB to be managed as per protocols
  - If cough persists after 2–3 weeks, to be tested for TB
  - Follow up COVID-19 patients post-treatment and periodically screen for TB

While the COVID-19 pandemic has had an adverse impact on the overall case finding of TB, it also presented us with many opportunities. Utilizing this opportunity in areas like lab strengthening - platform technology, surveillance, strengthening of currently existing treatment centres, further expansion of the network, and airborne infection control measures will play an important role in ending TB by 2025 *(43)*.

THE END TB STRATEGY

Measured by the number of people who die each year due to tuberculosis, it is the deadliest infectious disease. It claims 3 lives every minute. Of the 9 million people who become ill with TB each year, more than 3 million are not diagnosed, treated or officially registered by national TB programmes. Collectively, these "missed" millions are a global public health failure. This is especially the case considering that TB is airborne and that each undiagnosed and untreated person can infect as many as 15 individuals per year. Moreover, TB continues to be leading cause of death among people living with HIV. Likewise drug resistant TB poses a grave challenge.

Many of history's greatest successes in the fight against preventable diseases have been characterized by momentous shift in peoples belief of what is possible. A paradigm shift is needed now – a change in the way we fight TB at every level, in every community, in every health facility, in every country *(75)*. The global resolve for intensifying the fight against TB and achieving an end to the global epidemic is illustrated by adoption of WHO's End TB Strategy by World Health Assembly and the inclusion of "ending the TB epidemic" as a target within the health related Sustainable Development Goal 3 by the United Nations General Assembly in September 2015.

Evolution of End TB Strategy *(76)*

The End TB Strategy, developed in the context of the UN Sustainable Development Goals, is a logical evolution and a paradigm shift from past global TB strategies. The DOTS strategy of 1994 helped revitalize national tuberculosis programmes and equivalent entities by putting in place the essential basics to address the TB epidemic. The stop TB strategy of 2006 broadened the response by addressing the emerging challenges of HIV associated TB and MDR-TB. It aimed to improve access to quality TB care by engaging all public and private care providers, civil society organizations and communities. The stop TB strategy also encouraged investment in research for better tools and approaches. The End TB Strategy encompasses a package of interventions that can be fully adopted at country level. It has ten components organized under 3 pillars and four underlying principles. Fig. 6 summarizes the evolution of WHO global TB strategies.

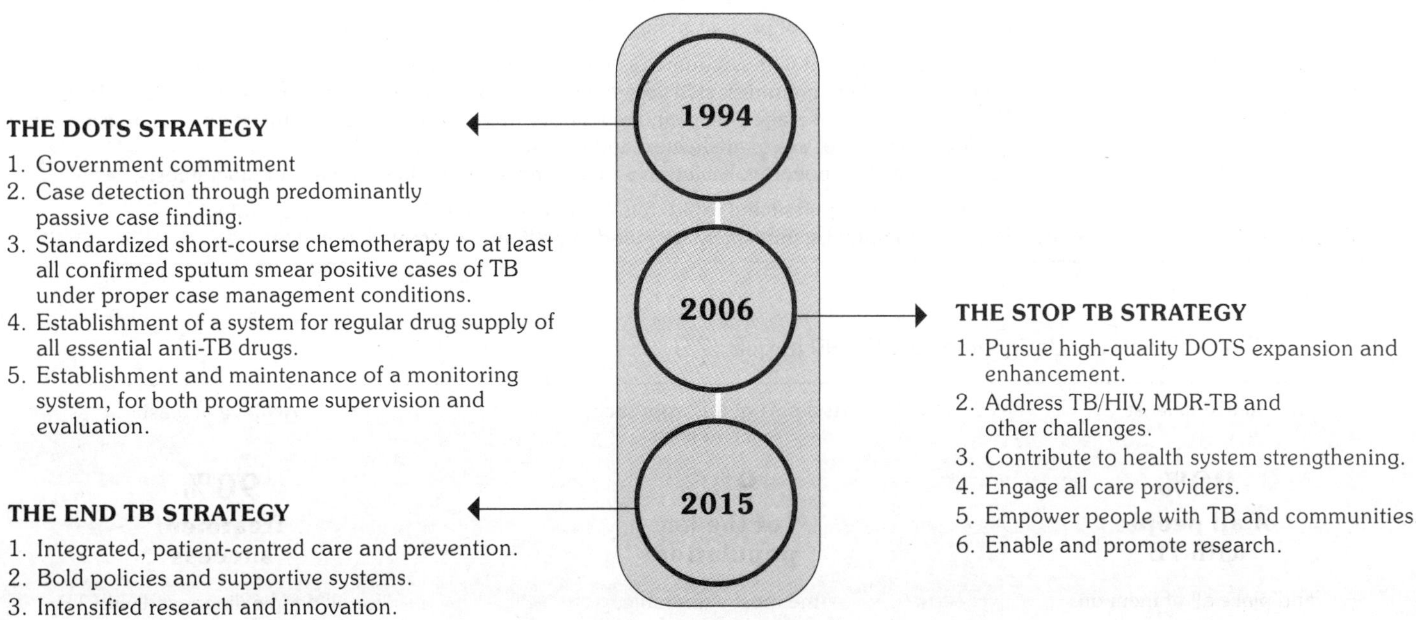

FIG. 6
Evolution of WHO Global TB Strategies.

Source : *(76)*

Through the implementation of the DOTS strategy (1994–2005) and the Stop TB Strategy (2006–2015), countries – especially those with a high burden of TB – established the basics required for providing high-quality TB diagnosis and treatment. These efforts contributed greatly to meeting the TB-related target of the Millennium Development Goals (MDGs) of halting and beginning to reverse the TB epidemic. Between year 2000 and 2014, improvements in quality-assured diagnosis and treatment of TB contributed to saving 43 million lives worldwide. It was apparent, however, that while enhancing access to diagnosis and treatment remarkably improved outcomes in terms of reducing suffering and death, it had very little effect on achieving the desired impact in terms of declining the incidence rates and driving down the TB epidemic. This is not entirely surprising: TB is not only a biomedical and a public health problem but also a disease associated with poverty; TB will continue thriving as long as poverty persists. The End TB strategy, whose aim is to end the TB epidemic, therefore combines a holistic mix of health and social interventions.

The strategy envisions universal access to high-quality TB care and goes beyond it to promote TB prevention. Ending the TB epidemic will also require new tools – a point-of-care test for diagnosing infection and disease; shorter and better regimens to treat disease and infection; and ideally, a pre and post-exposure vaccine.

The End TB Strategy identifies four barriers to achieving progress in the fight against TB. They are : (1) weak health system; (2) underlying determinants of TB such as poverty, undernutrition, migration and ageing population and risk factors such as diabetes, silicosis and smoking; (3) lack of effective tools; and (4) continuous unmet-funding needs.

The strategy is summarized as below :

END TB STRATEGY

VISION A world free of tuberculosis–zero deaths; disease and suffering due to tuberculosis.

GOAL End the global tuberculosis epidemic.

INDICATORS	**MILESTONES** 2020	2025	**TARGETS** SDG 2030	End TB 2035
Reduction in number of TB deaths compared with 2015 (%)	35%	75%	90%	95%
Reduction in TB incidence rate compared with 2015 (%)	20% (<85/100 000)	50% (<55/100 000)	80% (<20/100 000)	90% (<10/100 000)
TB-affected families facing catastrophic costs due to TB (%)	zero	zero	zero	zero

PRINCIPLES

1. Government stewardship and accountability, with monitoring and evaluation.
2. Strong coalition with civil society organizations and communities.
3. Protection and promotion of human rights, ethics and equity.
4. Adaptation of the strategy and targets at country level, with global collaboration.

PILLARS AND COMPONENTS

1. Integrated, patient-centred care and prevention
   - A. Early diagnosis of tuberculosis including universal drug-susceptibility testing, and systematic screening of contacts and high-risk groups.
   - B. Treatment of all people with tuberculosis including drug-resistant tuberculosis, and patient support.
   - C. Collaborative tuberculosis/HIV activities, and management of co-morbidities.
   - D. Preventive treatment of persons at high risk and vaccination against tuberculosis.
2. Bold policies and supportive systems
   - A. Political commitment with adequate resources for tuberculosis care and prevention.
   - B. Engagement of communities, civil society organizations, and public and private care providers.
   - C. Universal health coverage policy, and regulatory frameworks for case notification, vital registration, quality and rational use of medicines, and infection control.
   - D. Social protection, poverty alleviation and actions on other determinants of tuberculosis.
3. Intensified research and innovation
   - A. Discovery, development and rapid uptake of new tools, interventions and strategies.
   - B. Research to optimize implementation and impact, and promote innovations.

Source : *(75)*

The Global Plan's targets are designed as 90–90–90 targets *(75)*.

Reach at least	As a part of this approach, reach at least	Achieve at least
90%	**90%**	**90%**
of all people with TB	**of the key populations**	**Treatment success**
and place all of them on appropriate therapy– first-line, second-line and preventive therapy as required	the most vulnerable, underserved, at-risk populations	for all people diagnosed with TB through affordable treatment services, adherence to complete and correct treatment, and social support.

Key Population Groups *(75)*

The Global Plan defines "Key populations" as people who are vulnerable, underserved or at-risk of TB infection and illness. For purpose of the global plan, three key population groups are further expanded as shown below, along with examples of population within these groups. It is important to note that people who are likely to fall into one of these categories are also likely to be part of one or both of the other groups.

Key Populations for TB *(75)*

People who have **Increased exposure** to TB due to where they live or work	Prisoners, sex workers, miners, hospital visitors, health care workers and community health workers. PEOPLE WHO : • live in urban slums • live in poorly ventilated or dusty conditions • are contacts of TB patients, including children • work in environments that are overcrowded • work in hospitals or are health care professionals.
People who have **limited access to quality TB Services**	Migrant workers, women in settings with gender disparity, children, refugees or internally displaced people, illegal miners, and undocumented migrants PEOPLE WHO : • are from tribal populations or indigenous groups • are homeless • live in hard-to-reach areas • live in homes for the elderly • have mental or physical disabilities • face legal barriers to access care • are lesbian, gay, bisxeual or transgender.
People at **increased risk** of TB because of biological or behavioural factors that compromise immune function	PEOPLE WHO : • live with HIV • have diabetes or silicosis • undergo immunosuppressive therapy • are undernourished • use tobacco • suffer from alcohol-use disorders • inject drugs.

UN General Assembly Political Declaration

Please refer to page 208 for details.

Despite effective case-finding and therapeutic tools and declines in mortality and morbidity rates in some countries, tuberculosis appears to continue as an important communicable disease problem, worldwide, for several decades to come. The chronic nature of the disease, the ability of the tubercle bacilli to remain alive in the human body for years, the concentration of the disease in the older age-groups, the increased expectation of life, the high prevalence of infection rates in some countries, the relatively high reactivation rate, the emergence of drug-resistant strains, association of tuberculosis and HIV infection, and above all, the perpetuation of the "non-specific determinants" of the disease in the third world countries impede a rapid conquest of the disease.

References

1. WHO (2020), *Global Tuberculosis Report 2020.*
2. WHO (2004), *Weekly Epidemiological Record,* 23rd Jan 2004, No. 4.
3. WHO (2021), *Global Tuberculosis Report, 2021.*
4. WHO (2022), *Weekly Epidemiological Record,* No. 28, 15th July 2022.
5. WHO (2018), *Global Tuberculosis Report 2018.*
6. Govt. of India (2014), *TB India 2014,* RNTCP Annual Status Report, DGHS, Ministry of Health and Family Welfare, New Delhi.
7. WHO (2015), *Health in 2015, From MDGs (Millennium Development Goals) to SDGs* (Sustainable Development Goals).
8. WHO (2016), *Fact Sheet No. 104,* March 2016.
9. WHO (2022), *Teams/Global-Tuberculosis Programme/data,* 28.9.2022.
10. Govt. of India (2020), *India TB Report 2020, National Tuberculosis Elimination Programme Annual Report,* 2020.
11. Govt. of India (2010), *TB India 2010,* RNTCP Status Report, Central TB Division, Ministry of Health and Family Welfare, New Delhi.
12. Govt. of India (2008), *TB India 2008,* RNTCP Status Report, I am stopping TB, Ministry of Health and Family Welfare, New Delhi.
13. WHO (2014), *Standards for TB care in India.*
14. WHO (2016), *Global Tuberculosis Report 2016.*
15. WHO (1974). *Techn. Rep. Ser.,* No.552.
16. Styblo K. (1976). *Int. J. Epi.* 5 : 63.
17. WHO (1981). *Wkly Epi Rec.,* 56 (50) 393–400.
18. WHO (1967). *WHO Chronicle,* 21 : 156.
19. WHO (2013), *Definitions and Reporting Framework for Tuberculosis-* 2013 revision.
20. Youmans, G.P. et al (1980). *The Biological and Clinical Basis of Infectious Diseases,* 2nd ed, Saunders.
21. Gangadharan, P.R.J. (1980). *Ind. J. Tuberculosis,* 27 (3) 108.
22. Pamra, S.P. (1976), *Ind. J. Tuberculosis,* 23, No.2 Supplement.
23. American Thoracic Society (1976) *Ann Rev, of Resp. Disease* 114 : 459.
24. Comstock, G.W. (1978). *Am. Rev, Res. Dis.,* 117 : 621.
25. Govt. of India (2021), *India TB Report, 2021,* National Tuberculosis Elimination Programme Annual Report, Central TB Division.
26. Govt. of India (2020), *Training Modules for Programme Managers and Medical Officers,* National TB Elimination Programme, Central TB Division, New Delhi.
27. Govt. of India (2012), *Guidelines on Programmatic Management of Drug Resistant TB in India,* Ministry of Health and Family Welfare, New Delhi.
28. WHO (2004), *TB / HIV, A Clinical Manual,* 2nd Ed.
29. WHO (2010), *Policy Framework for Implementing New Tuberculosis Diagnostics,* March 2010.
30. Reichman, L.B. and Mc Donald R.J. (1977). *Med. Clin. N.A.* Nov. 1977, p.1185.
31. Maxine, A, Papadakis, Stephen J., Mcphee (2014), *Current Medical Diagnosis and Treatment,* 2014 Ed., Lange Publication.
32. CDC *Fact Sheet* for Parents.
33. TB Facts.ORG (2020), *Information about tuberculosis tests for TB-Sputum microscopy,* skin test, IGRAs.
34. WHO (1980). *WHO Chronicle,* 34 : 101.
35. Toman, K. (1979). *Tuberculosis : Case finding and Chemotherapy,* Questions and Answers, WHO, Geneva.
36. Govt. of India (2016), *Revised National TB Control Programme Technical and Operational Guidelines for Tuberculosis Control in India,* 2016, Ministry of Health and Family Welfare, New Delhi.
37. RNTCP (2018), *India TB Report 2018,* Annual Status Report, DGHS, Ministry of Health and Family Welfare, New Delhi.
38. Govt. of India (2010), *DOTS - Plus Guidelines,* Jan 2010, Ministry of Health and Family Welfare, New Delhi.
39. Govt. of India (2020), *Training modules (1–4) for Programme Managers and Medical Officers,* NTEP, Central TB Division, Ministry of Health and Family Welfare, New Delhi.
40. WHO (2019). *Consolidated guidelines on drug resistant TB treatment,* 2019.
41. Govt. of India (2021), *Guidelines for Programmatic Management of Drug Resistant Tuberculosis in India,* March 2021, NTEP, Ministry of Health and Family Welfare, New Delhi.
42. WHO (2020). *Operational handbook on tuberculosis, Module 4, Treatment, Drug resistant tuberculosis treatment.*
43. Govt. of India (2022), *India TB Report 2022, Coming together to End TB altogether,* Ministry of Health and Family Welfare, New Delhi.
44. RNTCP (2017), *Guidelines on Programmatic Management of drug-resistant tuberculosis in India, 2017.*
45. Suri, J.C. et al (1971). *Ind.J. Tuberculosis,* 18 : 48.
46. Snell, N.J.C. (1985). *P.G. Doctor* Middle East April 1985, 1232.
47. WHO (1980). *Tech.Rep Ser.,* No. 651.
48. WHO (1976). *The Work of WHO* Annual Rep. of the Director General for 1975, p. 73.
49. Humphrey, J.H. et al (1970). *Immunology for Students of Medicine,* Blackwell.

50. WHO (1982). *Tech. Rep. Ser.* No. 652.
51. Dam, H.G.T. et al (1976) *Bull WHO,* 54 (3) 255.
52. Galazka, A.M. et al (1984). *W.H. Forum* 5 (3) 269.
53. Any Questions (1981). *Brit. Med.J.* 282 : 1305, 18 April 1981.
54. Banker, D.D. (1969). *Modern Practice in Immunization.* Indian Journal of Medical Sciences, Mumbai.
55. Aronson, J.D. et al (1958) *Archieves of Int. Med.* 101 : 881.
56. WHO (1979). *Bull WHO,* 57 (5) 819–827.
57. Tuberculosis Prevention Trial, Madras (1979). *Ind. J. Med. Res.,* 70 : 349–363.
58. Baily, G.V.J. (1981). *Ind. J. Tuberculosis,* 28 (3) 117.
59. WHO (1980). *WHO Chronicle,* 34 : 119.
60. Gangadharan, P.R. (1981) *Tubercle* 62 : 223.
61. Wijsmuller, G. (1971). *Bull WHO* 45 : 633.
62. Dam, H.G.T. and Hitze, K.L. (1980). *Bull WHO,* 58 : 37.
63. WHO (1980). *Techn Rep Ser.,* No.652.
64. WHO (1982), *Tech. Rep. Ser.* No. 671.
65. WHO (2007), *Weekly Epidemiological Record* No. 21, May 25, 2007.
66. WHO (2004), Weekly Epidemiological Record, No. 4, 23rd Jan. 2004.
67. CDC (2014), *Centre for Disease Control and Prevention – Tuberculosis : Fact Sheet,* Oct. 2014.
68. TB Facts.ORG (2020), *Information about tuberculosis,* Jan. 2020.
69. Pamra, S.P. (1976). *Ind.J. Chest Dis and allied Sciences,* 23 : 152.
70. WHO, *Tuberculosis Control in South-East Asia Region,* Regional Report, 2017.
71. *AIDS Action,* Asia – Pacific edition, The international newsletter on HIV/AIDS prevention and cure, AHRTAG Issue 30, January – March 1996.
72. WHO (2006), Weekly Epidemiological Record, No. 41, 13th Oct. 2006
73. WHO (1996) TB *Groups At Risk,* WHO Report on the Tuberculosis Epidemic, Geneva.
74. WHO (2011), *Tuberculosis and diabetes,* The stop TB Department, Sept 2011.
75. Stop TB Partnership, UNOPS (2015), *The Paradigm shift 2016–2020, Global Plan to End TB.*
76. WHO (2015), Implementing the End TB Strategy: the Essentials.

II. INTESTINAL INFECTIONS

POLIOMYELITIS

Poliomyelitis is an acute viral infection caused by an RNA virus. It is primarily an infection of the human alimentary tract but the virus may infect the central nervous system in a very small percentage (about 1 per cent) of cases resulting in varying degrees of paralysis, and possibly death.

Problem statement

In the pre-vaccination era, poliomyelitis was found in all countries of the world. The extensive use of polio vaccines since 1954 eliminated the disease in developed countries. In 1988, the World Health Assembly resolved to eradicate poliomyelitis globally. Since then, implementation of the eradication strategies has reduced the number of polio endemic countries from more than 125 in 1988 to 2 in 2021. A total of 5 cases of wild poliovirus were reported globally in 2021. Afghanistan reported 4 cases and Pakistan reported 1 case. All the reported cases are of type1 wild poliovirus *(1, 2)*. India was certified as polio free since 27th March 2014.

Since the 1988 World Health Assembly resolution to eradicate poliomyelitis, transmission of all the 3 types of wild poliovirus (WPV) has been greately reduced. WPV type 2 has not been detected since 1999 and was declared eradicated in September 2015. Given that WPV type3 has not been detected since November 2012, WPV type 1 is likely to be the sole WPV remaining in circulation. This marked progress has been achieved through widespread use of trivalent oral polio vaccine (tOPV). The attenuated polioviruses in OPV can undergo genetic changes during replication, and in communities with low vaccination coverage, rarely, results in vaccine derived polioviruses (VDPV) that can cause paralytic polio indistinguishable from the disease caused by WPV (3). Eliminating the risk of polio caused by VDPVs requires stopping of all OPV use. Recognizing the epidemiological opportunity, a new Polio Eradication and Endgame Strategic Plan 2013–2018 was developed. The plan was to eradicate all types of polio disease simultaneously – both due to WPV and VDPV.

Polio Eradication and Endgame Strategic Plan

The Polio Eradication and Endgame Strategic Plan 2013–2018 represents a major milestone in polio eradication and describes specific steps to take to successfully achieve eradication. The plan has four objectives as summarized in Fig. 1.

Under this endgame plan to achieve and sustain a polio-free world, the use of oral polio vaccine (OPV) must eventually be stopped worldwide, starting with OPV that contains type 2 poliovirus (OPV type 2). At least one dose of inactivated polio vaccine (IPV) must be introduced as a risk mitigation measure. The steps involved are *(5)* :

1. By end 2015, introduce at least 1 dose of IPV into all routine immunization systems, at least 6 months before the switch from trivalent oral polio vaccine (tOPV) to bivalent oral polio vaccine (bOPV, containing types 1 and 3 poliovirus).
2. During 2016, switch from tOPV to bOPV, which does not contain type 2 virus, in routine immunization and polio campaigns, as before that bOPV was only licensed for use in SIAs.
3. Plan for the eventual withdrawal of all OPV.

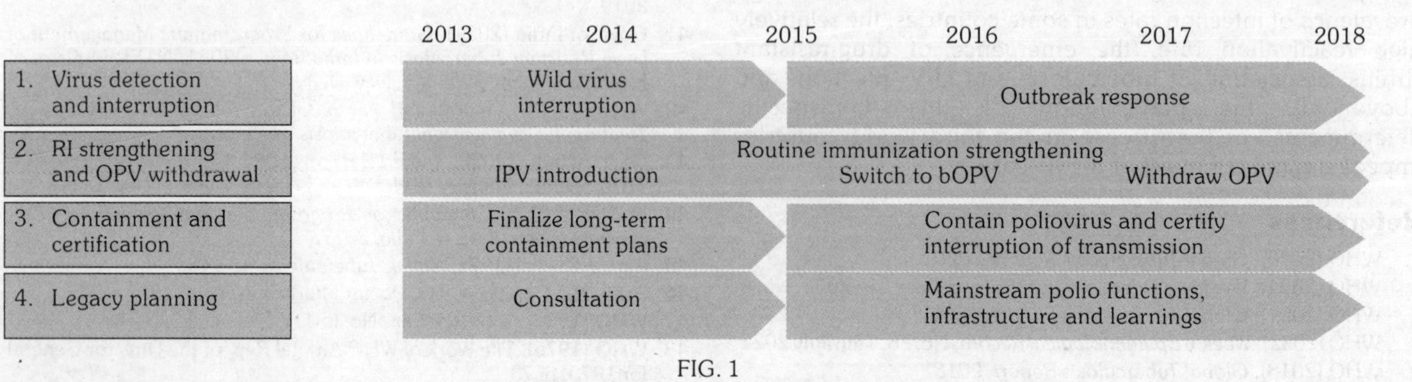

FIG. 1
The time–bound endgame objectives

Source : *(4)*

The first stage of OPV withdrawal involved a global synchronized cessation of tOPV use between 18th April and 1st May 2016, replacing tOPV with bOPV containing only type 1 and 3 poliovirus and withdrawing OPV type 2 from all immunization activities called **"the Switch"**. Once switch is made, tOPV will no longer be used anywhere in the world and manufacturers will no longer supply tOPV *(3, 6)*.

The tOPV to bOPV switch is necessary because no WPV type 2 has been recorded since 1999. The risk of vaccine associated paralytic poliomyelitis and cVDPV to type 2 component of OPV now out weighs its benefits. Replacing the tOPV with bOPV is key to ensuring the eradication of type 2 poliovirus. The switch will serve as a dry run for withdrawal of other type of OPV. It needed IPV to be introduced on an accelerated timeline i.e. by end of 2015, so that OPV2 can be withdrawn. Introducing atleast one dose of IPV will ensure that a substantial proportion of the population is protected against type 2 serotype. It will also boost immunity to the remaining type 1 and 3 serotypes. It will mitigate paralysis risks in case of outbreak by priming the population against type 2 poliovirus and ensure better immune response to OPV if needed. IPV introduction sets the stage for ending OPV use entirely in 2019–2020 *(5)*.

In the endgame, polio eradication activities and strengthening routine immunization can be mutually beneficial as : (1) IPV will be introduced through routine immunization delivery systems; (2) Strengthening routine immunization is necessary to achieve and maintain high population immunity against polioviruses, especially type 2, after OPV type 2 is withdrawn. The magnitude, number and length of both wild poliovirus (WPV) and cVDPV outbreaks are closely correlated with weaknesses in routine immunization systems; (3) This is an opportunity for the global polio eradication initiative to use its infrastructure to contribute more systematically to strengthening routine immunization systems; and (4) One of the goals is to improve infant routine immunization coverage in a group of focus countries which have some of the lowest routine immunization coverage levels in the world and the greatest proportion of the world's unvaccinated children. The third dose of DPT-containing vaccine will be used to measure routine immunization coverage improvements.

It is recommended that the dose of IPV be added at 14 weeks when the 3rd dose of DPT or pentavalent vaccine is given or at the contact soon thereafter *(5)*.

Containment : The eradication of WPV2 means it does not circulate in human population any longer and it is not detectable in environment sample either. However, the virus is still present in a number of facilities including research laboratories and vaccine producing sites. The identification and destruction of any unneeded type 2 poliovirus or appropriate containment of needed type 2 poliovirus is now critical to sustain polio eradication efforts and to prevent accidental or malicious release of these viruses from facility and their subsequent transmission to people. Within two weeks of national switch date, the Ministry of Health of all countries were to submit a report confirming the withdrawal of tOPV *(7)*.

The Polio Eradication Strategy 2022–2026

Over the last decade, the Global Polio Eradication Initiative made steady progress for the eradication of polio, to achieve a polio-free world. The Polio Eradication Strategy 2022–2026 offers a comprehensive set of actions to permanently interrupt all poliovirus transmission in the final wild polio virus endemic countries of Afghanistan and Pakistan, and to stop circulating vaccine-derived poliovirus transmission and prevent outbreaks in non-endemic countries *(2)*.

Fractional dose IPV

As an alternative to the full dose intramuscular injection of IPV, countries may consider using fractional dose of IPV (FIPV) via intradermal route. Studies have demonstrated that 2 FIPV doses intradermally at 6th and 14th weeks provide higher seroconversion rates than a single full dose of IPV given intramuscularly at 14 weeks. Table 1 shows comparison between IPV full dose and FIPV.

TABLE 1
Comparing IPV and FIPV

	IPV	Fractional IPV (fIPV)
Volume per dose	0.5 mL	0.1 mL
Schedule	1 dose : 14 weeks	2 doses : 6 and 14 weeks
Administration	Intramuscular (IM) injection	Intradermal (ID) injection
Site of administration	Thigh	Upper arm
Syringe	0.5 mL AD syringe	0.1 mL AD syringe
Are two fractional doses as effective as a single standard dose ?	Two fractional doses of IPV (ID) given at 6 and 14 weeks produces better immunogenicity than a single standard dose (IM) given at 14 weeks	

Source : *(8)*

In response to an isolation of VDPV2 from a sewage sample taken in Telangana state, India conducted a massive compaign in June 2016, using an intradermal fractional dose (0.1 ml) of IPV over a period of 6 days. The campaign vaccinated 311,064 children aged from 6 weeks to 3 years, reaching an estimated coverage of 94 per cent. The campaign was implemented using fixed site approach. The success of the campaign indicates that with appropriate preparation, an emergency response using FIPV can be implemented promptly and effectively *(9)*. In April 2016, India introduced FIPV into routine immunization programme in 8 states. In August 2016, the use of FIVP was expanded to another 8 states *(8)*. Presently it covers the whole country.

Polio Surveillance *(10)*

Surveillance is the most important part of the whole polio eradication initiative. Without surveillance, it would be impossible to pinpoint where and how wild poliovirus is still circulating, or to verify that the virus has been eradicated. Surveillance identifies new cases and detects importation of wild poliovirus.

Acute flaccid paralysis surveillance

There are four steps of acute flaccid paralysis (AFP) surveillance:

1. *Finding and reporting children with acute flaccid paralysis (AFP)* : The first links in the surveillance chain are staff in all health facilities – from district health centres to large hospitals. They must promptly report every case of acute flaccid paralysis (AFP) in any child under 15 years of

age. In addition, public health staff make regular visits to hospitals and rehabilitation centres to search for AFP cases which may have been overlooked or misdiagnosed. The number of AFP cases reported each year is used as an indicator of a country's ability to detect polio – even in countries where the disease no longer occurs. A country's surveillance system needs to be sensitive enough to detect at least one case of AFP for every 100,000 children under 15 years, even in the absence of polio.

2. *Transporting stool samples for analysis* : In the early stages, polio may be difficult to differentiate from other forms of acute flaccid paralysis, such as Guillain-Barre Syndrome, transverse myelitis, or traumatic neuritis. All children with acute flaccid paralysis (AFP) should be reported and tested for wild poliovirus within 48 hours of onset, even if doctors are confident on clinical grounds that the child does not have polio. To test for polio, faecal specimens are analyzed for the presence of poliovirus. Because shedding of the virus is variable, two specimens – taken 24–48 hours apart are required. Speed is essential, since the highest concentrations of poliovirus in the stools of infected individuals are found during the first two weeks after onset of paralysis.

Stool specimens have to be sealed in containers and stored immediately inside a refrigerator or packed between frozen ice packs at 4–8°C in a cold box, ready for shipment to a laboratory. Undue delays or prolonged exposure to heat on the way to the laboratory may destroy the virus. Specimens should arrive at the laboratory within 72 hours of collection.

3. *Isolating poliovirus* : In a laboratory, virologists begin the task of isolating poliovirus from the stool samples. If poliovirus is isolated, the next step is to distinguish between wild (naturally occurring) and vaccine-related poliovirus. This is necessary because the oral vaccine consists of attenuated live polioviruses and resembles wild virus in the laboratory. If wild poliovirus is isolated, the virologists identify which of the two surviving types of wild virus is involved. Wild poliovirus type 2 has not been recorded since 1999.

4. *Mapping the virus* : Once wild poliovirus has been identified, further tests are carried out to determine where the strain may have originated. By determining the exact genetic make-up of the virus, wild viruses can be compared to others and classified into genetic families which cluster in defined geographical areas. The newly-found poliovirus sequence is checked against a reference bank of known polioviruses, allowing inferences about the geographical origin of the newly found virus. When polio has been pinpointed to a precise geographical area, it is possible to identify the source of importation of poliovirus – both long-range and cross-border. Appropriate immunization strategies can then be determined to prevent further spread of the poliovirus.

Environmental surveillance

Environmental surveillance involves testing sewage or other environmental samples for the presence of poliovirus. Environmental surveillance often confirms wild poliovirus infections in the absence of cases of paralysis. Systematic environmental sampling (e.g. in Egypt and Mumbai, India) provides important supplementary surveillance data. Ad-hoc environmental surveillance elsewhere (especially in polio-free regions) provides insights into the international spread of poliovirus.

Surveillance indicators (10)

Indicator	Minimum levels for certification standard surveillance
Completeness of reporting	At least 80% of expected routine (weekly or monthly) AFP surveillance reports should be received on time, including zero reports where no AFP cases are seen. The distribution of reporting sites should be representative of the geography and demography of the country.
Sensitivity of surveillance	At least one case of non-polio AFP should be detected annually per 100,000 population aged less than 15 years. In endemic regions, to ensure even higher sensitivity, this rate should be two per 100,000.
Completeness of case investigation	All AFP cases should have a full clinical and virological investigation with at least 80% of AFP cases having 'adequate' stool specimens collected. 'Adequate' stool specimens are two stool specimens of sufficient quantity for laboratory analysis, collected at least 24 hours apart, within 14 days after the onset of paralysis, and arriving in the laboratory by reverse cold chain and with proper documentation.
Completeness of follow-up	At least 80% of AFP cases should have a follow-up examination for residual paralysis at 60 days after the onset of paralysis.
Laboratory performance	All AFP case specimens must be processed in a WHO accredited laboratory within the Global Polio Laboratory Network (GPLN).

VACCINE DERIVED POLIOVIRUS (VDPV) (11)

Although OPV is a safe vaccine, on rare occasions adverse events may occur. Vaccine-associated paralytic poliomyelitis (VAPP) is the most important of these rare adverse events. Cases of VAPP are clinically indistinguishable from poliomyelitis caused by WPV, but can be distinguished by laboratory analysis. The incidence of VAPP has been estimated at 4 cases/1000,000 birth cohort per year in countries using OPV. VAPP occurs in both OPV recipients and their unimmunized contacts; it is most frequently associated with Sabin 3 (60% of cases), followed by Sabin 2 and Sabin 1.

VDPVs resemble WPVs biologically and differ from the majority of vaccine-related poliovirus (VRPV) isolates in that they have genetic properties consistent with prolonged replication or transmission, which is substantially longer than the normal period of vaccine virus replication of 4–6 weeks in the OPV recipient *(12)*. All poliovirus isolates are characterized by Global Polio Laboratory Network. The diagnosis is made by real-time reverse transcription-polymerase chain reaction (rRT-PCR) nucleic acid amplification targetted to nucleotide substitution that occur early in VDPV emergence.

VDPVs are divided into three categories as (1) cVDPVs, when evidence of person-to-person transmission in the community exists; (2) immunodeficiency-associated VDPVs (iVDPVs), which are isolates from persons with primary immunodeficiencies, who have prolonged VDPV infections; and (3) ambiguous VDPVs (aVDPVs), which are either clinical isolates from person with no known immunodeficiency or sewage isolates whose source is unknown *(12)*.

The prolonged large outbreak of $cVDPV_2$ in Nigeria and D.R. of Congo, the increased detection of iVDPV infection in developing countries and continued detection of aVDPVs that resemble cVDPV and iVDPV reaffirm the following points *(12)*:

1. The clinical signs and severity of paralysis associated with VDPV and WPV infections are indistinguishable.
2. cVDPVs pose the same public health threat as WPVs and require the same control measures.
3. Surveillance for WPVs and VDPVs should continue to be strengthened.
4. Environmental surveillance to detect VDPVs and WPV infection can serve as an important, sensitive supplement to AFP surveillance in many settings.
5. Persons with prolonged iVDPV infection may transmit poliovirus to others, raising the risk of VDPV circulation in settings of low population immunity to the corresponding poliovirus serotype.
6. Prolonged iVDPV excretion is uncommon among persons with primary immunodeficiencies exposed to OPV.
7. The prevalence of long-term iVDPV excretors may be higher than suggested.

Because of these risks of emergence of vaccine-derived polioviruses, OPV use will be discontinued worldwide once all WPV transmission has been interrupted (i.e. inactivated polio vaccine (IPV) will replace OPV) and strategies to strengthen global polio immunization and surveillance are needed to limit the emergence of VDPVs.

Epidemiological determinants

Agent factors

(a) AGENT : The causative agent is the poliovirus which has three serotypes 1,2 and 3. Most outbreaks of paralytic polio are due to type–1 virus. Poliovirus can survive for long periods in the external environment. In a cold environment, it can live in water for 4 months and in faeces for 6 months *(13)*. It is, therefore, well-adapted for the faecal–oral route of transmission *(14)*. However, the virus may be rapidly inactivated by pasteurization, and a variety of physical and chemical agents. (b) RESERVOIR OF INFECTION : Man is the only known reservoir of infection. Most infections are subclinical. It is the mild and subclinical infections that play a dominant role in the spread of infection; they constitute the submerged portion of the iceberg. It is estimated that for every clinical case, there may be 1000 subclinical cases in children and 75 in adults *(15)*. There are no chronic carriers. No animal source has yet been demonstrated. (c) INFECTIOUS MATERIAL : The virus is found in the faeces and oropharyngeal secretions of an infected person. (d) PERIOD OF COMMUNICABILITY : The cases are most infectious 7 to 10 days before and after onset of symptoms. In the faeces, the virus is excreted commonly for 2 to 3 weeks, sometimes as long as 3 to 4 months.

Host factors

(a) AGE : The disease occurs in all age groups, but children are usually more susceptible than adults because of the acquired immunity of the adult population. In developed countries, before the advent of vaccination, the age distribution shifted so that most patients were over the age of 5 years, and 25 per cent were over age 15 years *(16)*. In India, polio is essentially a disease of infancy and childhood. About 50 per cent of cases are reported in infancy. The most vulnerable age is between 6 months and 3 years. (b) SEX : Sex differences have been noted in the ratio of 3 males to one female. (c) RISK FACTORS : Several provocative or risk factors have been found to precipitate an attack of paralytic polio in individuals already infected with polio viruses. They include fatigue, trauma, intramuscular injections, operative procedures such as tonsillectomy undertaken especially during epidemics of polio and administration of immunizing agents particularly alum-containing DPT. (d) IMMUNITY : The maternal antibodies gradually disappear during the first 6 months of life. Immunity following infection is fairly solid although reinfection can occur since infection with one type does not protect completely against the other two types of viruses. Type–2 virus appears to be the most effective antigen. Neutralizing antibody is widely recognized as an important index of immunity to polio after infection *(17)*.

Environmental factors

Polio is more likely to occur during the rainy season. Approximately 60 per cent of cases recorded in India were during June to September *(18)*. The environmental sources of infection are contaminated water, food and flies. Polio virus survives for a long time in a cold environment. Overcrowding and poor sanitation provide opportunities for exposure to infection.

Mode of transmission

(a) FAECAL–ORAL ROUTE : This is the main route of spread in developing countries. The infection may spread *directly* through contaminated fingers where hygiene is poor, or *indirectly* through contaminated water, milk, foods, flies and articles of daily use. (b) DROPLET INFECTION : This may occur in the acute phase of disease when the virus occurs in the throat. Close personal contact with an infected person facilitates droplet spread. This mode of transmission may be relatively more important in developed countries where faecal transmission is remote.

Incubation period

Usually 7 to 14 days (range 3 to 35 days).

Clinical spectrum

When an individual susceptible to polio is exposed to infection, one of the following responses may occur (Fig. 2) (a) INAPPARENT (SUBCLINICAL) INFECTION : This occurs approximately in 91–96 per cent of poliovirus infections *(19)*. There are no presenting symptoms. Recognition only by virus isolation or rising antibody titres. (b) ABORTIVE POLIO OR MINOR ILLNESS : Occurs in approximately 4 to 8 per cent of the infections *(20)*. It causes only a mild or self–limiting illness due to viraemia. The patient recovers quickly. The diagnosis cannot be made clinically. Recognition only by virus isolation or rising antibody titre. (c) NON-PARALYTIC POLIO : Occurs in approximately 1 per cent of all infections *(21)*. The presenting features are stiffness and pain in the neck and

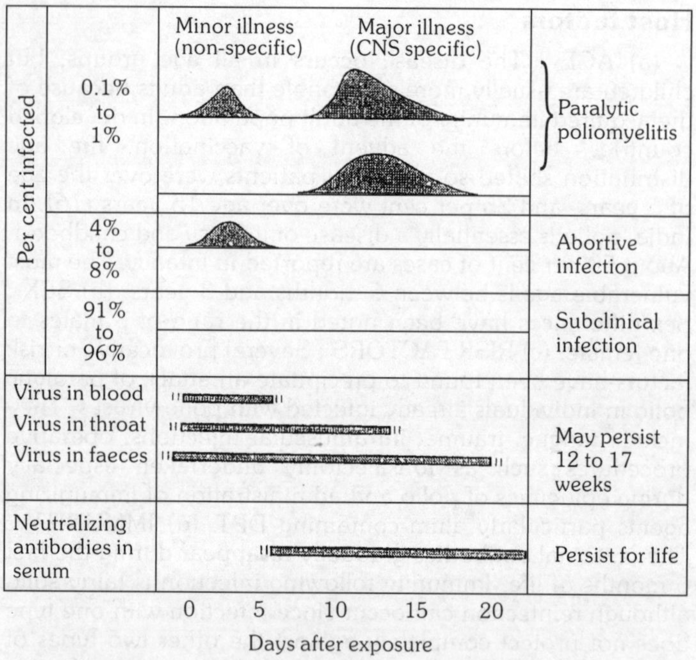

FIG. 2
Time course of events in infection with poliovirus.
Source : *(23)*

back. The disease lasts 2 to 10 days. Recovery is rapid. The disease is synonymous with aseptic meningitis. (d) PARALYTIC POLIO : Occurs in less than one per cent of infections. The virus invades CNS and causes varying degrees of paralysis. The predominant sign is asymmetrical flaccid paralysis. A history of fever at the time of onset of paralysis is suggestive of polio. The other associated symptoms are malaise, anorexia, nausea, vomiting, headache, sore throat, constipation and abdominal pain. There might be signs of meningeal irritation, i.e., stiffness of neck and back muscles. Tripod sign may be present, i.e. the child finds difficulty in sitting and sits by supporting hands at the back and by partially flexing the hips and knees. Progression of the paralysis to reach its maximum in the majority of cases occurs in less than 4 days (may take 4–7 days). The paralysis is characterized as descending, i.e. starting at the hip and then moving down to the distal parts of the extremity. As it is asymmetrical patchy paralysis, muscle strength varies in different muscle groups of different limbs. However, proximal muscle groups are more involved as compared to distal ones. Deep tendon reflexes (DTRs) are diminished before the onset of paralysis. There is no sensory loss. Cranial nerve involvement is seen in bulbar and bulbospinal forms of paralytic poliomyelitis. There might be facial asymmetry, difficulty in swallowing, weakness or loss of voice. Respiratory insufficiency can be life–threatening and is usually the cause of death. After the acute phase, atrophy of the affected muscles lead to a life with residual paralysis which is typical and relatively easy to identify as poliomyelitis *(22)*.

Progressive paralysis, coma or convulsions usually indicate a cause other than polio, as does a very high case fatality rate *(21)*.

There is no specific treatment for polio. Good nursing care from the beginning of illness can minimize or even prevent crippling. Physiotherapy is of vital importance. It can be initiated in the affected limb immediately. It helps the weakened muscles to regain strength. Very probably, the child may have to put on metal callipers.

PREVENTION

Immunization is the sole effective means of preventing poliomyelitis. Both killed and live attenuated vaccines are available and both are safe and effective when used correctly. It is essential to immunize all infants by 6 months of age to protect them against polio. Two types of vaccines are used throughout the world; they are :

1. Inactivated (Salk) polio vaccine (IPV).
2. Oral (Sabin) polio vaccine (OPV).

1. Inactivated (Salk) polio vaccine

The vaccine mixture is formulated to contain at least 40 units of type-1, 8 units of type-2 and 32 units of type-3 D-antigen (D-antigen, which is expressed only on intact poliovirus particles, is used to adjust the concentration of the individual viruses included in the trivalent IPV). All versions of IPV have higher antigenicity than the first-generation vaccines, and they are sometimes referred to as IPVs of enhanced potency. IPV may contain trace amounts of formaldehyde, streptomycin, neomycin or polymyxin B; some versions of IPV contain the preservative phenoxy-ethanol (0.5%), but neither thiomersal (incompatible with IPV antigenicity) nor adjuvants are used *(11)*.

IPV is administered by intramuscular injection or fractional dose by intradermal injection. The vaccine is stable at ambient temperature, but should be refrigerated to ensure no loss of potency. Freezing should be avoided as it could diminish potency. IPV is available either as a stand-alone product or in combination with ≥1 other vaccine antigens including diphtheria, tetanus, whole-cell or acellular pertussis, hepatitis B, or *Haemophilus influenzae* type b. In the combination vaccines, the alum or the pertussis vaccine, or both, have an adjuvant effect.

The primary or initial course of immunization consists of 4 inoculations. The first 3 doses are given at intervals of 1–2 months and 4th dose 6–12 months after the third dose. First dose is usually given when the infant is 6 weeks old. Additional doses are recommended prior to school entry and then every 5 years until the age of 18. Alternatively, one or two doses of live vaccine (OPV) can be given safely as boosters after an initial course of immunization with inactivated vaccine.

IPV induces, humoral antibodies (IgM, IgG and IgA serum antibodies) but does not induce intestinal or local immunity. The circulating antibodies protect the individual against paralytic polio, but do not prevent reinfection of the gut by wild viruses. For the individual, it gives protection from paralysis and nothing more; for the community, it offers nothing because the wild viruses can still multiply in the gut and be a source of infection to others. This is a major drawback of IPV. Further, in the case of an epidemic, IPV is unsuitable because : (i) immunity is not rapidly achieved, as more than one dose is required to induce immunity, and (ii) injections are to be avoided during epidemic times as they are likely to precipitate paralysis *(24)*. Therefore, IPV is not efficacious in combating epidemics of polio.

Advantages : Inactivated polio vaccine, because it does not contain living virus, is safe to administer (i) to persons with immune deficiency diseases (ii) to persons undergoing corticosteroid and radiation therapy (iii) to those over 50 years who are receiving vaccine for the first time, and (iv) during pregnancy.

Associated risks : No serious adverse reactions to IPV

vaccines currently in use have been reported except minor local erythema (0.5–1 per cent), induration (3–11 per cent) and tenderness (14–29 per cent).

2. Oral (Sabin) polio vaccine (OPV)

Oral polio vaccine (OPV) was described by Sabin in 1957. It contains live attenuated virus (types 1, 2 and 3) grown in primary monkey kidney or human diploid cell cultures. Ideally each virus type should be given separately as monovalent vaccine, but for administrative convenience, rather than efficacy, it is given as *bivalent* (bOPV) vaccine. The vaccine contains not less than $10^{6.0}$ $CCID_{50}$ of type 1 poliomyelitis virus Sabin strain and not less than $10^{5.8}$ $CCID_{50}$ of type 3 poliomyelitis virus Sabin strain.

National Immunization Schedule

The WHO Programme on Immunization (EPI) and the National Immunization Programme in India recommends a primary course of 3 doses of OPV at one–month intervals, commencing the first dose when infant is 6 weeks old (see page 135). It is recommended that a dose of OPV (zero-dose) is required to be given to all children delivered in health institutions before their discharge from the hospital. The vaccine should be given in maternity wards, the newborn should not be taken to regular immunization sessions to avoid infection. OPV is given concurrently with DPT or pentavalent vaccine. BCG can be given simultaneously with the first dose of OPV. It is very important to complete vaccination of all infants before 6 months of age. This is because most polio cases occur between the ages of 6 months and 3 years. One booster dose of OPV is recommended 12 to 18 months later.

Dose and mode of administration

The dose is 2 drops or as stated on the label. WHO recommends that vaccinators use dropper supplied with the vial of oral polio vaccine. This is the most direct and effective way to deliver the correct drop size. Tilt the child's back, and gently squeeze the cheeks or pinch the nose to make the mouth open. Let the drops fall from the dropper onto the child's tongue. Repeat the process if the child spits out the vaccine. If the vaccine is spoon–fed there is a chance that it will not all be licked up by the child *(25)*.

Development of immunity

On administration, the live vaccine strains infect intestinal epithelial cells. After replication, the virus is transported to the Peyer's patches where a secondary multiplication with subsequent viraemia occurs. The virus spreads to other areas of the body, resulting in the production of circulating antibodies which prevent dissemination of the virus to the nervous system and prevent paralytic polio. Intestinal infection stimulates the production of IgA secretory antibodies which prevent subsequent infection of the alimentary tract with wild strains of poliovirus, and thus is effective in limiting virus transmission in the community. Thus OPV induces both local and systemic immunity.

The vaccine progeny is excreted in the faeces and secondary spread occurs to household contacts and susceptible contacts in the community. Non-immunized persons may therefore, be immunized. Thus widespread "herd immunity" results, even if only approximately 66 per cent of the community is immunized *(14)*. This property of OPV has been exploited in controlling epidemics of polio by administering the vaccine simultaneously in a short period to all susceptibles in a community. This procedure virtually eliminates the wild polio strains in the community and replaces them by attenuated strains *(26)*. The duration of immunity produced by the OPV is not known, it may possibly even be lifelong *(27)*.

Advantages

The advantages of OPV are : (i) since given orally, it is easy to administer and does not require the use of highly trained personnel (ii) induces both humoral and intestinal immunity. (iii) antibody is quickly produced in a large proportion of vaccinees, even a single dose elicits (except in tropical countries) substantial immunity (iv) the vaccinee excretes the virus and so infects others who are also immunized thereby (v) useful in controlling epidemics, and (vi) relatively inexpensive.

Complications

OPV is remarkably free from complications. However, being living viruses, the vaccine viruses, particularly type 3 do mutate in the course of their multiplication in vaccinated children, and rare cases of vaccine–associated paralytic polio have occurred in (a) recipients of the vaccine, and (b) their contacts. For details please refer to page 242.

Contraindications

Diarrhoea should not be considered a contraindication to OPV. However, to ensure full protection, a dose of OPV given to a child with diarrhoea should not be counted as part of the series and the child should receive another dose at the first available opportunity. Live vaccines are not usually given to immunocompromised individuals *(23)*. Patients suffering from leukaemias and malignancy and those receiving corticosteroids may not be given OPV. IPV is an alternative to OPV for immunization of children with HIV infection *(23)*. There is as yet no indication that polio immunization may pose any danger to a pregnant mother or developing foetus. However, OPV should be delayed until after pregnancy unless immediate protection is required, when IPV is indicated *(14)*.

Storage

(a) Stabilized vaccine : Recent oral polio vaccines are heat stabilized by adding magnesium chloride. They can be kept without losing potency for a year at 4 deg. C, and for a month at 25 deg. C temperature *(16)*. *(b) Non-stabilized vaccine :* The vaccine should be stored at –20 deg C in a deep freeze until used. In case a deep freeze is not available, it might be stored temporarily in the freezing chamber of the refrigerator. During transport, the vaccine must be kept either on dry ice (solid carbon dioxide) or a freezing mixture (equal quantities of wet ice and ammonium chloride) *(28)*.

At the vaccination clinic, the bottle containing the OPV should not be frozen and thawed repeatedly, since repeated freezing and thawing has a deleterious effect on the potency of live polio vaccine. It would be preferable to keep the vials of the vaccine in ice during its administration to children *(28)*.

Studies indicate that breast-feeding does not impede the effectiveness of oral poliovirus vaccine *(29)*. Breast milk can be given whenever the child is hungry. However, hot water, hot milk or hot fluids should be withheld for about half an hour after the administration of the vaccine. The vaccine should be administered preferably in a cool room, rather than in a hot, humid and crowded room.

The problems with OPV may be summarized as follows (a) A primary problem is the instability of the vaccine at high ambient temperatures. The vaccine has to be kept frozen during storage, and kept cold during transportation, right up to the point of administration. (b) A second problem is the frequent vaccine failures even with fully potent vaccines. (c) A third problem is the very small residual neurovirulence in OPV.

Sequential administration of IPV and OPV

Over the past decade, a number of countries in central and eastern Europe, the Middle East, the Far East, and southern Africa have adopted sequential schedules of 1–2 doses of IPV followed by ≥ 2 doses of OPV. Combined schedules of IPV and OPV appear to reduce or prevent VAPP while maintaining the high levels of intestinal mucosal immunity conferred by OPV. In addition, such schedules economize on limited resources by reducing the number of doses of IPV, and may optimize both the humoral and mucosal immunogenicity of polio vaccination. The effectiveness of this approach in preventing polio caused by WPV as well as VAPP has been documented by 2 large studies *(11)*.

The difference between IPV and OPV are given in Table 2.

TABLE 2
Differences between IPV and OPV

	IPV (Salk type)	OPV (Sabin type)
1	Killed formolized virus	Live attenuated virus
2	Given subcutaneously or IM	Given orally
3	Induces circulating antibody, but no local (intestinal) immunity	Immunity is both humoral and intestinal. Induces antibody quickly
4	Prevents paralysis, but does not prevent reinfection by wild polio viruses	Prevents not only paralysis, but also intestinal reinfection
5	Not useful in controlling epidemics	Can be effectively used in controlling epidemics. Even a single dose elicits substantial immunity (except in tropical countries)
6	More difficult to manufacture	Easy to manufacture
7	The virus content is 10,000 times more than OPV. Hence costlier	Cheaper
8	Does not require stringent conditions during storage and transportation. Has a longer shelf–life	Requires to be stored and transported at sub-zero temperatures, unless stabilized

Human Normal Ig

The current widespread practice of immunization has virtually eliminated the need for passive immunization. Normal human Ig in a dose of 0.25–0.3 ml per kg of body weight has been found to be protective for a few weeks against paralytic disease but does not prevent sub-clinical infections. Immunoglobulin is effective only if given shortly before infection, it is of no value after clinical symptoms develop *(17)*. The subject shall be actively immunized against polio after a few weeks.

Epidemiological Investigations

The occurrence of a single case of polio is now considered as an epidemic, and should prompt an immediate epidemiological investigation, including an active search for other cases. Samples of faeces from all cases or suspected cases of polio should be collected and forwarded to the laboratory for virus isolation. In addition, where possible, paired sera should be collected, the first specimen at the clinical suspicion of paralytic polio and the second at the period of convalescence. A rising titre of poliovirus neutralizing antibody provides useful confirmatory evidence. The Indian Council of Medical Research has set up National Enterovirus Units at Mumbai, Coonoor, Chennai, Delhi and Kasauli where samples may be sent for examination.

The following check-list indicates the essential data to be collected when investigating an outbreak *(30, 31)*.

1. Name of the administrative area and locality
2. Date first case reported from locality
3. Period of field investigation
   From..............to..............(dates)
4. No.of paralytic polio cases detected
   - 4.1 Clinical diagnosis only
   - 4.2 Laboratory confirmed
   - 4.3 Type(s) of virus isolated
5. No. of deaths from paralytic polio
6. No.of paralytic cases of polio by age
   -1 year — 10–14 years
   1–4 years — 15–19 years
   5–9 years — 20+ years
7. No.of contacts of paralytic polio examined :
   Household contacts
   Other. (specify)
8. Brief description of field investigation
9. History of previous vaccination practice in the locality including the dates of the last community vaccination programme, and the type of vaccine used.
10. Name of the principal investigator and laboratory.

Within an epidemic area, OPV should be provided for all persons over 6 weeks of age who have not been completely immunized or whose immune status is unknown.

Under the International Health Regulations, polio is subject to international surveillance. The WHO should be notified as soon as possible of the occurrence of paralytic polio and to supplement reports on such outbreaks with additional epidemiological information such as the type of virus, and the number of cases and deaths reported. In addition a quarterly report (on prescribed form) should be sent to WHO, Geneva. The WHO has prepared guidelines to poliovirus isolation and serological techniques for polio surveillance.

Strategies for polio eradication in India

(a) Conduct Pulse Polio Immunization days every year until poliomyelitis is eradicated.
(b) Sustain high levels of routine immunization coverage.
(c) Monitor OPV coverage at district level and below.
(d) Improve surveillance capable of detecting all cases of AFP due to polio and non-polio aetiology.
(e) Ensure rapid case investigation, including the collection of stool samples for virus isolation.
(f) Arrange follow-up of all cases of AFP at 60 days to check for residual paralysis.
(g) Conduct outbreak control for cases confirmed or suspected to be poliomyelitis to stop transmission.

Even a single case is treated as an outbreak and preventive measures are initiated, usually within 48 hours of notification of the case. The complete and timely reporting of cases of poliomyelitis is an important element for the eradication of poliomyelitis. Reporting of all cases of acute flaccid paralysis in children under 15 years of age is mandatory, and line lists of all reported cases of poliomyelitis are maintained. Since 1992, the active surveillance has been extended to all cases of acute flaccid paralysis, including causes other than poliomyelitis.

Line listing of cases

Line listing of reported cases was started in the year 1989 to check for duplication (same case reported more than once if the child visited more than one health facility), year of onset of illness (to screen children with residual paralysis who developed poliomyelitis prior to the year of reporting), identification of high risk pockets (by analysis of residential status) and documentation of high-risk age groups.

Line listing of cases made it possible to take appropriate follow-up action in areas from where the cases had been reported. The line lists have also provided useful epidemiological data for programme purposes. For example, it provided information on the age at onset of illness and to understand the urgency for the early completion of the OPV immunization schedule.

All cases of acute flaccid paralysis must be reported immediately to the chief medical officer/district immunization officer with the following details :

- Name, age and sex of the patient
- Father's name and complete address
- Vaccination status
- Date of onset of paralysis and date of reporting
- Clinical diagnosis
- Doctor's name, address and phone number

Mopping Up

Mopping up activities are usually the last stage in polio eradication. The strategy of "mopping up" involves door–to–door immunization in high-risk districts, where wild polio virus is known or suspected to be still circulating. This strategy is being implemented in India.

Pulse Polio Immunization

In India NIDs have become the largest public health campaigns ever conducted in a single country. Government of India conducted the first round of PPI consisting of two immunization days 6 weeks apart on 9th December 1995 and 20th January 1996. The first PPI conducted targeted all children under 3 years of age irrespective of their immunization status. Later on, as recommended by WHO, it was decided to increase the age group from under 3 to under 5 years.

The term "pulse" has been used to describe this sudden, simultaneous, mass administration of OPV on a single day to all children 0–5 years of age, regardless to previous immunization. PPIs occur as two rounds about 4 to 6 weeks apart during low transmission season of polio, i.e. between November to February. In India, the peak transmission is from June to September. The dose of OPV during PPIs are **extra** doses which supplement, and **do not** replace the doses received during routine immunization services. The children including 0–1 year old infants should receive all their scheduled doses and PPI doses. There is no minimum interval between PPI and scheduled OPV doses *(32)*.

An important improvement in PPI during 1998 has been the use of vaccine vial monitor. Colour monitors or labels are put on vaccine bottles. Each label has a circle of deep blue colour. Inside it is a white square which changes colour and gradually becomes blue, if vaccine bottle is exposed to higher temperature. When the colour of the white square becomes blue like that of surrounding circle, the vaccine should be considered ineffective. Thereby, the health worker can easily ascertain that the vaccine being given is effective or not. This mechanism has been made mandatory in all vaccine procurements since 1998. This quality assurance will ensure that the children will have better protection against polio in 1999 and thereafter.

Following recommendations from the India Expert Advisory Group on Polio Eradication (IEAG), several strategies were utilized during 2005 and early 2006 to improve the impact of SIAs : (i) development and licensure of monovalent OPV1 (mOPV1) and mOPV3 for targeted use during SIAs based on surveillance data; (ii) deployment of additional peronnel to assist with intensified SIAs in the States of Bihar and UP and in Mumbai City; (iii) social mobilization targeted at reaching population groups missed during previous SIAs; (iv) use of mobile teams to vaccinate children at transit points (e.g. railway and bus stations) and on moving trains; and (v) increased engagement and accountability of political leaders and of health staff at all levels. To further improve population immunity in the most critical age group, the IEAG added a specific recommendation at its May 2006 meeting to identify and target all neonates in high-risk areas of UP with a "birth dose" of mOPV1 *(33)*.

The last case of polio in the country was reported from Howrah of West Bengal with date of onset of disease on 13th January 2011. Thereafter no polio case has been reported in the country. On 27th March 2014, India was declared as non-endemic country for polio.

The steps taken by the Government to achieve the target of polio eradication and maintain the polio-free state are as follows *(34)* :

1. All states and union territories in the country have developed a Rapid Response Team (RRT) to respond to any polio outbreak in the country. An Emergency Preparedness and Response Plan (EPRP) has also been developed by all states indicating steps to be undertaken in case of detection of a polio case.
2. In the states of UP and Bihar every new born child is being identified and vaccinated during the polio immunization campaigns and is being tracked for 8 subsequent rounds.
3. In order to reach every eligible child during the pulse polio round, apart from the strategy of vaccinating children at fixed booths and house to house visit, efforts in vaccinating children in transit at railway stations, inside long distance trains, major bus stops, marker places, religious congregations, major road crossings etc. throughout the country have been intensified. Special booths are established in areas bordering neighbouring countries like Wagah border and Attari train station in Punjab and Munabao train station in Barmer district of Rajasthan, to ensure that all children under 5 years of age coming from across the border are given polio drops.
4. An extremely high level of vigilance through surveillance across the country for any importation or circulation of poliovirus and Vaccine Derived Polio Virus (VDPV) is being maintained. Environmental surveillance is continuing at four sites with establishment of two new sites in 2012.

5. Government of India has identified 107 high risk blocks for polio where a multi-pronged strategy is being implemented to ensure sanitation, hygiene and clean drinking water in addition to vaccinating each and every child oral polio vaccine (OPV).
6. Migratory population from UP and Bihar are being identified in the states of Punjab, Haryana, Gujarat and West Bengal and these migratory children are being covered during the Sub National Immunization Day (SNID) in UP and Bihar.
7. Social mobilization activities are being intensified by involving the local influencers, community and religious leaders to improve community participation and acceptance of polio vaccine.
8. A rolling emergency stock of oral polio vaccine (OPV) is being maintained to respond to any wild polio vaccine (WPV) or circulating vaccine derived polio virus (cVDPV) detection.

As part of the polio endgame strategic plan, India has introduced IVP in the national immunization programme from 30th November 2015 and tOPV – bOPV switch was carried out in April 2016 *(35)*.

AFP SURVEILLANCE : PPI is supported by AFP surveillance system since 1997. It is being conducted through a network of surveillance medical officers (SMOs), who are specially trained and are responsible for a defined area. A national surveillance team is positioned in Delhi. The SMOs are located at the state headquarters and at regional places in case of larger states. A regular weekly reporting system has been established. As a result of more meticulous search/reporting, the number of reported cases of AFP increased from 1,005 in 1996 to 11,675 and the completeness of stool specimen collection improved markedly from 59 per cent in 1998 to 82 per cent at the end of September 2020 *(36)*.

References

1. WHO (2022), *Weekly Epidemiological Record* No. 23, 2022.
2. WHO (2021), *Polio Global Eradication Initiative, Polio Eradication Strategy 2022–2026, Delivering on a promise*.
3. WHO (2016), *Weekly Epidemiological Record* No. 36/37, 9th Sept. 2016.
4. WHO, Immunization, Vaccines and Biologicals, *About the Polio Endgame Strategic Plan*.
5. EPI (2014), The Polio Eradication Endgame, Brief on *IPV introduction, OPV withdrawal and routine immunization strengthening*, March 2014.
6. EPI (2015), Polio–Global Eradication Initiative - *Preparing for withdrawal of all oral polio vaccine (OPV) : Replacing trivalent OPV with bivalent OPV frequently asked questions*, Feb. 2015.
7. EPI, Polio–Global Eradication Initiative - *Polio Today, Key Points about containment*.
8. WHO (2016), Immunization, Vaccine and Biologicals, *Fractional dose IPV*.
9. WHO (2016), *Weekly Epidemiological Record* No. 34, 26th Aug. 2016.
10. *Global Polio Eradication Initiative,* Data and Monitoring, Surveillance.
11. WHO (2010), *Weekly Epidemiological Record,* No. 23, 4th June, 2010.
12. WHO (2012), *Weekly Epidemiological Record* No. 38, 21st Sept. 2012.
13. Provoost, P. (1985). *Children in the Tropics* No. 156–157 P.58.
14. Ichout, B.D. (1988). *Med. Int.* 53 : 2189–2191.
15. Christie, A.B. (1980). *Infectious Diseases : Epidemiology and Clinical Practice,* 3rd ed, Churchill Livingstone.
16. Jewetz, Melnick and Adelberg's. *Medical Microbiology,* 26th Ed, 2013, A Lange Medical Book.
17. WHO (1983). *Tech.Rep.Ser.* No.693.
18. ICMR (1975). *ICMR Bulletin,* Jan. 1975.
19. Krishnan, R.et al (1983). *Bull WHO,* 61 (4) 689–692.
20. Young, N.A. (1979) in *Principles and Practice of Infectious Diseases,* Mandell, G.L. et al (eds), John Wiley, New York.
21. WHO (1981). *Wkly Epi.Rec.,* 56 (17) 131–132.
22. Govt. of India *CSSM review,* A Newsletter on the Child Survival and Safe Motherhood Programme, No.32, August 1995.
23. WHO (1993), *The Immunological Basis of Immunization Series, Module 6 : Poliomyelitis Global Programme for Vaccines and Immunization EPI, WHO.*
24. Galazka, A.M. et al (1984) *Bull WHO,* 62 : 357.
25. AHRTAG (1988) *Dialogue on diarrhoea* No. 33 June P.7.
26. Nightingale, E. (1977). *N.Eng.J.Med.,* 297 : 249.
27. WHO (2016), *Weekly Epidemiological Record* No. 12, 2016.
28. Ministry of Health, Govt. of India (1977). *Manual on Immunization,* Dept. of Family Welfare.
29. Sabin, A.B. (1980). *Bull WHO* 58 (1) 141.
30. WHO (1975). *Wkly Epi Rec.,* 50 : 205–209.
31. WHO (1976). *WHO Chronicle,* 30 : 72–75.
32. Govt. of India (1996), *Pulse Polio Immunization in India,* Operational Guide, MCH Division, Department of Family Welfare, New Delhi.
33. WHO (2006), *Weekly Epidemiological Record,* No. 29, 21st July, 2006.
34. Govt. of India (2013), *Annual Report 2012-2013,* Ministry of Health and Family Welfare, New Delhi
35. Govt. of India (2016), *Annual Report 2015–2016,* Ministry of Health and Family Welfare, New Delhi.
36. WHO (2020), *Weekly Epidemiological Record* No. 38, 2020.

VIRAL HEPATITIS

Viral hepatitis is a term commonly used for several clinically similar yet aetiologically and epidemiologically distinct diseases. It is caused by five different viruses with transmission either through contaminated food or water (hepatitis A and E) or through exposure to blood or body fluids (hepatitis B, C and D). Hepatitis A and hepatitis B have been recognized as separate entities since early 1940s and can be diagnosed with specific serological tests. Delta hepatitis is an infection dependent on the hepatitis B virus. It may occur as a coinfection with acute HBV infection or as superinfection of an HBV carrier.

HEPATITIS A

Hepatitis A (formerly known as "infectious" hepatitis or epidemic jaundice) is an acute infectious disease caused by hepatitis A virus (HAV). The disease is heralded by non-specific symptoms such as fever, chills, headache, fatigue, generalized weakness and aches and pains, followed by anorexia, nausea, vomiting, dark urine and jaundice. The disease spectrum is characterized by the occurrence of numerous subclinical or asymptomatic cases. The disease is benign with complete recovery in several weeks. The case fatality rate of icteric cases is less than 0.1 per cent, usually from acute liver failure and mainly affects older adults. Although the disease has, in general, a low mortality, patients may be incapacitated for many weeks.

Problem statement

Being an enterovirus infection like poliomyelitis, hepatitis A is endemic in most developing countries, with frequent outbursts of minor or major outbreaks. The exact incidence of the disease is difficult to estimate because of the high proportion of asymptomatic cases. However, based on an ongoing reassessment of the global burden of hepatitis A, WHO estimates suggest that about 1.4 million cases occur every year world-wide *(1)*.

Geographical areas can be characterized as having high, intermediate or low levels of hepatitis A infection *(2)*.

Areas with high levels of infection

In developing countries with very poor sanitary conditions and hygienic practices, most children (90%) have been infected with the hepatitis A virus before the age of 10 years. Those infected in childhood do not experience any noticeable symptoms. Epidemics are uncommon because older children and adults are generally immune. Symptomatic disease rates in these areas are low and outbreaks are rare.

Areas with intermediate levels of infection

In developing countries, countries with transitional economies, and regions where sanitary conditions are variable, children often escape infection in early childhood. Ironically, these improved economic and sanitary conditions may lead to a higher susceptibility in older age groups and higher disease rates, as infections occur in adolescents and adults, and large outbreaks can occur. Thus, paradoxically, with the transition from high to intermediate endemicity, the incidence of clinically significant hepatitis A increases *(2)*.

Areas with low levels of infection

In developed countries with good sanitary and hygienic conditions, infection rates are low. Disease may occur among adolescents and adults in high-risk groups, such as injecting-drug users, homosexual men, people travelling to areas of high endemicity, and in isolated populations such as closed religious communities *(2)*.

The exact incidence of HAV in India is not known. The Indian literature is replete with numerous reports of sporadic and epidemic occurrence of this disease in various cities, residential colonies and campuses. Epidemics of hepatitis A often evolve slowly, involve wide geographic areas and last many months, but, common source epidemics (e.g., faecal contamination of drinking water) may evolve explosively.

Epidemiological determinants

Agent factors

(a) AGENT : The causative agent, the hepatitis A virus, is an enterovirus (type 72) of the Picornaviridae family *(3)*. It multiplies only in hepatocytes. Faecal shedding of the virus is at its highest during the later part of the incubation period and early acute phase of illness. Only one serotype is known. (b) RESISTANCE : The virus is fairly resistant to low pH, heat and chemicals. It has been shown to survive more than 10 weeks in well water *(4)*. It withstands heating to 60 deg C for one hour, and is not affected by chlorine in doses usually employed for chlorination. Formalin is stated to be an effective disinfectant. The virus is inactivated by ultraviolet rays and by boiling for 5 minutes or autoclaving. In short the virus survives for long periods under variable conditions and resists many procedures that eliminate or inactivate most bacterial agents. (c) RESERVOIR OF INFECTION : The human cases are the only reservoir of infection. The cases range from asymptomatic infections to severe ones. Asymptomatic (anicteric) infections are especially common in children. These cases play an important role in maintaining the chain of transmission in the community. There is no evidence of a chronic carrier state. (d) PERIOD OF INFECTIVITY : The risk of transmitting HAV is greatest from 2 weeks before to 1 week after the onset of jaundice. Infectivity falls rapidly with the onset of jaundice *(2)*. (e) INFECTIVE MATERIAL : Mainly man's faeces. Blood, serum and other fluids are infective during the brief stage of viraemia. (f) VIRUS EXCRETION : HAV is excreted in the faeces for about 2 weeks before the onset of jaundice and for up to 2 weeks thereafter. There is little evidence for HAV transmission by exposure to urine or naso-pharyngeal secretions of infected patients. Haemodialysis plays no role in the spread of hepatitis A infections to either patients or the staff *(5)*.

Host factors

(a) AGE : Infection with HAV is more frequent among children than in adults. However, people from all ages may be infected if susceptible. In young children, infections tend to be mild or subclinical; the clinical severity increases with age. The ratio of anicteric to icteric cases in adults is about 1:3; in children, it may be as high as 12:1. However, faecal excretion of HAV antigen and RNA persists longer in the young than in adults *(5)*. (b) SEX : Both sexes are equally susceptible. (c) IMMUNITY : Immunity after attack probably lasts for life; second attacks have been reported in about 5 per cent of patients. Most people in endemic areas acquire immunity through subclinical infection. The IgM antibody appears early in the illness and persists for over 90 days. IgG appears more slowly, and persists for many years.

Environmental factors

Cases may occur throughout the year. In India the disease tends to be associated with periods of heavy rainfall *(9)*. Poor sanitation and overcrowding favour the spread of infection, giving rise to water-borne and food-borne epidemics. Paradoxically, when standards of hygiene and sanitation are improved, morbidity from infection with enteric viruses may increase. This is what happened with hepatitis A *(6)*.

Modes of transmission

(a) *FAECAL–ORAL ROUTE* : This is the major route of transmission. It may occur by direct (person-to-person) contact or indirectly by way of contaminated water, food or milk. Water-borne transmission, is not a major factor in developed countries, where food-borne outbreaks are becoming more frequent. For example, consumption of salads and vegetables, and of raw or inadequately cooked shellfish and oyesters cultivated in sewage polluted water is associated with epidemic outbreaks of hepatitis A *(5)*. Direct transmission comprises an array of routes such as contaminated hands or objects such as eating utensils. Direct infection occurs readily under conditions of poor sanitation and overcrowding.

(b) *PARENTERAL ROUTE* : Hepatitis A is rarely, if ever, transmitted by the parenteral route (i.e., by blood and blood products or by skin penetration through contaminated needles). This may occur during the stage of viraemia. This mode of transmission is of minor importance as viraemic stage of infection occurs during prodromal phase and there is no carrier state *(5)*.

(c) *SEXUAL TRANSMISSION* : As a sexually transmitted infection hepatitis A may occur mainly among homosexual men because of oral–anal contact *(7)*.

Food handlers are not at increased risk for hepatitis A, because of their occupation, but are noteworthy because of their critical role in common-source food-borne HAV transmission. Health care personnel do not have an increased prevalence of HAV infection and nosocomial HAV transmission is rare. Children play an important role in HAV transmission as they generally have asymptomatic or unrecognized illness *(8)*.

Incubation period

10 to 50 days (usually 14–28 days). The length of the incubation period is proportional to the dose of the virus ingested *(4)*.

Clinical spectrum

The onset of jaundice is often preceded by gastrointestinal symptoms such as nausea, vomiting, anorexia, and mild fever. Jaundice may appear within a few days of the prodromal period, but anicteric hepatitis is more common. Hepatitis A resolves completely in 98 per cent of cases but relapse of symptoms are noted in 3–20 per cent cases *(10)*. The outcome of infection with HAV is as shown in Table 1.

TABLE 1
Outcomes of infection with hepatitis A virus

Outcome	Children	Adults
Inapparent (sub-clinical) infection	80-95%	10-25%
Icteric disease	5-20%	75-90%
Complete recovery	>98%	>98%
Chronic disease	None	None
Mortality rate	0.1%	0.3-2.1%

Source : *(5)*

Diagnosis

Tests for abnormal liver function, such as serum alanine aminotransferase (ALT) and bilirubin, supplement the clinical, pathologic, and epidemiologic findings.

A specific laboratory diagnosis of hepatitis A can be obtained by :

a. Demonstration of HAV particles or specific viral antigens in the faeces, bile and blood. HAV is detected in the stool from about 2 weeks prior to the onset of jaundice, up to 2 weeks after.
b. Anti-HAV appears in the IgM fraction during the acute phase, peaking about 2 weeks after elevation of liver enzymes. Anti-HAV IgM usually declines to non–detectable levels within 3–6 months. Anti-HAV IgG appears soon after the onset of disease and persists for decades. Thus, detection of IgM-specific anti-HAV in the blood of an acutely infected patient confirms the diagnosis of hepatitis A. ELISA is the method of choice for measuring HAV antibodies *(5)*.

The clinical, virologic and serological events following exposure to HAV are as shown in Fig. 1.

Prevention and containment

a. Control of reservoir

Control of reservoir is difficult because of the following factors: (a) faecal shedding of the virus is at its height during the incubation period and early phase of illness (b) the occurrence of large number of subclinical cases (c) absence of specific treatment, and (d) low socio-economic profile of the population usually involved. Strict isolation of cases is not a useful control measure because of (a) and (b). However, attention should be paid to the usual control measures such as complete bed rest and disinfection of faeces and fomites. The use of 0.5 per cent sodium hypochlorite has been strongly recommended as an effective disinfectant *(11)*.

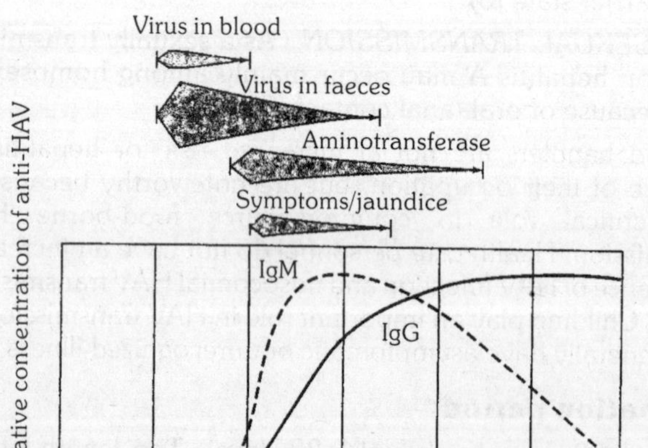

FIG. 1
Immunologic and biologic events associated with human infection with hepatitis A virus.

Source : *(5)*

b. Control of transmission

The best means of reducing the spread of infection is by promoting simple measures of personal and community hygiene, e.g., hand washing before eating and after toilet; the sanitary disposal of excreta which will prevent contamination of water, food and milk; and purification of community water supplies by flocculation, filtration and adequate chlorination. A question is often asked how much chlorine is needed to inactivate the virus. Studies indicated that 1 mg/L of free residual chlorine can cause destruction of the virus in 30 minutes at pH values of 8.5 or less *(12)*. The water treatment and distribution system should be improved. During epidemics, boiled water should be advocated for drinking purposes. Several countries of the world have achieved control of water-borne HAV infection. Other control measures include proper disposal of sewage within communities. If all these measures are properly implemented, a substantial reduction of HAV infection can be expected.

c. Control of susceptible population

Targeted protection of high-risk groups should be considered in low and very low endemicity, settings. Groups at increased risk of hepatitis A include travellers to areas of intermediate or high endemicity, those requiring life-long treatment with blood products, men having sex with men, workers in contact with non-human primates, and injection drug users. In addition, patients with chronic liver disease are at increased risk for fulminant hepatitis A and should be vaccinated *(10)*. Use of hepatitis A vaccine rather than passive prophylaxis with immune globuline should be considered for pre-exposure prophylaxis (e.g. for travellers) and post-exposure prophylaxis (e.g. for close contacts of acute cases of hepatitis A.

1. *Vaccines* : Two types of hepatitis A vaccines are currently used worldwide:

(a) Formaldehyde inactivated vaccines – produced in several countries and which are most commonly used worldwide.
(b) Live attenuated vaccinces – which are manufactured in China and are available in several countries.

Inactivated hepatitis A vaccine are licensed for use in persons ≥12 months of age. The complete vaccination schedule consists of 2 dose administration into the deltoid muscle. The interval between the first (primary) dose and second (booster) dose is commonly 6–12 months; however, the interval between the doses is flexible and can be extended to 18–36 months. It can be administered simultaneously with other vaccines. Following 2 doses of vaccine the protective efficacy is about 94 per cent.

The live attenuated vaccine is administered as a single subcutaneous dose.

Both inactivated and live attenuated hepatitis A vaccines are highly immunogenic and immunization will generate long-lasting, possibly life-long, protection against the disease in children and adults.

Recommendations for hepatitis A vaccination in outbreak situation depend on the epidemiologic features of disease in the community and the feasibility of rapidly implementing a widespread vaccination programme. National immunization programmes may consider inclusion of single-dose inactivated hepatitis A vaccine in immunization schedule *(10)*.

Combination of hepatitis A and B, or hepatitis A and typhoid vaccines have been developed, mainly intended for use in adult travellers.

2. *Human immunoglobulin :* The protective efficacy of immune globulin (Ig) against HAV infection is well documented. The duration of protection is, however, limited to approximately 1–2 months and 3–5 months following administration of IgG at dose of 0.02 and 0.06 ml/kg body weight, respectively. Prophylaxis is achieved within hours of injection and is 80 to 90 per cent effective when administered before or no later than 14 days after exposure. The use of Ig worldwide is now declining because of insufficient concentration of anti–HAV IgG in non-specific Ig preparations, the high cost of specific HAV IgG preparations, the limited duration of protection following passive IgG prophylaxis against HAV infection, and because hepatitis A vaccines have been shown to induce rapid protection against HAV after first dose *(10)*.

HEPATITIS B

Hepatitis B (formerly known as "serum" hepatitis) is an acute systemic infection with major pathology in the liver, caused by hepatitis B virus (HBV). HBV infection can be either acute or chronic, and may range from asymptomatic infection or mild disease, to severe, or rarely fulminant hepatitis. Acute hepatitis B is usually a self-limiting disease marked by acute inflammation and hepatocellular necrosis with case fatality rate of 0.5 to 1 per cent. Chronic hepatitis B infection encompasses a spectrum of disease and is defined as persistent HBV infection with or without associated active viral replication and evidence of hepatocellular injury and inflammation. Age is a key factor in determining the risk of chronic infection. Worldwide, the majority of persons with CHB were infected at birth or in early childhood *(13)*. Hepatitis B virus can form a dangerous alliance with delta virus and produce a new form of virulent hepatitis which is considered to be widespread threat for much of the world.

Problem statement

WORLD

Hepatitis B is endemic throughout the world, especially in tropical and developing countries and also in some regions of Europe *(8)*. Its prevalence varies from country to country and depends upon a complex mix of behavioural, environmental and host factors. In general, it is lowest in countries or areas with high standards of living.

The HBV infection is a global problem, with 60 per cent of all the world's population living in areas where there are high levels of infection. The endemicity of active HBV infection is reflected in the serologic prevalence of the hepatitis B surface antigen (HBsAg) in the general population of a defined geographical area. HBsAg prevalence of ≥8% defines highly endemic areas, prevalence of 5%–7% defines high intermediate, 2%–4% low intermediate, and <2% defines low endemic areas.

WHO estimated that, in 2019, 296 million people were living with chronic hepatitis B infection (defined as hepatitis B surface antigen positive), including about 1.5 million people newly infected with the virus during that year. Hepatitis B prevalence is highest in the WHO African and Western Pacific regions where an estimated 7.5 per cent and 5.9 per cent, respectively, of the adult population have acquired the virus. Prevalence is lower in the South-East Asia (3.0%), Eastern Mediterranean (2.5%) and European regions (1.5%), and in the Region of the Americas (0.5%).

Only 30.4 million people with chronic hepatitis B infection knew their hepatitis B status and 6.6 million were receiving treatment. The infection caused an estimated 8,20,000 deaths in 2019, mostly from cirrhosis and hepatocellular carcinoma. Globally in 2019, 36,000 people died from acute hepatitis B *(2)*, with the South-East Asia Region accounting about one third of those deaths (12,600).

Safe and effective vaccines exist for preventing hepatitis B infection. Their widening use has reduced the global proportion of children under five years of age who are chronically infected with hepatitis B virus to just under 1 per cent in 2019, down from around 5 per cent from the 1980s to the early 2000s before vaccines were available.

Most of the burden of HBV-related disease results from infections acquired in infancy through perinatal or early childhood exposure to HBV because infection acquired at an early age is more likely to become chronic than infection acquired later in life. The risk of chronic infection remains high until after 5 years of age when the rate stabilizes at around 5%.

Co-infections with other viral infections occur most frequently in high HBV endemic areas. About 2.7 million of the 36.7 million people infected with HIV worldwide are co-infected with HBV. Approximately 10%–15% of patients with chronic HBV infection are co-infected with HCV. HDV infection occurs exclusively in HBV-infected individuals, as the virus is deficient, requiring HBV surface proteins to form its envelope in HDV/HBV co-infected hepatocytes. Approximately 5% of HBV-infected persons are infected with HDV *(14)*.

Major progress in the global response to viral hepatitis has been achieved through the expansion of routine hepatitis B vaccination, which was facilitated by the introduction of new combination vaccines. In 2015, global coverage with 3 doses of hepatitis B vaccine during infancy reached 84 per cent *(14)*. By the year 2015, 185 countries had incorporated hepatitis B vaccination in the national infant immunization schedule, and 97 countries had introduced the recommended birth dose. In the absence of the universal birth dose or other effective interventions, the transmission HBV infection from mother-to-child remains a major source of chronic liver disease when infected children become adults *(14)*.

HBV infection also causes a significant economic burden in terms of years of life lost from liver disease in high-income settings as well as in developing countries and accounts for 5–10 per cent of liver transplants *(13)*.

Epidemiological determinants

Agent factors

(a) AGENT : Hepatitis B virus was discovered by Blumberg in 1963. Efforts to grow this virus have been so far unsuccessful *(15)*. HBV is a complex, 42–nm, double–shelled DNA virus, originally known as the **"Dane particle".** It replicates in the liver cells. HBV occurs in three morphological forms in the serum of a patient: (a) small spherical particles with an average diameter of 22–nm. These particles are antigenic and stimulate production of surface antibodies; (b) tubules of varying length and diameter, and (c) the Dane particle which corresponds morphologically to hepatitis B virus. A person who is serologically positive for the surface antigen is circulating all morphological forms, of which 22–nm particles constitute the bulk. Of the three morphological forms, only the Dane particle is considered infectious, the other circulating morphological forms are not infectious.

(b) RESERVOIR OF INFECTION : Man is the only reservoir of infection which can be spread either from **carriers** or from **cases.** The continued survival of infection is due to the large number of individuals who are carriers of the virus. The persistent carrier state has been defined as the presence of HBsAg (with or without concurrent HBeAg) for more than 6 months. Cases may range from inapparent to symptomatic cases.

(c) INFECTIVE MATERIAL : Contaminated blood is the main source of infection, although the virus has been found in body secretions such as saliva, vaginal secretions and semen of infected persons.

(d) RESISTANCE : The virus is quite stable and capable of surviving for at least 7 days on environmental surfaces. It can be readily destroyed by sodium hypochlorite, as is by heat sterilization in an autoclave for 30 to 60 minutes.

(e) PERIOD OF COMMUNICABILITY : The virus is present in the blood during the incubation period (for a month before jaundice) and acute phase of the disease. Period of communicability is usually several months (occasionally years in chronic carriers) or until disappearance of HBsAg and appearance of surface antibody.

Host factors

(a) AGE : The outcomes of HBV infection are age-dependent. Acute hepatitis B occurs in approximately 1 per cent of perinatal, 10 per cent of early childhood (1–5 years of age), and 30 per cent of late (>5 years age) HBV infections. Mortality from fulminant hepatitis B is approximately 70 per cent. The development of chronic HBV infection is inversely related to age and occurs in approximately 80–90 per cent of persons infected perinatally, in 30–50 per cent infected in early childhood (less than 6 years of age) and in <5 per cent occurring in otherwise healthy adults *(14)*.

(b) HIGH-RISK GROUPS : Certain groups carry higher risks. The annual incidence of HBV infection in surgeons is estimated to be 50 times greater than that in the general population, and is more than twice that of other physicians. Other high risk groups comprise recipients of blood transfusions, health care and laboratory personnel, homosexuals, prostitutes, percutaneous drug abusers, infants of HBV carrier mothers, recipients of solid organ transplants and patients who are immunocompromised. Serological screening and vaccination of high-risk groups is highly recommended.

(c) HEPATITIS B AND HIV INFECTION : It is estimated that 10 per cent of the 40 million people infected with HIV worldwide are coinfected with HBV. Although HBV infection appears to have a minimal effect on the progression of HIV, the presence of HIV markedly increases the risk of developing HBV-associated liver cirrhosis and hepatocellular carcinoma. The mortality rate increases among HIV-positive people due to HBV coinfection both before and after commencement of highly active anti-retroviral therapy *(15)*.

(d) HUMORAL AND CELLULAR RESPONSES *(16)*: Hepatitis B virus has three distinct antigens – a surface antigen, also known as "Australia antigen" (HBsAg), a core antigen (HBcAg), and an "e" antigen (HBeAg). They stimulate the production of corresponding antibodies e.g., surface antibody (anti-HBs), core antibody (anti-HBc) and "e" antibody (anti-HBe). These antibodies and their antigens constitute very useful markers of HBV infection. Patients with HBV infection are expected to have one or more HBV markers. The course of a typical acute hepatitis is outlined in Fig. 2.

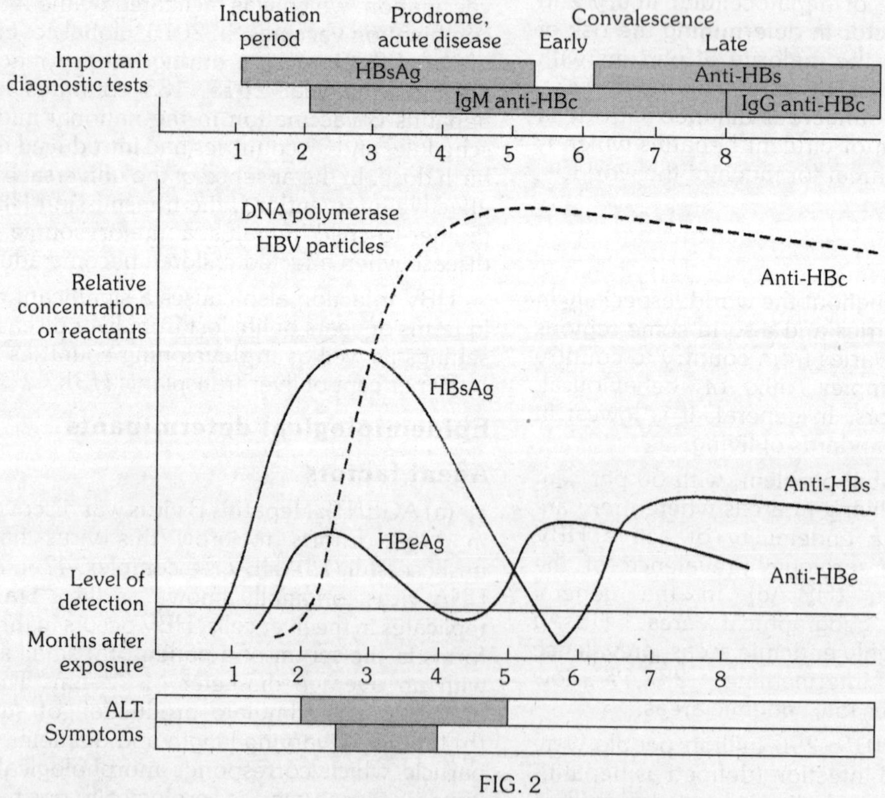

FIG. 2
Course of a typical acute hepatitis

ALT – alanine aminotransferase; anti-HBc – antibody to hepatitis B core antigen; anti-HBe – antibody to hepatitis Be antigen; anti-HBs – antibody to hepatitis B surface antigen; HBeAg – hepatitis B e antigen; HBsAg – hepatitis B surface antigen; HBV – hepatitis B virus; IgG – immunoglobulin G; IgM – immunoglobulin M.

Source : *(5)*

Modes of transmission

a. *Parenteral route*

Hepatitis B is essentially a blood-borne infection. It is transmitted by infected blood and blood products through transfusions, dialysis, contaminated syringes and needles, pricks of skin, handling of infected blood, accidental inoculation of minute quantities of blood such as may occur during surgical and dental procedures, immunization, traditional tattooing, ear piercing, nose piercing, ritual circumcision, accupuncture, etc. Accidental percutaneous inoculations by shared razors and tooth brushes have been implicated as occasional causes of hepatitis B *(13)*.

b. *Perinatal transmission*

Spread of infection from HBV carrier mothers to their babies appears to be an important factor for the high prevalence of HBV infection in some regions, particularly China and SE Asia. The risk of infection varies from country to country and unless vaccinated at birth, the majority of children born to mothers who are HBeAg–positive become chronically infected. The mechanism of perinatal infection is uncertain. Although HBV can infect the foetus *in utero*, this rarely happens and most infections appear to occur at birth, as a result of a leak of maternal blood into the baby's circulation, or ingestion or accidental inoculation of blood *(17)*. Infection of the baby is usually anicteric and is recognized by the appearance of surface antigen between 60–120 days after birth *(9)*.

c. *Sexual transmission*

There is ample evidence for the spread of infection by intimate contact or by sexual route. Various body fluids including saliva, vaginal, menstrual and seminal fluids have been implicated as vehicles of human transmission. The sexually promiscuous, particularly male homosexuals, are at very high risk of infection with hepatitis B.

d. *Other routes*

Transmission from child–to–child, often called horizontal transmission, is responsible for a majority of HBV infections and carriers in parts of the world other than Asia. The researchers believe that the spread occurs through physical contact between children with skin conditions such as cuts or grazes. Often transmission occurs when children play together or share the same bed *(18)*.

In short, transmission occurs in a wide variety of epidemiological settings. It can spread either from carriers or from people with no apparent infection, or during the incubation period, illness or early convalescence.

Incubation period

30 to 180 days. Lower doses of the virus result often in longer incubation period. The average incubation period is about 75 days *(15)*.

Clinical picture

The symptoms and manifestations of hepatitis B are similar to those of other types of viral hepatitis. The picture is complicated by the carrier state and by chronic liver disease, which may follow the infection. The spectrum of disease and natural history of chronic HBV infection are diverse. In some people, CHB is inactive and does not lead to significant liver disease. In others, it may cause progressive liver fibrosis, leading to cirrhosis with end-stage liver disease, and markedly increased risk of hepatocellular carcinoma, independent of the presence of cirrhosis – usually many years after initial infection. Longitudinal studies of untreated persons with CHB show 8–20 per cent cumulation risk of developing cirrhosis over 5 years. In those with cirrhosis, there is an approximately 20 per cent annual risk of hepatic decompensation and the annual incidence of hepatic B related HCC is high, ranging from 1 to 5 per cent. Untreated patients with decompensated cirrhosis have poor prognosis, with 15–40 per cent survival at 5 years. Several host and viral factors, especially coinfections with HIV, HCV and hepatitis D virus together with other cofactors such as alcohol use, may increase the rate of disease progression and risk of developing HCC *(13)*.

Diagnosis

There are three distinct antigen antibody systems that relate to HBV infection and a variety of circulating markers that are useful in diagnosis. The assays that detect the presence of either antigens or antibodies, typically in serum or plasma but also in capillary blood and oral fluid. These include rapid diagnostic tests (RDTs), and laboratory-based immunoassays. e.g. enzyme immunoassays (EIAs), chemiluminescence immunoassays (CLIAs), and electro-chemiluminescence immunoassays (ECLs). Interpretation of common serological patterns is as shown in Table 2.

TABLE 2

Common serologic patterns in hepatitis B virus infection and their interpretation

HBsAg	Anti-HBs	Anti-HBc	HBeAg	Anti-HBe	Interpretation
+	–	IgM	+	–	Acute hepatitis B
+	–	IgG[1]	+	–	Chronic hepatitis B with active viral replication
+	–	IgG	–	+	Chronic hepatitis B with low viral replication
+	+	IgG	+ or –	+ or –	Chronic hepatitis B with heterotypic anti-HBs (about 10% of cases)
–	–	IgM	+ or –	–	Acute hepatitis B
–	+	IgG	–	+ or –	Recovery from hepatitis B (immunity)
–	+	–	–	–	Vaccination (immunity)
–	–	IgG	–	–	False-positive, less commonly, infection in remote past

[1] Low levels of IgM anti-HBc may also be detected.

Source : *(16)*

PREVENTION AND CONTAINMENT

Since there is no specific treatment, prevention has been the major aim in managing viral hepatitis B. The following measures are available :

a. Hepatitis B vaccine

The recombinant hepatitis B vaccine was introduced in 1986 and has gradually replaced the plasma–derived hepatitis B vaccine. The active substance in recombinant hepatitis B vaccine is HBsAg.

Hepatitis B vaccine is available as monovalent formulation, or in fixed combination with other vaccines, including DPT, Hib, hepatitis A and inactivated polio. The immune response and safety of these combinations of vaccines are comparable to those observed when the vaccines are administered separately. When immunizing against HBV at birth, only monovalent hepatitis B vaccine should be used. Internationally marketed hepatitis B vaccines are considered immunologically comparable and can be used interchangeably *(19)*.

The dose for adults is 10–20 micrograms initially (depending on the formulation) and again at 1 and 6 months. Children under 10 years of age should be given half of the adult dose at the same time intervals. For greatest reliability of absorption, the deltoid muscle is preferred for injection as gluteal injection often results in deposition of vaccine in fat rather than muscle, with fewer serologic conversion. For infants and children under 2 years, anterolateral aspect of thigh is used as vaccination site. Intradermal administration is not recommended because the immune response is less reliable particularly in children. The hepatitis B vaccine does not interfere with immune response to any other vaccine and vice-versa. The birth dose of hepatitis B can be given safely together with BCG vaccine. However, the vaccines should be given at different sites.

There are multiple options for incorporating the hepatitis B vaccine into national immunization programmes. The choice of schedule depends on the local epidemiological situation and programme considerations. The recommended schedule for vaccination can be divided into those that include a birth-dose and those that do not. Schedules with a birth-dose call for the first dose at birth, followed by a second dose and third dose at the time of the first and third dose of DPT vaccination respectively. Alternatively, a four-dose schedule may be used (as in India) where the dose at birth is followed by three additional doses at 6, 10 and 14 weeks with DPT vaccination. These doses may be given either as monovalent vaccine or as a combination (eg. with DPT and/or Hib) following the schedules commonly used for these vaccines. The minimum recommended interval between the doses is four weeks. Longer dose intervals may increase the final anti-HBs titres but not the sero-conversion rates. These schedules will prevent most perinatally acquired infection. In countries where a high proportion of HBV infection is acquired perinatally, specifically in countries where the prevalence in the general population of chronic HBV infection is more than 8 per cent, the first dose of hepatitis B vaccine should be given within 24 hours after birth to prevent perinatal transmission *(20)*.

The complete vaccine series induces protective antibody levels in more than 95 per cent of infants, children and young adults. After the age of 40 years, protection following the primary vaccination series drops below 90 per cent; by 60 years, protective antibody levels are achieved in only 65–75 per cent of the vaccinees. The duration of protection is at least 15 years and based on current scientific evidence, life long *(20)*. Some infants born prematurely with low birth weight (< 2000 g) may not respond well to vaccination at birth. However, by one month of chronological age, all premature infants, regardless of initial birth weight or gestational age, are likely to respond adequately. In such cases the vaccine dose given at birth should not be counted towards the primary series and 3 additional doses should be given according to the national immunization schedule *(15)*. Immunosuppressive illness such as advanced HIV infection, chronic liver disease, chronic renal failure, and diabetes are associated with reduced immunogenicity of the vaccine.

Data on immunogenecity suggest that in any age group, interruption of the vaccination schedule does not require restarting of the vaccine series. If the primary series is interrupted after the first dose, the second dose should be administered as soon as possible and the second and the third doses separated by a minimum interval of 4 weeks; if only the third dose is delayed, it should be administered as soon as possible *(15)*.

Immunization in adults : Routine pre-exposure vaccination should be considered for groups of adults who are at increased risk of HBV infection. Adults 20 years of age and older should receive 1 ml of adult formulation. The usual schedule for adults is two doses separated by no less than 4 weeks, and a third dose 4 to 6 months after the second dose. If an accelerated schedule is needed, the minimum interval between first and second dose is 4 weeks and the minimum interval between the second and third dose is 8 weeks. However, the first and the third doses should be separated by no less than 16 weeks. Doses given at less than these minimum intervals should not be counted as part of the vaccination series. It is not necessary to restart the series or add doses because of an extended interval between doses *(8)*.

The high-risk persons for whom the vaccination is recommended are persons with high-risk sexual behaviour, partners and household contacts of HBsAg–positive persons, injecting drug users, persons who frequently require blood or blood products, recipients of solid organ transplantation, those at occupational risk of HBV infection, including health care workers, as well as for international travellers to HBV endemic countries.

Hepatitis B vaccine is contraindicated for individuals with a history of allergic reactions to any of the vaccine's components. Neither pregnancy nor lactation is a contraindication for use of this vaccine *(20)*.

The vaccine should be stored at 2–8°C. Freezing must be avoided as it dissociates antigen from the alum adjuvant.

Pentavalent Vaccine

It is a combined vaccine giving protection against diphtheria, pertussis, tetanus, hepatitis B and Hib. Kindly refer to page 181 for details.

b. Hepatitis B immunoglobulin (HBIG)

For immediate protection, HBIG is used for those acutely exposed to HBsAg–positive blood, for example (a) surgeons, nurses or laboratory workers (b) newborn infants of carrier mothers (c) sexual contacts of acute hepatitis B patients, and (d) patients who need protection against HBV infection after liver transplantation. The HBIG should be given as soon as possible after an accidental inoculation (ideally within 6 hours and preferably not later than 48 hours). At the same time the victim's blood is drawn for HBsAg testing. If the test is negative, vaccination should be started immediately and a full course given. If the test is positive for surface antibody, no further action is needed *(21)*.

The recommended dose is 0.05 to 0.07 ml/kg of body weight *(22)*; two doses should be given 30 days apart *(22, 23)*. HBIG provides short-term passive protection which lasts approximately 3 months. Since the median incubation period is said to be lower than 100 days *(24)*, two doses of HBIG given one month apart should suffice. The general use of HBIG for long-term prophylaxis has not been recommended because of its limited availability, its high cost and risk (although remote) of complications through repeated use over a long period of time *(25)*.

c. Passive–active immunization

The simultaneous administration of HBIG and hepatitis B vaccine is more efficacious than HBIG alone. HBIG does not interfere with the antibody response to the hepatitis B vaccine. This combined procedure is ideal both for prophylaxis of persons accidentally exposed to blood known to contain hepatitis B virus, and for prevention of the carrier state in the newborn babies of carrier mothers. HBIG (0.05–0.07 ml/kg) should be given as soon as possible and within 24 hours, if possible. Hepatitis B virus vaccine 1.0 ml (20 mcg/1.0 ml) should be given intramuscularly within 7 days of exposure, and second and third doses should be given one and six months, respectively, after the first dose.

d. Other measures

All blood donors should be screened for HBV infection, and those positive for HBsAg also known as Australia antigen should be rejected. Voluntary blood donation should be encouraged because purchased blood has shown a higher risk of post–transfusion hepatitis *(8)*. Health personnel should be alerted to the importance of adequate sterilization of all instruments and to the practice of simple hygienic measures. Carriers should be told not to share razors or tooth brushes and use barrier methods of contraception; they should not donate blood.

Most international guidelines recommend that several high-risk groups be screened for HBsAg, and that those at risk and not immune should be offered hepatitis B vaccination. These include: household and sexual contacts of persons with CHB, HIV-infected persons, persons who inject drugs (PWID), men who have sex with men, sex workers, as well as other groups such as indigenous people, persons who are imprisoned, and persons of transgender. Blood and organ donors should also be screened for HBsAg and other bloodborne pathogens in accordance with WHO recommendations to prevent HBV transmission *(13)*.

Treatment

There is no specific treatment for acute hepatitis B. Care is aimed at maintaining comfort and adequate nutritional balance, including replacement of fluids lost from vomiting and diarrhoea.

CHRONIC HEPATITIS B AND HEPATITIS C INFECTION

Chronic HBV infection is defined as persistence of hepatitis B surface antigen (HBsAg) for six months or more after acute infection with HBV. Worldwide, there are an estimated 257 million people living with chronic HBV infection and 110 million persons are HCV-antibody positive, and 80 million have chronic viraemic HCV infection.

Despite the high global burden of disease due to chronic hepatitis B and C infection, and the advances and opportunities for treatment, most people infected with HBV and/or HCV remain unaware of their infection and therefore frequently present with advance disease. Early identification of the infection would enable infected persons to receive the necessary care and treatment to prevent or delay the onset of liver disease and in addition, prevent transmission by HBV vaccination of the non-immune household contacts and sex partners *(26)*.

The WHO "5Cs"

The WHO "5Cs" are principles that apply to all models of hepatitis testing and in all settings : Consent, Confidentiality, Correct test results, Counselling and Connection (linkage to prevention, treatment and care services). This means hepatitis testing for diagnosis must always be voluntary, and consent for testing informed by pre-test information *(26)*.

Fig. 3 and 4 show summary algorithm for diagnosis, treatment and monitoring of chronic HBV and HCV infection respectively.

Chronic hepatitis B infection can be treated with drugs. Treatment can slow the progression of cirrhosis, reduce incidence of liver cancer and improve long term survival. WHO recommends the use of oral treatments - tenofovir or entecavir, as these are the most potent drugs to suppress hepatitis B virus. They rarely lead to drug resistance as compared with other drugs, are simple to take (1 pill a day), and have few side effects so require only limited monitoring. In most people, however, the treatment only supresses the replication of the virus. Therefore, people who start hepatitis B treatment must continue it for life. Treatment using interferon injections may be considered in some people in certain high-income settings, as this may shorten treatment duration. But its use is less feasible in low-resource settings due to high cost and significant adverse effects requiring careful monitoring *(27)*.

In March 2015, WHO launched its first "Guidelines for the prevention, care and treatment of persons living with chronic hepatitis B infection". The recommendations are *(27)* :

- promote the use of simple, non-invasive diagnostic tests to assess the stage of liver disease and eligibility for treatment;
- prioritize treatment for those with most advanced liver disease and at greatest risk of mortality; and
- recommend the preferred use of the nucleotide/nucleoside analogues with a high barrier to drug resistance (tenofovir and entecavir, and entecavir in children aged between 2–11 years) for first and second-line treatment.

These guidelines also recommend lifelong treatment in those with cirrhosis; and regular monitoring for disease progression, toxicity of drugs and early detection of liver cancer *(27)*.

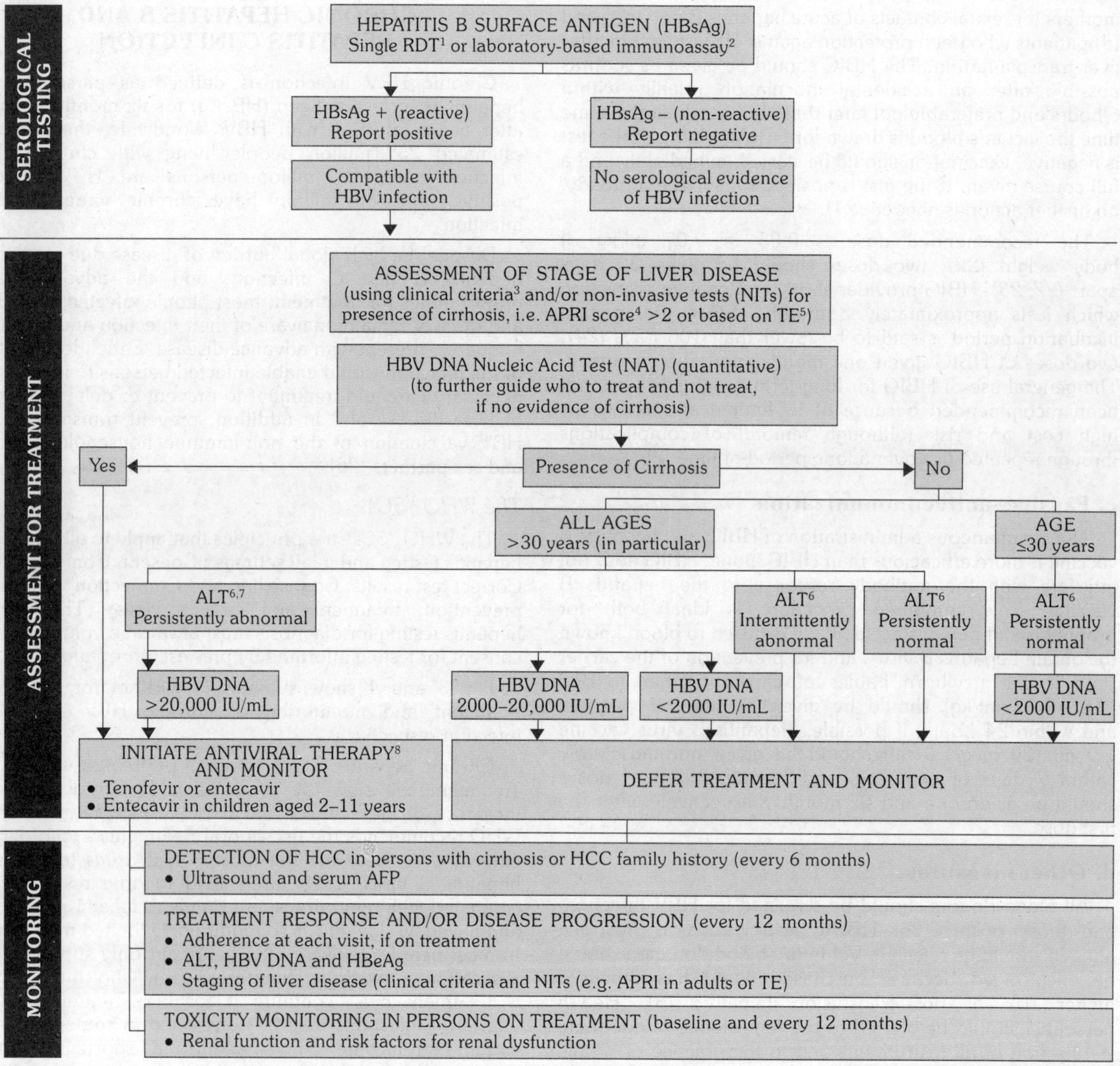

FIG. 3

Summary algorithm for diagnosis, treatment and monitoring of chronic HBV infection

Abbreviations : RDT: rapid diagnostic test; ALT: alanine aminotranferase: APRI: aspartase aminotransferase-to-platelet ratio index; TE: transient elastography; HCC: hepatocellular carcinoma: AFP: apha fetoprotein

[1] In settings or populations with a low HBsAg seroprevalence <0.4%, confirmation of HBsAg positivity on the same immunoassay with a neutralization step or a second different RDT assay for detection of HBsAg may be considered.

[2] Laboratory-based Immunoassays include enzyme immunoassay (EIA), chemoluminescence immunoassay (CLIA), and electrochemoluminescence assay (ECL)

[3] Decompensated cirrhosis is defined by the development of portal hypertension (ascites, variceal haemorrhage and hepatic encephalopathy), coagulopathy, or liver insufficiency (jaundice). Other clinical features of advanced liver disease/cirrhosis may include: hepatomegaly, splenomegaly, pruritus, fatigue, arthralgia, palmar erythema, and oedema.

[4] Aspartate aminotransferase (AST)-to-platelet ratio index (APRI) is a simple index for estimating hepatic fibrosis based on a formula derived from AST and platelet concentrations.
The formula for calculating the APRI score is : APRI = (AST/AST ULN) x 100)/platelet count (10^9/L). Most recommend using 40 IU/L as the value for AST upper limit of normal (ULN).

[5] Transient elastography (Fibroscan): a technique to measure liver stiffness (as a surrogate for fibrosis)

[6] ALT levels fluctuate in persons with chronic hepatitis B and require longitudinal monitoring to determine the trend. Upper limits for normal ALT have been defined as below 30 U/L for men and 19 U/L for women, though local laboratory normal ranges should be applied. Persistently normal/abnormal may be defined as three ALT determinations below or above the upper limit or normal, made at unspecified intervals during a 6–12 month period or predefined intervals during a 12 month period.

[7] Where HBV DNA testing is not available, treatment may be considered based on persistently abnormal ALT levels, such as impaired glucose tolerance, dyslipidaemia and fatty liver should be excluded.

[8] Initiate antiviral therapy with tenofovir alone only after exclusion of HIV coinfection.

Source : *(26)*

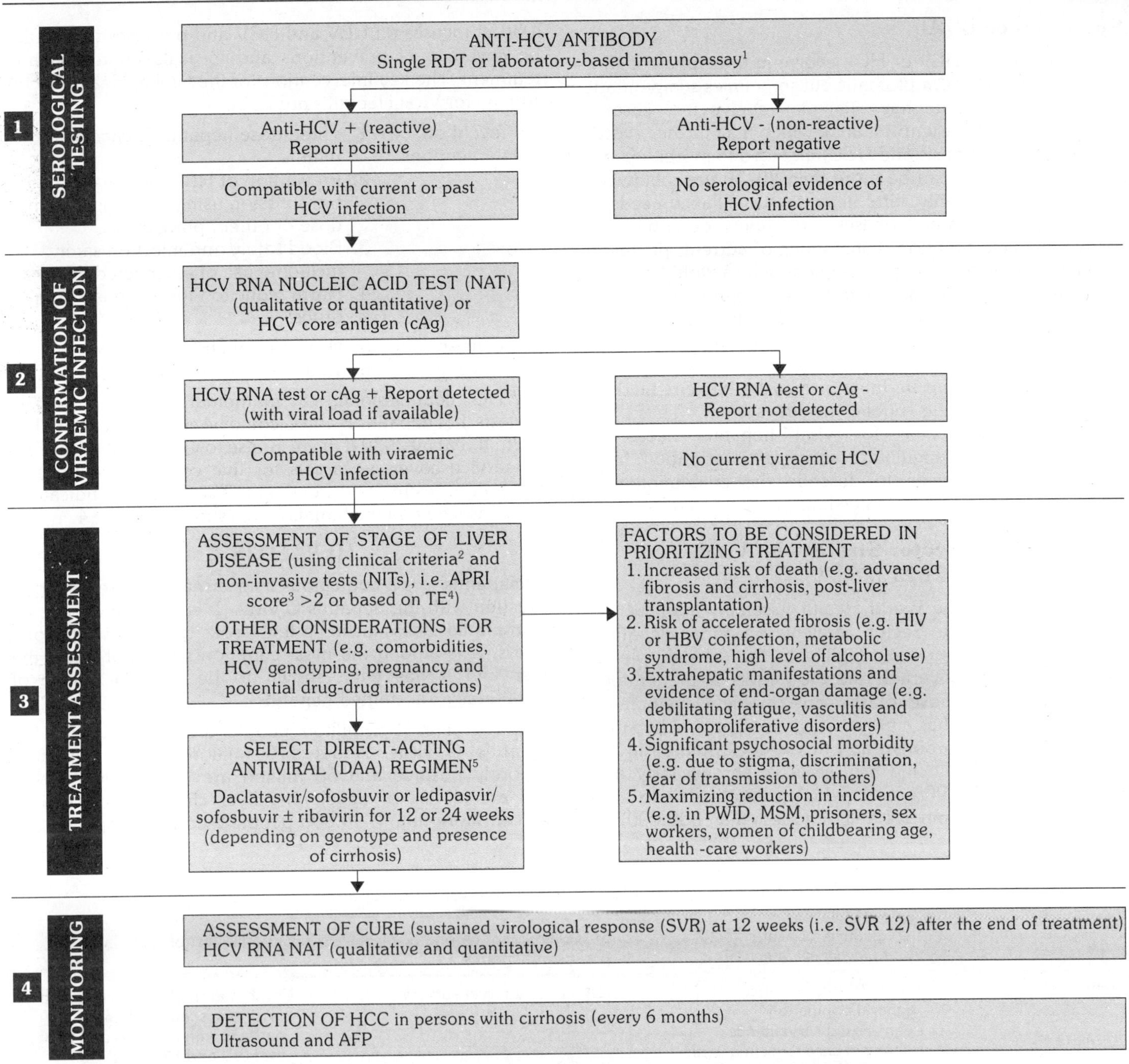

FIG. 4

Summary algorithm for diagnosis, treatment and monitoring of chronic HCV infection

Abbreviations: RDT: rapid diagnostic test: APRI: aspartase aminotransferase-to-platelet ratio index, TE: transient elastography; PWID: people who inject drugs; MSM: men who have sex with men; HCC: hepatocellular carcinoma; AFP: alpha fetoprotein

1 Laboratory-based immunoassays include enzyme immunoassay (EIA), chemoluminescence immunoassay (CLIA), and electrochemoluminescence assay (ECL).

2 Decompensated cirrhosis is defined by the development of portal hypertension (ascites, variceal haemorrhage and hepatic encephalopathy), coagulopathy , or liver insufficiency (jaundice). Other clinical features of advanced liver disease/cirrhosis may include: hepatomegaly, splenomegaly, pruritus, fatigue, arthralgia, palmar erythema, and oedema.

3 Aspartate aminotransferase (AST)-to-platelet ratio index (APRI) is a simple index for estimating hepatic fibrosis based on a formula derived from AST and platelet concentrations. The formula for calculating the APRI score is: APRI = (AST/AST ULN) x 100)/platelet count (10^9/L). Most recommend using 40 IU/L as the value for AST upper limit of normal (ULN).

4 Transient elastography (Fibroscan) is a technique to measure liver stiffness (as a surrogate for fibrosis).

5 Caution: there is a potential but uncertain risk of HBV reactivation during or after HCV clearance. Prior to starting DAA therapy, test for HBV infection (HBsAg, HBeAg, and HBV DNA) to assess indication for HBV treatment. Continue careful monitoring after completion of DAA therapy, including for HCC.

Source : *(26)*

Surveillance *(27A)*

Infections with HBV or HCV evolve in three phases. New infections (mostly asymptomatic but sometimes symptomatic in the form of acute hepatitis) may evolve into chronic infections (usually asymptomatic), which may further evolve into sequelae (cirrhosis and HCC) that lead to morbidity and mortality. As there can be more than 20–30 years between infection and mortality, viral hepatitis surveillance needs to capture these three phases to fully describe the epidemiological situation. Estimations of current, prevalent infections guide testing and treatment, which would prevent future morbidity and mortality. Current mortality from the sequelae of chronic infections acquired in the past quantifies the baseline burden and evaluates the impact of past interventions. The three components of viral hepatitis surveillance as shown in Table 3, may be implemented by different acts of the public health system. Thus, the programme responsible for viral hepatitis needs to consolidate and triangulate sources of information from these different systems to describe the epidemiological situation of HBV and HCV infection.

Global Health Sector Strategy on Viral Hepatitis 2016–2021 *(28, 29)*

In May 2016, The World Health Assembly adopted the first "Global Health Sector Strategy on Viral Hepatitis, 2016–2021". The strategy highlights the critical role of Universal Health Coverage and the targets of the strategy are aligned with those of the Sustainable Development Goals. The strategy has a vision of eliminating viral hepatitis as a public health problem and this is encapsulated in the global targets of reducing new cases of chronic HBV and HCV infections by 90% and reducing deaths due to viral hepatitis by 65% (from 1.4 million to less than 500,000) by 2030. It focuses on HBV and HCV and proposes to increase the coverage of preventions and to scale up testing and treatment. The key interventions of the Global Health Sector strategy for Viral Hepatitis are :

Prevention Interventions
1. Three-dose hepatitis B vaccine for infants.
2. Prevention of HBV mother-to-child transmission using hepatitis B birth dose or other approaches.
3. Blood safety and injection safety, including use of engineered devices.
4. Harm reduction for persons who use drugs.

Treatment Interventions
5. Diagnosis of HBV and HCV.
6. Treatment of HBV and HCV.

WHO commissioned a mathematical model, which suggests that hepatitis B and C could be eliminated as a public health threat by 2030 if the response to viral hepatitis reaches the service coverage targets for five core interventions of prevention, testing and treatment. The standard indicators, 2015 baseline and the targets are as shown in Table 4.

HEPATITIS C

Hepatitis C is a contagious liver disease that results from infection with the hepatitis C virus. It can range in severity from a mild illness lasting a few weeks to a serious, lifelong illness. It is among the most common virus that infect the liver and it has been shown to be a major cause of parenterally transmitted hepatitis.

Every year, 1.5 million people are infected with the hepatitis C virus. About 110 million people are HCV antibody positive and 58 million are chronically infected and are at risk of developing liver cirrhosis and/or liver cancer. More than 2,90,000 people died from hepatitis C –

TABLE 3

Activities that contribute to surveillance for viral hepatitis

	1. Surveillance for acute hepatitis that reflects new infections	2. Surveillance for chronic, prevalent hepatitis	3. Surveillance for sequelae
Activities	– Syndromic surveillance in the general population – Event-based surveillance – Enhanced case reporting (with in-vitro diagnosis and collection of information on risk factors)	– Regular biomarker surveys	– Combination of data from death certificates, and testing of patients with cirrhosis and HCC for HBV and HCV infection
Population under surveillance	– Persons presenting with acute hepatitis to health-care facilities (discrete onset of symptoms)	– Persons without acute symptoms tested during population surveys	– Persons diagnosed with cirrhosis and HCC
Usual implementer	– Communicable disease surveillance – Communicable disease surveillance (if countrywide) – Hepatitis programme (if sentinel sites)	– Hepatitis programme in coordination with the other actors implementing biomarker surveys	– Vital registration – Sentinel sites caring for patients with cirrhosis and HCC – Cancer registries
Case definitions to use	– Presumptive case of acute hepatitis – Confirmed case of acute hepatitis (by type)	– Chronic HBV and HCV infection – Serological evidence of past or present HCV infection	– Cases of cirrhosis or HCC – Chronic HBV or HCV infection
Objective of the surveillance activity	– Detect outbreaks – Describe trends in type-specific acute hepatitis and identify risk factors	– Estimate the prevalence of infections – Model incidence trends	– Estimate mortality from HBV- or HCV-associated HCC and cirrhosis

HBV: hepatitis B virus; HCC: hepatocellular carcinoma; HCV: hepatitis C virus

Source : *(27A)*

TABLE 4
Service coverage indicators : 2015 baseline and targets

Level	Areas	Indicators	Baseline 2015	2020 target	2030 target
Service coverage	Prevention	1. Three-dose hepatitis B vaccine for infants (coverage %)	82%	90%	90%
		2. Prevention of mother-to-child transmission of HBV: hepatitis B birth-dose vaccination or other approaches (coverage %)	38%	50%	90%
		3a. Blood safety: donations screened with quality assurance (coverage %)	89%	95%	100%
		3b. Injection safety: use of engineered devices (coverage %)*	5%	50%	90%
		4. Harm reduction (sterile syringe/needle sets distributed per person per year for PWID)	20	200	300
	Testing and treatment	5a. Diagnosis of HBV and HCV (coverage %)	<5%	30%	90%
		5b. Treatment of HBV and HCV (coverage %)	<1%	5 million (HBV) 3 million (HCV)	80% eligible treated
Impact leading to elimination	Incidence	Incidence of chronic HBV and HCV infections	6–10 million	–30%	–90%
	Mortality	Mortality from chronic HBV and HCV infections	1.46 million	–10%	–65%

HBV: hepatitis B virus; HCV: hepatitis C virus; PWID: persons who inject drugs

* While the service coverage target is about output (adoption of reuse-prevention injection devices), the C.5 indicator focusses on outcome (provision of safe injections).

Source : *(27A)*

related liver diseases in 2019. It is estimated that about 2.3 million people were co-infected with HCV and HIV *(31)*.

Transmission

The hepatitis C virus is most commonly transmitted through exposure to infectious blood. This can occur through: (a) receipt of contaminated blood transfusions, blood products and organ transplants; (b) injections given with contaminated syringes and needle-stick injuries in health-care settings; (c) injection drug use; and (d) being born to a hepatitis C-infected mother.

Hepatitis C may be transmitted through sex with an infected person or sharing of personal items contaminated with infectious blood, but these are less common. Hepatitis C is not spread through breast milk, food or water, or by casual contact such as hugging, kissing and sharing food or drinks with an infected person.

Incubation period

The incubation period for hepatitis C is 2 weeks to 6 months.

Symptoms

Following initial infection, approximately 80 per cent of people do not exhibit any symptoms. Those people who are acutely symptomatic may exhibit fever, fatigue, decreased appetite, nausea, vomiting, abdominal pain, dark urine, grey-coloured faeces, joint pain and jaundice. About 15–45 per cent of infected persons spontaneously clear the virus within 6 months of infection without any treatment. The remaining 55–85 per cent of persons will develop chronic HCV infection. Of those with chronic HCV infection, the risk of cirrhosis of liver is 15–30 per cent within 20 years *(31)*.

Diagnosis *(32)*

Diagnosis of acute infection is often missed because a majority of infected people have no symptoms. Common methods of antibody detection cannot differentiate between acute and chronic infection. The presence of antibodies against the hepatitis C virus indicates that a person is or has been infected. The hepatitis C virus recombinant immunoblot assay (RIBA) and hepatitis C virus RNA testing are used to confirm the diagnosis. Diagnosis of chronic infection is made when antibodies to the hepatitis C virus are present in the blood for more than six months. Similar to acute infections, diagnosis is confirmed with an additional test. Specialized tests are often used to evaluate patients for liver disease, including cirrhosis and liver cancer

Early diagnosis can prevent health problems that may result from infection and prevent transmission to family members and other close contacts. Some countries recommend screening for people who may be at risk for infection. These include: (a) people who recevied blood, blood products or organs before screening for hepatitis C virus was implemented, or where screening was not yet widespread. (b) current or former injecting drug users (even those who injected drugs once many years ago); (c) people on long-term haemodialysis; (d) health–care workers; (e) people living with HIV; (f) people with abnormal liver tests or liver disease, and (g) infants born to infected mothers; people having invasive procedures in health care facilities with inadequate infection control; people who have had tattoos and piercings; and people with sexual partners who are HCV infected *(31)*.

Treatment *(31)*

Hepatitis C does not always require treatment as the immune response in some people will clear the infection, and some people with chronic infection do not develop liver damage. When treatment is necessary, the goal of hepatitis C treatment is cure. The cure rate depends on several factors including the strain of the virus and the type of treatment given. The standard of care for hepatitis C is changing rapidly. Until recently, hepatitis C treatment was based on therapy with interferon and ribavirin, which required weekly injections for 48 weeks, cured approximately half of treated patients, but caused frequent and sometimes life-threatening adverse reactions. Recently, new antiviral drugs have been developed. These medicines, called direct antiviral agents (DAA) are much more effective, safer and better-tolerated than the older therapies. Therapy with DAAs can cure most persons with HCV infection and treatment is shorter (usually 12 weeks) and safer. Although the production cost of DAAs is low, these medicines remain very expensive in many high- and middle-income countries. The cost of generic version of these medicines are low.

Prevention

Primary prevention

1. Hand hygiene: including surgical hand preparation, hand washing and use of gloves;
2. Safe and appropriate use of health care injections;
3. Safe handling and disposal of sharps and waste;
4. Provision of comprehensive harm-reduction services to people who inject drugs including sterile injecting equipment;
5. Testing of donated blood for hepatitis B and C;
6. Training of health personnel; and
7. Promotion of correct and consistent use of condoms.

Secondary and tertiary prevention

For people infected with the hepatitis C virus, WHO recommends:

- education and counselling on options for care and treatment;
- immunization with the hepatitis A and B vaccines to prevent coinfection from these hepatitis viruses to protect their liver,
- early and appropriate medical management including antiviral therapy if appropriate; and
- regular monitoring for early diagnosis of chronic liver disease.

For a number of technical reasons, the development of a vaccine to prevent HCV infection is unlikely for many years.

The epidemiologic and clinical features of hepatitis A, hepatitis B and hepatitis C are summarized in Table 5.

HEPATITIS E

The infection caused by the hepatitis E virus (HEV) which was discovered in 1980, is essentially a water-borne disease. Formerly termed enterically transmitted hepatitis non–A, non–B (HNANB), HEV is a 29–nm to 32–nm RNA virus with 4 genotypes (type 1, 2, 3 and 4).

TABLE 5

Epidemiologic and clinical features of viral hepatitis types A, B and C

	Viral Hepatitis Type A	Viral Hepatitis Type B	Viral Hepatitis Type C
Incubation period	10–50 days (avg. 25–30)	50–180 days (avg. 60–90)	2 weeks–6 months (avg. 40–120 days)
Principal age distribution	Children[1], young adults	15–29 years[2]	Adults[2]
Seasonal incidence	Throughout the year but tends to peak in autumn	Throughout the year	Throughout the year
Route of infection	Predominantly faecal-oral	Predominantly parenteral	Predominantly parenteral
Occurrence of virus :			
Blood	2 weeks before to ≤ 1 week after jaundice	Months to years	Months to years
Stool	2 weeks before to 2 weeks after jaundice	Absent	Probably absent
Urine	Rare	Absent	Probably absent
Saliva, semen	Rare (saliva)	Frequently present	Unknown
Clinical and laboratory features :			
Onset	Abrupt	Insidious	Insidious
Fever > 38°C (100.4°F)	Common	Less common	Less common
Duration of aminotransferase elevation	1–3 weeks	1–6+ months	1–6+ months
Immunoglobulins (IgM levels)	Elevated	Normal to slightly elevated	Normal to slightly elevated
Complications	Uncommon, no chronicity	Chronicity in 5–10%	Chronicity in 50% or more
Mortality rate (icteric cases)	< 0.5%	< 1–2%	0.5–1%
HBsAg	Absent	Present	Absent
Immunity :			
Homologous	Yes	Yes	?
Heterologous	No	No	No
Duration	Probably lifetime	Probably lifetime	?
Immune globulin intramuscular (IG, gammaglobulin, ISG)	Regularly prevents jaundice	Prevents jaundice only if immunoglobulin is of sufficient potency against HBV	?

[1] Non-icteric hepatitis is common in children.

[2] Among the age group 15-29 years, hepatitis B and C are often associated with drug abuse or promiscuous sexual behaviour. Patients with transfusion-associated HBV or HCV are generally over age 29.

Source : *(5)*

Hepatitis E is found worldwide and different genotypes of the hepatitis E virus determine differences in epidemiology. For example, genotype 1 is usually seen in developing countries and causes community-level outbreaks while genotype 3 is usually seen in the developed countries, and does not cause outbreaks. Hepatitis E prevalence is highest in East and South Asia with genotype 1 most commonly found in India. Countries with limited resources, i.e., limited access to essential water, sanitation, hygiene and health services are frequently affected. In recent years, some of these outbreaks have occurred in areas of conflict and humanitarian emergencies, such as war zones, and in camps for refugees or internally displaced populations. An estimated 20 million infections and 3.3 million acute cases occur annually worldwide. An estimated 44,000 deaths occurred in 2015 *(33)*. Over 60 per cent of all hepatitis E infections and 65 per cent of hepatitis deaths occur in East and South Asia, where seroprevalence rate of 25 per cent are common in some age groups *(34)*.

Transmission

The hepatitis E virus is transmitted mainly through the faecal-oral route, due to faecal contamination of drinking water. Other transmission routes have been identified, which include : (a) food-borne transmission from ingestion of products derived from infected animals; (b) transfusion of infected blood products; and (c) vertical transmission from a pregnant woman to her foetus.

Incubation period

The incubation period following exposure to the hepatitis E virus ranges from three to eight weeks, with a mean of 40 days. The period of communicability is unknown.

Symptoms

Symptomatic infection is more common in young adults aged 15–40 years. Although infection is frequent in children, the disease is mostly asymptomatic or causes a very mild illness without jaundice that goes undiagnosed. The typical symptoms are jaundice, loss of appetite, abdominal pain and tenderness, nausea and vomiting, fever and enlarged and tender liver. The symptoms are largely indistinguishable from those experienced during any acute phase of hepatic illness and last for one or two weeks.

In rare cases, acute hepatitis E can result in fulminant hepatitis (acute liver failure) and death. Fulminant hepatitis occurs more frequently during pregnancy. Pregnant women are at greater risk of obstetrical complications and mortality from hepatitis E, which can induce a mortality rate of 20 per cent among pregnant women in their third trimester.

Cases of chronic hepatitis E infection have been reported in immunosuppressed people. Reactivation of hepatitis E infection has also been reported in immunocompromised people.

Diagnosis

Cases of hepatitis E are not clinically distinguishable from other types of acute viral hepatitis. Diagnosis of hepatitis E infection is, therefore, usually based on the detection of specific IgM and IgG antibodies to the virus in the blood. Additional tests include reverse transcriptase polymerase chain reaction (RT-PCR) to detect the hepatitis E virus RNA in blood and/or stool, but this assay may require specialized laboratory facilities.

Treatment

Hepatitis E is usually self-limiting. Prevention is the most effective approach against the disease as there is no specific treatment for altering the course of acute hepatitis. Hospitalization is required for fulminant cases and in symptomatic pregnant women. Recovery from disease is always complete. No specific immunoglobulin prophylaxis is available.

Prevention

The risk of infection and transmission can be reduced by maintaining quality standards for public water supplies and establishing proper disposal systems to eliminate sanitary waste. On an individual level, infection risk can be reduced by : (a) maintaining hygienic practices such as hand washing with safe water, particularly before handling food; (b) avoiding drinking water and/or ice of unknown purity; and (c) adhering to WHO safe food practices.

In 2011, the first vaccine to prevent hepatitis E infection was registered in China, although it is not available globally.

HEPATITIS D *(35)*

Hepatitis D is caused by hepatitis D virus that requires HBV for its replication. Hepatitis D cannot occur in the absence of HBV. The coinfection or super infection of HDV with HBV causes a more severe disease than HBV monoinfection.

Geographic distribution

It is estimated that globally, 5% of HBsAg positive people are coinfected with HDV and the distribution is resulting in a total of 15–20 million persons infected with HDV world-wide. High-prevalence areas include the Mediterranean, Middle East, Pakistan, Central and Northern Asia, Japan, Taiwan, Greenland and parts of Africa (mainly the horn of Africa and West Africa), the Amazon Basin and certain areas of the Pacific. Prevalence is low in North America and Northern Europe, South Africa, and Eastern Asia.

Route of transmission

The route of HDV transmission are the same as for HBV: percutaneously or sexually through contact with infected blood or blood products. Vertical transmission is possible but rare. Vaccination against HBV prevents HDV coinfection, and hence expansion of childhood HBV immunization programmes has resulted in a decline in hepatitis D incidence worldwide. However, in some settings, the increase of hepatitis D prevalence has been observed in people who inject drugs, or as a result of migration from areas where HDV is endemic.

Diagnosis

HDV infection is diagnosed by high titres of Immunoglobulin G (IgG) and Immunoglobulin M (IgM) anti-HDV, and confirmed by detection of HDV RNA in serum.

However, HDV diagnostics are not widely available and there is no standardization for HDV RNA assays, which are used for monitoring response to antiviral therapy.

Treatment

There is no specific treatment for acute or chronic HDV infection. Persistent HDV replication is the most important predictor of mortality and the need for antiviral therapy. *Pegylated* interferon alpha is the only drug effective against HDV; antiviral nucleotide analogues for HBV have no or limited effect on HDV replication. The optimal duration of therapy is not well defined, nor how long patients need to be HDV RNA negative after the end of therapy to achieve a sustained virological response. More than 1 year of therapy may be necessary.

The overall rate of sustained virological response remains low, including in children, and most patients relapse after discontinuation of therapy. Liver transplantation may be considered for cases of fulminant hepatitis and end-stage liver disease. New therapeutic agents and strategies are needed, and novel drugs, such as prenylation inhibitor or HBV entry inhibitors, have shown early promise.

Prevention

Prevention and control of HDV infection requires prevention of HBV transmission through hepatitis B immunization, blood safety, injection safety, and harm reduction services. Hepatitis B immunization does not provide protection against HDV for those already HBV infected.

HEPATITIS G

Hepatitis G virus HGV was discovered in 1996. The prevalence of this infection is still not known. A few publications provide information on the association of this infection with blood transfusion in India *(16)*.

The nomenclature and definitions used in the disease are shown in Table 6.

References

1. WHO (2014), *Fact Sheet Hepatitis A*, No. 328, June 2014.
2. WHO (2022), *Fact sheet*, 24th June 2022.
3. WHO (1989), *Techn.Rep.Ser.* No.784 Page 25.
4. Change, S.L. *Bull WHO* : 38, 401–414.
5. Jawetz et al (2013), *Medical Microbiology*, 26th ed., 2013, A Lange Medical Book.
6. Dientardt, F. (1983). *WHO Chr* 37 (6) 203–207.
7. Weller, Ian. (1984), *Brit Med.J.*, 288 : 47–49.
8. Centre for Disease Control and Prevention (2012), *Epidemiology and Prevention of Vaccine, Preventable Diseases*, 12th ed., May 2012.
9. WHO (1977), *Techn.Rep.Ser.* No : 602.
10. WHO (2012), *Weekly Epidemiological Record*, No. 28-29, 13th July 2012.
11. Jawetz, J.L. (2019), *Review of Medical Microbiology*, 28th ed, Lange Medical Publications, California.
12. *JAMA*, 1975 : 233 : 1316.
13. WHO (2016), *Guidelines for prevention care and treatment of persons with chronic hepatitis B infection*, March 2016.
14. WHO (2017), *Weekly Epidemiological Record*, 7th July 2017.
15. WHO (2009), *Weekly Epidemiological Record*, No. 40, 2nd Oct. 2009.
16. Lawrence M. Tierney, Jr., Stephen J. McPhee, and Maxine A. Papadakis, *Current Medical Diagnosis and Treatment*, 49th Ed. (2010), a Lange medical book.
17. Dienhardt, F et al (1982). *Bull WHO*, 60 : 661.
18. WHO (1996), *The World Health Report 1996*, Fighting disease Fostering development, Report of the Director–General.
19. WHO (2000), *Weekly Epidemiological Record*, No. 5, 4th June, 2000.

TABLE 6

Nomenclature and definitions of hepatitis viruses, antigens and antibodies

Disease	Component of system	Definition
Hepatitis A	HAV	Hepatitis A virus. Etiologic agent of infectious hepatitis. A *picornavirus*, the prototype of a new genus, *Hepatovirus*.
	Anti-HAV	Antibody to HAV. Detectable at onset of symptoms; lifetime persistence.
	IgM Anti-HAV	IgM class antibody to HAV. Indicates recent infection with hepatitis A; positive up to 4-6 months after infection.
Hepatitis B	HBV	Hepatitis B virus. Etiologic agent of serum hepatitis. A *hepadnavirus*.
	HBsAg	Hepatitis B surface antigen. Surface antigen(s) of HBV detectable in large quantity in serum; several sub-types identified.
	HBeAg	Hepatitis Be antigen. Soluble antigen ; associated with HBV replication, with high titers of HBV in serum, and with infectivity of serum.
	HBcAg	Hepatitis B core antigen.
	Anti-HBs	Antibody to HBsAg. Indicates past infection with and immunity to HBV, presence of passive antibody from HBIG, or immune response from HBV vaccine.
	Anti-HBe	Antibody to HBeAg. Presence in serum of HBsAg carrier suggests lower titer of HBV.
	Anti-HBc	Antibody to HBcAg. Indicates infection with HBV at some undefined time in the past.
	IgM Anti-HBc	IgM class antibody to HBcAg. Indicates recent infection with HBV ; positive for 4-6 months after infection.
Hepatitis C	HCV	Hepatitis C virus, a common etiologic agent of post-transfusion hepatitis. A flavivirus, genus *Hepacivirus*.
	Anti-HCV	Antibody to HCV.
Hepatitis D	HDV	Hepatitis D virus. Etiologic agent of delta hepatitis ; causes infection only in presence of HBV.
	HDAg	Delta antigen (delta-Ag). Detectable in early acute HDV infection.
	Anti-HDV	Antibody to delta-Ag (anti-delta). Indicates past or present infection with HDV.
Hepatitis E	HEV	Hepatitis E virus. Enterically transmitted hepatitis virus. Causes large epidemics in Asia and North Africa ; faecal–oral or waterborne transmission. Perhaps a *calicivirus*.
Hepatitis G	HGV	Hepatitis G virus, a *flavivirus*.
Immune globulins	IG	Immune globulin USP. Contains antibodies to HAV ; no antibodies to HBsAg, HCV, or HIV.
	HBIG	Hepatitis B immune globulin. Contains high titers of antibodies to HBV.

Source : *(5)*

20. WHO (2008), *Weekly Epidemiological Record* No. 48, 28th Nov. 2008.
21. Sherlock, S. (1984) *Post Graduate Doctor Middle East*, 7 (1) 49–56.
22. WHO (1982), *Bull WHO*, 60 (1) 43–47.
23. WHO (1983), *Tech.Rep.Ser.* No.693.
24. Krugman, S. et al (1979) *N.Eng.J.Med.*, 300 : 101 : 106.
25. WHO (1983), World Health Forum, 4 (2) 135–141.
26. WHO (2017), *Guidelines on Hepatitis B and C Testing*, Feb. 2017.
27. WHO (2020), *Fact Sheet Hepatitis B*, July 2020.
27A. WHO (2019), *Consolidated Strategic Information Guidelines for Viral Hepatitis*, Planning and tracking progress towards elimination.
28. WHO (2016), *Global Health Sector Strategy on Viral Hepatitis 2016–2021, Towards Ending Viral Hepatitis*, June 2016.
29. WHO (2016), *World Health Statistics 2016*, Monitoring Health for the SDGs, 2016.
30. WHO (2017), *Global Hepatitis Report*, 2017.
31. WHO (2022), *Fact Sheet Hepatitis C*, 24th June 2022.
32. WHO (2012), *Weekly Epidemiological Record*, No. 41 7th Oct, 2011.
33. WHO (2017), *Hepatitis E Fact Sheet*, 3rd July 2017.
34. WHO (2014), *Fact Sheet Hepatitis E*, No. 280, June 2014.
35. WHO (2018), *Hepatitis D Fact Sheet*, 23rd July 2018.

ACUTE DIARRHOEAL DISEASES

Diarrhoea is defined as the passage of loose, liquid or watery stools. These liquid stools are usually passed more than three times a day. However, it is the recent change in consistency and character of stools rather than the number of stools that is more important.

The term "diarrhoeal diseases" should be considered only as a convenient expression – not as a nosological or epidemiological entity – for a group of diseases in which the predominant symptom is diarrhoea.

CLINICAL TYPES OF DIARRHOEAL DISEASE *(1)*

It is most practical to base treatment of diarrhoea on the clinical type of illness, which can easily be determined. Four clinical types of diarrhoea can be recognized, each reflecting the basic underlying pathology and altered physiology :

(1) *Acute watery diarrhoea* – which lasts several hours to days; the main danger is dehydration, weight loss also occurs if feeding is not continued. The pathogens that usually cause acute diarrhoea include *V. cholerae* or *E. coli* bacteria, as well as rotavirus.

(2) *Acute bloody diarrhoea* – which is also called dysentery – the main dangers are damage of the intestinal mucosa, sepsis and malnutrition; other complications including dehydration, may also occur. It is marked by visible blood in the stools. (The most common cause of bloody diarrhoea is *shigella*, a bacteria that is also a most common cause of severe cases).

(3) *Persistent diarrhoea* – which lasts 14 days or longer. The main danger is malnutrition and serious non-intestinal infection, dehydration may also occur. Persons with other illness, such as AIDS, are more likely to develop persistent diarrhoea.

(4) *Diarrhoea with severe malnutrition (marasmus and Kwashiorkor)* – The main dangers are severe systemic infection, dehydration, heart failure, and vitamin and mineral deficiency.

Problem statement

Acute diarrhoea is rivalled in importance only by respiratory infection, as a cause of morbidity on a worldwide scale. When the WHO initiated the Diarrhoeal Diseases Control Programme in 1980, approximately 4.6 million children used to die each year of the dehydration caused by diarrhoea. Diarrhoea is still a major killer of children under 5 years of age, although its toll has dropped by a third over the past decade. It killed more than 3,70,000 children under 5 years of age in 2019. It accounts for 8 per cent of all under-five deaths. Most of these deaths occur among children less than 2 years of age *(2)*.

Comparing estimates of the current global burden of diarrhoeal disease with previously published estimates, highlights that the incidence of diarrhoea have not changed much, although overall diarrhoeal mortality has declined. For children aged under 5 years, a median of 3 episodes of diarrhoea occurred per child-year, which is similar to that reported previously. The current estimates in under-five children suggest that there are about 2.5 billion episodes of diarrhoea per year with 123 million clinic visits annually and 9 million hospitalizations worldwide, with a loss of 62 million disability-adjusted life years (DALYs) *(3)*.

In India, acute diarrhoeal disease accounts for about 10 per cent of deaths in under–5 years age group. During the year 2020, about 7.20 million cases with 1,606 deaths were reported in India *(4)*.

Diarrhoea is a leading cause of death during complex emergencies and natural disasters. Displacement of population into temporary, overcrowded shelters is often associated with polluted water sources, inadequate sanitation, poor hygiene practices, contaminated food and malnutrition – all of which affect the spread and severity of diarrhoea. At the same time, the lack of adequate health services and transport reduces the likelihood of prompt and appropriate treatment of diarrhoea cases.

Diarrhoeal disease causes a heavy economic burden on the health services. Much attention has been given to acute diarrhoeal disease and its management over the last decade, which is dominated by advances in oral rehydration technique and through integrated management of childhood illness. The treatment recommendations reflect a better understanding of what works to reduce child death from diarrhoea, as well as new insights into treatment feasibility. These changes in treatment recommendations and preventive measures have subsequently led to monitorable treatment and diarrhoea prevention indicators. They are as follows *(5)* :

(A) *Diarrhoea prevention indicators*

(1) Percentage of population using :
  (a) improved drinking water sources (urban, rural, total);
  (b) improved sanitation facilities (urban, rural, total);
(2) Percentage of one year old immunized against measles;
(3) Percentage of children who are :
  - under-weight (moderate and severe) – 0 to 59 months age
  - stunted (moderate and severe) – 0 to 59 months age
  - exclusively breast-fed – 0 to 5 months age
  - breast-fed with complementary food – 6 to 9 months age
  - still breast-feeding – 20 to 23 months age
(4) Vitamin A supplementation coverage rate (per cent full coverage) – 6 to 59 months (India–53%)

(B) *Diarrhoea treatment Indicators*

Percentage of children under-five years with diarrhoea receiving :

(1) ORT with continuous feeding
(2) ORS packet
(3) Recommended home made fluids
(4) Increased fluids
(5) Continued feeding

(C) *Use of oral rehydration therapy*

Percentage of children under-five years with diarrhoea receiving oral rehydration therapy (ORS packet or recommended home-made fluids or increased fluids with continued feeding)

(1) Gender – male, female
(2) Residence – Urban, rural
(3) Wealth index quintiles – poorest, second, middle, fourth, richest

Epidemiological determinants

Agent factors

In developing countries, diarrhoea is almost universally infectious in origin. A wide assortment of organisms cause acute diarrhoea, and many of them have been discovered only in recent years such as rotaviruses and campylobacters (Table 1).

TABLE 1
Infections causing diarrhoea

1. Viruses :	3. Others :
Rotaviruses	*Entamoeba histolytica*
Astroviruses	Giardia intestinalis
Adenoviruses	Trichuriasis
Calciviruses	Cryptosporidium SPP
Coronaviruses	Intestinal worms
Norwalk group viruses	*Cyclospora*
Enteroviruses	
Cytomegalovirus	
2. Bacteria :	
Campylobacter jejuni	
Enterotoxigenic Escherichia coli	
Shigella	
Salmonella	
Vibrio cholerae	
Vibrio parahaemolyticus	
Bacillus cereus	
Staphylococcus aureus	
Clostridium perfringens	
Enterohaemorrhagic E. coli	
Clostridium difficile	
Enteroinvasive E. coli	
Aeromonas	
Yersinia enterocolitica	
Chlamydia	
Neisseria gonorrhoeae	

Source : *(6)*

Until recent years, the identification of pathogens in the stool was only feasible in about 25 per cent of patients with acute diarrhoea. At present, new techniques enable competent laboratories to identify these pathogens in about 75 per cent of cases. The infectious agents most often connected with diarrhoea in young children, in developing countries, are as shown in Table 2.

TABLE 2
Pathogens frequently identified in children with acute diarrhoea in treatment centres in developing countries

Pathogen		% of cases
Viruses	Rotavirus	15–25
Bacteria	Enterotoxigenic *Escherichia coli*	10–20
	Shigella	5–15
	Campylobacter jejuni	10–15
	Vibrio cholerae 01	5–10
	Salmonella (non-typhoid)	1–5
	Enteropathogenic *Escherichia coli*	1–5
Protozoans	*Cryptosporidium*	5–15
No pathogen found	–	20–30

Source : *(7)*

(a) *VIRUSES*

A great many diarrhoeal diseases are caused by viruses (Table 1).

ROTAVIRUSES : The rotavirus, first discovered in 1973, has emerged as the leading cause of severe, dehydrating diarrhoea in children aged <5 years globally, with an estimated more than 25 million out-patient visits and more than 2 million hospitalizations attributable to rotavirus infections each year. In developing countries, three-quarters of children acquire their first episode of rotavirus diarrhoea before the age of 12 months, whereas in developed countries the first episode is frequently delayed until the age of 2–5 years. Severe rotavirus gastroenteritis is largely limited to children aged 6–24 months. Fatal outcomes in children, estimated to be approximately 420,000–494,000 in 2008 *(8)*, occur predominantly in low-income countries. Rotavirus reinfection is common, although the primary infection is usually the most significant clinically. In temperate climates, the incidence of rotavirus gastroenteritis typically peaks during the winter season, whereas in tropical settings rotavirus occurs year round and a marked seasonality may be masked by high background levels *(9)*.

Rotaviruses are shed in very high concentrations (>10^{12} particles/gram) and for many days in the stools and vomit of infected individuals. Transmission occurs primarily by the faecal-oral route, directly from person to person or indirectly *via* contaminated fomites. The universal occurrence of rotavirus infections shows that clean water supplies and good hygiene are unlikely to have a substantial effect on virus transmission *(9)*.

(b) *BACTERIAL CAUSES*

Besides the well–known bacterial causes of enteric infections and diarrhoeal diseases such as *V. cholerae* O1, Salmonella, *Shigella*, enterotoxigenic *E.coli* and *Campylobacter jejuni* are the most frequent cause of diarrhoea. They produce a potent enterotoxin similar to that produced by *V. cholerae*. The less–known pathogens which cause diarrhoea are *Yersinia enterocolitica*, and *V. parahaemolyticus*.

Enterotoxigenic *Escherichia coli* (ETEC) is an important cause of acute watery diarrhoea in adults and children in developing countries causing annually 280–400 million diarrhoeal episodes in children under 5 years of age, and an additional 100 million episodes in children aged 5–14 years. In adults it causes substantial disease (about 400 million cases per year). It is also the most common cause of traveller's diarrhoea. Being responsible for one-third to one-half of all diarrhoeal episodes in travellers to Africa, Asia and Latin America, the illness results in 0.3 to 0.5 million deaths per year mostly in young children *(10)*. ETEC does not invade the bowel mucosa and the diarrhoea it causes is mediated by toxins. There are two ETEC toxins, heat labile (LT) and heat stable (ST). Some strains produce only one type of toxin, some both. The LT toxin is closely related to cholera toxin. ETEC is spread mostly by means of contaminated food and water.

Salmonella cause inflammation of the bowel epithelium; *Vibrio cholerae* O1 do not. Both are endemic diseases in India. In cholera–endemic areas, cholera probably accounts for not more than 5 to 10 per cent of all acute diarrhoeas yearly, and in more than 90 per cent of instances is clinically indistinguishable from other acute diarrhoeas. *Campylobacters* are slim, highly motile, S-shaped, gram-negative rods, formerly classed as vibrios. They are one of the commonest causes of enteritis. They do not seem to produce any toxin. It is not clear how they cause diarrhoea *(11)*.

Shigella accounts for a high percentage of mortality due to diarrhoeal disease. The estimates suggest that it causes about 1 million deaths every year in children aged under-5 years, mostly in the developing countries. In addition about 164.7 million *Shigella* episodes are estimated worldwide, with 69 per cent of all episodes in young children *(12)*. It is a major cause of diarrhoea in India.

(c) *OTHERS*

Amoebiasis, giardiasis and other intestinal parasitic infections are associated with diarrhoea *(13)*. Giardiasis is a recognized cause of diarrhoea. It flourishes in the duodenum and jejunum. The organisms can be present in very large numbers, the lumen of the intestine teeming with them and the epithelial surfaces almost smothered with them *(14)*.

Cryptosporidium is a coccidian parasite that causes diarrhoea in infants, immunodeficient patients, and a variety of domestic animals. In developing countries most episodes of illness occur in the first year of life. Thereafter, infections are usually asymptomatic. Diarrhoea is usually neither severe nor prolonged, except in immunodeficient patients, such as those with severe malnutrition or AIDS. In such individuals cryptosporidium is an important cause of persistent diarrhoea with wasting *(14)*.

The enumeration of the germs causing the enteric infections which lead to acute diarrhoea should not overshadow the fact that diarrhoea may be caused by a parenteral infection (non-digestive origin) and particularly so in younger children. These include ENT infections, respiratory or urinary infections, malaria, bacterial meningitis, or even simple teething *(7)*.

Besides the above causes, malnutrition may lead to certain nutritional diseases such as kwashiorkor, sprue, coeliac disease and pellagra which are all associated with diarrhoea. In the developed countries, the causes of diarrhoea may be slightly different. Diarrhoea in the newborn is unusual and may be due to inborn errors of metabolism such as congenital enzyme deficiencies. It may also be associated with severe infections like septicaemia or necrotizing enterocolitis *(15)*.

Persistent diarrhoea is one of the main clinical signs of AIDS in the tropics (an episode of diarrhoea lasting more than 30 days, according to the WHO definition of AIDS in children). This is associated with one or several other signs of the disease. Children with measles or who have had measles recently, run a high risk of developing severe or fatal diarrhoea *(7)*.

Reservoir of infection

For some enteric pathogens, man is the principal reservoir and thus most transmission originates from human factors ; examples are enterotoxigenic *E. coli*, *shigella spp.*, *V. cholerae*, *Giardia lamblia* and *E. histolytica*. For other enteric pathogens, animals are important reservoirs and transmission originates from both human and animal faeces; examples are *Campylobacter jejuni*, *Salmonella spp* and *Y. enterocolitica*. For viral agents of diarrhoea, the role of animal reservoirs in human disease remains uncertain.

Host factors

Diarrhoea is most common in children especially those between 6 months and 2 years. Incidence is highest in the age group 6–11 months, when weaning occurs. It reflects the combined effects of declining levels of maternally acquired antibodies, the lack of active immunity in the infant, the introduction of contaminated food, and direct contact with human or animal faeces when the infant starts to crawl. It is also common in babies under 6 months of age fed on cow's milk or infant feeding formulas *(16)*. Diarrhoea is more common in persons with malnutrition. Malnutrition leads to infection and infection to diarrhoea which is a well known vicious circle. Poverty, prematurity, reduced gastric acidity, immunodeficiency, lack of personal and domestic hygiene and incorrect feeding practices are all contributory factors.

Environmental factors

Distinct seasonal patterns of diarrhoea occur in many geographical areas. In temperature climates, bacterial diarrhoea occur more frequently during the warm season, whereas viral diarrhoea, particularly diarrhoea caused by rotavirus peak during the winter. In tropical areas, rotavirus diarrhoea occurs throughout the year, increasing in frequency during the drier, cool months, whereas bacterial diarrhoeas peak during the warmer, rainy season. The incidence of persistent diarrhoea follows the same seasonal patterns as that of acute watery diarrhoea *(14)*.

Mode of transmission

Most of the pathogenic organisms that cause diarrhoea and all the pathogens that are known to be major causes of diarrhoea in many countries, are transmitted primarily or exclusively by the **faecal–oral route**. Faecal–oral transmission may be water-borne; food-borne, or direct transmission which implies an array of other faecal–oral routes such as *via* fingers, or fomites, or dirt which may be ingested by young children *(17)*.

CONTROL OF DIARRHOEAL DISEASES

It is now obvious that many different organisms – some known, probably many unknown – cause diarrhoea. It is also clear that they do not act in the same way to cause diarrhoea. But from an epidemiological point of view, they are considered together because of the common symptom, diarrhoea. It is now firmly established that regardless of the causative agent or the age of the patient, the sheet anchor of treatment is oral rehydration therapy such as the one advocated by WHO/UNICEF.

The Diarrhoeal Diseases Control (DDC) Programme of WHO has since its inception in 1980, advocated several interventional measures to be implemented simultaneously with mutually reinforcing and complementary impacts. These measures centre round the widespread practice of "oral rehydration therapy".

Components of a Diarrhoeal Diseases Control Programme

The intervention measures recommended by WHO *(15)* may be classified as below :

1. Short-term

a. Appropriate clinical management.

2. Long-term

b. Better MCH care practices.

c. Preventive strategies.

d. Preventing diarrhoeal epidemics.

a. Appropriate clinical management

(I) ORAL REHYDRATION THERAPY : With introduction of oral rehydration by WHO it is now firmly established that oral rehydration treatment can be safely and successfully used in treating acute diarrhoeas due to all aetiologies, in all age groups, and in all countries. The aim of oral fluid therapy is to prevent dehydration and reduce mortality. It has been the experience of workers at Kolkata that as many as 90–95 per cent of all cases of cholera and acute diarrhoea can be treated by oral fluids alone *(18)*. Oral fluid therapy is based on the observation that glucose given orally enhances the intestinal absorption of salt and water, and is capable of correcting the electrolyte and water deficit.

At first the composition of oral rehydration salt (ORS) recommended by WHO was sodium bicarbonate based. Inclusion of trisodium citrate in place of sodium bicarbonate made the product more stable and it resulted in less stool output especially in high-output diarrhoea as in cholera, probably because of direct effect of trisodium citrate in increasing intestinal absorption of sodium and water.

More recently an improved ORS formulation has been developed which is as safe and effective as the original in preventing and treating diarrhoeal dehydration but also reduced stool output or offers additional clinical benefit or both. It is focussed on reducing the osmolarity of ORS solution to avoid possible adverse effects of hypertonicity on net fluid absorption by reducing the concentration of glucose and sodium chloride in the solution. Decreasing the sodium concentration of ORS solution to 75 mOsm/l improved the efficacy of the ORS regimen for children with acute non-cholera diarrhoea. The need for unscheduled supplemental intravenous therapy in children given the new ORS fell by 33 per cent, the stool output decreased by 20 per cent and vomiting was reduced by 30 per cent. The reduced osmolarity (245 mOsm/l) solution also appears to be as safe and effective as standard ORS for use in children with cholera *(19)*.

Recommended formulation : Because of the improved effectiveness of reduced osmolarity ORS solution, WHO and UNICEF are recommending that countries manufacture and use the following formulation in place of the previously recommended ORS solution. Since January 2004, the new ORS formulation is the only one procured by UNICEF. India was the first country in the world to launch this ORS formulation since June 2004.

Composition of reduced osmolarity ORS

Reduced osmolarity ORS	**grams / litre**
Sodium chloride	2.6
Glucose, anhydrous	13.5
Potassium chloride	1.5
Trisodium citrate, dihydrate	2.9
Total weight	20.5
Reduced osmolarity ORS	**mmol / litre**
Sodium	75
Chloride	65
Glucose, anhydrous	75
Potassium	20
Citrate	10
Total osmolarity	245

Source : *(19)*

Guidelines for assessing dehydration and oral rehydration : The guidelines for assessing dehydration and oral rehydration are given in Tables 3 and 4 *(20, 21)*.

TABLE 3

Assessment of dehydration

	DEHYDRATION	
	Mild	Severe
(1) Patient's appearance	Thirsty; alert, restless	Drowsy; limp, cold, sweaty; may be comatose
(2) Radial pulse	Normal rate and volume	Rapid, feeble, sometimes impalpable
(3) Blood pressure	Normal	Less than 80 mm Hg; may be unrecordable
(4) Skin elasticity	Pinch retracts immediately	Pinch retracts very slowly (more than 2 seconds)
(5) Tongue	Moist	Very dry
(6) Ant. fontanelle	Normal	Very sunken
(7) Urine flow	Normal	Little or none
% body weight loss	4–5%	10% or more
Estimated fluid deficit	40–50 ml/kg	100–110 ml/kg

When obvious signs of dehydration exist, the water deficit is somewhere between 50 and 100 ml per kg of body weight. If the child's weight is known, the amount of ORS solution required for rehydration during the first four hours may be calculated by setting the deficit at approximately 75 ml/kg. If the child's weight is not known, the approximate deficit may be determined on the basis of age, although this procedure is less accurate. The guidelines for oral rehydration are given in Table 4.

TABLE 4

Guidelines for oral rehydration therapy (for all ages) during the first four hours

Age (*)	under 4 months	4–11 months	1–2 yrs.	2–4 yrs.	5–14 yrs.	15 yrs or over
Weight (kg)	under 5	5–7.9	8–10.9	11–15.9	16–29.9	30 or over
ORS solution (ml)	200–400	400–600	600–800	800–1200	1200–2200	2200–4000

(*) The patient's age should only be used if weight is not known. The approximate amount of ORS required in ml. may also be calculated by multiplying the patient's weight (expressed in kg) by 75.

Source : *(1)*

The actual amount given will depend on the patients desire to drink and by surveillance of signs of dehydration, keeping in mind the fact that greater amounts should be given to heavier patients, those with greater signs of dehydration and those who still have watery diarrhoea during rehydration. The general rule is that patients should be given as much ORS solution as they want, and that signs of dehydration should be checked until they subside.

Older children and adults should be given as much water as they want, in addition to the ORS solution.

Mothers should be taught how to administer ORS solution to their children. It is best for a demonstration to be given by a nurse or by a health worker following which the mother feeds the solution to her child under their supervision respecting the following rules :

- for children under age 2 years, give a teaspoon every 1 to 2 minutes, and offer frequent sips out of a cup for older children. Adults may drink as much as they like. Try to give the estimated required amount within a 4–hour period. As a general guide, after each loose stool, give – children under 2 years of age : 50–100 ml (a quarter to half a large cup) of fluid; children aged 2 up to 10 years : 100–200 ml (a half to one large cup); and older children and adults : as much fluid as they want.
- if the child vomits, wait for 10 minutes, then try again, giving the solution slowly – a spoonful every 2 to 3 minutes.
- if the child wants to drink more ORS solution than the estimated amount, and does not vomit, there can be no harm in feeding him/her more. If the child refuses to drink the required amount and signs of dehydration have disappeared, rehydration is completed. The treatment plan for non-dehydrated diarrhoeic children is then resumed.
- if the child is breast-fed, nursing should be pursued during treatment with ORS solution.

The introduction of oral rehydration fluid has not only reduced the cost of treatment, but also made possible treatment of patients in their own homes by primary health workers or relatives of patient. The ingredients required for the preparation of oral fluid are inexpensive and readily available, and the solution can be prepared with ordinary drinking water. The development of oral rehydration therapy is a major breakthrough in the fight against cholera and other diarrhoeal diseases.

Packets of "oral rehydration mixture" are now freely available at all primary health centres, sub-centres, hospitals and chemist shops. The contents of the packet are to be dissolved in one litre of drinking water. The solution should be made fresh daily and used within 24 hours. It should not be boiled or otherwise sterilized.

If the WHO mixture of salts is not available, a simple mixture consisting of table salt (one level teaspoon) and sugar (6 level teaspoon) dissolved in one litre of drinking water may be safely used until the proper mixture is obtained. The earlier the treatment is instituted the better it is for the patient.

Many countries have designated recommended house fluids. Wherever possible these should include at least one fluid that contains salt. Fluids that do not contain salt are water in which a cereal has been cooked e.g. rice water; unsalted soup, yogurt drinks, green coconut water, weak tea etc. The mothers should be taught to add salt about 3 g/litre to an unsalted drink or soup during diarrhoea. A few fluids are potentially dangerous and should be avoided during diarrhoea. Especially important are drinks sweetened with sugar, which can cause osmotic diarrhoea and hypernatremia. Examples are commercial carbonated beverages, commercial fruit juices and sweetened tea. Other fluids to be avoided are those with stimulant diuretic or purgative effect, e.g. coffee and some medicinal tea or infusions *(1)*.

The infant's usual diet of cereals, vegetables and other foods should be continued during diarrhoea, and increased afterwards. Food should never be withheld and the child's usual food should never be diluted. The aim is to give as much nutrient rich food as the child will accept. Most children with watery diarrhoea regain their appetite after dehydration is corrected, whereas those with bloody diarrhoea often eat poorly until the illness resolves. These children should be encouraged to resume normal feeding as soon as possible.

Please refer to end of Chapter 11, Annexure A for plan A, Plan B and Plan C for the management of dehydration due to diarrhoea.

(II) INTRAVENOUS REHYDRATION

Intravenous infusion is usually required only for the *initial* rehydration of severely dehydrated patients who are in shock or unable to drink. Such patients are best transferred to the nearest hospital or treatment centre.

The solutions recommended by WHO for intravenous infusion are: (a) *Ringer's lactate solution* (also called Hartmann's solution for injection) : It is the best commercially available solution. It supplies adequate concentrations of sodium and potassium and the lactate yields bicarbonate for correction of the acidosis. It can be used to correct dehydration due to acute diarrhoeas of all causes. (b) *Diarrhoea Treatment Solution (DTS):* Also recommended by WHO as an ideal polyelectrolyte solution for intravenous infusion. It contains in one litre, sodium chloride 4 g sodium acetate 6.5 g potassium chloride 1g and glucose 10g *(21)*. It must meet purity and sterility requirements of fluid for injection.

If nothing else is available, *normal saline* can be given because it is often readily available. Normal saline is the poorest fluid because it will not correct the acidosis and will not replace potassium losses. It should be replaced by the above solutions as early as possible. Plain glucose and dextrose solutions should not be used as they provide only water and glucose.

The recommended dose of the IV fluid to be given is 100 ml/kg, divided as follows (Table 5) :

TABLE 5

Treatment plan for rehydration therapy

Age	First give 30 ml/kg in	Then give 70 ml/kg in
Infants (under 12 months)	1 hour	5 hours
Older	30 minutes	$2^1/_2$ hours

The initial rehydration should be fast until an easily palpable pulse is present. Reassess the patient every

1–2 hours. If dehydration is not improving give the IV drip more rapidly. The use of large-bore needle (No.18) will permit rapid infusion. After infusing 1–2 litres of fluid, rehydration should be carried out at a somewhat slower rate until pulse and blood pressure return to normal. When the patient can drink the oral fluids give ORS about 5 ml/kg/hour.

The patient must be examined at intervals during rehydration. After 4–6 hours of satisfactory treatment, all signs of dehydration should have disappeared except that the urine flow may not have yet started. Sometimes if too much rehydration fluid is given, the eyelids become puffy; if this occurs, IV fluid should be stopped. It is most helpful to examine skin elasticity and pulse strength, both of which should be normal. Rehydration must continue until all signs of dehydration have disappeared.

(III) MAINTENANCE THERAPY

After the initial fluid and electrolyte deficit has been corrected (i.e., the signs of dehydration (Table 3) have gone) oral fluid should be used for maintenance therapy. In adults and older children, thirst is an adequate guide for fluid needs; they can be told to drink as much as they want to satisfy their thirst. The guidelines for maintenance therapy are given in Table 6. The general principle is that the oral fluid intake should equal the rate of continuing stool loss, which should be measured. Diarrhoea usually lasts for 1 or 2 days.

TABLE 6

Maintenance therapy

Amount of diarrhoea	Amount of oral fluid
Mild diarrhoea (not more than one stool every 2 hours or longer, or less than 5 ml stool per kg per hour)	100 ml/kg body weight per day until diarrhoea stops
Severe diarrhoea (more than one stool every 2 hours, or more than 5 ml of stool per kg per hour)	Replace stool losses volume for volume; if not measurable give 10–15 ml/kg body weight per hour

(IV) APPROPRIATE FEEDING : Medical profession has reeled for centuries under the mistaken assumption that it is important to "rest the gut" during diarrhoea. The current view is that during episodes of diarrhoea, normal food intake should be promoted as soon as the child whatever its age, is able to eat. This is especially relevant for the exclusively breast-fed infants. Newborn infants with diarrhoea who show little or no signs of dehydration can be treated by breast-feeding alone. Those with moderate or severe dehydration should receive oral rehydration solution. Breast-feeding is continued along with oral rehydration solution given after each liquid stool. Not only breast milk helps the infant to recover from an attack of diarrhoea both in terms of the nutrients it supplies, and its rehydrating effect, but it helps to prevent further infection because it has protective properties.

(V) CHEMOTHERAPY : Unnecessary prescription of antibiotics and other drugs will do more harm than good in the treatment of diarrhoea. Antibiotics should be considered where the cause of diarrhoea has been clearly identified as shigella, typhoid or cholera. The symptomatic differential diagnosis of *shigella* and cholera are as shown in Table 7.

TABLE 7

Symptomatic differential diagnosis of *shigella* and cholera

Symptoms	Cholera	*Shigella*
Diarrhoea	Acute watery diarrhoea	Acute bloody diarrhoea
Fever	No	Yes
Abdominal cramps	Yes	Yes
Vomiting	Yes	No
Rectal pain	No	Yes
Stool	> 3 loose stools per day, watery like rice water	> 3 stools per day, with blood or pus

For diarrhoea due to cholera the drug of choice is doxycycline, tetracycline, TMP-SMX and erythromycin. For diarrhoea due to *shigella*, the drug of choice is ciprofloxacin as *shigella* is usually resistant to ampicillin and TMP-SMX.

The medicines that should not be used in the treatment of diarrhoea are as follows *(16)* :

- neomycin (damages the intestinal mucosa and can cause malabsorption);
- purgatives (worsen diarrhoea and dehydration);
- tincture of opium or atropine (dangerous for children and dysentery patients because of decreased intestinal transit time);
- cardiotonics such as Coramine; shock in diarrhoea must be corrected by intravenous fluids and not by drugs;
- steroids (expensive, useless, and may cause adverse effects);
- oxygen (expensive, unnecessary);
- charcoal, kaolin, pectin, bismuth (no value);
- mexaform (no value and can be dangerous).

(VI) ZINC SUPPLEMENTATION : When a zinc supplement is given during an episode of acute diarrhoea, it reduces the episode's duration and severity. In addition, zinc supplements given for 10 to 14 days lower the incidence of diarrhoea in the following 2 to 3 months. WHO and UNICEF therefore recommend daily 10 mg of zinc for infants under 6 months of age, and 20 mg for children older than 6 months for 10–14 days *(19)*.

b. Better MCH care practices

(a) MATERNAL NUTRITION : Improving prenatal nutrition will reduce the low birth weight problem. Prenatal and postnatal nutrition will improve the quality of breast milk.

(b) CHILD NUTRITION : *(i) Promotion of breast-feeding :* Any measures to promote breast-feeding are likely to reduce the diarrhoeal diseases in infants. The breast-fed child is at very much less risk of severe diarrhoea and death than the bottlefed child. Promotion of breast-feeding should include strong efforts to limit the use of commercial and artificial formulas. Breast-feeding should be continued as long as possible. *(ii) Appropriate weaning practices :* Poor weaning practices are a major risk factor for diarrhoea. The child should be weaned neither too soon, nor too late, in any case not earlier than the sixth month of life using nutritious and locally available foods, and the foods should be hygienically prepared and given. *(iii) Supplementary feeding :* This is necessary to improve the nutritional status of children aged 6–59 months. As soon as the supplementary food is introduced, the child enters the high-risk category. *(iv) Vitamin A supplementation :* Vitamin A supplementation is a critical preventive measure, and studies have shown mortality reductions ranging from 19 per cent to 54 per cent in children receiving supplements. This reduction is associated in large part with decline in deaths due to diarrhoeal diseases and measles. It also reduces the duration, severity and complications associated with diarrhoea *(2)*.

c. Preventive strategies

(i) SANITATION : Measures to reduce transmission emphasize the traditional improved water supply, improved excreta disposal and improved domestic and food hygiene. Without an adequate supply of clean water close to their homes, it is extremely difficult to promote personal and domestic hygiene. Simple hygienic measures like hand washing with soap before preparing food, before eating, before feeding a child, after defecation, after cleaning a child who has defecated, and after disposing off a child's stool should be promoted. All families should have a clean and functioning latrine. The latrine should be kept clean by regular washing of dirty surface. If there is no latrine, family members should defecate at a distance from the house, paths or areas where children play and at least 10 metres away from the water supply source. It should be recognized that in many communities, young children are often permitted to defecate indiscriminately. Because diarrhoea attack rates are higher among children, it is the defecation in this age group that deserves the most attention. Contaminated foods of all sorts have been identified as major vehicles for the transmission of faecal pathogens during early infancy, e.g., diluted milk, cereal gruels, etc. Delays in consumption add to the problem.

(ii) HEALTH EDUCATION : Environmental sanitation measures require educational support, to ensure their proper use and maintenance of such facilities. An important part of health worker's job is to help prevent diarrhoea by convincing and helping community members to adopt and maintain certain preventive practices such as breast-feeding, improved weaning, clean drinking water, use of plenty of water for hygiene, use of latrine, proper disposal of stools of young children etc.

(iii) IMMUNIZATION : Immunization against measles is a potential intervention for diarrhoea control. When administered at the recommended age, the measles vaccine can prevent upto 25 per cent of diarrhoeal deaths in children under 5 years of age.

The protect, prevent and treat framework of integrated global action plan for prevention and control of pneumonia and diarrhoea is summarized in Fig. 1.

Rotavirus vaccine *(9)*

Two live, oral, attenuated rotavirus vaccines were licensed in 2006 : the monovalent human rotavirus vaccine (Rotarix™) and the pentavalent bovine-human, reassortant vaccine (Rota Teq™). Both vaccines have demonstrated very good safety and efficacy profiles in large clinical trials. The rotavirus vaccines are now introduced for routine use in a number of industrialized and developing

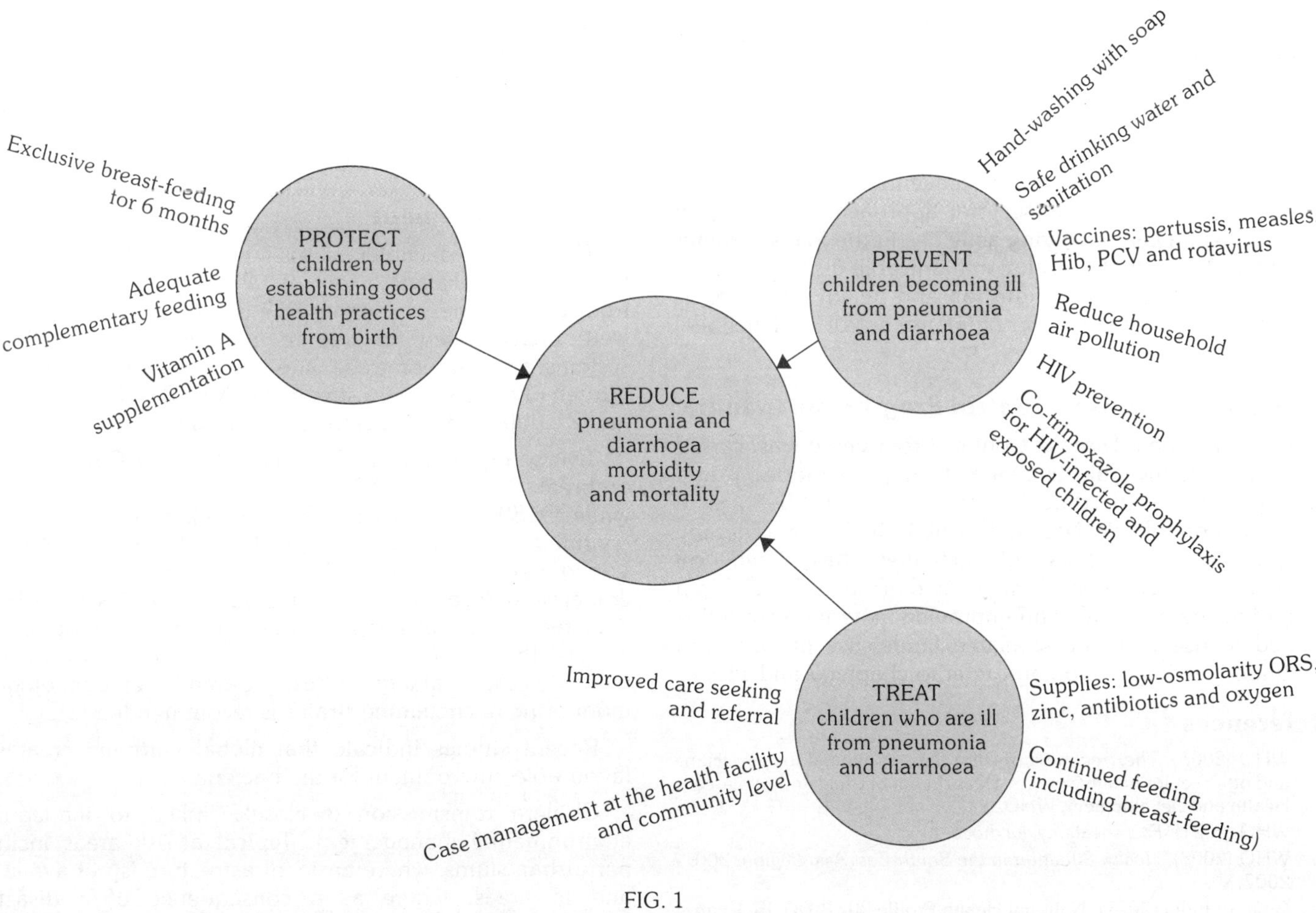

FIG. 1

Integrated global action plan for the prevention and control of pneumonia and diarrhoea

Source: *(2)*

countries.

The Rotarix™ vaccine is administered orally in a 2-dose schedule to infants of approximately 2 and 4 months of age. The first dose can already be administered at the age of 6 weeks and should be given no later than at the age of 12 weeks. The interval between the 2 doses should be at least 4 weeks. The 2-dose schedule should be completed by age 16 weeks, and no later than by 24 weeks of age.

For RotaTeq™, the recommended schedule is 3 oral doses at ages 2, 4 and 6 months. The first dose should be administered between ages 6–12 weeks and subsequent doses at intervals of 4–10 weeks. Vaccination should not be initiated for infants aged >12 weeks. All 3 doses should be administered before the age of 32 weeks.

There is a potentially higher risk of intussusception when the first dose of these vaccines is given to infants aged >12 weeks; consequently, current rotavirus vaccines should not be used in catch-up vaccination campaigns, where the exact age of the vaccinees may be difficult to ascertain.

(iv) FLY CONTROL : Flies breeding in association with human or animal faeces should be controlled.

d. Control and/or prevention of diarrhoeal epidemics

This requires strengthening of epidemiological surveillance systems.

e. The Integrated Global Action Plan for the Prevention and Control of Pneumonia and Diarrhoea (GAPPD)

Please refer to page 190 for details.

PRIMARY HEALTH CARE

The concept of primary health care involves the delivery of a package of curative and preventive services at the community level. An intersectoral approach centred upon primary health care involving activities in the fields of water supply and excreta disposal, communicable disease control, mother and child health, nutrition and health education is regarded as essential for the ultimate control of diarrhoeal diseases.

Diarrhoeal Diseases Control Programme in India

The Diarrhoeal Disease Control Programme was started in 1978 with the objective of reducing the mortality and morbidity due to diarrhoeal diseases. Since 1985–86, with the inception of the National Oral Rehydration Therapy Programme, the focus of activities has been on strengthening case management of diarrhoea for children under the age of 5 years and improving maternal knowledge related to use of home available fluids, use of ORS and continued feeding. For details, refer to chapter 7 and 11.

References

1. WHO (2005), *The Treatment of Diarrhoea,* A manual for physicians and other senior health workers, Department of Child and Adolescent Health and Development, WHO.
2. WHO (2021), *Fact sheet on Diarrhoea.*
3. WHO (2008), *Health Situation in the South-East Asia Region,* 2001-2007.
4. Govt. of India (2021), National Health Profile 2021, DGHS, Central Bureau of Health Intelligence, Ministry of Health and Family Welfare, New Delhi.
5. WHO, UNICEF (2009), *Diarrhoea : Why children are still dying and what can be done.*
6. Stephen J. McPHEE, MAXINEA (2010), *Current Medical Diagnosis and Treatment,* 49th Ed., A Lange publication.
7. Fricker, J., *Children in the Tropics* 1993 – No.204.
8. UNICEF (2012), *Pneumonia and Diarrhoea, tackling the deadliest disease for the world's poorest children.*
9. WHO (2007), *Weekly Epidemiological Record,* No. 37, 10th Oct, 2007.
10. WHO (2006), *Weekly Epidemiological Record,* No. 11, 17 March, 2006.
11. Christie, A.B. (1980) *Infectious Diseases : Epidemiology and Clinical Practice* (3rd Ed), Churchill Livingstone.
12. WHO (2006), *Weekly Epidemiological Record* No. 6, 10th Feb., 2006.
13. WHO (1980) *Bull WHO,* 58 (6) 819–830.
14. WHO (1992) *Readings on diarrhoea,* Student Manual.
15. Pizzarro, D. (1985). *Dialogue on Diarrhoea,* Issue No.22 Sept.1985, AHRTAG, 85 Marylebone High Street, London.
16. WHO (1981). Surveillance and control of acute diarrhoeal diseases. *EURO Reports.* Ser.No.44 Copenhagen, WHO.
17. R.G. Feachem (1984) *Bull WHO* 62 (3) 467–476.
18. De, S. et al (1975), *J. Com. Dis.,* 7 : 124 - 128.
19. WHO, UNICEF (2004), *Clinical Management of Acute Diarrhoea,* WHO / UNICEF Joint Statement.
20. Govt. of India (1998), *Health Information of India* 1995 and 1996, Ministry of Health and Family Welfare, New Delhi.
21. WHO (1980), *A Manual for the treatment of Acute Diarrhoea,* WHO / CDD / SER / 80.2.

CHOLERA

Cholera is an acute diarrhoeal disease caused by *V. Cholerae* O1 (classical or El Tor) and O139. It is now commonly due to the El Tor biotype and O139. Cases range from symptomless to severe infections. The majority of infections are mild or asymptomatic. Typical cases are characterized by the sudden onset of profuse, effortless, watery diarrhoea followed by vomiting, rapid dehydration, muscular cramps and suppression of urine. Unless there is rapid replacement of fluid and electrolytes, the case fatality may be as high as 30 to 40 per cent.

Problem statement

The number of cholera cases reported to WHO continues to rise. For 2020 alone, a total of 3,23,320 cases were notified from 27 countries, including 857 deaths. Many more cases were unaccounted for due to limitations in surveillance systems and fear of trade and travel sanctions. The true burden of the disease is estimated to be 1.3–4.0 million cases and 21,000–143,000 deaths annually *(1).*

Two serogroups of *V. cholerae* – O1 and O139 – cause outbreaks. *V. cholerae* O1 causes the majority of outbreaks, while O139 – first identified in Bangladesh in 1992 – is confined to South-East Asia. Non-O1 and non-O139 *V. cholerae* can cause mild diarrhoea but do not generate epidemics. Recently, new El Tor variant strains have been detected in several parts of Asia and Africa. Observations suggest that these strains cause more severe cholera with higher case fatality rates. Careful epidemiological monitoring of circulating strains is recommended *(2).*

Recent studies indicate that global warming creates a favourable environment for the bacteria.

Cholera transmission is closely linked to inadequate environmental management. Typical at-risk areas include peri-urban slums, where basic infrastructure is not available and in areas, where as a consequence of a disaster, disruption of water and sanitation system takes place, or the displacement of population to inadequate and overcrowded camps. Risk of cholera transmission increases, should the bacteria be present or introduced. Epidemics have never arisen from dead bodies *(2)*.

Cholera remains a global threat to public health and a key indicator of lack of social development.

The dynamics of cholera occurrences since 2005, combined with the emergence of new strains that lead to a more severe clinical presentation; increased antimicrobial resistance and climate change, suggest that cholera may well return to the forefront of the global public health agenda *(3)*.

INDIA

Since the introduction of Cholera El Tor biotype in 1964, the geographic distribution of cholera in India has considerably changed. West Bengal has lost its reputation as the "home" of cholera. Many of the States which never had cholera or were free from it for a long time, got infected and became endemic foci of El Tor infection. In several of the recently invaded areas, the disease is seen persisting as a smouldering infection. The classical severe epidemics with high mortality are now uncommon. Explosive outbreaks, particularly following large fairs and festivals are also now rare.

The bacteriology of cholera also presents a changed picture. For reasons that are not known, there has been no large scale epidemic of classical cholera since 1964. In short, the El Tor biotype of *V. Cholerae* O1 has rapidly replaced the classical biotype in all parts of the country. Most of the El Tor biotype isolated today belong to the serotype Ogawa.

During 2018, about 651 cholera cases were reported in India with 6 deaths. Majority of the cases were reported from Uttar Pradesh (153) followed by Delhi (134), West Bengal (126) and Gujarat (106) *(4)*.

Epidemiological features

Cholera is both an epidemic and endemic disease. The epidemicity and endemicity of a disease will depend on the *characteristics* of the agent, and those of the *system* (environment). Characteristics of the agent which influence its distribution include its ability to survive in a given environment, its virulence, the average number of organisms required to cause infection, etc. Characteristics of the system which affect the distribution of the agent include the number of susceptibles, and the opportunities it provides for transmission of the infection. Global experience has shown that the introduction of cholera into any country cannot be prevented, but cholera can create a problem only in areas where sanitation is defective.

Epidemics of cholera are characteristically abrupt and often create an acute public health problem. They have a high potential to spread fast and cause deaths. The epidemic reaches a peak and subsides gradually as the "force of infection" declines. Often–times, by the time control measures are instituted the epidemic has already reached its peak and is waning. Thus, cholera epidemic in a community is self–limiting. This is attributed to the acquisition of temporary immunity, as well as due to the occurrence of a large number of subclinical cases.

The "force of infection" is composed of 2 components, namely the force of infection through water and the force of infection through contacts *(5)*. It is well-known that the elimination of contaminated water does not immediately bring an outbreak to an end, but a so-called "tail" of the epidemic is produced. This is due to the continuation of transmission through contacts *(5)*.

In areas where cholera is endemic, it does not show a stable endemicity like typhoid fever *(5)*. It undergoes seasonal fluctuations as well as epidemic outbreaks. The seasonal variation differs between countries and even between regions of the same country. The seasonal incidence is also subject to change. For example, the disease used to be most common in the summer in Kolkata and in the early winter in Bangladesh; now in both places, it is most frequent in the autumn *(6)*. In some parts of India, the peak incidence is in August.

The El Tor biotype, wherever it has spread, has become endemic with periodic outbreaks. It appears to have greater "endemic tendency" than its classical counterpart in that it causes a higher infection–to–case ratio (i.e., inapparent infections and mild cases).

Cholera occurs at intervals even in endemic areas. A question that is frequently asked is about the fate of *V. cholerae* in the inter–epidemic periods. Three explanations are offered : (a) the existence of long-term carriers *(7)*; (b) the existence of diminished but continuous transmission involving asymptomatic cases *(8)*, and (c) the persistence of the organism in a free–living, perhaps altered form in the environment *(9, 10)*. The existence of a free–living cycle may explain why cholera became endemic for varying periods in certain areas after introduction of the current pandemic strains *(9, 10)*. Atypical non-toxigenic *V. cholerae* O1 of the El Tor biotype have sometimes been found in surface waters in endemic and non-endemic areas without any related human infection or disease *(11)*. A question of considerable epidemiological significance is whether "transmission" of somatic antigen can occur in the natural environment, i.e., can non–O1 *V. cholerae* become *V. cholerae* O1 *(12)*. Such "transformation" has been claimed by many workers *(13)*.

Epidemiological determinants

Agent factors

(a) AGENT : The organism that causes cholera is labelled as *V. cholerae* O Group 1 or *Vibrio cholerae* O1 and O139. The term "epidemic strain" has also been used for these vibrios. Vibrios that are biochemically similar to the epidemic strains (*V. cholerae* O1 and O139) but do not agglutinate in *V. cholerae* O1 and O139 antiserum have been referred to in the past as non–agglutinating (NAG) vibrios or as non–cholera vibrios (NCV). These are now included in the species *V. cholerae* and are referred to as non–O Group 1V/ O139 *cholerae* (non-epidemic strains). It is now recognized that the NCV/NAG vibrios include some species that are pathogenic for humans (e.g., *Vibrio parahaemolyticus*) which have caused outbreaks of cholera-like diarrhoea. It is, therefore, necessary to identify *V. cholerae* O1 and O139 for specific diagnosis of cholera. Within the O–Group 1, two biotypes – classical and El Tor, have been differentiated. It may be mentioned that the El Tor biotype was first isolated at the El Tor quarantine station in Egypt in 1905. Cholera is now caused mostly by the El Tor biotype and O139. Classical and El Tor vibrios are further divided each into 3 serological types namely Inaba, Ogawa and Hikojima. Most of the El Tor vibrios isolated in India belong to the Ogawa serotype. The El Tor biotype which are known for their haemolytic property, lost this property as the pandemic progressed. They may be distinguished from classical vibrios by the following tests :

(1) El Tor vibrio agglutinate chicken and sheep erythrocytes
(2) they are resistant to classical phage IV
(3) they are resistant to polymyxin B–50–unit disc, and
(4) the VP reaction and haemolytic test do not give consistent results.

(b) RESISTANCE : *V. cholerae* are killed within 30 minutes by heating at 56 deg.C or within a few seconds by boiling. They remain in ice for 4–6 weeks or longer. Drying and sunshine will kill them in a few hours. They are easily destroyed by coal tar disinfectants such as cresol. Bleaching powder is another good disinfectant which kills vibrios instantly at 6 mg/litre. The El Tor biotype tends to be more resistant than do classical vibrios. (c) TOXIN PRODUCTION : The vibrios multiply in the lumen of the small intestine and produce an exotoxin (enterotoxin). This toxin produces diarrhoea through its effect on the adenylate cyclase–cyclic AMP system of mucosal cells of the small intestine. The exotoxin has no effect on any other tissue except the intestinal epithelial cells. (d) RESERVOIR OF INFECTION: The human being is the only known reservoir of cholera infection. He may be a case or carrier. *(i) Cases :* Cases range from inapparent infections to severe ones. About 75 per cent of people infected with *V. cholerae* do not develop any symptoms, although the bacteria are present in their faeces for 7–14 days after infection and are shed back into the environment, potentially infecting other people. Among people who develop symptoms, about 20 per cent develop acute watery diarrhoea with severe dehydration. People with low immunity, e.g., malnourished children and people living with HIV are at a greater risk of death if infected *(1)*. It is the mild and asymptomatic cases that play a significant role in maintaining endemic reservoir. *(ii) Carriers :* The carriers are usually temporary, rarely chronic. They also make an important contribution to the reservoir of infection. Since carriers excrete fewer vibrios than clinical cases, carriers are best detected by bacteriological examination of the purged stool induced by the administration of 30–60 gram of magnesium sulphate in 100 ml of water by mouth. (e) INFECTIVE MATERIAL : The immediate sources of infection are the stools and vomit of cases and carriers. Large numbers of vibrios (about 10^7–10^9 vibrios per ml of fluid) are present in the watery stools of cholera patients; and an average patient excretes 10–20 litres of fluid. Carriers excrete fewer vibrios than cases, 10^2–10^5 vibrios per gram of stools. (f) INFECTIVE DOSE : Cholera is dose–related. Infection occurs when the number of vibrios ingested exceeds the dose that is infective for the individual. Experimental work suggests that in the normal person a very high dose–something like 10^{11} organisms – is required to produce the clinical disease *(14)*. (g) PERIOD OF COMMUNICABILITY : A case of cholera is infectious for a period of 7–10 days. Convalescent carriers are infectious for 2–3 weeks. The chronic carrier state may last from a month up to 10 years or more.

Carriers in cholera *(15)*

A cholera carrier may be defined as an apparently healthy person who is excreting *V. cholerae* O1 (classical or El Tor) in stools. Four types of cholera carriers have been described *(16)* : (a) PRECLINICAL OR INCUBATORY CARRIERS : Since the incubation period of cholera is short (1–5 days), incubatory carriage is of short duration. The incubatory carriers are potential patients. (b) CONVALESCENT CARRIER : The patient who has recovered from an attack of cholera may continue to excrete vibrios, during his convalescence for 2–3 weeks. Convalescent state has been found to occur in patients who have not received effective antibiotic treatment. The convalescent carriers can often become chronic or long-term carriers. (c) CONTACT OR HEALTHY CARRIER : This is the result of subclinical infection contracted through association with a source of infection, be it a case or infected environment. The duration of contact carrier state is usually less than 10 days; the gall bladder is not infected, and the stool culture is frequently positive for *V. cholerae* O1. Contact carriers probably play an important role in the spread of cholera. (d) CHRONIC CARRIER : A chronic carrier state occurs infrequently. The longest carrier state was found to be over 10 years *(16)*. Studies indicate that gall bladder is infected in chronic carriers. Since carriers excrete fewer vibrios than cases, selective media and proper enrichment are important for their diagnosis. In carriers, the antibody titre against *V. cholerae* O1 rises and remains positive as long as the person harbours the organism. This method may be used to detect long-term carriers along with bacteriological examination of stools.

Host factors

(a) AGE AND SEX : Cholera affects all ages and both sexes. In endemic areas, attack rate is highest in children. (b) GASTRIC ACIDITY : An effective barrier. The vibrio is destroyed in an acidity of pH 5 or lower. Conditions that reduce gastric acidity may influence individual susceptibility *(19)*. (c) POPULATION MOBILITY : Movement of population (e.g., pilgrimages, marriages, fairs and festivals) results in increased risk of exposure to infection. In this jet age, cases and carriers can easily transfer infection to other countries. (d) ECONOMIC STATUS : The incidence of cholera tends to be the highest in the lower socio-economic groups, and this is attributable mainly to poor hygiene. (e) IMMUNITY : An attack of cholera is followed by immunity to reinfection, but the duration and degree of immunity are not known. In experimental animals specific IgA antibodies occur in the lumen of the intestine. Similar antibodies in serum develop after the infection but only last a few months. Vibriocidal antibodies in serum (titer $\geq$ 1:20) have been associated with protection against colonization and disease. The presence of antitoxin antibodies has not been associated with protection *(17)*. Vaccination gives only temporary, partial immunity for 3–6 months.

Environmental factors

Vibrio transmission is readily possible in a community with poor environmental sanitation. The environmental factors of importance include contaminated water and food. Flies may carry *V. cholerae* but not vectors of proven importance. Numerous social factors have also been responsible for the endemicity of cholera in India. These comprise certain human habits favouring water and soil pollution, low standards of personal hygiene, lack of education and poor quality of life.

Mode of transmission

Transmission occurs from man to man *via* (a) FAECALLY CONTAMINATED WATER : Uncontrolled water sources such as wells, lakes, ponds, streams and rivers pose a great threat. (b) CONTAMINATED FOOD AND DRINKS : Ingestion of contaminated food and drinks have been associated with outbreaks of cholera. Bottle feeding could be a significant risk factor for infants. Fruits and vegetables washed with contaminated water can be a source of infection. After preparation, cooked food may be contaminated through contaminated hands and flies. There is growing opinion that El Tor cholera may in some instances be transmitted through a complex interaction of contaminated food, water and environment rather than through public drinking water supplies *(18)*. (c) DIRECT CONTACT : In developing countries, a considerable proportion of cases may result from secondary transmission, i.e., person to person transmission through contaminated fingers while carelessly handling excreta and vomit of patients and contaminated linen and fomites.

Incubation period

From a few hours upto 5 days, but commonly 1–2 days.

Pathogenesis

The main symptom of cholera is diarrhoea. Diarrhoea in cholera was attributed in the past to such factors as increased permeability of the intestinal epithelial cells, increased peristalsis, mucosal damage, an increase in mesenteric blood flow and failure of the "sodium pump", i.e., interference with the passage of sodium from the lumen to the plasma. None of these theories stood the test of time *(19)*.

According to current concepts, the cholera vibrio get through the mucus which overlies the intestinal epithelium. It probably secretes mucinase, which helps it move rapidly through the mucus. Then it gets attached or *adhered* to the intestinal epithelial cells, and this it probably does by an adherence factor on its surface. When the vibrio becomes *adherent* to the mucosa, it produces its enterotoxin which consists of 2 parts – the light or L toxin and the heavy or H toxin. The L toxin combines with substances in the epithelial cell membrane called *gangliosides* and this binds the vibrio to the cell wall. Binding is irreversible. The mode of action of H toxin is not fully clear. What we know is that there is a substance called "adenyl cyclase" in the intestinal epithelial cells, and H toxin activates this substance. The activated adenyl cyclase causes a rise in another substance, called 3, 5–adenosine monophosphate, better known as cyclic or cAMP (A physiologist got Noble Prize for describing this substance). cAMP provides energy which drives fluid and ions into the lumen of the intestine. This fluid is isotonic and is secreted by all segments of small intestine. The increase in fluid is the cause of diarrhoea, and not increased peristalsis. There is no evidence that *V. cholerae* invades any tissue, nor the enterotoxin to have any direct effect on any organ other than the small intestine *(19)*.

Clinical features

The severity of cholera is dependent on the rapidity and duration of fluid loss. Epidemiological studies have shown that more than 90 per cent of El Tor cholera cases are mild and clinically indistinguishable from other acute diarrhoeas *(20)*. However, a typical case of cholera shows 3 stages : (a) STAGE OF EVACUATION : The onset is abrupt with profuse, painless, watery diarrhoea followed by vomiting. The patient may pass as many as 40 stools in a day. The stools may have a "rice water" appearance. (b) STAGE OF COLLAPSE : The patient soon passes into a stage of collapse because of dehydration. The classical signs are : sunken eyes, hollow cheeks, scaphoid abdomen, sub–normal temperature, washerman's hands and feet, absent pulse, unrecordable blood pressure, loss of skin elasticity, shallow and quick respirations. The output of urine decreases and may ultimately cease. The patient becomes restless, and complains of intense thirst and cramps in legs and abdomen. Death may occur at this stage, due to dehydration and acidosis resulting from diarrhoea. (c) STAGE OF RECOVERY : If death does not occur, the patient begins to show signs of clinical improvement. The blood pressure begins to rise, the temperature returns to normal, and urine secretion is re-established. If anuria persists, the patient may die of renal failure. The classical form of severe cholera occurs in only 5–10 per cent of cases. In the rest, the disease tends to be mild characterized by diarrhoea with or without vomiting or marked dehydration. As a rule, mild cases recover in 1–3 days.

Epidemiologically, cholera due to El Tor biotype differs from classical cholera in the following respects : (a) a higher incidence of mild and asymptomatic infection. This implies that the characteristic picture of rice–water stools and other signs of classical cholera described above may not be seen often; (b) fewer secondary cases in the affected families; (c) occurrence of chronic carriers, and (d) since El Tor vibrios are more resistant than classical cholera vibrios, they survive longer in the extra–intestinal environment.

Laboratory diagnosis of cholera *(21)*

The diagnosis of cholera can never be made with certainty on clinical grounds. Laboratory methods of diagnosis are required to confirm the diagnosis : (a) COLLECTION OF STOOLS : A fresh specimen of stool should be collected for laboratory examination. Sample should be collected before the person is treated with antibiotics. Collection may be made generally in one of the following ways : *(i) Rubber catheter :* Collection by the catheter is the best method but is complicated under field conditions. Soft rubber catheter (No.26–28) sterilized by boiling should be used. The catheter is introduced (after lubrication with liquid paraffin) for at least 4–5 cm into the rectum. The specimen voided may be collected directly into a transport (holding) media, e.g., Venkatraman–Ramakrishnan (VR) medium, alkaline peptone water. *(ii) Rectal swab :* Swabs consisting of 15–20 cm long wooden sticks, with one end wrapped with absorbent cotton, sterilized by autoclaving have been found to be satisfactory. Rectal swabs should be dipped into the holding medium before being introduced into the rectum. (iii) If no transport medium is available, a cotton–tipped rectal swab should be soaked in the liquid stool, placed in a sterile plastic bag, tightly sealed and sent to the testing laboratory *(22)*. (b) VOMITUS : This is practically never used as the chances of isolating vibrios are much less and there is no advantage. (c) WATER : Samples containing 1–3 litres of suspect water should be collected in sterile bottles (for the filter method), or 9 volumes of the sample water added to 1 volume of 10 per cent peptone water, and despatched to the laboratory by the quickest method of transport. (d) FOOD SAMPLES : Samples of food suspected to be contaminated with *V. cholerae* (or other enteric bacteria) amounting to 1 to 3 g are collected in transport media and sent to the laboratory. (e) TRANSPORTATION : (i) The stools should be transported in sterilized McCartney bottles, 30 ml capacity containing alkaline peptone water or VR medium. VR medium can be used if larger stool specimens can be collected. The specimen should be transported in alkaline peptone water or Cary–Blair medium if it is collected by a rectal swab. One gram or one ml of faeces in 10 ml of the holding medium will suffice. Rectal swabs should have their tops broken off so that caps of the containers can be replaced (ii) If suitable plating media are available (e.g., bile salt agar) at the bed-side, the stools should be streaked on to the media and forwarded to the laboratory with the transport media. (f) DIRECT EXAMINATION : If a microscope with dark field illumination is available, it may be possible to diagnose about 80 per cent of the cases within a few minutes, and more cases after 5–6 hours of incubation in alkaline peptone water. In the dark field, the vibrios evoke the image of many shooting stars in a dark sky. If motility ceases on mixing with polyvalent anti–cholera diagnostic serum, the organisms are presumed to be cholera vibrios. A presumptive diagnosis of cholera can thus be established. (g) CULTURE METHODS : On arrival at the laboratory, the specimen in holding fluid is well shaken, and about 0.5 to 1.0 ml of material is inoculated into Peptone Water Tellurite (PWT) medium for enrichment. After 4 to 6 hours incubation at 37 deg. C, a loopful of the culture from the surface is subcultured on Bile Salt Agar medium (BSA, pH 8.6). After overnight incubation, the plates are screened under oblique light illumination for vibrio colonies. (h) CHARACTERIZATION : *V. cholerae* usually appears on bile salt agar (BSA) as translucent, moist, raised, smooth and easily emulsifiable colonies about 1 mm in diameter. The typical colonies are picked up and tested as follows : *(i) Gram's stain and motility* : Gram negative and curved rods with characteristic scintillating type of movement in hanging drop preparations are very characteristic of *V. cholerae* *(ii) Serological test:* Slide agglutination test is done by picking up suspected colonies and making a homogeneous suspension in 0.85 per cent sterile saline and adding one drop of polyvalent anti–cholera diagnostic serum. If agglutination is positive, the test is repeated with *Inaba* and *Ogawa* antisera, to determine the subtype. (i) BIOCHEMICAL TESTS : Serologically positive colonies should be subcultured in one tube each of the sugar broths (mannose, sucrose, arabinose) and a tube of peptone water pH 7.2 for the cholera red reaction. Production of acid in sucrose and mannose, but not arabinose is characteristic of *V. cholerae.* (j) FURTHER CHARACTERIZATION : For further characterization of biotypes of *V. cholerae* organisms are identified by slide agglutination tests using anti–O1 or group 139 antisera and by biochemical reaction patterns.

Suspicious colonies that do not agglutinate with anticholera sera are tested further by the oxidase and string tests *(19)*.

CONTROL OF CHOLERA

It is now considered that the best way to control cholera is to develop and implement a national programme for the control of ALL diarrhoeal diseases because of similarities in the epidemiology, pathophysiology, treatment and control of cholera and other acute diarrhoeal diseases *(23)*. The following account is based on the "Guidelines for Cholera Control" proposed by the WHO *(11)*.

1. Verification of the diagnosis

It is important to have confirmation of the outbreak as quickly as possible. All cases of diarrhoea should be investigated even on the slightest suspicion. For the specific diagnosis of cholera, it is important to identify *V. cholerae* O1 in the stools of the patient. Once the presence of cholera has been proved, it is not necessary to culture stools of all cases or contacts. Bacteriological diagnosis of cholera envisages a well–organized system of laboratory services in the community.

2. Notification

Cholera is a notifiable disease locally and nationally. Since 2005 cholera notification is no longer mandatory internationally. Health workers at all levels (particularly those who are closest to the community such as the community health workers and the multi-purpose workers) should be trained to identify and notify cases immediately to the local health authority. Under the International Health Regulations, cholera is notifiable to the WHO within 24 hours of its occurrence by the National Government; the number of cases and deaths are also to be reported daily and weekly till the area is declared free of cholera. An area is declared free of cholera when twice the incubation period (i.e., 10 days) has elapsed since the death, recovery or isolation of the last case *(24)*.

3. Early case-finding

An aggressive search for cases (mild, moderate, severe) should be made in the community to be able to initiate prompt treatment. Early detection of cases also permits the detection of infected household contacts and helps the epidemiologist in investigating the means of spread for deciding on specific intervention.

4. Establishment of treatment centres

In the control of cholera, no time should be lost in providing treatment for the patients. To achieve this objective, it is necessary to establish easily accessible treatment facilities in the community.

The *mildly dehydrated* patients (which account for over 90 per cent of cases) should be treated at home with oral rehydration fluid. *Severely dehydrated* patients, requiring intravenous fluids, should be transferred to the nearest treatment centre or hospital; if possible, they should receive oral rehydration on the way to the hospital or treatment centre. If there is no hospital or treatment centre within a convenient distance, a local school or public building should be taken over and converted into a temporary treatment centre, as close to the site of epidemic as possible. Transportation of cases over long distances is not desirable; it has been linked with the spread of the disease.

In areas where peripheral health services are poor and cholera is endemic or threatening, mobile teams should be established at the district level. When needed, these teams should be brought promptly into the epidemic area to assist the local workers.

5. Rehydration therapy

Cholera is now the most effectively treated disease. Mortality rates have been brought down to less than 1 per cent by effective rehydration therapy. The rehydration may be oral or intravenous. The guidelines for ORT and intravenous rehydration are discussed in detail on page 266, 267.

6. Adjuncts to therapy

Antibiotics should be given as soon as vomiting has stopped, which is usually after 3 to 4 hours of oral rehydration. Injectable antibiotics have no special advantages. The commonly used antibiotics for the treatment of cholera are flouroquinolones, tetracycline, Azithromycin, ampicilline and Trimethoprim TMP-Sulfamethoxazole (SMX). No other medication should be given to treat cholera, like antidiarrhoeals, antiemetics, antispasmodics, cardiotonics and corticosteroids. In regions where cholera is present, it is important to identify those antibiotics to which the vibrio cholerae O1 is resistant. If diarrhoea persists after 48 hours of treatment, resistance to antibiotic should be suspected.

7. Epidemiological investigations

General sanitation measures must be applied at the onset of an outbreak (see under sanitation measures). At the same time, epidemiological studies must be undertaken to define the extent of the outbreak and identify the modes of transmission so that more effective and specific control measures can be applied. The epidemiologist must maintain contact with all health and civic units in his area to ensure detection of new foci of disease.

There are certain institutions which are able to assist in investigating outbreaks. These include the National Institute of Communicable Diseases, Delhi and the All India Institute of Hygiene and Public Health, Kolkata, where epidemiological teams are available for investigating epidemics. In addition, stools for phage typing may be sent to the National Institute of Cholera and Enteric Diseases, 3, Dr Isaque Road, Kolkata–700016, where the WHO International Centre for Vibrios is located.

8. Sanitation measures

(a) *WATER CONTROL* : As water is the most important vehicle of transmission of cholera, all steps must be taken to provide properly treated or otherwise safe water to the community for all purposes (drinking, washing and cooking).

Various approaches have been described for supplying safe water quickly and with limited resources *(25)*. Facilities selected and installed should be appropriate and acceptable to the community. The ultimate aim should be provision of piped water supply on a permanent basis and elimination of alternative unsafe water sources. Because of financial limitations and other competitive priorities, this measure cannot be applied immediately on a large scale in developing countries, such as India. As an emergency measure, in urban areas, properly treated drinking water containing free residual chlorine should be made available to all families; this water should be stored in the household in narrow–mouthed, covered containers. In rural areas, water can be made safe by boiling or by chlorination. The emergency measures should be followed by the development of more permanent facilities.

(b) *EXCRETA DISPOSAL* : Provision of simple, cheap and effective excreta disposal system (sanitary latrines) is a basic need of all human settlements. When cholera appears in a community, the need for these facilities becomes vital. With the cooperation of the community, sanitary system should be selected and constructed *(25)*, taking into consideration the customs and practices of the population, the existing terrain and geology, and the available resources. Simultaneously, health education messages should stress the proper use of such facilities, the dangers involved in depositing faeces on the ground, and in or near water, and the importance of handwashing with soap after defecation.

(c) *FOOD SANITATION* : Since food may be an important vehicle of infection, steps should be taken to improve food sanitation, particularly sale of foods under hygienic conditions. Health education must stress the importance of eating cooked hot food and of proper individual food handling techniques. Cooking utensils should be cleaned and dried after use.

The housefly plays a relatively small role in transmitting cholera, but its prevalence is a general indicator of the level of sanitation.

(d) *DISINFECTION* : Disinfection should be both concurrent and terminal. The most effective disinfectant for general use is a coal tar disinfectant with a Rideal–Walker (RW) coefficient of 10 or more such as cresol. A disinfectant with a RW coefficient of less than 5 should not be used *(26)*. Bleaching powder, if used, should be of good quality. For disinfection, attention should be paid to the following : patient's stools and vomit; clothes and other personal items that may have been contaminated; the latrine, if any; the patient's house and neighbourhood.

9. Chemoprophylaxis

Studies have shown that approximately 10–12 per cent of close household contacts of a cholera case may be bacteriologically positive, and some of these develop clinical illness. In contrast, a very small proportion (0.6–1 per cent) in the community may be excreting vibrios. Mass chemoprophylaxis is not advised for the total community because in order to prevent one serious case of cholera, some 10,000 persons must be given the drug. Further, the drug's effect is only short–lived for a few days. Whenever mass chemoprophylaxis was attempted, it failed to stop the spread of cholera. Because of these reasons, chemoprophylaxis is advised only for household contacts or of a closed community in which cholera has occurred.

Tetracycline is the drug of choice for chemoprophylaxis. It has to be given over a 3–day period in a twice–daily dose of 500 mg for adults, 125 mg for children aged 4–13 years, and 50 mg for children aged 0–3 years. Alternatively, the long–acting tetracycline (doxycycline) may be used for chemoprophylaxis, if the prevailing strains are not resistant. A single oral dose of doxycycline (300 mg for adults and 6 mg/kg for children under 15 years) has proved to be effective.

10. Vaccination

ORAL VACCINE (27)

Three types of oral cholera vaccines are available : (a) Dukoral (WC-rBS), (b) Sanchol and mORCVAX and (c) Euvichol. The live attenuated single-dose vaccine (CVD103-HgR) is no longer produced.

(a) Dukoral (WC-rBS)

Dukoral is a monovalent vaccine based on formalin and heat-killed whole cells (WC) of *V. cholerae* O1 (classical and El Tor, Inaba and Ogawa) plus recombinant cholera toxin B subunit. The vaccine is provided in 3 ml single-dose vials together with the bicarbonate buffer (effervescent granules in sachets to protect the toxin B subunit from being destroyed by gastric acid). Vaccine and buffer are mixed in 150 ml of water (chlorinated or not) for persons aged >5 years and in 75 ml of water for children aged 2–5 years. The vaccine has a shelf life of 3 years at 2–8°C and remains stable for 1 month at 37°C.

Vaccine schedule and administration

According to the manufacturer, primary immunization consists of 2 oral doses given ≥7 days apart (but <6 weeks apart) for adults and children aged ≥6 years. Children aged 2–5 years should receive 3 doses ≥7 days apart (but <6 weeks apart). Intake of food and drink should be avoided for 1 hour before and after vaccination. If the interval between the primary immunization doses is delayed for >6 weeks, primary immunization should be restarted. Protection may be expected about 1 week after the last scheduled dose.

Provided there is continued risk of *V. cholerae* infection, 1 booster dose is recommended by manufacturer, after 2 years for adults and children aged ≥6 years. If the interval between the primary series and booster immunization is >2 years, primary immunization must be repeated. For children aged 2–5 years 1 booster dose is recommended every 6 months, and if the interval between primary immunization and the booster is >6 months, primary immunization must be repeated.

Dukoral is not licensed for children aged <2 years.

(b) Sanchol and mORCVAX

The closely related bivalent oral cholera vaccines are based on serogroups O1 and O139. Unlike Dukoral, these vaccines do not contain the bacterial toxin B subunit therefore it does not require buffer. According to the manufacturer, vaccine should be administered orally in 2 liquid doses 14 days apart for individuals aged ≥1 year. A booster dose is recommended after 2 years *(27)*.

(c) Euvichol

It was prequalified in December 2015 and has same characteristics as Sanchol *(2)*.

11. Health education

The most effective prophylactic measure is perhaps health education. It should be directed mainly to (a) the effectiveness and simplicity of oral rehydration therapy (b) the benefits of early reporting for prompt treatment (c) food hygiene practices (d) hand washing after defecation and before eating, and (e) the benefit of cooked, hot foods and safe water. Since cholera is mainly a disease of the poor and ignorant, these groups should be tackled first.

Diarrhoeal Diseases Control Programme

The incidence of cholera cases and deaths has decreased in recent years. During the year 1980–81, strategy of the National Cholera Control Programme has undergone changes *(28)*. It is now termed as Diarrhoeal Diseases Control Programme *(29)*. Oral Rehydration Therapy Programme was started in 1986–87 in a phased manner. The main objective of the programme is to prevent diarrhoea–associated deaths in children due to dehydration. The training programme and health education material highlight the rational management of diarrhoea in children, including increased intake of home available fluids and breast feeding. ORS is promoted as first line of treatment. ORS is being supplied as a part of the sub-centre kits *(30)*.

References

1. WHO (2020), *Weekly Epidemiological Record*, No. 37, 11th Sep. 2020.
2. WHO (2016), *Weekly Epidemiological Record*, No. 38, 23rd Sep. 2016.
3. WHO (2010), *Weekly Epidemiological Record*, No. 31, 30th July 2010.
4. Govt. of India (2021), *National Health Profile 2021*, Central Bureau of Health Intelligence, DGHS, Ministry of Health and Family Welfare, New Delhi.
5. Cvjetanovic, B. et al (1978). *Bull WHO*, 56 Supplement No.1, p. 76.
6. WHO (1980) *Programme for Control of Diarrhoeal Diseases*, Scientific Working Group Reports 1978–1980, CDD/80.1, WHO, Geneva.
7. Azurin, J.C. et al (1967). *Bull WHO*, 37 : 745–749.
8. Sinha, R. et al (1967). *Bull WHO*, 37 : 89–100.
9. Nalin, D.R. (1976). *Lancet*, 2 : 958.
10. Levine, M.M. (1980). *N. Eng.J.Med.*, 302 (6) 345.
11. WHO (1980). *Guidelines for Cholera Control*, WHO/CDD/SER/80.4, Geneva.
12. Blake, Paul A (1980). in *Annual Review of Microbiology*, 34 : 351.
13. Seal, S.C. (1977). Ind. *J. Pub. Health*, 21 (2) 48.
14. Mackay, D.M. (1979). *Trans. Roy.Soc.Trop.Med & Hyg.*, 73 (1) 1.
15. Seal, S.C. (1977). *Ind. J. Pub. Health*, 21 (2) 48.
16. Shrivastava, D.L. (1968).*J.Indian M.A.*, 50 : 581.
17. Jawetz. Melnick & Adelberg's *Medical Microbiology*, 25th Ed. 2010, A Lange Publications.
18. Gunn, R.A. et al (1981). *Bull WHO*, 59 (1) 65.
19. Christie, A.B. (1980). *Infectious Diseases : Epidemiology and Clinical Practice*, 3rd ed., Churchill Livingstone.
20. WHO (2004), *Weekly Epidemiological Record*, No.31, July 30, 2004.
21. WHO (1974). *Guidelines for the Laboratory Diagnosis of Cholera.*
22. WHO (2001), *Weekly Epidemiological Record*, No. 31, 3 Aug. 2001.
23. WHO (1978). *Development of a Programme for Diarrhoeal Diseases Control*, Report of an Advisory Group, WHO/DDC/78.1.
24. Delon, P.J. (1975). *International Health Regulations*, A Practical Guide, WHO, Geneva.
25. Rajagopalan, S. and Shiffman, M.A. (1974). *Guide to Simple Sanitary Measures for the Control of Enteric Diseases*, Geneva, WHO.
26. ICMR (1959). *Report of the Central Expert Committee on Smallpox and Cholera*, New Delhi.
27. WHO (2010), *Weekly Epidemiological Record*, No. 13, 26th March 2010.
28. Govt. of India, Ministry of Health and Family Welfare (1981). *Report 1980–81*, Department of Health and Family Welfare, New Delhi.
29. Govt. of India, Ministry of Health & Family Welfare (1982). *Annual Report 1981–1982.*
30. Govt. of India, *Annual Report 1993–94*, DGHS, New Delhi.

TYPHOID FEVER

Typhoid fever is the result of systemic infection mainly by *S. typhi* found only in man. The disease is clinically characterized by a typical continuous fever for 3 to 4 weeks, relative bradycardia with involvement of lymphoid tissues and considerable constitutional symptoms. The term ***"enteric fever"*** includes both typhoid and paratyphoid fevers. The disease may occur sporadically, epidemically or endemically.

Problem statement

WORLD

Typhoid fever occurs in all parts of the world where water supplies and sanitation are sub-standard. The disease is now uncommon in the developed countries where most of the cases that occur are either acquired abroad or imported by immigrants *(1)*. Improved living conditions and the introduction of antibiotics in the late 1940s resulted in drastic reduction of typhoid fever morbidity and mortality in industrialized countries. In developing areas of Asia, Africa, Latin America, however, the disease continues to be a public health problem, albeit with incidence rate that vary considerably between and within countries. WHO estimated the global typhoid fever disease burden at 11–20 million cases annually, resulting in an estimated 128,000–161,000 deaths per year, predominantly in children of school age or younger. Majority of this burden occurs in Asia *(2)*.

Since 1950, the organism's resistance to antibiotics has also been a growing problem; by 1989 resistance was reported in a number of countries, particularly in Asia and Middle East. Resistant strains have caused outbreaks of the disease in India and Pakistan in recent years. In South–East Asia, 50 per cent or more of the strains of the bacteria may already be resistant to several antibiotics *(3)*. Typhoid fever caused by multidrug-resistant (MDR) strains of *S. typhi* – that is resistant to all 3 of the first line of antibiotics (chloramphenicol, ampicillin and cotrimoxazole) – is associated with more severe illness and higher rates of complications and death, especially in children aged less than 2 years. Also, compared with typhoid fever caused by sensitive strains, a ten-fold higher rate of post-treatment symptomatic bacterial carriers has been reported with MDR *S. typhi* infection *(2)*. Without effective treatment, typhoid fever kills almost 10 per cent of those infected *(3)*.

The socio-economic impact of the disease is huge, because typhoid survivors may take several months to recover and resume work.

INDIA

Typhoid fever is endemic in India. Reported data for the year 2020 shows 1.069 million cases and 126 deaths. Maximum cases were reported from Uttar Pradesh (297,170 cases) West Bengal (117,842 cases and 9 deaths), Karnataka (88,558 cases), Telangana (68,280 cases) and Andhra Pradesh (65,068 cases and 9 deaths) *(5)*.

Epidemiological determinants

Agent factors

(a) AGENT : *S. typhi* is the major cause of enteric fever. *S. para A and S. para B* are relatively infrequent *(6)*. *S. typhi* has three main antigens – O, H and Vi and a number of phage types (at least 80). Phage typing has proved a useful epidemiological tool in tracing the source of epidemics. *S. typhi* survives intracellularly in the tissues of various organs. It is readily killed by drying, pasteurization, and common disinfectants. The factors which influence the onset of typhoid fever in man are the infecting dose and virulence of the organism.

(b) RESERVOIR OF INFECTION : Man is the only known reservoir of infection, viz. cases and carriers. (i) CASES : The case may be mild, missed or severe. A case (or carrier) is infectious as long as bacilli appear in stools or urine. (ii) CARRIERS : The carriers may be temporary (incubatory, convalescent) or chronic. *Convalescent carriers* excrete the bacilli for 6 to 8 weeks, after which their numbers diminish rapidly. By the end of three months, not more than 4 per cent of cases are still excreting the organisms; and by the end of one year, the average carrier rate is around 3 per cent *(7)*. Persons who excrete the bacilli for more than a year after a clinical attack are called chronic carriers. In most chronic carriers, the organisms persist in the gall bladder and in the biliary tract. A chronic carrier state may be expected to develop in 2 to 5 per cent of cases. A chronic carrier may excrete the bacilli for several years (may be as long as 50 years) either continuously or intermittently. The famous case of "Typhoid Mary" who gave rise to more than 1300 cases in her life time is a good example of a chronic carrier. Faecal carriers are more frequent than urinary carriers. Chronic urinary carrier state is often associated with some abnormality of the urinary tract.

(c) SOURCE OF INFECTION : The primary sources of infection are faeces and urine of cases or carriers; the secondary sources contaminated water, food, fingers and flies. There is no evidence that typhoid bacilli are excreted in sputum or milk.

Host factors

(a) Age : Typhoid fever may occur at any age. Highest incidence of this disease occurs in the 5–19 years of age group. Prospective population-based surveillance in some Asian urban slum areas has shown that in the age group 5–15 years, the annual incidence of blood culture-confirmed typhoid fever may reach 180–494 per 100,000. In some of these areas, pre-school-age children less than 5 years, show incidence rates similar to those of school-age children *(2)*. After the age of 20 years, the incidence falls probably due to acquisition of immunity from clinical or subclinical infection. *(b) Sex :* More cases are reported among males than females, probably as a result of increased exposure to infection. But carrier rate is more in females. *(c) Immunity:* All ages are susceptible to infection. Antibody may be stimulated by the infection or by immunization; however, the antibody to the somatic antigen (O) is usually higher in the patient with the disease, and the antibody to the flagellar antigen(H) is usually higher in immunized individuals. Serum antibodies are not the primary defences against infection; *S. typhi* being an intracellular organism, cell–mediated immunity plays a major role in combating the infection. Natural typhoid fever does not always confer solid immunity; second attacks may occur when challenged with a large oral dose. Among the host factors that contribute to resistance to *S. typhi are* gastric acidity and local intestinal immunity.

Environmental and social factors

Enteric fevers are observed all through the year. The peak incidence is reported during July–September *(8)*. This period coincides with the rainy season and an increase in fly population.

Outside the human body, the bacilli are found in water, ice, food, milk and soil for varying periods of time. Typhoid bacilli do not multiply in water; many of them perish within 48 hours, but some may survive for about 7 days. They may survive for over a month in ice and icecream. They may survive for up to 70 days in soil irrigated with sewage under moist winter conditions, and for half that period under drier summer conditions *(9)*. Food being a bad conductor of heat, provides shelter to the bacilli which may multiply and survive for sometime in food. Typhoid bacilli grow rapidly in milk without altering its taste or appearance in anyway. Vegetables grown in sewage farms or washed in contaminated water are a positive health hazard. These factors are compounded by such social factors as pollution of drinking water supplies, open air defecation and urination, low standards of food and personal hygiene and health ignorance. Typhoid fever may therefore be regarded as an index of general sanitation in any country.

Incubation period

Usually 10–14 days. But it may be as short as 3 days or as long as three weeks depending upon the dose of the bacilli ingested.

Modes of transmission

Typhoid fever is transmitted *via* the faecal–oral route or urine–oral routes. This may take place *directly* through soiled hands contaminated with faeces or urine of cases or carriers, or *indirectly* by the ingestion of contaminated water, milk and/or food, or through flies.

Fig. 1 shows the dynamics of transmission. There are numerous sources of infection and many vehicles of transmission, each making its own contribution to the total magnitude of the problem. The situation is rendered more complex by the web of social, cultural and economic factors which determine the quality of life of the people.

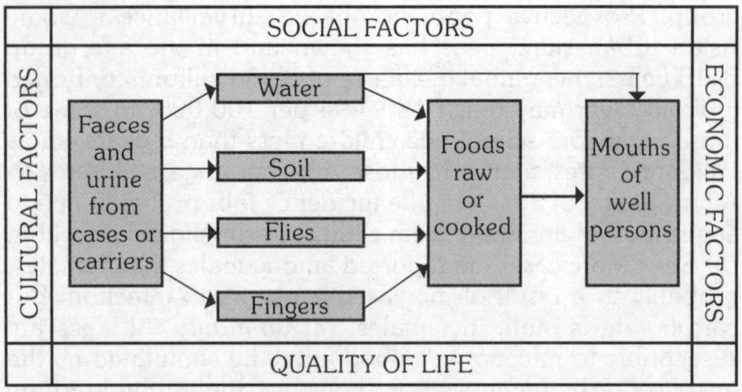

FIG.1
Dynamics of typhoid fever transmission

Clinical features

The onset is usually insidious but in children may be abrupt, with chills and high fever. During the prodromal stage, there is malaise, headache, cough and sore throat, often with abdominal pain and constipation. The fever ascends in a step–ladder fashion. After about 7–10 days, the fever reaches a plateau and the patient looks toxic, appearing exhausted and often prostrated. There may be marked constipation, especially in early stage or "pea soup" diarrhoea. There is marked abdominal distention. There is leukopenia and blood, urine and stool culture is positive for salmonella. If there are no complications the patient's condition improves over 7–10 days. However, relapse may occur for upto 2 weeks after termination of therapy.

During the early phase, physical findings are few. Later, splenomegaly, abdominal distension and tenderness, relative bradycardia, dicrotic pulse, and occasionally meningismus appear. The rash (rose spots) commonly appears during the second week of disease. The individual spot, found principally on the trunk, is a pink papule 2–3 mm in diameter that fades on pressure. It disappears in 3–4 days.

Serious complications occur in up to 10 per cent of typhoid fever patients, especially in those who have been ill longer than 2 weeks, and who have not received proper treatment. Intestinal haemorrhage is manifested by a sudden drop in temperature and signs of shock, followed by dark or fresh blood in the stool. Intestinal perforation is most likely to occur during the third week. Less frequent complications are urinary retention, pneumonia, thrombophlebitis, myocarditis, psychosis, cholecystitis, nephritis and osteomyelitis.

Estimates of case-fatality rates of typhoid fever range from 1 per cent to 4 per cent; fatality rates in children aged less than 4 years being 10 times higher (4.0%) than in older children (0.4%). In untreated cases, the fatality rates may rise to 10–20 per cent *(2)*.

Laboratory diagnosis of typhoid *(3)*

(a) MICROBIOLOGICAL PROCEDURES : The definitive diagnosis of typhoid fever depends on the isolation of *S. typhi* from blood, bone marrow and stools. Blood culture is the mainstay of diagnosis of this disease.

(b) SEROLOGICAL PROCEDURE : Felix-Widal test measures agglutinating antibody levels against O and H antigens. Usually, O antibodies appear on day 6–8 and H antibodies on day 10–12 after the onset of disease. The test is usually performed on an acute serum (at first contact with the patient). The test has only moderate sensitivity and specificity. It can be negative in upto 30 per cent of culture – proven cases of typhoid fever. This may be because of prior antibiotic therapy that has blunted the antibody response. On the other hand, *S. typhi* shares O and H antigens with other *salmonella* serotypes and has cross-reacting epitopes with other Enterobacteriacae, and this can lead to false-positive results. Such results may also occur in other clinical conditions, e.g. malaria, typhus, bacteraemia caused by other organisms, and cirrhosis.

(c) NEW DIAGNOSTIC TESTS : The recent advances for quick and reliable diagnostic tests for typhoid fever as an alternative to the Widal test include the IDL Tubex® test marketed by a Swedish company, which reportedly can detect IgM09 antibodies from patient within a few minutes. Another rapid serological test, Typhidot®, takes three hours to perform. It was developed in Malaysia for the detection of specific IgM and IgG antibodies against a 50 kD antigen of *S. typhi*. A newer version of the test, Typhidot-M®, was recently developed to detect specific IgM antibodies only. The dipstick test, developed in the Netherlands, is based on the binding of *S. typhi* – specific IgM antibodies in samples to *S. typhi lipopolysaccharide* (LPS) antigen and the staining of bound antibodies by an anti-human IgM antibody conjugated to colloidal dye particles.

CONTROL OF TYPHOID FEVER

The control or elimination of typhoid fever is well within the scope of modern public health. This is an accomplished fact in many developed countries. There are generally three lines of defence against typhoid fever :

1. control of reservoir
2. control of sanitation, and
3. immunization.

The weakest link in the chain of transmission is sanitation which is amenable to control.

1. Control of reservoir

The usual methods of control of reservoir are their identification, isolation, treatment and disinfection.

a. CASES

(i) Early diagnosis : This is of vital importance as the early symptoms are non-specific. Culture of blood and stools are important investigations in the diagnosis of cases. *(ii) Notification:* This should be done where such notification is mandatory. *(iii) Isolation :* Since typhoid fever is infectious and has a prolonged course, the cases are better transferred to a hospital for proper treatment, as well as to prevent the spread of infection. As a rule, cases should be isolated till three bacteriologically negative stools and urine reports, are obtained on three separate days. *(iv) Treatment :* The fluoroquinolones are widely regarded as the drug of choice for the treatment of typhoid fever. They are relatively inexpensive, well tolerated and more rapidly and reliably effective than the former first-line drugs, viz. chloramphenicol, ampicillin, amoxicillin and trimethoprim – sulfamethoxazole (TMP-SMX). The antibiotics used in uncomplicated typhoid fever are as shown in Table 1. Patients seriously ill and profoundly toxic may be given an injection of hydrocortisone 100 mg daily for 3 to 4 days. *(v) Disinfection :* Stools and urine are the sole sources of infection. They should be received in closed containers and disinfected with 5 per cent cresol for at least 2 hours. All soiled clothes and

TABLE 1

Treatment of uncomplicated typhoid fever

Susceptibility	Optimal therapy			Alternative effective drugs		
	Antibiotic	Daily dose mg/kg	Days	Antibiotic	Daily dose mg/kg	Days
Fully sensitive	Fluoroquinolone e.g. ofloxacin or ciprofloxacin	15	5–7 [a]	Chloramphenicol Amoxicillin TMP-SMX	50–75 75–100 8–40	14–21 14 14
Multidrug resistance	Fluoroquinolone or cefixime	15 15–20	5–7 7–14	Azithromycin Cefixime	8–10 15–20	7 7–14
Quinolone resistance [b]	Azithromycin or ceftriaxone	8–10 75	7 10–14	Cefixime	20	7–14

a Three-day courses are also effective and are particularly so in epidemic containment.

b The optimum treatment for quinolone-resistant typhoid fever has not been determined. Azithromycin, the third-generation cephalosporins, or a 10–14 days course of high-dose fluoroquinolones, is effective. Combinations of these are now being evaluated.

Source : *(10)*

linen should be soaked in a solution of 2 per cent chlorine and steam–sterilized. Nurses and doctors should not forget to disinfect their hands. *(vi) Follow-up :* Follow-up examination of stools and urine should be done for *S. typhi* 3 to 4 months after discharge of the patient, and again after 12 months to prevent the development of the carrier state. With early diagnosis and appropriate treatment, mortality has been reduced to about 1 per cent as compared to about 30 per cent in untreated cases.

(b) CARRIERS

Since carriers are the ultimate source of typhoid fever, their identification and treatment is one of the most radical ways of controlling typhoid fever. The measures recommended are : *(i) Identification :* Carriers are identified by cultural and serological examinations. Duodenal drainage establishes the presence of salmonella in the biliary tract in carriers. The Vi antibodies are present in about 80 per cent of chronic carriers. *(ii) Treatment :* The carrier should be given an intensive course of ampicillin or amoxycillin (4–6 g a day) together with Probenecid (2 g/day) for 6 weeks. These drugs are concentrated in the bile and may achieve eradication of the carrier state in about 70 per cent of carriers. Chloromycetin is considered worthless for clearing the carrier state. *(iii) Surgery :* Cholecystectomy with concomitant ampicillin therapy has been regarded as the most successful approach to the treatment of carriers. Cure rate may be as high as 80 per cent. Urinary carriers are easy to treat, but refractory cases may need nephrectomy when one kidney is damaged and the other healthy. *(iv) Surveillance :* The carriers should be kept under surveillance. They should be prevented from handling food, milk or water for others. *(v) Health education :* Health education regarding washing of hands with soap, after defecation or urination, and before preparing food is an essential element. In short, the management of carriers continues to be an unsolved problem. This is the crux of the problem, in the elimination of typhoid fever.

2. Control of sanitation

Protection and purification of drinking water supplies, improvement of basic sanitation, and promotion of food hygiene are essential measures to interrupt transmission of typhoid fever. For instance, typhoid fever is never a major problem where there is a clean domestic water supply. Sanitary measures, not followed by health education may produce only temporary results. However, when sanitation is combined with health education, the effects tend to be cumulative, resulting in a steady reduction of typhoid morbidity *(11)*.

3. Immunization

While ultimately, control of typhoid fever must take the form of improved sanitation and domestic and personal hygiene, these are long-term objectives in many developing countries. A complementary approach to prevention is immunization, which is the only specific preventive measure, likely to yield the highest benefit for the money spent. Immunization against typhoid does not give 100 per cent protection, but it definitely lowers both the incidence and seriousness of the infection. It can be given at any age upwards of two years. It is recommended to : (i) those living in endemic areas (ii) household contacts (iii) groups at risk of infection such as school children and hospital staff (iv) travellers proceeding to endemic areas, and (v) those attending *melas* and *yatras*.

ANTI-TYPHOID VACCINES *(2)*

The old parenteral killed whole-cell vaccine was effective but produced strong side-effects. Two safe and effective vaccines are now licensed and available. One is based on defined subunit antigens, the other on whole-cell live attenuated bacteria.

The Vi polysaccharide vaccine

This subunit vaccine was first licensed in the United States in 1994. It is composed of purified Vi capsular polysaccharide from the Ty2 S. Typhi strain and elicits a T-cell independent IgG response that is not boosted by additional doses. The vaccine is administered subcutaneously or intramuscularly. The target value for each single human dose is about 25μg of the antigen. The vaccine is stable for 6 months at 37°C, and for 2 years at 22°C. The recommended storage temperature is 2–8°C. The Vi vaccine does not elicit adequate immune responses in children aged less than 2 years.

Schedule

The vaccine is licensed for individuals aged ≥2 years. Only 1 dose is required, and the vaccine confers protection 7 days after injection. To maintain protection, re-vaccination is recommended every 3 years. The Vi polysaccharide vaccine can be co-administered with other vaccines relevant for international travellers, such as yellow fever and hepatitis A, and with vaccines of the routine childhood immunization programmes.

Safety

No serious adverse events and a minimum of local side-effects are associated with Vi vaccination. There are no contraindications to the use of this vaccine other than previous severe hypersensitivity reaction to vaccine components. Although the Vi polysaccharide vaccine is safe for HIV-infected individuals, the induction of protective antibodies is directly correlated to the levels of CD4 positive T-cells.

The Ty21a vaccine

This vaccine, which was first licensed in Europe in 1983 and in the USA in 1989, is an orally administered, live-attenuated Ty2 strain of *S. Typhi* in which multiple genes, including the genes responsible for the production of Vi, have been mutated chemically. The lyophilized vaccine is available as enteric coated capsules. Protection is markedly influenced by the number of doses and their spacing. There are currently no field trials to document the efficacy of Ty21a vaccine in children aged <3 years. Ty21a requires storage at 2–8°C; it retains potency for approximately 14 days at 25°C.

Schedule

The capsules are licensed for use in individuals aged ≥5 years. The vaccine is administered every other day; on 1, 3, and 5th day; a 3–dose regimen is recommended. With the 3–dose regimen, protective immunity is achieved 7 days after the last dose. The recommendation is to repeat this series every 3 years for people living in endemic areas, and every year for individuals travelling; from non-endemic to endemic countries. The Ty21a vaccine may be given simultaneously with other vaccines, including live vaccines against polio, cholera, and yellow fever, or the measles, mumps and rubella (MMR) combination.

Safety and precautions

Proguanil and antibacterial drugs should be stopped from 3 days before until 3 days after giving Ty21a, as such drugs may harm live bacterial vaccines. The vaccine is unlikely to be efficacious if administrated at the time of ongoing diarrhoea. It is not known whether this live attenuated vaccine may cause foetal harm when administered to pregnant women. Ty21a can be administered to HIV-positive, asymptomatic individuals as long as the T-cell count (CD_4) is >200/mm^3.

Ty21a is remarkably well tolerated and has low rates of adverse events.

The vaccine is not recommended in congenital or acquired immunodeficiency including treatment with immuno-suppressive and antimitotic drugs, acute febrile illness and acute intestinal infection.

References

1. Anderson, E.S. and Smith, H.P. (1972). *Brit. Med.J.*, 3 : 329–331.
2. WHO (2018) *Fact Sheet*, 31st Jan. 2018.
3. WHO (1996), The *World Health Report*, Report of the Director General WHO.
4. Ramesh Kumar, et al (1988). *Ann–Nat. Aced.Med.* Sc. (INDIA) 24 (4) 255–257.
5. Govt. of India (2021), *National Health Profile 2021*, DGHS, Ministry of Health and Family Welfare, New Delhi.
6. Basu, S. et al (1975). *Bull WHO*, 52 (3) 333.
7. Christie, A.B. (1974). *Infectious Diseases : Epidemiology and Clinical Practice*, 2nd ed., Churchill Livingstone.
8. Mangal, H.N. et al (1967). *Indian J. Med.* Res., 55 : 219.
9. WHO (1969), *Public Health Papers* No.38, p. 78.
10. WHO (2003), Background document : *The diagnosis, treatment and prevention of typhoid fever*, Communicable Disease Surveillance and Response Vaccines and Biologicals.
11. Cvjetanovic, B. et al (1978). *Bull WHO*, Supplement No. 1 56 : 45.

FOOD POISONING

Food poisoning is an acute gastroenteritis caused by ingestion of food or drink contaminated with either living bacteria or their toxins or inorganic chemical substances and poisons derived from plants and animals. The condition is characterized by: (a) history of ingestion of a common food (b) attack of many persons at the same time, and (c) similarity of signs and symptoms in the majority of cases.

High risk people

Some group of people are more likely to get sick and have a more serious illness. These groups include :

a. Adults age 65 and older;
b. Children younger than age 5 years;
c. Pregnant women; and
d. People whose immune systems are weekened by health conditions or medicines used to treat them including people with diabetes, liver or kidney disease, HIV/AIDS or cancer.

People who are more likely to get food poisoning should not eat undercooked food from animals, raw or lightly cooked sprouts, unpasteurized (raw) milk and juices and soft cheese (such as queso freso), unless it is labled as made with pasteurized milk *(2)*.

Types of food poisoning

Food poisoning may be of two types : non-bacterial and bacterial. *(a) Non-bacterial :* Caused by chemicals such as arsenic, certain plant and sea foods. In recent years, there has been a growing concern about contamination of food by chemicals, e.g., fertilizers, pesticides, cadmium, mercury etc. *(b) Bacterial :* Caused by the ingestion of foods contaminated by living bacteria or their toxins. The conventional classification of bacterial food poisoning into toxic and infective types is becoming increasingly blurred with the knowledge that in some types, both multiplication and toxin production are involved *(1)*. Bacterial food poisoning may be of the following types : Salmonellosis, Staphylococcal intoxication, *C. perfringens* illness, Botulism, B. cereus food poisoning, *E. coli* diarrhoea, Non-cholera vibrio illness, V. parahaemolyticus infection, streptococcal infection, Shigellosis Brucellosis. *(c) Viral diseases :* hepatitis A and E, Norovirus Gastroenteritis, Rotavirus. Some viruses can be transmitted by food consumption. It is characterized by nausea, explosive vomiting, watery diarrhoea and abdominal pain *(1)*. *(d) Parasites :* Taeniasis Hydatidosis, Trichinosis, Ascariasis, Amoebiasis, Oxyuriasis. Some parasites, such as fish-borne trematodes, are only transmitted through food. Others, for example tapeworms like *Echinococcus* spp, or *Taenia* spp, may infect people through food or direct contact with animals. Other parasites, such as *Ascaris*, *Cryptosporidium*, *Entamoeba histolytica* or *Giardia*, enter the food chain via water or soil and can contaminate fresh produce *(1)*.

1. Salmonella food poisoning

An extremely common form of food poisoning. Five reasons have been given for its increase in recent years : (a) an increase in community feeding (b) increase in international trade in human food (c) a higher incidence of salmonellosis in farm animals (d) widespread use of household detergents interfering with sewage treatment, and (e) wide distribution of "prepared foods" *(4)*.

(a) AGENT(S) : The species most often incriminated in human outbreaks are *S. typhimurium, S. cholera–suis* and *S. enteritidis,* besides many others. (b) SOURCE : Salmonellosis is primarily a disease of animals. Man gets the infection from *farm animals* and *poultry* – through contaminated meat, milk and milk products, sausages, custards, egg and egg products. Rats and mice are another source; they are often heavily infected and contaminate foodstuffs by their urine and faeces. Temporary human carriers can also contribute to the problem. (c) INCUBATION PERIOD : 12 to 24 hours commonly. (d) MECHANISM OF FOOD POISONING : The causative organisms, on ingestion, multiply in the intestine and give rise to acute enteritis and colitis. The onset is generally sudden with chills, fever, nausea, vomiting, and a profuse watery diarrhoea which usually lasts 2–3 days. Mortality is about 1 per cent. A convalescent carrier state lasting for several weeks may occur *(3)*.

Salmonellosis is described in detail separately, (Page 280).

2. Staphylococcal food poisoning

It is about as common as salmonella food poisoning. (a) AGENT : Enterotoxins of certain strains of coagulase–positive *Staphylococcus aureus.* At least 5 different enterotoxins have been identified, and a sixth may exist *(5)*. Toxins can be formed at optimum temperatures of 35 deg. to 37 deg. C. These toxins are relatively heat stable and resist boiling for 30 minutes or more. (b) SOURCE : Staphylococci are ubiquitous in nature, and are found on the skin and in the nose and throat of men and animals. They are a common agent of boils and pyogenic infections of man and animals. Cows suffering from mastitis have been responsible for outbreaks of food poisoning involving milk and milk products. The foods involved are salads, custards, milk and milk products which get contaminated by staphylococci. (c) INCUBATION PERIOD : 1–8 hours. The incubation period is short because of "preformed" toxin. (d) MECHANISM OF FOOD POISONING : Food poisoning results from ingestion of toxins preformed in the food in which bacteria have grown ("intradietetic" toxins). Since the toxin is heat–resistant, it can remain in food after the organisms have died. The toxins act directly on the intestine and CNS. The illness becomes manifest by the sudden onset of vomiting, abdominal cramps and diarrhoea. In severe cases, blood and mucus may appear. Unlike salmonella food poisoning, staphylococcal food poisoning rarely causes fever. Death is uncommon.

Botulism

Most serious but rare. It kills two-thirds of its victims. (a) AGENT : Exotoxin of *Clostridium botulinum* generally Type A, B or E. (b) SOURCE : The organism is widely distributed in soil, dust and the intestinal tract of animals and enters food as spores. The foods most frequently responsible for botulism are home preserved foods such as home–canned vegetables, smoked or pickled fish, home–made cheese and similar low acid foods. In fact, botulism derives its name from the Latin word for sausage (botulus). (c) INCUBATION PERIOD : 18 to 36 hours. (d) MECHANISM OF FOOD POISONING : The toxin is preformed in food ("intradietetic") under suitable anaerobic conditions. It acts on the parasympathetic nervous system. Botulism differs from other forms of food poisoning in that the gastrointestinal symptoms are very slight. The prominent symptoms are dysphagia, diplopia, ptosis, dysarthria, blurring of vision, muscle weakness and even quadriplegia. Fever is generally absent, and consciousness is retained. The condition is frequently fatal, death occurring 4–8 days later due to respiratory or cardiac failure. Patients who recover do not develop antitoxin in the blood. Since the toxin is thermolabile, the heating of food which may be subjected to 100 deg. C for a few minutes before use will make it quite safe for consumption *(6)*.

Botulism occurring in infants is called "infant botulism". It is due to infection of the gut by *C. botulinum* with subsequent in vivo production of toxin *(7)*.

Antitoxin is of considerable value in the prophylaxis of botulism. When a case of botulism has occurred, antitoxin should be given to all individuals partaking of the food. The dose varies from 50,000 to 100,000 units IV *(8)*. The antitoxin will be of no avail if the toxin is already fixed to the nervous tissue. Guanidine hydrochloride given orally in doses of 15 to 40 mg/kg of body weight has been shown to reverse the neuromuscular block of botulism. When combined with good medical and nursing care, the drug can be a useful adjunct in the treatment of botulism *(9)*. Active immunization with botulinum toxoid to prevent botulism is also available *(10)*.

C. perfringens food poisoning

(a) AGENT : *Clostridium (C.) perfringens (welchii)*. (b) SOURCE : The organism has been found in faeces of humans and animals, and in soil, water and air. The majority of outbreaks have been associated with the ingestion of meat, meat dishes and poultry. The usual story is that the food has been prepared and cooked 24 hours or more before consumption, and allowed to cool slowly at room temperature and then heated immediately prior to serving. (c) INCUBATION PERIOD : 6 to 24 hours, with a peak from 10 to 14 hours (d) MECHANISM OF FOOD POISONING : The spores are able to survive cooking, and if the cooked meat and poultry are not cooled enough, they will germinate. The organisms multiply between 30 deg. and 50 deg. C and produce a variety of toxins, e.g., alpha toxin, theta toxin, etc. Prevention consists either by cooking food just prior to its consumption or, if it has to be stored, by rapid and adequate cooling *(11)*. (e) CLINICAL SYMPTOMS : The most common symptoms are diarrhoea, abdominal cramps and little or no fever, occurring 8 to 24 hours after consumption of the food. Nausea and vomiting are rare. Illness is usually of short duration, usually 1 day or less. Recovery is rapid and no deaths have been reported.

B. cereus food poisoning

Bacillus cereus is an aerobic, spore–bearing, motile, gram positive rod. It is ubiquitous in soil, and in raw, dried and processed foods. The spores can survive cooking and germinate and multiply rapidly when the food is held at favourable temperatures. *B. cereus* has been recognized as a cause of food poisoning, with increasing frequency in recent years.

Recent work has shown that *B. cereus* produces at least 2 distinct enterotoxins, causing 2 distinct forms of food poisoning. One, the *emetic form* with a short incubation period (1–6 hours) characterized by predominantly upper gastro-intestinal tract symptoms, rather like staphylococcal food poisoning. The other, the *diarrhoeal* form, with a longer incubation period (12–24 hours) characterized by predominantly lower intestinal tract symptoms like *C. perfringens* food poisoning (diarrhoea, abdominal pain, nausea with little or no vomiting and no fever. Recovery within 24 hours is usual). The toxins are preformed and stable.

Diagnosis can be confirmed by isolation of 10^5 or more *B. cereus* organisms per gram of epidemiologically incriminated food. Treatment is symptomatic.

Differential diagnosis

Food poisoning may be mistaken for cholera, acute bacillary dysentery and chemical (arsenic) poisoning. The differentiating points between cholera and food poisoning are given in Table 1.

INVESTIGATION OF FOOD POISONING

(a) Secure complete list of people involved and their history : All the people who have shared part of the food should be interviewed. They may be supplied questionnaires concerning the foods eaten during the previous 2 days, and place of consumption; time of onset of symptoms; symptoms of illness (e.g., nausea, vomiting, diarrhoea, abdominal pain, headache, fever, prostration, etc.) in order of occurrence; personal data such as age, sex, residence, occupation, and any other helpful information. Questionnaires may be administered to kitchen employees and those working in the dining halls. *(b) Laboratory investigations* : An important part of the investigation. The object is not only to incriminate the causative agent from stool, vomit or remnants of food by inoculating into appropriate media, but also to determine the total number of bacteria and the relative numbers of each kind involved. This will give a better indication of the organism involved. Stool samples of the kitchen employees and food handlers should also be investigated. The samples should be examined aerobically and anaerobically. Phage typing of the organisms should be done to complete the laboratory investigation. *(c) Animal experiments* : It may be necessary to feed rhesus monkeys with the remnants of food. Protection tests are useful in the case of botulism; in this, a saline filtrate of food-stuff is injected subcutaneously into mice protected with antitoxic sera, keeping suitable controls. *(d) Blood for antibodies* : This is useful for retrospective diagnosis. *(e) Environmental study* : This includes inspection of the eating place(s), kitchen(s), and questioning of food handlers regarding food preparation. *(f) Data analysis* : The data should be analyzed according to the descriptive methods of time, place and person distribution. Food–specific attack rates should be calculated. A case control study may be undertaken to establish the epidemiologic association between, illness and the intake of a particular food.

PREVENTION AND CONTROL

(a) FOOD SANITATION : *(i) Meat inspection* : The food animals must be free from infection. This can be ensured by their examination by veterinary staff, both before and after slaughter. *(ii) Personal hygiene* : A high standard of personal hygiene among individuals engaged in the handling, preparation and cooking of food is needed. *(iii) Food handlers* : Those suffering from infected wounds, boils, diarrhoea, dysentery, throat infection, etc should be excluded from food handling. The medical inspection of food handlers is required in many countries; this is of limited value in the detection of carriers, although it will remove some sources of infection *(12)*. *(iv) Food handling techniques* : The handling of ready-to-eat foods with bare hands should be reduced to a minimum. Time between preparation and consumption of food should be kept short. The importance of rapid cooling and cold storage must be stressed. Milk, milk products and egg products should be pasteurized. Food must be thoroughly cooked. The heat must penetrate the centre of the food leaving thereby no cool spots. Most food poisoning organisms are killed at temperatures over 60 deg. C. Separate raw meat, poultry, seafood and eggs from ready to

TABLE 1

Differential diagnosis of cholera and food poisoning

		Cholera	Food poisoning
1.	Epidemiology	Occurs often in epidemic form associated with other cases in the neighbourhood Secondary cases occur	Often a single group of persons who shared a common meal No secondary cases
2.	Incubation	From a few hours upto 5 days	1 to 24 hours
3.	Onset	With purging	With vomiting
4.	Nausea and retching	None	Present
5.	Vomiting	Projectile, effortless, watery and continuous	Often single, severe vomit, mucus and blood streaked
6.	Stools	Copious rice watery, inoffensive	Frequent, may contain mucus and blood, offensive
7.	Tenesmus	None	Yes
8.	Abdominal tenderness	None	Yes
9.	Dehydration	Very marked	Distinct
10.	Muscular cramps	Constant and severe	Less constant
11.	Surface temperature	Subnormal	Often upto 100–102 deg.F.
12.	Headache	None	Often
13.	Urine	Suppressed	Seldom suppressed
14.	Blood	Leucocytosis	Normal

eat foods. Use separate cutting boards and keep raw meat away from other foods in shopping cart and refrigerator *(2)*. *(v) Sanitary improvements :* Sanitization of all work surfaces, utensils and equipments must be ensured. Food premises should be kept free from rats, mice, flies and dust. *(vi) Health education :* Food handlers should be educated in matters of clean habits and personal hygiene, such as frequent and thorough hand washing.

(b) REFRIGERATION : In the prevention of bacterial food poisoning, emphasis must be placed on proper temperature control. Food should not be left in warm pantries; a few germs can multiply to millions by the next morning. Foods not eaten immediately should be kept in cold storage to prevent bacterial multiplication and toxin production. "Cook and eat the same day" is a golden rule. When foods are held between 10 deg. C (50 deg. F) and 49 deg. C (120 deg.F) they are in the danger zone for bacterial growth. Cold is bacteriostatic at temperature below 4 deg. C (40 deg.F), and refrigeration temperature should not exceed this level.

SURVEILLANCE : Food samples must be obtained from the food establishments periodically and subjected to laboratory analysis if they were unsatisfactory. Continuing surveillance is necessary to avoid outbreaks of food-borne diseases.

References

1. WHO (2022), *Fact sheet on food safety,* 19th May 2022.
2. CDC (2022), *Food facts,* Feb. 2022.
3. Mandal, B.K. (1981). *Medicine International,* 2 : 56.
4. Beveridge, W.I.B. (1967). in *Health of Mankind,* 100th Symposium, Ciba Foundation, Churchill, London.
5. Werner, S.B. (1980). in *Maxcy–Rosenau : Public Health and Preventive Medicine,* 11th ed, John M. Last (ed), Appleton–Century Crofts, New York.
6. Jawetz, Melnick and Adelberg's *Medical Microbiology,* 26th ed., A Lange Publication.
7. Arnon, S.S. et al (1977). *JAMA,* 237 : 1946–1951.
8. Christie, A.B. (1980). *Infectious Diseases : Epidemiology and Clinical Practice,* 3rd ed., Churchill Livingstone.
9. Ryan, D.W. et al (1971). *JAMA,* 216 : 513.
10. Stuart, P.F. et al (1970). *Cand. J. Pub. Health,* 61 (6) 509.
11. Bailey, J. (1977). *Guide to Hygiene and Sanitation in Aviation,* WHO, Geneva.
12. WHO (1980). *WHO Chronicle,* 34 (2) 83.

AMOEBIASIS

The term "amoebiasis" has been defined by WHO as the condition of harbouring the protozoan parasite *Entamoeba histolytica* with or without clinical manifestations. The symptomatic disease occurs in less than 10 per cent of infected individuals *(2)*. The symptomatic group has been further subdivided into intestinal and extraintestinal amoebiasis. Only a small percentage of those having intestinal infection will develop invasive amoebiasis. The intestinal disease varies from mild abdominal discomfort and diarrhoea to acute fulminating dysentery. Extraintestinal amoebiasis includes involvement of liver (liver abscess), lungs, brain, spleen, skin, etc. Amoebiasis is a potentially lethal disease. It carries substantial morbidity and mortality.

Problem statement

WORLD : Amoebiasis is a common infection of the human gastro-intestinal tract. It has a worldwide distribution. It is a major health problem in the whole of China, South East and West Asia and Latin America, especially Mexico. Globally it is estimated that 50 million people carry *E. histolytica* in their intestinal tract and approximately one-tenth of infected people suffer from invasive amoebiasis. It is probable that invasive amoebiasis, accounted for about 50,000 deaths in the world *(3)*. Prevalence rates vary from as low as 2 per cent to 60 per cent or more in areas devoid of sanitation *(4)*. In areas of high prevalence, amoebiasis occurs in endemic forms as a result of high levels of transmission and constant reinfection. Epidemic water-borne infections can occur if there is heavy contamination of drinking water supply.

INDIA : It is generally agreed that amoebiasis affects about 15 per cent of the Indian population *(5)*. Amoebiasis has been reported throughout India : the prevalence rate is about 15% ranging from 3.6 to 47.4 per cent in different areas *(4)*. The reported variations in prevalence are attributed to variations in clinical diagnostic criteria *(6)* and to technical difficulties in establishing a correct diagnosis and lack of sampling criteria *(7)*.

Epidemiological determinants

Agent factors

(a) AGENT : Amoebiasis is caused by potentially pathogenic strains of *E. histolytica.* Studies have shown that *E. histolytica* can be differentiated into at least 18 zymodemes (a zymodeme is a population of organisms differing from similar population in the electrophoretic mobilities of one or more enzymes). It has furthermore been shown that pathogenic strains are all from particular zymodemes; that non-invasive strains are from quite distinct zymodemes; that invasive strains can give rise to faecal cysts, and the organisms breed true *(8)*. The iso-enzyme characteristics do not, however, determine why a particular zymodeme is able to invade. Isoenzyme electrophoretic mobility analysis have so far identified 7 potentially pathogenic and 11 non-pathogenic zymodems *(9)*.

E. histolytica exists in two forms – vegetative (trophozoite) and cystic forms. Trophozoites dwell in the colon where they multiply and encyst. The cysts are excreted in stool. Ingested cysts release trophozoites which colonize the large intestine. Some trophozoites invade the bowel and cause ulceration, mainly in the caecum and ascending colon; then in the rectum and sigmoid. Some may enter a vein and reach the liver and other organs.

The trophozoites are short-lived outside the human body; they are not important in the transmission of the disease. In contrast the cysts are infective to man and remain viable and infective for several days in faeces, water, sewage and soil in the presence of moisture and low temperature. The cysts are not affected by chlorine in the amounts normally used in water purification, but they are readily killed if dried, heated (to about 55 deg C) or frozen.

(b) RESERVOIR OF INFECTION : Man is the only reservoir of infection. The immediate source of infection is the faeces containing the cysts. Most individuals infected with *E. Histolytica* remain symptom free and are healthy carriers of the parasite *(12)*. The carriers can discharge upto 1.5 x 10^7 cysts daily *(6)*. The greatest risk is associated with carriers engaged in the preparation and handling of food *(6)*.

(c) PERIOD OF COMMUNICABILITY : As long as cysts are excreted; the period may be several years, if cases are unrecognized and untreated.

Host factors

Amoebiasis may occur at any age. There is no sex or racial difference in the occurrence of the disease. Amoebiasis is frequently a household infection. When an individual in a family is infected, others in the family may also be affected. Specific antiamoebic antibodies are produced when tissue invasion takes place. There is strong evidence that cell-mediated immunity plays an important part in controlling the recurrence of invasive amoebiasis *(10)*.

Environmental factors

Amoebiasis is more closely related to poor sanitation and socio-economic status than to climate. The use of nightsoil for agricultural purposes favours the spread of the disease. In countries with marked wet–dry seasons, infection rates are higher during rains, presumably since cysts may survive longer and the potential for transmission is thereby increased. Epidemic outbreaks are usually associated with sewage seepage into the water supply.

Mode of transmission

(i) Faecal–oral route : This may readily take place through intake of contaminated water or food. Epidemic water-borne infections can occur if there is heavy contamination of drinking water supply. Vegetables, especially those eaten raw, from fields irrigated with sewage polluted water can readily convey infection. Viable cysts have been found on the hands and under finger nails. This may lead to direct hand to mouth transmission. **(ii) Sexual transmission:** by oral–rectal contact is also recognized, especially among male homosexuals. **(iii) Vectors :** such as flies, cockroaches and rodents are capable of carrying cysts and contaminating food and drink.

Incubation period

About 2 to 4 weeks or longer.

PREVENTION AND CONTROL

1. Primary prevention

The measures aimed at primary prevention centre round preventing contamination of water, food, vegetables and fruits with human faeces. (a) **Sanitation :** Safe disposal of human excreta coupled with the elementary sanitary practice of washing hands after defecation and before eating is a crucial factor in the prevention and control of amoebiasis. But there are too many hurdles (both social and economic) in enforcing it in many developing countries. With the cooperation of the local community, the sanitary systems should be selected and constructed *(14)* taking into consideration the customs and practices of the population and the available resources. (b) **Water supply :** The protection of water supplies against faecal contamination is equally important because amoebic cysts may survive for several days and weeks in water. The cysts are not killed by chlorine in amounts used for water disinfection. Sand filters are quite effective in removing amoebic cysts. Therefore water filtration and boiling are more effective than chemical treatment of water against amoebiasis. (c) **Food hygiene :** Environmental measures should also include the protection of food and drink against faecal contamination. Uncooked vegetables and fruits can be disinfected with aqueous solution of acetic acid (5–10 per cent) or full strength vinegar *(1)*. In most instances, thorough washing with detergents in running water will remove amoebic cysts from fruits and vegetables. Since food handlers are major transmitters of amoebiasis, they should be periodically examined, treated and educated in food hygiene practices such as hand washing. (d) **Health education :** In the long-term, a great deal can be accomplished through health education of the public.

2. Secondary prevention

(a) **Early diagnosis :** Demonstration of trophozoites containing red cells is diagnostic. They are most readily seen in fresh mucus passed per rectum. Microscopy should be performed immediately before its cooling results. The absence of pus cells in the stool may be helpful in the differential diagnosis with shigellosis. Serological tests are often negative in intestinal amoebiaşis, but if positive, they provide a clue to extraintestinal amoebiasis. Indirect haemagglutination test (IHA) is regarded as the most sensitive serological test. Newer techniques include counter immuno-electrophoresis (CIE) and ELISA technique *(11)*.

(b) **Treatment :** *(i) Symptomatic cases :* At the health centre level, symptomatic cases can be treated effectively with metronidazole orally and the clinical response in 48 hours may confirm the suspected diagnosis. The dose is 30 mg/kg of body weight/day, divided into 3 doses after meals, for 8–10 days. Tinidazole can be used instead of metronidazole. Suspected cases of liver abscess should be referred to the nearest hospital. *(ii) Asymptomatic infections :* In an endemic area, the consensus is not to treat such persons because the probability of reinfection is very high *(10)*. They may, however, be treated, if the carrier is a food handler. In non-endemic areas they are always likely to be treated. They should be treated with oral diiodohyroxyquin, 650 mg TDS (adults) or 30–40 mg/kg of body weight/day (children) for 20 days, or oral diloxanide furoate, 500 mg TDS for 10 days (adults) *(3)*.

At present there is no acceptable chemoprophylaxis for amoebiasis. Mass examination and treatment cannot be considered as a solution for the control of amoebiasis *(10)*.

References

1. WHO (1969). *Techn. Rep. Ser.*, 421.
2. Jawetz (2010), Melnick and Adelberg's. *Medical Microbiology*, 25th Ed., A Lange Publication.
3. STEPHEN J. McPHEE and MAXINE A (2010), *Current Medical Diagnosis and Treatment*, 49th Ed., A Lange Publication.
4. *Bull WHO* (1980) 58 (6) 819-830.
5. Vakil, B.J. (1973), *Medical Times*, Aug. 1973, Sandoz Publications, Mumbai.
6. WHO (1987). *Techn. Rep. Ser.* No. 749.
7. WHO (1981). *Techn. Rep. Ser.* No. 666.
8. Ree, G.H. (1983). *Post Graduate Doctor*, Middle East Dec. 1983 P. 626.
9. Sargeaunt, P.G. et al (1982) *Lancet* 1 : 1386 - 1388.
10. *Bull WHO* (1985) 63 (3) 417-426.
11. WHO (1980), *Scientific Working Group Reports* 1978-1980, WHO/CDD/80. 1.
12. Nanda, R. et al (1984). *Lancet* 2 : 301.
13. Palmo, A.M. (1988). *Medicine International* 54 : 22, 16 June 1988.
14. Rajagopalan, S. and Shiffman, M.A. (1974). *Guide to Simple Sanitary Measures for the control of Enteric Diseases*, Geneva, WHO.

SOIL-TRANSMITTED HELMINTHIASIS

Soil-transmitted helminth (STHs) infections refer to a group of parasitic diseases in humans caused by intestinal roundworms (ascariasis), hookworms (*Necator americanus* and *Ancylostoma duodenale*) and whipworm (*Trichuris trichiura*). They are the most common infections worldwide.

More than 1.5 billion people, or about 24 per cent of the world's population are infected. Infections are widely distributed in tropical and subtropical areas, with the greatest numbers occurring in sub-Saharan Africa, the Americas, China and east Asia *(1)*. Over 267 million pre-school children and over 568 million school-age children and 250 million girls and adult women live in areas where these parasites are intensively transmitted and are in need of treatment and preventive interventions *(1)*.

Mode of transmission

Soil-transmitted helminths are transmitted by eggs that are passed in the faeces of infected people, as adult worms live in the intestine where they produce thousands of eggs each day. In areas that lack adequate sanitation, these eggs contaminate the soil. This can happen in several ways : (a) eggs that are attached to vegetables and salads are ingested when the vegetables are not carefully cooked, washed or peeled; (b) eggs are ingested from contaminated water sources; and (c) eggs are ingested by children who play in contaminated soil and then put their hands in their mouth without washing them.

In addition, hookworm eggs hatch in the soil, releasing larvae that mature into a form that can actively penetrate the skin. People become infected with hookworm primarily by walking barefoot on contaminated soil.

There is no direct person-to-person transmission, or infection from fresh faeces, because eggs passed in faeces need about three weeks to mature in the soil before they become infective. Since these worms do not multiply in the human host, reinfection occurs only as a result of contact with infective stages in the environment.

ASCARIASIS

An infection of the intestinal tract caused by the adult, *Ascaris lumbricoides* and clinically manifested by vague symptoms of nausea, abdominal pain and cough. Live worms are passed in the stool or vomited. Occasionally, they may produce intestinal obstruction or may migrate into the peritoneal cavity.

Geographic distribution and prevalence

Ascaris is cosmopolitan in distribution. It is the most common helminthic infestation. It is estimated that about 820 million people are infected world-wide annually with about 12 million acute cases and 20,000 or more deaths. Heavy infection is common in children aged 3–8 years *(2)*.

Epidemiological features

(a) AGENT : *Ascaris lumbricoides* lives in the lumen of small intestine, where it moves freely. Sexes are separate. The female measures 20–35 cm in length, and the male 12–30 cm. Egg production is very heavy – an estimated 2,40,000 eggs per day by each female, which counterbalances the heavy losses in the environment. The eggs are excreted in the faeces. They become embryonated in the external environment and become infective in 2–3 weeks. On ingestion by man, the embryonated eggs hatch in the small intestine. The resulting larvae penetrate the gut wall and are carried to the liver and then to the lungs *via* the blood stream. In the lungs, they moult twice. They break through the alveolar walls and migrate into the bronchioles. They are coughed up through the trachea and then swallowed by the human host. On reaching the intestine, they become mature into adults in 60–80 days. The life span of an adult is between 6–12 months, maximum reported being 1.5 years. (b) RESERVOIR OF INFECTION : Man is the only reservoir. (c) INFECTIVE MATERIAL : Faeces containing the fertilized eggs. (d) HOST : Infection rates are high in children; they are the most important disseminators of infection. Adults seem to acquire some resistance. There is a high degree of host–parasite tolerance. Roundworms rob man of his food and may possibly compete for vitamin A in the intestine *(3)*. They contribute to malnutrition especially in children who may show growth retardation. (e) ENVIRONMENT : Ascaris is a "soil–transmitted" helminth. The eggs remain viable in the soil for months or years under favourable conditions. Of the various ecological factors regulating the population of *Ascaris* eggs, the most important ones are the temperature, moisture, oxygen pressure and ultra-violet radiation from the sunlight *(4)*. A low temperature inhibits the development of eggs. Clay soils are most favourable for the development of ascariasis eggs, in contrast to moist porous soils for those of hookworms. (f) HUMAN HABITS : Seeding of the soil by ascariasis eggs takes place by the human habit of indiscriminate open air defecation. It is the most important factor responsible for the widespread distribution of ascariasis in the world *(4)*. Soil pollution is usually concentrated around houses where small children who have no regular habits pollute the house and surrounding areas. Infective eggs can then easily reach other children who play on the ground and contaminate their hands and food *(4)*. (g) PERIOD OF COMMUNICABILITY: Until all fertile females are destroyed and stools are negative.

Incubation period

18 days to several weeks.

Symptoms

The symptoms are related to the number of the worms harboured. People with light infection usually have no symptoms. Heavier infections can cause a range of symptoms including intestinal manifestations like diarrhoea, abdominal pain; general malaise, weakness, impaired cognitive and physical development. The WHO definition of heavy infection of roundworm is ≥ 50,000 eggs per gram of faeces *(5)*.

The larvae migration may cause fever, cough, sputum formation, asthma, skin rash, eosinophilia. The adult roundworm aggregate masses can cause volvulus, intestinal obstruction or intessusception; and wandering worm can cause bowel perforation in the ileococcal region, blocking of common bile duct or may come out with vomit *(5)*.

HOOKWORM INFECTION

Hookworm infection is defined as "any infection caused by *Ancylostoma duodenale* or *Necator americanus*" *(6)*. They may occur as single or mixed infections in the same person.

Problem statement

Ancylostoma duodenale and *Necator americanus* are the main nematodes causing hookworm infection in man. Almost eradicated from Europe and the USA *(4)*, hookworm infection is still seen in warm, moist climates in tropical and subtropical regions between 45°N and 30°S of the equator (e.g., Asia, Africa, Central and South America and the South Pacific). The geographic distribution of these two hookworms used to be regarded as relatively distinct, the former being more prevalent in Europe and South–western Asia, and the latter in tropical Africa and in the Americas. However, over the past decades both parasites have become widely distributed throughout the tropics and subtropics, and rigid demarcations are no longer tenable *(7)*.

It is estimated that, the global prevalence of hookworm is about 460 million cases, and the number of years lost due to ill health or death is estimated to be about 3.2 million *(8)*.

Epidemiological determinants

Agent factors

(a) AGENT : Adult worms live in the small intestine, mainly jejunum where they attach themselves to the villi. Males measure 8 to 11 mm, and females 10 to 13 mm in length with dorsally curved anterior end. Eggs are passed in the faeces in thousands; one female *A. duodenale* produces about 10,000–30,000 eggs and one female *N. americanus* about 5,000–10,000 eggs per day *(7)*. High egg production ensures constant exposure to infection.

When deposited on warm, moist soil, a larva rapidly develops in the egg and hatches after 1 to 2 days. The newly hatched larva (rhabditiform larva) moults twice in the soil and becomes a skin–penetrating third stage infective larva within 5 to 10 days. These lie in wait in the soil to pierce the skin of the human host. They move very little horizontally, but migrate upwards on blades of grass *(4)*. They can survive in shaded, moist soil for up to one month. Infection occurs when the larva enters the body through the skin, most commonly through the feet. Larvae of *A. duodenale* are also infective by mouth. Once inside the body, they migrate via lymphatics and blood stream to the lungs. They break into the alveoli, ascend the bronchi and trachea and are coughed up and swallowed to reach the small intestine, where they become sexually mature. Adult *A. duodenale* and *N. americanus* are believed to be capable of surviving for an average about 1 and 4 years, respectively *(6)*. (b) RESERVOIR : Man is the only important reservoir of human hookworm infection. (c) INFECTIVE MATERIAL : Faeces containing the ova of hookworms. However, the immediate source of infection is the soil contaminated with infective larvae. (d) PERIOD OF INFECTIVITY : As long as the person harbours the parasite.

Host factors

(a) AGE AND SEX : All ages and both sexes are susceptible to infection. In endemic areas, the highest incidence is found in the age group, 15 to 25 years. (b) NUTRITION : Studies indicate that malnutrition is a predisposing factor; the chronic disabling disease does not occur in the otherwise healthy individual who is well–nourished and whose iron intake is adequate. (c) HOST–PARASITE BALANCE : In endemic areas, the inhabitants develop a host–parasite balance in which the worm load is limited. They harbour the parasite without manifesting clinical signs and symptoms. In some areas, the infection rate may be 100 per cent, but most infections are light and only a small proportion of the people are heavily infected *(6)*. This delicate balance may be upset by malnutrition and intercurrent infections. Little is known about host immunity. (d) OCCUPATION : It is to be expected that hookworm infection will have a higher prevalence in agricultural than in town workers, and in many tropical countries, it is an occupational disease of the farming community.

Environmental factors

Hookworm larvae live in the upper half-inch (1.2 cm.) of the soil. Favourable environmental conditions are, therefore, crucial for the survival of the hookworm larvae in the soil. These are : (a) SOIL : The soil must be suitable for the eggs and larvae. The type of soil that favours the survival of hookworm larvae is a damp, sandy or friable soil with decaying vegetation. In general, sandy soil is more favourable than clay soil. (b) TEMPERATURE : A temperature of 24 to 32 deg. C is considered favourable for the survival of the larvae. The eggs fail to develop at temperatures below 13 deg. C. Larvae are killed at 45 to 50 deg. C. (c) OXYGEN : This is required for the growth and development of the larvae. (d) MOISTURE : Moisture is necessary for survival; dryness is rapidly fatal. (e) RAINFALL : A rainfall of 40 inches (100 cm) and above is considered a favourable environmental factor. More important than the total annual rainfall is the number of rainy days spread out evenly throughout the year to keep up the moisture content of the soil. Flooding is an unfavourable factor. (f) SHADE : Direct sunlight kills the larvae whereas shade protects them. (g) HUMAN HABITS : The habits of the human host not only determine the mode and extent of soil pollution, but also the mode and extent of contact between infected soil and skin or mouth *(4)*. These include indiscriminate defecation, using the same places for defecation, going barefoot, farming practices using untreated sewage, children wading in the infected mud with bare–feet and hands. These habits are compounded by social factors such as illiteracy, ignorance and low standard of living.

Incubation period (prepatent period)

Following infection, the prepatent period for *N. americanus* is 7 weeks while that for *A. duodenale* is unpredictable, ranging from 5 weeks to 9 months *(6)*. This is because the invading larva of *A. duodenale* is capable of remaining arrested or dormant in the tissues of the host for as long as 9 months and then again resume development and migration.

Effects of the disease

(a) INDIVIDUAL : Hookworm infection causes chronic blood loss and depletion of body's iron stores leading to iron–deficiency anaemia. This has implications for child health in terms of retarded physical growth and development; for the health of mothers in terms of increased morbidity, low birth weight babies, abortion, stillbirths and impaired lactation; and for the health of adults in terms of diminished capacity for sustained hard work. Hookworm infection also causes a loss of blood plasma into the small intestine which can lead to hypoalbuminaemia in some subjects. (b) COMMUNITY : Hookworm infection exerts a significant and harmful effect on various aspects of the economy and quality of life of a community, especially in three major areas. These are nutrition, growth and development; work and productivity, and medical care costs.

WHIPWORM

Whipworm is the third most common soil-transmitted helminthiasis in the humans. According to current estimate, nearly 440 million people are infected, and majority of cases are children 4–10 years age. Heavy infection could lead to acute symptoms such as diarrhoea and anaemia, and chronic symptoms such as growth retardation and impaired cognitive development. It is quite common in United States, South-East Asia, to a lesser extent equatorial Africa, Central and South America *(5)*.

Agent factor

Whipworms live in the large intestine, Male worm measures about 30–45 mm long while female is about 30–35 mm long. Female worm produces about 200–10,000 eggs per day for more than 5 years. Embryonization takes 21 days. It can withstand cold temperatures but not desiccation. The infection is directly from the faeces. Eggs hatch after being swallowed in the intestine, where shell is digested by intestinal juices and the larva emerges in the small intestine. It penetrates the villi and develops for a week until it re-emerges and passes to the cecum and colorectum where it attaches itself to the mucosa and becomes adult *(5, 7)*.

Incubation period

Period from ingestion of egg to appearance of egg in stool is 60–90 days *(5, 7)*.

Effect of the disease

Majority of infections are mild or asymptomatic. It causes epigestric pain, nausea, vomiting, distension flatulence, weight loss. Moderate infection causes growth deficit and anaemia. Severe infection causes severe chronic diarrhoea or dysentery with blood and mucous in stool, dehydration, rectal prolapse, colonic obstruction, hypoproteinaemia, chronic iron deficiency, anaemia etc. *(5)*.

PREVENTION AND CONTROL OF SOIL-TRANSMITTED HELMINTHS

Primary prevention

Methods based on primary prevention are the most effective in interrupting transmission. These are : sanitary disposal of human excreta to prevent or reduce faecal contamination of the soil, provision of safe drinking water, food hygiene habits, and health education of the community in the use of sanitary latrines, personal hygiene and changing behavioural patterns, measures of personal protection such as wearing protective footwear and making use of health facilities for diagnosis and treatment. Prevention, to be effective, must take into consideration the life cycle of the parasite and the peculiar ecological, social and cultural circumstances that prevail in a community.

Secondary prevention

Effective drugs are available for the treatment of the human reservoir. These are piperazine, mebendazole, levamisole and pyrantel; the last two drugs are effective in a single dose. (a) *Albendazole :* The usual dose for adults and children over 2 years is 400 mg as a single dose. Contraindicated in children below 2 years and in pregnancy. (b) *Mebendazole :* The usual dose is 100 mg twice daily for 3 days for all ages above 2 years. (c) *Levamisole :* It is the levorotatory form of tetramisole and is more active than the parent compound. For many it is now the drug of choice. A single oral dose of 2.5 mg/kg of body weight (maximum 150 mg) has been recommended. There are usually no side effects. It has been used successfully in the mass treatment of ascariasis.(d) *Pyrantel :* Effective in a single dose of 10 mg/kg of body weight *(9)* with a maximum of 1g.

Treatment of anaemia and other complications

Anaemia should be treated with iron and folic acid. Patient should be treated for hypoproteinaemia and hypereosinophilia.

Preventive chemotherapy *(3)*

The WHO strategy for control of soil-transmitted helminth infection is to control morbidity through periodic treatment of at-risk people living in endemic areas. The people at risk are : (a) preschool-aged children; (b) school aged children; (c) women of childbearing age including pregnant women in second and third trimesters and breast-feeding mothers; and (d) adults in certain high-risk occupations, such as tea-pickers or miners.

WHO recommends periodic deworming without previous individual diagnosis to all at-risk people living in endemic areas. Treatment should be given once a year when prevalence of soil-transmitted helminth infection in the community is over 20 per cent and twice a year if the prevalence is over 50 per cent. This reduces the morbidity by reducing the worm burden. Periodic deworming can easily be integrated with child health days or supplementation programmes for pre-school children, or can be integrated with school health programmes. Schools provide a particularly good entry point for deworming activities, as they allow easy provision of the health and hygiene education component – such as promotion of hand washing and improved sanitation.

The recommended medicines are albendazole (400 mg) and mebendazole (500 mg). They are effective and can be easily administered by non-medical persons. The drugs are donated by WHO.

Approximately 267 million pre-school-aged children, 568 million school-aged children and 560 million women of reproductive age group in 103 countries or territories were estimated to be in need of preventive chemotherapy against soil transmitted helminthiasis. Of these 436 million children were treated by preventive chemotherapy; 127 million women of reproductive age group were treated in 2016 principally through the lymphatic filariasis programme *(1)*.

The global target is to eliminate morbidity due to soil-transmitted helminthiasis in children by year 2020. This will be achieved by regularly treating at least 75 per cent of the children in endemic areas – an estimated 873 million children *(3)*.

References

1. WHO (2022), *Fact Sheet, Soil-Transmitted Helminth Infections,* 10th January, 2022.
2. Maxine A., Papadakis, Stephen J. McPhee, *Current Medical Diagnosis and Treatment,* 53rd ed. 2014, A Lange Publication.
3. WHO (2016), *Fact Sheet,* No. 366, March 2016.
4. WHO (1981), Tech. Rep. Ser., No. 666.
5. Global Health Education Consortium (2012), Soil-Transmitted Helminths by Sina Helbig et al.
6. WHO (1987), Tech, Rep. Ser., No. 749.
7. Center for Disease Control and Prevention (2011), *Neglected Tropical Diseases.*
8. WHO (2017), *Guideline: Preventive Chemotherapy to Control Soil-Transmitted Helminth Infections in at-risk population groups,* 2017.
9. WHO (1998), *World Health Report 1998,* Report of the Director General WHO.
10. WHO (2017), *Weekly Epidemiological Record,* No. 49, 8th Dec., 2017.

DRACUNCULIASIS

Dracunculiasis or guineaworm disease is a vectorborne parasitic disease, mainly of the subcutaneous tissues (usually leg and foot) caused by the nematode parasite, *Dracunculus medinensis.* Although not lethal, this parasitic disease can disable its victim temporarily.

Problem statement

Progress towards the elimination of dracunculiasis in the past decade has been spectacular, with the number of cases falling worldwide from an estimated 892,005 in 1989 (when most endemic countries began to report monthly cases from each endemic village) to a total of 14 cases in 2021. Compared with 2012 (542 cases), the largest decline in the number of cases occurred in South Sudan (4). At present only Ethiopia (1), Chad (7) and Mali (2), are reporting cases *(1)*.

In India, the last reported case was in July 1996. On completion of three years of zero incidence, India was declared free of guineaworm disease *(2)*.

Natural history

(a) AGENT : The adult parasite inhabits the subcutaneous tissue mainly of the legs but also of other parts of the body, including the head and neck. The female grows to a length of 55 to 120 cm, and the male is very short (2–3 cm). The gravid female makes it's way down to the infected person's lower limbs near the skin surface. There it penetrates into the dermis and induces an inflammatory reaction and subsequent blister formation. Upon contact with water, the blister soon ruptures and the parasite releases up to one million, microscopic, free–swimming larvae into water. The larvae may remain active in water for 3–6 days. They are picked up by small fresh–water crustaceans called cyclops. The larvae require a period of about 15 days for development in cyclops, which is the intermediate host.

Man acquires infection by drinking water containing infected cyclops. In the human body, digested by gastric juice, the parasites are released. They penetrate the duodenal wall. Subsequently they migrate through the viscera to the subcutaneous tissues of various parts of the body. They grow into adults in 10–14 months.

(b) RESERVOIR OF INFECTION : An infected person harbouring the gravid female. The possibility of an animal reservoir exists but not proved *(3)*.

(c) HOST FACTORS : Host susceptibility is universal. Multiple and repeated infections may occur in the same individual. The habit of washing and bathing in surface water and using step–wells is important.

(d) ENVIRONMENTAL FACTORS : The main link in the transmission of guineaworm disease is water infested with cyclops. The risk of transmission exists where such cyclops–infested water–sources are frequented by infected persons. *Season :* The seasonal variations in the incidence of the disease are marked. Where the step-wells are the source of water supply, peak transmission occurs during the dry season (March–May) when the contact between open cases of gunieaworm disease and the drinking water is the greatest; and there is little transmission when the wells are full during and after rains. Where the ponds are used, transmission appears to be confined to June–September, when the ponds contain water *(4, 5)*. *Temperature :* The larvae develop best between 25 and 30 deg C, and will not develop below 19 deg C. Therefore, the disease is limited to tropical and subtropical regions *(6)*.

Mode of transmission

The disease is transmitted entirely through the consumption of water containing cyclops harbouring the infective stages of the parasite. Guineaworm disease is a totally water–based disease and does not have an alternate pathway of transmission.

Treatment

No drug cures the infection but metronidazole and mebendazole are sometimes used to limit inflammation and facilitate worm removal. Wet compresses may relieve discomfort. Occlusive dressings improves hygiene and limit shedding of infectious larvae. Worms are removed by sequentially rolling them out over a small stick. When available simple surgical procedure can be used to remove worm. Topical antibiotics may limit bacterial superinfection.

Eradication

Guineaworm disease is amenable to eradication. The eradication strategy comprises the following elements :

i) Provision of safe drinking water (e.g., piped water, installation of hand pumps).
ii) Control of cyclops (See Chapter 15).
iii) Health education of the public in matters relating to boiling or sieving drinking water through a double–thickness cotton cloth for personal protection, and prevention of water contamination by infected persons.
iv) Surveillance : Active search for new cases, and

Guineaworm Eradication Programme

Refer to chapter 7 for details.

References

1. Centers for Disease Control and Prevention (2021), *Guineaworm Epidemiology and Risk Factors.*
2. WHO (2000), *Weekly Epidemiological Record* 2nd June 2000 No. 22.
3. WHO (1979). *Techn. Rep. Ser.*, No. 637.
4. Muller, R. (1979). *Bull WHO*, 57 (5) 683.
5. WHO (1980). *WHO Chr.*, 34 (4) 159.
6. *National Guineaworm Eradication Programme,* National Health Programme series 2, National Institute of Health and family welfare, New Mehrauli Road, New Delhi.

III. ARTHROPOD–BORNE INFECTIONS

THE DENGUE SYNDROME

Dengue viruses are arboviruses capable of infecting humans, and causing disease. These infections may be asymptomatic or may lead to (a) "classical" dengue fever, or (b) dengue haemorrhagic fever without shock, or (c) dengue haemorrhagic fever with shock. The manifestations of the dengue syndrome are as shown in Fig. 1.

Dengue fever is a self–limiting disease and represents the majority of cases of dengue infection. A prevalence of *Aedes aegypti* and *Aedes albopictus* together with the circulation of dengue virus of more than one type in any particular area tends to be associated with outbreaks of DHF/DSS *(1)*.

Problem statement

Dengue fever (DF) and its severe forms – dengue haemorrhagic fever (DHF) and dengue shock syndrome (DSS) – have become major international public health concerns. Over the past three decades, there has been dramatic global increase in the frequency of dengue fever, DHF and DSS and their epidemics. It is found in tropical and subtropical regions around the world, predominantly in urban and semi-urban areas, and are now spreading to rural areas.

About 3.9 billion people in 129 countries are at risk of infection with dengue viruses. A recent estimate indicates 390 million dengue infections per year, of which 96 million manifest clinically with any severity of disease. The number of reported cases have increased from over 2.4 million in 2010 to 5.2 million in 2019. Not only the number of cases are increasing as disease is spreading to new areas, but explosive outbreaks are occurring. The year 2016 was characterized by large dengue outbreaks worldwide. In 2015, Delhi, recorded its worst outbreak since 2006 with over 15,000 cases.

Worldwide, annually about 500,000 people with DHF require hospitalization. Approximately 90 per cent of them are children aged less than five years, and about 2.5 per cent of those affected die. During epidemics, infection rate among those who have not been previously exposed to the virus are often 40 to 50 per cent, but can also reach 80 to 90 per cent *(3)*. Co-circulation of multiple serotypes/genotypes is evident.

Dengue and DHF is endemic in more than 100 countries in the WHO regions of Africa, the Americas, Eastern Mediterranean, South-East Asia and Western Pacific. The South-East Asia and Western Pacific regions are most seriously affected. Detection of all four serotypes has now rendered the countries hyperendemic. The countries of South-East Asia region are divided into 3 categories *(3)*.

Category A (Bangladesh, India, Indonesia, Maldives, Myanmar, Sri Lanka, Thailand and Timor-Leste)

a. Major public health problem;
b. Leading cause of hospitalization and death among children;
c. Hyperendemicity with all 4 serotypes circulating in urban areas; and
d. Spreading to rural areas.

Category B (Bhutan, Nepal)

a. Endemicity uncertain;
b. Bhutan reported first outbreak in 2004; and
c. Nepal reported first indigenous case in 2004.

Category C (DPR Korea)

No evidence of endemicity.

INDIA

In India, the risk of dengue has shown an increase in recent years due to rapid urbanization, lifestyle changes and deficient water management including improper water storage practices in urban, peri-urban and rural areas, leading to proliferation of mosquito breeding sites. The disease has a seasonal pattern i.e. the cases peak after monsoon, and it is not uniformly distributed throughout the year. However, in the southern states and Gujarat the transmission is perennial *(4)*.

Dengue is endemic in 35 states/UTs. During 2020, about 44,585 cases were reported with 56 deaths. The case fatality rate was 0.12 per cent. As seen from Table 1, the highest number of cases were reported from Punjab (8,435) followed by West Bengal (5,166), Kerala (4,399), Karnataka (3,823), and Uttar Pradesh (3,715) *(5)*.

All the four serotypes i.e. dengue 1, 2, 3 and 4 have been isolated in India but at present DENV-1 and DENV-2 serotypes are widespread *(6)*.

TABLE 1

Dengue / DHF situation in India, 2019–2020 (P)

State/UT	2019		2020 (P)	
	Cases	Deaths	Cases	Deaths
Andhra Pradesh	5,286	0	925	0
Arunachal Pradesh	123	0	1	0
Assam	196	0	33	0
Bihar	6,712	0	493	2
Chhattisgarh	722	0	57	0
Goa	992	0	376	0
Gujarat	18,219	17	1,564	2
Haryana	1,207	0	1,377	0
Himachal Pradesh	344	2	21	0
J & K	439	0	53	0
Jharkhand	825	5	79	0
Karnataka	16,986	13	3,823	0
Kerala	4,652	16	4,399	5
Madhya Pradesh	4,189	2	806	0
Meghalaya	82	0	4	0
Maharashtra	14,907	29	3,356	10
Manipur	359	0	37	0
Mizoram	42	0	67	0
Nagaland	8	0	1	0
Odisha	3,758	4	496	0
Punjab	10,289	14	8,435	22
Rajasthan	13,706	17	2,023	7
Sikkim	444	0	11	0
Tamil Nadu	8,527	5	2,410	0
Tripura	114	0	24	0
Telangana	13,331	7	2,173	0
Uttar Pradesh	10,557	26	3,715	6
Uttarakhand	10,622	8	76	1
West Bengal	47,928	0	5,166	0
A&N Islands	168	0	98	0
Chandigarh	286	0	265	0
Delhi	5,077	0	1,269	0
D & N Haveli	1,491	2	319	0
Daman & Diu	625	2		
Lakshadweep	0	0	0	0
Puducherry	2,030	2	633	1
All India Total	2,05,243	166	44,585	56

P – Provisional
Source : *(5)*

Epidemiological determinants

Agent factors

(a) AGENT : The dengue virus forms a distinct complex within the genus *flavivirus* based on antigenic and biological characteristics. There are four virus serotypes which are designated as DENV-1, DENV-2, DENV-3 and DENV-4. Infection with any one serotype confers lifelong immunity to that virus serotype *(7)*. Although all four serotypes are antigenically similar, they are different enough to elicit cross-protection for only a few months after infection by any one of them. Secondary infection with dengue serotype 2 or multiple infection with different serotypes lead to severe form dengue DHF/DSS *(3)*. The first infection probably sensitizes the patient, while the second infection with different serotype appears to produce immunological catastrophy.

The pathogenesis of severe syndrome involves pre-existing dengue antibody. It is postulated that virus antibodies are formed within a few days of the second dengue infection and that the non-neutralizing enhancing antibodies promote infection of higher numbers of mononuclear cells, followed by the release of cytokines, vasoactive mediators, and procoagulants, leading to the disseminated intravascular coagulation seen in the haemorrhagic fever syndrome *(8)*.

All four serotypes have been associated with epidemics of dengue fever (with or without DHF) with varying degree of severity.

(b) VECTOR : *Aedes aegypti* and *Aedes albopictus* are the two most important vectors of dengue. They both carry high vectorial competency for dengue virus, i.e., high susceptibility to infecting virus, ability to replicate the virus and ability to transmit the virus to another host. *Aedes aegypti* is a highly domesticated, strongly anthropophilic, nervous feeder (i.e., it bites more than one host to complete one blood meal) and is a discordant species (i.e., it needs more than one feed for the completion of the gonotropic cycle). This habit results in the generation of multiple cases and the clustering of dengue cases in the cities. On the contrary, *Ae. albopictus* partly invades peripheral areas of urban cities. It is an aggressive feeder and concordant species, i.e., the species can complete its blood meal in one go on one person and also does not require a second blood meal for the completion of the gonotropic cycle.

Transmission of disease

The *Aedes* mosquito becomes infective by feeding on a patient from the day before onset to the 5th day (viraemia stage) of illness. After an extrinsic incubation period of 8 to 10 days, the mosquito becomes infective, and is able to transmit the infection. Once the mosquito becomes infective, it remains so for life. The genital tract of the mosquito gets infected and transovarian transmission of dengue virus occurs when virus enters fully developed eggs at the time of oviposition.

Environmental factors

The population of *Aedes aegypti* fluctuates with rainfall and water storage. Its life span is influenced by temperature and humidity, survives best between 16°C–30°C and a relative humidity of 60–80 per cent. It breeds in the containers in and around the houses. Being a domestic breeder, it is a endophagic and endophilic. However, even with a 2°C increase in temperature the extrinsic incubation period of DENV will be shortened and more infected mosquitoes are available for a longer duration. Besides that the mosquitoes will bite more frequently because of dehydration and thus increase man–mosquito contact *(3, 6)*.

The failure of urban authorities to provide civil amenities and poor public health infrastructure raises the potential for the vector to breed at high level and makes the environment transmission conducive. The rural spread of the vector is relatively recent occurrence associated with the development of rural water supply schemes, improved transport systems, scarcity of water and lifestyle changes *(6)*.

Dengue in the community *(3)*

A number of factors that contribute to initiation and maintenance of an epidemic include: (i) the strain of the virus, which may influence the magnitude and duration of the viraemia in humans; (ii) the density, behaviour and vectorial capacity of the vector population; (iii) the susceptibility of the human population (both genetic factors and pre-existing immune profile); and (iv) the introduction of the virus into a receptive community.

DF/DHF syndrome

DF/DHF is characterized by the "iceberg" or pyramid phenomenon. At the base of the pyramid, most of the cases are symptomless, followed by DF, DHF and DSS. Clusters of cases have been reported in particular households or neighbourhoods due to the feeding behaviour of the vector.

Affected population

The population affected varies from one outbreak to another. Actual estimates can be made by obtaining clinical/ subclinical ratios during epidemics. In a well-defined epidemic study in North Queensland, Australia, with primary infection, 20% to 50% of the population was found affected.

Severity of the disease

The serotype that produces the secondary infection and, in particular, the serotype sequence are important to ascertain the severity of the disease. All the four serotypes are able to produce DHF cases. However, during sequential infections, only 2% to 4% of individuals develop severe disease.

Studies in Thailand have revealed that the DENV-1/ DENV-2 sequence of infection was associated with a 500 fold risk of DHF compared with primary infection. For the DENV-3/DENV-2 sequence the risk was 150-fold, and a DENV-4/DENV-2 sequence had a 50-fold risk of DHF. There is no time-limit to sensitization after a primary infection. The 1997 Santiago de Cuba epidemic clearly demonstrated that with the introduction of DENV-2, DHF had occurred 16–20 years after the primary infection with DENV-1.

High-risk patients *(3)*

The following host factors contribute to more severe disease and its complications :

1. infants and elderly ;
2. obesity;
3. pregnancy;
4. peptic ulcer disease;

5. women who are in menstruation or have abnormal bleeding;
6. haemolytic disease such as G–6PD, thalassaemia and other haemoglobinopathies;
7. congenital heart disease;
8. chronic diseases such as diabetes mellitus, hypertension, asthma, ischaemic heart disease, chronic renal failure, liver cirrhosis; and
9. patients on steroid or NSAID treatment.

Clinical mainfestations

Dengue virus infection may be asymptomatic or may cause undifferientiated febrile illness (viral syndrome), dengue fever(DF), or dengue haemorrhagic fever (DHF) including dengue shock syndrome (DSS) as shown in Fig.1

1. Undifferentiated fever

Infants, children and adults who have been infected with denuge virus, especially for the first time (i.e. primary dengue infection), may develop a simple fever indistinguishable from other viral infection. Maculopapular rashes may accompany the fever or may appear during defervescence. Upper respiratory and gastrointestinal symptoms are common.

2. Classical dengue fever

All ages and both sexes are susceptible to dengue fever. Children usually have a milder disease than adults. The illness is characterized by an incubation period of 3 to 10 days (commonly 5–6 days). The onset is sudden, with chills and high fever, intense headache, muscle and joint pains, which prevent all movement. Within 24 hours retroorbital pain, particularly on eye movements or eye pressure and photophobia develops. Other common symptoms include extreme weakness, anorexia, constipation, altered taste sensation, colicky pain and abdominal tenderness, dragging pain in inguinal region, sore throat and general depression. Fever is usually between 39°C and 40°C. Fever is typically but not inevitably followed by a remission of a few hours to 2 days (biphasic curve). The skin eruptions appear in 80 per cent of cases during the remission or during second febrile phase, which lasts for 1–2 days. The rash is accompanied by similar but milder symptoms. The rash may be diffuse flushing, mottling or fleeting pin–point eruptions on the face, neck and chest during the first half of the febrile period and a conspicuous rash, that may be maculopapular or scarlatiniform on 3rd or 4th day. It starts on the chest and trunk and may spread to the extremities and rarely to the face. It may be accompanied by itching and hyperaesthesia. The rash lasts for 2 hours to several days and may be followed by desquamation *(1)*. Fever lasts for about 5 days, rarely more than 7 days after which recovery is usually complete although convalescence may be protracted *(8)*. The case fatality is exceedingly low.

3. Dengue haemorrhagic fever

Dengue haemorrhagic fever (DHF) is a severe form of dengue fever. The course of dengue illness can be divided into three phases–febrile phase, critical phase and recovery phase, as shown in Fig. 2 *(9)*.

1. Febrile phase

Following an incubation period of four to six days, the illness commonly begins abruptly with high fever accompanied by facial flushing and headache. Anorexia, vomiting, epigastric discomfort, tenderness at the right costal margin and generalized abdominal pain are common. During the first few days the illness usually resembles classical DF, but maculopapular rash usually rubelliform type, is less common. It may appear early or late in the course of the illness. Occasionally, the temperature may be 40°C to 41°C and febrile convulsions may occur particularly in infants *(1)*.

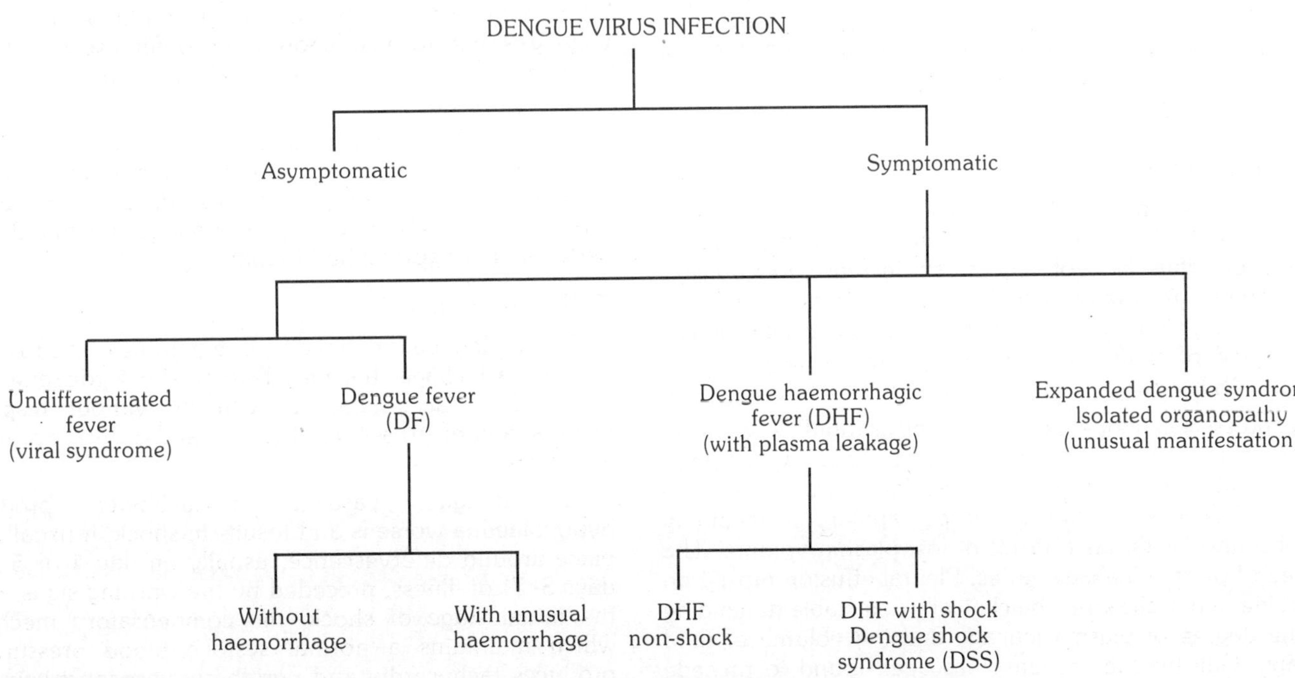

FIG. 1

Manifestations of the dengue virus infection

Source : *(3)*

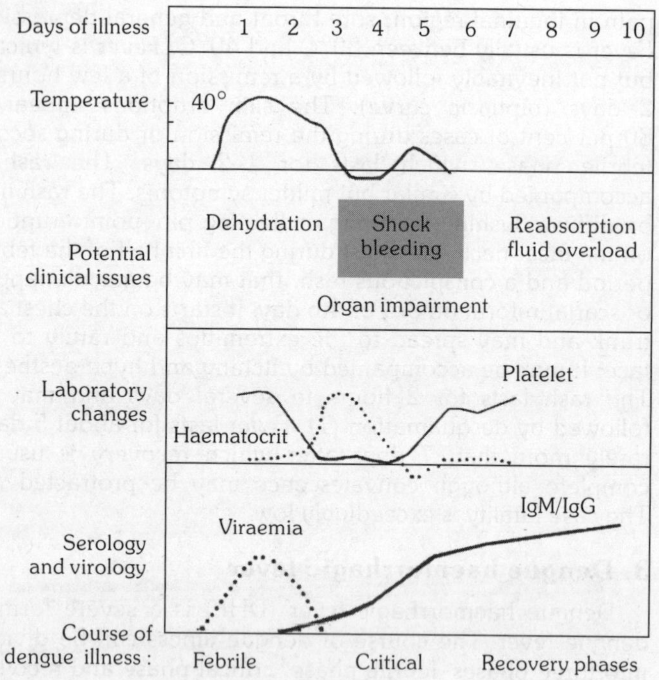

FIG. 2

The course of dengue illness

Source : *(10)*

The major pathophysiologic changes that determine the severity of disease in DHF and differentiate it from DF are plasma leakage and abnormal haemostasis, as manifested by a rising haematocrit value and moderate to marked thrombocytopenia. These two clinical laboratory changes are distinctive and constant findings.

A positive tournicate test is the most common haemorrhagic phenomenon. The test is performed by inflating a blood pressure cuff to a mid point between systolic and diastolic pressure for 5 minutes. The test is considered positive when 10 or more petechiae per 2.5×2.5 cm (1 inch square) are observed. In DHF, the test usually gives a definite positive with 20 petechiae or more *(6)*.

2. Critical phase (10)

Around the time of defervescence, when the temperature drops to 37.5–38°C or less, and remains below this level, usually on days 3–7 of illness, an increase in capillary permeability in parallel with increasing haematocrit levels may occur. This marks the beginning of the critical phase. The period of clinically significant plasma leakage usually lasts 24–48 hours.

Progressive leukopenia followed by a rapid decrease in platelet count usually precedes plasma leakage. At this point patients without an increase in capillary permeability will improve, while those with increased capillary permeability may become worse as a result of lost plasma volume. The degree of plasma leakage varies. Pleural effusion mostly on right side and ascites may be clinically detectable depending on the degree of plasma leakage and the volume of fluid therapy. Gall bladder oedema has been found to precede plasma leakage. Hence chest X-ray and abdominal ultrasound can be useful tools for diagnosis. The degree of increase above the baseline haematocrit often reflects the severity of plasma leakage.

Shock occurs when a critical volume of plasma is lost through leakage. It is often preceded by warning signs of abdominal pain or tenderness, persistent vomiting, clinical fluid accumulation, mucosal bleeding, lethargy, restlessness, liver enlargement more than 2 cm. and oliguria. The body temperature may be subnormal when shock occurs. With prolonged shock, the consequent organ hypoperfusion results in progressive organ impairment, metabolic acidosis and disseminated intravascular coagulation. This in turn leads to severe haemorrhage causing the haematocrit to decrease in severe shock. Instead of the leukopenia usually seen during this phase of dengue, the total white cell count may increase in patients with severe bleeding. In addition, severe organ impairment such as severe hepatits, encephalitis or myocarditis and/or severe bleeding may also develop without obvious plasma leakage or shock.

Those who improve after defervescence are said to have non-severe dengue. Some patients progress to the critical phase of plasma leakage without defervescence and, in these patients, changes in the full blood count should be used to guide the onset of the critical phase and plasma leakage. Those who deteriorate will manifest with warning signs. This is called dengue with warning signs. Cases of dengue with warning signs will probably recover with early intravenous rehydration. Some cases will deteriorate to severe dengue.

3. Recovery phase

If the patient survives the 24–48 hours critical phase, a gradual reabsorption of extravascular compartment fluid takes place in the following 48–72 hours. General well-being improves, appetite returns, gastrointestinal symptoms abate, haemodynamic status stabilizes and diuresis ensues. Some patients may have a rash of "isles of white in the sea of red". Some may experience generalized pruritus. Bradycardia and electrocardiographic changes are common during this stage.

The haematocrit stabilizes or may be lower due to the dilutional effect of reabsorbed fluid. White blood cell count usually starts to rise soon after defervescence but the recovery of platelet count is typically later than that of white blood cell count.

Respiratory distress from massive pleural effusion and ascites will occur at any time if excessive intravenous fluids have been administered. During the critical and/or recovery phases, excessive fluid therapy is associated with pulmonary oedema or congestive heart failure.

4. Severe dengue

Severe dengue is defined by one or more of the following : (i) plasma leakage that may lead to shock (dengue shock) and/or fluid accumulation, with or without respiratory distress, and/or (ii) severe bleeding, and/or (iii) severe organ impairment.

As dengue vascular permeability progresses, hypovolaemia worsens and results in shock. It usually takes place around defervescence, usually on day 4 or 5 (range days 3–7) of illness, preceded by the warning signs. During the initial stage of shock, the compensatory mechanism which maintains a normal systolic blood pressure also produces tachycardia and peripheral vasoconstriction with reduced skin perfusion, resulting in cold extremities and delayed capillary refill time. Uniquely, the diastolic pressure rises towards the systolic pressure and the pulse pressure narrows as the peripheral vascular resistance increases.

Patients in dengue shock often remain conscious and lucid. The inexperienced physician may measure a normal systolic pressure and misjudge the critical state of the patient. Finally, there is decompensation and both pressures disappear abruptly. Prolonged hypotensive shock and hypoxia may lead to multi-organ failure and an extremely difficult clinical course.

The patient is considered to have shock if the pulse pressure is ≤20 mm Hg in children or he/she has signs of poor capillary perfusion (cold extremities, delayed capillary refill, or rapid pulse rate). In adults, the pulse pressure of ≤20 mm Hg may indicate a more severe shock. Hypotension is usually associated with prolonged shock which is often complicated by major bleeding.

Patients with severe dengue may have coagulation abnormalities, but these are usually not sufficient to cause major bleeding. When major bleeding does occur, it is almost always associated with profound shock since this, in combination with thrombocytopenia, hypoxia and acidosis, can lead to multiple organ failure and advanced disseminated intravascular coagulation. Massive bleeding may occur without prolonged shock in instances when acetylsalicylic acid (aspirin), ibuprofen or corticosteriods have been taken.

Unusual manifestations, including acute liver failure and encephalopathy, may be present, even in the absence of severe plasma leakage or shock. Cardiomyopathy and encephalitis are also reported in a few dengue cases. However, most deaths from dengue occur in patients with profound shock, particularly if the situation is complicated by fluid overload.

CRITERIA FOR CLINICAL DIAGNOSIS *(3, 6, 11)*

A summary of clinical diagnosis of DF and DHF is as follows :

Dengue fever

Probable diagnosis

Acute febrile illness with two or more of the following;

- headache,
- retro-orbital pain,
- myalgia,
- arthralgia/bone pain,
- rash,
- haemorrhagic manifestations,
- leucopenia (wbc ≤ 5000 cells/mm^3),
- thrombocytopenia (platelet count <150,000 cells/mm^3),
- rising haematocrit (5–10%);

and at least one of the following :

- supportive serology on single serum sample: titre ≥ 1280 with haemagglutination inhibition test, comparable IgG titre with enzyme-linked immunosorbent assay, or testing positive in IgM antibody test, and
- occurrence at the same location and time as confirmed cases of dengue fever.

Confirmed diagnosis

Probable case with at least one of the following :

- isolation of dengue virus from serum, CSF or autopsy samples.
- fourfold or greater increase in serum IgG (by haemagglutination inhibition test) or increase in IgM antibody specific to dengue virus.
- detection of dengue virus or antigen in tissue, serum or cerebrospinal fluid by immunohistochemistry, immunofluorescence or enzyme-linked immunosorbent assay.
- detection of dengue virus genomic sequences by reverse transcription-polymerase chain reaction.

Dengue haemorrhagic fever

All of following :

- acute onset of fever of two to seven days duration.
- haemorrhagic manifestations, shown by any of the following; positive tourniquet test, petechiae, ecchymoses or purpura, or bleeding from mucosa, gastrointestinal tract, injection sites, or other locations.
- platelet count ≤ 100,000 cells/mm^3
- objective evidence of plasma leakage due to increased vascular permeability shown by any of the following :
  - Rising haematocrit/haemoconcentration ≥20% from baseline or evidence of plasma leakage such as pleural effusion, ascites or hypoproteinaemia/ albuminaemia.

Dengue shock syndrome

Criteria for dengue haemorrhagic fever as above with signs of shock including :

- tachycardia, cool extremities, delayed capillary refill, weak pulse, lethargy or restlessness, which may be a sign of reduced brain perfusion.
- pulse pressure ≤ 20 mmHg with increased diastolic pressure, e.g. 100/80 mmHg.
- hypotension by age, defined as systolic pressure <80 mmHg for those aged <5 years, or 80 to 90 mmHg for older children and adults.

Laboratory diagnosis *(3, 6)*

Rapid and accurate dengue diagnosis is of a paramount importance for : (1) clinical management; (2) epidemiological surveillance; (3) research; and (4) vaccine trials. Epidemiological surveillance requires early determination of dengue virus infection during the outbreak for urgent public health action towards control, as well as at sentinel sites for detection of circulating serotypes/genotypes during the inter-epidemic period for use in forecasting possible outbreak. The following laboratory tests are available to diagnose dengue fever and DHF :

1. *Virus isolation :* Isolation of dengue virus from clinical specimens is possible provided the specimen is taken during the first six days of illness and processed without delay. Specimen that are suitable for virus isolation are – acute phase serum, plasma or washed buffy coat from the patient,autopsy tissue from fatal case (especially liver, spleen, lymph nodes and thymus), and mosquitoes collected from the affected areas.

2. *Viral nucleic acid detection :* Dengue viral genome, which consists of RNA, can be detected by reverse transcriptase polymerase chain reaction (RT–PCR) assay and real time RT–PCR. In recent years, a number of

RT–PCR assays have been reported for detecting dengue virus. They offer better specificity and sensitivity compared to virus isolation with a much more rapid turnaround time.

3. *Immunological response and serological tests* : Following tests are available for diagnosis of dengue infection :

a. Haemagglutination Inhibition Assay (HIA);
b. Complement Fixation (CF);
c. Neutralization test (NT);
d. IgM capture enzyme-linked immunosorbent assay (MAC-ELISA);
e. Indirect IgG- ELISA, and
f. IgM/IgG ratio

4. *Viral antigen detection* : ELISA and dot blot assays directed against the envelop/membrane (EM) antigens and nonstructural protein 1 (NS1) can be detected in both patients with primary and secondary dengue infection upto 6 days after the onset of the illness. Commercial kits for the detection of NS1 antigens are now available; however, these kits do not differentiate between the serotypes. Besides providing an early diagnostic marker for clinical management, it may also facilitate the improvement of epidemiological surveys of dengue infection.

5. *Rapid diagnostic test (RDT)* : A number of commercial rapid format serological test-kits for anti-dengue IgM and IgG antibodies have become available in the past few years, some of these producing results within 15 minutes. Unfortunately, the accuracy of most of these tests is uncertain since they have not yet been properly validated.

6. *Analysis of haematological parameters* : Standard haematological parameters such as platelet count and haematocrit are important and are part of the diagnosis of dengue infection. They should be closely monitored.

The diagnostic tests are summarized in Table 2.

CLINICAL MANAGEMENT

Grading of the severity of dengue infection

To decide where to treat the patient, it is important to classify the severity of dengue infection. The presence of thrombocytopenia with concurrent haemoconcentration differentiates grade I and grade II DHF from DF. Table 3 shows grading of dengue infection.

Guidelines for treatment

A full blood count of the patient should be done at the first visit. A haematocrit test in the early febrile phase establishes the patient's own baseline haematocrit. A rapidly decreasing platelet count in parallel with a rising haematocrit compared to the baseline is suggestive of progress to the plasma leakage/critical phase of the disease. In the absence of the patients baseline, age specific population haematocrit levels could be used as a surrogate during the critical phase.

1. Management of dengue fever

These are patients who are able to tolerate adequate volumes of oral fluids and pass urine at least once every six hours, and do not have any of the warning signs, particularly when fever subsides. Those with stable haematocrit can be sent home after being advised to return to the hospital immediately if they develop any of the warning signs, and to adhere to the following action plan :

(1) Encourage intake of oral rehydration solution (ORS), fruit juice and other fluids containing electrolytes and sugar to replace losses from fever and vomiting. Adequate oral fluid intake may be able to reduce the number of hospitalizations. (Caution : fluids containing sugar/glucose may exacerbate hyperglycaemia of physiological stress from dengue and diabetes mellitus.)

(2) Give paracetamol for high fever if the patient is uncomfortable. The interval of paracetamol dosing

TABLE 2

Dengue diagnostics and sample characteristics

	Clinical sample	Diagnostic method	Methodology	Time to results
Virus detection and its components	Acute serum (1–5 days of fever) and necropsy tissues	Viral isolation	Mosquito or mosquito cell culture inoculation	One week or more
		Nucleic acid detection	RT-PCR and real time RT-PCR	1 or 2 days
		Antigen detection	NS1 Ag rapid tests	Minutes
			NS1 Ag ELISA	1 day
			Immuno-histochemistry	2–5 days
Serological response	Paired sera (acute serum from 1–5 days and second serum 15–21 days after)	IgM or IgG seroconversion	ELISA HIA	1–2 days
			Neutralization test	Minimum 7 days
	Serum after day 5 of fever	IgM detection (recent infection)	ELISA	1 or 2 days
			Rapid tests	Minutes
		IgG detection	IgG ELISA HIA	1 or 2 days

ELISA = enzyme-linked immunosorbent assay; HIA = haemagglutination inhibition assay; IgG = immunoglobulin G; IgM = immunoglobulin M; NS1 Ag = non-structural protein 1 antigen; RT-PCR = reverse transcriptase polymerase chain reaction.

Source : *(12)*

TABLE 3

WHO classification and grading of the severity of dengue infection

DF/DHF	Grade	Symptoms/signs	Laboratory findings
DF		Fever with two or more of the following – Headache – Retro-orbital pain – Myalgia – Arthralgia – Rash – Haemorrhagic manifestations – No evidence of plasma leakage	– Leucopenia (WBC ≤ 5000 cells/cu.mm), – Thrombocytopenia (platelet count < 150,000 cells/cu.mm), – Rising haematocrit (5–10 per cent)
DHF	I	Above criteria for DF and haemorrhagic manifestation plus positive tourniquet test, evidence of plasma leakage	Thrombocytopenia : Platelet count < 100,000/cu.mm. Haematorcit rise 20% or more
DHF	II	Above signs and symptoms plus some evidence of spontaneous bleeding in skin or other organs (black tarry stools, epistaxis, bleeding from gums, etc) and abdominal pain	Thrombocytopenia platelet count < 100,000/cu.mm. Haematocrit rise 20% or more
DHF	III	Above signs and symptoms plus circulating failure (weak rapid pulse, pulse pressure ≤ 20 mm Hg or high diastolic pressure, hypotension with the presence of cold clammy skin and restlessness)	Thrombocytopenia : Platelet count < 100,000/cu.mm. Haematocrit rise more than 20%
DHF	IV	Signs as grade III plus profound shock with undetectable blood pressure or pulse	Thrombocytopenia : Platelet count < 100,000/cu.mm. Haemotocrit rise more than 20%
DHF III and IV are Dengue Shock Syndrome			

Source : *(3, 6)*

should not be less than six hours. Tepid sponge if the patient still has high fever. Do not give acetylsalicylic acid (aspirin), ibuprofen or other non-steroidal anti-inflammatory agents (NSAIDs) as these drugs may aggravate gastritis or bleeding. Acetylsalicylic acid (aspirin) may be associated with Reye's Syndrome.

(3) Instruct the care-givers that the patient should be brought to hospital immediately if any of the following occur; no clinical improvement, deterioration around the time of defervescence, severe abdominal pain, persistent vomiting, cold and clammy extremities, lethargy or irritability/restlessness, bleeding (e.g. black stools or coffee–ground vomiting), not passing urine for more than 4–6 hours.

Patients who are sent home should be monitored daily by health care providers for temperature pattern, volume of fluid intake and losses, urine output (volume and frequency), warning signs, signs of plasma leakage and bleeding, haematocrit, and white blood cell and platelet counts.

2. Management of DHF (Febrile Phase) *(6, 11)*

The management of febrile phase is similar to that of DF. Paracetamol is recommended to keep the temperature below 39°C. Copious amount of fluid should be given orally, to the extent the patient tolerates, oral rehydration solution (ORS), such as those used for the treatment of diarrhoeal disesases and/or fruit juices are preferable to plain water. IV fluid may be administered, if the patient is vomiting persistently or refusing to feed.

Patients should be closely monitored for the initial signs of shock. The critical period is during the transition from the febrile to the afebrile stage and usually occurs after the third day of illness. Serial haematocrit determinations are essential guide for treatment, since they reflect the degree of plasma leakage and need for intravenous administration of fluids. Haematocrit should be determined daily from the third day until the temperature has remained normal for one or two days. If haematocrit determination is not possible, haemoglobin determination may be carried out as an alternative. The details of IV treatment when required for patients are given in Fig. 3.

3. Management of DHF Grade I and II

Any person who has dengue fever with thrombocytopenia and haemoconcentration and presents with abdominal pain, black tarry stools, epistaxis, bleeding from the gums and infection etc needs to be hospitalized. All these patients should be observed for signs of shock. The critical period for development of shock is transition from febrile to abferile phase of illness, which usually occurs after third day of illness. A rise of haemoconcentration indicates need for IV fluid therapy. If despite the treatment, the patient develops fall in BP, decrease in urine output or other features of shock, the management for Grade III/IV DHF/ DSS should be instituted.

Oral rehydration should be given along with antipyretics like paracetamol, sponging, etc. as described above. The detailed treatment for patients with DHF Grade I and II is given in Fig. 3.

4. Management of DHF Grade III and IV

Common signs of complication are observed during the afebrile phase of DHF. Immediately after hospitalization, the haematocrit, platelet count and vital signs should be examined to assess the patient's condition and intravenous fluid therapy should be started. The patient requires regular and sustained monitoring. If the patient has already received about 1000 ml of intravenous fluid, it should be changed to colloidal solution preferably Dextran 40/haemaccel or if haematocrit is decreasing, fresh whole blood transfusion 10–20 ml/kg/hour should be given.

However, in case of persistent shock when, after initial fluid replacement and resuscitation with plasma or plasma expanders, the haematocrit continues to decline, internal bleeding should be suspected. It may be difficult to recognize and estimate the degree of internal blood loss in the presence of haemoconcentration. It is thus recommended to give fresh whole blood in small volumes of 10 ml/kg/hour for all patients in shock as a routine precaution. Oxygen should be given to all patients in shock. The detailed graphical presentation of the treatment for patients with DHF Grades III and IV is given in Fig. 4 and 5.

Indications of red cell transfusion

1. Loss of blood (overt blood) – 10 per cent or more of total blood volume – preferably give whole blood or components to be used.
2. Refractory shock despite adequate fluid administration and declining haematocrit.
3. Replacement volume should be 10 ml/kg body weight at a time and coagulogram should be done.
4. If fluid overload is present packed cells are to be given.

Indications of platelet transfusion

In general there is no need to give prophylactic platelet even at < 20,000/cu.mm.

1. Prophylactic platelet transfusion may be given at level of < 10,000/cu.mm.
2. Prolonged shock; with coagulopathy and abnormal coagulogram.
3. In case of systemic massive bleeding, platelet transfusion may be needed in addition to red cell transfusion.

Criteria for discharge of patients

1. Absence of fever for atleast 24 hours without the use of anti-pyretic drugs.
2. Return of appetite.
3. Visible clinical improvement.
4. Good urine output.
5. Minimum of 2–3 days after recovery from shock.
6. No respiratory distress from pleural effusion or ascites.
7. Platelet count > 50,000/cu.mm.

Disease notification

In dengue-endemic countries, cases of suspected, probable and confirmed dengue should be notified as soon as possible so that appropriate health measures can be initiated.

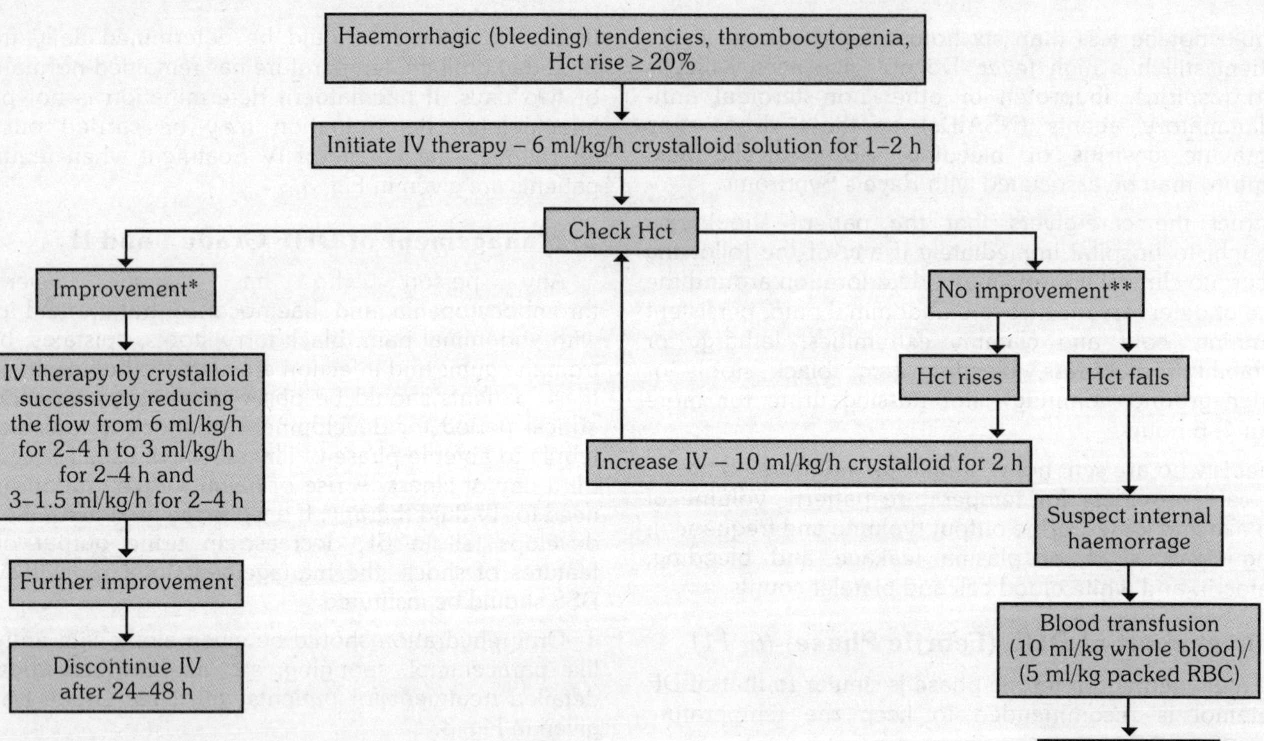

Note:

* Improvement : Hct falls, pulse rate and blood pressure stable, urine output rises

** No improvement : Hct or pulse rate rises, pulse pressure falls below 20 mmHg, urine output falls

FIG. 3
Volume replacement algorithm for patients with moderate dengue fever (DHF Grades I & II)

Source : *(11, 15)*

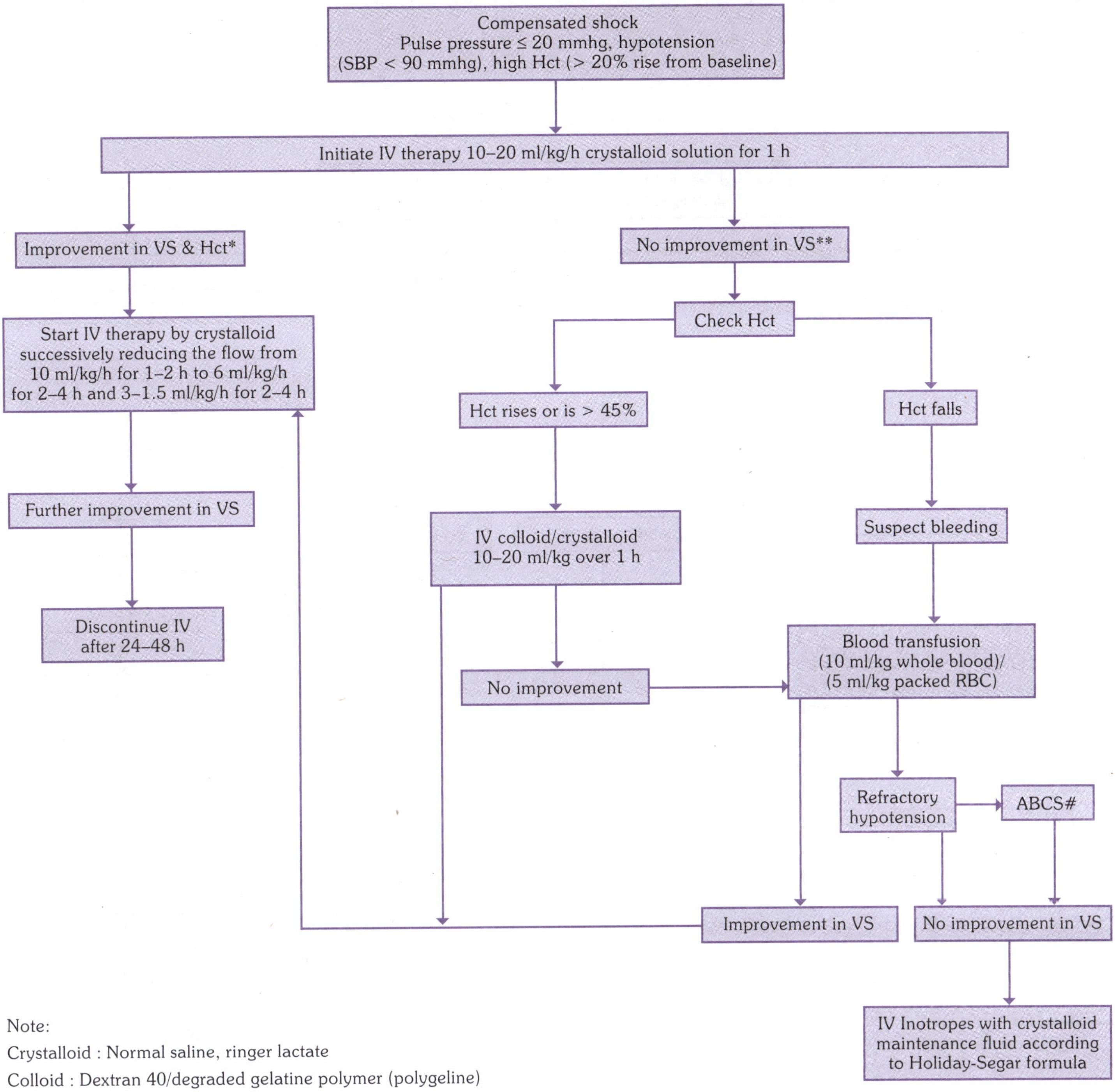

Note:

Crystalloid : Normal saline, ringer lactate

Colloid : Dextran 40/degraded gelatine polymer (polygeline)

ABCS = Acidosis, Bleeding, Calcium (Na++ & K+), Sugar

* Improvement: Hct falls, pulse rate and blood pressure stable, urine output rises

** No improvement: Hct or pulse rate rises, pulse pressure falls below 20 mmHg, urine output falls

- Unstable vital signs : urine output falls, signs of shock
- In cases of acidosis, hyperosmolar or Ringer's lactate solution should not be used
- Serial platelet and Hct determinations : drop in platelets and rise in Hct are essential for early diagnosis of DHF
- Cases of DHF should be observed every hour for vital signs and urine output

FIG. 4

Volume replacement algorithm for patients with severe dengue fever (DHF grade III)

Source : *(11, 15)*

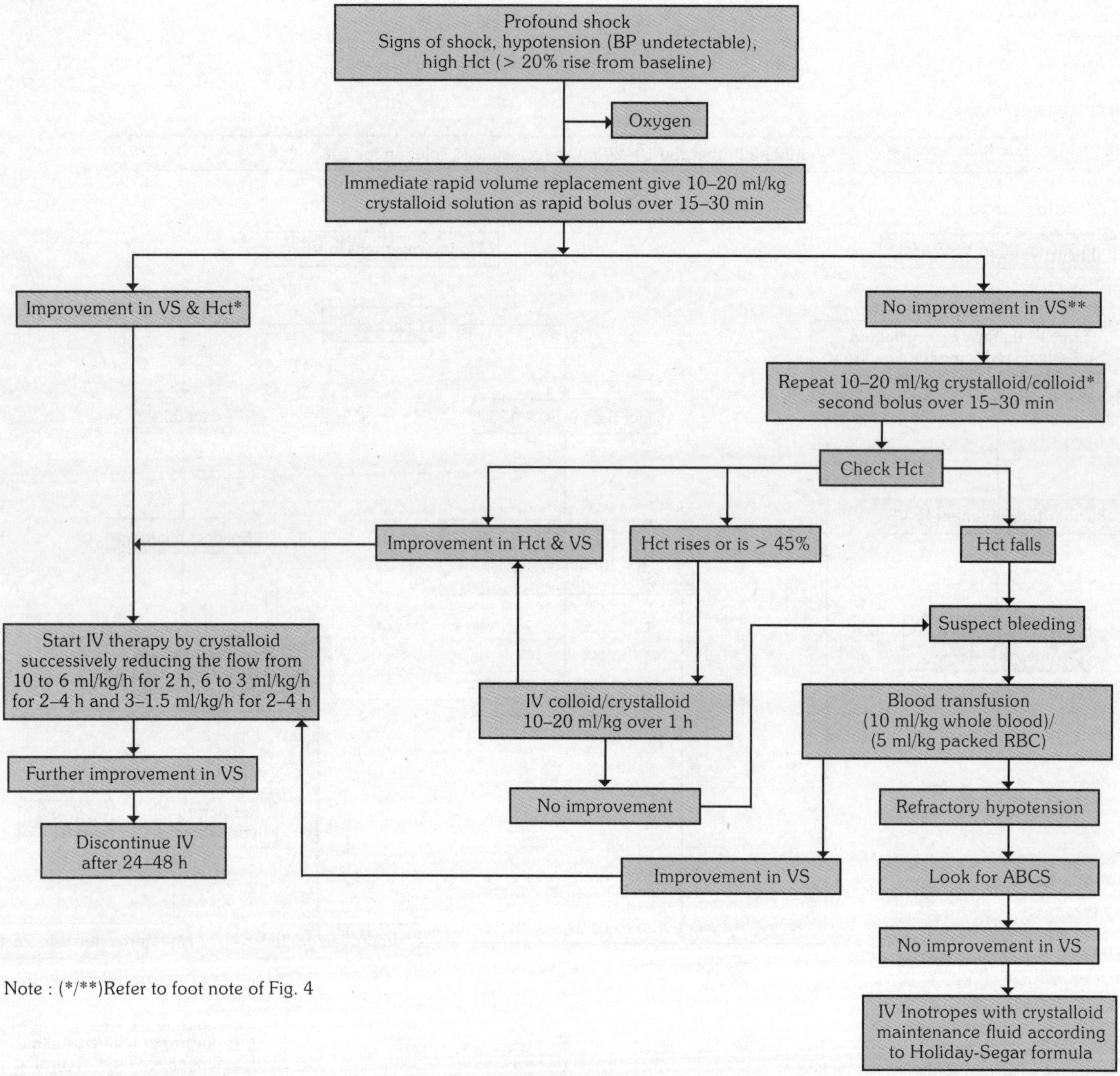

FIG. 5
Volume replacement algorithm for patients with decompensated shock in dengue (DHF IV (DSS))

Source : *(11, 15)*

CONTROL MEASURES

1. Mosquito control

The vectors of DF and DHF (e.g., *A. aegypti*) breed in and around houses and, in principle can be controlled by individual and community action, using antiadult and antilarval measures. These measures are outlined in chapter 14.

2. Vaccines *(13)*

CYD-TDV is a prophylactic, tetravalent, live attenuated viral vaccine developed by Sanofi Pasteur in December 2015. The vaccination schedule consists of 3 injections of 0.5 ml administered at 6-month intervals. The indication from the first licenses is for the prevention of dengue illness caused by dengue virus serotypes 1, 2, 3, and 4 in individuals 9–45 years or 9–60 years of age (depending on the license), living in dengue endemic areas. The lower limit of the indication at 9 years of age was chosen due to a safety concern in children aged 2–5 years identified in the Phase 3 clinical trials.

CYD-TDV is available in a single-dose vial or in a multidose (5–dose) vial. It is a freeze-dried product to be reconstituted before injection with either a sterile solution of 0.4% sodium chloride for the single-dose presentation or a sterile solution of 0.9% sodium chloride for the 5-dose presentation. After reconstitution, the 0.5 ml dose is to be administered by the subcutaneous route. The diluent is provided as a pre-filled syringe for single dose presentation or in a vial for the multi-dose presentation. The CYD-TDV dengue vaccine contains no adjuvant or preservatives. The shelf life of CYD-TDV is 36 months when stored between 2°C and 8°C. After reconstitution with the solvent provided, the vaccine must be kept at between 2°C and 8°C and protected from light. In accordance with the WHO multi-dose vial policy, any reconstituted doses remaining at the end of session should be discarded within 6 hours of opening/reconstitution or at the end of a vaccination session, whichever comes first.

The manufacturer stipulates that vaccination is contra-indicated in: (1) individuals with a history of severe allergic reaction to any component of the dengue vaccine or after prior administration of the dengue vaccine or a vaccine containing the same components; (2) individuals with congenital or acquired immune deficiency that impairs cell-mediated immunity; (3) individuals with symptomatic HIV infection or with asymptomatic HIV infection when accompanied by evidence of impaired immune function; (4) pregnant or breastfeeding women; and that vaccination should be postponed in individuals with moderate to severe febrile or acute disease.

3. Other measures

Isolation of the patient under bed-nets during the first few days; individual protection against mosquitoes.

The personal prophylactic measures are wearing of full sleeves shirts and full pants; use of mosquito repellent creams, liquids, coils, mats etc.; use of bed-nets for sleeping infants and young children during day time to prevent mosquito bite.

The environmental measurements are detection and elimination of mosquito breeding places, management of roof tops, porticos and sunshades, proper covering of stored water, observation of weekly dry day.

Global strategy for dengue prevention and control 2012–2020 *(14)*

Dengue is a global threat that requires a global response involving all possible partners. The global strategy promotes co-ordination and collaboration among multisectoral partners on integrated vector management approach and sustained control measures at all levels. The goals are :

a. to reduce dengue mortality by at least 50 per cent by 2020;
b. to reduce dengue morbidity by at least 25 per cent by 2020; and
c. to estimate the true burden of the disease by 2015.

References

1. WHO (1993), *Monograph on Dengue/Dengue Haemorrhagic Fever,* Compiled by Prasert Thongchroen, Regional Publication, SEARO No.22.
2. WHO (2022), *Fact Sheet on Dengue,* 10th January, 2022.
3. WHO (2011), *Comprehensive Guidelines for Prevention and Control of Dengue and Dengue Haemorrhagic Fever,* Revised and expanded edition, Regional office of SEAR.
4. Govt. of India (2018), *Annual Report 2017–2018,* DGHS, Ministry of Health and Family Welfare, New Delhi.
5. Govt. of India (2021), *National Health Profile 2021,* DGHS, Ministry of Health and Family Welfare, New Delhi.
6. Govt. of India (2008), *Guidelines for Clinical Management of Dengue Fever, Dengue Haemorrhagic Fever and Dengue Shock Syndrome,* Ministry of Health and Family Welfare, New Delhi.
7. WHO (2012), *Weekly Epidemiological Record,* No. 8, 24th Feb., 2012.
8. Jawetz, Melnick and Adelberg's *Medical Microbiology,* 24th International Ed. (2007), A Lange Medical Publication.
9. Govt. of India (2006), *National Vector Borne Disease Control Programme,* Ministry of Health and Family Welfare, New Delhi.
10. WHO (2009), *Dengue, Guidelines for Diagnosis, Treatment, Prevention and Control,* New edition.
11. Govt. of India (2014), *Operational Guidelines National Programme for Prevention and Control of Dengue,* Ministry of Health and Family Welfare, New Delhi.
12. WHO (2012), *Handbook for Clinical Management of Dengue.*
13. WHO (2016), *Weekly Epidemiological Record,* No. 30, 29th July, 2016.
14. WHO (2012), *Global Strategy for Dengue Prevention and Control,* 2012–2020.
15. Govt. of India (2020), *National Guidelines Dengue case management during COVID-19 Pandemic, 2020, NVBDCP,* Ministry of Health and Family Welfare, New Delhi.

MALARIA

Malaria is a protozoal disease caused by infection with parasites of the genus **Plasmodium** and transmitted to man by certain species of infected female Anopheline mosquito. A typical attack comprises three distinct stages : cold stage, hot stage and sweating stage. The clinical features of malaria vary from mild to severe, and complicated, according to the species of parasite present, the patient's state of immunity, the intensity of the infection and also the presence of concomitant conditions such as malnutrition or other diseases. The febrile paroxysms occur with definite intermittent periodicity repeating every third or fourth day depending upon the species of the parasite involved.

Problem statement

WORLD

It took almost 30 years from the end of the Global Malaria Eradication Programme (in 1969) for malaria to re-emerge as a public health priority in global health and development discourse. Although data from 1969 to 2000 are scarce, this period was characterized by a sense of failure and abandonment in the fight against malaria. During these 3 decades, hundreds of millions of people were infected with malaria, tens of millions – mostly in sub-Saharan Africa – died, millions of households failed to emerge out of poverty as they struggled with catastrophic health expenditures, hundreds of thousands of pregnant women died during delivery due to malaria-related complications, and millions of children were born with low birth-weight, potentially leading to early death or lifelong disability. Millions of children who survived, struggled with learning as they dealt with frequent absenteeism due to multiple episodes of malaria, chronic anaemia, seizures or cognitive impairment – consequences of infection and severe disease. Huge blows were dealt to the growth of already weak national economies, and their attempts to build viable health systems were hampered by lost productivity and high demand for health care.

Against this background, the first 2 decades of the 21st century represent a golden era in the history of malaria control. The world pulled together to fight malaria, delivering one of the biggest returns on investment in global health. The unprecedented scale-up of malaria interventions over this period has led to considerable reduction in disease incidence and mortality. These efforts coincided with other trends and changes that have had a positive impact on malaria, including a period of considerable economic growth and development, infrastructure and housing improvements, rapid urbanization, and general improvements in health systems and population health. The indirect effect of these gains on the overall health of populations and economies is substantial *(1)*.

Globally, there were an estimated 241 million cases of malaria in 2020 in 85 malaria endemic countries. Most of the increase (in 2019 there were 227 million cases) coming from countries in African region. At the Global Technical

Strategy for malaria 2016–2030 baseline of 2015, there were 224 million estimated malaria cases. The proportion of cases due to *P. vivax* reduced from about 8 per cent (18.5 million) in 2000 to 2 per cent (4.5 million) in 2020 *(2)*. Malaria case incidence rate reduced from 81 case/1000 population at risk in 2000 to 59/1000 population at risk. The case incidence in WHO African region was 222 per 1000 population at risk in 2019 but increased to 232 in 2020, mainly due to disruptions of services during the COVID-19 pandemic. WHO South-East Asia Region accounted for about 2 per cent of the burden of malaria cases globally, a reduction by 78 per cent, from 23 million in 2000 to about 5 million in 2020. Similarly incidence reduced by 83 per cent from 18 cases/1000 population at risk in 2000 to 3 cases per 1000 population at risk *(2)*. India accounted for 83 per cent of the cases in the region.

Globally, malaria deaths reduced steadily over the period 2000–2019, from 8,96,000 in 2000 to 5,58,000 in 2019. In 2020, malaria deaths increased by 12 per cent compared to 2019, to an estimated 6,27,000 due to disruptions of services because of COVID-19 pandemic *(2)*.

Approximately 95 per cent of malaria cases and deaths occur in sub-Saharan Africa, with the remainder occurring largely in South-East Asia and South America. Almost all malaria deaths are caused by *Plasmodium falciparum* and most occur in African children under 5 years of age. Adults who have lived in areas with high malaria transmission since childhood and remain resident in such areas are generally not at risk of death from malaria, as they usually have naturally acquired immunity as a result of repeated infections in childhood. *Plasmodium vivax* is an important cause of malaria morbidity outside sub-Saharan Africa. Vaccine development efforts have focused on preventing illness from *P. falciparum* and, to a lesser extent, *P. vivax*.

Current WHO guidance defines moderate to high malaria transmission settings as those with an annual incidence greater than around 250 cases per 1000 population or a prevalence of *P. falciparum* infection in children aged 2–10 years of approximately 10 per cent or more *(3)*.

In 2019, in 33 moderate to high transmission countries in African Region, there were an estimated 33 million pregnancies, of which 35 per cent (12 million) were exposed to malaria infection during pregnancy. It is estimated that malaria infection during pregnancy in these 33 countries resulted in 8,22,000 children with low birth-weight *(1)*.

The specific risk groups for malaria includes the following population *(4)* :

1. young children in stable transmission areas who have not yet developed protective immunity against the most severe forms of the disease;
2. non-immune pregnant women as malaria causes high rates of miscarriage and can lead to maternal death;
3. semi-immune pregnant women in areas of high transmission. Malaria can result in miscarriage and low birth weight, especially during first and second pregnancies;
4. semi-immune HIV-infected pregnant women in stable transmission areas, during all pregnancies. Women with malaria infection of the placenta also have a higher risk of passing HIV infection to their newborns;
5. people with HIV/AIDS;
6. international travellers from non-endemic areas because they lack immunity.
7. immigrants and their children living in non-endemic areas and returning to their home countries to visit friends and relatives are similarly at risk because of waning or absent immunity.

Acquired immunity

Natural immunity to malaria is acquired gradually with repeated exposure to *Plasmodium* infection. Immunity is acquired more rapidly against the more severe forms of the disease. Hence, with increasing age, there is progressive protection first against severe malaria and ensuing mortality, then against uncomplicated malaria and, much more slowly, asymptomatic parasitaemia. In areas of moderate to high transmission, malaria mortality rates begin to fall by around 2 years of age, with the incidence of acute febrile malaria falling later in childhood *(3)*.

Naturally acquired immunity is believed to wane substantially in people who migrate out of a malaria-endemic region and are no longer regularly exposed to malaria infection for a number of years. The use of available preventive interventions can delay the development of naturally acquired immunity. Significant roles for both humoral and cell-mediated effectors have been demonstrated in animal models, and both humoral and cell-mediated immune responses are induced in humans after natural malaria infection *(3)*.

Malaria affects mainly poor, underserved and marginalized populations in remote rural areas which are characterized by inadequate control measures and limited access to health care. Higher malaria prevalence has been reported among ethnic and tribal groups living in remote forested and border areas, as well as among mobile and migrant populations.

The childhood deaths result mainly from cerebral malaria and anaemia. Fatality rates of 10–30 per cent have been reported among children referred to hospital with severe malaria. However, these rates are even higher in rural and remote areas where patients have restricted access to adequate treatment. Malaria also contributes indirectly to illness and deaths from respiratory infections, diarrhoeal disease and malnutrition. Deaths from malaria in countries outside Sub-Saharan Africa occur principally in non-immune people who become infected with *P. falciparum*.

Underreporting of malaria cases and deaths remain a major challenge. Drug-resistant parasites, poor treatment-seeking behaviour and the presence of counterfeit antimalarial drugs further hinder control efforts. Resistance of *P. falciparum* to the 4–aminoquinolines and sulfadoxine–pyrimethamine is widespread in almost all countries of SEAR, with varying levels of severity. Resistance to mafloquine was reported from Myanmar and Thailand. Quinine has reduced susceptibility in Thailand. With progress from mono-to-multidrug resistance, all malaria-endemic countries that have *falciparum* malaria adopted the highly effective artemisinin – based combination therapy (ACT).

The coverage of indoor residual spraying with insecticides (IRS) remains low (42 per cent). Insecticide-treated nets have been introduced in almost all countries to supplement IRS efforts, but the coverage remains extremely low.

INDIA

Malaria is a public health problem in several parts of the country. About 95 per cent population in the country resides in malaria endemic areas and 80 per cent of malaria cases reported in the country are confined to areas consisting

20 per cent of population residing in tribal, hilly, difficult to reach areas.

Countrywide malaria situation is as reflected in surveillance data (as shown in Table 1). The cases have consistently declined from 2.09 million in 2001 to 0.161 million in 2021, similarly *Pf* cases have declined from 1.0 million to 0.10 million. Less than 2000 deaths were reported during all the years within this period with a peak in 2006 when an epidemic was reported in North East States. The country SPR has declined from 2.31 to 0.14 and SFR has declined from 1.11 in 2001 to 0.09 in 2021 *(5)*. This indicates declining overall endemicity of malaria in the country.

India is predominantly characterized by unstable malaria transmission. Transmission is seasonal with increased intensity related to rains. Due to the low and unstable transmission dynamics, most of the population has no or little immunity toward malaria. As a result, the majority of Indians living in malarious areas are at risk of infection with all age groups affected. However, surveys have shown that in some foci, mainly in forested areas, transmission is intense and the disease burden is to a large extent concentrated in children.

There are six primary vectors of malaria in India : (1) *An. culicifacies* is the main vector of rural and peri-urban areas and is widespread in peninsular India. It is found in a variety of natural and man-made breeding sites. It is highly zoophilic. Species A is an established vector for *P. Vivax* and *P. falciparum*, whereas species B is completely refractory to *P. Vivax* and partially refractory to *P. falciparum*. It has been demonstrated that species B, however, may play a role as a vector of *P. falciparum* in areas where the cattle population is very low or absent; (2) *An. stephensi* is responsible for malaria in urban and industrial areas. The type form is found in urban areas; intermediate form in urban and semi-urban localities and *mysorensis* form is present in rural areas (it is not a vector); (3) *An. fluviatilis* is the main vector in hilly areas, forests and forest fringes in many states, especially in the east; (4) *An. minimus* is the vector in the foot hills of North-Eastern states; (5) *An. dirus* is an important forest vector in the North-East; and (6) *An. epiroticus* is now restricted to the Andaman and Nicobar Islands *(6)*.

Prevalent major epidemiological types of malaria in India *(7)*

In the course of the stratification exercise, various problems and constraints responsible for the slow progress of malaria control have been identified. An analysis of these factors has resulted in the identification of malaria priority areas.

TRIBAL MALARIA : The population of tribal areas are contributing about 50 per cent of *P. falciparum* cases of the country *(6)*. Infants, young children and pregnant women have been identified as malaria high risk groups followed by mobile tribal population engaged in forest–related activities. Limited health infrastructure and lack of drugs at village level are the factors responsible for high morbidity and mortality due to malaria.

RURAL MALARIA : These include irrigated areas of arid and semiarid plains. Malaria is of moderate to low endemicity. *An. culicifacies* is the main vector and *P. vivax* is predominant during lean period and *P. falciparum* during periodic exacerbation. In these the health infrastructure is moderately developed.

URBAN MALARIA : 15 major cities including four metropolitans account for nearly 80 per cent of malaria cases covered under urban malaria control scheme. The health infrastructure is well developed. In peri-urban areas malaria situation is influenced by poor sanitary conditions and low socio-economic groups living in unplanned settlements prone to periodical epidemics.

MALARIA IN PROJECT AREAS : Project areas are those areas where construction and developmental activities are taken up and temporary tropical aggregation of labourers takes place bringing in different strains of malaria parasite and non-immune population. This results in disturbance in eco-system, prolific increase in vector breeding places and increased man–mosquito contact favouring high malaria transmission. These pockets contribute a large number of malaria cases which are highly disproportionate to the relatively small population groups inhabitating the area. One or more major vectors are involved in malaria transmission. Limited health facilities for prompt treatment is invariably associated with chloroquine resistant malaria parasite. Hence specific control strategy is required for such areas.

BORDER MALARIA : These are the high malaria transmission belts along the international borders and state borders. These areas have their own problems in regard to malaria control because of mixing of population and poor administrative control.

FOREST MALARIA : Forests and settlements in recently deforested areas are known to harbour very efficient malaria

TABLE 1

Countrywide malaria surveillance data 2015–2021

Year	BSE (in millions)	Total malaria cases (in millions)	*P. falciparum* cases (in millions)	Pf %	API	ABER	SPR	SFR	Deaths due to malaria
2001	90.389	2.085	1.005	–	2.12	9.18	2.31	1.11	1005
2015	121.14	1.17	0.78	66.61	0.92	9.58	0.97	0.64	384
2016	124.93	1.09	0.71	65.53	0.85	9.74	0.87	0.57	331
2017	125.97	0.84	0.53	62.70	0.64	9.58	0.67	0.42	194
2018	124.44	0.34	0.16	47.93	0.32	9.31	0.35	0.17	96
2019	134.23	0.34	0.16	46.36	0.25	9.95	0.25	0.12	77
2020	97.17	0.19	0.12	63.84	0.014	7.08	0.19	0.12	93
2021	114.293	0.16	0.10	63.10	0.12	8.25	0.14	0.09	90

Pf – Plasmodium falciparum   BSE – Blood smear examined
API – Annual parasite incidence   ABER – Annual blood examination rate
SPR – Slide positivity rate   SFR – Slide falciparum rate

Source : *(5)*

vectors. These vectors bite humans in their shelters, but return to rest in the forest, avoiding residual insecticides sprayed indoors in the shelters. Malaria transmission is therefore, more intense and more difficult to control in temporary or newly established forest settlements *(8)*.

FLOODS AND MALARIA : Floods may lead to a rise in incidence of malaria. Flooding may initially flush out mosquito breeding, but later result in pools of water creating mosquitogenic conditions. The lag time between the floods and possible malaria epidemic is estimated to be around 6–8 weeks *(8)*.

Some definitions *(8)*

Malaria control : reducing the malaria disease burden to a level at which it is no longer a public health problem.

Malaria elimination : the interruption of local mosquito-borne malaria transmission; reduction to 'zero' of the incidence of infection caused by human malaria parasites in a defined geographical area as a result of deliberate efforts; continued measures to prevent re-establishment of transmission are required.

Certification of malaria elimination : can be granted by WHO after it has been proven beyond reasonable doubt that the chain of local human malaria transmission by *Anopheles* mosquitoes has been fully interrupted in an entire country for at least 3 consecutive years.

Malaria eradication : permanent reduction to 'zero' of the worldwide incidence of infection caused by a specific agent; applies to a particular malaria parasite species. Intervention measures are no longer needed once eradication has been achieved.

Epidemiological determinants

Agent factors

(a) AGENT

Malaria in man is caused by four distinct species of the malaria parasite – *P. vivax, P. falciparum, P. malariae* and *P. ovale. Plasmodium vivax* has the widest geographic distribution throughout the world. In India, about 50 per cent of the infections are reported to be due to *P. falciparum* and 4–8 per cent due to mixed infection and rest due to *P. vivax. P. malariae* has a restricted distribution and is said to be responsible for less than 1 per cent of the infections in India. The largest focus of *P. malariae* in India is reported to be in Tumkur and Hassan districts in Karnataka. *P. ovale* is a very rare parasite of man, mostly confined to tropical Africa. It has also been reported in Vietnam. The severity of malaria is related to the species of the parasite.

Life history

The malaria parasite undergoes 2 cycles of development – the human cycle (asexual cycle) and the mosquito cycle (sexual cycle). Man is the intermediate host and mosquito the definitive host (Fig. 1).

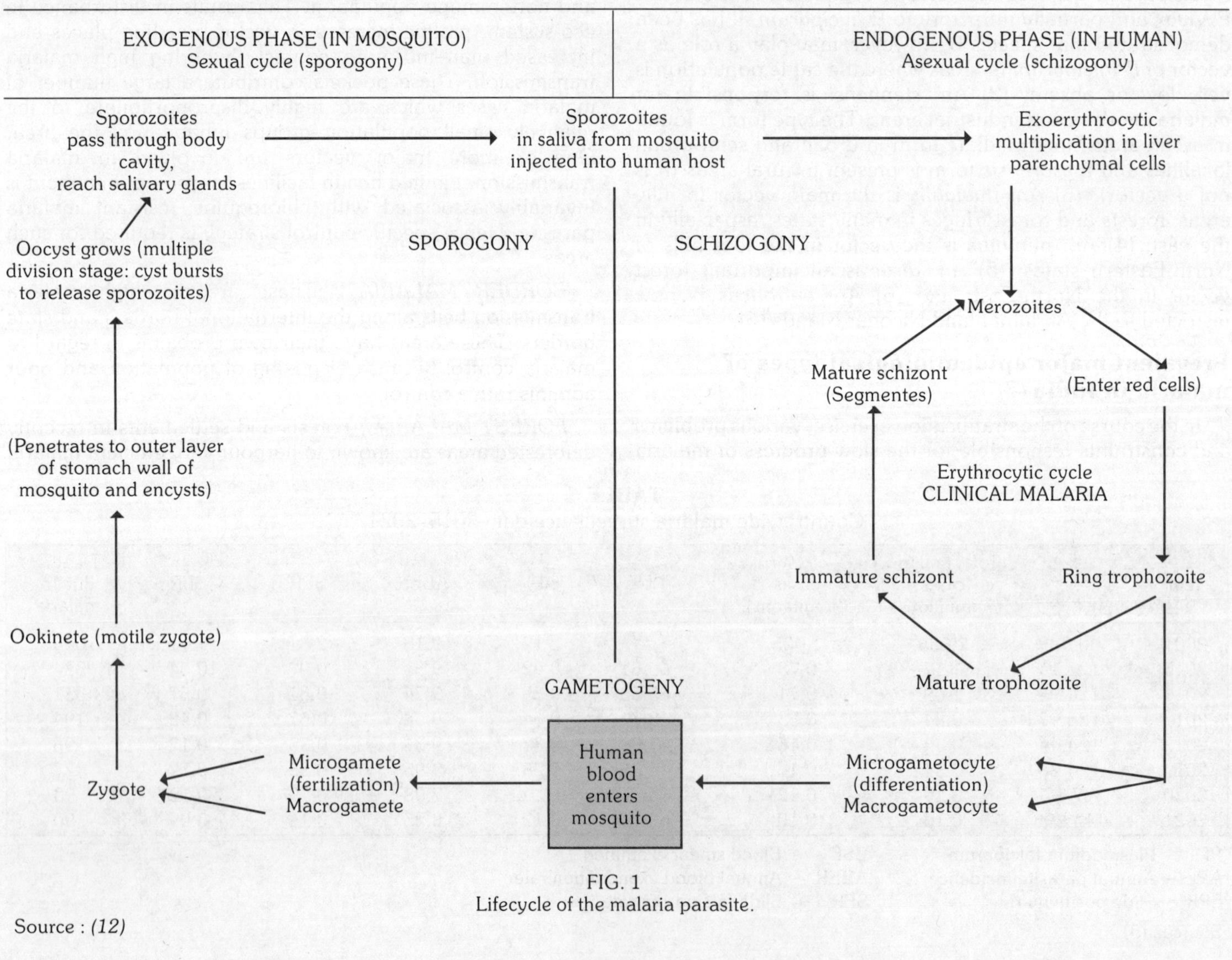

FIG. 1
Lifecycle of the malaria parasite.

Source : *(12)*

(i) *Asexual cycle:* The asexual cycle begins when an infected mosquito bites a person and injects sporozoites. A considerable amount of new knowledge about the parasite's life cycle has become available in recent years, concerning almost all phases of the cycle *(9)*. A brief description is as follows – four phases are described in the human cycle: (a) HEPATIC PHASE: The sporozoites disappear within 60 minutes from the peripheral circulation *(10)*. Many of them are destroyed by phagocytes, but some reach the liver cells. After 1–2 weeks of development (depending upon the species), they become hepatic schizonts, which eventually burst releasing a shower of merozoites. The number of merozoites produced from a single sporozoite varies considerably with the infecting species. A single *P. falciparum* sporozoite may form as many as 40,000 merozoites, whereas sporozoites from other species of plasmodia produce only 2,000 to 15,000 merozoites *(10)*. In the case of *P. falciparum,* the intrahepatic schizonts rupture almost simultaneously and there is no persistent tissue phase (the so-called exo-erythrocytic phase). On the contrary, the intrahepatic schizonts of the other plasmodia do not burst all at the same time. Some hepatic forms persist and remain dormant in the hepatocytes for considerable periods before they begin to grow and undergo pre-erythrocytic schizogony, thus liberating merozoites into the blood stream causing relapses of these infections. *P. vivax* and *P. ovale* may continue to relapse for 2 to 3 years and *P. malariae* may persist for 10 to 20 years or more. Once the parasites enter the RBC, they do not reinvade the liver. (b) ERYTHROCYTIC PHASE: Many of the merozoites are quickly destroyed, but a significant number attach to specific receptor sites on the RBC. The merozoites then penetrate the RBC and pass through the stages of trophozoite and schizont. The erythrocytic phase ends with the liberation of merozoites, which infect fresh red blood cells. The cycle is repeated over and over again until it is slowed down by the immune response of the host *(11)*. The duration of the erythrocytic cycle is constant for each species of malaria parasite – 48 hours for *P. falciparum, P. vivax* and *P. ovale*; and 72 hours for *P. malariae.* (c) GAMETOGENY: In all species of malaria some erythrocytic forms do not divide but become male and female gametocytes. These are the sexual forms of the parasite which are infective to mosquito.

(ii) *Sexual cycle:* The mosquito cycle (sporogony) begins when gametocytes are ingested by the vector mosquito when feeding on an infected person. The gametocytes continue further development in the mosquito. The first event to take place in the stomach of the mosquito is exflagellation of the male gametocyte; 4–8 thread–like filaments called "micro-gametes" are developed. The female gametocyte undergoes a process of maturation and becomes a female gamete or "macrogamete". By a process of chemotaxis, microgametes are attracted towards the female gamete, and one of which (microgamete) causes fertilization of the female gamete. The resulting zygote is at first a motionless body, but within 18–24 hours, it becomes motile. This is known as *Ookinete,* which penetrates the stomach wall of the mosquito and develops into an oocyst on the outer surface of the stomach. The oocyst grows rapidly and develops within it numerous sporozoites. When mature, the oocyst bursts and liberates sporozoites into the body cavity of mosquito. Many of the sporozoites migrate to the salivary glands of the mosquito, and the mosquito now becomes infective to man. The period of time required for the development of the parasite from the gametocyte to sporozoite stage in the body of the mosquito is about 10–20 days depending upon favourable conditions of atmospheric temperature and humidity. This period is also referred to as the "extrinsic incubation period".

(b) RESERVOIR OF INFECTION

With the possible exception of chimpanzees in tropical Africa, which may carry the infection with *P. malariae,* no other animal reservoir of human plasmodia is known to exist *(11)*. A human reservoir is one who harbours the sexual forms (gametocytes) of the parasite. A patient can be a carrier of several plasmodial species at the same time. Children are more likely to be gametocyte carriers than adults. The child is thus epidemiologically a better reservoir than the adult. Certain conditions must be met before a person can serve as a reservoir: (i) the person must harbour both the sexes of the gametocyte in his blood. If the person harbours only male or female gametocytes, further development cannot take place in the mosquito vector, (ii) the gametocytes must be mature; immature forms do not undergo further development. It may take 2–4 days for the gametocytes to attain maturity after their appearance in the blood, (iii) the gametocytes must be viable, i.e., if the patient receives an antimalarial drug, the gametocytes lose their viability or infectivity to mosquitoes (iv) the gametocytes must be present in sufficient density to infect mosquitoes. The number of gametocytes necessary to infect mosquitoes is not definitely known, but it is thought by some that there must be at least 12 per cubic mm of blood.

(c) PERIOD OF COMMUNICABILITY

Malaria is communicable as long as mature, viable gametocytes exist in the circulating blood in sufficient density to infect vector mosquitoes. In vivax infections, gametocytes appear in blood 4–5 days after the appearance of the asexual parasites; in falciparum infections, they do not appear until 10–12 days after the first appearance of asexual parasites. Gametocytes are the most numerous during the early stages of the infection when their density may exceed 1,000 per cubic mm of blood. They also tend to occur in waves in peripheral blood.

RELAPSES: It is usual for vivax and ovale malaria to relapse more than 3 years after the patient's first attack. Recurrences of falciparum malaria usually disappear within 1–2 years. *P. malariae* has a tendency to cause prolonged low–level, asymptomatic parasitaemia *(13)*. The infection is known to persist for 40 years or more. It is probable that persons harbouring such infections are at least occasionally infective to mosquitoes.

It is now considered more likely that vivax and ovale relapses are derived from original, sporozoite–induced, liver schizonts which have lain latent long before bursting. In *P. falciparum* and *P. malariae* infections latent liver schizonts do not appear to occur. Relapses in these species, most authorities maintain, are due to a chronic blood infection, i.e., erythrocytic schizogony persisting at a low level.

Host factors

The main variables of the human element that have an influence on malaria epidemiology include the following :

(a) AGE : Malaria affects all ages. Newborn infants have considerable resistance to infection with *P. falciparum.* This has been attributed to the high concentration of foetal haemoglobin during the first few months of life, which suppresses the development of *P. falciparum (14)*. (b) SEX : Males are more frequently exposed to the risk of acquiring malaria than females because of the outdoor life they lead. Further, females in India are usually better clothed than males. (c) RACE : Individuals with AS haemoglobin (sickle-cell trait) have a milder illness with falciparum infection than do those with normal (AA) haemoglobin *(10)*. Persons whose red blood cells are "Duffy negative" (a genetic trait) are resistant to *P. vivax* infection. (d) PREGNANCY : Pregnancy increases the risk of malaria in women. Malaria during pregnancy may cause intrauterine death of the foetus; it may also cause premature labour or abortion. Primigravid women are at greatest risk *(15)*. (e) SOCIO-ECONOMIC DEVELOPMENT : Malaria has demonstrated the relationship between health and socio-economic development. It is generally accepted that malaria has disappeared from most developed countries as a result of socio-economic development *(15)*. (f) HOUSING: Housing plays an important role in the epidemiology of malaria. The ill-ventilated and ill-lighted houses provide ideal indoor resting places for mosquitoes. Malaria is acquired in most instances by mosquito-bites within the houses. The site, type of construction, nature of the walls, etc. influence the selection of control measures *(16)*. (g) POPULATION MOBILITY : People migrate for one reason or other from one country to another or from one part of a country to another. Labourers connected with various engineering, irrigation, agricultural and other projects and periodic migration of nomads and wandering tribes are outstanding examples of internal migration. Some of them may import malaria parasites in their blood and reintroduce malaria into areas where malaria has been controlled or eliminated. Imported malaria has become quite a public health problem in Europe, North America, and other temperate parts of the world, owing to the rising tide of air travel, tourism and migration *(12)*. (h) OCCUPATION : Malaria is predominantly a rural disease and is closely related to agriculture practices. (i) HUMAN HABITS : Habits such as sleeping out of doors, nomadism, refusal to accept spraying of houses, replastering of walls after spraying and not using measures of personal protection (e.g. bed nets) influence man-vector contact, and obviously the choice of control measures. (j) IMMUNITY: The epidemic of malaria is influenced by the immune status of the population. Immunity to malaria in humans is acquired only after repeated exposure over several years. Thus in endemic malarious areas a state of collective immunity becomes established slowly, so that infants, young children, migrants and travellers from non-endemic areas suffer most from the disease. Those, however, who survive to the adult age show less evidence of adverse effects to the attenuated infection. Infants born of immune mothers are generally protected during the first 3–5 months by maternal IgG antibody; infants born of semi-immune mothers are only partially protected. Active immunity is species-specific, that is, immunity against one strain does not protect against another. People living in endemic areas exposed continually to malaria develop considerable degree of resistance to clinical disease, but their partial immunity to malaria declines with time after they leave their endemic countries. Semi-immune individuals may harbour malaria parasites without presenting any symptoms of disease. Both humoral and cellular factors play a role in this protection *(4)*.

Environmental factors

India's geographic position and climatic conditions had been, for long, favourable to the transmission of malaria. (a) SEASON : Malaria is a seasonal disease. In most parts of India, the maximum prevalence is from July to November. (b) TEMPERATURE: Temperature affects the life cycle of the malaria parasite. The optimum temperature for the development of the malaria parasite in the insect vector is between 20 deg. to 30 deg.C (68 deg. to 86 deg.F). The parasite ceases to undergo development in the mosquito if the mean temperature is below 16 deg.C (60.8 deg.F). Temperatures higher than 30 deg.C are lethal to the parasite. (c) HUMIDITY: The atmospheric humidity has a direct effect on the length of life of the mosquito, although it has no effect on the parasite. A relative humidity of 60 per cent is considered necessary for mosquitoes to live their normal span of life. When the relative humidity is high, mosquitoes are more active and they feed more voraciously. If the humidity is low, mosquitoes do not live long. (d) RAINFALL : Rain in general provides opportunities for the breeding of mosquitoes and may give rise to epidemics of malaria. Rain increases the atmospheric humidity which is necessary for the survival of mosquitoes. However, heavy rain may have an adverse affect in flushing out the breeding places. Paradoxically in some areas, (e.g., Sri Lanka) severe epidemics of malaria followed years of drought. It was because, the lesser monsoon rains led to the formation of small pools of water in river beds, which served as active breeding places for malaria vectors. The relationship between rainfall (total and its distribution) and mosquito breeding is of fundamental importance *(17)*. (e) ALTITUDE: As a rule, *Anophelines* are not found at altitudes above 2000–2500 metres, due to unfavourable climatic conditions. (f) MAN-MADE MALARIA: Burrow pits, garden pools, irrigation channels and engineering projects like construction of hydroelectric dams, roads, bridges have led to the breeding of mosquitoes and an increase in malaria. Malaria consequent on such human undertakings is called "man-made malaria".

Vector of malaria

Out of about 45 species of anopheline mosquitoes in India, only a few are regarded as the vectors of primary importance. These are: *An. culicifacies*, *An. fluviatilis*, *An. stephensi*, *An. minimus*, *An. philippinensis*, *An. sundaicus*, and *An. maculatus*. The vectors of major importance are *An. culicifacies* in rural areas and *An. stephensi* in urban areas.

In the absence of a vaccine, vector control is the only practical approach to malaria control. A knowledge of anopheline biology is essential for understanding the epidemiology of malaria and its prevention. The main factors which determine the vectorial importance of mosquitoes are: (a) DENSITY : To be an effective vector, a species must be present in adequate density in or near human habitations. A sudden increase in density of vectors, may be a cause of epidemic outbreaks. For each vector, there is what is known as "critical density" below which effective transmission cannot be maintained in a community. This level varies with different species. In the case of *An. culicifacies* a high density is required for the propagation of malaria; in the case of *An. fluviatilis* which is very efficient vector, a much lower density would suffice. (b) LIFE SPAN: The key factor in the transmission of malaria is the life span of the vector. The vector mosquito must live for at least 10–12 days after an infective blood meal to become infective. The strategy in malaria eradication is to shorten the life span of mosquitoes to less than 10 days by insecticides. (c) CHOICE OF HOST : Some mosquitoes prefer human blood, some animal blood, and some show great variation in their feeding habits. The percentage of human blood feeds in the case of *An. culicifacies*, an important vector in India, has been found to vary from 2–80 per cent *(10)*. In contrast, *An. fluviatilis* is a highly anthrophilic species. The anthrophilic species, i.e., those that have a high preference for human blood are better vectors of malaria than zoophilic species. (d) RESTING HABITS : After a blood meal, some mosquitoes rest indoors on the walls for quite sometime. This behaviour pattern is known as "endophily". But there are some species which rest outdoors (exophily). A knowledge of the resting habits (which must be under constant surveillance) is the basis for organizing rational anti–adult measures. In fact, the concept of malaria eradication is based on endophilism (indoor resting habits) of most malarial vectors. (e) BREEDING HABITS: The breeding habits of mosquitoes vary considerably. Some breed in moving water *(An. fluviatilis)*, some in brackish water *(An. sundaicus)* and some in wells, cisterns, fountains and overhead tanks *(An. stephensi)*. A knowledge of the breeding habits is required for conducting anti–larval operations. (f) TIME OF BITING : The majority of Indian mosquitoes bite at night excepting the Aedes mosquitoes. Anophiline mosquitoes have nocturnal feeding habits, between dusk and dawn. (g) VECTORIAL CAPACITY : The term vectorial capacity refers to the combined effect of the density of the vector population, its susceptibility to infection, life span and probability of feeding on man. It is distinct from physiological capacity to transmit infection. (h) RESISTANCE TO INSECTICIDES : A knowledge of the status of vector resistance to insecticides is also necessary. On this depends the choice of insecticides to be used. When an insect vector is resistant to a given insecticide, alternative insecticides have to be used.

Mode of transmission

(a) VECTOR TRANSMISSION: Malaria is transmitted by the bite of certain species of infected, female, anopheline mosquitoes. A single infected vector, during her life time, may infect several persons. The mosquito is not infective unless the sporozoites are present in its salivary glands. (b) DIRECT TRANSMISSION: Malaria may be induced accidentally by hypodermic intramuscular and intravenous injections of blood or plasma, e.g., blood transfusion, malaria in drug addicts *(18, 19)*. Blood transfusion poses a problem because the parasites keep their infective activity for at least 14 days in blood bottles stored at –4 deg. C *(18)*. Persons who have lived in an endemic area (including those who have been taking antimalarials prophylactically) and anyone who has had malaria should not be accepted as blood donor until 3 years afterwards *(20)*. (c) CONGENITAL MALARIA: Congenital infection of the newborn from an infected mother may also occur, but it is comparatively rare.

Incubation period

This is the length of time between the infective mosquito bite and the first appearance of clinical signs of which fever is most common. This period is usually not less than 10 days.

The duration of the incubation period varies with the species of the parasite, and in natural infections (in mosquito–transmitted malaria) this is 12 (9–14) days for falciparum malaria, 14 (8–17) days for vivax malaria, 28 (18–40) days for quartan malaria and 17 (16–18) days for ovale malaria. With some strains of *P. vivax*, the incubation period may be delayed for as long as 9 months; this may also occur with other species in persons who have been taking suppressive antimalarial drugs *(10)*.

Clinical features

The primary fever is marked by paroxysms which correspond to the development of the parasites in the red blood cells. The peaks of the fever coincide with the release into the blood stream of successive broods of merozites.

The typical attack comprises three distinct stages, i.e., the cold stage, the hot stage and the sweating stage. These are followed by an afebrile period in which the patient feels greately relieved.

COLD STAGE : The onset is with lassitude, headache, nausea and chilly sensation followed in an hour or so by rigors. The temperature rises rapidly to 39–41°C. Headache is often severe and commonly there is vomiting. In early part of this stage, skin feels cold; later it becomes hot. Parasites are usually demonstrable in the blood. The pulse is rapid and may be weak. This stage lasts for 1/4–1 hour.

HOT STAGE : The patient feels burning hot and casts off his clothes. The skin is hot and dry to touch. Headache is intense but nausea commonly diminishes. The pulse is full and respiration rapid. This stage lasts for 2 to 6 hours.

SWEATING STAGE : Fever comes down with profuse sweating. The temperature drops rapidly to normal and skin is cool and moist. The pulse rate becomes slower, patient feels relieved and often falls asleep. This stage lasts for 2–4 hours.

The febrile paroxysms occur with definite intermittent periodicity repeating every third or fourth day depending upon the species of the parasite involved. The classical 3 stages (cold, hot and sweating) may not always be observed due to maturation of generations of parasite at different times. Periods of latency may last several weeks or months *(10, 21)*. The disease has a tendency to relapse and is characterized by enlargement of the spleen and secondary anaemia. Febrile herpes is common in all malarial patients.

In patients with *P. falciparum* infection the primary fever in its first few days is usually irregular or even continuous and then the classical 48 hours periodicity becomes established or the fever may continue to be irregular and the hot and cold stages, so typical of other malarial infections are less clearly separated from one another. In persons with poor immunity the paroxysms are associated with marked prostration. Headache, nausea and vomiting are usually more severe, and there is greater tendency towards the development of delirium, haemolytic jaundice and anaemia. The mortality is much greater than in other forms of malaria.

With *P. vivax* infection, symptoms are same but are usually milder and more regularly divided into "hot" and "cold" stages than in *P. falciparum* infections.

P. ovale infections differ little from that of *P. vivax*. However, they tend to be milder than *P. vivax* and cease after a few paroxysms even if no treatment is given.

Clinically, *P. malariae* attacks resemble those of *P. vivax* but the cycle is of 72 hours instead of 48 hours. The tendency for long-term relapses to occur is marked.

The complications of *P. falciparum* malaria are cerebral malaria, acute renal failure, liver damage, gastro-intestinal symptoms, dehydration, collapse, anaemia, blackwater fever etc. The complications of *P. vivax, P. ovale* and *P. malariae* infections are anaemia, splenomegaly, enlargement of liver, herpes, renal complications etc.

Diagnosis

The diagnosis of malaria depends on demonstration of

the parasite in the blood. Suspicion of the diagnosis is aroused by epidemiological and clinical evidence.

1. Microscopy

Two types of blood films are useful in searching for and identification of malaria parasite. The "thin film" and the "thick film". It is recommended that both types of film be prepared on a single microscope glass slide. The thick film is more reliable in searching for parasite, as large volume of blood is examined under each microscope field. When scanty, parasite may be found about 20 times more rapidly in thick slide than in thin slide. The thin slide is more valuable for identifying the species of the parasite present. In it they are seen more clearly.

The advantage of microscopy are : The sensitivity is high. It is possible to detect malarial parasite at low densities. It also helps to quantify the parasite load; It is possible to distinguish the various species of malaria parasite and their different stages.

2. Serological test

The malarial fluorescent antibody test usually becomes positive two weeks or more after primary infection, by which time the infection may have been cured. A positive test is therefore, not necessarily an indication of current infection. The test is of the greatest value in epidemiological studies and in determining whether a person has had malaria in the past *(22)*.

3. Rapid diagnostic test (RDT)

Rapid Diagnostic Tests are based on the detection of circulating parasite antigens with a simple dipstick format. Several types of RDTs are available. Some of them can only detect *P. falciparum* while others can detect other parasites also. The latter kits are expensive and temperature sensitive. RDTs are produced by different companies, so there may be differences in the contents and in the manner in which the test is done. The users manual should always be read properly to avoid false negative results *(23)*.

Measurement of malaria

PRE-ERADICATION ERA

In the pre-eradication era, the magnitude of the malaria problem in a country used to be determined mostly from the reports of the *clinically diagnosed malaria cases.* The classical malariometric measures are spleen rate, average enlarged spleen, parasite rate etc. In a control programme, the case detection machinery is weak. Therefore, the classical malariometric measures may provide the needed information, i.e. the *trend of the disease.*

(a) SPLEEN RATE : It is defined as the percentage of children between 2 and 10 years of age showing enlargement of spleen. Adults are excluded from spleen surveys, because causes other than malaria frequently operate in causing splenic enlargement in them. The spleen rate is widely used for measuring the endemicity of malaria in a community. (b) AVERAGE ENLARGED SPLEEN : This is a further refinement of spleen rate, denoting the average size of the enlarged spleen *(24)*. It is a useful malariometric index. (c) PARASITE RATE : It is defined as the percentage of children between the ages 2 and 10 years showing malaria parasites in their blood films. (d) PARASITE DENSITY INDEX : It indicates the average degree of parasitaemia in a sample of well–defined group of the population. Only the positive slides are included in the denominator *(10)*. (e) INFANT PARASITE RATE : It is defined as the percentage of infants below the age of one year showing malaria parasites in their blood films. It is regarded as the most sensitive index of recent transmission of malaria in a locality. If the infant parasite rate is zero for 3 consecutive years in a locality, it is regarded as absence of malaria transmission even though, the Anopheline vectors responsible for previous transmission may remain. (f) PROPORTIONAL CASE RATE : Since the morbidity rate is difficult to determine, except in conditions when the diagnosis and reporting of each case is carried to perfection, proportional case rate is used *(10)*. It is defined as the number of cases diagnosed as clinical malaria for every 100 patients attending the hospitals and dispensaries. This is a crude index because the cases are not related to their time/space distribution.

ERADICATION ERA (current incidence levels)

During the eradication era, the *microscopic diagnosis* of malaria cases became the main method of diagnosis. The parameters used for the measurement of malaria were mostly parasitological in nature; the commonly used parameters were API, ABER, SPR and SFR. The same parameters are being used at the present time. These parameters are unlikely to reveal the true epidemiological picture, unless the case detection machinery is fully supervised and very efficient. The following parameters are in use at present :

a. Annual parasite incidence (API)
b. Annual blood examination rate (ABER)
c. Annual falciparum incidence (AFI)
d. Slide positivity rate (SPR)
e. Slide falciparum rate (SFR).

a. Annual parasite incidence (API)

API is given by the formula :

$$\text{API} = \frac{\text{Confirmed cases during one year}}{\text{Population under surveillance}} \times 1000$$

API is a sophisticated measure of malaria incidence in a community. It is based on intensive active and passive surveillance, and cases are confirmed by blood examination. Areas with API ≥ 2 per 1000 population per year have been classified as high risk areas in India, and thereby eligible for vector control.

b. Annual blood examination rate (ABER)

ABER is given by the formula :

$$\text{ABER} = \frac{\text{Number of slides examined}}{\text{Population}} \times 100$$

ABER is an index of operational efficiency. The annual parasite incidence (API) depends upon the annual blood collection and examination rates. A sufficient number of blood slides must be systematically obtained and examined for malaria parasite to work out accurately annual parasite incidence (API).

At present, about 100 million fever cases are screened every year in India. The aim is to screen 10 per cent of the population even though the disease transmission is expected to reduce. The surveillance system has not undergone any change *(6)*.

c. Annual falciparum incidence

Since the emergence of *P. falciparum* problem in India, data are collected separately for total malaria cases and *P. falciparum* cases.

d. Others

The slide positivity rate and slide falciparum rate are useful parameters. They provide information on the trend of malaria transmission.

Slide positivity rate : slide positivity rate is the percentage of slides found positive for malarial parasite, irrespective of the type of species.

Slide falciparum rate : It is the percentage of slides positive for *P. falciparum* parasite.

VECTOR INDICES

A malaria survey is not complete unless it includes investigations relating to the insect vector. Some of the important vector indices are: (a) HUMAN BLOOD INDEX : It is the proportion of freshly-fed female Anopheline mosquitoes whose stomach contains human blood. It indicates the degree of anthrophilism. (b) SPOROZOITE RATE : It is the percentage of female anophelines with sporozoites in their salivary glands. (c) MOSQUITO DENSITY : It is usually expressed as the number of mosquitoes per man-hour-catch. (d) MAN-BITING RATE (Biting density) : It is defined as the average incidence of anopheline bites per day per person. It is determined by standardized vector catches on human bait (e) INOCULATION RATE : The man-biting rate multiplied by the infective sporozoite rate is called the inoculation rate. All these rates are employed in the quantitative assessment of malaria and in building up a composite epidemiological picture of malaria.

APPROACHES AND STRATEGIES OF MALARIA CONTROL

As the concept of control replaces that of eradication in many national programmes, a reordering of priorities in the selection of control methods must occur. These priorities and approaches must be based on epidemiological considerations, adverse effects on health, economy, technical feasibility, functional resources, human resources and community participation. Recently WHO stressed a number of points relevant to future strategy of malaria control. The main emphasis is on the need to base it on an epidemiological approach. These aspects are discussed below.

APPROACHES TO MALARIA CONTROL

Strategic Action Plan for malaria control in India, 2007–2012, 2012–2017 and more recently 2017–2022 were developed by Directorate of National Vector Borne Disease Control Programme.

The strategies for prevention and control of malaria and its transmission are *(7)* :

(a) Surveillance and case management
  (1) Case detection (passive and active)
  (2) Early diagnosis and complete treatment
  (3) Sentinel surveillance.
(b) Integrated vector management
  (1) Indoor residual spray (IRS)
  (2) Insecticide treated bed-nets (ITNs) and long lasting insecticidal nets((LLINs)
  (3) Antilarval measures including source reduction.
(c) Epidemic preparedness and early response
(d) Supportive interventions
  (1) Capacity building
  (2) Behavioural change communication
  (3) Intersectoral collaboration
  (4) Monitoring and Evaluation
  (5) Operational research and applied field research.

Early diagnosis and treatment of malaria aims at :

(1) Complete cure;
(2) Prevention of progression of uncomplicated malaria to severe disease;
(3) Prevention of deaths;
(4) Interruption of transmission; and
(5) Minimizing risk of selection and spread of drug resistant malaria parasite.

GUIDELINES FOR DIAGNOSIS AND TREATMENT OF MALARIA IN INDIA–2013 *(25, 26)*

According to the revised drug policy 2013, there is no scope of presumptive treatment in malaria control. The recommended guidelines are as follows :

Treatment of Uncomplicated Malaria

All fever cases diagnosed as malaria by microscopy or RDT should promptly be given effective treatment.

TREATMENT OF P. VIVAX CASES

Positive *P. vivax* cases should be treated with chloroquine in full therapeutic dose of 25 mg/kg divided over three days. Vivax malaria relapses due to the presence of hypnozoites in the liver. The relapse rate in vivax malaria in India is around 30%. For its prevention, primaquine may be given at a dose of 0.25 mg/kg daily for 14 days under supervision. Primaquine is contraindicated in G6PD deficient patients, infants and pregnant women. Caution should be exercised before administering primaquine in areas known to have high prevalence of G6PD deficiency. Primaquine can lead to haemolysis in G6PD deficiency. Patient should be advised to stop primaquine immediately if he develops symptoms like dark coloured urine, yellow conjunctiva, bluish discolouration of lips, abdominal pain, nausea, vomiting etc. and should report to the doctor immediately.

TREATMENT OF P. FALCIPARUM CASES

Artemisinin Combination Therapy (ACT) (Artesunate 3 days + sulphadoxine-pyrimethamine 1 day) should be given to all confirmed *P. falciparum* cases found positive by microscopy or RDT. This is to be accompanied by single dose of primaquine (0.75 mg/kg body weight) on Day 2.

However, considering the reports of resistance to SP drug in North Eastern states, the Technical Advisory Committee has recommended to use the coformulated tablet of Artemether (20 mg) + Lumefantrine (120 mg) as per age-specific dose schedule for the treatment of *Pf* cases in North Eastern states. This drug is not recommended during the first trimester of pregnancy and for children weighing < 5 kg. Production and sale of Artemisinin monotherapy has been banned in India, as it can lead to development of parasite resistance to the drug.

TREATMENT OF MALARIA IN PREGNANCY

ACT should be given for treatment of *P. falciparum* malaria in second and third trimesters of pregnancy, while quinine is recommended in the first trimester. *P. vivax* malaria can be treated with chloroquine. Primaquine is contraindicated in pregnant woman.

TREATMENT OF MIXED INFECTIONS

Mixed infections with *P. falciparum* should be treated as falciparum malaria.

Resistance should be suspected if inspite of full treatment with no history of vomiting, diarrhoea, patient does not respond within 72 hours, clinically and parasitologically. Such cases not responding to ACT, should be treated with oral quinine with tetracycline/doxycycline. These instances should be reported to concerned District Malaria/State Malaria Officer/ROHFW for initiation of therapeutic efficacy studies.

Diagnosis and treatment of malaria *(25, 26)*

All fever cases diagnosed as malaria by either RDT or microscopy should be promptly given effective treatment. The medicines chosen will depend upon whether the patient has *vivax* malaria or *falciparum* malaria. The flow charts in different settings for diagnosis and drug selection for the treatment of malaria are shown in Fig. 2, 3 and 4.

A. *Where microscopy result is available within 24 hours*

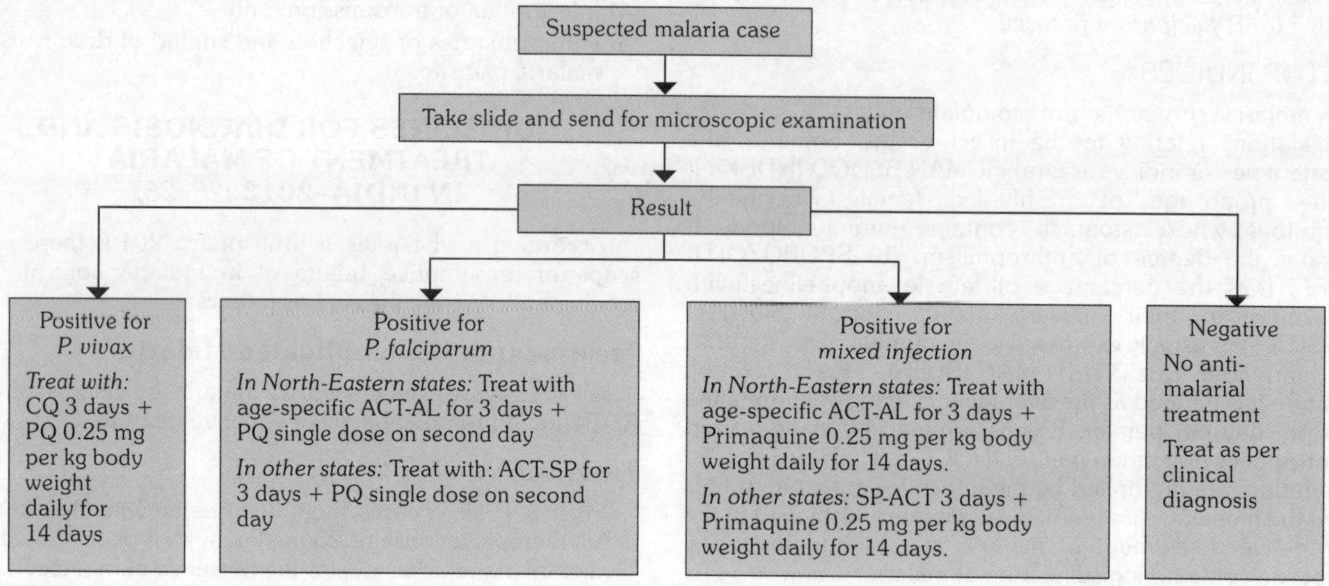

ACT-AL – Artemisinin-based combination therapy – Artemether – Lumefantrine
ACT-SP – Artemisinin-based combination therapy (Artesunate + Sulfadoxine-Pyrimethamine)

CQ – Chloroquine
PQ – Primaquine

FIG. 2

B. *Where microscopy result is not available within 24 hours and monovalent RDT is used*

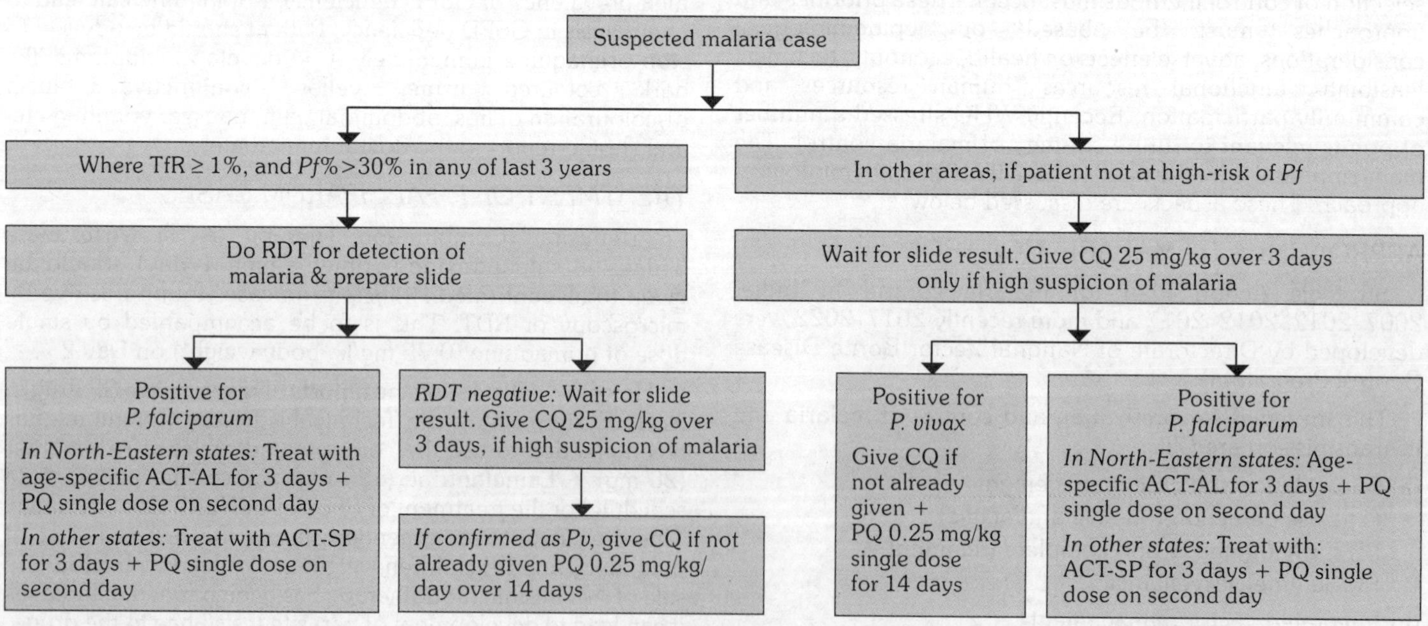

TfR = Test falciparum rate

Note : If a patient has severe symptoms at any stage, then immediately refer to a nearest PHC or other health facility with indoor patient management or a registered medical doctor.

FIG. 3

C. Where microscopy result is not available within 24 hours and bivalent RDT is used

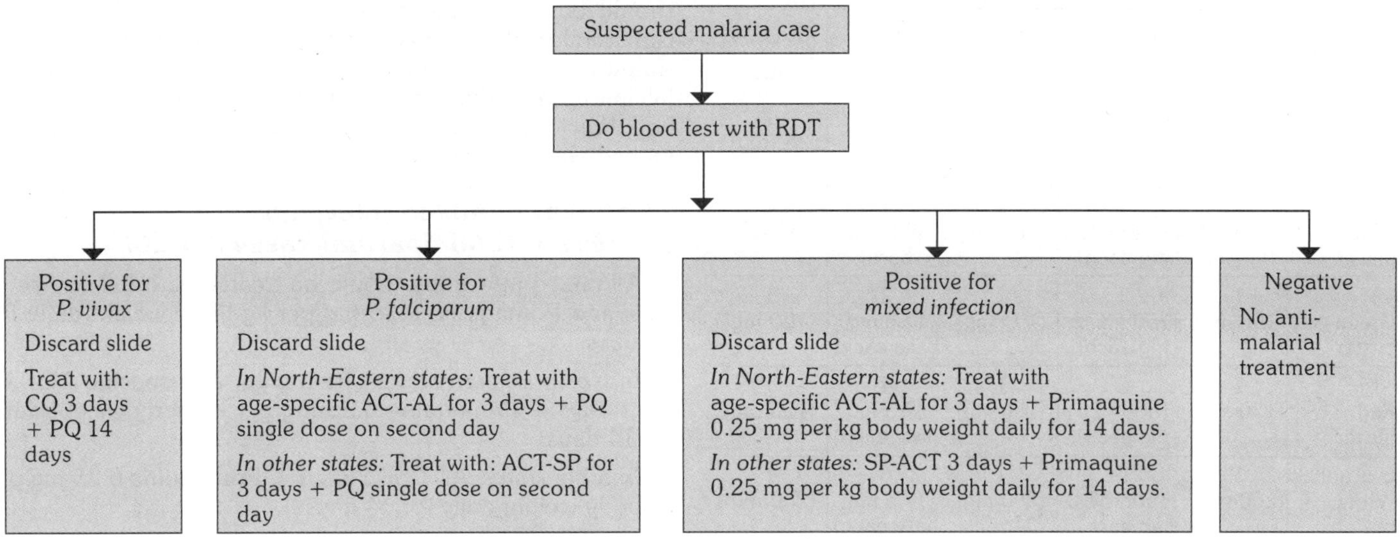

Note : (a) If a patient has severe symptoms at any stage, then immediately refer to a nearest PHC or other health facility with indoor patient management or a registered medical doctor.

(b) PQ is contra-indicated in pregnancy and in children under 1 year (Infant).

FIG. 4

Treatment of *vivax* malaria *(25, 26)*

Diagnosis of vivax malaria may be made by the used of RDT (Bivalent) or microscopic examination of the blood smear. On confirmation, following treatment is to be given :

Drug schedule for treatment of P. vivax malaria:

1. *Chloroquine:* 25 mg/kg body weight divided over three days i.e.

   10 mg/kg on day 1,

   10 mg/kg on day 2 and

   5 mg/kg on day 3.

2. *Primaquine:* 0.25 mg/kg body weight daily for 14 days.

   Primaquine is contraindicated in infants, pregnant women and individuals with G6PD deficiency.

   14 day regimen of Primaquine should be given under supervision.

Dosage chart for treatment of *vivax* malaria

Age	Day 1		Day 2		Day 3		Day 4 to 14
	CQ (150 mg base)	PQ (2.5 mg)	CQ (150 mg base)	PQ (2.5 mg)	CQ (150 mg base)	PQ (2.5 mg)	PQ (2.5 mg)
Less than 1 year	½	0	½	0	¼	0	0
1–4 years	1	1	1	1	½	1	1
5–8 years	2	2	2	2	1	2	2
9–14 years	3	4	3	4	1½	4	4
15 years or more*	4	6	4	6	2	6	6
Pregnancy	4	0	4	0	2	0	0

Note : CQ 250 mg tablet is having 150 mg base

Treatment of *falciparum* malaria *(25, 26)*

Diagnosis of falciparum malaria may be made by the use of RDT (monovalent or bivalent) or microscopic examination of the blood smear. It is imperative to start the treatment for falciparum malaria immediately on diagnosis. The treatment for falciparum malaria is as follows:

In other states (other than North-Eastern states):

1. Artemisinin based combination therapy (ACT-SP)*

   Artesunate (AS), available as 50 mg tablets are given for three days, and Sulfadoxine-Pyrimethamine (S-P) tablets, containing 500 mg Sulfadoxine and 25 mg pyrimethamine are given for one day, as shown in the dosage chart below.

   All tablets for a day should be taken together, swallowed with water.

   In addition, Primaquine (PQ large) tablets should be given on the second day.

Dose schedule for treatment of uncomplicated P. falciparum cases:

1. Artemisinin based combination therapy (ACT-SP) *

   Artesunate 4 mg/kg body weight daily for 3 days, plus

   Sulfadoxine (25 mg/kg body weight) – Pyrimethamine (1.25 mg/kg body weight) on first day.

   * ACT is not to be given in 1st trimester of pregnancy.

2. Primaquine * : 0.75 mg/kg body weight on day 2.

   With the introduction of different coloured blister packs for different age groups, treatment by the field level staff has been made easy. The colour code for different age groups for packing of tablet ACT+SP has been given as follows :

Dosage chart for treatment of *falciparum* malaria with ACT-SP

Age group (Years)	1st day AS	1st day SP	2nd day AS	2nd day PQ	3rd day AS
0–1* Pink blister	1 (25 mg)	1 (250+ 12.5 mg)	1 (25 mg)	Nil	1 25 (mg)
1–4 Yellow blister	1 (50 mg)	1 (500+25 mg each)	1 (50 mg)	1 (7.5 mg base)	1 (50 mg)
5–8 Green blister	1 (100 mg)	1 (750+37.5 mg each)	1 (100 mg)	2 (7.5 mg base each)	1 (100 mg)
9–14 Red blister	1 (150 mg)	2 (500+25 mg each)	1 (150 mg)	4 (7.5 mg base each)	1 (150 mg)
15 & above White blister	1 (200 mg)	2 (750+37.5 mg each)	1 (200 mg)	6 (7.5 mg base each)	1 (200 mg)

* SP is not to be prescribed for children <5 months of age and should be treated with alternate ACT

* ACT-AL is not to be prescribed for children weighing less than 5 kg.

In North-Eastern states (NE states):

1. ACT-AL co-formulated tablet of Artemether (20 mg) – Lumefantrine (120 mg)

   (Not recommended during the first trimester of pregnancy and for children weighing <5 kg)

   Recommended regimen by weight and age group The packing size for different age groups based on Kg body weight.

Co-formulated tablet ACT-AL	5–14 kg (>5 months to <3 years)	15–24 kg (>3 to 8 years)	25–34 kg (>9 to 14 years)	>34 kg (>14 years)
Total dose of ACT-AL	20 mg/ 120 mg twice daily for 3 days	40 mg/ 240 mg twice daily for 3 days	60 mg/ 360 mg twice daily for 3 days	80 mg/ 480 mg twice daily for 3 days
	Pack size			
No. of tablets in the packing	6	12	18	24
Give	1 tablet twice daily for 3 days	2 tablets twice daily for 3 days	3 tablets twice daily for 3 days	4 tablets twice daily for 3 days
Colour of the pack	Yellow	Green	Red	White

2. Primaquine * : 0.75 mg/kg body weight on day 2

Treatment of uncomplicated P. falciparum cases in pregnancy:

1st trimester : Quinine salt 10 mg/kg 3 times daily for 7 days.

Quinine may induce hypoglycaemia; pregnant women should not start taking quinine on an empty stomach and should eat regularly, while on quinine treatment.

2nd and 3rd trimester : Area-specific ACT as per dosage schedule given above i.e. ACT-AL in North-Eastern states, ACT-SP in other states.

Primaquine (PQ) prevents transmission of falciparum malaria to others by its ability to kill gametocytes. PQ tablets should be taken after a meal; not on an empty stomach. Children less than the age of one year and pregnant women should not be given primaquine. As pregnant women having falciparum malaria require different medicines, they should be directed to go to the nearest PHC or hospital immediately, without delay.

Treatment of mixed infections (*P. vivax* + *P. falciparum*) cases *(25, 26)*

All mixed infections should be treated with full course of ACT and Primaquine 0.25 mg per kg body weight daily for 14 days.

In North-Eastern states: Treat with: Age-specific ACT-AL for 3 days + Primaquine 0.25 mg per kg body weight daily for 14 days.

In other states: ACT-SP 3 days + Primaquine 0.25 mg per kg body weight daily for 14 days.

Dosage chart for treatment of mixed (*vivax* and *falciparum*) malaria with ACT-SP

Age	Day 1 AS tablet (50 mg)	Day 1 SP tablet	Day 1 PQ (2.5 mg)	Day 2 AS tablet (50 mg)	Day 2 PQ (2.5 mg)	Day 3 AS tablet (50 mg)	Day 3 PQ (2.5 mg)	Day 4-14 PQ (2.5 mg)
Less than 1 year	½	½	0	½	0	½	0	0
1–4 years	1	1	1	1	1	1	1	1
5–8 years	2	1½	2	2	2	2	2	2
9–14 years	3	2	4	3	4	3	4	4
15 years or more	4	3	6	4	6	4	6	6

Treatment of *P. ovale* and *P. malariae*

In India these species are very rarely found in few places. *P. ovale* should be treated as *P. vivax* and *P. malariae* should be treated as *P. falciparum*.

General recommendations for the management of uncomplicated malaria

1. Avoid starting treatment on an empty stomach. The first dose should be given under observation. Dose should be repeated if vomiting occurs within 15 minutes by opening a new blister pack (discard what remains of old pack). If the patient vomits the first dose again, it is considered a severe case of malaria and refer the patient immediately to the nearest Block PHC/CHC/Hospital. Special precaution should be taken in case of a child under-5 years of age, and in pregnant woman.
2. Explain to the patient or caretaker that : (a) if the treatment is not completed as prescribed, the disease may manifest again with more serious features and more difficult to treat; (b) to come back immediately, if there is no improvement after 24 hours, if the situation gets worse or the fever comes back; and (c) that regular use of a mosquito net (preferably insecticide treated net) is the best way to prevent malaria.
3. Patient should also be examined for concomitant illness.

Resistance to anti-malarial drugs

Resistance can be defined as either the ability of a parasite strain to survive and/or multiply despite the administration and absorption of a drug given in doses equal to or higher than those usually recommended, but within the limits of tolerance of the patient.

Drug resistance is a complex phenomenon, where, by genetic mutation, a parasite acquires the ability to resist, partly or fully, the effects of one or more anti-malarial drugs. When the resistant parasites are exposed to the drug, they multiply selectively. If parasites are resistant to the drug being used, the patient may not respond to treatment. One of the commonest reasons for the development of drug resistance is that the parasites are exposed to insufficient amount of the drug due to low prescription dosage, lesser amount of drug dispensed, incomplete treatment taken by the patient, drug vomited out or low absorption of drug due to any other reason e.g., diarrhoea, poorly stored drug, poor quality drug when supplied or expiry date medicine. In such cases, most of the sensitive parasites are killed by even these small doses, but resistant parasites survive, multiply and spread to other people by mosquitoes. The new patient then gets infection from the resistant malaria parasites and does not respond to the drug at all, or responds only partly. Meanwhile, the earlier patient may appear cured because most of the parasites were killed by the drug, and the symptoms abated.

It should be kept in mind that the patient might have had a fresh reinfection, or in the case of *vivax* malaria, there might have been a relapse of malaria *(25)*.

Treatment failure *(27)*

After treatment patient is considered cured if he/she does not have fever or parasitaemia till day 28th. Some patients may not respond to treatment which may be due to drug resistance or treatment failure, specially in falciparum malaria. If patient does not respond and presents with following, he/she should be given alternative treatment.

Early treatment failure (ETF) : Development of danger signs or severe malaria on Day 1, 2 or 3, in the presence of parasitaemia; parasitaemia on Day 2 higher than on Day 0, irrespective of axillary temperature; parasitaemia on Day 3 with axillary temperature >37.5°C; and parasitaemia on Day 3, >25% of count on Day 0.

Late clinical failure (LCF) : Development of danger signs or severe malaria in the presence of parasitaemia on any day between Day 4 and Day 28 in patients who did not previously meet any of the criteria of early treatment failure; and presence of parasitaemia on any day between Day 4 and Day 28 with axillary temperature >37.5°C in patients who did not previously meet any of the criteria of early treatment failure.

Late parasitological failure (LPF) : Presence of parasitaemia on any day between Day 7 and Day 28 with axillary temperature <37.5°C in patients who did not previously meet any of the criteria of early treatment failure or late clinical failure.

Such cases of falciparum malaria should be given alternative ACT or quinine with Doxycycline. Doxycycline is contraindicated in pregnancy, lactation and in children upto 8 years. Treatment failure with chloroquine in *P. vivax* malaria is rare in India.

Treatment of severe malaria

CLINICAL FEATURES *(25)*

Severe manifestations can develop in *P. falciparum* infection over a span of time as short as 12–24 hours and may lead to death, if not treated promptly and adequately. Severe malaria is characterized by one or more of the following features:

(1) Impaired consciousness/coma
(2) Repeated generalized convulsions
(3) Renal failure (Serum Creatinine >3 mg/dl)
(4) Jaundice (Serum Bilirubin >3 mg/dl)
(5) Severe anaemia (Hb <5 g/dl)
(6) Pulmonary oedema/acute respiratory distress syndrome
(7) Hypoglycaemia (Plasma glucose <40 mg/dl)
(8) Metabolic acidosis
(9) Circulatory collapse/shock (Systolic BP<80 mm Hg, < 50 mm Hg in children)
(10) Abnormal bleeding and disseminated intravascular coagulation.
(11) Haemoglobinuria
(12) Hyperthermia (Temperature >106°F or 42°C)
(13) Hyperparasitaemia (<5% parasitized RBCs in low endemic and >10% in hyperendemic areas)

Foetal and maternal complications are more common in pregnancy with severe malaria; therefore, they need prompt attention.

Microscopic evidence may be negative for asexual parasites in patients with severe infections due to sequestration and partial treatment. Efforts should be made to confirm these cases by RDT or repeat microscopy. However, if the symptoms clearly point to severe malaria and there is no alternative explanation, such a case should be treated accordingly.

Criteria for immediate referral are as follows: (a) Persistence of fever after 24 hours of initial treatment; (b) Continuous vomiting and inability to retain oral drug; (c) Headache continues to increase; (d) Severe dehydration (dry, parched skin, sunken eyes etc.); (e) Too weak to walk in the absence of any other obvious reason; (f) Change in sensorium e.g. confusion, drowsiness, blurring of vision, photophobia, disorientation; (g) Convulsion or muscle twitchings; (h) Bleeding and clotting disorder; (i) Suspicion of severe anaemia; (j) Jaundice; and (k) Hypothermia *(25)*.

Treatment of severe malaria cases *(25)*

Severe malaria is an emergency and treatment should be given as per severity and associated complications which can be best decided by the treating physicians. Before admitting or referring patients, the attending doctor or health worker, whoever is able to do it, should do RDT and take blood smear, give a parenteral dose of artemisinin derivative or quinine in suspected cerebral malaria cases and send case sheet, details of treatment history and blood slide with patient. Parenteral artemisinin derivatives or quinine should be used irrespective of chloroquine resistance status of the area with one of the following options:

Chemotherapy of severe and complicated malaria

Initial parenteral treatment for at least 48 hours: *Choose one of the following four options*	Follow-up treatment, when patient can take oral medication following parenteral treatment
Quinine : 20 mg quinine salt/kg body weight on admission (IV infusion or divided IM injection) followed by maintenance dose of 10 mg/kg 8 hourly; infusion rate should not exceed 5 mg/kg per hour. Loading dose of 20 mg/kg should not be given, if the patient has already received quinine.	*Quinine* 10 mg/kg three times a day with: doxycycline 100 mg once a day OR clindamycin in pregnant women and children under 8 years of age. – to complete 7 days of treatment.
Artesunate: 2.4 mg/kg IV or IM given on admission (time=0), then at 12 h and 24 h, then once a day. OR *Artemether:* 3.2 mg/kg bw IM given on admission then 1.6 mg/kg per day. OR *Arteether:* 150 mg daily IM for 3 days in adults only (not recommended for children).	Full oral course of area-specific ACT: *In North-Eastern states:* Age-specific ACT-AL for 3 days + PQ single dose on second day *In other states:* Treat with: ACT-SP for 3 days + PQ single dose on second day

Note : The parenteral treatment in severe malaria cases should be given for minimum of 24 hours once started (irrespective of the patient's ability to tolerate oral medication earlier than 24 hours).

After parenteral artemisinin therapy, patients will receive a full course of area-specific oral ACT for 3 days. Those patients who received parenteral Quinine therapy should receive oral Quinine 10 mg/kg body weight three times a day for 7 days (including the days when parenteral Quinine was administered) plus Doxycycline 3 mg/kg body weight once a day, or Clindamycin 10 mg/kg body weight 12-hourly for 7 days (Doxycycline is contraindicated in pregnant women and children under 8 years of age) or area-specific ACT as described.

Note :

- Pregnant women with severe malaria in any trimester can be treated with artemisinin derivatives, which, in contrast to quinine, do not risk aggravating hypoglycaemia.
- The parenteral treatment should be given for minimum of 24 hours.
- Once the patient can take oral therapy; give:
- Quinine 10 mg/kg three times a day with doxycycline 100 mg once a day or clindamycin in pregnant women and children under 8 years of age, to complete 7 days of treatment, in patients started on parenteral quinine.
- Full course of ACT to patients started on artemisinin derivatives.
- Use of mefloquine should be avoided in cerebral malaria due to neuropsychiatric complications associated with it.

Some don'ts in severe malaria case management

Do not use corticosteroids, do not give intravenous mannitol, do not use heparin as anticoagulant, do not administer adrenaline or do not overhydrate.

Toxic hazards of drugs

Chloroquine has few side-effects. Nausea, vomiting, blurring of vision and headaches may occur, but they are mild and transient. Cases of retinal damage have been reported but only in persons exposed to large cumulative doses over many years. It is important to remember that chloroquine should not be given on empty stomach. Despite reports of teratogenicity in experimental animals, most authorities accept that pyrimethamine can safely be taken alone during pregnancy *(28)*. The teratogenic effect of pyrimethamine in man is not proved. In regard to primaquine, although in recommended doses, no serious toxic manifestations have been encountered so far in India. It is useful to bear in mind the likely toxic symptoms, which may be of three types : *(a) Plasmocid types :* this is a rare toxic manifestation involving the CNS, *(b) Gastrointestinal* : cramps, nausea and vomiting, *(c) Cardiovascular :* This is probably the most serious toxic manifestation which is to be carefully observed during the administration of the drug. Even the first dose may bring about the warning sign of cyanosis. The surveillance worker/MPW must carefully check for all possible toxic symptoms before he administers the daily dose of primaquine. In the case of appearance of any of the toxic symptoms discussed above, primaquine treatment should be stopped immediately *(29)*.

Chemoprophylaxis

Chemoprophylaxis against malaria has, with the development of drug resistance, become unreliable. Experts disagree on whether well-conducted prophylaxis gives an additional benefit if effective treatment is readily available. However, experts feel that it can play a useful role in reducing the risk of fatal disease *(30)*.

Chemoprophylaxis is recommended for travellers from non-endemic areas and, as a short term measure for soldiers, police and labour forces serving in highly endemic areas. Chemoprophylaxis should be complemented by personal protection where feasible and by other methods of vector control *(30)*.

The recommendations for short-term chemoprophylaxis (less than 6 weeks) are as follows *(30)* :

(1) Dosing schedules for the children should be based on body weight.

(2) Antimalarials that have to be taken daily (e.g. Doxycycline) should be started the day before arrival in the risk area.

(3) Weekly chloroquine should be started 1 week before arrival.

(4) Weekly mefloquine should preferably be started 2–3 weeks before departure, to achieve higher pre–travel blood level and to allow side-effects to be detected before travel so that possible alternative can be considered.

(5) All prophylactic drugs should be taken with unfailing regularity for the duration of the stay in the malaria risk area, and should be continued for 4 weeks after the last possible exposure to infection, since parasites may still emerge from the liver during this period.

The recommendations for the long-term chemoprophylaxis (more than 6 weeks) are as follows :

(1) The risk of serious side-effects associated with long-term prohylactic use of chloroquine and proguanil is low. However, anyone who has taken 300 mg of chloroquine weekly for over five years and requires further prophylaxis should be screened twice-yearly for early retinal changes. If daily dose of 100 mg chloroquine have been taken, screening should start after three years *(30)*.

(2) Data indicate no increased risk of serious side-effects with long-term use of mefloquine if the drug is tolerated in the short-term, as mefloquine does not accumulate during long-term intake.

(3) Available data on long-term chemoprophylaxis with doxycycline is limited.

Mefloquine is contraindicated in cases with history of convulsions, neuropsychiatric problems and cardiac conditions.

Chemoprophylaxis is still desirable for pregnant women living in areas where transmission is very intense and leads to parasitaemias, causing low birth weight and anaemia, or to a high risk of life–threatening malaria attacks. However, the choice of safe drugs is becoming increasingly narrow, and it may be necessary to replace chemoprophylaxis by prompt treatment of clinical episodes or periodic treatments during pregnancy. While the choice of strategy should be guided by the national malaria control policy, its implementation should normally be part of antenatal care *(31)*.

The recommended regimens for chemoprophylaxis are as given in Table 2.

TABLE 2
Drug regimens for prophylaxis of malaria

Drugs		Usual amount	Adult dose
Generic name	Common trade names	per tablet or capsule	For prophylaxis
Chloroquine[a]	Aralen Avlochlor Nivaquine Resochin	100 or 150 mg (base)	300 mg (base) = 3 tablets of 100 mg or 2 tablets of 150 mg once a week, on the same day each week OR 100 mg (base) = 1 tablet of 100 mg daily for six days per week
Proguanil[b]	Paludrine	100 mg	200 mg = 2 tablets once a day
Mefloquine[c]	Lariam Eloquin Mephaquin	250 mg	250 mg = 1 tablet once a week, on the same day each week
Doxycycline[d]	Vibramycin	100 mg	100 mg=1 capsule once a day

a. Also available as suspension.
b. Recommended only in association with chloroquine.
c. The use of the higher treatment dose regimen is recommended for infections acquired in areas on the Thailand/Cambodia and Thailand / Myanmar borders only.
d. There is relatively little experience with this drug, and knowledge of its efficacy and toxicity is limited.

Source : *(30)*

ACTIVE INTERVENTION MEASURES

Neither chemotherapy nor chemoprophylaxis will be able to reduce significantly the malaria prevalence or transmission. It can be obtained only when proper anti–mosquito measures are introduced.

1. STRATIFICATION OF THE PROBLEM

Malaria is a complex disease, and its distribution and intensity vary from place to place. Stratification of the problem has become an essential feature for the planning and development of a sound control strategy to maximize the utilization of available resources. It can also provide guidelines as to which strategy could be most suited and economical under the existing conditions. For details please refer to chapter 7.

2. VECTOR CONTROL STRATEGIES

Vector control is still one of the primary weapons to control malaria in endemic areas. The methods used are as shown in Table 3.

(a) Anti–adult measures

(i) Residual spraying : The discovery of DDT in 1940s and followed by other insecticides revolutionized malaria control. The spraying of the indoor surfaces of houses with residual insecticides (e.g., DDT, malathion, fenitrothion) is still the most effective measure to kill the adult mosquito. It has been observed that discontinuation of spraying has very often led to the resurgence of malaria. This implies that spraying once applied may need to be continued for an indefinite period. If indoor spraying is to have any effect, then exhaustive coverage is needed. Indoor house spraying reduces the longevity of the vector.

Malathion and fenitrothion are organophosphate insecticides which are being used with increasing frequency for malaria control following the development of vector resistance to DDT *(33)*.

TABLE 3
Malaria vector control measures

Action	For individual and family protection	For community protection
Reduction of human-mosquito contact	Insecticide-treated nets, repellents, protective clothing, screening of houses	Insecticide-treated nets zoo-prophylaxis
Destruction of adult mosquitoes		Insecticide-treated nets, indoor residual spraying, space spraying, ultra low-volume sprays
Destruction of mosquito larvae	Peri-domestic sanitation	Larviciding of water surfaces, intermittent irrigation, sluicing, biological control
Source reduction	Small-scale drainage	Environmental sanitation, water management, drainage
Social participation	Motivation for personal and family protection	Health education, community participation

Source : *(32)*

1

(ii) Space application : This is a major anti–epidemic measure in mosquito–borne diseases. It involves the application of pesticides in the form of fog or mist using special equipment. The ultra–low–volume method of pesticide dispersion by air or by ground equipment has proved to be effective and economical. Outdoor space sprays reduce vector population quickly.

(iii) Individual protection : Man–vector contact can be reduced by other preventive measures such as the use of repellents, protective clothing, bed-nets (preferably impregnated with safe, long–acting repellent insecticides), mosquito coils, screening of houses etc. The methods of personal protection are of great value when properly employed. However, they have rarely been used on a large scale because of cost.

(b) Anti-larval measures

(i) Larvicides : During the first half of the 20th century, anti-larval measures such as oiling the collections of standing water or dusting them with paris green effectively controlled malaria (but the measures were eclipsed at the end of World War II). With the increase in insecticide resistance, the older methods of mosquito control have now become promising. Some modern larvicides such as temephos which confer long effect with low toxicity are more widely used. However larviciding must be repeated at frequent intervals and for this reason it is a comparatively costly operation.

(ii) Source reduction : Techniques to reduce mosquito breeding sites (often called source reduction) which include drainage or filling, deepening or flushing, management of water level, changing the salt content of water and intermittent irrigation are among the classical methods of malaria control to which attention is being paid again *(34)*. Whenever practicable, measures for the improvement of the environment by the permanent reduction of sources should be instituted.

(iii) Integrated control : In order to reduce too much dependance on residual insecticides, increasing emphasis is being put on "integrated" vector control methodology which includes bioenvironmental and personal protection measure *(35)*. This approach is important because there is no single and simple method that would ensure control of transmission.

By mid 1995 all malaria endemic countries in the region had adopted the revised malaria control strategy to reduce morbidity and mortality and to reduce its area of distribution, particularly of multidrug resistant malaria. The use of stratification approach by the majority of anti-malaria programmes in the Region has led to more cost-effective interventions. Vector resistance to insecticides has necessitated the use of more expensive pyrethroid, thereby limiting the coverage. Malaria control added impetus as **Roll Back Malaria** initiative was launched by WHO, UNICEF, UNDP and the World Bank in 1998.

The launch of Roll Back Back Malaria (RBM) in 1998, the United Nations Millenium Declaration in 2000, the Abuja Declaration by African Heads of State in 2000 (part of the African Summit on Roll Back Malaria), the World Health Assembly in 2005, and the RBM global strategic plan 2005–2015 have all contributed to the establishment of goals, indicators and targets for malaria control.

THE GLOBAL TECHNICAL STRATEGY FOR MALARIA (2016–2030)

Adopted by the World Health Assembly in May 2015, the strategy provides comprehensive technical guidance to countries and development partners for the next 15 years, emphasizing the importance of scaling up malaria responses and moving towards elimination. It also highlights the urgent need to increase investments across all interventions – including preventive measures, diagnostic testing, treatment and disease surveillance – as well as in harnessing innovation and expanding research. By adopting this strategy, WHO Member States have endorsed the bold vision of a world free of malaria and set the ambitious new target of reducing the global malaria burden by 90% by 2030. They also agreed to strengthen health systems, address emerging multi-drug and insecticide resistance, and intensify national, cross-border and regional efforts to scale up malaria responses to protect everyone at risk. By taking forward this strategy, countries will make a major contribution to implementing the post-2015 sustainable development framework. A major scale-up of malaria responses will not only help countries reach the health-related targets for 2030, but will contribute to poverty reduction and other development goals *(36)*.

The three pillars of Global Technical Strategy for malaria 2016–2030, and the goals, milestones and targets are as follows *(37)*:

Pillars	
Pillar 1	Ensure universal access to malaria prevention, diagnosis and treatment
Pillar 2	Accelerate efforts towards elimination and attainment of malaria free status
Pillar 3	Transform malaria surveillance into a core intervention

Goals	Milestones 2020	Milestones 2025	Targets 2030
1. Reduce malaria mortality rates globally compared with 2015	At least 40%	At least 75%	At least 90%
2. Reduce malaria case incidence globally compared with 2015	At least 40%	At least 75%	At least 90%
3. Eliminate malaria from countries in which malaria was transmitted in 2015	At least 10 countries	At least 20 countries	At least 35 countries
4. Prevent re-establishment of malaria in all countries that are malaria-free	Re-establishment prevented	Re-establishment prevented	Re-establishment prevented

Malaria vaccines *(3)*

The RTS,S/AS01 vaccine is the first and currently the only malaria vaccine to be recommended for use by WHO. It is a pre-erythrocytic recombinant protein vaccine. The vaccine should be used for the prevention of *P. falciparum* malaria in children living in region with moderate to high malaria transmission. Vaccine is provided in a 4 dose schedule in children from 5 months of age. There should be a minimum interval of 4 weeks between doses, 3 doses as primary schedule, with a fourth dose approximately 12–18 months after the 3rd dose to prolong the duration of protection.

The vaccine is currently produced as a 2-dose RTS,S powder to be reconstituted with a 2-dose AS01 adjuvant system suspension. After reconstitution the total volume is

1 ml (2 doses of 0.5 ml). No preservative is included in either the RTS,S formulation or the AS01 adjuvant system. The vials should therefore be discarded at the end of the vaccination session, or within 6 hours after opening, whichever comes first. The reconstituted vaccine should be administered by injection into the deltoid muscle in children aged 5 months or older. The vaccine should be stored at 2–8°C. The shelf life of the RTS,S/AS01 vaccine is 3 years. A vaccine vial monitor is on the AS01 vial.

National Malaria Control Progrmme

Please see chapter 7.

References

1. WHO (2020), *World Malaria Report,* 2020.
2. WHO (2021), *World Malaria Report,* 2021.
3. WHO (2022), *Weekly Epidemiological Record,* No. 9, 4th March 2022.
4. WHO (2014), *Fact Sheet Malaria,* No. 94, March 2014.
5. Govt. of India (2022), *National Vector Borne Disease Control Programme,* Dept. of Health and Family Welfare, New Delhi.
6. Govt. of India (2014), *Strategic Action Plan for Malaria Control in India 2012-2017,* DGHS, Ministry of Health and Family Welfare, New Delhi.
7. *National Malaria Control Strategy* (1995), Malaria Research Centre, 22 Sham Nath Marg, New Delhi.
8. Govt. of India (2016), *Operational Manual for Malaria Elimination in India,* Ministry of Health and Family Welfare, New Delhi.
9. WHO (1980). *Summary of Scientific Progress in the Field of Malaria published during the last Five Years,* MAP/80.1 VBC/80.2, WHO Geneva.
10. Youmans, G.P. et al (1980). *The Biological and Clinical Basis of Infectious Diseases,* 2nd ed. Saunders.
11. Bruce–Chwatt, LJ. (1980). *Essential Malariology,* William Heinemenn, London.
12. Jawetze et.al, 2007, *Medical Microbiology,* 24th Ed, A Lange Medical Book.
13. Hall, A. P. (1976) *Brit. Med. J.,* 1 : 323.
14. Pasrol, G. et al (1976) *Lancet,* 1, 1269.
15. WHO (1986). *Techn. Rept. Ser.* 735.
16. WHO (1979). *Tech Rep. Ser. No.* 640.
17. WHO (1995), *Tech. Rep. Ser., No.* 857.
18. Lariviere, M. (1977). *Children in the Tropics* No. 106, p. 9.
19. WHO (1984). *Techn. Rep.Ser.* No.712.
20. WHO (1995), *World Health,* March–April, 1995.
21. Council for International Organization of Medical Sciences (1973). *Communicable Diseases*, Provisional Nomenclature, CIOMS/WHO, Geneva.
22. WHO (1986). *The clinical Management of Acute Malaria,* SEARO, SEA Ser. No. 9. New Delhi.
23. Govt. of India (2009), *Guidelines for Diagnosis and Treatment of Malaria in India,* NVBDCP Division, Ministry of Health and Family Welfare, New Delhi.
24. WHO (1961) *Techn.Rep.Ser.* No.205.
25. Govt. of India (2013), *National Drug Policy on Malaria,* Directorate of NVBDCP, Ministry of Health and Family Welfare, New Delhi.
26. Malaria website (2019), *Treatment of malaria.*
27. Govt. of India (2011), *Guidelines for Diqgnosis and Treatment of Malaria in India,* NVBDCP, National Institute of Malaria Research, New Delhi.
28. Editorial (1976). *Lancet,* 2 :1005.
29. Govt. of India (1977), *Role of Medical Officer of PHC in Malaria Control,* Ministry of Dept. of Family Welfare, Health and Family Welfare, New Delhi. Mass Mailing Unit.
30. WHO (2010), *International Travel and Health.*
31. WHO (1993), *Tech. Rep. Ser.,* No.839.
32. WHO (2006), *Tech. Rep. Ser. No. 936.*
33. *WHO Bull* (1985) 63 (2) 353.
34. WHO (1991), *World Health,* Sept–Oct 1991.
35. WHO (1983). *Techn. Rep.Ser.* No.688.
36. WHO (2015), *Global Technical Strategy for Malaria 2016–2030.*
37. WHO (2019), *World Malaria Report,* 2019.

LYMPHATIC FILARIASIS

The term "lymphatic filariasis" covers infection with three closely related nematode worms – *W. bancrofti, B. malayi and B. timori.* All three infections are transmitted to man by the bites of infective mosquitoes. All three parasites have basically similar life cycles in man–adult worms living in lymphatic vessels whilst their offspring, the microfilariae circulate in peripheral blood and are available to infect mosquito vectors when they come to feed *(1).* The disease manifestations range from none to both acute and chronic manifestations such as lymphangitis, lymphadenitis, elephantiasis of genitals, legs and arms or as a hypersensitivity state such as tropical pulmonary eosinophilia or as an atypical form such as filarial arthritis. Though not fatal, the disease is responsible for considerable suffering, deformity and disability.

Problem statement

Filariasis is a global problem. It is a major social and economic scourage in the tropics and subtropics of Africa, Asia, Western Pacific and parts of the Americas, affecting over 47 countries. More than 863 million people live in areas where there is a risk of infection, of whom 120 million are infected and in need of treatment, including 40 million people with overt disease. This includes 15 million people with lymphoedema and 25 million men with urogenital swelling principally scrotal hydrocele. At least 36 million people remain with these chronic disease manifestations *(2, 3).*

About 90 per cent of cases of lymphatic filariasis are caused by infection with *W. bancrofti*; other related parasites that infect humans are *Brugia malayi* in South-East Asia and *B. timori* in Indonesia.

The formal goal of the global lymphatic filariasis programme is to eliminate the disease "as a public health problem" and 2020 is the informal target date for interrupting transmission. The strategy to interrupt transmission of the disease calls for mass administration of a 2-drug regimen (ivermectin or DEC plus albendazole) administration as a single dose annually for 4–6 years.

Since 2000, the global programme provided a cumulative total of nearly 6.7 billion treatments to at least 1 billion people. It represents about 73 per cent of the 1.4 billion people at risk *(2).*

The current hypothesis is that reducing the prevalence of microfilaraemia in humans to <1 per cent will stop transmission. One provisional set of guidelines for stopping treatment would require ≥ 5 annual rounds of MDA with coverage of ≥ 65 per cent of the total population *(4).*

INDIA

Lymphatic filariasis is a public health problem in 8 states of India. Heavily infected areas are found in Uttar Pradesh, Bihar, Jharkhand, Andhra Pradesh, Odisha, Telangana, Maharashtra and West Bengal *(5).*

An estimated 670 million people are at risk of lymphatic filariasis infection in 272 endemic districts in 16 states and 4 UTs in India. Mapping was carried out using epidemiological data supplemented by data from filaria control units, filaria clinics, and survey units under the national filaria control programme. Morbidity surveys of filaria cases in the states/UTs revealed 4.94 lakh cases of lymphoedema and 1.48 lakh cases of hydrocele till Dec. 2020 *(5).* The microfilaria survey reports received from 205 districts revealed microfilaria rate of about 0.45 per cent *(6).*

Mass drug administration (MDA) is being implemented in India since year 2004. In 2007 India changed its strategy from delivery of DEC alone to delivery of DEC plus albendazole; since that time, the number of people treated with combination therapy has increased steadily. In 2014, about 86 per cent people at risk were treated with combination drug *(4)*. India has reduced the prevalence of microfilaria to less than 1 per cent in 192 out of 250 implementation units.

Epidemiological determinants

Agent factors

There are at least 8 species of filarial parasites that are specific to man *(7)*. These are shown in Table 1. The first three worms are responsible for lymphatic filariasis; and the rest for "non–lymphatic filariasis". The parasites causing non–lymphatic filariasis will not be described as they are not found in India. Table 2 shows the differences between the microfilariae *(Mf)* of *W. bancrofti* and *B. malayi*.

TABLE 1
Human filarial infections

Organism	Vectors	Disease produced
1. *Wuchereria bancrofti*	Culex Mosquitoes	Lymphatic filariasis
2. *Brugia malayi*	Mansonia —"—	—"— —"—
3. *Brugia timori*	Anopheles —"— Mansonia —"—	—"— —"—
4. *Onchocerca volvulus*	Simulum flies	Subcutaneous; nodules; River blindness
5. *Loa loa*	Chrysops flies	Recurrent, transient subcutaneous swellings
6. *T. perstans*	Culicoides	Probably rarely any clinical illness
7. *T. streptocerca*	Culicoides	—"—
8. *Mansonella ozzardi*	Culicoides	—"—

TABLE 2
Differences between *Mf* of *W. bancrofti* and *B. malayi*

	Mf. W. bancrofti	*Mf. B. malayi*
1. General appearance	Graceful, sweeping curves	Crinkled, secondary curves
2. Length	244 to 296 μ	177 to 230 μ
3. Fee cephalic space	As long as broad	Nearly twice as long as broad
4. Excretory pore	Not prominent	Prominent
5. Caudal end	Uniformly tapering to a delicate point, No terminal nuclei present	Kinkled and two terminal nuclei present
6. Nuclear column	Nuclei discrete	Smudged

PERIODICITY

The *Mf* of *W. bancrofti* and *B.malayi* occurring in India display a nocturnal periodicity, i.e., they appear in large numbers at night and retreat from the blood stream during the day. This is a biological adaptation to the nocturnal biting habits of the vector mosquitoes. The maximum density of *Mf* in blood is reported between 10 pm and 2 am. When the sleeping habits of the host are altered, a reversal in periodicity has been observed.

In most parts of the world, *Mf* are nocturnally periodic but in the South Pacific islands and in limited foci in the Nicobar islands, Thailand and Vietnam, *W. bancrofti Mf* are non–periodic (sub-periodic), being detectable throughout the 24 hours with a slight peak during day or night. Sub-periodic *B.malayi* is found in parts of Malaysia and Indonesia.

LIFE CYCLE

Man is the definitive host and mosquito the intermediate host of Bancroftian and Brugian filariasis. The adult worms are usually found in the lymphatic system of man. The males are about 40 mm long and the females 50 to 100 mm long. The females are viviparous. They give birth to as many as 50,000 *Mf* per day *(8)* which find their way into blood circulation *via* the lymphatics. The life span of the *Mf* is not exactly known, probably up to a year or more. The adult worms may survive for 15 years or more *(8)*. There is a case on record of a woman, in whom live *Mf* were present 40 years after she left an endemic area *(9)*.

The mosquito cycle begins when the *Mf* are picked up by the vector mosquito during feeding. The following stages of development take place in the vector : *(a) Exsheathing :* The larva comes out of the sheath in which it is enclosed, within 1 to 2 hours of ingestion. This is known as exsheathing which takes place in the stomach of the mosquito. *(b) First stage larva :* After exsheathing, the larva is able to penetrate the stomach wall of the mosquito which it does in 6 to 12 hours and migrate to the thoracic muscles where it grows and develops into a sausage–shaped (short, thick) form. *(c) Second stage larva :* The larva moults and increases in length (long, thick form) with the development of an alimentary canal, but is relatively inactive. *(d) Third stage larva :* There is a final moult to the third stage or infective larva (long, thin form) which may be found in any part of the insect. It is highly active or motile. When it migrates to the proboscis of the mosquito, it is ready to be transmitted to a new host, and the mosquito is said to be infective. Under optimum conditions of temperature and humidity, the duration of mosquito cycle (extrinsic incubation period) is between 10 and 14 days. In the human host, the infective larvae develop into adult male and female worms.

RESERVOIR OF INFECTION

Although filarial infections occur in animals, human filariasis is not usually a zoonosis (sub-periodic *B. malayi* and *T. perstans* are exceptions). Animal reservoirs of Brugia are present in monkeys, cats and dogs *(8);* these animals are believed to acquire their infections from man, and they are not regarded as important sources of infection to man *(1)*. There is no evidence that *W. bancrofti* has animal reservoirs in India.

In humans the source of infection is a person with circulating *Mf* in peripheral blood. In filarial disease (late obstructive stages) *Mf* are not found in the blood.

The minimum level of *Mf* which will permit infection of mosquitoes is not known. It was reported that a man with one *Mf* per 40 cu. mm of blood was infective to 2.6 per cent of the mosquitoes which fed on him *(10)*. On the other hand, when mosquitoes were fed on carriers having as many as 80 or more *Mf* per 20 cu. mm of blood, the heavily infected mosquitoes did not survive when a number of *Mf* began to reach maturity *(11)*.

Host factors

Man is a natural host. (a) AGE: All ages are susceptible to infection. In endemic areas, filarial infection has been found even in infants aged less than 6 months. Infection rates rise with age up to the age of 20–30 years and then level off.

After a few years at this plateau level, *Mf* rates may decline in middle and old age. Filarial disease appears only in a small percentage of infected individuals, commonly in the age group over 10 years *(12)*, although there may be exceptions. (b) SEX : In most endemic areas the *Mf* rate is higher in men. (c) MIGRATION : The movement of people from one place to another has led to the extension of filariasis into areas previously non–endemic. (d) IMMUNITY : Man may develop resistance to infection only after many years of exposure *(8)*. The immunological basis of this resistance is not known *(13)*. (e) SOCIAL FACTORS : Lymphatic filariasis is often associated with urbanization, industrialization, migration of people, illiteracy, poverty and poor sanitation.

Environmental factors

(a) CLIMATE : Climate is an important factor in the epidemiology of filariasis. It influences the breeding of mosquitoes, their longevity and also determines the development of the parasite in the insect vector. The maximum prevalence of *Culex quinquefasciatus* (previously known as *C. fatigans*) was observed when the temperature was between 22 to 38 deg. C and optimum longevity when the relative humidity was 70 per cent. (b) DRAINAGE: Lymphatic filariasis is associated with bad drainage. The vectors breed profusely in polluted water. (c) TOWN PLANNING : Inadequate sewage disposal and lack of town planning have aggravated the problem of filariasis in India by increasing the facilities for the breeding of *C. quinquefasciatus (C. fatigans)*. The common breeding places are cesspools, soakage pits, ill–maintained drains, septic tanks, open ditches, burrow pits, etc.

Vectors of lymphatic filariasis

All three infections *(W. bancrofti, B. malayi and B. timori)* are transmitted to man by the bites of infective mosquitoes. No less than 5 genera are involved in different areas of the world – *Culex, Anopheles* and Aedes serve as vectors for *W. bancrofti;* and *Mansonia, Anopheles* and *Coquillettidia* serve as the vectors of the Brugia species.

The main vectors in India are : *C. quinquefasciatus (C. fatigans)* for Bancroftian filariasis, and *Mansonia (Mansonoides)* mosquitoes *(e.g., M. annulifers and M. uniformis)* for Brugian filariasis. The breeding of *Mansonia* mosquitoes is associated with certain aquatic plants such as *Pistia stratiotes.* In the absence of these plants, these mosquitoes cannot breed.

Mode of transmission

Filariasis is transmitted by the bite of infected vector mosquitoes. The parasite is deposited near the site of puncture. It passes through the punctured skin or may penetrate the skin on its own and finally reach the lymphatic system. The dynamics of transmission depends upon the man–mosquito contact (e.g., infective biting rate).

Incubation period

The time interval between inoculation of infective larvae and the first appearance of detectable *Mf* is known as "pre–patent period". Direct information on the duration of the prepatent period is lacking *(14)*.

The time interval from invasion of infective larvae to the development of clinical manifestations is known as the "clinical incubation period". This period, most commonly, is 8 to 16 months. This period may, however, be longer *(14)*.

Clinical manifestations

Only a small proportion of infected individuals exhibit clinical signs. The disease manifestations can be divided into two distinct clinical types : (a) *lymphatic filariasis* caused by the parasite in the lymphatic system, and (b) *occult filariasis* caused by an immune hyper-responsiveness of the human host (e.g., tropical pulmonary eosinophilia).

1. LYMPHATIC FILARIASIS

The following stages have been described *(14)*:

(i) Asymptomatic amicrofilaraemia : In all endemic areas a proportion of population does not show *Mf* or clinical manifestations of the disease although they have the same degree of exposure to infective larvae as those who become infected. With presently available diagnostic procedures it is not possible to determine whether persons in this group have detectable infections or whether they are free from infection.

(ii) Asymptomatic microfilaraemia : A considerable proportion of people are asymptomatic, although their blood is positive for *Mf.* They may remain without any symptoms for months – in some instances for years. They are an important source of infection in the community. These carriers are usually detected by night blood examination.

(iii) Stage of acute manifestations : In the first months and years there are recurrent episodes of acute inflammation in lymph glands and vessels. The clinical manifestations comprise filarial fever, lymphangitis, lymphadenitis, lymphoedema of the various parts of the body and of epididymo-orchitis in the male.

(iv) Stage of chronic obstructive lesions : The chronic stage usually develops 10–15 years from the onset of the first acute attack. This phase is due to fibrosis and obstruction of lymphatic vessels causing permanent structural changes.

In chronic Bancroftian filariasis, the main clinical features are hydrocele, elephantiasis and chyluria. Elephantiasis may affect the legs, scrotum, arms, penis, vulva and breasts, usually in that order of decreasing frequency. The prevalence of chyluria is usually very low.

The Brugian filariasis is generally similar to Bancroftian filariasis, but strangely the genitalia are rarely involved, except in areas where Brugian filariasis occurs together with Bancroftian filariasis.

Not all elephantiasis is caused by lymphatic filarial infection. Even in endemic areas, a small proportion of cases may be due to other causes – i.e., due to obstructions following infections (such as tuberculosis), tumours, surgery or irradiation *(14)*. In Ethiopia, endemic leg elephantiasis is caused by silica in the iliac lymph glands *(15)*.

2. OCCULT FILARIASIS

The term occult or cryptic filariasis refers to filarial infections in which the classical clinical manifestations are not present and *Mf* are not found in the blood. Occult filariasis is believed to result from a hypersensitivity reaction to filarial antigens derived from *Mf.* The best known example is tropical pulmonary eosinophilia.

Lymphoedema management *(16)*

The recommended management of lymphoedema in areas where lymphatic filariasis is endemic involves simple activities that have demonstrated their effectiveness in significantly improving the quality of life of patients. These activities include providing early detection of lymphoedema, caring for the skin by washing and drying the affected limb or area, preventing and treating entry lesions and providing lymph drainage by elevating the limb and exercising. These are the minimum activities that need to be undertaken, and there is a standard care beyond this that can be accessed where available.

Since the prevention and management of disability caused by lymphatic filariasis is now viewed as public health issue, the guidelines for the first level care worker developed by WHO to manage acute dermato-lymphangio adenitis (ADLA) are as follows:

1. TREATMENT FOR UNCOMPLICATED ADLA

a. Give analgesic such as paracetamol (1g given 3–4 times a day);
b. Give oral antibiotic such as amoxicillin (1.5g in 3 divided doses or oral penicillin) for at least 8 days. In case of allergy to penicillin, oral erythromycin (1g given 3 times a day) can be used;
c. Clean the limb with antiseptic;
d. Check for any wounds, cuts, abscesses and interdigital infection (especially between the toes). Clean with antiseptic, if any present. If local superficial skin infection is found give antibiotic cream, apply antifungal cream if interdigital infection is present;
e. Give advice about prevention of chronic lymphoedema caused by lymphatic filariasis;
f. Do not give antifilarial medicine.
g. Home management includes drinking plenty of water, rest, elevation of the limb, wriggling the toes, cooling the limb with cold water and washing the limb if the patient can do it; and
h. Follow-up after 2 days at home. If situation does not improve, then refer the patient to physician.

2. MANAGEMENT OF SEVERE ADLA

a. Refer the patient to physician immediately to receive recommended antibiotic treatment
   - Intravenous benzylpenicillin (Penicillin G) 5 million units given 3 times a day or intramuscular procain benzylpenicillin 5 million units given 2 times/day until fever subsides, then give oral phenoxymethylpenicillin (penicillin V) 750 mg (1.2 million units) to 1g (1.6 million units) given 3 times/day. The minimum total treatment is atleast for 8 days.
   - In case of allergy to penicillin give IV erythromycin 1g 3 times/day until fever subsides, then give oral erythromycin 1g given 3 times/day or give other antibiotic according to local situation.
b. Give analgesic / antipyretic such as paracetamol;
c. Do not give any antifilarial medicine.

Hydrocele management

In the management of hydrocele, the objective of any lymphatic filariasis disability prevention programme should be to increase access to hydrocelectomy. One of the first activities of the programme should be to detect scrotal swelling using an existing community survey (such as enumeration of mass drug administration or other health initiatives). Individuals with scrotal swelling should be referred to a facililty for diagnosis, and if necessary for surgery.

FILARIA SURVEY

The size of the sample to be examined in a filaria survey varies with the type of survey, whether it is a routine survey or survey for evaluation. The NICD (National Institute of Communicable Diseases, Delhi) standard is to examine 5–7 per cent of the population for routine surveys, and at least 20 per cent for evaluation studies. The sample must be random, representative and cover all ages and both sexes. Statistical advice should be obtained when surveys are being planned. A standardized schedule for conducting filaria surveys is given in a WHO Expert Committee Report on Filariasis *(17)*. A filaria survey comprises the following elements :

1. MASS BLOOD SURVEY

The definitive diagnosis of lymphatic filariasis depends upon the demonstration of living parasites in the human body. This calls for a night blood survey.

(i) The thick film : The thick film made from capillary blood is still the most commonly used method for epidemiological assessment. 20 cu. mm of blood is collected by a deep finger prick between 8.30 pm and 12 mid-night. A thick smear is prepared on a glass slide, and the slide is dried and serially numbered. The age, sex and other host factors are recorded on the survey card or register. On the next day or so, the blood films are dehaemoglobanized, stained, dried and examined for *Mf* under low power. The usual technique for enumeration of *Mf* on slides is to start at one end of the smear and work across to the other end, moving the slide field by field till the smear is covered.

(ii) Membrane filter concentration (MFC) methods : The most sensitive method currently available for detecting low-density microfilaraemia in the blood is by concentration techniques. It requires collection of blood by venepuncture and filtering large volumes of blood. Although MFC is the most sensitive method available, some very-low-density carriers will still not be detected *(14)*.

(iii) DEC provocation test : Mf can be induced to appear in blood in the daytime by administering diethylcarbamazine (DEC) 100 mg orally. *Mf* begin to reach their peak within 15 minutes and begin to decrease 2 hours later. The blood may be examined one hour after administration of DEC.

2. CLINICAL SURVEY

At the same time when blood is collected, the people are examined for clinical manifestations of filariasis which should be recorded in the suggested schedule.

3. SEROLOGICAL TESTS

Serological tests to detect antibodies to *Mf* and adults using immunofluorescent and complement–fixing techniques cannot distinguish between past and present infection, and heavy and light parasite loads in the human hosts *(18)*. Recent interest has focussed on the direct detection of parasite antigens in patient's blood or urine *(14)*.

4. XENODIAGNOSIS

The mosquitoes are allowed to feed on the patient, and then dissected 2 weeks later *(9)*. Where other techniques may fail, this may succeed in detecting low–density microfilaraemia.

5. ENTOMOLOGICAL SURVEY

This comprises of general mosquito collection from houses, dissection of female vector species for detection of developmental forms of the parasite, a study of the extent and type of breeding places and other bionomics of mosquitoes.

The data are assembled, analyzed and the results are expressed in terms of certain parameters (clinical, parasitological and entomological) as described below.

ASSESSMENT OF FILARIA CONTROL PROGRAMMES

The effect of filariasis control can be assessed using clinical, parasitological and entomological methods. These are :

1. CLINICAL PARAMETERS

The clinical parameters measured are the incidence of acute manifestations (adeno-lymphangitis, epididymo-orchitis, etc), and the prevalence of chronic manifestations (lymphoedema, elephantiasis, hydrocele, chyluria, etc).

2. PARASITOLOGICAL PARAMETERS

These are : (a) MICROFILARIA RATE : It is the percentage of persons showing *Mf* in their peripheral blood (20 cu. mm) in the sample population, one slide being taken from each person. Specify the species of the parasite. (b) FILARIAL ENDEMICITY RATE : It is the percentage of persons examined showing microfilariae in their blood, or disease manifestation or both. (c) MICROFILARIAL DENSITY : It is the number of *Mf* per unit volume (20 cu. mm) of blood in samples from individual persons. It indicates the intensity of infection. (d) AVERAGE INFESTATION RATE : It is the average number of *Mf* per positive slide, each slide being made from 20 cu.mm of blood. It indicates the prevalence of microfilaraemia in the population.

3. ENTOMOLOGICAL PARAMETERS

These comprise : (a) vector density per 10 man–hour catch (b) percentage of mosquitoes positive for all stages of development (c) percentage of mosquitoes positive for infective (stage III) larvae (d) the annual biting rate – for assessment of transmission (e) types of larval breeding places, etc.

The above parameters help to measure the conditions existing before and after control procedures began, and also to measure the progress of the control campaign against vectors from time to time.

CONTROL MEASURES

The current strategy of filariasis control is based on :

1. Chemotherapy
2. Vector control

Many years of experience with DEC chemotherapy has shown that, even after the full regimen of treatment, some microfilariae still persist in the body. Due to this and other reasons (e.g., toxic effects), it has not been possible to prevent the spread of filariasis by the administration of DEC alone. Chemotherapy must, therefore, be supplemented by an effective vector control programme, if the disease transmission has to be effectively prevented.

1. Chemotherapy

a. Diethylcarbamazine

Diethylcarbamazine (DEC) is both safe and effective. The dose of DEC that is most generally accepted for the treatment of Bancroftian filariasis is 6 mg/kg body weight per day orally for 12 days, given preferably in divided doses after meals. This amounts to a total of 72 mg of DEC per kg of body weight as a full treatment. For Brugian filariasis, recommended doses range from 3 to 6 mg of DEC/kg body weight per day, up to a total dose of 36–72 mg DEC/kg body weight as a full treatment *(14)*.

DEC is rapidly absorbed after oral administration, reaching peak blood levels in 1–2 hours. It is also rapidly excreted – the blood half-life is only 2–3 hours in alkaline urine and about 10–20 hours in acid urine.

DEC causes rapid disappearance of *Mf* from the circulation. It is effective in killing *Mf* The effect of the drug on the adult worm is uncertain. It has probably no effect on the infective stage larvae.

Toxic reactions :

DEC may produce severe side reactions. The reactions may be of two kinds : (a) those due to the drug itself, e.g., headache, nausea, vomiting, dizziness, etc, These reactions are observed a few hours after the first dose of DEC and generally do not last for more than 3 days, and (b) those which are allergic reactions due to destruction of microfilariae and adult worms, e.g., fever, local inflammations around dead worms, orchitis, lymphadenitis, transient lymphoedema and hydrocele. The local reactions tend to occur later in the course of treatment and to last longer. If the drug is given in spaced doses, systemic reactions are much less frequent and less intense after the second dose and are rare after subsequent doses. These reactions disappear spontaneously and interruption of treatment is not necessary.

b. Filaria control in the community

There are three reasons why filariasis never causes explosive epidemics : (a) the parasite does not multiply in the insect vector, (b) the infective larvae do not multiply in the human host, and (c) the life cycle of the parasite is relatively long, 15 years or more. These factors favour the success of control programme *(14)*.

The administration of DEC can be carried out in various ways :

(i) Preventive chemotherapy (2)

Elimination of lymphatic filariasis is possible by stopping the spread of the infection. Large-scale treatment involves a single dose of 2 medicines given annually to an entire at-risk population in the following way: albendazole (400 mg) together with either ivermectin (150–200 mcg/kg) or with diethylcarbamazine citrate (DEC) (6 mg/kg). These medicines have a limited effect on adult parasites but effectively reduce the density of microfilariae in the bloodstream and prevent the spread of parasites to mosquitoes. This recommended large-scale treatment strategy is called preventive chemotherapy when conducted annually for 4–6 years, and it can interrupt the transmission cycle.

(ii) Selective treatment

DEC is given only to those who are *Mf* positive. It is generally accepted that selective treatment may be more suitable in areas of low endemicity than in highly endemic areas.

The strategy is based on detection and treatment of human carriers and filaria cases. The recommended dose is 6 mg DEC per kg of body weight daily for 12 doses, to be completed in 2 weeks (i.e., 6 days in a week). In endemic areas, treatment must be repeated at specified intervals, usually every 2 years. This is partly because, despite remarkable antimicrofilarial properties, expected microfilaria clearance with DEC is incomplete at times even after adequate treatment. The other reason is that people living in endemic areas are exposed to reinfection.

(iii) DEC–medicated salt

The use of DEC–medicated salt is a special form of mass treatment using very low doses of the drug over a long period of time. Common salt medicated with 1–4 g of DEC per kg has been used for filariasis control in some endemic areas of *W. bancrofti* and *B. malayi*, particularly after an initial reduction in prevalence has been achieved by mass or selective treatment of *Mf* carriers. Treatment should be continued for at least 6 to 9 months. In the Lakshadweep islands, this regimen has been shown to be safe, cheap and effective *(14)*.

The combination of the long life of the adult parasite for several years and infectiousness of a patient with low parasitaemia represents a serious obstacle to control programmes based on chemotherapy alone *(19)*.

c. Ivermectin

Ivermectin is a semisynthetic macrolide antibiotic with a broad spectrum of activity against a variety of nematodes and ectoparasites. The dose is 150–200 μg/kg of body weight

There is no drug toxicity in normal persons. However, in microfilaraemic patients there may be a variety of reactions as a result of inflammatory response triggered by the cleared and dying microfilariae.

2. Vector control

Where mass treatment with DEC is impracticable, the control of filariasis must depend upon vector control. Vector control may also be beneficial when used in conjunction with mass treatment. The most important element in vector control is the reduction of the target mosquito population in order to stop or reduce transmission quickly. The techniques for controlling mosquitoes are given in chapter 14. Briefly they are :

I. Antilarval measures

The ideal method of vector control would be elimination of breeding places by providing adequate sanitation and underground waste-water disposal system. This involves considerable expenditure amounting to several crores of rupees. Because of financial constraints, this may not be feasible in developing countries such as India in the near future. For the time being, therefore, vector control must be based on temporary or recurrent methods.

The current approach in India is to restrict the antilarval measures to urban areas, because it is operationally difficult and very costly to cover the vast rural areas of the country. The urban areas include an extra 3–km peripheral belt because the flight range of *Culex quinquefasciatus (C. fatigans)* is about 3 km.

The anti-larval activities comprise the following *(20)*.

(1) CHEMICAL CONTROL : *(a) Mosquito larvicidal oil :* Mosquito larvicidal oil (MLO) is active against all preadult stages. It has been the main chemical used to control *C. quinquefasciatus* for some time. Since it has proved to be less efficient under field conditions and more expensive than other chemical preparations, it is being replaced by pyrethrum oil, temephos and fenthion. *(b) Pyrosene oil– E :* This is a pyrethrum–based emulsifiable larvicide. The emulsion concentrate contains 0.1 to 0.2 per cent pyrethrins by weight and is required to be diluted with water before use. The emulsion is diluted in the ratio of 1:4, *(c) Organophosphorus larvicides :* During the past 10 years, organophosphorus larvicides (e.g., temephos, fenthion) have been widely used with successful results. However, the vector mosquito has developed resistance to many of these chemicals. The frequency of application is once weekly on all breeding places.

(2) REMOVAL OF PISTIA PLANT : In the case of Mansonia mosquitoes, breeding is best controlled by removing the supporting aquatic vegetation such as the pistia plant from all water collections and converting the ponds to fish or lotus culture. Alternatively, certain herbicides such as phenoxylene 30 or Shell Weed Killer D may be used for destroying the aquatic vegetation.

(3) MINOR ENVIRONMENTAL MEASURES : Larvicidal operations are complemented by minor engineering operations such as filling up of ditches and cesspools, drainage of stagnant water, adequate maintenance of septic tanks and soakage pits, etc. Environmental management is the most efficient approach to the problem of controlling mosquito breeding.

II. Anti-adult measures

The vector mosquitoes of filariasis have become resistant to DDT, HCH and dieldrin. The use of these compounds for indoor residual spraying, tried earlier, has been discontinued. Pyrethrum, as a space spray, still holds promise. It is useful as a temporary means of personal protection, but has no practical value in present–day vector control programmes.

III. Personal prophylaxis

The most effective preventive measure is avoidance of mosquito bites (reduction of man–mosquito contact) by using mosquito nets. Screening of houses can substantially reduce transmission, but it is expensive.

Integrated vector control

None of the above vector control measures applied alone is likely to bring about sustained control of filariasis vectors. An integrated or combined approach is needed to control filariasis using all the above strategies and approaches in optimum combination.

In filariasis four major breakthroughs have occurred. The first of these is the development of safe, single dose, annual drug treatment. Trials have proved that a single dose of DEC is very effective even two years after treatment. A single dose of ivermectin has proved to be equally effective. A combination of single dose of both drugs reduced microfilaraemia more than 95 per cent, 2 years after treatment. Secondly, intensive local hygiene on the affected limb, with or without the use of antibiotic and antifungal creams, has shown to have dramatic effects by halting the progression of, or even reversing elephantiasis and lymphoedema. Thirdly, DEC–medicated tablet or cooking salt has been introduced in India. The carefully controlled addition of very low concentration of DEC has long been recognized as an effective means of eliminating lymphatic filariasis infections in communities. However, the addition increases the price of the salt. During 1994, the first commercially prepared DEC salt went on sale in India, at about twice the price of ordinary salt. Finally, there has been the development of insecticide sprays and polystyrene beads to seal latrines and roof-top water-storage tanks, to eliminate or reduce populations of urban culex mosquitoes.

National Filaria Control Programme

Please see chapter 7 for details.

References

1. *Lancet* (1985), i : 1135.
2. WHO (2018), *Fact Sheet*, 8th Oct., 2018.
3. WHO (2019), *Fact Sheet lymphatic filariasis*, 6th Oct., 2019.
4. WHO (2012), *Weekly Epidemiological Record*, No. 37, 14th Sept., 2012.
5. Govt. of India (2022), *Annual Report 2021–2022*, Ministry of Health and Family Welfare, New Delhi.
6. Govt. of India (2016), *Annual Report 2015–2016*, Ministry of Health and Family Welfare, New Delhi.
7. Dissanaike, A.S. (1979). *Bull WHO*, 57 (3) 349.
8. Nelson, G.S. (1981). *Medicine International*, 2 : 77.
9. Carme, B. et al. (1979).*Am. J. Trop. Med. Hyg.*, 28 : 53.
10. Hawking, F. (1962). *Bull WHO*, 27 : 566.
11. Omri, N. (1962). *Bull WHO*, 27 : 586.
12. Raghavan, N.G.S. (1969). *J. Com. Dis.*, 1 (2) 75–98.
13. Subramanyam, D. (1976). *J. Com. Dis.*, 8 : 137–141.
14. WHO (1984). *Techn. Rep. Ser.*, No.702.
15. Price, E.W. and Henderson, W.J. (1979). *Trans. R. Soc. Trop. Med. Hyg.*, 73 : 640–7.
16. WHO (2006), *Weekly Epidemiological Record* No. 40, 6th Oct 2006.
17. WHO (1974). *Techn. Rep. Ser.*, No.542.
18. Ottesen, E.A. (1984). *Trans. R. Soc. Trop. Med. Hyg.*, 78 (Suppl) 9–18.
19. Tmeuse and McMahon, J.E. (1981). *Trans. Roy. Soc. Trop. Med. Hyg.*, 75 : 835.
20. Govt. of India (2008), *Annual Report 2007-08*, Ministry of Health and Family Welfare, New Delhi.

ZIKA VIRUS DISEASE

Zika virus is a mosquito-borne flavivirus that was first identified in Uganda in 1947 through a network that monitored yellow fever. The first large outbreak of disease caused by Zika infection was reported from Island of Yap in 2007. In July 2015, Brazil reported an association between Zika virus infection and Guillain–Barre Syndrome. In October 2015, Brazil reported an association between Zika virus infection and microcephaly *(1)*.

Problem statement

Currently, WHO has reported 22 countries and territories in Americas from where local transmission of Zika virus has been reported. Zika virus disease has the potential for further international spread given the wide geographical distribution of the mosquito vector, a lack of immunity among population in newly affected areas and the high volume of international travel. As of now, the disease has not been reported in India. However, the mosquito that transmits Zika virus, namely Aedes aegypti, that also transmits dengue virus, is widely prevalent in India *(1, 2)*.

Agent factor

Zika virus disease is caused by Zika virus which belongs to the genre Flavivirus. This virus is transmitted by the bite from an infected mosquito hence also called arbovirus. The reservoir of infection is not known *(3)*.

Mode of transmission

Zika virus is transmitted through the bite of an infected mosquito from the Aedes genus, mainly Aedes aegypti, which usually bite during the morning and late afternoon hours. Transmission from an infected pregnant mother to her baby during pregnancy or around the time of birth is also now being seen as a distinct possibility.

Clinical picture

The incubation period of Zika virus disease is not clear, but is likely to be a few days. The symptoms are similar to other arbovirus infections such as dengue, and include fever, skin rashes, conjunctivitis, muscle and joint pain, malaise, and headache. These symptoms are usually mild and last for 2–7 days. Only one out of four infected people develops symptoms of the disease. Zika virus disease should be suspected in patients reporting with acute onset of fever, maculo-papular rash and arthralgia, among those individuals who travelled to areas with ongoing transmission during the two weeks preceding the onset of illness. Based on the available information of previous outbreaks, severe forms of disease requiring hospitalization is uncommon and fatalities are rare *(1, 3)*.

Diagnosis

Zika virus is diagnosed through PCR(polymerase chain reaction) and virus isolation from blood samples. Diagnosis by serology is not recommended.

Prevention

Aedes mosquitoes and their breeding sites pose a significant risk factor for Zika virus infection. Prevention and control relies on reducing mosquitoes through source reduction (removal and modification of breeding sites) and reducing contact between mosquitoes and people.

Treatment

Zika virus disease is usually relatively mild and requires no specific treatment. People sick with Zika virus should get plenty of rest, drink enough fluids, and treat pain and fever with paracetamol. If symptoms worsen, they should seek medical care and advice. There is currently no vaccine available.

NCDC, Delhi and National Institute of Virology (NIV), Pune, have the capacity to provide laboratory diagnosis of Zika virus disease in acute febrile stage. These two institutions would be the apex laboratories to support the outbreak investigation and for confirmation of laboratory diagnosis. Ten additional laboratories would be strengthened by ICMR to expand the scope of laboratory diagnosis. RT–PCR test would remain the standard test. As of now there is no commercially available test for Zika virus disease *(2)*.

References

1. WHO (2016), *Weekly Epidemiological Record*, No. 24, 17th June 2016.
2. Govt. of India (2016), *Guidelines on Zika Virus Disease*, 2nd Feb. 2016, Ministry of Health and Family Welfare, New Delhi.
3. WHO (2016), *Fact sheet on Zika Virus Disease*, Feb. 2016.

IV. ZOONOSES

Zoonotic diseases have been known since antiquity. Bubonic plague and rabies were known since biblical times. The discovery of causative agents during the "golden era" of microbiology called attention principally to diseases exclusively pathogenic to man. Zoonotic diseases were overshadowed by diseases peculiar to man alone. Only as human infections came under better control was attention drawn to zoonotic diseases.

More than 150 zoonoses have been recognized. In recent years, several new zoonotic diseases have emerged e.g. KFD, Monkey Pox etc., Quite apart from the morbidity and mortality they cause, zoonoses are responsible for great economic losses, particularly in animals, meat, milk and other foods and products of animal origin. The developing countries suffer much more severe losses than do the industrialized countries, partly because they have less well–developed public health and veterinary services and partly because of their unfavourable climatic and environmental conditions.

Zoonoses and human health are matters of particular concern in India – because nearly 68.86% of India's population is rural and live in close contact with domestic animals, and often not far from wild ones.

Zoonoses have been defined as "Those diseases and infections [the agents of] which are naturally transmitted between [other] vertebrate animals and man." G.S. Nelson has pointed out that it is essential to discuss the direction of transmission, as it is of little value to know that a particular organism is found in both man and animals. What one is really concerned about is its relative significance of man and animals, as maintenance hosts of the particular infection.

The zoonoses have been classified in terms of their reservoir hosts, whether these are men or lower vertebrate animals. Thus, the term anthropo-zoonoses has been applied to infections transmitted to man from lower vertebrate animals. The term zooanthroponoses is applied to infections transmitted from man to lower vertebrate animals; however, these terms have also been used interchangeably for all diseases found in both animals and man. A third term, amphixenoses, has been used for infections maintained in both man and lower vertebrate animals that may be transmitted in either direction.

A classification that is based upon the type of life cycle of the infecting organism and that divides the zoonoses into four categories, each with important shared epidemiologic features, has considerable teaching value.

The four categories are :

(1) Direct zoonoses are transmitted from an infected vertebrate host to a susceptible vertebrate host by direct contact, by contact with a fomite, or by a mechanical vector. The agent itself undergoes little or no propagative changes and no essential developmental change during transmission. Examples are rabies, trichinosis, and brucellosis.

(2) Cyclo–zoonoses require more than one vertebrate host species, but no invertebrate host, in order to complete the developmental cycle of the agent. Examples are the human taeniases, echinococcosis, and pentastomida infections.

(3) Meta-zoonoses are transmitted biologically by invertebrate vectors. In the invertebrate, the agent multiplies or develops, or both, and there is always an extrinsic incubation (prepatent) period before transmission to another vertebrate host is possible. Examples are numerous and include arbovirus infections, plague, and schistosomiasis.

(4) Sapro–zoonoses have both a vertebrate host and a non–animal developmental site or reservoir. Organic matter (including food), soil, and plants are considered to be non–animal. Examples include the various forms of larva migrants and some of the mycoses.

RABIES

Definition

Rabies, also known as *hydrophobia* is an acute, highly fatal viral disease of the central nervous system, caused by *Lyssavirus* type 1. It is primarily a zoonotic disease of warm–blooded animals, particularly carnivorous such as dogs, cats, jackals and wolves. It is transmitted to man usually by bites or licks of rabid animals. Classical hydrophobia is clinically characterized by a long and variable incubation period, a short period of illness due to encephalomyelitis ending in death, despite intensive care. It is the only communicable disease of man that is always fatal.

Problem statement

(i) GEOGRAPHIC DISTRIBUTION

Rabies is an enzootic and epizootic disease of worldwide importance. Some countries have achieved "rabies free" status by vigorous campaigns of elimination, while in others the disease has never been introduced. Geographic boundaries seem to play an important role here. Water appears to be the most effective natural barrier to rabies. Australia, China (Taiwan), Cyprus, Iceland, Ireland, Japan, Malta, New Zealand, the U.K. and the islands of Western Pacific are all free of the disease. The Liberian peninsula and Finland, Norway and Sweden are also rabies free *(1)*. In India, Union Territory of Lakshadweep and Andman and Nicobar islands are free of the disease *(2)*. A "Rabies-free" area has been defined as one in which no case of indigenously acquired rabies has occurred in man or any animal species for 2 years *(3)*. According to WHO reports, in many countries rabies is spreading inspite of great advances in research and field control methods.

Rabies occurs in more than 150 countries and territories. Although a number of carnivorous and bat species serve as natural reservoir, rabies in dogs is the source of 99 per cent of human infection, and posses a potential threat to more than 3.3 billion people.

In a number of countries, human deaths from rabies are likely to be grossly underreported, particularly in the youngest age groups. Vast majority of the estimated 55,000 deaths caused by rabies each year occur in rural areas of Africa and Asia. In India alone, 20,000 deaths (that is, about 2 per lac population at risk) are estimated to occur annually; in Africa, the corresponding figure is 24,000 (about 4 per lac population at risk) *(4)*.

Although all age groups are susceptible, rabies is most common in children aged less than 15 years; on an average, 40 per cent of post–exposure immunization are given to children aged 5–14 years, and the majority of those immunized are male. In the north–western part of the United Republic of Tanzania, the incidence of rabies was upto 5 times higher in children aged less than 15 years than in adults *(4)*. At the global level, more than 15 million people receive rabies prophylaxis annually, the majority of whom live in China and India. It is estimated that in the absence of post–exposure prophylaxis, about 327,000 persons would die from rabies in Africa and Asia each year *(4)*.

Epidemiological determinants

Agent factors

AGENT : The causative agent (*Lyssavirus* type 1) is a bullet shaped neurotropic RNA containing virus. It belongs to the family rhabdoviridae – serotype 1 (*Lyssavirus,* type 1) and is the causative agent of rabies. Serotype 2, 3 and 4 are *rabies–related* but antigenically distinct viruses; they cause rabies like disease in man and animals *(5)*. Available anti-rabies vaccines may not be effective against the rabies–related viruses *(6)*.

Rabies virus particles contain two distinct, major antigens : a glycoprotein (G protein) antigen from the virus membrane and an internal nucleoprotein antigen. The glycoprotein seems to be the only antigen capable of inducing the formation of virus–neutralizing antibodies *(7)*. The presence of neutralizing antibodies in the blood of man and animals is considered an index of protection against infection with rabies virus *(8)*. Recently, surface glycoprotein of rabies virus has been cloned and expressed in *E. coli* in a bid to develop genetically engineered rabies vaccine.

The virus is excreted in the saliva of the affected animals. The virus recovered from naturally occurring cases of rabies is called *"street virus"*. It is pathogenic for all mammals and shows a long variable incubation period (20–60 days in dogs). Serial brain–to–brain passage of the street virus in rabbits modifies the virus such that its incubation period is progressively reduced until it becomes constant between 4–6 days. Virus isolated at this stage is called a *fixed virus.* A "fixed" strain of virus may be defined as one that has a short, fixed and reproducible incubation period (4–6 days) when injected intracerebrally into suitable animals. It does not form Negri bodies. It no longer multiplies in extra–neural tissues. The *fixed virus* is used in the preparation of antirabies vaccine. There is evidence that *fixed virus* can be pathogenic for humans and mammals under certain conditions, as for example parenteral injection of antirabies vaccine inadequately inactivated *(7)*.

SOURCE OF INFECTION : The source of infection to man is the saliva of rabid animals. In dogs and cats, the virus may be present in the saliva for 3–4 days (occasionally 5–6 days) before the onset of clinical symptoms and during the course of illness till death *(9, 10)*.

Host factors

All warm blooded animals including man are susceptible to rabies. Rabies in man is a dead-end infection, and has no survival value for the virus. The overwhelming number of victims in India belong to the age group 1–24 years *(2)*. Laboratory staff working with rabies virus, veterinarians, dog handlers, hunters and field naturalists face bigger risks of rabies than do general public.

Mode of transmission *(11)*

People are infected following a deep bite or scratch by an infected animal. Dogs are the main host and transmitter of rabies. They are the source of infection in almost all the rabies deaths annually in Asia and Africa.

Bats are the source of most human rabies deaths in the United States of America and Canada. Bat rabies has also recently emerged as a public health threat in Australia, Latin America and western Europe. However in these regions the number of human deaths due to bat rabies remains small compared to deaths following dog bites. Human deaths following exposure to foxes, raccoons, skunks, jackals, mongooses and other wild carnivore host species are very rare.

Transmission can also occur when infectious material – usually saliva – comes into direct contact with human mucosa or fresh skin wounds. Human-to-human transmission by bite is theoretically possible but has never been confirmed.

Rarely, rabies may be contracted by inhalation of virus-containing aerosol or *via* transplantation of an infected organ. Ingestion of raw meat or other tissues from animals infected with rabies is not a source of human infection.

Incubation period

The incubation period in man is highly variable, commonly 1–3 months following exposure but may vary from 7 days to many years *(4)*. The incubation period depends on the site of the bite, severity of the bite, number of wounds, amount of virus injected, species of the biting animal, protection provided by the clothing and treatment undertaken, if any. In general, incubation period tends to be shorter in severe exposures and bites on face, head, neck and upper extremities and bites by wild animals. In no other specific communicable disease is the incubation period so variable and dependant on so many factors as in rabies.

Pathogenesis

Rabies virus replicates in muscle or connective tissue cells at or near the site of introduction before it attaches to nerve endings and enters peripheral nerves. It spreads from the site of infection centripetally *via* the peripheral nerves towards the central nervous system; most likely it "ascends" passively through the nerve associated tissue space *(7)*. Following infection of the central nervous system, the virus spreads centrifugally in peripheral nerves to many tissues, including skeletal and myocardial muscle, adrenal glands and skin. The salivary glands invasion is crucial for the transmission of the virus to another animal or human *(5)*.

RABIES IN MAN

Clinical picture

Rabies in man is called hydrophobia. The disease begins with *prodromal symptoms* such as headache, malaise, sore throat and slight fever lasting for 3–4 days. About 80% of patients complain of pain or tingling at the site of the bite. This is the only prodromal symptom which is considered reasonably specific *(12)*.

The prodromal stage is followed by widespread excitation and stimulation of all parts of nervous system usually involving, in order, the sensory system, the motor system, the sympathetic and mental system. The patient is intolerant to noise, bright light or a cold draught of air (sensory). Aerophobia (fear of air) may be present and is considered by some to be pathognomonic of rabies *(13)*. It can be elicited by fanning a current of air across the face which causes violent spasms of the pharyngeal and neck muscles. Examination may show increased reflexes and muscle spasms (motor) along with dilatation of the pupils and increased perspiration, salivation and lachrimation (sympathetic). Mental changes include fear of death, anger, irritability and depression.

The symptoms are progressively aggravated and all attempts at swallowing liquid become unsuccessful. At later stage the mere sight or sound of water may provoke spasm of the muscles of deglutition. This characteristic symptom of hydrophobia (fear of water) is pathognomonic of rabies and is absent in animals. The duration of illness is 2 to 3 days, but may be prolonged to 5–6 days in exceptional cases. The patient may die abruptly during one of the convulsions or may pass on to the stage of paralysis and coma. Intensive care may allow an occasional patient to survive *(10)*. To-date, only three people are on record who have been stricken with rabies and have survived *(1)*.

Diagnosis

A clinical diagnosis of hydrophobia can be made on the basis of history of bite by a rabid animal and characteristic signs and symptoms.

Rabies can be confirmed in patients early in the illness by antigen detection using immunofluorescence of skin biopsy, and by virus isolation from saliva and other secretions. Immunofluorescence of corneal impression smears has proved unreliable. Neutralizing antibodies are not usually detectable in serum or CSF before the eighth day *(5)*.

Treatment

There is no specific treatment for rabies. Case management includes the following procedure :

(a) The patient should be isolated in a quiet room protected as far as possible from external stimuli such as bright light, noise or cold draughts which may precipitate spasms or convulsions. (b) Relieve anxiety and pain by liberal use of sedatives. Morphia in doses of 30–45 mg may be given repeatedly. The drug is well tolerated and once the diagnosis is established there appears to be no reason to restrict the administration of a drug which does so much to allay acute suffering. (c) If spastic muscular contractions are present use drugs with curare–like action. (d) Ensure hydration and diuresis. (e) Intensive therapy in the form of respiratory and cardiac support may be given.

Patients with rabies are potentially infectious because the virus may be present in the saliva, vomits, tears, urine or other body fluids. Nursing personnel attending rabid patients should be warned against possible risk of contamination and should wear face masks, gloves, goggles and aprons to protect themselves. Persons having bruises, cuts or open wounds should not be entrusted to look after the patient. Where human cases of rabies are encountered frequently pre-exposure prophylaxis is recommended.

PREVENTION OF HUMAN RABIES

This may be considered under 3 heads.

a. Post-exposure prophylaxis.
b. Pre-exposure prophylaxis.
c. Post-exposure treatment of persons who have been vaccinated previously.

POST-EXPOSURE PROPHYLAXIS

1. General consideration

The vast majority of persons requiring anti-rabies treatment are those who were bitten by a suspected rabid animal. The aim of post-exposure prophylaxis is to neutralize the inoculated virus before it can enter the nervous system. Every instance of human exposure should be treated as a medical emergency. It is now well established that irrespective of the class of wound, the combined administration of a single dose of rabies immunoglobulin if indicated with a course of vaccine, together with local treatment of the wound is the best specific prophylactic treatment after exposure of man to rabies.

2. Local treatment of wound

Prompt and adequate local treatment of all bite wounds and scratches is the first requisite and is of utmost importance. The purpose of local treatment is to remove as much virus as possible from the site of inoculation before it can be absorbed on nerve endings. Local treatment of wounds is of maximal value when applied immediately after exposure (within minutes if possible) but it should not be neglected if several hours or days have elapsed *(3)*. Animal experiments have shown that local wound treatment can reduce the chances of developing rabies by upto 80% *(6)*. The local treatment comprises the following measures :

(a) Cleansing : Immediate flushing and washing the wound(s), scratches and the adjoining areas with plenty of soap and water, preferably under a running tap, for at least 15 minutes is of paramount importance in the prevention of human rabies. If soap is not available, simple flushing of the wounds with plenty of water should be done as first-aid. In case of punctured wounds, catheters, should be used to irrigate the wounds. This procedure is now standard worldwide. It does minimize the risk of contracting rabies. Unfortunately, very few patients get it in right time.

(b) Chemical treatment : Whatever residual virus remains in the wound(s), after cleansing, should be inactivated by irrigation with *virucidal* agents – either alcohol (400–700 ml/litre), tincture or 0.01% aqueous solution of iodine or povidone iodine.

(c) Suturing : Bite wounds should not be immediately sutured to prevent additional trauma which may help spread the virus into deeper tissues. If suturing is necessary, it should be done 24–48 hours later, applying minimum possible stitches, under the cover of rabies immunoglobulin locally.

(d) Antibiotics and anti-tetanus measure : The application of antibiotics and antitetanus procedures when indicated should follow the local treatment recommended above.

3. Immunization

Since their development more than four decades ago, concentrated and purified cell-culture vaccine (CCV) and embryonated egg-based vaccine (EEV) have proved to be safe and effective in preventing rabies. These vaccines are intended for pre-exposure as well as post-exposure prophylaxis.

The internationally available cell-culture and embryonated egg-based vaccines (CCEEVs) consist of rabies virus that has been propagated in cell substrates such as human diploid cells (embryonic fibroblast cells), fetal rhesus diploid cells, Vero cells (kidney cells from the African green monkey), primary Syrian hamster kidney cells, primary chick embryo cells or in embryonated duck eggs. The more recently developed vaccines based on chick embryo cells and Vero cells have safety and efficacy records comparable to those of the human diploid cell vaccines and are less expensive *(4)*.

Rabies vaccines prequalified by WHO do not contain preservatives such as thimerosal. The shelf-life of these vaccines is ≥ 3 years, provided they are stored at +2°C to +8°C and protected from sunlight. Following reconstitution with the accompanying sterile diluent, the vaccines should be used immediately, or within 6–8 hours if kept at the correct temperature.

All CCEEVs should comply with the WHO recommended potency of ≥ 2.5 IU per single intramuscular dose (0.5 ml or 1.0 ml volume after reconstitution, depending on the type of vaccine).

The guidelines for the post–exposure treatment by the WHO are given in Table 1.

TABLE 1

Categories of contact and recommended post-exposure prophylaxis (PEP)

Categories of contact with suspect rabid animal	Post–exposure prophylaxis measures
Category I – touching or feeding animals, licks on intact skin	None
Category II – nibbling of uncovered skin, minor scratches or abrasions without bleeding	Immediate vaccination and local treatment of the wound
Category III – single or multiple transdermal bites or scratches, licks on broken skin; contamination of mucous membrane with saliva from licks, contacts with bats.	Immediate vaccination and administration of rabies immunoglobulin; local treatment of the wound

Source: *(11)*

All category II and III exposures assessed as carrying a risk of developing rabies require PEP. This risk is increased if *(11)*:

- the biting mammal is a known rabies reservoir or vector species;
- the animal looks sick or has an abnormal behaviour;
- a wound or mucous membrane was contaminated by the animal's saliva;
- the bite was unprovoked;
- the animal has not been vaccinated; and
- if biting animal cannot be traced or identified.

In developing countries, the vaccination status of the suspected animal alone should not be considered when deciding whether to initiate prophylaxis or not.

Post-exposure prophylaxis may be discontinued if the suspected animal is proved by appropriate laboratory examination to be free of rabies or, in the case of domestic dogs, cats or ferrets, the animal remains healthy throughout a 10 day observation period starting from the date of the bite *(4)*.

Intramuscular administration of vaccine for post-exposure prophylaxis

The post-exposure vaccination schedule is based on injecting 1 ml or 0.5 ml (the volume depends on the type of vaccine) into the deltoid muscle (or anterolateral thigh in children aged <2 years) of patients with category II and III exposures. The recommended regimen consists of either a 5-dose or a 4-dose schedule:

(i) *Essen regimen:* the 5-dose regimen prescribes 1 dose on each of days 0, 3, 7, 14, and 28; as shown below

Dose : one IM dose (1.0 or 0.5 ml) into deltoid (or thigh)

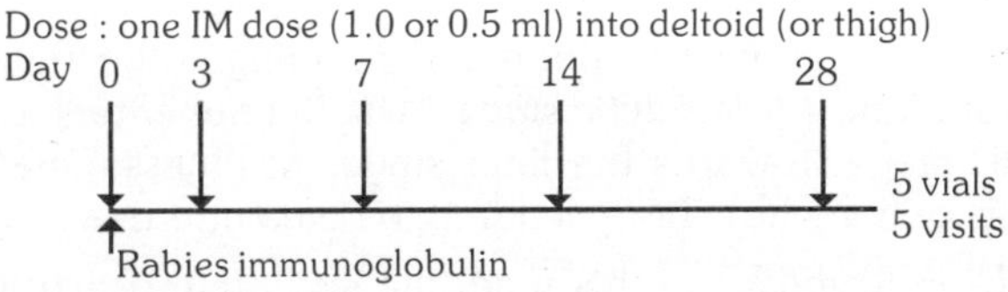

(ii) *Zareb regimen:* the 4-dose abbreviated multisite regimen prescribes 2 doses on day 0 (1 in each of the 2 deltoid or thigh sites) followed by 1 dose on each of days 7 and 21, as shown below.

Abbreviated multisite intramuscular regimen (2-1-1)

Dose : one IM dose (1.0 or 0.5 ml) into deltoid (or thigh)

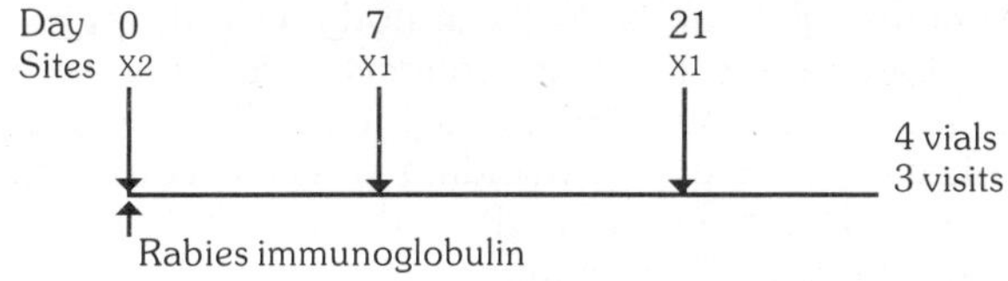

An alternative for healthy, fully immunocompetent, exposed people who receive wound care plus high quality rabies immunoglobulin plus WHO prequalified rabies vaccines, is a post-exposure regimen consisting of 4 doses administered intramuscularly on days 0, 3, 7 and 14.

Intradermal administration for post-exposure prophylaxis

The 2-site regimen prescribes injection of 0.1 ml at 2 sites (deltoid or thigh) on days 0, 3, 7 and 28. The day 14 dose is missed. This regimen may be used for people with category II and III exposures in countries where the intradermal route has been endorsed by national health authorities. The regimen is as shown below:

2-site intradermal regimen (2+2+2+0+2)

Dose : one ID dose = one fifth of IM dose (0.1 ml) ID per site

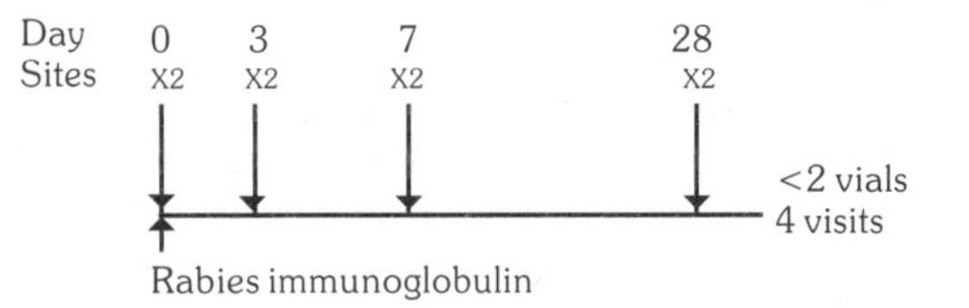

Post-exposure prophylaxis for previously vaccinated individuals

For rabies-exposed patients who can document previous complete pre-exposure vaccination or complete post-exposure prophylaxis with a CCEEV, 1 dose delivered intramuscularly or a CVV delivered intradermally on days 0 and 3 is sufficient. Rabies immunoglobulin is not indicated in such cases. This 1-site 2-day intradermal or intramuscular regimen also applies to people vaccinated against rabies who have demonstrated rabies-virus neutralizing antibody titres of ≥0.5 IU/ml . As an alternative to this regimen, the patient may be offered a single-visit 4-site intradermal regimen consisting of 4 injections of 0.1 ml equally distributed over left and right deltoids or thighs. Vaccination cards recording previous immunizations are invaluable for making correct decisions.

Immunization of immunocompromised individuals

In immunocompromised individuals including patients with HIV/AIDS, a complete series of 5 doses of intramuscular CCEEV in combination with comprehensive wound management and local infiltration with human rabies immunoglobulin is required for patients with category II and III exposures. When feasible, the rabies-virus neutralizing antibody response should be determined 2–4 weeks following vaccination to assess the possible need for an additional dose of the vaccine.

Rabies immunoglobulin for passive immunization

Rabies immunoglobulin for passive immunization is administered only once, preferably at, or as soon as possible after, the initiation of post-exposure vaccination. Beyond the seventh day after the first dose, rabies immunoglobulin is not indicated because an active antibody response to the CCEEV is presumed to have occurred. The dose of human rabies immunoglobulin is 20 IU/kg body weight; for equine immunoglobulin and F (ab')2 products, it is 40 IU/kg body weight. All of the rabies immunoglobulin, or as much as anatomically possible (but avoiding possible compartment syndrome), should be administered into or around the wound site or sites. The remaining immunoglobulin, if any, should be injected intramuscularly at a site distant from the site of vaccine administration. Rabies immunoglobulin may be diluted to a volume sufficient for all wounds to be effectively and safely infiltrated.

Most of the new equine immunoglobulin preparations are potent, highly purified, safe and considerably less expensive than human rabies immunoglobulin. However they are of heterologous origin and carry a small risk of anaphylactic reaction (1/45,000 cases). There are no scientific grounds for performing a skin test prior to administering equine immunoglobulin because testing does not predict reactions, and it should be given whatever the result of the test. The treating physician should be prepared to manage anaphylaxis which, although rare, could occur during any stage of administration *(14)*.

Guide for pre-exposure prophylaxis (PrEP) *(14)*

PrEP may be performed with any of the modern cell-derived vaccines and is recommended for anyone at increased risk of exposure to rabies virus. Traditionally, PrEP is recommended for anyone who is at continual, frequent or increased risk of exposure to the rabies virus either as a result of their residence or occupation (for example laboratory workers dealing with rabies virus and other lyssaviruses, veterinarians and animal handlers). Travellers with extensive outdoor exposure and children living in rural high-risk areas are at particular risk.

PrEP schedule requires intramuscular doses of 1ml or 0.5 ml, depending on the vaccine type, or intradermal administration of 0.1 ml volume per site (one site each day) given on days 0, 7 and 21 or 28. To lead to significant savings, intradermal PrEP sessions should involve enough individuals to utilize all opened vials within 6–8 hours.

Booster doses of rabies vaccines are not required for individuals living in or travelling to high-risk areas who have received a complete primary series of pre-exposure or post–exposure prophylaxis with a CCV. Periodic booster injections are recommended as an extra precaution only for people whose occupation puts them at continual or frequent risk of exposure. If available, antibody monitoring of personnel at risk is preferred to the administration of routine boosters. For people who are potentially at risk of laboratory exposure to high concentrations of live rabies virus, antibody testing should be done every 6 months. Those professionals who are not at continual risk of exposure through their activities, such as certain categories of veterinarians and animal health officers, should have serological monitoring every 2 years. Because vaccine-induced immunity persists in most cases for years, a booster would be recommended only if rabies virus neutralizing antibody titres fall to <0.5 IU/ml.

Adverse events following immunization *(4)*

In general, CCEEVs have been shown to be safe and well tolerated. However, in 35–45% of vaccinees, minor and transient erythema, pain and/or swelling may occur at the site of injection, particularly following intradermal administration of a booster. Mild systemic adverse events following immunization (AEFI), such as transient fever, headache, dizziness and gastrointestinal symptoms, have been observed in 5–15% of vaccinees.

Contraindications and precautions *(4)*

For pre-exposure prophylaxis, previous severe reaction to any components of the vaccine is a contraindication to further use of the same vaccine. Because rabies is a lethal disease, no contraindications exist to post-exposure prophylaxis following high-risk exposure. This is also the case for post-exposure prophylaxis during infancy or pregnancy, and for immunocompromised individuals, including children with HIV/AIDS. People taking chloroquine for malaria treatment or prophylaxis may have a reduced response to intradermal rabies vaccination. These patients should receive the vaccine intramuscularly.

NERVOUS TISSUE VACCINES

Nervous tissue vaccines are crude products capable of causing severe and even fatal reactions. Although apparently effective, they are generally of low or variable potency and are usually administered to exposed subjects in a large number of doses. The current trend is to limit or abandon completely the production of nervous tissue vaccines and replace them by safer and more effective inactivated cell-culture vaccines in both developed and developing countries. Government of India has stopped producing nervous tissue vaccine since 2004.

RABIES IN DOGS

In developing countries over 90% of human deaths from rabies are caused by dog bites and dog rabies control is the key that can lock the door against human rabies.

INCUBATION PERIOD

The incubation period in dogs ranges from 3–8 weeks, but it may be as short as 10 days or as long as a year or more *(15)*.

CLINICAL PICTURE

Rabies in dogs may manifest itself in two forms – Furious rabies and Dumb rabies.

(a) Furious rabies : This is the typical "mad-dog syndrome", characterized by *(i) a change in behaviour :* In animals, the cardinal sign is a change in behaviour. The animal loses its fear of people, becomes very aggressive, bites without provocation and bites unusual objects like sticks, straw and mud *(ii) running amuck:* i.e., tendency to run away from home and wander aimlessly and biting humans and animals who may come in its way *(iii) change in voice :* i.e., the dog barks or growls in a hoarse voice or often unable to bark because of paralysis of laryngeal muscles *(iv) excessive salivation* and foaming at the angle of the mouth, and *(v) Paralytic stage :* The animal enters into a paralytic stage, towards the later stages of illness. There is paralysis of the whole body leading to coma and death.

(b) Dumb rabies : In this type, the excitative or irritative stage is lacking. The disease is predominantly paralytic. The dog withdraws itself from being seen or disturbed. It lapses in to a stage of sleepiness and dies in about 3 days.

Once the symptoms of rabies develop in an animal, it rarely survives more than a week *(16)*.

LABORATORY DIAGNOSIS

The head of the animal is cut off and sent to the nearest testing laboratory, duly packed in ice in an airtight container. Alternatively, the brain may be removed with anti-septic precautions and sent in 50% glycerol–saline for examination *(17)*. This should be done by a qualified or trained person soon after the death of the animal.

Laboratory examination is made by : (a) FLUORESCENT ANTIBODY TEST : This is a highly reliable and the best single test currently available for the rapid diagnosis of rabies viral antigen in infected specimens. This test can establish a highly specific diagnosis within a few hours *(3)*. The accuracy of the test is considered equal to that of isolation of the virus by animal inoculation. If the brain is negative by FRA test, one can assume that the saliva contains no virus, and the bitten person need not be treated. Further, fluorescent antibody titres in clinical rabies have been well in excess of 1:10,000 a feature which helps to distinguish between rabies and vaccine reaction *(18)*. (b) MICROSCOPIC EXAMINATION : Although FRA test has largely supplanted other methods of diagnosis, the microscopic examination of brain tissue for Negri bodies is still a useful method for rapid diagnosis of rabies. The microscopic examination for Negri bodies identifies 75–90% of cases of rabies in dogs. (c) MOUSE INOCULATION TEST : Intracerebral mouse inoculation is still one of the most useful tests in the laboratory diagnosis of rabies. Suckling mice are generally more sensitive for virus isolation. A 10% emulsion of suspected brain tissue is prepared in normal saline and centrifuged at 2000 rpm for 5–10 minutes. 0.03 ml of the supernatant fluid is injected intracerebrally using a tuberculin syringe into at least 4 mice. If infected they show signs of rabies between 6–8 days. The virus can be identified by the FRA test or by the presence of Negri bodies. (d) CORNEAL TEST : Rabies virus antigen can be detected in live animals in corneal impressions or in frozen sections of skin biopsies by the FRA test. A positive result is indicative of rabies, but a negative result does not rule out the possibility of infection *(3)*.

Immunization of dogs

Prophylactic vaccination of dogs against rabies is one of the most important weapons in rabies control *(7)*. Studies have shown that, in general, 80–90% of the dog population is accessible for vaccination, thus confirming that the concept of controlling rabies through mass vaccination is a sound one *(19)*. All dogs should receive primary immunization at the age of 3–4 months and booster doses should be given at regular intervals, according to the type of vaccine used.

(1) *BPL inactivated nervous tissue vaccine (Single dose) :* This is based on 20% suspension of infected sheep brain. The dose is 5 ml for dogs and 3 ml for cats. Revaccination is advised after 6 months, and subsequently every year.

(2) *Modified live virus vaccine :* This is based on 33% chick embryo suspension infected with modified virus. The dose is 3 ml by single injection, and boosters every 3 years. As with the vaccines for human use, the adult-brain vaccines for use in animals should be replaced as soon as possible by cell-culture vaccines *(20)*.

Control of urban rabies

Since dog is the major source of infection, the most logical and cost-effective approach is elimination of stray and ownerless dogs combined with a programme of swift mass immunization, in the shortest possible time, of at least 80% of the entire dog population of the area.

Other methods include (i) registration and licensing of all domestic dogs (ii) restraint of dogs in public places (iii) immediate destruction of dogs and cats bitten by rabid animals (iv) quarantine for about 6 months of imported dogs and (v) health education of people regarding the care of dogs and prevention of rabies.

The discovery that foxes could be immunized against rabies by placing modified live virus vaccine directly into the mouths has generated a new control technique. So far no suitable oral bait is developed for use in dogs *(1)*.

Oral vaccines

The successful introduction of oral vaccines for the immunization of foxes is a great advancement in the rabies prophylaxis of wild life. An attempted live rabies vaccine harmless but immunizing to foxes, is placed in baits and distributed over the foxes habitat. Successful control of wild animal's rabies particularly foxes has been achieved in Canada, Germany and Switzerland by the use of "oral vaccine baits." The technique holds much promise for the future control of rabies not only in foxes but also in other wild life species.

References

1. Debbie, J.G. (1988). *W.H. forum,* 9 (4) 536.
2. Sehgal and R. Bhatia (1985) Rabies : *Current Status and Proposed Control Programmes in India, NICD,* Delhi.
3. WHO (1984). Techn. Rep. Ser. No.709.
4. WHO (2010), *Weekly Epidemiological Record,* No. 32, 6th Aug., 2010.
5. Warrell, D.A., and M.J. Warell (1988) *Medicine International 53 : 2194 May 1988.*
6. Molyneux M.E. (1985) *Medicine Digest* 11 (4) 5; York house, 37 Queen square London, U.K.
7. WHO (1973) *Techn. Rep. Ser.* No. 523.
8. J.B. Campbell, et al (1968). *Bull WHO,* 38 : 373.
9. Christie, A.B. (1980). *Infectious Diseases : Epidemiology and Clinical Practice,* Churchill Livingstone.
10. Vaughn, J.B. et al (1965). *JAMA,* 193 : 363.
11. WHO (2018), *Rabies Fact Sheet No. 99,* 13 Sept. 2018.
12. Warrel, D.A. (1976). *Tr. Roy. Soc. Trop. Med. and Hyg.* 70 : 188.
13. Plokin, S.A. (1979) in *Nelson's Textbook of Paediatrics,* 11th ed, Saunders.
14. WHO (2010), *Current Strategies for Human Rabies Pre and Post-Exposure Prophylaxis,* 3rd Sept, 2010.
15. Kaplan, M.M. and Koprowski, H. (1980). *Sci American,* 242 (1) 120.
16. Central Research Institute, Kasauli (1979) *Principles and Practice of Antirabies Treatment and Control of Rabies,* Govt. of India.
17. Fischman, H.R. (1980) in *Maxcy–Rosenau : Public Health and Preventive Medicine,* 11th ed, Appleton – Century Crofts, New York.
18. WHO (1975) *Wkly Epi Rec.* No.33.
19. *The work of WHO* 1986–87 P – 176.
20. *Bull WHO* (1985) 63 (4) 661.

YELLOW FEVER

Yellow fever is a zoonotic disease caused by an arbovirus. It affects principally monkeys and other vertebrates in tropical America and Africa and is transmitted to man by certain culicine mosquitoes. It shares clinical features with other viral haemorrhagic fevers (e.g., dengue HF, Lassa fever) but is characterized by more severe hepatic and renal involvement. The spectrum of disease varies from clinically indeterminate to severe cases. Severe cases develop jaundice with haemorrhagic manifestations (black vomit, epistaxis, melena) and albuminuria or anuria, shock, agitation, stupor and coma *(1)*. In general death occurs between the fifth and tenth day of illness. The case fatality rate may reach 80 per cent in severe cases. Survivors exhibit long–lasting immunity.

Problem statement

47 countries in Africa and Latin America, with a combined population of more than 900 million, are at risk of yellow fever. In Africa, an estimated 508 million people live in 32 countries at risk. The remaining are in 13 countries of Latin America, with Bolivia, Brazil, Colombia, Ecuador and Peru at greatest risk *(2)*.

There were an estimated 84,000–170,000 cases and 29,000–60,000 deaths worldwide in the year 2013. Small number of imported cases occur in countries free of yellow fever. Although disease has never been reported in Asia, the region is at risk because the conditions required for transmission are present there *(2)*.

Epidemiological determinants

Agent factors

(a) AGENT : The causative agent, *Flavivirus fibricus* formerly classified as a group B arbovirus, is a member of the togavirus family. It shares group–specific antigens with other members of the genus (e.g., West Nile, dengue). Under natural conditions, the virus is pantropic but after continued culture in tissues, as in chick embryo, it loses all its pathogenic properties but retains its antigenicity. (b) RESERVOIR OF INFECTION : In forest areas, the reservoir of infection is mainly monkeys and forest mosquitoes. In urban areas, the reservoir is man (subclinical and clinical cases) besides *Aedes aegypti* mosquitoes. (c) PERIOD OF COMMUNICABILITY : (i) MAN : Blood of patients is infective during the first 3 to 4 days of illness. (ii) MOSQUITOES : After an "extrinsic incubation period" of 8 to 12 days, the mosquito becomes infective. The virus multiplies in the insect vector. After becoming infective, the mosquito remains so for life. Transovarian transmission of the virus in mosquitoes has been shown to occur in adverse conditions (e.g., during extended dry seasons), in the absence of susceptible hosts *(1)*.

Host factors

(a) AGE AND SEX : All ages and both sexes are susceptible to yellow fever in the absence of immunity (b) OCCUPATION : Persons whose occupation brings them in contact with forests (wood cutters, hunters) where yellow fever is endemic are exposed to the risk of infection (c) IMMUNITY : One attack of yellow fever gives lifelong immunity; second attacks are unknown. Infants born of immune mothers have antibodies up to 6 months of life.

Environmental factors

(a) CLIMATE : A temperature of 24 deg.C or over is required for the multiplication of the virus in the mosquito. It should be accompanied by a relative humidity of over 60 per cent for the mosquitoes to live long enough to convey the disease. (b) SOCIAL FACTORS : In Africa, urbanization is leading to the extension of yellow fever. In addition, the expanding population is encroaching on areas that were previously sparsely populated, thereby bringing man closer to the jungle cycles of yellow fever. The increasing number of people who travel and the greater speed with which they are transported from endemic areas to receptive areas, also gives a cause for concern *(3)*.

Modes of transmission

There are three known cycles of transmission, the jungle, intermediate and the urban cycles *(2)*.

- *Sylvatic (or jungle) yellow fever.* In tropical rainforests, yellow fever occurs in monkeys that are infected by wild mosquitoes. The infected monkeys then pass the virus to other mosquitoes that feed on them. The infected mosquitoes bite humans entering the forest, resulting in occasional cases of yellow fever. The majority of infections occur in young men working in the forest (e.g. for logging).
- *Intermediate yellow fever.* In humid or semi-humid parts of Africa, small-scale epidemics occur, Semi-domestic mosquitoes (that breed in the wild and around households) infect both monkeys and humans. Increased contact between people and infected mosquitoes leads to transmission. Many separate villages in an area can suffer cases simultaneously. This is the most common type of outbreak in Africa. An outbreak can become a more severe epidemic if the infection is carried into an area populated with both domestic mosquitoes and unvaccinated people.
- *Urban yellow fever.* Large epidemics occur when infected people introduce the virus into densely populated areas with a high number of non-immune people and Aedes mosquitoes. Infected mosquitoes transmit the virus from person to person.

Treatment

There is no specific treatment for yellow fever, only supportive care to treat dehydration and fever. Associated bacterial infections can be treated with antibiotics. Supportive care may improve outcomes for seriously ill patients, but it is rarely available in poorer areas.

Incubation period

3 to 6 days (6 days recognized under International Health Regulations).

CONTROL OF YELLOW FEVER

Jungle yellow fever

Jungle yellow fever continues to be an uncontrollable disease. The virus maintains itself in the animal kingdom. Mosquito control is difficult and can be considered only in restricted areas. Vaccination of humans with 17D vaccine is the only control measure.

Urban yellow fever

(1) VACCINATION : Rapid immunization of the population at risk is the most effective control strategy for yellow fever. For international use, the approved vaccine is the ***17D vaccine.*** It is a live attenuated vaccine prepared from a non–virulent strain (17D strain), which is grown in chick embryo and subsequently freeze–dried.

The sensitivity of the lyophilized 17D vaccine to heat is a major drawback to the use of this vaccine, in mass campaigns in tropical countries. It has to be stored between +5 and –30 deg.C, preferably below zero deg. C until reconstituted with the sterile, cold physiological saline diluent provided. Reconstituted vaccine should be kept on ice, away from sunlight, and discarded if not used within half an hour.

The vaccine is administered subcutaneously at the insertion of deltoid in a single dose of 0.5 ml irrespective of age. Immunity begins to appear on the 7th day and lasts possibly for life *(2)*.

The risk of death from yellow fever is much higher than the risks related to the vaccine. People who should not be vaccinated include *(2)* :

(a) children aged under 9 months for routine immunization (or under 6 months during an epidemic);

(b) pregnant women – except during a yellow fever outbreak when the risk of infection is high;

(c) people with severe allergies to egg protein; and

(d) people with severe immunodeficiency caused by symptomatic HIV/AIDS or other causes, or in the presence of thymus disorder.

Mild post-vaccinial reactions (e.g., myalgia, headache, low–grade fever) may occur in 2–5 per cent of vaccinees, 5 to 10 days after vaccination. Anaphylaxis is very rare, occurring mainly in those allergic to eggs *(4)*.

Cholera and yellow fever vaccines together or within 3 weeks interfere with each other, so whenever possible, they should be given 3 weeks or more apart *(5)*.

(2) VECTOR CONTROL : The other principal method of preventing yellow fever is through intensive vector control. The objective of vector control is to reduce rapidly the vector population to the lowest possible level and thereby stop or reduce transmission quickly. This approach has proved successful in the Americas to prevent urban epidemics.

The vector, *Aedes* mosquito is peri-domestic in habits. It can be controlled by vigorous anti-adult and anti-larval measures. The long-term policy should be based on organized "source reduction" methods (e.g., elimination of breeding places) supported by health education aimed at securing community participation.

Personal protection against contact with insects is of major importance in integrated vector control. Such protection may include the use of repellents, mosquito nets, mosquito coils and fumigation mats *(7)*.

(3) SURVEILLANCE : A programme of surveillance (clinical, serological, histopathological and entomological) should be instituted in countries where the disease is endemic, for the early detection of the presence of the virus in human populations or in animals that may contribute to its dissemination.

For the surveillance of Aedes mosquitoes, the WHO uses an index known as ***Aedes aegypti index.*** This is a house index and is defined as "the percentage of houses and their premises, in a limited well-defined area, showing actual breeding of *Aedes aegypti larvae" (8)*. This index should not be more than 1 per cent in towns and seaports in endemic areas to ensure freedom from yellow fever *(9)*.

International measures

India is a yellow fever "receptive" area, that is, "an area in which yellow fever does not exist, but where conditions would permit its development if introduced". The population of India is unvaccinated and susceptible to yellow fever. The vector, *Aedes aegypti* is found in abundance. The climatic conditions are favourable in most parts of India for its transmission. The common monkey of India *(Macacus spp)* is susceptible to yellow fever. The missing link in the chain of transmission is the virus of yellow fever which does not seem to occur in India.

The virus of yellow fever could get imported into India in two ways: (i) through infected travellers (clinical and subclinical cases), and (ii) through infected mosquitoes. Measures designed to restrict the spread of yellow fever are specified in the "International Health Regulations" of WHO *(8)*. These are implemented by the Government of India through stringent aerial and maritime traffic regulations. Broadly these comprise :

(i) TRAVELLERS : All travellers (including infants) exposed to the risk of yellow fever or passing through endemic zones of yellow fever must possess a valid international certificate of vaccination against yellow fever before they are allowed to enter yellow fever "receptive" areas. If no such certificate is available, the traveller is placed on quarantine, in a mosquito–proof ward, for 6 days from the date of leaving an infected area. If the traveller arrives before the certificate becomes "valid", he is isolated till the certificate becomes valid.

(ii) MOSQUITOES : The aircraft and ships arriving from endemic areas are subjected to aerosol spraying with prescribed insecticides on arrival for destruction of insect vectors. Further, airports and seaports are kept free from the breeding of insect vectors over an area extending at least 400 metres around their perimeters. The *"aedes aegypti index"* is kept below 1.

International certificate of vaccination *(10)*

India and most other countries require a valid certificate of vaccination against yellow fever from travellers coming from infected areas. A few countries (including India) require this even if the traveller has been in transit. It rests with each country to decide whether a certificate of vaccination against yellow fever shall be required for infants under one year of age, after weighing the risk of importation of yellow fever by unvaccinated infants against the risk to the infant arising from vaccination. In this regard, India requires vaccination of infants (≥ 9 months of age) too. The validity of the certificate begins 10 days after the date of vaccination. For the purpose of international travel, the vaccination must be given at an officially designated centre, and the certificate must be validated with the official stamp of the Ministry of Health, Government of India. The certificate is valid only if it conforms with the model prescribed under the International Health Regulations. On the other hand, for their own protection, travellers who enter endemic areas should receive vaccination against yellow fever *(10)*.

New yellow fever vaccination requirement for travellers

In May 2014, the World Health Assembly adopted an amendment of International Health Regulations (2005), which stipulates that the period of protection afforded by yellow fever vaccination, and the term of validity of the certificate will change from 10 years to the duration of the life of the person vaccinated. On 11th July 2016, the amendment entered into force and is legally binding upon all IHR states. This lifetime validity applies automatically to all existing and new certificates, beginning 10 days after the date of vaccination. Accordingly, as of 11th July 2016, revaccination or a booster dose of yellow fever vaccine will not be required for international travellers as a condition of entry into a State Party, regardless of the date that their international certificate of vaccination was initially issued *(11)*.

In India, the lifetime validity of yellow fever vaccination applies automatically. The list of yellow fever endemic countries are as follows:

In Africa : Angola, Benin, Burkina Faso, Burundi, Cameroon, Central African Republic, Chad, Congo, Cote d'Ivoire, Democratic Republic of the Congo, Equatorial Guinea, Ethiopia, Gabon, Gambia, Ghana, Guinea, Guinea-Bissau, Kenya, Liberia, Mali, Mauritania, Niger, Nigeria, Rwanda, Senegal, Sierra Leone, Sudan, South Sudan, Togo and Uganda; and in the Americas: Argentina, Bolivia, Brazil, Colombia, Ecuador, French Guiana, Guyana, Panama, Paraguay, Peru, Suriname, Trinidad and Tobago (Trinidad only), and Venezuela (Bolivarian Republic of). *Note* : When a case of yellow fever is reported from any country, that country is regarded by the Government of India as a country with risk of yellow fever transmission and is added to the above list *(10)*.

Epidemic preparedness and response

WHO recommends that every at-risk country have at least one national laboratory where basic yellow fever blood tests can be performed. A confirmed case of yellow fever in an unvaccinated population is considered as an outbreak. A confirmed case in any context must be fully investigated. Investigation teams must assess and respond to the outbreak with both emergency vaccination campaigns and longer-term immunization plans *(2)*.

The Elimination of Yellow Fever Epidemic (EYE) Strategy *(2)*

The EYE Strategy was developed by WHO, UNICEF and GAVI, in response to increased threat of yellow fever urban outbreaks with international spread. It is guided by three strategic objectives :

1. Protect at-risk populations ;
2. Prevent international spread of yellow fever; and
3. Contain outbreaks rapidly.

These objectives are underpinned by five competencies of success :

1. Affordable vaccines and sustained vaccine market;
2. Strong political commitment at global, regional and country levels;
3. High-level governance with long-term partnerships;
4. Synergies with other health programmes and sectors; and
5. Research and development for better tools and practices.

References

1. WHO (1986). *Bull WHO* 64 (4) 511–524.
2. WHO (2018). *Fact Sheet Yellow Fever*, 1st May 2018.
3. WHO (1972). *WHO. Chr.*, 26 (2) 60–65.
4. WHO (2010), *Weekly Epidemiological Record*, No. 5, 29th Jan., 2010.
5. Immunization Practices. Advisory Committee, US countries for Disease Control (1984) *Ann. Int. Med.*, 100 : 540–42.
6. *Med Digest* (1985) Feb. P.29.
7. WHO (1985) *Tech. Rep. Ser.*, No. 720 P.31.
8. WHO (2005). *International Health Regulations*, Second Annotated Edition.
9. WHO (1971). *Tech. Rep. Ser.*, No.479.
10. Govt. of India (2013), *Bureau of Immigration, Health Regulation*, Ministry of Home Affairs, Immigration Visa – Foreigners Registration and Tracking.
11. WHO (2016). *International Travel and Health*, New Yellow Fever Vaccination Requirements for Travellers.

NIPAH VIRUS INFECTION

Nipah Virus is a zoonotic virus, an emerging infectious disease caused by virus of the family Paramyxoviridae, genus Henipavirus. It gets its name from the village in Malaysia where the person from whom the virus was first isolated succumbed to the disease in the year 1999 *(1)*.

Problem statement

Nipah virus infection was initially isolated and identified in 1999 during an outbreak of encephalitis and respiratory illness among pig farmers in Malaysia and Singapore. In 2001, it was again identified as the causative agent in the outbreak of human disease in Bangladesh and India. Since then it has been reported almost annually in Bangladesh and many times in India. A recent outbreak in India was in Kerala in the month of May 2018, recorded 19 cases with 17 deaths *(2)*.

Mode of transmission

Transmission of nipah virus to humans may occur after direct contact with infected bats, infected pigs or from other nipah virus infected people (as reported in Bangladesh and India), where it is seen in the family and caregivers of the infected patients. Transmission also occurs from direct exposure to infected bats. Example is consumption of raw date palm sap contaminated with infectious bat secretions, and excretions *(3)*.

Fruit bats of the family *Pteropodidae*, particularly species belonging to *Pteropus genus* are the natural host for nipah virus. There is no apparent disease in fruit bats *(1)*.

Incubation period

Usually 4 to 14 days.

Clinical manifestations

Human infection ranges from asymptomatic infection to acute respiratory infection and fatal encephalitis. Infected people initially develop fever, headache, myalgia, vomiting and sore throat. This can be followed by dizziness, drowsiness, altered consciousness and neurological signs that indicate acute encephalitis. Some people can also experience atypical pneumonia and severe respiratory problems, including acute respiratory distress. Encephalitis and seizures occur in severe cases, progressing to coma within 24 to 48 hours. Most people who survive acute encephalitis make a full recovery. Long term neurologic conditions have been reported in survivors. Approximately 20% of patients are left with residual neurological consequences such as seizure disorder and personality changes. A small number of people who recover subsequently relapse or develop delayed onset encephalitis. The case fatality rate is estimated at 40% to 75%. This rate can vary by outbreak depending on local capabilities for epidemiological surveillance and clinical management *(2)*.

Diagnosis

The main tests are real time polymerase chain reaction (RT-PCR) from bodily fluids and antibody detection via ELISA. Other tests used include polymerase chain reaction assay, and virus isolation by cell culture *(1)*.

Treatment

No drug or vaccine specific to nipah virus is available.

Intensive supportive care is recommended to treat severe respiratory and neurological complications.

Prevention

In the absence of a vaccine, the only way to reduce or prevent infection in people is by raising awareness of the risk factors and educating people about the measures they can take to reduce exposure to nipah virus.

References

1. WHO (2018), *Fact sheet Nipah Virus*, 30th May 2018.
2. *Communicable Disease Watch*, 3 June - 16 July 2018, vol.15.
3. *Centers for Disease Control and Prevention*, Saving lives, Protecting people.

OTHER ARBOVIRAL DISEASES

During the past few years, a large number of arthropod–borne viruses (arboviruses) have been isolated from sick persons, animals and arthropods throughout the world. Arthropod-borne viruses are defined as viruses "which are maintained in nature principally, or to an important extent through biological transmission between susceptible vertebrate hosts by haematophagous arthropods; they multiply in the tissues of arthropods, and are passed on to new vertebrates by the bites of arthropod after a period of extrinsic incubation" *(1)*.

Yellow fever is historically the most prominent among the diseases in this group. In recent years, a number of other arboviruses have emerged as important public health problems in both tropical and temperate zones. The number of arboviruses known in India had risen from two (dengue and sandfly fever) in 1951 to over 40 *(2)*.

CLASSIFICATION

The huge family of heterogeneous arboviruses is divided into no less than 7 major groups, and 18 smaller groups *(3)*. Many remain unclassified. The current trend is to name the viruses after the places where they were discovered. Some of the arboviruses known to be prevalent in India are as shown in Table 1.

TABLE 1
Some Arboviruses known to be prevalent in India

Group A	**OTHERS**
(Alphaviruses)	*Umbre*
Sindbis	Sathuperi
Chikungunya	Chandipura
	Chittor
	Ganjam
Group B	Minnal
(Flaviviruses)	Venkatapuram
Dengue	Dhori
KFD	Kaisodi
JE	Sandfly fever
West Nile	African Horse sickness
	Vellore

CLINICAL SYNDROMES

Although arboviruses are many, only a small number of them are known to be capable of infecting man, and a much smaller number capable of producing disease. A high proportion of the infections is inapparent. For convenience, three clinical syndromes have been described : (a) FEBRILE GROUP : This is the most common group which comprises a large number of relatively undifferentiated fevers, generally benign with or without rashes and joint pains. Viruses responsible for this group of illness in India are the sindbis, chikungunya and dengue viruses. (b) HAEMORRHAGIC FEVERS : The second group is that of haemorrhagic fevers, generally associated with moderate or high mortality. Viruses responsible for haemorrhagic fevers in India are the dengue, chikungunya and KFD viruses. (c) ENCEPHALITIDIS : The third group is that of encephalitidis or meningoencephalitis which is associated with a considerable and sometimes high mortality. The disease reported now frequently in some parts of India is the Japanese encephalitis.

1. The dengue syndrome

This is detailed separately at page 288.

2. Japanese encephalitis

Japanese encephalitis (JE) is a mosquito–borne encephalitis caused by a group B arbovirus (Flavivirus) and transmitted by culicine mosquitoes. It is a zoonotic disease, i.e., infecting mainly animals and incidentally man. The envelope glycoprotein of the JE virus contains specific as well as cross-reactive, neutralizing epitopes. The major genotypes of this virus have different geographical distribution, but all belong to the same serotype and are similar in terms of virulence and host preference. Following an infectious mosquito bite, the initial viral replication occurs in local and regional lymph nodes. Viral invasion of the central nervous system occurs probably *via* blood.

JE is the leading cause of viral encephalitis in Asia and occurs in almost 24 Asian and Western Pacific countries. Largely as a result of immunization, its incidence has been declining in Japan, the Korean peninsula and in some regions of China, but the disease is increasingly reported from Bangladesh, India, Nepal, Pakistan, northern Thailand and Vietnam. Transmission occurs principally in rural agricultural location where flooding irrigation is practised. Transmission is seasonal and mainly related to the rainy season in South-East Asia Region *(2)*.

The annual incidence of clinical disease varies both across and within countries, ranging from <10 to >100 per 100,000 population. A recent estimate puts nearly 68,000 clinical cases of JE globally each year, with upto 20,400 deaths due to JE *(3)*. The vast majority of cases occur among children less than 15 years of age. Nearly 10 per cent of cases are among those above 60 years, perhaps reflecting waning protective immunity.

The disease is rare in other parts of the world, and when seen, is generally associated with travellers returning from endemic areas *(3)*.

Major outbreaks of JE occur every 2–15 years. JE transmission intensifies during the rainy season, when vector population increases. However, there has not yet been any evidence of increased JE transmission following major floods. The spread of JE in new areas has been correlated with agricultural development supported by irrigation programmes *(3)*.

PROBLEM IN INDIA

Recognition of JE, based on serological surveys, was first made in 1955 in Tamil Nadu. JE has been reported from different parts of the country. The disease is endemic in 21 states. Assam, Bihar, Uttar Pradesh, Karnataka, West Bengal, Tripura and Tamil Nadu report out-breaks every year and contribute about 55 per cent of cases and deaths. In India about 375 million population is at risk. JE is reported under the umbrella of Acute Encephalitis Syndrome

(AES), therefore, the data reported from states are for total AES including JE cases *(4)*. The state-wise reported cases of Acute encephalitis syndrome are as shown in Table 2.

TABLE 2
State-wise reported cases and deaths due to Acute encephalitis syndrome in India 2018–2020 (P)

State	2018		2019		2020 (P)	
	Cases	Deaths	Cases	Deaths	Cases	Deaths
Assam	1492	183	2652	353	595	96
Bihar	124	33	292	82	172	23
Jharkhand	544	0	912	3	485	0
Karnataka	380	5	397	4	310	0
Manipur	283	3	1177	6	29	4
Meghalya	243	6	711	9	230	1
Odisha	1720	10	1962	8	373	3
Tamil Nadu	1287	5	1007	2	333	4
Tripura	311	0	325	2	244	0
Uttar Pradesh	3080	230	2185	126	1646	83
West Bengal	1762	146	1618	89	867	26
India Total	11,388	636	14,995	710	5,487	248

P – Provisional

Source : *(5)*

Epidemiological features

Unlike the dengue viruses, JE virus infects several extrahuman hosts, e.g., animals and birds. Available evidence indicates that the basic cycles of transmission are :

(a) Pig → Mosquito → Pig

(b) The Ardeid bird → Mosquito → Ardeid bird

The disease is transmitted to man by the bite of infected mosquitoes. Man is an incidental "dead–end" host. Man to man transmission has not so far been recorded.

(a) Animal hosts : Among the animal hosts, pigs have been incriminated as the major vertebrate hosts for JE virus. In some places, upto 100 per cent of pigs may be infected with JE virus. Infected pigs do not manifest any overt symptoms of illness but circulate the virus so that mosquitoes get infected and can transmit the virus to man. The pigs are thus considered as "amplifiers" of the virus *(6)*. Cattle and buffaloes may also be infected with the JE virus; although they may not be natural hosts of JE virus, they act as "mosquito attractants." Horses are the only domestic animals so far known which show signs of encephalitis due to JE virus infection. *(b) Birds :* Some species of birds such as pond herons; cattle egrets and perhaps poultry and ducks appear to be involved in the natural history of JE virus *(6)*.

MOSQUITO VECTORS

Culicine mosquitoes, notably *C.tritaeniorhynchus, C. vishnui* and *C. gelidus* along with some anophelines have been incriminated as the vectors of JE. Among these, *C.tritaeniorhynchus* and *vishnui* has been implicated as the most important vector in South India *(7)*. These mosquitoes generally breed in irrigated rice fields, shallow ditches and pools. The rice fields are probably the most important breeding places. These mosquitoes are zoophilic, feeding primarily on vertebrate hosts. Female mosquitoes get infected after feeding on a viraemic host, and after 9–12 days incubation period, they can transmit the virus to other hosts.

JE IN MAN

The incubation period in man, following mosquito bite is not exactly known. Probably, it varies from 5–15 days. Not all individuals bitten by infected mosquitoes develop disease. The ratio of overt disease to inapparent infection is about 1:250. Thus cases of encephalitis represent only the tip of the iceberg compared to the large number of inapparent infections. Encephalitis cases due to JE may show a scattered distribution.

The course of the disease in man may be divided into three stages : *(a) PRODROMAL STAGE :* The onset of illness is usually acute and is heralded by fever, headache, gastrointestinal disturbances, lethargy and malaise. The duration of this stage is usually 1–6 days. *(b) ACUTE ENCEPHALITIC STAGE :* Fever is usually high, 38 to 40.7 deg. C. The prominent features are fever, nuchal rigidity, focal CNS signs, convulsions signs of raised intra-cranial pressure, difficulty of speech, dystonia, ocular palsies, hemiplegia, quadriplegia, extra-pyramidal signs like coarse tremors and altered sensorium progressing in many cases to coma. *(c) LATE STAGE AND SEQUELAE :* This stage begins when active inflammation is at an end, i.e., the temperature and ESR touch normal. Neurological signs become stationary or tend to improve. Convalescence may be prolonged and residual neurological deficits may not be uncommon *(3)*. The case fatality rate varies between 20–40 per cent. The average period between the onset of illness and death is about 9 days *(3)*.

Confirmation of a suspected case of JE requires laboratory diagnosis. The aetiological diagnosis of JE is mainly based on serology using IgM-capture ELISA which detects specific IgM in the cerebrospinal fluid or in the blood of almost all patients within 7 days of onset of disease. Other methods include conventional antibody assays on paired sera for the demonstration of a significant rise in total JE–specific antibody, as well as a dot-blot IgM assay, suitable for use in the field. The virus is rarely recovered in tissue culture from blood or CSF, but may be found in encephalitic brain at autopsy. JE-viral RNA is rarely demonstrated in the CSF *(8)*.

Control of JE

(a) VACCINATION : Vaccination of population at risk has been recommended. Currently, the three types of JE vaccines in large-scale use are : (i) the mouse brain-derived, purified and inactivated vaccine, which is based on either the Nakayama or Beijing strains of the JE virus and produced in several Asian countries; (ii) the cell culture-derived, inactivated JE vaccine based on the Beijing P-3 strain, and (iii) the cell culture-derived, live attenuated vaccine based on the SA 14-14-2 strain of the JE virus. The mouse-brain derived, inactivated vaccine has been used successfully to reduce the incidence of JE in a number of countries, and is likely to be used nationally and internationally for some more years. Drawbacks of the mouse-brain vaccine are the limited duration of the induced protection, the need for multiple doses, and, in most countries, the relatively high price per dose. The cell culture-derived vaccines are manufactured and widely used in China, where the inactivated vaccine is gradually being replaced by the live attenuated vaccine. Several other promising JE vaccine candidates are in advanced stages of development.

The immunization schedules of the 3 licensed JE vaccines

that are currently in large-scale use vary with the profile of the respective vaccines and depend on local epidemiological circumstances and recommended schedules of other childhood vaccines. When immunizing children 1–3 years of age the mouse brain-derived vaccine provides adequate protection throughout childhood following 2 primary doses 4 weeks apart, and boosters after 1 year and subsequently at 3-yearly intervals until the age of 10–15 years. The vaccine is given subcutaneously in doses of 0.5 ml for children under 3 years and one ml for children more than 3 years of age. Protective immunity develops in about one month time after the second dose. The vaccine is best used in the inter-epidemic period. It should be offered to the most vulnerable and high-risk groups *(6, 7)*. Equally good childhood protection is obtained by a single dose of the cell-culture based, live attenuated vaccine (SA-14-14-2) followed by a single booster given at an interval of about 1 year. This vaccine is available in India and is an integral part of Universal Immunization Programme in 83 endemic districts in Uttar Pradesh, Assam, West Bengal and Karnataka targeting children in age group 1–15 years *(9)*. The importance of achieving long-term protection is underlined by the observation that in some areas an increasing proportion of the JE cases occur in individuals older than 10 years of age *(8)*.

Given the most infrequent occurrence of JE in infancy and the likely interference with passively acquired maternal antibodies during the first months of life, vaccination is not recommended for children before the age of 6 months *(8)*.

For travellers aged more than one year, visiting rural areas of endemic countries for at least 2 weeks, the established current practice is to administer 3 primary doses at days 0, 7 and 28; alternatively 2 primary doses preferably 4 weeks apart. When continued protection is required, boosters should be given after one year and then every 3 years *(8, 10)*.

The vaccination of swine is extremely important for both public health and economic reasons. It prevents viraemia in these animals, and hence eliminates their role as amplifiers of the virus. An inactivated vaccine and more recent modified live virus vaccines are all in current use. However, it is difficult to maintain vaccination coverage in the swine of a given region because the population is renewed so rapidly *(11)*.

(b) VECTOR CONTROL : The vector mosquito(es) of JE are widely scattered and not easily amenable to control. An effective way to deal with them is to resort to aerial or ground fogging with ultra–low–volume (ULV) insecticides (e.g., malathion, fenitrothion). All the villages reporting cases should be brought under indoor residual spray. The spraying should cover the vegetation around the houses, breeding sites and animal shelters in the affected villages. Uninfected villages falling within 2 to 3 km radius of the infected villages should also receive spraying as a preventive measure. Villages within the proximity of infected villages should be kept under surveillance. The use of mosquito nets should be advocated.

GUIDELINES FOR MANAGEMENT OF AES INCLUDING JAPANESE ENCEPHALITIS IN INDIA (2014) *(12)*

Following an outbreak of JE in Gorakhpur and Basti divisions in eastern Uttar Pradesh during 2005, Directorate of NVBDCP developed surveillance guidelines for endemic states and advised that all the JE cases be reported under Acute Encephalitis Syndrome (AES) as they have common similar clinical manifestations. Their case management usually follows a common protocol along with situation specific treatment. Diagnosis of JE will depend on laboratory investigations. The case definitions and case classification in the programme are as follows *(12)* :

Case definition of suspected case

- Acute onset of fever, not more than 5–7 days duration.
- Change in mental status with/without
  - New onset of seizures (excluding febrile seizures)
  - Other early clinical findings – may include irritability, somnolence or abnormal behaviour greater than that seen with usual febrile illness.

Case classification

Laboratory-confirmed case

A suspected case with any one of the following markers:

- Presence of IgM antibody in serum and/or CSF to a specific virus including JE/Enterovirus or others
- Four fold difference in IgG antibody titre in paired sera
- Virus isolation from brain tissue
- Antigen detection by immunofluroscence
- Nucleic acid detection by PCR

In the sentinel surveillance network, AES/JE is to be diagnosed by IgM Capture ELISA, and virus isolation to be done in National Reference Laboratory.

Probable cases

Suspected case in close geographic and temporal relationship to a laboratory-confirmed case of AES/JE in an outbreak.

Acute Encephalitis Syndrome (AES) due to other agent

A suspected case in which diagnostic testing is performed and an aetiological agent other than AES/JE is identified.

Acute Encephalitis Syndrome (AES) due to unknown agent

A suspected case in which no diagnostic testing is performed/no aetiological agent is identified/test results are indeterminate.

While the above classifications are useful for clearer definitions of AES cases, for practical purposes, the two key definitions to be used are "suspected JE cases" for those that meet the criteria for AES, and "confirmed JE cases" for those AES cases which have laboratory confirmation for JE. In an epidemic situation fever with altered sensorium persisting for more than two hours with a focal seizure or paralysis of any part of body, is encephalitis. Presence of rash on body excludes Japanese Encephalitis. AES with symmetrical signs and fever is likely to be cerebral Malaria.

The causes of AES are as shown in Fig. 1.

Management of Acute Encephalitis Syndrome, including Japanese Encephalitis, is essentially symptomatic. To reduce severe morbidity and mortality, it is important to identify early warning signs and refer patients to health facility and to educate the health workers about the first line of treatment for management of the case at the grassroot level.

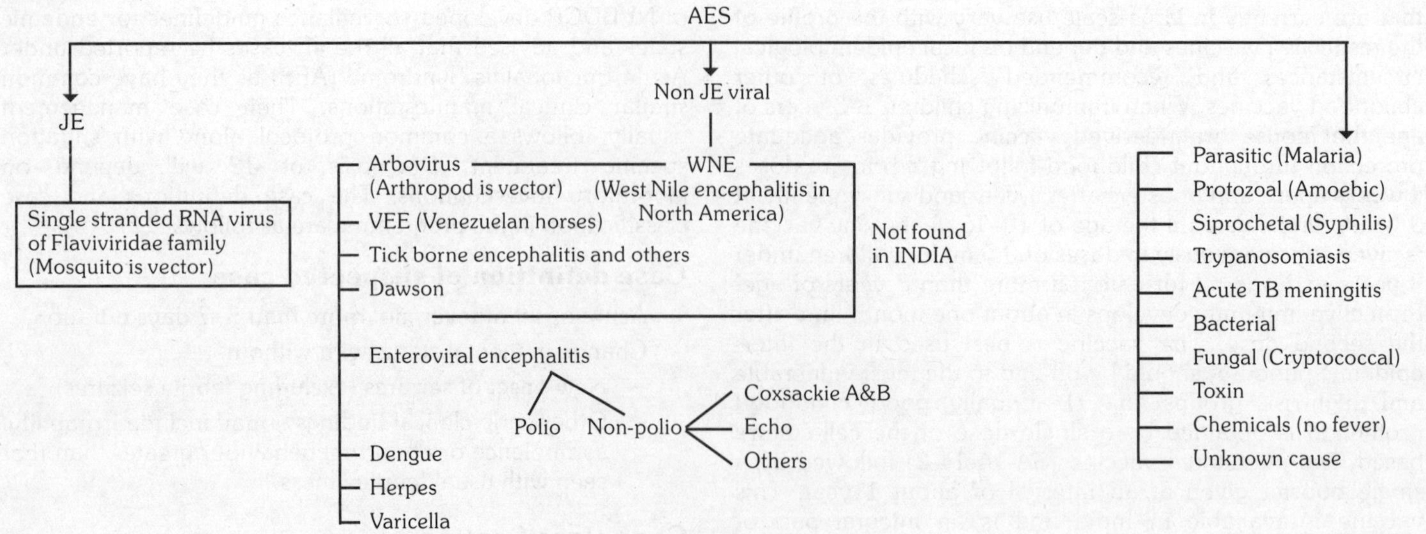

FIG. 1
Causes of Acute Encephalitis Syndrome

Source : *(13)*

Fig. 2 summarizes the guidelines for management of a case of AES at PHC and FRU level and management of circulation as blood pressure should be maintained at about 95th centile for the age of the patient with the help of dopamine drip. Failure of autoregulation of the brain makes the cerebral circulation depend solely on systemic blood pressure. Avoid fluid overload. The ultimate decision regarding the management depends upon the attending physician.

Treatment of specific cause

If laboratory investigation shows a non–JE cause, like herpes-zoster, varicella, malaria, pyogenic meningitis, tubercular meningitis, toxoplasmosis, amoebiasis, fungal infection or neurocysticercosis; the patient should be given specific treatment for that particular disease.

3. Kyasanur forest disease

Kyasanur forest disease (KFD) is a febrile disease associated with haemorrhages caused by an arbovirus flavivirus and transmitted to man by bite of infective ticks.

HISTORY

KFD was first recognized in 1957 in Shimoga district of Karnataka State in South India. Local inhabitants called the disease "monkey disease" because of its association with

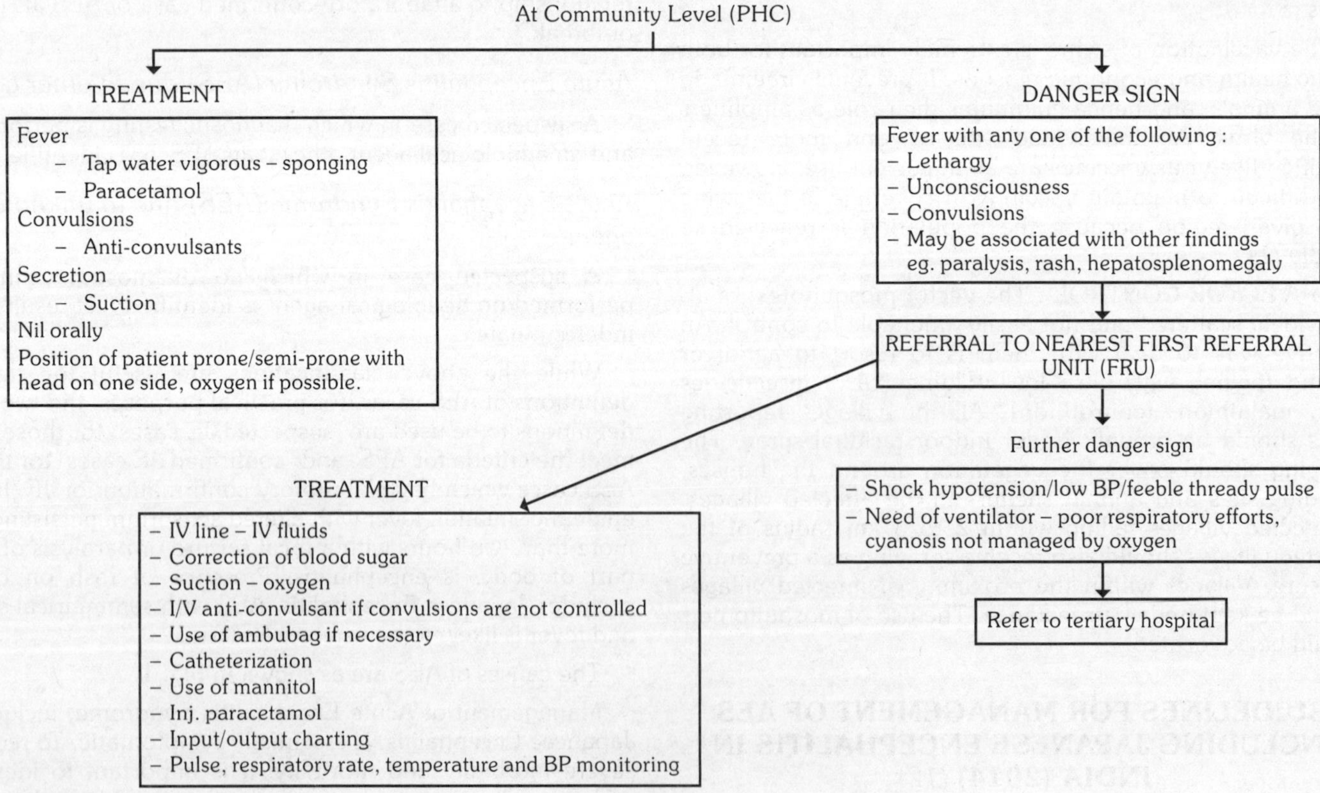

FIG. 2
Management of AES including Japanese Encephalitis

Source : *(12)*

dead monkeys. The disease was later named after the locality – Kyasanur Forest – from where the virus was first isolated.

PROBLEM STATEMENT

Earlier the disease was found to be limited mainly to an area around the original focus (Shimoga district) covering about 800 sq.km. Newer foci have since been recognized. The disease is now restricted to four districts (Shimoga, North Kannada, South Kannada and Chikamagaluru) in Karnataka State in India covering over 6,000 sq.km. *(14)*. Serological surveys in different parts of India revealed antibodies to KFD or a closely related virus in human and animals, particularly in cattle in Kutch and Saurashtra *(15)*.

According to the reports, the disease continues to be active in its endemic foci. About 400–500 cases occur every year. The Karnataka Government has established a surveillance system which monitors the occurrence of KFD in humans and mortality in monkeys in known epidemic areas, as well as neighbouring areas. Deaths of monkeys are considered as heralders of this disease in endemic areas *(16)*.

Epidemiological determinants

(a) AGENT

The agent KFD virus is a member of group B togaviruses (flaviviruses). It is antigenically related to other tick-borne flaviviruses, particularly the Far Eastern tick-borne encephalitis and Omsk haemorrhagic fever. Unlike in many other arbovirus infections, KFD has a prolonged viraemia in man for about 10 days or more.

(b) NATURAL HOSTS AND RESERVOIRS

Small mammals particularly rats and squirrels are the main reservoirs of the virus *(14)*. Birds and bats are less important hosts. The monkeys are recognized as amplifying hosts for the virus. However, they are not effective maintenance hosts because most of them die from KFD infection. Cattle provide *Haemaphysalis* ticks with a plentiful source of blood meals, which in turn leads to a population explosion among the ticks. Thus cattle are very important in maintaining tick populations but play no part in virus maintenance *(14)*. Man is an incidental or dead-end host, and plays no part in virus transmission.

(c) VECTORS

The virus has a complex life cycle involving a wide variety of tick–species. At least 15 species of hard ticks of the genus *Haemaphysalis*, particularly *H. spinigera* and *H. turtura* are known to transmit the disease. KFD has also been isolated from soft ticks *(17)*. The highest number of human and monkey infections occur during drier months, particularly from January to June. This period coincides with the peak nymphal activity of ticks.

(d) HOST FACTORS

(i) Age : Majority of cases affected were between 20 and 40 years. *(ii) Sex* : Attack rate was greater in males than in females. *(iii) Occupation* : The attacked people were mostly cultivators who visited forests accompanying their cattle or cutting woods and *(iv) Human activity* : The epidemic period correlates well with the period of greatest human activity in the forest, i.e., from January until the onset of rains in June.

(e) MODE OF TRANSMISSION

The transmission cycle involves mainly monkeys and ticks. The disease is transmitted by the bite of infective ticks, especially nymphal stages. There is no evidence of man to man transmission.

(f) INCUBATION PERIOD

Estimated to be between 3 and 8 days.

CLINICAL FEATURES

The disease appears with a sudden onset of fever, headache and severe myalgia, with prostration in some patients. The acute phase lasts for about 2 weeks. Gastrointestinal disturbances and haemorrhages from nose, gums, stomach and intestine may occur in severe cases.

In a number of cases, there is a second phase characterized by mild meningoencephalitis after an afebrile period of 7 to 21 days. It is manifested by a return of fever, severe headache followed by neck stiffness, coarse tremors, abnormal reflexes and mental disturbances. The case fatality rate has been estimated to be 5 to 10 per cent *(14)*.

Diagnosis is established only after detecting the presence of the virus in the blood and/or serological evidence.

CONTROL

(a) CONTROL OF TICKS : Since KFD is a tick–borne disease, control of ticks should be undertaken. For control of ticks in forests, application can be made by power equipment or by aircraft–mounted equipment to dispense carbaryl, fenthion, naled or propoxur at 2.24 kg of active ingredient per hectare *(18)*. The spraying must be carried out in "hot spots", i.e., in areas where monkey deaths have been reported, within 50 metres around the spot of the monkey deaths, besides the endemic foci. Since the heavy tick population in the forest areas is attributed partly to the free roaming cattle, restriction of cattle movement is thought to bring about a reduction in vector population. (b) VACCINATION : The population at risk should be immunized with killed KFD vaccine. (c) PERSONAL PROTECTION : Protection of individuals exposed to the risk of infection by adequate clothing and insect repellents such as dimethylphthalate (DMP, DEET) should be encouraged. They should examine their bodies at the end of each day for ticks and remove them promptly. The habit of sitting or lying down on the ground should be discouraged through health education.

4. Chikungunya fever

A dengue-like disease caused by a group A virus, the chikungunya virus and transmitted by *Aedes* mosquitoes. It is manifested by high fever and severe articular pains in the limbs and spinal column. The virus was first isolated from patients and mosquitoes during an epidemic in Tanzania in 1952–53. Chikungunya is a local word meaning "doubling up" owing to excruciating joint pains. The virus occurs widely in sub-Saharan Africa, India and in many areas in Asia.

After re-emergence of chikungunya in the year 2006, clinically suspected cases declined till the year 2014. However, the disease shows an upward trend since 2015. Chikungunya is endemic in 24 states and 6 UTs. During 2020, a total of 43,424 suspected cases were reported from 28 states. The maximum number of cases were from states as shown in Table 3.

The incubation period of chikungunya fever is 4–7 days, following which the disease has a sudden onset with fever, chills, cephalalgia, anorexia, lumbago and conjunctivitis. Adenopathy is also common. 60 to 80 per cent patients have a morbilliform rash, occasionally with purpura, on the trunk and limbs. The cutaneous eruption may recur every 3 to

TABLE 3
Top 10 states reporting suspected cases of Chikungunya, India (2018–2020)

States	2018 Cases	2019 Cases	2020 (P) Cases
Karnataka	20,411	43,698	16,111
Gujarat	10,601	8,084	8,120
Maharashtra	9,884	5,150	4,258
Puducherry	2,876	7,084	3,980
Kerala	77	109	2,302
Rajasthan	254	365	1,015
Tamil Nadu	284	623	1,461
Telangana	1,954	5,352	364
Madhya Pradesh	3,211	2,749	1,871
Tripura	683	1,105	454
India	57,813	81,914	43,424

P – Provisional

Source : *(5)*

7 days. Other symptoms are coffee-coloured vomiting, epistaxis and petechiae. A prominent symptom, seen especially in adult patients is arthropathy, from which the disease gets its name. The arthropathy is manifested by pain, swelling and stiffness, especially of the metacarpophalangeal, wrist, elbow, shoulder, knee, ankle and metatarsal joints. It appears between 3rd and 5th day after the onset of clinical symptoms, and it can persist for many months and even years. No deaths have been attributed to chikungunya fever *(11)*.

There is no specific treatment of chikungunya infection and it is usually self limiting. Analgesics, antipyretics like paracetamol, diclofenac sodium, chloroquine along with fluid supplementation are recommended to manage infection and relieve fever, joint pains and swelling. Drugs like aspirin and steroids should be avoided.

The disease occurs in the rainy season, when the mosquito vector population is at its peak. Research suggests that the virus has a wild cycle, similar to that of yellow fever, operating between jungle primates and mosquitoes, including *Aedes africanus* and members of the *A. furcifer-taylori* group.

DIAGONSIS

The virus can be isolated from the blood of febrile patients by the intracerebral inoculation in suckling mice or on VERO cells.

In serologic diagnosis, which is the approach most commonly used, sero-conversion is demonstrated by comparing acute – and convalescent – phase sera in the haemagglutination inhibition, serum neutralization, or complement fixation test. The enzyme-linked immunosorbent assay (ELISA) is used to detect IgM. A reverse-transcription polymerase chain reaction (RT-PCR) / nested PCR technique has also been shown to be useful in rapidly diagnosing the disease *(11)*.

CONTROL

(a) VECTOR CONTROL : The *Aedes aegypti* mosquito should be the main target of control activities. It requires active community involvement to keep water storage containers free of mosquitoes and to eliminate the other breeding places of mosquitoes in and around houses and dwellings *(4)*. Vector control strategies should address all life stages of the *Aedes* mosquito from the egg to larva and adult. Targeted residual spraying and space spraying/fogging when there is an outbreak is recommended to rapidly reduce the adult mosquito population. *(b) PERSONAL PROTECTION* : Personal preventive measures to avoid mosquito bites include clothing minimizing skin exposure, use of repellents, as well as window screens. The use of insecticide - treated bed nets is limited by the fact that *Aedes* mosquito bites during daytime. Eventually economic development will reduce mosquito-borne diseases by improving standard of living (e.g. people living in houses with solid floors and roofs, window screen and air conditioning) *(20)*. *(c) VACCINE* : No vaccine has yet been developed that is considered suitable for use.

5. West nile fever

An acute febrile illness caused by a group B arbovirus. The disease is endemic in Africa, the Middle East, South–West Asia and India, and transmitted by certain species of Culex mosquitoes. Clinically, it is manifested by a sudden onset of fever, severe headache and malaise lasting several days. In children, a maculopapular rash of short duration may appear. In the aged, a fatal meningo-encephalitis may be produced.

6. Sandfly fever

Sandfly fever is known to occur in the arid regions of West Pakistan and Middle East. Its occurrence in India was thought to be doubtful. However, in 1967, the sandfly fever virus was isolated in Aurangabad (Maharashtra) from febrile cases. The virus was also isolated from sandflies *(21)*. The control of sandfly fever is based on the control of insect vector.

References

1. WHO (1967), *Tech. Rep. Ser.*, No.369.
2. WHO (2010), *International travel and Health*, 2010.
3. WHO (2019), *Fact Sheet Japanese Encephalitis*, May 2019.
4. Govt. of India (2020), *Annual Report 2019–2020*, Ministry of Health and Family Welfare, New Delhi.
5. Govt. of India (2021), *National Health Profile 2021*, Ministry of Health and Family Welfare, New Delhi.
6. WHO (1979), *Japanese Encephalitis*, Technical Information and Guidelines for Treatment, SEA/CD/79, WHO, New Delhi.
7. National Institute of Virology, Pune (1980). *Japanese Encephalitis in India*, ICMR, New Delhi.
8. WHO (2006), *Weekly Epidemiological Record*, No. 34/35, 25th Aug. 2006.
9. Govt. of India (2012), *Annual Report 2011–2012*, DGHS, Ministry of Health and Family Welfare, New Delhi.
10. WHO (2005), *International travel and health 2005*.
11. Pan American Health Organization (2003), *Zoonoses and Communicable Diseases Common to Man and Animal* 3rd Ed., Vol. II.
12. Govt. of India, WHO (2014), *Operational Guidelines National Programme for Prevention and Control of Japanese Encephalitis/ Acute Encephalitis Syndrome*, Ministry of Health and Family Welfare, New Delhi.
13. Govt. of India (2009), *Guidelines, Clinical Management of Acute Encephalitis syndrome including Japanese Encephalitis*, DNVBDCP, DGHS, Ministry of Health and Family Welfare, New Delhi.
14. WHO (1985), *Tech. Rep. Ser.*, 721.
15. NICD (1985), *Manual of Zoonosis*.
16. Govt. of India (2006), *Health Information of India 2005*, Ministry of Health and Family Welfare, New Delhi.
17. Singh K.R.P. (1971), *Indian. J. Med. Res.*, 59 : 312.
18. WHO (1984), *Chemical methods for the Control of arthropod vectors and pests of Public Health importance*.
19. WHO (2006), *Weekly Epidemiological Record* No. 43, 27th Oct. 2006.
20. WHO (2018), *Managing epidemics, Key facts about major deadly diseases*, Version 1.
21. WHO (1975), *Wkly Epid Rec.*, No. 23, 6 June 1975.

BRUCELLOSIS

Brucellosis is one of the major bacterial zoonoses, and in humans is also known as Undulent fever, Malta fever or Mediterranean fever. It is occasionally transmitted to man by direct or indirect contact with infected animals. It is caused by different species of the brucella group of organisms and characterized by intermittent or irregular febrile attacks, with profuse sweating, arthritis and an enlarged spleen. The disease may last for several days, months or occasionally years. Brucellosis is both a severe human disease and a disease of animals with serious economic consequences.

Problem statement

Brucellosis is a recognized public health problem with worldwide distribution. It is endemic wherever cattle, pigs, goats and sheep are raised in large numbers. Important endemic areas for brucellosis exist in Mediterranean zones, Europe, Central Asia, Mexico and South America. Eastern Mediterranean countries have experienced an increase in the number of cases. The disease is now rare in most European countries, North America and Australia *(1)*.

Animal brucellosis is reported from practically every State in India. However, no statistical information is available about extent of infection in man in various parts of the country *(2)*.

The prevalence of human brucellosis is difficult to estimate. Many cases remain undiagnosed either because they are inapparent or because physicians in many countries are unfamiliar with the disease.

Epidemiological determinants

Agent factors

(a) AGENT : The agents are small, gram-negative rod-shaped, non-motile, non-sporing and intracellular coccobacilli of the genus *Brucella*. Four species infect man : *B.melitensis, B.abortus, B.suis,* and *B.canis. B.melitensis* is the most virulent and invasive species; it usually infects goats and occasionally sheep. *B.abortus* is less virulent and is primarily a disease of cattle. *B.suis* is of intermediate virulence and chiefly infects pigs. *B.canis* is a parasite of dogs. (b) RESERVOIR OF INFECTION : Main reservoirs of human infection are cattle, sheep, goats, swine, buffaloes, horses and dogs. In animals the disease can cause abortion, premature expulsion of the foetus or death. Cross infections can often occur between animal species. The infected animals excrete Brucella in the urine, milk, placenta, uterine and vaginal discharges particularly during a birth or abortion. The animals may remain infected for life.

Host factors

Human brucellosis is predominantly a disease of adult males. Farmers, shepherds, butchers, and abattoir workers, veterinarians and laboratory workers are particularly at special risk because of occupational exposure. Immunity follows infection.

Environmental factors

Brucellosis is most prevalent under conditions of advanced domestication of animals in the absence of correspondingly advanced standards of hygiene. Overcrowding of herds, high rainfall, lack of exposure to sunlight, unhygienic practices in milk and meat production, all favour the spread of brucellosis. The infection can travel long distances in milk and dust. The environment of a cowshed may be heavily infected. The organism can survive for weeks, or months in favourable conditions of water, urine, faeces, damp soil and manure.

Mode of transmission

Transmission is usually from infected animals to man. There is no evidence of transmission from man to man *(3)*. The routes of spread are :

(a) Contact infection : Most commonly, infection occurs by direct contact with infected tissues, blood, urine, vaginal discharge, aborted foetuses and especially placenta. Infection takes place through abraded skin, mucosa or conjunctiva (mucocutaneous route). This type of spread is largely occupational and occurs in persons involved in handling livestock and slaughter house workers.

(b) Food-borne infection : Infection may take place indirectly by the ingestion of raw milk or dairy products (cheese) from infected animals. Fresh raw vegetables can also carry infection if grown on soil containing manure from infected farms. Water contaminated with the excreta of infected animals may also serve as a source of infection.

(c) Air-borne infection : The environment of a cowshed may be heavily infected. Few people living in such an environment can escape inhalation of infected dust or aerosols. Brucellae may be inhaled in aerosol form in slaughter houses and laboratories, so these infections are notified as occupational.

Incubation period

Highly variable. Usually 1–3 weeks, but may be as long as 6 months or more.

Pattern of disease

Brucella infection in man can vary from an acute febrile disease to a chronic low–grade ill–defined disease, lasting for several days, months or occasionally years.

The acute phase is characterized by a sudden or insidious onset of illness with (i) swinging pyrexia (upto 40–41 deg C), rigors and sweating. (ii) arthralgia/arthritis (usually monoarticular) involving larger joints such as hip, knee, shoulder and ankle. (iii) low back pain. (iv) headache, insomnia. (v) small firm splenomegaly and hepatomegaly. (vi) leucopenia with relative lymphocytosis *(4)*. The most striking aspect of the clinical picture is the severity of the illness and the absence of clinical signs. The acute phase subsides within 2–3 weeks. If the patient is treated with tetracycline, the symptoms may disappear quickly, but the infection, being intracellular, may persist giving rise to subacute or relapsing disease.

In a few patients (upto 20 per cent), symptoms recur for prolonged periods. Diagnosis is established by isolation of the organism from cultures of blood, bone marrow, exudates and biopsy specimens during the acute phase of the disease; and by serological tests.

Control of brucellosis

(a) IN THE ANIMALS

The most rational approach for preventing human brucellosis is the control and eradication of the infection from animal reservoirs which is based on the combination of the following measures : *(a) Test and slaughter :* Case finding is done by mass surveys. Skin tests are available. The complement fixation test is also recommended. Those animals infected with brucellosis are slaughtered, with full compensation paid to farmers. This is the only satisfactory solution aimed at eradication of the disease. *(b) Vaccination :* Vaccine of *B. abortus* strain 19 is commonly used for young animals. A compulsory vaccination programme for all heifers in a given community on a yearly basis can considerably reduce the rate of infection. Systematic vaccination for a period of 7 to 10 years may result in the elimination of the disease. Control of the infection caused by *B. melitensis* in goats and sheep has to be based mainly on vaccination *(5)*. *(c) Hygienic measures :* These comprise provision of a clean sanitary environment for animals, sanitary disposal of urine and faeces, veterinary care of animals and health education of all those who are occupationally involved.

(b) IN THE HUMANS

(a) Early diagnosis and treatment : In uncomplicated cases the antibiotic of choice is tetracycline. For adults in the acute stage, the dose is 500 mg every 6 hours for about 3 weeks. In patients with skeletal or other complications, intramuscular streptomycin 1 g daily in addition to tetracycline usually achieves a cure. *(b) Pasteurization of milk :* This is a useful preventive measure which will render milk and milk products safe for consumption. Boiling of milk is effective when pasteurization is not possible. *(c) Protective measures :* The aim is to prevent direct contact with infected animals. Persons at risk such as farmers, shepherds, milkmen, abattoir workers should observe high standards of personal hygiene. They should exercise care in handling and disposal of placenta, discharges and foetuses from an aborted animal. They should wear protective clothing when handling carcasses. Exposed areas of the skin should be washed and soiled clothing renewed. *(d) Vaccination :* Human live vaccine of *B. abortus strain* 19–BA is available *(5)*.

Brucellosis would disappear if it were eradicated from animals. The national and international centre for brucellosis is located at FAO/WHO Brucella Reference Centre, Indian Veterinary Research Institute, Izatnagar, (Uttar Pradesh).

References

1. WHO (1996). *World Health Report 1996,* Report of the Director–General WHO.
2. DGHS, NICD (1985) *Manual on Zoonoses.*
3. WHO (1976) *Techn. Rep. Ser.,* No.598.
4. J.V. Zammit Maempel (1984). *Med Int* 2 : 85 Feb 1984 Middle Eastern edition.
5. T. Fujlkuva (1985) *World Health* July, 1985 P. 13.

LEPTOSPIROSIS

Leptospirosis is essentially animal infection by several serotypes of *Leptospira* (Spirocheates) and transmitted to man under certain environmental conditions. The disease manifestations are many and varied, ranging in severity from a mild febrile illness to severe, and sometimes fatal disease with liver and kidney involvement. Weils disease is one of the many manifestations of human leptospirosis.

Problem statement

Leptospirosis is considered to be the most widespread of the disease transmissible from animal to man *(1)*. It has high prevalence in warm humid tropical countries. Out breaks mostly occur as a result of heavy rainfall and consequent floodings *(2)*. Although the global burden of disease is unknown, more than 1 million cases of leptospirosis are estimated to occur worldwide each year including almost 60,000 deaths *(3)*. The incidence in some areas may be as high as 975 cases per lac population. During the past decade, the occurrence of outbreak has highlighted the strong links between leptospirosis and extreme weather events in Guyana, India, Philippines and Thailand etc *(4)*.

Epidemiological determinants

Agent factors

(a) AGENT : Leptospira are thin and light motile spirocheates 0.1–0.2 μm wide and 5–15 μm long with hooked ends. Only the strains of *L. interrogans* are pathogenic. The organisms are visible by dark–field illumination and silver staining. At present, 23 sero-groups and 200 serovars have been recognized from various parts of the world. They are serologically related with cross reactivity. (b) SOURCE OF INFECTION : Leptospira are excreted in the urine of infected animals for a long time, often for an entire life time in cases of rodents. (c) ANIMAL RESERVOIRS : Leptospirosis affects wild and domestic animals worldwide especially rodents such as rats, mice and voles. Most domestic animals including cattle, sheep, goats, water buffalo, pigs and horses may be infected through grazing in areas contaminated by the urine of the carrier host. Pet animals, particularly dogs may also be infected. Infection may spread from wild animals to domestic livestock, and then to humans. Rats and small rodents – particularly *R. norvegicus* and *Mus musculus* are the most important reservoirs *(5)*.

Host factors

(a) AGE AND SEX : Males suffer more frequently from leptospirosis than females because of greater occupational exposure to infected animals and contaminated environment. Leptospirosis infections occur more frequently in persons 20–45 years of age group. Leptospirosis rarely occurs in young children and infants, possibly, because of minimal exposure *(6)*. (b) OCCUPATION : Human infections are usually due to occupational exposure to the urine of infected animals, e.g, agricultural and livestock farmers, workers in rice fields, sugarcane fields, and underground sewers, abattoir workers, meat and animal handlers, veterinarians etc. *(5)*. Leisure time activities such as swimming and fishing may also carry risks. (c) IMMUNITY : A solid serovar specific immunity follows infection.

Environmental factors

Leptospirosis infection is unique in that it is acquired through contact with an environment contaminated by urine and faeces from carrier (reservoir) animal or other infected animals. Leptospira shed in the urine can survive for weeks in soil and water, so environmental contamination may reach high levels in areas where carrier animals frequently urinate *(7)*. The association of poor housing, limited water supply, inadequate method of waste disposal, all combine to make the disease a significant risk for the poor population in both urban and rural areas. Soil salinity and water logging are inter-linked problems. The salinity of the soil and alkaline pH provides favourable environment for survival of leptospires for months. The soil of endemic areas in general has lower base saturation and mean annual soil temperature at the depth of 50 cm is 22°C or more and the difference between mean summer (June–August) and mean winter (December–February) temperature is less than 5°C. This favours the survival of leptospires for long duration *(6)*.

Mode of transmission

(a) DIRECT CONTACT : Leptospira can enter the body through skin abrasions or through intact mucous membrane by direct contact with urine or tissue of infected animal. (b) INDIRECT CONTACT : Through the contact of the broken skin with soil, water or vegetation contaminated by urine of infected animals or through ingestion of food or water contaminated with leptospirae. (c) DROPLET INFECTION : Infection may also occur through inhalation as when milking infected cows or goats by breathing air polluted with droplets of urine *(8)*.

Direct man to man infection is rare *(5)*.

Incubation period

Usually 10 days with a range of 4 to 20 days.

Clinical picture *(6)*

The clinical spectrum of leptospirosis is very wide, with mild anicteric presentation at one end to severe leptospirosis with severe jaundice and multiple organ involvement on the other. Many infections may go unnoticed because of lack of significant clinical illness.

Clinical types of leptospirosis are as follows:

1. *Anicteric leptospirosis :* It is the milder form of the disease. Patient presents with fever with chills, myalgia, conjunctival suffusion, headache, renal manifestation (some form of renal involvement is invariable), pulmonary manifestations (cough and chest pain are primary manifestations and haemoptysis may occur), and haemorrhagic tendencies. All the clinical features either decrease or disappear within two or three days, and then they may reappear and may progress to severe disease *(6)*.
2. *Icteric leptospirosis :* It is the more severe form of leptospirosis. The patient has jaundice and presents with fever, myalgia (calf muscle tenderness becomes more evident), headache, conjunctival suffussion, acute renal failure, nausea, vomiting, diarrhoea, abdominal pain, hypotension and circulatory collapse, pulmonary insufficiency. Combined renal and liver failure associated with leptospirosis is referred to as Weil's disease *(6)*.

Leptospirosis during pregnancy can cause foetal complications including foetal death or abortion. The case fatality rate for leptospirosis is approximately 5 per cent to 15 per cent among patients with severe illness. Among patients with severe pulmonary haemorrhagic syndrome, the case fatality can exceed 50 per cent *(3)*.

Diagnosis

It is not possible to diagnose leptospirosis with certainty on clinical grounds alone. Because of the wide spectrum of signs and symptoms, the diagnosis is made by isolation of leptospires from blood during the acute illness and from urine after the first week *(8)*. Early in the disease, the organism may be identified by dark–field examination of the patient's blood or by culture on a semisolid medium. Culture takes 1–6 weeks to become positive. The organism may also be grown from the urine from 10th day to 6 weeks. Diagnosis is usually made by means of serological tests, of which several are available. Agglutination tests (microscopic using live organism, and macroscopic using killed antigen) become positive after 7–10 days of illness and peak at 3–4 weeks and may persist at high level for many years. Indirect haemagglutination, immunoflourescent antibody and ELISA tests are also available. The IgM ELISA is particularly useful in making an early diagnosis, as it is positive as early as 2 days into illness *(9)*. Now Leptodipstick test is also available.

Control

(a) ANTIBIOTICS : Penicillin is the drug of choice but other antibiotics (tetracycline, amoxycillin, ampicillin and doxycycline) are also effective. The dosage of penicillin is 6 million units daily intravenously.

(b) ENVIRONMENTAL MEASURES : This includes preventing exposure to potentially contaminated water, reducing contamination by rodent control and protection of workers in hazardous occupation. Measures should be taken to control rodents, proper disposal of wastes and health education etc.

Vaccination

Immunization of farmers and pets prevent disease. In some countries for instance Italy, USSR and China, where certain occupations carry a high risk of infection, vaccines are available. It is important that they should incorporate strains of the serotypes that predominate in the particular area since immunity to one type of *Leptospira* may not protect against infection by another *(8)*.

References

1. WHO (1978), *World Health,* Oct. 1978.
2. WHO (2000), *Weekly Epidemiological Record,* No. 27, 7th July 2000.
3. CDC (2018), Center for Disease Control and Prevention, *Fact Sheet,* 30th Jan. 2018.
4. WHO (2011), *Weekly Epidemiological Record,* No. 6, 4th Feb 2011.
5. WHO (2018), *Managing epidemics, Key facts about major deadly diseases,* Version 1.
6. National Centre for Disease Control (2015), *Programme for Prevention and Control of Leptospirosis. National Guidelines, Diagnosis, Case Management, Prevention and Control of Leptospirosis,* DGHS, New Delhi.
7. WHO (1985), *World Health,* July 1985.
8. Coghlan, J.D., *Post Graduate Doctor,* May 1983
9. Lawrence M. Tierney, Jr. et al. *Current Medical Diagnosis and Treatment,* 38th Ed. 1999, International edition.

PLAGUE

Plague is primarily and basically a zoonoses, caused by *Y. pestis,* involving rodents and fleas. It exists in natural foci, and is transmitted by infected flea bites to humans living or intruding into the same ecological environment. Plague occurs in many forms – enzootically, epizootically, sporadically and in epidemics of all types including anthroponotic and primary pneumonic forms. Despite the enormous body of knowledge regarding plague, this communicable disease continues to pose a threat in many areas.

Problem statement

WORLD

Plague is often seen as a problem of the past or an ancient disease that is unlikely to reappear. But continued outbreaks throughout the world attest to its tenacious presence. Plague continues to be a threat because vast areas exist where wild rodents are infected, particularly in endemic countries in Africa, Asia and the Americas. Although plague is predominantly a rural disease, there have been outbreaks among urban populations in Madagascar, Democratic

Republic of Congo and Peru. Plague is a major concern in countries where it remains endemic given its inherent communicability, its rapid clinical course and high mortality if left untreated.

The development of rapid diagnostic tests have contributed to better case-management and surveillane in Africa and other continents.

The data shows that from 2010 to 2015, a total of 3,248 cases of human plague, including 584 deaths, were reported globally *(1)*.

In 2004, India reported a localized outbreak of bubonic plague (8 cases and 3 deaths) in the Dangud village, District of Uttarkashi.

Absence of human plague may simply mean that there has been reduced human contact with plague bacteria circulating in nature. Therefore, there is a need to continue to make concerted effort to strengthen surveillance and improve control measures in order to manage human plague in endemic countries.

Epidemiological determinants

Agent factors

(a) AGENT : The causative agent, *Y. pestis* is a gram-negative, non-motile, cocco-bacillus that exhibits bipolar staining with special stains (e.g., Wayson's stain). The bacilli occur in great abundance in the buboes, blood, spleen, liver and other viscera of infected persons, and in the sputum of cases of pneumonic plague. The virulence of the organism is related to its ability to produce exotoxin, endotoxin, fraction 1 and many other antigens and toxins. It has been shown that plague bacilli can survive, and indeed multiply in the soil of rodent burrows where micro-climate and other conditions are favourable *(2)*.

(b) RESERVOIR OF INFECTION : Wild rodents (e.g., field mice, gerbils, skunks and other small animals) are the natural reservoirs of plague. These are found in mountains, deserts, cultivated areas and forests in temperate and tropical regions. Over 200 species of these small animals may carry plague *(3)*. In any given focus, rodent reservoirs may vary.

In India, the wild rodent, *Tatera indica* has been incriminated as the main reservoir, not the domestic rat, *Rattus rattus*, as once thought. Generally the disease is maintained and spread by the resistant species of wild rodents, i.e., rodents which have become immune to plague. The susceptible rodents die of the disease.

(c) SOURCE OF INFECTION : Infected rodents and fleas and case of pneumonic plague.

Host factors

(a) AGE AND SEX : All ages and both sexes are susceptible. (b)HUMAN ACTIVITIES : Man may come into contact with natural foci in the course of hunting, grazing, cultivation, harvesting and construction activities or while engaging in outdoor recreation. These activities offer numerous opportunities to flea–man contact. Social upheavals like war may also account for outbreaks, as had happened in Vietnam. (c) MOVEMENT OF PEOPLE : Plague is associated with movement of people and cargo by sea or land. Rats and rat fleas are transported in this way. Further, in these days of jet travel, it is possible for a person to acquire the disease and become ill thousands of miles away where plague would be least suspected.

(d) IMMUNITY : Man has no natural immunity. Immunity after recovery is relative.

Environmental factors

(a) SEASON : Outbreaks of plague are usually seasonal in nature. In northern India, the "plague season" starts from September until May. The disease tends to die out with the onset of hot weather. Researches indicated that the curious phenomenon of "plague season" depended primarily on the field rodent factors; from May onwards all species of rodents in the fields commenced aestivation, closing themselves in their burrows and living on stored food reserves. Then the epizootic ceased to advance and at the same time infection of village rats came to an end. When the field rodents again became active, that is mid-October, when the monsoon floods had dried up, the epizootic revived in the fields followed by human plague *(4)*. On the contrary, in south India, there was no definite plague season. The disease was found to be active all the year round. This is attributed partly to the topographic and climatic conditions in the south, favourable for the breeding of the field rodents. (b) TEMPERATURE AND HUMIDITY : A mean temperature of 20 to 25 deg. C, and a relative humidity of 60 per cent and above are considered favourable for the spread of plague. (c) RAINFALL : Heavy rainfall, especially in the flat fields tend to flood the rat burrows. This factor may be responsible for keeping certain states (e.g., Bengal) free from plague *(5)*. (d) URBAN AND RURAL AREAS: Plague had failed to gain a foothold in many towns of India perhaps due to untoward ecological conditions and lack of efficient flea vectors (as in Chennai and Assam) *(5)*. (e) HUMAN DWELLINGS: Rats, frequent dwelling houses and where housing conditions are poor, there may be an abundance of rats and rat fleas all the year round, and contact with man occurs readily.

Vectors of plague

The commonest and the most efficient vector of plague is the rat flea, *X. cheopis,* but other fleas may also transmit the infection, e.g., *X. astia, X. brasiliensis* and *Pulex irritans* (human flea). Both sexes of the flea bite and transmit the disease.

Blocked flea

A flea may ingest upto 0.5 cu.mm of blood which may contain as many as 5,000 plague bacilli. The bacilli multiply enormously in the gut of the rat flea and may block the proventriculus so that no food can pass through. Such a flea is called a "blocked flea". A blocked flea eventually faces starvation and death because it is unable to obtain a blood meal. It makes frantic efforts to bite and suck blood over and over again; and in so doing, it inoculates (regurgitates) plague bacilli into the bite wound each time it bites. A blocked flea, therefore, becomes an efficient transmitter of plague. A partially blocked flea is more dangerous than a completely blocked flea because it can live longer. Infected fleas may live upto an year, and certain species survive in the burrow micro-climate for as long as 4 years *(2)*.

Flea indices

Flea indices are useful measurements of the density of fleas. They are also useful in evaluating the effectiveness of a spraying programme. The following flea indices are widely used in rat flea surveys : (a) TOTAL FLEA INDEX : It is the average number of fleas of all species per rat.

(b) CHEOPIS INDEX : It is the average number of X. *cheopis* per rat. It is a specific flea index. It is a more significant index than the total flea index. If this index is more than 'one', it is regarded as indicative of potential explosiveness of the situation, should a plague outbreak occur *(6)*. (c) SPECIFIC PERCENTAGE OF FLEAS : It is the percentage of different species of fleas that are found on rats. (d) BURROW INDEX : It is the average number of free–living fleas per species per rodent burrow *(7)*.

Flea indices do not in themselves indicate an imminent plague epidemic. They serve as a warning that more stringent control measures are needed to protect the human population.

PLAGUE IN RODENTS

1. Rodents

Plague is primarily a disease of rodents in which man becomes accidentally involved. Approximately, 1,700 species of rodents are known, of which over 200 species are associated with plague. These are found in mountains, deserts, cultivated areas and forests throughout the world *(8)*.

Rodents may be classified into two distinct groups :

(a) WILD RODENTS : They are the reservoir of plague in nature. The common wild rodents in India are : *Tatera indica, Bandicota bengalensis varius, B. bengalensis kok (Gunomys kok), B. indica, Millardia meltada, M. gleadowi and Mus booduga*. In India, *tatera indica* has been incriminated as the main reservoir of plague, not the domestic rat (*R. rattus*) as once thought.

(b) COMMENSAL RODENTS : These are the rodents which live close to man. They may be further divided into domestic and peridomestic species. The domestic species include *Rattus rattus, Rattus norvegicus and Mus musculus.* The domestic species seldom live in fields. The peridomestic species live in both fields and houses; *R. norvegicus* which frequents sewers, drains as well as houses is a typical example of a peri-domestic species in India. Characteristics which are easily ascertainable of *Rattus rattus and R. norvegicus* are given elsewhere (see chapter 15).

2. Epizootiology

Plague is epizootic and enzootic in wild rodents. ***Two ecological cycles*** have been described :

a. WILD PLAGUE : Wild plague is defined as "plague existing in nature, independent of human populations and their activities" *(2)*. The disease spreads among wild rodents by wild rodent fleas. The epizootic wipes out the susceptible population. Those that survive (i.e., resistant species) maintain the enzootic in natural foci.

b. DOMESTIC PLAGUE : Is defined as "plague that is intimately associated with man and rodents living with him, and has a definite potential for producing epidemics *(2)*.

3. Natural foci

Worldwide, rodent plague is still firmly entrenched in its natural foci. A "natural focus" of plague has been defined as "a strictly delimited area where ecological conditions ensure the persistence of the aetiological agent for considerable periods of time, and where epizootics and periods of quiescence alternate, without introduction of infection from outside" *(2)*.

The long persistence of plague in some natural foci is not achieved through the usual simple chain of "Rat–flea–rat" transmission. Probably several other mechanisms are involved. They include : (a) latent infection in rodents, especially hibernating rodents, has been demonstrated; such animals may relapse and become bacteraemic, so initiating an epizootic. (b) development of resistance to plague infection by some rodents with subsequent localization of plague bacillus in some organ; such an animal may become a source of infection if eaten by another susceptible rodent. (c) survival of rat fleas for as long as 4 years in rat burrows under optimum micro-climatic conditions. This is considered the most likely mechanism of maintaining the natural focus. (d) variations in the pathogenecity of *Y. pestis,* and (e) survival and even multiplication of plague bacilli in the soil of rodent burrows. All these factors may combine to keep the infection alive in natural foci.

4. Epizootic process

The epizootic and enzootic process in each natural plague focus has its specific cyclic and periodical pattern. Researches into the epidemicity of plague indicated that the field rodents spread the infection very slowly from burrow to burrow, and from field to field taking months to cover several miles. In this process they infect the village rats (commensal rodents). The commensal rodents especially the peridomestic species (e.g., *R. norvegicus*) act as "Liaison rodents" between man and field rodents. An outbreak of human plague is always preceded by rodent plague. After the death of house rats, the fleas leave the dead rats and are forced to seek man for food. An unusual mortality among rodents should arouse suspicion of plague and should be investigated immediately.

5. Silent periods

Silences of long duration (10 years or more) followed by sudden explosive outbreaks of rodent or human plague have been repeatedly confirmed in some natural foci *(9)*. A number of explanations for this phenomenon have been put forward. It has been suggested that plague disappears completely for long periods and that it is reintroduced from other areas by infected rodents, fleas or migrating birds. On the other hand, the plague bacillus can survive and indeed multiply in the soil of rodent burrows, where micro-climatic conditions are suitable. It has been demonstrated that healthy rodents re-occupying and excavating such burrows may become infected through contact with contaminated soil *(2, 10)*.

6. Plague in rodents

Animal disease is similar to that in man. The disease is inapparent or mild in resistant species *(11)*.

7. Investigations

(1) COLLECTION AND FORWARDING OF DEAD RATS : Rodents (house or field) found dead regardless of its stage of decomposition should be carefully packed in several layers of packing paper or preferably in plastic bags. Such rodents should not be handled with naked hands. The neck of the bag should be tied to avoid escape of ectoparasites. The bag should then be placed in a wooden box or tin. The empty space left in the box or tin should be filled with absorbent cotton or sawdust to eliminate chances of leakage of effluents outside the box. The box is labelled giving details of collection and sent to the nearest laboratory. (2) AUTOPSY AND COLLECTION OF SMEARS : The rat is

held with a pair of tongs, and dipped in a solution of 5 per cent cresol. The animal is laid on its dorsum, stretched and the limbs nailed on a wooden board. The abdomen is swabbed with lysol or spirit. The skin is lifted and cut up to the chest. The instruments used are then put back into boiling water. Using another set of instruments, small portions of the viscera (spleen, liver, lungs, bubo) are cut and the freshly cut surface is first blotted on a blotting paper so as to remove excess of blood or plasma. Then the same surface of the tissue is gently pressed on the glass slides so as to make thin impressions (never rub the tissue on the slides). If the rat is completely decomposed and no tissue is left, smears should be obtained from the bone marrow. The smears are dried, treated with alcohol for three minutes and fixed by exposure to open flame. The fixed smears may be sent for examination. Persons handling infected rats are exposed to the risk of pneumonic plague and this danger should be borne in mind. (3) ANIMAL INOCULATION : It may be difficult to isolate the plague bacilli by cultural methods owing to gross contamination of the carcass. In such cases, small portions of liver or spleen are taken, ground in a mortar with a little saline and inoculated into a guinea pig or a white mouse. If there is plague infection, the guinea pig will die in 7 days and the white mouse in 48 hours. (4) PATHOLOGICAL CHANGES : The pathological changes in an animal infected with plague are as follows: (a) there is oedema and necrosis at the site of injection, (b) the lymph nodes are enlarged, (c) the spleen is enlarged and congested, and shows necrotic patches, (d) liver shows mottling, (e) lungs also show necrotic lesions, and (f) there is subcutaneous congestion and haemorrhages.

HUMAN PLAGUE

Mode of transmission

Human plague is most frequently contracted from : (a) the bite of an infected flea, (b) occasionally by direct contact with the tissues of the infected animal or (c) by droplet infection from cases of pneumonic plague. The dissemination of plague by plague patients (by the bite of the human flea, *Pulex irritans*) is a rare and exceptional occurrence.

There are at least 5 basic types of transmission cycles in plague. These cycles are as follows *(8)* :

1. *Commensal rats → rat fleas → man*

   This is the basic cycle in epidemic bubonic plague.

2. *Wild rodents → wild rodent fleas or direct contact → man*

   The disease is transmitted from rodent to rodent *via* wild rodent fleas or contaminated soil. Man contracts the infection from infectious wild rodent fleas or by direct contact with infected rodents.

3. *Wild rodents, peridomestic rodents, commensal rodents → wild rodent fleas, peridomestic rodent fleas, commensal rodent fleas → man*

   Plague foci impinge upon the habitats of peri-domestic or commensal rodents. Interaction of the rodents and their fleas convey the infection to man.

4. *Man → human flea (Pulex irritans) → man*

   This variety may be encountered in certain areas.

5. *Man → man*

   This results when a primary case of bubonic plague develops secondary pneumonic plague and infects contacts *via* the respiratory route.

Incubation period

(a)	bubonic plague	.....	2 to 7 days
(b)	septicaemic plague	.....	2 to 7 days
(c)	pneumonic plague	.....	1 to 3 days

Disease in man

There are three main clinical forms : ***(a) Bubonic plague :*** This is the most common type of the disease. The infected rat fleas usually bite on the lower extremities and inoculate the bacilli. The bacilli are intercepted by the regional lymphatic glands where they proliferate. Typically the patient develops sudden fever, chills, headache, prostration and painful lymphadenitis. Usually within a few days greatly enlarged tender lymph nodes (buboes) develop in the groin and less often in the axilla or neck, depending upon the site of the bite by the flea. When suppuration takes place it is considered a favourable sign. Bubonic plague cannot spread from person to person as the bacilli are locked up in the buboes and do not find a way or easy exit. ***(b) Pneumonic plague :*** Primary pneumonic plague is rare; it generally follows as a complication of bubonic–septicaemic plague. The incidence of pneumonic plague is usually below 1 per cent *(5)*. Pneumonic plague is highly infectious and spreads from man to man by droplet infection. The plague bacilli are present in the sputum. ***(c) Septicaemic plague :*** Primary septicaemic plague is rare except for accidental laboratory infections. However, bubonic plague may develop into septicaemic plague in the face of an overwhelming infection.

Laboratory investigations

The absolute confirmation of plague infection in human beings, rodents or fleas requires the isolation and identification of the plague bacillus. The important laboratory methods of diagnosis include the following : ***(a) Staining :*** It is important to prepare smears of the clinical material (e.g., bubo fluid, sputum) which should be fixed with alcohol and then stained with Giemsa's or Wayson's stain to demonstrate bipolar bacilli in the specimen. ***(b) Culture :*** Blood for culture should be collected from all patients. Under ideal circumstances, appropriate culture media should be inoculated on the spot with blood, bubo fluid or sputum to ensure speedy isolation of the plague bacilli. When this is not possible, the specimen must be transported to the laboratory in Cary–Blair transport medium. ***(c) Serology :*** Acute and convalescent specimens of blood sera should be collected for antibody studies. ***(d) Other methods :*** These include inoculation of guinea pigs or mice or immunofluorescent microscopic test.

PREVENTION AND CONTROL

1. Control of cases

(a) EARLY DIAGNOSIS : During epidemic situations, diagnosis of plague can be made readily on clinical grounds, e.g., acute fever and painful lymph node enlargement developing into buboes in the inguinal and other regions of the body. In other situations, "rat falls" (dead rats) provide a

useful warning of a possible outbreak. It is essential that plague–suspected humans and rodents be examined bacteriologically to confirm the presence of plague. It is often possible to arrive at a *prima facie* diagnosis by the examination of smears that show the characteristic bipolar stained plague bacilli *(8)*. *(b) NOTIFICATION* : If a human or rodent case is diagnosed, health authorities must be notified promptly. Case notification is required by International Health Regulations *(13)*. *(c) ISOLATION* : Although most bubonic plague patients are non–infectious, isolation is recommended whenever possible. All patients with pneumonic plague including suspected cases should be isolated. *(d) TREATMENT* : Treatment must be started without waiting for confirmation of the diagnosis *(2)*. Unless promptly treated, plague may have a mortality of nearly 50 per cent, and pneumonic plague 100 per cent. The drug of choice is streptomycin (30 mg per kg of body weight daily) administered intramuscularly in two divided doses for 7 to 10 days. Tetracycline orally (30–40 mg per kg of body weight daily) is an alternative drug, and is sometimes given in combination with streptomycin *(12)*. Gentamycin administered as a 2 mg/kg body wt. loading dose, then 1.7 mg/kg body wt. every 8 hours intravenously is effective. Penicillin is rather ineffective. Sulphonamides may be used if other drugs are not available. *(e) DISINFECTION* : Disinfection of sputum, discharges and articles soiled by the patient should be carried out. Dead bodies should be handled with aseptic precautions.

2. Control of fleas

The most effective method to break the chain of transmission (rodent → flea → man) is the destruction of rat fleas by the proper application of an effective insecticide. Flea control must precede or coincide anti-rodent measures. The choice of insecticide is dictated by the results of prior susceptibility tests. In general DDT and BHC should be used as dusts containing 10 per cent and 3 per cent of the active ingredient respectively. In areas where resistance to one or both of these insecticides occurs, dusts of carbaryl (2%) or malathion (5%) should prove effective. About 2 to 3 g of insecticide formulation will be needed for each sq. metre of surface requiring treatment *(8)*. Generally the organochlorine insecticides remain effective for 2 to 4 months.

Before spraying is to be done, the inhabitants of premises should be asked to remove all foodstuffs and eating and cooking vessels from their houses. Spraying is done inside the houses covering the entire floor area, bottoms of all walls up to 3 feet above floor level, back of the doors, roofing of thatched houses, crevices of walls, rat runs, clothing, bedding, cats, dogs and other pets. Rat burrows should be insufflated with the insecticidal dust with the help of a dust blower. Insecticidal spraying up to a radius of 5 miles around each infected locality is considered adequate *(8)*. Within 48 hours of application, the "flea index" should drop down to zero *(8)*.

3. Control of rodents

Continuous mass destruction of rodents is an important plague–preventive measure. The long-term policy for the control of rodents should be based on improvement of general sanitation, improvement of housing and quality of life. The various antirodent measures are given elsewhere.

4. Vaccination

Immunization with plague vaccine is a valuable preventive measure. The WHO recommends that under all circumstances, vaccination should be only for the prevention, not the control of human plague *(2)*. To be effective, vaccination should be carried out at least a week before an anticipated outbreak, and the vaccine should be given in 2 doses.

In 1897, Haffkine developed a killed plague vaccine while working in India and inoculated himself with his experimental vaccine *(14)*. The vaccine used currently is that of Haffkine, modified by Sokhey. It is a formalin–killed vaccine. Virulent strains of *Y. pestis* are grown in casein hydrolysate broth for 2 weeks at 27 deg. C and killed by treatment with 0.1 per cent formalin for 3 days at 37 deg. C. The final vaccine is a suspension of 2000 million killed organisms per ml *(15)*.

The vaccine is given subcutaneously in two doses of 0.5 and 1.0 ml at an interval of 7 to 14 days. A single dose will not result in dependable protection. However, in an emergency, when it is desired to carry out primary immunization by means of a single injection, the dose should be double the second dose, that is, 3 ml for adult males *(15)*. Immunity starts 5 to 7 days after inoculation, and lasts for about 6 months. Booster doses are recommended six–monthly for persons at continuing risk of infection (e.g., geologists, biologists and anthropologists). The recommended doses of the vaccine are given in Table 3. The reactions after inoculation (pain, tenderness, headache, etc) appear in a few hours and subside in 1 to 2 days. The vaccine is indicated for travellers to hyperendemic areas besides persons at special risk.

TABLE 3
Dosage of plague vaccine

Age and Sex	Primary inoculation		Booster dose six–monthly
	1st dose	2nd dose	
Adult males	1.0 ml	1.5 ml	1.0 ml
Adult females	0.75 ml	1.0 ml	0.75ml
Children			
1–4 years	0.2 ml		
5–10 years	0.3 ml	Double the first dose	Same as the first dose
11–16 years	0.4 ml		
Infants under 6 months are not immunized.			

Source : *(15)*

5. Chemoprophylaxis

Chemoprophylaxis is a valuable preventive measure, highly recommended. It should be offered to all plague contacts, medical, nursing and public health personnel exposed to the risk of infection. The drug of choice is tetracycline. For adults, the dose is 500 mg 6–hourly for 5 days *(16)*. A cheaper alternative is sulfonamide, 2 to 3 gram daily for 5 to 7 days.

6. Surveillance

Plague has a potential for spread into susceptible areas. Therefore, in areas where natural plague foci exist or where there is a history of past infection, surveillance is essential. Surveillance should cover all aspects of rodent and human plague, e.g., microbiology, serology, entomology, mammalogy, epidemiology and ecology. On the basis of information provided by surveillance, effective control measures must be established *(14)*. Surveillance of plague in its natural foci should, therefore, replace quarantine measures which have been shown to be ineffective *(2)*.

7. Health education

Health education is an essential part of any plague control programme. Education should aim at providing the public with the facts about plague and at enlisting their cooperation. Emphasis must be placed on the need for the prompt reporting of dead rats and suspected human cases so that preventive measures can be taken. Medical practitioners should keep plague in mind in differential diagnosis of any cases of fever with lymphadeno-pathy, or when multiple cases of pneumonia occur *(2)*.

Epidemiological investigations *(17)*

The determination of the source of infection and the distribution, prevalence, and potential spread of plague in human population is the main objective of epidemiological surveillance. This means that those engaged in surveillance must evaluate human plague in its relationship with epizootic factors and that the investigations must be based on direct contact with villages and other communities affected by plague. While the collection of demographic data and information on such subjects as population movements and local occupations, customs, and habits is important, special attention must be given to the factors bringing man into contact with the vertebrate reservoirs and vectors of *y. pestis.*

Some of the responsibilities of the surveillance team are as follows :

(1) to make a detailed study of all cases of human plague, giving special attention to dwellings where cases have occurred, in order to establish the rodent/vector source of the infection or the occurrence of man-to-man transmission;

(2) to keep complete and uniform records of each case of plague, using standardized forms, and to issue questionnaires to the population at risk;

(3) to isolate strains of *Y. pestis* and subject them to detailed biochemical analysis, samples being lyophilized for later study;

(4) to make a serological survey of the target population; such surveys are of value in investigation of possible cases of subclinical plague, of recovered untreated infections, and of asymptomatic pharyngeal infection in "carriers";

(5) to investigate changes in the human population, social or economic activities, and other features of natural foci where there is close contact between human populations and commensal rodents;

(6) to keep a watch on containerized cargoes of grain and other food crops originating in areas with natural plague foci and destined for national or international trade;

(7) to undertake surveillance in cooperation with adjacent countries when natural foci are common to two or more countries;

(8) to give special attention, in the case of seaports or airports, to the proximity of natural foci where there is contact between wild and commensal rodents, the proximity of epidemics, and the transport of cargo from enzootic areas.

The surveillance team should also be prepared to assist the national or community health service in organizing and carrying out the treatment of human cases and measures for the control and prevention of plague. An organizational basis should be established for rapid emergency services in the event of an epidemic.

Reporting of cases and outbreaks of plague *(17)*

The WHO should be informed promptly of the occurrence of any epidemic or isolated case of plague. The report should include details about the administrative area and exact locality involved. This preliminary notification should be followed up as soon as possible by a more detailed report containing the following information :

(a) The locality and administrative area, shown on a map if possible

(b) The date, the first case was noticed

(c) The period during which field investigations were made

(d) The number and types of cases of plague detected :
- clinical diagnosis only (presumptive)
- laboratory diagnosis (confirmed)
- recovered and confirmed serologically
- types of cases – bubonic, pneumonic, etc.
- age of patient with a confirmed diagnosis of plague
- number of deaths

(e) The contacts of known cases
- serological test results
- throat swab results

(f) Chemotherapy applied
- number of frank cases
- number of contacts

(g) Vertebrate host population
- identification of domestic rodents
- identification of wild rodents
- results of laboratory test for plague

(h) Vector population
- identification of *X. cheopis*
- identification of other species of flea
- results of laboratory tests for infection
- results of insecticide resistance tests
- control measures applied.

References

1. WHO (2017), *Fact Sheet on Plague,* Oct., 2017.
2. WHO (1970). *Tech. Rep. Ser. No.* 447.
3. WHO (1982). *Vol. 60.*
4. WHO (1960). *WHO Chr.* 14 : 422.
5. Seal, S.C. (1960). *Bull WHO* 23 : 286.
6. WHO (1974). *Tech. Rep. Ser.* No. 553.
7. WHO (1972). *Tech. Rep. Ser.* No. 501.
8. Bahmanyar, M. et al (1976). *Plague manual Geneva,* WHO.
9. WHO (2002), *Weekly Epidemiological Record,* No. 9, 1st March, 2002.
10. WHO (1970). *WHO Chr.* 24 (8) 371–373.
11. WHO (1982). *Tech. Rep. Ser.* No. 682.
12. Akier, A.K. (1982). *Bull WHO,* 62 (2) 165–169.
13. WHO (1983). *Int Health 3rd annotrated ed Geneva,* WHO.
14. WHO (1980). *Bull WHO* P.753.
15. Banker, D.D. (1969). *Modern Practice in Immunization,* The Indian Journal of Medical Sciences Mumbai.
16. Issacson, M. (1981). *Medicine International,* 3 : 127.
17. WHO (1974), *WHO Chronicle,* Vol.28, No.2, February 1974, p.71.

HUMAN SALMONELLOSIS

The term "salmonellosis" covers a complex group of foodborne infections affecting both man and animals *(1)*. The disease causes illness and even death in humans, as well as economic losses in the animal and food industries. The term "food poisoning" is also commonly applied to salmonellosis.

Problem statement

Salmonellosis is a global problem *(2)*. Human salmonellosis represents 60 to 80 per cent of all reported cases of foodborne diseases *(3)*.

While the incidence of typhoid fever has declined, the incidence of other *Salmonella* infections has increased in the developed countries. The problem is aggravated by the widespread use of animal feeds containing antimicrobial drugs that favour drug–resistant salmonellae and their potential transmission to humans. The disease can occur sporadically or in small outbreaks in the general population and usually from food contaminated at its source. The extent of the problem is not clear in developing countries where diarrhoeal diseases are widespread *(2)*.

Epidemiological determinants

Agent factors

AGENT : Salmonellae comprise a large and important group of bacteria. This group is now known to comprise more than 2,500 serotypes capable of infecting humans *(4)*, but in most countries only a small number of them (usually about 10) are endemic at any one time *(5)*.

Compared with other gram-negative rods, salmonellae are relatively resistant to various environmental factors. They have been shown to be resistant to drying, salting, smoking and freezing even for years. This explains why these organisms survive in many kinds of food. As a result, salmonellae have been isolated from divergent foods such as chocolates, biscuits, coconuts and spices. The bacterium is sensitive to heat and will not survive temperatures above 70 deg C.

From an epidemiological point of view, salmonellae can be classified into three main groups *(2)*.

(i) those which infect only man – e.g., *S. typhi, S. paratyphi A* and *C*.

(ii) those that are host–adapted for particular species of animals, e.g., *S. cholera–suis* in swine, *S. dublin* in cattle, *S. abortus equi* in horses, *S. gallinarum* in poultry, etc. Some of these are also pathogenic for man, e.g., *S. cholera–suis, S. dublin*.

(iii) those with no particular host preference and can infect both man and animals – e.g., *S. typhimurium, S.enteritidis*. In this group (approximately 2,200 serovars) are the principal agents of salmonellosis that occurs today *(2)*. They can be transmitted from animals to man and vice versa. *S. typhimurium* is responsible for upto 50 per cent or more of all human salmonella infections all over the world. *S. enteritidis* has also emerged as an important pathogen.

RESERVOIR AND SOURCES OF INFECTION : The main reservoir of Salmonella is the intestinal tract of man and animals. The source of the infecting agent could be contaminated food, animals, man or the environment.

(a) Foods

Foods of animal origin, particularly commercially prepared foods such as meat, poultry and egg products are considered to be the primary sources of salmonellosis. Most of these foods, e.g., meat and poultry become contaminated during slaughter. Every food that is produced or processed (including chocolates, spices, coconut) in a contaminated environment may become contaminated. Cross-contamination of cooked foods from raw ingredients, kitchen utensils or surfaces has been described frequently as a cause of salmonellosis *(5)*. Eggs may be infected directly through shell–cracks. Recent investigations suggest that salmonellae may penetrate the ovaries of egg–laying chickens. What food will ultimately become the vehicle varies from country to country *(6)*. For example, in the USA, beef is the main source of salmonella infection, while in England and Wales poultry accounts for more than 50 per cent of Salmonellosis outbreaks *(2)*.

(b) Animals

Animals are the hosts and the principal vectors of zoonotic salmonellosis. Many animals including cattle, swine, rodents and fowl are naturally infected with a variety of salmonellae and have the bacilli in their tissues (meat), eggs or excreta. Carriers occur among both man and animals.

(c) Environment

Salmonellae are widely distributed in the environment – in dust, water, manure, sewage, sludge, vegetables, insects, birds, fish, rodents and other mammals. They can survive in soil for months *(6)*. They may even multiply in the warm environment provided by the high ambient temperatures of many countries. Man may be infected from these sources.

Multidrug resistant strains of *salmonella* are now encountered frequently. Resistance to fluoroquinolones and third generation cephalosporins is a serious development, which results in severe limitation of the possibilities for effective treatment of human infections *(4)*.

Mode of transmission

By ingestion of contaminated food or drink. In addition, man can contract infection following direct contact with domestic animals especially such as dogs, pigeons, rats, mice and insects. Once man is infected, he becomes a source (case or carrier) and the infection may spread to others by the faecal–oral route.

Transmission is facilitated by food handling methods, local customs, cooking and food habits, food processing, storage and distribution methods, and prevailing sanitary conditions.

Incubation period

6 to 72 hours (usually).

Clinical features

The disease arises from the ingestion of the living organisms. Recent studies indicate that *Salmonella spp.* possess both invasive and cholera–like enterotoxic properties *(6)*. Clinically, the disease may manifest by one of the three syndromes :

3

(i) Enteric fever : S. typhi, S. paratyphi A and *C* are human pathogens, and are not considered zoonotic agents *(2)*. *S. paratyphi B,* while predominantly found in man has also been isolated from turkeys, chickens, cattle, sheep, swine, mice and monkeys. This syndrome (enteric fever) is dealt with separately (see page 276 under typhoid fever).

(ii) Salmonella enterocolitis (gastroenteritis) : This is the most common manifestation of *Salmonella* infection. 6 to 48 hours after ingestion of *Salmonellae* there is nausea, headache, vomiting and diarrhoea. Low grade fever is common. Most infections are mild with diarrhoea as the only symptom. In severe cases there may be dehydration requiring replacement of fluids and electrolytes. The episode usually resolves in 2 to 3 days, but the stools often remain loose for several weeks. The excretion of salmonella may be prolonged by antimicrobial therapy. Blood cultures are usually negative but stool cultures are positive for salmonella and may remain positive for several weeks after clinical recovery. Death is rare and occurs primarily in neonates, infants and elderly.

(iii) Septicaemia with focal lesions : Non–typhoid salmonellae (e.g., *S. cholera–suis*) may occasionally invade the blood stream leading to generalized or localized infection presenting itself as pyrexia of unknown origin. Focal infection may result in osteomyelitis, pyelonephritis, arthritis, meningitis, cholecystitis and endocarditis. Stool cultures are negative but blood cultures are positive.

Prevention and control

Since salmonellosis is zoonotic in origin, preventive measures should begin at the farm and embrace all the elements of the food chain through live animals, animal products, processing, final food preparation to consumption. Approaches indicated at the farm level are : (i) disease control, e.g., immunization of farm animals against salmonellosis. (ii) the use of hygienic animal feed, and (iii) ensuring a sanitary environment for the animals. The aim is to raise "salmonella–free" animals.

The other approaches include : hygienic slaughtering and milking, pasteurization of milk and eggs; proper disposal of liquid and solid wastes, cold storage facilities, and health education and training.

Since the health sector alone cannot solve the problem of salmonellosis, responsibility for prevention and control measures may fall to agriculture, veterinary and other ministries, outside the health sector *(1, 7)*.

References

1. WHO (1982). *Economic aspects of communicable diseases,* EURO 68.
2. WHO (1988). *Salmonellosis control : the role of animals and product hygiene,* TRS 774.
3. WHO (1988). *WH Forum;* 9 (1) 123.
4. WHO (2005). Fact Sheet No. 139, *Drug-resistant Salmonella.*
5. WHO (1976). TRS 598 *(Microbiological aspects of food hygiene).*
6. Velimirovic, B. et al (1984). *Infectious diseases in Europe, A fresh look WHO, Copenhagen.*
7. WHO (1984) TRS 705 *(The role of food safety in health and develop).*

RICKETTSIAL ZOONOSES
(Rickettsial diseases)

Rickettsial zoonoses are a group of specific communicable diseases caused by rickettsial organisms and transmitted to man by arthropod vectors, (Q fever excepted). Increasingly, it is realized that rickettsial diseases are under-diagnosed and that they contribute substantially to the acute febrile burden and preventive illness in many populations *(1)*.

Classification

Rickettsial diseases may be grouped on the basis of clinical features and epidemiological aspects as follows (Table 1).

TABLE 1
Rickettsial diseases

Diseases	Rickettsial agent	Insect vectors	Mammalian reservoirs
1. Typhus group			
a. Epidemic typhus	*R. prowazekii*	Louse	Humans
b. Murine typhus	*R. typhi*	Flea	Rodents
c. Scrub typhus	*R. tsutsugamushi*	Mite*	Rodents
2. Spotted fever group			
a. Indian tick typhus	*R. conorii*	Tick*	Rodents, dogs
b. Rocky mountain spotted fever	*R. rickettsii*	Tick*	Rodents, dogs
c. Rickettsial pox	*R. akari*	Mite*	Mice
3. Others			
a. Q fever	*C. burnetii*	Nil	Cattle, sheep, goats
b. Trench fever	*Rochalimaea quintana*	Louse	Humans

*Also serves as arthropod reservoir, by maintaining the rickettsiae through ovarian transmission.

Source : *(2)*

Causal agents

Rickettsiae are small bacteria that are obligate intracellular parasites. They are pleomorphic, appearing either as short rods, or as cocci and they occur singly, in pairs, in short chains, or in filaments. With Giemsa's stain they stain blue and are readily visible under microscope. They grow readily in the yolk sac of the embryonated egg. Rickettsial growth is enhanced by the presence of sulfonamides.

Clinical features

Excepting for Q fever, in which there is no skin lesion, rickettsial infections are characterized by fever, headache, malaise, prostration, skin rash and enlargement of the spleen and liver. Tetracycline is the drug of choice for specific treatment of all rickettsial diseases. Long–acting antibiotics (doxycycline, minocycline) now make single dose treatment possible *(3)*.

Diagnostic procedures

These include : (a) isolation of rickettsiae. (b) established serological tests such as indirect fluorescent antibody (IFA) test, the complement fixation test, and the Weil Felix reaction. The newer techniques include ELISA and the fluorescent antibody staining of frozen tissue sections from rickettsial lesions.

Among the major groups of rickettioses, the commonly reported diseases in India are scrub typhus, murine flea–born typhus, Indian tick typhus and Q fever. These are considered in more detail :

SCRUB TYPHUS

Distribution

Of the diseases caused by rickettsiae in man, the most widespread is scrub typhus. It exists as a zoonoses in nature between certain species of trombiculid mites and their small mammals (e.g., field mice, rats, shrews). Scrub typhus is endemic in Northern Japan, South East Asia, the Western Pacific Islands, Eastern Australia, China, Maritime areas and several parts of South-Central Russia, India and Sri Lanka. More than 1 million cases occur annually. Most travel-acquired cases of scrub typhus occur during visits to rural areas in endemic countries for activities such as camping, hiking or rafting, but urban cases have also been described *(4)*.

Epidemiological determinants

Agent factors

(a) AGENT : The causative agent of scrub typhus is *Rickettsia tsutsugamushi*. There are several serologically distinct strains. (b) RESERVOIR : The true reservoir of infection is the trombiculid mite *(Leptotrombidium delinese* and *L.akamushi)*. The infection is maintained in nature transovarially from one generation of mite to the next. The nymphal and adult stages of the mite are free–living in the soil; they do not feed on vertebrate hosts. It is the larva (chigger) that feed on vertebrate hosts and picks up the rickettsiae. The larval stage serves both as a reservoir, through ovarian transmission, and as a vector for infecting humans and rodents.

Mode of transmission

By the bite of infected larval mites. The transmission cycle may be depicted as below :

Mite → Rats and mice → Mite → Rats and mice

↓

Man

The disease is not directly transmitted from person to person.

Incubation period

Usually 10 to 12 days; varies from 6 to 21 days.

Clinical features

Scrub typhus resembles epidemic typhus clinically. The onset is acute with chills and fever (104°–105°F), headache, malaise, prostration and a macular rash appearing around the 5th day of illness. Generalized lymphadenopathy and lymphocytosis are common. One typical feature is the punched–out ulcer covered with a blackened scab (eschar) which indicates the location of the mite bite. The pyrexia falls by lysis in the 3rd week in untreated cases. The Weil Felix reaction is strongly positive with the *Proteus* strain OXK.

Control measures

(a) TREATMENT : Tetracycline is the drug of choice. With proper therapy the mortality is nil. (b) VECTOR CONTROL : Clearing the vegetation where rats and mice live; application of insecticides such as lindane or chlordane to ground and vegetation. (c) PERSONAL PROPHYLAXIS : Impregnating clothes and blankets with miticial chemicals (benzyl benzoate) and application of mite repellents (diethyltoluamide) to exposed skin surfaces *(5)*. No vaccine exists at present.

MURINE TYPHUS

(Endemic or flea–borne typhus)

Distribution

Murine typhus (MT) is a zoonoses. It is worldwide in distribution especially in areas of high rat infestation. It appears to be more prevalent in South-East Asian and Western Pacific countries than previously recognized. In USA, cases tend to be scattered. Successful isolation of the causative agent from rats, fleas and bandicoots was made at many places in India. Focal infections are often associated with docks and shipping places where rats abound.

Agent factors

(a) AGENT : *Rickettsia typhi* (*R. mooseri*). (b) RESERVOIR OF INFECTION : Rats are the reservoir *(Rattus rattus and R.norvegicus)*. Infection in rats is inapparent, long–lasting and non–fatal.

Mode of transmission

The infection spreads from rat to rat *(X. cheopis)* and possibly by the rat louse *(6)*. The actual mode of transmission is not by the bite of the rat flea, but by (i) inoculation into skin of faeces of infected fleas, and (ii) possibly by inhalation of dried infective faeces. There is no direct man to man transmission. Once infected the flea remains so for life. The flea cannot transmit the rickettsiae transovarially. The transmission cycle may be shown as below :

Rat → Rat flea → Rat → Rat flea → Rat

↓

Man

Incubation period

1 to 2 weeks, commonly 12 days.

Clinical features

The clinical features resemble that of louse–borne typhus, but milder and rarely fatal. The Weil Felix reaction with Proteus OX–19 becomes positive in the 2nd week.

Control measures

(a) TREATMENT : Tetracycline is the only drug of choice. Since rickettsial growth is enhanced in the presence of sulfonamides, these drugs should not be given. *(b) CONTROL OF FLEAS* : Residual insecticides (e.g., BHC, malathion) are effective against rat fleas. Rodent control measures should be implemented in the affected areas. No murine typhus vaccine is currently available.

INDIAN TICK TYPHUS

Epidemiological determinants

Agent factors

(a) AGENT : The causative agent is *Rickettsia conorii*, a member of the spotted fever group of rickettsiae, the best known member of which is *R. rickettsii* the causative agent of Rocky Mountain spotted fever. (b) RESERVOIR OF

INFECTION : The tick is the reservoir of infection. It is infective at all stages of its life cycle and remains infective for life (commonly 18 months). Various tick genera *(e.g., Rhipicephalus, Ixodes, Boophilus, Haemaphysalis)* have been incriminated as vectors. Infection in nature is maintained by transovarian and trans-stadial passage. The rickettsiae can be transmitted to dogs, various rodents and other animals, which assist in maintaining the disease cycle.

Mode of transmission

Man is only an accidental host. He acquires infection by the bite of an infected tick. Contamination of skin with crushed tissues or faeces of an infected tick may also cause infection. The cycle of transmission is as follows :

```
Tick → Tick → Tick → Tick
        ↓      ↓
       Dog    Man
        ↓
       Tick → Man
```

Incubation period

Usually 3 to 7 days.

Clinical features

The patient usually gives history of a recent tick–bite and a careful examination will reveal a lesion or eschar at the site of the bite. After an interval of 3 to 7 days, there is an acute onset of fever, which may persist for 2 to 3 weeks, malaise and headache. A maculopapular rash appears on the third day. Unlike the rash in other rickettsial diseases, the rash appears first on the extremities (ankles and wrist), moves centripetally and involves the rest of the body. The clinical syndrome may be confused with atypical measles.

Control measures

(a) TREATMENT : Broad spectrum antibiotics have proved to be effective. (b) PERSONAL PROPHYLAXIS : Known tick–infested areas should be avoided. Daily inspection of the body for ticks is particularly important for those who are exposed to the risk of infection. Disinfection of dogs will minimize the tick population. Health education of the people in the mode of transmission by ticks, and the means of personal protection is equally important.

Q FEVER

Distribution

Q fever is a highly infectious zoonotic disease with world-wide distribution. It occurs mainly in persons associated with sheep, goats, cattle or other domestic animals.

Agent factors

(a) AGENT : The causative agent is *Coxiella burnetii.* It is found in ticks which act as vectors as well as reservoir. (b) ANIMAL HOSTS : Cattle, sheep, goats, ticks and some wild animals are natural reservoirs. Infected animals shed the disease agent in the faeces and urine and heavily contaminate the soil. The placenta of infected cows and sheep contains the infectious agent which may create infectious aerosols during parturition. Camels, horses, dogs and many other domestic animals have been shown to be capable of acting as maintenance hosts *(7)*.

Mode of transmission

Q fever differs from other rickettsial infections in that there is no arthropod involved in its transmission to man. Transmission results from : (i) inhalation of infected dust from soil previously contaminated by urine or faeces of diseased animals. The organism can also be transmitted through aerosols. (ii) the organism can also gain entry into the body through abrasions, conjunctivae or ingestion of contaminated foods such as meat, milk and milk products. In most countries, the respiratory route is regarded as most important.

Incubation period

Usually 2 to 3 weeks.

Clinical features

The disease has an acute onset with fever, chills, general malaise and headache. The clinical picture is one of influenza or non–bacterial pneumonia rather than a typhus fever. There is no rash or local lesion. The infection can cause pneumonia, hepatitis, encephalitis and rarely endocarditis. Inapparent infections also occur.

Control measures

(a) TREATMENT : Chronic Q fever requires prolonged treatment for 18 months or longer. Doxycycline is the drug of choice. *(b) PREVENTIVE MEASURES* **:** Pasteurization or boiling of milk to inactivate the causative agent; providing sanitary cattle sheds; adequate disinfection and disposal of products. An inactivated *Coxiella* vaccine has also been prepared to protect occupationally exposed workers. Several purified vaccines are under development *(8)*.

OTHER RICKETTSIAL INFECTIONS

1. Epidemic typhus

Epidemic or louse borne typhus was in the past the most formidable disease caused by rickettsiae. It was the cause of devastating epidemics among military and refugee populations and in areas affected by famine. The advent of modern insecticides has considerably reduced the prevalence of epidemic typhus today.

No cases of this disease have been reported from South East Asia since 1978 or from the Western Pacific since 1969 *(1)*. It is still endemic in Africa (notably Burundi, Rwanda and Ethiopia) and South America (notably Peru, Bolivia, and Ecuador). All of them are known endemic areas of the disease.

The infection is transmitted from man to man by the infected louse *(P. corporis and P. capitis)*. The louse gets infected by feeding on an infectious patient during the febrile stage. The organisms multiply in the cells lining the intestinal tract of the louse and begin to appear in 3 to 5 days in the louse faeces. Man acquires the disease not by the bite of the louse, but : (i) by scratching and inoculating himself with the infected louse faeces (ii) by crushing an infected louse on his person, and (iii) possibly by inhalation of infected louse faeces or dust. The infected louse after 10–14 days of existence dies of the infection. In humans, the organisms can persist for many years as latent infection without any symptoms, and the disease may appear later as ***Brill–Zinsser disease,*** and can be transmitted to other humans by the louse.

The control measures comprise anti–louse measures and improvements in personal hygiene and living conditions. Under the International Health Regulations, louse–borne typhus is subject to international surveillance.

2. Rickettsialpox

Man gets the infection through the bite of certain infected mites, which are found on mice *(Mus musculus)*. Transovarial transmission occurs in the mite. The mouse acts as true reservoir as well as vector. Rickettsialpox may be confused with atypical cases of chickenpox.

3. Trench fever

This disease is limited to central Europe. The vector is louse and the disease is transmitted by louse faeces. Man is the only known reservoir.

References

1. WHO (1983). *Bull WHO* 61 : 443.
2. Jawetz E et al (1986). *Reivew of Medical Microbiology* 17th ed. Lange Med. Publ. California.
3. WHO (1975). *The work of WHO,* Geneva.
4. *Current Medical Diagnosis and Treatment,* by Maxine A Padakis etc., 2014 ed., A Lange Publication.
5. WHO (1982). Bull WHO, P.162.
6. Saah, J.J. and Hormick, R.B. (1979). In *Principles and Practice of Infectious Diseases,* G.L. Mandell et al (eds), John Wiley, New York.
7. Sehgal, S and R. Bhatia eds (1985). *Manual on Zoonosis* NICD, 29–Sham Nath Marg, Delhi–54.
8. Kazar, J. et al (1982). *Bull WHO,* 60 (3) 389–394.

TAENIASIS

A group of cestode infections which are important zoonotic diseases. Three parasites of importance in taeniasis are *Taenia saginata, T. solium* and *T. asiatica*. These are classified as "cyclo–zoonoses" because they require more than one vertebrate host species (but no invertebrate host) to complete their developmental cycles.

Humans can become infected with *T. saginata* or *T. asiatica* when they consume beef meat or pig liver tissue, respectively, which has not been adequately cooked. Infection with the *T. solium* tapeworm occurs when humans eat raw or undercooked, infected pork. Tapeworm eggs pass with the faeces and are infective for pigs. Infection in humans with the *T. Solium* causes few clinical symptoms. However, infection with the larval parasite in the tissue (human cysticercosis) can result in devastating effect on human health. The larvae may develop in the muscle, skin, eyes and the central nervous system (neurocysticercosis). Neurocysticercosis is the most frequent preventable cause of epilepsy worldwide, and is estimated to cause 30 per cent of all epilepsy cases in countries where the parasite is endemic *(1)*.

Cysticercosis mainly affects the health and livelihood of communities in developing countries of Africa, Asia and Latin America. In 2010, the WHO added *T. solium* cysticercosis to the list of major Neglected Tropical Diseases. In 2015, the WHO Foodborne Disease Burden Epidemiology Reference Group identified *T. solium* as a leading cause of deaths from food-borne diseases resulting in a considerable total of 2.8 million DALYs lost and an estimated 2.56–8.30 million symptomatic and asymptomatic neurocysticercosis *(1)*.

Hosts of infection

T. saginata and *T. solium* pass their life cycles in two hosts. In man, the adult parasites live in the small intestine. The adult *T. saginata* measures 5 to 12 metres in length, and may be up to 24 metres; *T. solium* measures 2 to 6 metres.

TABLE 1

Hosts of infection

	Parasite	Definitive	Intermediate host
1.	*T. saginata*	Man	Cattle *(C. bovis)*
2.	*T. solium*	Man	Pig *(C. cellulosae)*

The larval stage of *T. saginata (C. bovis)* mainly occurs in cattle. The pig is the main host for the larval stage of *T. solium (C. cellulosae)* but man may also be infected. This may lead to muscular, ocular and cerebral cysticercosis.

The adult stages of *T. saginata* and *T. solium* may persist for several years in infected humans. Mixed infections of both the parasites can occur. Although the life span of *C. cellulosae* in man is not known, it is suspected to be some years.

Mode of transmission

These infections are acquired : (a) through the ingestion of infective cysticerci in undercooked beef *(T. saginata)* or pork *(T. solium)*; (b) through ingestion of food, water or vegetables contaminated with eggs; and (c) reinfection by the transport of eggs from the bowel to the stomach by retroperistalsis is considered to be rare.

Incubation period

For the adult tapeworm, from 8 to 14 weeks.

Clinical illness

The impact of tapeworm infection in man is difficult to quantify because in the vast majority of cases, they do not lead to clinical illhealth, except occasional abdominal discomfort, anorexia and chronic indigestion.

Straying of proglottids may sporadically cause appendicitis or cholangitis. The most serious risk of *T. solium* infection is cysticercosis.

Human cysticercosis

Human infection is caused by the ingestion of eggs of *T. solium* in contaminated water or food (hetero–infection) or regurgitated eggs from the small intestine (auto–infection). The eggs disintegrate and the infective stages leave the intestine via the hepatic portal system, and are dispersed throughout the body where they develop to form cysticerci. Cysticerci that develop in the central nervous system (neuro-cysticercosis), represent a serious threat to the individual and even to the community, if this condition is prevalent. As a result of mechanical pressure, obstruction or inflammation, a variety of pathological changes are produced, leading to epilepsy, intracranial hypertensive syndromes, hydrocephalus, psychiatric diseases or death *(2)*.

Control measures

The methods usually employed for control are : (a) treatment of infected persons, (b) meat inspection, (c) health education, and (d) adequate sewage treatment and disposal *(1, 2)*. Early detection and early treatment of *T. solium* cases is essential to prevent human cysticercosis.

Effective drugs (e.g., praziquantel and niclosamide) are available for the treatment of these infections. Surgical removal of symptom-producing cysts is indicated although cure can seldom, if ever, be complete. In many countries, *T. solium* has been controlled by meat inspection and by the proper housing and feeding of pigs. Thorough cooking of beef and pork is the most effective method to prevent food–borne infections. Education of the public to prevent pollution of soil, water and food with human faeces, and washing of hands before eating and after defecation, are important health educational messages. Improvement of living conditions, especially safe treatment of sewage used for farming, should be aimed at.

Treatment

Praziquantel and niclosamide have replaced former taenicides (i.e., mepacrine). They are safe and effective in more than 90 per cent of patients. Praziquantel is given in a single dose of 10 mg/kg. body wt. It achieves cure rates of about 99 per cent. At this dose, side effects are minimal. With a single dose of 4 tablets (2 grams) of niclosamide, cure rates are over 90 per cent. This drug is given in the morning–empty stomach. The tablets must be chewed thoroughly and swallowed with water. Eating may be resumed after 2 hours. It usually produces no side effects. Pre and post-treatment purges are not used for either drug to treat *T. saginata*. For the treatment of *T. solium*, give moderate purgative 2–3 hours after the drug to rapidly eliminate segments and eggs from the bowels to avoid–theoretical possibility of cysticercosis *(3)*.

TREATMENT FOR CYSTICERCOSIS *(3)* : The treatment should be individualized, based on the number and location of cysts and their viability. Medical treatment is more effective for parenchymal cysts and less effective for intraventricular, subarachnoid, or recemose cysts. Albendazole and praziquantel are both effective in the treatment. 10–15 mg/kg body wt/day of albendazole is given twice daily with a fatty meal. The duration of treatment is unsettled. Seven to 14 days may be sufficient for some patients, but a longer course (up to 28 days) is advisable at present. It can be repeated as necessary. Up to 3 months of treatment may be needed for ventricular and subarachnoid cysts. Praziquantel is given in 50 mg/kg/day in three divided doses for 15 days.

Albendazole is the drug of choice because co-administration of albendazole and a steroid (to treat inflammation) results in increased albendazole absorption, whereas combined use of praziquantel and steroid greatly decreases plasma level of praziquantel. Both the drugs are given with fatty meals as this increases absorption four-fold to five-fold.

References

1. WHO (2018) *Fact Sheet Taeniasis/Cysticercosis*, 15th February 2018.
2. WHO (1981) *Tech. Rep. Ser.* 666.
3. *Current Medical Diagnosis and Treatment 2004*, Ed. by Lawrence M. Tierney, Jr. Stephen J. Mcphee, Maxine A. Papadakis, Lange publication.

HYDATID DISEASE

Hydatid disease is a zoonoses – a group of cestode infections which are important zoonotic diseases of man. The disease in man is caused by the metacystode stage (infective larva) of the canine intestinal tapeworm *Echinococcus;* the adult worms are found in dogs and other carnivores.

Geographic distribution

Hydatidosis has been recognized as a public health problem of nearly global dimensions. It is found in all sheep–raising countries, e.g., Australia, New Zealand, Tasmania, Middle East countries, Turkey, Greece, USSR, Cyprus, Latin America and the Far East etc. It is believed that there are relatively few countries in which cestodes of the genus *Echinococcus* are entirely absent *(1)*. Foci are also known to exist in India where the highest prevalence is reported in Andhra Pradesh and Tamil Nadu, than in other parts of the country. The prevalence of the disease is reported to be high in food animals in India.

More than 1 million people are living with cystic echinococcosis and alveolar echinococcosis worldwide at any one time. For cystic echinococcosis, there is an average of 2.2 per cent post-operative death rate for surgical patients and about 6.5 per cent of cases relapse after the interventions, thereby requiring prolonged recovery time. In 2015, WHO Foodborne Disease Burden Epidemiology Reference Group estimated echinococcosis to be the cause of 19,300 deaths and around 871,000 DALYs lost globally each year. Annual cost associated with cystic echinococcosis are estimated to be US $ 3 billion for treating the cases and losses to the livestock industry *(1)*.

Epidemiological determinants

Agent factors

Echinococcus species are small tapeworms, rarely more than 7 mm in length. The scolex bears four suckers, and there are two rows of hooks, one small and one large on the rostellum. The number of proglottids varies from 2 to 6. At present four species are regarded as valid.

(a) E. granulosus : of worldwide distribution, is for the most part, maintained in the domestic transmission cycle involving the dog as final host. In man the infective larva causes hydatidosis, the "unilocular" type of echinococcosis. *(b) E. multilocularis* : is restricted to the northern hemisphere. It has been detected increasingly in various countries (e.g. Iran, Turkey). In man, the metacystode causes the "alveolar" type of the disease. *(c) E. oligarthus* : a species occurring in Central and South America is suspected to cause disease in man, and *(d) E. Vogeli* : a species occurring in Central and South America, has been shown to cause polycystic hydatidosis.

Life cycle

Basically it is a "dog–sheep" cycle with man as an accidental, intermediate host. The adult tapeworm lives in the small intestine of dogs (definitive host) for 2 to 4 years. The eggs are voided in the faeces and contaminate the soil, vegetation and drinking water. They are highly resistant and can survive for several months in pastures, gardens and around households. Sheep, cattle and other intermediate hosts become infected when they ingest vegetation which has become contaminated with faeces from infected dogs. Ingested eggs hatch in the intestine and the larvae penetrate the intestinal lining and migrate to various organs of the body. Most frequently, they lodge in such organs as liver, lungs and brain and develop into hydatid cysts. The life cycle is completed when sheep (cattle) viscera containing hydatid cysts are eaten by dogs. Infected dogs begin to pass eggs of the parasite approximately 7 weeks after infection. Man does not harbour the adult worm *(1)*.

Host factors

It is becoming increasingly evident that human behaviour, especially in relation to dogs and cats, uncontrolled slaughter of food animals, indiscriminate disposal of offal and carcasses, and eating habits of the people play an important part in the epidemiology of the disease. Human infection is acquired usually in childhood through contact with infected dogs. The impact of hydatidosis can be described only in terms of human suffering, cost of medical diagnosis, hospitalization and surgery, man–hours lost, as well as in terms of temporary or permanent incapacity. The retarded growth of animals, and reduction in the quality and yield of meat, milk and wool and condemnation of offal are also very great *(2)*. Hydatid disease is an occupational disease of certain groups, e.g., shepherds and their families in endemic areas and shoe–makers.

Mode of transmission

Human infection occurs by ingestion of the eggs of *Echinococcus* inadvertently with food, unwashed vegetables or water contaminated with faeces from infected dogs. Infection can also take place while handling or playing with infected dogs, e.g., hand to mouth transfer of eggs, or by inhalation of dust contaminated with infected eggs. The disease is not directly transmissible from person to person.

The disease is maintained in the "dog–sheep" cycle. Other animal combinations may also be involved, e.g., dog–goat, dog–cattle, and dog–camel. Carnivores get infected by eating viscera containing hydatid cysts. The disease is not directly transmissible from one intermediate host to another.

Incubation period

Variable, from months to years depending upon the number and location of cysts and how rapidly they grow.

Clinical features

In man, symptoms of hydatid disease are usually manifested several years after exposure. The cysts grow slowly from 5 to 20 years before they are diagnosed. The size of the cyst may vary from a pinhead to that of a small football. It has been estimated that more than 70 per cent of the cysts become located in the right lobe of the liver, and the rest in lungs, brain, peritoneum, long bones and kidney. The cysts are filled with watery fluid and contain a large number of tapeworm heads. If the cyst ruptures, the brood capsules can spill out of the cyst, metastasize to other sites and develops into a hydatid, thus ingestion of a single egg can give rise to several hydatid cysts, each containing several brood capsules *(3)*.

Cysts of small size are generally asymptomatic. Large cysts, however, cause pressure symptoms (e.g., jaundice in liver cysts). In vital organs they may cause severe symptoms and death.

Diagnosis

(a) Clinical : Based on the history of residence in an endemic area, close association with dogs and the presence of a slowly growing cystic tumour. *(b) X-ray :* A plain X-ray permits the location of the cyst. Modern techniques of diagnosis include ultrasonography, MRI and CAT scan. *(c) Serological :* Serological tests with a high degree of sensitivity and specificity have been introduced such as the indirect immunofluorescent test. ELISA is regarded as a relatively simple method with a high sensitivity superior to that of some other serological procedures *(1)*. The intradermal (Casoni) test is still in wide use, since it is simple to perform. This test often lacks specificity.

Treatment

There is no specific treatment excepting surgical removal of cysts which is not without considerable risk in as much as the accidental penetration of one of the cysts can lead to anaphylactic shock which may prove fatal.

Mebendazole (Vermox) has been tried and found very effective in mice. It may well become the drug of choice.

Prevention and control *(4)*

1. Wash fruits and raw vegetables before eating.
2. Wash hands before eating or smoking, after handling dogs and after contact with items that are likely to be soiled with dog faeces.
3. Discourage dogs from licking people's faces, and do not kiss dogs.
4. Do not allow dogs to defecate near vegetable gardens or children's play areas.
5. Reduce the amount of disease in dogs
   - Ensure dogs are kept away from the areas where animals are slaughtered and are not allowed to scavenge on carcasses.
   - Prevent dogs from eating uncooked offal.
   - Dispose of infected offal by deep burial or burning to prevent it from being consumed by dogs or other canines.
   - Reduce dog populations on farms to the occupational need for them.
   - Seek advice from your veterinarian about effective treatment to prevent infection in working, pet or visiting dogs. This is particularly important for dogs in rural areas or those that may have contact with wildlife or feral animals.

References

1. WHO (2018), *Fact Sheet, Echinococcosis,* 8th February, 2018
2. WHO (1974). *WHO Chr.* 28 (3) 110.
3. Jawetz, Melnick and Adelberg's *Medical Microbiology (2014),* 26th Ed., A Lange Publication.
4. Queensland Govt. (2017), *Health Condition/14/165/81/ Hydatid-Disease.*

LEISHMANIASIS

Leishmaniasis are a group of protozoal diseases caused by parasites of the genus *Leishmania,* and transmitted to man by the bite of female phlebotomine sandfly. They are responsible for various syndromes in humans – kala-azar or visceral leishmaniasis (VL), cutaneous leishmaniasis (CL), muco–cutaneous leishmaniasis (MCL), anthroponotic cutaneous leishmaniasis (ACL), zoonotic cutaneous leishmaniasis (ZCL), post–kala-azar dermal leishmaniasis (PKDL), etc *(1)*. The visceral type of disease, kala-azar, is still an important disease in India. The majority of the leishmaniasis are zoonoses involving wild or domestic mammals (rodents, canines). Some forms (e.g., Indian kala-azar) are considered to be nonzoonotic infections *(2)*.

Problem statement

WORLD

Leishmaniasis is endemic in many countries in tropical and subtropical regions. The 3 main forms of the disease are distributed as follows (3):

1. *Visceral leishmaniasis (VL),* also known as Kala-azar is fatal if left untreated in over 95% of cases. It is characterized by irregular bouts of fever, weight loss, enlargement of the spleen and liver, and anaemia. Most cases occur in Brazil, East Africa and in South-East Asia. An estimated 50,000 to 90,000 new cases of VL occur worldwide each year. In 2020, more than 95% of new cases reported to WHO occurred in 10 countries : Brazil, Ethiopia, India, Kenya, Somalia, South Sudan, Sudan, China, Yemen and Eritrea.
2. *Cutaneous leishmaniasis (CL),* is the most common form of leishmaniasis and causes skin lesions, mainly ulcers, on exposed parts of the body, leaving life-long scars and serious disability. About 95% of CL cases occur in the Americas, the Mediterranean basin, the Middle East and Central Asia. In 2020 over 85 per cent of new CL cases occurred in 8 countries: Afghanistan, Algeria, Brazil, Colombia, Iraq, Libya, Peru, Pakistan, Tunisia and the Syrian Arab Republic. It is estimated that between 600,000 to 1 million new cases occur worldwide annually.
3. *Muco-cutaneous lesihmaniasis* leads to partial or total destruction of mucous membranes of the nose, mouth and throat. Over 90% of muco-cutaneous leishmaniasis cases occur in Bolivia (the Plurinational State of) Brazil, Ethiopia and Peru.

Kala-azar situation is worsening due to the occurrence of asymptomatic cases, post-kala-azar dermal leishmaniasis (PKDL), undernutrition, and kala-azar/HIV coinfection. Case fatality rate has decreased perhaps due to improved case management in endemic countries.

INDIA

Kala-azar is endemic in 54 districts in Bihar (33), Jharkhand (4), West Bengal (11) and Uttar Pradesh (6). About 130 million population is at risk of the disease. The present situation is shown in Table 1. While both cutaneous (ZCL and ACL) and visceral (VL) disease occur in India, kala-azar is by far the most important leishmaniasis in India *(5)*. Kala-azar has been declared as notifiable disease in Bihar and West Bengal *(5)*.

TABLE 1

State-wise Kala-azar cases and deaths in India (2018–2020)

State	2020		2019		2018	
	Cases	Deaths	Cases	Deaths	Cases	Deaths
Bihar	1,502	0	2,537	0	3,569	0
West Bengal	60	3	87	6	96	3
Uttar Pradesh	55	3	97	0	110	0
Jharkhand	431	0	544	0	758	0
India	2,052	6	3,269	6	4,539	3

Source : *(4)*

The epidemiological profile of VL and PKDL cases in these 4 endemic states are as shown in Table 2.

TABLE 2

The epidemiological profile of VL and PKDL cases in endemic states (India-2016)

Particulars	Jharkhand		West Bengal		Uttar Pradesh		Bihar	
	VL	PKDL	VL	PKDL	VL	PKDL	VL	PKDL
Female proportion	40%	43%	39.7%	40.8%	40%	50%	43%	NA
<15 years (Child proportion)	35%	29%	25%	18%	37%	0	39%	NA

Source : *(2)*

Epidemiological determinants

Agent factors

(a) AGENTS : The leishmania are intracellular parasites. They infect and divide within macrophages. At least nineteen different leishmania parasites have been associated with human infection. Further, the majority of these offer no cross immunity of one against the other *(6)*. *Leishmania donovani* is the causative agent of kala-azar (VL); *L. tropica* is the causative agent of cutaneous leishmaniasis (oriental sore); and, *L. braziliensis* is the causative agent of muco-cutaneous leishmaniasis. But this distinction is not absolute; visceral forms may produce cutaneous lesions, and cutaneous forms may visceralize *(7)*. The life cycle is completed in two different hosts – a vertebrate and an insect; in the former, it occurs in an amastigote form (called "leishmania bodies") and in the latter as a flagellated promastigote. *(b) RESERVOIRS OF INFECTION :* There is a variety of animal reservoirs, e.g., dogs, jackals, foxes, rodents and other mammals. Indian kala-azar is considered to be a non–zoonotic infection with man as the sole reservoir. This assumption is based largely on the absence of evidence *(8)*.

Host factors

(a) AGE : Kala-azar can occur in all age groups including infants below the age of one year. In India, the peak age is 5 to 9 years *(1)*. *(b) SEX :* Males are affected twice as often as females. *(c) POPULATION MOVEMENT :* Movement of population (migrants, labourers, tourists) between endemic and non–endemic areas can result in the spread of infection. *(d) SOCIO-ECONOMIC STATUS :* Kala-azar usually strikes the poorest of the poor. Poverty increases the risk for kala-azar. Poor housing and domestic sanitary conditions (e.g. lack of waste management, open sewerage) may increase sandfly breeding and resting sites, as well as their access to humans. Sandflies are attracted to crowded housing as these provide a good source of blood-meal. Human behaviour, such as sleeping outside or on the ground, may increase risk. As a disease it more often debilitate than kills, and makes people become dependants on others; *(e) MALNUTRITION :* Diets lacking protein-energy; iron, vitamin A and zinc increases the risk that an infection will progress to kala-azar *(3)*. *(f) OCCUPATION :* The disease strongly associates with occupation. People who work in various farming practices, forestry, mining and fishing have a great risk of being bitten by sandflies. *(g) IMMUNITY :* Recovery from kala-azar and oriental sore gives a lasting immunity. During the active phase of kala-azar, there is impairment of cell mediated immunity, this is reflected in the negative skin reaction to leishmanin test.

Environmental factors

(a) ALTITUDE : Kala-azar is mostly confined to the plains; it does not occur in altitudes over 2000 feet (600 metres). (b) SEASON : In the past epidemics, two peaks, one in November and another in March–April were reported. Generally there is high prevalence during and after rains. (c) CLIMATE CHANGES : Kala-azar is climate sensitive, and is strongly affected by changes in rainfall, temperature and humidity. Global warming and land degradation together affect the epidemiology of kala-azar in many ways. It can have strong effects on vector and reservoir hosts by altering their distribution and influence their survival. Drought famine and flood resulting from climate changes can lead to massive displacement and migration of people to areas with transmission of kala-azar, and poor nutrition could compromise their immunity *(3)*. (d) RURAL AREAS : The disease is generally confined to rural areas, where conditions for the breeding of sandflies readily exist compared to urban areas. (e) VECTORS : In India, *P. argentipes* is a proven vector of kala-azar. Cutaneous leishmaniasis is transmitted by *P. papatasi* and *P. sergenti*. Sandflies breed in cracks and crevices in the soil and buildings, tree holes, caves etc. Overcrowding, ill-ventilation and accumulation of organic matter in the environment facilitate transmission. Their habits are primarily nocturnal. Only the females bite. (f) DEVELOPMENT PROJECTS : Ironically many development projects are exposing more people to leishmaniasis. Forest clearing, and cultivation projects, large water resource schemes, and colonization and resettlement programmes are bringing human beings into areas of high vector and reservoir concentration *(3)*.

Mode of transmission

In India, Kala-azar is transmitted from person to person by the bite of the female phlebotomine sandfly, *P. argentipes* which is a highly anthrophilic species. Transmission may also take place by contamination of the bite wound or by contact when the insect is crushed during the act of feeding. Cutaneous leishmaniasis is transmitted by *P. papatasi* and *P. sergenti*.

After an infective blood meal, the sandfly becomes infective in 4 to 25 days (extrinsic incubation period). This is the time required for the development of the parasite in the insect vector. Transmission of kala-azar has also been recorded by blood transfusion *(7)*, and is also possible by contaminated syringes and needles *(9)*.

Incubation period

The incubation period in man is quite variable, generally 1 to 4 months; range is 10 days to 2 years.

Clinical features

1. Kala-azar (VL)

The classical features of kala-azar are fever, splenomegaly and hepatomegaly accompanied by anaemia and weight–loss. A family history of the disease is also common. Darkening of the skin of the face, hands, feet and abdomen is common in India (kala-azar = black sickness). Atypical features of the disease (e.g., lymphadenopathy) may also occur. Kala-azar, if left untreated, has a high mortality.

PKDL : Post-kala-azar dermal leishmaniasis, caused by *L. donovani*, is common in India. It appears one to several years after apparent cure of kala-azar. The lesions consist of multiple nodular infiltrations of the skin, usually without ulceration. Parasites are numerous in the lesion.

2. Cutaneous leishmaniasis

Several forms of cutaneous leishmaniasis have been described – Anthroponotic or urban cutaneous leishmaniasis (ACL), Zoonotic or rural cutaneous leishmaniasis (ZCL), Diffuse cutaneous leishmaniasis (DCL), etc *(1)*. The disease may be mistaken for leprosy. The agent is restricted to skin. The disease is characterized by painful ulcers in the parts of the body exposed to sandfly bites (e.g., legs, arms or face) reducing the victim's ability to work.

3. Muco-cutaneous leishmaniasis

Ulcers similar to the oriental sore (CL) appear around the margins of mouth and nose. It can mutilate the face so badly that victims may become social outcasts.

Laboratory diagnosis

1. Rapid diagnostic test

The rapid dipstick test has become the mainstay in the serological diagnosis of Kala-azar, and is the method of choice for diagnosis of the disease.

The rk39 – rapid diagnostic test is based on the recombinant k39 protein. It is an epitope apparently conserved on amastigotes of *Leishmania* species that cause visceral infection. The test is simple to perform and yields result within five minutes. However, the test should not be used in Kala-azar relapse cases, Kala-azar reinfection cases and Kala-azar and HIV co-infection cases.

Kala-azar dipstick test strip is a membrane, pre-coated with a recombinant VL antigen on the test line region and chicken anti-protein A on the control line region. It is a immunochromatographic assay for qualitative detection of antibodies to *L. donovani* in human serum. During testing the serum sample reacts with the dye conjugate. The mixture then migrates upwards on the membrane chromatographically by capillary action to react with rk39 antigen on the membrane and generates a red line. Presence of this red line indicates a positive result while its absence indicates a negative result.

Regardless of the presence of antibody to VL antigen, as the mixture continues to migrate across the membrane to the immobilized chicken antiprotien A region, a red line at the control line will always appear. The presence of this red line serves as a verification for sufficient sample volume and proper flow, and is a control for the reagent. If no lines appear at control and test line areas, the test is invalid. The test is also invalid if no control line appears, even though a test line is seen *(10)*.

2. Parasitological diagnosis

The demonstration of the parasite LD bodies in the aspirates of the spleen, liver, bone marrow, lymph nodes or in the skin (in the case of CL) is the only way to confirm VL or CL conclusively. The parasite must be isolated in culture to confirm the identity of the parasite.

3. Aldehyde test

The aldehyde test of Napier is a simple test widely used in India for the diagnosis of kala-azar. 1 to 2 ml of serum from a case of kala-azar is taken and a drop or two of 40 per cent formalin is added. A positive test is indicated by jellification to milk–white opacity like the white of a hard–boiled egg so that in ordinary light newsprint is invisible through it. If it occurs within 2 to 20 minutes, it is said to be strongly positive. Reaction after 30 minutes is not significant. The test usually becomes positive 2 to 3 months after onset of the disease, and reverts to negative 6 months after cure. Therefore, this test is good for surveillance but not for diagnosis. The test is non–specific and demands the use of venous blood. Further, the test is positive in many other chronic infections in which albumin to globulin ratio is reversed.

4. Serological tests

Of the numerous serological tests available, Direct Aggutination test (DAT), rk39 dipstick test, ELISA and the indirect fluorescent antibody test (IFAT) are considered most suitable *(10)*. Being a simple test where blood samples can be collected on a filter paper strip and examined at leisure in laboratory, the ELISA test has a wide potential both for diagnosis as well as for epidemiological field surveys.

5. Leishmanin (Montenegro) test

This test is based on skin reaction. Leishmanin is a preparation of 10^6 per ml washed promastigotes of leishmania, suspended in 0.5 per cent phenol saline or merthiolate. Sterile and standardized preparations are available commercially. An intradermal injection of 0.1 ml on the flexor surface of the forearm is given and examined after 48 to 72 hours. Induration is measured and recorded. An induration of 5 mm or more is considered positive. The test is usually positive 4 to 6 weeks after onset in the case of CL and MCL. It is usually negative in the active phase of kala-azar and becomes positive in 75 per cent patients within one year of recovery. The test is not species–specific. The test remains a valuable tool for distinguishing immune from non–immune subjects. From this information, it may be possible to infer the endemicity or epidemicity of the infection and to identify groups at risk of infection *(10)*.

6. Haematological findings

These include progressive leucopenia, anaemia and reversed albumin–globulin ratio, with greatly increased IgG. The WBC:RBC ratio is 1:1500 or even 1:2000 (normal 1:750). ESR is increased.

ICMR has developed a new kit to diagnose Kala-azar, which was launched on 3rd Sept. 2014. The test needs the sample of urine or oral fluid of the subject in question. It is mixed with the given solution in the 'tube' - part of the kit. Dip the stipulated strip in the solution thus created. Those infected would get two or one red bond on the strip once it comes out. Absence of the red bond means negative result.

Some definitions *(11)*

1. *Case definition of kala-azar* : A case of kala-azar is defined as a person from an endemic area with fever of more than 2 weeks duration and with splenomegaly, who is confirmed by an RDT or a biopsy.
2. *Treatment outcome definitions of kala-azar*
   a. *Cure* : a patient is considered clinically cured if he/she has completed full treatment and there are no signs and symptoms of kala-azar.
   b. *Non-response* : Signs and symptoms persist or recur despite satisfactory treatment for more than two weeks.
   c. *Relapse* : any reappearance of kala-azar signs and symptoms within a period of six months after the end of treatment.
   d. *Treatment failure* : non-response or relapse.
   e. *Final cure* : an initially cured patient who is symptom-free at six months after the end of treatment.
3. *Case definition of PKDL*
   a. *Probable PKDL* : a patient from kala-azar endemic area with multiple hypopigmented macules, papules or nodules, who is RDT positive.
   b. *Confirmed PKDL* : a patient from kala-azar endemic area with multiple hypopigmented macules, papules, plaques or nodules, who is parasite positive in slit-skin smear (SSS) or biopsy.

Treatment outcome in PKDL

a. *Initial cure* : Clinical improvement at the end of treatment – defined as a considerable reduction in the number and size of skin lesions.

b. *Final cure* : Clinical cure 12 months after the end of treatment – defined as a complete resolution of macules, papules, plaques and nodules.

Key indicators in the kala-azar elimination initiative *(11)*

1. *Detection rate (%)*

$$= \frac{\text{Number of new cases of KA detected per year in the district, UHC or subdistrict}}{\text{Total population in the same area}} \times 100$$

2. *Treatment completion rate (%)*

$$= \frac{\text{Number of patients that took a full course of first-line drugs}}{\text{All new KA cases that started treatment in a given period}} \times 100$$

3. *Coverage rate of vector control (%)*

$$= \frac{\text{Number of households protected}}{\text{All households at risk}} \times 100$$

Monitoring clinical outcomes *(11)*

1. *Final cure rate (%)*

$$= \frac{\text{Number of patients with final cure}}{\text{Total number who started treatment}} \times 100$$

2. *Treatment failure rate (%)*

$$= \frac{\text{Total number of non-response + relapse + KA - related deaths}}{\text{Total number who started treatment}} \times 100$$

3. *Loss to follow-up rate (%)*

$$= \frac{\text{Number of defaulters + Number of loss to follow-up}}{\text{Total number who started treatment}} \times 100$$

4. *Mortality (%)*

$$= \frac{\text{Number of deaths}}{\text{Total number who started treatment}} \times 100$$

CONTROL MEASURES

In the absence of an effective vaccine, the control measures comprise the following :

1. Control of reservoir

Since man is the only reservoir of kala-azar in India, active and passive case detection and treatment of those found to be infected (including PKDL) may be sufficient to abolish the human reservoir and control the disease. House-to-house visits and mass surveys may be undertaken in endemic areas for early detection of cases.

TREATMENT GUIDELINES (2017)

Following drugs are used for the treatment of kala-azar in Indian programme *(2, 7)* :

- Single dose Liposomal Amphotericin B (LAMB) injection intravenously across all age groups in dose of 10 mg/kg bw including paediatric, pregnant & elderly patients.
- Miltefosine capsules of 10 mg (paediatric) and 50 mg (adults) in the age group between 2–65 years. Not to be given to pregnant and lactating women and women who refuse contraception during treatment with Miltefosine. Dosages are: patients > 12 years, weight > 25 kgs–100 mg daily in two doses of 50 mg each after meals for 28 days, and patients > 12 years, weight < 25 kgs, only one capsule of 50 mg daily × 28 days. Children 2–11 years miltefosine to be given at 2.5 mg/kg once daily after meals × 28 days.
- Amphotericin B deoxycholate injection intravenously at a dose of 1 mg/kg b.w. on alternate days × 15 doses.
- Combination of Paromomycin injection intramuscular & Miltefosine in a dose of 11mg/kg b.w. × 10 days together with Miltefosine for 10 days. Not to be given to chronic kidney patients, pregnant and lactating women, and those not inclined to contraception during treatment.
- HIV–coinfected patients – LAMB 40 mg /kg b.w as total dose of 3–5 mg/kg bw daily or intermittently for 10 doses, on days 1–5, 10, 17, 24, 31 and 38.
- PKDL – In order of preference: First drug of choice, miltefosine 100 mg orally per day × 12 weeks.
- Amphotericin 'B' deoxycholate injection 1 mg/kg bw over 4 months in 60–80 doses.

Given the high efficacy, safety, ease of use and assured compliance, Liposomal Amphotericin B (LAMB) is used as the first line of treatment. The drugs used in order of preference at all levels are:

- Liposomal Amphotericin B intra venous (LAMB) single dose 10 mg/kg bw
- Combination regimens (e.g. Miltefosine capsules plus Paromomycin inj IM)
- Amphotericin B emulsion
- Miltefosine capsule
- Amphotericin B deoxycholate inj in multiple doses
- Amphotericin B emulsion inj in selected districts on pilot project.

Miltefosine is relatively safe oral drug for the treatment of Kala-azar. The treatment is provided as Directly Observed Treatment (DOT) with patient coding system being followed for each patient registered at the treatment centre. The dose guide is as follows :

Dosage guide for children (2–11 years)

Body weight	Daily dosage (after meal)	Number of capsules
9–11 kg	20 mg	2 capsules of Miltefosine 10 mg
12–16 kg	30 mg	3 capsules of Miltefosine 10 mg
17–20 kg	40 mg	4 capsules of Miltefosine 10 mg
21–25 kg	50 mg	1 capsule of Miltefosine 50 mg
26–31 kg	60 mg	1 capsule of Miltefosine 50 mg & 1 capsule of Miltefosine 10 mg
32–39 kg	80 mg	1 capsule of Miltefosine 50 mg & 3 capsules of Miltefosine 10 mg
40 kg and above	100 mg	2 capsules of Miltefosine 50 mg

Miltefosine dosage guide for persons (>12 years)

Weight	Morning dose (after meal)	Evening dose (after meal)
More than 25 kg	1 capsule of Miltefosine 50 mg	1 capsule of Miltefosine 50 mg
Less than 25 kg	1 capsule of Miltefosine 50 mg	Drug not to be given at evening

National Road Map on Kala-azar elimination was developed in August 2014 with specific time line, roles and responsibility for states and district level vector borne diseases consultants and technical supervisors.

Animal reservoirs

If animal reservoirs (e.g., dogs) are involved, appropriate control measures against them should be undertaken. In many endemic countries, extensive dog and rodent control programmes have contributed greatly to the reduction in the number of human cases.

2. Sandfly control

The application of residual insecticides has proved effective in the control of sandflies. DDT is the first choice since the vector of kala-azar, *P. argentipes* is susceptible to DDT. (*P. papatasi* in north Bihar has been shown to be resistant to DDT, but fortunately, it is not the vector of kala-azar in India). Insecticide spraying should be undertaken in human dwellings, animal shelters and all other resting places upto a height of 6 feet (2 metres) from floor level. DDT (two rounds per year) at the rate of 1–2 g per sq. metre is considered sufficient to control transmission. Spraying should be preceded and followed by an assessment of susceptibility. Any sign of resistance in vector should lead to an immediate change in insecticide. BHC should be kept as a second line of defence.

Spraying should be repeated at regular intervals to keep down the density of sandflies. For long-lasting results, insecticidal spraying should be combined with **sanitation measures,** viz elimination of breeding places (e.g., cracks in mud or stone walls, rodent burrows, removal of firewood, bricks or rubbish around houses), location of cattle sheds and poultry at a fair distance from human dwellings, and improvement of housing and general sanitation.

3. Personal prophylaxis

The risk of infection can be reduced through health education and by the use of individual protective measures such as avoiding sleeping on floor, using fine-mesh nets around the bed. Insect repellents (in the form of lotions, creams, or sticks) for temporary protection and keeping the environment clean. There are no drugs for personal prophylaxis.

References

1. WHO (1984). *Tech. Rep. Ser.*, No.701.
2. Govt. of India (2017), *Accelerated Plan for the Kala-azar elimination 2017*, Directorate NVBDCP.
3. WHO (2022), *Fact Sheet, Leishmaniasis*, 8th January, 2022.
4. Govt. of India (2021), *National Health Profile 2021*, Ministry of Health and Family Welfare, New Delhi.
5. Govt. of India (2020), *Annual Report 2019–2020*, Ministry of Health and Family Welfare, New Delhi.
6. Lainson, R. (1983). In *Proceedings of the Indo–UK Workshop on Leishmaniasis* ICMR, N.D.
7. Govt. of India (2015), *Operational Guidelines on Kala-azar visceral Leishmaniasis*, Elimination in India - 2015, Ministry of Health and Family Welfare, New Delhi.
8. Sanyal, R.K. et al (1979). *J. Comm Dis*, 11 (4) 149–169.
9. WHO (2010), *International travel and Health*, 2010.
10. Govt. of India (2010), *Guidelines of Kala-azar*, Division of National Vector Borne Disease Control Programme, Ministry of Health and Family Welfare, New Delhi.
11. WHO, TDR (2010), *Indicators for Monitoring and Evaluation of Kala-azar Elimination Programme*, Aug. 2010, for Bangladesh, India and Nepal.

V. SURFACE INFECTIONS

TRACHOMA

Trachoma is a chronic infectious disease of the conjunctiva and cornea, caused by *Chlamydia trachomatis*, but other pathogenic microorganisms often contribute to the disease. Trachoma inflammation may undergo spontaneous resolution or may progress to conjunctival scarring which can cause inward deviation of eyelashes (trichiasis) or of the lid margin (entropion). The abrasion of the cornea by eyelashes frequently result in corneal ulceration, followed by scarring and visual loss.

From the public health point of view, trachoma is classified as blinding and non-blinding *(1)*. A community with blinding trachoma can be recognized by the presence of persons with lesions such as entropion, trichiasis and corneal ulcers. It is the blinding trachoma that requires urgent control measures. Non-blinding trachoma often becomes blinding trachoma when other ocular pathogens interact synergistically and enhance the risk of damage to eye sight *(2)*.

Diagnosis

In epidemiological studies, more stress is now put on the upper tarsal conjunctiva as a convenient index of trachomatous inflammation in the eye as a whole *(2)*. For the purpose of diagnosis in the field, cases must have at least 2 of the following diagnostic criteria *(3)*.

a. follicles on the upper tarsal conjunctiva
b. limbal follicles or their sequelae, Herbert's pits
c. typical conjunctival scarring (trichiasis, entropion)
d. vascular pannus, most marked at the superior limbus

Problem statement

Trachoma is a major preventable cause of blindness in developing countries. According to recent estimates, in 41 endemic countries about 1.9 million people suffer from visual impairment due to trachoma, of these 1.2 million are irreversibly blind, and about 190.2 million are at risk of infection *(4)*. In 2016, more than 260,000 people with trachoma were provided with curative surgery and 85 million in endemic communities were treated with antibiotics to eliminate trachoma *(4)*.

The incidence and prevalence of trachoma has shown a significant decrease in many endemic countries of SEAR during the past few decades. This decrease has been mainly due to improved sanitation, water and housing, and implementation of control measures. However, trachoma, particularly in its active form, still remains a public health concern in some parts of Myanmar, in the western region of Nepal and in a few rural areas in India *(5)*. It is estimated to be responsible for 0.1 per cent of visual impairment and blindness in India *(6)*.

Epidemiological determinants

Agent factors

(a) AGENT : The classical endemic trachoma of developing countries is caused by *C. trachomatis* of immune types A, B, or C. The sexually-transmitted *C. trachomatis* (serotypes D,E,F,G,H,I,J or K) may also infect, causing an eye disease difficult to differentiate from endemic trachoma. Milder cases of this are usually called "inclusion conjunctivitis". These strains rarely produce permanent visual loss – but they cause respiratory infections (pneumonia) in infants and genital tract infections in adults *(2)*. Other pathogenic organisms (e.g., Morax–Axenfeld diplobacillus, the Koch–Weeks bacillus, the gonococcus) often contribute to the disease process. The Morax–Axenfeld diplobacillus is the most innocuos; the Koch–Weeks bacillus is the most widespread, and the gonococcus the most dangerous *(7)*. *C. trachomatis,* originally believed to be a virus, is an obligatory intracellular bacteria, now classified as Chlamydia. (b) RESERVOIR : Children with active disease, chronically infected older children and adults. (c) SOURCE OF INFECTION : Ocular discharges of infected persons and fomites, and (d) COMMUNICABILITY: Trachoma is a disease of low infectivity. It is infective as long as active lesions are present in the conjunctiva, but not after complete cicatrization.

Host factors

(a) AGE : In endemic areas, children may show signs of the disease at the age of only a few months. But typically, children from the age of two to five years are the most infected, and this contributes not only to the high rate of blindness but also to the rate of occurrence among children. (b) SEX : Prevalence equal in younger age groups. In older age groups, females have been found to be affected more than males. The explanation for this may be that women remain more in contact with children who infect them. Further, females are more exposed to irritating factors such as smoke than males. (c) PRE-DISPOSING FACTORS : Direct sunlight, dust, smoke and irritants such as *kajal* or *surma* may predispose to infection.

Environmental factors

(a) SEASON : Seasonal epidemics are associated with vastly increased number of eye–seeking flies. The incidence of active trachoma is found generally high in India during April–May and again during July–September. The higher temperature and rainfall favours the increase in fly population.

(b) QUALITY OF LIFE : Trachoma is associated with poor quality of life. The disease thrives in conditions of poverty, crowding, ignorance, poor personal hygiene, squalor, illiteracy and poor housing. As living conditions improve the disease tends to regress. (c) CUSTOMS : The custom of applying *kajal* or *surma* to the eyes is a positive risk factor.

Mode of transmission

In communities where trachoma is endemic, eye-to-eye transmission can be considered as a rule *(8)*. This may occur by direct or indirect contact with ocular discharges of infected persons or fomites, e.g., infected fingers, towels, *kajal* or *surma*. Eye-seeking flies (e.g., *Musca* spp., *Hippelatus* spp.) play some role in spreading the infection by mechanical transmission. In countries where only sporadic cases of trachoma occur, genital localization of *C. trachomatis* (urethral, cervical) may lead to venereal transmission *(7)*.

It has been shown that trachoma is a familial disease. When one case is detected, others will almost certainly be found in the family group. There is a continuous feedback of infection, partly as a result of grandfathers or sisters and brothers tending small children *(8)*.

Incubation period

5 to 12 days.

CONTROL OF TRACHOMA

Trachoma control still requires long-term efforts. It requires proper planning and organization, which should include the following elements :

1. Assessment of the problem

The primary objective of a programme for the control of trachoma is the prevention of blindness. Control programmes should be focussed on communities with a substantial prevalence of "blinding trachoma" – as indicated by the presence of : (a) corneal blindness (b) trachomatous trichiasis and entropion, and (c) moderate and severe trachomatous inflammation. Such communities are likely to be found in countries with blindness rates that are above 0.5 per cent. The first task, therefore, is to undertake an epidemiological survey to identify and delimit communities with blinding trachoma; assess the magnitude of the problem, local conditions and other causes of blindness and to obtain information on existing facilities. The basic principles of these surveys are set out in the WHO publication : "Methods of Assessment of Avoidable Blindness" *(9)*.

2. Chemotherapy

In trachoma control, the main activity is chemotherapeutic intervention. The objective of chemotherapy is to reduce severity, lower the incidence and in the long run decrease the prevalence of trachoma. The antibiotic of choice is 1 per cent ophthalmic ointment or oily suspension of tetracyclines. Erythromycin and rifampicin have also been used in the treatment of trachoma. Treatment may be given to the entire community – this is known as **mass treatment** (or blanket treatment). In some programmes, **selective treatment** is chosen, in which case, the whole population at risk is screened, and treatment is applied only to persons with active trachoma *(10)*.

(a) Mass treatment

A prevalence of more than 5 per cent severe and moderate trachoma in children under 10 years is an indication for mass or blanket treatment. The treatment consists of the application twice daily of tetracycline 1 per cent ointment to all children, for 5 consecutive days each month or once daily for 10 days each month for 6 consecutive months, or for 60 consecutive days *(2)*. An alternative antibiotic is erythromycin.

From the practical point of view, one of the main difficulties is the need for repeated applications of the antibiotic over long periods of time. Emphasis is now being placed on the active participation of the community itself in trachoma control activities and on the utilization of primary health care workers. This makes possible a wider coverage and a greater efficacy of the programme.

(b) Selective treatment

In communities with a low to medium prevalence, treatment should be applied to individuals by *case finding* rather than by community–wide coverage, the principals of treatment remaining the same. For the selective treatment to be effective, the whole population at risk must be screened for case finding.

3. Surgical correction

Antibiotic ointment is just one component of a trachoma control programme. Individuals with lid deformities (trichiasis, entropion) should be actively sought out, so that necessary surgical procedures can be performed and followed-up. It has an immediate impact on preventing blindness.

4. Surveillance

Once control of blinding trachoma has been achieved, provision must be made to maintain surveillance, which may be necessary for several years after active inflammatory trachoma has been controlled. Since trachoma is a familial disease, the whole family group should be under surveillance.

5. Health education

In the long run, most of the antibiotic treatment must be carried out by the affected population itself. To do this, the population needs to be educated. The mothers of young children should be the target for health education. Measures of personal and community hygiene should also be incorporated in programmes of health education. Thus real primary prevention could only come through health education for the total elimination of transmission. This would require a permanent change in the behaviour patterns and in environmental factors. The final solution would be the improvement of living conditions and quality of life of the people *(10)*.

6. Evaluation

Lastly evaluation. Trachoma control programme must be evaluated at frequent intervals. The effect of intervention can be judged by the changes in the age-specific rates of active trachoma and in the prevention of trichiasis and entropion.

The 28th World Health Assembly in 1975, in a resolution requested the Director General of WHO "to encourage Member countries to develop national programmes for the prevention of blindness especially aimed at the control of trachoma, xerophthalmia, onchocerciasis and other causes". With this came the re-orientation of strategies away from single cause prevention, to the adoption of the concept of integrated delivery of eye care as part of primary health care. In this context, many countries have now integrated their trachoma control programmes into National Programmes for the Prevention of Blindness, to give simultaneous introduction of other specific measures for dealing with all causes of avoidable blindness.

The trachoma control programme in India which was launched in 1963. Later on, it was integrated with the National Programme for Control of Blindness (see chapter 7).

References

1. Dawson, C.R. et al (1975). *Bull WHO,* 52 : 279.
2. WHO (1984). *Strategies for the Prevention of Blindness in National Programmes.* A Primary Health Care Approach.
3. WHO (1962). *Techn. Rep. Ser.,* No. 234.
4. WHO (2018), *Fact sheet Trachoma,* 16th Feb., 2018.
5. WHO (1996), *World Health Report 1996,* Fighting Disease, Fostering Development, Report of the Director General, WHO.
6. Govt. of India (2018), *Annual Report 2017–2018,* Ministry of Health and Family Welfare, New Delhi.
7. Govt of India (1992), *Present Status of National Programme for control of Blindness (NPCB) 1992,* Ophthalmology Section, DGHS, New Delhi.
8. Tarizzo, M.L. (1973). *Field Methods for the Control of Trachoma,* WHO, Geneva.
9. Tarizzo, M.L. (1976). *World Health,* Feb–March, 1976.
10. WHO (1980). *Methods of Assessment of Avoidable Blindness,* WHO Offset Publ. No.54.

TETANUS

An acute disease induced by the exotoxin of *Clostridium tetani* and clinically characterized by muscular rigidity which persists throughout illness punctuated by painful paroxysmal spasms of the voluntary muscles, especially the masseters (trismus or "lock–jaw"), the facial muscles (risus sardonicus), the muscles of the back and neck (opisthotonos), and those of the lower limbs and abdomen *(1).* The mortality tends to be very high, varying from 40 to 80 per cent.

Problem statement

WORLD

Tetanus is now comparatively rare disease in the developed countries. Neonatal tetanus (NT) is a killer disease, second only to measles among the nine target diseases of the EPI. In the absence of high quality treatment, the case–fatality rate can be as high as 80–90 per cent. It tends to occur in areas with poor access to health care, hence it often remains hidden within the community.

Maternal and neonatal tetanus (MNT) is an important preventable cause of neonatal and maternal mortality, particularly in developing countries. Although easily prevented by maternal immunization with tetanus toxoid containing vaccines (TTCV) and aseptic obstetric and postnatal umbilical cord care practices, both maternal and neonatal tetanus persist as public health problems. Most cases occur in poor, remote and isolated communities where unhygienic obstetric and postnatal practices prevail along with poor access to health services.

The spores of tetanus are very resistant and remain in the environment in extremes of temperature for long periods. Hence, technically it is not possible to eradicate tetanus, including NT. However, MNT can be eliminated by reducing the disease incidence to such low levels that it ceases to be a public health problem. The disease is easily preventable through *(2)* :- (1) clean delivery and umbilical cord care practices to ensure infection is not contracted by mother or newborn during the delivery process; (2) delivery of appropriate doses of TTCV to pregnant women through antenatal care services and other routine contacts; (3) vaccination campaigns with TTCV targeting all women of reproductive age in high-risk areas; and (4) strengthening surveillance to identify women at risk, reasons for the risk, and potential clustering.

In the 1980s, over 1 million deaths every year were attributable to tetanus, with an estimated 787,000 deaths in 1988 from NT alone. Recognizing, the substantial burden of NT in developing countries, the 42nd World Health Assembly adopted a resolution to eliminate NT by 1995, through the increased availability of TTCV, clean deliveries and improved surveillance. The elimination of NT was defined as <1 case per 1000 live births in every district. In the early 1990s, it was estimated that maternal tetanus accounted for about 5% of maternal mortality, or 15,000– 30,000 deaths every year. As a result, in 1999, the elimination of maternal tetanus (MT) was added to the goals of the elimination programme for neonatal tetanus, and the programme title was changed to Maternal and Neonatal Tetanus Elimination (MNTE). Since NT is linked to the immunization status of mothers, elimination of NT has been adopted as a proxy for the elimination of MT *(2).*

The implementation of various initiatives under the MNTE programme led to a significant reduction in cases of MNT. These initiatives included promotion of maternal tetanus immunization along with safe delivery and avoidance of unsafe abortion and umbilical cord care practices. According to WHO estimates, substantial progress has been made in the past decade in reducing neonatal incidence and deaths from an estimated 787,000 deaths in 1988 to 34,000 in 2015, a reduction of about 96 per cent *(3).*

Maternal and Neonatal tetanus elimination in India *(2)*

A mix of strategies has been implemented in India to facilitate clean deliveries by training auxiliary nurse, midwives and other cadres of trained birth attendants who work at the village level, in addition to increasing routine TT protection. The Indian Ministry of Health & Family Welfare in collaboration with WHO India, UNICEF and other partners, designed and implemented the following strategies to control neonatal tetanus:

- acceleration of TT immunization coverage through the WHO-recommended high risk approach, and strengthening routine TT immunization of pregnant women, and supplemental TT immunization activities targeting women of child-bearing age in high-risk districts;
- systematic vaccination of pregnant women attending antenatal care (ANC) with TT vaccine;
- promotion of institutional deliveries focusing on poor pregnant women with an institutional stay for 48 hours, through training of traditional birth attendants;
- intensive communication programme targeting communities to reduce harmful cord care practices (promotion of the 5 cleans – hand, delivery surfaces, instruments for cutting the umbilical cord, cord tie and caring of the umbilical cord); and

- distribution of disposable delivery kits to skilled birth attendants for each pregnancy.

The launch of the national rural health mission (NRHM) in 2005 also helped to strengthen these initiatives. Strategies to improve clean delivery included the innovative Janani Suraksha Yojana (JSY), a conditional cash transfer scheme, to encourage women to give birth in a health facility. Other interventions to improve TT protection and reduce maternal and neonatal mortality under the NRHM included:

- Integrating and extending outreach services through village health and nutrition days, including vaccination of children, adolescents and pregnant women with TT containing vaccines;
- Intense 3–week refresher training for all skilled birth attendants;
- Operationalization of selected sub-centres and community health centres to provide 24–hour services 7 days per week for obstetric and neonatal care;
- Strengthening of facility-based neonatal care by setting up newborn care corners in health facilities where deliveries take place, special neonatal care units in district hospitals and new born stabilization units in first referral units for the care of sick neonates;
- Engagement of more than 896,411 accredited social health activists (ASHA) to generate demand and facilitate use of health-care services by communities and poor women.

As a result, safe deliveries rose from 52 per cent in 2007 to 76 per cent in 2009. Janani Shishu Suraksha Karyakram, launched in 2011 also helped. India's successful implementation of a mix of strategies, and experience and knowledge gained from polio eradication efforts has led to a substantial decline in the number of MNT cases in the country. As of December 2014, 30 of the 36 states/UTs were validated as having achieved MNT elimination and in May 2015, India was officially certified as achieving maternal and neonatal elimination *(4)*.

Epidemiological determinants

Agent factors

(a) AGENT : *C. tetani* is a gram–positive, anaerobic, spore–bearing organism. The spores are terminal and give the organism a drum-stick appearance. The spores are highly resistant to a number of injurious agents, including boiling, phenol, cresol and autoclaving for 15 minutes at 120 deg. Centigrade *(5)*. They germinate under anaerobic conditions and produce a potent exotoxin ("tetanospasmin"). The spores are best destroyed by steam under pressure at 120 deg. C for 20 minutes or by gamma irradiation. (b) RESERVOIR OF INFECTION : The natural habitat of the organism is soil and dust. The bacilli are found in the intestine of many herbivorous animals, e.g., cattle, horses, goats and sheep and are excreted in their faeces. The spores survive for years in nature. The bacilli may be found frequently in the intestine of man without causing ill-effects. The spores are blown about in dust and may occur in a wide variety of situations, including operation theatres. (c) EXOTOXIN : Tetanus bacilli produce a soluble exotoxin. It has an astounding lethal toxicity, exceeded only by botulinum toxin. The lethal dose for a 70 kg man is about 0.1 mg *(6)*. The toxin acts on 4 areas of the nervous system : (a) the motor end plates in skeletal system (b) the spinal cord (c) the brain, and (d) the sympathetic system *(5)*. Its principal action is to block inhibition of spinal reflexes *(7)*. (d) PERIOD OF COMMUNICABILITY : None. Not transmitted from person to person.

Host factors

(a) AGE : Commonly, tetanus is a disease of the active age (5 to 40 years). This period predisposes to all kinds of trauma and therefore, the risk of acquiring the disease is pretty high. Tetanus occurring in the new-born is known as "neonatal tetanus". Infants typically contact the disease at birth, when delivered in non–aseptic conditions – especially when the umbilical cord is cut with unclean instruments or when the umbilical stump is dressed with ashes, soil or cowdung. (b) SEX : Although a higher incidence is found in males, females are more exposed to the risk of tetanus, especially during delivery or abortion leading to "puerperal tetanus". Males appear to be more sensitive to tetanus toxin than females *(8)*. (c) OCCUPATION : Agricultural workers are at special risk because of their contact with soil. (d) RURAL–URBAN DIFFERENCES : The incidence of tetanus is much lower in urban than in rural areas. Within the urban areas, there may be vast differences in the incidence of tetanus. For example, it was observed in one town that tetanus was more frequent on the outskirts where floors were earthen and animals lived close to human beings, than in the centre of the town where there were paved and mosaic floors. (e) IMMUNITY : No age is immune unless protected by previous immunization. The immunity resulting from 2 injections of tetanus toxoid is highly effective and lasts for several years. As a general rule, patients who have recovered from tetanus must be actively immunized, because the amounts of toxin responsible for the disease in man do not stimulate protective immunity *(7)*. Immunity lasting for a few weeks (less than 6 months) can be transferred to the baby, if the mother is immunized during pregnancy or if she already has a high level of immunity at the time she becomes pregnant. Tetanus is one disease in which herd immunity does not protect the individual.

Environmental and social factors

Tetanus is a positive environmental hazard *(9)*. Its occurrence depends upon man's physical and ecological surroundings – the soil, agriculture, animal husbandry – and not on the presence or absence of infection in the population. The environmental factors are compounded by social factors such as unhygienic customs and habits (e.g., application of dust or animal dung to wounds); unhygienic delivery practices (e.g., using unsterilized instruments for cutting the umbilical cord); ignorance of infection and lack of primary health care services. In the developed countries, urbanization, industrialization and mechanization of agriculture have interfered with the normal process of distribution of *C. tetani* and have reduced the morbidity rate, as has occurred, for example in UK, USA and Germany during the last 40 years *(8)*.

Mode of transmission

Infection is acquired by contamination of wounds with tetanus spores. The range of injuries and accidents which may lead to tetanus – comprise a trivial pin prick, skin abrasion, puncture wounds, burns, human bites, animal bites and stings, unsterile surgery, intra-uterine death, bowel surgery, dental extractions, injections, unsterile division of umbilical cord, compound fractures, otitis media, chronic skin ulcers, eye infections, and gangrenous limbs *(7)*.

The sequence of events are : introduction of spores, germination and elaboration of the exotoxin and binding to the receptor.

Incubation period

The incubation period is usually 6 to 10 days. However, it may be as short as one day or as long as several months *(5)*. Long incubation is probably explained by the spores lying dormant in the wounds. Incubation is also prolonged by prophylaxis *(7)*.

Types of tetanus

(a) TRAUMATIC : Trauma is a major and important cause of tetanus. Sometimes tetanus may result from most trivial or even unnoticed wounds. (b) PUERPERAL : Tetanus follows abortion more frequently than a normal labour. A post–abortal uterus is a favourable site for the germination of tetanus spores. (c) OTOGENIC : Ear may be a rare portal of entry. Foreign bodies such as infected pencils, matches, and beads may introduce the infection. Otogenic tetanus is a paediatric problem, but cases, may occur in adults also. (d) IDIOPATHIC : In these cases there is no definite history of sustaining an injury. Some consider it to be the result of microscopic trauma. Others hold the view that it is due to the absorption of tetanus toxin from the intestinal tract. A third view is that the tetanus spores may be inhaled and may start the infection. (e) TETANUS NEONATORUM : In many countries, neonatal tetanus kills about 85 per cent of those afflicted. The common cause is infection of the umbilical stump after birth, the first symptom being seen about the 7th day. Therefore, tetanus is known as "8th day disease" in Punjab *(6)*. In any country where hygiene is poor, neonatal tetanus may be common.

PREVENTION

1. Active immunization (10, 11, 12)

Tetanus is best prevented by active immunization with tetanus toxoid. It stimulates the production of the protective antitoxin. The aim should be to vaccinate the entire community and ensure a protective level of antitoxin approximately 0.01 IU/ml serum throughout life. All persons should be immunized regardless of age.

Two preparations are available for active immunization

a. *Combined vaccine – DPT*
b. *Monovalent vaccines*
   i) Plain or fluid (formal) toxoid
   ii) Tetanus vaccine, adsorbed (PTAP, APT)

a. COMBINED VACCINE

Tetanus vaccine is offered routinely to infants (Expanded Immunization Programme) in combination with diphtheria vaccine and killed *B. pertussis* organisms as DPT vaccine. According to the National Immunization Schedule (see page 135), the primary course of immunization consists of 3 doses of DPT, at intervals of 4–8 weeks, starting at 6 weeks of age, followed by a booster at 18 months of age, and a second booster at 5–6 years of age and a third booster (Only TT) after 10 years of age.

Pentavalent vaccine: At present pentavalent vaccine is being given at 6th, 10th and 14th weeks of age instead of DPT vaccine. The DPT vaccine is used for booster dose.

b. MONOVALENT VACCINES

Purified tetanus toxoid (adsorbed) has largely supplanted plain toxoid because it stimulates a higher and longer–lasting immunity response than plain toxoid *(13)*. However, the latter may be employed for purposes of booster injection when rapid protection is indicated.

A primary course of immunization consists of two doses of tetanus toxoid adsorbed (each dose 0.5 ml, injected into the arm) given at intervals of 1–2 months. The longer the intervals between the two doses, the better is the immune response. The first booster dose (the third in order) should be given a year after the initial two doses. The opinion was expressed that no more than one additional booster dose (a total of 4 doses altogether) given 5 years after the third dose is required in adults (including pregnant women) in developing countries *(14)*. Frequent boosters must be avoided.

Reactions following the injections of tetanus toxoid are uncommon. They are less likely to occur with a refined and adsorbed toxoid such as Purified Tetanus Toxoid (Aluminium Phosphate Adsorbed). However, in persons giving history of allergy usual precautions should be observed. Purified tetanus toxoid should be stored between 2 and 8 deg. C. It must not be allowed to freeze at any time.

2. Passive immunization (10, 11)

Temporary protection against tetanus can be provided by an injection of human tetanus hyperimmunoglobulin (TIG) or ATS. (i) HUMAN TETANUS HYPERIMMUNOGLOBULIN : It is the best prophylactic to use. The dose for all ages is 250 IU. It does not cause serum reactions. It gives a longer passive protection upto 30 days or more compared with 7–10 days for horse ATS. Human tetanus Ig is now available in India – it is produced by the Serum Institute of India, Pune. (ii) ATS (EQUINE) : If human antitoxin is not available, equine antitoxin (anti-tetanus serum or ATS) should be used. The standard dose is 1500 IU, injected subcutaneously after sensitivity testing. ATS gives passive protection for about 7–10 days. Being a foreign protein, ATS is rapidly excreted from the body and there may be very little antibody at the end of 2 weeks. Because of this drawback, ATS may not cover the tetanus incubation period in all cases. Horse ATS has other disadvantages too – (i) It causes sensitivity reaction in many people because it contains foreign proteins. A person receiving ATS for the first time may tolerate it well, but there is a possibility that subsequent injections of horse serum may lead to allergic reactions varying in severity from rash to anaphylactic shock. It is estimated that the incidence of serious systemic reactions to ATS is 5 to 10 per cent of the persons who receive it. It is well to remember that local tests for sensitivity are unreliable as to general sensitivity to horse serum. (ii) Another drawback of ATS is that it stimulates the formation of antibodies to it and hence a person who has once received ATS tends to rapidly eliminate subsequent doses. As such the value of second and subsequent doses of ATS becomes questionable. In practice, therefore, ATS becomes less and less reliable as a prophylactic. These drawbacks have been responsible for the growing unpopularity of ATS as an agent for immediate protection against tetanus.

3. Active and passive immunization

Simultaneous active and passive immunization is widely carried out in non-immune persons. The patient is given 1500 units of ATS or 250 units of Human Ig in one arm, and 0.5 ml of adsorbed tetanus toxoid (PTAP or APT) into the other arm or gluteal region. This should be followed 6 weeks later by another dose of 0.5 ml of tetanus toxoid, and a third dose one year later. The purpose of antitoxin is for immediate temporary protection, and the purpose of toxoid is for long–lasting protection.

4. Antibiotics

Active immunization with tetanus toxoid is the ideal method of tetanus prophylaxis, but it is of no immediate avail to a person who is non-immune and has sustained injury. ATS as an agent for immediate protection against tetanus has its drawbacks. For these reasons, antibiotics are indicated in the prophylaxis against tetanus. A single intramuscular injection of 1.2 mega units of a long–acting penicillin (e.g., benzathine penicillin) will provide a sustained concentration of the drug for 3 to 4 weeks, which is sufficient to kill any vegetative forms of tetanus bacilli that may emerge from the sporulating stage. Penicillin has no effect on tetanus spores. For patients who are sensitive to penicillin, a 7–day course of erythromycin estolate 500 mg 6–hourly by mouth will kill vegetative forms of *C. tetani* but not spores. Antibiotics should be given as soon as possible after an injury, before a lethal dose of toxin is produced in the wound, which may be as soon as 6 hours after injury. Antibiotic prophylaxis should not be relied upon for patients seen later than 6 hours after injury. Moreover, it is not certain whether the antibiotic can reach the bacilli, if there is dead tissue present in the wound. Therefore, antibiotic alone is ineffective in the prevention of tetanus; it is not a substitute to immunization.

Prevention of neonatal tetanus

Neonatal tetanus is well controlled in some industrialized countries through clean delivery practices alone. Over the last decade, most programmes in developing countries have concentrated on training the traditional birth attendants, providing home delivery kits and educating pregnant women about the "five cleans" – clean hands, clean delivery surface and clean cord care i.e., clean blade for cutting the cord, clean tie for the cord and no application on the cord stump. Operational research has shown that training of birth attendants alone can reduce death due to neonatal tetanus by 90 per cent *(15)*.

Tetanus toxoid will protect both the mother and her child. In **unimmunized** pregnant women, two doses of tetanus toxoid should be given, the first as early as possible during pregnancy and the second at least a month later and at least 3 weeks before delivery. According to the National Immunization Schedule (see page 135), these doses may be given between 16–36 weeks of pregnancy, allowing an interval of 1–2 months between the 2 doses. In previously **immunized** pregnant women, a booster dose is considered sufficient. There is no need for a booster at every consecutive pregnancy, because of the risk of hyper-immunization and side-effects.

In areas where the incidence of neonatal tetanus is high, the primary 2–dose course can be extended to all women of child-bearing age, particularly if the present coverage of antenatal care is low.

In developing countries, the majority of pregnant women are not seen antenatally. Since a pregnant woman coming for an antenatal visit may in fact never return again, immunization should be given regardless of the month of pregnancy as there is no evidence to suggest that tetanus toxoids are dangerous or harmful to the foetus. The golden rule is that no pregnant mother should be denied even one dose of tetanus toxoid if she is seen late in pregnancy.

The infants born to the mothers who have not previously received 2–doses of tetanus toxoid are exposed to the risk of neonatal tetanus. They can be protected by injection of antitoxin (heterologous serum, 750 IU), if it is administered within 6 hours of birth.

Prevention of tetanus after injury *(12)*

All wounds must be thoroughly cleaned soon after injury – removal of foreign bodies, soil, dust, necrotic tissue. This procedure will abolish anaerobic conditions which favour germination of tetanus spores.

A useful scheme for the prevention of tetanus in the wounded is given in Fig. 1.

All wounds receive surgical toilet

Wounds less than 6 hours old, clean, non-penetrating and with negligible tissue damage.

Immunity category	*Treatment*
A	Nothing more required
B	Toxoid 1 dose
C	Toxoid 1 dose
D	Toxoid complete course

Other wounds

Immunity category	*Treatment*
A	Nothing more required
B	Toxoid 1 dose
C	Toxoid 1 dose + Human Tet. Ig.
D	Toxoid complete course + Human Tet. Ig

A = Has had a complete course of toxoid or a booster dose within the past 5 years.
B = Has had a complete course of toxoid or a booster dose more than 5 years ago and less than 10 years ago.
C = Has had a complete course of toxoid or a booster dose more than 10 years ago.
D = Has not had a complete course of toxoid or immunity status is unknown.

FIG. 1
Recommendations for prevention of tetanus in the wounded

When ATS is given, adrenaline solution 1 in 1000 for intramuscular injection in the dosage of 0.5 to 1 ml and hydrocortisone 100 mg for intravenous injection must be kept available in case of a generalized anaphylactoid reaction *(11)*. A test dose of ATS (0.1 ml in a tuberculin syringe) should be given subcutaneously (not intradermally) and the patient observed carefully (not casually) at least for half an hour for any evidence of general reaction (not only local reaction), e.g., alteration in pulse, fall in blood pressure, dyspnoea and distress. If there is reaction, the rest of the antitoxin should be given in gradually increasing fractions after treatment with adrenaline. In patients with history of allergy, e.g., asthma, eczema, food or drug idiosyncracy, the above test should be preceded by a dose of 0.05 ml of 1 in 10 dilution of the ATS. If there is reaction, ATS should be withheld.

Lastly, it should be pointed out that tetanus may occasionally occur inspite of active or passive immunization or both. Nevertheless, the aim is to provide as much protection as possible in the light of our present scientific knowledge.

References

1. WHO (1973), Council for International Organizations of Medical Sciences (1973). *Communicable Diseases,* Provisional International Nomenclature, c/o WHO, Geneva.
2. WHO (2016), *Weekly Epidemiological Record,* No. 44, 30th Oct., 2016.
3. WHO (2018), *Fact sheet Tetanus,* 9th May, 2018.
4. Govt. of India (2016), *Annual Report 2015–2016,* Ministry of Health and Family Welfare, New Delhi.
5. Weinstein, Louis (1973). *N. Eng. J. Med.,* 289 : 1293.
6. Gordon, J.E. et al (1961). *J. Indian M.A.,* 37 : 157.
7. Warrel, David A (1981). *Medicine International,* 3 : 118.
8. Bytchenko, B. (1966). *Bull WHO,* 34 : 71.
9. Cvetanovic, B. et al (1978). *Bull WHO,* Supplement No.1 to Vol 56, p.29.
10. Adams, E.B. et al (1969). *Tetanus,* Blackwell.
11. Sen, B. (1972). *J. Indian M.A.,* 59 : 294.
12. Smith, J.W.G. et al (1975). *Brit. Med. J.* 3 : 453–455.
13. White, W.G. et al (1969). *Lancet, 2 : 94.*
14. WHO (1982). *Prevention of Neonatal Tetanus,* SEARO Tech. Publ. No.3.
15. WHO (1992), *World Health Statistics,* Quarterly Report, Communicable Disease, Vol. 45, No. 2/3.

LEPROSY

Leprosy (Hansen's disease) is a chronic infectious disease caused by *M. leprae.* It affects mainly the peripheral nerves. It also affects the skin, muscles, eyes, bones, testes and internal organs. The disease manifests itself in two polar forms, namely the lepromatous leprosy and tuberculoid leprosy, lying at the two ends of a long spectrum of the disease. Between these two polar types occur the borderline and indeterminate forms depending upon the host response to infection.

Leprosy is clinically characterized by one or more of the following cardinal features :

a. hypopigmented patches
b. partial or total loss of cutaneous sensation in the affected areas (the earliest sensation to be affected is usually light touch)
c. presence of thickened nerves, and
d. presence of acid–fast bacilli in the skin or nasal smears.

The signs of advanced disease are striking : presence of nodules or lumps especially in the skin of the face and ears; plantar ulcers; loss of fingers or toes, nasal depression, foot-drop, claw toes and other deformities.

Problem statement

WORLD

In 1991, WHO member states resolved to decrease the level of leprosy in the world by over 90 per cent. This has now been accomplished, and the overall target for the global elimination of leprosy as a public health problem has been attained *(1)*. The fall in prevalence rate is largely explained by an improvement in the management of cases, very low rates of relapse, high cure rates, absence of drug resistance and shorter duration of treatment with MDT *(2)*.

The achievement can be summarized as follows *(3)* :

(1) Over the past 20 years, more than 16 million leprosy patients have been cured.
(2) The prevalence rate of the disease has dropped from 21.1 cases per 10,000 population in 1985 to 16.6 per million population by end of 2020.
(3) The global burden of leprosy has declined dramatically from 5.2 million cases in 1985 to 127,558 cases at the end of 2020.
(4) The new case detection rate was 16.4 per million population at the end of 2020. The ten year trend shows a slow decrease in detection rate of new cases globally.
(5) Currently the emphasis is on 23 countries of global priority.

Although significant progress has been made in controlling the disease and reducing the disease burden, much remains to be done in order to sustain the gains and further reduce the impact of the disease, especially the burden due to the physical, mental and socio-economic consequences of leprosy on persons affected and their families. There is a growing need to develop more effective tools and procedures for early recognition and management of leprosy reactions and nerve damage. Most programmes need to initiate activities to improve the quality of life of persons affected by leprosy through prevention of disability and community-based rehabilitation measures. One of the long-term needs is to develop reliable diagnostic tests for early diagnosis and an effective vaccine for the prevention of leprosy.

WHO has been regularly collecting data on several indicators from various WHO regions and member states. The indicators and reported data is as follows *(3)* :

1. 127,396 new cases of leprosy were detected during 2020. As in previous years, SEAR accounted for 66.6 per cent of the global leprosy burden, where India and Indonesia contributed 72.5 per cent of the new leprosy cases globally and 91.725 per cent regionally.
2. Among the new cases detected in 2020, the proportion of multibacillary cases of leprosy was about 67.3 per cent.
3. The proportion of female cases among newly detected cases in 2020 was 38.6 per cent (49,208 cases).
4. The proportion of children below 15 years of age was 6.8 per cent (8,629 cases).
5. The number of new cases with grade-2 disabilities were 7,198 (0.9 per cent).
6. The number of new child cases with grade-2 disabilities were 308.
7. The number of relapse cases in 2020 were 2,990.
8. The number of retreatment cases were 10,432.

In view of the changing trends in leprosy, the Director General of WHO placed the management of the Global Leprosy Programme under the Regional Director, SEAR, considering that this region has the highest burden of disease globally. The office and staff of the Global Leprosy Programme moved from Geneva to New Delhi on July 1st 2005. The WHO has evolved the Global Strategy for further reducing the leprosy burden and sustaining leprosy control activities 2010–2015, and more recently Global Leprosy Strategy 2016–2020: "Accelerating towards a leprosy-free world".

The Global leprosy strategy 2016–2020: "Accelerating towards a leprosy-free world"

The Global Leprosy Strategy 2016–2020: "Accelerating towards a leprosy-free world" was released in April 2016. The strategy is based on the principles of initiating action, ensuring accountability and promoting inclusion. It is built around 3 pillars: to strengthen government ownership, coordination and partnership; to stop leprosy and its complications; and to stop discrimination and promote inclusion. In endorsing the global strategy, 3 key targets have been agreed by all national programmes : (1) zero grade 2 disability (G2D) among children diagnosed with leprosy; (2) the reduction of new leprosy cases with G2D to <1 case per million population and (3) zero countries with legislation allowing discrimination on the basis of leprosy *(3)*. Early detection and complete treatment with MDT remains the fundamental principle of leprosy control.

INDIA

Leprosy is widely prevalent in India. Although the disease is present throughout the country, the distribution is uneven. After introduction of MDT in the country, the recorded leprosy case load has come down from 57.6 cases per 10,000 population in 1981 to less than one case per 10,000 population at national level in December 2005, and the country achieved the goal of leprosy elimination at national level.

Based on the reports received from the states/UTs for the year 2020–2021, the current leprosy situation in the country is as follows *(4A)* :

A total of 65,147 new cases were detected during the year 2020, which gives annual new case detection rate (ANCDR) of 4.56 per lakh population. A total of 79,898 cases were on record as on March 2021, giving a prevalence rate (PR) of 0.41 per 10,000 population. The detailed information on new leprosy cases detected during 2020–21 indicates the proportion of multibacillary cases was 58.1 per cent, proportion of female cases was 39 per cent, child case proportion was 5.8 per cent, 2.41 per cent patients were with grade-II disability, giving disability rate of 1.1 per million population).

34 states/UTs had already achieved the level of leprosy elimination i.e. PR of less than 1 case per 10,000 population. Chhattisgarh and Dadra & Nagar Haveli has PR of 2–5 per 10,000 population.

As on 31st March 2019, 514 districts out of 708 have ANCDR less than 10 per lakh population, 72 districts have more than 20 per lakh population, and only 12 districts are with more than 50 per lakh population (of which 3 are in Chhattisgarh, 1 in Gujarat, 2 in Maharashtra, 1 in Dadra & Nagar Haveli and 5 in Odisha. Three districts reported ANCDR of more than 90 per lakh population.

Out of the total 65,147 new cases detected, a total of 79,898 cases were recorded under treatment during 2020.

Epidemiological determinants

Agent factors

(a) AGENT : Leprosy is caused by *M. leprae*. They are acid–fast and occur in the human host both intracellularly and extracellularly. They occur characteristically in clumps or bundles (called globi). They have an affinity for Schwann cells and cells of the reticulo–endothelial system. They remain dormant in various sites and cause relapse. The bacterial load is the highest in the lepromatous cases. As many as 2 to 7 billion were estimated in one gram of leproma *(5)*. Numerous antigens (more than 20) have been detected in *M. leprae* by electrophoretic techniques. Some of these are shared by those of pathogenic and non–pathogenic mycobacteria, e.g., BCG, *M. smegmatis, M. vaccae, M. tuberculosis,* etc. Most interesting of these antigens is the phenolic glycolipid (PGL) which may be the specific *M. leprae* antigen. Recent years have witnessed the successful transmission of *M. leprae* to some experimental animals. Currently large quantities of *M. leprae* are being produced by multiplication in the 9–banded armadillo and nude mouse. Despite repeated claims, *M. leprae* has not yet been conclusively shown to grow in artificial medium *(6)*. It is perhaps mainly for this reason that progress in research has lagged behind than that of many other diseases.

(b) SOURCE OF INFECTION : It is generally agreed that multibacillary cases (lepromatous and borderline lepromatous cases) are the most important source of infection in the community. The inapparent infections are also source of infection. The role of individuals with tuberculoid forms of the disease as sources of infection is not clear. The current view is that all patients with "active leprosy" must be considered infectious *(7)*. Until recently man was considered to be the only host and source of infection. There is now evidence that natural infections with *M. leprae* are present in wild animals, e.g., armadillos, mangabey monkeys and chimpanzees. It is not yet known if leprosy in wild animals is a threat to public health.

(c) PORTAL OF EXIT : It is widely accepted that the nose is a major portal of exit. Lepromatous cases harbour millions of *M. leprae* in their nasal mucosa which are discharged when they sneeze or blow the nose. The bacilli can also exit through ulcerated or broken skin of bacteriologically positive cases of leprosy *(8)*.

(d) INFECTIVITY : Leprosy is a highly infectious disease but of low pathogenicity *(9)*. It is claimed that an infectious patient can be rendered non-infectious by treatment with dapsone for about 90 days *(10)* or with rifampicin for 3 weeks *(12)*. Local application of rifampicin (drops or spray) might destroy all the bacilli within 8 days *(11)*.

(e) ATTACK RATES : Among household contacts of lepromatous cases, a varying proportion – 4.4 per cent to 12 per cent – is expected to show signs of leprosy within 5 years *(11)*. This occurs despite treatment of the index case, most, if not all, cases having been infectious for long periods, before treatment is sought.

Host factors

(a) AGE : Infection can take place at any time depending upon the opportunities for exposure. Incidence rates generally rise to a peak between 20 and 30 years of age and then fall *(12)*. In areas where leprosy is rare, the first contact may not take place early in life and consequently, the disease may appear late. However, the presence of leprosy in child population is of considerable epidemiological importance. A high prevalence of infection among children means that the disease is active and spreading.

(b) SEX : Both the incidence and prevalence of leprosy appear to be higher in males than in females in most regions of the world. Sex difference is found least in children below 15 years, and more marked among adults; more marked among lepromatous cases than among non-lepromatous cases. The excess of cases in males has sometimes been attributed to their greater mobility and increased opportunities for contact in many populations.

(c) MIGRATION : In India leprosy was considered to be mostly a rural problem. However, because of the movement of population from rural to urban areas, leprosy is creating a problem in the urban areas also *(13)*.

(d) THE PREVALENCE POOL *(14)*: The prevalence pool of leprosy in a population in general is in a constant flux resulting from inflow and outflow. The inflow is contributed by the occurrence of new cases, relapse of cured cases, and immigration of cases. The outflow is mainly through cure or inactivation of cases, death of cases, and emigration of cases. Of the various factors that influence the prevalence pool, the importance of inactivation of disease and mortality are less well recognized.

(e) INACTIVATION OF DISEASE *(14)* : Where leprosy treatment facilities exist, inactivation or cure due to specific treatment is an important mode of elimination of cases from the prevalence pool. Even in the absence of specific treatment, a majority of patients, particularly of the tuberculoid and indeterminate types, tend to get cured spontaneously. An earlier study in India had shown that over a period of 20 years, the extent of spontaneous regression among children with tuberculoid leprosy was about 90%. A study in Culion Island in the Philippines showed that among children self-healing occurred in 77.7% of cases (Lara & Nolasco, 1956). A later study in South India involving long-term follow-up of a high endemic population showed that among newly detected tuberculoid cases of all ages and both sexes, the rate of inactivation was 10.9% per year, the bulk of inactivation in the study being spontaneous (Noordeen, 1975).

(f) IMMUNITY : It is a well-established fact that only a few persons exposed to infection develop the disease. A large proportion of early lesions that occur in leprosy heal spontaneously. Such abortive and self-healing lesions suggest immunity acquired through such lesions. Subclinical infections are far more common than was thought earlier; they are also believed to contribute to active immunity. A certain degree of immunity is also probable through infections with other related mycobacteria *(15)*.

It is now recognized that cell-mediated immunity (CMI) is responsible for resistance to infection with *M. leprae*. In lepromatous leprosy, there is a complete breakdown of CMI; in these cases the lepromin test is negative. CMI does not however, exclude the participation of humoral response. Antibodies have been demonstrated throughout the spectrum of leprosy; they are more pronounced at the lepromatous end. Similarly an increase of immunoglobulins of IgG and IgM classes is noted towards the lepromatous end *(16)*. Leprosy workers have found that the anergy of lepromatous leprosy is due to suppression of T cell production of interleukin–2 (T–cell growth factor). This is normally secreted by activated T cells to make other T cells proliferate. If exogenous interleukin–2 is added, the process may be reversed. However, further studies are needed to find out whether administration of IL–2 would benefit the lepromatous patient *(16)*.

(g) GENETIC FACTORS : There is now evidence that human lymphocyte antigen (HLA) linked genes influence the type of immune response that develops *(6)*.

Environmental factors

The risk of transmission is predominantly controlled by environmental factors *(10)* : (a) the presence of infectious cases in that environment. There is evidence that humidity favours the survival of *M. leprae* in the environment. *M. leprae* can remain viable in dried nasal secretions for at least 9 days and in moist soil at room temperature for 46 days *(6)*, (b) overcrowding and lack of ventilation within households.

Mode of transmission

The mode of transmission of leprosy has not been established with certainty. The following theories are frequently debated :

(A) DROPLET INFECTION : There is more and more evidence that leprosy may be transmitted *via* aerosols containing *M. leprae* (droplet infection). With the realization of the importance of the nose as a portal of exit, there has been increased emphasis on the respiratory tract as the portal of entry. The possibility of this route of transmission is based on (a) the inability of the organisms to be found on the surface of the skin; (b) the demonstration of a large number of organisms in the nasal discharge; (c) the high proportion of morphologically intact bacilli in the nasal secretions; and (d) the evidence that *M. leprae* could survive outside the human host for several hours or days *(14)*.

(B) CONTACT TRANSMISSION : Numerous studies indicate that leprosy is transmitted from person-to-person by close contact between an infectious patient and a healthy but susceptible person. This contact may be direct or indirect (e.g., contact with soil, and fomites such as contaminated clothes and linen).

Now that it is known that leprosy bacilli can survive for long periods of time in the soil under favourable environmental conditions, the hypothesis that leprosy can be transmitted by indirect contact has been strengthened *(17)*. In epidemiological studies, the first lesions were found in feet and legs of patients from hilly areas in India, where injury to the skin is common. In the Philippines 91 per cent of the first lesions were seen in extremities open to injury *(13)*. These observations lend support to indirect transmission. Although contact transmission has been a long-favoured hypothesis, leprologists opine that skin–to–skin contact is really not necessary to acquire infection, and that the disease is transmissible with far less than intimate contact *(7, 9)*.

(C) OTHER ROUTES : Bacilli may also be transmitted by insect vectors, or by tattooing needles. These transmission channels cannot be ruled out *(17)*. However, there is no evidence that any of these transmission routes is important in nature *(6)*.

Incubation period

Leprosy has a long incubation period, an average of 3 to 5 years or more. Symptoms can take as long as 20 years to appear. Failure to recognize early symptoms or signs may contribute to an assumed prolonged incubation period in some patients. Some leprologists prefer the term "latent period" to incubation period because of the long duration of the incubation period.

Knowledge of incubation period of relapses is also essential, as this will define the duration of surveillance after treatment has been stopped.

Pathogenesis of leprosy *(12)*

Onset of leprosy is insidious. It affects nerves, skin and the eyes, it may also affect mucosa (mouth, nose, pharynx), testis, kidney, voluntary/smooth muscles, reticulo-endothelial system and vascular endothelium.

Bacilli enter the body usually through respiratory system. It has low pathogenicity, only a small proportion of infected people develop signs of the disease. Though infected, majority of the population do not develop the disease. After entering the body, bacilli migrate towards the neural tissue and enter Schwann cells. Bacteria can also be found in macrophages, muscles cells and endothelial cells of blood vessels.

After entering Schwann cells or macrophages, fate of the bacterium depends on the resistance of the infected individual towards the organism. Bacilli start multiplying slowly (about 12–14 days for one bacterium to divide into two) within the cells, get released from the destroyed cells and enter other unaffected cells. During this state, person remains free from signs and symptoms of leprosy.

As the bacilli multiply, bacterial load increases in the body and infection is recognized by the immunological system. Lymphocytes and histiocytes (macrophages) invade the infected tissue. At this stage, clinical manifestation may appear as involvement of nerves with impairment of sensation and/or skin patch. If it is not diagnosed and treated in the early stages, further progress of the disease is determined by the strength of the patient's immune response.

Specific and effective cell mediated immunity (CMI) provides protection to a person against leprosy. When specific CMI is effective in elimination/controlling the infection in the body, lesions heal spontaneously or it produces pauci-bacillary (PB) type of leprosy. If CMI is deficient; the disease spreads uncontrolled and produces multi bacillary (MB) leprosy with multiple system involvement. Sometimes, the immune response is abruptly altered, either following treatment (MDT) or due to improvement of immunological status, which results in the inflammation of skin or nerves and even other tissues, called as Lepra reaction leading to temporary and permanent disabilities/deformities. Pathogenesis of leprosy is summarized in Fig. 1.

Classification

Leprosy is a disease bedevilled by classifications, e.g., the Madrid classification *(18)*, Ridley–Jopling classification *(19)*, the Indian classification *(20)*, etc. These classifications are based on clinical, bacteriological, immunological and histological status of patients.

The Indian and Madrid classification systems are the most widely used in field leprosy programmes; they are not essentially different, as the following comparison shows :

Indian classification	*Madrid classification*
indeterminate type	indeterminate
tuberculoid type	tuberculoid; flat; raised
borderline type	borderline
lepromatous type	lepromatous
pure neuritic type	

The Indian classification has an additional form, the pure neuritic in which no skin lesions exist.

The classification system of Ridley and Jopling *(21)* divides leprosy cases into five groups according to their position on an immuno-histological scale : tuberculoid (TT), borderline tuberculoid (BL), borderline (BB), borderline lepromatous (BL) and lepromatous (LL). The neuritic type of leprosy does not find a place in the Ridley and Jopling classification. This classification can be used only when full research facilities are available.

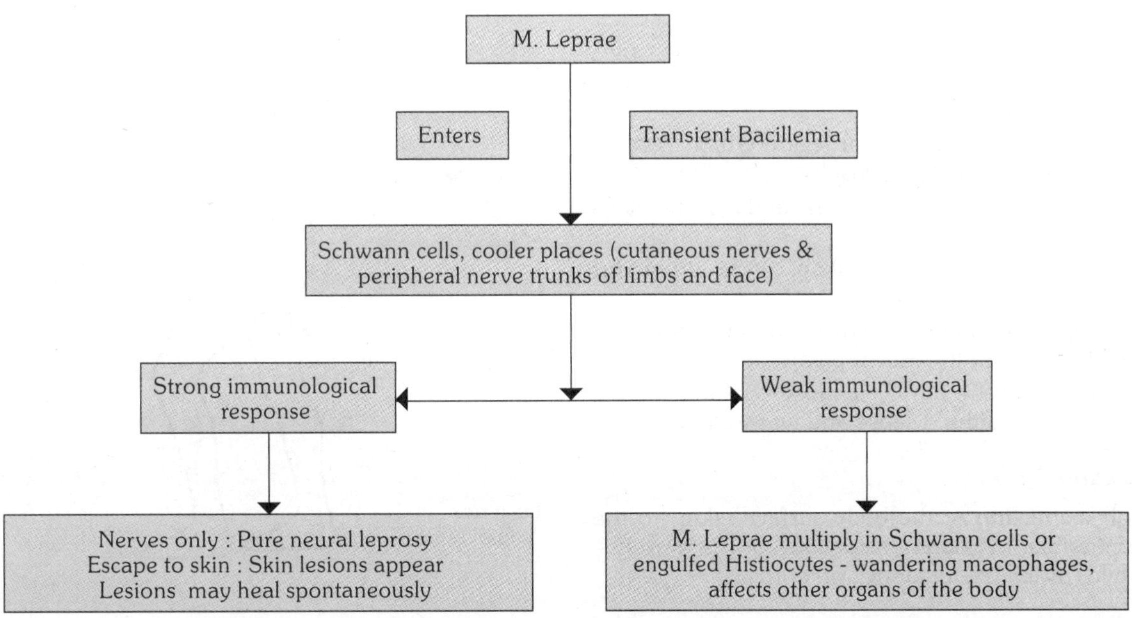

FIG. 1
Pathogenesis of leprosy

Clinical classification for control programme

After making a diagnosis of leprosy, one should group the patient based on certain characteristics. This is important because, it helps in selecting the correct combination of drugs for a given patient.

Criteria for classification (12)

Characteristics	PB (Pauci-bacillary)	MB (Multi-bacillary)
Skin lesions	1–5 lesions	6 and above
Peripheral nerve	No nerve / only one nerve involvement	More than one nerve involvement
Skin smear	Negative at all sites	Positive at any site

Diagnosis of leprosy *(12)*

A case of leprosy is diagnosed by eliciting cardinal signs of leprosy through systematic clinical (and wherever required bacteriological) examination. At least one of the following cardinal (unique and very important) signs must be present to diagnose leprosy.

a. Hypo-pigmented or reddish skin lesion(s) with definite sensory deficit;
b. Involvement of the peripheral nerves, as demonstrated by definite thickening with loss of sensation and weakness /paralysis of the corresponding muscles of the hands, feet or eyes;
c. Demonstration of *M. leprae* in the lesions.

The first two cardinal signs can be identified by clinical examination alone, while the third can be identified by examination of the slit skin smear.

1. CLINICAL EXAMINATION

Clinical examination includes careful interview of the patient to get detailed history and examination of skin and nerves.

a. Case history

The leprosy history should elicit the following :

- Name, sex, age (year of birth), address, occupation etc.;
- Presenting complaints and their duration (A patch of a few days or that which is present since birth or an itchy patch is unlikely to be leprosy);
- History of recurrence (a recurrent lesion which "comes and goes" will not be due to leprosy);
- Any deformity, the time of its onset, and nature of its progress;
- Treatment history - treatment taken, what drugs for leprosy and how long;
- Any other associated illness (jaundice, cough, swelling of the feet at present or in the recent past);
- Any other person in the family or close contacts having similar disease or had the disease and was treated.

b. Physical examination

(i) A thorough inspection of the body surface (skin) to the extent permissible, in good natural light for the presence of suggestive, or tell tale evidence of leprosy

Testing the sensation over skin *(12)* :

It is very important to pick up the skill of eliciting sensory loss in skin patch. A light ballpoint pen (with plastic body) without cap will be needed. Explain to the person what you are going to do and demonstrate it. Touch the skin with the tip of the pen lightly and ask the individual to point to the spot touched with his index finger. Repeat this procedure a few times until the patient is familiar and comfortable with the procedure. Now ask the patient to close his eyes and repeat the procedure (first on the normal skin then over the affected area). While testing lesions over inaccessible areas (back, buttocks) the patient may be asked to count on each touch. Do not use other "instruments" like pin, cotton wool, feather, etc. When testing for sensation, touch the skin lightly with the pen. Do not stroke. The pen should be perpendicular to the surface of the skin. Do not keep asking the patient whether he feels the touch. You may get misleading results. Proceed from the normal skin to the patch. Give only one stimulus at a time. Vary the pace of testing.

c. Nerve examination (12)

Resource person should demonstrate nerve examination from head to toe and also use video clips. The cardinal sign is : "Involvement of the peripheral nerves, as demonstrated by definite thickening with a loss of sensation with or without weakness/paralysis of the corresponding muscles of the hands, feet or eyes". Examination of nerves in all the patients is very important for diagnosis, grouping and for prevention of deformity. This involves two aspects : (a) palpation of the nerves for thickening, tenderness and consistency; and (b) assessment of nerve function – sensory and motor. The commonly affected nerves are as shown in Fig. 2.

Before the introduction of MDT, most leprosy cases were diagnosed by medical officer or specialized leprosy workers, and it often led to delay in diagnosis and initiation of treatment. Since the introduction of MDT, many procedures have been simplified, so that leprosy patients can be detected by health workers in the field.

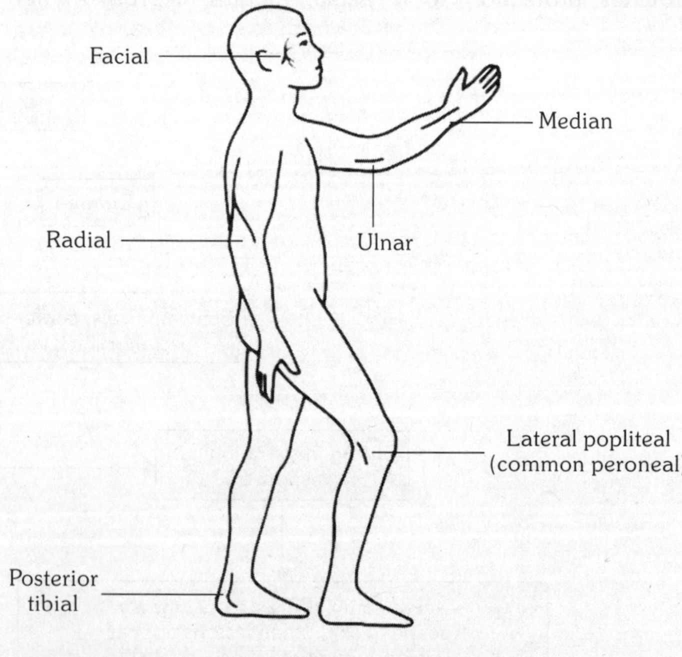

FIG. 2

Sites of nerve involvement

Source : *(21)*

2. *BACTERIOLOGICAL EXAMINATION*

Skin smears are useful for diagnosing multibacillary leprosy and were originally used for distinguishing between paucibacillary and multibacillary leprosy. However, the quality of skin smears and of microscopy is probably the weakest link in most leprosy elimination programmes. In view of this situation, and since it is possible to classify leprosy without skin smear results, it should not be a pre-requisite for implementing the MDT *(22)*.

A brief account of method of skin smear and nasal smear examination is as follows :

(i) Skin smears : Material from the skin is obtained from an active lesion, and also from one of the ear lobe by the "slit and scrape" method. Conventionally, two sites are examined. The skin is cleaned with ether or spirit and allowed to dry. A fold of the skin is nipped between the thumb and forefinger (of left hand in an operator). Enough pressure should be applied to stop or minimize bleeding. Holding the point of knife vertical to the apex of the skin fold, it is pushed into the skin to a depth of about 2 mm or so, to reach the dermis. A tiny incision is made 5 mm or so in length. If blood exudes, it should be wiped off with a small dry cotton-wool swab. The knife blade is rotated transversely to the line of the cut 90° and the knife point is used to scrape first on one side and then on the other side of the incision 2 or 3 times to obtain a tissue pulp from below the epidermis. This material is transferred on to a glass slide and spread over an area of about 8 mm diameter. Six smears can conveniently be made on one microscopic slide. The sites of the smear should be accurately recorded so that the same sites can be used for successive sets of smears made for assesing the effect of treatment. The wound is dressed and closed with a piece of sticking tape applied over the site.

(ii) Nasal smears or blows : Nasal smears can be best prepared from early morning mucus material. The patient blows his nose into a clean dry sheet of cellophane or plastic. The smear should be made straightaway and fixed. This should be done in the early morning from the first blowing of the nose. Nose-blowing smears are used for assessing the patient's infectivity. In patients with untreated lepromatous leprosy, nose-blow smears may show a higher percentage of solid-staining bacilli than skin smears.

(iii) Nasal scrapings : An alternative is to use a nasal mucosal scrapper. After going in 4.5 cm, the blade is rotated towards the septum and scraped a few times and withdrawn. A small ball of cotton is introduced into the nostril to absorb any blood that may ooze out. Nasal scrapings are not recommended as a routine, because they are painful, and non-pathogenic atypical mycobacteria may be present in the nose of healthy persons. Leprosy bacilli are not found in nasal mucosa if they are absent in skin lesions. During treatment, *M. leprae* may disappear from the nasal mucosa before they disappear from the skin lesions *(23)*.

The skin or nasal smear is immediately fixed by lightly passing the underside of the slide over the spirit lamp flame and transported to the laboratory for staining with Ziehl–Neelsen method.

The glass slides used should be absolutely clean. They should not be reused for making smears a second time as organisms from a previous examination may give a false positive result *(20)*. Before a smear is declared negative, at least 200 fields should be examined *(7)*.

Bacterial index *(12)*

Bacterial index (BI) is the only objective way of monitoring the benefit of treatment. The Bacteriological (or Bacterial) Index indicates the density of leprosy bacilli in smears and includes both living (solid-staining) and dead (fragmented or granular) bacilli. According to **Ridley's logarithmic scale,** it ranges from zero to 6+ and is based on the number of bacilli seen in an average microscopic field of the smear using an oil-immersion objective.

- 0 No bacilli in any of the 100 oil-immersion fields
- 1+ 1–10 bacilli, on average, in 100 oil-immersion fields
- 2+ 1–10 bacilli on average, in 10 oil-immersion fields
- 3+ 1–10 bacilli, on average, in each oil-immersion field
- 4+ 10–100 bacilli, on average, in each oil-immersion field
- 5+ 100–1000 bacilli, on average, in each oil-immersion field
- 6+ More than 1000 bacilli, on average, in each oil-immersion field

The BI of the patient is calculated by adding up the index from each site examined and dividing the total by the number of sites examined.

(e.g. Right ear 5+ Left ear 5+
Back 4+ Chin 4+

$$\text{Bacteriological Index} = \frac{5+5+4+4}{4} = \frac{18}{4} = 4.5+$$

When the bacteriological Index is BI 1+ and BI 2+, at least 100 oil immersion fields should be examined. When the index is BI 3+, BI 4+, BI 5+ and BI 6+, at least 25 oil-immersion fields should be examined *(23)*.

Morphological index

During the course of microscopic examination of smears, it is possible to distinguish and count the number of solid staining organisms (organisms that stain completely) and irregularly staining bacilli. The MI is calculated after examining 200 pink–stained free standing (i.e. not in clumps) bacilli. The percentage of solid staining bacilli in a stained smear is referred to as morphological index (MI). The total of the MIs for all sites divided by the number of sites gives the average MI for the body. The criteria for calling the bacilli solid rods are *(20)* :

a. uniform staining of the entire organism
b. parallel sides
c. rounded ends, and
d. length 5 times that of the width.

It has been widely believed that only solid–staining organisms are viable. Accurate evaluation of the MI requires much skill and experience. It is a valuable indicator of the patient's response to treatment with drugs, during the first few months and helps to signal drug resistance.

Solid-fragmented-granular (SFG) percentage (23)

The procedure for recording the percentages of solid, fragmented and granular bacilli is basically the same as that used for determining the MI. Since percentages of solid, fragmented and granular bacilli are mentioned separately. SFG percentages give a better picture of the bacterial morphology than the MI, and are a more sensitive indicator of the patient's response to treatment.

3. FOOT-PAD CULTURE

The only certain way to identify *M. leprae* is to inoculate the material into the foot-pads of mice and demonstrate its multiplication. Mouse foot-pad inoculation is 10 times more sensitive at detecting *M. leprae* than are slit–skin smears *(24)*.

The drawback of this technique is that it is time consuming and requires 6 to 9 months before the results are obtained. Newer *In vitro* methods such as macrophage culture have been evolved, which take only 3 to 4 weeks to obtain results.

Mouse foot–pad technique has been successfully used for (i) detecting drug resistance (ii) evaluating the potency of anti-leprosy drugs, and (iii) detecting the viability of the bacilli during treatment.

4. HISTAMINE TEST

The histamine test is a very reliable method for detecting at an early stage peripheral nerve damage due to leprosy. The test is carried out by injecting intradermally 0.1 ml of a 1:1000 solution of histamine phosphate or chlorohydrate into hypopigmented patches or in areas of anaesthesia. In normal persons, it gives rise to a wheal surrounded by an erythematous flare within a few minutes (Lewis triple response). In cases of leprosy where the nerve supply is destroyed, flare response is lost. Histamine test is recommended when difficulty is experienced in the diagnosis, as for example, indeterminate leprosy *(25)*.

5. BIOPSY

When the examinations detailed above do not yield diagnosis, histopathological examination may be necessary. It allows a more accurate classification of the disease. It also gives information about the bacterial content of the skin.

6. IMMUNOLOGICAL TESTS

There are now available different kinds of immunological tests. These may be classified as *(26)* :

a. tests for detecting cell mediated immunity (CMI)
b. tests for humoral antibodies (serological tests).

a. TESTS FOR DETECTING CMI

(i) LEPROMIN TEST

The test is performed by injecting intradermally 0.1 ml of lepromin into the inner aspect of the forearm of the individual. As a routine, the reaction is read at 48 hours and 21 days *(7)*. Two types of positive reactions have been described :

(a) EARLY REACTION : The early reaction is also known as Fernandez reaction. An inflammatory response develops within 24 to 48 hours and this tends to disappear after 3 to 4 days. It is evidenced by redness and induration at the site of inoculation. If the diameter of the *red area* is more than 10 mm at the end of 48 hours, the test is considered positive.

The early positive reaction indicates whether or not a person has been previously sensitized by exposure to and infection by the leprosy bacilli. In this sense, the early reaction is much superior to the late reaction. The early reaction has been described as delayed hypersensitivity reaction to "soluble" constituents of the leprosy bacilli. The reaction corresponds to the Mantoux reaction in tuberculosis, caused by the soluble antigens (PPD) of the tubercle bacilli.

(b) LATE REACTION : This is the classical Mitsuda reaction. The reaction develops late, becomes apparent in 7–10 days following the injection and reaching its maximum in 3 or 4 weeks. The test is read at 21 days. At the end of 21 days, if there is a *nodule* more than 5 mm in diameter at the site of inoculation, the reaction is said to be positive. The nodule may even ulcerate and heal with scarring if the antigen is crude.

It may be noted that the diameter of the *red area* in the early reaction, and the diameter of the *nodule* in the late reaction are measured. The early reaction is induced by the soluble constituents of the leprosy bacilli; and the late reaction by the bacillary component of the antigen. It indicates cell–mediated immunity.

In the first 6 months of life, most children are lepromin negative; some may become positive by the end of first year. Data obtained from different parts of the world indicate that in endemic areas, lepromin reaction is already positive in 20 per cent of children under 5 years of age, and this proportion increases to around 60 per cent or more in the 10–14 years age group, and to 80 per cent or more in persons over 19 years of age *(27)*. BCG vaccination is capable of converting the lepra reaction from negative to positive in a large proportion of individuals.

Value of the lepromin test

Lepromin test is not a diagnostic test. The two drawbacks that stand in the way of this test being used for diagnosis are : (i) positive results in non-cases, and (ii) negative results in lepromatous and near–lepromatous cases *(13)*.

The test has been generally accepted as a useful tool in evaluating the immune status (CMI) of leprosy patients. It is of considerable value in confirming the results of classification of cases of leprosy on clinical and bacteriological grounds. In other words, the test is widely used as an aid to classify the type of disease.

The test is also of great value in estimating the *prognosis* in cases of leprosy of all types. The test is usually strongly positive in the typical tuberculoid cases, and the positivity getting weaker as one passes through the spectrum to the lepromatous end, the typical lepromatous cases being lepromin negative indicating a failure of CMI. It is known that lepromin negative individuals are at a higher risk of developing progressive multibacillary leprosy, but those who are lepromin positive either escape the clinical disease (the majority) or develop paucibacillary disease (the minority).

(ii) LTT and LMIT

In recent years, newer *In vitro* tests such as lymphocyte transformation test (LTT) and leucocyte migration inhibition test (LMIT) have been developed. They give a measure of the cell mediated immunity. These tests have been used to detect subclinical infection. A disadvantage of these highly sophisticated tests is that they cannot be applied on a mass scale under field conditions *(28)*.

b. TESTS FOR HUMORAL RESPONSES TO M. LEPRAE

Probably the most important recent advance in the study of the epidemiology of leprosy is the development of serological tests. These tests are expected to have value in detecting subclinical infections, preclinical manifestations and follow-up efficacy of drug treatment. These tests include :

(i) FLA–ABS test

The Fluorescent Leprosy Antibody Absorption Test is now widely used for identification of subclinical infection.

Studies revealed that FLA–ABS test is 92.3 per cent sensitive and 100 per cent specific in detecting *M. leprae* specific antibodies in all types of leprosy irrespective of the type and duration of the disease *(29)*.

(ii) Monoclonal antibodies

Monoclonal antibodies against *M. leprae* antigens have been produced. It has been shown that these antibodies recognize specific and non-specific epitopes of *M. leprae* antigens. If antibodies against specific antigens are found, they will become reagents of choice for identifying *M. leprae*. An antibody competition test (SACT) based on this approach has been found to be quite sensitive for detection of *M.leprae* antibody *(30)*.

(iii) Others

There are numerous other sensitive tests which include the radio-immune assay and ELISA tests. The ELISA test is based on a phenolic glycolipid (PGL) antigen.

For the present, the only practical approach is to use FLA–ABS test till some other more sensitive and specific tests are available for use on a large scale *(31)*.

LEPROSY CONTROL

The introduction of multidrug therapy has infused a new hope that the disease could be brought under effective control in the not too distant future. A revised strategy of leprosy control has emerged based on multidrug therapy. The following elements are considered as a minimum requirement for all leprosy control programmes :

1. *Medical measures*
    - I. estimation of the problem
    - II. early case detection
    - III. multidrug therapy
    - IV. surveillance
    - V. immunoprophylaxis
    - VI. chemoprophylaxis
    - VII. deformities
    - VIII. rehabilitation
    - IX. health education
2. *Social support*
3. *Programme management*
4. *Evaluation*

The three main goals of leprosy control are *(7)* : (a) to interrupt transmission of the infection, thereby reduce the incidence of the disease so that it no longer constitutes a public health problem; (b) to treat patients in order to achieve their cure and where possible, complete rehabilitation; and (c) to prevent the development of associated deformities. Ultimate prevention is achieved by breaking the chain of transmission.

1. MEDICAL MEASURES

I. Estimation of the problem

The first step in a leprosy control programme is to define the size of the problem or disease load in the community by means of epidemiological surveys. Random sample surveys are good enough to collect baseline data. The survey should bring out not merely the prevalence of leprosy, but also the age and sex distribution of cases, the various forms of leprosy and the facilities available for providing the needed health care. A rough estimate of the prevalence can be determined by examining all school-age children; the total prevalence will be about 4 times the number of cases found *(26)*. Estimates of the prevalence of leprosy are essential for planning and implementing an anti-leprosy programme and also for evaluating the results of the programme.

II. Early case detection

The aim of case detection is to identify and to register all cases of leprosy as soon as possible after they become evident *(6)*. Ideally, patients should seek medical care voluntarily. However, because leprosy is frequently symptomless in the early stages, patients do not know they have the disease. By the time patient becomes aware of the disease and reports voluntarily, there is usually a lag period of 2 to 3 years *(32)*. Because of the social stigma, some patients are afraid to disclose themselves. It is, therefore, necessary to devise active methods of case detection *(7)*. Even in countries, with a satisfactory case-finding programme, new cases could still be found *(9)*. The current trend is to involve the primary health care workers (village health guides, multipurpose workers) in case detection with the active participation of the community *(9)*. These workers need to be adequately trained to make a tentative diagnosis of leprosy. The desirability of confirming the diagnosis by laboratory methods is not mandatory. It is important that criteria for identifying cases are valid, unambiguous and reproducible as far as possible. If data are to be compared between different areas and different times, it is important that diagnostic criteria used for leprosy around the world is standardized.

Case-finding methods : The choice of case-finding methods should be related to the prevalence rate of leprosy in the region : (a) CONTACT SURVEY : In areas where the prevalence of leprosy is generally low, (less than 1 case per 1000 population), the technique of choice is examination of all contacts (e.g., household contacts, especially children and persons reported to be suspected cases). These examinations will have to be arranged with discretion so as not to cause alarm. (b) GROUP SURVEYS : When the prevalence is about 1 per 1000 or higher, additional case finding methods should be employed such as screening of preschool and school children, people living in slums, military recruits, industrial labour and other selected groups for all types of skin diseases; this technique ("skin camps") may bring out additional cases of leprosy. It should be noted that the value of school surveys as a case finding method will be considerably diminished if the school enrolment is less than 70 per cent of all children in the 6–14 years age group *(11)*. (c) MASS SURVEYS : Total population surveys for examination of each and every individual, family by family by house-to-house visits are recommended only in hyperendemic areas, i.e., areas where the prevalence of leprosy is about 10 or more per 1000 population. In mass surveys, a coverage of not less than 95 per cent of the population should be obtained *(9)*. Mass surveys require high quality team work. They should be multipurpose covering not only leprosy but also possibly other diseases. They should have the full backing of the administration and whole-hearted participation of the local community.

Records : The case information should be collected for all patients in a standardized manner. The WHO has already a standard computer-based proforma for data collection from individual patients (see Annex 3 of WHO Expert Committee Report No. 716, page 58) which should be followed or suitably adapted. The Government of India had also approved a set of forms for keeping records and submitting reports.

Leprosy is an "iceberg" disease. The problem is one of discovering the subclinical cases, as considerable proportion of these cases lie outside the scope of existing case detection technology.

III. Multidrug therapy

In the absence of primary prevention by a leprosy vaccine, the strategy of leprosy control is based on effective chemotherapy (secondary prevention). Till recently, chemotherapy of leprosy has relied almost entirely on dapsone (DDS). Due to dependence on dapsone monotherapy for many years, drug-resistant leprosy bacilli (both primary and secondary resistance) have emerged in all parts of the world. This has led to relapse of the disease even in those in whom the disease had been arrested and the spread of dapsone-resistant strains to susceptibles jeopardizing the whole strategy of leprosy control *(33)*. In order to cope with this problem, a WHO Study Group on Chemotherapy of Leprosy, has recommended multiple drug therapy for both multibacillary and paucibacillary leprosy *(33)*.

OBJECTIVES

The main objectives of multidrug chemotherapy of leprosy are *(33)*

a. to interrupt transmission of the infection in the community by sterilizing infectious patients as rapidly as possible with bactericidal drugs;
b. to ensure early detection and treatment of cases to prevent deformities, and
c. to prevent drug resistance.

The multidrug treatment has the additional advantage of curtailing the duration of treatment of leprosy considerably. Shorter therapy has the added advantages of patient compliance, cost-effectiveness and decreased work load.

DEFINITIONS

Following the introduction of multidrug therapy, some changes in terminology have taken place. The following working definitions have been proposed by WHO *(6)*.

(i) Case of leprosy : A "case" of leprosy is a person showing clinical signs of leprosy with or without bacteriological confirmation of the diagnosis, and who has not yet completed a full course of treatment with MDT. This definition is for estimating the prevalence of leprosy.

(ii) Paucibacillary leprosy : A person having 1–5 skin lesions and/or only one nerve involvement *(34)*.

(iii) Multibacillary leprosy : A person having 6 or more skin lesions and/or more than one nerve involvement *(34)*.

(iv) Adequate treatment : Adequate treatment implies the completion of a regimen of multidrug therapy within a reasonably short period of time : (a) for paucibacillary cases, adequate treatment implies that the patient has received 6 monthly doses of combined therapy within 9 months. (b) for multibacillary cases, adequate treatment implies that the patient has received 12 monthly doses of combined therapy within 18 months.

(v) Regular treatment : A patient may be considered to have had regular treatment if he or she has received MDT for at least two-thirds of the months in any interval of time. For example, regular treatment for 12 months, implies that the patient has had at least 8 full months of combined therapy during that 12–month period.

(vi) Newly diagnosed case : A person who has been diagnosed as a leprosy case, and who has not taken MDT in the past.

(vii) Defaulter case : A defaulter is a leprosy patient on MDT, who has not collected treatment for 12 consecutive months.

Any patient who has been categorized as a defaulter should be removed from the register *(36)*.

(viii) Relapsed case : A patient whose therapy was terminated, having successfully completed an adequate course of multidrug therapy, but who subsequently develops new signs and symptoms of the disease, either during the surveillance period or thereafter, is considered to have "relapsed" *(6)*.

Drugs

In multidrug regimens, only bactericidal drugs are used. At present, only a small number of such drugs are available : these are rifampicin, dapsone, clofazimine, ethionamide and protionamide. A brief account of these drugs is given below :

(a) Rifampicin

Rifampicin (RMP) is the only drug that is highly bactericidal against *M. leprae*. A single dose of 1500 mg or 3–4 consecutive daily doses of 600 mg appear to kill 99 per cent of viable organisms *(35)*. Further the drug is effective when given at monthly intervals, which is a big advantage. The drug is expensive but safe.

The toxic effects of RMP are anorexia, nausea, abdominal pain and occasionally vomiting. It is hepatotoxic. The patient should be kept under supervision for 1 hour, after the administration of the drug since shock and collapse are known to occur.

RMP is now an essential drug in the chemotherapy of leprosy. Given alone, resistance to the drug develops. Hence it is given in combination with other anti-leprosy drugs.

(b) Dapsone

Dapsone (DDS) has been in use all over the world for the control of leprosy for more than 30 years. It continues to be an important drug in the multidrug chemotherapy of leprosy. It is cheap and effective in the dosage employed (1–2 mg/kg of body weight). When given orally, it is completely absorbed from the gut and fairly well tolerated. It has shown to be weak bactericidal against *M. leprae (37)*.

The common adverse effects following DDS administration are haemolytic anaemia, methaemoglobinaemia, agranulocytosis, hepatitis, peripheral neuropathy, psychosis and lepra reaction. A rare syndrome, known as *DDS–syndrome* consisting of fever, enlarged lymph glands, exfoliative dermatitis, hepatitis and maculopapular rash has also been reported. Since dapsone is a haemolytic drug, care should be taken that the haemoglobin level is not less than 60 per cent, and the dosage of DDS is strictly weight-based. Iron tablets are prescribed routinely to correct anaemia.

(c) Clofazimine

Clofazimine (CLF) was originally synthesized for the treatment of tuberculosis, but was subsequently found to have far greater value in leprosy. It has both anti–leprosy and anti–inflammatory properties. CLF though less effective than dapsone has the added advantage in suppressing and preventing reactions. CLF is relatively expensive and is reasonably free from toxic effects in the usual dosage. It is used as the third drug, whenever possible in leprosy chemotherapy.

Clofazimine may be unacceptable to some patients because it may give rise to darkish red coloration to skin, mucous membranes, urine and sweat. These symptoms are not serious. They would disappear after the drug is stopped. If totally unacceptable, it may be replaced by ethionamide or protionamide.

(d) Ethionamide and protionamide

These are bactericidal drugs killing 98 per cent of viable bacilli in 4 to 5 days. They are virtually interchangeable and gives rise to cross-resistance with each other. They are both more expensive and more toxic than dapsone. The WHO *(30)* has recommended that ethionamide or protionamide should be used as the third drug in the treatment of multibacillary leprosy in those patients, who find clofazimine unacceptable.

(e) Quinolones

These drugs work by inhibiting DNA synthesis during bacterial replication. Ofloxacin, a fluorinated quinolone is the most preferred drug in this group. Oral ofloxacin is 98 per cent bioavailable with elimination half-life of about 5 to 8 hours. 22 doses of ofloxacin kill about 99.9 per cent of viable *M. leprae (38)*. This is the basis of very short term clinical trials of a combination of 400 mg ofloxacin and 600 mg rifampicin daily for 28 days.

Side-effects include nausea, diarrhoea and other gastrointestinal complaints and a variety of central nervous system complaints.

(f) Minocycline

This is the most lipid–soluble of the tetracyclines and inhibits bacterial protein synthesis. In clinical trials, the clearance of viable *M. leprae* from the skin by minocycline was faster than that reported from dapsone or clofazimine and similar to that for ofloxacin. Minocycline may strengthen MDT, for multibacillary patients and thereby shorten the duration of treatment needed to treat leprosy effectively *(33)*. The standard dose is 100 mg daily. The side-effects include discoloration of teeth in infants and children, occasional pigmentation of the skin and mucous membrane, various gastrointestinal symptoms and central nervous system complaints. It should not be given to infants, children and during pregnancy *(22)*.

(g) Clarithromycin

Clarithromycin is a member of the macrolid group of antibiotics and displays a significant bactericidal activity against *M. leprae*. In patients with lepromatous leprosy, daily administration of 500 mg of clarithromycin killed 99 per cent of viable *M. leprae* within 28 days, and 99.9 per cent by 56 days. Side-effects include nausea, vomiting and diarrhoea.

RECOMMENDED REGIMENS OF CHEMOTHERAPY

The proper application of multidrug therapy is crucial to the success of leprosy control. The regimens recommended by WHO have been widely accepted in many countries. They are as below *(12)*.

a. Multibacillary leprosy

The WHO has recommended the following combination of drugs for treatment of adult multibacillary cases of leprosy :

- Rifampicin ..... 600 mg, once monthly, given under supervision
- Dapsone ..... 100 mg daily, self–administered
- Clofazimine ..... 300 mg once monthly supervised; and 50 mg daily, self–administered.

Where clofazimine is totally unacceptable owing to the colouration of skin, its replacement by 250 to 375 mg self–administered daily doses of ethionamide or protionamide has been suggested.

b. Paucibacillary leprosy

Paucibacillary cases should also receive combined therapy in view of primary dapsone resistance which is becoming widespread. The recommended standard regimen for adults is :

- Rifampicin ..... 600 mg once a month, supervised
- Dapsone ..... 100 mg (1–2 mg/kg of body weight) daily, self–administered

The standard treatment regimen for children aged 10–14 years is as follows :

a. Multibacillary leprosy

- Rifampicin ..... 450 mg once a month, given under supervision
- Dapsone ..... 50 mg daily, self administered
- Clofazimine ..... 150 mg once a month supervised; and 50 mg every other day.

b. Paucibacillary leprosy

- Rifampicin ..... 450 mg once a month, supervised
- Dapsone ..... 50 mg daily, self administered

Children under the age of 10 years should receive appropriately reduced doses of the above drugs.

Duration of treatment

The treatment duration varies according to the type of disease. The recommendations are as follows :

Multibacillary leprosy – MB blisterpacks for 12 months, within 18 months

Paucibacillary leprosy – PB blisterpacks for 6 months, within 9 months

A defaulter who returns to the health centre for treatment should be given a new course of MDT when he or she shows one or more of the following signs *(36)*:

- reddish and/or raised skin lesions;
- appearance of new skin lesions (since the previous examination);

- new nerve involvement (e.g. changes in skin sensation) since the previous examination;
- lepromatous nodules;
- signs of reversal reaction or ENL.

For registration purposes, returning defaulters are not considered as newly detected cases.

MDT is not contraindicated in patients with HIV infection. Management of leprosy and of lepra reactions is same as that of any other leprosy patient. The response of such patients to MDT is also similar *(36)*.

Since leprosy is exacerbated during pregnancy, it is important that MDT be continued. The evidence so far indicates that MDT is safe during pregnancy. Small quantities of anti-leprosy drugs are excreted through breast milk, but there is no report of adverse reaction as a result of this, except for mild discolouration of the infant's skin caused by clofazimine *(39)*.

Lepra reaction *(40)*

During the course of leprosy, immunologically mediated episodes of acute or subacute inflammation known as reactions may occur. Because peripheral nerve trunks are often involved, unless reactions are promptly and adequately treated, such episodes can result in permanent deformities.

Lepra reactions are usually diagnosed by clinical examination only. Inflammatory changes in skin lesions or appearance of new lesions, patches or nodules with acute onset, draw the attention of patient to report. Some cases develop signs of nerve damage without changes in skin lesions.

There are two types of reaction : Reversal reaction (or Type 1) and Erythema Nodosum Leprosum (ENL or Type 2). Both types can occur before the start of multi-drug treatment, during treatment, or after treatment has been completed. Both types can be mild or severe. Only severe reactions are treated with corticosteroids.

Distinguishing between the two types of reactions is usually not difficult. In a reversal reaction, the leprosy skin lesions themselves become inflamed, red and swollen. In an ENL reaction, new inflamed, red nodules (about 1–2 cm across) appear under the skin of the limbs or trunk, while the original leprosy skin patches remain as they were. In addition, ENL reactions cause a general feeling of fever and malaise, while reversal reactions cause less systemic upset. Common differentiating features are as shown in Table 1.

Because of the high risk of permanent damage to the peripheral nerve trunks, reversal reaction needs to be diagnosed as soon as possible, and treated adequately. The drug of choice is prednisolone, the cheapest and most widely available corticosteroid.

Most reversal reactions and neuritis can be treated successfully under field conditions, with a standard 12–week course of prednisolone. The potential risk of serious adverse effects caused by long-term corticosteroid therapy must not be ignored, particularly under field conditions. The more common problems of prolonged steroid therapy include weight gain, peptic ulcer, diabetes, hypertension, reactivation of tuberculosis, osteoporosis and psychiatric disorders.

ENL varies in severity, duration and organ involvement. Acute or subacute neuritis, with or without loss of nerve function, is one of the major criteria in distinguishing mild and severe ENL. Mild ENL can be treated with analgesic or antipyretic drugs such as aspirin, while severe ENL can be treated with prednisolone, as for reversal reaction.

Clofazimine is also effective for ENL, but is less potent than cortico-steroids and often takes 4–6 weeks to develop its full effects, so it should never be started as the sole agent for the treatment of severe ENL.

Signs of a severe reversal reaction

If any of the following signs are found, the reaction should be treated as severe :

- Loss of nerve function – that is, loss of sensation or muscle weakness in the area supplied by nerve.
- Pain or tenderness in one or more nerves.
- Silent neuritis/quiet nerve paralysis i.e. signs of nerve damage without symptoms.
- A red, swollen skin patch on the face, or overlying another major nerve trunk.
- A skin lesion anywhere that becomes ulcerated.
- Marked oedema of the hands, feet or face.

TABLE 1

Difference between reversal reaction and ENL

Type I (Reversal Reaction)	Type II (ENL)
1. Delayed hypersensitivity.	1. Antigen antibody reaction.
2. Occurs in both PB and MB cases in unstable types like BT.BB.BL.	2. Seen in MB cases only (BL and LL type).
3. Skin lesions suddenly become reddish, swollen, warm, painful, and tender. New lesions may appear.	3. Red, painful, tender, sub-cutaneous nodules – ENL may appear, commonly on face, arms, legs, bilaterally symmetrical. They appear in crops and subside within few days even without treatment (Evanescent skin nodules). Nodules are better felt than seen and these are recurrent (episodic).
4. Nerves close to skin may be enlarged, tender and painful (neuritis) with loss of its functions (loss of sensory, motor or autonomic) which may appear suddenly.	4. Nerves may be affected but not as common or severe and acute as in Type I.
5. Other organs – not affected.	5. Other organs like eyes, testis, and kidney may be affected.
6. General symptoms – not common.	6. Fever, joints pain, red eyes with watering may be associated.
7. Eye-Lagophthalmos and corneal anaesthesia due to neuritis.	7. Iritis/iridocyclitis

Source : *(12, 40)*

Signs of a severe ENL reaction

If any of the following signs is found, the reaction should be treated as severe :

- Pain or tenderness in one or more nerves, with or without loss of nerve function.
- Ulceration of ENL nodules.
- Pain of eyes with or without redness and loss of visual acuity.
- Painful swelling of the testes (orchitis) or of the fingers (dactylitis).
- Marked arthritis or lymphadenitis.

Treatment of Lepra reactions (moderate to severe cases)

It includes bed rest, rest to affected nerves by splint, analgesics, prednisolone. Each case of reaction should be assessed for his/her fitness to put on prednisolone as per check list given above *(12, 40)*.

Prednisolone regimen	Add Clofazimine in ENL
40 mg daily for first 2 weeks 30 mg daily for weeks 3 and 4	One capsule (100 mg) 3 times a day × 4 weeks
20 mg daily for weeks 5 and 6 15 mg daily for weeks 7 and 8	One capsule (100 mg) 2 times a day × next 4 weeks
10 mg daily for weeks 9 and 10 5 mg daily for weeks 11 and 12	One capsule (100 mg) once a day × third month
For neuritis, treatment with Prednisolone should be prolonged to four weeks from 20 mg onwards	

Prednisolone tablets issued must be entered in 'Prednisolone card'. Tapering of prednisolone may be done according to its response. Patient must be instructed on salt restriction, no prednisolone intake on empty stomach and reporting adverse effects/symptoms immediately.

Adding Clofazimine for Type II reaction may be extremely useful for reducing or withdrawing corticosteroids in patients who have become dependent on them. Total duration of Clofazimine therapy should not exceed 12 months.

If a patient develops lepra reaction during the treatment, do not stop MDT (rather complete the course of MDT). Lepra reactions, which occur after completion of treatment, should also be managed as mentioned earlier. MDT should not be restarted for such cases. Response to treatment should be monitored and assessed, including check on adverse effects of prednisolone.

Before starting the steroid treatment, the patient should be asked questions about epigastric pain and diarrhoea, with or without blood and or mucous; and examined for fungal infection, scabies, and worm infestations, as all these conditions may be made worse by steroids. Treatment of all these conditions can be started at the same time as steroids are started *(40)*.

Before starting the steroid treatment the patient should be explained the reason for treatment; the duration of the treatment; importance of taking daily dose and that the treatment should not be stopped suddenly (the dosage is decreased gradually) and importance of completing the full course of treatment; and possible side-effects.

Follow-up after treatment with steroids

People who have been given a course of steroids for reaction or nerve damage should be followed up closely because of the risk of recurrence. Each person must understand that a reaction or new nerve damage may recur. They must know how to recognize the early signs of nerve damage and be aware of how important it is to return promptly to the clinic for treatment. These signs include pain or tingling sensations, further loss of feeling or loss of muscle strength and inability to close the eye.

Patients still on MDT should have their nerve function checked monthly by the health worker when they come to collect their treatment. Any deterioration should be noted and the person referred. Patients who have already completed MDT, by the time they come to the end of a course of steroids, should be asked to come back three months and six months after the end of the course for review and nerve function assessment. Patients who still have lagophthalmos (weakness of eyelids) after completion of treatment with steroids should be referred to ophthalmic surgeon.

Groups requiring special precautions when prescribing steroids

The following groups of people require special precautions when steroids are prescribed. One must not give steroids to people with tuberculosis, diabetes, deep ulcers, osteomyelitis, corneal ulcers or other serious conditions without starting treatment for the underlying condition.

Pregnant women

All pregnant women should be treated at referral level, so as to minimize the steroid dose they are given and thus avoid harmful effects, such as growth retardation on the foetus. If steroids are given in the third trimester, this may cause adrenal suppression in the newborn infant. Ideally, such infants should be monitored in a referral centre for a few days after birth. The dose of prednisolone to be given during pregnancy are as follows :

- PB cases : start at 30 mg daily instead of 40 mg and limit the course to ten weeks rather than the usual twelve weeks regime.
- MB cases : starting at 30 mg daily but lasting for twenty weeks.

Children

All children under the age of twelve should be treated at referral level, so as to minimize the effects of steroids on their growth. Children can be given a course similar to that for pregnant women, but the starting dose of prednisolone should not exceed 1 mg per kilogram of body weight per day. Giving children steroids on alternate days may reduce the effect on their growth. A suitable regimen for PB cases would be 30 mg of prednisolone daily for two weeks, then 30 mg on alternate days for two weeks with a gradually reducing dose over the total course of ten weeks. For MB cases, one should double the duration of each stage of the course.

Diabetes

Patients who show symptoms that suggest diabetes or whose urine tests positive for glucose should be referred to confirm whether the diagnosis is correct and, if it is confirmed, for management of the diabetes condition. Steroids may increase the diabetic's requirement for insulin.

A person taking steroids may also develop diabetes for the first time. This possibility must be considered when patient develops typical symptoms of diabetes during the treatment with steroids. The condition usually resolves itself when steroids are stopped.

Ulcers or osteomyelitis

Patients with deep or dirty ulcers or osteomyelitis should be referred for surgical treatment and antibiotics. Starting steroids before such treatment may lead to a worsening of the sepsis and more permanent damage, including the need for amputation. One should suspect osteomyelitis if the person's hand or foot is warmer than normal, with or without swelling. Any person with a wound discharging pus should be referred for surgical advice and debridement (removal of dead and infected tissue) before taking steroids, or osteomyelitis may develop.

Eye involvement

Patients who have corneal damage or iritis should be referred for specialist diagnosis and management at a centre properly equipped for eye care. Corneal ulcers and keratitis are inflammatory conditions of the cornea. They are often caused by exposure, as a result of the person being unable to close the eye properly. Steroids, whether taken by mouth or locally applied, may make these conditions worse. Iritis, uveitis, iridocyclitis and scleritis are all types of inflammation inside the eye and they can all occur as part of a Type-2 reaction. These conditions cause pain, redness, photophobia and loss of vision, although the symptoms are not always severe. The treatment includes atropine eye ointment to prevent adhesion.

Tuberculosis

If tuberculosis is suspected, the diagnosis must be confirmed and treatment started before giving steroids.

The crucial elements in the management of leprosy reactions and thereby, the prevention of disabilities are early diagnosis of reactions together with prompt and adequate treatment. Usually the diagnosis of leprosy reactions is relatively straightforward, but occasionally, in paucibacillary patients who have completed treatment, differentiation of a reversal reaction from relapse may be difficult. Nevertheless, it is essential that this distinction must be made correctly. The differences are as summarized in Table 2.

As a consequence of all these factors, the diagnosis and treatment of leprosy reactions may often be delayed and, by the time the patients arrive at the referral centres, they may have already developed permanent deformities. In order to avoid these problems, national leprosy programmes should try to ensure that patients are taught to recognize the early signs of reactions, and to report promptly for treatment; health workers are able to diagnose and treat reactions and to refer patients when necessary; and adequate stocks of prednisolone are maintained at the peripheral level *(22)*.

IV. Surveillance

Clinical surveillance of cases after completion of treatment is an important part of the current recommendations for multidrug therapy; it is essential for the assurance of long-term success of treatment and for the early detection of any relapses.

(a) Paucibacillary leprosy : It is recommended that paucibacillary cases be examined clinically at least once a year for a minimum of 2 years after completion of treatment *(6)*.

(b) Multibacillary leprosy : It is recommended that multibacillary cases be examined clinically at least once a year for a minimum period of 5 years after completion of therapy *(8)*.

A patient who has completed the required period of surveillance following the course of multidrug therapy and shows no evidence of relapse is considered to have completed surveillance. The phrase "release from control" should not be applied in the context of multidrug therapy *(6)*.

V. Immunoprophylaxis

The fact that a scientifically valid tool for the detection of infection is not yet available which could deepen the understanding of how leprosy is transmitted, and could lead to the development of an effective vaccine and other interventions. Trials in different population groups with BCG vaccine either alone or in combination with other vaccine (from killed *Mycobacterium leprae* or atypical *Mycobacteria*), have shown protective efficacy ranging between 28 per cent and 60 per cent. High BCG coverage remains an important contribution to reducing the disease burden due to leprosy *(41)*.

VI. Chemoprophylaxis

Chemoprophylaxis in chronic infectious diseases has an established benefit, particularly when given to persons who are known to be at higher risk of developing the disease. The

TABLE 2
Differences between reversal reaction and relapse

	Reversal reaction	Relapse
Time interval	Generally occurs during chemotherapy or within 3 years of stopping treatment	Usually occurs only when chemotherapy has been discontinued, after an interval of usually more than 3 years
Onset	Abrupt and sudden	Slow and insidious
Old lesions	Existing lesions become oedematous, erythematous or tender	Lesion may show erythema and infiltration, but no tenderness
New lesions	Several new lesions appear	New lesions are minimal
Ulceration	Lesions may ulcerate	Ulceration does not occur
Nerve involvement	Multiple nerve involvement common, painful and tender	Nerve involvement may occur only in a single nerve; usually no pain or tenderness
General condition	May have fever, joint pains, malaise	Not usually affected
Response to steroid treatment	Rapid	Nil

Source : *(24, 41)*

immediate contacts of a case of leprosy, especially multibacillary, are known to have a higher risk of developing the disease than compared to the general population. It is important, therefore, to consider possible interventions to prevent the occurrence of leprosy among household contacts. However, there must be robust trial evidence to demonstrate that the drug/s used for chemoprophylaxis are safe, effective and cost-efficient in terms of the number of new cases prevented.

On account of lack of consistent results from various studies using various drugs (dapsone, acedapsone, rifampicin) it is too premature to advise chemoprophylaxis as a public health measure. Further research is needed to use this as a routine tool to prevent the occurrence of disease among contacts *(41)*.

VII. Disability

It is estimated that approximately 25 per cent of the patients who are not treated at an early stage of disease develop anaesthesia and/or deformities of the hands and feet. As a single disease entity, leprosy is one of the foremost causes of deformities and crippling.

The deformities may result due to the disease process (e.g. loss of eye brows, other facial deformities), or those resulting from paralysis of some muslces due to damage to peripheral nerve trunk (e.g. claw-hand, foot-drop, lagophthalmos), or those resulting from injuries or infections to hands and feet (e.g. scar contractures of fingers, mutilation of hands and feet, corneal ulceration). Fig. 3 shows the process of disability in hands, feet and eyes.

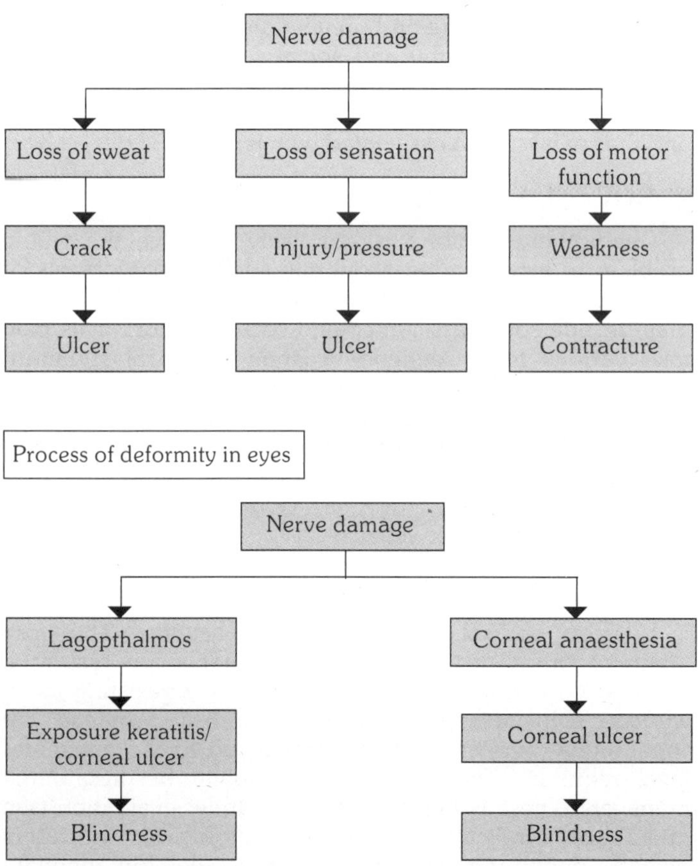

FIG. 3
Process of deformity in hands, feet and eyes
Source : *(12)*

Patients at high risk of developing disability :

People with the following features are more likely to develop lepra reaction and neuritis compared to others and thus subjected to developing disability -

- Multi-bacillary leprosy
- Past or present thickened/painful/tender nerve trunk
- Skin lesion on face
- Adolescents, pregnancy, old age
- Any inter-current infection

Stages of involvement of nerve

Stage I : *Stage of nerve involvement* – Nerves become swollen (thickened) due to inflammatory response and tender, but no loss of function. This condition is reversible if action is taken early.

Stage II : *Stage of nerve damage* – Along with thickened and painful peripheral nerves, associated with loss of function (loss of autonomic, sensory and motor functions). This condition is reversible if suitable action is taken early preferably within 6 months.

Stage III : *Stage of nerve destruction* – In long standing case of nerve involvement (usually more than one year) nerve may become fibrosed, thin and atrophic. Involved nerve is completely destroyed and its function cannot be recovered to any useful degree.

There are two types of disabilities in leprosy :

1. *Primary* : These disabilities occur as a result of nerve damage – e.g. loss of sensation, paralysis, dryness
2. *Secondary* : These occur as a result of neglected primary disability – e.g. ulcer, contracture.

A **disability** is defined as lack of ability to perform an activity.

A **deformity** is a visible consequence of an impairment inside the body.

The findings of the examination are first noted in the Disability Assessment Form separately for right and left eyes, hands and feet. Thereafter each eye, each hand and each foot is given its own grade. Deformities are classified into three grades. The criterias are as follows *(12, 42)* :

Examination of parts	WHO Disability Grades	Sensory testing	Voluntary muscle testing	
Hands	0	Sensation present	Muscle power normal	
	1	Sensation absent	Muscle power normal	
	2	Sensation absent	Muscle power weak or paralyzed	
Feet	0	Sensation present	Muscle power normal	
	1	Sensation absent	Muscle power normal	
	2	Sensation absent	Muscle power weak or paralyzed	
Eye		Vision	Lid Gap	Blinking
	0	Normal	No lid gap	Present
	2	Cannot count fingers at 6 metres	Gap present/ red eye/ corneal ulcer or opacity	Absent

The highest grade given in any of the part is used as the Disability Grade for that patient. Eye, hand and feet score i.e. sum of all the individual disability grades for two eyes, two hands and two feet 0–12, should be recorded at each examination.

Table 3 shows deformities occurring in patients with leprosy.

TABLE 3
Deformities occurring in leprosy

Face	Mask face, facies leonina, sagging face, lagophthalmos, loss of eyebrows (superciliary madarosis) and eyelashes (ciliary madarosis), corneal ulcers and opacities, perforated nose, depressed nose, ear deformities, e.g. nodules on the ear and elongated lobules.
Hands	Claw hand, wrist–drop, ulcers, absorption of digits, thumb–web contracture, hollowing of the interosseous spaces and swollen hand.
Feet	Plantar ulcers, foot–drop, inversion of the foot, clawing of the toes, absorption of the toes, collapsed foot, swollen foot and callosities.
Other deformities	Gynaecomastia and perforation of the palate.

Source : *(21, 23)*

The measures to prevent disabilities include actions to take care of the dry, denervated skin of palms and soles, heal the wounds, ulcers and skin cracks in palms and soles, prevent injuries to hands and feet by using protective gloves and footwear, prevent joint stiffness in cases of paralytic deformities, protect the eyes, and assess periodically the commonly damaged nerves for loss of nerve function and its progression, using simple tests that can be carried out in the field.

Improvement of disabilities is achieved through the use of prostheses and orthopaedic devices, including corrective splints, as well as by corrective surgery. All these measures, however, require special expertise and facilities.

VIII. Rehabilitation

The WHO Expert Committee on Leprosy in its Second Report *(43)* defined rehabilitation as :

> *"the physical and mental restoration, as far as possible, of all treated patients to normal activity, so that they may be able to resume their place in the home, society and industry".*

Rehabilitation is, therefore, an integral part of leprosy control. It must begin as soon as the disease is diagnosed. The cheapest and surest rehabilitation is to prevent physical deformities and social and vocational disruption by early diagnosis and adequate treatment. The measures that are taken in this direction are known as "preventive rehabilitation". The approach to rehabilitation should, therefore, begin with preventing dehabilitation. We should never allow dehabilitation to take place and afterwards take up the uphill task of rehabilitation *(44)*.

Community-based rehabilitation defined by WHO and major NGOs is as follows (41) :

"Community-based rehabilitation is a strategy within general community development for the rehabilitation, equalization of opportunities and social inclusion of all people with disabilities. Community-based rehabilitation is implemented through the combined efforts of the people with disabilities themselves, their families, organizations and communities, and the relevant governmental and non-governmental health, education, vocational, social and other services".

Rehabilitation measures may appear to be simple; they require planned and systematic actions – medical, surgical, social, educational and vocational – consistently over years with sustained counselling and health education for training or retraining of the individual to the highest possible level of functional ability. For this purpose, coordinated efforts by the Departments of Health, Education and Social Welfare, as well as voluntary organizations are necessary.

IX. Health education

No anti-leprosy campaign is complete without health education. Health education aims at helping people develop attitudes and behaviour by their own actions and efforts and seeking professional help when needed. Health education should be directed towards the patient and his family and the general public. *(a) Patient and his family :* The main problem in leprosy control is poor patient compliance with the drug regimen and high drop-out rates. The patient and his family should be educated about the need for regular treatment, repeated examination of contacts, self care regarding prevention of disabilities and protection of children. Health education thus minimizes hurdles in implementing the leprosy control programme. *(b) General public :* There is a growing realization that technological advances alone cannot solve the leprosy problem, unless we succeed in involving the people in the control programme. Health education aims at ensuring community participation. The public should be made aware that leprosy is not a hereditary disease; it is a bacterial disease like tuberculosis; it is curable; not all leprosy patients are infectious; regular and adequate treatment is essential to obtain cure and prevent disabilities, and that the patient needs sympathy and social support. A nationwide mass education is needed to educate people on the true facts about leprosy and remove superstitions and wrong beliefs and the social stigma associated with leprosy *(32)*.

2. SOCIAL SUPPORT

Chemotherapy alone is not likely to solve the whole problem of leprosy. The economic and social problems of the patient and his family should be identified and met. This may include social assistance and social support. This may take various forms depending upon the local situation, e.g., assistance to the patient to travel to and from the clinic; help to the needy families in terms of foodgrains, clothes, care of children and their education, and job placement; programmes such as slum improvement, etc. Such care should be provided through voluntary agencies and Departments of Social Welfare.

3. PROGRAMME MANAGEMENT

Leprosy control is a long-term activity. Therefore planning and programme management are essential ingredients. It is generally assumed that with existing tools, we can achieve rapid control of leprosy, provided the "operational performance" is stepped up to the maximum level required. This is the responsibility of programme managers. These issues are discussed under evaluation (see operational indicators and epidemiological indicators below). Among the resources that are needed are adequate infrastructure, trained health personnel, adequate supply of drugs and vehicles, and financial allocation. The National Leprosy Eradication Programme incorporates all these elements (see chapter 7).

4. EVALUATION

An important aspect of leprosy control is to assess the impact of the control operations on the endemicity of the disease, and to compare results between different times and places. Indicators are required for such an evaluation. It is important that these indicators can be easily used and satisfy the criteria of repeatability and validity. Ideally they should be conceived and treated as signals for action by programme managers *(6)*. There are two main types of indicators in leprosy control.

I. Epidemiological indicators

These are required to evaluate the effectiveness of the programme, that is to assess the impact of the action taken with regard to the problem reduction. These indices are : (a) INCIDENCE : Incidence rates are often calculated separately for different subgroups of population, e.g., age, sex, frequency of household contact. It is the most sensitive index of transmission of the disease. It is the only index for measuring the effectiveness of the measures taken, i.e., reduction of transmission. Thus they are useful in monitoring the success of a control programme. (b) PREVALENCE : This provides a measure of the "case load" and is useful in the planning of the treatment services. The continued reduction in the prevalence could also give information about the downward trend of the disease. It is often useful to calculate prevalence rates for different subgroups, e.g., age sex, geographic area. The fact that leprosy is not uniformly distributed should be borne in mind when these statistics are interpreted *(6)*.

A. Main or core indicators for monitoring progress *(41)*

(1) The number and rate of new cases detected per 100,000 population per year.
(2) Rate of new cases with grade-2 disabilities per 100,000 population per year.
(3) Treatment completion/cure rate.
(4) Prevalence rate

B. Additional epidemiological indicators *(12)*

- Proportion of grade II disabilities among new cases
- Proportion of females among new cases
- Proportion of MB among new cases
- Proportion of child (0–14 years) among new cases
- Child rate per 1,00,000 population
- Scheduled caste new case detection rate
- Scheduled tribe new case detection rate

C. Quality of service indicators *(12)*

- Patient month blister calendar pack stock
- Absolute number of patients made RFT
- Number of relapse reported
- Proportion of cases who developed new or additional disability after starting MDT
- Proportion of treatment defaulters
- Proportion of new cases correctly diagnosed

Definitions

Indicators and formula to be used for their calculation are indicated below :

(1) Annual new case detection rate (ANCDR)

Definition : It is the rate at which new cases (never treated before) are detected in a defined geographical area (block, district) in a year (April-March).

$$\text{ANCDR} = \frac{\text{No. of new leprosy cases detected in one year}}{\text{Total population of the area (as on 31st March)}} \times 100{,}000$$

(2) Rate of new cases with Grade-2 disabilities per 10,00,000 population per year

Definition : It is the rate at which new cases with disability grade 2 are detected in the defined geographical population (area) in a given year.

$$\text{RNCWG2D} = \frac{\text{Total no. of new cases detected with Gr II disability}}{\text{Total population of the area (as on 31st March)}} \times 10{,}00{,}000$$

(3) Treatment completion rate

Definition : It is the rate of patients who complete their treatment on time as a proxy for cure rate. Cohort analysis of PB and MB cases are done separately.

$$\text{PB TCR} = \frac{\text{Number of new PB cases who completed MDT in 9 months}}{\text{Number of new PB cases who started MDT in a year}} \times 100$$

$$\text{MB TCR} = \frac{\text{Number of new MB cases who completed MDT in 18 months}}{\text{Number of new MB cases who started MDT in a year}} \times 100$$

4. Prevalence rate (PR)

Definition : It is the total number of leprosy cases on record/under treatment per 10,000 population at a given point of time in an area.

$$\text{PR} = \frac{\text{Total number of leprosy cases on record}}{\text{Total population of the area (as on 31st March)}} \times 10{,}000$$

(A case of leprosy is a person with clinical signs of leprosy, who requires MDT)

5. Proportion of Grade II disability among new cases (PG2DANC)

Definition : It is the proportion (%) of new leprosy patients with grade II disability among total new cases detected.

$$\text{PG2DANC} = \frac{\text{No. of Grade II disabled cases detected in a year}}{\text{Total new cases detected in a year}} \times 100$$

6. Proportion of female among new cases (PFANC)

Definition : It is the proportion (%) of new female patients among total newly detected cases.

$$\text{PFANC} = \frac{\text{Number of new female patients}}{\text{Total no. of newly detected cases}} \times 100$$

7. Proportion of Multi-bacillary (MB) among new cases (PMBANC)

Definition : It is the proportion (%) of new patients diagnosed as MB among newly detected cases.

$$\text{PMBANC} = \frac{\text{Number of new MB cases}}{\text{Total no. of newly detected cases}} \times 100$$

8. Proportion of child among new cases (PCANC)

Definition : proportion (%) of new leprosy patients upto 14 years of age among newly detected patients.

$$\text{PCANC} = \frac{\text{Number of child leprosy cases detected}}{\text{Total no. of newly detected leprosy cases}} \times 100$$

9. Child rate (CR) per 100,000 population

Definition : The rate of new child leprosy cases (0–14 yrs of age) detected among the population of the area in a year.

$$\text{CR} = \frac{\text{No. of new child cases (0–14 yrs) detected in a year}}{\text{Population of the area (as on 31st March)}} \times 100{,}000$$

10. Scheduled caste (SC) new cases detection rate

Definition : Total number of new cases detected among the SC population in a given time in an area.

$$\text{SCNCDR} = \frac{\text{Total number of SC cases newly detected}}{\text{Total SC population in an area}} \times 10{,}000$$

11. Scheduled tribe (ST) new cases detection rate

Definition : Total number of new ST cases detected among the ST population in given time in an area.

$$\text{STNCDR} = \frac{\text{Total number of ST cases newly detected}}{\text{Total ST population in an area}} \times 10{,}000$$

12. Patients month blister calendar pack (BCP) stock (PMBCP)

Definition : Stock of BCPs in months, according to the number of patients expected to be treated in the next quarter.

$$\text{PMBCP} = \frac{\text{Number of blister packs of each category [PB(A/C), MB(A/C)]}}{\text{No. of cases under treatment in each category [PB(A/C), MB(A/C)]}}$$

13. Absolute number of patients made RFT

Definition : Number of patients released from treatment during the year. The number should include both the new and the other cases treated in a year.

14. Number of relapses reported

Definition : No. of relapse cases recorded in (and reported by) the PHC, District Hospitals, Medical colleges and other institutions in the district during the given time.

15. Proportion of cases with new disability after starting MDT (PCWNDASMDT)

Definition : Proportion (%) of cases who developed new or additional disability after starting MDT (new disability includes new nerve damage or new secondary impairment).

$$\text{PCWNDASMDT} = \frac{\text{No. of cases developed new or additional disability during treatment}}{\text{No. of cases put under MDT during the year}} \times 100$$

16. Proportion of new cases correctly diagnosed (PNCCD)

$$\text{PNCCD} = \frac{\text{No. of new cases correctly diagnosed}}{\text{No. of cases validated (DNT team)}} \times 100$$

Anti-leprosy activities in India

The history of anti-leprosy work in India goes back to 1874 when the Mission to Lepers (now Leprosy Mission) was founded by Baily at Chamba, in the Himachal Pradesh. The headquarters of this organization later moved to Purulia in West Bengal. Since then, many voluntary organizations (now about 150) have sprung up in the cause of leprosy. Important among these are the Hind Kusht Nivaran Sangh (formerly the British Empire Leprosy Relief Association); Gandhi Memorial Leprosy Foundation, Sevagram, Wardha; the German Leprosy Relief Association; the Damien Foundation; the Danish Save the Child Fund; and the more recent JALMA which was taken over by the ICMR in 1975. A federation body, "National Leprosy Organization" came into being in 1965 to provide a common platform to discuss their problems and share their experiences. The campaign against leprosy in India is accomplished through an official programme, the National Leprosy Control Programme which was initiated in the middle of 1954. In 1983, it was converted into an eradication programme.

An account of the National Leprosy Eradication Programme is given in chapter 7.

References

1. WHO (2001), *Weekly Epidemiolgical Record,* No. 20, 18 May, 2001.
2. WHO (2000), *Weekly Epidemiological Record,* No. 28 14th July, 2000.
3. WHO (2021), *Weekly Epidemiological Record,* No. 36, 10th Sep., 2021.
4. Govt. of India (2020), *Annual Report 2019–20,* Ministry of Health and Family Welfare, New Delhi.

4A. Govt. of India (2022), *Annual Report 2021–22,* Ministry of Health and Family Welfare, New Delhi.

5. Dharmendra (1985), *Leprosy* Vol III, Samant and Company, Bombay.
6. WHO (1988). Techn. Rep. Ser., No. 768.
7. Job, C.K. et al (1975). *Leprosy : Diagnosis and Management,* Hind Kusht Nivaran Sangh, New Delhi.
8. Periaswamy, V. (1984). *Ind. J. Lepr,* 56, No.1 (suppl).
9. WHO (1980). *A Guide to Leprosy Control.*
10. Last, J.M. ed (1980). *Maxcy–Rosenau : Public Health and Preventive Medicine, 11th ed.,* Appleton Century Crofts.
11. Prabhakar, M.C. et al (1984). *Ind. J. Lepr,* 56 No.1 (Suppl).
12. NLEP (2019), *Training Manual for Medical Officers,* 2019.
13. Van Braket, W.H. et al. (1992). *Leprosy review,* 63:231 – 245.
14. WHO (2009), Transmission of Leprosy.
15. Noordeen, S.K. (1980). In : *A Manual of Leprosy,* R.H. Thangaraj (ed) The Leprosy Mission, New Delhi.
16. Desikan, K.V. (1985). *Ann. Natl. Acad. Med. Sci, India,* 21 (4) 207, The Times of India, New Delhi 30 Jan. 1991.
17. Job, C.K. (1987). *Ind. J. Lepr.,* 59 (1) 1–8.
18. International Leprosy Congress, Madrid (1953). *Int. J. Lepr.,* 21 : 504.
19. Ridley, D.S. and Jopling, W.H. (1966). *Int. J. Lepr.,* 34, 255.
20. Chacko, C.J.G. (1980). In : *A Manual of Leprosy,* R.H. Thangaraj (ed). The Leprosy Mission, New Delhi.
21. NLEP (2012). *Disability Prevention & Medical Rehabilitation, Guidelines for primary, secondary and tertiary level care,* June, 2012
22. WHO (1998), *Tech. Rep. Ser.* No. 874.
23. Yawalkar, S.I. (1994). *Leprosy for medical practitioners and paramedical workers,* Sixth Edition, CIBA–GEIGY Ltd.
24. Bryceson, A. and Roy, E.P. (1979). *Leprosy,* 2nd ed., Churchill Livingstone.
25. Van Brakel, W.H. et al. (1992). Leprosy review, 63:231-245.
26. Bharadwaj, V.P. (1985). *Ann. Natl. Acad. Med. Sci,* 21 (3) 128.
27. Noussitou, F.M. et al (1976). *Leprosy in Children* WHO.
28. Ramu, G. et al (1980). *Lepr India,* 52 (3) 390.
29. Bharadwaj, V.P. et al (1981). *Lepr India,* 53 : 518.
30. Sinha, S. et al (1985). *Ind. J. Lepr.,* 53 : 33–38.
31. Dharmendra (1982). *Lepr India,* 54 : 193.
32. Govt. of India (1982). *Report of the Working Group on the Eradication of Leprosy,* Ministry of Health and Family Welfare, New Delhi.
33. WHO (1982). *Techn. Rep. Ser.,* No.675.
34. WHO and NLEP India (2000), *Guide to Eliminate Leprosy as a Public Health Problem.*
35. Katochi, K. et al (1985). *Ind. J. Lepr.,* 57 (3) 499.
36. WHO (2003), *The Final Push strategy to Eliminate Leprosy as a Public Health Problem,* Questions and Answers, 2nd Ed. 2003.

37. Ramu, G. (1985). *Ind. J. Lepr.*, 57 (3) 465.
38. Ganpati, R., *Leprosy – A Glimpse at the Changing Scenario* (1996), Published by Acworth Leprosy Hospital Society for Research, Rehabilitation and Education in Leprosy and Bombay Leprosy Project.
39. *Indian Journal of Leprosy*, Oct-Dec. 2003, Vol 75 (4).
40. Govt. of India (2007), *Operational Guidelines (Secondary Level), Disability Prevention and Medical Rehabilitation*, 2007, National Leprosy Eradication Programme, Central Leprosy Division, Ministry of Health and Family Welfare, New Delhi.
41. WHO (2009), *Enhanced Global Strategy for Further Reducing the Disease Burden due to Leprosy* (Plan period 2011–2015).
42. Govt. of India (2007), *Operational Guidelines (Primay Level), Disability Prevention and Medical Rehabilitation*, 2007, National Leprosy Eradication Programme, Central Leprosy Division, Ministry of Health and Family Welfare, New Delhi.
43. WHO (1960). *Techn. Rep. Ser.*, No.189.
44. Bhowmick, A. (1987). *Ind. J. Lepr.*, 59 (1) 92.

SEXUALLY TRANSMITTED DISEASES

The sexually transmitted diseases (STD) are a group of communicable diseases that are transmitted predominantly by sexual contact and caused by a wide range of bacterial, viral, protozoal and fungal agents and ectoparasites.

During the past few decades, STDs have undergone a dramatic transformation *(1)*. First, the change in name from venereal diseases (V.D.) to sexually transmitted diseases (STD) indicates this transformation. The list of pathogens which are sexually transmissible has expanded from the 5 "classical" venereal diseases (syphilis, gonorrhoea, chancroid, lymphogranuloma venereum and donovanosis) to include more than 20 agents, as shown in Table 1 *(2)*. Secondly, attention is now given not only to specific diseases, but also to clinical syndromes associated with STDs as shown in Table 3 *(1)*. Most of the recently recognized STDs are now referred to as **second generation STDs**. AIDS, the most recently recognized, is a totally new disease.

TABLE 1

Classification of sexually transmitted disease agents

A. Bacterial agents
- *Neisseria gonorrhoeae*
- *Chlamydia trachomatis*
- *Treponema pallidum*
- *Haemophilus ducreyi*
- *Mycoplasma hominis*
- *Ureaplasma urealyticum*
- *Calymmatobacterium granulomatis*
- *Shigella spp.*
- *Campylobacter spp.*
- Group B streptococcus
- *Bacterial vaginosis–associated organisms*

B. Viral agents
- Human (alpha) herpesvirus 1 or 2 (herpes simplex virus)
- Human (beta) herpesvirus 5 (formerly cytomegalovirus)
- Hepatitis virus B
- Human papilloma viruses
- Molluscum contagiosum virus
- Human immunodeficiency virus

C. Protozoal agents
- *Entamoeba histolytica*
- *Giardia lamblia*
- *Trichomonas vaginalis*

D. Fungal agents
- *Candida albicans*

E. Ectoparasites
- *Phthirus pubis*
- *Sarcoptes scabiei*

Extent of the problem

WORLD

The true incidence of STDs will never be known not only because of inadequate reporting but because of the secrecy that surrounds them. Most of them are not even notifiable. All available data, however, indicate a very high prevalence of STD.

STDs have a profound impact on sexual and reproductive health worldwide, and rank among the top 5 disease categories for which adults seek health care.

More than 1 million STIs are acquired every day. Each year, there are an estimated 374 million new infections with 1 of 4 STIs. During 2020, there were about chlamydia (129 million), gonorrhoea (82 million), syphilis (7.1 million) and trichomoniasis (156 million). More than 500 million people are living with genital HSV (herpes) infections. At any point in time, more than 300 million women have an HPV (Human Papilloma Virus) infection, one of the most common STIs. An estimated 296 million people are living with chronic hapatitis B globally *(3)*.

STIs can have serious consequences beyond the immediate impact of the infection itself. STIs like herpes and syphilis can increase the risk of HIV acquisition three-fold or more. Mother-to-child transmission of STIs can result in stillbirth, neonatal death, low-birth-weight and prematurity, sepsis, pneumonia, neonatal conjunctivitis, and congenital deformities. Over 900,000 pregnant women were infected with syphilis resulting in approximately 350,000 adverse birth outcomes including stillbirth in 2012. HPV infection causes about 528,000 cases of cervical cancer and 266,000 cervical cancer deaths each year. STIs such as gonorrhoea and Chlamydia are major causes of pelvic inflammatory disease (PID) and infertility in women *(4)*.

INDIA

Sexually transmitted diseases are becoming a major public health problem in India.

(a) Syphilis : Serological surveys continue to be the best source of information on the prevalence of syphilis. During 2020, about 17,787 cases of syphilis (6,088 males and 11,699 females) were reported in the country with 40 death *(5)*.

(b) Gonorrhoea : Information on the morbidity of gonorrhoea is notoriously lacking as most cases are not reported. The general impression is that gonorrhoea is more widely prevalent than syphilis. During 2020, about 27,582 gonorrhoea cases (8,669 males and 18,903 females) were reported in the country with 5 deaths *(5)*.

(c) Chancroid : Chancroid or soft sore is reported to be fairly widely prevalent in India.

(d) LGV : It is reported to be more prevalent in the southern states of Tamil Nadu, Andhra Pradesh, Maharashtra and Karnataka than in the northern states.

(e) Donovanosis : Donovanosis or granuloma inguinale is endemic in Tamil Nadu, Andhra Pradesh, Orissa, Karnataka and Maharashtra. A greater prevalence along the coastal areas has been reported.

(f) Other STDs : Information on the other STDs is not readily available, as there is no reporting system for these diseases.

Epidemiological determinants

Agent factors

Over 20 pathogens have been found to be spread by sexual contact. A classification of these agents and the diseases caused by them are as shown in Table 2.

TABLE 2
Important sexually transmitted pathogens and the diseases caused by them

Pathogen	Disease or syndrome
Neisseria gonorrhoeae	Gonorrhoea, urethritis, cervicitis, epididymitis, salpingitis, PID, neonatal conjunctivitis
Treponema pallidum	Syphilis
Haemophilus ducreyi	Chancroid
Chlamydia trachomatis	LGV, urethritis, cervicitis, proctitis, epididymitis, infant pneumonia, Reiter's syndrome, PID, neonatal conjunctivitis
Calymmatobacterium granulomatis	Donovanosis (granuloma inguinale)
Herpes simplex virus	Genital herpes
Hepatitis B virus	Acute and chronic hepatitis
Human papillomaviruses	Genital and anal warts
Human immuno-deficiency virus (HIV)	AIDS
Molluscum contagiosum	Genital molluscum contagiosum
Candida albicans	Vaginitis
Trichomonas vaginalis	Vaginitis

Source : *(2, 6)*

Host factors

(a) Age : For most notifiable STDs, the highest rates of incidence are observed in 20–24 year-olds, followed by the 25–29 and 15–19 years age groups. The most serious morbidity is observed during foetal development and in the neonate *(2)*. *(b) Sex* : For most STDs, the overall morbidity rate is higher for men than for women, but the morbidity caused by infection is generally much more severe in women, as for example, pelvic inflammatory disease. *(c) Marital status* : The frequency of STD infection is higher among single, divorced and separated persons than among married couples. *(d) Socio-economic status* : Individuals from the lowest socio–economic groups have the highest morbidity rate.

Demographic factors

Certain demographic factors will undoubtedly contribute to increase in STDs in the developing countries. These include population explosion and marked increase in the number of young people, the group at high risk for STD in the population; rural to urban migration; increasing educational opportunities for women delaying their marriage and increasing STD risks.

Social factors

Numerous social and behavioural factors are involved in the spread of STDs. These include : *(a) Prostitution* : This is a major factor in the spread of STDs. The prostitute acts as a reservoir of infection. In Asia, most STDs are contracted from prostitutes, whereas in many developed countries, the professional prostitute has largely been replaced by the "good–time girl". The male component of prostitution – the prostituant is equally important. Prostitution supplies a demand; if there were no prostituants, there would be no prostitutes. *(b) Broken homes* : Social studies indicate the promiscuous women are usually drawn from broken homes, e.g., homes which are broken either due to death of one or both parents or their separation. The atmosphere in such homes is unhappy, and children reared in such an atmosphere are likely to go astray in search of other avenues of happiness. *(c) Sexual disharmony* : Married people with strained relations, divorced and separated persons are often victims of STDs. *(d) Easy money* : In most of the developing world, prostitution is simply a reflection of poverty. It provides an occupation for earning easy money. It is fostered by lack of female employment and the prospect of a financial return impossible to achieve by other means *(7)*. *(e) Emotional immaturity* : This has been often stressed as a social factor in acquiring STDs. *(f) Urbanization and industrialization* : These are conductive to the type of lifestyle that contributes to high levels of infection, since long working hours, relative isolation from the family and geographical and social mobility foster casual sexual relationships. *(g) Social disruption* : Caused by disasters, wars and civil unrest have always caused an increase in the spread of STDs. *(h) International travel* : Travellers can import as well as export infection and their important role in the transmission of STD is exemplified by the rapid spread throughout the world of resistant strains of *N. gonorrhoea* and AIDS *(2)*. *(i) Changing behavioural patterns* : In modern society, the value traditionally set on chastity is in conflict with the more recent ideas of independence, freedom from supervision, and equal rights for both sexes. There has been a relaxation of moral and cultural values in present–day society. The tendency to break away from traditional ways of life is particularly marked among young people. *(j) Social stigma* : The social stigma attached to STDs accounts for the non–detection of cases, not disclosing the sources of contact, dropping out before treatment is complete, going to quacks for treatment, and self-treatment. *(k) Alcoholism* : The effect of alcohol seems to be more indirect than direct. Alcohol may encourage prostitution and conversely, prostitution may boost the sale of alcohol.

Clinical spectrum *(8)*

GONOCOCCAL INFECTION : Gonococcal infection causes inflammation of the genital tract involving the urethra in men and women, the cervix and rectum in women, and the rectum in men who have sex with men. Other sites are the throat (pharyngitis) and the eyes. The possible complications in women include pelvic inflammatory disease (PID). Long-term sequelae of PID are increased risk of ectopic pregnancy, infertility and chronic pelvic pain. In men, complications include inflammation of the epididymis. Long term consequences are sub-fertility and possibly urethral strictures. Serious consequences in infants include eye infection which can lead to blindness if not treated promptly. The antibiotics of choice are ciprofloxacin, ceftriaxone, cefixime or spectinomycin.

SYPHILIS : Syphilis causes ulceration of the uro-genital tract, mouth or rectum. Other signs of this infection, occurring in later stages, range from skin eruptions to complications of the cardiovascular and nervous system.

Congenital syphilis is an important cause of stillbirth. The antibiotics used to treat syphilis are penicillin, doxycycline and erythromycin.

CHLAMYDIAL INFECTION : A high percentage of individuals have no obvious clinical manifestations of this infection. If symptoms occur they are similar to those caused by gonorrhoea. Complications, which are similar to those of gonorrhoea, can result in steriltiy in women or vertical transmission during childbirth, leading to conjunctivitis or eye inflammation in the newborn. In men it can cause urethritis with possible epididymitis. The antibiotics used are doxycycline or azithromycin. The alternatives are amoxycillin, ofloxacin, erythromycin or tetracycline.

TRICHOMONIASIS : This parasitic infection leads to vaginitis and vaginal discharge in women. Usually, there are no symptoms. In most men there are no symptoms but it may cause urethritis. There is increasing evidence that *T. Vaginalis* may cause adverse outcomes in pregnancy, e.g. low birth weight and premature rupture of the membranes. The treatment option is metronidazole or tinidazole.

CHANCROID : After infection a small papule develops at the site of inoculation, normally within 2–3 days. The lesion then erodes into a deep ulcer that is extremely painful. In about 25 per cent of patients there is a painful swelling of one or the other inguinal lymph nodes (bubo). The antibiotics used are ciprofloxacin, erythromycin, ciftriaxone and azithromycin.

LYMPHOGRANULOMA VENEREUM : It commonly presents with swelling of lymph nodes in the groin. Although initially there is a small, painless ulcer of the genitalia 3–30 days after exposure it may pass unrecognized and resolve spontaneously. Untreated, the disease may cause extensive lymphatic damage resulting in elephantiasis of the genitalia. The antibiotics used are doxycycline, erythromycin and tetracycline. Benefit in late cases, e.g. with rectal stricture is slight. Surgical operation may be of benefit in cases with extensive elephantiasis or deformity.

DONOVANOSIS : Synonyms are granuloma inguinale, granuloma venereum. The first manifestation, appearing after a 3–40 days incubation period, is usually a small papule which ruptures to form a granulomatous lesion that is characteristically pain free and bleeds readily on contact, often elevated above the level of the surrounding skin. Antibiotics used are azithromycin and doxycycline, or alterantively erythromycin, tetracycline, trimethoprim–sulfamethoxazole.

GENITAL HERPES : Herpes simplex virus type 2 (HSV-2) is the primary cause of genital herpes. Classical genital herpes can be recognized by the presence of typical papular lesions that progress to multiple blisters and ulcers. However, the features can be variable in many people and the appearance can easily be confused with other genital infections. First episode of disease manifestation are frequently associated with a prolonged course of ulceration, lasting up to three to four weeks. Antiviral treatment of these episodes can be very effective in shortening the duration and alleviating pain. HSV-2 infection is life-long and recurrent ulcerative episodes occur. The median recurrence rate after a symptomatic first episode of genital herpes is four to five episodes per year. Asymptomatic or subclinical infection does occur, as do subclinical recurrences, accompanied by viral shedding without a visible ulcer. These subclinical episodes can be infectious to sexual partners. There is no cure for HSV-2 infection. However, oral antiviral medications such as acyclovir, valacyclovir and famciclovir are all effective in reducing the severity and duration of first-episode genital herpes. Topical creams are less effective. Episodic treatment has a limited role in reducing the duration of lesions as they tend to last less than a week.

HUMAN PAPILLOMA VIRUS : Human papilloma virus (HPV) causes ano-genital warts, which vary from the common soft, flesh-coloured protuberances which may become exuberant (cauliflower like) to papular flat warts on drier areas (eg. shaft of penis), which resemble those seen on other parts of the body. They can be seen anywhere in the genitalia including in the perianal region, even in those denying anal sexual intercourse. The other commonly recognized manifestation of genital HPV infection is cervical cancer, caused by some sub-types of HPV. Treatment is generally reserved for large lesions because sub-clinical infection tend to resolve on their own. For any viral infection the mainstay of control is prevention, especially in young sexually active individuals. Regular examination of the cervix and cervical cytology using Papanicolaou staining method is recommended for female patients and female contacts in order to detect progression of lesions to cervical cancer. Detection programmes based on cervical cytology screening and colposcopy services have been successful in curbing the incidence of, and mortality from cervical cancers in industrialized countries, but are expensive to run in developing countries.

Syndromic approach to STD

Many different agents cause sexually transmitted diseases. However, some of these agents give rise to similar or overlapping clinical manifestations. Common syndromes and sequelae are as shown in Table 3.

TABLE 3

Common syndromes and sequelae for which sexual transmission is of epidemiological importance

Male urethritis
Lower genital syndromes in women : vaginitis/cervicitis/urethritis
Genital ulceration
Proctitis/colitis
Salpingitis
Epididymitis/orchitis
Infertility/ectopic pregnancy
Postnatal and perinatal morbidity
Hepatitis/hepatic carcinoma
Genital carcinoma
Acquired Immuno Deficiency Syndrome (AIDS)

Source : *(1)*

The traditional method of diagnosing STD is by laboratory tests. However, these are often not available or are expensive. Since 1990 WHO has recommended syndromic management of STDs in patients presenting with consistently recognized signs and symptoms of STD. The syndromic approach is a scientifically derived approach and offers accessible and immediate treatment, that is effective and efficient, management of STD using flowcharts (as shown in Fig. 1, 2, 3, 4, 5 and 6) is more cost-effective than diagnosis based on laboratory tests *(9)*.

1. Syndromic management of urethral discharge in males

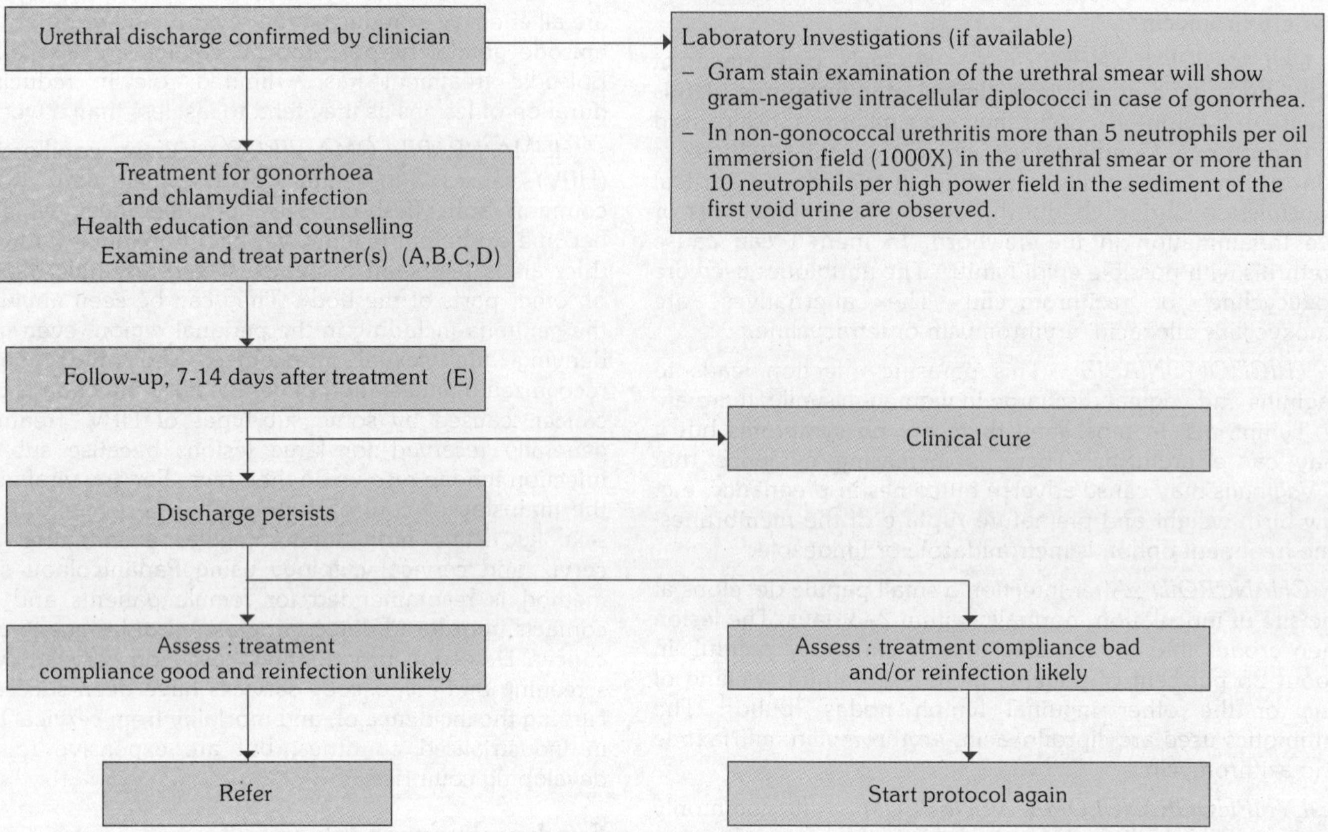

(A) Notification and treatment of female partners of men with urethritis are of the highest priority as one of the best ways of identifying women at high risk of having asymptomatic gonococcal and chlamydial infections.

(B) Treatment :

As dual infection is common, the treatment for urethral discharge should adequately cover therapy for both, gonorrhea and chlamydial infections.

Recommended regimen for uncomplicated gonorrhea + chlamydia.

Uncomplicated infections indicate that the disease is limited to the anogenital region (anterior urethritis and proctitis).

– Tab. Cefixime 400 mg orally, single dose Plus Tab Azithromycin 1 gram orally single dose, under supervision.

– Advise the patient to return after 7 days of start of therapy.

When symptoms persist or recur after adequate treatment for gonorrhea and chlamydia in the index patient and partner(s), they should be treated for *Trichomonas vaginalis*.

If discharge or only dysuria persists after 7 days – Tab. Secnidazole 2 gm orally, single dose (to treat for T. vaginalis).

If the symptoms still persists – Refer to higher centre as early as possible.

If individuals are allergic to Azithromycin, give Erythromycin 500 mg four times a day for 7 days.

(C) Syndrome specific guidelines for partner management :

Treat all recent partners; Treat female partners (for gonorrhea and chlamydia) on same lines after ruling out pregnancy and history of allergies; advise sexual abstinence during the course of treatment; provide condoms, educate about correct and consistent use; refer for voluntary counselling and testing for HIV, syphilis and Hepatitis B, and schedule return visit after 7 days.

(D) Management of pregnant partner :

Pregnant partners of male clients with urethral discharge should be examined by doing as per speculum as well as per vaginal examination and should be treated for gonococcal as well as chlamydial infections.

– Cephalosporins to cover gonococcal infection are safe and effective in pregnancy.

– Tab. Cefixime 400 mg orally, single dose OR Ceftriaxone 125 mg by intramuscular injection.

+

– Tab. Erythromycin 500 mg orally four times a day for seven days OR Cap Amoxicillin 500 mg orally, three times a day for seven days to cover chlamydial infection.

– Quinolones (like ofloxacin, ciprofloxacin), doxycycline are contraindicated in pregnant women.

(E) Follow up after seven days to see reports of tests done for HIV, syphilis and Hepatitis B; if symptoms persist, to assess whether it is due to treatment failure or re-infection; and for prompt referral if required.

FIG. 1

Syndromic management of urethral discharge (in the absence of laboratory support)

Source : *(9)*

2. Syndromic management of vaginal discharge

Causative Organisms

Vaginitis : Trichomonas vaginalis (Tv); Candida albicans; and Gardnerella vaginalis, Mycoplasma causing bacterial vaginosis (Bv).

Cervicitis : Neisseria gonorrhoeae, Chlamydia trachomatis, Trichomonas vaginalis, and Herpes simplex virus.

History:

- Menstrual history to rule out pregnancy.
- Nature and type of discharge (amount, smell, color, consistency).
- Genital itching
- Burning while passing urine, increased frequency.
- Presence of any ulcer, swelling on the vulval or inguinal region.
- Genital complaints in sexual partners.
- Low backache.

→

Examination:

- Per speculum examination to differentiate between vaginitis and cervicitis.
  - (a) Vaginitis:
    - Trichomoniasis – greenish frothy discharge
    - Candidiasis – curdy white discharge
    - Bacterial vaginosis – adherent discharge
    - Mixed infections may present with atypical discharge.
  - (b) Cervicitis :
- Cervical erosion / cervical ulcer / mucopurulent cervical discharge.
- Bimanual pelvic examination to rule out pelvic inflammatory disease.
- If speculum examination is not possible or client is hesitant, treat both for vaginitis and cervicitis.

→

Laboratory investigations (if available):

- Wet mount microscopy of the discharge for Trichomonas vaginalis and clue cells.
- 10% KOH preparation for candida albicans.
- Gram's stain of vaginal smear for clue cells seen in bacterial vaginosis.
- Gram's stain of endocervical smear to detect gonococci.

↓

Treatment:

Vaginitis (TV+BV+Candida)

- Tab. Secnidazole 2 gm orally, single dose OR Tab. Tinidazole 500 mg orally, twice daily for 5 days.
- Tab. Metoclopropramide taken 30 minutes before Tab. Secnidazole, to prevent gastric intolerance.
- Treat for candidiasis with Tab Fluconazole 150 mg orally single dose OR local Clotrimazole 500 mg vaginal pessaries once.

Treatment for cervical infection (chlamydia and gonorrhea):

- Tab cefixime 400 mg orally, single dose.

  Plus – Azithromycin 1 gram, 1 hour before lunch. If vomiting within 1 hour, give anti-emetic and repeat
  - If vaginitis and cervicitis are present treat for both.
  - Instruct client to avoid douching.
  - Pregnancy, diabetes, HIV may also be influencing factors and should be considered in recurrent infections.
  - Follow-up after one week.

↓

Management in pregnant women:

Per speculum examination should be done to rule out pregnancy complications like abortion, premature rupture of membranes.

Treatment for vaginitis (TV+BV+Candida):

In first trimester of pregnancy

- Local treatment with Clotrimazole vaginal pessary/cream only for candidiasis. Oral Flucanozole is contraindicated in pregnancy.
- Metronidazole pessaries or cream intravaginally if trichomoniasis or BV is suspected.

In second and third trimester oral metronidazole can be given

- Tab. Secnidazole 2 gm orally, single dose or Tab. Tinidazole 500 mg orally, twice daily for 5 days.
- Tab. Metoclopropramide taken 30 minutes before Tab. Metronidazole, to prevent gastric intolerance.

↓

Specific guidelines for partner management:

- Treat current partner only if no improvement after initial treatment.
- If partner is symptomatic, treat client and partner using above protocols.
- Advise sexual abstinence during the course of treatment.
- Provide condoms, educate about correct and consistent use.
- Schedule return visit after 7 days.

FIG. 2

Syndromic management of vaginal discharge

Source : *(9)*

3. Management of lower abdominal pain in females

Causative organisms:
Neisseria gonorrhoeae; Chlamydia trachomatis; and Mycoplasma, Gardnerella, Anaerobic bacteria (Bacteroides specially gram positive cocci).
Differential diagnosis : ectopic pregnancy, twisted ovarian cyst, ovarian tumor, appendicitis, and abdominal tuberculosis.

History:
- Lower abdominal pain
- Fever
- Vaginal discharge
- Menstrual irregularities like heavy, irregular vaginal bleeding.
- Dysmenorrhea
- Dyspareunia
- Dysuria, tenesmus
- Low backache
- Contraceptive use like IUD.

→

Examination:
- General examination : temperature, pulse, blood pressure.
- Per speculum examination : vaginal/cervical discharge, congestion or ulcers.
- Per abdominal examination : lower abdominal tenderness or guarding.
- Pelvic examination :
  Uterine/adnexal tenderness, cervical movement tenderness.

Note : A urine pregnancy test should be done in all women suspected of having PID to rule out ectopic pregnancy.

→

Laboratory investigations (if available):
- Wet smear examination
- Gram stain for gonorrhea
- Complete blood count and ESR
- Urine microscopy for pus cells

↓

Treatment (out patient treatment):
In mild or moderate PID (in the absence of tubo ovarian abscess), out patient treatment can be given. Therapy is required to cover *Neisseria gonorrhoeae, Chlamydia trachomatis and anaerobes.*
- Tab. Cefixime 400 mg orally twice daily for 7 days + Tab. Metronidazole 400 mg orally, twice daily for 14 days.
  +
- Doxycycline, 100 mg orally, twice a day for 2 weeks (to treat chlamydial infection).
- Tab. Ibuprofen 400 mg orally, three times a day for 3-5 days.
- Tab. Ranitidine 150 mg orally, twice daily to prevent gastritis.
- Remove intra uterine device, if present, under antibiotic cover of 24-48 hours.
- Advise abstinence during the course of treatment and educate on correct and consistent use of condoms.
- Observe for 3 days. If no improvement (i.e. absence of fever, reduction in abdominal tenderness, reduction in cervical movement, adnexal and uterine tenderness) or if symptoms worsen, refer for In patient treatment.

Caution : PID can be a serious condition. Refer the patient to the hospital if she does not respond to treatment within 3 days and even earlier if her condition worsens.

→

Syndrome specific guidelines for partner management:
- Treat all partners in past 2 months.
- Treat male partners for urethral discharge (gonorrhea and chlamydia).
- Advise sexual abstinence during the course of treatment.
- Provide condoms, educate on correct and consistent use.
- Refer for voluntary counselling and testing for HIV, syphilis and Hepatitis B.
- Inform about the complications if left untreated and sequelae.
- Schedule return visit after 3 days, 7 days and 14 days to ensure compliance.

Management of pregnant women:
Though PID is rare in pregnancy,
- Any pregnant woman suspected to have PID should be referred to district hospital for hospitalization and treated with a parenteral regimen which would be safe in pregnancy.
- Doxycycline is contraindicated in pregnancy.
- Note : Metronidazole is generally not recommended during the first three months of pregnancy. However, it should not be withheld for a severly acute PID, which represents an emergency.

↓

Hospitalization of clients with acute PID should be seriously considered when:
- The diagnosis is uncertain.
- Surgical emergencies e.g. appendicitis or ectopic pregnancy can not be excluded.
- A pelvic abscess is suspected.
- Severe illness precludes management on an out patient basis.
- The woman is pregnant.
- The patient is unable to follow or tolerate an out patient regimen.
- The patient has failed to respond to out patient therapy.

Note : All patients requiring hospitalization should be referred to the district hospital.

FIG. 3
Management of lower abdominal pain in females

Source : *(9)*

4. Management of genital ulcers

Causative organisms :
Treponema pallidum (syphilis),
Haemophilus ducreyi (chancroid),
Klebsiella granulomatis (granuloma inguinale),
Chlamydia trachomatis (lymphogranuloma venerum),
Herpes simplex (genital herpes)

History:
- Genital ulcer/vesicles
- Burning sensation in the genital region.
- Sexual exposure of either partner to high risk practices including orogenital sex.

→

Examination:
- Presence of vesicles.
- Presence of genital ulcer-single or multiple.
- Associated inguinal lymph node swelling and if present refer to respective flowchart.

Ulcer characteristics:
- Painful vesicles/ulcers, single or multiple – herpes simplex.
- Painless ulcer with shotty lymph node – syphilis.
- Painless ulcer with inguinal lymph nodes – granuloma inguinale and LGV.
- Painful ulcer usually single, sometimes – chancroid associated with painful bubo.

→

Laboratory investigations:
- RPR test for syphilis.
- For further investigations refer to higher centre.

↓

Treatment:
- If vesicles or multiple painful ulcers are present treat for herpes with Tab. Acyclovir 400 mg orally, three times a day for 7 days.
- If vesicles are not seen and only ulcer is seen, treat for syphilis and chancroid and counsel on herpes genitalis.

To cover syphilis give

Inj Benzathine penicillin 2.4 million IU IM after test dose in two divided doses (with emergency tray ready).

(In individuals allergic or intolerant to penicillin, Doxycycline 100 mg orally, twice daily for 14 days).

\+

Tab. Azithromycin 1g orally single dose OR

Tab. Ciprofloxacin 500 mg orally, twice a day for three days to cover chancroid.

Treatment should be extended beyond 7 days if ulcers have not epithelialized i.e. formed a new layer of skin over the sore.

Refer to higher centre
- If not responding to treatment.
- Genital ulcers co-existent with HIV.
- Recurrent lesion.

↓

Syndrome specific guidelines for partner management:
- Treat all partners who are in contact with patient in last 3 months.
- Partners should be treated for syphilis and chancroid.
- Advise sexual abstinence during the course of treatment.
- Provide condoms, educate about correct and consistent use.
- Refer for voluntary counselling and testing for HIV, Syphilis and Hepatitis B.
- Schedule return visit after 7 days.

Management of pregnant women:
- Quinolones (like ofloxacin, ciprofloxacin), doxycycline, sulfonamides are contraindicated in pregnant women.
- Pregnant women who test positive for RPR should be considered infected unless adequate treatment is documented in the medical records and sequential serologic antibody titers have declined.
- Inj Benzathine penicillin 2.4 million IU IM after test dose (with emergency tray ready).
- A second dose of benzathine penicillin 2.4 million units IM should be administered 1 week after the initial dose for women who have primary, secondary, or early latent syphilis.
- Pregnant women who are allergic to penicillin should be treated with erythromycin and the neonate should be treated for syphilis after delivery.
- Tab. Erythromycin 500 mg orally four times a day for 15 days.
- (Note : Erthromycin estolate is contraindicated in pregnancy because of drug related hepatotoxicity. Only Erythromycin base or Erythromycin ethyl succinate should be used in pregnancy).
- All pregnant women should be asked history of genital herpes and examined carefully for herpetic lesions.
- Women without symptoms or signs of genital herpes or its prodrome can deliver vaginally.
- Women with genital herpetic lesions at the onset of labour should be delivered by caesarean section to prevent neonatal herpes.
- Acyclovir may be administered orally to pregnant women with first episode genital herpes or severe recurrent herpes.

FIG. 4

Management of genital ulcers

Source : *(9)*

5. Management of scrotal swelling

Causative Organisms
Neisseria gonorrhoeae
Chlamydia trachomatis.

Differential diagnosis (non RTIs/STIs)
Infections causing scrotal swelling : tuberculosis, filariasis, coliforms, pseudomonas, mumps virus infection.
Non infectious causes : trauma, hernia, hydrocele, testicular torsion, and testicular tumors.

History of
- Swelling and pain in scrotal region.
- Pain or burning while passing urine.
- Systemic symptoms like malaise, fever.
- Sexual exposure of either partner to high risk practices including oro-genital sex.

Examination
Look for
- Scrotal swelling.
- Redness and edema of the overlying skin.
- Tenderness of the epididymis and vas deferens.
- Associated urethral discharge/genital ulcer/inguinal lymph nodes and if present refer to the respective flowchart.
- A transillumination test to rule out hydrocele should be done.

Laboratory Investigations
(If available)
- Gram's stain examination of the urethral smear will show gram-negative intracellular diplococci in case of complicated gonococcal infection.
- In non-gonococcal urethritis more than 5 neutrophils per oil immersion field in the urethral smear or more than 10 neutrophils per high power field in the sediment of the first void urine are observed.

Treatment
- Treat for both gonococcal and chlamydial infections
  Tab Cefixime 400 mg orally twice daily for 7 days, Plus
  Cap. Doxycycline 100 mg orally, twice daily for 14 days and refer to higher centre as early as possible since complicated gonococcal infection needs parenteral and longer duration of treatment.
- Supportive therapy to reduce pain
  (bed rest, scrotal elevation with T-bandage and analgesics)

Note :
If quick and effective therapy is not given, damage and scarring of testicular tissues may result, causing sub-fertility.

Syndrome specific guidelines for partner management.
Partner needs to be treated depending on the clinical findings.

Management protocol in case the partner is pregnant
- Depending on the clinical findings in the pregnant partner (whether vaginal discharge or endocervical discharge or PID is present) the drug regimens should be used.
- Doxycycline is contraindicated in pregnancy.
- Erythromycin base/Amoxicillin can be used in pregnancy.

(Erythromycin estolate is contraindicated in pregnancy due to hepatotoxicity.
Erythromycin base or erythromycin ethyl succinate should be given).

FIG. 5

Syndromic management of scrotal swelling

Source : *(9)*

6. Management of inguinal bubo

Causative organisms
- Chlamydia trachomatis serovars L1, L2, L3, causative agent of lympho granuloma venerum (LGV).
- Haemophilus ducreyi causative agent of chancroid.

Differential diagnosis
- Mycobacterium tuberculosis, filarisis.
- Any acute infection of skin of pubic area, genitals, buttocks, anus and lower limbs can also cause inguinal swelling.

If malignancy or tuberculosis is suspected refer to higher centre for biopsy.

History
- Swelling in inguinal region which may be painful.
- Preceding history of genital ulcer or discharge.
- Sexual exposure of either partner to high risk practices including oro-genital sex.
- Systemic symptoms like malaise, fever.

Examination

Look for
- Localized enlargement of lymph nodes in groin which may be tender and fluctuant.
- Inflammation of skin over the swelling.
- Presence of multiple sinuses.
- Edema of genitals and lower limbs
- Presence of genital ulcer or urethral discharge, and if present refer to respective flowchart.

Laboratory Investigations.
Diagnosis is on clinical grounds.

Treatment
- Start Cap. Doxycycline 100 mg orally twice daily for 21 days (to cover LGV)
  Plus
- Tab Azithromycin 1g orally single dose OR
- Tab. Ciprofloxacin 500 mg orally, twice a day for three days to cover chancroid.
- Refer to higher centre as early as possible.

Note :
- A bubo should never be incised and drained at the primary health centre, even if it is fluctuant, as there is a high risk of a fistula formation and chronicity. If bubo becomes fluctuant always refer for aspiration to higher centre.
- In severe cases with vulval edema in females, surgical intervention may be required for which they should be referred to higher centre.

Syndrome specific guidelines for partner management
- Treat all partners who are in contact with patient in last 3 months.
- Partners should be treated for chancroid and LGV.
- Tab Azithromycin 1 g orally single dose to cover chancroid
  +
  Cap Doxycycline 100 mg orally, twice daily for 21 days to cover LGV
- Advise sexual abstinence during the course of treatment.
- Provide condoms, educate on correct and consistent use.
- Refer for voluntary counselling and testing for HIV, syphilis and Hepatitis B.
- Schedule return visit after 7 days and 21 days.

Management of Pregnant partner
- Quinolones (like ofloxacin, ciprofloxacin), doxycycline, sulfonamides are contraindicated in pregnant women.
- Pregnant and lactating women should be treated with the erythromycin regimen, and consideration should be given to the addition of a parenteral amino glycoside (e.g., gentamicin)

Tab. Erythromycin base, 500 mg orally, 4 times daily for 21 days and refer to higher centre. (Erythromycin estolate is contraindicated in pregnancy due to hepatotoxicity. Erythromycin base or erythromycin ethyl succinate should be given)

FIG. 6

Syndrome management of inguinal bubo

Source : *(9)*

Control of STDs

The aim of the control programme for STDs is the prevention of ill-health resulting from the above conditions through various interventions. These interventions may have a primary prevention focus (the prevention of infection), a secondary prevention focus (minimizing the adverse health effects of infection), or usually a combination of the two. The control of STD may be considered under the following heads *(10)*.

1. Initial planning
2. Intervention strategies
3. Support components
4. Monitoring and evaluation

INITIAL PLANNING

Control programmes have to be designed to meet the unique needs of each country and to be in line with that country's health care system, its resources and priorities. This requires initial planning which comprises the following steps : (1) PROBLEM DEFINITION : The disease problem must be defined in terms of prevalence, psychosocial consequences and other health effects – by geographic areas and population groups, with the aid of sero–epidemiological surveys and population surveys. This is an important first step, since such information is usually inadequate or non-existent in most cases. (2) ESTABLISHING PRIORITIES : Rational planning requires establishment of priorities. This will depend upon health problem considerations (e.g., magnitude, consequences) and feasibility of control (e.g., availability of adequate resources, social and political commitment). Priority groups may be categorized on the basis of age, sex, place of residence, occupation, drug addiction, etc. (3) SETTING OBJECTIVES : Priorities must be converted into discrete, achievable and measurable objectives. That is, to reduce the magnitude of the problem, in a given population and a stated time. To be most useful, objectives should be unambiguous and quantifiable. Broad coverage of the population is crucial for effective STD control. (4) CONSIDERING STRATEGIES : A variety of intervention strategies are available. Planners must define the mixture of strategies that appears to be most appropriate to the setting. (The reader is referred to chapter 23 for a broad discussion of the planning cycle).

INTERVENTION STRATEGIES

1. Case detection

Case detection is an essential part of any control programme. The usual methods of early detection in a STD control programme are :

(a) SCREENING : Screening is the testing of apparently healthy volunteers from the general population for the early detection of disease. High priority is given to screening of special groups, viz. pregnant women, blood donors, industrial workers, army, police, refugees, prostitutes, convicts, restaurant and hotel staff etc. The availability of an appropriate test is critical for screening purposes. The sensitivity, specificity, and the predictive value of a test are important considerations (see Chapter 4).

(b) CONTACT TRACING : Contact tracing is the term used for the technique by which the sexual partners of diagnosed patients are identified, located, investigated, and treated *(11)*. This is one of the best methods of controlling the spread of infection. Patients are interviewed for their sexual contacts by specially trained staff. The key to success in contact tracing is the patient himself who must disclose all sex contacts voluntarily. In some parts of USA, contacts are sought as quickly as possible using telephone, telegram and other rapid means of communication. The contacts are then persuaded to attend a STD clinic for examination and treatment. Where prevalence is low, contact tracing is relatively expensive.

(c) CLUSTER TESTING : Here the patients are asked to name other persons of either sex who move in the same socio–sexual environment. These persons are then screened (e.g., blood testing). This technique has been shown almost to double the number of cases found *(12)*.

2. Case holding and treatment

Adequate treatment of patients and their contacts is the mainstay of STD control. There is a tendency on the part of patients suffering from STDs to disappear or drop out before treatment is complete. Therefore every effort should be made to ensure complete and adequate treatment. A recent WHO Expert Committee *(2)* drew up a list of recommended regimens for treating STDs. Not less than the recommended dosages should be used.

3. Epidemiological treatment

What is known as epidemiological treatment or more appropriately **contact treatment** has become a keystone of the control campaigns *(11)*. It consists of the administration of full therapeutic dose of treatment to persons recently exposed to STD while awaiting the results of laboratory tests *(13)*. Epidemiological treatment should not be an end in itself. Its effects are not lasting unless it is combined with a venereological examination and the tracing of contacts revealed by that examination.

4. Personal prophylaxis

(i) Contraceptives : Mechanical barriers (e.g., condoms and the diaphragms) can be recommended for personal prophylaxis against STDs. These barrier methods, especially when used with spermicides, will minimize the risk of acquiring STD infections. However, their use is limited by lack of motivation, acceptability and convenience. The effectiveness of most of the prophylactic techniques available is poorly documented since few controlled studies have been carried out *(2)*. The exposed parts should be washed with soap and water as soon after contact as possible. *(ii) Vaccines* : The development of a vaccine for hepatitis B has raised hopes that vaccines will be found for other STDs.

5. Health education

Health education is an integral part of STD control programmes. The principal aim of educational intervention is to help individuals alter their behaviour in an effort to avoid STDs, that is, to minimize disease acquisition and transmission. The target groups may include the general public, patients, priority groups, community leaders, etc. The primary health care of WHO also underlines the importance of health education.

SUPPORT COMPONENTS

1. STD clinic

The starting point for the control of STDs is the establishment of STD clinics where all consultation, investigations and treatment, contact tracing and all other relevant services are available. An ideal service is one that is free, easily accessible to patients and available for long hours each day. There should be suitable arrangements for treating female patients separately. Since the patients desire anonymity, the STD clinic should try to maintain it.

Because of the stigma attached to the STD clinics, many patients seek alternative sources of medical care, including self-medication. It is now considered that the key to the success of a STD control programme is the integration of its essential elements into the primary health care services.

However, it is essential to have in each administrative unit one specialized centre, which should provide the necessary clinical, and laboratory expertise and coordinate control activities at all levels of the health care system. The centre should be housed adjacent to other medical facilities and training centres.

2. Laboratory services

Adequate laboratory facilities and trained staff are essential for proper patient management. It provides a basis for correct aetiological diagnosis and treatment decisions; for contact tracing; surveillance of morbidity and detection of antimicrobial resistance. The diagnostic tests that should be available for the important sexually transmitted pathogens are given in a WHO report *(10)*.

3. Primary health care

The current trend is to integrate STD control activities into primary health care system. This will imply inclusion of primary health care workers (e.g., ASHA, multipurpose workers) in the STD "health team". Then only it will be possible to provide effective treatment to the greatest number of cases in the community. Such management limits further disease transmission. Primary health care which is based on the principles of universal coverage, community participation, equity and intersectoral coordination is ideally suited to control STD in the community.

4. Information system

The basis of an effective control programme of any communicable disease is the existence of an information system. It is a prerequisite for effective programme planning, coordination, monitoring and evaluation. Three types of data requirement are relevant in the control of STDs: these are clinical notification, laboratory notification, and sentinel and *adhoc* surveillance.

National notification system, at best, includes only the "classical" venereal diseases, where existing, reporting systems suffer from undernotification, inaccurate diagnosis and concealment of cases owing to social stigma. Without a notification system, it is not possible to assess the magnitude of the problem, to allocate resources and to evaluate the impact of control measures. There is an urgent need to develop an effective and detailed reporting system of STDs in countries where it does not exist. Sentinel surveillance systems and/or *adhoc* surveys can be used to supplement the routine reporting system. Population–based sample surveys may also be used to identify the true distribution of disease in a particular setting. Such surveys are very expensive and are generally of limited use for sexually transmitted disease programmes *(10)*.

The information system should be built around a small number of questions : How many cases were interviewed ? How many villages were visited ? How many cultures were examined? The system should provide information on activities, resource utilization and task accomplishment of programme personnel *(10)*.

5. Legislation

Many countries are still far away in enacting suitable legislation for the control of STDs *(14)*. Although legislations and regulations cannot wipe out STDs, they are nonetheless needed, particularly to establish responsibilities and define standards. The purpose of legislation should be to encourage patients to seek early treatment and name their sexual contacts, to screen high risk groups, to improve notification by general practitioners, health education of the public, etc. The Immoral Traffic (Prevention) Act, 1986 (which replaced the earlier Suppression of the Immoral Traffic Act, 1956) covers all persons, whether male or female, who are exploited sexually for commercial purposes. It makes punishment for the offences under the Act more stringent than the previous Act.

6. Social welfare measures

STDs are social problems with medical aspects. It implies there should be "social therapy" which would prevent or control the conditions leading to promiscuity and STDs. The various social measures include : rehabilitation of prostitutes; provision of recreation facilities in the community; provision of decent living conditions; marriage counselling; prohibiting the sale of sexually stimulating literature, pornographic books and photographs, etc.

MONITORING AND EVALUATION

A critical aspect of effective management is the monitoring of disease trends and evaluating programme activities. Evaluation will show if the activities have been performed in a satisfactory way. Ongoing evaluation of disease trends provides a more direct measure of programme effectiveness and may be used to determine the appropriateness of the selected intervention strategies for a particular setting *(10)*.

Global health sector strategy on HIV, hepatitis and sexually transmitted infections, 2022–2030

With this framework, WHO :

1. develops global targets, norms and standards for STI prevention, testing and treatment;
2. supports the estimation and economic burden of STIs and the strengthening of STI surveillance;
3. globally monitors anti microbial resistance (AMR) to gonorrhoea; and
4. leads the setting of the global research agenda on STIs, including the development of diagnostic tests, vaccines and additional drugs for gonorrhoea and syphilis *(3)*.

National STD Control Programme

See chapter 7 for details.

References

1. Brown, S.T. et al (1985). *Int. J. Epidemiology,* 14 (4) 505.
2. WHO (1986). *Techn. Rep. Ser.*, No. 736.
3. WHO (2022), *Fact Sheet on STIs,* 22nd Aug. 2022.
4. WHO (2017), *Prevention, Diagnosis and Treatment of Sexually Transmitted Infections,* 27th Dec. 2017.
5. Govt. of India (2021), *National Health Profile 2021,* Ministry of Health and Family Welfare, New Delhi.
6. WHO (1981). Techn. *Rep. Ser.*, No. 660.
7. Willcox, R.R. (1976). *Sexually Transmitted Diseases,* R.D. Catterall and C.S. Nicol (eds). Academic Press.
8. *WHO Fact Sheet,* 2006, on STD.
9. Govt. of India (2007), *National Guidelines on Prevention, Management and Control of Reproductive Tract Infections including Sexually Transmitted Infections,* NACO, Ministry of Health and Family Welfare, New Delhi.

10. WHO (1985). *Control of Sexually Transmitted Diseases,* WHO, Geneva.
11. WHO (1982). *Techn. Rep. Ser.*, No. 674.
12. WHO (1963). *Techn. Rep. Ser.*, No. 262.
13. WHO (1978). *Techn. Rep. Ser.*, No. 616.
14. WHO (1975). VD Control : *A Survey of Recent Legislation,* Geneva.

ENDEMIC TREPONEMATOSIS

Endemic treponematoses (pinta, endemic syphilis (Bejel, yaws) continue to be public health problems in some tropical countries. Of these, yaws and endemic syphilis still constitute a considerable health hazard to the child population in medically under–served areas, particularly in West and Central Africa and, the Americas *(1)*. These diseases are caused by agents which are microscopically indistinguishable. Typically these diseases have a patchy distribution in population groups away from the network of health centres *(1)*. They are usually contracted in childhood, non–venereally. Intrauterine transmission is absent. The late cardiac and cerebral manifestations of venereal syphilis which are particularly severe in that disease, do not occur in these infections (excepting scanty or mild lesions in endemic syphilis). In most countries, the prevalence of these diseases was reduced to low levels, and in some areas their transmission was interrupted due to mass–treatment campaigns. However, complacency after successful mass campaigns and the premature discontinuation of surveillance activities have led to resurgence of these infections in a number of countries *(1)*.

PINTA

A chronic infectious disease caused by *T. carateum*. Reports suggest that pinta has virtually disappeared from countries of Latin America *(1, 2)*. The disease is now restricted to the Philippines and some areas of the Pacific. The disease is essentially one of childhood, often beginning after the age of 10 to 15 years. Transmission is non-venereal, by direct contact with infectious lesions. After an incubation period of 7 to 21 days, an initial papular lesion appears on the hands and legs, followed by a maculo-papular, erythematous rash (pintides) lasting for years. A late stage is characterized by depigmented, leukodermic patches which may be permanent. Individuals with late pinta are resistant to infection with *T. pallidum*. In the treatment of pinta, the antibiotic of choice is benzathine penicillin G (BPG) which has replaced PAM. The dose for patients under 10 years is 0.6 mega units, and for those 10 years and over 1.2 mega units *(3)*.

ENDEMIC SYPHILIS

Endemic syphilis (Bejel is a local name for this disease in Syria) occurs in the arid areas of Syria, Saudi Arabia, Iraq, Iran, Yugoslavia, northern and southern Africa and Australia. It does not occur in the Americas. The causative agent is difficult to differentiate from *T. pallidum*. The claim that it is the same microorganism has yet to be substantiated *(4)*. It is transmitted non–venereally by direct or indirect contact – among children and adolescents through their play or by drinking vessels and common eating and other household utensils under primitive, crowded and substandard conditions of living. It is thought that poor hygiene rather than climatic conditions is a major factor in the continued transmission of Bejel. It is thought that 25 per cent of children acquire the infection before the age of 10 years. The figure is increased to 60 per cent before the age of 16 years *(4)*. Endemic syphilis produces highly infectious skin lesions. Late manifestations include gumatous lesions of the skin, nasopharynx and bones *(5)*. A single injection of benzathine penicillin G is the treatment of choice. For patients under 10 years the dose is 0.6 mega units, and for patients age 10 years and over, the dose is 1.2 mega units *(3)*.

YAWS

Yaws is a chronic contagious non-venereal disease caused by *T. pertenue*, usually beginning in early childhood. It resembles syphilis in its clinical course and is characterized by a primary skin lesion (mother yaw) followed by a generalized eruption and a late stage of destructive lesions of the skin and bone. Yaws is also known as pian, bubas or framboesia.

Geographic distribution

The disease is found primarily in poor communities in warm, humid and tropical forest areas of Africa, Asia, Latin America and the Pacific. The majority of affected populations live at the "end of the road" and therefore have limited access to basic social amenities and health care.

A review of historic documents from the 1950s shows that at least 88 countries and territories within the tropical belt 20 degrees north and south of the equator were endemic for yaws. Only 13 countries are known to be currently endemic for yaws. However, these countries need support to implement the WHO "Yaws Eradication Strategy" (the Morges Strategy). Recent estimates indicate that about 89 million people live in the 13 countries endemic for yaws.

Ecuador and India have reported no cases of yaws since 2003. A WHO International Verification Team (IVT) visited India in October 2015 to assess the status of interruption of transmission. Based on the report of the IVT and endorsed by the WHO NTD Strategic and Technical Advisory Group (STAG); WHO declared India free of yaws in May 2016 *(6)*.

Epidemiological determinants

Agent factors

(a) AGENT : Yaws is caused by *T. pertenue* which closely resembles *T. pallidum* culturally and morphologically. It measures 20μ in length with 8 to 12 rigid spirals. The agent occurs in the epidermis of the lesions, lymph glands, spleen and bone marrow. The organism rapidly dies outside the tissues. (b) RESERVOIR OF INFECTION : Man is the only known reservoir of yaws. He is an infected person. Clinical lesions may relapse 2 to 3 times or more during the first 5 years of infection, and serve as source for new infections *(1)*. Most latent cases are found in clusters centred around an infectious case. There are frequent relapses in latent cases within the first 3 to 5 years of infection. The source of infection is usually the skin lesions and the exudates from early lesions. (c) COMMUNICABILITY : Variable, and may extend over several years intermittently as moist lesions break out. Treponema are usually not found in late lesions.

Host factors

(a) AGE : Yaws is primarily a disease of childhood and adolescence. Over 75 per cent of cases occur before the age of 15 years, but the disease can occur at any age *(9)*. (b) SEX : Generally, the prevalence among males is greater than among females. (c) IMMUNITY : Man has no natural immunity. Acquired resistance develops slowly and may take months or years to develop fully unless suppressed by treatment. There is considerable experimental and epidemiological evidence *(3)* that yaws provides partial immunity to venereal syphilis. The near eradication of yaws in Haiti has been followed by a high prevalence of venereal syphilis.

Environmental factors

(a) CLIMATE : Yaws is endemic in warm and humid regions. High humidity for at least 6 months of the year and an average rainfall of at least 40 inches are considered favourable for the transmission of yaws. (b) SOCIAL FACTORS : Social factors are even more important than biological factors in the perpetuation of yaws in the endemic areas. Yaws is mostly endemic among the tribal people, whose ways of living favour its transmission. Scanty clothing, poor personal cleanliness, overcrowding, bad housing, low standard of living and the absence of soap are important socio-economic factors in the epidemiology of yaws. Yaws is a crippling disease; lesions on palms and soles may disable a person for long periods making him dependant on others.

Mode of transmission

Yaws is transmitted non–venereally by : (a) DIRECT CONTACT : That is, by contact with secretions from infectious lesions. (b) FOMITES : Yaws may also be transmitted by indirect contact. The organism may remain alive on fomites or on the earthen floor in hot and humid conditions long enough to cause infection, and (c) VECTOR : There is some evidence that small flies and other insects feeding on the lesion may possibly convey the infection mechanically for brief periods.

Transplacental, congenital transmission does not occur.

Incubation period

9–90 days (average 21 days).

Clinical features

(a) EARLY YAWS : The primary lesion or "mother yaw" appears at the site of inoculation after an incubation period of 3 to 5 weeks. The lesion is extra-genital and is seen on exposed parts of the body such as legs, arms, buttocks or face. The local lymph glands are enlarged and the blood becomes positive for STS. Within the next 3 to 6 weeks, a generalized eruption appears consisting of large, yellow, crusted, granulomatous eruptions often resembling condylomata lata in secondary syphilis. During the next 5 years skin, mucous membrane, periosteal and bone lesions may develop, subside and relapse at irregular intervals. The early lesions are highly infectious.

(b) LATE YAWS : By the end of 5 years, destructive and often deforming lesions of the skin, bone and periosteum appear. The lesions of sole and palms are called "crab yaws". The destructive lesions of soft palate, hard palate, and nose are called "Gangosa". Swelling by the side of the nose due to osteo–periostitis of the superior maxillary bone is called "Goundu".

CONTROL OF YAWS

The control of yaws is based on the following principles :

1. Survey

A clinical survey of all the families in endemic areas is made. The survey should cover not less than 95 per cent of the total population. During the survey, persons suffering from yaws and their contacts are listed.

2. Treatment

Treatment is based on the following observations : (a) treatment with a single dose of Azithromycin oral or a single injection of long-acting penicillin will cure infection. (b) the simultaneous treatment of all clinical cases and their likely contacts in the community will interrupt transmission in the community *(9)*.

Benzathine penicillin G is the penicillin of choice. It has now replaced PAM *(3)*. The dose of BPG is 1.2 million units for all cases and contacts, and half that dose (0.6 million units) for children under 10 years of age. Azithromycin is given as a single oral dose at 30 mg/kg body weight (maximum 2 gm).

The WHO *(3)* has recommended three treatment policies : (a) TOTAL MASS TREATMENT : In areas where yaws is hyperendemic (i.e., more than 10 per cent prevalence of clinically active yaws), a great part of the population is at risk. The entire population including the cases should be given penicillin in the doses mentioned above. (b) JUVENILE MASS TREATMENT : In meso-endemic communities (5 to 10 per cent prevalence), treatment is given to all cases and to all children under 15 years of age and other obvious contacts of infectious cases. (c) SELECTIVE MASS TREATMENT : In hypo-endemic or areas of low prevalence (less than 5 per cent) treatment is confined to cases, their household, and other obvious contacts of infectious cases.

3. Resurvey and treatment

It is unlikely that a single round of survey and treatment will cover the entire population. In order to interrupt transmission, it is necessary to find out and treat the missed cases and new cases. Resurveys should be undertaken every 6 to 12 months. Several such follow-ups may be needed before eradication is achieved.

4. Surveillance

With the decline of yaws to very low levels, emphasis has shifted to "Surveillance and containment" – a technique which has proved highly successful in the eradication of smallpox. The surveillance and containment measures would be concentrated on affected villages, households and other contacts of known yaws cases. The measures comprise epidemiological investigation of cases to identify probable source(s) of infection and contacts of each known case so as to discover previously unknown cases and prevent new cases; treatment of cases; prophylactic treatment of contacts with BPG; and, monthly follow-up of households with confirmed cases for at least 3 to 4 months after treatment of the last active case to assure interruption of transmission.

5. Environmental Improvement

In a disease like yaws, an attack on social and economic conditions of life is as important as an attack on the biological cause. Recrudescence of the disease is apt to occur unless environmental improvement is promoted, e.g., improvement of personal and domestic hygiene, adequate water supply, liberal use of soap, better housing conditions and improvement of the quality of life.

6. Renewed eradication efforts *(9)*

The WHO roadmap for neglected tropical diseases (NTDs) have set 2020 target for the eradication of yaws from the remaining countries.

Since January 2012, when the WHO roadmap for NTDs were set and an article in the Lancet on the efficacy of a single-dose azithromycin in the treatment of yaws was published, WHO has taken steps to move the renewed eradication efforts by developing a new eradication strategy based on single dose treatment with azithromycin. These are:

a. *Total community treatment (TCT)* – treatment of the endemic community, irrespective of the number of active clinical cases;

b. *Total targeted treatment (TTT)* – treatment of all active clinical cases and their contacts (household, school, playmates).

As a first step in implemeting the new eradication strategy, 7 countries were selected for the initial pilot treatment campaigns. In 2012 it was implemented in Betou and Enyelle districts of Congo. In 2013, implementation was carried out in Ghana, Papua New Guinea and Vanuatu, achieving a coverage of more than 90 per cent. In 2014, Cameroon, Indonesia, and Solomon Islands are to implement mass treatment activities *(9)*.

7. Evaluation

To determine whether or not yaws has really been brought under control, serological studies are needed. Ideally if no yaws antibodies were found among children born since the yaws mass campaign was completed, it would mean that the campaign had been totally successful. The actual sample of the population to be tested may be as low as 1 or 2 per cent.

References

1. WHO (1981). *Wkly. Epi. Rec.*, 56 : 241–248.
2. WHO (1982). *The Work of WHO, 1980–81*.
3. WHO (1982). *Techn. Rep. Ser.*, 674.
4. Wasley, G.D. (1980). *Middle East Health*, 4 (7) 33.
5. Chulay, J.D. (1979). *Principles and Practice of Infectious Diseases*, Mandell, G.L. et al (eds), John Wiley, New York.
6. WHO (2016), *Yaws Fact sheet*, June 2016.
7. WHO (1968). *The Second Ten Years of the WHO, 1958–1967*.
8. Hopkins, D.R. (1976). *Am. J. Trop. Med & Hyg.*, 25 : 860.
9. WHO (2014), *Fact Sheet*, No. 316, Feb. 2, 2014.

AIDS

AIDS, the acquired immuno-deficiency syndrome (sometimes called "slim disease") is a fatal illness caused by a retrovirus known as the human immuno-deficiency virus (HIV) which breaks down the body's immune system, leaving the victim vulnerable to a host of life–threatening opportunistic infections, neurological disorders, or unusual malignancies *(1)*. Among the special features of HIV infection are that once infected, it is probable that a person will be infected for life. Strictly speaking, the term AIDS refers only to the last stage of the HIV infection. AIDS can be called our modern pandemic, affecting both industrialized and developing countries.

Problem statement

WORLD

Recognized as an emerging disease only in the early 1980s, AIDS has rapidly established itself throughout the world, and is likely to endure and persist well into the 21st century. AIDS has evolved from a mysterious illness to a global pandemic which has infected tens of millions people.

Promising development have been seen in recent years in global efforts to address the AIDS epidemic, including increased access to effective treatment and prevention programmes. However, the number of people living with HIV continues to grow, as does the number of deaths due to AIDS. Of particular concern are trends affecting Eastern Europe and Central Asia, where the numbers of people acquiring HIV infection and dying from HIV-related causes continue to increase. The global HIV epidemic during 2019 is summarized in Table 1.

WHO and UNAIDS has defined different types of HIV epidemics. They are as follows *(3)* :

Low-level HIV epidemics

Although HIV may have existed for many years, it has never spread to substantial levels in any sub-population. Recorded infection is largely confined to individuals with higher risk behaviour e.g. sex workers, drug injectors, men having sex with other men. Numerical proxy : HIV prevalence has not consistently exceeded 5% in any defined sub-population.

Concentrated HIV epidemics

HIV has spread rapidly in a defined sub-population, but is not well-established in the general population. This epidemic state suggests active networks of risk within the sub-population. The future course of the epidemic is determined by the frequency and nature of links between highly infected sub-populations and the general population. Numerical proxy : HIV prevalence is consistently over 5% in at least one defined sub-population but is below 1% in pregnant women in urban areas.

Generalized HIV epidemics

In generalized epidemics, HIV is firmly established in the general population. Although sub-populations at high risk may contribute disproportionately to the spread of HIV, sexual networking in the general population is sufficient to sustain an epidemic independent of sub–populations at higher risk of infection. Numerical proxy : HIV prevalence consistently over 1% in pregnant women.

On the verge of fourth decade of the AIDS epidemic, the world has turned the corner – it has halted and begun to reverse the spread of HIV. The question remains how quickly the response can chart a new course towards vision zero discrimination, zero new HIV infection and zero AIDS–related deaths through universal access to effective HIV – prevention, treatment, care and support.

HIV incidence (the number of new HIV infections in a population per year) is the key parameter that prevention efforts aim to reduce, since newly infected persons contribute to the total number of persons living with HIV; they will progress to disease and death over time; and are a potential source of further transmission. Since 1997, the year in which annual new infections peaked to 3.2 million cases globally, the number of new infections has fallen to 1.5 million in 2021. This reduction in HIV incidence reflects natural trend of epidemic, as well as the result of prevention programmes resulting in behavioural changes in different contexts, like changes in sexual behavior; programmes targeting key populations such as harm-reducing programmes for people who inject drugs; maximizing the prevention benefits of ARVs, including for the prevention of mother-to-child transmission of HIV; and voluntary medical male circumcision in high HIV-prevalence settings *(4)*.

Women represent about half of all people living with HIV worldwide, and more than half (about 63 per cent) in sub–Saharan Africa. HIV is the leading cause of death among women in reproductive age. Gender inequalities, differential access to services and sexual violence increase women's

TABLE 1
Global HIV statistics (2021)

Global HIV statistics *(2)*	– 38.4 million (33.9 million–43.8 million) people globally were living with HIV in 2021. – 1.5 million (1.1 million–2.0 million) people became newly infected with HIV in 2021. – 6,50,000 (5,10,000–8,60,000) people died from AIDS-related illnesses in 2021. – 28.7 million people were accessing antiretroviral therapy in 2021. – 84.2 million (64.0 million–113.0 million) people have become infected with HIV since the start of the epidemic. – 40.1 million (33.6 million–48.6million) people have died from AIDS-related illnesses since the start of the epidemic.
People living with HIV	– In 2021, there were 38.4 million (33.9 million–43.8 million) people living with HIV. • 36.7 million (32.3 million–41.9 million) adults (15 years or older) . • 1.7 million (1.3 million–2.1 million) children (0–14 years). • 54% of all people living with HIV were women and girls. – 85% (75–97%) of all people living with HIV knew their HIV status in 2021. – About 5.9 million people did not know that they were living with HIV in 2021.
People living with HIV accessing antiretroviral therapy	– As of the end of December 2021, 28.7 million people were accessing antiretroviral therapy, up from 7.8 million in 2010. – In 2021, 75% (66–85%) of all people living with HIV were accessing treatment. • 76% (67–87%) of adults aged 15 years and older living with HIV had access to treatment, as did 52% (42–65%) of children aged 0–14 years. • 80% (72–91%) of female adults aged 15 years and older had access to treatment; however, just 70% (61–82%) of male adults aged 15 years and older had access. – 81% (63–97%) of pregnant women living with HIV had access to antiretroviral medicines to prevent transmission of HIV to their child in 2021.
New HIV infections	– New HIV infections have been reduced by 54% since the peak in 1996. • In 2021, around 1.5 million (1.1 million–2.0 million) people were newly infected with HIV, compared to 3.2 million (2.4 million–4.3 million) people in 1996. • Women and girls accounted for 49% of all new infections in 2021. – Since 2010, new HIV infections have declined by 32%, from 2.2 million (1.7 million–2.9 million) to 1.5 million (1.1 million–2.0 million) in 2021. • Since 2010, new HIV infections among children have declined by 52%, from 3,20,000 (2,20,000–4,80,000) in 2010 to 1,60,000 (1,10,000–2,30,000) in 2021.
AIDS-related deaths	– AIDS-related deaths have been reduced by 68% since the peak in 2004 and by 52% since 2010. • In 2021, around 6,50,000 (5,10,000–8,60,000) people died from AIDS-related illnesses worldwide, compared to 2.0 million (1.6 million–2.7 million) people in 2004 and 1.4 million (1.1 million–1.8 million) people in 2010. – AIDS-related mortality has declined by 57% among women and girls and by 47% among men and boys since 2010.
Key populations	– In 2021, key populations (sex workers and their clients, gay men and other men who have sex with men, people who inject drugs, transgender people) and their sexual partners accounted for 70% of HIV infections globally : – 94% of new HIV infections outside of sub-Saharan Africa. – 51% of new HIV infections in sub-Saharan Africa. – The risk of acquiring HIV is : – 35 times higher among people who inject drugs than adults who do not inject drugs. – 30 times higher for female sex workers than adult women. – 28 times higher among gay men and other men who have sex with men than adult men. – 14 times higher for transgender women than adult women.
Women	– Every week, around 4,900 young women aged 15–24 years become infected with HIV. – In sub-Saharan Africa, six in seven new HIV infections among adolescents aged 15–19 years are among girls. Girls and young women aged 15–24 years are twice as likely to be living with HIV than young men. – In sub-Saharan Africa, women and girls accounted for 63% of all new HIV infections in 2021
95–95–95	– In 2021, 85% (75–97%) of people living with HIV knew their HIV status. – Among people who knew their status, 88% (78–>98%) were accessing treatment. – And among people accessing treatment, 92% (81–>98%) were virally suppressed. – Of all people living with HIV, 85% (75–97%) knew their status, 75% (66–85%) were accessing treatment and 68% (60–78%) were virally suppressed in 2021.

Source : *(2)*

vulnerability to HIV, and women, especially younger women, are biologically more susceptible to HIV *(5)*.

The UNAIDS 2016–2021 strategy is a bold call to action to get on the "Fast-Track" and reach people being left behind. The strategy focuses on the unfinished agenda. It is a call to reach the 90–90–90 treatment targets, to close the testing gap and to protect the health of the people living with HIV. It calls for 90 per cent of the people with HIV being aware of their infection, 90 per cent of people aware that they have HIV initiating ART and 90 per cent of those receiving ART having undetectable levels of HIV in their blood by 2020. Milestone targets also include a 75 per cent reduction in new infection between 2010 and 2020, achieving zero discrimination and reducing annual HIV-related deaths to less than 500,000 by 2020 globally *(6)*.

Only when above targets are met, the next set of goals will be 95–95–95 for treatment, i.e., 95 per cent of people living with HIV knowing their HIV status; 95 per cent of people who know their status on treatment; and 95 per cent of people on treatment with suppressed viral loads. Reduce the annual number of new HIV infection among adults to 200,000 and achieving zero discrimination *(7)*.

The Sustainable Development Goal target is to end the AIDS epidemic by 2030. UNAIDS has led the development of a global strategy, "Fast Track : Ending the AIDS Epidemic by 2030", while more detailed, sectoral strategy such as the WHO sector strategy on HIV 2016–2021 are under development. The main areas of focus post-2015 include *(4)* :

1. A focus on population left behind by the HIV response, such as adolescent girls, key population (sex workers, men who have sex with men, people who inject drugs and transgender people), migrants and children;
2. A focus on locations where the greatest HIV transmission is occurring and with the greatest HIV burden, and the use of data to support the impact of programmes;
3. An integrated HIV response that expands the contribution towards universal health care, including health workforce, procurement systems, injection and blood safety, and treatment of coinfections; and
4. Sustainable programmes with transitioning to domestic funding of essential HIV services.

The interaction of HIV/AIDS with other infectious diseases is an increasing public health concern. Tuberculosis, bacterial infection and malaria have been identified as the leading cause of HIV-related morbidity in Sub-Saharan Africa. HIV infection increases the incidence and severity of clinical malaria in adults *(8)*.

The national HIV strategic plans in most SEAR countries accord priority to prevention, care and treatment interventions to high-risk populations; however coverage of a comprehensive package of HIV interventions for sex workers, men having sex with men, transgender persons and injecting drug users remains low in all countries.

INDIA

Now into its fifth decade, India's epidemic is marked by heterogeneity – not a single epidemic but made up of a number of distinct epidemics, in some places within the same state.

Latest 2021 HIV estimates for India are as shown in Table 2. The HIV prevalence trend has been declining since the epidemic's peak in the year 2000.

At the national level, estimated adult HIV prevalence (15–49 years) is the highest in the north-east region states followed by southern states. AIDS related deaths (ARD) are estimated at 41.97 thousand in 2021. A decline of 76.5 per cent in ARD has been estimated at national level from 2010 to 2021. The declining trend is noted in all states/UTs excluding Puducherry, Arunachal Pradesh, Meghalaya, and Tripura. The highest decline in ARD is estimated in Chandigarh, Telangana, and West Bengal. Fig. 1 and Fig. 2 shows estimated prevalence percentage state-wise and ARD state-wise respectively *(9)*.

TABLE 2

HIV estimates, summary for the year 2021 (India)

Indicators		Value
Adult (15–49 years) Prevalence (in %)	Total	0.21 (0.17–0.25)
	Male	0.22 (0.18–0.28)
	Female	0.19 (0.15–0.23)
Number of people living with HIV (in lakh)	Total	24.01 (19.92–29.07)
	Adult (15+ years)	23.31 (19.38–28.19)
	Women (15+ years)	10.50 (8.73–12.69)
	Children (<15 years)	0.70 (0.54–0.89)
	Young people (15–24)	1.70 (1.30–2.26)
HIV incidence per 1000 uninfected population	Total	0.05 (0.03–0.08)
	Male	0.05 (0.03–0.09)
	Female	0.04 (0.02–0.07)
New HIV Infections (in thousand)	Total	62.97 (36.72–104.06)
	Adults (15+ years)	57.97 (33.49–96.53)
	Women (15+ years)	24.55 (14.27–40.69)
	Young people (15–24)	15.08 (8.60–25.17)
Decline in new HIV infections since 2010 (%)	Total	46.25
	Adults (15+ years)	44.48
	Female (15+ years)	43.75
	Children (<15 years)	60.82
AIDS-related deaths (in thousand)	Total	41.97 (26.50–67.45)
	Adults (15+ years)	39.46 (25.14–63.26)
	Women (15+ years)	11.26 (5.79–20.46)
	Children (<15 years)	2.51 (1.13–4.39)
	Young people (15–24)	1.12 (0.64–1.95)
AIDS-related deaths per 100,000 population	Total	3.08 (1.94–4.95)
	Male	4.21 (2.77–6.41)
	Female	1.88 (0.97–3.40)
Decline in AIDS related deaths since 2010 (%)	Total	76.54
	Adults (15+ years)	76.44
	Female (15+ years)	82.74
	Children (<15 years)	77.92
PMTCT need	Total	20.61 (16.38–26.36)
Final MTCT rate of HIV (%)	Total	24.25 (18.50–29.50)

Source : *(9)*

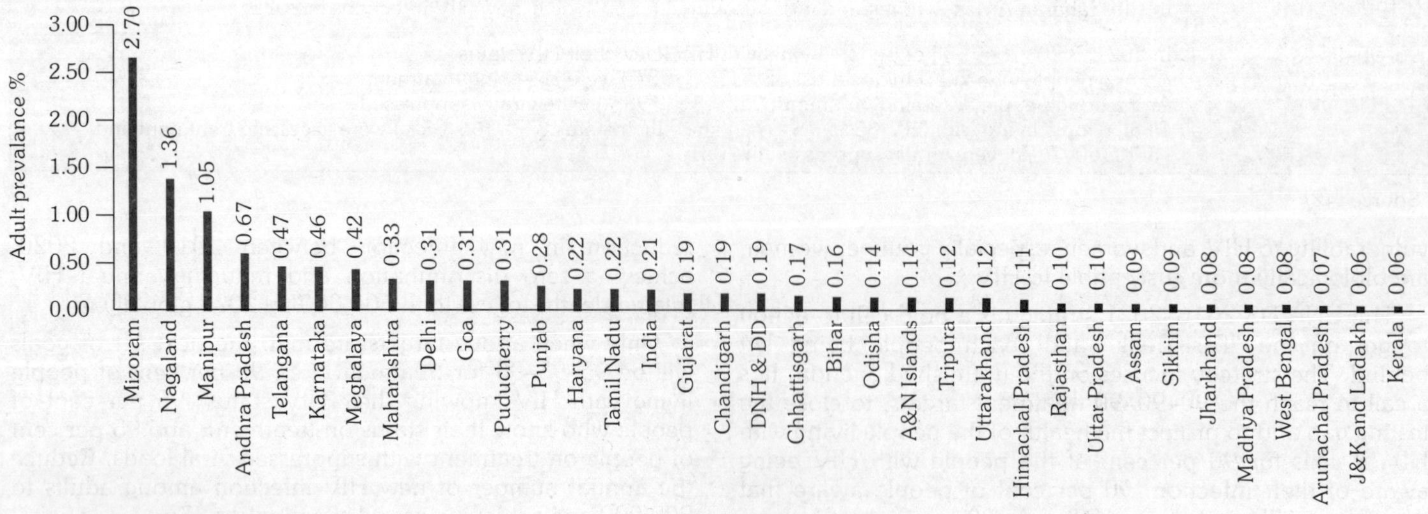

FIG. 1
State/UT wise adult HIV prevalence (%), 2021

Source : *(9)*

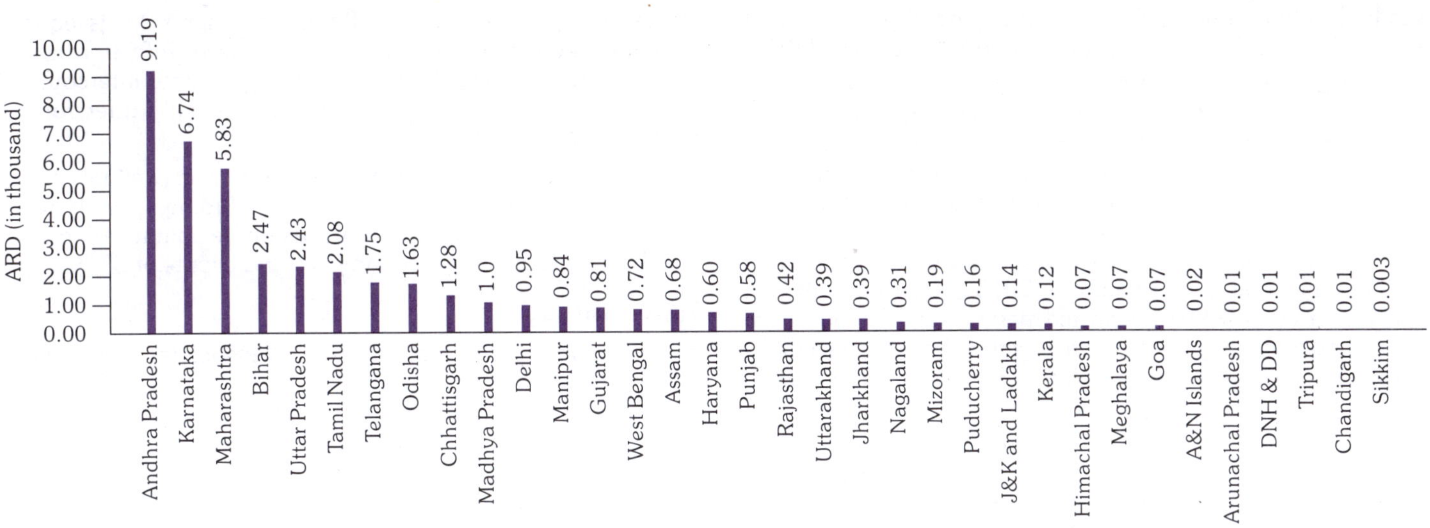

FIG. 2
State/UT wise Estimated Annual AIDS related deaths (in thousand), 2021

Source : *(9)*

Key population affected in India

The HIV epidemic in India is driven by sexual transmission, which accounts for 86 per cent of new infections in 2017. It is followed by parent-to-child, injecting drug users, homosexuals and blood and blood products use etc.

According to HIV sentinel surveillance during 2019, the overall HIV prevalence among ANC clinic attendees (considered as proxy for prevalence among general population) continues to be low at 0.24 per cent, with an overall declining trend at national level. India continues to portray a concentrated epidemic. HIV prevalence among different risk groups is as shown in Fig. 3.

Sex workers and HIV (FSW) : In 2017, an estimated 1.6 per cent of female sex workers in India were living with HIV, although this figure varies between states. For example, prevalence among FSW is estimated at 7.4 per cent in Maharashtra and 6.3 per cent in Andhra Pradesh. Stigma and discrimination against sex workers restrict their access to healthcare. NACO reported reaching 77.4 per cent of sex workers with HIV prevention activities in the year 2015. In the year 2017, around 67 per cent of HIV positive sex workers were aware of their status and 91 per cent of sex workers (HIV positive and negative) reported using condom *(10)*.

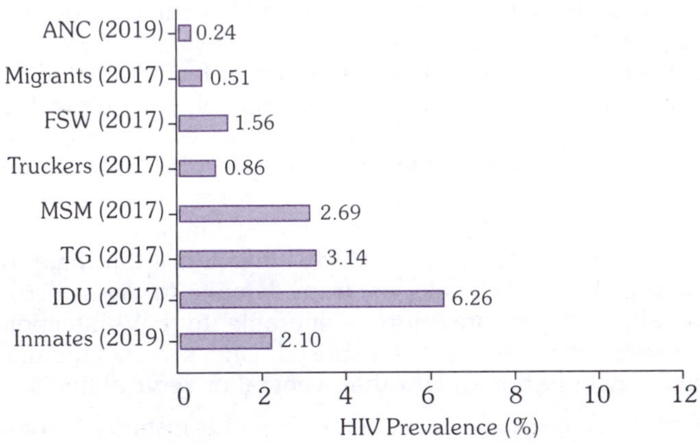

FIG. 3
HIV prevalence for ANC attendees and among different high risk groups, India, (2017–2019)

Source : *(11)*

People who inject drugs and HIV : Prevalence of HIV among injecting drug users (IDU) is high and major route of HIV transmission in India's north-eastern states. In 2016, 1.7 million people in India were estimated to be injecting drug users. In 2017, 6.3 per cent of people who inject drugs were thought to be living with HIV, of whom half were aware of their status. Prevalence varies with states e.g., 12.1 per cent in Manipur, 10 per cent in Mizoram and 3.2 per cent in Nagaland. A 2018 study analyzed unsafe injecting and sexual risk behaviours among about 20,000 Indian men who injected drugs. Results suggest that beginning drug use at age 25 years or below, engagement in drug use for longer time, injecting three times or more per day, sharing needles and syringes, and sufferers of sexually transmitted diseases were all linked to an increased likelihood of HIV infection *(10)*.

HIV prevention efforts in the north-east of the country have been effective in reducing the number of new infections. However, there is evidence that the number of people who inject drugs is growing. In addition, evidence of higher HIV prevalence among sub-populations of people who inject drugs is also emerging. For instance, a 2015 study found prevalence to be more than three times higher among women who inject drugs than men *(10)*.

Hijras/transgender people and HIV : HIV prevalence among transgender people in India was estimated to be 3.1% in 2017, the second highest prevalence among all key populations in the country. Around 68% of HIV positive transgender people are aware of their status. In 2017, NACO reported around 45 per cent of transgender people and hijras were receiving targetted interventions *(10)*.

Migrant workers and HIV : Research worldwide has linked migration to increase in HIV transmission. There are an estimated 7.2 million migrant workers in India, of whom 0.2% are living with HIV. NACO categorizes groups of migrants as 'bridge populations', as they form links between urban and rural areas, and between groups that are at high-and low-risk of HIV transmission. HIV testing among these groups remains low, standing at 11.32% in 2016. Despite being an important driver of the HIV epidemic in India, data on migrant sexual behaviour is limited. In 2014, UNAIDS reported that 75% of women testing positive in India have a husband who is a migrant labourer. A 2017 study found that HIV prevalence among the wives of migrant workers in rural northern India was higher than among women in the general population at 0.59%. Only 15.5% of those questioned had heard of HIV.

Truck drivers and HIV : A number of studies have reported high vulnerability of truckers to HIV transmission in India. NACO estimated that 0.2% of truck drivers were living with HIV in 2017–18. NACO also categorizes truck drivers as a bridge population because they often have unprotected sex with high-risk groups such as female sex workers as well as their regular sex partners, which increases the risk of transmitting HIV into the general population. A 2015 study found 49% of truckers in central India reported paying for sex, of whom 21.5% had a sexually transmitted infection. HIV testing among truck drivers remains low, standing at 21.74% in 2016 *(10)*.

Impoverished, unemployed, under employed, mobile and migrant youth, and street children are particularly vulnerable to HIV, as they are less likely to have information about HIV or access to preventive measures, and they may face repeated risks of HIV infection.

EPIDEMIOLOGICAL FEATURES

1. Agent factors

(a) AGENT : When the virus was first identified it was called "lymphadenopathy–associated virus (LAV)" by the French scientists. Researchers in USA called it "human T–cell lymphotropic virus III (HTLV–III)". In May 1986, the International Committee on the Taxonomy gave it a new name : human immunodeficiency virus (HIV).

The virus is 1/10,000th of a millimetre in diametre. It is a protein capsule containing two short strands of genetic material (RNA) and enzymes. The virus replicates in actively dividing T4 lymphocytes and like other retroviruses can remain in lymphoid cells in a latent state that can be activated. The virus has the unique ability to destroy human T4 helper cells, a subset of the human T–lymphocytes. The virus is able to spread throughout the body. It can pass through the blood–brain barrier and can then destroy some brain cells. This may account for certain of the neurological and psychomotor abnormalities, observed in AIDS patients. HIV mutates rapidly, new strains are continually developing. There are two types of HIV – HIV 1 and HIV 2, which exceeds 50 per cent.

The virus is easily killed by heat. It is readily inactivated by ether, acetone, ethanol (20 per cent) and beta–propiolactone (1:400 dilution), but is relatively resistant to ionizing radiation and ultraviolet light *(12)*.

(b) RESERVOIR OF INFECTION : These are cases and carriers. Once a person is infected, the virus remains in the body life-long. The risk of developing AIDS increases with time. Since HIV infection can take years to manifest itself, the symptomless carrier can infect other people for years.

(c) SOURCE OF INFECTION : The virus has been found in greatest concentration in blood, semen and CSF. Lower concentrations have been detected in tears, saliva, breast milk, urine, and cervical and vaginal secretions. HIV has also been isolated in brain tissue, lymph nodes, bone marrow cells and skin *(13)*.

2. Host factors

(a) AGE : Most cases have occurred among sexually active persons aged 20–49 years. This group represents the most productive members of the society, and those responsible for child-bearing and child-rearing.

(b) SEX : In North America, Europe and Australia, about 51 per cent of cases are homosexual or bisexual men. In Africa, the picture is very different; the sex ratio is equal. Certain sexual practices increase the risk of infection more than others, e.g., multiple sexual partners, anal intercourse, and male homosexuality. Higher rate of HIV infection is found in prostitutes.

(c) HIGH-RISK GROUPS : Male homosexuals and bisexuals, heterosexual partners (including prostitutes), intravenous drug abusers, transfusion recipients of blood and blood products, haemophiliacs and clients of STD.

Immunology

The immune system disorders associated with HIV infection/AIDS are considered to occur primarily from the gradual depletion in a specialised group of white blood cells (lymphocytes) called T–helper or T–4 cells. The full name of T–helper cell is CD4 + T lymphocyte and is also commonly known as CD4 + cell. These cells play a key role in regulating the immune response.

HIV selectively infects T–helper cells apart from several other cells in the immune system such as B–cells, microphages and nerve cells. When the virus reproduces, the infected T–helper cells are destroyed. Consequently people with AIDS tend to have low overall white blood cell count *(14)*. Whereas healthy individuals have twice as many "helper" cells as "suppressor" cells, in the AIDS patients the ratio is reversed. A decreased ratio of T–helper to T–suppressor cells may be an indirect indicator of reduced cellular immunity. One of the most striking features of the immune system of patients with AIDS is profound lymphopenia, with a total lymphocyte count often below 500/cu. mm. It is the alteration in T–cell function that is responsible for the development of neoplasms, the development of opportunistic infections, or the inability to mount a delayed–type hypersensitivity response. The lack of an obvious immunological response by the host to the virus is one of the problems confronting scientists *(15)*. That is, those with antibodies to HIV, usually will have too few of HIV antibodies, and these antibodies are also ineffective against the virus.

Mode of transmission

The causative virus is transmitted from person-to-person, most frequently through sexual activity. The basic modes of transmission are :

(a) Sexual transmission

AIDS is first and foremost a sexually transmitted disease. Any vaginal, anal or oral sex can spread AIDS. Every single act of unprotected intercourse with an HIV–infected person exposes the uninfected partner to the risk of infection. The size of the risk is affected by a number of factors, including the presence of STD, the sex and age of the uninfected partner, the type of sexual act, the stage of illness of the infected partner, and the virulence of the HIV strain involved. A European study of heterosexual couples in which only one partner was infected at the start, suggests that chances of transmission of HIV infection from male to female is twice as likely as from female to male *(16)*. Generally, women are more vulnerable to HIV infection because a larger surface is exposed, and semen contains higher concentration of HIV than vaginal or cervical fluids.

Anal intercourse carries a higher risk of transmission than vaginal intercourse because it is more likely to injure tissues of the receptive partner. For all forms of sex, the risk of transmission is greater where there are abrasions of the skin or mucous membrane. For vaginal sex the risk is greater when woman is menstruating.

Exposed adolescent girls and women above 45 years of age are more prone to get HIV infection. In teenagers the cervix is thought to be less efficient barrier to HIV than in mature genital tract of adult women. The thinning of mucosa at menopause is believed to lessen the protective effect. The production of mucus in the genital tract of adolescent girls and in postmenopausal women is not as prolific as in women between these life stages and this may also enhance their susceptibility to HIV infection.

An STD in either the HIV–negative or the HIV–positive partner facilitates the transmission of HIV. The risk of transmission is 8–10 times higher. If an STD, such as syphilis, chancroid or herpes, causes ulceration in the genital or perineal region of the uninfected partner, it becomes far easier for HIV to pass into his or her tissues. An STD causes inflammation. T–cells and monocytes/macrophages, get concentrated in the genital area. In a person already infected with HIV, some of these key cells of the immune system will be carrying the virus – which magnifies the risk of transmission to the uninfected partner.

As for HIV–infected people, they are more infectious to others in the very early stages, before antibody production i.e. during the "window period", and when the infection is well advanced, because levels of virus in the blood at that time is higher than at other times.

(b) Blood contact

AIDS is also transmitted by contaminated blood – transfusion of whole blood cells, platelets and factors VIII and IX derived from human plasma. There is no evidence that transmission ever occurred through blood products such as albumin, immunoglobulins or hepatitis vaccines that meet WHO requirements *(12)*. Contaminated blood is highly infective when introduced in large quantities directly into the blood stream. The risk of contracting HIV infection from transfusion of a unit of infected blood is estimated to be over 95 per cent. Since the likelihood of HIV transmission through blood depends on the "dose" of virus injected, the risk of getting infected through a contaminated needle, syringe or any other skin–piercing instrument is very much lower than with transfusion. Nevertheless, among drug users who inject heroin, cocaine or other drugs, this route of transmission is significant because exposure is repeated so often, in some cases, several times a day. As a result, needle–sharing by drug users is a major cause of AIDS in many countries, both developed and developing, and in some it is the predominant cause. Any skin piercing (including injections, ear-piercing, tattooing, accupuncture or scarification) can transmit the virus, if the instruments used have not been sterilized and have previously been used on an infected person. It may be mentioned that transfusion of blood and blood products has played a minor role in the spread of AIDS in the developed countries.

(c) Maternal–foetal transmission : mother-to child transmission

HIV may pass from an infected mother to her foetus, through the placenta or to her infant during delivery or by breast-feeding. In the absence of any intervention, rates of this form of transmission can vary from 20–25 per cent. Transmission during the peripartum period accounts for one-third to two-thirds of overall numbers infected, depending on whether breast-feeding transmission occurs or not, and this period has, therefore, become a focus of prevention efforts. The risk of infection is higher if the mother is newly infected, or if she has already developed AIDS. HIV infected infants and children progress rapidly to AIDS.

Transmission of HIV from mother to child can be prevented almost entirely by anti-retroviral drug prophylaxis, elective caesarean section before onset of labour and rupture of membranes, and by refraining from breast-feeding. However, in economically poor countries, elective caesarean section is not a safe option. A substantial efficacy of triple combination of drugs has been shown in industrialized countries, where the rate of transmission is now below 2 per cent in the absence of breast-feeding *(8)*.

There is no evidence that HIV is transmitted through mosquitoes or any other insect, casual social contact with infected persons including within households, or by food or water. There is no evidence of spread to health care workers in their professional contact with people with AIDS *(17)*.

Incubation period

While the natural history of HIV infection is not yet fully known, current data suggest that the incubation period is uncertain, (from a few months to 10 years or even more) from HIV infection to the development of AIDS. The virus can lie silent in the body for many years. The percentage of people infected with HIV, who will develop clinical disease remains uncertain – possibly 10–30 per cent will develop AIDS, and another 25–30 per cent will develop AIDS–related complex. However, it is estimated that 75 per cent of those infected with HIV will develop AIDS by the end of ten years *(18)*.

Clinical manifestations

The clinical features of HIV infection have been classified into four broad categories *(15)* :

I. Initial infection with the virus and development of antibodies
II. Asymptomatic carrier state
III. AIDS–related complex (ARC)
IV. AIDS.

(I) INITIAL INFECTION

Except for a generally mild illness (fever, sore throat and rash) which about 70 per cent of people experience a few weeks after initial infection with the virus, most HIV – infected people have no symptoms for the first five years or so. They look healthy and feel well although right from the start they can transmit the virus to others. Once infected, people are infected for life. Scientists have not found as yet, a way of curing them, or making them uninfectious to others.

HIV antibodies usually take between 2 to 12 weeks to appear in the blood-stream, though they have been known to take longer. The period before antibodies are produced is the "window period" during which, although the person is particularly infectious because of the high concentration of virus in the blood, he will test negative on the standard antibody blood test. Though the body's immune system reacts to the invasion of HIV by producing antibodies, these do not inactivate the virus in the usual way.

(II) ASYMPTOMATIC CARRIER STATE

Infected people have antibodies, but no overt signs of disease, except persistent generalized lymphadenopathy. It is not clear how long the asymptomatic carrier state lasts.

(III) AIDS-RELATED COMPLEX

A person with ARC has illnesses caused by damage to the immune system, but without the opportunistic infections (Fig. 4) and cancers associated with AIDS, they may exhibit

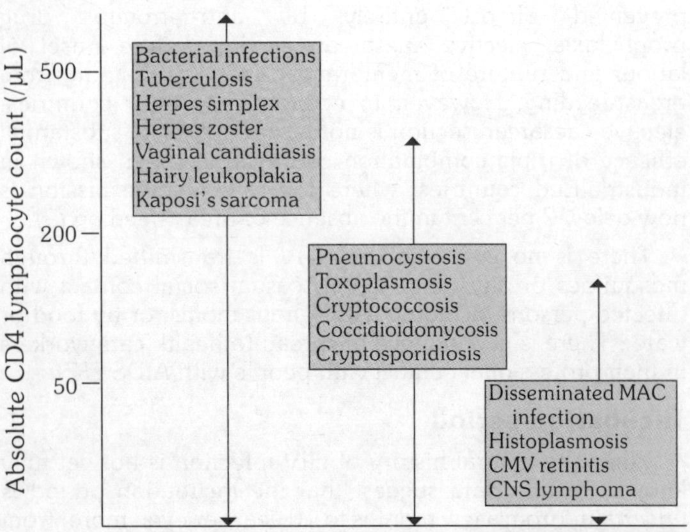

FIG. 4
Relationship of CD4 count to development of opportunistic infection

Source : *(19)*

one or more of the following clinical signs; unexplained diarrhoea lasting longer than a month, fatigue, malaise, loss of more than 10 per cent body weight, fever, night sweats, or other milder opportunistic infections such as oral thrush, generalized lymphadenopathy or enlarged spleen. Patients from high-risk groups who have two or more of these manifestations (typically including generalised lymphadenopathy), and who have a decreased number of T–helper lymphocytes are considered to have AIDS-related complex *(1)*. Some patients with AIDS-related complex, subsequently develop AIDS.

(IV) AIDS

AIDS is the end–stage of HIV infection. A number of opportunist infections commonly occur at this stage (Fig. 2), and/or cancers that occur in people with otherwise unexplained defects in immunity. Death is due to uncontrolled or untreatable infection. Tuberculosis and Kaposi sarcoma are usually seen relatively early. Serious fungal infections such as *Candida oesophagitis*, *Cryptococcus meningitis* and *penicillosis,* and parasitic infections such as *Pneumocystis carinni* pneumonia or *Toxoplasma gondii* encephalitis tend to occur, when T–helper cell count has dropped to around 100. People whose counts are below 50 have the late opportunistic infections such as *cytomegaloviral retinitis.*

Many people with AIDS are affected by a wasting syndrome that is known, especially in Africa, as "slim disease". It involves chronic diarrhoea and severe weight loss. Another condition, seen worldwide, is AIDS encephalopathy or AIDS dementia, which is caused by HIV crossing "blood–brain barrier". In its late stages, AIDS encephalopathy resembles senile dementia or Alzheimer's disease. AIDS dementia appears to result not from opportunistic infection, but from the action of the virus itself.

TUBERCULOSIS. An alarming factor in the AIDS epidemic is the increasing link between HIV infection and tuberculosis. In countries where tuberculosis is endemic, many people are infected in childhood. When the immune system breaks down, as in HIV infection, tuberculosis becomes active and the person becomes contagious to others. Studies in Rwanda, the USA, Zaire and Zambia found that HIV–positive individuals were 30–50 times more likely to develop active tuberculosis than HIV–negative people. As a consequence, AIDS is reviving an old problem in developed countries e.g. in the USA, where there was sudden increase in tuberculosis cases. The situation in developing countries is still worst.

The emergence of drug resistance makes it essential that antibiotic sensitivity be performed on all positive cultures. Drug therapy should be individualized. Patients with multi drug resistance should receive atleast three drugs to which their organism is sensitive *(19)*.

PERSISTENT GENERALIZED LYMPHADENOPATHY. Lymph nodes are larger than one centimetre in diameter, in two or more sites other than the groin area for a period of at least three months.

KAPOSI SARCOMA. A tumour featuring reddish brown or purplish plaques or nodules on the skin and mucous membranes. Endemic in Africa prior to HIV, it used to affect mainly older men. With HIV infection it affects a wider age range and both sexes, and is characterized by lesions in the mouth or gut; or lesions are generalized (in two or more places) or rapidly progressive or invasive.

OROPHARYNGEAL CANDIDIASIS. Caused by a common yeast fungus, oral thrush presents with soreness and redness, with white plaques on the tongue, and in the mouth and throat; and sometimes a white fibrous layer covering the tonsils and back of the mouth. Infection of the oesophagus presents with pain behind the breastbone.

CYTOMEGALOVIRUS RETINITIS. Inflammation of the eye retina which may lead to blindness.

PNEUMOCYSTOSIS CARINII PNEUMONIA. Symptoms can include a dry, non-productive cough; inability to take a full breath and occasional pain on breathing; and weight loss and fever.

TOXOPLASMA ENCEPHALITIS. Protozoal infection in the central nervous system, presenting with focal neurological signs such as mild hemiplegia or stroke, resulting from damage to part of the brain, seizures or altered mental status.

HAIRY LEUKOPLAKIA. White patches on the sides of the tongue, in vertical folds resembling corrugations.

CRYPTOCOCCAL MENINGITIS. A fungal infection in the central nervous system which usually presents with fever, headache, vomiting and neck stiffness.

HERPES-ZOSTER OR SHINGLES. Viral inflammation of the central nervous system, presenting with localised pain and burning sensations, followed by vesicle eruption (skin blistering) and ulceration.

SEVERE PRURIGO OR PRURITIC DERMATITIS. Chronic skin inflammation in the form of a very itchy rash of small flat spots developing into blisters.

SEVERE OR RECURRENT SKIN INFECTIONS. Warts; dermatophytosis or ringworm; and folliculitis (inflammation of hair follicles).

DIAGNOSIS OF AIDS

CLINICAL

I. WHO case definition for AIDS surveillance

For the purposes of AIDS surveillance an adult or adolescent (>12 years of age) is considered to have AIDS if at least 2 of the following major signs are present in combination with at least 1 of the minor signs listed below, and if these signs are not known to be due to a condition unrelated to HIV infection *(20)*.

Major signs
- weight loss ≥ 10% of body weight
- chronic diarrhoea for more than 1 month
- prolonged fever for more than 1 month (intermittent or constant).

Minor signs
- persistent cough for more than 1 month[a, b]
- generalized pruritic dermatitis
- history of herpes zoster[b]
- oropharyngeal candidiasis
- chronic progressive or disseminated herpes simplex infection
- generalized lymphadenopathy.

The presence of either generalized Kaposi sarcoma or cryptococcal meningitis is sufficient for the diagnosis of AIDS for surveillance purposes.

a. For patients with tuberculosis, persistent cough for more than 1 month should not be considered as a minor sign
b. Indicates changes from the 1985 provisional WHO clinical case definition for AIDS ("Bangui definition")

The clinical definition is relatively *specific* (if used correctly), meaning that the vast majority of people diagnosed as having AIDS will have been correctly assessed. However, studies show that the definition is relatively *insensitive*, meaning that only half the patients who have severe illness related to HIV infection are included. This is because not all HIV–related opportunistic diseases are in the AIDS definition. Tuberculosis is widely recognized as the commonest opportunistic disease associated with HIV in Africa. But because TB causes wasting, cough and fever in most patients, the AIDS clinical case definition cannot reliably distinguish between HIV–positive and HIV–negative TB patients.

The clinical case definition was developed to enable reporting of the number of people with AIDS for the purposes of public health surveillance, rather than for patient care. However, for the purpose of individual case management, it is useful to be able to diagnose whether illnesses may be related to HIV infection (symptomatic HIV infection) because :

- clinical manifestations can be a reliable indicator of underlying HIV infection;
- over-use of HIV testing is avoided, testing is used to confirm suspected HIV infection, rather than as a diagnostic tool in the first instance;
- a patient with suspected HIV infection can be counselled about having an HIV test, the implications for them and their sexual partners, self-care and nutrition;
- many HIV–related illnesses can be treated, improving the patient's quality of life;
- certain drugs (such as thiacetazone) cause severe side effects in people with HIV infection, and should not be prescribed for them.

Children *(21)*

The case definition for AIDS is fulfilled if at least 2 major signs and 2 minor signs are present (if there is no other known cause of immunosuppression).

Major signs
- weight loss or abnormally slow growth
- chronic diarrhoea for more than 1 month
- prolonged fever for more than 1 month.

Minor signs
- generalized lymph node enlargement
- oropharyngeal candidiasis
- recurrent common infections, e.g. ear infection, pharyngitis
- persistent cough
- generalized rash

Confirmed HIV infection in the mother counts as a minor criterion.

The definition for children is not very specific, particularly in poor regions where childhood malnutrition and TB are common. Further, many children present with acute HIV-related illness such as *pneumocystis carinii pneumonia* without any clinical evidence of AIDS.

II. Expanded WHO case definition for AIDS surveillance

For the purposes of AIDS surveillance an adult or adolescent (>12 years of age) is considered to have AIDS if a test for HIV antibody gives a positive result, and one or more of the following conditions are present :

- ≥ 10% body weight loss or cachexia, with diarrhoea or fever, or both, intermittent or constant, for at least 1 month, not known to be due to a condition unrelated to HIV infection
- cryptococcal meningitis
- pulmonary or extra–pulmonary tuberculosis
- Kaposi sarcoma
- neurological impairment that is sufficient to prevent independent daily activities, not known to be due to a condition unrelated to HIV infection (for example, trauma or cerebrovascular accident)
- candidiasis of the oesophagus (which may be presumptively diagnosed based on the presence of oral candidiasis accompanied by dysphagia)
- clinically diagnosed life–threatening or recurrent episodes of pneumonia, with or without aetiological confirmation
- invasive cervical cancer.

Major features of this expanded surveillance case definition are that it requires an *HIV serological test,* and includes a broader spectrum of clinical manifestations of HIV such as tuberculosis, neurological impairment, pneumonia, and invasive cervical cancer. The expanded definition is simple to use and has a higher specificity *(20)*.

CLINICAL STAGING

WHO clinical staging system for HIV infection and HIV-related disease *(21)*

WHO has developed a clinical staging system (originally for prognosis), based on clinical criteria. The definition of symptoms, signs and diseases is according to clinical judgement. Clinical condition or performance score, whichever is the higher, determines whether a patient is at clinical stage 1, 2, 3, or 4 as shown in Table 3. Clinical stage is important as a criterion for starting antiretroviral (ARV) therapy.

TABLE 3

WHO clinical staging of HIV disease in adults and adolescents

Clinical stage 1

Asymptomatic
Persistent generalized lymphadenopathy

Clinical stage 2

Moderate unexplained weight loss (under 10% of presumed or measured body weight)
Recurrent respiratory tract infections (sinusitis, tonsillitis, otitis media, pharyngitis)
Herpes zoster
Angular cheilitis
Recurrent oral ulcerations
Papular pruritic eruptions
Seborrheic dermatitis
Fungal nail infections

Clinical stage 3

Unexplained severe weight loss (over 10% of presumed or measured body weight)
Unexplained chronic diarrhoea for longer than 1 month
Unexplained persistent fever (intermittent or constant for longer than 1 month)
Persistent oral candidiasis
Oral hairy leukoplakia
Pulmonary tuberculosis
Severe bacterial infections (e.g. pneumonia, empyema, meningitis, pyomyositis, bone or joint infection, bacteraemia, severe pelvic inflammatory disease)
Acute necrotizing ulcerative stomatitis, gingivitis or periodontitis
Unexplained anaemia (below 8 g/dl), neutropenia (below 0.5 x 10^9/l) and/or chronic thrombocytopenia (below 50 x 10^9/l)

Clinical stage 4

HIV wasting syndrome[a]
Pneumocystis jiroveci pneumonia
Recurrent severe bacterial pneumonia
Chronic herpes simplex infection (orolabial, genital or anorectal of more than 1 month's duration or visceral at any site
Oesophageal candidiasis (or candidiasis of trachea, bronchi or lungs)
Extrapulmonary tuberculosis
Kaposi sarcoma
Cytomegalovirus disease (retinitis or infection of other organs, excluding liver, spleen and lymph nodes)
Central nervous system toxoplasmosis
HIV encephalopathy[b]
Extrapulmonary cryptococcosis including meningitis
Disseminated non-tuberculous mycobacteria infection
Progressive multifocal leukoencephalopathy
Chronic cryptosporidiosis
Chronic isosporiasis
Disseminated mycosis (histoplasmosis, coccidiomycosis)
Recurrent septicaemia (including nontyphoidal Salmonella)
Lymphoma (cerebral or B cell non-Hodgkin)
Invasive cervical carcinoma
Atypical disseminated leishmaniasis
Symptomatic HIV-associated nephropathy or HIV-associated cardiomyopathy

[a] HIV wasting syndrome : weight loss > 10% of body weight, plus either unexplained diarrhoea for more than one month or chronic weakness, and unexplained fever for more than one month.

[b] HIV encephalopathy : clinical findings of disabling mental or motor dysfunction, interfering with activities of daily living, progressing over weeks and months, in the absence of a concurrent illness or condition other than HIV infection which could explain the findings.

Source : *(22, 23)*

Children

WHO clinical staging system for HIV infection and related disease in children

Stage 1 :
- Asymptomatic
- Persistent generalized lymphadenopathy

Stage 2 :
- Unexplained chronic diarrhoea
- Severe persistent or recurrent candidiasis outside the neonatal period
- Weight loss or failure to thrive
- Persistent fever
- Recurrent severe bacterial infections

Stage 3 :
- AIDS-defining opportunistic infections
- Severe failure to thrive
- Progressive encephalopathy
- Malignancy
- Recurrent septicaemia or meningitis.

Source : *(21)*

LABORATORY DIAGNOSIS

SCREENING TESTS : As antibodies to HIV are far easier to detect than the virus itself, their presence or absence in blood–stream is the basis for the most widely used test of HIV infection. A person whose blood contains HIV antibodies is said to be HIV–positive, or seropositive, meaning that he or she is infected with HIV. There is now a wide range of screening tests based on detection of HIV–antibodies. To be reliable, a screening test must be ***sensitive*** enough to identify all "true positives", while being ***specific*** enough to record few "false positives". The ideal test needs both the attributes.

At present, to ensure accuracy, two different tests are commonly applied. At first a sensitive test is used to detect the HIV–antibodies, while a second **confirmatory test** is used to weed out any false positive results. The first kind of test is normally the **ELISA**. The confirmatory test, usually a **Western Blot** is a highly specific test; it is based on detecting specific antibody to viral core protein (p24) and envelop glycoprotein (gp 41). This is a more difficult test to perform and requires trained and experienced laboratory workers to interpret the test.

VIRUS ISOLATION : A test for the virus itself would eliminate the painful uncertainty of AIDS infection. HIV can be recovered from cultured lymphocytes *(22)*. This type of testing is very expensive and requires extensive laboratory support.

The current trend in HIV–antibody tests is towards simple, cheap, reliable kits whose results can be read on the spot without much waiting and without the need for laboratory backup. HIV self testing kits are available in the market.

Non-specific laboratory findings with HIV infection may include anaemia, leukopenia (particularly lymphocytopenia) and thrombocytopenia in any combination, polyclonal hypergammaglobulinaemia. Cutaneous energy is frequent early in the course, and becomes universal as the disease progresses *(19)*.

Several laboratory markers are available to provide prognostic information and guide therapy decisions. The most widely used marker is the absolute CD4 lymphocyte count. As the count decreases, the risk of opportunistic infection increases. People with healthy immune system usually have more than 950 CD4 cells/μL of blood. The number falls over the course of HIV infection. People with

AIDS usually have CD4 cell count below 200 (USA makes CD cell count below 200 in an HIV–infected person a definition of AIDS). The trend of the count is much more important than any single reading. The frequency of performance of counts depends on the patient's health system. Some studies suggest that the percentage of CD4 lymphocytes is more reliable indicator of prognosis than the absolute count because the percentage does not depend on calculating a manual differential. Risk of progression to AIDS is high with percentage of CD4 lymphocyte less than 20 *(19)*.

The laboratory tests and their significance are as summarized in Table 4.

TABLE 4

Laboratory findings with HIV infection

Test	Significance
HIV enzyme-linked immunosorbent assay (ELISA)	Screening test for HIV infection. Sensitivity > 99.9%; to avoid false-positive results, repeatedly reactive results must be confirmed with Western blot.
Western blot	Confirmatory test for HIV. Specificity when combined with ELISA>99.99%. Indeterminate results with early HIV infection, HIV-2 infection, autoimmune disease, pregnancy and recent tetanus toxoid administration.
CBC	Anaemia, neutropenia, and thrombocytopenia common with advanced HIV infection.
Absolute CD4 lymphocyte count	Most widely used predictor of HIV progression. Risk of progression to an AIDS opportunistic infection or malignancy is high with CD4 < 200 cells/μL.
CD4 lymphocyte percentage	Percentage may be more reliable than the CD4 count. Risk of progression to an AIDS opportunistic infection or malignancy is high with percentage < 14%.
HIV viral load tests	These tests measure the amount of actively replicating HIV virus. Correlates with disease progression and response to antiretroviral drugs.
β_2 - Microglobulin	Cell surface protein indicative of macrophage – monocyte stimulation. Levels >3.5 mg/dL associated with rapid progression of disease. Not useful with intravenous drug users.
p24 antigen	Indicates active HIV replication. Tends to be positive prior to seroconversion and with advanced disease.

Source : *(19)*

The WHO has pointed out the danger of compulsory testing programmes in their tendency to social rejection of HIV–carrier and the resulting social and psychological consequences. Diagnostic testing may be useful in gauging the magnitude and course of the epidemic. It is a gateway to HIV prevention, treatment, care and other support services, including pre-test information and post-test counselling. The WHO five C's – consent, confidentiality, counselling, correct test results and connection to care and treatment – are principles that apply to all models of HIV testing services and in all circumstances.

Control of AIDS

There are four basic approaches to the control of AIDS :

1. Prevention

(a) EDUCATION

Until a vaccine or cure for AIDS is found, the only means at present available is health education to enable people to make life-saving choices (e.g., avoiding indiscriminate sex, using condoms). There is, however, no guarantee that the use of condoms will give full protection. One should also avoid the use of shared razors and toothbrushes. Intravenous drug users should be informed that the sharing of needles and syringes involves special risk. Women suffering from AIDS or who are at high risk of infection should avoid becoming pregnant, since infection can be transmitted to the unborn or newborn. Educational material and guidelines for prevention should be made widely available. All mass media channels should be involved in educating the people on AIDS, its nature, transmission and prevention; this includes international travellers.

(b) COMBINATION HIV PREVENTION *(24)*

Combination prevention programmes use a mix of biomedical, behavioural and structural interventions to meet the current HIV prevention needs of particular individuals and communities so as to have the greatest possible impact on reducing new infections.

ARV drugs play a key role in HIV prevention. People taking ART who achieve optimal viral suppression are extremely unlikely to pass HIV to sexual partners. ARV drugs taken by people without HIV as PrEP or PEP are highly effective in preventing HIV acquisition.

Other biomedical interventions that reduce HIV risk practices and/or the probability of HIV transmission per contact event include the following:

- *Male and female condoms and condom compatible lubricant* : male condoms are estimated to reduce heterosexual transmission by at least 80% and to offer 64% protection in anal sex among men who have sex with men, if used consistently and correctly. Fewer data are available for the efficacy of female condoms, but evidence suggests they can have a similar prevention effect.
- *Needle and syringe programmes* are highly associated with a reduction in HIV transmission through injecting drug use.
- *Opioid substitution therapy* with methadone or buprenorphine is the most effective form of treatment for opioid dependence and has the additional benefit of effectively reducing HIV risk behaviour and transmission through injecting drug use. Opioid substitution therapy also provides adherence support to people on ART.
- *Voluntary medical male circumcision (VMMC)* : three randomized clinical trials in Africa demonstrated an approximately 60% reduction in the risk of female-to-male sexual transmission. For high-burden settings, joint programme of WHO and United Nations on HIV/AIDS (UNAIDS) recommended the inclusion of VMMC as an additional important strategy for prevention of heterosexually acquired HIV infection in men.

(c) PREVENTION OF BLOOD-BORNE HIV TRANSMISSION

People in high-risk groups should be urged to refrain from donating blood, body organs, sperm or other tissues. All blood should be screened for HIV 1 & HIV 2 before transfusion. Transmission of infection to haemophiliacs can be reduced by introducing heat treatment of factors VIII and IX. Strict sterilization practices should be ensured in hospitals and clinics. Pre-sterilized disposable syringes and needles should be used as far as possible. One should avoid injections unless they are absolutely necessary.

2. Antiretroviral treatment

At present there is no vaccine or cure for treatment of HIV infection/AIDS. However, the development of drugs that suppress the HIV infection itself rather than its complications has been important development. These antiviral chemotherapy have proved to be useful in prolonging the life of severely ill patients.

The availability of agents in combination suppress HIV replication. It has a profound impact on the natural history of HIV infection. Patients who achieve excellent suppression of HIV generally have stabilization or improvement of their clinical course which results from partial immunologic reconstitution and a subsequent decrease in complications of immunosuppression. Concept about the timing of such therapy have changed considerably.

Classification of drugs used for ART *(19)*

The drugs used for ART are classified as :

Nucleoside reverse transcriptase inhibitors (NRTIs)
Abacavir (ABC) Didanosine (ddl) Emtricitabine (FTC) Lamivudine (3TC) Stavudine (d4T) Zidovudine (AZT)
Nucleotide reverse transcriptase inhibitors (NtRTIs)
Tenofovir (TDF)
Non-nucleoside reverese transcriptase inhibitors (NNRTIs)
Efavirenz (EFV) Etravirine (ETV) Nevirapine (NVP)
Protease inhibitors (PIs)
Atazanavir + ritonavir (ATV/r) Darunavir + ritonavir (DRV)r) Fos-amprenavir + ritonavir (FPV/r) Indinavir + ritonavir (IDV/r) Lopinavir/ritonavir (LPV/r) Saquinavir + ritonavir (SQV/r)
Integrase strand transfer inhibitors (INSTIs)
Raltegravir (RAL) Dolutegravir (DTG)
Fusion inhibitors
Enfuvirtide (T-20, Fuzeon)

HIV care and management recommendations (NACO 2021) *(23)*

Antiretroviral therapy (ART) in adults and adolescents

There has been a rapid decline in HIV-related mortality and morbidity due to the wider availability of affordable, more efficacious and less toxic ARVs over the last two decades. ART consists of the use of a combination of at least three ARV drugs from different classes to inhibit the replication of HIV and reduce viraemia to undetectable levels. Continued suppression of viral replication leads to the restoration of immune response, reflected by an increase in the CD4 count. Increase in CD4 count leads to slowing of the disease progression, reduced frequency of OIs, improvement in the quality of life and increased longevity. Successes achieved by ART have now transformed the perception about HIV infection from being a 'virtual death sentence' to a 'chronic manageable illness'. ART was earlier known as Highly Active ART (HAART) and as combination ART (cART).

Since 2016, WHO recommended that all people living with HIV be provided with lifelong ART, including children, adolescents and adults, pregnant and breast-feeding women, regardless of clinical status or CD4 cell count. The current HIV treatment guidelines include new ARV options with better tolerability, higher efficacy, and lower rates of treatment discontinuation when compared with previous recommended medicines.

The goals of ART are as follows (23) :

Clinical goals	Increased survival and improvement in quality of life
Virological goals	Greatest possible sustained reduction in viral load
Immunological goals	Immune reconstitution, that is, both quantitative and qualitative
Therapeutic goals	Rational sequencing of drugs in a manner that achieves clinical, virological and immunological goals while maintaining future treatment options, limiting drug toxicity and facilitating adherence
Preventive goals	Reduction of HIV transmission by suppression of viral load

Rapid ART initiation for newly diagnosed PLHIV at ART centre

The introduction of the 'Treat All' recommendation supports the rapid initiation of ART, including the offer of same-day initiation where there is no clinical contraindication. Rapid ART initiation is defined as "ART initiation within seven days from the day of HIV diagnosis". Following a confirmed HIV diagnosis and clinical assessment, same-day /rapid ART initiation should be offered to all PLHIV adequately prepared and ready for initiation. However, if an active OI is present, ART initiation may be deferred as required.

PLHIV should be assessed for readiness for ART initiation using the algorithm provided in Fig. 5 (with concurrent sample collection for CD4 testing and baseline investigation). This algorithm focusses on clinical screening of PLHIV for potential presence of common OIs/advanced HIV disease/comorbid conditions.

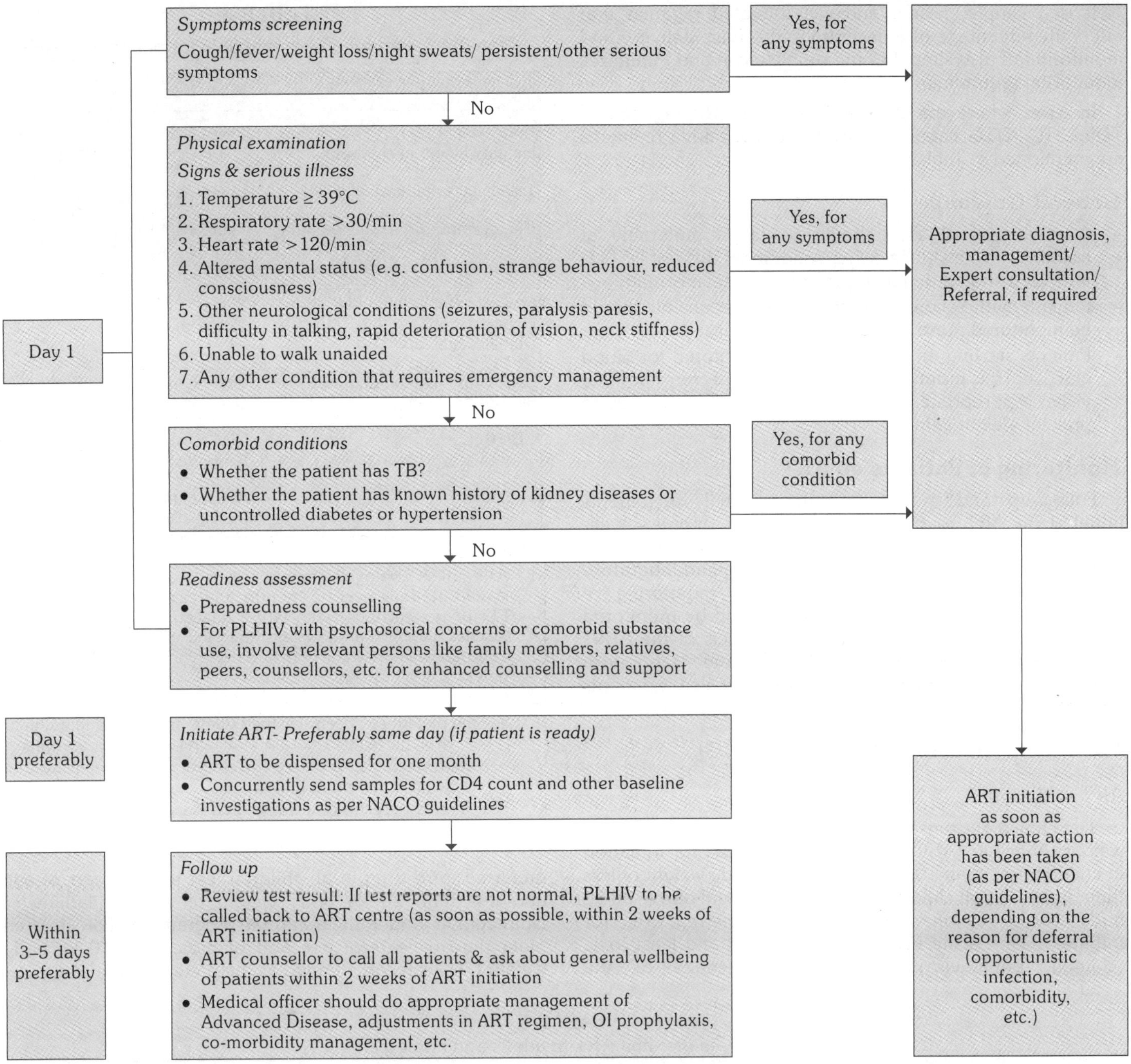

FIG. 5

Rapid ART initiation algorithm in PLHIV

Source : *(23)*

Antiretroviral Therapy Regimens *(23)*

Fixed-dose combinations (FDCs) of ARVs are preferred because they are easy to prescribe and easy for patients to take, thereby facilitating improved and desirable treatment adherence. This is essential for PLHIV as the treatment is life-long and we need to minimize the chance of developing drug-resistant mutants in their body and the resultant treatment failure. Further, FDCs have distinct advantages in drug procurement and distribution, essentially the drug stock management itself. National experience has shown that regimens with FDCs are more acceptable, well tolerated and adequately complied with.

The basic principle for first-line ART for treatment-naive adult and adolescent patients is to use a triple drug combination from two different classes of ARVs.

The first-line ART essentially comprises of a NRTI backbone, preferably Non-Thymidine (Tenofovir plus Lamivudine) and one INSTI, preferably DTG. Based on the evidence supporting better efficacy and fewer side effects, the preferred first-line ART regimen for all PLHIV with age >10 years and weight >30kg is as follows :

Tenofovir (TDF 300 mg) + Lamivudine (3TC 300 mg) + Dolutegravir (DTG 50 mg) regimen (TLD) as FDC in a single pill once a day (at a fixed time every day as per patient's convenience).

This regimen has the advantage of harmonization in the treatment of all adults, adolescents, pregnant women including those with HIV-1, HIV-2, HIV-1 & 2, women exposed to single dose nevirapine in the past and those co-infected with TB or Hepatitis.

It is a simple, potent and well-tolerated regimen that offers the advantage of a decentralized service delivery and monitoring. It also simplifies the supply chain and minimizes monitoring requirements.

In cases where the preferred first-line ARV regimen of TDF+3TC+DTG cannot be used, the alternative regimens are mentioned in Table 5.

General Guidance

- A single pill of TLD should be taken preferably at bedtime, and instances where additional dose of DTG is indicated should be taken preferably in the morning.
- Patients with severe Diabetes and Hypertension should be monitored more closely for TDF toxicity.
- Patients starting on DTG should be monitored for blood glucose (six monthly) and weight gain (on monthly visits). Appropriate physical activity should be advised to prevent weight gain.

Monitoring of Patients on ART

Follow-up and monitoring are essential in patients initiated on ART to track clinical progress, monitor well-being and to identify adverse drug reactions and toxicities. ART monitoring includes clinical monitoring and laboratory monitoring. Clinical monitoring includes monitoring of adherence to ART as well. The client should be monitored every month for clinical progress, side effects of the ARVs and treatment adherence. Clinical and laboratory evaluations are carried out at specified intervals for patients on ART. Table 6 summarizes the monitoring tools *(23)*.

TABLE 6

Monitoring and follow-up schedule for patients on ART

Monitoring Tool	When to Monitor
Body weight Height / length in children	Every visit
Treatment adherence	Every visit
Clinical monitoring and T-staging	Every visit
4-symptom TB screening	Every visit
Screening for common NCD; Hypertension, Diabetes mellitus	Every 6 months or symptom directed
Laboratory evaluation based on ART regimen	Every 6 months or symptom directed
CD4 Count	CD4 must be done every 6 months*
Viral load	At 6 months, 12 months and then every 12 months**

**CD4 Count :*

1. As routine virological monitoring is available, CD4 testing should be done every 6 months and can be discontinued in PLHIV (except those with HIV-2 infection) when CD4 count reaches greater than 350 cells/mm^3 and viral load is less than 1000 copies/ml (when both tests are conducted at the same time).
2. CD4 monitoring should be restarted for any patient if
   a. the patient has been switched due to treatment failure, that is, virologic failure (Plasma Viral Load ≥ 1000 copies/ml); or
   b. when deemed necessary for clinical management by the clinician at any point in time.

** For patients on second/third-line ART, Plasma Viral Load testing to be done every 6 months.

Paediatric first-line ART regimens *(23)*

ART initiation

The choice of drugs depends on the child's age and body weight. Abacavir (ABC) is the preferred NRTI for initiation in children less than 10 years of age and body weight of less than 30 kg. For all children above 10 years and above 30 kg body weight, Tenofovir (TDF) is the preferred drug for initiation. This is the simplest, most potent and least toxic regimen. Lopinavir/ritonavir is recommended as the preferred third drug in all children less than 6 years of age and less than 20 kg body weight till the availability of Dolutegravir under the national programme. For children older than 6 years of age and of more than 20 kg body weight DTG is recommended as the preferred third drug.

TABLE 5

Alternate first-line ART in adults and adolescents

Condition	Alternate First-line Regimen
PLHIV with body weight <30 kg	ABC 600 mg + Lamivudine 300 mg, one tablet + DTG (50 mg) once daily in the morning or any fixed time every day as per patient's convenience
All patients with high (above ULN for laboratory) serum creatinine values (Calculate Creatinine clearance)	ABC 600 mg OD, Lamivudine (as per creatinine clearance**) and DTG 50 mg once daily in the morning or any fixed time every day as per patient's convenience
PLHIV on Rifampicin-containing ATT regimen	Tenofovir (300 mg) + Lamivudine (300 mg) + Dolutegravir (50 mg) - FDC one tablet once daily (in the morning or any fixed time every day as per patient's convenience) + Additional dose of DTG 50 mg to be provided (12 hours after taking their regular dose) until 2 weeks after completion of ATT
Women of childbearing potential who do not wish to take DTG-based ART after adequate and optimal counselling***	Tenofovir (300 mg) + Lamivudine (300 mg) + Efavirenz (600 mg) If Efavirenz is contraindicated (HIV-2/HIV-1&2/prior NNRTI exposure) then Tenofovir (300 mg) + Lamivudine (300 mg) + [Lopinavir (200 mg) + ritonavir (50 mg) twice daily]

* For all patients with high serum creatinine values (above ULN for laboratory), calculate creatinine clearance.

** Lamivudine, along with Abacavir, may be used in full dose if creatinine clearance is more than 30 ml per minute, with patient being closely monitored.

*** Women of childbearing potential receive full information and medical guidance that is appropriate to their situation and are supported in making an informed decision.

Source : *(23)*

First-line ART regimens for infants and children with HIV-1 and HIV-2 infection are as follows :

Particulars	Recommended Regimen
1. Age less than 6 years and body weight less than 20 kg	Abacavir + Lamivudine + Lopinavir/ritonavir (AL+LPV/r)
2. Age between 6 and 10 years and body weight between 20 kg and 30 kg	Abacavir + Lamivudine + Dolutegravir (ALD)
3. Age more than 10 years and body weight more than 30 kg	Tenofovir + Lamivudine + Dolutegravir (TLD)

Important considerations for ART regimens for infants and children include the availability of suitable paediatric drug formulations that can be taken in appropriate doses; simplicity of dose schedule; and the taste and palatability. All these are potential factors for better treatment adherence in young children. Fixed-dose combinations are increasingly available for younger children *(23)*.

Occupational HIV postexposure prophylaxis *(25)*

Postexposure prophylaxis (PEP) is recommended for healthcare personnel who have an occupational exposure to blood, tissue, or other body fluids that may contain human immunodeficiency virus (HIV). Types of exposure that might place healthcare personnel at risk for HIV infection include any of the following : (1) Percutaneous injury (e.g., a needlestick or cut with a sharp object); and (2) Contact of mucous membranes or non-intact skin (e.g., exposed skin that is chapped, abraded, or irritated due to dermatitis) with blood, tissue, or body fluids that are potentially infectious.

The following fluids are considered potentially infectious : (a) Semen and vaginal secretions; (b) Cerebrospinal fluid; (c) Synovial fluid; (d) Pleural fluid; (e) Peritoneal fluid; (f) Pericardial fluid; and (g) Amniotic fluid.

The following are not considered potentially infectious unless they are visibly bloody : (a) Faeces; (b) Nasal secretions; (c) Saliva; (d) Sputum; (e) Sweat; (f) Tears; (g) Urine; and (h) Vomitus.

Treatment recommendations

HIV PEP should be initiated as soon as possible after the exposure, preferably within hours. Do not delay administration of PEP while awaiting HIV test results of the source patient. The rationale behind this practice includes the following : (a) Animal studies demonstrate that PEP is likely to be less effective when started more than 72 hours after exposure; (b) In the abscence of PEP, HIV replication occurs within 48 to 72 hours in regional lymph nodes close to the site of exposure, followed by viremia within 72 to 120 hours of virus inoculation; (c) If PEP initiation is delayed, the benefits might not outweigh the risks inherent in taking antiretroviral medications; and (d) Initiating therapy after a longer interval (eg, 1 week) might still be considered for exposures that represent an extremely high risk for transmission.

Preferred regimens

- Raltegravir 400 mg twice daily plus tenofovir disoproxil fumarate/emtricitabine (300 mg–200 mg) once daily for 4 weeks.
- Dolutegravir 50 mg once daily plus tenofovir disoproxial fumarate/emtricitabine (300 mg–200 mg) once daily for 4 weeks.

Lamivudine may be substituted for tenofovir disoproxial fumarate/emtricitabine in either regimen.

Since August 2019, dolutegravir has been considered an acceptable alternative to raltegravir in patients who intend to become pregnant and those who initiate therapy during the first trimester. However, patients should be advised of the small risk for teratogenicity when administered in the first trimester. There is no known elevated risk beyond the first trimester of pregnancy. Non-pregnant individuals of childbearing potential should be counseled about the need for birth control while completing a PEP regimen.

Use of co-trimoxazole prophylaxis for HIV-related infections *(24)*

Co-trimoxazole is a fixed dose combination of two antimicrobial drugs (sulfamethoxazole and trimethoprim) that covers a variety of bacterial, fungal and protozoan infections. The therapy is feasible, well tolerated and inexpensive intervention for people living with HIV to reduce HIV-related morbidity and mortality. The WHO recommendations (2016) for the use of co-trimoxazole is summarized in Table 7.

TABLE 7

Use of co-trimoxazole for HIV related infections, WHO (2016)

Adults (including pregnant women)
Co-trimoxazole prophylaxis is recommended for severe or advanced HIV clinical disease (WHO stage 3 or 4) and/or for a CD4 count ≤ 350 cells/mm³. – In settings where malaria and/or severe bacterial infections are highly prevalent, co-trimoxazole prophylaxis should be initiated regardless of CD4 cell count or WHO stage. Co-trimoxazole prophylaxis may be discontinued in adults (including pregnant women) with HIV infection who are clinically stable on antiretroviral therapy, with evidence of immune recovery and viral suppression. – In settings where malaria and/or severe bacterial infections are highly prevalent, co-trimoxazole prophylaxis should be continued regardless of CD4 cell count or WHO clinical stage.
Infants, children and adolescents
Co-trimoxazole prophylaxis is recommended for infants, children, and adolescents with HIV, irrespective of clinical and immune conditions. Priority should be given to all children younger than 5 years old regardless of CD4 cell count or clinical stage and to children with severe or advanced HIV clinical disease (WHO clinical stage 3 or 4) and/or those with CD4 ≤ 350 cells/mm³. – In settings with a high prevalence of malaria and/or severe bacterial infections, co-trimoxazole prophylaxis should be continued until adulthood irrespective of antiretroviral therapy provision. – In settings with low prevalence for both malaria and bacterial infections, co-trimoxazole prophylaxis may be discontinued for children 5 years of age and older who are clinically stable and/or virally suppressed on antiretroviral therapy for at least 6 months and CD4 > 350 cells/mm³.
HIV-exposed infants
Co-trimoxazole prophylaxis is recommended for HIV-exposed infants from 4–6 weeks of age and should be continued until HIV infection has been excluded by an age-appropriate HIV test to establish final diagnosis after complete cessation of breast-feeding. LPV/r is recommended as the preferred third drug for HIV post-exposure prophylaxis among children younger than 10 years. An age-appropriate alternative regimen can be identified among ATV/r, RAL, DRV, EFV and NVP.
HIV and TB coinfection
Routine co-trimoxazole prophylaxis should be administered to all HIV-infected people with active TB disease regardless of CD4 cell counts.

Source : *(24)*

HIV and Tuberculosis

Despite being preventable and curable, TB is the leading cause of HIV-associated mortality. Xpert MTB/RIF should be used rather than conventional microscopy, culture and drug susceptibility testing (DST) as the initial diagnostic test in adults and children suspected of having HIV-associated TB or multidrug resistant TB. Isoniazid preventive therapy and ART, given together, can reduce the risk of TB among people living with HIV by upto 97 per cent. For details, refer to page 235.

Monitoring the efficacy of ART

Efficacy is monitored by (20)

(a) clinical improvement
- gain in body weight,
- decrease in occurrence and severity of HIV-related diseases (infections and malignancies),

(b) increase in total lymphocyte count,

(c) improvement in biological markers of HIV (when available)
- CD4 + T-lymphocyte counts,
- plasma HIV RNA levels.

3. Specific prophylaxis

Until more effective antiviral therapy becomes available, the main aim of existing therapies will be to treat the manifestations of AIDS. Primary prophylaxis against *P. carinii* pneumonia should be offered to patients with CD4 count below 200 cells/μL. The regimens available are trimethoprim – sulfamethoxazole, aerosolized pentamidine and dapsone. Patients who develop *P. carinii* infection on a particular prophylactic regimen should be switched to the other drug or should receive a combination regimen.

M. avium complex occurs in at least one-third of AIDS patients. Rifabutin has been shown in a randomized trial to decrease the incidence of disseminated *Mavium–intracellulare* in persons with less than 200 CD4 cell/μL. Clinicians should make certain that patients do not have active *M. tuberculosis* infection before starting Rifabutin. Prophylaxis against *M. tuberculosis* is 300 mg isoniazid daily for 9 months to one year. It should be given to all HIV–infected patients with positive PPD reactions (defined for HIV–infected patients as more than 5 mm in induration). Kaposi's sarcoma might be treated in some stage with interferon, chemotherapy or radiation. Cytomegalovirus retinitis can be controlled by ganciclovir, cryptococcal meningitis with fluconazole. Esophageal candidiasis or recurrent vaginal candidiasis can be treated by fluconazole or ketoconazole. Herpes simplex infection and herpes zoster can be treated with acyclovir or foscamet.

4. Primary health care

Because of its wide–ranging health implications, AIDS touches all aspects of primary health care, including mother and child health, family planning and education. It is important, therefore, that AIDS control programmes are not developed in isolation. Integration into country's primary health care system is essential.

National AIDS Control Programme

Refer to chapter 7 for details.

References

1. WHO (1986). *Techn. Rep. Ser.*, 736.
2. UNAIDS (2022), *Fact Sheet, Global HIV statistics, 2022.*
3. WHO (2008), *Priority Interventions, HIV/AIDS Prevention Treatment and Care in the Health Sector,* August 2008, WHO HIV/AIDS Department.
4. WHO (2015), *From MDGs (Millennium Development Goals) to SDGs (Sustainable Development Goals).*
5. U.S. Global Health Policy (2012), *The Global HIV/AIDS Epidemic,* Fact Sheet, July 2012.
6. WHO (2016), *World Health Statistics,* 2016.
7. UNAIDS (2014), *Fast-Track : Ending the AIDS Epidemic by 2030,* Nov. 18, 2014.
8. WHO (2004), *The World Health Report 2004*, Changing History.
9. NACO/ICMR (2022), *India HIV estimates 2021*, Fact Sheet, Ministry of Health and Family Welfare, New Delhi.
10. UNAIDS (2018), *Country Fact Sheet, HIV/AIDS in India,* 2018.
11. Govt. of India (2022), *Annual Report 2021–2022,* Ministry of Health and Family Welfare, New Delhi.
12. WHO (1994), *AIDS,* Images of the Epidemics.
13. Population Reports (1986). *AIDS : A Public Health Crisis,* Sr. L, No.6, July–Aug 1986. The John Hopkins University, Baltimore, Maryland, USA.
14. Internet website :www.naco.nic.in/vsnaco/indiascene/update.
15. WHO (1985). *WHO Chronicle* 39 (6) 207–211 .
16. *British Medical Journal,* 1992, 304:809–813 .
17. WHO (1986). *Guidelines on AIDS in Europe,* WHO, Copenhagen .
18. P.N. Sehgal *Health For The Millions* Aug. 91 P–1, 8, 26.
19. Lawrence M. Tiercy et al. (2014), *Current Medical Diagnosis and Treatment,* 47th Ed., 2014, A Lange Medical Publication.
20. WHO (1994), *Weekly Epidemiological Record,* No.37, 16 Sept., 1994.
21. WHO (2004), *TB / HIV, A Clinical Manual,* 2nd Ed., Stop TB Department, Department of HIV / AIDS & Department of Child and Adolescent Health and Development.
22. WHO (2010), *Antiretroviral Therapy for HIV infection in Adults and Adolescents*, 2010 Revision, Recommendations for a Public Health Approach.
23. Govt. of India (2022), *National Guidelines for HIV care and Treatment 2021*, NACO, Ministry of Health and Family Welfare, New Delhi.
24. WHO (2016), *Consolidated Guidelines on the use of Antiretroviral Drugs for Treating and Preventing HIV Infection,* Recommendation for a Public Health Approach, 2nd Edition, 2016.
25. Medscape (2022), *HIV Postexposure prophylaxis occupational,* June 27, 2022.

EMERGING AND RE-EMERGING INFECTIOUS DISEASES

Today the world stands on the threshold of a new era in which hundreds of millions of people will be safe from some of the most terrible diseases. Soon poliomyelitis, neonatal tetanus, guineaworm disease, river blindness, Chagas' disease will join smallpox as diseases of the past. On the other hand, the world also stands on the brink of a global crisis in infectious diseases. No country is safe from them and no country can afford to ignore their threat any longer. The optimism of a relatively few years ago that many of these diseases could easily be brought under control has led to a tragic complacency among the international community. This complacency is now costing millions of lives. Today the infectious diseases are not only a health issue; they have become a social problem with tremendous consequences for the well-being of the individual and the world we live in.

Some infectious diseases once thought to be all but conquered, have returned with a vengeance. Others have developed stubborn resistance to antibiotic drugs. New and previously unknown diseases continue to emerge (Table 1). Together, these trends amount to a crisis for today and a challenge for the future.

The factors responsible for emergence and re-emergence of infectious diseases are : (1) unplanned and under-planned urbanization; (2) overcrowding and rapid population growth; (3) poor sanitation; (4) inadequate public health infrastructure; (5) resistance to antibiotics; (6) increased exposure of humans to disease vectors and reservoirs of infection in nature; (7) rapid and intense international travel; and (8) microbial genetic mutation.

Emerging diseases

During the past 30 years, at least 30 new diseases have emerged to threaten the health of hundreds of millions of people. For many of these diseases there is no treatment, cure or vaccine and the possibility of preventing or controlling them is limited.

Emerging infectious diseases are those whose incidence in humans has increased during the last two decades or which threaten to increase in the near future. The term also refers to newly–appearing infectious diseases, or diseases that are spreading to new geographical areas – such as cholera in South America and yellow fever in Kenya.

The diseases in question involve all the major modes of transmission – they are spread either from person to person, by insects or animals, or through contaminated water or food. The most dramatic example of a new disease is **COVID-19** in the year 2019. The ongoing COVID-19 pandemic has changed the whole world with virtual global lockdown, social distancing and use of mask as the only weapon against the uncontrolled spread of the disease. First case of COVID-19 was reported in the month of November, 2019 and on 11th March, 2020, it was declared a pandemic by the WHO. As of 20th Sept., 2022 about 618,141,427 cases with 6,533,467 deaths were reported worldwide. Although, now vaccines are available against COVID-19, the disease is yet to come under control. New strains of the virus are also now in circulation *(1)*.

Human Monkey pox, in May 2022 multiple cases of monkey pox were reported from several non-endemic countries. Studies are currently underway to further understand the epidemiology, source of infection and transmission patterns of the disease.

Tomato fever (tomatoflu), a virus infection has emerged in India in the state of Kerala in children younger than 5 years of age. It was first identified in Kollam district on May 6, 2022. Till date, this infection has been seen in the state of Odisha and Tamil Nadu along with Kerala. Tomato fever is so called because of the eruptions of red and painful blisters throughout the body. In the year 2007 also cases of tomato fever were reported in the state of Kerala.

AIDS, caused by the human immunodeficiency virus (HIV). The existence of the virus was unknown until 1983. About 38.4 million people are living with HIV globally in 2021. 1.5 million cases with 650,000 deaths were reported worldwide in 2021 *(2)*.

A new breed of deadly haemorrhagic fevers, of which **Ebola virus disease** (previously known as Ebola haemorrhagic fever) is the most notorious, has struck in Africa. Ebola appeared for the first time in Zaire and Sudan in 1976. Since then it has appeared periodically. Ebola virus is a member of Filoviridae family and comprises of 5 distinct species – Zaire ebolavirus; Reston ebolavirus; Sudan ebolavirus; Tai ebolavirus; and Bundibugyo ebolavirus. The recent epidemic started in December 2013 in Guinea and spread to South Africa. By 8th April 2015, a total of 25,515 cases have been reported with over 10,000 deaths. Case fatality rate may be as high as 70 per cent. Ebola has incubation period of 2–21 days, and is not infective during this period. Asymptomatic cases are also not infective. The virus is transmitted through direct contact with the blood, organs, body secretions or other body fluids of infected animals like chimpanzees, gorillas, monkeys, fruit bats etc. Human to human transmission is through blood or body fluids of an infected symptomatic person or through exposure to objects (such as needles) that have been contaminated with infected secretions. It is not transmitted through air, water or food. The illness is characterized by sudden onset of fever, intense weakness, muscle pain, headache, sore throat, vomiting, diarrhoea, rash, impaired kidney and liver functions and in some cases both internal and external bleeding. Currently there is no specific treatment for this disease. However, by intensive supportive care, the mortality can be reduced and spread of the disease can be prevented by instituting specific infection control measures. There is no vaccine against ebola *(3)*.

The United States has seen the emergence of **hantavirus** pulmonary syndrome, characterized by respiratory failure and a case fatality rate of over 50%. Since it was first recognized in 1993, this type of hantavirus infection has been detected in more than 20 states in that country, and has also surfaced in Argentina and Brazil. This hantavirus is carried by rodents, particularly deer mice. Other hantaviruses have been recognized for many years in Asia, where they cause haemorrhagic fever with renal involvement in humans.

Epidemics of foodborne and waterborne diseases due to new organisms such as cryptosporidium or new strains of bacteria such as ***Escherichia coli*** have hit industrialized and developing countries alike. The O157:H7 strain of *E.coli* was first reported in 1982 and has since then been implicated in many serious outbreaks of diarrhoeal illness, sometimes leading to kidney failure. The strain has been linked to undercooked hamburger beef and unpasteurized milk. A completely new strain of cholera, 0139, appeared in south–eastern India in 1992 and has since spread north and west to other areas of India, into western China, Thailand and other parts of South-East Asia.

The threat of a new global **influenza pandemic** is increasing. Major shifts in the make-up of influenza viruses occur every 20 years or so, triggering large epidemics in many parts of the world, and causing many thousands of deaths. The next such shift is expected to take place very soon. Epidemic strains of influenza viruses originate from China. The influenza virus is carried by ducks, chickens and pigs raised in close proximity to one another on farms. The exchange of genetic material between these viruses produces new strains, leading to epidemics of human influenza, each epidemic being due to a different strain. Currently avian H5N1 is the strain with pandemic potential, since it might adapt into a strain that is contagious among humans. Since 1997, 478 cases with 286 deaths have been reported to WHO. The first case was from Hong Kong. Other countries involved are Cambodia, Indonesia, Thailand and Viet Nam *(6)*. In late 2002, a new disease called **SARS** was reported from China with rapid spread to Hong Kong, Singapore, Viet Nam, Taiwan, and Toronto. During 2003, 8,422 SARS cases were reported from 30 countries with 916 fatalities *(7)*. More recently, pandemic due to influenza A (H1N1) 2009 strain is continuing worldwide involving 214 countries, already taking 18,156 lives. New strains such as those of cholera and influenza do not follow the usual pattern of being more common in younger people. They affect all age groups, since older people have not acquired immunity to them from previous infection.

Table 1 summarizes the aetiological agents and infectious diseases in humans and/or animals recognized since 1973. The year may differ from first appearance and first identification of cases.

TABLE 1

New infectious diseases recognized since 1973

Year	Agent	Type	Disease/Comments
1973	Rotavirus	Virus	Major cause of infantile diarrhoea worldwide
1975	Parvovirus B19	Virus	Aplastic crisis in chronic haemolytic anaemia
1976	*Cryptosporidium parvum*	Parasite	Acute and chronic diarrhoea
1977	*Ebola virus*	Virus	Ebola haemorrhagic fever
1977	*Legionella pneumophila*	Bacterium	Legionnaires' disease
1977	Hantaan virus	Virus	Haemorrhagic fever with renal syndrome (HRFS)
1977	*Campylobacter jejuni*	Bacterium	Enteric pathogen distributed globally
1980	Human T-lymphotropic virus 1 (HTLV-1)	Virus	T-cell lymphoma-leukaemia
1981	Toxin-producing strains of *Staphylococcus aureus*	Bacterium	Toxic shock syndrome
1982	*Escherichia coli 0157:H7*	Bacterium	Haemorrhagic colitis; haemolytic uraemic syndrome
1982	*Borrelia burgdorferi*	Bacterium	Lyme disease
1982	HTLV-2	Virus	Hairy cell leukaemia
1983	Human immunodeficiency virus (HIV)	Virus	Acquired immunodeficiency syndrome (AIDS)
1983	*Helicobacter pylori*	Bacterium	Peptic ulcer disease
1985	*Enterocytozoon bieneusi*	Parasite	Persistent diarrhoea
1986	*Cyclospara cayetanensis*	Parasite	Persistent diarrhoea
1986	BSE agent	Non-conventional agent	Bovine spongiform encephalopathy in cattle (Mad cow disease)
1988	Human herpes virus 6 (HHV-6)	Virus	Exanthem subitum
1988	*Hepatitis E virus*	Virus	Enterically transmitted non-A, non-B hepatitis
1989	Ehrlichia chaffeensis	Bacterium	Human ehrlichiosis
1989	*Hepatitis C virus*	Virus	Parenterally transmitted non-A, non-B liver hepatitis
1991	Guanarito virus	Virus	Venezuelan haemorrhagic fever
1991	*Encephalitozoon hellem*	Parasite	Conjunctivitis, disseminated disease
1991	*New species of Babesia*	Parasite	Atypical babesiosis
1992	*Vibrio cholerae 0139*	Bacterium	New strain associated with epidemic cholera
1992	*Bartonella henselae*	Bacterium	Cat-scratch disease; bacillary angiomatosis
1993	Sin Nambre virus	Virus	Hantavirus pulmonary syndrome
1993	*Encephalitozoon cuniculi*	Parasite	Disseminated disease
1994	Sabia virus	Virus	Brazilian haemorrhagic fever
1995	Human herpes virus 8	Virus	Associated with Kaposi's sarcoma in AIDS patients
1996	nvCJD Australian bat lyssavirus	Virus	–
1997	H5N1	Virus	Avian flu (Bird flu)
1999	Nipah virus	Virus	–
2003	Corona virus	Virus	SARS
2009	H1N1	Virus	Pandemic A (H1N1) 2009 influenza
2019	Corona virus	Virus	COVID-19 (SARS-CoV-2)

Source : *(4, 5)*

Re-emerging diseases

The term re-emerging diseases refers to the diseases which were previously easily controlled by chemotherapy and antibiotics, but now they have developed antimicrobial resistance and are often appearing in epidemic form.

The emergence of drug–resistant strains of microorganisms or parasites is promoted by treatments that do not result in cure. The increasing use of antimicrobials worldwide, often in subtherapeutic doses and sometimes in counterfeit form, indicates that this problem will increase in the foreseeable future. Changes in lifestyle, behaviour (including injecting and non–injecting drug use) and cultural or social values are behind the emergence of some infectious diseases such as syphilis. Increases in the number of sexual partners have been the main factor in the spread of HIV infection and other sexually transmitted diseases. Travel, including tourism, also plays a role. The spread of syphilis in the 18th and 19th centuries was related to the movement of armies. Today, the introduction of HIV in many parts of the world is due to greatly increased human mobility. Studies show that whereas only a few generations ago most people in their lifetime travelled no further than 40 kilometres from their birthplace, many today go up to 1,000 times further, travelling the whole world.

The practices of modern medicine also contribute. The spread of viral hepatitis is related in part to techniques such as kidney dialysis and multiple blood transfusions, as well as to other forms of transmission. Relaxation in immunization practices can quickly result in the resurgence of diseases, as, for example, the recent spread of diphtheria in the Russian Federation and other former republics of the USSR.

New animal diseases pose potential foodborne risks to human health that are sometimes difficult to evaluate or predict. An example that has caused much public concern in Europe is bovine spongiform encephalopathy ("mad cow disease"). Fears have grown that the infectious agent responsible may be passed through the food chain to cause a variant of the incurable Creutzfeldt–Jakob disease in humans, in which the brain is attacked. The British beef market has been seriously affected and stringent public health safeguards have been introduced.

The reasons for outbreaks of new diseases, or sharp increases in those once believed to be under control, are complex and still not fully understood. The fact is however, that national health has become an international challenge. An outbreak anywhere must now be seen as a threat to virtually all countries, especially those that serve as major hubs of international travel. Despite the emergence of new diseases in the last 30 years, there is still a lack of national and international political will and resources to develop and support the systems that are necessary to detect them and stop their spread. Without doubt diseases as yet unknown, but with the potential to be the AIDS of tomorrow, lurk in the shadows.

Antimicrobial resistance

Resistance by disease–causing organisms to antimicrobial drugs and other agents is a major public health problem worldwide. It is making a growing number of infections virtually untreatable, both in hospitals and in the general community. It is having a deadly impact on the control of diseases such as tuberculosis, malaria, cholera, dysentery and pneumonia.

Antimicrobial resistance is not a new problem, but it has worsened dramatically in the last decade. During that time, the pace of development of new antimicrobials has slowed down while the prevalence of resistance has grown at an alarming rate. The increase in the number of drug–resistant bacteria is no longer matched by a parallel expansion in the arsenal of agents used to treat infections. There is strong evidence that a major cause of the current crisis in antimicrobial resistance is the uncontrolled and inappropriate use of antibiotic drugs, in both industrialized and developing countries. They are used by too many people to treat the wrong kind of infection, in the wrong dosage and for the wrong period of time. The implications are awesome : drugs that cost tens of millions of dollars to produce, and take perhaps 10 years to reach the market, have only a limited life span in which they are effective. As resistance spreads, the life span shrinks; as fewer new drugs appear, the gulf widens between infection and control. So far, the pattern of excessive or inappropriate use and the development of resistance has been repeated after the introduction of each new antimicrobial. The over-use of expensive drugs designed to cover a range of infections is a particularly serious problem in industrialized countries. In developing countries, the problem is compounded by the ready availability of over-the-counter drugs. This allows patients to treat themselves, either with the wrong medicine, or in quantities that are too small to be effective. Sub-standard and counterfeit drugs which lack adequate amounts of active ingredients further exacerbate the resistance problem.

The examples of bacterial resistance are as follows :

Strains of *M.tuberculosis* resistant to anti-tuberculosis drugs are widespread, although attention has recently focused on the alarming outbreaks of tuberculosis caused by multidrug-resistant strains in the United States. Drug resistance is the result of poor prescribing practices, or poor patient compliance with treatment. It is low in the few countries with effective tuberculosis programmes. The most dangerous form of the multidrug-resistant disease occurs when cases become virtually incurable and doctors face situations similar to those of the pre-antibiotic era.

Malaria presents a double resistance problem : resistance of the *Plasmodium* parasites, which cause the disease, to antimalarial drugs; and resistance of the *Anopheles* mosquitoes, the vectors of the disease, to insecticides. The arsenal of antimalarial drugs is limited. Most of them act by killing parasites when they are multiplying in the blood stream of the human host. Unfortunately, due to inadequate regimens, poor drug supply, and poor quality and misuse of drugs, rapid development of drug resistance has occurred in most areas of the world. Drug resistance is particularly important in falciparum malaria, the most severe form of the disease. Resistance to chloroquine, the most commonly used drug, has been found in all endemic countries except those of Central America and the Caribbean. Resistance to multiple drugs is common in South–East Asia. This serious obstacle to malaria control efforts is further complicated by mosquito resistance to insecticides. Many mosquitoes are reported to be resistant to the three classes of insecticides available for public health use, and some are becoming resistant to pyrethroids, widely promoted for bed-net and curtain impregnation.

Enterococci contribute to some of the most common infections acquired in hospitals, causing intra-abdominal abscesses, endocarditis, and infections of the urinary tract and soft tissues. In some countries, infections resulting from strains resistant to the main groups of antibiotics, such as the beta–lactams and the aminoglycosides, can only be treated with vancomycin, an expensive intravenous drug. Even resistance to vancomycin has developed in the last 10 years or so. Staphylococci, which can contribute to skin infections, endocarditis, osteomyelitis, food poisoning and other serious disorders, have developed resistance to all antibiotics except vancomycin. If vancomycin–resistant strains were to emerge, some of the most prevalent hospital–acquired infections would become virtually untreatable.

Streptococci have become increasingly resistant to some antibiotics. They are among the most common disease–causing bacteria, responsible for infections of the throat, middle ear, skin and wounds, and also necrotizing fasciitis and gangrene. Pneumococci and *Haemophilus influenzae* are the most common bacteria causing acute respiratory infections in children, particularly pneumonia. Both of these organisms are becoming more and more resistant to drugs. Strains of pneumococci, once uniformly susceptible to penicillin, are currently resistant to it in up to 18% of cases in the United States and, 40% in South Africa. In addition, they are becoming resistant to many other commonly used antibiotics, including cotrimoxazole, the drug recommended by WHO for treatment of pneumonia. The most virulent type of *Haemophilus influenzae* is today frequently resistant to ampicillin, and strains have been identified that are resistant to other drugs, including cotrimoxazole. In brief, doctors worldwide are losing some of the most useful and affordable antibiotics against the two bacteria which are the major cause of death in children.

Neisseria gonorrhoeae, cause of one of the most common sexually transmitted diseases, has acquired such resistance to penicillin and tetracyclines in most countries that the use of these antibiotics to treat it has become unacceptable and this infection now requires the use of much more expensive drugs which are often unavailable.

Shigella dysenteriae has been causing outbreaks of severe diarrhoeal disease in central and southern Africa in recent years, including those in refugee camps, with the epidemic strain acquiring increasing resistance to standard antibiotics. Epidemic dysentery caused by this strain results in the death of up to 15% of those infected. *Salmonella typhi,* the bacterium responsible for typhoid fever, has developed resistance to antibiotics commonly used in the past for treatment. Resistant strains have caused outbreaks of the disease in India and Pakistan. Without effective antibiotic treatment, typhoid fever kills almost 10% of those infected. In South–East Asia, 50% or more of the strains of the bacteria may already be resistant to several antibiotics.

More than half of the antibiotics produced worldwide are used in animals, largely in subtherapeutic concentrations which favour the onset of drug resistance. As a result, two important human pathogens of animal origin, *E.coli* and salmonellae, are today highly resistant to antibiotics in both industrialized and developing countries. For instance, in the United Kingdom, the increase of multidrug–resistant strains of *Salmonella typhimurium* isolated from cattle is paralleled by increasing resistance among strains of human origin. In Thailand, salmonellae isolated from food animals are also highly resistant to the common antibiotics. These bacteria cause diarrhoeal disease and can lead to life-threatening complications. Due to the globalization of food supply and international travel, antimicrobial resistance among animal bacteria can affect consumers anywhere in the world.

Together, these factors have created perhaps the richest opportunities ever for the spread of infections, many of which become global problems that make the first line of defence – early recognition and adequate and timely response – essential.

Responding to epidemics

The process of response encompasses a multitude of activities including : diagnosis of the disease; investigation to understand the source of transmission; implementation of control strategies and programmes; research to develop adequate means to treat the disease and prevent its spread; and the production and distribution of the necessary drugs and vaccines.

The strategy for controlling re-emerging diseases is through available cost-effective interventions such as early diagnosis and prompt treatment, vector control measures and the prevention of epidemics, for malaria; and DOTS– directly observed treatment, short–course – for tuberculosis; by launching research initiatives for treatment regimens and improved diagnostics, drugs and vaccines; and above all by strengthening epidemiological surveillance and drug–resistance surveillance mechanisms and procedures with appropriate laboratory support for early detection, confirmation and communication.

The category of diseases – **"new diseases – new problems"**– such as Ebola and other viral haemorrhagic fevers, is probably the most frightening. The need, therefore, is for expanding research on infectious disease agents, their evolution, the vectors of disease spread and methods of controlling them, and vaccines and drug development. Much of this already applies to HIV/AIDS, one of the most serious diseases to emerge in recent decades.

References

1. Worldometer.info, *COVID-19 Corona virus pandemic*, 20th Sept. 2022.
2. UNAIDS (2022), *Fact Sheet, Global HIV Statistics*, 2022.
3. WHO (2014), *Fact Sheet on Ebola Viral Disease*, No. 103, Sept. 2014.
4. WHO (1996), *The World Health Report 1996*.
5. WHO (1999), *Removing Obstacles to Healthy Development*, WHO Report on Infectious Diseases.
6. WHO (2005), *Weekly Epidemiological Record* No. 49/50, 14th Oct., 2005.
7. WHO (2003), *World Health Report 2003*, Shaping the Future.

HOSPITAL-ACQUIRED INFECTION

Hospital-acquired infection is cross infection of one patient by another or by doctors, nurses and other hospital staff, while in hospital. A high frequency of nosocomial infection is evidence of a poor quality of health service delivery. Many factors contribute to the frequency of nosocomial infections: hospitalized patients are often immunocompromised, they undergo invasive examinations and treatments, and patient care practices and the hospital environment may facilitate the transmission of microorganisms among patients. The selective pressure of intense antibiotic use promotes antibiotic resistance. While progress in the prevention of nosocomial infections has been made, changes in medical practice continually present new opportunities for development of infection.

Definition of nosocomial infections

Nosocomial infections, also called "hospital-acquired infections", are infections acquired during hospital care which are not present or incubating at admission. Infections occurring more than 48 hours after admission are usually considered nosocomial. Definitions to identify nosocomial infections have been developed for specific infection sites (e.g. urinary, pulmonary).

Nosocomial infections may also be considered either endemic or epidemic. Endemic infections are most common. Epidemic infections occur during outbreaks, defined as an unusual increase above the baseline of a specific infection or infecting organism.

Changes in health care delivery have resulted in shorter hospital stays and increased outpatient care. It has been suggested that the term nosocomial infections should encompass infections occurring in patients receiving treatment in any health care setting. Infections acquired by staff or visitors to the hospital or other health care setting may also be considered nosocomial infections.

Simplified definitions may be helpful for some facilities without access to full diagnostic techniques. Table 1 provides definitions for common infections that could be used for surveys in facilities with limited access to sophisticated diagnostic techniques.

TABLE 1

Simplified criteria for surveillance of nosocomial infections

Type of nosocomial infection	Simplified criteria
Surgical site infection	Any purulent discharge, abscess, or spreading cellulitis at the surgical site during the month after the operation.
Urinary infection	Positive urine culture (1 or 2 species) with at least 10^5 bacteria/ml, with or without clinical symptoms.
Respiratory infection	Respiratory symptoms with at least two of the following signs appearing during hospitalization : – cough – purulent sputum – new infiltrate on chest radiograph consistent with infection.
Vascular catheter infection	Inflammation, lymphangitis or purulent discharge at the insertion site of the catheter.
Septicaemia	Fever or rigors and at least one positive blood culture.

Source : *(1)*

According to a French National Prevalence Survey the distribtution of sites of nosocomial infection are as shown in Fig. 1.

Hospital–acquired infection may be considered from three angles :

1. Source
2. Routes of spread; and
3. Recipients.

1. Sources

The sources are patients, hospital staff and the environment. (a) PATIENTS : Patients suffering from infectious diseases are potential sources of infection. These cases may be certain **viral infections** (measles, german measles, influenza, viral hepatitis); **Skin infections** (discharging wounds, infected skin lesions, eczema, psoriasis, boils, bed sores); **respiratory infections** (sore throat, pulmonary tuberculosis, chest infection); and **urinary tract infection** (*B. coli* infection). All these are very common sources of hospital acquired infection. (b) STAFF: The hospital staff (viz doctors, nurses, ward boys) who come in close contact with patients may often be an important source of cross infection. For example, staphylococcus aureus is commonly carried in the nose or on the skin. *Haemolytic streptococci* may be carried in the throat and *salmonella* in the gut. (c) ENVIRONMENT : The hospital environment (viz. hospital dust, linen, bed clothes, furniture, sinks, basins, door handles and even the air) is laden with microorganisms, and is thus an important source of infection.

2. Routes of spread

The common routes of spread of cross infection are : (a) Direct contact, i.e. the organism may be transferred directly from the hands of a nurse or doctor to a susceptible patient; (b) Droplet infection, e.g. droplets released from nose and throat through coughing or sneezing; (c) Air-borne particles ; (d) Release of hospital dust into the air; (e) Through various hospital procedures, viz, catheterization, intravenous procedures, infected cat gut, dressings, sputum cups, bed pans, urinals etc.

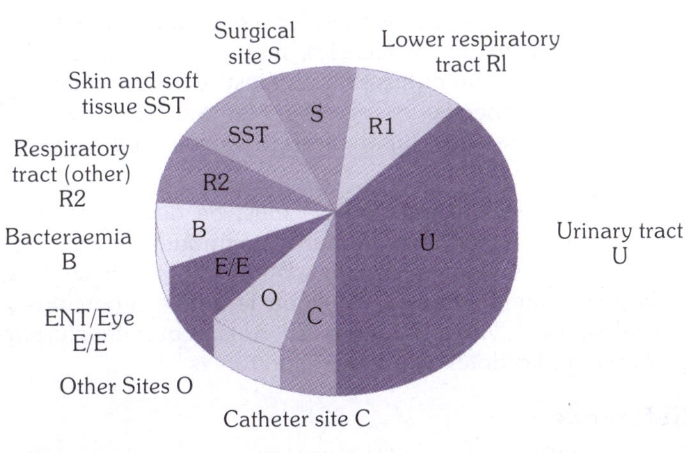

FIG. 1

Sites of the most common nosocomial infections

Source : *(1)*

3. Recipients

All patients in hospitals are potential recipients of cross infection. Some patients are more susceptible than others, especially those who are severely ill and those under corticosteroid therapy. Cross infection is greater in intensive care units, urological and geriatric wards and in special baby care units.

Preventive measures

The main preventive measures are : (a) Isolation : Infectious patients must be isolated. Patients who are susceptible to infection should not be placed in beds next to patients who are a source of infection. (b) Hospital staff : Those who are suffering from skin diseases, sore throat, common cold, ear infection, diarrhoea or dysentery and other infectious ailments should be kept away from work until completely cured. They should be careful about personal hygiene and in regular changes of aprons and outer clothing. (c) Hand-washing : The most common route of infection is *via* the hands. When dealing with patients, hand-washing must be thorough. When hand-washing with soap and water is not sufficient, a suitable alcohol-based disinfectant must be employed for hand-washing. In the year 2009, WHO developed guidelines for hand hygiene known as *"Clean Care is Safer Care"*. It should be followed to improve the standards of hand hygiene practices *(2)*. (d) Dust control : Hospital dust contains numerous bacteria and viruses. The dust is released during sweeping, dusting and bed making. Suppression of dust by wet dusting and vacuum cleaning are important control measures. (e) Disinfection : The articles used by the patient as well as patient's urine, faeces, sputum should be properly disinfected. Proper sterilization of instruments should be enforced. (f) Control of droplet infection : Use of face masks, proper bed spacing, prevention of overcrowding and ensuring adequate lighting and ventilation are important control measures. (g) Nursing techniques : Barrier nursing and task nursing have also been recommended to minimize cross infection. (h) Administrative measures : There should be a hospital "Control of Infection Committee" to formulate policies regarding admission of infectious cases, isolation facilities, disinfection procedures, and in fact all matters relating to control of hospital acquired infection.

The four most common nosocomial infections are urinary tract infections, surgical wound infections, pneumonia, and primary bloodstream infection. Each of these is associated with an invasive medical device or invasive procedure. Specific policies and practices to minimize these infections must be established, reviewed and updated regularly, and compliance monitored, as shown in Table 2.

Standard (routine) precautions

Standard precautions should be applied to the care of all patients. This includes limiting health care worker contact with all secretions or biological fluids; skin lesions, mucous membranes, and blood or body fluids. Health care workers must wear gloves for each contact which may lead to contamination, and also gown, mask and eye protection where contamination of clothes or the face is anticipated.

Considerations for protective clothing include :

- gown: should be of washable material, buttoned or tied at the back and protected, if necessary, by a plastic apron

TABLE 2

Measures for prevention of infection

Infection	Proven effective	Proven not effective
Urinary tract infections	Limit duration of catheter Aseptic technique at insertion Maintain closed drainage Antiseptic added to drainage bag Antimicrobial-coated catheter Daily antiseptic perineal cleaning.	Systemic antibiotic prophylaxis Bladder irrigation or instillation of normal saline antiseptic or antibiotic
Surgical site infections	Surgical technique Clean operating environment Staff attire Limiting preoperative hospital stay Preoperative shower and local skin preparation of patient Optimal antibiotic prophylaxis Aseptic practice in operating room Surgical wound surveillance.	Fumigation Preoperative shaving
Pneumonia	Ventilator-associated Aseptic intubation and suctioning Limit duration Non-invasive ventilation Others Influenza vaccination for staff Isolation policy Sterile water for oxygen and aerosol therapy Prevention of *Legionella* and *Aspergillus* during renovations.	Digestive decontamination for all patients Changes of ventilator circuit every 48 or 72 hours
Vascular device infections	All catheters Closed system Limit duration Local skin preparation Aseptic technique at insertion Removal if infection suspected Central lines Surgical asepsis for insertion Limitation of frequency of dressing change Antibiotic-coated catheter for short term.	Antimicrobial creams for skin preparation

- gloves: inexpensive plastic gloves are available and usually sufficient
- mask : surgical masks made of cloth or paper may be used to protect from splashes.

Standard precautions for all patients are as follows :

- Wash hands promptly after contact with infective material.
- Use no touch technique wherever possible.
- Wear gloves when in contact with blood, body fluids, secretions, excretions, mucous membranes and contaminated items.
- Wash hands immediately after removing gloves.
- All sharps should be handled with extreme care.
- Clean up spills of infective material promptly.
- Ensure that patient-care equipment, supplies and linen contaminated with infective material is either discarded, or disinfected or sterilized between each patient use.
- Ensure appropriate waste handling.
- If no washing machine is available for linen soiled with infective material, the linen can be boiled.

Health care workers are at risk of acquiring infection through occupational exposure. Hospital employees can also transmit infections to patients and other employees. Thus, a programme must be in place to prevent and manage infections in hospital staff.

Employee's health should be reviewed at recruitment, including immunization history and previous exposure to communicable diseases (e.g. tuberculosis) and immune status. Some previous infections (e.g. varicella-zoster virus (VZV) may be assessed by serological tests.

Immunizations recommended for staff include: hepatitis A and B, yearly influenza, measles, mumps, rubella, tetanus, and diphtheria. Immunization against varicella may be considered in specific cases. The Mantoux skin test will document a previous tuberculosis infection and must be obtained as a base-line.

Specific postexposure policies must be developed, and compliance ensured for: human immunodeficiency virus (HIV), hepatitis A virus, hepatitis B virus, hepatitis C virus, Neisseria meningitidis, Mycobacterium tuberculosis, varicella-zoster virus, hepatitis E virus, corynebacterium *diphtheriae*, bordetella *pertussis*, and rabies.

Reference

1. WHO(2002), *Prevention of Hospital-Acquired Infections: A practical guide,* 2nd edition, Department of Communicable Disease, Surveillance and Response.
2. WHO (2009), *WHO Guidelines on Hand Hygiene in Health Care,* First Global Patient Safety Challenge Clean Care is Safer Care.

6 Epidemiology of Chronic Non-communicable Diseases and Conditions

"While there are many diseases, there is, in a sense, only one health"

Chronic diseases and conditions have been variously defined. An EURO symposium in 1957 *(1)* gave the following definition :

> "An impairment of bodily structure and/or function that necessitates a modification of the patient's normal life, and has persisted over an extended period of time".

Another EURO symposium in 1965 *(2)* observed:

> "Upto now no widely acceptable definition (of acute or chronic patients) has been found. Some authors maintain that an acute illness usually consists of a simple episode of fairly short duration from which the patient returns to normal activity, whereas a chronic illness is one of long duration in which the patient is permanently incapacitated to a more or less marked degree. There is also the view that progress in the technology of resuscitation and haemobiology has blurred the borderline between acute and chronic conditions".

The Commission on Chronic Illness in USA *(3)* has defined "chronic diseases" as "comprising all impairments or deviations from normal, which have one or more of the following characteristics :

a. are permanent
b. leave residual disability
c. are caused by non-reversible pathological alteration
d. require special training of the patient for rehabilitation
e. may be expected to require a long period of supervision, observation or care.''

In short, there is no international definition of what duration should be considered long-term *(4)*, although many consider that chronic conditions are generally those, that have had a duration of at least 3 months *(5)*. A practical definition should be established which will suit the particular conditions of the community *(4)*.

Non-communicable diseases (NCDs) include cardiovascular, renal, nervous and mental diseases, musculo-skeletal conditions such as arthritis and allied diseases, chronic non-specific respiratory diseases (e.g., chronic bronchitis, emphysema, asthma), permanent results of accidents, senility, blindness, cancer, diabetes, obesity and various other metabolic and degenerative diseases and chronic results of communicable diseases. Disorders of unknown cause and progressive course are often labelled "degenerative".

The problem

Chronic non-communicable diseases are assuming increasing importance among the adult population in both developed and developing countries. Cardiovascular diseases and cancer are at present the leading causes of death in developed countries. The prevalence of chronic disease is showing an upward trend in most countries, and for several reasons this trend is likely to increase. For one reason, life expectancy is increasing in most countries and a greater number of people are living to older ages, and are at greater risk to chronic diseases of various kinds. For another, the life-styles and behavioural patterns of people are changing rapidly, these being favourable to the onset of chronic diseases. Modern medical care is now enabling many with chronic diseases to survive. The impact of chronic diseases on the lives of people is serious when measured in terms of loss of life, disablement, family hardship and poverty, and economic loss to the country. Developing countries are now warned to take appropriate steps to avoid the "epidemics" of non-communicable diseases likely to come with socio-economic and health developments.

A total of 55.4 million deaths occurred worldwide during 2019. Of these, 41 million were due to NCDs, principally cardiovascular diseases, cancer and chronic respiratory diseases. Nearly three quarters of these NCD deaths (31.4 million about 77 per cent) occurred in low-and middle-income countries. The number of NCD deaths has increased worldwide and in every region since year 2000, when there were 31 million NCD deaths. The leading cause of NCD death in 2019 were: cardiovascular diseases (17.9 million deaths or 44 per cent of NCD deaths), cancers (9.3 million or 16 per cent of NCD deaths), respiratory disease, including asthma and chronic obstructive pulmonary disease (4.1 million or 9 per cent of NCD deaths), and diabetes (2.0 million or 4 per cent of NCD deaths) *(6)*. In 2016, the age standardized NCD death rate was 539 per 100,000 population globally. The rate was lowest in high-income countries (397 per 100,000) and highest in low-income countries (625 per 100,000) and lower-middle income countries (673 per 100,000) *(7)*. Approximately 17 million of the deaths were before the age of 70 years *(6)*.

India is experiencing a rapid health transition with a rising burden of NCDs causing significant morbidity and mortality, both in urban and rural population, with considerable loss in potentially productive years (age 35–64 years) of life. NCDs are estimated to account for about 63 per cent of all deaths. India shares more than two-thirds of the total deaths due to NCDs in the SEAR of WHO. Four types of NCDs – cardiovascular diseases, cancer, chronic respiratory diseases and diabetes make the largest contribution to morbidity and mortality due to NCDs. Four behavioural risk factors are responsible for significant proportions of these diseases – tobacco use, unhealthy diet, physical inactivity and harmful use of alcohol. Major metabolic risk factors are obesity, raised blood pressure, raised blood glucose and raised total cholesterol levels *(8)*. The probability of dying between ages 30 and 70 years from four major NCDs is 23 per cent (27 per cent in men and 20 per cent in women), which means that a 30 year old individual has a one-fourth chance of dying from these diseases before the age of 70 years *(8)*. Fig. 1 shows the proportional mortality in the country.

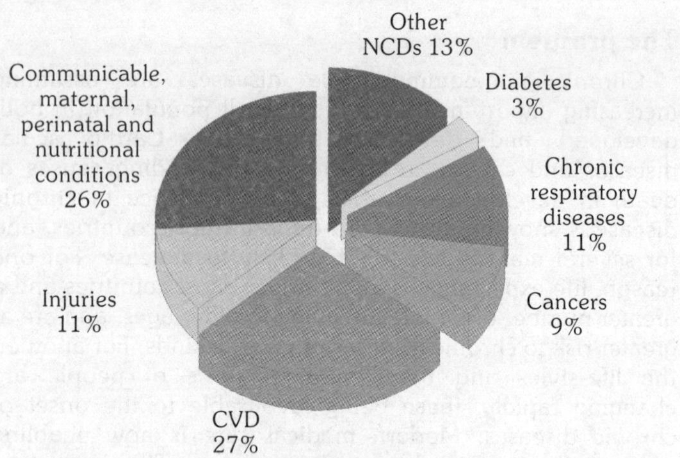

FIG. 1
Proportional mortality in India (% of total deaths, all ages) 2016
Total deaths 9,569,000

Source : *(9)*

Epidemiological transition ratio *(10)*

Epidemiological transition ratio is defined as the ratio of DALYs caused by CMNNDs (Communicable, Maternal, Neonatal and Nutritional Diseases) to those caused by NCDs and injuries. A ratio greater than one indicates a higher burden of CMNNDs than NCDs and injuries, while a ratio less than one indicates the opposite. The lower the ratio, the greater the contribution of NCDs and injuries to a state's overall disease burden. Most of the states had ratios more than one in 1990, whereas all states had ratios less than one in 2016. This means that the proportion of DALYs caused by NCDs and injuries has increased heavily across the country since 1990, and in 2016 accounted for the majority of premature death and disability for all states – a major shift in drivers of health loss.

There are wide variations in the epidemiological transition ratio between individual states, ranging from 0.16 in Kerala, which is far along in this progression, to 0.74 in Bihar, where the challenge of the double burden of diseases is more acute. The states with ratio 0.56–0.75 in 2016 were considered as having the lowest epidemiological transition level (ETL), those with ratio 0.41–0.55 as lower-middle ETL, those with ratio 0.31–0.40 as higher-middle ETL, and those with ratio 0.30 or less as highest ETL.

India's health system therefore faces a dual challenge. Although the absolute burden from diseases such as diarrhoea, lower respiratory infections, tuberculosis, and neonatal disorders is being reduced, it remains high. At the same time, the contribution to health loss of non-communicable conditions such as heart disease, stroke and diabetes is rising. The precise nature of this challenge varies across the country. While all states have experienced a change in disease patterns to some degree, clear differences emerge both in terms of the extent of this change and the rate at which it has occurred *(10)*.

Non-communicable disease risk factors *(7)*

Most epidemiologists accept that a sets of "risk factors" are responsible for a major share of adult non-communicable disease morbidity and premature mortality. A large percentage of NCDs are preventable through the changes in these factors. The influences of these risk factors and other underlying metabolic/physiological causes, on the non-communicable disease epidemic include *(7)* :

Tobacco : Almost 8 million people die from tobacco use each year, both from direct tobacco use and second-hand smoke. About 600,000 deaths are caused by second hand smoke, of these 170,000 are children. In 2016, there were 1.1 billion smokers worldwide with over 80% every day smokers *(11)*. By 2020, this number will increase to 7.5 million, accounting for 10% of all deaths. Smoking is estimated to cause about 71% of lung cancer, 42% of chronic respiratory disease and nearly 10% of cardiovascular disease. The highest incidence of smoking among men is in lower-middle-income countries; for total population, smoking prevalence is highest among upper–middle–income countries.

Insufficient physical activity : WHO defines physical activity as any bodily movement produced by skeletal muscles that requires energy expenditure. Physical activity refers to all movement including during leisure time, for transport to get to and from places, or as part of a person's work. Both moderate - and vigorous-intensity physical activity improve health. Physical activity has significant health benefits for heart, body and mind; it contributes to preventing and managing noncommunicable diseases such as cardiovascular diseases, cancer and diabetes; it reduces symptoms of depression and anxiety; it enhances thinking, learning, and judgment skills; it ensures healthy growth and development in young people; it improves overall well-being.

Globally, 1 in 4 adults do not meet the global recommended levels of physical activity. Upto 5 million deaths a year could be averted if the global population was more active. People who are insufficiently active have a 20 per cent to 30 per cent increased risk of death compared to people who are sufficiently active. More than 80 per cent of the world's adolescent population is insufficiently physically active.

People living with chronic conditions (hypertension, type 2 diabetes, HIV and cancer survivors), should do at least 150–300 minutes of moderate-intensity aerobic physical activity or at least 75–150 minutes of vigorous-intensity aerobic physical activity; or an equivalent combination of moderate- and vigorous-intensity activity throughout the week. They should also do muscle-strengthening activities at moderate or greater intensity that involve all major muscle groups on 2 or more days a week, as these provide additional health benefits. As part of their weekly physical activity, older adults should do varied multicomponent physical activity that emphasizes functional balance and strength training at moderate or greater intensity, on 3 or more days a week, to enhance functional capacity and to prevent falls. They may increase moderate-intensity aerobic physical activity to more than 300 minutes; or do more than

150 minutes of vigorous-intensity aerobic physical activity; or an equivalent combination of moderate - and vigorous-intensity activity throughout the week for additional health benefits. They should limit the amount of time spent being sedentary. Replacing sedentary time with physical activity of any intensity (including light intensity) provides health benefits, and to help reduce the detrimental effects of high levels of sedentary behaviour on health, all adults and older adults should aim to do more than the recommended levels of moderate - to vigorous-intensity physical activity *(12)*.

Harmful use of alcohol : Approximately 3.3 million people die each year from the harmful use of alcohol, accounting for about 5.9% of all deaths in the world and 5.1 per cent DALYs were attributable to alcoholism *(11)*. More than half of these deaths occur from NCDs including cancers, cardiovascular disease and liver cirrhosis. Moreover there is a close relationship between drinking and violent crime including domestic violence. Alcohol related harm is determined by three related dimensions : the volume of alcohol consumed, the pattern of drinking and quality of alcohol consumed *(11)*. While adult per capita consumption is highest in high-income countries, it is nearly as high in the populous upper-middle-income countries.

Unhealthy diet : Adequate consumption of fruit and vegetables reduces the risk for cardiovascular diseases, stomach cancer and colorectal cancer. Most populations consume much higher levels of salt than recommended by WHO for disease prevention; high salt consumption is an important determinant of high blood pressure and cardiovascular risk. 1.8 million deaths from CVD causes have been attributed to excess salt/sodium intake *(6)*. High consumption of saturated fats and trans-fatty acids is linked to heart disease. Unhealthy diet is rising quickly in lower-resource settings. Available data suggest that fat intake has been rising rapidly in lower-middle-income countries since the 1980s. Fat intake, especially saturated fat and industrially-produced trans-fat intake, can be reduced by : (a) steaming or boiling instead of frying when cooking; (b) replacing butter, lard and ghee with oils rich in polyunsaturated fats, such as soybean, canola (rapeseed), corn, safflower and sunflower oils; (c) eating reduced-fat dairy foods and lean meats, or trimming visible fat from meat; and (d) limiting the consumption of baked and fried foods, and pre-packaged snacks and foods (e.g. doughnuts, cakes, pies, cookies, biscuits and wafers) that contain industrially-produced trans-fats.

In both adults and children, the intake of free sugars should be reduced to less than 10 per cent of total energy intake. A reduction to less than 5 per cent of total energy intake would provide additional health benefits. Sugar intake can be reduced by : (a) limiting the consumption of foods and drinks containing high amounts of sugars, such as sugary snacks, candies and sugar-sweetened beverages (i.e. all types of beverages containing free sugars - these include carbonated or non-carbonated soft drinks, fruit or vegetable juices and drinks, liquid and powder concentrates, flavoured water, energy and sports drinks, ready-to-drink tea, ready-to-drink coffee and flavoured milk drinks); and (b) eating fresh fruit and raw vegetables as snacks instead of sugary snacks *(13)*.

Raised blood pressure : Raised blood pressure is estimated to cause 9.4 million deaths, about 12.8% of all deaths. It is a major risk factor for cardiovascular disease. The prevalence of raised blood pressure is similar across all income groups. During the year 2015, the global prevalence of raised blood pressure in adults 18 year and above was around 22 per cent *(11)*.

Overweight and obesity : At least 2.8 million people die each year as a result of being overweight or obese. Risks of heart disease, stroke and diabetes increase steadily with increasing body mass index (BMI). Raised BMI also increases the risk of certain cancers. The prevalence of overweight is highest in upper-middle-income countries, but very high levels are also reported from some lower-middle income countries. In the year 2016, 11% of men and 15% of women aged 18 years and above were obese. More than 42 million children under the age of 5 years were overweight in 2015 *(11)*. Factors driving this rise include poor diet and lack of exercise. Many children are growing up in a society which promotes high energy intake while encouraging physical inactivity. Most of these children will become obese adults, which makes them more susceptible to develop NCDs *(11)*.

Raised cholesterol : Raised cholesterol is estimated to cause 2.6 million deaths annually; it increases the risk of heart disease and stroke. Raised cholesterol is highest in high-income countries.

Cancer-associated infections : At least 2 million cancer cases per year, 18% of the global cancer burden, are attributable to a few specific chronic infections, and this fraction is substantially larger in low-income countries. The principal infectious agents are human papillomavirus, Hepatitis B virus, Hepatitis C virus and *Helicobacter pylori*. These infections are largely preventable through vaccinations and measures to avoid transmission, or treatable. For example, transmission of Hepatitis C virus has been largely stopped among high–income populations, but not in many low–resource countries.

Environmental risk factors : occupational hazards, air and water pollution, and possession of destructive weapons in case of injuries.

Gaps in natural history

There are many gaps in our knowledge about the natural history of chronic diseases. These gaps cause difficulties in aetiological investigations and research *(14)*. These are :–

1. *Absence of a known agent*

There is much to learn about the cause of chronic diseases. Whereas in some chronic diseases the cause is known (e.g., silica in silicosis, asbestos in mesothelioma), for many chronic diseases the causative agent is not known. The absence of a known agent makes both diagnosis and specific prevention difficult.

2. *Multifactorial causation*

Most chronic diseases are the result of multiple causes – rarely is there a simple one-to-one cause-effect relationship. In the absence of a known agent, the term "risk factor(s)" is used to describe certain factors in a person's background or life-style that make, the likelihood of the chronic condition more probable. Further, chronic diseases appear to result from the cumulative effects of multiple risk factors. These factors may be both environmental and behavioural, or constitutional. Epidemiology has contributed massively in the identification of risk factors of chronic diseases. Many more are yet to be identified and evaluated.

3. *Long latent period*

A further obstacle to our understanding of the natural history of chronic disease is the long latent (or incubation) period between the first exposure to "suspected cause" and the eventual development of disease (e.g., cervical cancer). This makes it difficult to link suspected causes (antecedent events) with outcomes, e.g., the possible relation between oral contraceptives and the occurrence of cervical cancer. In an attempt to overcome this problem, a search has been made for precursor lesions in, for example, cancer cervix, oral cancer and gastric cancer. But this is not possible in all chronic diseases. However, it has now become increasingly evident that the factors favouring the development of chronic disease are often present early in life, preceding the appearance of chronic disease by many years. Examples include hypertension, diabetes, stroke, etc.

4. Indefinite onset

Most chronic diseases are slow in onset and development, and the distinction between diseased and non-diseased states may be difficult to establish (e.g., diabetes and hypertension). In many chronic diseases (e.g., cancer) the underlying pathological processes are well established long before the disease manifests itself. By the time the patient seeks medical advice, the damage already caused may be irreversible or difficult to treat.

Prevention

The preventive attack on chronic diseases is based on the knowledge that they are multifactorial in causation, so their prevention demands a complex mix of interventions. Previously only tertiary prevention seemed possible to prevent or delay the development of further disability or the occurrence of premature death. But, now, with the identification of risk factors, health promotion activities aimed at primary prevention are being increasingly applied in the control of chronic diseases. Some of the interventions that should be undertaken immediately to produce accelerated results in terms of lives saved, disease prevented and heavy cost avoided are as follows *(15)* :

1. Protecting people from tobacco smoke and banning smoking in public places, warning about the dangers of tobacco use, enforcing bans on tobacco advertising, promotion and sponsorships and raising taxes on tobacco;
2. Restricting access to retailed alcohol, enforcing bans on alcohol advertising and raising taxes on alcohol;
3. Reduce salt intake and salt content of food;
4. Replacing trans-fat in food with polyunsaturated fat; and
5. Promoting public awareness about diet and physical activity, including through mass media.

In addition, there are many other cost-effective and low-cost population-wide interventions that can reduce risk factors for NCDs. These include :

1. Nicotine dependence treatment;
2. Enforcing drink-driving laws;
3. Restrictions on marketing of foods and beverages high in salt, fats and sugar;
4. Food taxes and subsidies to promote healthy diets;
5. Healthy nutrition environments in schools;
6. Nutrition information and counselling in health care; and
7. National physical activity guidelines (school based physical activity programmes for children and workplace programmes for physical activity and healthy diets).

There also are population-wide interventions that focus on cancer prevention, like vaccination against Hepatitis B, a major cause of liver cancer. Vaccination against human papillomavirus (HPV), the main cause of cervical cancer, is also recommended. Protection against environmental or occupational risk factors for cancer, such as aflatoxin, asbestos and contaminants in drinking-water can be included in effective prevention strategies.

Present knowledge indicates that the chronically ill require a wide spectrum of services – case finding through screening and health examination techniques; application of improved methods of diagnosis, treatment and rehabilitation; control of food, water and air pollution; reducing accidents; influencing patterns of human behaviour and life-styles through intensive education; upgrading standards of institutional care and developing and applying better methods of comprehensive medical care including primary health care. Political approaches are also needed as in the case of smoking control, control of alcohol and drug abuse. The approach should be holistic in handling the complex medical and social needs of the chronically ill and should always be considered in relation to the family and community.

Integrated approach

It is now felt that the principles of prevention of CHD can be applied also to other major non-communicable diseases (NCDs) because of common risk factors. A broader concept is emerging, that is, to develop an overall integrated programme for the **Prevention and Control of NCDs** as part of primary health care systems, simultaneously attacking several risk factors known to be implicated in the development of non-communicable diseases. Such concerted preventive action should reduce not only cardiovascular diseases but also other major NCDs, with an overall improvement in health and length of life *(16)*.

The WHO has developed a survey methodology known as *"the STEPS Non-communicable Disease Risk Factors Survey"* to help countries establish NCD surveillance system. Some surveys are conducted at the country level and others at the subnational level. The methodology prescribes three steps – questionnaire, physical measurements, and biochemical measurements. The core topics covered by most surveys are demographic, health status and health behaviours. These provide data on socio-economic risk factors and metabolic, nutritional and lifestyle risk factors. Details may differ from country to country and from year to year *(17)*.

In India, the survey was conducted from April 2003 to March 2005 in 6 states and again in 2007 in 7 states.

WHO Global Action Plan for the Prevention and Control of NCDs (2013–2020)

The Global Action Plan provides member states with a road map and menu of policy options which, when implemented collectively between 2013 and 2020, will contribute to progress on 9 global NCD targets including that of 25 per cent relative reduction in premature mortality from cardiovascular diseases, cancer, diabetes and chronic respiratory diseases by 2025. These four diseases make the largest contribution to mortality and morbidity due to NCDs. It will target four behavioural risk factors – tobacco use, unhealthy diet, physical inactivity and harmful use of alcohol. The voluntary global targets are *(18)* :

1. A 25 per cent relative reduction in risk of premature mortality from cardiovascular diseases, cancer, diabetes and chronic respiratory disease;
2. At least 10 per cent relative reduction in the harmful use of alcohol as appropriate within national context;
3. A 10 per cent relative reduction in prevalence of insufficient physical activity;

4. A 10 per cent relative reduction in mean population intake of salt/sodium;
5. A 30 per cent relative reduction in prevalence of current tobacco use in persons aged 15+ years;
6. A 25 per cent relative reduction in prevalence of raised blood pressure;
7. Halt the rise of diabetes and obesity;
8. At least 50 per cent of eligible people receive drug therapy and counselling (including glycaemic control) to prevent heart attacks and strokes; and
9. An 80 per cent availability of the affordable basic technology and essential medicines including generics, required to treat major NCDs in both public and private facilities.

2030 Agenda for Sustainable Development

The Sustainable Development Goals include a specific target for NCDs and several NCD – related targets. Target 3.4 calls for a one third reduction in premature mortality from NCDs by year 2030 and is an extension of the global NCD mortality target. For further details, please refer to chapter 14.

References

1. Amsterdam (1956), Report on a Symposium, *The Public Health Aspects of Chronic Diseases.* EURO 111.1, p. 9 WHO. Copenhagen.
2. Hogarth, J. (1978) *Glossary of Health Care Terminology.* WHO, Copenhagen.
3. Commission on Chronic illness (1956) *Chronic illness in the US*. Vol II, Care of the long-term patient. Cambridge, Mass, Harvard University Press.
4. WHO (1981). *Health for All,* Sr. No. 4, p. 80.
5. Wilson, R.W. and T.F. Drury (1984), *Annual Review of Public Health,* 5: 83–106.
6. WHO (2022), *Fact sheet, Non-communicable diseases,* 16th Sept. 2022.
7. WHO (2014), *Global Status Report on Non-communicable Diseases,* 2014.
8. WHO (2014), *Non-communicable Diseases by Country Profile,* India.
9. WHO (2018), *Non-communicable Disease, Country Profiles 2018.*
10. ICMR (2017), *India : Health of the Nation's States,* The India State - Level Disease Burden Initiative, Dec. 2017.
11. JFMJA (2018), *Non-communicable Diseases and the 4 Most Common Shared risk factors,* March meeting 2018 in Hurghada, Egypt.
12. WHO (2020), *Fact sheet, Physical Activity,* 26th Nov. 2020.
13. WHO (2020), *Fact sheet, Healthy Diet,* 29th April 2020.
14. Mausner, J.S. and Kramer, K. (1985), *Epidemiology–An Introductory Text,* Saunders.
15. WHO (2011), *Global Status Report on Non-communicable Diseases 2010.*
16. WHO (1986), *Techn. Rep. Ser.,* No. 732.
17. WHO (2011), *STEPS : A Framework for Surveillance of NCD Risk Factors.*
18. WHO (2013), *Global Action Plan for the Prevention and Control of NCD,* 2013–2020.

CARDIOVASCULAR DISEASES

Cardiovascular diseases (CVD) comprise of a group of diseases of the heart and the vascular system. The major conditions are ischaemic heart disease (IHD), hypertension, cerebrovascular disease (stroke) and congenital heart disease. Rheumatic heart disease (RHD) continues to be an important health problem in many developing countries.

Problem statement

WORLD

CVDs are the number one cause of death globally, more people die annually from CVD than any other cause. An estimated 17.9 million people died from CVD in 2019, representing 32 per cent of all global deaths. Of these global deaths, an estimated 7.4 million were due to coronary heart disease and 6.7 million were due to stroke *(1)*. At least 82 per cent of the world's deaths from CVDs occur in low and middle-income countries, where people do not have the benefit of integrated primary health care programmes for early detection and treatment of risk factors compared to people in high-income countries. As a result, many cases in these countries are detected late in the course of the disease and die younger from CVDs and other NCDs, often in their most productive years. The poorest people are affected most. At the household level, CVD and other NCDs contribute to poverty due to catastrophic health spending and high out-of-pocket expenditure *(2)*.

The incidence of CVD is greater in urban areas than in rural areas reflecting the acquisition of several risk factors such as tobacco consumption, lack of physical activity, unhealthy diet (today's fast food habits) and obesity. A peculiar cause of concern is the relative early age of CVD deaths in the developing countries. Ironically CVDs are now in decline in the industrialized countries first associated with them. They seem to have crossed the peak of the epidemic by now. The decline is largely a result of the success of primary prevention and to a lesser extent, treatment. The middle and low-income countries are at the mid-point of the emerging epidemic and will face its full impact in the coming years. These countries can be benefitted from the strategy of primary prevention.

INDIA

An estimated 2.59 million people died of CVD in India during 2016, Table 1 shows the break-up of the cases and crude death rate per 100,000 population as reported to WHO.

Compared with all other countries, India suffers the highest loss in potentially productive years of life, due to deaths from CVD in people aged 35–64 years. The

TABLE 1

Estimated deaths (000) and crude death rate by cause and sex (2016)

Disease	Men		Women		Total	
	Number	CDR	Number	CDR	Number	CDR
CVD	15,04,400	219.2	10,85,700	170.2	2,59,100	195.6
Rheumatic Heart Disease	41,800	6.1	55,300	8.7	97,100	7.3
Hypertension	54,100	7.9	60,500	9.5	1,14,600	8.7
Ischaemic Heart Disease	10,00,800	145.8	6,07,800	95.3	16,08,700	121.5
Stroke	3,72,000	54.2	3,34,200	52.4	7,06,200	53.3

Source : *(4, 5)*

prevalence of CVD is reported to be 2–3 times higher in the urban population as compared to the rural population. In one study, the prevalence of IHD among adults (based on clinical and ECG criteria) was estimated at 96.7 per 1000 population in the urban and 27.1 per 1000 in rural areas *(3)*.

The contribution of risk factors to the CVD have increased massively since last couple of decades. These risk factors are summarized in Table 2 *(4)*.

TABLE 2
Risk factors contributing to CVD, India (2016)

Risk factors	Data year	Males	Females	Total
Total alcohol per capita consumption per year, adults aged 15+ (litres of pure alcohol)	2016	9	2	6
Physical inactivity, adults aged 18+ (%)	2016	24	43	33
Mean population salt intake, adults aged 20+ (g/day)	2010	10	9	9
Current tobacco smoking, adults aged 15+ (%)	2016	20	2	11
Raised blood pressure, adults aged 18+ (%)	2015	24	23	24
Raised blood glucose, adults aged 18+ (%)	2014	8	8	8
Obesity, adults aged 18+ (%)	2016	3	5	4
Obesity, adolescents aged 10–19(%)	2016	2	1	2

Source : *(4, 5)*

Risk factors

The present mortality rates are the consequence of previous exposure to behavioural risk factors such as inappropriate nutrition, insufficient physical activity and increased tobacco consumption. It is called the "lag-time" effect of risk factors for CVD. Overweight, central obesity, high blood pressure, dyslipidaemia, diabetes and low cardio-respiratory fitness are among the biological factors contributing principally to increased risk.

It is now well established fact that a persistently high cholesterol level can almost certainly precipitate a cardiac event such as CHD. Still most people do not have an idea of nutritional requirements and a balanced diet. Unhealthy dietary practices include a high consumption of saturated fats, salt and refined carbohydrates, as well as a low consumption of vegetables and fruits and these tend to cluster together.

Cessation of tobacco use, reduction of salt in the diet, consuming fruits and vegetables, regular physical activity and avoiding harmful use of alcohol have been shown to reduce the risk of cardiovascular disease. In addition, drug treatment of diabetes, hypertension and high blood lipids may be necessary to reduce cardiovascular risk and prevent heart attacks and strokes. Health policies that create conducive environment for making healthy choices affordable and available are essential for motivating people to adopt and sustain healthy behaviour.

There are also a number of underlying determinants of CVDs or "the causes of the causes". These are a reflection of the major forces driving social, economic and cultural change - globalization, urbanization and population ageing. Other determinants of CVDs include poverty, stress and hereditary factors.

Symptoms of heart attack and stroke

Often, there are no symptoms of the underlying disease of the blood vessels. A heart attack or stroke may be the first warning of underlying disease. Symptoms of a heart attack include:

- pain or discomfort in the centre of the chest; and
- pain or discomfort in the arms, the left shoulder, elbows, jaw, or back.

In addition, the person may experience difficulty in breathing or shortness of breath; feeling sick or vomiting; feeling light-headed or faint; breaking into a cold sweat; and becoming pale. Women are more likely to have shortness of breath, nausea, vomiting, and back or jaw pain.

The most common symptom of a stroke is sudden weakness of the face, arm, or leg, most often on one side of the body. Other symptoms include sudden onset of:

1. numbness of the face, arm, or leg, especially on one side of the body;
2. confusion, difficulty in speaking or understanding speech;
3. difficulty in seeing with one or both eyes;
4. difficulty in walking, dizziness, loss of balance or coordination;
5. severe headache with no known cause; and
6. fainting or unconsciousness.

People experiencing these symptoms should seek medical care immediately.

Symptoms of rheumatic heart disease include: shortness of breath, fatigue, irregular heart beats, chest pain and fainting. Symptoms of rheumatic fever include: fever, pain and swelling of the joints, nausea, stomach cramps and vomiting.

Interventions to reduce cardiovascular disease burden *(3)*

PRIMARY PREVENTION

The cost effective interventions that are feasible to be implemented include population-wide interventions and individual level interventions, which are recommended to be used in combination to reduce the CVDs.

The example of population- wide intervention are:

- comprehensive tobacco control policies;
- taxation to reduce the intake of foods that are high in fat, sugar and salt;
- building walking and cycle paths to increase physical activity;
- strategies to reduce harmful use of alcohol; and
- providing healthy school meals to children.

At the individual level, for prevention of first heart attacks and strokes, individual health-care interventions need to be targeted to those at high total cardiovascular risk or those with single risk factor level above traditional thresholds, such as hypertension and hypercholesterolemia. The former approach is more cost-effective than the later and has the potential to substantially reduce cardiovascular events. This approach is feasible in primary care in low- resource settings, including by non-physician health workers.

SECONDARY PREVENTION

For secondary prevention of cardiovascular disease in those with established disease, including diabetes, treatment with the following medications are necessary:

- aspirin;

- beta-blockers;
- angiotensin-converting enzyme inhibitors; and
- statins.

The benefits of these interventions are largely independent, but when used together with smoking cessation, nearly 75% of recurrent vascular events may be prevented. Currently there are major gaps in the implementation of these interventions particularly at the primary health care level.

In addition costly surgical operations are sometimes required to treat CVDs. They include:

- coronary artery bypass;
- balloon angioplasty (where a small balloon-like device is threaded through an artery to open the blockage);
- valve repair and replacement; and
- heart transplantation.

References

1. WHO (2022), *Fact Sheet, Cardiovascular Diseases,* 11th June, 2022.
2. WHO (2016), *Fact Sheet Cardiovascular Diseases,* Sept. 2016.
3. WHO (2002), *Health Situation in South East Asia Region 1998–2000,* New Delhi.
4. WHO (2018), *Estimated deaths (000) by cause and sex in WHO Member States, 2016.*
5. WHO (2018), *Crude Death Rate per 100,000 population by cause and sex in WHO Member States, 2016.*

CORONARY HEART DISEASE

Coronary heart disease (syn : ischaemic heart disease) has been defined as "impairment of heart function due to inadequate blood flow to the heart compared to its needs, caused by obstructive changes in the coronary circulation to the heart" *(1)*. It is the cause of 25–30 per cent of deaths in most industrialized countries. The WHO has drawn attention to the fact that CHD is our modern "epidemic", i.e., a disease that affects populations, not an unavoidable attribute of ageing. CHD may manifest itself in many presentations :

a. angina pectoris of effort
b. myocardial infarction
c. irregularities of the heart
d. cardiac failure
e. sudden death.

Myocardial infarction is specific to CHD; angina pectoris and sudden death are not. Rheumatic heart disease and cardiomyopathy are potential sources of diagnostic confusion *(2)*. The natural history of CHD is very variable. Death may occur in the first episode or after a long history of disease.

Measuring the burden of disease

The burden of CHD may be estimated in various ways, each illustrating a different aspect of the picture *(3)*.

(a) Proportional mortality ratio : The simplest measure is the proportional mortality ratio, i.e., the proportion of all deaths currently attributed to it. For example, CHD is held responsible for about 30 per cent of deaths in men and 25 per cent of deaths in women in most western countries.

(b) Loss of life expectancy : CHD cuts short the life expectancy. Calculations have been made *(4)* for the average gain in life expectation that would follow a complete elimination of all cardiovascular deaths if other mortality rates remain unchanged. The benefit would range for men from 3.4 years to 9.4 years, and even greater for women.

(c) CHD incidence rate: This is the sum of fatal and non-fatal attack rates *(5)*. Because of its different manifestations, accurate incidence of CHD rates are difficult to compute. Mortality rates can be used as a crude indicator of incidence.

(d) Age-specific death rates : When analysis is planned to throw light on aetiology, it is essential to study the age-specific rates. Age-specific death rates suggest a true increase in incidence.

(e) Prevalence rate : The prevalence of CHD can be estimated from cross-sectional surveys using ECG for evidence of infarction and history of prolonged chest pain. A useful publication to conduct such surveys is "Cardiovascular Survey Methods" by Rose and Blackburn *(6)*.

(f) Case fatality rate : This is defined as the proportion of attacks that are fatal within 28 days of onset. The International Society and Federation of Cardiology has suggested that "sudden deaths" be defined to include deaths "occurring instantly or within an estimated 24 hours of the onset of acute symptoms or signs". Data collected in many industrialized countries indicate that 25–28 per cent of patients who suffer a heart attack die suddenly. In about 55 per cent of all cardiac deaths mortality occurs within the first hour *(7)*.

(g) Measurement of risk factor levels : These include measurement of levels of cigarette smoking, blood pressure, alcohol consumption and serum cholesterol in the community *(8)*.

(h) Medical care : Measurement of levels of medical care in the community are also pertinent.

Epidemicity

"Epidemics" of CHD began at different times in different countries. In United States, epidemics began in the early 1920s *(9)*; in Britain in the 1930s *(10)*; in several European countries, still later. And now the developing countries are catching up. Countries where the epidemic began earlier are now showing a decline. For example, in United States, where the epidemic began in early 1920s, a steady decline was evident by 1968, and a 25 per cent fall in mortality (not morbidity) by 1980 *(9)*. Substantial declines in mortality have also occurred in Australia, Canada and New Zealand.

The decline in CHD mortality in US and other countries has been attributed to changes in life-styles and related risk factors (e.g., diet and diet-dependent serum cholesterol, cigarette use and exercise habits) plus better control of hypertension *(11)*.

The reasons for the changing trends in CHD are not precisely known. The WHO has completed a project known as MONICA "(multinational monitoring of trends and determinants in cardiovascular diseases)" to elucidate this issue. Forty-one centres in 26 countries were participating in this project, which was planned to continue for a 10 year period ending in 1994 *(12)*.

When CHD emerged as the modern epidemic, it was the disease of the higher social classes in the most affluent societies. Fifty years later the situation is changing; there is a strong inverse relation between social class and CHD in developed countries *(13)*.

To summarize, in many developed countries, CHD still poses the largest public health problem. But even in those showing a decline, CHD is still the most frequent single cause of death among men under 65 *(13)*.

International variations

With 7.2 million deaths and 12.8 per cent of total deaths, CHD is a worldwide disease. Mortality rates vary widely in different parts of the world (Table 1).

TABLE 1
Mortality due to CHD, global estimates for 2016

Region	Deaths (000)	Per cent of total CHD deaths
Africa	512	5.8
SEAR	2,234	16.2
Americas	1,091	15.9
East Mediterranean	835	20.3
Europe	2,342	25.4
Western Pacific	2,393	17.4
World	9,433*	100

* 16.6 per cent of all deaths.

Source : *(14)*

The highest coronary mortality is seen at present in the Western Pacific Region followed by European Region. On the other hand rates in Americas and Eastern Mediterranean countries are much lower.

Coronary heart disease in India

Coronary heart disease is assuming serious dimension in developing countries. There is a considerable increase in prevalence of CHD in urban areas in India during the last decade. Although there is increase in prevalence of CHD in rural areas also, but it is not that steep because life-style changes have affected people in urban areas more than in rural areas.

The pooled estimates from studies carried out in 1990s upto 2002 shows the prevalent rate of CHD in urban areas as 6.4 per cent and 2.5 per cent in rural areas. In urban areas the pooled estimate was 6.1 per cent for males and 6.7 per cent for females. In rural areas the estimate was 2.1 per cent for males and 2.7 per cent for females *(15)*. According to medical certification of cause of death data, 25.1 per cent of total deaths in urban areas are attributable to diseases of the circulatory system. Therefore, it was assumed that mortality rates due to CHD (which forms an important disease entity and the diseases of circulatory system) in rural areas are expected to be half of CHD specific mortality rates in urban areas.

It is estimated that 16,08,700 people died of CHD during 2016, of which 10,00,800 were men and 6,07,800 women. The crude death rate was 121.5/100,000 population.

Risk factors

The aetiology of CHD is multifactorial. Apart from the obvious ones such as increasing age and male sex, studies have identified several important "risk" factors (i.e., factors that make the occurrence of the disease more probable). Some of the risk factors are modifiable, others immutable (Table 2). Presence of any one of the risk factors places an individual in a high-risk category for developing CHD. The greater the number of risk factors present, the more likely one is to develop CHD. The principal risk factors are discussed below:

TABLE 2
Risk factors for CHD

Not modifiable	Modifiable
Age	Cigarette smoking
Sex	High blood pressure
Family history	Elevated serum cholesterol
Genetic factors	Diabetes
Personality	Obesity
	Sedentary habits
	Stress

1. Smoking

Some people commit suicide by drowning, but many by smoking. A uniquely human habit, smoking has been identified as a major CHD risk factor *(16, 17)* with several possible mechanisms – carbon monoxide induced atherogenesis; nicotine stimulation of adrenergic drive raising both blood pressure and myocardial oxygen demand; lipid metabolism with fall in "protective" high-density lipoproteins, etc.

It has been calculated that in countries where smoking has been a widespread habit, it is responsible for 25 per cent of CHD deaths under 65 years of age in men *(18)*. Cigarettes seem to be particularly important in causing sudden death from CHD especially in men under 50 years of age *(18)*.

The degree of risk of developing CHD is directly related to the number of cigarettes smoked per day *(20)*. Filter cigarettes are probably not protective *(21)*. There is evidence that the influence of smoking is not only independent of, but also synergistic with other risk factors such as hypertension and elevated serum cholesterol (Fig. 1). This means that the effects are more than additive *(18)*.

The risk of death from CHD decreases on cessation of smoking. The risk declines quite substantially within one year of stopping smoking and more gradually thereafter until, after 10–20 years, it is the same as that of non-smokers *(18)*. For those who have had a myocardial infarction, the risk of a fatal recurrence may be reduced by 50 per cent after giving up smoking *(18)*.

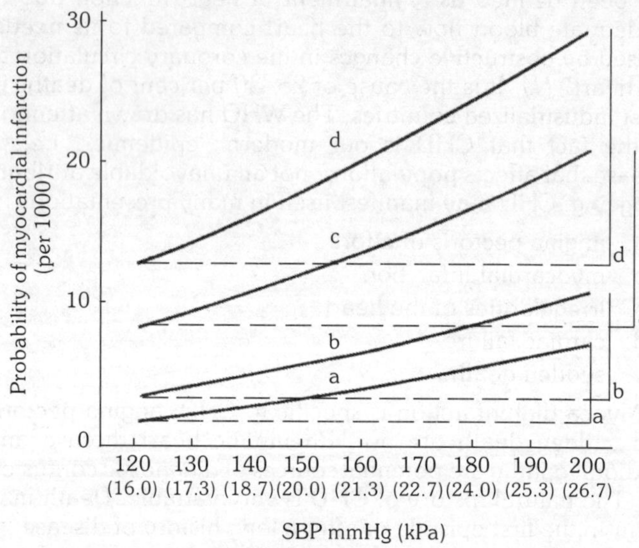

FIG. 1

The importance of risk-factor combinations, illustrated by the six-year risk of myocardial infarction at various levels of SBP and serum cholesterol in smokers and non-smokers

The vertical axis gives the probability of myocardial infarction occuring in the next 6 years per 1000 men with a given SBP.

Curve a : risk in the absence of smoking and elevated serum cholesterol.

Curve b : risk in smokers.

Curve c : risk with elevated serum cholesterol.

Curve d : risk with smoking and elevated serum cholesterol.

The vertical bars a–d show how the increment in the risk of myocardial infarction associated with a given SBP elevation depends on the various "constellations" (combinations) of risk factors. The ratios of the length of the bars provide a measure of the risk due to a particular risk-factor constellation.

Source : *(19)*

2. Hypertension

The blood pressure is the single most useful test for identifying individuals at a high risk of developing CHD. Hypertension accelerates the atherosclerotic process, especially if hyperlipidaemia is also present and contributes importantly to CHD. In the past, emphasis was placed on the importance of diastolic blood pressure. Many investigators feel that systolic blood pressure is a better predictor of CHD than is the diastolic. However, both components are significant risk factors. The risk role of "mild" hypertension is generally accepted *(13)*.

3. Serum cholesterol

It is nearly three decades since it became clear that elevation of serum cholesterol was one of the factors which carried an increased risk for the development of myocardial infarction. Today, there is a vast body of evidence showing a triangular relationship between habitual diet, blood cholesterol–lipoprotein levels and CHD, and that these relationships are judged to be causal *(1)*. There is no population, in which CHD is common, that does not also have a relatively high mean level of cholesterol (i.e. greater than 200 mg/dl in adults). This is illustrated in Fig. 2 *(1)* which shows the cultural differences in serum cholesterol levels between two countries, Japan and Finland – Japan having the lowest incidence and Finland the highest incidence of CHD.

Fig. 3 shows that the risk of CHD rises steadily with the serum cholesterol concentration *(22)*. The 14–years experience of the Seven Countries Study *(23)* showed that serum cholesterol concentration is an important risk factor for the incidence of CHD at levels perhaps 220 mg/dl or more. This supports the notion of a "threshold level" of cholesterol, that is, a certain level beyond which there is an association.

The *strength* of the dietary-fat hypothesis is that observations in the Seven Countries Study (among others) fitted it well – that is, the Japanese had low fat diets, low serum cholesterol and low incidence of CHD while the East Fins were at the other extreme (Fig. 2). The weakness of the hypothesis is that studies of individuals have not shown such a relationship. This has been attributed to genetic and dietary intake differences between individuals *(1)*.

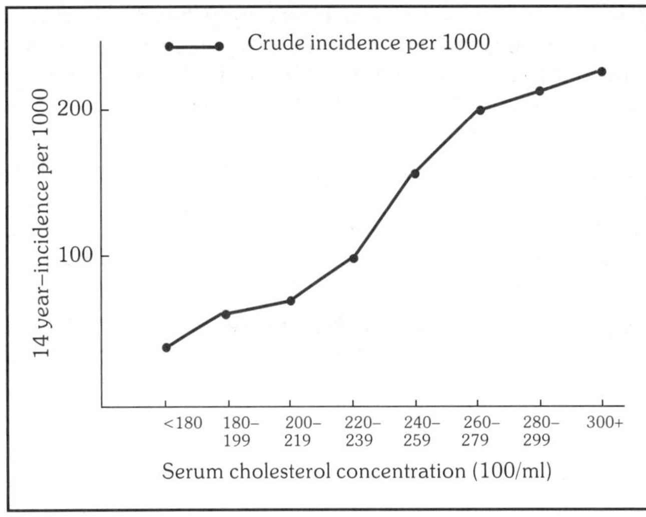

FIG. 3
The risk of CHD and serum cholesterol levels

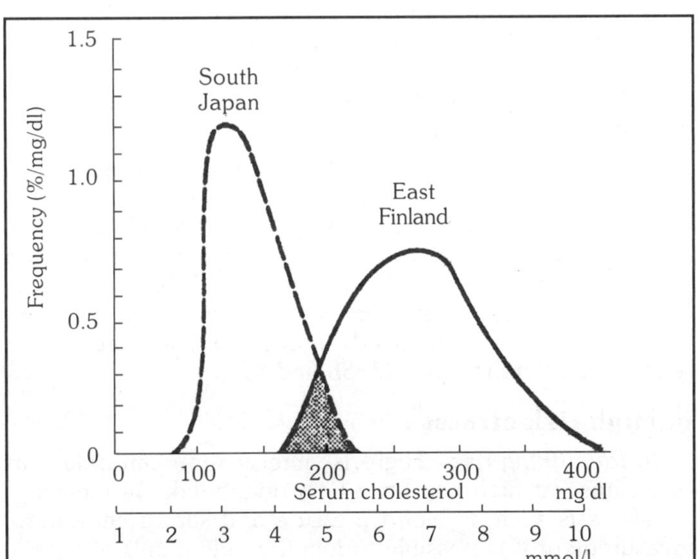

FIG. 2
Cultural differences in serum cholesterol levels

When we look at the various types of lipoproteins, it is the level of low-density lipoprotein (LDL) cholesterol that is most directly associated with CHD *(24)*. While very low-density lipoprotein (VLDL) has also been shown to be associated with premature atherosclerosis, it is more strongly associated with peripheral vascular disease (e.g., intermittent claudication) than with CHD. High-density lipoprotein (HDL) cholesterol is protective against the development of CHD – the higher its mean level in a group of individuals, the lower the incidence of infarction in that group *(24)*. HDL should be more than 40 mg/dl.

To further refine CHD risk prediction based on serum lipid levels, a total "cholesterol/HDL ratio" has been developed. A ratio of less than 3.5 has been recommended as a clinical goal for CHD prevention *(25)*.

With newer techniques, high-density and low-density lipoproteins have been further subdivided into sub-fractions. Recent evidence indicates that levels of plasma apolipoprotein–A–I (the major HDL protein) and apolipoprotein–B (the major LDL protein) are better predictors of CHD than HDL cholesterol or LDL cholesterol respectively. Therefore, measurement of apolipoproteins may replace lipoprotein cholesterol determinations in assessing the risk of CHD *(26)*.

4. Other risk factors

(i) Diabetes : The risk of CHD is 2–3 times higher in diabetics than in non-diabetics. CHD is responsible for 30 to 50 per cent of deaths in diabetics over the age of 40 years in industrialized countries *(27)*.

(ii) Genetic factors : A family history of CHD is known to increase the risk of premature death. Genetic factors are probably the most important determinants of a given individual's TC and LDL levels. However, the importance of genetic factors in the majority of cases is largely unknown.

(iii) Physical activity : Sedentary life-style is associated with a greater risk of the development of early CHD. There is evidence that regular physical exercise increases the concentration of HDL *(28)* and decreases both body weight and blood pressure which are beneficial to cardiovascular health.

(iv) Hormones : The pronounced difference in the mortality rates for CHD between male and female subjects

suggests that the underlying factor may have a hormonal basis. It has been hypothesized that hyperestrogenemia may be the common underlying factor that leads both to atherosclerosis and its complications such as CHD, stroke and peripheral vascular disease *(29)*.

(v) Type A personality : Type A behaviour is associated with competitive drive, restlessness, hostility and a sense of urgency or impatience. Type–A individuals are more coronary prone to CHD than the calmer, more philosophical Type B individuals *(30)*.

(vi) Alcohol : High alcohol intake, defined as 75g or more per day is an independent risk factor for CHD, hypertension and all cardiovascular diseases *(13)*. The evidence that moderate alcohol intake leads to a reduction in the risk of CHD is un-substantiated *(31)*.

(vii) Oral contraceptives : Women using oral contraceptives have higher systolic and diastolic blood pressure. The risk of myocardial infarction in women seems to be increased by oral contraceptives, and the risk is compounded by cigarette smoking *(32)*.

(viii) *Miscellaneous* : The possible role of dietary fibre, sucrose and soft water have been debated *(5)*. Dyspnoea on exertion and low vital capacity have also been cited as possible risk factors.

PREVENTION OF CHD

In the 1960s the issue was whether CHD could be prevented or not. Studies were launched, reported and debated. The accumulated evidence led to a broad consensus of expert opinion that CHD is preventable *(13)*. This is best expressed in a report of the WHO Expert Committee on the Prevention of CHD *(1)* which recommended the following strategies :

a. Population strategy
   (i) prevention in whole populations
   (ii) primordial prevention in whole populations
b. High risk strategy
c. Secondary prevention.

a. Population strategy

CHD is primarily a mass disease. The strategy should therefore be based on mass approach focusing mainly on the control of underlying causes (risk factors) in *whole populations,* not merely in individuals. This approach is based on the principle that small changes in risk factor levels in total populations can achieve the biggest reduction in mortality *(33)*. That is, the aim should be to shift the whole risk-factor distribution in the direction of "biological normality" *(1)*. This cannot obviously be done by medical means alone; it requires the mobilization and involvement of the whole community to alter its lifestyle practices that are associated with CHD.

Specific interventions

The population strategy centres round the following key areas:

1. Dietary changes : Dietary modification is the principal preventive strategy in the prevention of CHD. The WHO Expert Committee *(1)* considered the following dietary changes to be appropriate for high incidence populations :

- reduction of fat intake to 20–30 per cent of total energy intake
- consumption of saturated fats must be limited to less than 10 per cent of total energy intake; some of the reduction in saturated fat may be made up by mono and poly-unsaturated fats
- a reduction of dietary cholesterol to below 100 mg per 1000 kcal per day
- an increase in complex carbohydrate consumption (i.e., vegetables, fruits, whole grains and legumes)
- avoidance of alcohol consumption; reduction of salt intake to 5 g daily or less.

2. Smoking : As far as CHD is concerned, present evidence does not support promotion of the so-called "safer cigarette" *(13)*. The goal should be to achieve a smoke-free society, and several countries are progressing towards this goal.

To achieve the goal of a smoke-free society, a comprehensive health programme would be required which includes effective information and education activities, legislative restrictions, fiscal measures and smoking cessation programmes.

3. Blood pressure : It has been estimated that even a small reduction in the average blood pressure of the whole population by a mere 2 or 3 mm Hg would produce a large reduction in the incidence of cardiovascular complications *(34, 35)*. The goal of the population approach to high blood pressure would thus be to reduce mean population blood pressure levels. This involves a multifactorial approach based on a "prudent diet" (reduced salt intake and avoidance of a high alcohol intake), regular physical activity and weight control. The potential benefits and the safety and low cost of this advice would justify its implementation.

4. Physical activity : Regular physical activity should be a part of normal daily life. It is particularly important to encourage children to take up physical activities that they can continue throughout their lives *(1)*.

PRIMORDIAL PREVENTION

A novel approach to primary prevention of CHD is **primordial prevention** *(1)*. It involves preventing the emergence and spread of CHD risk factors and life-styles that have not yet appeared or become endemic. This applies to developing countries in particular. These countries should seek to preserve their traditional eating patterns and life-styles associated with low levels of CHD risk factors.

Since the aetiology of CHD is multifactorial the approach to prevention should be multifactorial aimed at controlling or modifying as many risk factors as possible. The aim should be to change the community as a whole, not the individual subjects living in it *(36)*.

Several well-planned risk factor intervention trials (e.g., The Multiple Risk Factor Intervention Trial (MRFIT) in the US *(37)*, The Stanford Heart Disease Prevention Programme in California *(38)*, and The North Kerelia Project in Finland *(39)* have demonstrated that primary prevention can achieve substantial reduction in the incidence of coronary heart disease. For detailed information, the reader is referred to references no. *37*, *38* and *39*.

b. High risk strategy

(i) Identifying risk : High-risk intervention can only start once those at high risk have been identified. By means of simple tests such as blood pressure and serum cholesterol measurement it is possible to identify individuals at special risk *(1)*. Individuals at special risk also include those who smoke, those with a strong family history of CHD, diabetes and obesity and young women using oral contraceptives.

(ii) Specific advice : Having identified those at high risk, the next step will be to bring them under preventive care and motivate them to take positive action against all the identified risk factors, e.g., an elevated blood pressure should be treated; the patient should be helped to break the smoking habit permanently – nicotine chewing gum can be tried to wean patients from smoking *(40)*; serum cholesterol concentration should be reduced in those in whom it is raised, etc.

Several well planned high-risk intervention studies (e.g., Oslo Heart Study *(41)*, Lipid Research Clinics Study *(42)*, in US have shown that it is feasible to reduce the CHD risk factors.

From a methodological point of view, however, high-risk approach suffers from the disadvantage that the intervention (e.g., treatment) may be effective in reducing the disease in a high-risk group, but it may not reduce the disease to the same extent in the general population which consists of symptomatic, asymptomatic, high-risk, low-risk and healthy people *(43)*. Further, unfortunately, more than half of the CHD cases occur in those who are *not* apparently at special risk, and this is one limitation of the high-risk strategy *(1)*. Nevertheless, recognition and treatment of high-risk cases do make an important contribution to prevention *(1)*.

c. Secondary prevention

Secondary prevention must be seen as a continuation of primary prevention. It forms an important part of an overall strategy. The aim of secondary prevention is to prevent the recurrence and progression of CHD. Secondary prevention is a rapidly expanding field with much research in progress (e.g., drug trials, coronary surgery, use of pace makers).

The principles governing secondary prevention are the same as those already set out in the above sections, e.g., cessation of smoking, control of hypertension and diabetes, healthy nutrition, exercise promotion, etc. The most promising results to date have come from beta-blockers which appear to reduce the risk of CHD mortality in patients who have already suffered at least one infarct in the order of 25 per cent. None of the preventive measures discussed earlier lose their importance even after the first attack. For example, cessation of smoking is the most effective single means of intervention currently available in the management of patients after a heart attack. The risk of fatal infarction or sudden death is reduced by 20–50 per cent. If the patient does not stop smoking, nothing else is worth doing *(44)*.

Despite advances in treatment, the mortality of an acute heart attack is still high among survivors, around 10 per cent in the first year, and 5 per cent yearly thereafter. Delay in reaching hospital is still considerable even in big cities in the West and may be as much as 3.5 hours. About 30 per cent of all deaths occur within 30 minutes of onset. This is one of the reasons why coronary care units have failed to make impact on the total coronary mortality in the community *(45, 46)*.

Each strategy – population strategy, high-risk strategy, secondary prevention – has its advantages and disadvantages, but the population strategy has the greatest potential.

Revascularization procedures for patients with angina pectoris *(47)*

The indications for coronary artery revascularization i.e. coronary artery bypass grafting (CABG) and percutaneous transluminal coronary angioplasty (PTCA) in patients with angina pectoris are often debated. There is general agreement that otherwise healthy patients in the following groups should undergo revascularization. (a) patients with unacceptable symptoms despite medical therapy to its tolerable limits; (b) patients with left main coronary artery stenosis greater than 50 per cent with or without symptoms; (c) patients with three-vessel disease with left ventricular dysfunction (ejection fraction <50 per cent or previous transmural infarction); (d) patients with unstable angina who after symptom control by medical therapy continue to exhibit ischaemia on exercise testing or monitoring; and (e) post-myocardial infarction patients with continuing angina or severe ischaemia on noninvasive testing.

CABG can be accomplished with a very low mortality rate (1–3 per cent) in otherwise healthy patients with preserved cardiac function. However, the mortality rate of this procedure rises to 4–8 per cent in older individuals and in patients who have had a prior CABG. Increasingly, younger individuals with focal lesions of one or more vessels are undergoing coronary angioplasty as the initial revascularization procedure, where coronary artery stenosis can be effectively dilated by inflation of a balloon under high pressure. PTCA is also possible but less successful in bypass graft stenosis.

The incidents of restenosis appears to be reduced with intracoronary stent placement and may be as low as 15–20 per cent. The number of PTCA and stent procedure now exceeds that of CABG operations. Several studies have shown PTCA to be superior to medical therapy for symptom relief but not in preventing infarction or death. In patients with no or only mild symptoms, aggressive lipid-lowering and anti-anginal therapy may be preferable to PTCA.

RISK FACTOR INTERVENTION TRIALS

Since 1951, one of the best known large prospective studies, the **Framingham Study,** has played a major role in establishing the nature of CHD risk factors and their relative importance *(48, 49)*. The major risk factors of CHD are elevated serum cholesterol, smoking, hypertension and sedentary habits. Accordingly, the four main possibilities of intervention in CHD prevention are: reduction of serum cholesterol, the cessation of smoking, control of hypertension and promotion of physical activity.

Risk factor trials can be "single factor" trials or "multi-factor" trials. Both the approaches are complementary and both are needed. Early trials of CHD prevention concentrated on one factor (e.g., dietary cholesterol). Later emphasis swung away from unifactorial to multifactorial approach.

The widely reported intervention trials are : (a) The Stanford Heart Disease Prevention Programme in California, (b) The North Kerelia Project in Finland, (c) The Oslo Study, (d) The Multiple Risk Factor Intervention Trial (MRFIT) in USA, and (e) The Lipid Research Clinics Study. A brief account of these trials is given below. For more details the reader is referred to the references cited in the text.

1. The Stanford–Three–Community Study *(38)*.

To determine whether community health education can reduce the risk of cardiovascular disease, a field experiment was undertaken in 1972 in three northern California towns with populations varying between 12,000 and 15,000. In two of these towns intensive mass education campaigns were conducted against cardiovascular risk factors over a period of 2 years. The third community served as a control. People from each community were interviewed and examined before the campaign began and one and two years afterwards to assess knowledge and behaviour related to cardiovascular diseases (e.g., diet and smoking) and also to measure physiological indicators of risk (e.g., blood pressure, serum cholesterol, relative weight). In the control community, the risk of cardiovascular disease increased over the two years, but in the intervention communities there was a substantial and sustained decrease in risk. The net difference in estimated total risk between control and intervention samples was 23–28 per cent.

2. The North Kerelia Project *(36, 39)*

North Kerelia is a county in the eastern part of Finland, where CHD is particularly common. Its 185,000 inhabitants work mostly in farming and forestry and live in the countryside.

A multiple risk factor intervention trial was started in 1972. The project had two aims : (a) to reduce the high levels of risk factors for cardiovascular disease (e.g., smoking, blood pressure and serum cholesterol), and (b) to promote the early diagnosis, treatment and rehabilitation of patients with CV disease. A control population was established in a neighbouring county which has similar CV mortality. The main strategy employed was mass community action against risk factors and advice on their avoidance.

Follow-up surveys at 5–years demonstrated a significant reduction in all three major risk factors. By 1979, mortality began to decline by 24 per cent in men and 51 per cent in women in North Kerelia, compared with 12 per cent in men and 26 per cent in women in rest of Finland. A further representative sample (8000) was studied in 1982. It exhibited its effect on CHD deaths – more than twice the reduction achieved in the rest of Finland during the same period. Thus it took 10 years (Rose's 10–years incubation period) to exhibit its effect on CHD deaths.

3. MRFIT *(37)*

The multiple risk factor intervention trial (MRFIT) carried out in USA was aimed at high risk adult males aged 35–57 years. A total of 12,866 men who showed no evidence of CHD either clinically or on ECG were enrolled for the study. Half the group was randomly allocated to an intensive intervention programme, being seen at least every four months to ensure adequate control of risk factors. The other half (control group) received a medical examination once yearly, and no specific advice was given to them about the control of risk factors. The intervention procedures included cessation of smoking, controlling blood pressure and altering diet to reduce hypercholesterolemia.

Over the 7 year follow-up period, IHD mortality was reduced by 22 per cent more in the intervention group but this was not statistically significant. This was because the control group had also changed their habits and lifestyle to a far greater extent than anticipated by the designers of the trial. The trial produced no significant changes at all in mortality or risk factors in as much as the control group was not properly chosen.

4. Oslow diet/smoking Intervention Study *(41)*

This study began in 1973. 16,202 Norwegian men aged 40–49 years were screened for coronary risk factors; of these 1,232 healthy normotensive men at high risk (total serum cholesterol 290–379 mg/dl; smoking) of CHD were selected for a 5 year randomized trial. The aim of the study was to determine whether lowering of serum lipids and cessation of smoking would reduce the incidence of first attack of CHD in males aged 40–50.

The intervention group underwent techniques designed to lower serum cholesterol level through dietary means (e.g., a polyunsaturated fat diet), and to decrease or eliminate smoking. At the end of 5 years, the incidence of myocardial infarction (fatal and nonfatal) was lower by 47 per cent in the intervention group than in the control group.

With this study, primary prevention of CHD entered the practical field of preventive medicine in an impressive manner.

5. Lipid Research Clinics Study *(42)*

This double-blind, randomized clinical trial involved 3,806 asymptomatic "high-risk" American men aged 35–59 years with type II hyperlipoproteinaemia. The trial was designed to test whether reducing serum cholesterol would prevent CHD events.

The men were randomized into two groups, one receiving cholestyramine and the other receiving a placebo. Both the groups were followed for an average of 7.4 years.

The treatment group had an 8.5 per cent and 12.6 per cent greater reduction in total cholesterol and LDL–cholesterol levels respectively than the placebo–treated group. This difference resulted in a 24 per cent reduction in death from definite CHD and a 19 per cent reduction in non-fatal myocardial infarction. The findings of this study have resulted in enthusiasm for the drug treatment of those men with considerably elevated serum cholesterol levels.

Secondary prevention trials

Secondary prevention trials are aimed at preventing a subsequent coronary attack or sudden death. A wide range of clinical trials have been performed with four main groups of drugs – anti-coagulants, lipid-lowering agents (e.g., clofibrate), anti-thrombotic agents (e.g., aspirin) and beta-blockers. The most promising results to date have come from beta blockers.

In general the above studies and similar others show that it is feasible through well-planned intervention programmes to reduce the risk factors in the populations studied. The primary and secondary prevention studies promise at present to be the main contribution of epidemiology to the conquest of chronic diseases.

References

1. WHO (1982) . *Techn Rep. Ser.* No. 678.
2. Pedoe, H.T. (1982). In *Epidemiology of Diseases,* D.L. Miller and R.T.D. Farmer (eds), Blackwell, Oxford.
3. Rose, G.A. (1973). In : *Chronic Diseases,* Public Health in Europe No. 2, Regional Office of WHO, Copenhagen.
4. WHO (1972). *WHO Statis Rep.,* 25:430.
5. Oliver, M.F. (1981). *Br. Med. Bull.,* 37 (1) 49.
6. Rose, G.A. and Blackburn, H. (1968). *Cardiovascular Survey Methods,* Geneva, WHO.
7. WHO (1985). *Techn. Rep. Ser. No 726.*
8. Hetzel, B.S. (1979). In : *Measurement of Levels of Health,* WHO. Copenhagen.
9. Rose, G. (1985) In : *Oxford Textbook of Public Health,* Vol. 4, p. 133.
10. Hart, J.T. (1983). In : *Practising Prevention,* British Medical Association.
11. Stamler, J. (1985). *N. Eng. J. Med.,* 312 : 1053.
12. WHO (1983). *Bull WHO,* 61: 45.
13. WHO (1985). *Primary Prevention of CHD* EURO Rep and Studies 98. Copenhagen.
14. WHO (2018), *World Health Estimates by cause and WHO Regions,* 2018.
15. ICMR (2004). *Assessment of Burden of Non-Communicable Diseases,* Final Report.
16. Slone, D. et al (1978). *N. Eng. J. Med.* 298 : 1273.

17. Shaper A.G. et al (1981). *Brit. Med. J.* 283 : 179.
18. WHO (1979). *Tech. Rep. Ser.*, No. 636.
19. WHO (1996). *Tech. Rep. Ser. No. 862,* Hypertension control.
20. Bain, C. et al (1978). *Lancet,* 1 : 1087.
21. Wald, N.J. (1976). *Lancet,* 1 : 136.
22. Kannel, W.B. (1976). *Am. J. Cardiol.*, 37 : 269.
23. Keys, A. (1980). *Seven Countries : A Multivariate Analysis of Death and CHD,* Harvard University Press, Cambridge, M.A.
24. Gordon, T. et al (1977). *Am. J. Med.*, 62 : 707.
25. Superko, H.R. et al (1985). *Am. J. Med.*, 78 : 826.
26. Schaefer, E.J. (1985). *N. Eng. J. Med.*, 312 : 1300.
27. WHO (1985). *Techn. Rep. Ser.*, 727.
28. Miller, N.E. et al (1979) *Lancet,* 1 : 111.
29. Phillips, G.B. (1985). *Am. J. Med.*, 78 (3) 363.
30. Jenkins, C.D. et al (1974). *N. Eng. J. Med.*, 290 : 1271.
31. WHO (1986). *Techn. Rep. Ser.*, No. 732.
32. Mann, J.I. et al (1976). *Brit. Med. J.*, 2 : 445.
33. WHO (2008). *The Global Burden of Disease, 2004* update.
34. WHO (1986). *Techn. Rep. Ser.*, No. 732.
35. Rose, G. (1981). *Brit. Med. J.,* 282 : 1847.
36. Puska, P. et al (1979). *Brit. Med. J.*, 2 : 1173.
37. Multiple Risk Factor Intervention Trial Research Group (1982). *JAMA,* 248 : 1465.
38. Farquhar, J. et al (1977). *Lancet.*, 1 : 1192.
39. Salonen, J.T. et al (1983). *Brit. Med. J.*, 286 : 1857.
40. *Lancet* (1985). 1 : 320.
41. Hjermann. I. et al (1981). *Lancet,* 2 : 1303.
42. Lipid Research Clinics Programme (1984). *JAMA,* 251 : 351.
43. Glasunov, I. et al (1973). *Int. J. Epi.*, 2 (2) 137.
44. Bradely, N. (1984). In : *Medical Annual,* D.J.P. Gray (ed). John Wright and Sons.
45. Rose, G. (1975). *Brit. J. PSM,* 29 : 147.
46. G. Lamm (1979) In : *Measurement of Levels of Health,* WHO Reg. Publ. EURO Ser. No. 7.
47. Lawrence M. Tierney, Jr. Stephen J. Mcphee Maxine A. Papadakis (2002), *Current Medical Diagnosis and Treatment,* 41st Ed., 2002, Large Publication.
48. Dawber, T.R. (1980). *The Framingham Study,* Cambridge, M.A., Harvard University Press.
49. Kannel, W.B. et al (1976). *Am. J. Cardiol.*, 38 : 46.

HYPERTENSION

Hypertension is a chronic condition of concern due to its role in the causation of coronary heart disease, stroke and other vascular complications. It is the commonest cardiovascular disorder, posing a major public health challenge to population in socio-economic and epidemiological transition. It is one of the major risk factors for cardiovascular mortality, which accounts for 20–50 per cent of all deaths.

Definition of hypertension is difficult and, by necessity arbitrary. Sir George Peckering first fomulated a concept that blood pressure in a population is distributed continuously as a bell-shaped curve with no real separation between normotension and hypertension *(1)*. There is also a direct relation between cardiovascular risk and blood pressure : the higher the blood pressure, the higher the risk of both stroke and coronary events *(1)*. As a consequence, the dividing line between normal and high blood pressure can be defined only in an operational way.

As intervention trials included only adults aged 18 years or older, definition and classification of hypertension refers to adults not taking anti-hypertensive drugs and not actually ill, and based on the average of two or more readings on two or more occasions after initial screening. Table 1 shows the classification of hypertension by blood pressure level.

TABLE 1
Classification of blood pressure measurements

Category	Systolic (mm of Hg)		Diastolic (mm of Hg)
Optimal	< 120	and	< 80
Normal	< 130	and/or	< 85
High normal	130–139	and/or	85–89
Grade 1 Hypertension	140–159	and/or	90–99
Grade 2 Hypertension	> 160	and/or	> 100
Hypertensive crisis	≥180	and/or	> 110
Isolated systolic hypertension	≥140	and	< 90

Source : *(2)*

When systolic and diastolic blood pressure fall into different categories, the higher category should be selected to classify the individual's blood pressure. *"Isolated systolic hypertension"* is defined as a systolic blood pressure of 140 mm of Hg or more and a diastolic blood pressure of less than 90 mm of Hg.

Organ damage

Although the extent of organ damage often correlates with the level of blood pressure, it is not always the case. In addition the rate of progression of organ damage varies from one individual to another depending on many influences, most of which are incompletely understood. Therefore, blood pressure and organ impairment should be evaluated separately, since markedly high pressures may be seen without organ damage and, conversely, organ damage may be present with only moderate elevation of blood pressure. The presence of signs of organ damage confers an increased cardiovascular risk to any level of blood pressure.

Blood pressure measurement

Despite more than 75 years of experience with the measurement of blood pressure, discussion continues about its reliability and wide variability in individual subjects. Accurate measurements are essential under standardized conditions for valid comparison between persons or groups over time. Three sources of errors have been identified in the recording of blood pressure : *(a) Observer errors :* e.g., hearing acuity, interpretation of Korotkow sounds. *(b) Instrumental errors* : e.g., leaking valve, cuffs that do not encircle the arm. If the cuff is too small and fails to encircle the arm properly then too high a reading will be obtained; and *(c) Subject errors :* e.g., the circumstances of examination. These include the physical environment, the position of the subject, external stimuli such as fear, anxiety, and so on *(3)*.

A few salient points need be mentioned about measuring blood pressure. A WHO Study Group *(4)* recommended the sitting position than the supine position for recording blood pressure. In any clinic a uniform policy should be adopted, using either the right or left arm consistently. The pressure at which the sounds are first heard (phase I) is taken to indicate the systolic pressure. Near the diastolic pressure the sounds first become muffled (phase IV) and then disappear (phase V). Most of the studies have used phase V to measure diastolic blood pressure. The systolic and diastolic pressures should be measured at least three times over a period of at least 3 minutes and the lowest reading recorded. For reasons of comparability, the data should be recorded everywhere in a uniform way.

Classification

Hypertension is divided into primary (essential) and

secondary. Hypertension is classified as "essential" when the causes are generally unknown. Essential hypertension is the most prevalent form of hypertension accounting for 90 per cent of all cases of hypertension. Hypertension is classified as "secondary" when some other disease process or abnormality is involved in its causation. Prominent among these are diseases of kidney (chronic glomerulo-nephritis and chronic pyelonephritis), tumours of the adrenal glands, congenital narrowing of the aorta and toxemias of pregnancy. Altogether, these are estimated to account for about 10 per cent or less of the cases of hypertension.

Magnitude of the problem

Although blood pressure is easily measured, it had taken several decades to realise that arterial hypertension is a frequent, worldwide health disorder *(5)*.

"Rule of halves"

Hypertension is an "iceberg" disease. It became evident in the early 1970s that only about half of the hypertensive subjects in the general population of most developed countries were aware of the condition, only about half of those aware of the problem were being treated, and only about half of those treated were considered adequately treated *(6)*. Fig. 1 illustrates this situation *(7)*. If this was the situation in countries with highly developed medical services, in the developing countries, the proportion treated would be far too less.

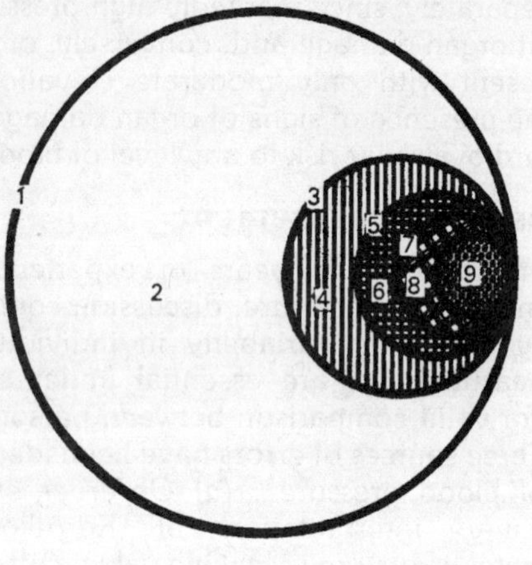

FIG. 1
Hypertension in the community

The areas of the circles shown in Fig. 1 correspond to the actual proportions observed in several population based studies and number-wise represent the following : *(6)*.

1. The whole community
2. Normotensive subjects
3. Hypertensive subjects
4. Undiagnosed hypertension
5. Diagnosed hypertension
6. Diagnosed but untreated
7. Diagnosed and treated
8. Inadequately treated
9. Adequately treated

INCIDENCE : The concept of incidence has limited value in hypertension because of the variability of consecutive readings in individuals, ambiguity of what is "normal" blood pressure and the insidious nature of the condition *(8)*.

The global prevalence of hypertension was estimated to be 1.13 billion killing 10 million people every year. The overall prevalence of hypertension in adults is around 30–40 per cent, with a global age standardized prevalence of 24 and 20 per cent in men and women respectively. This high prevalence of hypertension across the world is irrespective of income status i.e., in lower, middle and higher income countries. Hypertension becomes progressively more common with advancing age, with a prevalence of >60 per cent in people aged >60 years. As populations age, they adopt more sedentary life styles and increase in their body weight. It is estimated that the number of people with hypertension will increase by 15–20 per cent by year 2025 *(2)*. Elevated blood pressure is a leading cause of premature death in 2015, accounting to almost 10 million deaths and over 200 million DALYs. Despite advances in diagnosis and treatment over the past 30 years, the DALYs have increased by 40 per cent since 1990. Systolic blood pressure ≥140 mmHg accounts for most of the mortality and disability burden. The largest number of systolic blood pressure related deaths per year are due to IHD (4.9 million), haemorrhagic stroke (2 million) and ischaemic stroke (1.5 million) *(2)*.

Prevalence in India

In India an individual is classified as having hypertension if that individual has a systolic blood pressure level greater than or equal to 140 mmHg or a diastolic blood pressure level greater than or equal to 90 mmHg or that individual is currently taking antihypertensive medication to lower his/ her blood pressure.

Based on blood pressure measurement during the NFHS-5 21 per cent of women age 15 years and over have hypertension, including 12 per cent with mildly elevated blood pressure, 4 per cent with moderately elevated blood pressure, and 2 per cent with severely elevated blood pressure. Forty-four per cent of women have blood pressure within the normal range. Almost two-fifths (39%) of women are pre-hypertensive. One per cent of women are currently taking antihypertensive medicine and have their blood pressure in the normal range.

The prevalence of hypertension is higher among men age 15 years and over than among women age 15 years and over. Twentyfour per cent of men age 15 years and over have hypertension, including 16 per cent with mildly elevated blood pressure, 4 per cent with moderately elevate blood pressure, and 2 per cent with severely elevated blood pressure. Thirty per cent of men have normal blood pressure and 49 per cent are pre-hypertensive. About one per cent of men are currently taking antihypertensive medicine and have their blood pressure in the normal range.

Patterns by background characteristics

1. For both women and men, the prevalence of hypertension increases sharply with age. This increase is for all categories of hypertension, including pre-hypertension, for both women and men. About one-fourth of women and men age 40–49 have hypertension. Even at an earlier age, one in eight women and more than one in five men age 30–39 have hypertension as seen in Fig. 2.
2. The prevalence of hypertension is higher among Sikhs (37% for men and 31% for women), Jains (30% for men and 25% for women), and Christians (29% for men and 26% for women) than the rest of the religions.
3. There is a consistent and steep increase in the prevalence of hypertension with increases in the body mass index (BMI) for both women and men. Forty percent of obese men and 28 per cent of obese women are hypertensive.

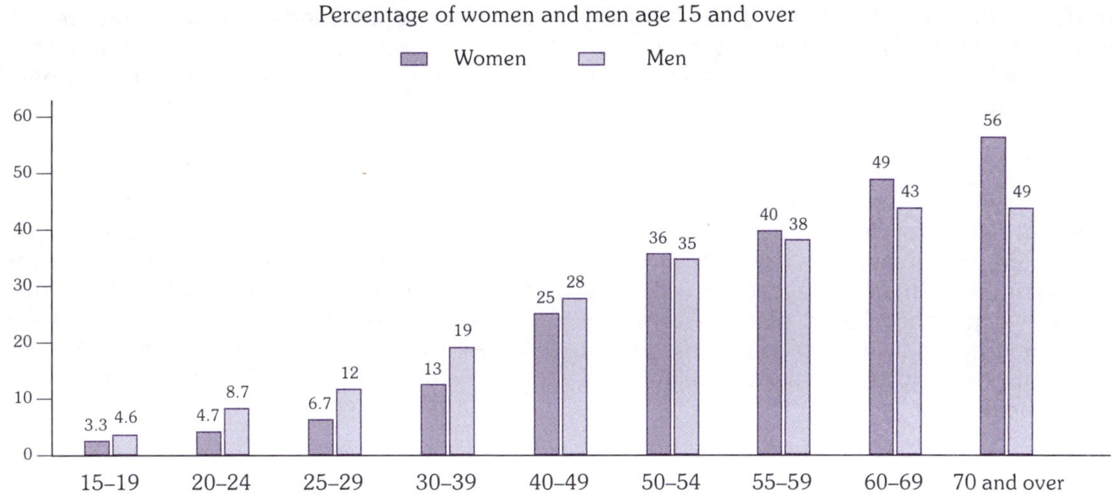

FIG. 2
Prevalence of Hypertension by Age and Sex

4. The prevalence of hypertension among women is highest (35%) in Sikkim. The prevalence of hypertension among men age 15 and over ranges from 15 per cent in Dadra & Nagar Haveli and Daman & Diu to 42 per cent in Sikkim.
5. For both women and men, the southern states have a higher prevalence of hypertension than the national average.

"Tracking" of blood pressure

If blood pressure levels of individuals were followed up over a period of years from early childhood into adult life, then those individuals whose pressures were initially high in the distribution, would probably continue in the same "track" as adults. In other words, low blood pressure levels tend to remain low, and high levels tend to become higher as individuals grow older (Fig. 3). This phenomenon of persistence of rank order of blood pressure has been described as "tracking" *(9)*. This knowledge can be applied in identifying children and adolescents "at risk" of developing hypertension at a future date.

Risk factors for hypertension

Hypertension is not only one of the major risk factors for most forms of cardiovascular disease, but that it is a condition with its own risk factors. A WHO Scientific Group *(5)* has recently reviewed the risk factors for essential hypertension. These may be classified as :

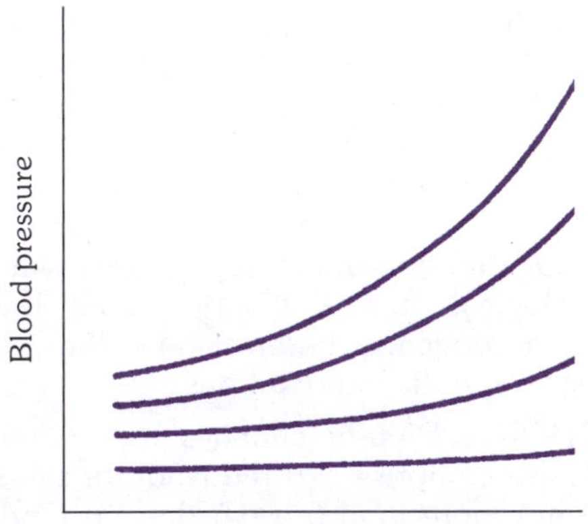

FIG. 3
Tracking of blood pressure

1. Non-modifiable risk factors

(a) AGE : Blood pressure rises with age in both sexes and the rise is greater in those with higher initial blood pressure. Age probably represents an accumulation of environmental influences and the effects of genetically programmed senescence in body systems *(3)*. Some populations have now been identified whose mean blood pressure does not rise with age *(10)*. These communities are for the most part primitive societies with calorie and often salt intakes at subsistence level.

(b) SEX : Early in life there is little evidence of a difference in blood pressure between the sexes. However, at adolescence, men display a higher average level. This difference is most evident in young and middle aged adults. Late in life the difference narrows and the pattern may even be reversed *(1)*. Post-menopausal changes in women may be the contributory factor for this change. Studies are in progress to evaluate whether oestrogen supplementation protects against the late relative rise of blood pressure in women *(1)*.

(c) GENETIC FACTORS : There is considerable evidence that blood pressure levels are determined in part by genetic factors, and that the inheritance is polygenic. The evidence is based on twin and family studies. *Twin studies* have confirmed the importance of genetic factors in hypertension. The blood pressure values of monozygotic twins are usually more strongly correlated than those of zygotic twins. In contrast, no significant correlation has been noted between husbands and wives, and between adopted children and their adoptive parents *(5)*.

Family studies have shown that the children of two normotensive parents have 3 per cent possibility of developing hypertension, whereas this possibility is 45 per cent in children of two hypertensive parents *(11)*. Blood pressure levels among first degree adult relatives have also been noted to be statistically significant *(5)*.

Attempts to find genetic markers that are associated with hypertension have been largely unsuccessful. The detailed mechanism of heredity, i.e., how many genes and loci are involved and their mode of inheritance have not yet been conclusively elucidated.

(d) ETHNICITY : Population studies have consistently revealed higher blood pressure levels in black communities than other ethnic groups *(1)*. Average difference in blood pressure between the two groups vary from slightly less than 5 mm Hg during the second decade of life to nearly 20 mm Hg during the sixth. Black Americans of African origin have been demonstrated to have higher blood pressure levels than whites.

2. *Modifiable risk factors*

(a) OBESITY : Epidemiological observations have identified obesity as a risk factor for hypertension *(12)*. The greater the weight gain, the greater the risk of high blood pressure. Data also indicate that when people with high blood pressure lose weight, their blood pressure generally decreases. "Central obesity" indicated by an increased waist to hip ratio, has been positively correlated with high blood pressure in several populations.

(b) SALT INTAKE : There is an increasing body of evidence to the effect that a high salt intake (i.e., 7–8 g per day) increases blood pressure proportionately. Low sodium intake has been found to lower the blood pressure *(13)*. For instance, the higher incidence of hypertension is found in Japan where sodium intake is above 400 mmol/day while primitive societies ingesting less than 60 mmol/day have virtually no hypertension *(14)*. It has been postulated that essential hypertensives have a genetic abnormality of the kidney which makes salt excretion difficult except at raised levels of arterial pressure *(5)*.

Besides sodium, there are other mineral elements such as potassium which are determinants of blood pressure. Potassium antagonizes the biological effects of sodium, and thereby reduces blood pressure. Potassium supplements have been found to lower blood pressure of mild to moderate hypertensives. Other cations such as calcium, cadmium and magnesium have also been suggested as of importance in reducing blood pressure levels.

(c) SATURATED FAT : The evidences suggest that saturated fat raises blood pressure as well as serum cholesterol *(15)*. For further details refer to chapter 11.

(d) DIETARY FIBRE : Several studies indicate that the risk of CHD and hypertension is inversely related to the consumption of dietary fibre. Most fibres reduce plasma total and LDL cholesterol *(1)*.

(e) ALCOHOL : High alcohol intake is associated with an increased risk of high blood pressure. It appears that alcohol consumption raises systolic pressure more than the diastolic. But the finding that blood pressure returns to normal with abstinence suggests that alcohol–induced elevations may not be fixed, and do not necessarily lead to sustained blood pressure elevation *(3)*.

(f) HEART RATE : When groups of normotensive and untreated hypertensive subjects, matched for age and sex, are compared, the heart rate of the hypertensive group is invariably higher. This may reflect a resetting of sympathetic activity at a higher level. The role of heart variability in blood pressure needs further research to elucidate whether the relation is casual or prognostic *(1)*.

(g) PHYSICAL ACTIVITY : Physical activity by reducing body weight may have an indirect effect on blood pressure.

(h) ENVIRONMENTAL STRESS : The term hypertension itself implies a disorder initiated by tension or stress. Since stress is nowhere defined, the hypothesis is untestable *(3)*. However, it is an accepted fact that psychosocial factors operate through mental processes, consciously or unconsciously, to produce hypertension. Virtually all studies on blood pressure and catecholamine levels in young people revealed significantly higher noradrenaline levels in hypertensives than in normotensives. This supports the contention that over-activity of the sympathetic nervous system has an important part to play in the pathogenesis of hypertension *(9)*.

(i) SOCIO-ECONOMIC STATUS : In countries that are in post-transitional stage of economic and epidemiological change, consistently higher levels of blood pressure have been noted in lower socio-economic groups. This inverse relation has been noted with levels of education, income and occupation. However, in societies that are transitional or pre-transitional, a higher prevalence of hypertension have been noted in upper socio-economic groups. This probably represents the initial stage of the epidemic of CVD *(1)*.

(j) OTHER FACTORS : The commonest present cause of secondary hypertension is oral contraception, because of the oestrogen component in combined preparations. Other factors such as noise, vibration, temperature and humidity require further investigation *(5)*.

PREVENTION OF HYPERTENSION

The low prevalence of hypertension in some communities indicates that hypertension is potentially preventable *(16)*. The WHO has recommended the following approaches in the prevention of hypertension :

1. Primary prevention
   (a) Population strategy
   (b) High-risk strategy
2. Secondary prevention

1. PRIMARY PREVENTION

Although control of hypertension can be successfully achieved by medication (secondary prevention) the ultimate goal in general is primary prevention. Primary prevention has been defined as "all measures to reduce the incidence of disease in a population by reducing the risk of onset" *(17)*. The earlier the prevention starts the more likely it is to be effective.

In connection with primary prevention, terms such as "population strategy" and "high-risk strategy" have become established *(5, 18)*. The WHO has recommended these approaches in the prevention of hypertension. Both the approaches are complementary.

a. POPULATION STRATEGY

The population approach is directed at the whole population, irrespective of individual risk levels. The concept of population approach is based on the fact that even a small reduction in the average blood pressure of a population would produce a large reduction in the incidence of cardiovascular complications such as stroke and CHD *(16)*. The goal of the population approach is to shift the community distribution of blood pressure towards lower levels or "biological normality" *(9)*. This involves a multifactorial approach, based on the following non-pharmacotherapeutic interventions :

(a) NUTRITION : Dietary changes are of paramount importance. These comprise : (i) reduction of salt intake to an average of not more than 5 g per day (ii) moderate fat intake (iii) the avoidance of a high alcohol intake, and (iv) restriction of energy intake appropriate to body needs.
(b) WEIGHT REDUCTION : The prevention and correction

of over weight/obesity (Body Mass Index greater than 25) is a prudent way of reducing the risk of hypertension and indirectly CHD; it goes with dietary changes. (c) EXERCISE PROMOTION : The evidence that regular physical activity leads to a fall in body weight, blood lipids and blood pressure goes to suggest that regular physical activity should be encouraged as part of the strategy for risk-factor control. (d) BEHAVIOURAL CHANGES : Reduction of stress and smoking, modification of personal life-style, yoga and transcendental meditation could be profitable. (e) HEALTH EDUCATION : The general public require preventive advice on all risk factors and related health behaviour. The whole community must be mobilized and made aware of the possibility of primary prevention, and (f) SELF-CARE : An important element in community–based health programmes is patient participation. The patient is taught self-care, i.e., to take his own blood pressure and keep a log–book of his readings. By doing so, the burden on the official health services would be considerably reduced. Log–books can also be useful for statistical purposes and for the long-term follow-up of cases *(19)*.

Table 2 shows some of the lifestyle modifications to manage hypertension.

b. HIGH-RISK STRATEGY

This is also part of primary prevention. The aim of this approach is "to prevent the attainment of levels of blood pressure at which the institution of treatment would be considered" *(3)*. This approach is appropriate if the risk factors occur with very low prevalence in the community *(3)*.

Detection of high-risk subjects should be encouraged by the optimum use of clinical methods. Since hypertension tends to cluster in families, the family history of hypertension and "tracking" of blood pressure from childhood may be used to identify individuals at risk.

2. SECONDARY PREVENTION

The goal of secondary prevention is to detect and control high blood pressure in affected individuals. Modern anti-hypertensive drug therapy can effectively reduce high blood pressure and consequently, the excess risk of morbidity and mortality from coronary, cerebrovascular and kidney disease. The control measures comprise:

(i) EARLY CASE DETECTION : Early detection is a major problem. This is because high blood pressure rarely causes symptoms until organ damage has already occurred, and our aim should be to control it before this happens. The only effective method of diagnosis of hypertension is to screen the population. But screening, that is not linked to follow-up and sustained care, is a fruitless exercise. It is emphasized that screening should not be initiated if health resources for treatment and follow-up are not adequate.

In the developed countries, mass screening is not considered essential for the adequate control of blood pressure in the population. In Europe, the large majority of people have at least one contact in every 2 years with the health service. If blood pressure is measured at each such contact, the bulk of the problem of detecting those in need of intervention is solved.

(ii) TREATMENT : In essential hypertension, as in diabetes, we cannot treat the cause, because we do not know what it is. Instead, we try to scale down the high blood pressure to acceptable levels. The aim of treatment should be to obtain a blood pressure below 140/90 mm Hg, and ideally a blood pressure of 120/80 mm Hg. Control of hypertension has been shown to reduce the incidence of stroke and other complications. This is a major reason for identifying and treating asymptomatic hypertension. Care of hypertensives should also involve attention to other risk factors such as smoking and elevated blood cholesterol levels *(16)*.

(iii) PATIENT COMPLIANCE : The treatment of high blood pressure must normally be life-long and this presents problems of patient compliance, which is defined as "the extent to which patient behaviour (in terms of taking medicines, following diets or executing other lifestyle changes) coincides with clinical prescription". The compliance rates can be improved through education directed to patients, families and the community.

Intensive research carried out during the past decade, aiming at control of hypertension at the community level, has already provided valuable results. The studies have shown that control of hypertension in a population is

TABLE 2
Lifestyle modifications to manage hypertension

Modification	Recommendation Reduction, Range	Approximate systolic BP
Weight reduction	Maintain normal body weight (BMI, 18.5–24.9)	5–20 mm Hg/10 kg weight loss
Adopt DASH eating plan	Consume a diet rich in fruits, vegetables and low-fat dairy products with a reduced content of saturated fat and total fat	8–14 mm Hg
Dietary sodium reduction	Reduce dietary sodium intake to no more than 100 mEq/d (2.4 g sodium or 6 g sodium chloride)	2–8 mm Hg
Physical activity	Engage in regular aerobic physical activity such as brisk walking (at least 30 minutes per day, most days of the week)	4–9 mm Hg
Moderation of alcohol consumption	Limit consumption to no more than two drinks per day (1 oz or 30 ml ethanol eg, 24 oz beer, 10 oz wine, or 3 oz 80- proof whisky) in most men, and no more than one drink per day in women and lighter-weight persons	2–4 mm Hg

For overall cardiovascular risk reduction, stop smoking.
The effects of implementing these modifications are dose and time dependent and could be higher for some individuals.
BMI – body mass index calculated as weight in kilograms divided by the square of height in metres;
DASH – Dietary Approaches to Stop Hypertension.
Source : *(20)*

feasible, that it can be carried out through the existing system of health services in different countries, and that the control of blood pressure leads to a reduction of complications of high blood pressure – namely stroke, heart failure and renal failure. In some of the projects the incidence of myocardial infarction was also reduced. As a result of these findings some countries have launched nationwide control programmes in the field of hypertension *(21)*.

References

1. WHO (1996). *Techn. Rep. Ser.*, No. 862.
2. European Heart Journal (2018), *Guidelines for the management of arterial hypertension*, Vol. 39 issue 33, 25 Aug. 2018.
3. Hart, J.T. (1980). *Hypertension*, Library of General Practitioner Series, Churchill Livingstone.
4. WHO (1983). *Bull WHO*, 61 (1) 53.
5. WHO (1983). *Techn. Rep. Ser.*, No. 686.
6. Strasser, T. (1972). *WHO Chronicle*, 26 : 451.
7. WHO (1974). *WHO Chronicle*, 28 (3) 11.
8. Govt. of India (2022), *National Family Health Survey-5 (2019–2021)*, Ministry of Health and Family welfare, New Delhi.
9. WHO (1985). *Techn. Rep. Ser.*, No. 715.
10. Marmot, M.G. (1984). *Brit. Med. Bulletin*, 40 (4) 380.
11. Bianchi, G. et al (1979). *Lancet*, 1 : 173–177.
12. Stamler, R. et al (1978). *JAMA*, 240 : 1607.
13. Beard, T.C. et al (1982). *Lancet*, 2 : 455.
14. Oliver, M.F. (1981). *Br. Med. Bull.*, 37 (1) 49.
15. Puska, P. et al (1983). *Lancet*, 1 : 1–5.
16. WHO (1986). *Techn. Rep. Ser.*, No. 732.
17. Hogarth, J. (1978). *Glossary Health Care Terminology*, WHO, Copenhagen.
18. Rose, G. (1981). Brit.Med.J., 1: 1847.
19. WHO (1978). *WHO Chronicle*, 32 (11) 448.
20. STEPHEN J. McPHEE, MAXINE A. PAPADAKIS (2010). *Current Medical Diagnosis and Treatment*, 49th Ed. A Lange Publication.
21. WHO (1980). *Sixth Report World Health Situation*, Part I.

STROKE

The term "stroke" (syn : apoplexy) is applied to acute severe manifestations of cerebrovascular disease. It causes both physical and mental crippling. WHO defined stroke as "rapidly developed clinical signs of focal disturbance of cerebral function; lasting more than 24 hours or leading to death, with no apparent cause other than vascular origin" *(1)*. The 24 hours threshold in the definition excludes transcient ischaemic attacks (TIA) which is defined to last less than 24 hours, and patients with stroke symptoms caused by subdural haemorrhage, tumours, poisoning or trauma are excluded.

The disturbance of cerebral function is caused by three morphological abnormalities, i.e., stenosis, occlusion or rupture of the arteries. Dysfunction of the brain ("neurological deficit") manifests itself by various neurological signs and symptoms that are related to extent and site of the area involved and to the underlying causes. These include coma, hemiplegia, paraplegia, monoplegia, multiple paralysis, speech disturbances, nerve paresis, sensory impairment, etc. Of these hemiplegia constitutes the main somatoneurological disorder in about 90 per cent of patients *(2)*.

Stroke includes a number of syndromes with differing aetiologies, epidemiology, prognosis and treatment. These are listed below :

A. Ischaemic stroke
   a. Lacunar infarct
   b. Carotid circulation obstruction
   c. Vertebro-basilar obstruction

B. Haemorrhagic stroke
   a. Spontaneous intracerebral haemorrhage
   b. Subarachnoid haemorrhage
   c. Intracranial aneurysm
   d. Arteriovenous malformations.

Problem

Stroke is a worldwide health problem. It makes an important contribution to morbidity, mortality and disability in developed as well as developing countries. Although there are substantial differences in frequency from place to place, cerebral thrombosis is usually the most frequent form of stroke encountered in clinical studies, followed by haemorrhage. Subarachnoid haemorrhage and cerebral embolism come next as regards both mortality and morbidity *(2)*. However, stroke from cerebral haemorrhage is more common in Japan than elsewhere *(1)*.

MORBIDITY AND MORTALITY

Cerebrovascular disease remain a leading cause of death from NCDs. In 2016 it was estimated that cerebrovascular disease accounted for 5.78 million deaths worldwide, equivalent to 10.2 per cent of all deaths. Majority of these deaths occurred in people living in developing countries and 33.72 per cent of the subjects were aged less than 70 years *(3)*. Additionally, cerebrovascular disease is the leading cause of disability in adults and each year millions of stroke survivors have to adopt life with restriction in activities of daily living as a consequence of stroke. Many surviving stroke patients will often depend on other people's continuous support to live *(4)*.

In demographically developed countries, the average age at which stroke occurs is around 73 years reflecting the older age structure of these countries. The probability of a first stroke or first TIA is around 1.6 per 1000 and 0.42 per 1000 respectively. In less developed regions, the average age of stroke is less due to the different population age structure, resulting from higher mortality rates.

Stroke patients are at highest risk of death in the first weeks after the event, and between 20–50 per cent die within first month depending on type, severity, age, co-morbidity and effectiveness of treatment of complications. Patients who survive may be left with no disability or with mild, moderate or severe disability. Considerable spontaneous recovery occurs upto about 6 months. However, patients with history of stroke are at high risk of a subsequent event of around 10 per cent in the first year and 5 per cent year thereafter *(4)*.

The proportion of patients achieving independence in self-care by one year after a stroke range from around 60 to 83 per cent. This depends on whether the studies are community-based or hospital-based, which activity is considered in estimating independence, and the methods used to rate ability *(4)*.

There is evidence that mortality from stroke has been declining in many countries for several years. Some of the decline occurred before modern treatment methods became available, indicating that the decline in stroke was associated with social and economic changes.

INDIA

Although the prevalence of stroke appears to be comparatively less in India than in developed countries, it is likely to increase proportionally with the increase in life expectancy. The proportion of stroke in the young population is significantly more in India than in developed countries; some of the more important causes for this are likely to be rheumatic heart disease, ischaemic strokes in peripartum period and arteriopathies as a sequale of CNS infections like bacterial and tubercular meningitis etc. *(5)*.

In India 0.706 million people died of stroke in 2016 of which 0.372 million were men and 0.334 million were women. The crude death rate of stroke was about 54.2 per 100,000 population *(3)*. More recently, in 2020, 73,349 people were diagnosed as having stroke *(7)*.

1. RISK FACTORS

Epidemiological studies have indicated that stroke does not occur at random, and there are factors (risk factors) which precede stroke by several years. These are : *(a) Hypertension:* This is considered the main risk factor for cerebral thrombosis as well as cerebral haemorrhage; *(b) Other factors:* Additional factors contributing to risk are cardiac abnormalities (i.e., left ventricular hypertrophy, cardiac dilatation), diabetes, elevated blood lipids, obesity, smoking, glucose intolerance, blood clotting and viscosity, oral contraceptives, etc. The importance of these factors is not clearly defined. Although the risk factors for stroke are similar to those for CHD, their relative importance differs *(6)*.

2. TRANSCIENT ISCHAEMIC ATTACKS (TIA)

One phenomenon that has received increasing attention is the occurrence of TIA in a fair proportion of cases. These are episodes of focal, reversible, neurological deficit of sudden onset and of less than 24 hours duration. They show a tendency to recurrence. They are due to microemboli, and are a warning sign of stroke.

HOST FACTORS

(i) Age : Stroke can occur at any age. Usually incidence rates rise steeply with age. Globally about 47 per cent of all stroke deaths occur in persons over 70 years. In India, about one fifth of all strokes occur below the age of 40 (called "strokes in the young"). This is attributed to our "young population", and shorter life expectancy.

(ii) Sex : The incidence rates are higher in males than females at all ages.

(iii) Personal history : The WHO Study showed that nearly three-quarters of all registered stroke patients had associated diseases, mostly in the cardiovascular system or of diabetes. This supports the view that in most cases stroke is merely an incident in the slowly progressive course of a generalized vascular disease.

Stroke control programme

The aim of a stroke control programme is to apply at community level effective measures for the prevention of stroke. The first priority goes to control of arterial hypertension which is a major cause of stroke. As transcient ischaemic attacks (TIA) may be one of the earliest manifestations of stroke, their early detection and treatment is important for the prevention of stroke *(2)*. Control of diabetes, elimination of smoking, and prevention and management of other risk factors at the population level are new approaches. Treatment for acute stroke is largely the control of complications. Facilities for the long-term follow-up of patients are essential. The education and training of health personnel and of the public form an integral part of the programme. For any such programme, reliable knowledge of the extent of the problem in the community concerned is essential *(2)*.

In summary, control of stroke that was once considered an inevitable accompaniment to ageing is now being approached through primary prevention. It has generated the hope that stroke can be tackled by community health action.

References

1. WHO (1980). *Bull WHO,* 58 : 113–130.
2. WHO (1971). *Techn. Rep. Ser.*, No. 469.
3. WHO (2018). *Global Health Estimates,* April 2018.
4. WHO (2011). *Related Article to the Global Burden of Cerebrovascular Disease* by Truelse T.
5. ICMR (2004). *Assessment of Burden of Non-Communicable Diseases,* Final Report.
6. Pedoe, H.T. (1982). In : *Epidemiology of Diseases,* Miller, D.L. and R.D.T. Farmer (eds), Blackwell, Oxford.
7. Govt. of India (2021), *National Health Profile 2021*.

RHEUMATIC HEART DISEASE

Rheumatic fever (RF) and rheumatic heart disease (RHD) cannot be separated from an epidemiological point of view *(1)*. Rheumatic fever is a febrile disease affecting connective tissues particularly in the heart and joints initiated by infection of the throat by group A β *haemolytic streptococci*. Although RF is not a communicable disease, it results from a communicable disease (streptococcal pharyngitis). Rheumatic fever often leads to RHD which is a crippling disease. The consequences of RHD include : continuing damage to the heart; increasing disabilities; repeated hospitalization, and premature death usually by the age of 35 years or even earlier. RHD is one of the most readily preventable chronic disease.

Problem

WORLD

The incidence of rheumatic fever and rheumatic heart disease has not decreased in developing countries. Retrospective studies reveal developing countries to have the highest figures for cardiac involvement and recurrence rates of rheumatic fever. Worldwide, there are over 15 million cases of RHD with 500,000 new cases. During 2008, 230,000 deaths from this disease occurred which is about 0.4 per cent of total deaths *(2)*.

RHD is a major cause of morbidity and a major cause of mitral insufficiency and stenosis in the world. Variables that correlate with the severity of valve disease include the number of previous attacks of RF, the length of time between the onset of disease and start of therapy, and sex (the disease is more severe in females than in males). Insufficiency from acute rheumatic valve disease resolves in 60–80 per cent of patients who adhere to antibiotic prophylaxis *(3)*.

In a number of affluent countries (North America, Western Europe and in Japan) the incidence of RF and the prevalence of and mortality from RHD have fallen during the last two decades, where the disease is now generally uncommon. Some of this decline occurred before modern treatment methods became available, indicating that the fall in prevalence and incidence was associated with social and economic changes *(4)*.

As a result of the above decline, there has been a tendency to minimize the public health importance of RF – the assumption being that the disease may subside or even vanish spontaneously as living standards rise. However, even in the most affluent countries, there remain pockets of poverty where socio-economic conditions continue to favour the persistence of RF *(5)*.

INDIA

In India, RHD is prevalent in the range of 5–7 per thousand in 5–15 years age group and there are about 1 million RHD cases in India. RHD constitutes 20–30% of hospital admissions due to CVD in India *(6)*. Streptococcal infections are very common especially in children living in under-privileged conditions, and RF is reported to occur in 1–3 per cent of those infections *(7)*.

Jai Vigyan Mission Mode project on Community Control of RF/RHD in India is being carried out with four main components, viz. to study the epidemiology of streptococcal sore throats, establish registries for RF and RHD, vaccine development for streptococcal infection and conducting advanced studies on pathological aspects of RF and RHD *(7)*.

Epidemiological factors

1. AGENT FACTORS

(a) AGENT : The onset of RF is usually preceded by a streptococcal sore throat. Of the streptococci, it is the group A streptococcus that has been incriminated as the causative agent. It has been suggested that not all strains of group A streptococci lead to RF; it is believed that there might be some strains with "rheumatogenic potential". The serotype that has attracted special emphasis is M type 5 which is frequently associated with RF *(8)*. All group A streptococci are sensitive to penicillin. Unfortunately, the group consists of a great number of immunologically different types with little cross immunity, defying all attempts to produce an effective vaccine. Recently the virus (coxsackie B4) has been suggested as a causative factor and streptococcus acting as a conditioning agent. There are many gaps in our knowledge about the causative agent and underlying pathogenic mechanisms. (b) CARRIERS : Carriers of group A streptococcus are frequent, e.g., convalescent, transcient and chronic carriers. In view of the high carrier rate, their eradication is not even theoretically possible *(9)*.

2. HOST AND ENVIRONMENTAL FACTORS

(a) AGE : RF is typically a disease of childhood and adolescence (5–15 years) although it also occured in adults (20 per cent cases). Mention has already been made about the high incidence of "juvenile mitral stenosis" in India *(9, 10)*. The initial attack of RF occurs at a young age, progresses to valvular lesions faster and is associated with pulmonary arterial hypertension. The cause of the "juvenile" disease in India is not known. (b) SEX : The disease affects both sexes equally but prognosis is worse for females than for males. (c) IMMUNITY : An immunological basis for RF and RHD has been proposed. The most prevalent concept is the toxic–immunological hypothesis. According to this theory, group A streptococcal products have certain toxic products, and components of the streptococcus and of host tissues have an antigenic cross-relationship, leading to immunological processes that result in an attack of RF *(11)*. (d) SOCIO-ECONOMIC STATUS : RF is a social disease linked to poverty, overcrowding, poor housing conditions, inadequate health services, inadequate expertise of health-care providers and a low level of awareness of the disease in the community. It declines sharply when the standard of living is improved, but even in the most affluent countries, there are areas where the disease still exists. (e) HIGH-RISK GROUPS : The school-age children between 5 and 15 years; slum dwellers; and those living in a closed community (e.g., barracks).

Table 1 summarizes the effects of environmental factors on RF and RHD.

Clinical features

(a) FEVER : Fever is present at the onset of acute illness and may be accompanied by profuse sweating. It may last for about 12 weeks or longer and has a tendency to recur. (b) POLYARTHRITIS: This occurs in 90 per cent of cases. Large joints like ankles, knees, elbows and wrists are involved; uncommonly smaller joints of hands and feet may be involved. The pain and swelling come on quickly and also subside spontaneously within 5–7 days. There is no residual damage to the joint. (c) CARDITIS : Occurs in 60–70 per cent of cases. It starts early in the course of RF. Moreover RHD may not be preceded by a clinically apparent attack of RF. All layers of the heart– pericardium, myocardium and the heart valves – are involved. The involvement of heart is manifested by tachycardia, cardiac murmurs, cardiac enlargement, pericarditis and heart failure. The most common ECG finding is the first degree AV block. (d) NODULES : Nodules below the skin tend to

TABLE 1
Direct and indirect results of enviromental and health-system determinants on rheumatic fever and rheumatic heart disease

Determinants	Effects	Impact on RF and RHD burden
Socio-economic and environmental factors : (poverty, undernutrition, overcrowding, poor housing).	Rapid spread of group A streptococcal strains. Difficulties in accessing health care.	Higher incidence of acute streptococcal-pharyngitis and suppurative complications. Higher incidence of acute RF. Higher rates of recurrent attacks.
Health-system related factors : – shortage of resources for health care;	Inadequate diagnosis and treatment of streptococcal pharyngitis.	Higher incidence of acute RF and its recurrence.
– inadequate expertise of health-care providers;	Misdiagnosis or late diagnosis of acute RF.	Patients unaware of the first RF episode. More severe evolution of disease.
– Low-level awareness of the disease in the community.	Inadequate secondary prophylaxis and/or non-compliance with secondary prophylaxis.	Untimely initiation or lack of secondary prophylaxis. Higher rates of recurrent attacks with more frequent and severe heart valve involvement, and higher rates of repeated hospital admissions and expensive surgical interventions.

Source : *(12)*

appear 4 weeks after the onset of RF. They are small, painless and non-tender. They last for a variable period of time and then disappear leaving no residual damage. (e) BRAIN INVOLVEMENT: This manifests as abnormal jerky purposeless movements of the arms, legs and the body. It gradually disappears leaving no residual damage. (f) SKIN : Various types of skin rash are known to occur. It is thus obvious that except carditis all other manifestations of RF do not cause permanent damage.

Diagnosis

The 2015 WHO criteria for the diagnosis of RF and RHD are based on revised Jones criteria (Table 2).

In the revised 2015 Jones criteria, a low, medium and high-risk population was identified. A low risk population is one in which cases of acute RF occur in ≤ 2/100 000 school-age children or rheumatic heart disease is diagnosed in ≤ 1/ 1000 patients at any age during one year.

The modifications introduced in 2015 in the Jones criteria are as follows :

1. In the major criteria:
   - *Low risk population* : clinical and/or subclinical carditis. AHA recommends that all the patients with suspected RF undergo Doppler echocardiographic examination, even if no clinical signs of carditis are present. In doubtful cases it is recommended that echocardiography is repeated.
   - *Medium and high risk population* : also clinical and/or subclinical carditis and arthritis - monoarthritis or polyarthritis, possibly also with polyarthralgia.
2. In the minor criteria:
   - *Low risk population* : the parameters of inflammation and the level of fever were defined precisely.
   - *Medium and high risk population* : monoarthralgia, also with defined parameters of inflammation and the level of fever.

TABLE 2
Diagnostic criteria for rheumatic fever modified 2015 Jones criteria

Major criteria	
Low risk population	High risk population
Carditis (clinical or subclinical) Arthritis - only polyarthritis Chorea Erythema marginatum Subcutaneous nodules	Carditis (clinical or subclinical) Arthritis - monoarthritis or polyarthritis Polyarthralgia Chorea Erythema marginatum Subcutaneous nodules
Minor criteria	
Low risk population	High risk population
Polyarthralgia	Monoarthralgia
Hyperpyrexia (≥ 38.5°C)	Hyperpyrexia (≥ 38.0°C)
ESR ≥ 60 mm/h and/or CRP ≥ 3.0 mg/dl	ESR ≥ 30 mm/h and/or CRP ≥ 3.0 mg/dl
Prolonged PR interval (after taking into account the differences related to age; if there is no carditis as a major criterion)	Prolonged PR interval (after taking into account the differences related to age; if there is no carditis as a major criterion)

ESR - erythrocyte sedimentation rate; CRP - C-reactive protein
Source : *(13)*

The diagnosis of RF in the whole population with evidence of antecedent group A β-hemolytic streptococcal infection requires a confirmation of two major criteria or one major and two minor criteria – the first episode of the disease.

Diagnosis of subsequent episodes of the disease requires a confirmation of two major criteria or one major and two minor criteria or three minor criteria.

Echocardiographic examination is currently the main diagnostic tool used for confirmation, diagnosis and monitoring of valvular lesions in the course of RF, especially in cases of subclinical carditis.

Subclinical carditis is one in which physical examination does not confirm any lesions in auscultation over the heart. Only echocardiography (Doppler) reveals mitral or aortic valve pathology.

The echocardiographic criteria developed by AHA in 2012 are as follows *(13)* :

I. Echocardiographic (Doppler) criteria :

- Pathological mitral regurgitation–4 criteria (all must be met) :
  1. Visible at least in 2 projections.
  2. Regurgitation jet length ≥ 2 cm at least in 1 projection.
  3. Regurgitation peak velocity > 3 m/s.
  4. Regurgitation pansystolic.
- Pathological aortic regurgitation–4 criteria (all must be met) :
  1. Visible at least in 2 projections.
  2. Regurgitation jet length ≥ 1 cm at least in 1 projection.
  3. Regurgitation peak velocity > 3 m/s.
  4. Regurgitation pandiastolic.

Prevention

Two preventive approaches are possible :

a. PRIMARY PREVENTION

The aim of primary prevention is to prevent the first attack of RF, by identifying all patients with streptococcal throat infection and treating them with penicillin. While this approach is theoretically simple, in practice, it is difficult to achieve and may not be feasible in many developing countries *(4)*. In order to prevent a single case of RHD, several thousand cases of streptococcal throat infection must be identified and treated. Many infections are inapparent or if apparent are not brought to the attention of the health services; even if they are reported, quick and reliable laboratory services are needed to confirm the diagnosis.

A viable approach is to concentrate on "high-risk" groups such as school-age children. They should be kept under surveillance for streptococcal pharyngitis. Ideally a sore throat should be swabbed and cultured. If streptococci are present, the child should be put on penicillin. Since facilities for throat swab culture are not easily available, it is justified to treat a sore throat with penicillin even without having the culture. For this purpose, a single intramuscular injection of 1.2 million units of benzathine benzyl penicillin for adults and 600,000 units for children is adequate, or oral penicillin (Penicillin V or Penicillin G) should be given for 10 days. This is the least expensive method of giving penicillin for eradication of streptococci from the throat. For patients with allergy to penicillin, first generation cephalosporins i.e., cefodroxil or cefalexin is used. The other drugs used – erythromycin, clarithromycin and azithromycin *(13)*. The MCH and school health services should be utilized for this purpose.

In short, the impossible logistics of primary prevention coupled with enormous financial constraints force us to concentrate on secondary prevention *(10)*.

b. SECONDARY PREVENTION

Secondary prevention (i.e., the prevention of recurrences of RF) is a more practicable approach, especially in developing countries. It consists in identifying those who have had RF and giving them one intramuscular injection of benzathine benzyl penicillin (1.2 million units in adults and 600,000 units in children) at intervals of 3 weeks *(12)*. This must be continued for at least 5 years or until the child reaches 21 years whichever is later. For patients with carditis (mild mitral regurgitation or healed carditis) the treatment should continue for 10 years after the last attack, or at least until 40 years of age, which ever is longer. More severe valvular disease or post-valve surgery cases need life-long treatment *(13)*. This prevents streptococcal sore throat and therefore recurrence of RF and RHD.

However, the crucial problem is one of patient compliance as penicillin prophylaxis is a long-term affair. Studies have shown that secondary prevention is feasible, inexpensive and cost-effective, when implemented through primary health care systems *(13)*.

c. NON-MEDICAL MEASURES

Non-medical measures for the prevention/control of RF are related to improving living conditions, and breaking the poverty–disease–poverty cycle. Improvements in socio-economic conditions (particularly better housing) will in the long term reduce the incidence of RF.

Objective evaluation of available data indicates that penicillin alone will not lead to effective control. Predictions suggest that many of the countries which suffer severe economic constraints will not be likely to be able to raise their standards of living in the foreseeable future to significantly alter the incidence of this disease *(9)*.

d. EVALUATION

In the evaluation of the programme, the prevalence of RHD in school children from periodic surveys of random samples is probably the best indicator. It is suggested that surveys should be carried out on samples of schools (not individuals) in the 6–14 years age group at 5–year intervals. The recommended sample size is 20,000 to 30,000 children depending upon the expected prevalence *(14)*.

References

1. WHO (1969). *WHO Chronicle*, 28:345.
2. WHO (2011). *Disease and Injuries, Regional Estimates, Cause Specific Mortality, Estimates for 2008*.
3. Medscape (2012). Thomas K Chin, *Paediatric Rheumatic Heart Disease Overview Epidemiology*, May 30th, 2012.
4. WHO (1986). *Techn Rep. Ser.* No. 732.
5. Strasser, T. and Rotta J. (1973) *WHO Chronicle*, 27 (2) 49–54.
6. Govt. of India (2006). *Health Information of India*, 2005, Min. of Health and Family Welfare New Delhi.
7. Govt of India (2004). *Annual Report 2003-2004*, Ministry of Health and Family Welfare, New Delhi.
8. Kaplan, E.L. (1985). *Int. J. Epi*, 14 (4) 499.
9. Strasser, T. (1978). *WHO Chronicle*, 32 (1) 18–25.
10. Wahi, P.L. (1984). *Ann Acad. Med. Sci. (India)* 20 (4) 199–215.
11. El Kholy, A. et al (1978). *Bull WHO*, 56:887.
12. WHO (2004), *Tech. Rep. Ser.* No. 923.
13. Szczgielska Izabela et.al. (2018), *Rheumatic fever-new diagnostic criteria*, Rheumatologia 2018 : 56 (1) : 37–41.
14. Strasser, T. et al (1981), *Bull WHO*, 59 : 285–294.

CANCER

Cancer may be regarded as a group of diseases characterized by an (i) abnormal growth of cells (ii) ability to invade adjacent tissues and even distant organs, and (iii) the eventual death of the affected patient if the tumour has progressed beyond that stage when it can be successfully removed. Cancer can occur at any site or tissue of the body and may involve any type of cells.

The major categories of cancer are : *(a) Carcinomas*, which arise from epithelial cells lining the internal surfaces of the various organs (e.g. mouth, oesophagus, intestines, uterus) and from the skin epithelium; *(b) Sarcomas*, which arise from mesodermal cells constituting the various connective tissues (e.g. fibrous tissue, fat and bone); and *(c) Lymphomas, myeloma* and *leukaemias* arising from the cells of bone marrow and immune systems.

The term "primary tumour" is used to denote cancer in the organ of origin, while "secondary tumour" denotes cancer that has spread to regional lymph nodes and distant organs. When cancer cells multiply and reach a critical size, the cancer is clinically evident as a lump or ulcer localized to the organ of origin in early stages. As the disease advances, symptoms and signs of invasion and distant metastases become clinically evident *(1)*.

Problem statement

WORLD

In the year 2020, the global burden of cancer rose to an estimated 19.292 million new cases with 9.958 million deaths. The most common cancer diagnosed were cancer breast followed by cancer lung, prostate, colon and stomach. The most common cause of death due to cancer was cancer lung, cancer liver, cancer stomach and cancer breast. The summary statistics for the year 2020 is as follows *(2)* :

	Males	Females	Both sexes
Population	3,929,973,836	3,864,824,712	7,794,798,844
Number of new cancer cases	10,065,305	9,227,484	19,292,789
Age-standardized incidence rate (World)	222.0	186.0	201.0
Risk of developing cancer before the age of 75 years (%)	22.6	18.6	20.4
Number of cancer deaths	5,528,810	4,429,323	9,958,133
Age-standardized mortality rate (World)	120.8	84.2	100.7
Risk of dying from cancer before the age of 75 years (%)	12.6	8.9	10.7
5-year prevalent cases	24,828,480	25,721,807	50,550,287
Top 5 most frequent cancers excluding non-melanoma skin cancer (ranked by cases)	Lung Prostate Colorectum Stomach Liver	Breast Colorectum Lung Cervix uteri Thyroid	Breast Lung Colorectum Prostate Stomach

The age standardized incidence rate of top 10 cancers by sex, and age standardized incidence and mortality rate of top 10 cancers worldwide are as shown in Fig. 1 and 2.

As a consequence of growing and ageing populations, as well as changes in the prevalence and distribution of main risk factors for cancer, several of which are associated with

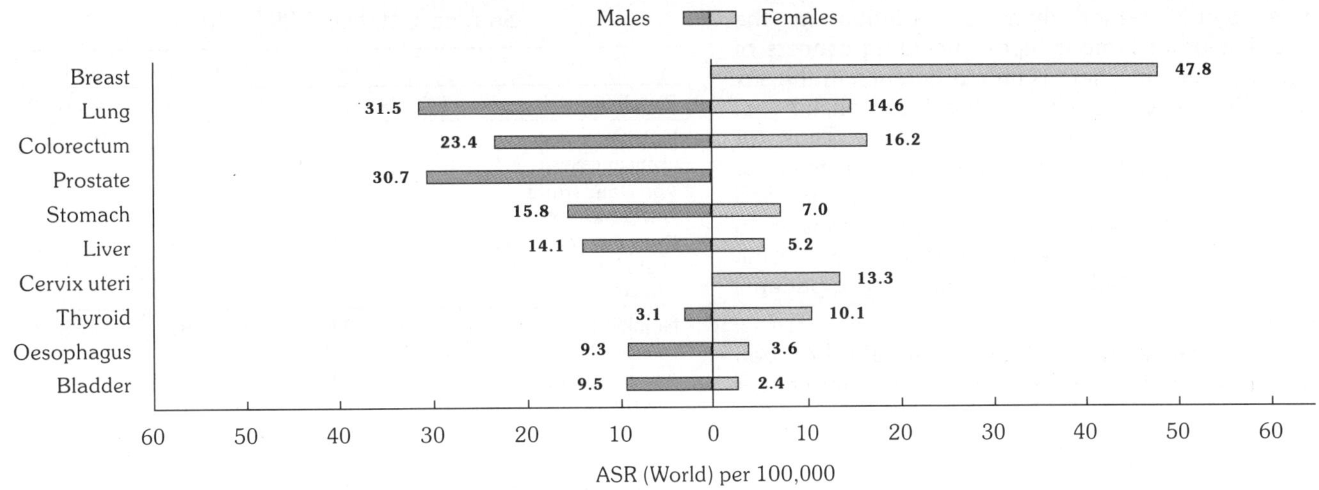

FIG. 1
Age standardized (World) incidence rates by sex, top 10 cancers

Source : *(2)*

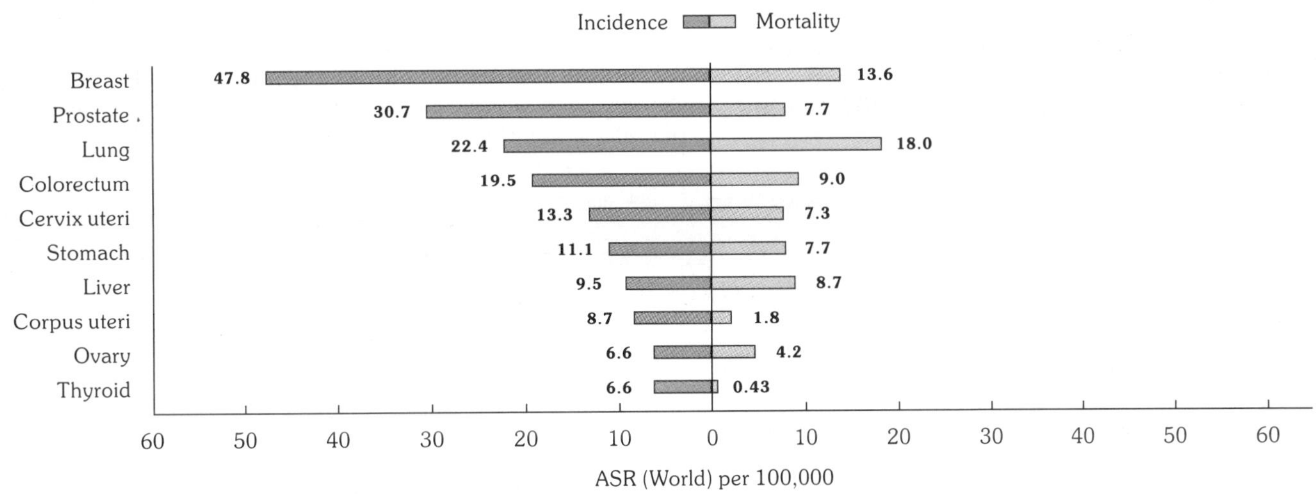

FIG. 2
Age standardized (World) incidence and mortality rates, top 10 cancers

Source : *(2)*

socio-economic development, developing countries are disproportionately affected by the increasing numbers of cancers.

For both sexes combined, one-half of all cases and 58.3 per cent of cancer deaths are estimated to occur in Asia in 2020, where 59.5 per cent of the global population resides. Europe accounts for 22.8 per cent of the total cancer cases and 19.6 per cent of the cancer deaths, although it represents 9.7 per cent of the global population, followed by the Americas' 20.9 per cent of incidence and 14.2 per cent of mortality worldwide. In contrast to other regions, the share of cancer deaths in Asia (58.3 per cent) and Africa (7.2 per cent) are higher than the share of incidence (49.3 per cent and 5.7 per cent, respectively) because of the different distribution of cancer types and higher case fatality rates in these regions *(3)*.

The "Westernization" trends : As low human-development index (HDI) countries become more developed through rapid societal and economic changes, they are likely to become "westernized". As such, the pattern of cancer incidence is likely to follow that seen in high HDI settings, with likely decline in cancer incidence rate of cervix uteri and stomach, and increasing incidence rates of breast, prostate and colorectal cancers. This westernization effect is a result of reduction in infection-related cancers and increase in cancers associated with reproductive, dietary and hormonal risk factors *(4)*.

For any disease, the relationship of incidence to mortality is an indication of prognosis. Similar incidence and mortality rates being indicative of an essentially fatal condition. Thus, lung cancer accounts for most deaths from cancer in the world (1.7 million) annually, since it is most invariably associated with poor prognosis. On the other hand, appropriate intervention is often effective in avoiding fatal outcome following diagnosis of breast cancer. Hence this particular cancer, which rank second in terms of incidence, is not among the top three causes of death from cancer, which are respectively cancers of the lung, stomach, and liver.

The most conspicuous feature of the distribution of cancers between the sexes is the male predominance of lung cancer. Prostate, colorectal, stomach and liver cancer are also much more common in males. Cancer of breast, colorectum, lung, cervix, uteri and stomach are common in females *(5)*. For the most part, differences in distribution between the sexes are attributable to differences in exposure to causative agents rather than to variation in the susceptibility. For other tumour types, including cancers of pancreas and colorectum, there is little difference in the sex distribution. Generally speaking, the relationship of incidence to mortality is not affected by sex. Thus for example, the prognosis following diagnosis of liver or pancreatic cancer is dismal for both males and females. Many other tumour types are more responsive to therapy, so that cancers of breast, prostate and uterine cervix are the cause of death in only a minority of patients diagnosed *(6)*.

The burden of cancer is distributed unequally between developed and developing countries, with particular cancer types exhibiting different patterns of distribution.

INDIA

In India, the National Cancer Registry Programme of the ICMR provides data on incidence, mortality and distribution of cancer from 28 population-based registries and 5 hospital based registries.

In India, in the year 2020, the number of prevalent cases (5 years) is about 2,720,251, the number of new cases 1,324,413 and the number of deaths 851,678. The summary statistical situation for the year 2020 in the country is as follows :

Summary statistics 2020, India

	Males	Females	Both sexes
Population	717,100,976	662,903,415	1,380,004,378
Number of new cancer cases	646,030	678,383	1,324,413
Age-standardized incidence rate	95.7	99.3	97.1
Risk of developing cancer before the age of 75 years (%)	10.4	10.5	10.4
Number of cancer deaths	438,297	413,381	851,678
Age-standardized mortality rate	65.4	61.0	63.1
Risk of dying from cancer before the age of 75 years (%)	7.4	6.7	7.1
5-year prevalent cases	1,208,835	1,511,416	2,720,251
Top 5 most frequent cancers excluding non-melanoma skin cancer (ranked by cases)	Lip, oral cavity Lung Stomach Colorectum Oesophagus	Breast Cervix uteri Ovary Lip, oral cavity Colorectum	Breast Lip, oral cavity Cervix uteri Lung Colorectum

Source : *(7)*

The age standardized incidence rate of top 10 cancers by sex, and age standardized mortality rate and incidence rate per lakh population in India is as shown in Fig. 3 and 4 *(7)*.

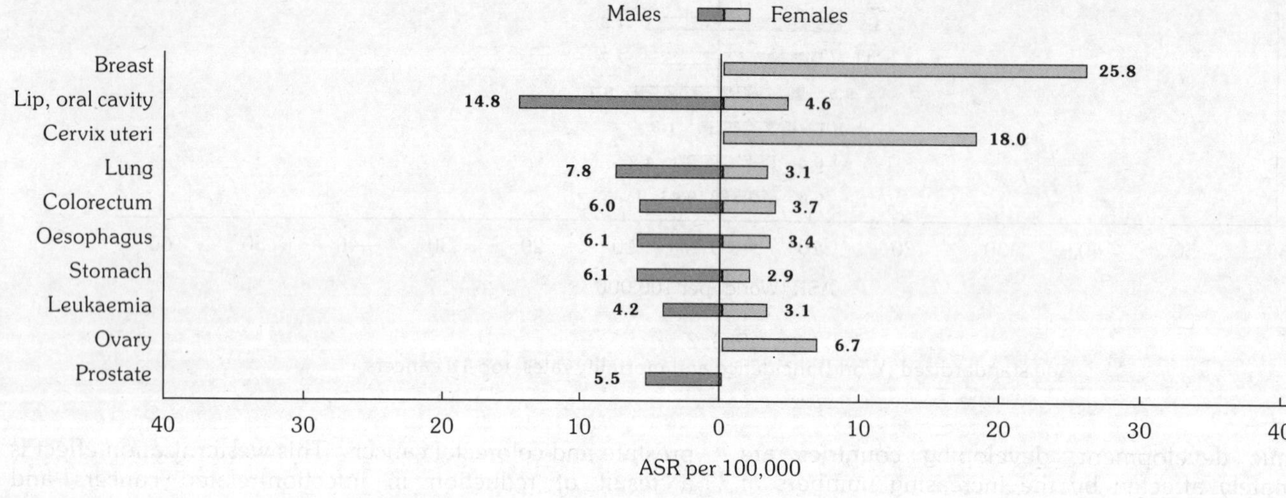

FIG. 3
Age standardized incidence rates by sex, top 10 cancers in India (2020)

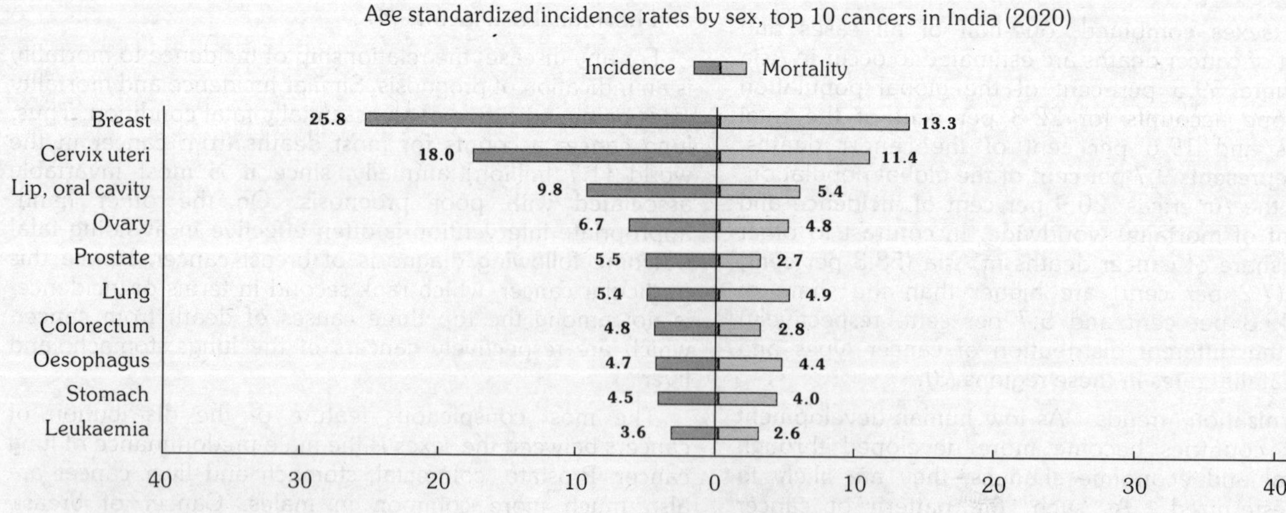

FIG. 4
Age standardized incidence and mortality rates, top 10 cancers in India (2020)

The five most frequent cancers in men were cancer lip and oral cavity, lung, stomach, colorectum and oesophagus, and in women, cancer breast, cervix uteri, ovary, lip, oral cavity and colorectum. Cancer in males were mostly tobacco related. In women, cervical cancer is closely associated with poor genital hygiene, early consummation of marriage, multiple pregnancies, and contact with multiple sexual partners. It is also reported that breast cancer is proportionately on the increase in a few metropolitan areas of India. This appears to be related to late marriage, birth of the first child at a late age, fewer children, and shorter periods of breast-feeding, which are increasingly common practice among the educated urban women *(8)*.

Facilities for screening and proper management of cancer patients are grossly limited in India. More than two-thirds of cancer patients are already in an advanced and incurable stage at the time of diagnosis. Appropriate strategies are being developed, including creating public awareness about cancer, tobacco control and application of self or assisted screening technique for oral, cervical, and breast cancers.

Time trends

Few decades ago, cancer was the sixth leading cause of death in industrialized countries; today, it is the second leading cause of death. There are a number of reasons for this increase, the three main ones being a longer life expectancy, more accurate diagnosis and the rise in cigarette smoking, especially among males. The overall rates do not reflect the different trends according to the type of cancer. For example, there has been a large increase in lung cancer incidence and the stomach cancer has shown a declining trend in most developed countries for reasons not understood.

Cancer patterns

There are wide variations in the distribution of cancer throughout the world. That cancer of the stomach is very common in Japan, and has a low incidence in United States. The cervical cancer is high in Columbia and has a low incidence in Japan. In the South-East Asia Region of WHO, the great majority are cancers of the oral cavity and uterine cervix. These and other international variations in the pattern of cancer are attributed to multiple factors such as environmental factors, food habits, lifestyle, genetic factors or even inadequacy in detection and reporting of cases.

Hospital data clearly indicates that the two organ sites most commonly involved are: (i) the uterine cervix in women, and (ii) the oropharynx in both sexes. These two sites represent approximately 50 per cent of all cancer cases. Both these cancers are predominantly environment related and have a strong socio-cultural relationship. It is also important to note that these two kinds of cancer are easily accessible for physical examination and amenable to early diagnosis by knowledge already available. i.e., good clinical examination and exfoliative cytology. The cure rate for these neoplasma is also very high if they are treated surgically at stages I and II. But unfortunately, in most cases, the patients present themselves to a medical facility when the disease is far advanced and is not amenable to treatment. This is the crux of the problem.

Causes of cancer

As with other chronic diseases, cancer has a multifactorial aetiology.

1. ENVIRONMENTAL FACTORS

Environmental factors are generally held responsible for 80 to 90 per cent of all human cancers. The major environmental factors identified so far include : *(a) TOBACCO* : Tobacco in various forms of its usage (e.g., smoking, chewing) is the major environmental cause of cancers of the lung, larynx, mouth, pharynx, oesophagus, bladder, pancreas and probably kidney. It has been estimated that, in the world as a whole, cigarette smoking is now responsible for more than one million premature deaths each year *(9)*. *(b) ALCOHOL* : Excessive intake of alcoholic beverages is associated with oesophageal and liver cancer. Some recent studies have suggested that beer consumption may be associated with rectal cancer *(10)*. It is estimated that alcohol contributed to about 3 per cent of all cancer deaths *(11)*. *(c) DIETARY FACTORS* : Dietary factors are also related to cancer. Smoked fish is related to stomach cancer, dietary fibre to intestinal cancer, beef consumption to bowel cancer and a high fat diet to breast cancer. A variety of other dietary factors such as food additives and contaminants have fallen under suspicion as causative agents. (Refer to chapter 12 for further details.) *(d) OCCUPATIONAL EXPOSURES* : These include exposure to benzene, arsenic, cadmium, chromium, vinyl chloride, asbestos, polycyclic hydrocarbons, etc. Many others remain to be identified. The risk of occupational exposure is considerably increased if the individuals also smoke cigarettes. Occupational exposures are usually reported to account for 1 to 5 per cent of all human cancers *(12)*. *(e) VIRUSES* : An intensive search for a viral origin of human cancers revealed that hepatitis B and C virus is causally related to hepatocellular carcinoma. The relative risk of Kaposi's sarcoma occurring in patients with HIV infection is so high that it was the first manifestation of the AIDS epidemic to be recognized. Non–Hodgkin's lymphoma, a cancer of the lymph nodes and spleen is a late complication of AIDS. The Epstein-Barr virus (EBV) is associated with 2 human malignancies, viz. Burkitt's lymphoma and nasopharyngeal carcinoma. *Cytomegalovirus* (CMV) is a suspected oncogenic agent and classical Kaposi's sarcoma is associated with a higher prevalence of antibodies to CMV. *Human papilloma virus* (HPV) is a chief suspect in cancer cervix. Hodgkin's disease is also believed to be of viral origin. The human T–cell leukaemia virus is associated with adult T–cell leukaemia/lymphoma in the United States and southern parts of Japan *(6, 13)*. *(f) PARASITES* : Parasitic infections may also increase the risk of cancer, as for example, schistosomiasis in Middle East producing carcinoma of the bladder. *(g) CUSTOMS, HABITS AND LIFESTYLES* : To the above causes must be added customs, habits and lifestyles of people which may be associated with an increased risk for certain cancers. The familiar examples are the demonstrated association between smoking and lung cancer, tobacco and betel chewing and oral cancer, etc *(14)*. *(h) OTHERS* : There are numerous other environmental factors such as sunlight, radiation, air and water pollution, medications (e.g., oestrogen) and pesticides which are related to cancer.

2. GENETIC FACTORS

Genetic influences have long been suspected. For example, retinoblastoma occurs in children of the same parent. Mongols are more likely to develop cancer (leukaemia) than normal children. However, genetic factors are less conspicuous and more difficult to identify. There is probably a complex interrelationship between hereditary susceptibility and environmental carcinogenic stimuli in the causation of a number of cancers.

Cancer control

Cancer control consists of a series of measures based on present medical knowledge in the fields of prevention, detection, diagnosis, treatment, after care and rehabilitation, aimed at reducing significantly the number of new cases, increasing the number of cures and reducing the invalidism due to cancer.

The basic approach to the control of cancer is through primary and secondary prevention. It is estimated that at least one-third of all cancers are preventable *(15)*.

1. PRIMARY PREVENTION

Cancer prevention until recently was mainly concerned with the early diagnosis of the disease (secondary prevention), preferably at a precancerous stage. Advancing knowledge has increased our understanding of causative factors of some cancers and it is now possible to control these factors in the general population as well as in particular occupational groups. They include the following :

(a) CONTROL OF TOBACCO AND ALCOHOL CONSUMPTION : Primary prevention offers the greatest hope for reducing the number of tobacco–induced and alcohol related cancer deaths. It has been estimated that control of tobacco smoking alone would reduce the total burden of cancer by over a million cancers each year *(16)*. *(b) PERSONAL HYGIENE:* Improvements in personal hygiene may lead to declines in the incidence of certain types of cancer, e.g., cancer cervix. *(c) RADIATION:* Special efforts should be made to reduce the amount of radiation (including medical radiation) received by each individual to a minimum without reducing the benefits. *(d) OCCUPATIONAL EXPOSURES :* The occupational aspects of cancer are frequently neglected. Measures to protect workers from exposure to industrial carcinogens should be enforced in industries. *(e) IMMUNIZATION :* In the case of primary liver cancer, immunization against hepatitis B virus and for prevention of cancer cervix immunization against HPV presents an exciting prospect. *(f) FOODS, DRUGS AND COSMETICS:* These should be tested for carcinogens. *(g) AIR POLLUTION :* Control of air pollution is another preventive measure. *(h) TREATMENT OF PRECANCEROUS LESIONS :* Early detection and prompt treatment of precancerous lesions such as cervical tears, intestinal polyposis, warts, chronic gastritis, chronic cervicitis, and adenomata is one of the cornerstones of cancer prevention. *(i) LEGISLATION :* Legislation has also a role in primary prevention. For example, legislation to control known environmental carcinogens (e.g., tobacco, alcohol, air pollution). *(j) CANCER EDUCATION :* An important area of primary prevention is cancer education. It should be directed at "high-risk" groups. The aim of cancer education is to motivate people to seek early diagnosis and early treatment. Cancer organizations in many countries remind the public of the early warning signs ("danger signals") of cancer. These are :

- *a.* a lump or hard area in the breast
- *b.* a change in a wart or mole
- *c.* a persistent change in digestive and bowel habits
- *d.* a persistent cough or hoarseness
- *e.* excessive loss of blood at the monthly period or loss of blood outside the usual dates
- *f.* blood loss from any natural orifice
- *g.* a swelling or sore that does not get better
- *h.* unexplained loss of weight.

There is no doubt that the possibilities for primary prevention are many. Since primary prevention is directed at large population groups (e.g., high risk groups, school children, occupational groups, youth clubs), the cost can be high and programmes difficult to conduct. Primary prevention, although a hopeful approach, is still in its early stages. Major risk factors have been identified for a small number of cancers only and far more research is needed in that direction.

2. SECONDARY PREVENTION

Secondary prevention comprises the following measures :

i) CANCER REGISTRATION

Cancer registration is a *sine qua non* for any cancer control programme. It provides a base for assessing the magnitude of the problem and for planning the necessary services. Cancer registries are basically of two types : hospital–based and population based. *(a) HOSPITAL-BASED REGISTRIES:* The hospital-based registry includes all patients treated by a particular institution, whether in-patients or out-patients. Registries should collect the uniform minimum set of data recommended in the "WHO Handbook for Standardized Cancer Registers" *(17)*. If there is a long-term follow-up of patients, hospital-based registries can be of considerable value in the evaluation of diagnostic and treatment programmes. Since hospital population will always be a selected population, the use of these registries for epidemiological purposes is thus limited. *(b) POPULATION-BASED REGISTRIES :* A right step is to set up a "hospital–based cancer registry" and extend the same to a "population-based cancer registry". The aim is to cover the complete cancer situation in a given geographic area. The optimum size of base population for a population based cancer registry is in the range of 2–7 million *(18)*. The data from such registries alone can provide the incidence rate of cancer and serve as a useful tool for initiating epidemiological enquiries into causes of cancer, surveillance of time trends, and planning and evaluation of operational activities in all main areas of cancer control.

ii) EARLY DETECTION OF CASES

Cancer screening is the main weapon for early detection of cancer at a pre-invasive *(in situ)* or pre-malignant stage. Effective screening programmes have been developed for cervical cancer, breast cancer and oral cancer. Like primary prevention, early diagnosis has to be conducted on a large scale; however, it may be possible to increase the efficiency of screening programmes by focussing on high-risk groups. Clearly, there is no point in detecting cancer at an early stage unless facilities for treatment and after-care are available. Early detection programmes will require mobilization of all available resources and development of a cancer infrastructure starting at the level of primary health care, ending with complex cancer centres or institutions at the state or national levels.

iii) TREATMENT

Treatment facilities should be available to all cancer patients. Certain forms of cancer are amenable to surgical removal, while some others respond favourably to radiation or chemotherapy or both. Since most of the known methods of treatment have complementary effect on the ultimate outcome of the patient, multi-modality approach to cancer control has become a standard practice in cancer centres all over the world. In the developed countries today, cancer treatment is geared to high technology. For those who are beyond the curable stage, the goal must be to provide pain relief. A largely neglected problem in cancer care is the management of pain. The WHO has developed guidelines on relief of cancer pain *(19)*. "Freedom from cancer pain" is now considered a right of cancer patients.

CANCER SCREENING

In the light of present knowledge, early detection and prompt treatment of early cancer and precancerous conditions provide the best possible protection against cancer for the individual and the community. Now a good deal of attention is being paid to screening for early detection of cancer. This approach, that is, cancer screening may be defined as the "search for unrecognized malignancy by means of rapidly applied tests".

Cancer screening is possible because : (a) in many instances, malignant disease is preceded for a period of months or years by a premalignant lesion, removal of which prevents subsequent development of cancer; (b) most cancers begin as localized lesions and if found at this stage a high rate of cure is obtainable; and (c) as much as 75 per cent of all cancers occur in body sites that are accessible.

METHODS OF CANCER SCREENING

(a) Mass screening by comprehensive cancer detection examination: A rapid clinical examination, and examination of one or more body sites by the physician is one of the important approaches for screening for cancer. *(b) Mass screening at single sites :* This comprises examination of single sites such as uterine cervix, breast or lung. *(c) Selective screening :* This refers to examination of those people thought to be at special risk, for example, parous women of lower socio-economic strata upwards of 30 years of age for detection of cancer cervix, chronic smokers for lung cancer, etc.

1. Screening for cancer cervix

Screening for cervical cancer has become an accepted clinical practice. The prolonged early phase of cancer in situ can be detected by the Pap smear. Current policy suggests that all women should have a Pap test (cervical smear) at the age of 30 years, and then every 3 years thereafter. A periodic pelvic examination is also recommended. Organized population based screening programmes have reduced the incidence and mortality from cervical cancer in many developed countries.

However, screening for cancer cervix using Pap smear requires excessive resources in terms of laboratories, equipments and trained personnels. This has led to search for an alternative screening method that can be more cost-effective. Visual inspection based screening tests such as visual inspection with 5 per cent acetic acid (VIA), VIA with magnification (VIAM), and visual inspection post application of Lugol's iodine (VILI) are some of the alternative screening tests, which have been studied for their effectiveness in India. Sensitivity of VIA tends to be similar to cytology based screening. It is easy to carry out and easy to train appropriate health workers *(21)*.

The strategy is to screen women using visual inspection after application of freshly prepared 5 per cent acetic acid solution (5 ml of glacial acetic acid mixed with 95 ml distilled water). Detection of well-defined opaque acetowhite lesions close to the squamo-columnar junction, well defined circum-orificial acetowhite lesion or dense acetowhitening of ulceroproliferative growth on the cervix constiute a positive VIA or VIAM. The test is followed by a single visit approach for further investigation and management at district hospital. The management at district hospital is planned in such a way that the treatment based on colposcopy is offered in the same visit. Pap smear and biopsy are the investigations that are done to ensure that there are cytological and histopathological back-up for the interventions *(21)*.

With its updated guidelines, WHO now encourages countries to use HPV tests for cervical screening, including HPV DNA and HPV mRNA tests. HPV-DNA testing detects high-risk strains of HPV, which cause almost all cervical cancers; and HPV mRNA detects HPV infections leading to cellular transformation. Unlike tests that rely on visual inspection, HPV-testing is an objective test. It has been shown to be simpler, prevents more pre-cancers and cancer, and saves more lives. It is also more cost-effective than visual inspection techniques or cytology (commonly known as 'pap smears'). Screening should start from 30 years of age in the general population of women, with regular screening with a validated HPV test every 5 to 10 years, and from 25 years of age for women living with HIV. Women living with HIV also need to be screened more frequently, every 3 to 5 years. Screening must be linked to treatment and management of positive screening tests. HPV positive women may be treated without diagnostic verification in limited resourced settings. A test to triage the HPV positive women (e.g. VIA) is essential for treating HIV positive women *(20)*.

Intensive information, education and communication activities are required to sensitize the community about the significance of the disease and its early detection through screening.

2. Screening for breast cancer

There is evidence that screening for breast cancer has a favourable effect on mortality from breast cancer. The basic techniques for early detection of breast cancer are : (a) breast self-examination (BSE) by the patient (b) palpation by a physician (c) thermography, and (d) mammography.

All women should be encouraged to perform breast self-examination. Breast cancers are more frequently found by women themselves than by a physician during a routine examination. Although the effectiveness of BSE has not been adequately quantified, it is a useful adjuvant to early case detection. In many countries, BSE will probably be the only feasible approach to wide population coverage for a long time to come. *Palpation* is unreliable for large fatty breasts. *Thermography* has the advantage that the patient is not exposed to radiation. Unfortunately, it is not a sensitive tool. *Mammography* is most sensitive and specific in detecting small tumours that are sometimes missed on palpation. The use of mammography has three potential drawbacks: (i) exposure to radiation. This may amount to a dose of 500 milliroentgen compared to a 30–40 milliroentgen dose received in chest X-ray. Therefore, there has been concern about exposure to radiation from repeated mammographies and the risk of breast cancer developing as a result (ii) mammography requires technical equipment of a high standard and radiologists with very considerable experience – these two factors limit its more widespread use for mass screening purposes, and (iii) biopsy from a suspicious lesion may end up in a false-positive in as many as 5–10 cases for each case of cancer detected.

Although recent evidence points to the superiority of mammography over clinical examination in terms of sensitivity and specificity *(22)*, medical opinion is against routine mammography on the very young. Women under 35 years of age should not have X-rays unless they are symptomatic or a family history of early onset of breast cancer *(23)*.

3. Screening for lung cancer

At present there are only two techniques for screening for lung cancer, viz. chest radiograph and sputum cytology. Mass radiography has been suggested for early diagnosis at six monthly intervals, but the evidence in support of this is not convincing. So it is not recommended. It is doubtful whether the disease satisfies the criteria of suitability for screening (see chapter 4).

EPIDEMIOLOGY OF SELECTED CANCERS

1. Oral cancer

Oral cancer is one of the ten most common cancers in the world. Its high frequency in Central and South East Asian countries (e.g., India, Bangladesh, Sri Lanka, Thailand, Indonesia, Pakistan) has been well documented. It is estimated that during the year 2020, about 2,64,211 men and 1,13,502 women were having oral cancer. About 1,77,757 persons (1.8 per cent of all cancers) died of oral cancer worldwide.

Oral cancer is a major problem in India. It is estimated that in 2020 it caused 5.4 deaths per 100,000 population (total 75,290 deaths), 57,380 cases in men and 22,483 cases in women. The age standardized incidence rate was 14.8 per 100,000 population in men and 4.6 per 100,000 population in women *(7)*.

EPIDEMIOLOGICAL FEATURES

(a) Tobacco : Approximately 90 per cent of oral cancers in South East Asia are linked to tobacco chewing and tobacco smoking. During 1966–1977, a large epidemiological survey was carried out in different parts of the country. In this 10–year follow-up study of 30,000 individuals in the three districts of Ernakulam (Kerala), Srikakulam (Andhra), and Bhavnagar (Gujarat), the results indicated that (i) oral cancer and precancerous lesions occurred almost solely among those who smoked or chewed tobacco, and (ii) oral cancer was almost always preceded by some type of precancerous lesion *(24, 25)*. The case about tobacco is further strengthened by the findings that the cancer almost always occurred on the side of the mouth where the tobacco quid was kept *(26)*, and the risk was 36 times higher than for non–chewers if the quid was kept in the mouth during sleep *(27)*.

(b) Alcohol : Data indicates that oral cancer can also be caused by high concentrations of alcohol, and that alcohol appears to have a synergistic effect in tobacco users *(26)*.

(c) Pre-cancerous stage : The natural history of oral cancer shows that often a precancerous stage precedes the development of cancer. The pre-cancerous lesions (leukoplakia, erythroplakia) can be detected for upto 15 years prior to their change to an invasive carcinoma *(26)*. Intervention at this stage may result in regression of the lesion.

(d) High-risk groups : These include tobacco chewers and smokers, bidi smokers, people using tobacco in other forms such as betel quid; people who sleep with the tobacco quid in the mouth *(28)*.

(e) Cultural patterns : In studying the tobacco habits in developing countries, indigenous forms of smoking, as well as chewing, which are characteristic of certain regions have to be taken into account *(9)*. Tobacco is smoked in the form of manufactured cigarettes. The indigenous forms of smoking are : *bidi*, *chutta* (cigar), *chilum*, *hookah* (hubble–bubble). Tobacco in powdered form is inhaled as snuff.

The most common form of tobacco chewing in India is the betel quid which usually consists of the betel leaf, arecanut, lime and tobacco. It is common for the poorer people to rub with the thumb flakes of sun-dried tobacco and slaked lime in the palm of their left hand until the desired mixture is obtained. The mixture *(khaini)* is then put into the mouth in small amounts and at frequent intervals during the day and slowly sucked and swallowed after dilution with saliva.

Cancer of the oral cavity is also very prevalent in Central Asian districts of USSR, where people chew "nass" or "nasswar" – a mixture of tobacco, ashes, lime and cotton-seed oil.

Another type of cancer common in the eastern coastal regions of Andhra Pradesh state in India is the epidermoid carcinoma of the hard palate. It is associated with the habit of reverse smoking of cigar *(chutta)*, i.e., smoking with the burning end inside the mouth *(29)*.

PREVENTION

a. PRIMARY PREVENTION

Oral cancer is amenable to primary prevention. If the tobacco habits are eliminated from the community, a great deal of reduction in the incidence of oral cancer can be achieved. This requires intensive public education and motivation for changing lifestyles supported by legislative measures like banning or restricting the sale of tobacco.

b. SECONDARY PREVENTION

Oral cancers are easily accessible for inspection allowing early detection. If detected early, possibly at the precancerous stage, they can be treated or cured. The precancerous lesions can be detected for up to 15 years, prior to their change to an invasive carcinoma. Leukoplakia can be cured by cessation of tobacco use. The main treatment modalities that offer hope are surgery and radiotherapy *(30)*. In developing countries over 50 per cent of oral cancers are detected only after they have reached an advanced stage *(15)*.

The primary health care workers (village health guides, and multi-purpose workers) are in a strategic position to detect oral cancers at an early stage during home visits. They can prove to be a vital link and a key instrument in the control of oral cancer in developing countries *(31)*.

2. Cancer of the cervix

Cervical cancer is the fourth most frequent cancer in women with an estimated 6,04,000 new cases in 2020 representing 6.6 per cent of all female cancers *(3)*. During the year about 3,42,000 women died of cervical cancer, which comes to 3.1 per cent of all deaths due to cancer in women *(3)*. Approximately 90 per cent of deaths from cervical cancer occurred in low and middle income countries. Wide variations in incidence and mortality from the disease exist between countries. Cases and deaths have declined markedly in the last 40 years in most industrialized countries, partly owing to a reduction in risk factors, but mainly as a result of extensive screening programmes. More limited improvements have been observed in developing countries, where persistently high rates tend to be the rule *(1)*.

In India, cancer cervix constitutes 9.4 per cent of all cancer incidence among women. The age standardized incidence rate is about 18.0 per 100,000 population. The estimated deaths were 77,348 in 2020 *(7)*.

NATURAL HISTORY

(a) The disease: Cancer cervix seems to follow a progressive course from epithelial dysplasia to carcinoma *in situ* to invasive carcinoma (Fig. 5). There is good evidence that carcinoma *in situ* persists for a long time, more than 8 years on an average *(32)*. The proportion of cases progressing to invasive carcinoma from preinvasive stage is not known – it may average 15 to 20 years or longer. The duration of the preinvasive stage is also not known. There is evidence that some *in situ* cases will spontaneously regress without treatment. Once the invasive stage is reached, the disease spreads by direct extension into the lymph nodes and pelvic organs.

Normal epithelium	↔	Dysplasia	↔	Cancer *in situ*	→	Invasive cancer

FIG. 5
Hypothetical model of the natural history of cancer cervix

When a woman presents symptoms of suspicion for cervical cancer, she must be referred to an appropriate facility for further evaluation, diagnosis and treatment. The symptoms of early-stage cervical cancer may include : (a) irregular blood spotting or light bleeding between periods in women of reproductive age; (b) postmenopausal spotting or bleeding; (c) bleeding after sexual intercourse; and (d) increased vaginal discharge, sometimes foul smelling.

As cervical cancer advances, more severe symptoms may appear including : (a) persistent back, leg or pelvic pain; (b) weight loss, fatigue, loss of appetite; (c) foul-smell discharge and vaginal discomfort; and (d) swelling of a leg or both lower extremities.

Other severe symptoms may arise at advanced stages depending on which organs the cancer has spread to.

(b) Causative agent : There is evidence pointing to Human papilloma virus (HPV) – sexually transmitted – as the cause of cervical cancer *(33)*. This virus was once supposed to produce only vegetant warts. More than 90 per cent of the infected population eventually clear the infection. But now virus is acknowledged as responsible for a much wider clinical and subclinical lesions. The virus is found in more than 95% of the cancers. Current evidence suggests that the virus is a necessary cause of the disease. It takes 15–20 years for cervical cancer to develop in women with normal immune system. It can take only 5–10 years in women with weakened immune system, such as those with untreated HIV infection *(20)*.

RISK FACTORS

(a) AGE : Cancer cervix affects relatively young women with incidence increasing rapidly from the age of 25 to 45, then levelling off, and finally falling again. *(b) GENITAL WARTS :* Past and/or present occurrence of clinical genital warts has been found to be an important risk factor *(33)*. *(c) MARITAL STATUS :* Cases are less likely to be single, more likely to be widowed, divorced or separated and having multiple sexual partners. The fact that cancer of the cervix is very common in prostitutes and practically unknown among virgins suggests that the disease could be linked with sexual intercourse. *(d) EARLY MARRIAGE:* Early marriage, early coitus, early childbearing and repeated childbirth have been associated with increasing risk. *(e) ORAL CONTRACEPTIVE PILLS :* There is renewed concern about the possible relationship between pill use and the development of invasive cervical cancer *(34)*. A recent WHO study finds an increased risk with increased duration of pill use and with the use of oral contraceptives high in oestrogen *(35)*. *(f) SOCIO-ECONOMIC CLASS :* Cancer cervix is more common in the lower socio-economic groups reflecting probably poor genital hygiene.

PREVENTION AND CONTROL

The Global strategy towards eliminating cervical cancer as a public health problem, adopted by the World Health Assembly in 2020, recommends a comprehensive approach to cervical cancer prevention and control. The recommended actions include interventions across the life course *(20)*.

Primary prevention	Secondary prevention	Tertiary prevention
Girls 9–14 years • HPV vaccination	From 30 years of age for women from the general population and 25 years of age for women living with HIV	All women as needed
Girls and boys should also be offered, as appropriate • Health information and warnings about tobacco use • Sex education tailored to age and culture • Condom promotion and provision for those engaged in sexual activity • Male circumcision	• Screening with a high-performance test equivalent or better than HPV test • Followed by immediate treatment or as quickly as possible after an HPV molecular positive test.	Treatment of invasive cancer at any age • Surgery • Radiotherapy • Chemotherapy • Palliative care

Cervical cancer prevention should encompass a multidisciplinary, including components from community education, social mobilization, vaccination, screening, treatment and palliative care.

HPV vaccination

HPV vaccines work best if administered prior to exposure to HPV. Therefore, to prevent cervical cancer WHO recommends vaccinating girls aged 9 to 14 years, when most have not started sexual activity. Some countries have started to vaccinate boys as the vaccination prevents HPV related cancers in males as well HPV vaccination does not replace cervical cancer screening. In countries where HPV vaccine is introduced, population-based screening programmes are still needed to identify and treat cervical pre-cancer and cancer to reduce cervical cancer incidence and deaths.

3. Breast cancer

Female breast cancer has now surpassed lung cancer as the leading cause of global cancer incidence in 2020, with an estimated 2.3 million new cases, representing 11.7 per cent of all cancer cases. It is the fifth leading cause of cancer mortality worldwide, with 6,85,000 deaths. Among women, breast cancer accounts for 1 in 4 cancer cases and for 1 in 6 cancer deaths, ranking first for incidence in the vast majority of countries (159 of 185 countries), and for mortality in 110 countries. There are exceptions, most notably in terms of deaths, with the disease preceded by lung cancer in Australia/New Zealand, Northern Europe, Northern America, and China (part of Eastern Asia) and by cervical cancer in many countries in sub-Saharan Africa *(3)*.

Incidence rates are 88 per cent higher in transitioned countries than in transitioning countries (55.9 and 29.7 per 100,000, respectively), with the highest incidence rates (>80 per 100,000) in Australia/New Zealand, Western Europe (Belgium has the world's highest incidence), Northern America, and Northern Europe, and the lowest rates (<40 per 100,000) in Central America, Eastern and Middle Africa, and South Central Asia. However, women living in transitioning countries have 17 per cent higher mortality rates compared with women in transitioned countries (15.0 and 12.8 per 100,000, respectively) because of high fatality rates, with the highest mortality rates found in Melanesia, Western Africa, Micronesia/Polynesia, and the Caribbean (Barbados has the world's highest mortality) *(3)*.

In India, breast cancer is the top most cancer with about 178,361 (13.6 per cent) new cases diagnosed in 2020. The incidence rate is about 25.8 per 100,000 population.

In India, breast cancer was estimated to cause 13.3 deaths per 100,000 population in the year 2020. The survival rate decreased by 2.7 times for breast cancer, in case of detection at stage IV as against stage I. A total of 90,408 women died of cancer breast in 2020 in India *(7)*.

THE DISEASE *(36)*

Breast cancer most commonly presents as a painless lump or thickening in the breast. It is important that women finding an abnormal lump in the breast consult a health practitioner without a delay of more than 1–2 months even when there is no pain associated with it. Seeking medical attention at the first sign of a potential symptom allows for more successful treatment.

Generally, symptoms of breast cancer include:

- a breast lump or thickening;
- alteration in size, shape or appearance of a breast;
- dimpling, redness, pitting or other alteration in the skin;
- change in nipple appearance or alteration in the skin surrounding the nipple (areola); and/or
- abnormal nipple discharge.

There are many reasons for lumps to develop in the breast, most of which are not cancer. As many as 90% of breast masses are not cancerous. Non-cancerous breast abnormalities include benign masses like fibroadenomas and cysts as well as infections.

Breast cancer can present in a wide variety of ways, which is why a complete medical examination is important. Women with persistent abnormalities (generally lasting more than one month) should undergo tests including imaging of the breast and in some cases tissue biopsy to determine if a mass is malignant or benign.

Advanced cancers can erode through the skin to cause ulceration but are not necessarily painful. Women with breast wounds that do not heal should have a biopsy performed.

Breast cancers may spread to other areas of the body and trigger other symptoms. Often, the most common first detectable site of spread is to the lymph nodes under the arm although it is possible to have cancer-bearing lymph nodes that cannot be felt.

Over time, cancerous cells may spread to other organs including the lungs, liver, brain and bones. Once they reach these sites, new cancer-related symptoms such as bone pain or headaches may appear.

RISK FACTORS

The established risk factors of breast cancer include the following:

(a) AGE : Breast cancer is uncommon below the age of 35, the incidence increasing rapidly between the ages of 35 and 50. A slight bimodal trend in the age distribution has been observed *(37)* with a dip in incidence at the time of menopause. A secondary rise in frequency often occurs after the age of 65. Women who developed their first breast cancer under the age of 40, had three times the risk of developing a second breast cancer than did those who developed their first cancer after the age of 40 *(38)*. Indeed the aetiologies of pre-menopausal and post-menopausal breast cancer appears to be different *(39)*.

Breast cancer is not only infrequent in Indian women, but also it occurs in them a decade earlier than in Western women – the mean age of occurrence is about 42 in India, as compared to 53 in the white women.

(b) FAMILY HISTORY : The risk is high in those with a positive family history of breast cancer, especially if a mother or sister developed breast cancer when premenopausal.

(c) PARITY : MacMahon, *et al (40)* in their international case–control study found that the risk of breast cancer is directly related to the age at which women bear the first child. An early first, full-term pregnancy seems to have a protective effect. Those whose first pregnancy is delayed to their late thirties are at a higher risk than multiparous women. Unmarried women tend to have more breast tumours than married single women, and nulliparous women had the same risk.

(d) AGE AT MENARCHE AND MENOPAUSE : Early menarche and late menopause are established risk factors *(41)*. The risk is reduced for those with a surgically induced menopause. Forty or more years of menstruation doubles the risk of breast cancer as compared with 30 years *(42)*.

(e) HORMONAL FACTORS : The association of breast cancer with early menarche and late menopause suggests that ovary appears to play a crucial role in the development of breast cancer. Evidence suggests that both elevated oestrogen as well as progesterone are important factors in increasing breast cancer risk *(43)*. In short, hormones appear to hold the key to the understanding of breast cancer.

(f) PRIOR BREAST BIOPSY : Prior breast biopsy for benign breast disease is associated with an increased risk of breast cancer.

(g) DIET : Current aetiological hypotheses suggest that cancer of the breast is linked with a high fat diet and obesity. It is not known how dietary fat influences breast cancer risk at a cellular level *(43)*.

(h) SOCIO-ECONOMIC STATUS : Breast cancer is common in higher socio-economic groups. This is explained by the risk factor of higher age at first birth.

(i) OTHERS : *(i) Radiation* : An increased incidence of breast cancer has been observed in women exposed to radiation. *(ii) Oral contraceptives* : Oral contraceptive appears to have little overall effect on breast cancer, although prolonged use of oral pills before the first pregnancy or before the age of 25 may increase the risk in younger women *(44)*.

PREVENTION

Behavioural choices and related interventions that reduce the risk of breast cancer include *(36)* :

- prolonged breastfeeding;
- regular physical activity;
- weight control;
- avoidance of harmful use of alcohol;
- avoidance of exposure to tobacco smoke;
- avoidance of prolonged use of hormones; and
- avoidance of excessive radiation exposure.

Unfortunately, even if all of the potentially modifiable risk factors could be controlled, this would only reduce the risk of developing breast cancer by at most 30 per cent.

Female gender is the strongest breast cancer risk factor. Approximately 0.5–1 per cent of breast cancers occur in men. The treatment of breast cancer in men follows the same principles of management as for women.

In the past, all breast cancers were treated surgically by mastectomy (complete removal of the breast). When cancers are large, mastectomy may still be required. Today, the majority of breast cancers can be treated with a smaller procedure called a "lumpectomy" or partial mastectomy, in which only the tumor is removed from the breast. In these cases, radiation therapy to the breast is generally required to minimize the chances of recurrence in the breast.

Lymph nodes are removed at the time of cancer surgery for invasive cancers. Complete removal of the lymph node bed under the arm (complete axillary dissection) in the past was thought to be necessary to prevent the spread of cancer. A smaller lymph node procedure called "sentinel node biopsy" is now preferred as it has fewer complications. It uses dye and/or a radioactive tracer to find the first few lymph nodes to which cancer could spread from the breast.

Medical treatments for breast cancer, which may be given before ("neoadjuvant") or after ("adjuvant") surgery, is based on the biological subtyping of the cancer. Cancers that express the estrogen receptor (ER) and/or progesterone receptor (PR) are likely to respond to endocrine (hormone) therapies such as tamoxifen or aromatase inhibitors. These medicines are taken orally for 5–10 years, and reduce the chance of recurrence of these "hormone-positive" cancers by nearly half. Endocrine therapies can cause symptoms of menopause but are generally well tolerated.

Cancers that do not express ER or PR are "hormone receptor negative" and need to be treated with chemotherapy unless the cancer is very small. The chemotherapy regimens available today are very effective in reducing the chances of cancer spread or recurrence and are generally given as outpatient therapy. Chemotherapy for breast cancer generally does not require hospital admission in the absence of complications.

Breast cancers may independently overexpress a molecule called the HER2/neu oncogene. These "HER2 positive" cancers are amenable to treatment with targeted biological agents such as trastuzumab. These biological agents are very effective but also very expensive, because they are antibodies rather than chemicals. When targeted biological therapies are given, they are combined with chemotherapy to make them effective at killing cancer cells.

Radiotherapy also plays a very important role in treating breast cancer. With early stage breast cancer, radiation can prevent a woman having to undergo a mastectomy. With later stage cancer, radiotherapy can reduce cancer recurrence risk even when a mastectomy has been performed. For advanced stage of breast cancer, in some circumstances, radiation therapy may reduce the likelihood of dying of the disease.

The effectiveness of breast cancer therapies depends on the full course of treatment. Partial treatment is less likely to lead to a positive outcome.

The strategies for improving breast cancer outcomes depend on fundamental health system strengthening to deliver the treatments that are already known to work. For example, having reliable referral pathways from primary care facilities to district hospitals to dedicated cancer centres.

GLOBAL BREAST CANCER INITIATIVE *(36)*

The objective of the WHO Global Breast Cancer Initiative (GBCI) is to reduce global breast cancer mortality by 2.5 per cent per year, thereby averting 2.5 million breast cancer deaths globally between 2020 and 2040. Reducing global breast cancer mortality by 2.5 per cent per year would avert 25% of breast cancer deaths by 2030 and 40 per cent by 2040 among women under 70 years of age. The three pillars toward achieving these objectives are: health promotion for early detection; timely diagnosis; and comprehensive breast cancer management.

4. Lung cancer

MAGNITUDE OF THE PROBLEM

Lung cancer has been known in industrial workers from the late 19th century. It came into prominence as a public health problem in the Western world in 1930s – at first in men, and later (in 1960s) among women *(45)*, and has followed the increasing adoption of cigarette smoking first by men and later by women. According to WHO reports, between 1960 and 1980, the death rate due to lung cancer increased by 76 per cent in men and by 135 per cent in women *(46, 28)*. In countries where cigarette smoking has only recently begun to be widely adopted, lung cancer deaths still remain low, but it may be expected that they will rise soon. In others, such as Poland, where the use of cigarettes began earlier, the rise is already occurring. The total burden of lung cancer in any country is directly related to the amount and duration of cigarette smoking.

With an estimated 2.2 million new cancer cases and 1.8 million deaths, lung cancer is the second most commonly diagnosed cancer and the leading cause of cancer deaths in 2020, representing approximately one in 10 (11.4 per cent) cancers diagnosed and one in 5 (18.0 per cent) deaths. Lung cancer is the leading cause of cancer morbidity and mortality in men, whereas, in women, it ranks third for incidence, after breast and colorectal cancer, and second for mortality, after breast cancer. Incidence and mortality rates are roughly 2 times higher in men than in women, although the male-to-female ratio varies widely across regions, ranging from 1.2 in Northern America to 5.6 in Northern Africa. Lung cancer incidence and mortality rates are 3 to 4 times higher in transitioned countries than in transitioning countries; this pattern may well change as the tobacco epidemic evolves given that 80% of smokers aged ≥15 years resided in low-income and middle-income countries *(3)*.

In India, the age standardized incidence rate for the year 2020 was : total 8.4 per 100,000 population; for men 7.8 per 100,000 population and women 3.1 per 100,000 population. The estimated deaths were 66,279. The rate was 4.9 per 100,000 population *(7)*.

EPIDEMIOLOGICAL FEATURES

a. AGE AND SEX

About a third of all lung cancer deaths occur below the age of 65. In many industrialized countries, the incidence of lung cancer is at present increasing more in females than in males *(47)*.

b. RISK FACTORS

(i) Smoking : Tobacco smoking was first suggested as a cause of lung cancer in the 1920s. Subsequent studies proved the causal relationship between cigarette smoking and lung cancer. Two studies in India showed that the lung cancer risk for cigarette smokers is 8.6 times the risk for non-smokers *(48, 49)*. The risk is strongly related to the number of cigarettes smoked, the age of starting to smoke and smoking habits, such as inhalation and the number of puffs and the nicotine, the tar content and the length of cigarettes. Those who are highly exposed to "passive smoking" (somebody else's smoke) are at an increased risk of developing lung cancer. It has been calculated that in countries where smoking has been a widespread habit, it is responsible for 90 per cent of lung cancer deaths *(50)*. The strongest evidence that cigarette smoking is responsible for lung cancer is the incidence reduction that occurs after cessation of smoking. This has been convincingly demonstrated in a 20 year prospective study on male British doctors *(51)*.

The most noxious components of tobacco smoke are tar, carbon monoxide and nicotine. The carcinogenic role of tar is well established. Nicotine and carbon monoxide, particularly, contribute to increased risk of cardiovascular diseases through enhancement of blood coagulation in the vessels, interference with myocardial oxygen delivery, and reduction of the threshold for ventricular fibrillation *(9)*.

A study in India has shown that there is no difference between the tar and nicotine delivery of the filter and non-filter cigarettes smoked in India, so that a filter gives no protection to Indian smokers. The "king-size" filter cigarettes deliver more tar and nicotine than ordinary cigarettes. *Bidi* smoking appears to carry a higher lung cancer risk than cigarette smoking owing to the higher concentration of carcinogenic hydrocarbons in the smoke *(9)*.

(ii) Other factors : Besides cigarette smoking, there are other factors which are implicated in the aetiology of lung cancer. These include air pollution, radioactivity, and occupational exposure to asbestos, arsenic and its compounds, chromates, particles containing polycyclic aromatic hydrocarbons and certain nickel–bearing dusts. A number of studies have shown an interaction between smoking and asbestos exposure.

PREVENTION

1. PRIMARY PREVENTION

In lung cancer control, primary prevention is of greatest importance. The most promising approach is to control the "smoking epidemic", because 80 to 90 per cent of all cases of lung cancer in developed countries are due to smoking of cigarettes. Methods of controlling the smoking epidemic have been described by the WHO expert committees in their reports. Broadly these methods include :

a. Public information and education
b. Legislative and restrictive measures
c. Smoking cessation activities
d. National and international coordination

a. Public information and education

The need of the hour is to create public awareness about the hazards of smoking through mass media. The target population should be the entire population with greater emphasis laid on young people and school children. Nothing less than a national anti-smoking campaign will be needed to change human behaviour or life styles associated with smoking. Curtailment of smoking must be an essential part of national health policy.

b. Legislative and restrictive measures

Legislation and restrictive measures have been suggested in the following areas : control of sales promotion; health warnings on cigarette packets and advertisements; product description showing yield of harmful substances; imposition of upper limits for harmful substances in smoking materials; taxation; sales restrictions; restriction on smoking in public places; restriction on smoking in places of work, etc.

The Government of India have provided legislative support to the anti-smoking campaign. "The Cigarettes (Regulation of production, supply and distribution) Act of 1975" which came into force from 1 April 1976, requires all manufacturers or persons trading in cigarettes to display prominently the statutory warning "Cigarette Smoking is Injurious to Health" on all cartons or packets of cigarettes that are put on sale. Most of the State Governments in India have promulgated laws prohibiting smoking in closed areas, e.g., cinemas, buses, educational institutions, and hospitals. Again in the year 2003, a comprehensive tobacco control legislation titled "The Cigarettes And Other Tobacco Products (Prohibition of Advertisement and Regulation of Trade and Commerce, Production, Supply and Distribution) Act 2003 was passed by the Govt of India. Refer to chapter 7 "National cancer control programme" for the details.

c. Smoking cessation activities

Research continues on different methods of smoking cessation. In all countries well over 90 per cent of those who give up smoking do so of their own volition, i.e., without use of any specific therapy. The basic role of most treatments for smoking cessation would be to relieve the smoker of "abstinence symptoms" (e.g., sleeplessness, craving for smoking, dizziness, constipation, etc). The report of the WHO expert committee on smoking control contains information on specific smoking cessation methods such as smoking cessation clinics, nicotine substitutes, hypnosis, etc.

d. National and International coordination

Since smoking is a worldwide epidemic, it requires coordinated political and non-political approaches at local, national and international levels to contain the smoking epidemic.

2. SECONDARY PREVENTION

This rests on early detection of cases and their treatment.

At present, there are only two procedures capable of detecting presymptomatic, early-stage lung cancer. These are the chest X-ray and sputum cytology. But screening for early–stage lung cancer is less attractive, more expensive and appears to have less potential for reducing mortality than primary prevention. Therefore, mass screening for lung cancer is not recommended as a routine public health policy *(47)*.

Efforts to find effective treatment for lung cancer have met with only limited success. For untreated patients, the median survival is 2 to 3 months, compared to 10–14 months for patients receiving combined chemotherapy. In view of these limitations, primary prevention merits greater attention. An important part of treatment is relief of pain so that each dying patient has the right to spend his last days as pain-free as possible.

5. Stomach cancer

Stomach cancer remains an important cancer worldwide and is responsible for over 1.089 million new cases in 2020 and an estimated 768,793 deaths, equating to 7.7 per cent of all cancer deaths, making it the fifth most frequently diagnosed cancer, and third leading cause of cancer deaths. The rates are 2-fold higher in men than women.

Although they are often reported as a single entity, gastric cancer can generally be classified into 2 topographical categories. Rates of noncardia gastric cancer (arising from distal regions) have steadily declined over the last 50 years in most populations. Cancers of the gastric cardia (arising in the area adjoining the oesophageal-gastric junction) have epidemiological characteristics more similar to those of oesophageal adenocarcinoma and important risk factors include obesity and gastroesophageal reflux disease. The incidence of these cancers are increasing particularly in high-income countries *(3)*.

In India the age-standardized incidence rate for stomach cancer in 2020 was 6.1 per 100,000 population in men, and 3.4 per 100,000 population in women. The crude mortality rate was 6.3 per 100,000 population. As a total, 53,253 people died of cancer stomach in 2020 *(7)*.

The constant decline of stomach cancer in industrialized countries is linked to improved food preservation practices; better nutrition more rich in vitamins from fresh vegetables and fruits; and less consumption of preserved, cured and salted foods. Infection with the bacterium *Helicobacter pylori* contributes to the risk, probably by interacting with the other factors.

Symptoms are non-specific, which explains why most of the cases are diagnosed when the disease is at an advanced stage. Patients may complain of weight loss, fatigue or gastric discomfort. Diagnosis is performed by barium X-rays and with biopsy.

This cancer is treated by surgical removal of the tumour, with or without adjuvant chemotherapy.

Stomach cancer cases have a generally poor survival prognosis, averaging no more than 20% survival after five years. If the tumour is localized to the stomach, about 60% of patients survive five years or more. However, only about 18% of all cases are diagnosed at this early stage. Screening by photofluoroscopy has been widespread in Japan since the late 1960s and mortality rates are declining. It is unclear whether this trend can be attributed to mass screening alone.

References

1. WHO (1997). *The World Health Report 1997,* Report of the Director General WHO.
2. WHO (2020). *Global Cancer Observatory,* Nov. 2020.
3. Hyuna Sung et al (2021), *Global Cancer Statistics 2020, Globocan estimates of incidence and mortality worldwide for 36 cancers in 185 countries.*
4. WHO (2014), *World Cancer Fact Sheet,* Cancer Research UK, January 2014.
5. Freddie Bray et. al. (2018), *Global Cancer Statistics 2018,* Globocan estimates of incidence and mortality worldwide for 36 cancers in 185 countries.
6. WHO (2003), *World Cancer Report,* Ed. by Bernard W. Stewart and Paul Kleihues.
7. Globocan (2020), *The Global Cancer Observatory, Fact Sheet, India,* Dec. 2020.
8. WHO (1999). *Health Situation in the South-East Asia Region 1994-1997,* Regional office for SEAR, New Delhi.
9. WHO (1983). *Techn. Rep. Ser.,* No. 695.
10. Kabat, G.C. et al (1986). *Int. J. Epi.,* 15 (4) 494–501.
11. Rothman, K.J. (1980). *Preventive Medicine,* 9 : 174–179.
12. Doll, R and R. Peto (1981). *J. Natl. Cancer Inst.,* 61 : 1191–1308.
13. Broder, S. et al (1984). *Ann. Int. Med.,* 100 : 543.
14. Reddy, D.J. (1968). *Cancer, Customs, Habits, Usages and Environment,* Current Technical Literature, Mumbai.
15. WHO (1985). *World Health Forum,* 6 (2) 160–164.
16. WHO (1986). *Techn. Rep. Ser.,* No. 731.
17. WHO (1976). *WHO Handbook for Standardized Cancer Registers* (hospital based). WHO Offset Publ No. 25.
18. WHO (1979). *Techn. Rep. Ser.,* No. 632.
19. WHO (1986). *Cancer Pain Relief,* WHO, Geneva.
20. WHO (2022), *Fact sheet, Cervical cancer,* 22nd Feb. 2022.
21. Govt. of India, WHO (2006), *Guidelines for Cervical Cancer Screening Programme,* Department of Cytology and Gynaecological Pathology, Postgraduate Institute of Medical Education and Research, Chandigarh, India.
22. Editorial (1985). *Lancet,* 1 : 851.
23. Tucker, A.K. (1985). *Practitioner,* 229–217.
24. Mehta, F.S. et al (1982), *Bull WHO,* 60 (3) 441 - 446.
25. Gupta, P.C. et al (1980), *Community Dentistry and Oral Epidemiology,* 8 : 287 - 333.
26. WHO (1984). *Bull WHO,* 62 (6) 817–830.
27. Wahi, P.N. (1968), *Bull WHO,* 38 : 495.
28. WHO (1985). *Wkly Epi,Rec.,* 60 (17). 125–129.
29. Reddy, C.R.R.M. et al (1976). *Ind.J.Cancer,* 13 : 161.
30. WHO (1984). *Bull WHO,* 62 (6) 861–869.
31. Warnakulasuriya, K.A.A.S. et al (1984). *Bull WHO,* 62 (2) 243–250.
32. Ken, Stanley (1981). *World Health,* Sept–Oct, pp 21–23.
33. Zaninetti, P. et al (1986). *Int.J.Epi.* 15 (4) 477.
34. Brinton, L.A. et al (1986). *Int.J.Cancer,* 38 : 339.
35. The WHO Collaborative Study of Neoplasis and Steroid Contraceptives (1985). *Brit.Med.J.,* 290 : 961–965.
36. WHO (2021), *Fact sheet, Breast cancer,* 26th March 2021.
37. Clemmesen, J. (1979). In: *Measurement of Levels of Health,* WHO Reg.Publ.EURO Ser.No.7, p. 199.
38. Hughes L.E. and Courtney, S.P. (1985). *Brit.Med.J.* 290 : 1229 (editorial).
39. Hislop, T.G. et al (1986). *Int.J.Epi.,* 15 (4) 469.
40. MacMahon, B. et al (1970). *Bull WHO,* 43 : 209–217.
41. Miller, A.B. and Bulbrook, R.D. (1980). *N.Eng.J.Med.,* 303 : 1246–1248.
42. Marks, M. (1985). *Practitioner,* 229 : 225.
43. Pike, M.C. and R.K. Ross (1984). *Br.Med.Bull.,* 40 (4) 351–354.
44. Pike, M.C. et al (1983). *Lancet,* 2 : 926–929.
45. Muir, C.S. (1981). *World Health,* Sept–Oct, pp 8–11.
46. WHO (1985). *WHO Chronicle,* 39 (3) 109–111.
47. WHO (1982). *Bull WHO,* 60 (6) 809–819.
48. Notani, P.N. et al (1977). *Int.J.Cancer,* 14 : 115.
49. Jussawalla, D.J. and Jain, D.K. (1979). *Brit.J.Cancer* 40 : 437.
50. WHO (1979). *Techn.Rep.Ser.,* No. 636.
51. Doll, R. and Peto, R. (1976). *Brit.Med.J.,* 2 : 1525.

DIABETES MELLITUS

The term diabetes describes a group of metabolic disorders characterized and identified by the presence of hyperglycaemia in the absence of treatment. The heterogeneous aetio-pathology includes defects in insulin secretion, insulin action, or both, and disturbances of carbohydrate, fat and protein metabolism. The long-term specific effects of diabetes include retinopathy, nephropathy and neuropathy, among other complications. People with diabetes are also at increased risk of other diseases including heart, peripheral arterial and cerebrovascular disease, obesity, cataracts, erectile dysfunction, and non-alcoholic fatty liver disease. They are also at increased risk of some infectious diseases, such as tuberculosis *(1)*.

Classification of diabetes (2019)

Ideally a single classification system for diabetes would facilitate three primary purposes: clinical care, aetio-pathology and epidemiology. With this in mind, the Expert group considered it best to define a classification system that prioritizes clinical care and helps health professionals choose appropriate treatment, and whether or not to start treatment with insulin, particularly at the time of diagnosis. The WHO classification of diabetes is as shown in Table 1 *(2)*.

Type 1 diabetes (Insulin-dependent diabetes mellitus) is the most severe form of the disease. Its onset is typically abrupt and is usually seen in individuals less than 30 years of age. It is lethal unless promptly diagnosed and treated. This form of diabetes is immune-mediated in over 90 per cent of

TABLE 1

Types of diabetes

Type of diabetes	Brief description	Change from previous classification
Type 1 diabetes	β-cell destruction (mostly immune-mediated) and absolute insulin deficiency; onset most common in childhood and early adulthood	Type 1 sub-classes removed
Type 2 diabetes	Most common type, various degrees of β-cell dysfunction and insulin resistance; commonly associated with overweight and obesity	Type 2 sub-classes removed
Hybrid forms of diabetes		New type of diabetes
Slowly evolving, immune-mediated diabetes of adults	Similar to slowly evolving type 1 in adults but more often has features of the metabolic syndrome, a single GAD autoantibody and retains greater β-cell function	Nomenclature changed - previously referred to as latent autoimmune diabetes of adults (LADA)
Ketosis-prone type 2 diabetes	Presents with ketosis and insulin deficiency but later does not require insulin; common episodes of ketosis, not immune-mediated	No change
Other specific types		
Monogenic diabetes – Monogenic defects of β-cell function – Monogenic defects in insulin action	Caused by specific gene mutations, has several clinical manifestations requiring different treatment, some occurring in the neonatal period, others by early adulthood Caused by specific gene mutations; has features of severe insulin resistance without obesity; diabetes develops when β-cells do not compensate for insulin resistance	Updated nomenclature for specific genetic defects
Diseases of the exocrine pancreas	Various conditions that affect the pancreas can result in hyperglycaemia (trauma, tumor, inflammation, etc.)	No change
Endocrine disorders	Occurs in diseases with excess secretion of hormones that are insulin antagonists	No change
Drug- or chemical-induced	Some medicines and chemicals impair insulin secretion or action, some can destroy β-cells	No change
Infection-related diabetes	Some viruses have been associated with direct ß-cell destruction	No change
Uncommon specific forms of immune-mediated diabetes	Associated with rare immune-mediated diseases	No change
Other genetic syndromes sometimes associated with diabetes	Many genetic disorders and chromosomal abnormalities increase the risk of diabetes	No change
Unclassified diabetes	Used to describe diabetes that does not clearly fit into other categories. This category should be used temporarily when there is not a clear diagnostic category especially close to the time of diagnosis	New types of diabetes
Hyperglycaemia first detected during pregnancy		
Diabetes mellitus in pregnancy	Type 1 or type 2 diabetes first diagnosed during pregnancy	No change
Gestational diabetes mellitus	Hyperglycaemia below diagnostic thresholds for diabetes in pregnancy	Defined by 2013 diagnostic criteria
Diagnostic criteria for diabetes : fasting plasma glucose ≥7.0 mmol/L or 2-hour post-load plasma glucose ≥11.1 mmol/L or Hba1c ≥48 mmol/mol		
Diagnostic criteria for gestational diabetes : fasting plasma glucose 5.1–6.9 mmol/L or 1-hour post-load plasma glucose ≥10.0 mmol/L or 2-hour post-load plasma glucose 8.5–11.0 mmol/L		

Source : *(2)*

cases and idiopathic in less than 10 per cent cases. The rate of destruction of pancreatic β cell is quite variable. Rapid in some individuals and slow in others. Type 1 diabetes is usually associated with ketosis in its untreated state. It occurs mostly in children, the incidence is highest among 10–14 year old group, but occasionally occur in adults. It is catabolic disorder in which circulating insulin is virtually absent, plasma glucagon is elevated, and the pancreatic β cells fail to respond to all insulinogenic stimuli. Exogenous insulin is therefore required to reverse the catabolic state, prevent ketosis, reduce the hyperglucagonaemia, and reduce blood glucose *(3)*.

Type 2 diabetes is much more common than type 1 diabetes. It is often discovered by chance. It is typically gradual in onset and occurs mainly in the middle-aged and elderly, frequently mild, slow to ketosis and is compatible with long survival if given adequate treatment. Its clinical picture is usually complicated by the presence of other disease processes.

Gestational diabetes is hyperglycaemia with blood glucose values above normal but below those diagnostic of diabetes, occurring during pregnancy. Women with gastational diabetes are at an increased risk of complications during pregnancy and at delivery. They and their children are also at increased risk of type 2 diabetes in the future.

Impaired glucose tolerance (IGT) describes a state intermediate– "at-risk" group – between diabetes mellitus and normality. It can only be defined by the oral glucose tolerance test (see Table 3).

Insulin resistance syndrome (Syndrome X)

In obese patients with type 2 diabetes, the association of hyperglycaemia, hyperinsulinaemia, dyslipidaemia and hypertension, which leads to coronary artery disease and stroke, may result from a genetic defect producing insulin resistance, with the latter being exaggerated by obesity. It has been proposed that insulin resistance predisposes to hyperglycaemia, which results in hyperinsulinaemia (which may or may not be of sufficient magnitude to correct the hyperglycaemia) and this excessive insulin level then contributes to high levels of triglycerides and increased sodium retention by renal tubules, thus inducing hypertension. High levels of insulin can stimulate endothelial proliferation to initiate atherosclerosis *(3)*.

Problem statement

WORLD

Diabetes is an "iceberg" disease. Although increase in both the prevalence and incidence of type 2 diabetes have occurred gloablly, they have been especially dramatic in societies in economic transition, in newly industrialized countries and in developing countries. During year 2014, the number of cases of diabetes worlwide is estimated to be around 422 million, of these more than 90 per cent are type 2 diabetes. In 2019, an estimated 1.5 million people died from consequences of high blood sugar *(4)*. More than 80 per cent diabetes deaths occur in low and middle income countries.

The apparent prevalence of hyperglycaemia depends on the diagnostic criteria used in epidemiological surveys. The global prevalence of diabetes in 2014 was estimated to be 8.5% in adults aged 18+ years *(4)*. The prevalence of diabetes was highest in the Eastern Mediterranean Region and the Region of the Americas (11% for both sexes) and lowest in the WHO European and Western Pacific Regions (9% for both sexes). The magnitude of diabetes and other abnormalities of glucose tolerance are considerably higher than the above estimates if the categories of 'impaired fasting' and 'impaired glucose tolerance' are also included. The estimated prevalence of diabetes was relatively consistent across the income groupings of countries. Low-income countries showed the lowest prevalence (8% for both sexes), and the upper-middle-income countries showed the highest (10% for both sexes) *(5)*.

Unfavourable modification of lifestyle and dietary habits that are associated with urbanization are believed to be the most important factors for the development of diabetes. The prevalence of diabetes is approximately twice in urban areas than in rural population.

A bulk of evidence from studies on migrants indicates that the ethnic, presumably genetic, vulnerability of Asians manifests into diabetes when subjected to unfavourable life-styles. Population-based surveys completed recently in Bangladesh, India and Indonesia have shown considerable increase in the prevalence rate of the disease in both urban and rural dwellers when compared to results obtained earlier.

Diabetic patients, if undiagnosed or inadequately treated, develop multiple chronic complications leading to irreversible disability and death. Coronary heart disease and stroke are more common in diabetics than in the general population. Microvascular complications like diabetic renal disease and diabetic retinopathy and neuropathy are serious health problems resulting in deterioration of the quality of life and premature death. In fact, diabetes is listed among the five most important determinants of the cardiovascular disease epidemic in Asia. Lower limb amputation are at least 10 times more common in diabetic than in non-diabetic individuals in developed countries, more than half of all non-traumatic lower limb amputations are due to diabetes *(5)*. Metabolic disorders in pregnant diabetic women as well as those caused by gestational diabetes (diabetes diagnosed for the first time during pregnancy) pose a high health risk, to both the mother and foetus.

Unfortunately, there is still inadequate awareness about the real dimension of the problem among the general public. There is also a lack of awareness about the existing interventions for preventing diabetes and the management of complications. Inadequacies in primary health care systems, which are not designed to cope with the additional challenges posed by the chronic non-communicable diseases, result in poor detection of cases, suboptimal treatment and insufficient follow-up leading to unnecessary disabilities and severe complications, often resulting in early death.

The age-adjusted mortality rates among the people with diabetes are 1.5 to 2.5 times higher than in the general population *(6)*. In Caucassian population, much of the excess mortality is attributable to cardiovascular disease, especially coronary heart disease; amongst Asian and American Indian population, renal disease is a major contributor *(6)*; whereas in some developing societies, infections are an important cause of death. It is conceivable that the decline in mortality due to coronary heart disease which has occurred in many affluent countries may be halted or even reversed if rates of type 2 diabetes continue to rise. This may occur if the coronary risk factors associated with diabetes increase to the extent that the risk they mediate outweighs the benefit accrued from improvements in conventional cardiovascular risk factors, and the improved care of patients with established cardiovascular disease *(6)*.

In addition to non-insulin dependent diabetes, which is rather silent, chronic, often unidentified killer mostly among the adult population, the insulin dependent form of the disease (type 1) makes an even more dramatic appearance in affected children. They develop symptoms of ketoacidosis and often die, since the majority do not have access to adequate medical care, and since insulin is not available or too expensive. It is estimated that the prevalence of type 1 diabetes in Asia is relatively low, accounting for about 9.7 per cent of all diabetes mellitus cases in the Region. The insulin dependent diabetes registry at Chennai (India) reported an incidence of 10.5 per 100,000 children in the age group of 10–12 years *(7)*.

INDIA

The population in India has an increased susceptibility to diabetes mellitus. This propensity was demonstrated by multiple surveys of migrant Indians residing in Fiji, Singapore, South Africa, U.K. and USA. The rates of diabetes in migrants from the Indian subcontinent have consistently shown to exceed those of the local population.

India is home to 77 million diabetics, second only to China in the world. The Govt. of India and diabetic retinopathy survey 2019 found 11.8 per cent prevalence of diabetes in India. Males showed prevalence of 12 per cent and females 11.7 per cent. There is no sex difference. Nearly 40 per cent of known diabetics were diagnosed 1 to 4 years back, while 5.3 per cent of known diabetics reported diagnosis within one-year *(8)*. Majority of cases are of type 2 diabetes. In the year 2016, about 2 per cent deaths were attributable to diabetes. In the age group 30–69 years, 75,900 males and 51,700 females died of diabetes and in the age group 75 and above, about 46,800 males and 45,600 females died of diabetes *(9)*. The prevalence was higher in urban areas ranging between 10.9 to 14.2 per cent. In rural areas it was 3.0 to 7.8 per cent in population aged 20 years and above.

National programme for prevention and control of non-communicable diseases are operational in India and it includes diabetes and diabetes registry. For details please refer to chapter 7.

Natural history

Epidemiological determinants

1. AGENT

The underlying cause of diabetes is insulin deficiency which is absolute in type 1 diabetes and partial in type 2 diabetes. This may be due to a wide variety of mechanisms: (a) pancreatic disorders – inflammatory, neoplastic and other disorders such as cystic fibrosis, (b) defects in the formation of insulin, e.g., synthesis of an abnormal, biologically less active insulin molecule; (c) destruction of beta cells, e.g., viral infections and chemical agents, (d) decreased insulin sensitivity, due to decreased numbers of adipocyte and monocyte insulin receptors. (e) genetic defects, e.g., mutation of insulin gene; and (f) auto-immunity. Evidence is accumulating that the insulin response to glucose is genetically controlled. The overall effect of these mechanisms is reduced utilization of glucose which leads to hyperglycaemia accompanied by glycosuria.

2. HOST FACTORS

(a) AGE : Although diabetes may occur at any age, surveys indicate that prevalence rises steeply with age. Type 2 diabetes usually comes to light in the middle years of life and thereafter begins to rise in frequency. Malnutrition related diabetes affects large number of young people. The prognosis is worse in younger diabetics who tend to develop complications earlier than older diabetics. *(b) SEX* : In some countries (e.g., UK) the overall male–female ratio is about equal *(10)*. In south-east Asia, an excess of male diabetics has been observed, but this is open to question. *(c) GENETIC FACTORS:* The genetic nature of diabetes is undisputed. Twin studies showed that in identical twins who developed type 2 diabetes, concordance was approximately 90 per cent *(11)*, thus demonstrating a strong genetic component. In type 1 diabetes, the concordance was only about 50 per cent indicating that type 1 diabetes is not totally a genetic entity. *(d) GENETIC MARKERS* : Type 1 diabetes is associated with HLA–B8 and B15, and more powerfully with HLA–DR3 and DR4. The highest risk of type 1 diabetes is carried by individuals with both DR3 and DR4. On the other hand type 2 diabetes is not HLA–associated *(11)*. *(e) IMMUNE MECHANISMS* : There is some evidence of both cell–mediated and of humoral activity against islet cells. Some people appear to have defective immunological mechanisms, and under the influence of some environmental "trigger", attack their own insulin producing cells. *(f) OBESITY* : Obesity particularly central adiposity has long been accepted as a risk factor for type 2 diabetes and the risk is related to both the duration and degree of obesity. The association has been repeatedly demonstrated in longitudinal studies in different populations, with a striking gradient of risk apparent with increasing level of BMI, adult weight gain, waist circumference or waist to hip ratio. Indeed waist circumference or waist to hip ratio (reflecting abdominal or visceral adiposity) are more powerful determinants of subsequent risk of type 2 diabetes than BMI *(6)*. Central obesity is also an important determinant of insulin resistance, the underlying abnormality in most cases of type 2 diabetes. In some instances obesity reduces the number of insulin receptors on target cells. Voluntary weight loss improves insulin sensitivity and in several randomized controlled trials has shown to reduce the risk of progression from impaired glucose tolerence to type 2 diabetes *(12, 13)*. However, many obese subjects are not diabetic. Thus obesity by itself is inadequate to account for all, or even most, cases of type 2 diabetes; physical inactivity and/or deficiencies of specific nutrients may also be involved *(11)*. Obesity appears to play no role in type 1 diabetes pathogenesis *(14)*. *(g) MATERNAL DIABETES* : Offsprings of diabetic pregnancies including gestational diabetes are often large and heavy at birth, tend to develop obesity in childhood and are at high risk of developing type 2 diabetes at an early age. Those born to mothers after they have developed diabetes have a three-fold higher risk of developing diabetes than those born before. Maternal diabetes associated with intrauterine growth retardation and low birth weight, when associated with rapid growth catch-up later on, appears to increase the risk of subsequent diabetes in the child *(6)*.

3. ENVIRONMENTAL RISK FACTORS

Susceptibility to diabetes appears to be unmasked by a number of environmental factors acting on genetically susceptible individuals. They include : *(a) SEDENTARY LIFESTYLE* : Sedentary life style appears to be an important risk factor for the development of type 2 diabetes.

Lack of exercise may alter the interaction between insulin and its receptors and subsequently lead to type 2 diabetes *(11)*. *(b) DIET* : A high saturated fat intake has been associated with a higher risk of impaired glucose tolerance, and higher fasting glucose and insulin levels *(6)*. Higher proportions of saturated fatty acids in serum lipid or muscle phospholipid have been associated with higher fasting insulin, lower insulin sensitivity and a higher risk of type 2 diabetes. Higher unsaturated fatty acids from vegetable sources and polyunsaturated fatty acids have been associated with reduced risk of type 2 diabetes and lower fasting and 2-hour glucose concentrations. Higher proportions of long-chain polyunsaturated fatty acids in skeletal muscle phospholipids have been associated with increased insulin sensitivity *(6)*. In human intervention studies, replacement of saturated by unsaturated fatty acids leads to improved glucose tolerence and enhanced insulin sensitivity. However, long chain polyunsaturated fatty acids do not appear to confer additional benefit over monounsaturated fatty acids. When total fat intake is high (greater than 37 per cent of total energy), altering the quality of dietary fat appears to have little effect *(15)*. *(c) DIETARY FIBRE* : In many controlled experimental studies, high intakes of dietary fibre have been shown to result in reduced blood glucose and insulin levels in people with type 2 diabetes and impaired glucose tolerance *(16)*. Moreover an increased intake of wholegrain cereals, vegetables and fruits (all rich in NSP) was a feature of diets in randomized controlled trials. Thus the evidence for a potential protective effect of dietary fibre appears strong. A minimum daily intake of 20 grams of dietary fibre is recommended *(6)*. Table 2 shows a summary of lifestyle and dietary factors associated with diabetes.*(d) MALNUTRITION* : Malnutrition (PEM) in early infancy and childhood may result in partial failure of β–cell function. Damage to beta cells may well explain the associated impaired carbohydrate tolerance in kwashiorkor *(11)*. *(e) ALCOHOL* : Excessive intake of alcohol can increase the risk of diabetes by damaging the pancreas and liver and by promoting obesity *(11)*. *(f) VIRAL INFECTIONS:* Among the viruses that have been implicated are rubella, mumps, and human coxsackie virus B4. Viral infections may trigger in immunogenetically susceptible people a sequence of events resulting in β–cell destruction. *(g) CHEMICAL AGENTS* : A number of chemical agents are known to be toxic to beta cells, e.g., alloxan, streptozotocin, the rodenticide VALCOR, etc *(17)*. A high intake of cyanide producing foods (e.g., cassava and certain beans) may also have toxic effects on β–cells. *(h) STRESS* : Surgery, trauma, and stress of situations, internal or external, may "bring out" the disease. *(i) OTHER FACTORS* : High and low rates of diabetes have been linked to a number of social factors such as occupation, marital status, religion, economic status, education, urbanization and changes in life style which are elements of what is broadly known as **social class.** One of the most important epidemiological features of diabetes is that it is now common in the lower social classes whereas 50 years ago, the gradient was the reverse. One reason could be rapid changes in lifestyle in lower classes.

TABLE 2

Summary of strength of evidence on lifestyle factors and risk of developing type 2 diabetes

Evidence	Decreased risk	Increased risk
Convincing	Voluntary weight loss in overweight and obese people Physical activity	Overweight and obesity Abdominal obesity Physical inactivity Maternal diabetes[a]
Probable	NSP[1]	Saturated fats Intrauterine growth retardation
Possible	η-3 fatty acids Low glycaemic index foods Exclusive breast-feeding[b]	Total fat intake Trans-fatty acids
Insufficient	Vitamin E Chromium Magnesium Moderate alcohol	Excess alcohol

1 NSP = Non-starch Polysaccharides.
a Includes gestational diabetes.
b As a global public health recommendation, infants should be exclusively breast-fed for the first six months of life to achieve optimal growth, development and health.

Source : *(6)*

SCREENING FOR DIABETES

In the past, the commonest approach to diabetes screening was a preliminary, semi–quantitative test for glucose in a urine sample, followed by an oral glucose tolerance test for those found to have glycosuria. The underlying assumption is that early detection and effective control of hyperglycaemia in asymptomatic diabetics reduces morbidity.

1. Urine examination

Urine test for glucose, 2 hours after a meal, is commonly used in medical practice for detecting cases of diabetes. All those with glycosuria are considered diabetic unless otherwise proved by a standard oral glucose tolerance test. Most studies now confirm that although glucose is found in urine in the most severe cases of diabetes, it is often absent in milder forms of the disease, and such cases are likely to be missed by urine test. This is known as lack of "sensitivity". To be more precise, the sensitivity of the test (i.e., proportion of people with disease who have a positive test) varies between 10–50 per cent. The lack of sensitivity means that many diabetics would have been missed if this had been the only test. That is, the test yields too many "false-negatives". Further, glycosuria may be found in perfectly normal people; this gives rise to "false-positives". Since the specificity of the test is over 90 per cent, the yield of false-positives is not very high. For these reasons, urine testing is not considered an appropriate tool for case-finding or epidemiological surveys of the population *(11)*.

2. Blood sugar testing

Because of the inadequacies of urine examination, "standard oral glucose test" remains the cornerstone of diagnosis of diabetes. Mass screening programmes have used glucose measurements of fasting, postprandial or random blood sample. The measurement of glucose levels in random blood samples is considered unsatisfactory for epidemiological use; at the most, it can give only a crude estimate of the frequency of diabetes in a population *(11)*. The fasting value alone is considered less reliable since true fasting cannot be assured and spurious diagnosis of diabetes may more readily occur. Therefore, for epidemiological purposes, the 2-hour value after 75 g oral glucose may be used either alone or with the fasting value *(11)*. Automated biochemistry has now made it possible to screen thousands of samples for glucose estimation. The criteria for the diagnosis of diabetes, proposed by WHO, are given in Table 3.

Target population

Screening of the whole population for diabetes is not considered a rewarding exercise *(18, 19)*. However, screening of "high-risk" groups is considered more appropriate. These groups are: (i) those in the age group 40 and over; (ii) those with a family history of diabetes; (iii) the obese; (iv) women who have had a baby weighing more than 4.5 kg (or 3.5 kg in constitutionally small populations); (v) women who show excess weight gain during pregnancy; and (vi) patients with premature atherosclerosis.

PREVENTION AND CARE

1. Primary prevention

Two strategies for primary prevention have been suggested: (a) population strategy, and (b) high-risk strategy *(11)*.

a. POPULATION STRATEGY

The scope for primary prevention of type 1 diabetes is limited on the basis of current knowledge and is probably not appropriate *(11)*. However, the development of prevention programmes for type 2 diabetes based on elimination of environmental risk factors is possible. There is pressing need for **primordial prevention** – that is, prevention of the emergence of risk factors in countries in which they have not yet appeared. The preventive measures comprise maintenance of normal body weight through adoption of healthy nutritional habits and physical exercise. The nutritional habits include an adequate protein intake, a high intake of dietary fibre and avoidance of sweet foods. Elimination of other less well defined factors such as protein deficiency and food toxins may be considered in some populations. These measures should be fully integrated into other community–based programmes for the prevention of non-communicable diseases (e.g., coronary heart disease).

TABLE 3

The WHO recommendations for the diagnostic criteria for diabetes (2019)

Measurement	Diagnostic cut-off value
Fasting venous or capillary* plasma glucose	≥7.0 mmol/L (126 mg/dL)
2-hour post-load venous plasma glucose	≥11.1 mol/L (200 mg/dL)
2-hour post-load capillary** plasma glucose	≥12.2 mmol/L (220 mg/dL)
Random plasma glucose	≥11.1 mmol/L (200 mg/dL)
HbA1c***	6.5% (48 mmol/mol)

* Overnight fast of 8–14 hours.

** If laboratory measurement is not available, point of care, ("finger stick") devices can be used (they report glucose values in capillary plasma).

*** Plasma glucose is preferred in people with symptoms who are suspected of having type 1 diabetes.

Source : *(1)*

b. HIGH-RISK STRATEGY

There is no special high-risk strategy for type 1 diabetes. At present, there is no practical justification for genetic counselling as a method of prevention *(11)*.

Since NIDDM appears to be linked with sedentary life-style, over-nutrition and obesity, correction of these may reduce the risk of diabetes and its complications. Since alcohol can indirectly increase the risk of diabetes, it should be avoided. Subjects at risk should avoid diabetogenic drugs like oral contraceptives. It is wise to reduce factors that promote atherosclerosis, e.g., smoking, high blood pressure, elevated cholesterol and high triglyceride levels. These programmes may most effectively be directed at target population groups.

2. Secondary prevention

When diabetes is detected, it must be adequately treated. The aims of treatment are : (a) to maintain blood glucose levels as close within the normal limits as is practicable (see Table 3), and (b) to maintain ideal body weight. Treatment is based on (a) diet alone – small balanced meals more frequently, (b) diet and oral antidiabetic drugs, or (c) diet and insulin. Good control of blood glucose protects against the development of complications. Please see in chapter 10 "Nutrition and health" under title "Nutritional factors in selected diseases" for details.

Proper management of the diabetic is most important to prevent complications. Routine checking of blood sugar, of urine for proteins and ketones, of blood pressure, visual acuity and weight should be done periodically. The feet should be examined for any defective blood circulation (Doppler ultrasound probes are advised), loss of sensation and the health of the skin. Primary health care is of great importance to diabetic patients since most care is obtained at this level.

Glycosylated haemoglobin : There should be an estimation of glycated (glycosylated) haemoglobin at half–yearly intervals. This test provides a long-term index of glucose control. This test is based on the following rationale: glucose in the blood is complexed to a certain fraction of haemoglobin to an extent proportional to the blood glucose concentration. The percentage of such glycosylated haemoglobin reflects the mean blood glucose levels during the red cell life-time (i.e., about the previous 2–3 months) *(20)*.

Self-care : A crucial element in secondary prevention is self care. That is, the diabetic should take a major responsibility for his own care with medical guidance – e.g., adherence to diet and drug regimens, examination of his own urine and where possible blood glucose monitoring; self administration of insulin, abstinence from alcohol, maintenance of optimum weight, attending periodic check–ups, recognition of symptoms associated with glycosuria and hypoglycaemia, etc.

Table 4 shows some of the individual interventions in diabetes with evidence of efficacy.

Home blood glucose monitoring : Assessment of control has been greatly aided by the recent facility of immediate, reasonably accurate, capillary blood glucose measurements either by one of the many meters now available or the direct reading Haemoglucotest strips *(21)*.

The patient should carry an identification card showing his name, address, telephone number (if any) and the details of treatment he is receiving. In short, he must have a working knowledge of diabetes. All these mean education of patients and their families to optimize the effectiveness of primary health care services.

TABLE 4

Individual interventions in diabetes with evidence of efficacy

Interventions with evidence of efficacy	Benefit
Lifestyle interventions for preventing type 2 diabetes in people of high risk	Reduction of 35–58% in incidence
Metformin for preventing type 2 diabetes for people at high risk	Reduction of 25–31% in incidence
Glycaemic control in people with HbA1c greater than 9%	Reduction of 30% in microvascular disease per 1 percent drop in HbA1c
Blood pressure control in people whose pressure is higher than 130/80 mmHg	Reduction of 35% in macrovascular and microvascular disease per 10 mmHg drop in blood pressure
Annual eye examinations	Reduction of 60 to 70% in serious vision loss
Foot care in people with high risk of ulcers	Reduction of 50 to 60% in serious foot disease
Angiotensin converting enzyme inhibitor use in all people with diabetes	Reduction of 42% in nephropathy; 22% drop in cardiovascular disease

Source : *(5)*

3. Tertiary prevention

Diabetes is major cause of disability through its complications, e.g., blindness, kidney failure, coronary thrombosis, gangrene of the lower extremities, etc. The main objective at the tertiary level is to organize specialized clinics (Diabetic clinics) and units capable of providing diagnostic and management skills of a high order. There is a great need to establish such clinics in large towns and cities *(22)*. The tertiary level should also be involved in basic, clinical and epidemiological research. It has also been recommended that local and national registries for diabetics should be established *(11)*.

References

1. WHO (2020). *Diagnosis and Management of Type 2 Diabetes.*
2. WHO (2019). *Classification of Diabetes Mellitus*, 2019.
3. Lawrence M. Tierney, Jr. Stephen J. McPhee Maxine A. Papadakis (2002), *Current Medical Diagnosis and Treatment*, 41st ed., Lange Publication.
4. WHO (2022), *Diabetes Fact Sheet*, 16th Sept. 2022.
5. WHO (2011), *Global Status Report on Non-communicable Diseases*, 2010.
6. WHO (2003), *Tech. Rep. Ser.*, N 916.
7. WHO (2002), *Health Situation in the South-East Asia Region 1998-2000*, New Delhi.
8. Govt. of India (2019), *Govt. of India Survey 2018–2019 for Diabetes.*
9. WHO (2016), *Diabetes Country Profile, India*, 2016.
10. Drury, M.I. (1979). *Diabetes Mellitus*, Blackwell, Oxford.
11. WHO (1985). *Techn. Rep. Ser.*, No. 727.
12. Tuomilento J. et al. (2002), Prevention of type 2 diabetes Mellitus by changes in lifestyle among subjects with impaired glucose tolerance, *New England Journal of Medicine, 2002*, 344 : 1343-1350.
13. Knowler WC et al. (2002), Reduction in the incidence of type 2 diabetes with lifestyle intervention of metformin, *New England Journal of Medicine, 2002*, 346 : 393-403.
14. Keen, H. (1985). In: *Oxford Textbook of Public Health*, Vol.4, p.268.
15. Vessby B. et al. (2001), Substituting dietary saturated for monounsaturated fat impairs insuline sensitivity in healthy men and women : the KANWU study. *Diabetologia, 2001*, 44 : 312-319.
16. Marshal JA et al. (1994), Dietary fat predicts conversion from impaired glucose tolerance to NIDDM, The San Luis Valley Diabetes Study, *Diabetes Care, 1994*, 17 : 50-56.
17. Arky, R.A. (1983). *Nutrition Reviews*, 41 (6) 165.
18. Melins, J.M. (1974). *Lancet*, 2 : 1367.
19. Redhead, I.H. (1975). In: *Screening in General Practice*, C.R. Hart (ed), Churchill Livingstone.
20. Anonymous (1978). *Glycosylated Haemoglobin and Diabetic Control*, Brit, Med. J., 1: 1373–4.
21. Sonksen, P.H. et al (1978). Home Monitoring of Blood Glucose. *Lancet*, 1 : 729–32.
22. Diabetic Clinics Today and Tomorrow : *Brit. Med. J.* (1973) 2 : 534 and *Brit. Med. J.* (1971) 4 : 161.

OBESITY

Obesity may be defined as an abnormal growth of the adipose tissue due to an enlargement of fat cell size (hypertrophic obesity) or an increase in fat cell number (hyperplastic obesity) or a combination of both *(1)*. Obesity is often expressed in terms of body mass index (BMI) (see Table 1). Overweight is usually due to obesity but can arise from other causes such as abnormal muscle development or fluid retention *(2)*.

TABLE 1

Adult weights and heights corresponding to recommended cut-off values for body mass index

	BMI							
	16.0	17.0	18.5	20.0	22.0	25.0	30.0	40.0
Height (cm)	Thinness					Overweight		
	Body weight (kg)							
140	31.4	33.3	36.2	39.2	43.1	49.0	58.8	78.4
142	32.3	34.3	37.3	40.3	44.4	50.4	60.5	80.7
144	33.2	35.3	38.4	41.5	45.6	51.8	62.2	82.9
146	34.1	36.2	39.4	42.6	46.9	53.3	63.9	85.3
148	35.0	37.2	40.5	43.8	48.2	54.8	65.7	87.6
150	36.0	38.2	41.6	45.0	49.5	56.3	67.5	90.0
152	37.0	39.3	42.7	46.2	50.8	57.8	69.3	92.4
154	37.9	40.3	43.9	47.4	52.2	59.3	71.1	94.9
156	38.9	41.4	45.0	48.7	53.5	60.8	73.0	97.3
158	39.9	42.4	46.2	49.9	54.9	62.4	74.9	99.9
160	41.0	43.5	47.4	51.2	56.3	64.0	76.8	102.4
162	42.0	44.6	48.3	52.5	57.7	65.6	78.7	105.0
164	43.0	45.7	49.8	53.8	59.2	67.2	80.7	107.6
166	44.1	46.8	51.0	55.1	60.6	68.9	82.7	110.2
168	45.2	48.0	52.2	56.4	62.1	70.6	84.7	112.9
170	46.2	49.1	53.5	57.8	63.6	72.3	86.7	115.6
172	47.3	50.3	54.7	59.2	65.1	74.0	88.8	118.3
174	48.4	51.5	56.0	60.6	66.6	75.7	90.8	121.1
176	49.6	52.7	57.3	62.0	68.1	77.4	92.9	123.9
178	50.7	53.9	58.6	63.4	69.7	79.2	95.0	126.7
180	51.9	55.1	59.9	64.8	71.3	81.0	97.2	129.6
182	53.0	56.3	61.3	66.2	72.9	82.8	99.4	132.5
184	54.2	57.6	62.6	67.7	74.5	84.6	101.6	135.4
186	55.5	58.8	64.0	69.2	76.1	86.5	103.8	138.4
188	56.6	60.1	65.4	70.7	77.8	88.4	106.0	141.4
190	57.8	61.4	66.8	72.2	79.4	90.3	108.3	144.4

For easy reference and calculation of BMI values corresponding to recommended cut-offs, first find the height of the individual in the left hand column. The weights given in the row for that height correspond to various recommended cut-off values for adult BMI. Weight for two normal BMI values are also included.

Source : *(5)*

However, obese individuals differ not only in the amount of excess fat that they store, but also in the regional distribution of the fat within the body. The distribution of fat induced by the weight gain affects the risk associated with obesity, and the kind of disease that results. It is useful therefore, to be able to distinguish between those at increased risk as a result of "abdominal fat distribution" or "android obesity" from those with the less serious "gynoid" fat distribution, in which fat is more evenly and peripherally distributed around the body.

Prevalence

Obesity is perhaps the most prevalent form of malnutrition. As a chronic disease, prevalent in both developed and developing countries, and affecting children as well as adults, it is now so common that it is replacing the more traditional public health concerns including undernutrition. It is one of the most significant contributors to ill health. For industrialized countries, it has been suggested that such increase in body weight have been caused primarily by reduced levels of physical activity, rather than by changes in food intake or by other factors. It is extremely difficult to assess the size of the problem and compare the prevalence rates in different countries as no exact figures are available and also because the definitions of obesity are not standardized.

Overweight and obesity are the fifth leading risk of global deaths. Worldwide, obesity has more than doubled since 1980. In 2016, more than 1.9 billion adults, 18 years and older, were overweight. Of these over 650 million men and women were obese *(3)*.

In 2019, more than 38.2 million children under 5 years of age were overweight or obese. Once considered a high-income country problem, overweight and obesity are now rising in low-and middle-income countries, particularly in urban settings *(3)*. Close to 30 million overweight children are living in developing and 10 million in developed countries *(3)*. Childhood obesity is associated with a higher chance of obesity, premature death and disability in adulthood. In addition, it is associated with future risk of increased breathing difficulties, increased risk of fractures, hypertension, early markers of cardiovascular disease, insulin resistance and psychological effects.

At least 3.4 million adults die each year as a result of being overweight or obese. In addition, 44 per cent of the diabetes burden, 23 per cent of ischaemic heart disease burden and between 7 to 41 per cent of certain cancer burdens are attributable to overweight and obesity *(3)*. Overweight and obesity are linked to more deaths worldwide than underweight.

INDIA

The National Family Health Survey-5 (2019–2021) calculated Body Mass Index (BMI) of men and women (aged 15–49 years) interviewed to know the trend of nutritional status of the population. The trend of obesity and overweight persons are as follows :

(a) 19 per cent of women age 15–49 are thin, 24 per cent are overweight or obese, and 57 per cent are in the normal range. The patterns by background characteristics are *(4)* :

- The proportion of thin women decreases with age, from 40 per cent for women age 15–19 to 9 per cent for women age 40–49, whereas the proportion of overweight or obese women increases steadily, from 5 per cent of women age 15–49 to 37 per cent of women age 40–49.
- The proportion of thin women is higher in rural areas (21%) than in urban areas (13%) and the reverse is observed for the prevalence of overweight or obesity (33% in urban areas and 20% in rural areas).
- There is a steady decrease in the proportion of thin women as household wealth increases (from 28% in the lowest wealth quintile to 10% in the highest wealth quintile), which is accompanied by a steady increase in the proportion of overweight or obese women (from 10% in the lowest wealth quintile to 39% in the highest wealth quintile).
- The highest proportion of thin women is observed in Jharkhand and Bihar (26% each), followed by Gujarat and Dadra & Nagar Haveli and Daman & Diu (25% each). The highest proportion of overweight or obese women is found in Puducherry (46%), Chandigarh (44%), Delhi, Tamil Nadu, and Punjab (41% each), and Kerala and Andaman & Nicobar Islands (38% each).

(b) 16 per cent of men age 15–49 are thin, 23 per cent are overweight and obese, and 61 per cent have BMI in normal range. The patterns by background characteristics are *(4)* :

- The patterns of nutritional status by background characteristics among men are similar to those among women.
- The proportion of thin men decreases with age, from 41 per cent of men age 15–19 to 8 per cent of men age 40–49, whereas the proportion of overweight or obese men increases from 7 per cent of men age 15–19 to 32 per cent of men age 40–49.
- The proportion of thin men is higher in rural areas (18%) than in urban areas (13%), whereas 30 per cent of men are overweight or obese in urban areas, compared with 19 per cent in rural areas.
- There is steady decrease in the proportion of thin men with increasing household wealth (from 24% in the lowest wealth quintile to 9% in the highest wealth quintile), and a steady increase in the proportion of overweight or obese men (from 10% in the lowest wealth quintile to 37% in the highest wealth quintile).
- The proportion of thin men is highest in Bihar (22%), followed by Madhya Pradesh and Gujarat (21% each). The highest proportion of overweight or obese men is observed in Andaman & Nicobar Island (45%), followed by Puducherry (43%) and Lakshadweep (41%).

As obesity is a key risk factor in natural history of other chronic and non-communicable diseases, the typical time sequence of emergence of chronic diseases following the increased prevalence of obesity is important in public health planning. The first adverse effects of obesity to emerge in population in transition are hypertension, hyperlipidaemia and glucose intolerence, while coronary heart disease and the long-term complications of diabetes, such as renal failure begin to emerge several years (or decades) later *(6)*. It is matter of time before same mortality rates for such diseases will be seen in developing countries as those prevailing 30 years ago in industrialized countries *(7)*.

Epidemiological determinants

The aetiology of obesity is complex, and is one of multiple causation :

(a) AGE : Obesity can occur at any age, and generally increases with age. Infants with excessive weight gain have an increased incidence of obesity in later life *(8)*. About one-third of obese adults have been so since childhood *(1)*. It has been well established that most adipose cells are formed early in life and the obese infant lays down more of these cells (hyperplastic obesity) than the normal infant. Hyperplastic obesity in adults is extremely difficult to treat with conventional methods.

(b) SEX : Women generally have higher rate of obesity than men, although men may have higher rates of overweight. In the Framingham, USA study, men were found to gain most weight between the ages of 29 and 35 years, while women gain most between 45 and 49 years of age *(9)*, i.e. at menopausal age. It has been claimed that woman's BMI increases with successive pregnancies. The recent evidence suggested that this increase is likely to be, on an average, about 1 kg per pregnancy. On the other hand in many developing countries, consecutive pregnancies at short intervals are often associated with weight loss rather than weight gain *(7)*.

(c) GENETIC FACTORS : There is a genetic component in the aetiology of obesity. Twin studies have shown a close correlation between the weights of identical twins even when they are reared in dissimilar environments *(10)*. The profile of fat distribution is also characterized by a significant heritability level of the order of about 50 per cent of the total human variation. Recent studies have shown that the amount of abdominal fat was influenced by a genetic component accounting for 50–60 per cent of the individual differences *(7)*.

(d) PHYSICAL INACTIVITY : There is convincing evidence that regular physical activity is protective against unhealthy weight gain. Where as sedentary lifestyle particularly sedentary occupation and inactive recreation such as watching television promote it, physical activity and physical fitness are important modifiers of mortality and morbildity related to overweight and obesity *(11)*. In some individuals a major reduction in activity without the compensatory decrease in habitual energy intake may be the major cause of increased obesity, e.g. in athletes when they retire and in young people who sustain injuries etc. Physical inactivity may cause obesity, which in turn restricts activity. This is a vicious circle. It is the reduced energy output that is probably more important in the aetiology of obesity than used to be thought *(10)*.

(e) SOCIO-ECONOMIC STATUS : The relationship of obesity to social class has been studied in some detail. There is a clear direct relationship between socio-economic status and obesity. Within some affluent countries, however, obesity has been found to be more prevalent in the lower socio-economic groups.

(f) EATING HABITS : Eating habits (e.g., eating in between meals, preference to sweets, refined foods and fats) are established very early in life. The composition of the diet, the periodicity with which it is eaten and the amount of energy derived from it are all relevant to the aetiology of obesity. A diet containing more energy than needed may lead to prolonged post-prandial hyperlipidaemia and to deposition of triglycerides in the adipose tissue resulting in obesity *(12)*. Nowadays television and print media is playing an important role in producing obesity by heavy advertisement of fast food outlets of energy-dense, micronutrient poor food and beverages (usually classified under the "eat least" category in diet guidelines) of multinational corporations, which influence the daily eating habits. The consumer demand by itself may be influenced by advertising, marketing, culture, fashion and convenience *(7)*. It has been calculated that a child whose energy requirement is 2000 kcal/day and who consumes 100 kcal/day extra will gain about 5 kg a year *(9)*. The accumulation of one kilo of fat corresponds to 7,700 kcal of energy *(14)*.

(g) PSYCHOSOCIAL FACTORS : Psychosocial factors (e.g., emotional disturbances) are deeply involved in the aetiology of obesity. Overeating may be a symptom of depression, anxiety, frustration and loneliness in childhood as it is in adult life. Excessively obese individuals are usually withdrawn, self-conscious, lonely and secret eaters. An insight into the circumstances in which the obesity has developed is essential for planning the most suitable management.

(h) FAMILIAL TENDENCY : Obesity frequently runs in families (obese parents frequently having obese children), but this is not necessarily explained solely by the influence of genes.

(i) ENDOCRINE FACTORS : These may be involved in occasional cases, e.g., Cushing's syndrome, growth hormone deficiency.

(j) ALCOHOL : A recent review of studies concluded that the relationship between alcohol consumption and adiposity was generally positive for men and negative for women *(6)*.

(k) EDUCATION : In most affluent societies, there is an inverse relationship between educational level and prevalence of overweight *(5)*.

(l) SMOKING : Reports that the use of tobacco lowers body weight began to appear more than 100 years ago, but detailed studies have been reported only during the past 10 years or so. In most populations, smokers weigh somewhat less than ex-smokers; individuals who have never smoked fall somewhat between the two.

(m) ETHNICITY : Ethnic groups in many industrialized countries appear to be especially susceptible to the development of obesity and its complications. Evidence suggests that this may be due to a genetic predisposition to obesity that only become apparent when such groups are exposed to a more affluent lifestyle *(7)*.

(n) DRUGS : Use of certain drugs, e.g., cortico-steroids, contraceptives, insulin, β-adrenergic blockers, etc. can promote weight gain *(7)*.

Use of BMI to classify obesity

Body mass index (BMI) is a simple index of weight-for-height that is commonly used to classify underweight, overweight and obesity in adults. It is defined as the weight in kilograms divided by the square of the height in metres (kg/m^2).

For example, an adult who weighs 70 kg and whose height is 1.75 m will have a BMI of 22.9 :

$$BMI = 70\ (kg)/1.75^2\ (m^2) = 22.9$$

The classification of overweight and obesity, according to BMI, is shown in Table 2. Obesity is classified as a BMI ≥ 30.0. The classification shown is in agreement with that recommended by WHO *(11)*, but includes an additional subdivision at BMI 35.0–39.9 in recognition of the fact that management options for dealing with obesity differ above a BMI of 35. The WHO classification is based primarily on the association between BMI and mortality.

TABLE 2

Classification of adults according to BMI

Classification	BMI	Risk of comorbidities
Underweight	< 18.50	Low (but risk of other clinical problems increased)
Normal range	18.50-24.99	Average
Overweight :	≥ 25.00	
Pre-obese	25.00-29.99	Increased
Obese class I	30.00-34.99	Moderate
Obese class II	35.00-39.99	Severe
Obese class III	≥ 40.00	Very severe

Source : *(11)*

These BMI values are age-independent and the same for both sexes. The table shows a simplistic relationship between BMI and the risk of comorbidity, which can be affected by a range of factors, including the nature of the diet, ethnic group and activity level. The risks associated with increasing BMI are continuous and graded and begin at a BMI above 25.

Although it can generally be assumed that individuals with a BMI of 30 or above have an excess fat mass in their body, BMI does not distinguish between weight associated with muscle and weight associated with fat. As a result, the relationship between BMI and body fat content varies according to body build and proportion, and it has been shown repeatedly that a given BMI may not correspond to the same degree of fatness across populations. Polynesians, for example, tend to have a lower fat percentage than Caucasian Australians at an identical BMI. In addition, the percentage of body fat mass increases with age up to 60–65 years in both sexes, and is higher in women than in men of equivalent BMI. In cross-sectional comparisons, therefore, BMI values should be interpreted with caution if estimates of body fat are required.

INTRA-ABDOMINAL (CENTRAL) FAT ACCUMULATION AND INCREASED RISK

Compared with subcutaneous adipose tissue, intra-abdominal adipose tissue has more cells per unit mass, higher blood flow, more glucocorticoid (cortisol) receptors, probably more androgen (testosterone) receptors, and greater catecholamine-induced lipolysis. These differences make intra-abdominal adipose tissue more susceptible to both normal stimulation and changes in lipid accumulation and metabolism. Furthermore, intra-abdominal adipocytes are located upstream from liver in the portal circulation. This means that there is a marked increase in the flux of nonesterified fatty acid to the liver *via* the portal blood in patients with abdominal obesity.

There is good evidence that abdominal obesity is important in the development of insulin resistance, and in the metabolic syndrome (hyperinsulinaemia, dyslipidaemia, glucose intolerance, and hypertension) that link obesity with CHD *(7)*. Premenopausal women have quantitatively more lipoprotein lipase (LPL) and higher LPL activity in the gluteal and femoral subcutaneous regions, which contain fat cells larger than those in men, but these differences disappear after menopause *(7)*.

Assessment of obesity

Before we consider assessment of obesity, it will be useful to first look at body composition as under;

a. the active mass (muscle, liver, heart etc.)
b. the fatty mass (fat)
c. the extracellular fluid (blood, lymph, etc.)
d. the connective tissue (skin, bones, connective tissue)

Structurally speaking, the state of obesity is characterized by an increase in the fatty mass at the expense of the other parts of the body. The water content of the body is never increased in case of obesity.

Although obesity can easily be identified at first sight, a precise assessment requires measurements and reference standards. The most widely used criteria are :

1. BODY WEIGHT

Body weight, though not an accurate measure of excess fat, is a widely used index. In epidemiological studies it is conventional to accept + 2 SD (standard deviations) from the median weight for height as a cut-off point for overweight and + 3 SD for obesity.

For adults, some people calculate various other indicators such as *(9)* :

(1) *Body mass index* (Quetelet's index)

$$= \frac{\text{Weight (kg)}}{\text{Height}^2\text{(m)}}$$

(2) *Ponderal index*

$$= \frac{\text{Height (cm)}}{\text{Cube root of body weight (kg)}}$$

(3) *Brocca index*

= Height (cm) *minus* 100

For example, if a person's height is 160 cm, his ideal weight is (160−100) = 60 kg

(4) *Lorentz's formula*

$$= \text{Ht (cm)} - 100 - \frac{\text{Ht (cm)} - 150}{\text{2 (women) or 4 (men)}}$$

(5) *Corpulence index*

$$= \frac{\text{Actual weight}}{\text{Desirable weight}}$$

This should not exceed 1.2

The body mass index (BMI) and the Brocca index are widely used. A FAO/WHO/UNU Report gives the much needed reference tables for body mass index (see Table 1) which can be used internationally as reference standards for assessing the prevalence of obesity in a community.

2. SKINFOLD THICKNESS

A large proportion of total body fat is located just under the skin. Since it is most accessible, the method most used is the measurement of skinfold thickness. It is a rapid and "non–invasive" method for assessing body fat. Several varieties of callipers (e.g., Harpenden skin callipers) are available for the purpose. The measurement may be taken at all the four sites – mid-triceps, biceps, subscapular and suprailiac regions. The sum of the measurements should be less than 40 mm in boys and 50 mm in girls *(14)*. Unfortunately standards for subcutaneous fat do not exist for comparison. Further, in extreme obesity, measurements may be impossible. The main drawback of skinfold measurements is their poor repeatability.

3. WAIST CIRCUMFERENCE AND WAIST : HIP RATIO (WHR)

Waist circumference is measured at the mid point between the lower border of the rib cage and the iliac crest. It is a convenient and simple measurement that is unrelated to height, correlates closely with BMI and WHR and is an approximate index of intra-abdominal fat mass and total body fat. Changes in waist circumference reflect changes in risk factors for cardiovascular disease and other forms of chronic diseases. There is an increased risk of metabolic complications for men with a waist circumference ≥ 102 cm, and women with a waist circumference ≥ 88 cm *(11)*.

According to WHO guidelines, it has become accepted that a high WHR (> 0.9 in men and > 0.85 in women) indicates abdominal fat accumulation *(4)*.

4. OTHERS

In addition to the above, three well-established and more accurate measurements are used for the estimation of body fat. They are measurement of total body water, of total body potassium and of body density. The techniques involved are relatively complex and cannot be used for routine clinical purposes or for epidemiological studies *(7)*. The introduction of measuring fat cells has opened up a new field in obesity research.

Hazards of obesity

Obesity is a health hazard and a detriment to well-being which is reflected in the increased morbidity and mortality: (a) INCREASED MORBIDITY : Obesity is a positive risk factor in the development of hypertension, diabetes, gall bladder disease and coronary heart disease and certain types of cancers, especially the hormonally related and large bowel cancers. There are in addition, several associated diseases, which, although not usually fatal, cause a great deal of morbidity in the community, e.g., varicose veins, abdominal hernia, osteoarthritis of the knees, hips and lumbar spine, flat feet and psychological stresses particularly during adolescence. Obese persons are exposed to increased risk from surgery. Obesity may lead to lowered fertility. Table 3 shows the relative risk of health problems associated with obesity. (b) INCREASED MORTALITY : The Framingham Heart Study in United States showed a dramatic increase in sudden death among men more than 20 per cent overweight as compared with those with normal weight. The increased mortality is brought about mainly by the increased incidence of hypertension and coronary heart disease. There is also an excess number of deaths from renal diseases. Obesity lowers life expectancy. More information is needed about the relationship between different degrees of obesity and morbidity and mortality. Please see in chapter 11 under heading "Nutritional factors in selected diseases" for dietary factors of obesity.

TABLE 3

Relative risk of health problems associated with obesity[a]

Greatly increased	Moderately increased	Slightly increased
Type 2 diabetes	CHD	Cancer (breast cancer in postmenopausal women, endometrial cancer, colon cancer)
Gall bladder disease	Hypertension	Reproductive hormone abnormalities
Dyslipidaemia	Osteoarthritis (knees)	Polycystic ovary syndrome
Insulin resistance	Hyperuricaemia and gout	Impaired fertility
Breathlessness		Low back pain due to obesity
Sleep apnea		Increased risk of anaesthesia complications
		Fetal defects associated with maternal obesity

[a] All relative risk values are approximate.

Source : *(7)*

Prevention and control

Weight control is widely defined as approaches to maintaining weight within the 'healthy' (i.e. 'normal' or 'acceptable') range of body mass index of 18.5 to 24.9 kg/m^2 throughout adulthood (WHO Expert Committee, 1995). It should also include prevention of weight gain of more than 5 kg in all people. In those who are already overweight, a reduction of 5–10 per cent of body weight is recommended as an initial goal *(6)*.

Prevention of obesity should begin in early childhood. Obesity is harder to treat in adults than it is in children. The control of obesity centres around weight reduction. This can be achieved by dietary changes, increased physical activity and a combination of both. (a) DIETARY CHANGES: The following dietary principles apply both to prevention and treatment : the proportion of energy-dense foods such as simple carbohydrates and fats should be reduced; the fibre content in the diet should be increased through the consumption of common un-refined foods; adequate levels of essential nutrients in the low energy diets (most conventional diets for weight reduction are based on 1000 kcal daily model for an adult) should be ensured, and reducing diets should be as close as possible to existing nutritional patterns *(15)*. The most basic consideration is that the food energy intake should not be greater than what is necessary for energy expenditure. It requires modification of the patient's behaviour and strong motivation to lose weight and maintain ideal weight. Unfortunately, most attempts to reduce weight in obese persons by dietary advice remain unsuccessful. (b) INCREASED PHYSICAL ACTIVITY: This is an important part of weight reducing programme. Regular physical exercise is the key to an increased energy expenditure. (c) OTHERS: Appetite suppressing drugs have been tried in the control of obesity. They are generally inadequate to produce massive weight loss in severely obese patients. Surgical treatment (e.g., gastric bypass, gastroplasty, jaw-wiring, to eliminate the eating of solid food have all been tried with limited success *(16)*. In short, one should not expect quick or even tangible results in all cases from obesity prevention programmes. Health education has an important role to play in teaching the people how to reduce overweight and prevent obesity. A fruitful approach will be to identify those children who are at risk of becoming obese and find way of preventing it.

References

1. Hager, A. (1981). *Br. Med. Bull.*, 37 (3) 287.
2. Aykroyd, W.R. and J.Mayer (1968). *Food and Nutrition Terminology.* In : WHO Doc NUT/68.6, Geneva.
3. WHO (2021), *Obesity and Overweight,* Fact sheet, 9th June 2021.
4. Govt. of India (2022), *National Family Health Survey-5,* Ministry of Health and Family Welfare, New Delhi.
5. WHO (1995). Tech. Rep. Ser. No. 854.
6. WHO (2002), International Agency for Research on Cancer, *IARC Handbooks of Cancer Prevention - Weight Control and Physical Acitivity,* IARC Press, Lyon 2002.
7. WHO (2000). Tech. Rep. Ser. No. 894.
8. Charney, E. et al (1976). *N. Eng. J. Med.*, 295 : 6.
9. International Children's Centre, Paris (1984). *Children in the Tropics,* No.151.
10. Falkner, F.ed (1980). *Prevention in Childhood of Health Problems in Adult Life,* WHO, Geneva.
11. WHO (2003), *Tech. Rep. Ser. No.* 916.
12. Oliver, M.F. (1981). *Br. Med. Bull.*, 37 (1) 49.
13. Beaton, G.H. (1976). In: *Nutrition in Preventive Medicine* Annex 2, P. 482. Beaton, G.H. and J.M. Bengoa (eds). WHO, Geneva, Monograph Ser.No. 62.
14. James, W.P.T. (1982). *Medicine International,* 1 (15) 664.
15. Tasher, T. (1986). *Food and Nutrition Bull.*, 8 (3) 12. The United Nations University.
16. Garrow, J.S. (1981). In : *Recent Advances in Medicine,* Vol 18, Churchill Livingstone.

VISUAL IMPAIRMENT AND BLINDNESS

A compilation published by WHO in 1966 *(1)* lists 65 definitions of blindness. As might be expected the definitions differed widely. Terms such as total blindness, economic blindness, and social blindness were in vogue. The 25th World Health Assembly in 1972 noted the complexity of the problem and considered the need for a generally accepted definition of blindness and visual impairment for national and international comparability. Taking into consideration existing definitions, the WHO proposed a uniform criterion and defined blindness as "visual acuity of less than 3/60 (Snellen) or its equivalent" *(2)*.

The International Classification of Disease 11 (2018) classifies vision impairment into two groups, distance and near presenting vision impairment.

Distance vision impairment:

Mild – Presenting visual acuity worse than 6/12

Moderate – Presenting visual acuity worse than 6/18

Severe – Presenting visual acuity worse than 6/60

Blindness – Presenting visual acuity worse than 3/60

Near vision impairment :

Presenting near vision acuity worse than N6 or M0.8 at 40 cm with existing correction.

A person's experience of vision impairment varies depending upon many different factors. This includes, for example, the availability of prevention and treatment interventions, access to vision rehabilitation (including assistive products such as glasses or white canes), and whether the person experiences problems with inaccessible buildings, transport information etc. *(3)*.

The problem

WORLD

Globally, 2.2 billion people have a near or distance visual impairment. In at least 1 billion people impairment could have been prevented or has yet to be addressed. This 1 billion people includes those with moderate or severe distance vision impairment or blindness due to unaddressed refractive error (88.4 million), cataract (94 million), glaucoma (7.7 million), corneal opacities (4.2 million), diabetic retinopathy (3.2 million), and trachoma (2 million), as well as near vision impairment caused by unaddressed presbyopia (826 million) *(4)*.

About 80 per cent of blindness is avoidable (treatable or potentially preventable). However, a large proportion of those affected remain blind for want of access to affordable eye care. Blindness leads not only to reduced economic and social status but may also result in premature death. The major causes of moderate to severe vision impairment are as follows *(5)*:

1. Uncorrected refractive errors, 53 per cent;
2. Un-operated cataract, 25 per cent;
3. Age-related macular degeneration, 4 per cent;
4. Glaucoma, 2 per cent; and
5. Diabetic retinopathy 1 per cent.

The major causes of blindness are *(5)*.

1. Un-operated cataract 35 per cent;
2. Un-corrected refractive error 21 per cent; and
3. Glaucoma 8 per cent.

About 82 per cent of all people who are visually impaired are aged 50 years and older, while this age group comprises about 20 per cent of the world's population. With an increasing elderly population in many countries, more people will be at risk of age-related visual impairment. An estimated 19 million children are visually impaired. Of these, 12 million children are visually impaired due to refractory errors, a condition that could be easily diagnosed and corrected. 1.4 million are irreversibly blind for the rest of their lives *(5)*.

The most frequent causes of blindness in developed countries are accidents, glaucoma, diabetes, vascular diseases (hypertension), cataract and degeneration of ocular tissues especially of the retina, and hereditary conditions.

In South–East Asia Region, cataract is the single most common cause of blindness being responsible for 50–80 per cent of all blindness. Uncorrected refractive errors are being increasingly recognized as a cause of blindness and low vision. Vitamin A deficiency, which has been responsible for most childhood blindness in the Region is gradually declining. The emerging causes of blindness include glaucoma, age-related macular degeneration, diabetic retinopathy, corneal ulcer and ocular trauma *(6)*.

Among the leading causes of childhood blindness in the region are xerophthalmia, congenital cataract, congenital glaucoma and optic atrophy due to meningitis, retinopathy of prematurity, and uncorrected refractive errors. Xerophthalmia is largely under control with vitamin A distribution in immunization programmes.

There are an estimated 3–4 million persons blind, due to corneal opacity. With declining incidence of trachoma and xerophthalmia, the consequences of ocular trauma and corneal ulceration are emerging as important causes. According to an estimate, 6.5 million people are affected with, and 1.3 million eyes become blind due to corneal ulcer every year in the region *(6)*. Trachoma remains an important cause in pockets in some countries although its importance as a cause of blindness has declined over the years *(7)*.

Overall, visual impairment worldwide has decreased since the early 1990s. This decrease is principally the result of a reduction of visual impairment from infectious diseases through public health action, overall socio-economic development, increased availability of eye care services and awareness of the general population about solution to the problems related to vision impairment (surgery, refraction devices, etc.). However, it is estimated that the number of people with vision impairment could triple due to population growth and ageing *(5)*.

INDIA

India has changed its over four-decade-old definition of blindness, bringing it in line with the WHO criteria. According to the new definition, a person who is unable to count fingers from a distance of three meters would be considered blind as against the earlier stipulation of six meters, which was adopted in 1976. The notification in this regard has been issued by the Union Health Ministry.

According to this definition, the population of blind people in India will reduce from 1.20 crore (as per National Blindness Survey 2007 data) to 80 Lacs *(8)*.

The nomenclature of the programme is also changed from "National Programme for Control of Blindness" to "National Programme for Control of Blindness and visual impairment" *(8)*.

The prevalence of blindness according to rapid national survey on blindness 2006–2007 was 1.0 per cent. In the current survey (2015–2019) the projected prevalence rate is 0.36 per cent *(10)*.

The National Survey on Blindness 2015–19 conducted in the country recognized the main causes responsible for visual impairment and blindness. As shown in Table 1, the principal cause of blindness in India today is cataract, responsible for about 66.2 per cent of all cases. Cataract occurs more frequently with advancing age. Senile cataract occurs a decade earlier in India relative to Europe and America. Uncorrected refractive error are responsible for about 0.1 per cent of blindness; overall prevalence of glaucoma was about 5.5 per cent; posterior segment pathology accounts for about 5.9 per cent cases *(10)*. In a camp based study, glaucoma prevalence was found to be about 3.07 per cent with a slight female preponderance (males 2.9 per cent and females 3.19 per cent). Primary open angle glaucoma was more common (about 1.7 per cent) than primary angle closure glaucoma (0.73 per cent) *(9)*. In the others group, injuries as a cause of blindness accounts for 1.2 per cent *(11)*. There is evidence that injuries are on the increase due to increase in cottage industry (e.g. carpentry, black smithy, stone crushing, chiselling and hammering and chopping wood), and rapid industrialization in the country. The other causes in this group includes congenital disorder, uveitis, retina detachment, tumours, diabetes, hypertension, diseases of the nervous system, leprosy, etc.

TABLE 1

Causes of blindness in India
(2015–19 National survey on blindness)

Refractive error	0.1 per cent
Aphakia uncorrected	1.7 per cent
Cataract untreated	66.2 per cent
Cataract surgical complications	7.2 per cent
Trachomatous corneal opacity	0.8 per cent
Non-trachomatous corneal opacity	7.4 per cent
Phthisis	2.8 per cent
Glaucoma	5.5 per cent
Diabetic retinopathy	1.2 per cent
ARMD	0.7 per cent
Other posterior segment disease	5.9 per cent
All other globe/CNS abnormalities	0.5 per cent

Source : *(10)*

Retinopathy of prematurity (ROP) is emerging as an important cause of childhood blindness. With the advent of hyperbaric oxygen and opening of large number of private and governmnet NICUs, the survival of the premature babies (born before 30 weeks of gestation and 1500 grams of weight at birth) has improved considerably. These babies are at risk of developing ROP and there is dire necessity to create awareness not only in public but also amongst opthalmologists and paediatricians to detect and treat ROP in time.

Epidemiological determinants

(a) AGE : About 30 per cent of the blind in India are said to lose their eyesight before they reach the age of 20 years, and many under the age of 5 years. Refractive error, trachoma, conjunctivitis and malnutrition (vitamin A deficiency) are important causes of blindness among children and the younger age groups; cataract, refractive error, glaucoma and diabetes are causes of blindness in middle age; accidents and injuries can occur in all age groups, but more importantly in the age group 20 to 40 years. (b) SEX : A higher prevalence of blindness is reported in females than in males in India. This has been attributed to a higher prevalence of trachoma, conjunctivitis and cataract among females than in males *(12)*. (c) MALNUTRITION : Malnutrition as a cause of blindness was hardly recognized a few years ago. It is closely related not only with low vitamin A intake, but also with infectious diseases of childhood especially measles and diarrhoea (which precipitate malnutrition). In many cases protein energy malnutrition (PEM) is also associated with blindness. Severe blinding corneal destruction due to vitamin A deficiency (e.g., keratomalacia) is largely limited to the first 4–6 years of life and is especially frequent among those 6 months to 3 years of life. (d) OCCUPATION : It has long been recognized that people working in factories, workshops and cottage industries are prone to eye injuries because of exposure to dust, airborne particles, flying objects, gases, fumes, radiation (usually welding flash), electrical flash, etc. Many workers including doctors are known to have developed premature cataracts while exposed to X-rays, ultraviolet rays or heat waves. (e) SOCIAL CLASS : There is a close relationship between the incidence of blindness and socio-economic status. Surveys indicate that blindness is twice more prevalent in the poorer classes than in the well-to-do *(12)*. (f) SOCIAL FACTORS: Many people lose their eyesight because of meddlesome ophthalmology by quacks. The basic social factors are ignorance, poverty, low standard of personal and community hygiene, and inadequate health care services.

Changing concepts in eye health care

Recent years have witnessed a change from acute intervention (cure) typical of clinical ophthalmology to comprehensive eye-health care which includes the following concepts :

1. Primary eye care

One of the most significant developments in the field of eye health care over the last few years has been the concept of *primary eye care,* that is, the inclusion of an eye-care component in primary health care system. The idea of primary eye care, as one of the main ingredients of a primary health care approach to blindness, has rapidly gained acceptance the world over. It is today recognized as a model for eye care at the community level. The promotion and protection of eye health, together with on-the-spot treatment for the commonest eye diseases, are its cornerstones. The final objective of primary eye care is to increase the coverage and quality of eye health care through primary health care approach and thereby improve the utilization of existing resources.

2. Epidemiological approach

The epidemiological approach which involves studies at the population level has been recognized. It focuses, among other things, on the measurement of the incidence, prevalence of diseases and their risk factors. The local epidemiological situation will determine the action needed.

3. Team concept

In many developing countries, there is only one eye specialist for more than a million people. Increasingly, therefore, health care leans on the use of auxiliary health personnel to fill many gaps. In India this gap is filled by village health workers, ophthalmic assistants, multi-purpose workers, and voluntary agencies.

4. Establishment of national programmes

Another important development in connection with the prevention of blindness has been the establishment of national programmes. Many of these programmes were first started by voluntary agencies concerned with blindness prevention (e.g., eye camps) and some of them focused on a single disease, such as trachoma. The increasing recognition of the primary health care approach to blindness resulted in comprehensive national programmes for the prevention of blindness *(13)* from all causes.

Prevention of blindness

The concept of **avoidable blindness** (i.e., preventable or curable blindness) has gained increasing recognition during recent years. A great many of the causes of blindness lend themselves to prevention and/or control – whether by improving nutrition, by treating cases of infectious diseases, or by controlling the organisms which cause infection, or by improving safety conditions – particularly on the roads, at work or in the home *(14)*.

The components for action in national programmes for the prevention of blindness comprise the following :

1. INITIAL ASSESSMENT

The first step is to assess the magnitude, geographic distribution and causes of blindness within the country or region by prevalence surveys. This knowledge is essential for setting priorities and development of appropriate intervention programmes.

2. METHODS OF INTERVENTION *(15)*

(a) Primary eye care

A wide range of eye conditions (e.g., acute conjunctivitis, ophthalmia neonatorum, trachoma, superficial foreign bodies, xerophthalmia) can be treated/prevented at the grass-root level by locally trained primary health workers (e.g., village health guides, multi-purpose workers) who are the first to make contact with the community. For this purpose, they are provided with essential drugs such as topical tetracycline, vitamin A capsules, eye bandages, shields, etc. They are also trained to refer difficult cases (e.g., corneal ulcer, penetrating foreign bodies, painful eye conditions and infections which do not respond to treatment) to the nearest PHC or district hospital. Their activities also involve promotion of personal hygiene, sanitation, good dietary habits and safety in general. Currently, there is one village health guide for 1000 population and 2 multipurpose workers for 5000 population in India.

In short, primary eye care is based firmly in primary health care which is ".....essential health care......made universally accessible to individuals and families in the community through their full participation and at a cost that the community and country can afford ...." (Article VI of the Declaration of Alma Ata, 1978).

(b) Secondary care

Secondary care involves definitive management of common blinding conditions such as cataract, trichiasis, entropion, ocular trauma, glaucoma, etc. This care is provided in PHCs and district hospitals where eye departments or eye clinics are established. The secondary care may involve the use of mobile eye clinics. For instance, cataract accounts for over 62 per cent of blindness in India. The eye camp approach to make cataract surgery available has been highly successful, and has received wide popular support. Apart from cataract operations, these camps undertake general health surveys for the early detection of visual defects as well as education of the masses. For mobile services to be effective, there must be good community participation in the programme. Adequate follow-up and evaluation must also be provided. The "mobile units", though valuable, lack permanence and are being utilized as part of a comprehensive strategy for eye care. The great advantage of this strategy is, it is problem-specific and makes the best use of local resources and provides inexpensive eye care to the population at the peripheral level *(16)*.

(c) Tertiary care

These services are usually established in the national or regional capitals and are often associated with Medical Colleges and Institutes of Medicine. They provide sophisticated eye care such as retinal detachment surgery, corneal grafting and other complex forms of management not available in secondary centres. The majority of States in India has passed the Corneal Grafting Acts which have helped the establishment of Eye Banks. Other measures of rehabilitation comprise education of the blind in special schools and utilization of their services in gainful employment. The central government has established National Institute for the Blind in Dehradun (U.P.) to work out new approaches and strategies for solving the problems of the blind.

(d) Specific programmes

(i) *Trachoma control :* Endemic trachoma and associated infections are a major cause of preventable blindness in many developing countries. Early diagnosis and treatment will cure trachoma. National programmes have been mounted against trachoma in many countries. Mass campaigns with topical tetracycline and the improvement of socio-economic conditions have markedly reduced the severity of trachoma and associated bacterial conjunctival infections. The Trachoma Control Programme launched in India in 1963 was merged with the National Programme for the Control of Blindness in 1976.

(ii) *School eye health services :* This is another useful approach to the eye health problems in the community. School children who form a sizable segment of the community can be screened and treated for defects such as refraction errors, squint, amblyopia, trachoma, etc. Health education is an important component of school health service. Students should be taught to practise the principles of good posture, proper lighting, avoidance of glare, proper distance and angle between the books and the eyes. Use of suitably readable type style in textbooks should be encouraged.

(iii) *Vitamin A prophylaxis :* Under the vitamin A distribution scheme in India, 200,000 IU of vitamin A are given orally at 6–monthly intervals between the ages 1–6 years. To be able to control xerophthalmia, the whole family should be kept under surveillance for one year and children for 5 years *(17)*.

(iv) *Occupational eye health services:* This is to prevent/ treat eye hazards in industries. Education on the prevention of occupational eye hazards and the use of protective devices in some occupations (like welding) is essential. The key to the prevention of accidents in factories is to improve the safety features of machines, to have proper illumination of the working area, to select workers with the requisite alertness and good vision, and to encourage the use of protective devices *(15)*.

3. LONG-TERM MEASURES

Long-term measures also have a part to play in controlling eye infections. Broadly these measures are aimed at improving the quality of life and modifying or attacking the factors responsible for the persistence of eye health problems, e.g., poor sanitation, lack of adequate safe water supplies, little intake of foods rich in vitamin A, lack of personal hygiene, etc. Health education is an important long-term measure in order to create community awareness of the problem; to motivate the community, to accept total eye health care programmes, and to secure community participation.

4. EVALUATION

Evaluation should be an integral part of intervention programmes to measure the extent to which ocular diseases and blindness have been alleviated, assess the manner and degree to which programme activities have been carried out, and determine the nature of other changes that may have been produced *(18)*.

National and International agencies

The National Association for the Blind (NAB), a voluntary organization which came into existence in 1952 has been active in the field of providing welfare services to the blind throughout India. The Royal Commonwealth Society for the Blind has been working in the field since 1950. In 1974, by invitation of WHO, the organizations concerned with blindness and with its prevention came together to build a new agency, the "International Agency for Prevention of Blindness". The Agency's primary task is to prevent blindness. There is a growing movement for direct technical cooperation among the developing countries. Neighbouring countries may provide training, exchange workers, share plans, and, in a variety of ways enrich and stimulate their programmes *(18)*.

National Programme for the Control of Blindness and Visual Impairment

See chapter 7 for details.

Vision 2020 : The Right to Sight

Vision 2020 : The Right to Sight, a global initiative to eliminate avoidable blindness was launched by WHO on 18th Feb. 1999. One significant way in which this initiative differs from previous ones is that the concept centres around Rights issues. Recognition of sight as a fundamental human right by all countries can be an important catalyst of initiatives for the prevention and control of blindness. The objective of Vision 2020 is to assist member countries in developing sustainable systems which will enable them to eliminate avoidable blindness from major causes, i.e. cataract, xerophthalmia and other causes of childhood blindness, refractive error and low vision, trachoma and other causes of corneal blindness by the year 2020 *(10, 6)*.

Global eye health action plan 2014–2019 *(19)*

The global eye health action plan 2014–2019 aims to reduce avoidable visual impairment as a global public health problem and to secure access to rehabilitation services for the visually impaired.

The global eye health action plan is based on five principles and approaches which underpin the plan: universal access and equity, human rights, evidence-based practice, a life course approach, and empowerment of people with visual impairment. As there have been significant shifts in the pattern of causes of visual impairment, the action plan is structured to particularly address the global trend towards an increasing incidence of chronic eye diseases related to ageing . These are expected to be the most prevalent causes of avoidable visual impairment in the next decades.

The global eye health action plan is built using the health system approach, which encompasses the integration of eye care programmes into the wider health care system at all levels (primary, secondary and tertiary). As a global target, the reduction in prevalence of avoidable visual impairment by 25 per cent by 2019, from the baseline of 2010 has been selected for this action plan.

There are three indicators at the goal and purpose levels to measure progress at the national level : (1) The prevalence and causes of visual impairment; (2) The number of eye care personnel; and (3) Cataract surgery.

References

1. WHO (1966). *Epi and Vital Statis Rep.*, 19 : 437.
2. WHO (2011), *Change the Definition of Blindness.*
3. WHO (2018), *Visual Impairment and Blindness, fact sheet,* 18th Oct. 2018.
4. WHO (2021), *Fact sheet,* 14th Oct. 2021.
5. WHO (2017), *Blindness and visual impairment, Fact sheet,* 11th Oct. 2017.

6. WHO (2002), *Health Situation in the South-East Asia Region 1998-2000*, New Delhi.
7. WHO (2000), *Strategic Plan for Vision 2020 : The Right to sight*, Elimination of Avoidable Blindness in the South-East Asia Region, New Delhi.
8. Govt. of India (2018), *National Programme for Control of Blindness and Visual Impairment, 2017–2018*, Ministry of Health and Family welfare, New Delhi.
9. Govt. of India (2018), *Annual Report 2017–2018*, Ministry of Health and Family Welfare, New Delhi.
10. Govt. of India (2020), *Annual Report 2019–20*, Ministry of Health and Family Welfare, New Delhi.
11. Kapoor, P.M. and A.K. Kundu (1985). *J. Com. Dis.*, 17 (2) 118.
12. Sharma, K.L. and B.G. Prasad (1962). *Ind. J. Med. Res.*, 50 : 842.
13. Thylefors, B. (1987). *World Health*, May.
14. Bietti, G.B. (1976). *World Health*, Feb–March.
15. WHO (1984). *Strategies for the Prevention of Blindness in National Programmes*, WHO, Geneva.
16. WHO (1980). *WHO Chronicle*, 34 (9) 332.
17. Madan Mohan (1984). *Swasth Hind*, 28 (5) 105.
18. WHO (1979). *Guidelines for Programmes for the Prevention of Blindness*, WHO, Geneva.
19. WHO (2013), *Universal eye health, A global action plan 2014–2019*.

ORAL DISEASES

Oral diseases are the most common non-communicable diseases and affect people throughout their lifetime, causing pain, discomfort, disfigurement and even death. Oral health is a key indicator of overall health, wellbeing and quality of life. WHO defines oral health as "a state of being free from chronic mouth and facial pain, oral and throat cancer, oral infection and sores, periodontal (gum) disease, tooth decay, tooth loss, and other diseases and disorders that limit an individual's capacity in biting, chewing, smiling, speaking, and psychosocial wellbeing" *(1)*.

Problem Statement

WORLD

Seven oral diseases and conditions account for most of the oral disease burden. They include dental caries (tooth decay), periodontal (gum) diseases, oral cancers, oral manifestations of HIV, oro-dental trauma, cleft lip and palate, and noma. Almost all diseases and conditions are either largely preventable or can be treated in their early stages. It is estimated that oral diseases affected at least 3.58 billion people in 2016 worldwide, with caries of the permanent teeth being the most prevalent of all conditions assessed. Globally, it is estimated that 2.4 billion people suffer from caries of permanent teeth and 486 million children suffer from caries of primary teeth. In most middle and low income countries, with increasing urbanization and changes in living conditions, the prevalence of oral diseases continues to increase notably due to inadequate exposure to fluoride and poor access to primary oral health care services. Heavy marketing of sugars, tobacco and alcohol leads to growing consumption of unhealthy products.

INDIA

Two large scale oral health surveys have been conducted in India: (i) National Oral Health Survey & Fluoride Mapping by Dental Council of India in 2003; and (ii) Oral Health in India : Report of multi-centric oral health survey by Ministry of Health and Family Welfare in collaboration with dental department of AIIMS in 2007. These two surveys indicate the prevalence of some of the oral diseases and conditions in the country. The burden of diseases are as shown in Table 1.

TABLE 1

Burden of oral diseases (Multi-centric survey 2007), India

Disease	Prevalence
Dental Caries	40–45%
Periodontal diseases	>90% (Advanced disease in 40%)
Malocclusion	30% of children
Cleft lip and palate	1.7 per 1000 live births
Oral cancer	12.6 per lakh population
Oral submucous fibrosis (premalignant and crippling condition of mouth)	4 per 1000 adults in rural India
Dental fluorosis	Endemic in 230 districts of 19 States
Edentulousness (tooth loss)	19–32% of elderly population >65 years
Oral lesions due to HIV/AIDS	72% of HIV/AIDS patients
Birth defects involving oro-facial complex	0.82 to 3.36 per 1000 live births
Others: Traumatic injuries, • Mucosal lesions associated with radiation and chemotherapy • Morbidity and deformity following oral cancer surgery.	

Source : *(2)*

Taking into account the oral health situation in the country, Govt. of India has initiated a National Oral Health Programme during the year 2014–2015, to provide integrated and comprehensive oral health care in the existing health care facilities *(3)*.

RISK FACTORS

Most oral diseases and conditions share modifiable risk factors (such as tobacco use, alcohol consumption and unhealthy diets high in free sugars) common to the four leading NCDs (cardiovascular diseases, cancer, chronic respiratory diseases and diabetes). In addition, it is reported that diabetes mellitus is linked in a reciprocal way with the development and progression of periodontitis. Moreover, there is a causal link between high sugars consumption and diabetes, obesity and dental caries.

Oral health inequalities :

Oral health inequalities are caused by a broad range of interacting biological, socio-behavioural, psychosocial, societal and political factors that create 'the conditions in which people are born, grow, live, work and age' - the so-called social determinants. Oral diseases disproportionally affect the poor and socially-disadvantaged members of society. There is a very strong and consistent association between socioeconomic status (income, occupation and educational level) and the prevalence and severity of oral diseases. This association exists across the life course from early childhood to older age, and across populations in high, middle and low-income countries. Oral health inequalities are therefore considered as differences in oral health that are avoidable, and deemed both unfair and unjust in modern society *(1)*.

Oral diseases *(1)*

Dental caries (tooth decay)

Dental caries results when microbial biofilm (plaque) formed on the tooth surface converts the free sugars contained in foods and drinks into acids that dissolve tooth enamel and dentine over time. With continued high intake of free sugars, inadequate exposure to fluoride and without regular microbial biofilm removal, tooth structures are destroyed, resulting in development of cavities and pain, impacts on oral-health-related quality of life, and, in the advanced stage, tooth loss and systemic infection.

Periodontal (gum) disease

Periodontal disease affects the tissues that both surround and support the tooth. This often presents as bleeding or swollen gums (gingivitis), pain and sometimes as bad breath. In its more severe form, loss of gum attachment to the tooth and supporting bone causes "pockets" and loosening of teeth (periodontitis). Severe periodontal disease, which may result in tooth loss, was the 11th most prevalent disease globally in 2016. The main causes of periodontal disease are poor oral hygiene and tobacco use.

Tooth loss

Dental caries and periodontal diseases are major causes of tooth loss. Severe tooth loss and edentulism (no natural teeth remaining) are widespread and particularly seen among older people. Severe tooth loss and edentulism was one of the leading ten causes of years lived with disability (YLD) in some high income countries due to their aging populations.

Oral cancer

Oral cancer includes cancers of lip and all subsites of the oral cavity, and oropharynx. The age-adjusted incidence of oral cancer (cancers of the lip and oral cavity) in the world is estimated at 4 cases per 100,000 people. However, there is wide variation across the globe: from no recorded cases to around 20 cases per 100,000 people. Oral cancer is more common in men, in older people, and varies strongly by socio-economic condition. In some Asian-Pacific countries, the incidence of oral cancer ranks among the three top cancers. Tobacco, alcohol and areca nut (betel quid) use are among the leading causes of oral cancer. In regions like North America and Europe, "high risk" human papillomavirus infections are responsible for a growing percentage of oro-pharyngeal cancers among young people.

Oral manifestations of HIV infection

Oral manifestations occur in 30–80% of people with HIV, with considerable variations depending on the situations such as affordability of standard antiretroviral therapy (ART). Oral manifestations include fungal, bacterial or viral infections of which oral candidiasis is the most common and often the first symptom early in the course of the disease. Oral HIV lesions cause pain, discomfort, dry mouth, eating restrictions and are a constant source of opportunistic infection. Early detection of HIV-related oral lesions can be used to diagnose HIV infection, monitor the disease's progression, predict immune status and result in timely therapeutic intervention. The treatment and management of oral HIV lesions can considerably improve oral health, quality of life and wellbeing.

Oro-dental trauma

Oro-dental trauma is an impact injury to the teeth and/or other hard or soft tissues within and around the mouth and oral cavity. The world prevalence of traumatic dental injuries in either dentition (primary and permanent) is around 20%. Oro-dental trauma can be caused by oral factors (e.g. increased overjet); environmental factors (for example; unsafe playgrounds or schools); risk-taking behaviour; and violence. Treatment is costly and lengthy and sometimes can even lead to tooth loss, resulting in complications for facial and psychological development and quality of life.

Noma (1)

Noma is a necrotizing disease that affects children between the ages of 2 and 6 years suffering from malnutrition, affected by infectious disease, living in extreme poverty and with weakened immune systems.

Noma is mostly prevalent in sub-Saharan Africa, but rare cases are reported in Latin America and Asia. Noma starts as a soft tissue lesion (a sore) of the gums, inside the mouth. The initial gum lesion then develops into an ulcerative, necrotizing gingivitis that progresses rapidly, destroying the soft tissues and further progressing to involve the hard tissues and skin of the face.

In 1998, WHO estimated that there were 140,000 new cases of noma annually. Without treatment, noma is fatal in 90% of cases. Where noma is detected at an early stage, its progression can be rapidly halted, through basic hygiene, antibiotics and nutritional rehabilitation. Such early detection helps to prevent suffering, disability and death. Survivors suffer from severe facial disfigurement, have difficulty speaking and eating, face social stigma, and require complex surgery and rehabilitation.

Cleft lip and cleft palate

Clefts of the lip and palate are heterogeneous disorders that affect the lips and oral cavity, and occur either alone (70%) or as part of a syndrome, affecting more than 1 in 1000 newborns worldwide. Although genetic predisposition is an important factor for congenital anomalies, other modifiable risk factors such as poor maternal nutrition, tobacco consumption, alcohol and obesity during pregnancy also play a role. In low-income settings, there is a high mortality rate in the neonatal period. If lip and palate clefts are properly treated by surgery, complete rehabilitation is possible.

Prevention of oral diseases *(1)*

The burden of oral diseases can be reduced through public health interventions by addressing common risk factors. These are :

- Promoting a well-balanced diet:
  - Low in free sugars to prevent development of dental caries, premature tooth loss and other diet-related NCDs;
  - With adequate fruit and vegetable intake, which may have a protective role in oral cancer prevention;
- Reducing smoking, the use of smokeless tobacco including chewing of areca nuts, and alcohol consumption to reduce the risk of oral cancers, periodontal disease and tooth loss; and
- Encouraging use of protective equipment in sports and when traveling in motor vehicles, to reduce the risk of facial injuries.

Dental caries can be largely prevented by maintaining a constant low level of fluoride in the oral cavity. Optimal fluoride can be obtained from different sources such as fluoridated drinking water, salt, milk and toothpaste. Twice-daily tooth brushing with fluoride-containing toothpaste (1000 to 1500 ppm) should be encouraged. Long-term exposure to an optimal level of fluoride results in substantially lower incidence and prevalence of tooth decay across all ages.

Oral health inequalities must be reduced by tacking the broader social determinants through a range of complementary downstream, midstream and integrated upstream policies such as: water fluoridation; regulation of the marketing and promotion of sugary foods to children and taxes on sugar-sweetened beverages. Moreover, promoting healthy settings such as healthy workplaces and health promoting schools is critical to building comprehensive supporting environments to promote oral health.

References

1. WHO (2018), *Fact sheet on Oral Health*, 24th Sept. 2018.
2. Govt. of India (2015), *Operational guidelines, National Oral Health programme*, Ministry of Health and Family Welfare, New Delhi.
3. Govt. of India (2018), *Annual Report 2017–2018*, Ministry of Health and Family Welfare, New Delhi.

ACCIDENTS AND INJURIES

An accident has been defined as : "an unexpected, unplanned occurrence which may involve injury" *(1)*. A WHO Advisory Group in 1956 defined accident as an "unpremeditated event resulting in recognizable damage" *(2)*. According to another definition, an accident is that "occurrence in a sequence of events which usually produces unintended injury, death or property damage".

Accidents represent a major epidemic of non–communicable disease in the present century. They are no longer considered accidental. They are part of the price we pay for technological progress.

Accidents have their own natural history and follow the same epidemiological pattern as any other disease – that is, the agent, the host and the environment interacting together to produce injury or damage. They occur more frequently in certain age–groups, at certain times of day and week and at certain localities. Some people are more prone to accidents than others and susceptibility is increased by the effect of alcohol and other drugs as well as physiological state such as fatigue. Lastly, a majority of accidents are preventable.

Measurement of the problem

a. *MORTALITY*

The following epidemiological indices will be useful in assessing the magnitude of the problem : (i) Proportional mortality rate : That is, the number of deaths due to accidents per 100 (or 1000) total deaths. (ii) Number of deaths per million population : The term "killed" (in a road traffic accident) is defined as any person who was killed outright or who died within 30 days as a result of the accident *(3)*. (iii) Death rate per 1000 (or 100,000) registered vehicles per year. (iv) Number of accidents or fatalities as a ratio of the number of vehicles per kilometre or passengers per kilometre. (v) Deaths of vehicle occupants per 1000 vehicles per year, etc.

b. *MORBIDITY*

Morbidity is measured in terms of "serious injuries" and "slight injuries" *(4)*. The seriousness of the injury is assessed by a scale known as "Abbreviated Injury Scale" *(3)*. Morbidity rates are generally less reliable because of under-reporting and mis-reporting.

c. *DISABILITY*

An important outcome of the accident process is disability, which may be temporary or permanent, partial or total. Measurement of disability in terms of its duration is a limited concept; it does not take into consideration the psychological or social aspects of an accident or injury *(5)*. The International classification of "Functioning, Disability and Health" (ICF) is an attempt by WHO *(6)* to estimate the disability of individuals at a given moment.

The problem

WORLD

Injuries constitute a variable epidemic. Injuries are commonly classified based on "intentionality". Most road traffic injuries, poisoning, falls, fire and burn injuries and drowning are unintentional. Intentional injuries include interpersonal violence (homicide, sexual assault, neglect and abandonment, and other maltreatment), suicide and collective violence (war). Evidence suggests that some children and adolescents are more vulnerable to certain types of injuries. For example poisoning, drowning, burns and maltreatment by caregivers affects primarily small children, while road traffic accidents, interpersonal violence and sports injuries tend to affect older children, adolescents and adults *(7)*.

The leading cause of injury deaths is road traffic injury, followed by suicide, falls and interpersonal violence. Other important cause of injuries include drowning, fires and burns, poisoning, and war or conflict *(1)*. Table 1 shows the global estimated deaths by type of injury, percentage of total deaths, crude death rate per lakh population and age specific death rate per lakh population due to injuries during the year 2016 *(8)*.

TABLE 1
Leading causes of injuries and deaths worldwide, 2016

Type of injury	Deaths (000)	% of total deaths	Crude death rate (per lakh population)	Age specific death rate (per lakh population)
A. Unintentional injuries	3,429	6.0	46.0	45.0
1. Road injury	1,402	2.5	18.8	18.7
2. Poisonings	107	0.2	1.4	1.4
3. Falls	660	1.2	8.8	8.4
4. Fire, heat & hot substance	153	0.3	2.0	2.0
5. Drowning	322	0.6	4.3	4.3
6. Exposure to mechanical forces	150	0.3	2.0	2.0
7. Natural disasters	2	0.0	0.0	0.0
8. Other unintentional injuries	633	1.1	8.5	8.2
B. Intentional injuries	1,454	2.6	19.5	19.4
1. Self harm	793	1.4	10.6	10.5
2. Interpersonal violence	477	0.8	6.4	6.4
3. Collective violence and legal intervention	184	0.3	2.5	2.5
Total	4,883	8.6	65.4	64.4

Sources: *(8)*

Injuries and violence are included in multiple Sustainable Development Goals targets. Road traffic injuries and unintentional injuries are included in the health goal SDG 3 with targets related to violence and disasters part of other goals. Table 2 enumerates the indicators related to the goal targets, the global and Indian scenario.

TABLE 2

Selected indicators of SDG, global and India scenario

Cause	Global	India
Average death rate due to natural disaster (per 100,000 population) 2016	<0.1	<0.1
Mortality rate due to homicide (per 100,000 population) 2016	6.4	2.1
Estimated direct deaths from major conflicts (per 100,000 population) 2016	2.5	<0.1
Mortality rate unintentional poisoning (per 100,000 population) 2016	2.5	1.9
Suicide mortality rate (per 100,000 population) 2016	10.6	14.7
Road traffic mortality rate (per 100,000 population) 2016	18.8	8.0

Source : *(8)*

INDIA

Accidents are definitely on an increase in India. Increasing mechanization in agriculture and industry, induction of semi-skilled and unskilled workers in various operations and rapid increase in vehicular traffic have resulted in an increase in morbidity and mortality due to accidents. Overcrowding, lack of awareness and poor implementation of essential safety precautions result in an increasing number of accidents. Consumption of poisonous substances accidentally or intentionally is also on the rise. Deaths, disabilities and hospitalization due to injuries continue to have impact of socio-economic loss to individuals, families, society and infrastructure. The traditional view of injury as an accident, has resulted in the neglect of this aspect of public health. Today injuries are low in priority for policy makers, and only few plans are drawn for injury prevention.

Table 3 shows the reported number of accidental deaths by main causes in India.

TABLE 3

Reported number of accidental deaths in India by main cause (2018–2019)

Causes	No. of Deaths	
	2018	2019
A. Natural Calamity	6,891	8,145
B. Un-natural Causes		
Air-Crash	15	12
Collapse of Structures	2,017	1,929
Drowning	30,187	32,671
Electrocution	12,154	13,432
Explosions	696	655
Falls	20,201	20,901
Factory/Machine accidents	694	1,001
Fire	12,748	10,915
Fire Arms	528	320
Sudden Deaths	46,003	47,295
Killed by Animals	1,130	1,425
Mines or quarry disaster	125	82
Poisoning	21,646	21,196
Stampede	6	12
Suffocation	1,921	1,598
Traffic accidents	1,78,832	1,81,113
Causes Not Known	58,010	58,576
Other Causes	14,634	16,666
Total (B)	4,01,547	4,09,799
Total (A+B)	4,08,438	4,17,944

Source : *(9)*

TYPES OF ACCIDENTS

1. Road traffic accidents

The number of road traffic deaths continues to rise steadily, reaching 1.35 million in 2016. However, the rate of death relative to the size of the world's population has remained constant. When considered in context of the increasing global population and rapid motorization that has taken place over the same period. This suggest that existing road safety efforts may have mitigated the situation from getting worse.

As progress is made in the prevention and control of infectious diseases, the relative contribution of deaths from injuries have increased. Road traffic injuries are the 8th leading cause death for children and young adults aged 5–29 years. A number of countries have seen success in reducing road traffic deaths over the last few years, but progress varies significantly between different regions and countries of the world. With an average rate of 27.5 deaths per 100,000 population, the risk of a road traffic death is more than three times higher in low-income countries than in high-income countries where the average rate is 8.3 deaths per 100,000 population. The variation in rates of death observed corresponds with differences in the types of road users most affected. Vulnerable road users – pedestrians, cyclists and motor cyclists represent more than half of all global deaths. Pedestrians and cyclists represent 26 per cent of all deaths while those using motorized two or three wheelers comprise another 28 per cent. Car occupants make up 29 per cent of all deaths *(11)*.

In addition, there are as many as 20–50 million non-fatal injuries and 10–20 million serious injuries requiring long period of expensive care, nursing and treatment. From a young age, males are more likely to be involved in road traffic crashes than females. They are almost 3 times as likely to be killed in a car crash as young females *(10, 12)*.

INDIA *(13A)*

Road Accidents (55,442 cases) accounted for 97.4% of total traffic accidents in 53 mega cities during 2021. Chennai accounted for 9.1% (5,034 cases) of total road accidents reported, followed by Delhi City 8.1% (4,505 cases) and Bengaluru 5.8% (3,213 cases). However, the largest number of fatal road accidents were reported in Delhi City (1,172 deaths) followed by Chennai (998 deaths), accounting for 8.8% and 7.5% of total deaths due to road accidents respectively during 2021.

Cause-wise analysis of road accidents revealed that most of road accident deaths (including unmanned railway crossing) in 53 mega cities were due to over-speeding which accounted for 55.4% (7,415 out of 13,396 deaths) of total deaths due to road accidents during 2021. Dangerous or Careless driving/Over-taking etc. also caused 29.0% of total deaths due to road accidents. Driving under influence of drug/alcohol had caused 2.0% (262) of fatalities in road accidents. Most of fatalities due to driving under influence of drug/alcohol were reported in Ranchi (54 out of 262 deaths).

Place of occurrence-wise deaths in road accidents reveals that most of fatalities due to road accidents have taken place near residential area, contributing 30.2% (4,045 out of 13,396 deaths) of deaths, followed by 9.6% (1,281) near factory/industrial area and 7.4% near schools/ college/other educational institutions (987). Out of 53 mega cities, Ahmedabad (161 deaths) followed by Delhi City (63 deaths) have reported maximum cases of road accidents at pedestrian crossing. As per road-wise classification of road accidents, 21.5% of total road accidents were reported at the National Highways. 29.0% of fatalities in road accidents were reported at the National Highways during 2021.

Risk factors *(11)*

Speed

An increase in average speed is directly related both to the likelihood of a crash occurring and to the severity of the consequences of the crash. Some other facts are as below.

- Pedestrians have a 90% chance of surviving a car crash at 30 km/h or below, but less than a 50% chance of surviving an impact of 45 km/h or above.
- 30 km/h speed zones can reduce the risk of a crash and are recommended in areas where vulnerable road users are common (e.g. residential areas, around schools).
- Apart from reducing road traffic injuries, lower average traffic speeds can have other positive effects on health outcomes (e.g. by reducing respiratory problems associated with car emissions).

Drink-driving

Drinking and driving increases both the risk of a crash and the likelihood that death or serious injury will result.

- The risk of being involved in a crash increases significantly above a blood alcohol concentration (BAC) of 0.04 g/dl.
- Laws that establish BACs of 0.05 g/dl or below are effective at reducing the number of alcohol-related crashes.
- Enforcing sobriety check-points and random breath testing can lead to reductions in alcohol-related crashes by about 20%, and have shown to be very cost-effective.

Motorcycle helmets

- Wearing a motorcycle helmet correctly can reduce the risk of death by almost 42% and the risk of severe head injury by over 69%.
- When motorcycle helmet laws are enforced effectively, helmet wearing rates can increase to over 90%.
- Requiring helmets to meet a recognized safety standard is important to ensure that helmets can effectively reduce the impact of a collision to the head in the event of a crash.

Seat-belts and child restraints

- Wearing car seat-belt reduces the risk of fatality among front-seat passengers by 40–50% and of rear-seat passengers by between 25–75%.
- Mandatory seat-belt laws and their enforcement have been shown to be very effective at increasing seat-belt wearing rates.
- If correctly installed and used, child restraints reduce deaths among infants by approximately 70%, and deaths among small children by between 54% and 80%.

Distracted driving

There are many types of distractions that can lead to impaired driving, but recently there has been a marked increase around the world in the use of mobile phones by drivers that is becoming a growing concern for road safety. The distraction caused by mobile phones can impair driving performance in a number of ways, e.g. longer reaction times (notably braking reaction time, but also reaction to traffic signals), impaired ability to keep in the correct lane, and shorter following distances.

- Text messaging also results in considerably reduced driving performance, with young drivers at particular risk of the effects of distraction resulting from this use;
- Drivers using a mobile phone are approximately four times more likely to be involved in a crash than when a driver does not use a phone. Hands-free phones are not much safer than hand-held phone sets;
- While there is little concrete evidence yet on how to reduce mobile phone use while driving, governments need to be proactive. Actions that can be taken include adopting legislative measures, launching public awareness campaigns, and regularly collecting data on distracted driving to better understand the nature of this problem.

Developing countries are very different from the industrialized countries with regard to the environment and the mix of vehicles in the traffic stream. The following are the more important differences *(13)*:

1. Large numbers of pedestrians and animals share the roadway with fast-moving and slow-moving (e.g., bullock carts) vehicles. There is almost no segregation of pedestrians from wheeled traffic;
2. Large numbers of old, poorly maintained vehicles;
3. Large numbers of motor cycles, scooters, and mopeds;
4. Low driving standards;
5. Large numbers of buses, often overloaded;
6. Widespread disregard of traffic rules;
7. Defective roads, poor street lighting, defective lay-out of cross roads and speed breakers; and
8. Unusual behaviour of men and animals.

In South-East Asia region countries, semi-urban and rural areas contribute 60–80 per cent of road accident injuries, although all media attention is focussed on urban road accidents.

Road traffic injuries cause the considerable economic loss to victims, their families, and to the nation as a whole. These losses arise from the cost of treatment (including rehabilitation and incident investigation) as well as reduced/ lost productivity (e.g. in wages) for those killed or disabled by their injuries, and for family members who need to take time off work (or school) to care for the injured *(12)*.

Multiple causation

Accidents are a complex phenomena of multiple causation (Fig. 1). The aetiological factors may be classified into two broad categories – human and environmental. Upto 90 per cent of the factors responsible for accidents are attributed to human failure. Many of the psychological circumstances in which accidents occur are still poorly known *(5)*.

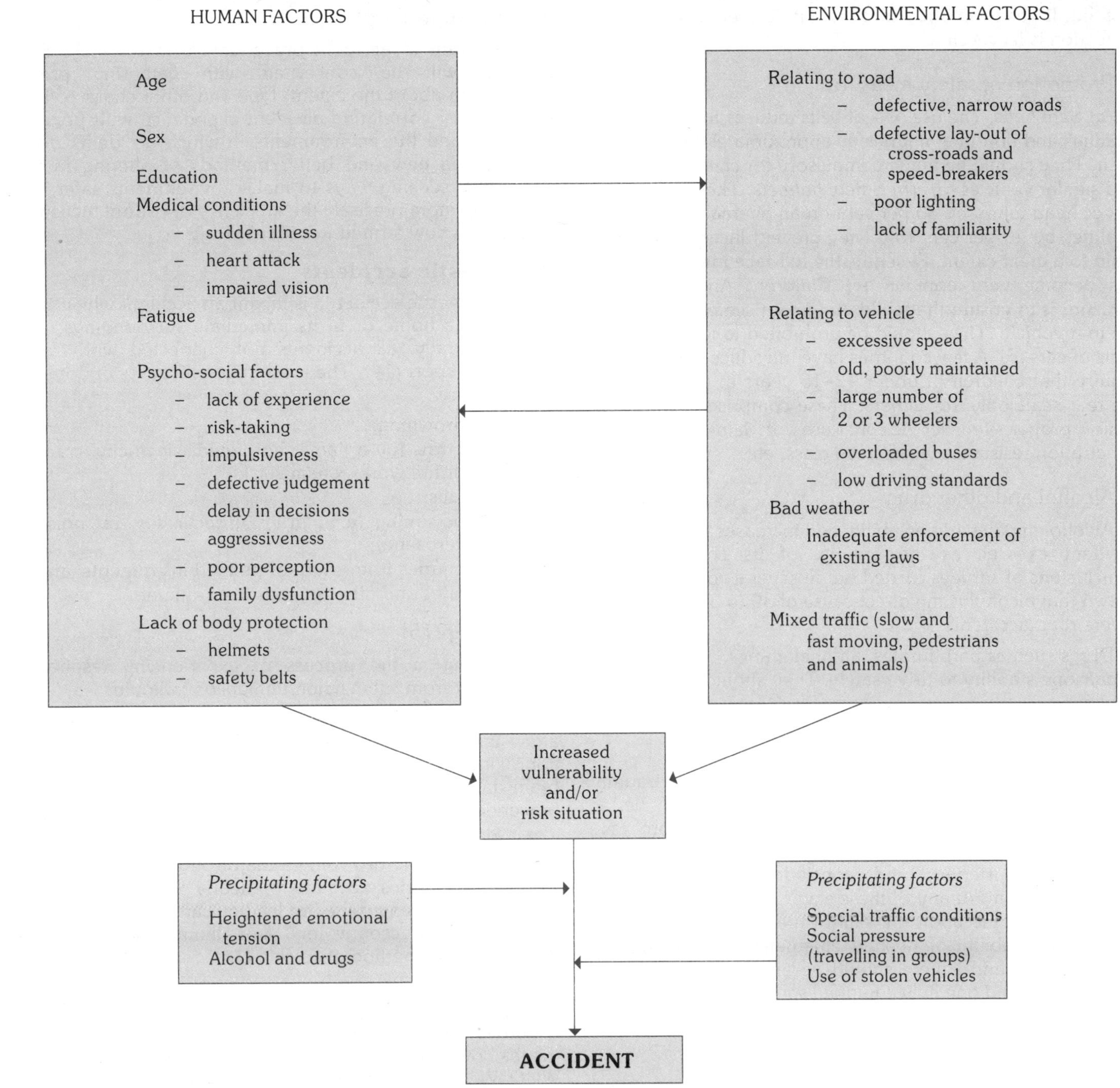

FIG. 1
Primary factors in accidents

PREVENTION

Accidents don't just happen; they are caused. The causes in a given situation must be identified by epidemiological methods. Since accidents are multifactorial, they call for an intersectoral approach to both prevention and care of the injured. The various measures comprise the following :

1. Data collection

There should be a basic reporting system of all accidents. The national data should be supplemented by special surveys and in-depth studies. These studies will bring out the risk factors, the circumstances and chain of events leading upto the accident. These details are rarely provided by the basic reporting system. Detailed environmental data relating to the road, vehicle, weather, etc must also be collected. The police have a statutory duty in many countries to investigate accidents, for legal as well as preventive purposes; the data collecting systems should recognize this and take police records as their starting point *(3)*. Without adequate data collection, analysis and interpretation there could be no effective counter–measures, evaluations and strategies for prevention.

2. Safety education

There is a widespread belief that accidents are inevitable; this fatalistic attitude must be curbed. Safety education must begin with school children. The drivers need to be trained in proper maintenance of vehicles and safe driving. Young people need to be educated regarding risk factors, traffic rules and safety precautions. They should also be trained in first aid. It has been aptly said that "if accident is a disease, education is its vaccine".

3. Promotion of safety measures

(a) Seat belts: The use of seat belts reduces the number of fatalities and non-fatal injuries by approximately 50 per cent each. They should be made compulsory for cars, light trucks and similar vehicles *(3)*. *(b) Safety helmets:* They reduce the risk of head injury by 30 per cent on an average and that of fatalities by 40 per cent *(5)*. They prevent laceration of the scalp to a great extent. Recently, the full-face integral helmet has become very popular. *(c) Children:* Another safety measure is to ensure that children remain seated when they are in a vehicle. They should be prohibited to take the front seats of cars *(5)*. A few countries have introduced laws which require that children of under 12–15 years in cars to be in the rear seats only. *(d) Others:* These comprise use of door locks, proper vehicle design, use of laminated high-penetration resistance windscreen glass, etc.

4. Alcohol and other drugs

Alcohol impairs driving ability and increases the risk of an accident as well as the severity of its consequences. Conclusions of surveys carried out in several countries have shown that alcohol is the direct cause of 30 to 50 per cent of severe road accidents.

Drugs such as barbiturates, amphetamines, and cannabis impair one's ability to drive safely. They should be avoided totally.

5. Primary care

Planning, organization and management of trauma treatment, and emergency care services should be a fundamental element of health service managerial process. Emergency care should begin at the accident site, continued during transportation, and conclude in the hospital emergency room. At any of these stages a life may be saved or lost, depending upon the skill of the health care worker and the availability of needed emergency equipment. To achieve these ends, there should be an Accident Services Organization and one fully equipped specialized trauma care hospital in all major cities.

6. Elimination of causative factors

The factors which tend to cause accidents must be sought out and eliminated, e.g., improvement of roads, imposition of speed limits and marking of danger points.

7. Enforcement of laws

Legislation embodies codified set of rules. These are enforced by the State to prevent accidents. These include driving tests, medical fitness to drive, enforcement of speed limits, compulsory wearing of seat-belts and crash-helmets, checking of blood alcohol concentration, road-side breath testing for alcohol, regular inspection of vehicles, periodic re-examination of drivers over the age of 55, etc.

8. Rehabilitation services

Rehabilitation consists of a number of elements which each injured person should benefit from. These are medical rehabilitation, social rehabilitation, occupational rehabilitation, etc. The aim of rehabilitation is to prevent, reduce or compensate disability and thereby handicap.

9. Accident research

The future of accident prevention is in research. Such research will be concerned with gathering precise information about the extent, type and other characteristics of accidents, correlating accident experience with personal attributes and the environments in which accidents occur, investigating new and better methods of altering human behaviour; seeking ways to make environments safer; and evaluating more precisely the efficiency of control measures. This area is now termed **accidentology**.

2. Domestic accidents

By "domestic accident" is meant an accident which takes place in the home or in its immediate surroundings, and, more generally, all accidents not connected with traffic, vehicles or sport *(14)*. The most frequent causes of domestic accidents are :

1. drowning;
2. burns (by a flame, hot liquid, electricity, crackers or fire works, chemicals);
3. falls;
4. poisoning (e.g., drugs, insecticides, rat poisons, kerosene);
5. injuries from sharp or pointed instruments; and
6. bites and other injuries from animals.

Drowning *(15)*

Drowning is the process of experiencing respiratory impairment from submersion/immersion in liquid.

Victims of drowning have a very slim chance of survival after immersion. The victim loses consciousness after approximately 2 minutes of immersion, and irreversible brain damage can take place after 4–6 minutes. Therefore, prevention strategies are very important.

In 2016, an estimated 322,000 people died from drowning, making drowning a major public health problem worldwide. Injuries account for nearly 9% of total global mortality. Drowning is the 3rd leading cause of unintentional injury/ death. It accounts for 7% of all injury-related deaths. It is a common method of suicide *(16)*.

The global burden and death from drowning is found in all economies and regions, however; low and middle-income countries account for 90% of unintentional drowning deaths; over 50% of the world's drowning occurs in the WHO Western Pacific Region and WHO South-East Asia Region; China and India have particularly high drowning mortality rates and together contribute 43% of the world's drowning deaths and 41% of the total global DALYs (disability-adjusted life years) lost related to drowning.

There is a wide range of uncertainty around the estimate of global drowning deaths. It is important to point out that the global problem is much greater than the above figures reveal; due to the way data are classified, global numbers exclude drowning due to floods (cataclysms), boating and water transport mishaps. Non-fatal drowning statistics in many countries are not readily available or are unreliable.

Risk factors *(15)*

1. *Age :* Age is one of the major risk factor for drowning. This relationship is often associated with a lapse in supervision. In general, children under 5 years of age have the highest drowning mortality rates worldwide. Canada and New Zealand are the only exceptions, where adult males drown at higher rates.

2. *Gender :* Males are especially at risk of drowning with twice the overall mortality rate of females. They are more likely to be hospitalized than females for non-fatal drowning. Studies suggest that the higher drowning rates among males are due to increased exposure to water and riskier behaviour such as swimming alone, drinking alcohol before swimming alone, and boating.

3. *Access to water :* Increased access to water is another risk factor for drowning. Individuals with occupations such as commercial fishing or fishing for subsistence, using small boats in low-income countries, are more prone to drowning. Children who live near open water sources, such as ditches, ponds, irrigation channels, or pools are especially at risk.

4. *Other risk factors :* There are other factors that are associated with an increased risk of drowning, such as :

a. infants left unsupervised or alone, or with another child in a bathtub;
b. unsafe or overcrowded transportation vessels lacking flotation devices;
c. alcohol use, near or in the water;
d. medical conditions, such as epilepsy;
e. tourists unfamiliar with local water risks and features; and
f. floods and other cataclysmic events like tsunamis.

Prevention *(15)*

Drowning prevention strategies should be comprehensive and include: engineering methods which help to remove the hazard, legislation to enforce prevention and assure decreased exposure, education for individuals and communities to build awareness of risk and to aid in response if a drowning occurs.

Engineering methods to eliminate exposure to water hazards are the most effective strategy for drowning prevention. Examples include :

- development and implementation of safe water systems, such as drainage systems, piped water systems, flood control embankments in flood prone areas;
- building four-sided pool fences or barriers preventing access to standing water;
- creating and maintaining safe water zones for recreation;
- covering of wells or open cisterns;
- emptying buckets and baths, and storing them upside-down.

Laws or regulations which target risk factors for drowning include laws requiring regular safety checks of transportation vessels, and laws on alcohol use while boating or swimming.

Individual and community education on drowning awareness, learning water survival skills and ensuring the presence of lifeguards at swimming areas are promising strategy to prevent drowning.

Burns *(17)*

A burn is an injury to the skin or other organic tissue primarily caused by heat or due to radiation, radioactivity, electricity, friction or contact with chemicals. Thermal (heat) burns occur when some or all of the cells in the skin or other tissues are destroyed by :

- hot liquids (scalds)
- hot solids (contact burns), or
- flames (flame burns).

The problem

Burns are a global public health problem, accounting for an estimated 180,000 deaths annually. About 11 million people worldwide require medical attention due to severe burns. The majority of these occur in low and middle-income countries and almost half occur in the South-East Asia Region.

In many high-income countries, burn death rates have been decreasing, and the rate of child deaths from burns is currently over seven times higher in low and middle-income countries than in high-income countries.

Non-fatal burns are a leading cause of morbidity, including prolonged hospitalization, disfigurement and disability, often with resulting stigma and rejection.

It is estimated that over one million people are moderately or severely burnt every year in India. In Bangladesh 1.73 lac children get moderate or severe burns every year with about 17 per cent getting temporary disability and 18 per cent permanent disability. Burns are the second most common injury in rural Nepal accounting for 5 per cent disabilities.

Risk factors *(17)*

Gender : Females suffer burns more frequently than males. Women in the South-East Asia Region have the highest rate of burns, accounting for 27% of global burn deaths and nearly 70% of burn deaths in the region. The high risk for females is associated with open fire cooking, or inherently unsafe cookstoves, which can ignite loose clothing. Open flames used for heating and lighting also pose risks, and self-directed or interpersonal violence are also important factors (although understudied).

Age : Along with adult women, children are particularly vulnerable to burns. Burns are the 11th leading cause of death of children aged 1–9 years and are also the fifth most common cause of non-fatal childhood injuries. While a major risk is improper adult supervision, a considerable number of burn injuries in children result from child maltreatment.

Socio-economic factors

People living in low and middle-income countries are at higher risk for burns than people living in high-income countries. Within the countries also, burn risk correlates with socio-economic status.

Other risk factors

There are a number of other risk factors for burns, including :

- occupations that increase exposure to fire;
- poverty, overcrowding and lack of proper safety measures;
- placement of young girls in household roles such as cooking and care of small children;
- underlying medical conditions, including epilepsy, peripheral neuropathy, and physical and cognitive disabilities;
- alcohol abuse and smoking;
- easy access to chemicals used for assault (such as in acid violence attacks);
- use of kerosene (paraffin) as a fuel source for non-electric domestic appliances;
- inadequate safety measures for liquefied petroleum gas and electricity.

Burns occur mainly in the home and workplace. Community surveys in Bangladesh and Ethiopia showed that 80–90% of burns occur at home. Children and women usually get burns in domestic kitchens, from upset receptacles containing hot liquids, or flames, or from cookstove explosions. Men are more likely to get burns in the workplace due to fire, scalds, chemicals and electricity.

Prevention *(17)*

Burns are preventable. High-income countries have made considerable progress in lowering rates of burn deaths, through a combination of prevention strategies and improvemetns in the care of people affected by burns. Most of these advances in prevention and care have been incompletely applied in low and middle-income countries. Increased efforts to do so would likely lead to significant reduction in rates of burn-related death and disability.

Prevention strategies should address the hazards for specific burn injuries, education for vulnerable populations and training of communities in first-aid. An effective burn prevention plan should be multisectoral. There are a number of specific recommendations for individuals, communities and public health officials to reduce burn risk.

FIRST-AID *(17)*

Do's

1. Stop the burning process by removing clothing and irrigating the burns.
2. Use cool running water to reduce the temperature of the burn.
3. Extinguish flames by allowing the person to roll on the ground, or by applying a blanket, or by using water or other fire-extinguishing liquids.
4. In chemical burns, remove or dilute the chemical agent by irrigating with large volumes of water.
5. Wrap the patient in a clean cloth or sheet and transport to the nearest appropriate facility for medical care.

Don'ts

1. Do not start first-aid before ensuring your own safety (switch off electrical current, wear gloves for chemicals etc.)
2. Do not apply paste, oil, haldi (turmeric) or raw cotton to the burn.
3. Do not apply ice because it deepens the injury.
4. Avoid prolonged cooling with water because it may lead to hypothermia.
5. Do not open blisters until topical antimicrobials can be applied, by a health-care provider.
6. Do not apply any material directly to the wound as it might become infected.
7. Avoid application of topical medication until the patient has been placed under appropriate medical care.

Falls

Globally, falls are a major public health problem. An estimated 646,000 fatal falls occur each year, making it the second leading cause of unintentional injury death, after road traffic injuries. Though not fatal 37.3 million falls are severe enough to require medical attention. Such falls are responsible for 17 million DALYs lost. Over 80% of fall-related fatalities occur in low and middle-income countries, with regions of the Western Pacific and South East Asia accounting for more than two-thirds of these deaths. In all regions of the world, death rates are highest among adults over the age of 65 years *(18)*.

Falls are responsible for the largest number of hospital visits for non-fatal injuries, especially for children and young adults. Falls from rooftops, balconies, windows and stair cases are common. Factors specific to SEAR countries are falls from trees of workers picking fruits or coconuts, tapping toddy, children falling from rooftops while flying kites, high incidence of falls among construction and forestry workers. As life expetancy increases in these countries, the incidence of hip and other fractures due to fall among the elderly are also assuming greater proportions *(19)*.

Some of the risk factors include *(18)* :

- occupations at elevated heights or other hazardous working conditions;
- alcohol or substance use;
- socio-economic factors including poverty, overcrowded housing, young maternal age;
- underlying medical conditions, such as neurological, cardiac or other disabling conditions;
- side-effects of medication, physical inactivity and loss of balance, particularly among older people;
- unsafe environments, particularly for those with poor balance and limited vision.

Prevention *(18)*

For children, effective interventions include multifaceted community programmes; engineering modifications of nursery furniture, playground equipment, and other products; and legislation for the use of window guard.

For older individuals, fall prevention programmes can include a number of components to identify and modify risk, such as :

- screening within living environments for risks for falls;
- clinical interventions to identify risk factors, such as medication review and modification, treatment of low blood pressure, Vitamin D and calcium supplementation, treatment of correctable visual impairment;
- home assessment and environmental modification for those with known risk factors or a history of falling;
- prescription of appropriate assistive devices to address physical and sensory impairments;
- muscle strengthening and balance retraining prescribed by a trained health professional;

Poisoning

Poisoning was responsible for an estimated 252,000 deaths during the year 2008 worldwide. In India about 28,012 poisoning deaths were reported during the year 2010 *(20)*. The most common agents responsible for poisoning are pesticides, kerosene, prescription drugs, and household chemicals. Pesticides are widely used in many countries where agriculture is an important part of the economy. Reports from India, Indonesia, Sri Lanka, and Thailand indicate that common availability and use of toxic pesticides is responsible for intentional and unintentional morbidity and mortality.

In Sri Lanka, pesticides are one of the main agents used in attempted suicide in rural areas. The use of organophosphorous insecticides in suicide events has been reported to be as high as 20–30 per cent. Paraquat intoxication is known to cause irreversible damage in patients. Many countries also report accidental ingestion of kerosene as a leading cause of poisoning, especially among children *(19)*. A study from Thailand revealed that 54 per cent of cases of poisoning among pre-school children involved therapeutic drugs.

Snake bite

Snake bite is a neglected public health issue in many tropical and subtropical countries. About 5 million snake bites occur each year, resulting in upto 2.4 million envenomings (poisoning from snake bites) at least 94,000–125,000 deaths and around 400,000 amputations and other permanent disabilities. Most of these occur in Africa, Asia and Latin America. In Africa alone there are an estimated 1 million snake bites annually with about half needing treatment. This type of injury is often found among women, children and farmers in poor rural communities in low and middle-income countries *(21)*.

The outcome of snake bite depends on numerous factors, including the species of snake, the area of the body bitten, the amount of venom injected, and the health condition of the victim. Feelings of terror and panic are common after a snake bite and can produce a characteristic set of symptoms mediated by the autonomic nervous system, such as a tachycardia and nausea. Bites from non-venomous snakes can also cause injury, often due to lacerations caused by the snake's teeth, or from a resulting infection. A bite may also trigger an anaphylactic reaction, which is potentially fatal. First-aid recommendations for bite depends on the snakes inhabiting the region, as effective treatment for bite inflicted by some species can be ineffective for others.

The venom of poisonous snakes may be predominantly neurotoxic or predominantly cytolytic. Neurotoxins cause respiratory paralysis and cytolytic venoms cause tissue destruction by digestion and haemorrhage due to haemolysis and destruction of the endothelial lining of the blood vessels. The manifestations of rattlesnake envenomation are mostly local pain, redness, swelling and extravasation of blood. Perioral tingling, metallic taste, nausea, and vomiting, hypotension and coagulopathy may also occur. Neurotoxic envenomation may cause ptosis, dysphagia, diplopia, and respiratory failure. Venom emitted from some types of cobras, almost all vipers cause necrosis of muscle tissue. Muscle tissues begin to die throughout the body and it results in accumulation of myoglobin in the renal tubules which leads to acute renal failure.

Early clues that a patient has severe envenoming *(22)* :

- Snake identified as a very dangerous one;
- Rapid early extension of local swelling from the site of the bite;
- Early tender enlargement of local lymph nodes, indicating spread of venom in the lymphatic system;
- Early systemic symptoms: collapse (hypotension, shock), nausea, vomiting, diarrhoea, severe headache, "heaviness" of the eyelids, inappropriate (pathological) drowsiness or early ptosis/ophthalmoplegia;
- Early spontaneous systemic bleeding;
- Passage of dark brown/black urine.

MANAGEMENT AT COMMUNITY OR VILLAGE LEVEL *(23)*

A. First-aid

The Government of India developed a national snake-bite protocol in 2007 which includes following advice :

1. Reassure the patient. 70% of all snake bites are from non-venomous species. Only 50% of bites by venomous species actually envenomate the patient;
2. Immobilize in the same way as a fractured limb. Use bandages or cloth to hold the splints, not to block the blood supply or apply pressure. Do not apply any compression in the form of tight ligatures, they don't work and can be dangerous;
3. Do not give alcoholic beverages or stimulants. They are known vasodilators and they speed up the absorption of venom;
4. Remove any items or clothings which may constrict the bitten limb if it swells (rings, bracelets, watches, footwear, etc.);
5. Do not incise or manipulate the bitten site. Do not apply ice; and
6. Transport the patient to a medical faculty for definitive treatment.

B. At the Rural Clinic, Dispensary, Health Post, or Primary Health Centre

1. *Assess for signs of local and systemic envenoming :* carry out a simple medical assessment including history and simple physical examination – local swelling, painful tender enlarged local lymph glands, persistent bleeding from the bite wound, blood pressure, pulse rate, bleeding (gums, nose, vomit, stool or urine), level of consciousness, drooping eyelids (ptosis) and other signs of paralysis. Monitor these signs hourly.
2. *Check :* 20 minute whole blood clotting test (20WBCT), urine examination (appearance, sticks testing for blood etc.). Identify the snake or a photo of it (if brought).
3. *Analgesia :* give analgesia by mouth if required: paracetamol (acetaminophen) (adult dose 500 mg to 1g maximum, 4g in 24 hours; children 10–15 mg/kg, maximum 100mg/kg/day) or codeine phosphate (adult dose 30–60 mg, maximum 240 mg in 24 hours; children more than 2 years old, 0.5 mg/kg, maximum 2 mg/kg/day) can be given every 4–6 hours by mouth as required (not aspirin or non-steroidal anti-inflammatory drugs which can cause bleeding).
4. *Antivenom :* if the patient fulfils criteria for antivenom treatment and if the necessary skills, equipment, antivenom, adrenaline and other necessary drugs are available, give antivenom. These skills include ability to diagnose local and systemic envenoming, set up intravenous infusion or intravenous injection, identify the early signs of anaphylaxis and treat it with intramuscular adrenaline. Re-assess for repeated dose(s) of antivenom. If no antivenom is available, transfer to a hospital.
5. *If the patient is in shock/hypotensive :* give cautious intravenous fluid challenge (adult 250–500 ml of 0.9% saline) to correct hypovolaemia shock.
6. *If the patient has evidence of respiratory paralysis :* give oxygen by mask, consider atropine and neostigmine,

and transfer to a hospital. It is assumed that assisted ventilation other than by a tight-fitting face mask connected to an anaesthetic (Ambu) bag will not be possible at this level.

7. *If the patient is oliguric* : initiate conservative management.
8. *The bite wound* : if necrotic, tampered with (incisions etc.) or obviously septic, give antibiotics and tetanus prophylaxis.
9. Assess the need and feasibility of transporting the patient to a higher level of the health service (see A above) especially in case of :
   a. Substantial bleeding, 20WBCT still positive (non-clotting) 6 hours after initial antivenom dose
   b. Progressive paralysis (muscle weakness) or respiratory difficulty
   c. Reduced urine output
   d. Anaphylaxis – unresponsive to adrenaline
   e. Shock/hypotension – unresponsive to fluids
   f. Severe local necrosis or signs suggestive of compartment syndrome
10. Discourage the use of ineffective and potentially harmful drugs (e.g. corticosteroids, antihistamines, and heparin).

C. At the District Hospital *(23)*

Proceed as in B above plus :

1. *Assessment* : carry out a more detailed clinical and laboratory assessment including biochemical and haematological measurements, ECG or radiography, as indicated.
2. *Antivenom* : if no antivenom is available, transfer to a hospital that has antivenom or treat conservatively; this may require transfusion of blood or fresh frozen plasma.
3. *Analgesia* : (see B above) and, if required, consider stronger parenteral opioid drugs as required, all with great caution (e.g. subcutanous, intramuscular or even intravenous pethidine, initial adult dose 50–100 mg; children 1–1.5 mg/kg; or morphine, initial adult dose 5–10 mg; children 0.03-0.05 mg/kg,).
4. *If the patient has evidence of local necrosis (gangrene)* : give tetanus toxoid booster, antibiotics and do surgical debridement of dead tissue.
5. *If the patient has evidence of bulbar or respiratory paralysis* : insert endotracheal tube, laryngeal mask airway or i-gel airway. If there is evidence of respiratory failure, assist ventilation manually by anaesthetic (Ambu) bag or mechanical ventilator.
6. *If the patient has evidence of acute kidney injury* : treat with peritoneal dialysis. If this is not available, transfer to a specialized hospital.
7. *If the patient is bleeding severely or is already seriously anaemic* : cross-match and transfuse.
8. *Rehabilitation* : encourage exercising of bitten limb.

D. At the Referral (Specialized) Hospital *(23)*

Proceed as in B and C above plus :

1. More advanced surgical management of local necrosis (e.g. split skin grafting).
2. More advanced investigations including bacterial cultures and imaging (CT scans) as indicated.
3. If the patient has evidence of acute renal failure peritoneal or haemodialysis or haemofiltration.
4. Implement rehabilitation by physiotherapists.

Strengthening of health system in managing snakebite

To reduce complications and deaths from snakebites, health systems need to be improved at various levels. The government must develop a policy for snakebite, making it a notifiable disease, developing a snakebite programme that includes standard treatment guidelines, training of health personnel and ensure an adequate supply, distribution and storage of good quality antivenom.

ANTIVENOM *(22)*

Until the advent of antivenom, bites from some species of snake were almost universally fatal. Despite huge advances in emergency therapy, antivenom is often still the only effective treatment for envenomation. The first antivenom was developed in 1895 by French physician Albert Calmette for the treatment of Indian cobra bites. Antivenom is made by injecting a small amount of venom into an animal (usually a horse or sheep) to initiate an immune system response. The resulting antibodies are then harvested from the animal's blood.

Antivenom is injected into the person intravenously, and works by binding to, and neutralizing venom enzymes. It cannot undo damage already caused by venom, so antivenom treatment should be sought as soon as possible. Modern antivenoms are usually polyvalent, making them effective against the venom of numerous snake species.

Pharmaceutical companies which produce antivenom target their products against the species native to a particular area. Although some people may develop serious adverse reactions to antivenom, such as anaphylaxis, in emergency situations this is usually treatable and hence the benefit outweighs the potential consequences of not using antivenom.

3. Industrial accidents

There are approximately 580 million workers in the South–East Asia Region. Approximately 60–80 per cent of these workers are employed in agriculture, fisheries, home industries, and small-scale units. Injuries due to these occupations result in an estimated 120 million injuries and 200,000 deaths per year *(19)*.

Though reliable estimates for work related injuries and deaths in the Region are not available, partly because a majority of the workers are employed in unorganized sectors, few studies indicate that nearly one per cent of deaths and 10 per cent of permanent impairment result from agricultural injuries. Agriculture workers are exposed to wide variety of physical, chemical (pesticide and fertilizers), biological (animal bites and animal related injuries) and mechanical injuries. The estimates from agriculture injury vary from 22–29 per 1000 workers. The incidence rate of injury among agriculture workers in India is estimated to be 116 per 100,000 workers. In a study population of 23,000 in rural Haryana, nearly 31 per cent of the injuries were related to agricultural activity *(24)*. Of these, serious injuries were caused by mechanized equipment and tractors *(19)*.

Rapid industrialization has also resulted in mortality and morbidity of many workers in hazardous industries.

The unique features common to the workplace in this region are that the manual labour content is high and the man–machine interaction is unsafe. In addition, there is greater emphasis on attempts to change the worker's behaviour, but designs that provide automatic protection are ignored. Children and people who are challenged physically as well as mentally are at a greater risk of encountering occupational injuries *(19)*.

4. Railway accidents

With the increase in number of trains and passengers, the increase in the number of accidents and casualties resulting therefrom is not unexpected. During 2020, about 8,700 people died of railway accidents in India *(9)*. The main factor involved in railway accidents is human failure.

5. Violence

Homicide and collective violence account for around 10% of global, injury-related death. In 2016, there were an estimated 477,000 murders. Four fifths of homicide victims are men, and 60% of victims, males age 15–44. The low- and middle-income countries of the Region of the Americas has the most homicides, with 28.5 per 100,000 population, while the lowest murder rate, almost 14 times lower (2.1 per 100,000 population), is found in the low- and middle-income countries of The Western Pacific Region *(25)*.

Violence is reported to be increasing rapidly. It also follow the same epidemiological pattern as any other disease (host, agent and environment), i.e. a motivated person who injures; a suitable target; and a suitable environment or the absence of a guardian, all coinciding in time and space. Often, it may only be possible to initiate steps for prevention after an episode of violence has already taken place.

Some of the risk factors for violent behaviour are *(19)* :

- Exposure to violence and societal acceptability of violence as a means to solve problems. The image of violence as an acceptable and effective tool for solving problems, whether across international borders, on the street, or around the home, may spill over into real behaviour;
- Availability of lethal weapons like fire-arms significantly increases the possibility of both fatal and non-fatal injuries;
- Consumption of alcohol and other drugs is linked to almost 2/3 of cases of violence according to several studies.

Violence due to war and political unrest is fairly common in several countries. Organized and unorganized, ethnic and communal violence are well known in some places.

Suicides have been increasing at an alarming rate in SEAR countries. Crude death rates of 8.7 per lac population in Bangladesh, 14.7 per lac population in India, 6.4 per lac in Sri Lanka, and 5.9 per lac in Thailand; per year have been reported in 2016 *(8)*. Nearly 70 per cent of suicides in all countries have been reported in the age group of 15–34 years with male-female ratio of 1:1.2 to 1:3 from different countries. Poisoning, hanging, self-immolation and drowning are the most commonly reported methods of suicide *(24)*.

In India, an average of 369 suicides take place every day, out of these 248 are committed by males and 121 by females (62 are house wives). Family problems (89) and illness (72) are the main cause of suicides. Majority cases are below 29 years of age (136) followed by 30–44 years of age group (125) *(26)*.

References

1. Hogarth, J. (1978). *Glossary of Health Care Terminology,* WHO, Copenhagen.
2. WHO (1957). *Techn. Rep. Ser.,* No.118.
3. WHO (1984). *Techn. Rep. Ser.,* 703.
4. WHO (1976). *The Epidemiology of Road Traffic Injuries,* European Sr. No.2, WHO Copenhagen.
5. WHO (1982). *The Epidemiology of Accident Traumas and Resulting Disabilities,* EURO Reports and Studies, 57, WHO, Copenhagen.
6. WHO (2013), *How to use the ICF, A Practical Manual for using the International Classification of Functioning, Disability and Health (ICF).*
7. WHO, *Children's Environmental Health, Injuries.*
8. WHO (2018), *Global Health Estimates 2016,* April 2018.
9. Govt. of India (2021), *National Health Profile 2021,* Ministry of Health and Family Welfare, New Delhi.
10. WHO (2022), *Fact Sheet, Road Traffic Injuries,* June 2022.
11. WHO (2018), *Global Status Report on Road Safety,* 2018.
12. WHO (2012), *Road Traffic Injuries,* Fact sheet No. 358, Sept 2012.
13. WHO (1981). *Seat belts and other devices to reduce injuries from traffic accidents,* EURO Reports and Studies 40, WHO, Copenhagen.

13A. Govt. of India (2021). *Accidental Deaths and Suicides in India,* 2021.

14. Govt. of India (1979). *Swasth Hind,* 25 (12) 329.
15. WHO (2020), *Drowning,* Fact Sheet 3rd Feb., 2020.
16. WHO (2018), *Fact Sheet or Drowning,* 15th Jan., 2018.
17. WHO (2018), *Burns,* Fact Sheet 6th. March, 2018.
18. WHO (2018), *Falls,* Fact Sheet 16th Jan., 2018.
19. WHO (2002), *Injuries in South-East Asia Region, Priorities for Policy and Action,* SEA / Injuries / A1.
20. WHO (2011), *Estimates of Deaths by Causes for the year 2008 Summary Tables.*
21. WHO (2018), *Snake envenoming,* Fact sheet, 5th Feb. 2018.
22. WHO (2016), *Guidelines for the Management of Snake-bites,* Regional Office of SEAR, New Delhi.
23. WHO (2010), *Guidelines for the Management of Snake-bites,* 2nd Ed., Regional Office for SEAR.
24. WHO (2002), *Health Situation in the South-East Asia Region 1998-2000,* Regional Office for SEAR, New Delhi.
25. WHO (2015), *Health in 2015 from MDGs. Millennium Development Goals to SDGs - Sustainable Development Goals.*
26. Lancet Public Health (2019), *India state-level disease burden initiative, Road Injury,* Dec. 24th, 2019.

7 Health Programmes in India

"Those who would benefit most from a service are least likely to obtain it"

Since India became independent, several measures have been undertaken by the National Government to improve the health of the people. Prominent among these measures are the NATIONAL HEALTH PROGRAMMES, which have been launched by the Central Government for the control/eradication of the communicable diseases, improvement of environmental sanitation, raising the standard of nutrition, control of population and improving rural health. Various international agencies like WHO, UNICEF, UNFPA, World Bank, as also a number of foreign agencies like SIDA, DANIDA, NORAD and USAID have been providing technical and material assistance in the implementation of these programmes. A brief account of these programmes which are currently in operation is given below :

NATIONAL VECTOR BORNE DISEASE CONTROL PROGRAMME

The National Vector Borne Disease Control Programme (NVBDCP) is implemented in the State/UT's for prevention and control of vector borne diseases namely Malaria, Filariasis, Kala-azar, Japanese Encephalitis (JE), Dengue and Chikungunya. The Directorate of NVBDCP is the nodal agency for planning, policy making and technical guidance and monitoring and evaluation of programme implementation in respect of prevention and control of these vector borne diseases under the overall umbrella of NRHM. The States are responsible for planning, implementation and supervision of the programme. The vector borne diseases are major public health problems in India. Chikungunya fever which has re-emerged as epidemic outbreaks after more than three decades has added to the problem. The prevention and control of vector borne diseases is complex; as their transmission depends on interaction of numerous ecological, biological, social and economic factors including migration *(1)*.

Out of the six vector borne diseases, malaria, filariasis, japanese encephalitis, dengue and chikungunya are transmitted by different kind of vector mosquitoes, while kala-azar is transmitted by sand flies. The transmission of vector borne diseases in any area is dependent on frequency of man-vector contact, which is further, influenced by various factors including vector density, biting time, etc. Mosquito density is directly related with water collection, clean or polluted, in which the mosquitoes breed.

Under NVBDCP, the three pronged strategy for prevention and control of VBDs is as follows : (i) Disease management including early case detection and complete treatment, strengthening of referral services, epidemic preparedness and rapid response; (ii) Integrated vector management (IVM) for transmission risk reduction including indoor residual spraying in selected high-risk areas, use of insecticide treated bed-nets, use of larvivorous fish, anti-larval measures in urban areas, source reduction and minor environmental engineering; and (iii) Supportive interventions including behaviour change communication (BCC), public private partnership and inter-sectoral convergence, human resource development through capacity building, operational research including studies on drug resistance and insecticide susceptibility, monitoring and evaluation through periodic reviews/field visits, web based management information system, vaccination against JE and annual mass drug administration against lymphatic filariasis *(1)*.

(A) MALARIA

The programme began originally as National Malaria Control Programme in 1953, during the First Five Year Plan. Because of the spectacular success achieved in the control of malaria, the control programme, was converted in 1958 into an eradication programme, with the objective of eradicating malaria once and for all from the country. Since then the programme has undergone many changes and the milestones of malaria control activities in India are as shown below *(2)* :

Milestones of malaria control activities in India

Year	Milestone
Prior to 1953	Estimated malaria cases in India – 75 million; Deaths due to malaria – 0.8 million.
1953	Launching of National Malaria Control Programme (NMCP).
1958	NMCP was changed to National Malaria Eradication Programme.
1965	Cases reduced to 0.1 million.
Early 1970's	Resurgence of malaria.
1976	Malaria cases – 6.46 million.
1977	Modified Plan of Operations implemented.
1997	World Bank assisted Enhanced Malaria Control Project (EMCP) launched.
1999	Renaming of programme to National Anti Malaria Programme (NAMP).
2002	Renaming of NAMP to National Vector Borne Disease Control Programme.
2005	Global Fund assisted Intensified Malaria Control Project (IMCP) launched.
2005	NVBDCP became integral part of NRHM.
2005	Introduction of RDT in the programme.
2006	ACT introduced in areas showing chloroquine resistance in falciparum malaria.

2008	ACT extended to high *Pf* predominant districts covering about 95% *Pf* cases.
2008	World Bank supported National Malaria Control Project launched.
2009	Introduction of LLINs.
2010	New drug policy 2010.
2012	Introduction of bivalent RDT.
2013	New drug policy 2013.
2016	National Framework for Malaria Elimination in India launched.
2017	National Strategic Plan for Malaria Elimination in India 2017–2022 launched.

The main activities of the programme are :

1. Formulating policies and guidelines.
2. Technical guidance.
3. Planning.
4. Logistics.
5. Monitoring and evaluation.
6. Coordination of activities through the States/Union Territories and in consultation with national organizations such as National Centre for Disease Control (NCDC), National Institute of Malaria Research (NIMR).
7. Collaboration with international organizations like the WHO, World Bank, GFATM and other donor agencies.
8. Training.
9. Facilitating research through NCDC, NIMR, Regional Medical Research Centres etc.
10. Coordinating control activities in the inter-state and inter-country border areas.

Organization *(2)*

There are 19 Regional Offices for Health and Family Welfare under Directorate General of Health Services, Ministry of Health and Family Welfare, located in 19 states, which play a crucial role in monitoring the activities under NVBDCP. These offices are equipped with malaria trained staff.

The state governments are required to plan and implement the malaria control operations in their respective states. Every state has a Vector Borne Disease Control Division under its Department of Health and Family Welfare. It is headed by the State Programme Officer (SPO) who is responsible for supervision, guidance and effective implementation of the programme and for coordination of the activities with the neighbouring States/UTs. States are responsible for the procurement of certain insecticides for indoor residual spray (IRS), spray equipment and certain anti-malarials, the central government supplies DDT and larvicides.

Each state has established a State Vector Borne Disease Control Society, which includes civil society and sometimes private sector representation. These are now merged with similar entities for other centrally sponsored schemes into a single state-level Health and Family Welfare Society. The main role of these societies is to channelize funds from GOI to the states and onwards to districts for financing of the programmes. They also play a role in district level planning and in monitoring of programme activities within districts.

At the divisional level, zonal officers have technical and administrative responsibilities of the programme in their areas under the overall supervision of Senior Divisional Officers (SDOs).

At the district level, the Chief Medical Officer (CMO)/ District Health Officer (DHO) has the overall responsibility of the programme. At the district level, district malaria offices have been established in many places headed by the DVBDC officer to assist the CMO/DHO. This office is the key unit for the planning and monitoring of the programme. Spray operations are the direct responsibility of DMO/DVBDC officer in the entire district under overall supervision of CMO and collaborative supervision/monitoring by PHC's Medical Officer. There is one Assistant Malaria Officer (AMO) and Malaria Inspectors (MIs) to assist him *(2)*.

In many districts, District Vector Borne Disease Control Societies (now merged with District Health Societies under NRHM) have been established to assist the management of funds and planning, and monitoring of programme activities.

The laboratories have been decentralized and positioned at the PHCs. The medical officer – PHC has the overall responsibility for surveillance and laboratory services, and also supervises the spray. Case detection management and community outreach services are carried out by MPWs as well as ASHAs and other community health volunteers.

DRUG DISTRIBUTION CENTRES AND FEVER TREATMENT DEPOTS

With the increasing number of malaria cases, the demand for antimalarial drugs has increased tremendously. It became clear that drug supply only through the surveillance workers and medical institutions was not enough. This led to the establishment of a wide network of Drug Distribution Centres and Fever Treatment Depots and malaria clinics at some sub-centres. Drug Distribution Centres are only to dispense the anti-malarial tablets as per NMEP schedules. Fever Treatment Depots collect the blood slides in addition to the distribution of antimalarial tablets. These centres are manned by voluntary workers from the community.

URBAN MALARIA SCHEME

The urban malaria scheme was launched in 1971 to reduce or interrupt malaria transmission in towns and cities. The methodology comprises vector control by intensive antilarval measures and drug treatment.

About 7.4 per cent of the total cases of malaria and 10.9 per cent of deaths due to malaria are reported from urban areas. Maximum cases are reported from Chennai, Vadodara, Visakhapatnam, Ahmedabad, Kolkata, New Mumbai, Vijayawada etc. *(3)*. The vector of malaria in the urban areas breeds largely in man-made containers including overhead tanks and underground water storage tanks, water coolers, cisterns, roof gutters, flower vases, bottles and ornamental ponds, old tyres etc., which can collect water. Large construction activities provide suitable breeding sites for the mosqitoes. Influx of migrant labour, from malarious zones contribute to increase in incidence. Control of urban malaria lies primarily in the implementation of civil bye-laws to prevent mosquito breeding in the domestic and peridomestic areas. Use of larvivorous fish in the water bodies such as slow moving streams, ornamental ponds etc. is recommended. Larvicides are used for water bodies which are unsuitable for fish use *(2)*. The urban malaria scheme under national vector disease control programme is presently protecting 130 million population from malaria and other mosquito borne diseases in 131 towns in 19 states and Union Territories. The civic bye-laws have been enacted and implemented in Delhi, Mumbai, Kolkata, Chandigarh, Bengaluru, Chennai, Ahmedabad and Goa etc *(3)*.

The Expert Committee on Malaria had recommended the inclusion of all urban areas with more than 50,000 population and reporting slide positivity rate of 5 per cent and above, under Urban Malaria Scheme and introduction of active surveillance under this scheme.

National Framework for Malaria Elimination in India (2016–2030) *(4)*

Encouraged by the success achieved in malaria control in recent years, the vision of India's malaria control programme has been now shifted to sustained malaria elimination to contribute more effectively to improved health and quality of life of the people. The National Framework for malaria elimination in India 2016–2030 was launched in February 2016.

Goals

In line with the WHO Global Technical Strategy (GTS) for Malaria 2016–2030 and the Asia Pacific Leaders Malaria Alliance Malaria Elimination Roadmap, the goals of the National Framework for Malaria Elimination in India 2016–2030 are:

- Eliminate malaria (zero indigenous cases) throughout the entire country by 2030; and
- Maintain malaria-free status in areas where malaria transmission has been interrupted and prevent re-introduction of malaria.

Objectives

The National Framework for Malaria Elimination in India has formulated the following objectives:

- By 2022, transmission of malaria interrupted and zero indigenous cases to be attained in all 26 States/UTs that were under Categories 1 and 2 in 2014;
- By 2024, incidence of malaria to be reduced to less than 1 case per 1000 population in all States and UTs, and their districts;
- By 2027, indigenous transmission of malaria to be interrupted in all States and UTs of India; and
- By 2030, malaria to be eliminated throughout the entire country, and re-establishment of transmission prevented.

Programme phasing

Malaria elimination in India will be carried out in a phased manner because the various States/UTs have different levels of malaria burden. While some low burden states are in a position to plan action for malaria elimination right now, the high burden states will need to reduce the malaria burden first before proceeding towards elimination. Therefore, states and UTs have been categorized into phases, based on their API as primary criterion with due consideration given to ABER and SPR as secondary criteria. The categorization is given in Table 1.

TABLE 1
Classification of States/UTs for malaria elimination in India (2014)

Category	Definition
Category 0 Prevention of re-establishment phase	States/UTs with zero indigenous cases of malaria (currently, no state/UT)
Category 1 Elimination phase	States/UTs with API less than one, and all their districts reporting API<1 (15 states/UTs)
Category 2 Pre-elimination phase	States/UTs with API < 1, but some of their districts reporting API ≥ 1 (11 states)
Category 3 Intensified control phase	States/UTs with API ≥ 1 (10 states/UTs)

Category 1 states/UTs are: Himachal Pradesh, Punjab, Jammu & Kashmir, Kerala, Manipur, Puducherry, Chandigarh, Uttarakhand, Haryana, Sikkim, Rajasthan, Daman & Diu, Goa, Delhi and Lakshadweep.

Category 2 states/UTs are: Bihar, Tamil Nadu, Telangana, Uttar Pradesh, Karnataka, West Bengal, Andhra Pradesh, Assam, Maharashtra, Gujarat and Nagaland.

Category 3 states/UTs are: Andaman & Nicobar islands, Madhya Pradesh, Dadar & Nagar Haveli, Jharkhand, Arunachal Pradesh, Chhattisgarh, Odisha, Meghalaya, Tripura and Mizoram.

Category 1 states/UTs generally have very low proportion of *P. falciparum* cases except Kerela, Manipur and Sikkim. On the other hand, category 3 states/UTs have a high proportion of *P. falciparum* except in Andaman & Nicobar islands and Dadar and Nagar Haveli *(4)*.

Milestones and targets *(4)*

The milestones and targets set for malaria elimination in India are as follows:

By the end of the year 2016

All states and UTs to have included malaria elimination in their broader health policies and planning framework.

By the year 2020

1. All 15 states/UTs that were under category 1 (elimination phase) in 2014 to completely interrupted malaria transmission and achieved zero indigenous cases and deaths due to malaria;
2. All 11 states/UTs under category 2 (pre-elimination phase) in 2014 to enter into category 1 (elimination phase);
3. 5 states/UTs under category 3 (intensified control phases) in 2014 to enter into category 2 (pre-elimination phase)
4. 5 states/UTs under category 3 (intensified control phase) in 2014 to reduce disease burden but continue to remain in category 3; and
5. Estimated malaria burden at national level to reduce by 15–20% as compared to 2014.

Additionally, states with stronger health systems such as Gujarat, Maharashtra and Karnataka may implement accelerated malaria elimination programmes to achieve interruption of transmission and demonstrate early elimination followed by sustenance of zero indigenous cases.

By the year 2022

1. All 26 states/UTs that were under categories 1 and 2 in 2014 to interrupt malaria transmission and achieved zero indigenous cases and deaths due to malaria;
2. 5 states/UTs which were under category 3 (intensified control phases) in 2014 to enter into category 1 (elimination phase);
3. 5 states/UTs which were under category 3 (intensified control phases) in 2014 to enter into category 2 (pre-elimination phase); and
4. Estimated malaria burden at national level reduced by 30–35% as compared to 2014.

By the year 2024

1. All states and UTs and their districts to reduce API to less than 1 case per 1000 population at risk, sustain zero

deaths due to malaria and establish fully functional malaria surveillance to track, investigate and respond to each case;
2. 31 states/UTs to interrupt transmission of malaria and zero indigineous cases and deaths attained; and
3. 5 states/UTs which were under category 3 (intensified control phases) in 2014 to enter into elimination phase.

By the year 2027

Indigenous transmission of malaria interrupted and the entire country to have no indigenous cases and no deaths due to malaria.

By the year 2030

The entire country to sustain status of zero indigenous cases and deaths due to malaria for 3 consecutive years; and India to initiate the processes for certification of malaria elimination status.

Focus on High-Endemic Areas and Tribal Population:

Most of the malaria cases in India are reported from Andhra Pradesh, Chhattisgarh, Jharkhand, Madhya Pradesh, Maharashtra, Meghalaya, Mizoram, Odisha, Telangana and Tripura. The high incidence in these states is particularly noted in tribal populations living in foothills forested or conflict - affected areas. The malaria programme plans to scale up interventions in these areas along with innovative strategies.

Special strategy for P. vivax elimination (4)

India accounts for more than 50% of the estimated *P. vivax* cases in the world. Elimination of *P. vivax* from India is a serious challenge due to its magnitude as well as the need for a special strategy as *P. vivax* usually disappears from an area much after *P. falciparum,* because: (1) *P. vivax* hypnozoites prolong the parasite's lifespan and are difficult to detect; (2) RDTs currently available to detect *P. vivax* are less sensitive than RDTs for *P. falciparum* detection; (3) Radical treatment for *P. vivax* requires 14 days of primaquine therapy to kill the hypnozoites whereas treatment for *P. falciparum* can be completed in only 3 days; and (4) *P. vivax* strains have a longer incubation period.

The states and UTs with *P. vivax* preponderance will now initiate special measures for elimination of *P. vivax* by expanding bivalent RDTs and quality microscopy services to detect all *P. vivax* infections; ensuring compliance of the 14–days radical treatment by affected individuals; and tackling urban malaria by targeting *An. stephensi* by antilarval measures.

District as the unit of planning and implementation:

States and UTs should categorize their districts so that even if the given state/UT is not yet in the elimination phase, their districts with API < 1 could be considered eligible for initiating elimination phase activities. In addition, each district may sub-categorize its blocks into different phases based on their API; and further each block into its PHCs, PHC into SCs and SC to villages. This would facilitate some category 2 districts to start elimination activities in their blocks falling in category 1. Stratification may be done in this manner up to the subcentre level *(4)*.

Each district should stratify its PHCs and sub-centres (with their population) into the following five strata, as those with:

1. Zero cases
2. API > 0 to < 1
3. API 1 to < 2
4. API 2 to < 5
5. API ≥ 5

Strategies *(4)*

The overall objectives of the malaria elimination programme are rapid reduction of transmission in areas with high malaria incidence; interruption of malaria transmission in low transmission areas; and prevention of re-establishment of malaria in areas where transmission has been interrupted.

The broad strategies of the malaria elimination framework are:

- Early diagnosis and radical treatment
- Case-based surveillance and rapid response
- Integrated vector management (IVM)
  - Indoor residual spray (IRS)
  - Long-lasting insecticidal nets (LLINs) / Insecticide treated bed nets (ITNs)
  - Larval source management (LSM)
- Epidemic preparedness and early response
- Monitoring and evaluation
- Advocacy, coordination and partnerships
- Behaviour change communication and community mobilization
- Programme planning and management

The key interventions recommended for each category of states/UTs are detailed below.

Category 3 (Intensified control phase: States/UTs with API ≥ 1)

1. Massive scaling up of existing disease management and preventive approaches and tools, aimed at a significant reduction in the prevalence and incidence of malaria as well as associated deaths.
2. Screening of all fever cases suspected for malaria.
3. Classification of areas as per local malaria epidemiology and grading of areas as per risk of malaria transmission followed by implementation of tailored interventions.
4. Strengthening of intersectoral collaboration. Special interventions for high-risk groups such as tribal populations and populations residing in conflict affected or hard-to-reach areas.
5. One-stop centres or mobile clinics on fixed days in tribal or conflict affected areas to provide malaria diagnosis and treatment, and increasing community awareness with the involvement of other agencies and service providers as required.
6. Timely referral and treatment of severe malaria cases to reduce malaria-related mortality. Strengthening all district and sub-district hospitals in malaria endemic areas as per Indian Public Health Standards with facilities for management of severe malaria cases.
7. Establishment of a robust supply chain management system.
8. Maintenance of an optimum level of surveillance using appropriate diagnostic measures.
9. Equipping all health institutions (primary health care level and above), especially in high-risk areas, with microscopy facilities and RDTs for emergency use and injectable artemisinin derivatives for treatment of severe malaria.

Category 2 (Pre-elimination phase : States/UTs with API < 1, but some of their districts reporting API ≥ 1)

The states/UTs in pre-elimination phase are those close to entering the elimination phase. Therefore, malaria elimination interventions will be introduced with particular focus on setting up an elimination surveillance system and initiating elimination phase activities in those districts where the API has been reduced to less than 1 case per 1000 population at risk per year. The planning of elimination measures will be based on epidemiological investigation and classification of each malaria case and focus.

Category 1 (Elimination phase : States/UTs with API<1, and all their districts reporting API < 1)

1. All efforts will be directed at interrupting local transmission in all active foci of malaria.
2. Mandatory notification of each case of malaria from the private sector, other organized government sectors or any other health facility.
3. Adequate case-based surveillance and complete case management established and fully functional across the entire country to handle each case of malaria.
4. Investigation and classification of all foci of malaria.
5. A strict total coverage of all active foci by effective vector control measures.
6. Early detection and treatment of all cases of malaria by means of ACD and/or PCD to prevent onward transmission.
7. State and national level malaria elimination database established and made operational.
8. Implementation of interventions for effective screening, management and prevention of malaria among mobile and migrant populations.
9. Establishment of an effective epidemic forecasting and response system.
10. Ensuring rigorous quality assurance of all medicines and diagnostics.
11. Setting up a national-level reference laboratory to serve following two functions:
    (a) All positive and a fixed percentage of negative slides will be referred to this laboratory for confirmation of diagnosis and cross-checking. After elimination has been achieved in each State/UT, 100% of cases will be notified to this laboratory for confirmation of diagnosis. The laboratory will be notified immediately on all positive cases of malaria by each state/UT through either SMS, e-mail or telephone with information on name, gender, address (village and district), date and type of testing and type of parasite for each positive case of malaria so that a national level database can be maintained.
    (b) Training of master trainers and accreditation/certification of microscopists as per Indian Public Health Standards shall also be undertaken at this laboratory.
12. During investigation of foci, all suspected cases of malaria are to be screened for malaria. These could include household members, neighbours, school children, workplace colleagues and relatives.
13. Surveillance of special groups, migrant populations or populations residing in the vicinity of industrial areas are also to be covered under surveillance operations.

Category 0 (prevention of re-establishment phase)

When any area, whether a state/UT or a district within a state/UT has, achieved malaria elimination, the specific objectives will be as follows:

1. Detect any re-introduced case of malaria;
2. Notify immediately all detected cases of malaria;
3. Determine the underlying causes of resumed local transmission;
4. Apply rapid curative and preventive measures;
5. Prevent re-introduction and possible re-establishment of malaria transmission; and
6. Maintain malaria-free status in these areas.

Surveillance *(2, 4)*

The malaria surveillance system in India was initially set up in the early 1960s. The system has since been adapted to the needs of control and now monitors malaria incidence trends and geographic distribution. The aim is to target control interventions in high transmission areas and assessing their impact. Surveillance also plays a key role in the early detection of outbreaks.

Active case detection (ACD) is carried out in rural areas with blood smears collected by MPWs/ANM during fortnightly house visits. Passive case detection (PCD) is done in fever cases reporting to peripheral health volunteers/ASHAs and at sub-centres, malaria clinic, CHC, and other secondary and tertiary level health institutions that patients visit for treatment. ASHA and other volunteer workers provide diagnostic services by RDTs, and at PHCs by examination of blood smears. In villages where no ASHA or other volunteer has been trained and deployed for providing early diagnosis and effective treatment, ACD and case management is done by the MPWs.

The surveillance data of NVBDCP reflects malaria trends reasonably well because the ABER in the country as a whole has remained relatively constant at about 10%, and the surveillance system has not undergone any major changes. The ABER is, however, low in a few states, while in most of the high endemic areas it is much above 10%. Microscopy remains the best method of diagnosis on account of its high sensitivity and specificity. It is also more economical in facilities where large number of slides are examined daily.

There are about 100 million blood slides collected from fever cases in India annually from which about 1.5 million malaria cases are detected. The new norms for case management emphasize quality care for patients. The implementation of use of Rapid Diagnostic Tests (RDTs) and Artesunate combination therapy (ACT) and the improvements in service delivery is expected to attract greater number of fever cases to the programme in the coming years. The programme also plans to supply RDT kits to private providers in return for data. The current level of screening of 100 million fever cases will not be reduced as it is aimed to screen 10% of the population, even though the disease transmission is expected to reduce.

During 2003, the NVBDCP introduced the use of RDT for early diagnosis of malaria. In the year 2012, bivalent RDT were introduced in the programme to detect *P. vivax* and *P. falciparum*. Since then, the programme has procured and distributed RDTs to community level workers/volunteers who have been trained to use them to enable timely diagnosis in these areas. In remote and inaccessible rural and tribal areas, RDTs are now the established method of choice for malaria diagnosis.

Parameters of malaria surveillance

By definition, surveillance also implies the continuing scrutiny of all aspects of occurrence and spread of a disease, that are pertinent to effective control. Included in these are the systematic collection and evaluation of field investigations, etc. The following parameters are widely used in the epidemiological surveillance of malaria : (a) Annual parasite incidence (API); (b) Annual blood examination rate (ABER); (c) Annual *falciparum* incidence (AFI); (d) Slide positivity rate (SPR); and (e) Slide *falciparum* rate (SFR).

Sentinel surveillance

One of the weakness of the existing malaria surveillance system is the lack of articulation with hospitals, which means that severe malaria cases are not reported separately and that only a small fraction of malaria deaths are recorded. Therefore, sentinel surveillance is being established in high endemic districts, by selecting in each district, depending on its size, 1–3 sentinel sites in large hospitals for recording of all out-patient and in-patient cases of malaria, and malaria related deaths.

Case management

According to the revised drug policy, there is no scope of presumptive treatment in malaria control. The new drug policy of 2013 is being followed in the country. For further details please refer to page 307, chapter 5.

Integrated vector management (IVM)

The NVBDCP aims to achieve effective vector control by the appropriate biological, chemical and environmental interventions of proven efficacy, separately or in combination as appropriate to the area through the optimal use of resources. Efforts are made for collaboration with various public and private agencies and community participation for vector control. Integration of IVM is done by using identical vector control methods to control malaria and leishmaniasis in rural areas, and malaria and dengue in urban areas, to achieve cost-effectiveness and synergy. The IVM includes safe use of insecticides and monitoring of insecticide resistance. The measures of vector control and protection include :

- Measures to control adult mosquitoes : Indoor Residual Spray (IRS).
- Antilarval measures : chemical, biological and environmental.
- Personal protection : use of bed-nets, including insecticide treated nets.

The national malaria control programme is currently using IRS as the primary method of vector control in rural settings, and anti-larval measures in the urban areas. Insecticide treated bed-nets have been introduced in the programme and the programme envisages a scale up in their use as vector control option for full population coverage, which will replace IRS in areas, where operational factors indicate that this method alone will give sufficient impact.

As much as possible, the village is to be the unit of intervention, but in some districts, data available with knowledge of ecological conditions may make it more rational to classify whole sub-centre areas as high-risk areas. High risk areas and populations will be re-defined at least annually. Such villages shall be protected by indoor residual spray and insecticide treated nets and the coverage will be more than 80 per cent, whatever may be the intervention.

The population living in areas with API ≥ 5 is planned to be covered by LLINs and population living in endemic areas registering API ≥ 2 is covered with conventional net treated with insecticides and IRS. Conventional nets treated with insecticides will continue to be used in areas registering API 2 to 5. IRS is still the preferred method of vector control in areas with very hot summers and where ITNs are not acceptable to population.

A population of about 80 million is at present being covered by IRS in the country *(2)*. DDT is the insecticide of choice; in areas where the vector has shown resistance to DDT, the alternatives are malathion and synthetic pyrethroids. Two rounds of spraying are done for DDT and synthetic pyrethroids to provide protection during the entire transmission season, and in the case of malathion, three rounds of spraying are required. About 60 per cent of the high risk areas targeted under IRS are under coverage with DDT. The real coverage by IRS is, however, limited by the low community acceptance due to the white marks left on plastered surface, acrid smell associated with malathion, re-plastering of walls after completion of IRS etc. *(4)*.

Malaria paradigms/ecotypes *(2)*

The association between malaria and various ecological situations have been studied in India since the early part of the 20th century. There is considerable heterogenicity in malaria transmission characteristics between and within the states of the country, and many ecotypes/paradigms of malaria have been recognized. They are discussed in detail on page 301 chapter 5.

Presently, malaria burden in the country is highly concentrated in a few forest-tribal states and areas. In most of these states, vector control interventions are limited to villages with API ≥ 5 or other high risk criteria, due to resource constraints. The North-East has specific difficulties in implementation and monitoring due to various reasons. A large section of tribal population lives in inaccessible terrains, forest, hilly and riverbed conditions, and characterized by high degree of mobility, poverty, inadequate clothing, outdoor sleeping habits, forest based economy etc. Presence of efficient vectors, triple insecticide resistance and innumerous breeding sites add to the problem. Moreover, health infrastructure is generally found to be inadequate in these areas. All these factors maintain malaria as one of the most important cause of morbidity and mortality affecting tribal populations. The predominant parasite species in tribal areas is *P. falciparum* which is known to cause severity and lead to mortality if timely treatment is not provided.

A tribal-specific strategy is being envisaged to be implemented through a Tribal Malaria Action Plan (TMAP). Category 2 and 3 districts are planned to be covered initially. This will enable concentration of available resources to high endemic areas. The key interventions are as follows *(4)* :

1. Strengthening surveillance : Introduction of mobile-based surveillance, where routine health services/ facilities are not available.
2. Provision of hamlet-wise ASHAs instead of village-wise.
3. Wherever engagement of ASHAs is not possible, anganwadi workers of ICDS, faith healers, local medical/ health care providers, village headmen, PRIs or school teachers may be trained and provided relevant logistics to diagnose and treat malaria cases. In forest areas, involvement of forest department in diagnosis and treatment may be done.

4. In areas with civic disturbance, provision of well-informed and pre-scheduled mobile health services.
5. Involvement of locally available, credible NGOs.
6. Strengthening of PHCs with quality microscopy facilities.
7. Provision of diagnosis and treatment facilities by contractors/owners of development projects to the labours on site, should be made mandatory.
8. On the spot, species-specific radical treatment of all positive cases of malaria.
9. Identification of serious cases and early referral to specialized health facilities, ensuring free transport services.
10. Follow up and epidemiological tracking of all positive cases.
11. Mass screening of migrants wherever necessary.
12. Integrated Vector Management (IVM) for appropriate vector control. Prioritization of villages according to degree of risk for taking appropriate vector control measures (IRS/LLINs or treatment of community- owned bed nets with insecticides).
13. Social marketing to increase usage of bed nets.
14. Minor environmental engineering like cleaning/de-silting of drainage, filling pits and ditches, solid waste management through Village Health, Sanitation and Nutrition Committee (VHSNC) as well as MNREGA.
15. Regular and efficient supply chain management.
16. Intensive training for all cadres of staff, ASHAs/ community volunteers.
17. Community mobilization by utilizing traditional IEC/BCC tools and practices.

Table 2 summarizes the key indicators that will be used to measure the country's progress towards elimination at national and sub-national level.

Behaviour change communication (BCC)

BCC is a systematic process that motivates individuals, families and communities to change their inappropriate or unhealthy behaviour, or to continue a healthy behaviour. BCC is a key supportive strategy for malaria prevention and treatment under NVBDCP.

BCC is directed at : (a) early recognition of signs and symptoms of malaria; (b) early treatment seeking from appropriate provider; (c) adherence to treatment regimens; (d) ensuring protection of children and pregnant women; (e) use of ITNs/LLINs; and (f) acceptance of IRS, etc.

Anti-malaria month campaign

Anti-malaria month is observed every year in the month of June throughout the country, prior to the onset of monsoon and transmission season, to enhance the level of awareness and encourage community participation through mass media campaign and inter-personal communication and consolidate inter-sectoral collaborative efforts with other government departments, corporate and voluntary agencies at national, state and district levels.

Interaction of malaria control with other health programmes

The other main public health programmes related to malaria control are :

(1) Integrated Disease Surveillance Project (IDSP) : The project, with weekly fever alerts is increasingly providing the early warning signals on malaria outbreaks.

(2) Other vector borne diseases : Dengue and malaria control activities overlap in many urban areas, malaria and kala-azar in a few districts of Jharkhand, and malaria and filariasis in some areas including a few districts of Odisha.

(3) Reproductive and child health : Antenatal care services are utilized in distribtuion of LLINs to pregnant women in some areas of the country. Janani Suraksha Yojana also makes provision of bed-nets distribution to pregnant women. Changes in the malaria case management norms have been included in the Integrated Management of Neonatal and Childhood Illness.

TABLE 2

Key indicators to measure progress towards malaria elimination

	IMPACT
1	Number and incidence rate of confirmed malaria cases classified according to sex, age, parasite species and other relevant parameters.
2	Number and incidence of severe malaria cases as well as case fatality rate.
3	Number of malaria cases in pregnancy.
4	Number and type of malaria foci(in areas eligible for elimination).
5	Number of confirmed deaths due to malaria.
6	Number of states/UTs which have eliminated malaria and are currently in the phase of prevention of re-establishment of local transmission.
7	Number of states/UTs which are in elimination phase.
8	Number of states/UTs which are in pre-elimination phase.
9	Number of states/UTs which are in intensified control phase.
	OUTCOME
1	Proportion of population at risk who slept under insecticide-treated net/LLIN in the previous night.
2	Proportion of population at risk protected by indoor residual spraying within the past 12 months.
3	Proportion of patients with confirmed malaria who received anti-malarial treatment as per national policy.
4	Proportion of cases investigated and classified(in areas eligible for elimination).
5	Proportion of foci investigated and classified(in areas eligible for elimination).
6	Proportion of expected monthly reports received from health facilities at the national and subnational level.

Source: *(5)*

Achievements under National Framework for Malaria Elimination in India *(6)* :

1. India has made considerable progress in malaria reduction. The country has achieved a reduction of 84% in malaria morbidity and 76% in malaria mortality between 2015 and 2020.
2. India has achieved National Annual Parasite Incidence (API) less than 1 per 1000 population in 2012. In 2020, National API was 0.14 per 1000 population. In 2020, total 34 States/UTs have achieved API less than 1 except Chhattisgarh (1.19) and Mizoram (6.82) have API more than 1. Only 32 districts have Annual Parasite Incidence (API) one and above. 116 districts in the country have reported 'zero malaria case'.
3. Among 177 tribal districts, there has been 86.6% reduction in malaria morbidity and 83.4% reduction in malaria mortality between 2015 and 2020.
4. Malaria has been made notifiable in 31 States/ UTs (Andhra Pradesh, Arunachal Pradesh, Assam, Chhattisgarh, Goa, Gujarat, Haryana, Himachal Pradesh, Jammu & Kashmir, Jharkhand, Karnataka, Kerala, Madhya Pradesh, Manipur, Mizoram, Nagaland, Odisha, Punjab, Rajasthan, Sikkim, Tamil Nadu, Telangana, Tripura Uttar Pradesh, Uttarakhand, West Bengal, Puducherry, Chandigarh, Daman & Diu, D&N Haveli and Lakshadweep).
5. Till September 2021, 28 States have constituted State Task Force and District Task Force for malaria elimination. Remaining States/UTs are under process of constituting State Task Force and District Task Force.
6. Malaria microscopy, the gold standard for malaria elimination, has also been strengthened by national refresher trainings and certification of a core group of laboratory technicians from different states.
7. Award to Districts/States for achieving 'Zero indigenous case status' and maintaining it for three consecutive years on attaining sub-national malaria elimination, instituted for Year 1 and Year 3.
8. Mass Screening and Treatment (MSAT) campaign has been initiated in the high burden districts of Tripura, Mizoram and Chhattisgarh to break the ongoing transmission cycle of malaria in asymptomatic carriers.
9. Availability of Bivalent Rapid Diagnostic Tests (RDTs) and anti-malarials with ASHAs for early diagnosis and prompt treatment at community level.

During the last 6 years, 9.7 crore LLINs have been distributed in the high malaria endemic areas of various states/UTs.

High Burden and High Impact (HBHI) initiative of WHO has been started in four states i.e. West Bengal, Jharkhand, Chhattisgarh and Madhya Pradesh in July, 2019 for intensification of malaria elimination activities in these states.

Setting up of health web based reporting system for the whole country on Integrated Health Information Platform (IHIP) - malaria included, and mapping of high malaria-prone areas using GIS maps and hotspots.

Global Fund Supported Malaria Elimination Project *(6)* :

The Global Fund to fight AIDS, Tuberculosis & Malaria (GFATM) is supporting malaria control in India since 2005. GF supported Intensified Malaria Control Projects (IMCP) I to III were implemented from July 2005–December 2017. From January 2018–March 2021 Intensified Malaria Elimination Project (IMEP) was implemented in 7 North-eastern states and Madhya Pradesh. At present, Intensified Malaria Elimination Project–2 is being implemented in 7 North-eastern states (Arunachal Pradesh, Assam, Meghalaya, Mizoram, Nagaland, Manipur& Tripura), Odisha, Jharkhand and Chhattisgarh, covering 166 million population in 155 districts within the existing framework of National Vector Borne Disease Control Programme. At present Global Fund supports for LLINs, human resources, monitoring etc.

(B) ELIMINATION OF LYMPHATIC FILARIASIS

The disease is endemic in 256 districts in 16 states and 5 UTs. According to recent estimates about 630 million people are exposed to the risk of infection *(7)*.

The National Filaria Control Programme has been in operation since 1955. In June 1978, the operational component of the NFCP was merged with the urban malaria scheme for maximum utilization of available resources. The training and research components, however, continue to be with the Director, National Institute of Communicable Diseases, Delhi.

Training in filariology is being given at three Regional Filaria Training and Research Centres situated at Calicut (Kerala), Rajahmundry (A.P.) and Varanasi (U.P.) under the National Institute of Communicable Diseases, Delhi. Besides, 12 headquarters bureaux are functioning at the state level.

Filaria control strategy includes vector control through anti larval operations, source reduction, detection and treatment of microfilaria carriers, morbidity management and IEC. National Filaria Control Programme is being implemented through 206 filaria control units, 199 filaria clinics and 27 survey units, primarily in endemic urban towns. In rural areas anti filaria medicines and morbidity management services are provided through primary health care system.

In India, the National Health Policy (2002), envisages elimination of lymphatic filariasis (ELF) by 2015 and National Health Policy 2017 to maintain elimination status. The elimination is defined as "lymphatic filariasis ceases to be public health problem, when the number of microfilaria carriers is less than 1 per cent and the children born after initiation of ELF are free from circulating antigenaemia (presence of adult filaria worm in human body).

The strategy of lymphatic filariasis elimination is through :

(a) Annual Mass Drug Administration (MDA) of single dose of antifilarial drug for 5 years or more to the eligible population (except pregnant women, children below 2 years of age and seriously ill persons) to interrupt transmission of the disease.

(b) Home based management of lymphoedema cases and up-scaling of hydrocele operations in identified CHCs/ district hospitals/medical colleges.

To achieve elimination of lymphatic filariasis, during 2004 the Govt. of India launched annual MDA with single dose of DEC tablets in addition to scaling-up home based foot care and hydrocele operation. The co-administration of DEC + Albendazole has been upscaled since 2007. The programme covered 202 districts in 2004 whereas by the year 2007, all the 250 LF endemic districts were covered. The mass drug administration starts in the month of November. Presently, antifilarial drug i.e., DEC + Albendazole (DA)/ Ivermectin + DEC + Albendazole (IDA) is administered.

The achievements of the programme are as follows :

Key achievements Status 2020

Stage in the programme	Total endemic districts in 2020
Total Lymphatic Filariasis endemic districts	272
Districts conducted MDA in 2020	97
DEC + Albendazole administered	89
Ivermectin + DEC + Albendazole administered	8
Districts cleared 1st Transmission Assessment Survey (TAS) and Stopped MDA	98
Districts cleared 2nd Transmission Assessment Survey (TAS)	88
Districts cleared 3rd Transmission Assessment Survey (TAS)	42

Source : *(6)*

The line listing of lymphoedema and hydrocele cases were initiated since 2004 by door-to-door survey in filaria endemic districts. The updated figure till December 2014 reveals about 12.5 lakh cases with clinical manifestation of filariasis were line listed which includes 8.7 lakh cases of lymphoedema and 3.8 lakh cases of hydrocele. Initiation has also been taken to demonstrate the simple washing of foot to maintain hygiene for prevention of secondary bacterial and fungal infection in chronic lymphoedema cases, so that the patients get relief from frequent acute attacks.

The microfilaria survey in all the implementation units is being done through night blood survey before MDA. The survey is done in 4 sentinel and 4 random sites collecting total 4000 slides (500 from each site). There is definite evidence of microfilaria reduction in the MDA districts. However, the coverage of population with MDA should be above 80 per cent persistently for 5–6 years, which would reduce microfilaria load in the community, and thereby, interrupt the transmission *(3)*.

(C) KALA-AZAR

Kala-azar is now endemic in 33 districts of Bihar, 4 districts of Jharkhand, 11 districts of West Bengal and 6 districts of Uttar Pradesh, besides sporadic cases in few other districts of Uttar Pradesh. A centrally sponsored programme was launched in 1990–91. This has brought down the incidence of the disease from 77,102 cases in 1992 to 2,052 cases in 2020 *(6)*.

The strategies for Kala-azar elmination are : (a) Enhanced case detection and complete treatment including introduction of rK39 rapid diagnostic kits and oral drug Miltefosine for treatment of Kala-azar cases; (b) Interruption of transmission through vector control. It has been decided to replace DDT with synthetic pyrethroid for the purpose of fogging to eliminate sandfly, as the insect is becoming resistant to DDT; (c) Communication for behavioural impact and intersectoral convergence; (d) Capacity building; (e) Monitoring, supervision and evaluation; and (f) Research guidelines on prevention and control of Kala-azar have been developed and circulated to the states.

ACTIVE CASE SEARCH : The frequency of case searches has been increased from a single annual case search to quarterly case searches. The active case searches are carried out during a fortnight designated as the "Kala-azar Fortnight", during which the peripheral health workers and volunteers are engaged to make door-to-door search and refer the cases conforming to the case definition of kala-azar and PKDL to the treatment centres for definitive diagnosis and treatment *(3)*.

An incentive amount of Rs. 300 is provided to ASHA for identifying each case of kala-azar and Rs. 100 for ensuring one round and Rs. 200 for two rounds of insecticide spraying. Even the patient being treated in the hospital will be given Rs. 500 as compensation of daily wage for the time he spends in the hospital during the treatment for kala-azar and Rs. 2,000 for PKDL. This revised strategy of total eradication of kala-azar was launched on 2nd September 2014.

The new strategy also includes introduction of Rapid Diagnostic Kit developed by ICMR into the programme and single dose treatment with Liposomal Amphotericin B, which is given intravenously in 10 mg/kgbw dose. It is to reduce the human reservoir of infection. WHO will supply the drug free of cost *(8)*.

Achievements *(6)*

In 2020, out of 633 endemic blocks, only 16 blocks (12 blocks in Jharkhand & 4 blocks in Bihar) reported above elimination threshold. Remaining 97.5 per cent blocks achieved the elimination target. Till August 2021, only two blocks of Jharkhand have reported above elimination threshold. West Bengal and Uttar Pradesh have sustained the elimination target since 2017 & 2019, respectively. There has been 40 per cent decline in KA cases up to August 2021, compared to corresponding period of 2020. PKDL cases have increased in (Aug) 2021 by 17 per cent compared to corresponding period of 2020.

(D) JAPANESE ENCEPHALITIS

Japanese encephalitis is a disease with high mortality rate and those who survive do so with various degrees of neurological complications. During the last few years it has become a major public health problem. States of Andhra Pradesh, West Bengal, Assam, Tamil Nadu, Karnataka, Bihar, Maharashtra, Manipur, Haryana, Kerala and Uttar Pradesh are reporting maximum number of cases.

The strategies for prevention and control of Japanese encephalitis include strengthening of the surveillance activities through sentinel sites in tertiary health care institutions, early diagnosis and proper case management, integrated vector control, particularly personal protection and use of larvivorous fishes, capacity building and behaviour change communication. As the JE vectors are outdoor resters, indoor residual spray is not effective. The government of India provides need–based assistance to the states, including support for training programmes and social mobilization.

As there is no specific cure for this disease, early case management is very important to minimize the risk of complications and death. JE vaccination is recommended for children between 1 to 15 years of age. In addition, health education through different media and interpersonal communication for the community is crucial. Emphasis should be given on keeping pigs away from human dwellings, or in pigsties, particularly during dusk to dawn, which is the biting time of vector mosquitoes. Use of clothes which cover the body fully to avoid mosquito bites are advocated. Use of bed-nets is also very important precaution. Since early reporting of case is important to avoid complications, the community should be given full information about the signs and symptoms of the disease, and the health facilities available at health centres/hospitals. The states are advised to use malathion for outdoor fogging as outbreak control measure in the affected areas *(9)*. Epidemiological monitoring of the disease for effective implementation of preventive and control measure and technical support is provided on request by the state health authorities.

(E) DENGUE FEVER/ DENGUE HAEMORRHAGIC FEVER

During 1996, an outbreak of dengue was reported in Delhi. Since then dengue has been reported from other states also. In view of this major outbreak of the disease a "Guideline of Preparation of Contingency Plan in case of outbreak/epidemic of Dengue/Dengue haemorrhagic fever'' was prepared and sent to all the states. It includes all the important aspects of control measures like identification of outbreak, demarcation of affected area, containment of outbreak, case management, vector control, IEC activities about Do's and Dont's for prevention of dengue, monitoring and reporting etc.

Since early reporting of cases is crucial to avoid any complication and mortality, the community is given full information about the signs and symptoms as well as availability of health services at health centres/hospitals. Alerting the hospitals for making adequate arrangements for management of dengue/dengue haemorrhagic fever cases has also been advised.

Government of India in consultation with states has identified 521 sentinel surveillance hospitals with laboratory support for augmentation of diagnostic facilities in the endemic states. Further, for advanced diagnosis and back-up support 14 Apex Referral Laboratories have been identified and linked with sentinel surveillance hospitals. To make these functional IgM capture ELISA test kits are provided through National Institute of Virology, Pune free of cost. Contingency grant is also provided to meet the operational costs.

For early diagnosis ELISA based NSI kits have been introduced under the programme which can detect the cases from 1st day of infection. IgM capture ELISA tests can detect the cases after 5th day of infection.

The GOI has taken the following steps for prevention and control of dengue *(6)* :

- Monitoring the situation through reports received from state health authorities.
- A mid-term plan for prevention and control of dengue has been developed in 2011 and circulated to the states for implementation. The main components of mid term plan for prevention and control of dengue are as follows :
  - (a) *Surveillance :* Disease and entomological surveillance.
  - (b) *Case mangement :* Laboratory diagnosis and clinical management.
  - (c) *Vector management :* Environmental management for source reduction, chemical control, personal protection and legislation.
  - (d) *Outbreak response :* Epidemic preparedness and media management.
  - (e) *Capacity building :* Training, strengthening human resource and operational research.
  - (f) *Behavioural change communication :* Social mobilization, and information, education and communication (IEC).
  - (g) *Inter-sectoral coordination :* with ministries of urban development, rural development, panchayati raj, surface transport and education sector.
  - (h) *Monitoring and supervision :* Analysis of reports, review, field visit and feed-back.

(F) CHIKUNGUNYA FEVER

Chikungunya fever is a debilitating non-fatal viral illness, re-emerging in the country after a gap of three decades. Govt. of India is continuously monitoring the situation. Guidelines for prevention and control of the disease have been prepared. Since same vector is involved in the transmission of dengue and chikungunya, strategies for transmission risk reduction by vector control are also the same. Support in the form of logistics and funds are provided to the states.

For carrying out proactive surveillance and enhancing diagnostic facilities for chikungunya, the 521 sentinel surveillance hospitals involved in dengue in the affected states also carry out chikungunya tests. The diagnostic kits are provided through National Institute of Virology, Pune, by the central government.

NATIONAL LEPROSY "ERADICATION" PROGRAMME

The National Leprosy Control Programme (NLCP) has been in operation since 1955, as a centrally aided programme to achieve control of leprosy through early detection of cases and DDS (dapsone) monotherapy on an ambulatory basis. The NLCP moved ahead initially at a slow pace, presumably for want of clear-cut policies or operational objectives for nearly two decades *(10)*. The programme gained momentum during the Fourth Five Year Plan after it was made a centrally-sponsored programme. In 1980 the Government of India declared its resolve to "eradicate" leprosy by the year 2000 and constituted a Working Group to advise accordingly. The Working Group submitted its report in 1982 and recommended a revised strategy based on multi-drug chemotherapy aimed at leprosy "eradication" through reduction in the quantum of infection in the population, reduction in the sources of infection, and breaking the chain of transmission of disease. In 1983 the control programme was redesignated National Leprosy "Eradication" Programme with the goal of eradicating the disease by the turn of the century. The aim was to reduce case load to 1 or less than 1 per 10,000 population.

To strengthen the process of elimination of leprosy in the country, the first World Bank supported project was introduced in 1993. On completion of this project, the 2nd phase of project with World Bank support was started in 2001–02 which ended in December 2004. Since then, the programme is being continued with Government of India funds with technical support from WHO and International Federation of Anti-Leprosy Association (ILEP) organizations. The programme has been integrated with general health care system in 2002–03, since then leprosy diagnosis and treatment services are available at all PHCs and government hospitals.

The components of the programme are as follows :

(1) Decentralized integrated leprosy services through general health care system;
(2) Capacity building of all general health services functionaries;
(3) Intensified information, education and communication;
(4) Prevention of disability and medical rehabilitation; and
(5) Intensified monitoring and supervision.

After introduction of MDT, the recorded case load of leprosy came down from 57.6 cases per 10,000 population in 1981 to less than one at the national level in December 2005, and the country could achieve the goal of leprosy elimination at national level as set by the National Health Policy (2002).

34 states/UTs achieved the status of leprosy elimination. Only 2 states/UTs viz. Chhattisgarh and Dadra & Nagar Haveli are yet to achieve elimination. Odisha, who has achieved elimination status earlier, show PR > 1 per 1000 population *(6)*.

A total of 209 high endemic districts were identified for special action during 2012–13. 1792 blocks and 150 urban areas were identified for special activities, i.e., house to house survey along with IEC and capacity building of the workers and volunteers *(1)*.

Major initiatives

Major initiatives taken are as follows :

(1) More focus has now been given to new case detection than prevalence which only gives the number of cases on record at a point in time. The new case detection rate is the main indicator for programme monitoring.

(2) Treatment completion rate has been taken as an important indicator, to be calculated by states at yearly basis.

(3) More emphasis is being given on providing disability prevention and medical rehabilitation (DPMR) services to leprosy affected persons. The aid provided is as follows :

(a) Dressing materials, supportive medicines and ulcer kits are provided to leprosy affected persons with ulcers and wounds. These services are also provided to leprosy affected persons residing in self settled colonies.

(b) Micro-cellular rubber footwear is provided for protection of insensitive feet. 41 NGOs in the country and 42 Government Medical Colleges have been strengthened for providing reconstructive surgery services to leprosy affected persons for correction of their disability, thus totalling to 83 centres for conducting reconstructive surgeries in the country.

(c) An amount of Rs. 8,000/- is provided as incentive to each leprosy affected person from BPL family undergoing reconstructive surgery in these identified institutions to compensate for loss of wages.

(d) Support is also provided to government institutions/ PMR centres in the form of Rs 5,000/- per reconstructive surgery conducted.

(4) ASHAs have been involved in bringing out suspected leprosy cases from their villages for diagnosis and treatment at PHC and follow-up of confirmed cases for their treatment completion. To facilitate the involvement of ASHA in the programme, they are being paid incentive money as below *(6)* :

(a) On confirmed diagnosis of case brought by them – Rs. 250/-.

(b) On completion of full course of treatment of the case within specified time – PB leprosy case – Rs. 400/-, and MB leprosy case – Rs. 600/-.

(c) An early case before onset of any visible deformity – Rs. 250/-.

(d) A new case with visible deformity in hands, feet or eye – Rs. 200/-.

Activities to be performed by ASHA are as follows :

(a) Search for suspected cases of leprosy i.e. before any sign of disability appears. Such early detection will help in prevention of disability and also cut down transmission potential. ASHA based surveillance for leprosy suspects (ABSULS) was launched on 1st July 2019 *(11)*.

(b) Follow-up all cases for completion of treatment in scheduled time. During follow up visit, also look for symptoms of any reaction due to leprosy and refer them to the Health Workers/PHC for treatment. This will again reduce chances of disability occurring in cases under treatment.

(c) Advise and motivate self-care practices by disabled cases for proper care of their hands and feet during the follow-up period. This will improve quality of life of the affected persons and prevent deterioration of disabilities.

(d) Spreading awareness.

(e) There are 612 self settled colonies in the country where more than 50,000 leprosy affected persons reside. Free medical facilities like care of ulcers, self care training, counselling and MCR footwear are provided to leprosy affected persons residing in these colonies through para-medical workers/NGOs on weekly/fortnightly basis.

6. Intensive IEC campaign with a theme "Towards Leprosy Free India" has been carried out towards further reduction of leprosy burden in the community, early reporting of cases and their treatment completion, provision of quality leprosy services and reduction of stigma and discrimination against leprosy affected persons. Awareness generation activities are carried out through mass media and local media.

Disability prevention and medical rehabilitation (DPMR)

The main activities carried out under DPMR are as follows *(12)* :

(1) Implementation of DPMR activities as per guidelines and reporting its outcome eg. treatment of leprosy reaction, ulcers, physiotherapy, reconstructive surgery and, providing MCR footwear.

(2) Integrating DPMR services – There are provision of services to persons with disability by various departments under different ministries. Convergence of NLEP services into NRHM facilitates this integration.

(3) To develop a referral system to provide prevention of disability services to all leprosy disabled persons in an integrated set-up.

The DPMR activities are planned to be carried out in a three tier system i.e. the primary level care (First level), secondary level care (Second level) and the tertiary level care (Third level). The primary level care institutions are all PHCs, CHCs, Sub-divisional hospitals and urban leprosy centres/dispensaries. The secondary level care institutions are all District Head Quarter Hospitals and District Nucleus Units. The tertiary level care institutions are :

1. Central Government Institutes (CLTRI Chengalpattu and RLTRI at Aska/Gauripur/Raipur).
2. ICMR Institute JALMA, Agra.
3. ILEP supported Leprosy Hospitals.
4. All PMR Institutes and departments of medical colleges.

The other support units are :

(1) Orthopaedics and plastic surgery departments of medical colleges.

(2) Identified NGO institutions.

(3) All National Institutes under Ministry of Social Justice and Empowerment.

(4) Contractual surgeons skilled in RCS and Rehabilitation Programmes.

The referral system in NLEP is as summarized in Fig. 1.

Decentralization and institutional development : Integration of leprosy services into the general health care system has been completed. Services are available from all PHCs, and other

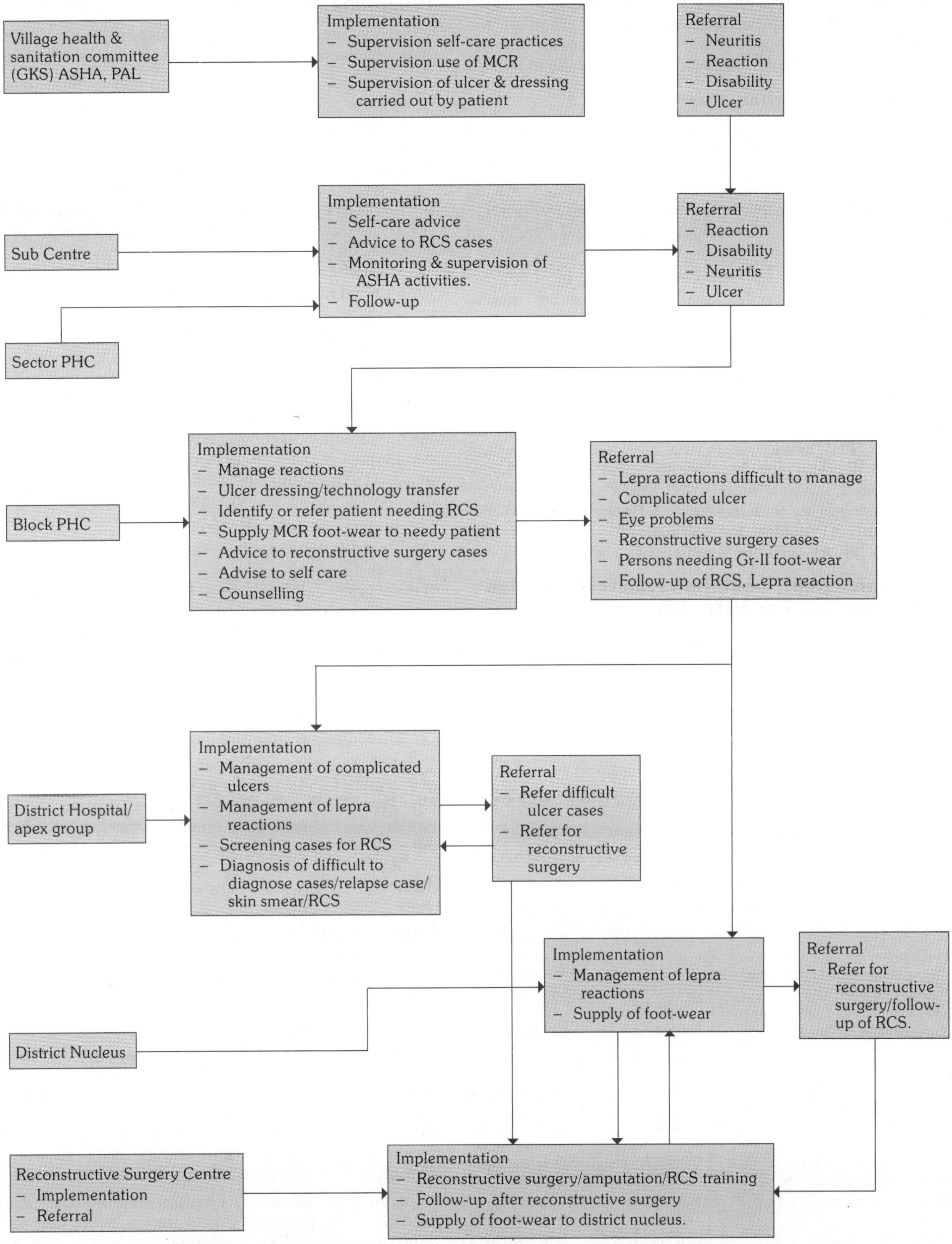

FIG. 1

Referral System in NLEP

Source : *(12)*

health centres where a medical officer is available. District nucleus has been formed to supervise and monitor the programme. State leprosy societies formed will merge with the state health society under the National Rural Health Mission.

Services in the urban areas *(13)*

The health services in the urban areas differ from the rural areas because of non-availability of infrastructure like PHC and manpower for providing services upto domiciliary level. The services in urban areas are provided mainly through institutional level. Multiple organizations provide health services in urban localities without much of coordination amongst them.

More number of cases are detected in urban localities due to migration of people,, availability of good quality institutions with easy accessibility, but treatment completion rate is less as compared to rural areas.

For the implementation of special action under the plan, about 524 urban localities have been identified out of 4,388 urban areas (census 2011). These localities are having population more than 100,000. Remaining areas will be covered by PHC services as in rural areas *(13)*. These urban areas are divided into 4 categories : (a) Town and city (population 1 lac to 5 lacs) – 432 areas; (b) Medium city (population >5 lac to 1 million) – 53 areas; (c) Mega city (population >1 million to 4.5 million) – 34 areas; and (d) Areas with >4.5 million population – 5 areas.

Programme Implementation Plan for 12th Plan period (2012–13 to 2016–17)

As the disease is still prevalent with moderate endemicity in about 15 per cent of the country, the plan objectives are set as follows *(13)*.

a. Elimination of leprosy i.e. prevalence of less than 1 case per 10,000 population in all districts of the country.
b. Strengthen disability prevention and medical rehabilitation of persons affected by leprosy.
c. Reduction in the level of stigma associated with leprosy.

Targets *(13)*

The plan targets are as shown in Table 3.

TABLE 3
Targets for the plan period 2012–13 to 2016–17

Indicator	Baseline (2011–12)	Targets (by March 2017)
Prevalence Rate (PR) < 1/10,000	543 districts (84.6%)	642 districts (100%)
Annual New Case Detection Rate (ANCDR) <10/100,000 population	445 districts (69.3%)	642 districts (100%)
Cure rate multi bacillary leprosy cases (MB)	90.56%	>95%
Cure rate pauci bacillary leprosy cases (PB)	95.28%	>97%
Gr.II disability rate in percentage of new cases	3.04% *	35% reduction 1.98%
Stigma reduction	Percentage reported (NSS 2010–11)**	50% reduction over the percentage reported by NSS

* Gr-II disability rate among new cases per million population to be reduced by 35% i.e. from 3 (2011–12) to 2 per million population by end of the 12th Plan.
** Based on the National Sample Survey (NSS) report, 2010–11.

Programme strategy *(13)*

To achieve the objectives of the plan, the main strategies to be followed are :

- Integrated leprosy services through general health care system.
- Early detection and complete treatment of new leprosy cases.
- Carrying out house-hold contact survey for early detection of cases.
- Involvement of Accredited Social Health Activist (ASHA) in the detection and completion of treatment of leprosy cases on time.
- Strengthening of disability prevention and medical rehabilitation (DPMR) services.

Case detection and management *(13)*

It is expected that the new cases will continue to occur regularly but the people are still hesitant to come forward to get themselves diagnosed and treated due to the stigma associated with the disease. Detection of the new cases at the early stage is the only solution to cut down the transmission potential in the community, and also to provide relief to the leprosy affected persons by preventing disabilities. It is therefore suggested that the states will draw up innovative plans :

(i) To improve access to services.
(ii) To involve women including leprosy affected persons in case detection.
(iii) To organize skin camps for detecting leprosy patients while providing services for other skin conditions.
(iv) To undertake contact survey to identify the source in the neighbourhood of each child or multibacillary case.
(v) To increase awareness through the ANM, AWW, ASHA and other health workers visiting the villages and people affected by leprosy, to motivate leprosy affected persons for early reporting to the medical officer.

Integrated leprosy services through all the primary health care facilities will continue to be provided in the rural areas. However, for providing technical support to the primary health care system, to strengthen the quality of services being provided, a team of dedicated workers including medical officer and para-medical workers are placed at district level. This will be known as "District Leprosy Cell".

Three pronged strategy was introduced in the National Leprosy Eradication Programme from 2016–2017. The components of the strategy are:

1. Leprosy Case Detection Campaign (LCDC);
2. Focused Leprosy Campaign; and
3. Special plan for hard to reach areas.

During 2016–17, LCDC was carried out in 163 districts of 20 states, wherein 34,672 cases were detected and were put on treatment. The activity was aimed at early case detection and timely treatment. The success of the campaign, as shown by the drastic decline of grade 2 disability, led to continuation of LCDC and during 2017–18 about 305 districts in 23 states were identified for LCDC phase I *(14)*.

In the year 2016–17, Focused Leprosy Campaign was carried out by house to house survey in the village/ urban areas (covering 300 households) wherein one case of grade 2 disability due to leprosy was detected.

The purpose of the special plan for hard to reach areas is to find the cases in population in areas of difficult terrains, naxalite affected areas and other geographically difficult locations *(14)*.

Sparsh leprosy awareness campaign

Sparsh leprosy awareness campaign was launched in the year 2017 through Gram Sabhas and carried out with the help of Panchayat and Village Health and Sanitation Community. The aim was to generate awareness, reduce stigma and improve self-reporting of the cases. The campaign activity was carried out in 60 per cent of the total villages across India *(7)*. The campaign continued during the year 2018.

Survey education and treatment (SET) scheme

Under the SET scheme, the NGOs are presently involved in disability prevention and ulcer care, IEC, referral of suspected cases, referral for reconstruction surgery (RCS), research and rehabilitation. NGO support is mainly required for follow-up of under treatment cases in urban locations and difficult to reach areas.

Incentive to patient *(7)*

An incentive of Rs. 8000/- will be paid to all patients affected by leprosy undergoing major reconstructive surgery irrespective of their financial status. The payment will be made by the district leprosy officer. As on January 2017, there were 115 recognized RCS centres (61 Government and 54 NGO) in the country.

Information, education and communication (IEC/BCC)

The IEC strategy during the 12th plan period was focus on communication for behavioural changes in general public against the stigma and discrimination against the leprosy affected persons. Making the public aware about the availability of MDT, correction of deformity through surgery and that the leprosy affected person can live a normal life with the family.

Research into the basic problems of leprosy is also part of the activities of the NLEP. This is mainly carried out in the Government sector, viz. the Central JALMA Institute of Leprosy at Agra and the Central Leprosy Teaching and Training Institute at Chengalpattu, Chennai supported by Regional Training and Referral Institutes at Aska (Orissa), Raipur (Chhattisgarh) and Gouripur (West Bengal).

The present day strategy *(6, 15)* :

1. A well laid out operational strategy for active case detection and regular surveillance has been put in place, both in rural and urban areas, through ASHAs and frontline workers in order to ensure detection of leprosy cases on regular basis and at an early stage in order to prevent grade II disabilities.
2. Leprosy screening has been integrated with Rashtriya Bal Swasthya Karyakram (RBSK) and Rashtriya Kishore Swasthya Karyakram (RKSK) for screening of children (0–18 years).
3. Leprosy screening has been integrated with the activities of Comprehensive Primary Health Care under Ayushman Bharat - Health and Wellness Centre (AB-HWC) for screening of people above 30 years of age.
4. Contact tracing is done and Post Exposure Prophylaxis (PEP) is administered to the eligible contacts of Index case (Person diagnosed with leprosy) in order to interrupt the chain of transmission at the community level.
5. Various services are provided under the programme for Disability Prevention and Medical Rehabilitation (DPMR) i.e., reaction management, provision of Microcellular Rubber (MCR) footwear, aids & appliances, self-care kits etc.
6. Reconstructive Surgeries (RCS) are conducted at District Hospitals/Medical Colleges/ Central Leprosy Institutes, and welfare allowance of Rs 8,000 is paid to each patient undergoing RCS.

ILEP Agencies

The International Federation of Anti-Leprosy Associations is actively involved as partner in NLEP. In India, ILEP is constituted by 10 agencies viz. The Leprosy Mission, Damien Foundation of India Trust, Netherland Leprosy Relief, German Leprosy Relief Association, Lepra India, ALES, AIFO, Fontilles–India, AERF–India and American Leprosy Mission. ILEP is providing support in the form of planning, monitoring and supervision of the programme, capacity building of general health care staff, IEC, providing re-constructive surgery services and socio-economic rehabilitation of persons affected with leprosy. 36 NGOs conducting re-constructive surgeries for disability correction in leprosy affected persons are also supported by ILEP *(1)*.

Non Government Organizations have been involved in the programme for many decades and have provided valuable contribution in reducing the burden of leprosy. Presently, 54 NGOs are getting grant-in-aid from Government of India under SET scheme. NGOs serve in remote, inaccessible areas, urban slums, industrial/labour population and other marginalized population groups. IEC, prevention of disability, case detection and referral, and follow-up for treatment completion are some important activities taken up by NGOs *(1)*.

The leprosy scene in India is passing through an important phase of transition – from a high burden country of leprosy to a relatively low burden country, from a partially vertical programme to a more integrated one, from a programme aimed at increase in coverage for leprosy services to one of sustaining quality services, and from centralization to decentralization *(16)*.

WHO has announced Global Leprosy Strategy 2016–2020 : "Accelerating towards a leprosy-free world" for further reducing the disease burden due to leprosy. Please refer to page 363 for details.

NATIONAL TB ELIMINATION PROGRAMME

National Tuberculosis Programme (NTP) has been in operation since 1962. However, the treatment success rates were unacceptably low and the death and default rates remained high. Spread of multidrug resistant TB was threatening to further worsen the situation.

In 1993, in order to overcome these lacunae, the Government of India decided to give a new thrust to TB control activities by revitalizing the NTP, with the assistance from international agencies. The Revised National TB Control Programme (RNTCP) thus formulated, adopted the internationally recommended Directly Observed Treatment Short-course (DOTS) strategy, as the most systematic and cost-effective approach to revitalize the TB control programme in India. Political and administrative commitment, to ensure the provision of organized and comprehensive TB control services was obtained. Adoption of smear microscopy for reliable and early diagnosis was introduced in a decentralized manner in the general health services. DOTS was adopted as a strategy for provision of treatment to increase the treatment completion rates. Supply of drugs was also strengthened to provide assured supply of drugs to meet the requirements of the system *(17)*.

The objectives of the RNTCP are :

1. Achievement of at least 85 per cent cure rate of infectious cases of tuberculosis, through DOTS involving peripheral health functionaries; and
2. Augmentation of case finding activities through quality sputum microscopy to detect at least 70 per cent of estimated cases.

The revised strategy was introduced in the country in a phased manner. The RNTCP has expanded rapidly over the years and since March 2006, it covers the whole country. The RNTCP has now entered into it's second phase in which the programme aims to consolidate the gains made to date, to widen services in terms of activities and access and to sustain the achievements. The new initiatives and the wider collaboration with other sectors aim to provide standardized treatment and diagnostic facilities to all TB patients irrespective of the health care facility from which they seek treatment. The RNTCP also envisages improved access to marginalized groups such as urban slum dwellers and tribal groups etc.

RNTCP is built upon infrastructure already established by the previous national tuberculosis programme, while incorporating the elements of the internationally recommended DOTS.

DOTS strategy adopted by Revised National TB Control Programme initially had the following five main components:

1. Political will and administrative commitment.
2. Diagnosis by quality assured sputum smear microscopy.
3. Adequate supply of quality assured short course chemotherapy drugs.
4. Directly observed treatment.
5. Systematic monitoring and accountability.

In 2006, STOP TB strategy was announced by WHO and adopted by RNTCP. The components are as follows :

- Pursuing quality DOTS – expansion and enhancement.
- Addressing TB/HIV and MDR-TB.
- Contributing to health system strengthening.
- Engaging all care providers.
- Empowering patients and communities.
- Enabling and promoting research (diagnosis, treatment, vaccine).

Many of the initiatives like developing and piloting the feasibility of National Airborne Infection Control Guidelines, developing and piloting strategy for 'Practical Approach to Lung Health' are the examples of initiatives taken by RNTCP under the comprehensive strategy of STOP TB *(17)*.

In 2014, the World Health Assembly unanimously approved to end global TB epidemic by **"End TB Strategy"**, a 20 year programme with vision of a world with zero death, disease and suffering due to TB. For details please refer to page 237.

In view of End TB targets, the programme has been renamed from Revised National Tuberculosis Control Programme (RNTCP) to National Tuberculosis Elimination Programme (NTEP).

NTEP Organogram *(18)*

NTEP structure comprises of five levels: National, state, district, sub-district and peripheral health institution levels as shown in Fig. 2 *(18)*.

National level

Central TB Division (CTD) manages the National TB Control Programme for the entire country at the central level under AS&DG (RNTCP & NACO) through a national programme manager, Deputy Director General TB (DDG TB). The financial and administrative control of the programe is managed by the Joint Secretary from the administrative arm of the MoHFW.

The CTD is supported by a National TB Institute (NTI) Bengaluru, six National Reference Laboratories (NRL) including NTI, National Institute for Research in Tuberculosis (NIRT), Chennai, National Institute of Tuberculosis and Respiratory Diseases (NITRD), Delhi, National Japanese Leprosy Mission for Asia (JALMA), Institute for Leprosy and other mycobacterial diseases, Agra, Regional Medical Research Centre, Bhubaneswar and Bhopal Memorial Hospital & Research Centre – (BMHRC), Bhopal. The CTD is also supported by National Task Force for collaboration of Medical Colleges activities in the country through ZTF/STF.

Various committees of experts to guide the programme at different levels on technical & policy matters are there supporting Central TB Division.

State Level

The states have total ownership and accountability for the TB control in their state. State health society or its equivalent under National Health Mission of the state manages the TB control programme. A full-time State Tuberculosis Officer (STO), trained at national level and based at the State TB Cell (STC), is responsible for planning, training, supervising and monitoring the programme in all the districts of their respective states. STO is administratively

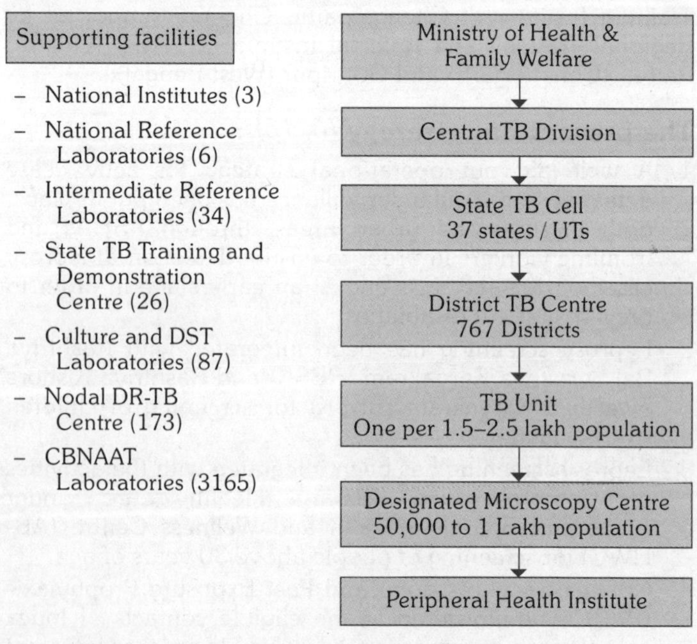

FIG. 2

Organization structure of NTEP

Source : *(6, 18)*

accountable to the state government, technically follows the instructions of the CTD, and coordinates with CTD and the districts, and is assisted by other technical & secretarial staff.

State TB cell is being supported by State TB Training and Demonstration Centre (STDC) in many states through its three units – a training unit, supervision and monitoring unit and an Intermediate Reference Laboratory (IRL) supporting an effective quality assurance system of the sputum smear microscopy network and laboratary services for PMDT (molecular DR testing and C&DST) in the State. Operational Research is also a component of STDC.

Each state also has one fully operational State Drug Store (SDS) for each 5 crore of population. It is responsible for effective management of medicines and other logistics, and ensuring uninterrupted supply of good quality 1st & 2nd line anti-TB medicines for adults and paediatric population.

District level

The key level for the management of primary health care services is the district. The Chief District Health Officer (CDHO)/Chief District Medical Officer (CDMO)/Civil Surgeon or an equivalent functionary in the district is responsible for all medical and public health activities including control of TB. The District Tuberculosis Centre (DTC) is the nodal point for TB control activities in the district. A full-time District Tuberculosis Officer (DTO), trained at national level & based at the DTC, is responsible for planning, training, supervising and monitoring the programme in the district. DTO is assisted by other technical & secretarial staff. The primary role of the DTC is a managerial one.

Sub-District Level (Tuberculosis Unit Level)

Integrating the TB control programme with the health system increases effectiveness and efficiency of TB care and control. India's TB control programme has been mainstreamed efficiently with National Health Mission (NHM).

A major organizational change in NTEP is the creation of a sub-district level (Tuberculosis Unit-TU). The TU is the nodal point for TB control activities in the sub-district. TUs are based mainly in NHM health blocks with the overall aim to align with NHM Block Programme Management Unit (BPMU) for optimum resource utilization and appropriate monitoring. In urban areas the TUs have been created based on a population of 1 per 2,00,000 (range 1.5–2.5 lakh) for rural and urban population and 1 per 1,00,000 (0.75–1.25 lakh) population in hilly/tribal/difficult areas. The Tuberculosis Unit (TU) consists of a designated Medical Officer - Tuberculosis Control (MO-TC), as well as one full-time supervisory staff – Senior Treatment Supervisor (STS). However, One Senior TB Laboratory Supervisor (STLS) will continue to be in 5 lakh population (one per 2.5 lakh population for tribal/hilly/difficult areas). There is a provision of additional STS if more than 300 TB cases are registered in public sector annually in a TU; additional STS if more than 50 private health establishments are registered in NIKSHAY in a TU and more than 200 TB patients are notified from these private health establishments annually in a TU.

The Block Medical Officer also functions as a Medical Officer TB Control (MO-TC). For the urban TB Units, a medical officer from the health facility where TU is located should be designated, in coordination with CMHO/DHO to function as a MO-TC. All MO-TCs should be trained in NTEP at a state level institution. MO-TC has the overall responsibility of management of TB Control Programme at the TU and is expected to undertake supervisory visits for seven days in a month. The team of STS and STLS are under the administrative supervision of the MO-TC and the DTO. The TU will have one Microscopy Centre for every 100,000 population (50,000 in tribal, desert, remote and hilly regions) referred to as the Designated Microscopy Centre (DMC, however, for complete geographic coverage National programme envisages to expand sputum smear microscopy services at PHC level). Microscopy Centres may also be established beyond population norms in Medical colleges, corporate hospitals, ESIC, railways, NGOs, private hospitals, etc.

Peripheral Health Institutions (PHIs)

For the purpose of NTEP, a PHI is a health facility which is manned by at least a medical officer. At this level, there are dispensaries, PHCs, CHCs, referral hospitals, major hospitals, speciality clinics or hospitals (including other health facilities), TB hospitals, ART Centres and medical colleges within the respective district. All health facilities in the private and NGO sectors participating in NTEP are also considered as PHIs by the programme. Some of these PHIs also function as DMCs. Peripheral health institution undertake tuberculosis case-finding and treatment activities as a part of the general health services. In situations where more than one MO is posted in any of the peripheral health centres, one of them may be identified and entrusted with the responsibilities of the NTEP. There is 1 TB Health Visitor (TBHV) per one lakh urban population to support the urban TB control activities *(18)*.

TB laboratory services *(18)*

The services of the laboratory are utilized for diagnosing TB & DR-TB cases and for monitoring of treatment of these patients. The laboratory network under NTEP is a 3-tier system for provision of diagnostic services and maintaining its quality.

A. *The peripheral laboratories* are situated in the public sector like the dispensaries, PHCs, CHCs, referral hospitals, major hospitals, specialty clinics/other sector hospitals/TB hospitals/medical colleges and in the private/NGO sectors. For establishment of microscopy centre in a lab, it must have adequate physical infrastructure, Binocular microscope and a trained LT. These laboratories are covered under quality assurance mechanisms

   i. Some of the labs not having facility for sputum microscopy, function as a sputum collection centres, and such facilities are also established in areas such as the tribal, hilly, desert and difficult to reach areas of the country for improving the access to diagnostic services.

   ii. In addition, large hospitals and medical colleges have facilities of digital X-Ray, rapid molecular test (Cartridge based nucleic acid amplification test – CBNAAT & Line Probe Assay-LPA), Fine Needle Aspiration Cytology (FNAC), histopathology, and culture & DST for diagnostic services of TB.

B. *At the state level* a nodal laboratory is designated as intermediate reference laboratory (IRL) which is usually situated in the State TB Training and Demonstration Centre (STDC)/medical college/public health laboratory.

The main functions of IRLs are monitoring of laboratory services across the state and maintenance of its quality through external quality assurance. There are 27 IRLs with facilities for culture & DST using Phenotypic (Solid – LJ & Liquid Culture – MGIT) and Genotypic technology (LPA & CBNAAT).

CBNAAT sites

In addition to the culture DST laboratories, CBNAAT centres are also established to diagnose Rifampicin resistance among all TB patients (Universal DST). Usually these are established in DTCs, TB units and medical colleges. The country is in the process of expanding CBNAAT site network. They also serve to diagnose TB among presumptive TB cases from key population.

DRTB Centres (18)

DRTB Centres are specialized centres for clinical management of drug resistant TB. At state/regional/division level, there are Nodal DRTB Centres (NDRTBC), to manage seriously ill DRTB cases, DRTB with extensive resistance and DRTB cases to be treated with regimes containing new drugs (Bedaquiline and Delamanid).

At the district level, there are district DRTB centres (DDRTBC), to manage DRTB cases with MDRTB, and H mono/poly-resistance. These centres will function under the guidance of NDRTBCs.

C. *At the central level* there are six designated National Reference Laboratories (NRLs) namely National Tuberculosis Institute, Bengaluru, National Institute for Research in Tuberculosis (NIRT), Chennai, National Institute of Tuberculosis and Respiratory Diseases (NITRD), Delhi, National JALMA Institute, Agra, Regional Medical Research Centre, Bhubaneswar and Bhopal Memorial Hospital & Research Centre (BMHRC), Bhopal. NIRT Chennai is also a Supra National Reference Lab (SNRL) for World Health Organization (WHO) for the South East Asia Region. NTI is a WHO collaborating centre for training, while NITRD is WHO centre of excellence in TB laboratory services. The NRLs are mainly responsible for external quality assurance of Lab network, drug resistance surveillance, training and research.

NTEP endorsed TB diagnostics *(1)*

1. Smear microscopy for acid fast bacilli.
   a. Sputum smear stained with Ziehl-Neelsen staining; or
   b. Fluoresence stains and examined under direct or indirect microscopy with or without LED.
2. Culture
   a. Solid (Lowenstein Jensen) media; or
   b. Liquid media (Middle Brook) using manual semi-automatic or automatic machines, e.g., Bactec, MGIT etc.
3. Rapid diagnostic molecular test
   a. Conventional PCR based Line Probe Assay for MTB complex; or
   b. Real-time PCR based Nucleic Acid Amplification Test NAAT for MTB complex, e.g. GeneXpert.
4. Radiography where available.
5. Tuberculin skin test.

New Initiatives

1. *NIKSHAY : TB surveillance using case based, web based IT system (19)*

Central TB Division in collaboration with National Informatics Centre has undertaken the initiative to develop a case based web based application named Nikshay. The word is combination of two Hindi words NI and KSHAY, meaning eradication of TB.

This software was launched in May 2012 and has following functional components.

– Master management
– User details
– TB patient registration and details of diagnosis, DOT provider, HIV status, follow-up, contact tracing, outcomes.
– Details of solid and liquid culture and DST, LPA, CBNAAT details.
– DR-TB patient registration with details.
– Referral and transfer of patients.
– Private health facility registration and TB notification.
– Mobile application for TB notification.
– SMS alerts to patients on registration.
– SMS alerts to programme officers.
– Automated periodic reports:
  a. Case finding
  b. Sputum conversion
  c. Treatment outcome.

The programme has started using IT enabled adherence tools like 99 DOTS for HIV-TB patients. This will be expanded to all TB patients with implementation of daily regimen *(7)*.

2. *TB Notification*

In order to ensure proper diagnosis and management of TB cases, and to reduce TB transmission and the emergence and spread of MDR-TB, it is essential to have complete information of all TB cases. According to the Government of India notification dated 7th May 2012, it is now mandatory for all healthcare providers to notify every TB case to local authorities i.e. District Health Officer/Chief Medical Officer of a district and Municipal health officer, every month in a given format *(20)*.

3. *Ban on TB Serology*

The serological tests are based on antibody response, which is highly variable in TB and may reflect remote infection rather than active disease. Currently available serological tests are having poor specificity and should not be used for the diagnosis of pulmonary or extra-pulmonary TB. Their import, manufacturing, sale, distribution and use is banned by the Government of India *(19)*.

4. *Direct benefit transfer schemes*

Direct beneficiary transfer systems are being established by linking TB patients reported in NIKSHAY with AADHAR and PEMS to effectively deliver benefits to TB patients and their providers *(7)*.

Initiation of treatment

Early identification of people with high probability of having active TB (presumptive TB) is the most important activity of the case finding strategy. Patients presenting themselves with symptoms suspicious of tuberculosis are screened through 2 sputum smear examinations. Sputum microscopic examination is done in designated RNTCP microscopy centres. They are located either in the CHC, PHC, Taluka Hospitals or in the TB dispensary. Each centre has a skilled technician to ensure quality control, a senior TB laboratory supervisor is appointed for every 5 microscopy centres. The senior TB laboratory supervisor rechecks all the positive slides and 10 per cent of the negative slides of these five microscopy centres. Thus the error in diagnosing a patient is minimized. It is essential to examine 2 sputum specimens of each patient before a conclusive diagnosis can be made. One sputum sample is not sufficient for diagnosis as the chance of detecting smear positive case is only 80 per cent. Sputum microscopy not only confirms the diagnosis, but also indicates the degree of infectivity and response to treatment. Fig. 1 on page number 206 shows the criteria of diagnosis and initiation of treatment.

All patients are provided short-course chemotherapy free of charge. During the intensive phase of chemotherapy all the drugs are administered under direct supervision called Direct Observed Therapy Short–term (DOTS). DOTS is a community based tuberculosis treatment and care strategy which combines the benefits of supervised treatment, and the benefits of community based care and support. It ensures high cure rates through its three components: appropriate medical treatment, supervision and motivation by a health or non-health worker, and monitoring of disease status by the health services. DOTS is given by peripheral health staff such as MPWs, or through voluntary workers such as teachers, anganwadi workers, dais, ex-patients, social workers etc. They are known as DOT 'Agent' and paid incentive/ honorarium of Rs 150 per patient completing the treatment.

Newer initiatives *(11)*

1. *Daily regimen for paediatric TB* : In order to transition the country to the updated guidelines for paediatric treatment in the STCI, which follow the current WHO dosing guidelines, the government has decided to introduce a daily dosing regimen using child-friendly fixed dosage combinations (FDCs). The procurement of anti-TB drugs in daily fixed dose combination (FDC) has been initiated. Treatment with FDCs of anti-Tb drugs will be in six weight bands for paediatric patients. An option for family members to provide Directly Observed Treatment (DOT) to paediatric patients has been incorporated in the guidelines.
2. Daily regimen for all forms of TB in the country.
3. Pilots for universal access to TB cases.
4. *Universal drug susceptibility testing (DST)* : Expansion of rapid molecular diagnostics have been scaled up to 3164 CBNAAT/TrueNat, covering all districts for decentralized diagnosis of drug resistant TB services. Nearly 55 per cent of all notified TB cases were offered universal drug susceptibility testing in 3rd quarter of 2019.
5. *Shorter regimen and Bedaquiline* : In 2018, shorter regimen and Bedaquiline for treatment of drug resistant TB patients have been expanded in the country. From 2018, more than 46,129 DR-TB patients have been initiated on shorter regimen and 7,973 DR-TB patients on newer drug containing regimen.
6. *Campaign mode* – Active case finding : To reach the unreached, the programme has carried out systematic active TB screening among high risk populations through house visits or targeted setting visit (tribal population, slums, old age homes, prisons, orphanages, transit camps etc.) The campaign was conducted in priority districts selected based on burden of TB, case finding efforts, HIV-TB and drug resistant TB in the respective districts *(7)*.

The drugs are supplied in patient-wise boxes containing the full course of treatment, and packaged in blister packs. For the intensive phase, each blister pack contains one day's medication. For the continuation phase, each blister pack contains one weeks supply of medication. The combipack drugs for extension of intensive phase are supplied separately. The boxes are coloured according to the category of the regimen, red for category I patients, blue for category II patients.

Paediatric tuberculosis

Please refer to page 221 for details.

Drug resistance surveillance (DRS) under NTEP (2014–2016) *(17)*

The prevalence of drug resistance to TB can be taken as an indicator of the effectiveness of the TB control activities over a period of time and, therefore, RNTCP has taken steps to measure this important indicator.

The aim of DRS is to determine the prevalence of antimycobacterial drug resistance among new sputum smear positive pulmonary tuberculosis (PTB) patients, and also amongst previously treated sputum smear positive PTB patients. Drug–resistant TB has frequently been encountered in India, and its presence has been known virtually from the time anti-TB drugs were introduced for the treatment of TB.

To obtain a more precise estimate of Multi-Drug Resistant TB (MDR-TB) burden in the country, RNTCP carried out drug resistance surveillance (DRS) surveys (2014–2016) in accordance with global guidelines in selected states. The results of these surveys indicate prevalence of MDR-TB to be about 2.84 per cent in new cases and 11.60 per cent in retreatment cases *(18)*.

MANAGEMENT OF DRUG RESISTANT TB

The services for quality diagnosis and treatment of drug resistant TB cases were initiated in 2007 in Gujarat and Maharashtra. These services since then have been scaled up and currently these services are available across the country from March 2013. For full details about the patient regimens, please refer to page 222. The milestones in the evolution of PMDT are as shown in Fig. 3.

State-level structure and responsibilities *(22)*

While a national expert technical working group has developed national policies, technical and operational guidelines, the state-level is where the majority of planning activities, implementation and monitoring occur. The state PMDT Committee is responsible for developing the plan of action for implementation, expansion, maintenance, supervision, monitoring and quality enhancement of PMDT services in the respective state.

Drug-resistant tuberculosis centre *(22)*

Programmatic and clinical management of DR-TB is complex but feasible when the health system is strengthened to effectively integrate what is necessary. Treatment of drug-resistant TB is not completely based on centralized and institutionalized care for the entire duration. In fact, clinical care needs the presence of a clinical and patient support expert

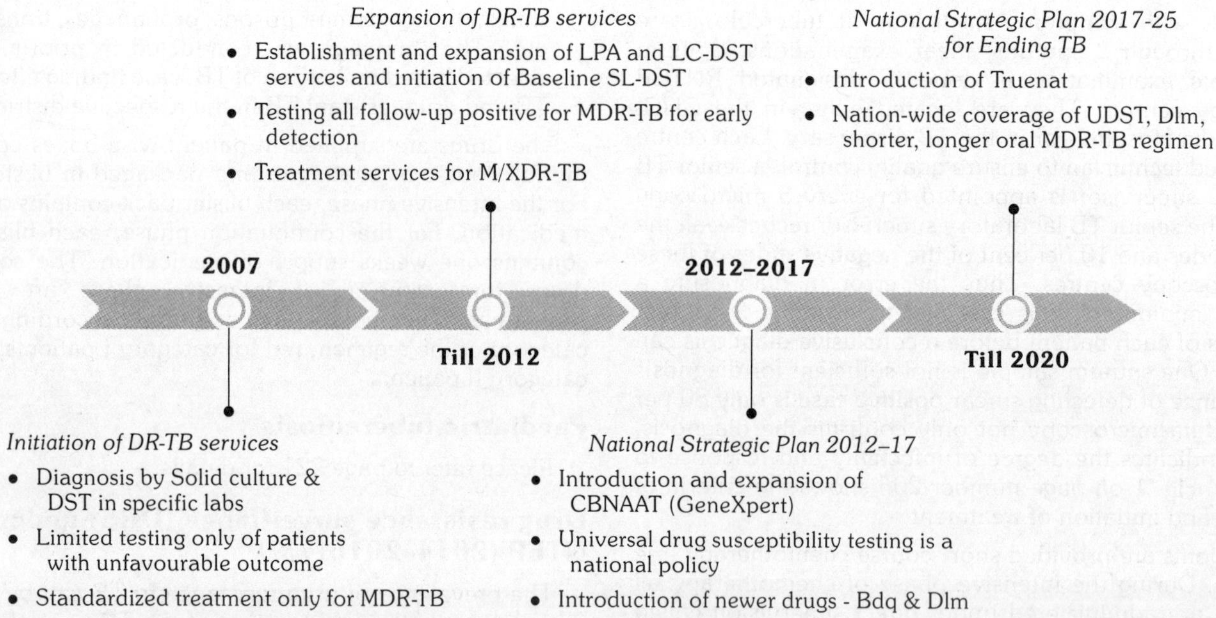

FIG. 3

Milestones in evolution of PMDT in India

Source : *(21)*

resource centre. This is the DR-TB Centre, which is a 20–30 bedded tertiary care facility established to serve a population of approximately 10 million, with an airborne infection control compliant ward, facilities for pretreatment evaluations, treatment initiations, follow-up monitoring and management of adverse drug reactions, prevention and relief of physical and social suffering caused by the disease and its treatment, complications and co-morbidities. All these activities are supported by the programme staff in addition to having counselling for patients and undertaking data management.

By 2017, 147 DR-TBCs were established across India, designated as Nodal DR-TB centre, one for approximately every 10 million population, including some in private institutes partnering with RNTCP. About 5 to 10 districts are attached to each centre. DR-TB patients are admitted for a short period and once stabilized on treatment, discharged with advance intimation to the districts and referred back to their districts for continuation and completion of treatment. During treatment they are referred back to DR-TBCs for change of regimens and management of adverse reactions.

To decentralize the pretreatment evaluation, treatment initiation of RR-TB or H mono/poly DR-TB and follow-up processes, two distinct types of DR-TBCs will be established. The existing nodal DR-TB centre (NDR-TBC) will continue for approximately 10 million population. One District DR-TB centre (DDR-TBC) will be established for every district. Some of the states have already established these centres.

The advantages of decentralized "test and treat approach" are *(22)*:

- Early and faster initiation of treatment of all diagnosed DR-TB patients;
- Bringing care closer to the residence of majority of the DR-TB patients;
- Significant reduction in catastrophic expenditure including loss of work hours and family income;
- Rationally minimizing the need and duration for hospitalization;
- Minimizing travel of patients, thereby transmission risks during travels;
- Accountability of the district programme management units; and
- Rationalizing utilization of existing DR-TBCs to enable them to concentrate in more complex clinical decisions and ensuring quality assurance of treatment and research.

1. District DR-TB centre *(22)*

The DDR-TBC is responsible for the initiation and management of uncomplicated DR-TB patients like RR-TB or H mono/poly DR-TB in a district, not only on inpatient basis, but also on outpatient basis, wherever advisable and possible. The DDR-TBC can be established at institutes in a certain order of preference, namely, medical colleges, district hospitals, TB hospitals and NGO/private/corporate institutes/other sector hospitals with the availability of required clinical expertise.

2. Nodal DR-TB centre *(22)*

Patients with additional resistance to second-line drugs, drug intolerance, contraindications, failing regimen, patients returning after treatment interruption of >1 month, emergence of any exclusion criteria for standard regimen for RR-TB or H mono/poly DR-TB regimen, non-TB mycobacterium (NTMs) and those needing palliative care would be managed at NDR-TBC.

The requirements for the NDR-TB centre are as follows:

- Should preferably be a tertiary care institute;
- Separate ward for male and female patients should be available with at least 10 beds in each;
- All PMDT services (beds, investigations, ECG and ancillary drugs for management of adverse drug reactions) to be provided free of cost to the patient;
- Relevant specialties including respiratory medicine, general medicine, psychiatry, dermatology, ENT,

ophthalmology, gynaecology, paediatrician, anaesthesiologist and cardiologist should be available directly or through linkages;

- NDR-TBC committee to be formed;
- National training of NDR-TBC committee members (including Chairperson);
- National AIC guidelines to be implemented in DR-TB wards and outpatients setting.
- Routine clinical laboratory investigation facility to be made available for pretreatment evaluation and monitoring;
- Ancillary drugs should be available;
- Management of adverse drug reaction as per PMDT guidelines;
- Doctors, nursing and support staff should be available from the institute;
- Reports and records to be maintained for PMDT; and
- Quarterly report to be submitted electronically.

The overall structure and roles of different level of PMDT services are summarized in Fig. 4.

TB care services in the private sector

The private sector is everything outside the ambit of the Government run public health services. It varies widely in its size, nature of service delivery and the socio-economic groups served. It holds a factual predominance of health care service delivery in India. As per National Sample Survey Organization report, about 70 per cent patients seek care in private clinics and hospitals *(23)*.

Delays in diagnosis, over-diagnosis of TB due to an over-dependence on X-rays, the use of multiple non-standard regimens for inappropriate durations, the lack of a mechanism to ensure full course of treatment and to record treatment outcomes are some issues of concern in the private sector. Similar problems in varying degrees are encountered in other health sectors as well. The advantages and disadvantages of public and private sector are as shown below:

	Public sector	Private sector
Advantages	• Free diagnosis • Free treatment • Standardized regimen • Referral and transfer system • Supervision and monitoring • Accountability of treatment outcome	• Wide choices (> 5 lakh practitioners) • Better access – Convenient timings – Shorter distances – Personal attention and care – Projected discounts • Faith and perceptions of better care
Disadvantages	• Staff's non-response to symptoms • Delays between tests and receiving results • Difficulty in transporting specimens • Financial expenditure on travel, food, daily necessities, extra medicines • Perceived low quality of services	• Cost of clinical examination fees • Cost of diagnostic tests • Cost of drugs • Irrational prescriptions • Infrequent use of quality sputum tests for diagnosis of TB • No adherence tracking mechanisms • Fear of losing patient if involved in RNTCP

Source : *(23)*

The strategic vision of RNTCP is to lay down guidelines and norms for TB care in country. The underlying principle is for RNTCP to extend public services to privately managed patients. Standards for TB care in India, mandatory TB notification, NIKSHAY, ban on serodiagnostics are among the tools to improve TB care services in private sector. Regulatory tools, however, are limited and partnership is preferred. Programme staff should understand that RNTCP needs private providers more than private providers need the RNTCP.

C & DST lab

- Receive diagnosis and FU specimens
- Provide rapid results to district, Field and DR-TB centre
- Maintain records in Nikshay (LIMS)
- Quality assurance of results

Nodal DR-TB Centre

- Maintain ward & AIC measures
- Undertake pre-treatment evaluation & initiate treatment
- Manage major ADR
- Mentor/supervise concerned DDR-TBC as expert resource

State drug store

- Prepare & ship drug boxes to district level
- Manage supply chain for diagnostics and drugs
- Maintain record in Nikshay Aushadh

NAAT sites

- Diagnose TB & RR-TB patients at district/sub-district level
- Maintain records & Nikshay
- Reflex transportation of 2nd sample to concerned C&DST Lab for FL-LPA & SL-LPA

District DR-TB

- Initiate DR-TB treatment regimen
- Manage ADR and Record ADR
- Consult for complications
- Maintain records and Nikshay
- Coordinate with NDR-TBC/ Field
- Monitor DR-TB treatment

District

- Coordinate for test results
- Refer patients to N/DDR-TBC
- Coordinate care and drug flow from district drug store to field level
- Maintain records, Nikshay, monitor & supervise

Health facility (HF)

- Identify presumptive case, Collect/transport specimens
- Identify treatment supporter
- Support, supervise DR-TB patients during treatment
- Communicate results to patients
- Manage minor adverse effects
- Refer patient for the treatment initiation
- Collect and refer follow-up specimens

FIG. 4
Overall PMDT structure and roles

Source : *(21)*

Monitoring *(24)*

The program is continuously monitored at the block, district, state, and national levels by the respective program managers, with the aid of the reports generated from Nikshay database The NTEP is also part of all the important health review meetings held under the chairpersonship of elected representatives, Principal Secretary (Health), Mission Directors and District Magistrates/Collectors.

The Central TB Division also releases quarterly, and bi-annual rankings of the states and districts based on the TB Score. This aids the states to identify the areas of lacunae, identify challenges and expedite their resolution on a real-time basis. Nikshay Dashboard plays an important role in real-time monitoring of the program performance.

TB Score

For continuous monitoring of the programme performance at the national, state as well as district level, a composite score calculated from a selected list of key performance indicators from various thematic areas in the National Tuberculosis Elimination Programme. Appropriate weightage has been given to each of these indicators and each state is scored for the performance in each indicator. The individual indicators sum up to a total of 100.

The TB index helps in objectively measuring the performance of the state, identify areas where guidance/ resolution of challenges are necessary as well as promote a healthy competition towards ending TB.

The achievements during COVID-19 pandemic *(6)*

The onset of the COVID-19 pandemic triggered lockdowns, restrictions in movement, repurposing of available NTEP and health system resources, infrastructure, diagnostics, treatment centers and manpower to fight this emerging threat, and disrupted ongoing TB elimination efforts and services all over the country. NTEP's response plan and mitigation efforts included integrated TB-COVID bi-directional screening, diagnostic and treatment capacity. Large scale active TB case finding campaigns were undertaken with massive screening and testing in communities, health outreach workers and community volunteers were engaged to facilitate surveillance of symptoms within households, doorstep collection of samples and delivery of monthly medicine stock to help patients stick to treatment regimens, and tele-consultations with patients. Private sector TB care facilities were reopened, call centres were fully activated, digital tools were rolled out along with support like direct cash transfers and supplementary food provisions were delivered to people's home. Contact tracing systems and testing for TB linked to COVID-19 contact tracing were also quickly set up throughout the country.

By December 2020, NTEP had managed notifying a total of 18,05,670 patients which was 11% more than the estimated projections made in April 2020 in view of the ongoing COVID-19 pandemic. The private sector too contributed notification of 5.49 lakh patients (31% of total notifications), 3% more than in 2019. Despite the pandemic, 95% of total patients notified were put on treatment during 2020. During the year 2021, a total of 15,79,410 (Jan-Sep) patients were notified with 95% of patients put on treatment. Treatment Success Rate of TB notified patients remains at 81% in 2021 despite the pandemic.

The NTEP has also initiated Sub-National Certification of Districts/States/UTs for achieving "Progress towards TB Free Status" under Bronze, Silver and Gold categories measured with graded milestones of decline in TB incidence compared to 2015 levels. Districts/States/UTs are certified under the categories upon independent verification by a national team comprising of National Institute of Epidemiology, WHO India and Indian Association of Preventive and Social Medicine.

TB-HIV coordination *(25)*

Since the advent of the collaborative efforts in 2001, TB-HIV activities have evolved to cover most of the recommendations as per the latest WHO policy statement issued in 2012. In 2007, the first national framework for joint TB-HIV collaborative activities was developed which

The TB Index currently in usage consists of 9 indicators

S.No.	Parameter	Indicator	Score allotted
1.	Achievement of TB notification among the target identified	% of Target TB notification achieved (Source: Nikshay)	20
2.	HIV testing/ screening of TB notified patients	% of net TB notified patients with known HIV status (Source: Nikshay)	10
3.	UDST coverage among the TB notified patients	% of net TB notified patients with UDST done (Source: Nikshay)	10
4.	Treatment Success Rate of TB notified patients	Treatment Success Rate for net TB patients (Source: Nikshay)	15
5.	Nikshay Poshan Yojana implementation Nikshay Poshan Yojana	% of Eligible beneficiaries paid at least once under (Source: Nikshay)	10
6.	DRTB treatment initiation among the diagnosed patients	% of MDR/ RR patients initiated on treatment out of net diagnosed (Source: PMDT Quarterly Reports)	15
7.	Utilisation of the allotted budget	% of expenditure amongst ROP (Source: PFMS)	10
8.	Latent TB infection management	% of children <5/<6 years given chemoprophylaxis against the total eligible children identified (Source: Nikshay)	5
		% of PLHIV given IPT against total eligible PLHIV (Source: NACP)	5

Source : *(24)*

endorsed a differential strategy reflective of the heterogeneity of TB-HIV epidemic. Coordinated TB-HIV interventions were implemented including establishment of a coordinating body at national and state level, dedicated human resources, integration of surveillance, joint monitoring and evaluation, capacity building and operational research.

The implementation of collaborative TB/HIV activities are as follows :

1. Intensified TB case finding has been implemented nationwide at all HIV testing centres (known as integrated counselling and testing centres, or ICTCs), and has now been extended to all ART centres.
2. HIV testing of TB patients is now routine through provider initiated testing and counselling (PITC), implemented in all states with the intensified TB-HIV package.
3. Persons found to be HIV-positive are eligible for free HIV care at a network of antiretroviral treatment (ART) centres. ART centres are located in medical colleges, mainly staffed and operated by the state AIDS control societies, and a few are situated within the facilities of private or NGO partners. As of December 2017, there were 536 ART centres operating in the country, 1120 link-ART centres and 158 link-ART plus centres. Ten Regional Centres of Excellence provide second-line ART services for PLHIV, and 24 centres provide second line ART (ART-plus centres). HIV-infected TB patients who are on protease inhibitor based second line ART are getting rifabutin-based TB treatment in place of Rifampicin.
4. Policy decision has been taken by National Technical Working Group on TB/HIV collaborative activities (NTWG on TB/HIV) to expand coverage of whole blood finger prick HIV screening test at all DMC without a stand-alone or F-ICTC.
5. Provider initiated HIV testing and counselling (PITC) among presumptive TB cases (TB suspects) is now a policy –
   a. In high HIV prevalent states/settings – The implementation will be done in a phased manner, starting with high prevalent states and then in A and B category districts in rest of the country.
   b. In low HIV prevalent states/settings – HIV testing among presumptive TB cases should be routinely implemented in the age-group of 25–54 years in low HIV prevalent districts (C & D) at places where there are co-located TB and HIV testing facilities.
6. Intensified case finding activities to be specifically monitored among HIV infected pregnant women and children living with HIV.
7. The National AIDS Control Programme (NACP) and RNTCP have taken the policy decision to adopt isoniazid prophylaxis therapy (IPT) as a strategy for prevention of TB among PLHIV. The implementation will be in a phased manner.
8. The RNTCP has prioritized presumptive TB cases among people living with HIV for diagnosis of TB and Rifampicin resistance with rapid diagnostic tools having high sensitivity e.g. Xpert MTB/RIF.

The treatment guidelines are discussed in detail on page 235.

Tuberculosis in pregnancy

Please refer to page 230 for details.

NATIONAL STRATEGIC PLAN (2017–2025) FOR TB ELIMINATION

The National Strategic Plan (NSP) 2017–2025 for TB elimination builds on the success of last NSP. It is a three year costed plan and an eight year strategic document. It provides goals and strategies for the country's response to the disease during the period 2017–2025 to bring about significant changes in the incidence, prevalence and mortality of TB, and attain the global End TB targets five years ahead of Sustainable Development Goals of TB free India. The VISION is – TB free India with zero deaths, disease and poverty due to TB *(26)*.

Objectives:

The main objectives of NPS are:

1. Find all drug sensitive TB and drug resistant TB cases with an emphasis on reaching TB patients seeking care from private providers, and undiagnosed TB in high-risk populations.
2. Initiate and sustain all patients on appropriate anti-TB treatment wherever they seek care, with patient friendly systems and social support.
3. Prevent the emergence of TB in susceptible populations.
4. Build and strengthen enabling policies, empowered institutions, additional human resources with enhanced capacities, and provide adequate financial resources.

The key strategies are as follows:

1. Private sector engagement
2. Active case finding
3. Drug resistant TB case management
4. Addressing social determinants including nutrition
5. Robust surveillance system
6. Community engagement and multi-sectoral approach

Expected outcome:

The aim of the National Strategic Plan is to achieve elimination of TB by 2025. During plan period, targets for TB are:

1. 80% reduction in TB incidence (i.e. reduction from 211 per lakh to 43 per lakh)
2. 90% reduction in TB mortality (i.e. reduction from 32 per lakh to 3 per lakh
3. 0% patient having catastrophic expenditure due to TB

New comprehensively deployed interventions are required to accelerate the rate of decline of incidence of TB to more than 10–15 per cent annually. The requirements of moving towards TB elimination have been integrated into four strategic pillars of Detect–Treat–Prevent–Build (DTPB). By taking the DTPB approach, the national programme can achieve significant positive change and make a real difference in the lives of many people it serves.

Table 4 highlights the core impact, outcome indicators and targets of the NSP. The four priority areas include private sector engagement, ensuring a seamless efficient TB care cascade, active TB case-finding among key population (socially vulnerable and clinically high risk), and preventing progression from latent TB infection (LTBI) to active TB in high risk groups.

TABLE 4

NSP 2017–25 results framework

Impact indicators	Baseline	Target		
	2015	2020	2023	2025
To reduce estimated TB incidence rate (per 100,000 population)	217 (112–355)	142 (76–255)	77 (49–185)	44 (36–158)
To reduce estimated TB prevalence (per 100,000 population)	320 (280–380)	170 (159–217)	90 (81–125)	65 (56–93)
To reduce estimated mortality due to TB (per 100,000 population)	32 (29–35)	15 (13–16)	6 (5–7)	3 (3–4)
To ensure no family should suffer catastrophic cost due to TB	35%	0%	0%	0%
Outcome Indicators				
Total TB patient notification (in millions)	1.74	3.6	2.7	2
Total patient private providers notification (in millions)	0.19	2	1.5	1.2
MDR/RR TB patients notified	28,096	92,000	69,000	55,000
Proportion of notified TB patients offered DST	25%	80%	98%	100%
Proportion of notified patients initiated on treatment	90%	95%	95%	95%
Treatment success rate among notified DSTB	75%	90%	92%	92%
Treatment success rate among notified DRTB	46%	65%	73%	75%
Proportion of identified targetted key affected population undergoing active case finding	0%	100%	100%	100%
Proportion of notified TB patients receiving financial support through Direct Benefit Transfers (DBT)	0%	80%	90%	90%
Proportion of identified/eligible individuals for preventive therapy/LTBIs - initiated on treatment	10%	60%	90%	95%

Source : *(23)*

Financial resources

The programme is being assisted by the World Bank and the Department for International Development (DFID) *via* WHO. In addition, the RNTCP is supported by the Global TB Drug Facility (GDF), Global Fund to Fight AIDS, Tuberculosis and Malaria (GFATM), the United States Agency for International Development (USAID) and DANIDA. Government of India provides 100 per cent grant-in-aid to the implementing agencies i.e., states/UTs, besides free drugs. The states are expected to use the existing infrastructure and also to provide some manpower resources.

NATIONAL AIDS CONTROL PROGRAMME

National AIDS Control Programme was launched in India in the year 1987. The Ministry of Health and Family Welfare has set up National AIDS Control Organization (NACO) as a separate wing to implement and closely monitor the various components of the programme. The aim of the programme is to prevent further transmission of HIV, to decrease morbidity and mortality associated with HIV infection and to minimize the socio-eonomic impact resulting from HIV infection.

The milestones of the programme are summarized as follows *(23A)* :

1986 – First case of HIV detected.
– AIDS Task Force set up by the ICMR.
– National AIDS Committee established under the Ministry of Health.

1990 – Medium Term Plan launched for four states and the four metros.

1992 – NACP–I launched to slow down the spread of HIV infection.
– National AIDS Control Board constituted.
– NACO set-up.

1999 – NACP–II begins, focussing on behaviour change, increased decentralization and NGO involvement.
– State AIDS Control Societies established.

2002 – National AIDS Control Policy adopted.
– National Blood Policy adopted.

2004 – Anti-retroviral treatment initiated.

2006 – National Council on AIDS constituted under chairmanship of the Prime Minister.
– National Policy on Paediatric ART formulated.

2007 – NACP–III launched for 5 years (2007–2012).

2014 – NACP–IV launched for 5 years (2012–2017).

2017 – National Strategic Plan for HIV/AIDS and STIs 2017–2024

The national strategy has the following components : establishment of surveillance centres to cover the whole country; identification of high-risk group and their screening; issuing specific guidelines for management of detected cases and their follow-up; formulating guidelines for blood bank, blood product manufacturers, blood donors and dialysis units; information, education, and communication activities by involving mass media and research for reduction of personal and social impact of the disease; control of sexually transmitted diseases; and condom programme.

The Government of India initiated programmes of prevention and raising awareness under the Medium Term Plan (1990–92), NACP–I (1992–99), NACP–II (1999–2006) and NACP–III (2007–2012). Based on the lessons learnt and achievements made in Phase I, II and III. India developed the Fourth National Programme Implementation Plan (NACP–IV, 2012–2017). The primary goal of NACP–IV is to halt and reverse the epidemic in India over the next 5 years by integrating programmes for prevention, care, support and treatment.

The package of services under NACP-IV are as follows *(27)* :

1. *Prevention services*
   - Targeted interventions for high-risk groups (female sex workers, men who have sex with men, transgenders/hijras, injecting drug users) and bridge population (truckers and migrants).
   - Needle-syringe exchange programme and opioid substitution therapy for IDUs.
   - Prevention interventions for migrant population at source, transit and destination.
   - Link worker scheme for HRGs and vulnerable population in rural areas.
   - Prevention and control of sexually transmitted infections/reproductive tract infections.
   - Blood safety.
   - HIV counselling and testing services.
   - Prevention of parent to child transmission.
   - Condom promotion.
   - Information, education and communication and behaviour change communication (BCC).
   - Social mobilization, youth interventions and adolescence education programme.
   - Mainstreaming HIV/AIDS response.
   - Work place interventions.
2. *Care, support and treatment services*
   - Laboratory services for CD4 testing and other investigations
   - Free first-line and second-line Anti-Retroviral Therapy (ART) through ART centres and Link ART Centres (LACs), Centres of Excellence (CoE) and ART plus centres.
   - Paediatric ART for children.
   - Early infant diagnosis for HIV exposed infants and children below 18 months.
   - Nutritional and psycho-social support through Care and Support Centres (CSC).
   - HIV/TB coordination (cross-referral, detection and treatment of co-infections).
   - Treatment of opportunistic infections.
   - Drop-in centres for PLHIV networks.

Organizational structure

The National AIDS Control Organization (NACO) is presently established as a division under the Ministry of Health and Family Welfare, headed by the Additional Secretary, Ministry of Health and Director General, NACO Govt. of India. The technical divisions are headed by officers at the level of Deputy Director General/DGHS. The finance division is headed by Director-Finance while Admin and Procurement is headed by the Joint Secretary, Ministry of Health. Fig. 5 shows the NACO structure.

Country scenario

Based on sentinel surveillance data, the HIV prevalence in adult population can be broadly classified into three groups of States/UTs in the country.

Group I High Prevalence States : includes states of Maharashtra, Tamil Nadu, Karnataka, Andhra Pradesh, Manipur and Nagaland where the HIV infection has crossed 5 per cent mark in high-risk group and 1% or more in antenatal women.

Group II Moderate Prevalence States : includes states of Gujarat, Goa and Puducherry where HIV infection has crossed 5% or more among high risk groups but the infection is below 1% in antenatal women.

Group III Low Prevalence States : includes remaining states where the HIV infection in any of the high risk groups is still less than 5% and is less than 1% among antenatal women.

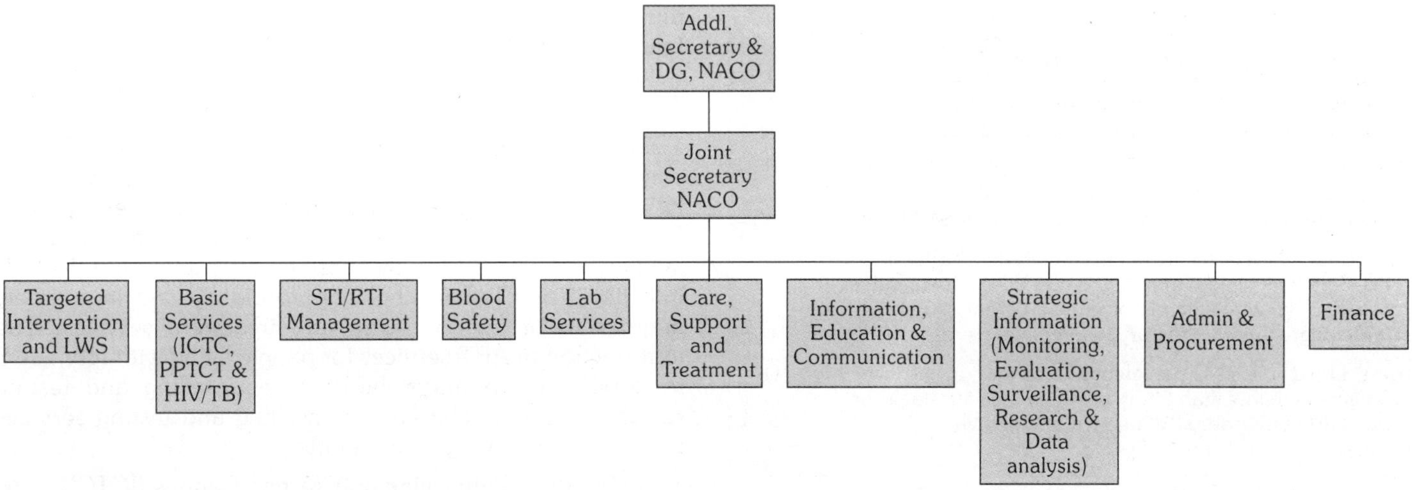

FIG. 5
NACO Structure

Source : *(28)*

Categories of Districts

In the country, the districts have been classified according to the epidemiological and vulnerability–criteria using the sentinel surveillance data for the last 3 years (Table 5). Accordingly, 156 districts have been classified as category A. 39 districts as category B, 296 as category C and 118 as category D districts. The planning for HIV related services has also been graded as per categorization of districts. This approach has been implemented since March 2007.

HIV surveillance

Different types of surveillance activities are being carried out in the country to detect the spread of the disease and to make appropriate strategy for prevention and control viz., area specific targeted intervention and best practice approach. The types of surveillance are : (a) HIV Sentinel Surveillance, (b) HIV Sero–Surveillance, (c) AIDS Case Surveillance, (d) STD Surveillance, (e) Behavioural Surveillance, and (f) Integration with surveillance of other diseases like tuberculosis etc.

HIV SENTINEL SURVEILLANCE : After the establishment of the fact that HIV infection is present in wide geographic areas, the aim of surveillance was redefined to monitor the trends of HIV infection. The objectives of the surveillance are as follows *(30)* :

1. To determine the level of HIV infection among general population as well as high-risk groups in different states;
2. To understand the trends of HIV epidemic among general population as well as high-risk groups in different states;
3. To understand the geographical spread of HIV infection and to identify emerging pockets;
4. To provide information for prioritization of programme resources and evaluation of programme impact; and
5. To estimate HIV prevalence and HIV burden in the country.

The objective of the surveillance is best achieved by annual cross-sectional survey of the risk group, in the same place over few years by unlinked anonymous serological testing procedures by two ERS (i.e., when HIV testing is carried out without indentification of name of samples collected for other purposes e.g., VDRL in STD clinics. The objective of surveillance may be fulfilled in this example whereas the positive person is not identified). The number of samples to be screened must represent the risk group under study and the sample size is determined accordingly. Clinical based approach for such collection has many advantages including the procedure for collection of samples which should be carried out on the above lines to avoid "selection bias" and "participation bias"

TABLE 5

Categories of districts

Category of Districts	
More than 1% ANC/PTCT prevalence in district at any time in any of the sites in the last 3 years.	A
Less than 1% ANC/PTCT prevalence in all the sites during last 3 years associated with more than 5% prevalence in any HRG group (STD/CSW/MSM/IDU).	B
Less than 1% in ANC prevalence in all sites during last 3 years with less than 5% in all STD clinic attendees or any HRG with known hot spots (Migrants, truckers, large aggregation of factory workers, tourist etc.).	C
Less than 1% in ANC prevalence in all sites during last 3 years with less than 5% in all STD clinic attendees or any HRG OR, poor HIV data with no known hot spots.	D

ANC – Antenatal clinic

PTCT – Parent to child transmission

Source : *(29)*

To start with, the HIV sentinel surveillance for HIV was taken up from 1994 in 55 sentinel sites attached to the existing surveillance centres and were increased to 180 in 1998. While the number of the high risk groups of HIV sentinel sites were increased every year, with change of sites, these 180 sites have remained consistent. Inclusion of data from high-risk population through targeted intervention sites and the additional sub–set of rural samples through ante-natal clinics are the key features of HIV sentinel surveillance. Pregnant women attending antenatal clinics are taken as proxy for general population. The number of HIV sentinel surveillance sites for different population groups during 2016–17 are as shown in Table 6.

TABLE 6

Number of HIV sentinel surveillance sites (2016–2017)

Site type	2016–2017
ANC	829
IDU	87
MSM	89
FSW	245
Migrant	27
TG	18
Truckers	28
Total	1,323

Source : *(31)*

The strategy adopted for collection and testing of samples during HIV Sentinel Surveillance Round 2016–2017 was as follows (Table 7).

Counselling and HIV testing services

The Basic Service Division of the department of AIDS control provides HIV counselling and testing services for HIV infection. The national programme is offering these services since 1997 with the goal to identify as many people living with HIV, as early as possible (after acquiring the HIV infection), and linking them appropriately and in a timely manner to prevention, care and treatment services. The introduction of ART services for people living with HIV/AIDS in 2004, gave a major boost to counselling and testing services in India. The HIV counselling and testing services include the following components:

1. Integrated Counselling and Testing Centres (ICTC).
2. Prevention of parent-to-child transmission of HIV (PPTCT).
3. HIV/tuberculosis collaborative activities.

TABLE 7
HIV sentinel surveillence round 2016–2017

	High risk groups: IDU/MSM/FSW/TG	Bridge population: SMM/LDT	General population: Pregnant women attending ANC clinics
Sentinel site	Targeted interventions (TI) projects	STD clinic, TI projects	Antenatal clinic
Sample size	250	250	400
Duration	3 months	3 months	3 months
Frequency	Once in 2 years	Once in 2 years	Once in 2 years
Sampling method	Consecutive/random	Consecutive	Consecutive
Age group	15–49 years	15–49 years	15–49 years
Testing strategy	Unlinked anonymous with informed consent	Unlinked anonymous at STD, with informed consent at TI sites	Unlinked anonymous
Blood specimen	Dried blood spot	Serum at STD, DBS at TI sites	Serum
Testing protocol	Two test protocol	Two test protocol	Two test protocol

SMM – Single male migrants, LDT – Long distance truckers

Source : *(31)*

INTEGRATED COUNSELLING AND TESTING CENTRES

Diverse models of HIV counselling and testing services are available to increase access to HIV diagnosis, these include testing services in health care facilities, standalone sites and community-based approaches at various levels of public health systems in India from state, district, sub-district and village/community levels as depicted in Fig. 6.

Types of facilities for HIV counselling and testing services

Integrated Counselling and Testing Centres (ICTC): A person is counselled and tested for HIV at ICTC, either of his own free will (client initiated) or as advised by a medical provider (provider initiated). Functions of ICTC include early detection of HIV, provision of basic information on modes of transmission and prevention of HIV/AIDS for promoting behavioural change and reducing vulnerability, and linking PLHIV with other HIV prevention, care and treatment services. The ICTC have been classified into two types: Fixed facility ICTC and Mobile ICTC.

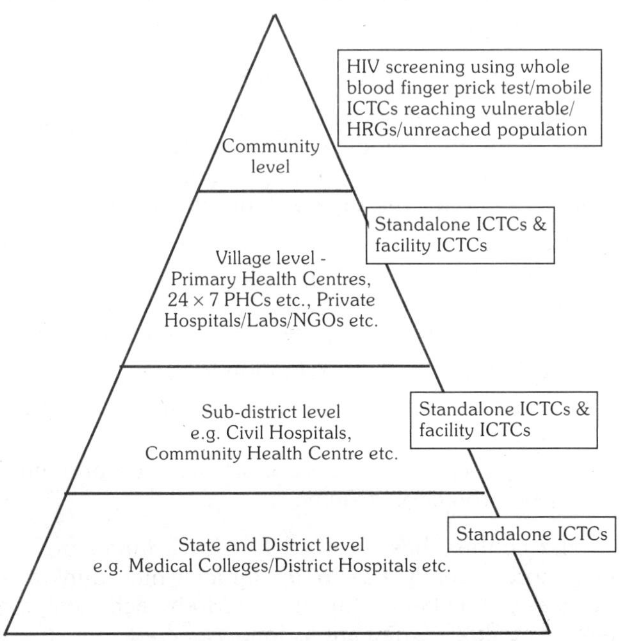

FIG. 6
Level of HIV counselling and testing services in India

Source : *(32)*

1. Fixed facility ICTCs are located within an existing healthcare facility/hospital/health centre, and are of two types – Standalone ICTC and Facility-integrated counselling and testing centres.
   a. *Standalone ICTC (SA-ICTC):* The client load is high in these centres, with full-time counsellor and laboratory technician who provide HIV counselling and testing services. SA-ICTC are located in medical colleges, district hospitals, sub-district hospitals, CHCs etc.
   b. *Facility-integrated counselling and testing centres (F-ICTCs):* Considering the need for rapid scale-up and sustainability of HIV counselling and testing services, the F-ICTCs have been set up below the block levels at 24 × 7 PHC, etc. Staff of the existing health facilities are trained in counselling and testing services of HIV. The HIV service delivery is ensured with logistic support from DAC. Similar to F-ICTC at 24 × 7 PHC, the Public Private Partnership (PPP)-ICTCs were established in private facilities (for profit/ not-for-profit hospitals, laboratories, non-governmental organizations etc.), and have been supported by DAC/SACs in supply of rapid HIV testing kits, training of existing staff, quality assurance, supply of protective kits and prophylactic drugs for post-exposure prophylaxis for staff, supply of IEC materials such as flip charts, posters etc. required for ICTC.
2. Mobile ICTC: Mobile counselling and testing centre is a van with a room to conduct general examination, counselling and space for collection and processing blood samples by a team of paramedical healthcare providers (a health educator/ANM, counsellor and laboratory technician). Mobile ICTC are set up as temporary clinics in hard-to-reach areas with flexible working hours and provide a wide range of services like

counselling and testing services for HIV, syndromic management of STI/RTI and other minor ailments, along with regular health check-ups, antenatal, immunization services etc.

Community based HIV screening: In order to offer HIV testing to every pregnant woman in the country, so as to detect all HIV positive pregnant women and eliminate transmission of HIV from parent to child, the community-based HIV screening is conducted by frontline health workers (Auxiliary Nurse Midwives) at the sub-centre level.

PREVENTION OF PARENT-TO-CHILD TRANSMISSION OF HIV

The prevention of parent-to-child transmission of HIV/AIDS (PPTCT) programme was started in the country in the year 2002. Currently there are more than 15,000 ICTCs in the country which offer PPTCT services to pregnant women. The aim of the PPTCT programme is to offer HIV testing to every pregnant woman (universal coverage) in the country, so as to cover all estimated HIV positive pregnant women and eliminate transmission of HIV from mother-to-child.

In India, PPTCT interventions under NACP was started in 2002, using SD-NVP prophylaxis for HIV positive pregnant women during labour and also for her new born child immediately after birth. With the department of AIDS control adopting "Option B" of the World Health Organization recommendations (2010), India has also transitioned from the single dose Nevirapine strategy to that of multi-drug ARV prophylaxis from September 2012. This strategy was executed in the three southern high HIV prevalence states of Andhra Pradesh, Karnataka and Tamil Nadu. The national strategic plan for PPTCT services using multi-drug ARVs in India was developed in May-June 2013 for nationwide implementation in a phased manner. Based on the new WHO guidelines (June 2013) and on the suggestions from the technical resource groups during December 2013, department of AIDS control has decided to initiate lifelong ART (using the triple drug regimen) for all pregnant and breast-feeding women living with HIV, regardless of CD4 count or WHO clinical stage, both for their own health and to prevent vertical HIV transmission, and for additional HIV prevention benefits.

The PPTCT services provide access to all pregnant women for HIV diagnostic, prevention, care and treatment services. As such, the key goal is to ensure the integrated PPTCT service delivery with the existing Reproductive and Child Health (RCH) programme.

The essential package of PPTCT services in India are as follows *(32)* :

1. Routine offer of HIV counselling and testing to all pregnant women enrolled into antenatal care, with an 'opt out' option.
2. Ensuring involvement of spouse and other family members, and move from an "ANC-Centric" to a "Family-Centric" approach.
3. Provision of life-long ART (TDF+3TC+EFV) to all pregnant and breast-feeding HIV infected women, regardless of CD4 count and clinical stage of HIV progression.
4. Promotion of institutional deliveries of all HIV infected pregnant women.
5. Provision of care for associated conditions (STI/RTI, TB and other opportunistic infections).
6. Provision of nutrition, counselling and psychosocial support for HIV infected pregnant women.
7. Provision of counselling and support for initiation of exclusive breast-feeds within an hour of delivery as the preferred option and continued for 6 months.
8. Provision of ARV prophylaxis to infants from birth upto a minimum of 6 months.
9. Integrating follow-up of HIV-exposed infants into routine healthcare services including immunization.
10. Ensuring initiation of Co-trimoxazole Prophylactic Therapy (CPT) and Early Infant Diagnosis (EID) using HIV-DNA PCR at 6 weeks of age onwards, as per the EID guidelines.
11. Strengthening community follow-up and outreach through local community networks to support HIV-positive pregnant women and their families.

HIV TESTING OF TB PATIENTS

Detection of HIV by offering HIV tests to diagnosed TB patients is being implemented by NACP and RNTCP jointly since 2007–08. States with high HIV prevalence cover about 90% TB patients for HIV testing, but case fatality rate among HIV infected TB cases remains 13–14%, as compared to less than 4% in HIV negative TB cases, indicating delayed detection of HIV/TB inspite of good coverage. Therefore, NACP and RNTCP have jointly decided to offer HIV testing upstream during evaluation of patients for TB when they present with TB symptoms. This activity is expected to expedite detection of HIV within 2–4 weeks of TB positivity, leading to early linkage to HIV treatment and hence reduction in mortality. HIV testing in presumptive TB cases was rolled-out in India in October 2012 in Karnataka, followed by Maharashtra, Andhra Pradesh and Tamil Nadu. It is planned to extend this strategy to high HIV prevalence districts i.e. A and B category districts. Further the NTWG has recommended implementation of this strategy among 25–54 years age group in the rest of the country.

The four pronged strategy for HIV–TB coordination activity to reduce mortality are summarized in Fig. 7.

Care, support and treatment

The care, support and treatment (CST) component of NACP aims to provide comprehensive services to people living with HIV (PLHIV) to improve the survival and quality of life. The policy package includes the following *(7)*:

- Free universal access to life long standardized antiretroviral therapy (ART);
- Free laboratory diagnostic and monitoring services (baseline tests, CD4 testing, targeted viral load);
- Facilitating long term retention in care;
- Prevention, diagnosis and management of opportunistic infection; and
- Linkage to care and support services and linkage to social protection scheme.

The country has adopted fast track target of 90–90–90 and more recently 95–95–95 target which aims at ending AIDS as public health threat by 2030 by achieving fast track targets by 2020. They are as follows:

1. 95 per cent of PLHIV know their status, of which
2. 95 per cent of PLHIV are on ART, of which
3. 95 per cent of PLHIV have viral suppression.

Prevention
1. Isoniazid preventive treatment
2. Air borne infection control
3. Awareness generation

Early detection of TB/HIV
1. 100% coverage of PITC in TB patients
2. PITC in presumptive TB cases
3. Rapid diagnostics for detection of TB and DR-TB in PLHIV
4. ICF activities at all HIV settings – ICTC, ART, LAC and TI settings

TB/HIV co-ordination to reduce mortality

Prompt treatment of TB/HIV
1. Early initiation of ART
2. Prompt initiation of TB treatment

Management of special TB/HIV cases
1. TB/HIV patients on PI based ARV
2. TB/HIV in children
3. TB/HIV pregnant women
4. Drug resistant TB/HIV

FIG. 7
Activities to reduce HIV–TB mortality

PITC – Provider initiated HIV testing and counselling; ICF – Intensified case finding; LAC – Link ART centres; TI – Targeted interventions

Source : *(33)*

A significant step of rolling out "test and treat" policy has been taken towards achieving these targets.

CST services are provided through ART centres established by DAC in health facilities across the country. These are linked to Centres of Excellence (CoE) and ART-Plus centres at selected institutions, while some of the services have been decentralized through Link ART Centres (LAC). ART centres are also linked to ICTCs, STI clinics, PPTCT services and other clinical departments in the institutions of their location, as well as with the Revised National Tuberculosis Programme (RNTCP), in order to ensure proper management of TB–HIV co-infected patients. Fig. 8 gives a graphic view of this service delivery model.

As of September 2021, about 645 ART centres, 1,261 link ART centres, 17 centres of excellence, 7 paediatric centres of excellence, 93 ART Plus centres and 310 care and support centres are functioning in the country *(6)*.

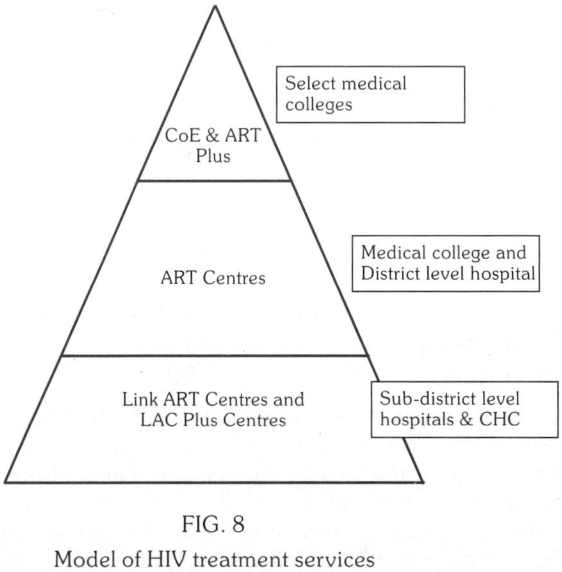

FIG. 8
Model of HIV treatment services

Source : *(32)*

Services provided

1. *First-line ART:* First-line ART is provided free of cost to all eligible PLHIV through ART centres. Positive cases referred by ICTCs are registered in ART centres for pre-ART and ART services. The assessment for eligibility for ART is done through clinical examination and CD4 count. Patients are also provided counselling on treatment adherence, nutrition, positive prevention and positive living. Follow-up of patients on ART is done by assessing drug adherence, regularity of visits, periodic examination and CD4 count (every six months). Treatment for opportunistic infections is also provided through ART centres. Till Sept. 2021, 14.06 lakh PLHIV were on first-line ART.
2. *Alternative first-line ART:* It has been observed that a small number of patients initiated on first-line ART experience acute/chronic toxicity/intolerance to first-line ARV drugs, thus necessitating change of ARV drugs to alternative first-line drugs. Presently, the provision of alternative first-line ART is done through the Centres of Excellence and ART-Plus centres across the country.
3. *Second-line ART:* The second-line ART began in January 2008 at two sites – GHTM, Tambaram, Chennai and JJ Hospital, Mumbai on a pilot basis, and was then further expanded to the other CoEs in January 2009. Further decentralization of second-line ART was done through capacitating and upgrading some well-functioning ART centres as 'ART-Plus Centres'. Till Sept. 2021, 1,01,069 patients were receiving second-line drugs at CoEs and ART-Plus centres. All ART centres are linked to CoE/ART-Plus centres. For the evaluation of patients for initiation on second-line and alternate first-line ART, a State AIDS Clinical Expert Panel (SACEP) has been constituted by DAC at all CoEs and ART-Plus centres. This panel meets once in a week for taking decisions on patients referred to them with treatment failure/major side effects.
4. *Third -Line ART:* Some patients on second-line ART also experience treatment failure. National programme rolled

out third-line regimen for them in 2015. Currently Raltegravir and Darunavir are used for third-line regimen *(7)* as on Sept. 2021, 4,528 patients were on 3rd line treatment *(34)*.

National paediatric HIV/AIDS initiative: The national paediatric HIV/AIDS initiative was launched on 30 November 2006. Till March 2014, nearly 1,06,824 children living with HIV/AIDS (CLHIV) were registered in HIV care at ART centres, of whom 42,015 were receiving free ART. Paediatric formulations of ARV drugs are available at all ART centres.

Paediatric second-line ART: While the first-line therapy is efficacious, certain proportion of children do show evidence of failure. There is not much data available on the failure rate of Nevirapine-based ART in children. However, WHO estimates that the average switch rate from first to second-line ART is 2–3% per year for adults. It is likely that similar rates are applicable for children as well. Currently, second-line ART for children has been made available at all CoE and ART-Plus centres.

Early infant diagnosis: In order to promote confirmatory diagnosis for HIV exposed children, a programme on Early Infant Diagnosis (EID) was launched by DAC. All children with HIV infection confirmed through EID have been linked to ART services.

Follow-up and monitoring: Patients initiated on ART are regularly followed up on monthly basis. The basic examination including weight measurement, clinical evaluation, and screening for opportunistic infections is done on every visit. Assessment of adherence is done by counsellor on every visit and necessary support is provided as per requirement. CD4 testing is done every six months to monitor the response of ART. During each visit, patients are encouraged to visit care and support centers for psycho-social support and availing various social beneficiary scheme *(7)*.

Management of Opportunistic infection (7): Screening prophylaxis and management of various opportunistic infections is an important part of comprehensive HIV care. Following intervention are done at ART centers for this:

a. HIV-TB: TB is the most common opportunistic infection among PLHIVs. All patients attending ART centers including new registrations, pre-ART and on ART patients are screened verbally for 4 symptom complex. In case any one of the symptom is present, patients are referred for TB testing. Those diagnosed with co-infection are initiated on Anti TB treatment from ART center followed by ART. When TB is ruled out, Isoniazid prophylaxis is offered. NACP works in close coordination with RNTCP for managing co-infections.
b. HIV-Hepatitis B and Hepatitis C: The PLHIV are at high risk of co-morbidity with hepatitis B and C. It is important to ensure timely detection and initiation of hepatitis B or C treatment in HIV/viral hepatitis co-infected patients to minimize hepatitis-related liver disease and its long-term negative impact on HIV outcomes. Hepatitis B and C detection and treatment for PLHIV will be provided at ART centers. Hepatitis B treatment is available as part of ART programme since ART regimens containing tenofovir (TDF) plus a second NRTI active against HBV (3TC/FTC) have been shown to suppress both HIV and HBV viral replication. Treatment for Hepatitis C needs direct acting antivirals (DAAs) such as sofosbuvir, grazoprevir, glecaprevir etc. *(28)*.
c. HIV - Kala-azar: Kala-azar or Visceral Leishmaniasis is endemic in some districts of states like UP, Bihar and Jharkhand. All PLHIVs with symptoms suggestive of Kala-azar are screened for Kala-azar and those found infected are referred for appropriate treatment.
d. Other opportunistic infection: PLHIVs are regularly screened for co-infection and co-morbidities. Those diagnosed having these are treated appropriately at ART center or are referred to concerned facility. Those who are vulnerable to opportunistic infections due to low CD4 count or any other reasons are provided with prophylaxis, for eg. Co-trimoxazole.

TARGETTED INTERVENTIONS FOR HIGH RISK GROUPS: The main objective of targeted interventions (TI) is to improve health-seeking behaviour of high risk groups (HRG) and reduce their risk of acquiring sexually transmitted infections (STI) and HIV infections. High risk groups under TI include female sex workers (FSW), men who have sex with men (MSM), transgenders (TG)/hijras and injecting drug users (IDU), and bridge populations include high risk behaviour migrants and long distance truckers. Targeted interventions provide the information, means and skills needed to prevent HIV transmission and improve their access to care, support and treatment services. These programmes also focus on improving sexual and reproductive health and general health of high-risk population.

The services offered through targeted interventions include:

- Detection and treatment for sexually transmitted infections.
- Condom distribution (except in TIs for bridge population).
- Condom promotion through social marketing (for HRG and bridge population).
- Behaviour change communication.
- Creating an enabling environment with community involvement and participation.
- Linkages to integrated counselling and testing centres.
- Linkages with care and support services for HIV positive HRGs.
- Community organization and ownership building.
- Specific interventions for IDUs.
  - Distribution of clean needles and syringes.
  - Abscess prevention and management.
  - Opioid substitution therapy.
  - Linkage with detoxification/rehabilitation services.
- Specific interventions for MSM/TGs.
  - Provision of lubricants.
  - Specific interventions for TG/hijra populations.
  - Provision of project-based STI clinics.

The targeted interventions (TIs) supported by NACO as on September 2021 are as follows *(6)* :

FSW	–	313
MSM	–	94
IDU	–	200
Transgender/Hijaras	–	40
Migrants	–	210
Truckers	–	70

Link worker scheme: The Link worker scheme is a community-based outreach strategy to address HIV prevention and care needs of HRG and vulnerable population in rural areas. The specific objectives of the scheme include reaching out to these groups with information and knowledge on prevention and risk reduction of HIV and STI, condom promotion and distribution, providing referral and follow-up linkages for various services. It includes counselling, testing and treatment of STI and opportunistic infections through link workers, creating an enabling environment for PLHIV and their families, and reducing stigma and discrimination against them. In partnership with various development partners, the link worker scheme has been expanded and as on September 2021, it is being implemented in 16 states covering 143 highly vulnerable districts covering 1500 villages.

The population covered under the link worker scheme from January to September 2021 are as follows *(6)* :

Population	Line Listed	Covered
FSW	55,448	49,990
IDU	8,573	7,573
MSM	8,543	7,676
TG	554	456
Migrant	4,38,043	2,10,368
Trucker	75,170	48,628
Other-Vul. Pop	5,85,151	3,34,107
TB cases	23,081	9,135
ANC	88,517	65,181
PLHIV	34,265	25,788

Blood transfusion services: The division of blood safety has been renamed as the division of blood transfusion services. The change in nomenclature is to broaden the horizon of blood safety to include transfusion transmitted infections, immuno-hematology, quality management systems, logistics and other processes involved to improve confidence in the "safe blood".

Blood transfusion services have been considered as an integral part of the health care system. Blood Transfusion Councils have been set-up at national and state levels. Professional blood donation has been prohibited in the country since 1st January 1998. Only licensed blood banks are permitted to operate in the country and voluntary blood donation is encouraged. The strategy is to ensure safe collection, processing, storage and distribution of blood and blood products. Zonal blood testing centres have been established to provide linkage with other blood banks affiliated to public, private and voluntary sectors. As per national blood safety policy, testing of every unit of blood is mandatory for detecting infections like HIV, hepatitis B, hepatitis C, malaria and syphilis.

Access to safe blood for the needy is the primary responsibility of NACO. It is supporting a network of 1,131 blood banks, including 590 Blood Component Separation Units (BCSU) and 34 Model Blood Banks, 108 major blood banks and 591 district level blood banks *(7)*. NACO supported the installation of BCSU and has given funds for modernization of all major blood banks at state and district levels. Besides enhancing awareness about the need to procure safe blood and blood products, NACO has supported the procurement of equipment, test kits and reagents, and is helping in the recurring expenditure of government blood banks and those run by voluntary/ charitable organizations, that were modernized.

In order to ease the situation of shortage of availability of blood in the rural areas, where it is not feasible to operate a blood bank, Govt. has decided to establish blood storage centres at First Referral Units (FRUs), at sub-district levels, for wider availability of safe blood, particularly for emergency obstetric care and trauma care services.

Condom promotion: Condom promotion strategies will be strengthened through free distribution and social marketing channels, non-traditional outlets, female condoms, etc. aided by an effective communication strategy. The programme will continue to link prevention with care, support and treatment. This will promote positive prevention.

On the basis of HIV prevalence and family planning needs, the districts have been mapped and classified into four categories: (a) High prevalence of HIV and high fertility (HPHF); (b) High prevalence of HIV and low fertility (HPLF); (c) Low prevalence of HIV and low fertility (LPLF); and (d) Low prevalence of HIV and high fertility (LPHF). During 2014 the coverage of condom social marketing programme implementation was spread across 395 districts, i.e. 141 HPHF, 84 HPLF and 170 LPHF districts in 11 states *(31)*.

STD CONTROL PROGRAMME : STD control is linked to HIV/AIDS control as behaviour resulting in the transmission of STD and HIV are same. HIV is transmitted more easily in the presence of another STD. Hence, early diagnosis and treatment of STD is now recognized as one of the major strategies to control spread of HIV infection. The following approach is adopted for the STD control *(35)* :

a. Management of STDs through syndromic approach (management of sexually transmitted diseases based on specific symptoms and signs and not dependent on laboratory investigations). Please refer to page 381 chapter 5 for details.
b. STDs among women, though highly prevalent, are suppressed because of the social stigma attached to the disease. It has, therefore, been decided to integrate services for treatment of reproductive tract infections (RTIs) and sexually transmitted diseases (STDs) at all levels of health care. Department of Family Welfare and NACO will coordinate their activities for an effective implementation of such integration. STDs Clinics at district / block/ First Referral Unit (FRU) level would function as referral centres for treatment of STDs referred from peripheries. STDs clinics in all district hospitals, medical colleges and other centres would be strengthened by providing technical support, equipment, reagents and drugs. A massive orientation-training programme would be undertaken to train all the medical and paramedical workers engaged in providing STDs/RTIs services through a syndromic approach. All STDs clinics would also provide counselling services and good quality condoms to the STD patients. Services of NGOs would be utilised for providing such counselling services at the STDs clinics.

NACO has branded the STI/RTI services as **"Suraksha Clinic"**, and has developed a communication strategy for generating demand for these services *(3)*.

PRE-PACKED STI/RTI COLOUR CODED KITS : Pre-packed colour coded STI/RTI kits have been provided for free supply to all designated STI/RTI clinics. These kits are being procured centrally and supplied to all State AIDS Control Societies.

The colour code is as follows *(36)* :

Kit 1 – grey, for urethral discharge, ano-rectal discharge and cervicitis.
Kit 2 – green, for vaginitis.
Kit 3 – white, for genital ulcers.
Kit 4 – blue, for genital ulcers.
Kit 5 – red, for genital ulcers.
Kit 6 – yellow, for lower abdominal pain.
Kit 7 – black, for inguinal bubo.

National Strategic Plan for HIV/AIDS and STI 2017–2024 *(28)*

The National Strategic Plan for HIV/AIDS and STI (2017–2024) is developed with a vision of an AIDS free India. The mission is to attain universal coverage of HIV prevention, testing, treatment to care continuum that is effective, inclusive, equitable and adapted to population and local needs.

Goal : The goal is to achieve zero new infection, zero AIDS-related deaths and zero AIDS related stigma and discrimination.

Strategic framework: The NSP is designed around a results-based framework that reflects the fast-track targets and the 'ending of AIDS' commitment. The framework is based on a causal relationship between the vision, mission, goal and the outcomes. This will be articulated in terms of inputs, outputs and costs in the implementation plan. While there are several external and internal risks that may positively or adversely affect results, the combination of strategies adopted will be calibrated according to the epidemiological, health priorities and resource scenarios of different State/UTs and in cognisance of needs of people living with HIV and the communities.

Based on this strategic framework, a specific planning approach is required which helps differentiate States and Union Territories (UT) according to three predominant epidemiological contexts *(28)*:

(i) States/UT with a 'mature' epidemic where HIV incidence and prevalence are high in key, bridge and other at-risk populations and, in some cases, in other segments of the general population.

(ii) Those States/UT where there are 'emerging' epidemics with relatively new and rising rates of infection among key, bridge and other at-risk populations.

(iii) States/UT with 'low' or stable epidemics where there is still a need to focus on potential risks among key, bridge and other at-risk populations, to maintain the low infection rates and eliminate HIV transmission.

While a range of services is needed in all the three case scenarios, the mix and relative weight of each set of interventions and service-delivery models may need to vary accordingly. The most critical interventions include prevention, outreach, testing and counselling, treatment, PPTCT, viral load suppression, care and support, as well as social protection. Programmatic support components (e.g. monitoring and evaluation, surveillance, research, laboratory services, procurement etc.) remain relevant across all three contexts. However, the service delivery modality, the level of integration into health systems and corresponding budget requirements will vary according to the epidemiological, social and demographic characteristics of the above three contexts.

Objectives: This NSP proposes six objectives towards fulfilling its vision of an AIDS free India. These are:

Objective 1 : Reduce 80% new infections by 2024 (Baseline 2010)

Objective 2 : Ensure 95% of estimated PLHIV know their status by 2024

Objective 3 : Ensure 95% PLHIV have ART initiation and retention by 2024, for sustained viral suppression

Objective 4 : Eliminate mother-to-child transmission of HIV and syphilis by 2020.

Objective 5 : Eliminate HIV/AIDS related stigma and discrimination by 2020

Objective 6 : Facilitate sustainable NACP service delivery by 2024

Achievement of these objectives by 2024 would result in the following: *(28)*:

1. Estimated new infections will reduce from 102,226 (2010) to < 21,000 per year
2. 2.14 million PLHIV of the total estimated PLHIV (2.25 million) would know their status
3. 2.03 million PLHIV would be put on ART
4. 1.93 million PLHIV would be retained on treatment and have HIV VL < 1000 copies/ml
5. Attainment of <50 cases of new paediatric HIV infections per 100,000 live births with a mother-to-child transmission rate <5% by 2020 and maintenance of same thereof
6. Attainment of <50 cases of congenital syphilis per 100,000 live births and maintenance of same thereof
7. HIV/AIDS will be perceived as chronic manageable disease with no stigma and discrimination attached to it.
8. Key components of the NACP such as prevention outreach, testing, treatment, prevention of mother-to-child transmission, viral load suppression, care and support, as well as social protection schemes will continue through 100% domestic funding.

Information, education and communication

Communication is the key to generating awareness on prevention as well as motivating access to testing, treatment, care and support. Communication in NACP-IV is directed at:

a. To increase knowledge among general population (especially youth and women) on safe sexual behaviour;
b. To sustain behaviour change in high risk groups and bridge populations;
c. To generate demand for care, support and treatment services; and
d. To make appropriate changes in societal norms that reinforce positive attitude, beliefs and practices to reduce stigma and discrimination.

Adolescence Education Programme: This programme runs in secondary and senior secondary schools to built up life skills of adolescents to cope with the physical and psychological changes associated with growing up. Under the programme, 16 hour sessions are scheduled during the academic terms of class IX and XI. State AIDS control society have further adapted the modules after state level consultations with NGOs, academicians, psychologists and parent-teacher bodies. This programme is being implemented in 23 states and currently 50,000 schools have been covered.

Red Ribbon Clubs: The purpose of Red Ribbon Club formation in colleges is to encourage peer-to-peer messaging on HIV prevention and to provide a safe space for young people to seek clarifications of their doubts and myths surrounding HIV/AIDS. The RRCs also promote voluntary blood donation among youth. Currently, 12,546 Red Ribbon Clubs are functioning under the programme.

Achievement on Key Indicators under NACP during FY 2021–22 :

The key indicators across the domain of Output, Outcome and Impact have been summarised below. These indicators are used to report to various forums including NITI Aayog's Output Outcome Monitoring Framework.

Achievement on Key Indicators under NACP during FY 2021–22 (April to November 2021)

Indicator(s)	Annual Target (2021–22)	Achievement (April- Nov. 2021)
No. of High-Risk Group and Bridge Population covered through Targeted Interventions	83.87 lakh	41.17 Lakh
No. of High-Risk Groups & Vulnerable Population covered through LWS	18.53 lakh	7.59 lakh
No. of STI/RTI patients managed as per national protocol	100.16 lakh	53.94 lakhs
No. of persons trained under mainstreaming training programmes	1.49 lakh	1.44 lakh
No. of condoms free distributed (in pieces)	30.19 crore pieces	17.02 crore pieces
No. of General Clients tested for HIV	252 lakh	145.0 lakhs
No. of Pregnant Women tested for HIV	252 lakh	162.2 lakhs
No. of HIV-TB cross referrals	35 lakh	18.32 lakh
No. of PLHIV on ART* (Cumulative)	15.30 lakh	15.21 lakh
No. of opportunistic infections treated	3.5 lakh	2.00 lakh
No. of viral load test conducted among PLHIV on ART	11.00 lakh	6.55 lakh

*Inclusive of 1.06 lakh PLHIV on ART in private sector

Progress on Output and Impact Indicators during 2020

Indicator(s)	Target	National Achievement	Global Achievement
Decline in annual new HIV infections (%)	75%	48%	31%
People living with HIV (PLHIV) who know their HIV status (%)	90%	78%	84%
PLHIV who know their HIV Positive status and are on Antiretroviral Therapy (%)	90%	83%	87%
PLHIV on Antiretroviral Therapy and virally suppressed (%)	90%	85%	90%
Decline in annual AIDS-related deaths (%)	75%	82%	42%
HIV positive mother on Antiretroviral Therapy (%)	95%	52%	85%

Source : *(6)*

NATIONAL PROGRAMME FOR CONTROL OF BLINDNESS

The National Programme for Control of Blindness was launched in the year 1976 as a 100 per cent centrally sponsored programme and incorporates the earlier trachoma control programme started in the year 1968. The programme was launched with the goal to reduce the prevalence of blindness from 1.4 to 0.3 per cent. As per 2015–19 survey the prevalence of blindness was 0.36 per cent *(11)*.

Main objectives of the programme in the 12th Five Year Plan period are:

1. To continue three ongoing signature activities, i.e., performance of 66 lacs cataract operations per year; school eye screening and distribution of 9 lacs free spectacles per year to school children suffering from refractive errors; and collection of 50,000 donated eyes per year for keratoplasty *(6)*.
2. To reduce the backlog of avoidable blindness through identification and treatment of curable blind at primary, secondary and tertiary levels, based on assessment of the overall burden of visual impairment in the country;
3. Develop and strengthen the strategy of NPCB for "Eye Health for All" and prevention of visual impairment, through provision of comprehensive universal eye-care services and quality service delivery;
4. Strengthening and upgradation of Regional Institutes of Ophthalmology (RIOs) to become centre of excellence in various sub-specialities of ophthalmology and also other partners like Medical Colleges, District Hospitals, Sub-district Hospitals, Vision Centres, NGO Eye Hospitals;
5. Strengthening the existing infrastructure facilities and developing additional human resources for providing high quality comprehensive eye care in all districts of the country;
6. To enhance community awareness on eye care and lay stress on preventive measures;
7. Increase and expand research for prevention of blindness and visual impairment; and
8. To secure participation of voluntary organizations/ private practitioners in delivering eye care.

Salient features/strategies adopted to achieve the objectives are:

1. Continued emphasis on free cataract surgery through the health care delivery system as well as by the involvement of NGO sector and private practitioners.
2. Emphasis on the comprehensive eye care programmes by covering diseases other than cataract, like diabetic retinopathy, glaucoma, corneal transplantation, vitreo-retinal surgery, treatment of childhood blindness etc. These emerging diseases need immediate attention to eliminate avoidable blindness from the country.
3. Reduction in the backlog of blind persons by active screening of population above 50 years age, organizing screening eye camps and transporting operable cases to fixed eye care facilities.
4. Refractive error comprises a major part of avoidable blindness. Screening of children for identification and treatment of refractive errors and provision of free glasses to those affected and belonging to poor socio-economic strata.
5. Coverage of underserved area for eye care services through public-private partnership.
6. Capacity building of health personnel for improving their knowledge and skill in delivery of high quality eye services.
7. Information Education Communication (IEC) activities for creating awareness on eye-care within the community.
8. Regional Institutes of Ophthalmology and Medical Colleges of the states to be strengthened in a phased manner with latest equipments and training of manpower so that they can be upgraded as Centres of Excellence in the regions.

9. The district hospitals to be strengthened by upgrading infrastructure, equipment and providing adequate manpower like ophthalmologists and PMOAs on contractual basis and provide earmarked funds for basic medicines and drugs.
10. Continuing emphasis on primary healthcare (eye care) by establishing vision centres in all PHCs with a PMOA in position.
11. Multipurpose District Mobile Ophthalmic Units for better coverage.

To avoid duplicity of work, State Ophthalmic Cell has been merged with State Blindness Control Society, and after the launch of NRHM, State Blindness Control Societies have been further merged with State Health Society. Likewise, District Blindness Control Societies have also been merged with District Health Societies. Facilities for intra-ocular lense implantation have been expanded to taluka level.

The problem of blindness is acute in rural areas, and hence the programme has tried to expand the accessibility of eye services in these areas. At present there are 80 central mobile units attached to medical colleges and 341 district mobile units to provide eye care in mobile eye camps. These units have a vehicle, ophthalmic surgeon and other paramedical staff. Most of the cataract surgeries in rural population are conducted through these mobile camps. Primary health centres are the basic units in the rural areas.

The findings of the survey conducted during 2001–2002, in randomly selected districts of the states covered by World Bank Project shows that dependence on eye camps has reduced, except in remote and tribal areas; involvement of PHC/CHC doctor in the programme has increased; higher percentage of cataract operated persons consult the doctor at an early stage; there is an increase in demand for modern techniques like intra-ocular lenses and suture-less surgeries; and about 84 per cent of cataract operated persons receive free spectacles from the health facilities.

The organizational structure for the national programme for control of blindness is as shown in Fig. 9.

Administration

Central	Ophthalmology Section, Directorate General of Health Services, Ministry of Health & FW, New Delhi
State	State Ophthalmic Cell, Directorate of Health Services, State Health Societies
District	District Blindness Control Society

Service Delivery and Referral System

Tertiary Level	Regional Institutes of Ophthalmology & Centres of Excellence in Eye Care Medical Colleges
Secondary Level	District Hospital and NGO Eye Hospital
Primary Level	Sub-district level hospitals/CHCs Mobile Ophthalmic Units Upgraded PHCs, Link Workers/Panchayats

FIG. 9
Organizational structure for national programme for control of blindness

Source : *(37)*

SCHOOL EYE SCREENING PROGRAMME : 6–7 per cent of children aged 10–14 years have problem with their eye sight affecting their learning at school. Children are being first screened by trained teachers. Children suspected to have refractive error are seen by ophthalmic assistants and corrective spectacles are prescribed or given free for persons below poverty line.

COLLECTION AND UTILIZATION OF DONATED EYES : During 2018–19 nearly 68,409 donated eyes were collected for corneal implantation *(11)*. Hospital retrieval programme is the major strategy for collection of donated eyes, which envisage motivation of relatives of terminally ill patients, accident victims and others with grave diseases to donate eyes. Eye donation fortnight is organized from 25th August to 8th September every year to promote eye donation/eye banking. Gujarat, Tamil Nadu, Maharashtra and Andhra Pradesh are leading states in this activity *(1)*.

The voluntary organizations such as Lions International and its branches, Rotary International and its branches, NSPB India etc. are encouraged to organize eye camps in remote rural and urban areas as per guidelines, with the permission from the state authorities. They have been active in providing eye health education, preventive, rehabilitative and surgical services for control of blindness.

Community health education is a built-in component at all levels of implementation of National Blindness Control Programme. The programme also includes regular eye check-up and provision of vitamin A prophylaxis and service facilities in rural areas.

WHO assistance for prevention of blindness : This includes intra-country fellowships in corneal transplantation, vitreo-retinal surgery, lasers in ophthalmology and paediatric ophthalmology; pilot survey on childhood blindness in Delhi; training in district programme management; study on situational analysis of eye care infrastructure and human resources in India; high quality workshops in eye care for faculty of medical colleges; and developement of plan of action for "Vision 2020 : The Right to Sight" initiative.

Vision 2020 : The Right to Sight

It is a global initiative to reduce avoidable (preventable and curable) blindness by the year 2020. India is also committed to this initiative. The plan of action for the country has been developed with following main features :

1. Target diseases are cataract, refractive errors, childhood blindness, corneal blindness, glaucoma, diabetic retinopathy.
2. Human resource development as well as infrastructure and technology development at various levels of health system. The proposed four tier structure includes Centres of Excellence (20), Training Centres (200), Service Centres (2000), and Vision Centres (20,000).

Fig. 10 shows the proposed structure for primary, secondary and tertiary eye care.

Universal eye health : a global action plan 2014–2019 *(38)*

WHO estimates that in 2010 there were 285 million people visually impaired, of which 39 million were blind. If

Proposed Structure

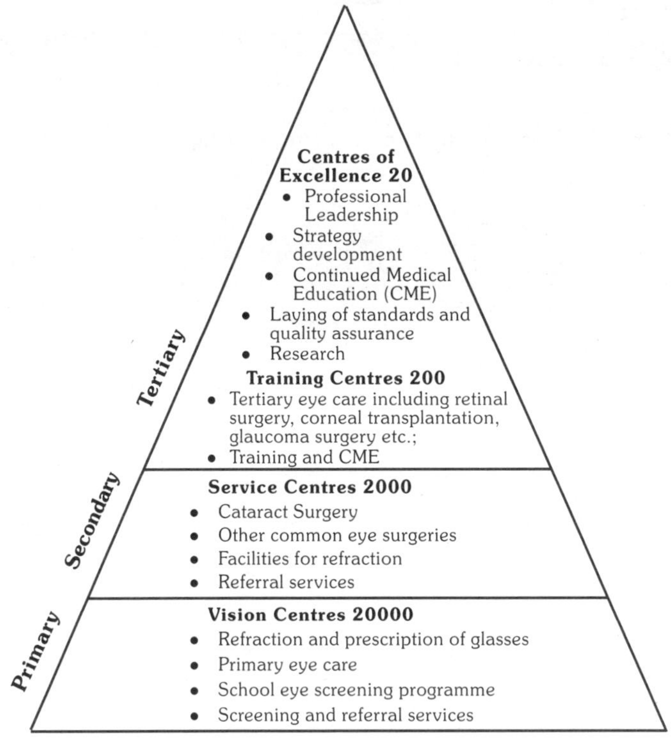

FIG. 10

Proposed structure for Vision 2020 : The Right to Sight

Source : *(37)*

just the two major causes of visual impairment were considered priorities and control measures were implemented consistently by providing refractive services and offering cataract surgery to the people in need, two-thirds of the visually impaired people could recover good eye sight.

Provision of effective and accessible eye care services is the key to control measures. The preference should be given to strengthening eye care services through their integration into the primary health care and health system development, as almost all causes of visual impairment are avoidable, e.g., diabetes mellitus, smoking, premature birth, rubella, vitamin A deficiency etc., and visual impairment is frequent among older age groups. Improvements in the areas of maternal, child and reproductive health and the provision of safe drinking water and basic sanitation are important. Eye health should be included in the broader non-communicable and communicable disease frameworks, as well as those addressing ageing populations. There are three indicators to measure progress at the national level. They are:

1. The prevalence and causes of visual impairment. As a global target, reduction in prevalence of avoidable visual impairment by 25 per cent by 2019 from the baseline of 2010 has been selected for this action plan;
2. The number of eye care personnel; and
3. Cataract surgical service delivery. The cataract surgical rate (number of surgeries performed per year, per million population) and cataract surgical coverage (number of individuals with bilateral cataract causing visual impairment, who have received cataract surgery on one or both eyes).

IODINE DEFICIENCY DISORDERS (IDD) PROGRAMME

India commenced a goitre control programme in 1962, based on iodized salt. At the end of three decades, the prevalence of the disease still remained high.

As a result, a major national programme – "The IDD Control Programme" was initiated in which nation-wide, rather than area-specific use of iodized salt is being promoted. It was decided as a national policy to fortify all edible salt in a phased manner by end of 8th Plan. The essential components of a national IDD programme are use of iodized salt in place of common salt, monitoring and surveillance, manpower training and mass communication.

The objectives of the programme are *(1)* :

1. Surveys to assess the magnitude of the Iodine Deficiency Disorders in districts.
2. Supply of iodized salt in place of common salt.
3. Resurveys to assess iodine deficiency disorders and the impact of iodized salt after every 5 years in districts.
4. Laboratory monitoring of iodized salt and urinary iodine excretion.
5. Health education and publicity.

Significant achievements

Consequent upon liberalization of iodized salt production, Salt Commissioner has issued licenses to 824 salt manufacturers out of which 777 units have commenced production. These units have an annual production capacity of 222 lakh metric tonnes of iodized salt.

The production/supply of iodized salt from April 2015 to August 2015 was 26.44 lakh tonnes and 25.12 lakh tonnes.

Notification banning the sale of non-iodized salt for different human consumption in the entire country is already issued under "Food Safety & Standards Act 2006 and Regulations 2011".

For effective implementation of National Iodine Deficiency Disorders Control Programme 34 States/UTs have established Iodine Deficiency Disorders Control Cells in their State Health Directorate.

UNIVERSAL IMMUNIZATION PROGRAMME

Experience with smallpox eradication programme showed the world that immunization was the most powerful and cost-effective weapon against vaccine preventable diseases. In 1974, the WHO launched its "Expanded Programme on Immunization" (EPI) against six, most common, preventable childhood diseases, viz. diphtheria, pertussis (whooping cough), tetanus, polio, tuberculosis and measles. From the beginning of the programme UNICEF has been providing significant support to EPI.

"Expanded" in the WHO definition meant adding more disease controlling antigens of vaccination schedules, extending coverage to all corners of a country and spreading services to reach the less privileged sectors of the society *(39)*.

The primary health care concept as enunciated in the 1978 Alma-Ata Declaration included immunization as one of the strategies for reaching the goal of "Health For All" by the year 2000. While the WHO's programme is called EPI, the UNICEF in 1985 renamed it as "Universal Child

TABLE 8
Immunization milestones - India

1978	Expanded programme of immunization BCG,DPT,OPV, typhoid (urban areas)
1983	TT vaccine for pregnant women
1985	Universal Immunization Programme - measles added, typhoid removed. Focus on children less than 1 yr of age
1990	Vitamin-A supplementation
1995	Polio National Immunization Days
1997	VVM introduced on vaccines in UIP
2002	Hep B introduced as pilot in 33 districts and cities of 10 states
2005	• National Rural Health Mission Launched • Auto disable (AD) syringes introduced into UIP
2006	JE vaccine introduced after campaigns in endemic districts
2007–08	Hep B expanded to all districts in 10 states and schedule revised to 4 dose from 3 dose
2010	Measles 2nd dose introduced in RI and MCUP (14 states)
2011	• Hepatitis B universalized and Haemophilus influenza type b introduced as pentavalent in 2 states • Open Vial Policy for vaccines in UIP
2013	• Pentavalent expanded to 9 states • Second dose of JE vaccine
2014	India and South East Asia Region certified POLIO-FREE
2015	• India validated for Maternal and Neonatal Tetanus elimination • Pentavalent expanded to all states • IPV Introduced
2016	• Rotavirus vaccine introduced in 4 states in Phase 1 • tOPV to bOPV Switch. • Switch to fractional IPV (Phased)
2017	• MR Vaccine introduced • PCV (Phased launch) • Use of adrenaline IM by ANM in AEFI (Adverse event following immunization)
2020	Covishield and Covaxin against COVID-19 introduced

Source : *(41)*

Immunization" (UCI). There was absolutely no difference between these two. The goal was the same, i.e., to achieve universal immunization by 1990. EPI is regarded as the instrument of UCI *(40)*.

The first vaccine to be introduced in India was BCG in 1962 as part of the National Tuberculosis Programme. Over the years, various new vaccines have been introduced and many milestones achieved. Table 8 gives a chronological listing of some important milestones in India's immunization programme.

The Government of India launched its EPI in 1978 with the objective of reducing the mortality and morbidity resulting from vaccine-preventable diseases of childhood, and to achieve self-sufficiency in the production of vaccines. Universal Immunization Programme was started in India in 1985. It has two vital components: immunization of pregnant women against tetanus, and immunization of children in their first year of life against the six EPI target diseases. The aim was to achieve 100 per cent coverage of pregnant women with 2 doses of tetanus toxoid (or a booster dose), and at least 85 per cent coverage of infants with 3 doses each of DPT, OPV, one dose of BCG and one dose of measles vaccine by 1990. Universal immunization was first taken up in 30 selected districts and catchment areas of 50 Medical Colleges in November 1985. The programme now covers entire country and practice areas of all the 242 Medical colleges, thus creating a base for wider coverage *(42)*. A "Technology Mission on Vaccination and Immunization of Vulnerable Population, specially Children" was set up to cover all aspects of the immunization activity from research and development to actual delivery of services to the target population *(43)*.

The immunization services are being provided through the existing health care delivery system (i.e., MCH centres, primary health centres and subcentres, hospitals, dispensaries and ICD units). There is no separate cadre of staff for EPI. The recommended immunization schedule is on page 136.

Although the target was "universal" immunization by 1990, in practice, no country, even in the industrialized world, has ever achieved 100 per cent immunization in children. 'Universal' immunization is, therefore, best interpreted as implying the ideal that no child should be denied immunization against tuberculosis, diphtheria, whooping cough, tetanus, polio and measles. It is, however, generally agreed that when immunization coverage reaches a figure of 80 per cent or more, then disease transmission patterns are so severely disrupted as to provide a degree of protection even for the remaining children who have not been immunized, because of "herd immunity" *(44)*. It is also important that children are immunized during the first year of life and that levels of immunization are sustained so that each new generation is protected.

Significant achievements have been made in India. At the beginning of the programme in 1985–86, vaccine coverage ranged between 29 per cent for BCG and 41 per cent for DPT. By the end of 2021, coverage levels had gone up significantly to about 85 per cent for tetanus toxoid for pregnant women, about 85 per cent for BCG, 85 per cent for DPT 3 doses, 85 per cent for OPV 3 doses, 85 per cent for $HepB_3$, 85 per cent for Hib_3 and 81 per cent for MCV_2. Since then, there is a significant decline in the reported incidence of the vaccine preventable diseases as compared to their incidence in 1987, as shown in Table 9.

TABLE 9
Decline in reported vaccine preventable diseases from year 1987 to 2020

Disease	1987	2020
Poliomyelitis	28,257	0
Diphtheria	12,952	1,991
Pertussis	163,786	11,985
NNT	11,849	1,159
Measles	247,519	12,081

To strengthen routine immunization, Government of India has planned the State Programme Implementation Plan (PIP) part C. It consists of : (a) Support for alternate vaccine delivery from PHC to sub-centre and outreach sessions; (b) Deploying retired manpower to carry out immunization activities in urban slums and underserved areas, where services are deficient; (c) Mobility support to district immunization officer as per state plan for monitoring and supportive supervision; (d) Review meeting at the state level with the districts at 6 monthly intervals; (e) Training of ANM, cold chain handlers, mid-level managers, refrigerator mechanics etc.; (f) Support for mobilization of children to immunization session sites by ASHA, women self-help groups etc.; (g) Printing of immunization cards, monitoring sheet, cold chain chart vaccine inventory charts etc.

In addition, central government is supporting in supplies of auto-disable syringes, downsizing the BCG vial from 20 doses to 10 doses to ensure that BCG vaccine is available in all immunization session sites, strengthening and maintenance of the cold chain system in the states, and supply of vaccines and vaccine van.

PULSE POLIO IMMUNIZATION PROGRAMME

Pulse Polio Immunization Programme was launched in the country in the year 1995. Under this programme children under five years of age are given additional oral polio drops in December and January every year on fixed days. From 1999–2000, house to house vaccination of missed children was also introduced. The NIDs rounds cover approximately 172 million children and SNIDs rounds cover 40–80 million children. In addition, large scale multi-district mop-ups have been conducted *(46)*. As a result only one case of polio was reported in 2011 in the month of January. As on 25th Feb 2012, India was removed from the list of polio endemic countries, and on 27th March 2014, India was certified as polio-free country. Please see page 242 for more details.

INTRODUCTION OF INACTIVATED POLIO VACCINE (IPV)

The last global case due to WPV type-2 was reported at Aligarh in India in 1999. Most of the global cases due to VDPVs (97%) as well as VAPP (40%) are due to type-2 virus. This necessitates the discontinuation of the use of type-2 component from OPV. Polio Endgame Strategic Plan thus recommends replacing tOPV with bOPV. However, this puts the recent birth cohort at the time of switch at risk of VDPV and wild polio virus type 2 due to silent/ongoing transmission of VDPV type-2 and also to potential leakage of wild polio virus type-2 in case of accidental/intended leakage of the virus from a laboratory. To mitigate this risk, inactivated polio virus vaccine was introduced prior to the tOPV–bOPV switch in April 2016. As part of this Polio Endgame Strategy, India has introduced Inactivated Polio Vaccine (IPV) from 30 November 2015. It is given as fractional IPV of 0.1 ml dose as intradermal injection at 6 and 14 weeks of life *(45)*.

INTRODUCTION OF MEASLES VACCINE SECOND OPPORTUNITY

In order to accelerate the reduction of measles related morbidity and mortality, second opportunity for measles vaccination is being implemented. The National Technical Advisory Group on immunization recommended introduction of 2nd dose of measles vaccine to children between 9 months and 10 years of age through supplementary immunization activity (SIA) for states where evaluated coverage of first dose of measles vaccination is less than 80 per cent. In states, with coverage of measles vaccination more than 80 per cent, the second dose of vaccine will be given through routine immunization at 16–24 months *(1)*.

INTRODUCTION OF PENTAVALENT VACCINE (DPT + Hep B + Hib)

The pentavalent vaccine contains five antigens i.e., hepatitis B, diphtheria, pertusis, tetanus and haemophilus influenza b (Hib) vaccine. Pentavalent vaccine is given at 6th, 10th and 14th weeks as primary dose. The vaccine has replaced DPT and hepatitis B vaccines in the immunization schedule. However, birth dose of hepatitis B and two booster doses of DPT will continue as before *(45)*.

Initially, India introduced pentavalent vaccine in two states – Kerala and Tamil Nadu. Presently it covers the whole country.

INTRODUCTION OF JAPANESE ENCEPHALITIS VACCINE

The programme was introduced in 2006 to cover 104 endemic districts in phased manner, using SA 14-14-2 vaccine, imported from China. Single dose of JE vaccine was given to all children between 1 to 15 years of age through campaigns *(3)*. The JE vaccine is being integrated into routine immunization in the districts where campaign had already been conducted to immunize the new cohort of children by vaccinating with two doses at 9–12 months and 16–24 months *(1)*.

21 high burden districts have been identified in Assam, Uttar Pradesh and West Bengal for adult JE vaccination in the age group of 15–65 years. This will cut down deaths and morbidity due to JE in adults as well *(45)*.

INTRODUCTION OF ROTA VIRUS VACCINE

Rota virus vaccine was introduced in 2016 in Odisha, Himachal Pradesh, Haryana and Andhra Pradesh, and now it covers the whole country. It is given under universal immunization programme as a 3 dose vaccine along with pentavalent 1st, 2nd and 3rd dose *(45)*.

RUBELLA VACCINE

To be initiated as Measles Rubella (MR) campaign

targeting 9 months to 15 years of age in a phased manner over a period of three years. Subsequently, the Rubella vaccine will be introduced as MR vaccine as two doses in the place of measles containing vaccine 1 and 2 at 9–12 months and 16–24 months as per NTAGI recommendations *(45)*.

MISSION INDRADHANUSH

The Ministry of Health & Family Welfare has launched "Mission Indradhanush", depicting seven colours of the rainbow, in December 2014, to fully immunize 90 per cent of children who are either unvaccinated or partially vaccinated; those that have not been covered during the rounds of routine immunization for various reasons, by 2020. The target has now been pre-poned to 2018 *(7)*.

Mission Indradhanush has completed six phases (from April 2015 to Dec. 2018) covering 681 districts wherein 3.39 crore children were reached; 81.79 lakh children were immunized; and 87.18 lakh pregnant women were immunized. The first two phases of Mission Indradhanush have led to an increase of 6.7 per cent in full immunization coverage in one year, as compared to 1 per cent in the past. This increase was more in rural areas (7.9 per cent) as compared to urban areas (3.1 per cent), hence shifting the focus of the programme towards urban areas *(11)*.

Intensified Mission Indradhanush: A total of 190 districts/ urban areas across 24 states have been identified where intensified mission indradhanush has started. It was launched in Oct 2017. It involves intensive preparation, implementation and integration of sessions into regular immunization microplans. The focus is an urban slum areas and districts with slowest progress and completion of due-list of beneficiaries on the basis of head count surveys. As on 15th Jan, 2018, number of children vaccinated were 49.30 lakh; number of children fully vaccinated was 12.02 lakh; and number of pregnant women vaccinated was 10.05 lakh *(7)*.

MEASLES–RUBELLA (MR) VACCINE

The WHO regional goal for SEAR is measles elimination and rubella/congenital rubella syndrome control by 2020. The MR vaccine is being introduced through campaign, targeting around 41 crore children in the age group of 9 months to 15 years in phased manner (covering 1/3rd of the total population of the country), followed by 2 doses in routine immunization at 9–12 months and 16–24 months, replacing the measles vaccine *(7)*.

MR campaign was launched in February 2017 from 5 States/UTs (Karnataka, Tamil Nadu, Goa, Lakshadweep and Puducherry) where 3.34 crore children were vaccinated against the target of 3.43 crore, with a coverage of 97 per cent. Campaign has completed 33 states and immunized 32.36 crore children (97.04 per cent of the target) *(11)*.

PNEUMOCOCCAL VACCINE (PCV)

PCV was launched in May 2017 for reducing infant mortality and morbidity caused by pneumococcal pneumonia. The vaccine was introduced in Himachal Pradesh, 6 districts of Uttar Pradesh and 17 districts of Bihar, Madhya Pradesh, and Haryana, in 2021 it covers whole country. Till September 2021, around 6.05 crore children were vaccinated *(6)*.

Very frequently queries come up about the vaccines and the vaccination schedule. It is important to have the exact answer to these questions.

Questions about all vaccines *(47)*

Q. If the mother/caregiver permits administration of only one injection during an infant's first visit at 9 months of age, which vaccine should be given ?

A. At 9 months of age, the priority is to give measles vaccine with OPV and Vitamin-A.

Q. Which vaccines can be given to a child between 1–5 years of age, who has never been vaccinated ?

A. The child should be given DPT1, OPV-1, measles and 2 ml of vitamin A solution. It should then be given the second and third doses of DPT and OPV at one month intervals. Measles second dose is also to be given as per the schedule. The booster dose of OPV/DPT can be given at a minimum of 6 months after administering OPV3/DPT3.

Q. Which vaccines can be given to a child between 5–7 years of age, who has never been vaccinated ?

A. The child should be given first, second and third doses of DPT at one month intervals. The booster dose of DPT can be given at a minimum of 6 months after administering DPT3 upto 7 years of age.

Q. Should one re-start with the first dose of a vaccine if a child is brought late for a dose ?

A. Do not start the schedule all over again even if the child is brought late for a dose. Pick up where the schedule was left off. For example: If a child who has received BCG, HepB-1, DPT-1 and OPV-1 at 5 months of age, returns at 11 months of age, vaccinate the child with DPT-2, HepB-2, OPV-2 and measles and do not start from DPT-1, HepB-1 again.

Q. Why it is not advisable to clean the injection site with a spirit swab before vaccination ?

A. This is because some of the live components of the vaccine are killed if they come in contact with spirit.

DPT vaccine

Q. If a child could not receive DPT1, 2, 3 and OPV 1, 2, 3 according to the schedule, upto what age can the vaccine be given ?

A. The DPT vaccine can be given upto 7 years of age and OPV can be given upto 5 years of age. If a child has received previous doses but not completed the schedule, do not restart the schedule and instead administer the remaining doses needed to complete the series.

Q. Why should there be a minimum gap of 4 weeks between two doses of DPT ?

A. This is because decreasing the interval between two doses may not obtain optimal antibody production for protection.

Q. Why give the DPT vaccine in the antero-lateral mid thigh and not the gluteal region ?

A. DPT is given in the antero-lateral mid-thigh and not the gluteal region to prevent damage to the sciatic nerve. Moreover, the vaccine deposited in the fat of gluteal region does not invoke the appropriate immune response.

Q. What should one do if the child is found allergic to DPT or develops encephalopathy after DPT ?

A. A child who is allergic to DPT or develops encephalopathy after DPT should be given the DTaP/DT vaccine instead of DPT for the remaining doses, as it is usually the P (whole cell Pertussis) component of the vaccine which causes the allergy/encephalopathy. It may be purchased with locally available resources.

Q. Why DT is replaced by DPT vaccine for children above 2 years of age ?

A. As pertussis cases were reported in higher age group children and the risk of AEFIs were not found to be more after DPT vaccine as compared to DT vaccine.

Measles vaccine

Q. Why give the measles vaccine only on the right upper arm ?

A. The measles vaccine is given on the right upper arm to maintain uniformity and to help surveyors in verifying the receipt of the vaccine.

Q. If a child has received the measles vaccine before 9 months of age, is it necessary to repeat the vaccine later ?

A. Yes, the measles vaccine needs to be administered, according to the National Immunization Schedule i.e. after the completion of 9 months until 12 months of age and at 16–24 months. If not administered in the ideal age for measles vaccine, it can be administered upto 5 years of age.

Q. What is measles catch-up campaign ?

A. A measles catch-up campaign is a special campaign to vaccinate all children in a wide age group in a state or a district with one dose of measles vaccine. The catch-up campaign dose is given to all children, both immunized and un-immunized, who belong to the target age group of 9 months to 10 years. The goal of a catch-up campaign is to quickly make the population immune from measles and reduce deaths from measles. A catch-up campaign must immunize nearly 100% of target age group children.

Q. Why 2nd dose of measles vaccine is introduced in the National Immunization Programme ?

A. Measles is highly infectious disease causing illness and death due to complications such as diarrhoea, pneumonia or brain infection. One dose of measles vaccine at 9 months of age protects 85% of infants. With 2nd dose the aim is to protect all the children who remain unprotected after first dose.

Q. If a child comes late for the first dose, then can it get the second dose ?

A. All efforts should be made to immunize the children at the right age i.e. first dose at completed 9 months to 12 months and second dose at 16–24 months. However if a child comes late then give two doses of measles vaccine at one month interval until 5 years of age.

Q. If a child received one dose of measles vaccine during an SIA campaign, should it receive the routine dose of measles vaccine ?

A. Yes, the child should receive routine doses of measles vaccine according to the Immunization Schedule irrespective of the measles SIA dose.

BCG vaccine

Q. Why give BCG vaccine only on the left upper arm ?

A. BCG is given on the left upper arm to maintain uniformity and for helping surveyors in verifying the receipt of the vaccine.

Q. Why do we give 0.05 ml dose of BCG to newborns (below 1 month of age) ?

A. This is because the skin of newborns is thin and an intradermal injection of 0.1 ml may break the skin or penetrate into the deeper tissue and cause local abscess and enlarged axillary lymph nodes. Dose of 0.05 ml is sufficient to elicit adequate protection.

Q. Why is BCG given only upto one year of age ?

A. Most children acquire natural clinical/sub-clinical tuberculosis infection by the age of one year. This too protects against severe forms of childhood tuberculosis e.g. TB meningitis and miliary disease.

Q. If no scar appears after administering BCG, should one re-vaccinate the child ?

A. There is no need to re-vaccinate the child, even if there is no scar.

OPV

Q. Till what age can a child be given OPV ?

A. OPV can be given to children till 5 years of age.

Q. Can OPV and vitamin A be given together with DPT-booster dose ?

A. Yes.

Q. Can an infant be breast-fed immediately after OPV ?

A. Yes.

TT vaccine

Q. If a girl has received all doses of DPT and TT as per the NIS till 16 years of age and she gets pregnant at 20 years, should she get one dose of TT during pregnancy ?

A. Give 2 doses of TT during the pregnancy as per the schedule.

Q. Is TT at 10 years and 16 years meant only for girls ?

A. No, it is to be given to both boys and girls.

Q. Can TT be given in the first trimester of pregnancy ?

A. Yes, it should be given as soon as pregnancy is diagnosed.

Hepatitis B vaccine

Q. Up to what age can hepatitis B vaccine be given ?

A. According to the National Immunization Schedule, Hepatitis B vaccine should be given with the first, second and third doses of DPT till one year of age.

Q. Why give the birth dose of hepatitis B vaccine only within 24 hours of birth ?

A. The birth dose of Hepatitis B vaccine is effective in preventing perinatal transmission of Hepatitis B if given within the first 24 hours.

JE vaccine

Q. If a child 16–24 months of age has been immunized with JE vaccine during an SIA, can it receive the JE vaccine again, as part of routine immunization ?

A. No, currently this is a single dose vaccine and should not be repeated.

Q. If a child above 2 years (24 months) of age has not received the JE vaccine through either RI or an SIA, should she/he be given the JE vaccine ?

A. Yes, the child is eligible to receive a dose of the JE vaccine, through RI, till the age of 15 years.

Following are some Do's and Don'ts during immunization sessions *(47)* :

Do's and Don'ts during immunization sessions

Do's	Don'ts
Vaccination schedule	
– It is safe and effective to give BCG, DPT, OPV and Measles vaccines at the same time to a child who has completed 9 months and never been vaccinated. – Give BCG to infants less than 1 year of age (never give BCG to children above 1 year of age). – If a child is brought late for a dose, pick up where the schedule was left off. For example, if a child left with DPT-2 and comes after 3 months give DPT-3.	– Withhold the vaccine in case of illness such as cold, cough, diarrhoea or fever.
Cold chain	
– Check expiry date and VVM label of vaccine vial before immunizing every child. – Keep the vaccines and diluents in a plastic bag/zipper bag in the centre of vaccine carrier with 4 conditioned ice-packs. Make sure that the diluents are also at +2 to +8 centigrade before reconstitution. – Take one ice pack from vaccine carrier and keep reconstituted BCG & Measles vaccines only on the top of the ice pack.	– Leave vaccine carrier in sunlight: this spoils vaccines that are sensitive to heat and light. – Leave the lid open, this can allow heat and light into the carrier, which can spoil vaccine. – Drop or sit on the vaccine carrier: this can damage the carrier. – Carry vaccines in handbag as this can spoil vaccines that are sensitive to heat. – Keep the DPT, DT, TT and Hep. B vaccines on the ice pack during the session.
Vaccine handling and administration	
– Welcome beneficiaries. – Wash hands before conducting the session. – Verify beneficiary's record and age of the child. – Screen for contraindications. – Check label of the vial and expiry date. – Lightly shake the vial of T-Series Vaccine before drawing the dose. – Use a new AD syringe for each injection and new disposable syringe for each reconstitution. – Use correct diluent for reconstitution of vaccine. – Give appropriate vaccine. – Inject vaccine using the correct site and route for the vaccine e.g. Intradermal in left arm for BCG; subcutaneous in right arm for Measles; intramuscular in anterolateral aspect of mid thigh for DPT and Hepatitis B. – Allow dose to self-disperse instead of massaging. – Explain potential adverse events following immunization and what to do. – Discuss with beneficiaries/parents about next visit.	– Use un-sterile syringe or needle for immunization. – Draw air into AD syringes. – Touch any part of the needle. – Recap the needle. – Leave the needle inside the vial. – Ever inject in the buttock, never do that. – Massage the vaccination site after vaccination. – Use reconstituted measles and BCG vaccine after 4hrs and JE after 2 hrs. – Use vaccine with VVM in unusable stage or with expiry date.
Recording and reporting	
– Fully document each immunization in the immunization card, tally sheet and immunization register. Ask parents/guardians to bring the card on next visit. – Retain the counterfoil.	– Turn away beneficiaries for not bringing the card. – Leave any cell blank in immunization card.
Adverse events following immunization (AEFI)	
– In case of serious AEFI refer the patient to appropriate health facility, inform your supervisor immediately – document the type of vaccine(s), batch number, expiry date, and full address of the child. – Report all serious AEFIs to the MOI/C.	– Report minor reaction following vaccination (mild fever of less than three days, redness and pain).
Social mobilization	
– Use vaccination card to remind parents when to return with their child. – Enlist community team like AWW, ASHA, NGOs and other community-based workers to remind parents of the importance of full immunization.	– Leave any community meeting without communicating about immunization session days.

Source : *(47)*

NATIONAL HEALTH MISSION

The Ministry of Health and Family Welfare is implementing various schemes and programmes and national initiatives to provide universal access to quality health care. The approach is to increase access to the decentralized health system by establishing new infrastructure in deficient areas and by upgrading the infrastructure in existing institutions. As part of the plan process, many different programmes have been brought together under the overarching umbrella of National Health Mission (NHM), with National Rural Health Mission (NRHM) and National Urban Health Mission (NUHM) as its two sub–Missions. The National Health Mission was approved in May 2013. The main programmatic components include health system strengthening in rural and urban areas; Reproductive – Maternal – Newborn – Child and Adolescent Health (RMNCH+A); and control of communicable and non-communicable diseases. An important achievement of NHM has been considerable reduction in out of pocket expenses from 72 per cent to 60 per cent *(1)*.

The Government of India has introduced a series of programmes over the past two decades to address maternal and newborn health. The major milestones so far include *(48)*

a. 1992 – Child Survival and Safe Motherhood Programme (CSSM)
b. 1997 – RCH I
c. 2005 – RCH II
d. 2005 – National Rural Health Mission
e. 2013 – RMNCH+A Strategy
f. 2013 – National Health Mission
g. 2014 – India Newborn Action Plan (INAP)
h. 2018 – Ayushman Bharat Programme
i. 2018 – Midwifery Initiative
j. 2018 – RMNACH+N Strategy

Under NHM, health interventions/ initiatives are regularly designed and implemented to address the healthcare needs of the country. A list of interventions currently being implemented under NHM to reduce IMR and MMR is given below *(49)*:

- Promotion of institutional deliveries through Janani Suraksha Yojana.
- Capacity building of health care providers in basic and comprehensive obstetric care.
- Operationalization of sub-centres, primary health centres, community health centres and district hospitals for providing 24 × 7 basic and comprehensive obstetric care services.
- Name based web enabled tracking of pregnant women to ensure antenatal, intranatal and postnatal care.
- Mother and child protection card in collaboration with the Ministry of Women and Child Development to monitor service delivery for mothers and children.
- Antenatal, intranatal and postnatal care including iron and folic acid supplementation to pregnant & lactating women for prevention and treatment of anaemia.
- Village health and nutrition days in rural areas as an outreach activity, for provision of maternal and child health services.
- Health and nutrition education to promote dietary diversification, inclusion of iron and folate rich food as well as food items that promote iron absorption.
- Janani Shishu Suraksha Karyakram (JSSK) entitles all pregnant women delivering in public health institutions to absolutely free and no expense delivery including caesarean section. The initiative stipulates free drugs, diagnostics, blood and diet, besides free transport from home to institution, between facilities in case of a referral, and drop back home. Similar entitlements have been put in place for all sick infants accessing public health institutions for treatment.
- To sharpen the focus on the low performing districts, 184 high priority districts have been prioritized for Reproductive Maternal Newborn Child Health+ Adolescent (RMNCH+A) interventions for achieving improved maternal and child health outcomes.
- Emphasis on facility based newborn care at different levels to reduce child morbidity and mortality: Setting up of facilities for care of sick newborn such as Special New Born Care Units (SNCUs), Newborn Stabilization Units (NBSUs) and Newborn Care Corners (NBCCs) at different levels is a thrust area under NHM.
- Capacity building of health care providers: Various trainings are being conducted under NHM to train doctors, nurses and ANMs for essential newborn care, early diagnosis and case management of common ailments of children. These trainings are on Navjaat Shishu Suraksha Karyakram (NSSK), Integrated Management of Neonatal and Childhood Illnesses (IMNCI), Facility Based Newborn Care (FBNC), Infant and Young Child Feeding practices (IYCF), etc.
- India Newborn Action Plan (INAP) has been launched with an aim to reduce neonatal mortality and stillbirths.
- Newer interventions to reduce newborn mortality - vitamin K injection at birth, antenatal corticosteroids for preterm labour, kangaroo mother care and injection gentamicin to young infants in cases of suspected sepsis.
- Home Based New Born Care (HBNC): Home based newborn care through ASHAs has been initiated to improve new born practices at the community level and early detection and referral of sick new born babies.
- Intensified Diarrhoea Control Fortnight (IDCF) to be observed in July-August focusing on ORS and Zinc distribution for management of diarrhoea and feeding practices.
- Integrated Action Plan for Pneumonia and Diarrhoea (IAPPD) launched in four states with highest infant mortality (Uttar Pradesh, Madhya Pradesh, Bihar and Rajasthan).
- Management of malnutrition: Nutritional Rehabilitation Centres (NRCs) have been established for management of severe acute malnutrition in children.
- Appropriate Infant and young child feeding practices are being promoted in convergence with Ministry of Woman and Child Development.
- Some programmes for control of communicable and non-communicable diseases are now under NHM.
- Universal Immunization Programme (UIP): Vaccination protects children against many life threatening diseases such as tuberculosis, diptheria, pertussis, polio, tetanus, hepatitis B, Hib, measles and Japanese encephalitis in endemic districts. Infants are thus immunized against nine vaccine preventable diseases every year. The Government of India supports the vaccine programme by supply of vaccines and syringes, cold chain equipment and provision of operational costs.
- Mission Indradhanush has been launched in 528 high focus districts to reach more than 2.5 crore children who are either unvaccinated or partially vaccinated; those that have not been covered during the rounds of routine immunization for various reasons. They will be fully immunized against eight life-threatening but vaccine preventable diseases which include diphtheria, whooping cough, tetanus, polio, tuberculosis, measles, haemophilus influenza type B and hepatitis-B. In addition, vaccination against japanese encephalitis will be provided in selected districts/states of the country. Pregnant women will also be immunized against tetanus.

- Mother and Child Tracking System (MCTS): A name based mother and child tracking system has been put in place which is web based to ensure registration and tracking of all pregnant women and new born babies so that provision of regular and complete services to them can be ensured.
- Rashtriya Bal Swasthya Karyakram (RBSK) for health screening and early intervention services has been launched to provide comprehensive care to all the children in the age group of 0–18 years in the community. The purpose of these services is to improve the overall quality of life of children through early detection of birth defects, diseases, deficiencies, development delays including disability.
- Under National Iron Plus Initiative (NIPI), through life cycle approach, age and dose specific IFA supplementation programme is being implemented for the prevention of anaemia among the vulnerable age groups like under-5 children, children of 6–10 years of age group, adolescents, pregnant and lactating women and women in reproductive age along with treatment of anaemic children and pregnant mothers at health facilities.
- Comprehensive primary health care through Ayushman Bharat - Health and Wellness Centres : Launched in 2018, Ayushman Bharat works a paradigm shift to move from sectoral and selective approach of health service delivery to a comprehensive range of health care service. Ayushman Bharat aims to cover preventive, promotive and ambulatory care at primary, secondary and tertiary level by adopting a continuum of care approach. Since the screening, prevention and management of chronic illnesses including non-communicable diseases, tuberculosis, and leprosy have been introduced at these centres, training skill upgradation of the primary health team in all functional Health and Wellness Centres on NCDs and use of information technology application is being done. For details, please refer to page 547.

The targets of National Health Mission

The National Health Mission was launched with targets as shown in Table 10.

TABLE 10
Targets for NHM

Targets (2012–17)
Reduce IMR to 25/1000 live births.
Reduce MMR to 1/1000 live births.
Reduce TFR to 2.1
Reduce annual incidence and mortality from tuberculosis by half.
Reduce prevalence of leprosy to <1/10,000 population and incidence to zero in all districts.
Annual malaria incidence to be <1/1000.
Less than 1% microfilaria prevalence in all districts.
Kala-azar elimination by 2015, <1 case per 10,000 population in all blocks.

NATIONAL URBAN HEALTH MISSION

NUHM seeks to improve the health status of the urban population particularly slum dwellers and other vulnerable section by facilitating their access to quality health care. NUHM would cover all state capitals, district headquarters and about 779 other cities/towns with a population of 50,000 and above (as per census 2011) in a phased manner. Cities and towns below 50,000 population will be covered by NRHM. The NUHM will focus on *(39)* :

1. Urban poor population living in listed and unlisted slums;
2. All other vulnerable population such as homeless, rag-pickers, street children, rickshaw pullers, construction and brick and lime-kiln workers, sex workers and other temporary migrants;
3. Public health thrust on sanitation, clean drinking water, vector control etc.; and
4. Strengthening public health capacity of urban local bodies.

The treatment of seven metropolitan cities, viz., Mumbai, New Delhi, Chennai, Kolkata, Hyderabad, Bengaluru and Ahmedabad will be different. These cities are expected to manage NUHM through their Municipal Corporation directly.

The NUHM will provide flexibility to the states to choose which model suits the needs and capacities of the states to best address the healthcare needs of the urban poor. Models will be decided through community led action. All the services delivered under the urban health delivery system through the urban PHCs and urban CHCs will be universal in nature, whereas the outreach services will be targetted to the target group (slum dwellers and other vulnerable groups). Outreach services will be provided through the Female Health Workers (FHWs), essentially ANMs with an induction training of three to six months, who will be placed at the Urban PHCs. These ANMs will report at the U-PHC and then move to their respective areas for outreach services on designated days. On other days, they will conduct immunization and ANC clinics etc. at the U-PHC itself.

The NUHM would encourage the effective participation of the community in planning and management of health care services. It would promote a community health volunteer – Accredited Social Health Activist (ASHA) or Link Worker (LW) in urban poor settlement (one ASHA for 1000–2500 urban poor population covering about 200 to 500 households); ensure the participation by creation of community based institutions like Mahila Arogya Samiti (MAS) (50–100 households) and Rogi Kalyan Samitis. However, the states will have the flexibility to either engage ASHA or entrust her responsibilities to MAS. In that case, the incentives accruing to ASHA would accrue to MAS *(50)*. The NUHM would provide annual grant of Rs. 5000/- to MAS every year.

Essential services to be rendered by the ASHA may be as follows *(50)*:

(i) Active promoter of good health practices and enjoying community support.

(ii) Facilitate awareness on essential RCH services, sexuality, gender equality, age at marriage/pregnancy; motivation on contraception adoption, medical termination of pregnancy, sterilization, spacing methods. Early registration of pregnancies, pregnancy care, clean and safe delivery, nutritional care during pregnancy, identification of danger signs during pregnancy; counselling on immunization, ANC, PNC etc., act as a depot holder for essential provisions like oral re-hydration therapy (ORS), Iron Folic Acid Tablet (IFA), chloroquine, oral pills and condoms, etc.; identification of target beneficiaries and support the ANM in conducting regular monthly outreach sessions and tracking service coverage.

(iii) Facilitate access to health related services available at the Anganwadi/Primary Urban Health Centres/Urban Local Body (ULBs) and other services being provided by the ULB/State/Central Government.

(iv) Formation and promotion of Mahila Arogya Samitis in her community.

(v) Arrange escort/accompany pregnant women and children requiring treatment to the nearest Urban Primary Health Centre, secondary/tertiary level health care facility.

(vi) Reinforcement of community action for immunization, prevention of water borne and other communicable diseases like TB (DOTS), Malaria, Chikungunya and Japanese Encephalitis.

(vii) Carrying out preventive and promotive health activities with AWW/Mahila Arogya Samiti.

(viii) Maintenance of necessary information and records about births and deaths, immunization, antenatal services in her assigned locality as also about any unusual health problem or disease outbreak in the slum, and share it with the ANM in charge of the area.

In return for the services rendered, she would receive a performance based incentive. For this purpose a revolving fund would be kept with the ANM at the U-PHC (in the PHC account), which would be replenished from time to time.

The urban health care facilities are as shown in Fig. 11.

Urban Primary Health Centre

Functional for a population of around approximately 30,000–50,000, the U-PHC may be located preferably within a slum or near a slum within half a kilometer radius, catering to a slum population of approximately 25,000–30,000, with provision for OPD. The cities, based upon the local situation may establish a U-PHC for 75,000 for areas with very high density and can also establish one for around 5,000–10,000, slum population for isolated slum clusters.

At the U-PHC level services provided will include OPD (consultation), basic laboratory diagnosis, drug/contraceptive dispensing, apart from distribution of health education material delivering RCH services and counselling for all communicable and non-communicable diseases. In order to ensure access to the urban slum population at convenient timings, the U-PHC may provide services from 12 noon to 8 pm. It will not include in-patient care. The staff pattern will be as shown in Fig. 11.

Referral unit

Urban Community Health Centre (U-CHC) may be set up as a satellite hospital for every 4–5 U-PHCs. The U-CHC would cater to a population of 2,50,000. It would provide in-patient services and would be a 30–50 bedded facility. U-CHCs would be set up in cities with a population of above 5 lakhs, wherever required. These facilities would be in addition to the existing facilities (SDH/DH) to cater to the urban population in the locality.

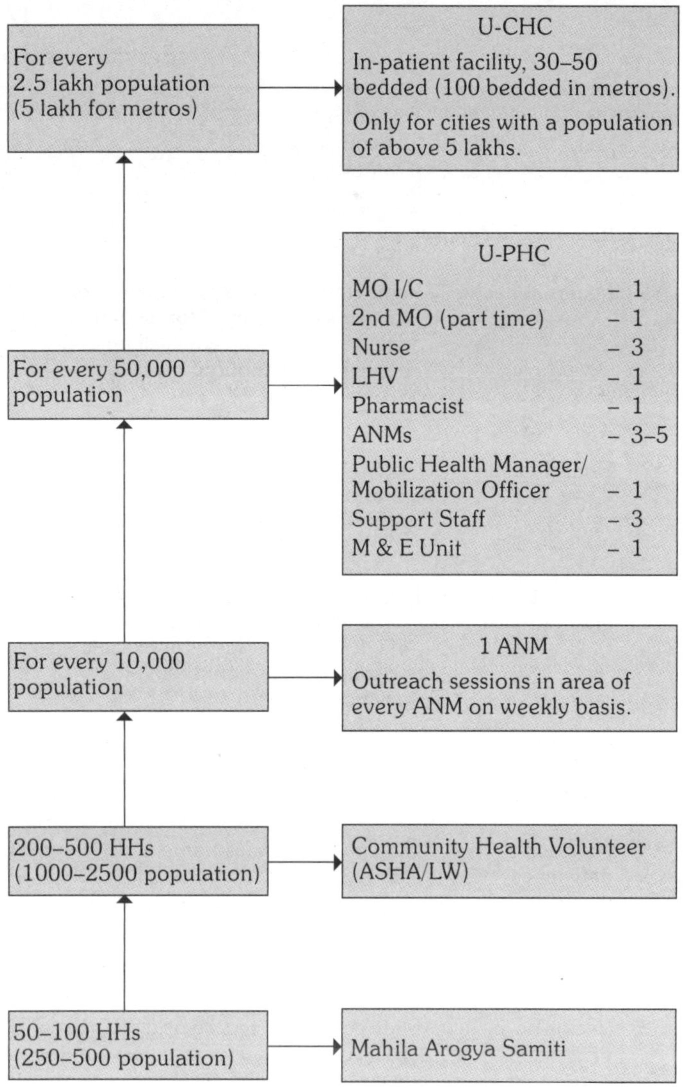

FIG. 11

Urban Health Care Facilities

Source : *(51)*

For the metro cities, the U-CHCs may be established for every 5 lakh population with 100 beds.

For setting up the U-CHCs the Central Government would provide only a one time capital cost, and the recurrent costs including the salary of the staff would be borne by the respective state governments.

The U-CHC would provide medical care, minor surgical facilities and facilities for institutional delivery.

Referral linkages

Existing hospitals, including ULB maternity homes, state government hospitals and medical colleges, apart from private hospitals will be empanelled/accredited to act as referral points for different types of healthcare services like maternal health, child health, diabetes, trauma care, orthopaedic complications, dental surgeries, mental health, critical illness, deafness control, cancer management, tobacco counselling/cessation, critical illness, surgical cases etc.

The services provided at different levels are as shown in Table 11 *(51)*.

TABLE 11

Service norm by level of care facility

Services	Levels of service delivery		
	Community (Outreach)	First point of service delivery (U-PHC)	Referral Centre - U-CHC (specialist services)
A. *Essential Health Services*			
A1. Maternal health	Registration, ANC, identification of danger signs, referral for institutional delivery, follow-up counselling and behaviour promotion.	ANC, PNC, initial management of complicated delivery cases and referral, management of regular maternal health conditions, referral of complicated cases.	Delivery (normal and complicated), management of complicated gynae/maternal health condition, hospitalization and surgical interventions, including blood transfusion.
A2. Family welfare	Counselling, distribution of OCP/CC, referral for sterilization, follow-up of contraceptive related complications.	Distribution of OCP/CC, IUD insertion, referral for sterilization, management of contraceptive related complications.	Sterilization operations, fertility treatment.
A3. Child health and nutrition	Immunization, identification of danger signs, referral, follow-up, distribution of ORS, paediatric cotrimoxazole, post-natal visits/counselling for newborn care.	Diagnosis and treatment of childhood illnesses, referral of acute cases/chronic illness, identification and referral of neonatal sickness.	Management of complicated paediatric/neo-natal cases, hospitalization, surgical interventions, blood transfusion.
A4. RTI/STI (including HIV/AIDS)	referral, community level follow-up for ensuring adherence to treatment regime of cases undergoing treatment.	Symptomatic diagnosis and primary treatment and referral of complicated cases.	Management of complicated cases, hospitalization (if needed).
A5. Nutrition deficiency disorders	Height/weight measurement, Hb testing, distribution of IFA tablets promotion of iodized salt, nutrition supplements to children and pregnant/lactating women, promotion of breast feeding.	Diagnosis and treatment of seriously deficient patients, referral of acute deficiency cases.	Management of acute deficiency cases, hospitalization, treatment and rehabilitation of severe under-nutrition.
A6. Vector-borne diseases	Slide collection, testing using RDKs, DDT, counselling for practices for vector control and protection.	Diagnosis and treatment, referral of terminally ill cases.	Management of terminally ill cases, hospitalization.
A7. Mental health	–	Initial screening and referral	Psychiatric, neurological services.
A7.1 Oral health	–	Diagnosis and referral	Management of complicated cases.
A7.2 Hearing Impairment/ deafness	–	–	Management of complicated cases.
A8. Chest infections (TB/asthma)	Symptomatic search and referral, ensuring adherence to DOTS, other treatment.	Diagnosis and treatment, referral of complicated cases.	Management of complicated cases.
A9. Cardiovascular diseases	BP measurement, symptomatic search and referral, follow-up of under-treatment patients.	Diagnosis and treatment and referral during specialist visits.	Management of emergency cases, hospitalization and surgical interventions (if needed).
A10. Diabetes	Blood/urine sugar test (using disposable kit), symptomatic search and referral.	Diagnosis and treatment, referral of complicated cases.	Management of complicated cases, hospitalization (if needed).
A11. Cancer	Symptomatic search and referral, follow-up of under-treatment patients.	Identification and referral, follow-up of under-treatment patients.	Diagnosis and treatment, hospitalization (if and when needed).
A12. Trauma care (burns and injuries)	First aid and referral	First-aid/emergency resuscitation, documentation for medicolegal case (if applicable) and referral.	Case management and hospitalization, physiotherapy and rehabilitation.
A13. Other surgical interventions	Not applicable	Identification and referral	Hospitalization and surgical intervention.
B. *Other support services like IEC, BCC, counselling and personal and social hygiene.*			

City level indicators

The city level indicators are as shown in Table 12.

TABLE 12

Process and input indicators in NUHM

Indicator
Community Processes
1. Number of Mahila Arogya Samiti (MAS) formed.*
2. Number of MAS members trained.*
3. Number of Accredited Social Health Activists (ASHAs). selected and trained.
Health Systems
4. Number of ANMs recruited *
5. No. of Special Outreach health camps organized in the slum/HFAs.*
6. No. of UHNDs organized in the slums and vulnerable areas.*
7. Number of UPHCs made operational.*
8. Number of UCHCs made operational.*
9. No. of RKS created at UPHC and UCHC.*
10. OPD attendance in the UPHCs.
11. No. of deliveries conducted in public health facilities.
RCH Services
12. ANC early registration in first trimester.
13. Number of women who had ANC check-up in their first trimester of pregnancy.
14. TT (2nd dose) coverage among pregnant women.
15. No. of children fully immunized (through public health facilities).
16. No. of Severely Acute Malnourished (SAM) children identified and referred for treatment.
Communicable Diseases
17. No. of malaria cases detected through blood examination.
18. No. of TB cases identified through chest symptomatic.
19. No. of suspected TB cases referred for sputum examination.
20. No. of MDR-TB cases put under DOTS plus.
Non-communicable Diseases
21. No. of diabetes cases screened in the city.
22. No. of cancer cases screened in the city.
23. No. of hypertension cases screened in the city.

* Year 2013–14 being the baseline year, the indicators for these NUHM components would be zero. For other indicators, the figure for 2012–13 will be the base line.

Source : *(50)*

Impact level targets of NUHM are as follows :

1. Reduce IMR by 40% (in urban areas) – National Urban IMR down to 20 per 1000 live births by 2017.
   40% reduction in U5MR and IMR.
   Achieve universal immunization in all urban areas.
2. Reduce MMR by 50%.
   50% reduction in MMR (among urban population of the state/country).
   100% ANC coverage (in urban areas).
3. Achieve universal access to reproductive health including 100% institutional delivery.
4. Achieve replacement level fertility (TFR 2.1).
5. Achieve all targets of disease control programmes.

Source : *(51)*

NATIONAL RURAL HEALTH MISSION

Recognizing the importance of health in the process of economic and social development and to improve the quality of life of its citizens, the government of India launched "National Rural Health Mission" (NRHM) on 5th April, 2005 for a period of 7 years (2005–2012) and recently extended upto year 2017. The mission seeks to improve rural health care delivery system. It is operational in the whole country with special focus on 18 states viz. 8 Empowered Action Group states (Bihar, Jharkhand, Madhya Pradesh, Chhattisgarh, Uttar Pradesh, Uttarakhand, Orissa and Rajasthan), 8 North East states (Assam, Arunachal Pradesh, Manipur, Meghalaya, Mizoram, Nagaland, Sikkim and Tripura), Himachal Pradesh and Jammu and Kashmir. By making necessary changes in the basic health care delivery system the mission adopts a synergic approach by relating health to determinants of good health viz. of nutrition, sanitation, hygiene and safe drinking water. It also brings the Indian system of medicine (AYUSH) to the mainstream of health care *(9)*.

The main aim of NRHM is to provide accessible, affordable, accountable, effective and reliable primary health care, and bridging the gap in rural health care through creation of a cadre of Accredited Social Health Activist (ASHA). The mission is an instrument to integrate multiple vertical programmes alongwith their funds at the district level. The programmes integrated into NRHM are existing programmes of health and family welfare including RCH II; national vector borne disease control programmes against malaria, filaria, kala-azar, dengue fever/DHF and Japanese encephalitis; national leprosy eradication programme; revised national tuberculosis control programme; national programme for control of blindness; iodine deficiency disorder control programme, and integrated disease surveillance project *(9)*.

PLAN OF ACTION TO STRENGTHEN INFRASTRUCTURE

1. Creation of a cadre of Accredited Social Health Activist (ASHA).
2. Strengthening sub-centres by : (a) Supply of essential drugs both allopathic and AYUSH to the sub-centre; (b) In case of additional outlay, provision of multipurpose worker (male)/additional ANMs wherever needed, sanction of new sub-centres and upgrading existing sub-centres; and (c) Strengthening sub-centres with untied funds of Rs. 10,000 per annum in all 18 states.
3. Strengthening Primary Health Centres : Mission aims at strengthening PHCs for quality preventive, promotive, curative, supervisory and outreach services through (a) Adequate and regular supply of essential drugs and equipment to PHCs (including supply of auto-disabled syringes for immunization); (b) Provision of 24 hours service in at least 50 per cent PHCs by including an AYUSH practitioner; (c) Following standard treatment guidelines; (d) Upgradation of all the PHCs for 24 hours referral service and provision of second doctor at PHC level (one male and one female) on the basis of felt need; strengthening the ongoing communicable disease control programmes and new programmes for control of non-communicable diseases.
4. Strengthening Community Health Centres for First Referral care by (a) Operating all existing CHCs (30–50 beds) as 24 hours first referral units, including

posting of an anaesthetist; (b) Codification of new "Indian Public Health Standards" (Refer to chapter 20 for more details) by setting up norms for infrastructure, staff, equipment, management etc. for CHCs; (c) Promotion of *"Rogi Kalyan Samiti"* for hospital management; and (d) Developing standards of services and costs in hospital care.

The NRHM infrastructure is as shown in Fig. 12.

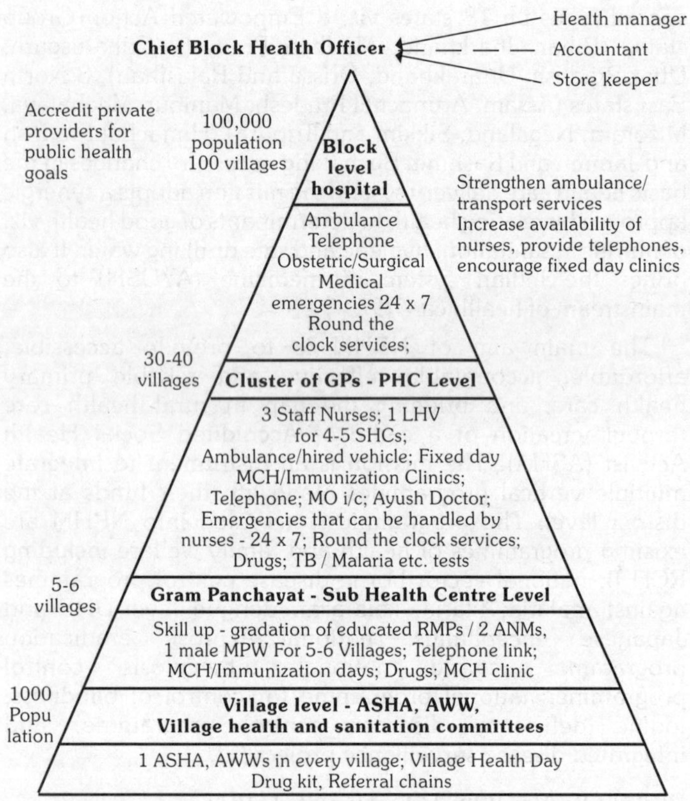

Fig. 12

The NRHM infrastructure

District is the core unit of planning, budgeting and implementation of the programme. All vertical health and family welfare programmes at district level have merged into one common "District Health Mission" and at state level into "State Health Mission". There is provision of a *"mobile medical unit"* at district level for improved outreach services.

Since almost 75 per cent of health services are being currently provided by the private sector, it is contemplated that involving the private sector as part of the RCH initiatives will provide more effective health care delivery system. Thus setting up of *"Public Private Partnership" (PPP)"* is to help to make the RCH II programme better, and ensure availability of preventive and curative reproductive and child health services to the community.

Major initiatives under NRHM

1. *Selection of ASHA:* ASHA must be the resident of the village – a woman (married / widow / divorced) preferably in the age group of 25 to 45 years with formal education up to eighth class, having communication skills and leadership qualities. Adequate representation from the disadvantaged population group will ensure to serve such groups better.

The general norm of selection is *one* ASHA *for 1000 population*. In tribal, hilly and desert areas the norm could be relaxed to one ASHA per habitation.

2. *Rogi Kalyan Samiti (Patient Welfare Committee/Hospital Management Society:* It is a simple yet effective management structure. This committee is a registered society whose members act as trustees to manage the affairs of the hospital and is responsible for upkeep of the facilities and ensure provision of better facilities to the patients in the hospital. Financial assistance is provided to these Committees through untied fund to undertake activities for patient welfare. 33,757 Rogi Kalyan Samities (RKS) have been set up involving the community members in almost all District Hospitals (DHs), Sub-District Hospitals (SDHs), Community Health Centres (CHCs) and Primary Health Centres (PHCs) till June 2021.

3. *The untied grants to sub-centres (SCs):* The SCs are far better equipped now with blood pressure measuring equipment, haemoglobin (Hb) measuring equipment, stethoscope, weighing machine etc. This has facilitated provision of quality antenatal care and other health care services.

4. *The Village Health Sanitation and Nutrition Committee (VHSNC):* It is an important tool of community empowerment and participation at the grassroots level. The VHSNC reflects the aspirations of the local community, especially the poor households and children by year 2021, 5.55 lakh VHSNCs have been set up across the country.

5. *Janani Suraksha Yojana (JSY):* aims to reduce maternal mortality among pregnant women by encouraging them to deliver in government health facilities. Under the scheme, cash assistance is provided to eligible pregnant women for giving birth in a government health facility. Since the inception of NRHM, 8.55 crore women have benefited under this scheme. For details please refer to page 521.

6. *Janani Shishu Suraksha Karyakarm (JSSK):* Launched on 1st June, 2011, JSSK entitles all pregnant women delivering in public health institutions to absolutely free and no expense delivery, including caesarean section. This marks a shift to an entitlement based approach. Please refer to page 522 for details.

7. *National Mobile Medical Units (NMMUs):* Support has been provided by 1,634 MMUs under NHM in the country. To increase visibility, awareness and accountability, all Mobile Medical Units have been repositioned as "National Mobile Medical Unit Service" with universal colour and design.

8. *National Ambulance Services:* NRHM has supported free ambulance services to provide patients transport in every nook and corner of the country connected with a toll free number. Currently, 35 states/UTs have the facility where people can dial 108 or 102 telephone number for calling an ambulance. Dial 108 is predominantly an emergency response system, primarily designed to attend to patients of critical care, trauma and accident victims etc. Dial 102 services essentially consist of basic patient transport aimed to cater the needs of pregnant women and children though other categories are also taking benefit and are not excluded. Janani Shishu Suraksha Karyakram (JSSK) entitlements e.g. free transport from home to facility, inter facility transfer in case of referral and drop back for mother and children are the key focus of 102 service. This service can be accessed through a toll free call to a Call Centre *(6)*.

Presently as on June 2021, 11,879 Dial-108 and 10,716 Dial-102/104 Emergency Response Service Vehicles are operational under NRHM, besides 5859 empaneled vehicles are for transportation of patients, particularly pregnant women and sick infants from home to public health facilities and back *(6)*.

9. *Web enabled Mother and Child Tracking System (MCTS):* The name-based tracking of pregnant women and children has been initiated under NRHM with an intention to track every pregnant woman, infant and child upto the age of three years by name, for ensuring delivery of services like timely antenatal care, institutional delivery and postnatal care for the mother, and immunization and other related services for the child. The MCTs is to be fully updated for regular and effective monitoring of service delivery, including tracking and monitoring of severely anaemic women, low birth weight babies and sick neonates. In the long run, it could be used for tracking the health status of the girl child and school health services. A more recent initiative is to link MCTS with AADHAR in order to track subsidies to eligible women *(52)*.

New initiatives *(46)*

The following are the major decisions of Mission Steering Group; taken since 2011 :

1. Home delivery of contraceptives (condoms, oral contraceptive pills, emergency contraceptive pills) by ASHA;
2. Conducting District Level Household Survey (DLHS) – 4 in 26 States/UTs where the Annual Health Survey (AHS) is not being done;
3. Modifications in the scheme for promotion of menstrual hygiene covering 152 districts and nearly 1.5 crores of adolescent girls in 20 states;
4. Differential financial approach for comprehensive health care by which allocation of Untied Funds and Rogi Kalyan Samiti grants will be made based on the case load and services provided by the health facility;
5. Involving ASHA in Home Based Newborn Care;
6. Revision in the criterion of allocation of funds to the states under NRHM based on the performance of the states against the monitorable targets and implementation of specific reform agenda in the health sector;
7. Expansion of Village Health and Sanitation Committees to include nutrition in its mandate and renaming it as Village Health, Sanitation and Nutrition Committee (VHSNC);
8. Partial modification of the centrally sponsored scheme for development of AYUSH hospitals and dispensaries for mainstreaming of AYUSH under NRHM;
9. Rashtriya Bal Swasthya Karyakram (RBSK): This initiative was launched in February 2013 and provides for Child Health Screening and Early Intervention Services through early detection and management of 4 Ds i.e., Defects at birth, Diseases, Deficiencies, Development delays including disability. For details please refer to page 529;
10. Rashtriya Kishor Swasthya Karyakram (RKSK): This is a new initiative, launched in January 2014 to reach out to 253 million adolescents in the country in their own spaces and introduces peer-led interventions at the community level, supported by augmentation of facility based services. This initiative broadens the focus of the adolescent health programme beyond reproductive and sexual health and brings in focus on life skills, nutrition, injuries and violence (including gender based violence), non-communicable diseases, mental health and substance misuse *(1)*;
11. Mother and Child Health Wings (MCH Wings): 100/50/30 bedded Maternal and Child Health (MCH) Wings have been sanctioned in public health facilities with high bed occupancy to cater to the increased demand for services. More than 32,000 additional beds have been sanctioned across 550 health facilities across 18 states;
12. Free drugs and free diagnostic service;
13. National Iron+ Initiative is another new initiative launched in 2013, to prevent and control iron deficiency anaemia, a grave public health challenge in India. Besides pregnant women and lactating mothers, it aims to provide IFA supplementation for children, adolescents and women in reproductive age group. Weekly Iron and Folic Acid Supplementation (WIFS) for adolescents is an important strategy under this initiative. WIFS (for 10–19 years age) has already been rolled out in 32 states and UTs under the National Iron Plus Initiative. WIFS covered around 3 crore beneficiaries in December 2013 *(1)*;
14. Reproductive, Maternal, Newborn, Child and Adolescent Health Services (RMNCH+A): A continuum of care approach has now been adopted under NRHM with the articulation of strategic approach to Reproductive Maternal, Newborn, Child and Adolescent Health (RMNCH+A) in India. This approach brings focus on adolescents as a critical life stage and linkages between child survival, maternal health and family planning efforts. It aims to strengthen the referral linkages between community and facility based health services and between the various levels of health system itself. Please refer to page 530 for details;
15. Delivery Points (DPs): Health facilities that have a high demand for services and performance above a certain benchmark have been identified as "Delivery Points" with the objective of providing comprehensive reproductive, maternal, newborn, child and adolescent health services (RMNCH+A) at these facilities. Funds have been allocated to strengthen these DPs in terms of infrastructure, human resource, drugs, equipments etc. Around 25,000 health facilities have been identified as "Delivery Points" for focussed support under NRHM;
16. Universal Health Coverage (UHC): Moving towards Universal Health Coverage (UHC) is a key goal of the 12th Five Year Plan. The National Health Mission is the primary vehicle to move towards this goal;
17. Comprehensive primary healthcare: Nine areas for action to make primary healthcare comprehensive and universal are proposed. They are *(45)* :
    a. Strengthen institutional structures and organization of primary healthcare services;
    b. Improve access to technologies, drugs and diagnostics for comprehensive primary healthcare;
    c. Increase utilization of Information, Communication and Technology (ICT) – empowering patients and providers;
    d. Promote continuity of care - making care patient centric;
    e. Enhance quality of care;
    f. Focus on social determinants of health;
    g. Emphasize community participation and address equity concerns in health;
    h. Develop a human resource policy to support primary healthcare;
    i. Strengthen governance including financing, partnerships and accountability; and
    j. States are also offered support through the PIPs of the NHM to strengthen existing sub-centres.
18. Kilkari: Kilkari is an Interactive Voice Response (IVR) based mobile service that delivers time- sensitive audio messages (voice call) about pregnancy and child health directly to the mobile phones of pregnant women, mothers of young children and their families. The service covers the critical time period– where the most maternal/

infant deaths occur from the 4th month of pregnancy until the child is one year old. Families which subscribe to the service receive one pre-recorded system generated call per week. Each call will be 2 minutes in length and serve as reminders for what the family should be doing that week depending on woman's stage of pregnancy or the child's age. Kilkari services will be available to states in regional dialect too *(45)*;

19. Launch of Nationwide anti-TB drug resistance survey: Drug resistance survey for 13 anti-tuberculosis drugs was launched to estimate the burden of MDR-TB within the community. It is the biggest ever such survey in the world; and
20. Kala- azar elimination plan: Kala- azar elimination plan for Uttar Pradesh, Bihar, West Bengal and Jharkhand was launched. It includes active search, new drug regimen, coordinated indoor residual spray and use of non-invasive diagnostic kit.
21. ANMOL: ANMOL is a tablet-based application which helps ANMs in carrying out their day to day work efficiently and effectively by entering and updating service records of beneficiaries on real time basis, provides them with readily available information. It was launched on 7th April, 2016, and is operational in 24 States/UTs. It is being used by more than 97,883 ANMs since its launch *(6)*.

REPRODUCTIVE AND CHILD HEALTH PROGRAMME

Reproductive and child health approach has been defined as "people have the ability to reproduce and regulate their fertility, women are able to go through pregnancy and child birth safely, the outcome of pregnancies is successful in terms of maternal and infant survival and well being, and couples are able to have sexual relations, free of fear of pregnancy and of contracting disease" *(53)*.

The concept is in keeping with the evolution of an integrated approach to the programme aimed at improving the health status of young women and young children which has been going on in the country namely family welfare programme, universal immunization programme, oral rehydration therapy, child survival and safe motherhood programme and acute respiratory infection control etc. It is obviously sensible that integrated RCH programme would help in reducing the cost inputs to some extent because overlapping of expenditure would not be necessary and integrated implementation would optimise outcomes at field level.

The RCH phase–I programme incorporated the components relating child survival and safe motherhood and included two additional components, one relating to sexually transmitted disease (STD) and other relating to reproductive tract infection (RTI).

The RCH programme was based on a differential approach. Inputs in all the districts were not kept uniform. While the care components was same for all districts, the weaker districts got more support and sophisticated facilities were proposed for relatively advanced districts. On the basis of crude birth rate and female literacy rate, all the districts were divided into three categories. Category A having 58 districts, category B having 184 districts and category C having 265 districts. All the districts were covered in a phased manner over a period of three years. The programme was formally launched on 15th October 1997.

RCH phase–I interventions at district level were as follows :

Interventions in all districts

- Child Survival interventions i.e. immunization, Vitamin A (to prevent blindness), oral rehydration therapy and prevention of deaths due to pneumonia.
- Safe Motherhood interventions e.g. antenatal check up, immunization for tetanus, safe delivery, anaemia control programme.
- Implementation of Target Free Approach.
- High quality training at all levels.
- IEC activities.
- Specially designed RCH package for urban slums and tribal areas.
- District sub-projects under Local Capacity Enhancement.
- RTI/STD Clinics at District Hospitals (where not available)
- Facility for safe abortions at PHCs by providing equipment, contractual doctors etc.
- Enhanced community participation through Panchayats, Women's Groups and NGOs.
- Adolescent health and reproductive hygiene.

Interventions in selected States/Distts.

- Screening and treatment of RTI/STD at sub-divisional level.
- Emergency obstetric care at selected FRUs by providing drugs.
- Essential obstetric care by providing drugs and PHN/ Staff Nurse at PHCs.
- Additional ANM at sub-centres in the weak districts for ensuring MCH care.
- Improved delivery services and emergency care by providing equipment kits, IUD insertions and ANM kits at sub-centres.
- Facility of referral transport for pregnant women during emergency to the nearest referral centre through Panchayat in weak districts.

The major interventions under RCH – Phase I

Essential obstetric care (54)

Essential obstetric care intends to provide the basic maternity services to all pregnant women through (1) early registration of pregnancy (within 12–16 weeks). (2) provision of minimum three antenatal check ups by ANM or medical officer to monitor progress of the pregnancy and to detect any risk/complication so that appropriate care including referral could be taken in time. (3) provision of safe delivery at home or in an institution, and (4) provision of three postnatal check ups to monitor the postnatal recovery and to detect complications.

Emergency obstetric care

Complications associated with pregnancy are not always predictable, hence, emergency obstetric care is an important intervention to prevent maternal morbidity and mortality. Under the CSSM programme 1748 Referral Units were identified and supported with equipment kit E to kit P. Under the RCH programme the FRUs were strengthened through supply of emergency obstetric kit, equipment kit and provision of skilled manpower on contract basis etc. Traditional Birth Attendant still plays an important role during deliveries in our society.

24-Hour delivery services at PHCs/CHCs

To promote institutional deliveries, provision has been made to give additional honorarium to the staff to encourage round the clock delivery facilities at health centres.

Medical Termination of Pregnancy

MTP is a reproductive health measure that enables a woman to opt out of an unwanted or unintended pregnancy in certain specified circumstances without endangering her life, through MTP Act 1971. The aim is to reduce maternal morbidity and mortality from unsafe abortions. The assistance from the Central Government is in the form of training of manpower, supply of MTP equipment and provision for engaging doctors trained in MTP to visit PHCs on fixed dates to perform MTP.

Control of reproductive tract infections (RTI) and sexually transmitted diseases (STD)

Under the RCH programme, the component of RTI/STD control is linked to HIV and AIDS control. It has been planned and implemented in close collaboration with National AIDS Control Organization (NACO). NACO provides assistance for setting up RTI/STD clinics upto the district level. The assistance from the Central Government is in the form of training of the manpower and drug kits including disposable equipment. Each district is assisted by two laboratory technicians on contract basis for testing blood, urine and RTI/STD tests.

Immunization

The Universal Immunization Programme (UIP) became a part of CSSM programme in 1992, RCH programme in 1997, and currently of National Health Mission.

Essential newborn care

The primary goal of essential newborn care is to reduce perinatal and neonatal mortality. The main components are resuscitation of newborn with asphyxia, prevention of hypothermia, prevention of infection, exclusive breast feeding and referral of sick newborn. The strategies are to train medical and other health personnel in essential newborn care, provide basic facilities for care of low birth weight and sick new borns in FRU and district hospitals etc.

Diarrhoeal disease control

In the districts not implementing Integrated Management of Neonatal and Childhood Illness, the vertical programme for control of diarrhoeal disease will continue. India is the first country in the world to introduce the low osmolarity Oral Rehydration Solution. Zinc is to be used as an adjunct to ORS for the management of diarrhoea. Addition of Zinc would result in reduction of the number and severity of episodes and the duration of diarrhoea. De-worming guidelines have been formulated. The incidence of diarrhoea is reduced by provision of safe drinking water.

Acute respiratory disease control

The standard case management of ARI and prevention of deaths due to pneumonia is now an integral part of RCH programme. Peripheral health workers are being trained to recognize and treat pneumonia. Cotrimoxazole is being supplied to the health workers through the drug kit.

Prevention and control of vitamin A deficiency in children

It is estimated that large number of children suffer from sub-clinical deficiency of vitamin A. Under the programme, doses of vitamin A are given to all children under 5 years of age. The first dose (1 lakh units) is given at nine months of age along with measles vaccination. The second dose (2 lakh units) is given after 9 months. Subsequent doses (2 lakh units each) are given at six months intervals upto 5 years of age *(3)*. All cases of severe malnutrition to be given one additional dose of vitamin A.

Prevention and control of anaemia in children

Iron deficiency anaemia is widely prevalent in young children. To manage anaemia, the policy has been revised. Infants from the age of 6 months onwards upto the age of 5 years are to receive iron supplements in liquid formulation in doses of 20 mg elemental iron and 100 mcg folic acid per day for 100 days in a year. Children 6 to 10 years of age will receive iron in the dose of 30 mg elemental iron and 250 mcg folic acid for 100 days in a year. Children above this age group would receive iron supplement in the adult dose *(3)*.

Training of dais

A scheme for training of dais was initiated during 2001–02. The scheme is being implemented in 156 districts in 18 states/UTs of the country. The districts have been selected on the basis of the safe delivery rates being less than 30 per cent. The scheme was extended to all the districts of EAG states. The aim was to train at least one Dai in every village, with the objective of making deliveries safe.

Empowered Action Group (EAG)

An Empowered Action Group has been constituted in the Ministry of Health and Family Welfare, with Union Minister for Health and Family Welfare as chairman on 20th March 2001. As 55 per cent of the increase in the population of India is anticipated in the states of Uttar Pradesh, Bihar, Madhya Pradesh, Rajasthan, Odisha, Chhattisgarh, Jharkhand and Uttarakhand, these states are perceived to be most deficient in critical socio–demographic indices. Through EAG, these states will get focussed attention for different health and family welfare programmes.

District Surveys

There is no regular source of data to indicate the reproductive health status of women. The RCH programme conducts district based rapid household survey to assess the reproductive health status of women. The key indicators are :

a. Percentage of pregnant women with full ANC;
b. Percentage of institutional deliveries and home deliveries;
c. Percentage of home deliveries by trained birth attendant;
d. Current contraceptive prevalence rate;
e. Percentage of children fully immunized;
f. Percentage of unmet need for family planning; and
g. Percentage of household reported visits by health worker in previous 3 months.

RCH – PHASE II

RCH–phase II began from 1st April, 2005. The focus of the programme is to reduce maternal and child morbidity and mortality with emphasis on rural health care.

The major strategies under the second phase of RCH are *(55)* :

- *Essential obstetric care*
  a. Institutional delivery.
  b. Skilled attendance at delivery.
- *Emergency obstetric care*
  a. Operationalizing First Referral Units.
  b. Operationalizing PHCs and CHCs for round the clock delivery services.
- *Strengthening referral system*

The Government of India has given some broad guidelines and strategies for achieving the reduction in maternal mortality rate and infant mortality rate. The initiatives which have been planned are :

Essential obstetric care

a. Institutional delivery – To promote institutional delivery in RCH Phase II, it was envisaged that fifty percent of the PHCs and all the CHCs would be made operational as 24–hour delivery centres, in a phased manner, by the year 2010. These centres would be responsible for providing basic emergency obstetric care and essential newborn care and basic newborn resuscitation services round the clock. The experience of RCH phase-I indicates that giving incentive to health workers for providing round the clock services did not function well in most of the states. On the contrary there is the experience from government of Andhra Pradesh and Tamil Nadu, where round the clock delivery and new born care services could be ensured by providing 3 to 4 staff nurses/ANM at the PHCs.

b. Skilled attendance at delivery – It is now recognized globally that the countries which have been successful in bringing down maternal mortality are the ones where the provision of skilled attendance at every birth and its linkage with appropriate referral services for complicated cases have been ensured. The WHO has also emphasized that skilled attendance at every birth is essential to reduce the maternal mortality in any country. Guidelines for normal delivery and management of obstetric complications at PHC/CHC for medical officers and for ANC and skilled attendance at birth for ANM/LHVs have been formulated and disseminated to the states.

c. The policy decisions : ANMs / LHVs / SNs have now been permitted to use drugs in specific emergency situations to reduce maternal mortality. They have also been permitted to carry out certain emergency interventions when the life of the mother is at stake.

Emergency obstetric care

Operationalization of FRUs and skilled attendance at birth are the two activities which go hand in hand. In view of this, simultaneous steps have been taken to ensure tackling obstetric emergencies. It has been decided that all the First Referral Units be made operational for providing emergency and essential obstetric care during the second phase of RCH.The minimum services to be provided by a fully functional FRU are *(56)* :

1. 24 hours delivery services including normal and assisted deliveries;
2. Emergency obstetric care including surgical interventions like caesarean sections;
3. New-born care;
4. Emergency care of sick children;
5. Full range of family planning services including laproscopic services;
6. Safe abortion services;
7. Treatment of STI/RTI;
8. Blood storage facility;
9. Essential laboratory services; and
10. Referral (transport) services.

There are three critical determinants of a facility being 'declared' as a FRU. They are : availability of surgical interventions, new-born care and blood storage facility on a 24 hours basis.

To be able to perform the full range of FRU function, a health facility must have the following facilities : (a) A minimum bed strength of 20–30. However, in difficult areas, as the North–East states and the underserved areas of EAG states, this could initially be relaxed to 10–12 beds; (b) A fully functional operation theatre; (c) A fully functional labour room; (d) An area earmarked and equipped for new-born care in the labour room, and in the ward; (e) A functional laboratory; (f) Blood storage facility; (g) 24 hour water supply and electricity supply; and (h) Arrangements for waste disposal; and (i) Ambulance facility.

Strengthening referral system

During RCH phase–I, funds were given to the Panchayat for providing assitance to poor people in the case of obstetric emergencies. Feedback from the states indicate that there was no active involvement of Panchayats in running the scheme. Based on these experiences different states have proposed different modes of referral linkage in RCH Phase II. Some of them have indicated to involve local self help groups, NGOs and women groups, whereas few others have indicated to outsource it.

New initiatives

1. Training of MBBS doctors in life saving anaesthetic skills for emergency obstetric care : Provision of adequate and timely emergency obstetric care (EmOC) has been recognized as the most important intervention for saving lives of pregnant women who may develop complications during pregnancy or childbirth. The operationalisation of First Referral Unit at sub-district/CHC level for providing EmOC to pregnant women is a crucial strategy of RCH-II, which needs focussed attention. The training of MBBS doctors will be undertaken for only such numbers who are required for the functioning of FRUs and CHCs, and shall be limited to the requirement of tackling emergency obstetric situations only. It is **not** the replacement of the specialist anaesthetist. Government of India is also introducing training of MBBS doctors in obstetric management skills. Federation of Obstetric and Gynaecology Society of India has prepared a training plan for 16 weeks in all obstetric management skills, including caesarean section operation.
2. Setting up of blood storage centres at FRUs according to government of India guidelines.

JANANI SURAKSHA YOJANA

The National Maternity Benefit scheme has been modified into a new scheme called *Janani Suraksha Yojana* (JSY). It was launched on 12th April, 2005. The objectives of the scheme are – reducing maternal mortality and neonatal mortality through encouraging delivery at health institutions, and focusing at institutional care among women in below poverty line families.

The salient features of *Janani Suraksha Yojana* are as follows *(7)* :

a. It is a 100 per cent centrally sponsored scheme;

b. Under National Rural Health Mission, it integrates the benefit of cash assistance with institutional care during antenatal, delivery and immediate post-partum care; This benefit will be given to all women, both rural and urban, belonging to below poverty line household. However, with a view to give special focus in 10 low performing states (states having low institutional delivery rate), namely Uttar Pradesh, Uttarakhand, Madhya Pradesh, Jharkhand, Bihar, Rajasthan, Chhattisgarh, Odisha, Assam and Jammu & Kashmir, the benefit will be extended upto the third child if the mother, of her own accord, chooses to undergo sterilization in the health facility where she delivered, immediately after delivery. The other states are called high performing states. The Accredited Social Health Activist (ASHA) would work as a link health worker between the poor pregnant women and public sector health insitution in the low performing states. ASHA would be responsible for making available institutional antenatal as well as postnatal care. She would also be responsible for escorting the pregnant women to the health centre. The scale of assistance under the scheme from 2012–13 would be as follows :

Category	Rural Area			Urban Area		
	Mother's package	ASHA's package*	Total Rs.	Mother's package	ASHA's package**	Total Rs.
LPS	1400	600	2000	1000	400	1400
HPS	700	600	1300	600	400	1000

LPS : Low performing states, HPS : High performing states

* ASHA incentive of Rs. 600/- in rural areas includes Rs. 300/- for ANC component and Rs. 300/- for accompanying pregnant woman for institutional delivery.

** ASHA incentive of Rs. 400/- in urban area includes Rs. 200/- for ANC component and Rs. 200/- for accompanying pregnant woman for institutional delivery.

Source : *(6)*

The eligibility of cash assistance is as follows *(6)* :

1. *In low performing states (LPS) :* All women, including those from SC and ST families, delivering in government health centres like sub-centre, primary health centre, community health centre, first referral unit, general wards of district and state hospitals or accredited private institutions.
2. *In high performing states (HPS) :* Below poverty line women, and the SC and ST pregnant women delivering in Govt. health centres or accredited private institutes.

The limitation of cash assistance for institutional delivery is as follows :

1. In low performing states : All births, delivered in health centre, government or accredited private health institutions will get the benefit.
2. In high performing states the benefit is only upto 2 live births.

ASHA package is available in all low performing states, North-East states and in tribal districts of all states and UTs. In rural areas it includes the following components : (a) Cash assistance for referral transport for pregnant women to go to the nearest health centre for delivery (should not be less than Rs. 250/-); (b) Cash incentive : This should not be less than Rs. 200/- per delivery. ASHA should get her money after her post-natal visit to the beneficiary, and when the child has been immunized for BCG; and (c) Balance amount to be paid to ASHA in lieu of her services rendered by her. The payment should be made at the hospital/health institution itself.

The Yojana subsidizes the cost of caesarean section and for management of obstetric complications, upto Rs. 1500 per delivery to the government institutions, where government specialists are not in position.

In low performing and high performing states, all below poverty line pregnant women preferring to deliver at home, are entitled to cash assistance of Rs. 500 per delivery, regardless of age and number of children *(1)*.

Direct benefit transfer under JSY: Payments under the JSY are being made through direct benefit transfer mode. Under this initiative, eligible pregnant women are entitled to get JSY benefit directly into their Aadhar linked bank account/electronic fund transfer *(7)*.

The year 2006–07 was declared as the year for institutional deliveries. During the year scope of the scheme was extended to the urban areas of high performing states and restriction of age and birth order were removed in the low performing states. The benefits of the scheme was also extended to all women belonging to SC/ST families for institutional deliveries.

During the year 2018–19, about 100.41 lakh pregnant women were benefitted from the scheme *(11)*.

Vandemataram scheme

This is a voluntary scheme wherein any obstetric and gynaec specialist, maternity home, nursing home, lady doctor/MBBS doctor can volunteer themselves for providing safe motherhood services. The enrolled doctors will display 'Vandemataram logo' at their clinic. Iron and Folic Acid tablets, oral pills, TT injections etc. will be provided by the respective District Medical Officers to the 'Vandemataram doctors/ clinics' for free distribution to beneficiaries. The cases needing special care and treatment can be referred to the government hospitals, who have been advised to take due care of the patients coming with Vandemataram cards.

Safe abortion services

In India, abortion is a major cause of maternal mortality and morbidity and accounts for nearly 8.9 per cent maternal deaths. Majority of abortions take place outside authorized health services and/or by unauthorized and unskilled persons. Whether spontaneous or induced, abortion is a matter of concern as it may lead to complications. Under RCH phase II following facilities are provided :

a. *Medical method of abortion :* Termination of early pregnancy with two drugs – Mifepristone (RU 486) followed by Misoprostol. They are considered safe under supervision, with appropriate counselling. Currently its use in India is recommended upto 7 weeks (49 days) of amenorrhoea in a facility with provision for safe abortion services and blood transfusion. Termination of pregnancy with RU 486 and Misoprostol is offered to women under the preview of the MTP Act, 1971.

b. *Manual Vacuum Aspiration (MVA)* : The department of family welfare has introduced Manual Vacuum Aspiration (MVA) technique in the family welfare programme. Manual Vacuum Aspiration is a safe and simple technique for termination of early pregnancy, makes it feasible to be used in primary health centres or comparable facilities, thereby increasing access to safe abortion services. The project of introducing the MVA technique has been piloted in coordination with FOGSI, WHO and respective state governments before being accepted for implementation by the ministry of health and family welfare.

Village Health and Nutrition Day

Organizing Village Health and Nutrition Day once a month at anganwadi centre to provide antenatal/post-partum care for pregnant women, promote institutional delivery, health education, immunization, family planning and nutrition services etc.

Maternal death review

Maternal death review as a strategy has been spelt out clearly in the RCH-II. Maternal death audit, both facility and community based, is an important strategy to improve the quality of obstetric care and reduce maternal mortality and morbidity. Guidelines and tools for initiating maternal death review have been formulated *(3)*.

Pregnancy tracking

The link between pregnancy-related care and maternal mortality is well established. RCH-II stresses the need for universal screening of pregnant women and providing essential and emergency obstetric care. Focussed antenatal care, birth preparedness and complication readiness, skilled attendance at birth, care within the first seven days etc. are the factors that can reduce the maternal mortality *(3)*.

JANANI-SHISHU SURAKSHA KARYAKRAM (JSSK)

Government of India launched the Janani-Shishu Suraksha Karyakram (JSSK) on 1st June 2011, a new national initiative, to make available better health facitlies for women and child. The new initiatives provide the following facilities to the pregnant women *(57)* :

- All pregnant women delivering in public health institutions to have absolutely free and no expense delivery, including caesarean section. The entitlements include free drugs and consumables, free diet upto 3 days during normal delivery and upto 7 days for C-section, free diagnostics, and free blood wherever required. This initiative would also provide for free transport from home to institution, between facilities in case of a referral and drop back home. Similar entitlements have been put in place for all sick newborns accessing public health institutions for treatment till 30 days after birth. The scheme has now been extended to cover the complications during ANC, PNC and also sick infants.
- The scheme is estimated to benefit more than 12 million pregnant women who access government health facilities for their delivery. Moreover, it will motivate those who still choose to deliver at their homes to opt for institutional deliveries.

PRADHAN MANTRI SURAKSHIT MATRITVA ABHIYAN (PMSMA)

The Pradhan Mantri Surakshit Matritva Abhiyan (PMSMA) has been launched by the Ministry in June, 2016. Under PMSMA, all pregnant women in the country are provided fixed day, free of cost assured and quality antenatal care. As part of the campaign, a minimum package of antenatal care services (including investigations and drugs) is being provided to the beneficiaries on the 9th day of every month. The Abhiyan also involves private sector's health care providers as volunteers to provide specialist care in government facilities. About 2.20 crore ANC check-ups were conducted by about 6,000 volunteers in more than 17,000 government facilities. Also, more than 11.66 lakh high risk pregnancy cases were identified across the country *(11)*.

SUMAN (Surakshit Matritva Aashwasan)

Ministry has launched a new initiative namely "SUMAN-Surakshit Matritva Aashwasan" on 10th October 2019 with an aim to provide assured, dignified, respectful and quality healthcare at no cost and zero tolerance for denial of services for every woman and newborn visiting the public health facility in order to end all preventable maternal and newborn deaths and morbidities and provide a positive birthing experience.

The expected outcome of this new initiative is "Zero preventable maternal and newborn deaths and high quality of maternity care delivered with dignity and respect" *(11)*.

LAQSHYA PROGRAMME (11)

MOHFW launched "LaQshya program" to improve quality of care in labour room and maternity OTs in public health facilities in 2017. The LaQshya programme is evidence based approach to improve quality of maternal and newborn care and provide respectful care, particularly during the intrapartum and postpartum periods, which are the most vulnerable periods for a woman and contribute to a significant proportion of maternal deaths.

Its implementation involves improving infrastructure upgradation, ensuring availability of essential equipment, providing adequate human resources, capacity building of health care workers, and adherence to clinical guidelines and improving quality processes in labour room and maternity OT.

LaQshya program is being implemented at District Hospital (DH), Sub district Hospital (SDH), high case load Community Health Centre (CHC) and First Referral Units (FRUs), and medical colleges. 2,445 public health facilities including 193 medical colleges have been identified under LaQshya. Out of these, 441 labour rooms and 392 OTs have achieved state certification. National certification for LaQshya has been achieved by 447 labour rooms and 365 OTs till Dec. 2021 *(6)*.

Regional trainings of trainers have been completed for all States/UTs across country to build a critical mass of trainers who took this training cascade further. State orientation and baseline assessment have been conducted for all State/UTs. Based on the gaps, the States have prepared gap closure plan. Onsite mentoring is being conducted in 24 identified medical colleges to accelerate process of certification in medical colleges. LaQshya portal has been finalized and operationalized. Data upload on LaQshya portal has been initiated to aid digitization of all LaQshya related data, readily available results and visualization through dashboard.

ANAEMIA MUKT BHARAT PROGRAMME (AMB) (6)

In 2018, Anaemia Mukt Bharat strategy was launched to achieve the envisaged target of 3% reduction in anaemia prevalence every year under the POSHAN Abhiyaan. The strategy recommends 6 × 6 × 6 strategy to reduce anaemia prevalence (nutritional and non-nutritional) in six age groups namely pre-school children (6–59 months), children (5–9 years), adolescent girls and boys (10–19 years), pregnant women, lactating women and in women of reproductive age group (15–49 years) in programme mode through life cycle approach.

The six interventions under Anaemia Mukt Bharat strategy are prophylactic iron folic acid supplementation, periodic deworming, intensified year-round behaviour change communication campaign including delayed cord clamping, testing and treatment of anaemia using digital methods and point of care treatment, mandatory provision of iron folic acid fortified foods in public health programmes and addressing non-nutritional causes of anaemia in endemic pockets, with special focus on malaria, haemoglobinopathies and fluorosis. The six institutional mechanisms are inter-ministerial coordination, national Anemia Mukt Bharat unit, national centre of excellence and advanced research on anaemia control, convergence with other ministries, strengthening supply chain and logistics, Anaemia Mukt Bharat dashboard and digital portal-one-stop shop for anaemia.

To address anaemia in children, bi-weekly IFA supplements are provided to children aged 6-59 months through ASHAs and Weekly IFA supplements to children of 5–10 years and adolescents 10–19 years of age. 180 doses of IFA supplements are also being provided to pregnant and lactating women during ANC and PNC period, respectively. Bi-annual Vitamin-A supplementation is being done for all children below five years of age. During FY 2021–22 (till September, 2021), the achievements under IFA supplementation is as follows :

a. 2 crore children of age group 6–59 months were provided 8–10 doses of Iron Folic Acid (IFA) Syrup every month.
b. 1.9 crore children of age group 5–9 years were provided 4–5 IFA Pink tablets every month.
c. 3 crore children of age group 10–19 years were provided 4–5 IFA Blue tablets every month.
d. 1.3 crore pregnant women and 0.6 crore lactating women were provided 180 IFA Red tablets during ANC and PNC respectively.

MOTHER'S ABSOLUTE AFFECTION (MAA) PROGRAMME :

Mother's Absolute Affection (MAA) programme focuses on promotion of optimum Infant and Young Child Feeding (IYCF) practices including early initiation of breastfeeding within one hour, exclusive breastfeeding up to six months, age appropriate and adequate complementary feeding after six months and continuation of breastfeeding for two years and beyond through capacity building of frontline health workers and comprehensive IEC campaigns. As per NFHS–5 (2019–21), only 41.8 per cent newborns initiated on breastfeed within one hour of birth while, 63.7 per cent children breastfed exclusively till 6 months of age *(6)*.

MIDWIFERY INITIATIVE :

The Government of India has taken a landmark policy decision to roll out midwifery services in the country in order to improve the quality of care and ensure respectful care to pregnant women and newborns. The initiative was launched in December 2018.

The initiative aims to create a cadre of Nurse Practitioners in Midwifery (NPMs) who are skilled in accordance to competencies prescribed by the International Confederation of Midwives (ICM) and are knowledgeable and capable of providing compassionate women-centred, reproductive, maternal and newborn health care services. In order to create a cadre of Nurse Practitioner Midwives, eighteen months training would be provided to GNM/BSc nurses having 2 years experience in conducting deliveries. Training Curriculum would be based on the 'Essential Competencies for Midwifery Practice' defined by International Confederation of Midwife. Midwifery practices intend to minimise unnecessary medical interventions and promote physiological birthing by adoption of alternate birthing positions during child birth *(6)*.

15 National Midwifery Training Centres are located in the country. They are as follows : Telangana (2), one each in Madhya Pradesh, Gujarat, Assam, Maharashtra, Uttar Pradesh, Rajasthan, West Bengal, Tamil Nadu, Karnataka, Delhi, Punjab, Jammu & Kashmir and Andhra Pradesh *(6)*.

Release of Scope of Practice : In July 2021, GoI released a "Scope of Practice document for Midwifery Educators (ME) and Nurse Practitioner Midwife (NPM)" in collaboration with the Indian Nursing Council (INC). It acts as a guiding document for their education, regulation and ongoing professional development.

Newer interventions to reduce newborn mortality have also been implemented, including Vitamin-K injection at birth, Antenatal corticosteroids in preterm labour, Kangaroo Mother Care and empowering ANMs to provide Injection Gentamycin to young infants for possible serious bacterial infection.

Social Awareness and Actions to Neutralize Pneumonia Successfully (SAANS) : SAANS (Social Awareness and Actions to Neutralize Pneumonia Successfully) Initiative was launched on 16th November 2019 to accelerate action to reduce deaths due to Childhood Pneumonia. SAANS Campaign rolled out in the States/ UTs from 12th November 2021–28th February 2022 with aims of accelerating action against Childhood Pneumonia by generating awareness around protect, prevent and treatment aspects of Childhood Pneumonia and to enhance early identification and care seeking behaviours among parents and caregivers *(6)*.

Child health components

The strategy for child health care, aims to reduce under-five child mortality through interventions at every level of service delivery and through improved child care practices and child nutrition.

Nutritional rehabilitation centres (NRCs)

Severe acute malnutrition is an important contributing factor for most deaths among children suffering from common childhood illness such as diarrhoea and pneumonia. Deaths among these malnourished children are preventable, provided timely and appropriate actions are taken. NRCs are facility based units providing medical and nutritional care to Severe Acute Malnutrition (SAM) children under 5 years of age who have medical complications. In addition special focus is on improving the skill of mothers on child care and feeding practices so that the child continues to get adequate care at home. The services provided at the NRCs include *(1)*:

a. 24 hours care and monitoring of the child;
b. Treatment of medical complication;
c. Therapeutic feeding;
d. Sensory stimulation and emotional care;

e. Counselling on appropriate feed, care and hygiene;
f. Demonstration and practice-by-doing on the preparation of energy dense food using locally available, culturally acceptable and affordable food items;
g. Social assessment of the family to identify and address contributory factors; and
h. Follow up of the children discharged from the facility.

Management of medical complications in a child with SAM at health facility *(58)*

A majority of the deaths in hospitals occur within 24 hours of admission, many of these deaths can be prevented if the critically ill children are identified as soon as they are admitted and their treatment is started immediately.

Triage

Triage is the process of rapidly screening sick children. Triage must be done for all paediatric patients coming to the health facility. The first step is to check every child for emergency signs and provide emergency treatment as necessary, keeping in mind the ABCD steps : Airway, Breathing, Circulation, Coma, Convulsion and Dehydration.

Assessment at admission *(58)*

The child should be assessed by taking detailed history and should be examined for the signs of under-nutrition.

Principles of hospital-based management *(58)*

The principles of management of SAM are based on 3 phases: stabilization phase, transition phase and rehabilitative phase.

Stabilization Phase: Children with SAM without an adequate appetite and/or a major medical complication are stabilized in an in-patient facility. This phase usually lasts for 1–2 days. The feeding formula used during this phase is Starter diet which promotes recovery of normal metabolic function and nutrition – electrolytic balance. All children must be carefully monitored for signs of overfeeding or over hydration in this phase.

Transition Phase: This phase is the subsequent part of the stabilization phase and usually lasts for 2–3 days. The transition phase is intended to ensure that the child is clinically stable and can tolerate an increased energy and protein intake. The child moves to the Transition Phase from Stabilization Phase when there is:

- At least the beginning of loss of oedema.
  AND
- Return of appetite.
  AND
- No nasogastric tube, infusions, no severe medical problems.
  AND
- Is alert and active?

The ONLY difference in management of the child in transition phase is the change in type of diet. There is gradual transition from starter diet to catch up diet. The quantity of catch up diet given is equal to the quantity of starter diet given in stabilization phase.

Rehabilitation Phase: Once children with SAM have recovered their appetite and received treatment for medical complications they enter Rehabilitation Phase. The aim is to promote rapid weight gain, stimulate emotional and physical development and prepare the child for normal feeding at home. The child progresses from transition phase to rehabilitation phase when:

- S/he has reasonable appetite; finishes > 90% of the feed that is given, without a significant pause.
- Major reduction or loss of oedema.
- No other medical problem.

Micronutrient supplementation *(58)*

Vitamin A: Give Vitamin A in a single dose to all SAM children unless there is evidence that child has received vitamin A dose in last 1 month.

Recommended oral dose of Vitamin A according to child's age:

Age	Vit. A dose
<6 months	50,000 IU
6–12 months or if weight <8 kg	100,000 IU
>12 months	200,000 IU

- Give same dose on Day 1, 2 and 14 if there is clinical evidence of vitamin A deficiency.
- Children more than twelve months but having weight less than 8 kg should be given 100,000 IU orally irrespective of age.
- Oral treatment with vitamin A is preferred. For oral administration, an oil-based formulation is preferred.

Take a history concerning	On examination, look for
• Recent intake of food and fluids • Usual diet (before the current illness) • Breastfeeding • Duration and frequency of diarrhoea and vomiting • Type of diarrhoea (watery/ bloody) • Chronic cough • Loss of appetite • Family circumstances (to understand the child's social background). • Contact with tuberculosis • Recent contact with measles • Known or suspected HIV infection • Immunizations	• Anthropometry– weight, height/length, mid arm circumference. • Oedema. • Pulse, heart rate, respiratory rate. • Signs of dehydration. • Shock (cold hands, slow capillary refill, weak and rapid pulse). • Palmar pallor. • Eye signs of vitamin A deficiency: – Dry conjunctiva or cornea, – Bitot's spots – Corneal ulceration – Keratomalacia • Localizing signs of infection, including ear and throat infections, skin infection or pneumonia. • Mouth ulcers. • Skin changes of kwashiorkor: – Hypo or hyperpigmentation – Desquamation – Ulceration (spreading over limbs, thighs, genitalia, groin, and behind the ears). – Exudative lesions (resembling severe burns) often with secondary infection (including candida).

- IM treatment should be used in children with severe anorexia, oedematous malnutrition, or septic shock. Only water based formulations and half of oral dose should be used.

Other micronutrients should be given daily for at least 2 weeks:

- *Multivitamin supplement* (should contain vitamin A, C, D, E and B_{12} and not just vitamin B complex): Twice recommended daily allowance.
- *Folic acid:* 5 mg on day 1, then 1 mg/day.
- *Elemental Zinc:* 2 mg/kg/day.
- *Copper:* 0.3 mg/kg/day (if separate preparation not available use commercial preparation containing copper).
- *Iron:* Start daily iron supplementation after two days of the child being on catch up diet. Give elemental iron in the dose of 3 mg/kg/day in two divided doses, preferably between meals. (DO not give iron in stabilization phase).

Follow-up of children discharged from NRC

Close collaboration and information sharing between NRC and community based care (at PHC, sub-centre and AWC) are essential. The list of SAM children discharged from NRC should be shared with area specific ANM and ICDS supervisors. These children should be enrolled in the anganwadi centre and given supplementary food as per the guidelines. The AWWs should prioritize these children for home visits, every week in the first 4 weeks and then once in 2 weeks till the child is discharged from the programme. During the home visits, AWW should observe feeding and provide appropriate counselling and support to the mother. These children should be weighed every week at AWC. The ASHA and AWW should ensure that these children should return for the scheduled follow-ups at the NRC *(58)*. Incentive of Rs 50 can be provided to ASHA for accompanying the child to the NRC and motivating the mother to stay at NRC for atleast 7 days till the child is stabilized and has started to eat. Additional incentive of Rs 50 may be given for each follow-up visit by the child, upto a maximum of three visits *(58)*.

Presently 1075 NRCs are functional across 17 states/UTs *(11)*.

Integrated Management of Neonatal and Childhood Illness (IMNCI)

IMNCI strategy is one of the main intervention under the RCH II/ NRHM. The strategy encompasses a range of interventions to prevent and manage the commonest major childhood diseases.

Pre-service IMNCI

Pre-service IMNCI has been accepted as an important strategy to scale up IMNCI by Govt. of India and is being included in the curriculum of medical colleges of the country. This will help in providing the much needed trained IMNCI manpower in the public and private sector.

Facility based IMNCI (F–IMNCI)

F–IMNCI is the integration of the facility based care package with the IMNCI package, to empower the health personnel with the skill to manage new born and childhood illness at the community level as well as the health facility. It focusses on providing appropriate in-patient management of the major causes of neonatal and childhood mortality such as asphyxia, sepsis, low birth weight, pneumonia, diarrhoea, malaria, meningitis and severe malnutrition in children. The master trainers at state and district level are paediatricians from tertiary hospitals and medical colleges *(3)*.

Facility based newborn care (59)

As more sick children are screened at the peripheries through IMNCI and referred to the health facilities, care of the sick newborn and child at CHCs, FRUs, district hospitals and medical college hospitals assumes priority. Equipping the facilities to provide the requisite level of care and simultaneously enhancing the capacity of the medical officers at these facilities to handle such cases thus becomes important. The setting up of SNCUs at district hospitals, stabilization units at CHCs, and newborn care corners at all facilities offering delivery facilities, is thus a key activity *(3)*.

In the overall planning of facility based care it is important to understand the level of care that is provided at the various facility levels. The newborn care facilities at different levels are as follows :

Health facility	All newborns at birth	Sick newborns
Primary health centre (PHC)/Sub-centre (SC) identified as MCH level I	Newborn care corner in labor rooms.	Prompt referral
Community health centre (CHC)/First referral unit (FRU) identified as MCH Level II	Newborn care corner in labor rooms and in operation theatre.	Newborn stabilization unit (NBSU).
District hospital identified as MCH Level III	Newborn care corner in labor rooms and in operation theatre.	Special newborn care unit (SNCU).

Newborn Care Corner (NBCC)

NBCC is a space within the delivery room in any health facility where immediate care is provided to all newborns at birth. This area is MANDATORY for all health facilities where deliveries are conducted. About 20,337 NBCCs are operational in the country *(6)*.

Newborn Stabilization Unit (NBSU)

NBSU is a facility within or in close proximity of the maternity ward where sick and low birth weight newborns can be cared for during short periods. All FRUs/CHCs need to have a neonatal stabilization unit, in addition to the newborn care corner. It requires space for 4 bedded unit and two beds in post-natal ward for rooming-in. About 2,579 NBSUs are functional in the country.

Special Newborn Care Unit (SNCU)

SNCU is a neonatal unit in the vicinity of the labor room which is to provide special care (all care except assisted ventilation and major surgery) for sick newborns. Any facility with more than 3,000 deliveries per year should have an SNCU (most district hospitals and some sub-district hospitals would fulfil this criteria).

The minimum recommended number of beds for an SNCU at a district hospital is 12. However, if the district hospital conducts more than 3,000 deliveries per year, 4 beds should be added for each 1,000 additional deliveries. A 12 bedded unit will require 4 additional adult beds for the step down. 894 SNCUs are functional in the country.

Triage of sick newborns (59)

Triage is sorting of neonates to rapidly screen sick neonates for prioritizing management. Fig. 13 summarizes the process.

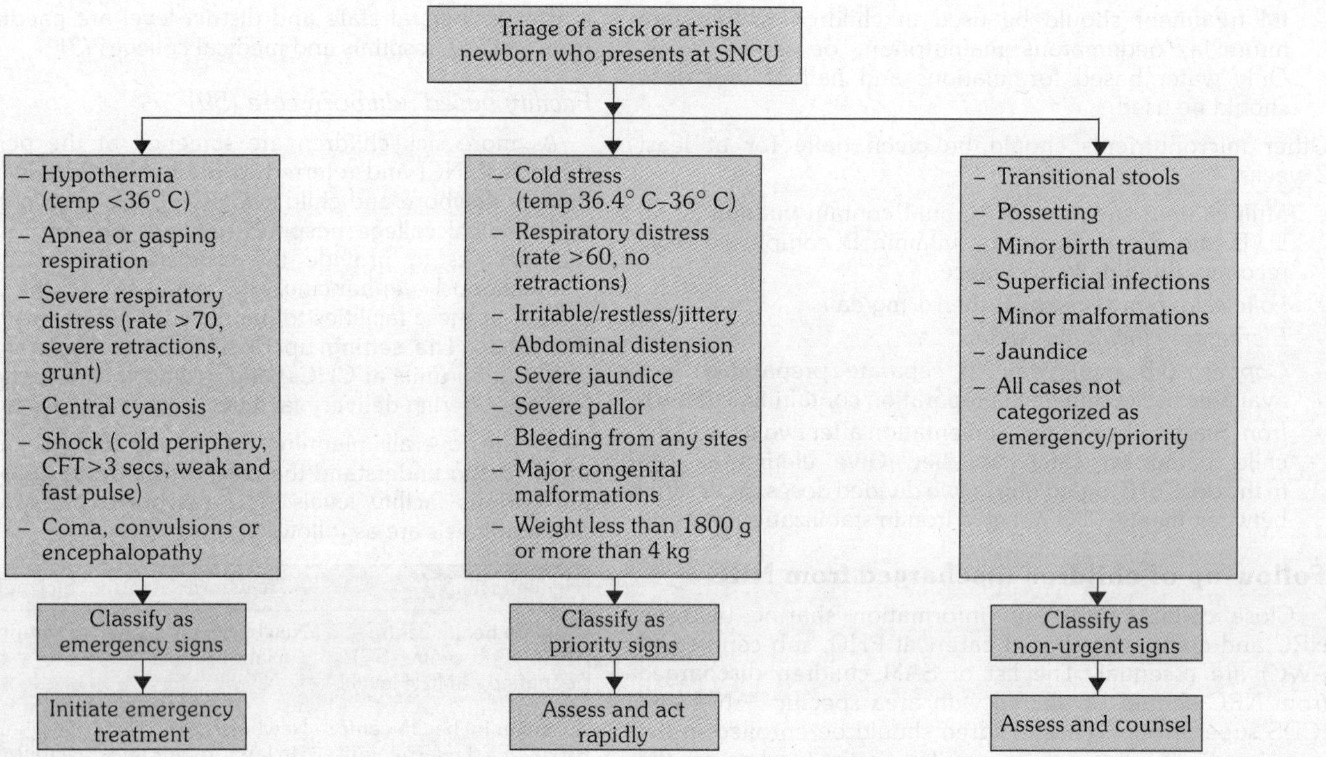

Newborns classified as "Emergency" require urgent intervention and emergency measures. All such newborns will be admitted to SNCU after initial stabilization.
Newborns classified as "Priority" are sick and need rapid assessment and admission to SNCU.
Newborns classified as non-urgent do not require urgent attention, but require further assessment and counselling.

FIG. 13

A. CRITERIA FOR ADMISSION TO NBSU *(59)* :

Newborn presenting with any of the following signs to a facility with neonatal stabilization unit requires admission for initial stabilization and transfer to SNCU :

- Apnea or gasping.
- Respiratory distress (Rate>70/min with severe retractions/grunt).
- Hypothermia <35.4°C
- Hyperthermia (>37.5°C)
- Central cyanosis.
- Shock (cold periphery with capillary filling time (CFT) more than 3 seconds and weak and fast pulse).
- Significant bleeding that requires blood or component transfusion.

Newborns, who after assessment and stabilization, can be managed at stabilization unit*.

- Newborns with respiratory distress, having respiratory rate 60–70/min without grunting or retractions (for observation and oxygen therapy).
- Newborns with gestation less than 34 weeks or weight <1800 g (for observation and assisted feeding).
- Newborns with hypothermia and hyperthermia who are haemodynamically stable after initial stabilization.
- Newborns with jaundice requiring phototherapy.
- Neonates with sepsis who are haemodynamically stable, for observation and antibiotic therapy.

* Others would require referral to an SNCU after stabilization, if an SNCU and appropriate referral is available in the district.

B. CRITERIA FOR ADMISSION TO SNCU *(59)* :

Criteria for admission to SNCU and criteria for transfer to step-down unit and discharge are as follows :

I. Any newborn with following criteria should be immediately admitted to the SNCU :
- Birth weight <1800 g or gestation <34 weeks.
- Large baby (>4.0 kg).
- Perinatal asphyxia.
- Apnea or gasping.
- Refusal to feed.
- Respiratory distress (rate>60/min or grunt/retractions).
- Severe jaundice (appears <24 hrs/stains palms and soles/lasts>2 weeks).
- Hypothermia <35.4°C, or hyperthermia (>37.5°C).
- Central cyanosis.
- Shock (cold periphery with CFT>3 seconds, and weak and fast pulse).
- Coma, convulsions or encephalopathy.
- Abdominal distension.
- Diarrhoea/dysentery.
- Bleeding.
- Major malformations.

II. Criteria for transfer from SNCU to the Step-Down :
- Newborn whose respiratory distress is improving and does not require oxygen supplementation to maintain saturation.
- Newborn on antibiotics for completion of duration of therapy.
- Low birth weight newborn (less than 1800 g), who are otherwise stable (for adequate weight gain).
- Newborn with jaundice requiring phototherapy but otherwise stable.
- Newborn admitted for any condition, but are now thermodynamically and hemodynamically stable.

III. Criteria for discharge from SNCU :
- Newborn is able to maintain temperature without radiant warmer.

- Newborn is haemodynamically stable (normal CFT, strong peripheral pulse).
- Newborn accepting breast-feeds well.
- Newborn has documented weight gain for 3 consecutive days; and the weight is more than 1.5 kg.
- Primary illness has resolved.

In addition to the above, mother should be confident of taking care of the newborn at home.

HOME BASED NEWBORN CARE (HBNC) (60) :

Home based newborn care is aimed at improving newborn survival. The strategy of universal access to home based newborn care must complement the strategy of institutional delivery to achieve significant reduction in postpartum and neonatal mortality and morbidity. The providers of service include anganwadi workers, ANM, ASHA and the medical officer. However, ASHA is the main person involved in home based newborn care.

The major objective of HBNC is to decrease neonatal mortality and morbidity through :

1. The provision of essential newborn care to all newborns and the prevention of complications.
2. Early detection and special care of preterm and low birth weight newborns.
3. Early identification of illness in the newborn and provision of appropriate care and referral.
4. Support the family for adoption of healthy practices and build confidence and skills of the mother to safeguard her health and that of the newborn.

The responsibilities of ASHA for home based newborn care are as follows *(60)* :

1. Mobilize all pregnant mothers and ensure that they receive the full package of antenatal care.
2. Undertake birth planning and birth preparedness with the mother and family to ensure access to safe delivery.
3. Provide newborn care through a series of home visits which include the skills for:
   a. Weighing the newborn;
   b. Measuring newborn temperature;
   c. Ensuring warmth;
   d. Supporting exclusive breast-feeding by teaching the mother proper positioning and attachment for initiating and maintaining breast-feeding;
   e. Diagnosing and counselling in case of problems with breast-feeding;
   f. Promoting hand-washing;
   g. Providing skin, cord and eye care;
   h. Health promotion and counselling mothers and families on key messages on newborn care which includes discouraging unhealthy practices such as early bathing, and bottle feeding; and
   i. Ensuring prompt identification of sepsis or other illnesses.
4. Assessing if the baby is high-risk (preterm or low birth weight), through the use of protocols and managing such LBW or preterm babies through :
   a. Increasing the number of home visits;
   b. Monitoring weight gain; and
   c. Supporting and counselling the mother and family to keep the baby warm and enabling frequent and exclusive breast-feeding.
5. Detect signs and symptoms of sepsis, provide first level care and refer the baby to an appropriate centre. If the family is unable to go, ASHA should ensure that the ANM visits sick newborn on a priority basis.
6. Recognize postpartum complications in the mother and refer appropriately.
7. Counsel the couple for family planning.
8. Provide immediate newborn care, in case of those deliveries that do not occur in institutions (home deliveries and deliveries occurring on the way to the institution).

ASHA will make visits to all newborns according to specified schedule upto 42 days of life. The schedule of visit is as follows :

a. Six visits in the case of institutional delivery – Day 3, 7, 14, 21, 28, and 42.
b. Seven visits in the case of home delivery (Day 1, 3, 7, 14, 21, 28 and 42).
c. In cases of Caesarean section delivery, where the mother returns home after 5–6 days, ASHAs are entitled to full incentive of Rs. 250 if she completes all five visits starting from Day 7 to Day 42.
d. In cases when a newborn is discharged from SNCU, ASHAs are eligible to full incentive amount of Rs. 250 for completing the remaining visits. In addition, ASHAs are also eligible for an incentive of Rs. 50 for monthly follow- up of low birth weight babies and newborns discharged from SNCU (as approved by MSG of the National Health Mission on 6th December 2013). The low birth weight are followed up for two years and SNCU discharged babies for one year.
e. In cases where the woman delivers at her maternal house and returns to her husband's house, two ASHAs undertake the HBNC visits, i.e., one at maternal house immediately after delivery, and another one at husband's house when the new-born returns home or vice versa. In such cases the HBNC incentive of Rs. 250 can be divided into two parts in a way that each ASHA who completes 3 visits or more is entitled to Rs. 125. In these instances, if an ASHA undertakes less than 3 visits, she would not be entitled to HBNC incentive.
f. In cases of twin or triples the incentive amount for ASHA would be two time of the regular HBNC incentive of Rs. 250/- (i.e., Rs. 500/-) or three times of Rs. 250/- (i.e., Rs. 750/-) respectively.

The incentive money is paid to ASHA on 45th day subject to the following :

a. Record of birth weight in the mother and child protection card;
b. Immunization of newborn with BCG, first dose of OPV, hep B and DPT/pentavalent vaccine and entry into the mother and child protection card;
c. Registration of birth; and
d. Both mother and newborn are safe until 42nd day of delivery.

Home-Based Care for Young Child (HBYC)

Under National Health Mission, Child Health division, MoHFW, GOI has rolled out Home-Based Care for Young Child (HBYC) Programme as an extension of the Home Based New Born Care (HBNC) programme to promote evidence based interventions delivered in four key domains namely nutrition, health, childhood development and WASH (Water, Sanitation and Hygiene). Under Home Based Care of Young Child (HBYC) programme, the additional five home visits will be carried out by ASHA with support from Anganwadi workers. ASHA will provide home visits on 3rd, 6th, 9th, 12th and 15th months to promote early initiation of breast feeding, exclusive breast feeding till 6 months and continued breast feeding till 2nd year of life along with adequate complementary feeding, prevention of childhood Pneumonia and Diarrhoea and to ensure age appropriate immunization and early childhood development. The quarterly home visits schedule for low birth weight babies, SNCU & NRC discharges will now be harmonized with the new HBYC schedule. ASHAs will be provided incentive of Rs. 250 for completion of 5 home visits under HBYC for each young child (Rs. 50 per visit) as per the recommended schedule and additional commodities namely ORS packet and Iron Folic Acid syrup will be provided in the kit.

Strengthening facility based paediatric care

Facility based care is complementary to community level interventions in bringing down childhood morbidity and mortality. Newborns and children referred from communities and primary healthcare facilities are often seriously ill and at high risk of dying. Those reaching health facilities need to be managed appropriately and without delay in instituting care. This objective can be achieved by establishing a well-organised unit, adequate human resources, drugs, equipment and other logistics that provides functional quality of care consistent with clinical standards.

The vision for paediatric care at District Hospital is to set up a comprehensive unit comprising of the following sub-units :

1. Paediatric Outpatient Facility (including immunization and counselling services).
2. Emergency Triage Assessment and Treatment (ETAT) Facility.
3. Paediatric Inpatient Facility.
   a. High Dependency Unit.
   b. Paediatric Ward.
   c. Diarrhoea Treatment Unit.
   d. Isolation Room.
4. Ancillary (e.g. laboratory, imaging, pharmacy) & Auxiliary Facilities (e.g. play area, hospital kitchen).

The general paediatric care facility will function in close coordination with specialised units that already have approved guidelines for operationalization and include the following : Newborn care facilities (Newborn Care Corners, Newborn Stabilisation Unit, Special Newborn Care Unit); Nutrition Rehabilitation Centre; and District Early Intervention Centre.

Navjat Shishu Suraksha Karyakram (NSSK)

NSSK is a programme aimed to train health personnel in basic newborn care and resuscitation. It has been launched to address care at birth issue i.e. prevention of hypothermia, prevention of infection, early initiation of breast-feeding and basic newborn resuscitation. The objective of the new initiative is to have a trained health person in basic newborn care and resuscitation unit at every delivery point *(46)*.

Integrated management of neonatal and childhood illness (IMNCI)

Integrated management of childhood illness (IMCI)

The extent of childhood morbidity and mortality caused by diarrhoea, ARI, malaria, measles and malnutrition is substantial. Most sick children present with signs and symptoms of more than one of these conditions. This overlap means that a single diagnosis may not be possible or appropriate, and treatment may be complicated by the need to combine for several conditions. An integrated approach to manage sick children is, therefore, necessary. IMCI is a strategy for an integrated approach to the management of childhood illness as it is important for child health programmes to look beyond the treatment of a single disease. This is cost effective and emphasizes prevention of disease and promotion of child health and development besides provision of standard case management of childhood illness.

In the Indian context this strategy is quite pertinent considering the evidence from NFHS–III report highlighting that ARI (17 per cent), diarrhoea (13 per cent), fever (27 per cent) and under–nutrition (43 per cent) were the commonest morbidities observed in the children aged under 3 years. Coverage of measles vaccination in children between 12–23 months was also low. An integrated approach to address these major childhood illnesses seems to be an effective strategy to promote child health in this country. The line of action is as shown in Fig. 14.

The Indian version of IMCI has been renamed as Integrated Management of Neonatal and Childhood Illness (IMNCI). It is the central pillar of child health interventions under the RCH II strategy. The major highlights of the Indian adaptation are :

a. Inclusion of 0–7 days age in the programme;

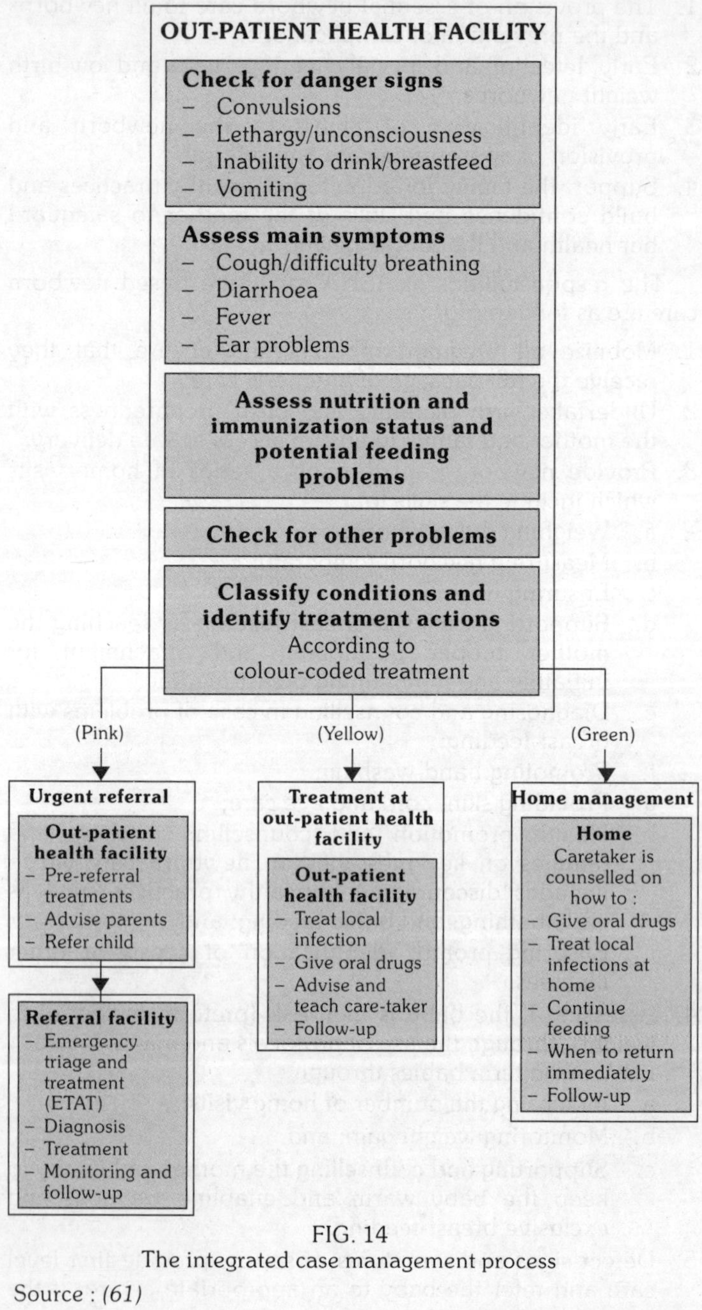

FIG. 14

The integrated case management process

Source : *(61)*

b. Incorporating national guidelines on malaria, anaemia, vitamin–A supplementation and immunization schedule;
c. Training of the health personnel begins with sick young infants upto 2 months;
d. Proportion of training time devoted to sick young infant and sick child is almost equal; and
e. Is skill based ?

For more details please refer to chapter 9.

IMNCI strategy is one of the main interventions under RCH-II/NRHM. It focusses on preventive, promotive and curative aspects of the programme. The objective is to implement IMNCI package at the level of household, and through ANMs at sub-centre level; through medical officers, nurses and LHVs at PHCs level.

Rashtriya Bal Swasthya Karyakram (RBSK) *(62)*

RBSK is a new initiative launched in February 2013. It includes provision for Child Health Screening and Early Intervention Services through early detection and management of 4 Ds, prevalent in children. These are defects at birth, diseases in children, deficiency conditions and development delays including disabilities. An estimated 27 crore children in the age group of 0–18 years are expected to be covered across the country in a phased manner.

Child Health Screening and Early Intervention Services under NRHM envisage to cover 30 identified health conditions for early detection, free treatment and management. Based on the high prevalence of diseases like hypothyroidism, sickle cell anaemia and beta thalassaemia in certain geographical pockets of some states/UTs, and availability of testing and specialized support facilities, these states and UTs may incorporate them as part of this initiative. The health conditions are as shown in Table 13.

TABLE 13

Identified health conditions for child health screening and early intervention services

Defects at Birth :
1. Neural tube defect
2. Down's Syndrome
3. Cleft Lip and Palate / cleft palate alone
4. Talipes (club foot)
5. Developmental dysplasia of the Hip
6. Congenital cataract
7. Congenital deafness
8. Congenital heart diseases
9. Retinopathy of prematurity
Deficiencies :
10. Anaemia especially severe anaemia
11. Vitamin A deficiency (Bitot's spots)
12. Vitamin D deficiency (Rickets)
13. Severe acute malnutrition
14. Goitre
Childhood Diseases :
15. Skin conditions (scabies, fungal infection and eczema)
16. Otitis media
17. Rheumatic Heart Disease
18. Reactive Airway Disease
19. Dental caries
20. Convulsive disorders
Developmental delays and disabilities :
21. Vision impairment
22. Hearing impairment
23. Neuro-motor impairment
24. Motor delay
25. Cognitive delay
26. Language delay
27. Behaviour disorder (Autism)
28. Learning disorder
29. Attention Deficit Hyperactivity Disorder
30. Congenital Hypothyroidism, Sickle Cell Anaemia, Beta Thalassaemia (Optional)

Source : *(62)*

Programme Implementation

1. For newborn :
   - Facility based newborn screening at public health facilities, by existing health manpower.
   - Community based newborn screening at home through ASHAs for newborn till 6 weeks of age during home visits.
2. For children 6 weeks to 6 years :
   - Anganwadi centre based screening by dedicated Mobile Health Teams.
3. For children 6 years to 18 years :
   - Government and Government aided school based screening by dedicated Mobile Health Teams.

Facility based newborn screening

This includes screening of birth defects in institutional deliveries at public health facilities, especially at the designated delivery points by ANMs, Medical Officers/ Gynaecologists. Existing health service providers at all designated delivery points will be trained to detect, register report and refer birth defects to the District Early Intervention Centres in District Hospitals.

Community based newborn screening (age 0–6 weeks) for birth defects

Accredited Social Health Activists (ASHAs) during home visits for newborn care will use the opportunity to screen the babies born at home and the institutions till 6 weeks of age. ASHAs will be trained with simple tools for detecting gross birth defects. Further ASHAs will mobilise caregivers of children to attend the local Anganwadi Centres for screening by the dedicated Mobile Health Team. For performing the above additional tasks, she would be equipped with a tool kit consisting of a pictorial reference book having self-explanatory pictures for identification of birth defects. Suitable performance based incentive may also be provided to ASHAs. In order to ensure improved outcome of the screening programme by Mobile Health Teams, ASHAs will give priority to the children with low birth weight, underweight and children from households known to have any chronic illness (e.g., tuberculosis, HIV, haemoglobinopathy etc.). Line lists maintained by the ANMs and AWWs would also be used to mobilise children.

Screening of children aged 6 weeks till 6 years attending Anganwadi Centres

Children in the age group 6 weeks to 6 years of age will be examined in the Anganwadi Centres by dedicated Mobile Health Teams.

Screening of children enrolled in Government and Government aided schools

For children in the age group 6 to 18 years, who will be screened in Government and Government aided schools, the block will be the hub of activity for the programme. At least two dedicated Mobile Health Teams in each block will be engaged to conduct screening of children. Villages within the jurisdiction of the block would be distributed amongst the mobile health teams. The number of teams may vary depending on the number of Anganwadi Centres, difficult to reach areas and children enrolled in the schools. The screening of children in the Anganwadi Centres would be conducted at least twice a year and at least once a year for school children to begin with.

In RCH Phase–II the other interventions of RCH Phase–I, e.g., additional ANMs, public health nurses, private anaesthetists, safe motherhood consultants, 24 hours delivery services at PHCs and CHCs, referral transports, integrated financial envelop, RCH camps, training of Dais, border district cluster strategy, and intervention for newborn care and child health (immunization, control of ARI and diarrhoea, vitamin A and iron suplementation etc.) will continue.

The quality indicators used to monitor and evaluate RCH programme through monthly reports are (63) :

1. Number of antenatal cases registered – total and at less than 12 weeks;
2. Number of pregnant women who had 3 antenatal check-ups;
3. Number of high-risk pregnant women referred;
4. Number of pregnant women who had two doses of tetanus toxoid injection;
5. Number of pregnant women under prophylaxis and treatment for anaemia;
6. Number of deliveries by trained and untrained birth attendant;
7. Number of cases with complications referred to PHC/FRU;
8. Number of new born with birth weight recorded;
9. Number of women given 3 post natal check-ups;
10. Number of RTI/STI cases detected, treated and referred;
11. Number of children fully immunized;
12. Number of adverse reactions reported after immunization;
13. Number of cases of ARI and diarrhoea under 5 years treated, referred PHC/FRU and deaths; and
14. Number of cases motivated and followed up for contraception.

REPRODUCTIVE, MATERNAL, NEWBORN, CHILD AND ADOLESCENT HEALTH (RMNCH+A) STRATEGY

In June 2012, the Government of India, Ethiopia, USA and the UNICEF convened the "Global Child Survival Call to Action : A Promise to Keep" summit in Washington, DC to energize the global fight to end preventable child deaths through targeted interventions in effective, life-saving interventions for children. More than 80 countries gathered at the Call to Action to pledge to reduce child mortality to ≤ 20 child deaths per 1000 live births in every country by 2035 *(57)*. Eight months after the event, in February 2013, the Government of India held its own historic Summit on the Call to Action for Child Survival, where it launched "A Strategic Approach to Reproductive, Maternal, Newborn, Child, and Adolescent Health (RMNCH+A) in India." Since that time, RMNCH+A has become the heart of the Government of India's flagship public health programme, the National Health Mission *(64)*.

With support from USAID and its Maternal Child Health Integrated Programme (MCHIP), as well as from UNICEF, UNFPA, NIPI and other development partners, the Government of India has taken important steps to introduce and support RMNCH+A implementation. This approach is likely to succeed given that India already has a community based programme with presence of 9.15 lakh ASHA workers, as well as the three tiered health system in place. These provide a strong platform for delivery of services. This integrated strategy can potentially promote greater efficiency while reducing duplication of resources and efforts in the ongoing programme.

The RMNCH+A strategy is based on provision of comprehensive care through the five pillars, or thematic areas, of reproductive, maternal, neonatal, child, and adolescent health, and is guided by central tenets of equity, universal care, entitlement, and accountability. The "plus" within the strategy focusses on :

- Including adolescence for the first time as a distinct life stage;
- Linking maternal and child health to reproductive health, family planning, adolescent health, HIV, gender, preconception and prenatal diagnostic techniques;
- Linking home and community-based services to facility-based care; and
- Ensuring linkages, referrals, and counter-referrals between and among health facilities at primary (primary health centre), secondary (community health centre), and tertiary levels (district hospital).

In developing the RMNCH+A strategy, the aim is to reach the maximum number of people in the remotest corners of the country through a continuum of services, constant innovation, and routine monitoring of interventions. In rolling out the new strategy, the emphasis is on high impact interventions in each of the five thematic areas of reproductive, maternal, newborn, child, and adolescent health, and then to focus its efforts, and those of its development partners, on improving the coverage and quality of those interventions in 184 high-priority districts (HPDs) across India. Guidelines and tools were developed and policies were adjusted.

1. *High-Priority Districts:* The RMNCH+A strategy addresses India's inter-state and inter-district variations. The districts with relatively weak performance against RMNCH+A indicators were identified. Uniform and clearly defined criteria were used to identify 184 high-priority districts across all 29 states. The RMNCH+A approach is a conscious articulation of the GOI's commitment to tailoring programmes to meet the needs of previously underserved groups, including adolescents, urban poor, and tribal populations.

2. *Management tools and job aids:* The RMNCH+A 5×5 matrix identifies five high-impact interventions across each of the five thematic areas, five cross-cutting and health systems strengthening interventions, and the minimum essential commodities. The 5×5 matrix as shown in Fig. 15, is an important tool for explaining the strategy in simple terms, organizing technical support, and monitoring progress with the states and high-priority districts.

Goals and targets *(52)*

Taking into account the progress made so far in maternal and child health, it is pertinent to establish the goals and targets for the implementation phase 2012–2017, after considering the main reasons for mortality and interventions

Reproductive Health

- Focus on spacing methods, particularly PPIUCD at high case load facilities.
- Focus on interval IUCD at all facilities including subcentres on fixed days.
- Home delivery of Contraceptives (HDC) and Ensuring Spacing at Birth (ESB) through ASHAs.
- Ensuring access to Pregnancy Testing Kits (PTK "Nischay Kits") and strengthening comprehensive abortion care services.
- Maintaining quality sterilization services.

Maternal Health

- Use MCTS to ensure early registration of pregnancy and full ANC.
- Detect high risk pregnancies and line list including severely anaemic mothers and ensure appropriate management.
- Equip delivery points with highly trained HR and ensure equitable access to EmOC services through FRUs, Add MCH wings as per need.
- Review maternal, infant and child deaths for corrective actions.
- Identify villages with high numbers of home deliveries and distribute Misoprostol to selected women in 8th month of pregnancy for consumption during 3rd stage of labour; Incentivize ANMs for home deliveries.

Newborn Health

- Early initiation and exclusive breast-feeding.
- Home based newborn care through ASHA.
- Essential Newborn Care and resuscitation services at all delivery points.
- Special Newborn Care Units with highly trained human resource and other infrastructure.
- Community level use of Gentamycin by ANM.

Child Health

- Complementary feeding, IFA supplementation and focus on nutrition.
- Diarrhoea management at community level using ORS and Zinc.
- Management of pneumonia.
- Full immunization coverage.
- Rashtriya Bal Swasthya Karyakram (RBSK); screening of children for 4Ds' (birth defects, development delays, deficiencies and disease) and its management.

Adolescent Health

- Address teenage pregnancy and increase contraceptive prevalence in adolescents.
- Introduce community based services through peer educators.
- Strengthen ARSH clinics.
- Roll out National Iron Plus Initiative including weekly IFA supplementation.
- Promote menstrual hygiene.

Health Systems Strengthening

- Cases load based deployment of HR at all levels.
- Ambulances, drugs, diagnostics, reproductive health commodities.
- Health education, demand promotion & behaviour change communication.
- Supportive supervision and use of data for monitoring and review, including scorecards based on HMIS.
- Public grievances redressal mechanism, client satisfaction and patient safety through all round quality assurance.

Cross Cutting Interventions

- Bring down out of pocket expenses by ensuring JSSK, RBSK and other free entitlements.
- ANMs & Nurses to provide specialized and quality care to pregnant women and children.
- Address social determinants of health through convergence.
- Focus on un-served and underserved villages, urban slums and blocks.
- Introduce difficult area and performance based incentives.

FIG. 15
5 × 5 matrix for high impact RMNCH+A interventions
To be Implemented with High Coverage and High Quality

proven to have an impact on them. The 12th Five Year Plan has defined the national health outcomes and the three goals that are relevant to RMNCH+A strategic approach are as follows :

- Reduction of Infant Mortality Rate (IMR) to 25 per 1,000 live births by 2017.
- Reduction in Maternal Mortality Ratio (MMR) to 100 per 100,000 live births by 2017.
- Reduction in Total Fertility Rate (TFR) to 2.1 by 2017.

For achieving these goals, variable increase in the coverage level for key interventions are required. These are defined in the Table 14.

TABLE 14

Coverage targets for key RMNCH+A interventions for 2017

- Increase facilities equipped for perinatal care (designated as 'delivery points') by 100%.
- Increase proportion of all births in government and accredited private institutions at annual rate of 5.6% from the baseline of 61% (SRS 2010).
- Increase proportion of pregnant women receiving antenatal care at annual rate of 6% from the baseline of 53% (CES 2009).
- Increase proportion of mothers and newborns receiving postnatal care at annual rate of 7.5% from the baseline of 45% (CES 2009).
- Increase proportion of deliveries conducted by skilled birth attendants at annual rate of 2% from the baseline of 76% (CES 2009).
- Increase exclusive breast-feeding rates at annual rate of 9.6% from the baseline of 35% (CES 2009).
- Reduce prevalence of under-five children who are underweight at annual rate of 5.5% from the baseline of 45% (NFHS-3).
- Increase coverage of three doses of combined diphtheria-tetanus-pertussis (DTP3) (12–23 months) at annual rate of 3.5% from the baseline of 7% (CES 2009).
- Increase ORS use in under-five children with diarrhoea at annual rate of 7.2% from the baseline of 43% (CES 2009).
- Reduce unmet need for family planning methods among eligible couples, married and unmarried, at annual rate of 8.8% from the baseline of 21% (DLHS 3).
- Increase met need for modern family planning methods among eligible couples at annual rate of 4.5% from the baseline of 47% (DLH 3).
- Reduce anaemia in adolescent girls and boys (15–19 years) at annual rate of 6% from the baseline of 56% and 30%, respectively (NFHS-3).
- Decrease the porportion of total fertility contributed by adolescents (15–19 years) at annual rate of 3.8% per year from the baseline of 16% (NFHS-3).
- Raise child sex ratio in the 0–6 years age group at annual rate of 0.6% per year from the baseline of 914 (Census 2011).

While the country aims to set one collective goal towards reducing preventable maternal, newborn and child deaths by 2017, it is increasingly becoming apparent that there is varied and unequal rate of progress within the states and districts. Therefore, state specific coverage targets should be established against existing baselines. The national and state 'scorecard' is being introduced as a tool to increase transparency and track progress against reproductive and maternal health and child survival indicators related with intervention coverage. For more details about the score cards please refer to page 534.

The implementation strategies of RMNCH+A *(52)*

The key interventions of RMNCH+A as a "Continuum of Care" are as shown in Fig. 16. The set of interventions are those that have high impact on reducing mortality and improving survival. Most of these interventions have been part of the previous phase of NRHM. The effectiveness of these will be determined by the coverage achieved among the affected fraction of population as also the availability, accessibility, actual utilization of services and quality of services delivered.

Adolescent Health Programme *(1, 52)*

Taking cognisance of the diverse nature of adolescent health needs, a comprehensive adolescent health strategy has been developed. The priority under adolescent health include nutrition, sexual and reproductive health, mental health, addressing gender-based violence, non-communicable diseases and substance use. The strategy proposes a set of interventions (health promotion, prevention, diagnosis, treatment and referral) across levels of care. These interventions and approaches work towards building protective factors that can help adolescents and young people develop 'resilience' to resist negative behaviours and operate at four major levels: individual, family, school and community by providing a comprehensive package of information, commodities and services.

The priority interventions are as follows :

1. Adolescent nutrition; iron and folic acid supplementation.
2. Facility-based adolescent reproductive and sexual health services (ARSH) (Adolescent health clinics).
3. Information and counselling on adolescent sexual reproductive health and other health issues.
4. Menstrual hygiene.
5. Preventive health check-ups.

Clinical

Reproductive care
- Comprehensive abortion care
- RTI/STI case management,
- Postpartum IUCD and sterilization; interval IUCD procedures
- Adolescent friendly health services

Pregnancy and child birth care
- Skilled obstetric care, immediate newborn care and resuscitation
- Emergency obstetric care
- Preventing Parent-to-Child Transmission (PPTCT) of HIV
- Postpartum sterilization

Newborn and childcare
- Essential newborn care
- Care of sick newborn (SNCU, NBSU)
- Facility-based care of childhood illnesses (IMNCI)
- Care of children with severe acute malnutrition (NRC)
- Immunization

Outreach/Sub-centre

Reproductive health care
- Family planning (including IUCD insertion, OCP and condoms)
- Prevention and management of STIs
- Peri-conception folic acid supplementation

Antenatal care
- Full antenatal care package
- PPTCT

Postnatal care
- Early detection and management of illnesses in mother and newborn.
- Immunization

Child health care
- First level assessment and care for newborn and childhood illnesses.
- Immunization
- Micro-nutrient supplementation

Family & Community

- Weekly IFA supplementation
- Information and counselling on sexual reproductive health and family planning.
- Community based promotion and delivery of contraceptives.
- Menstrual hygiene

- Counselling and preparation for newborn care, breast-feeding, birth preparedness.
- Demand generation for pregnancy care and institutional delivery (JSY, JSSK).

- Home-based newborn care and prompt referral (HBNC scheme).
- Antibiotic for suspected case of newborn sepsis.
- Infant and Young Child Feeding (IYCF), including exclusive breast-feeding and complementary feeding.
- Child health screening and early intervention services (0–18 years).
- Early childhood development
- Danger sign recognition and care-seeking for illness
- Use of ORS and Zinc in case of diarrhoea

Intersectoral : Water, sanitation, hygiene, nutrition, education, empowerment.

Adolescence/Pre-pregnancy → Pregnancy → Birth → Newborn/postnatal → Childhood

FIG. 16

Continuum of care across life cycle and different levels of health system

A. *Adolescent Reproductive and Sexual Health programme (ARSH)*

Adolescent Reproductive and Sexual Health programme (ARSH) focusses on reorganizing the existing public health system in order to meet service needs of adolescents. Steps are being taken to ensure improved service delivery for adolescents during routine sub-centre clinics and also to ensure service availability on fixed days and timings at the Primary Health Centre, Community Health Centre and District Hospital levels. Core package of services includes promotive, preventive, curative and counselling services being made available for all adolescents – married and unmarried, girls and boys through adolescent friendly health clinics. ARSH programme envisages creating an enabling environment for adolescents to seek health care services through a spectrum of programmatic approaches :

- Facility based health services–Adolescent Friendly Health Clinics;
- Counselling–Dedicated ARSH and ICTC counselling;
- Community based interventions–Outreach activities; and
- Capacity building for service providers.
  i. *Adolescent Friendly Health Clinics (AFHC):* Through Adolescent Friendly Health Clinics, routine check-up at primary, secondary and tertiary levels of care is provided on fixed day clinics. At present 6,302 AFHCs are functional across the country providing services, information and commodities to more than 2.5 million adolescents for varied health related needs such as contraceptives provision, management of menstrual problems, RTI/STI management, antenatal care and anaemia.
  ii. *Facility based counselling services:* Counselling services for adolescents on important issues such as nutrition, puberty, RTI/STI prevention and contraception, delaying marriage and childbearing, and concerns related to contraception, abortion services, pre-marital concerns, substance misuse, sexual abuse and mental health problems are being provided through recruitment and training of dedicated counsellors. At present 881 dedicated ARSH counsellors are providing comprehensive counselling services to adolescents across the country. In 23 States/UTs, 1439 ICTC counsellors have been enrolled to provide sexual and reproductive health counselling to adolescents.
  iii. *Outreach activities:* Outreach activities are being conducted in schools, colleges, teen clubs, vocational training centres, during Village Health Nutrition Day (VHND), health melas and in collaboration with self help groups to provide adequate and appropriate information to adolescents in spaces where they normally congregate.

B. *Weekly Iron and Folic Acid Supplementation (WIFS)*

Ministry of Health and Family Welfare has launched the Weekly Iron and Folic Acid Supplementation (WIFS) Programme to meet the challenge of high prevalence and incidence of anaemia amongst adolescent girls and boys. The long term goal is to break the intergenerational cycle of anaemia, the short term benefit is of a nutritionally improved human capital. The programme, implemented across the country, both in rural and urban areas, will cover 10.25 crore adolescents. The key interventions under this programme are as follows :

- Administration of supervised weekly iron-folic acid supplements of 100 mg elemental iron and 500 μg folic acid using a fixed day approach.
- Screening of target groups for moderate/severe anaemia and referring these cases to an appropriate health facility.
- Biannual de-worming (Albendazole 400 mg), six months apart, for control of helminths infestation.
- Information and counselling for improving dietary intake and for taking actions for prevention of intestinal worm infestation.

C. *Menstrual Hygiene Scheme (1)*

The Ministry of Health and Family Welfare has launched scheme for promotion of menstrual hygiene among adolescent girls in the age group of 10–19 years in rural areas. This programme aims at ensuring that girls have adequate knowledge and information about menstrual hygiene and have access to high quality sanitary napkins along with safe disposal mechanisms. Key activities under the scheme include :

- Community based health education and outreach in the target population to promote menstrual health;
- Ensuring regular availability of sanitary napkins to the adolescents;
- Sourcing and procurement of sanitary napkins;
- Storage and distribution of sanitary napkins to the adolescent girls;
- Training of ASHA and nodal teachers in menstrual health; and
- Safe disposal of sanitary napkins.

CARE DURING PREGNANCY AND CHILDBIRTH *(52)*

Pregnancy and childbirth are physiological events in the life of a woman. Though most pregnancies result in normal birth, it is estimated that about 15 per cent may develop complications, which cannot be predicted. Most of these complications can be averted by preventive care, skilled care at birth, early detection of risk, appropriate and timely management of obstetric complications and postnatal care.

The delivery of services during pregnancy and childbirth requires a strong element of continuum of care from community to facility level and vice versa. While the antenatal package, counselling and preparation for newborn care, breast-feeding, birth and emergency preparedness will mainly be delivered through community outreach; skilled birth attendance are to be provided at health facilities, primarily 24×7 PHC and FRU. These facilities are most likely to be the one that have been designated as "delivery points" and therefore have provision for full complement of RMNCH services. Following discharge from the health facilities, mothers and newborns will be provided postnatal care through home visits. Most of these services are already in place.

The priority interventions are as follows *(52)* :

1. Delivery of antenatal care package and tracking of high-risk pregnancies.
2. Skilled obstetric care.
3. Immediate essential newborn care and resuscitation.
4. Emergency obstetric and newborn care.
5. Postpartum care for mother and newborn.
6. Postpartum IUCD and sterilization.
7. Implementation of PC & PNDT Act.

NEWBORN AND CHILD CARE

The interventions in this phase of life mainly focus on children under 5 years of age. Given below are the priority child health interventions that are already in place under NRHM.

Priority Interventions (52) :

1. Home-based newborn care and prompt referral.
2. Facility-based care of the sick newborn.
3. Integrated management of common childhood illnesses (diarrhoea, pneumonia and malaria).
4. Child nutrition and essential micronutrients supplementation.
5. Immunization
6. Early detection and management of defects at birth, deficiencies, diseases and disability in children 0–18 years of age (Rashtriya Bal Swasthya Karyakram).

CARE THROUGH THE REPRODUCTIVE YEARS

Reproductive health needs to exist across the reproductive years and therefore access to these services is required in various life stages starting from the adolescence phase. Reproductive health services include the provision for contraceptives, access to comprehensive and safe abortion services, diagnosis and management of sexually transmitted infections, including HIV.

A new strategic direction has been developed for the family planning programme, wherein it has been repositioned to not only achieve population stabilisation but also to reduce maternal mortality as also infant and child mortality. A target-free approach based on unmet needs for contraception; equal emphasis on spacing and limiting methods; and promoting 'children by choice' in the context of reproductive health are the key approaches to be adopted for the promotion of family planning and improving reproductive health.

These services will be delivered at home, through community outreach and at all levels of health facilities and include adolescents and adults in the reproductive age group.

Priority interventions (52)

1. Community-based promotion and delivery of contraceptives.
2. Promotion of spacing methods (interval IUCD).
3. Sterilization services (vasectomies and tubectomies).
4. Comprehensive abortion care (includes MTP Act).
5. Prevention and management of sexually transmitted and reproductive infections (STI/RTI).

Delivery Points *(52)*

The provision of services for delivery care in a health facility generally serves as an important indicator to assess whether the facility is optimally functional or not. The concept of 'delivery point' emerges from this presumption. Among the health facilities designated as L1, L2 and L3, there are some facilities which are conducting deliveries above a minimum bench mark (minimum 3 normal deliveries per month at L1; minimum 10 deliveries per month, including management of complications, at L2; and minimum 20–50 deliveries per month including C-section at L3). These are designated as delivery points. According to the government mandate, these facilities should be the first to be strengthened for providing comprehensive RMNCH Services. This should be supported by a referral transport system that reaches the patient within 30 minutes of receiving a call and the health facility within the next 30 minutes. The long-term goal should be to establish and operationalize Basic Emergency Obstetric Care and Comprehensive Emergency Obstetric Care Centres as per the expected delivery load in the state and district.

Maternal and Child Health (MCH) Wing *(52)*

Most health facilities, especially those at secondary and tertiary level are having high case load of pregnant women and newborn due to increase in institutional deliveries following launch of JSY and JSSK. Therefore, it has been decided that dedicated Maternal and Child Health Wings will be established in high case load facilities with adequate provision of beds. The new MCH wings will be comprehensive units (30/50/100 bedded) with antenatal waiting rooms, labour wing, essential newborn care room, SNCU, operation theatre, blood storage units and a postnatal ward and an academic wing. This will ensure provision of emergency maternal and newborn care services as well as 48 hours stay, i.e., quality postnatal care to mothers and newborns *(52)*.

SCORE CARD *(52)*

A. Health Management Information System – based dashboard monitoring system:

The choice of indicators for dashboard monitoring system are based on life cycle approach, and are as shown in Fig. 17.

1. Steps underway to include proportion:
   - Pregnant women <19 yrs old to total women registered for ANC.
   - Home Based New born Care (HBNC) visit by ASHA to planned visits.
   - Children 9–11 months fully immunized to children 9–11 months due for immunization.
   - Children with diarrhoea who were treated with ORS to children reported with diarrhoea.
   - Children with diarrhoea who were treated with ORS and Zinc to children reported with diarrhoea.
   - Children discharged live from SNCUs to number of admissions in SNCUs.
   - Children with ARI who received treatment to children reported with ARI.
2. All India average for each indicator will be taken as the reference point.
3. States scores will be determined on the basis of the national average :
   - Positive scores from 1 to 4 for those above the national average (for positive indicators) and for those below the national average (for negative indicators).
   - Negative scores –1 to –4 for those below national average (for positive indicators) and for those above national average (for negative indicators).
4. All the indicator scores for each state will be consolidated as state score (all indicators have the same weightage).
5. States have been classified into four categories based on the state scores.

B. Survey based score card *(52)*

19 survey based outcome and coverage indicators related to health, nutrition and sanitation will be used for the score card. The indicators are as shown in Table 15.

Proportion of :

- 1st Trimester registration to total ANC registration.
- Pregnant women recieved 3 ANC to total ANC registration.
- Pregnant women given 100 IFA to total ANC registration.
- Cases of pregnant women with obstetric complications and attended to reported deliveries.
- Pregnant women receiving TT2 or Booster to total ANC registration.

Proportion of :

- Postpartum sterilization to total female sterilization.
- Male sterilization to total sterilization.
- IUD insertions in public plus private accredited institutions to all family planning methods (IUD plus permanent).

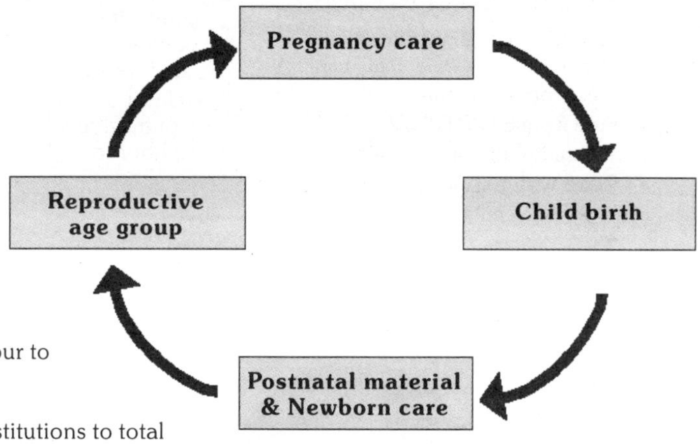

Proportion of :

- SBA attended home deliveries to total reported home deliveries.
- Institutional deliveries to total ANC registration.
- C-Section to reported deliveries.

Proportion of :

- Newborns breast-fed within 1 hour to total live births.
- Women discharged in less than 48 hours of delivery in public institutions to total number of deliveries in public institutions.
- Newborns weighing less than 2.5 kg to newborns weighed at birth.
- Newborns visited within 24 hrs of home delivery to total reported home deliveries.
- Infants 0 to 11 months old who received measles vaccine to reported live births.

FIG. 17

Choice of indicators for dash board

TABLE 15

Indicators for survey based score card

Mortality	– Under-five mortality rate – Infant mortality rate – Neonatal mortality rate – Maternal mortality ratio (per 100,000 live births)
Fertility	– Total fertility rate – Births to women during age 15–19 out of total births.
Nutrition	– Children with birth weight less than 2.5 kg – Children under 3 years who are underweight
Gender	– Child sex ratio 0–6
Cross-cutting	– Full Immunization Children (12–23 months) receiving 1 dose BCG, 3 doses of Pentavelent/OPV/ 1 dose IPV each and 2 measles vaccine. – Household having access to toilet facility – Couple using spacing method for more than 6 months.
Diarrhoea	– ORT or increased fluids for diarrhoea (among children <2 years of age who had diarrhoea in preceding 2 weeks).
Pneumonia	– Care seeking for ARI in any health facility (Among children <2 years of age who had ARI in preceding 2 weeks).
Service Delivery	– Woman who received 4 + ANC – Skilled Birth Attendance (delivery by doctor, ANM/Nurse/LHV). – Mothers who recieved postnatal care from a doctor/nurse/LHV/ANM/other health personnel within 2 days of delivery for their last birth (%). – Early initiation of breast-feeding (<1hr) – Exclusive breast-feeding for 6 months (among 6–9 months children).

Latest available data from national surveys will be taken into consideration including Sample Registration System, Coverage Evaluation Survey, District Level Household and Facility Survey, National Family Health Survey, Census, Annual Health Survey.

All India average for each indicator will be taken as a reference point. States will be colour coded based on :

- *Mortality indicators, nutrition, fertility:* Green – less than 20% of the national average, Yellow – 20% below and above national average, Red – more than 20% of the national average.
- *Remaining Indicators:* Green – more than 20% of the national average, Yellow – 20% below and above the national average, Red – less than 20% of the national average.

The score card will be updated as and when (every 1–2 years) new survey data is available.

REPRODUCTIVE, MATERNAL, NEWBORN, CHILD, ADOLESCENT HEALTH "PLUS" NUTRITION STRATEGY (RMNCAH+N)

Due to the importance of nutrition across all life stages, the strategy now includes nutrition as one of its important pillars. RMNCAH+N strategy thus covers Reproductive, Maternal, Newborn, Child and Adolescent Health and the "plus" within it focuses on Nutrition, as well as important linkages between these services and with other components like family planning, adolescent health, HIV, gender, and preconception and prenatal diagnostic techniques. It also focuses on linkages between community-based services and facility-based services and ensures referrals, and counter-referrals between various levels of health care system to create a continuous care pathway.

The life course approach determines equal care and interventions to address both men and women in the community addressing the gender disparity in health seeking behaviour and health education and promotion at all levels. The interlinkages between different life stages are summarized in Fig. 18.

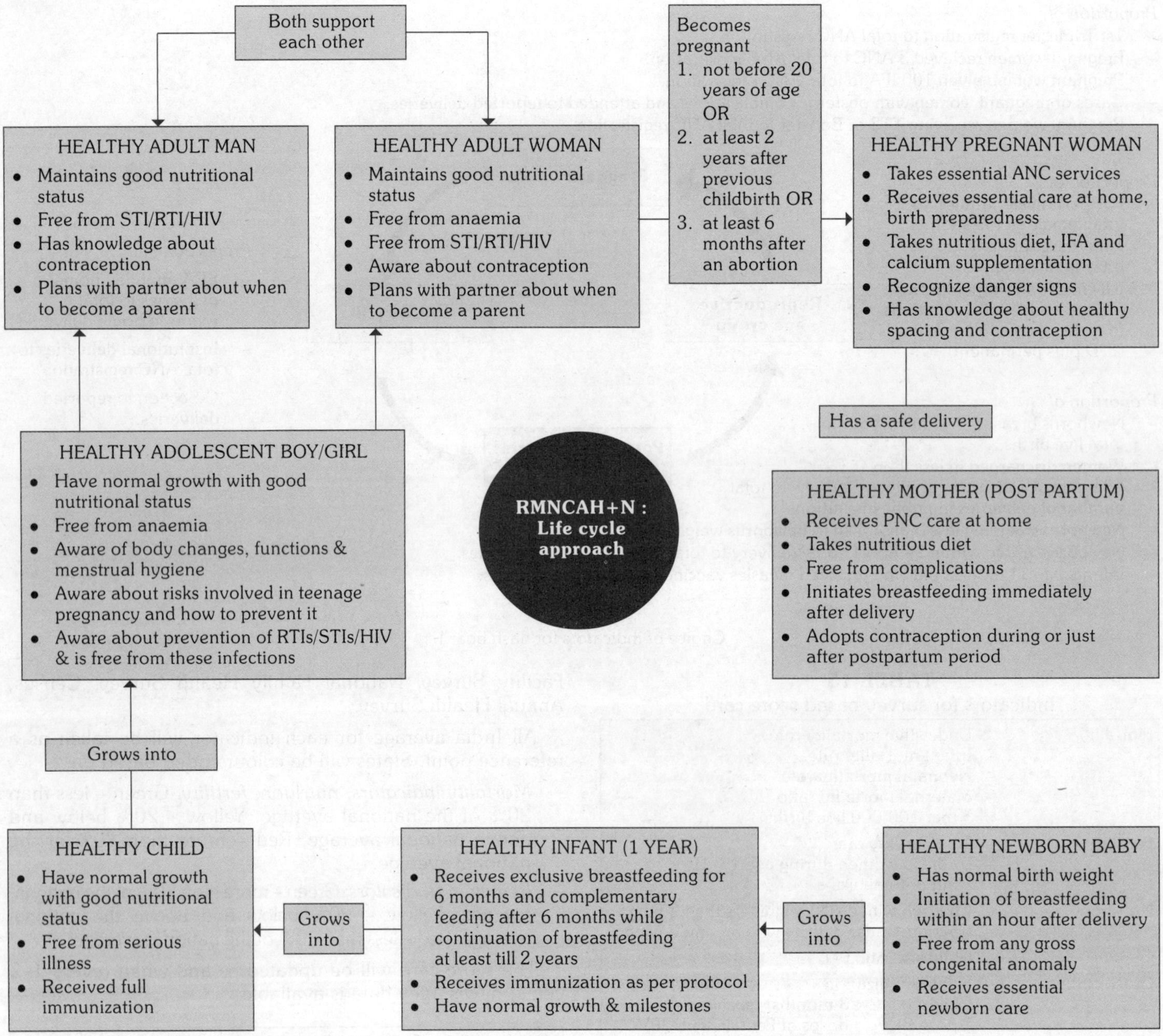

FIG. 18
Interlinkages between different life stages

Source : *(65)*

INDIA NEWBORN ACTION PLAN (INAP)

In the past two decades, there has been remarkable progress in the survival of mother and children beyond the newborn period. Presently, the newborn health has captured the attention of the policy makers and two important milestones in this direction have been the National Rural Health Mission and the Reproductive, Maternal, Newborn, Child and Adolescent Health Strategy (RMNCH+A Strategy), NRHM has provided unprecedented attention and resources for newborn health. By adopting RMNCH+A strategy in 2013, the country observed a paradigm shift in its approach towards health care. Newborn health occupies centre stage in the overall strategy as all the inter-linkages between various components have the greatest impact on the mortality and morbidity rates of the newborn.

In India, Newborn Action Plan (INAP) developed in response to the global Every Newborn Action Plan (ENAP), was launched in June 2014. The plan outlines a targetted strategy for accelerating the reduction of preventable newborn deaths and stillbirths in the country. INAP defines the latest evidence on effective interventions which will not only help in reducing the burden of stillbirths and neonatal mortality, but also maternal deaths. The goal is to attain "Single Digit Neonatal Mortality Rate by 2030" and "Single Digit Stillbirth Rate by 2030".

The INAP will be implemented within the existing RMNCH+A framework, and guided by the principles of integration, equity, gender, quality of care, convergence, accountability and partnerships. Its strength is built on its six pillars of intervention packages impacting stillbirths and newborn health, which includes : (a) Pre-conception and antenatal care; (b) Care during labour and childbirth; (c) Immediate newborn care; (d) Care of the healthy newborn; (e) Care of small and sick newborn; and (f) Care beyond newborn survival. For effective implementation, a systematic plan of monitoring and evaluation has been developed with a list of dashboard indicators *(48)*.

The interventions under the National Health Mission focussing on newborns are shown in Table 16.

Strategic Intervention Packages *(48)*

The interventions are grouped in six packages, corresponding to the various life stages of the newborn. It is estimated that high coverage of available intervention packages can prevent almost three-quarters of the newborn deaths, one-third of stillbirths and half of the maternal deaths by 2025.

The interventions have been categorized as :

a. Essential [E], to be implemented universally;
b. Situational [S], implementation dependent on epidemiological context; and
c. Advanced [A], implementation based on health-system capacity of the state/district.

The states are urged to develop their own action plans based on the six packages described below :

1. *Pre-conception and antenatal care*

Health interventions must start well before conception and their impact on the neonatal and stillbirth outcome requires equivalent consideration. The importance of antenatal care for improved neonatal and perinatal outcome is well established; however, coverage of a few salient interventions needs increased attention (e.g., use of long lasting insecticide treated nets and intermittent preventive treatment of malaria, antenatal syphilis screening combined with treatment and increased emphasis on early detection, and prompt treatment of complications in pregnancy such as pre-eclampsia, type-2 diabetes).

TABLE 16

Interventions under National Health Mission focussing on newborns

Programme (Year)	Objectives	Status
Janani Suraksha Yojana (JSY) (2005).	Safe motherhood intervention to increase institutional delivery through demand-side financing and conditional cash transfer.	– Implemented in all states and union territories (UTs). – Special focus on low-performing states.
Integrated Management of Neonatal and Childhood Illnesses (IMNCI) at the community level and F-IMNCI at health facilities (2007).	Standard case management of major causes of neonatal and childhood morbidity and mortality.	– Operationalised in more than 500 districts – 5.9 lakhs health and other functionaries, including physicians, nurses, AWWs, and ASHAs trained under IMNCI. – 26,800 medical officers and specialists placed at the CHCs/FRUs trained under F-IMNCI.
Navjat Shishu Suraksha Karyakram (NSSK) (2009).	Basic newborn care and resuscitation training programme.	– 1.3 lakh health providers trained to-date.
Janani Shishu Suraksha Karyakram (JSSK) (2011).	Zero out-of-pocket expenditure for maternal and infant health services through free healthcare and referral transport entitlements.	– Implemented in all states and UTs – Assured service package benefits extended to sick children upto age one.
Facility Based Newborn Care (FBNC) (2011).	Newborn care facilities at various levels of public health services that includes Newborn Care Corners (NBCCs) at all points of childbirth to provide immediate care; Newborn Stabilization Units (NBSUs) at CHC/FRUs for management of selected conditions and to stablize sick newborns before referral to higher centres; and Special Newborn Care Unit (SNCUs) at district/ sub-district hospitals to care for sick newborns (all types of care except assisted ventilation and major surgeries).	– 20,337 NBCCs established at delivery points to provide essential newborn care. – 2,579 NBSUs established at CHCs/FRUs. – 894 SNCUs established at district/sub-district hospitals or medical colleges. – More than 6,300 personnel provided FBNC training. – Online reporting system adapted and scaled up in seven states with 245 SNCUs made online and more than 2.5 lakhs newborns registered in the data base.
Home Based Newborn Care (HBNC) (2011).	Provision of essential newborn care to all newborns, special care of preterm and low-birth-weight newborns; early detection of illness followed by referral; and support to family for adoption of healthy practices, by ASHA worker.	– Implemented in all states and UTs. – Most of the ASHAs trained in newborn care. – ASHAs visited more than 12 lakhs newborns in 2013.
Rashtriya Bal Swasthya Karyakram (RBSK) (2013).	Screening of children with birth defects, diseases, deficiencies, and developmental delays (including disabilities).	– All children, ages 0 to 18 years targeted. – More than 8 crore children screened and more than 10 lakhs children identified for tertiary care in 2013.

Source : *(48)*

The strategic interventions for pre-conception and antenatal care for newborns are given below.

Pre-conception and antenatal care interventions package

Family and community
1. Reproductive health & family planning [E] : – Adolescent reproductive health – Delaying age of marriage and first pregnancy – Birth spacing 2. Nutrition related interventions [E] : – Balanced energy protein supplementation – Peri-conceptional folic acid – Maternal calcium supplementation – Multiple micronutrient supplementation (Iron, folic acid and iodine) – Nutrition counselling 3. Counselling and birth preparedness [E] 4. Prevention against malaria [S]
Outreach/Sub-centre
5. Antenatal screening for anaemia and hypertensive disorders of pregnancy (PIH, preeclampsia, eclampsia) [E] 6. Antenatal screening for malaria [S] 7. Prevention and management of mild to moderate anaemia [E] 8. Maternal tetanus immunization [E] 9. Adolescent friendly health services (nutrition and reproductive health counselling) [E] 10. Interval IUCD insertion [E]
Health facility
11. Antenatal screening and management of severe anaemia, hypertensive disorders of pregnancy (PIH, preeclampsia, eclampsia), gestational diabetes, syphilis [E] 12. Antenatal screening and management of hypothyroidism, hepatitis B, HIV, malaria [S] 13. Adolescent friendly health clinics (as per RKSK guidelines) [E] 14. Postpartum family planning services including PPIUCD insertion [E] 15. Prevention of Rh disease using anti D immunoglobulin [S]

2. *Care during labour and childbirth*

Intra-partum complications and preterm births remain a challenge to the neonatal survival. Care during labour and childbirth have the potential to reduce stillbirths by a third. It is important to emphasize that BEmOC can reduce intra-partum-related neonatal deaths by 40% and CEmOC can also reduce newborn mortality by 40%, whereas skilled attendance at birth alone without access to the emergency component has a smaller effect at 25%. Care at childbirth also has additional benefits on child survival, improved growth, reduced disability and non-communicable diseases.

Antenatal corticosteroids use to manage preterm labour not only reduces neonatal deaths by 31%, but this intervention is also associated with reduced need of specialized care for newborns, such as ventilators, etc. Antibiotics administration for pre-mature rupture of membranes (PROM) reduces early-onset postnatal sepsis. Clean birth practices especially hand-washing with soap and water by birth attendant has been found to reduce mortality due to sepsis in births at home (15%), facilities (27%), and during postnatal period (40%).

The strategic interventions for care during labour and child birth are given below :

Care during labour and childbirth

Family and community
1. Skilled birth attendance [E] 2. Clean birth practices [E]
Outreach/Sub-centre
3. Identification of complications and timely referral [E] 4. Pre-referral dose by ANM [E] : – Antenatal corticosteriods in preterm labour – Antibiotics for premature rupture of membranes
Health facility
5. Emergency obstetric care [E] : – Basic and comprehensive 6. Management of preterm labour [E] : – Antenatal corticosteroids in preterm labour – Antibiotics for premature rupture of membranes

3. *Immediate newborn care*

Immediate care is the basic right of every newborn baby. This package includes interventions such as immediate drying and stimulation, provision of warmth, hygienic care, early initiation of breast-feeding, and administration of vitamin K. For babies who do not breathe at birth, neonatal resuscitation is a crucial life-saving intervention. Resuscitation training of providers in facilities reduces intrapartum-related neonatal deaths and early neonatal deaths substantially. Hypothermia is a risk factor for neonatal mortality, especially in cases of preterm and low birth weight babies. All steps should be taken to prevent and manage hypothermia, and rooming-in of babies with mother must be universally practiced. Delayed cord clamping in newborns, including pre-term babies is associated with decreased risk of anaemia and intraventricular haemorrhage. Administration of vitamin K at birth prevents haemorrhagic disease of newborn.

The strategic interventions for immediate newborn care are given below :

Immediate newborn care

Family and community
1. Delayed cord clamping [E] 2. Interventions to prevent hypothermia [E] : – Immediate drying – Head covering – Skin-to-skin care – Delayed bathing 3. Early initiation and exclusive breast-feeding [E] 4. Hygiene to prevent infection [E]
Outreach/Sub-centre
5. Vitamin K at birth [E] 6. Neonatal resuscitation [E]
Health facility
7. Advanced neonatal resuscitation [E]

4. *Care of healthy newborn*

Evidence shows that community-based interventions can significantly improve child survival. A large number of ASHAs have been trained to perform various preventive and promotive health activities, such as counselling of mothers on breast-feeding, complementary feeding, immunization, care-seeking, promoting nutrition, sanitation, and safe drinking water, etc. Despite the significant increase in institutional deliveries, home deliveries persist to about 25% to 40% in pockets across states. Even in cases of institutional deliveries, most women tend to return home within a few hours after delivery. For women who stay at the institution for 48 hours or more, it is also important to provide care to the neonate at home for the remaining critical days of the first week and upto the 42nd day of life. Home visitation by ASHAs can contribute significantly to delivery of interventions with focus on the newborn period. Regular and timed contacts with the newborn are essential for ensuring continued exclusive breast-feeding, appropriate immunization, and care-seeking of children with danger signs.

The interventions for care of healthy newborn are given below :

Care of healthy newborn

Family and community
1. Home visits till six weeks by trained ASHA [E] : – Counselling – Prevention of hypothermia, cord care – Early identification of danger signs – Prompt and appropriate referral 2. Exclusive breast-feeding [E] 3. Clean postnatal practices [E]
Outreach/Sub-centre
4. Immunization [E] : – BCG – OPV – Hepatitis B – Pentavalent vaccine
Health facility
All the interventions (except home visits)

5. *Care of small and sick newborn*

Specific interventions for small and sick newborns include Kangaroo mother care (KMC). KMC involves package of early and continuous skin-to-skin contact, breast-feeding support, and supportive care in stable newborns weighing less than 2000 gm. KMC can be practiced even at home, thus improving chances of newborn survival.

Strategic interventions for care of small and sick newborn include :

Care of small and sick newborn

Family and community
1. Thermal care and feeding support (for home deliveries) [E]
Outreach/Sub-centre
2. Integrated management using IMNCI and use of oral antibiotics [E] 3. Injectable Gentamicin by ANMs for sepsis [E] : – Pre -referral – Completion of antibiotic course in case referral is refused/ not possible "OR" as advised by treating physician.
Health facility
4. Kangaroo mother care at facility [E] 5. Full supportive care at block and district level [E] : – NBSU at block level – SNCU at district level 6. Intensive care services (NICU) at regional level [A] for – – Assisted ventilation – Surfactant use – Surgery

6. *Care beyond newborn survival*

This is a new package considering the burden of birth defects and development delays in newborns. It is of particular significance for SGA and preterm newborns, as well as newborns discharged from SNCUs.

The table below lists the interventions to care for newborns beyond their survival.

Care beyond newborn survival

Family and community	*Outreach/Sub-centre*	*Health facility*
1. Screening for birth defects, failure to thrive and developmental delays [E] 2. Follow-up visits of [E] : – SNCU discharged babies till 1 year of age – Small and low birth weight babies till 2 years of age	3. As before	4. Newborn screening [A] 5. Management of birth defects [E] : – Diagnosis – Treatment, including surgery 6. Follow-up of high-risk infants (discharged from SNCUs and small newborns) for – – Developmental delay – Appropriate management

Monitoring and evaluation *(48)*

A comprehensive assessment of targets would be done in 2020, which will help plan course corrections, if any, in on-going interventions. Further, from the year 2020, the milestones will be reviewed every five years keeping in sync with ENAP – i.e., 2025, 2030, and 2035.

Following core indicators (dashboard indicators) have been selected for monitoring, based on direct relevance to the action plan framework, targets, goals, and review of current data availability.

Dashboard indicators for INAP

Level and focus areas	Indicators
Impact level indicators	– Birth registration – Stillbirth rate – Early neonatal mortality rate – Neonatal mortality rate – Percentage of neonatal deaths to under-5 deaths – Survival rate of newborns discharged from SNCU/NICU at one year of age – Cause-specific neonatal mortality
Pre-conception & antenatal care	– Births to women aged 15–19 years out of total births (teenage pregnancy) – Percentage of pregnant women who received full ANC – Percentage of pregnant women detected and treated with severe anaemia – Percentage of pregnant women detected and treated with PIH
Care during labour and child birth	– Percentage of safe deliveries (institutional + home deliveries by SBA) – Percentage of preterm births – Caesarean section rate – Percentage of women with preterm labour (< 34 weeks) receiving at least one dose of antenatal corticosteroid – Intra-partum stillbirth rate
Immediate newborn care	– Percentage of newborns breast-fed within one hour of birth – Percentage of newborns delivered at health facility receiving vitamin K at birth – Percentage of labour room staff trained in Navjat Shishu Suraksha Karyakram – Percentage of newborns weighed at birth – Percentage of low birth weight babies
Care of healthy newborn	– Percentage of newborns received complete schedule of home visits under HBNC by ASHAs – Percentage of sick newborns identified during home visits by ASHAs – Exclusive breast-feeding rate – Percentage of mothers stayed for 48 hrs in the facility – Percentage of newborn received birth dose of Hepatitis B, OPV and BCG
Care of small and sick newborn	– Percentage of district hospitals with functional SNCU – Percentage of facilities with SNCUs having functional KMC units – Percentage of female admissions in SNCU – Mortality rate in newborns with admission weight <1800 gm – Percentage of newborn deaths due to birth asphyxia – Percentage of newborns with suspected sepsis receiving pre-referral dose of gentamicin by ANM
Care beyond survival	– Percentage of newborns screened for birth defects (facility + community) – Percentage of newborns with any defect seen as birth – Percentage of newborns discharged from SNCU followed up till one year of age – Percentage of districts with functional District Early Intervention Centre (DEIC)

NATIONAL PROGRAMME FOR HEALTHCARE OF THE ELDERLY (NPHCE) *(45)*

Government of India has launched the "National Programme for Health Care of the Elderly" (NPHCE) to address health related problems of elderly people, in 100 identified districts of 21 states during the 11th Plan period. 8 regional geriatrics centres as referral units have also been developed in different regions of the country under the programme.

The basic aim of the NPHCE Programme is to provide separate, specialized and comprehensive healthcare to the senior citizens at various level of state healthcare delivery system including outreach services. Preventive and promotive care, management of illness, health manpower development for geriatric services, medical rehabilitation and therapeutic intervention and Information Education & Communication (IEC) are some of the strategies envisaged in the NPHCE.

It is expected to cover other districts in a phased manner. 12 regional geriatric centres in selected medical colleges of the country are expected to be developed under the programme. In addition, 2 National Centre of Ageing (NCA) are being established at AIIMS, New Delhi and Madras Medical College, Chennai, the core functions of which are training of health professionals, research activity and healthcare delivery in the field of geriatrics.

The details of the geriatric setup and activities undertaken so far under the programme at various healthcare levels are as below *(7)* :

Department of Geriatric at 20 Super Specialized Institutions : Geriatric Departments are being developed at 8 identified medical institution located in various regions of the country with 30 bedded in-patient facility. Apart from providing referral treatment, research and manpower development, these institutions are involved in developing and updating training materials for various levels of health functionaries, developing IEC material, guidelines, etc. Funds have been provided for manpower, equipments, medicines, construction of building, training etc.

Geriatric unit at district hospitals: The programme is approved for implementation in 2017–2018 in 520 districts, covering 35 states. There is provision for establishing 10 bedded geriatric wards and dedicated OPD services exclusively for geriatric patients. The grant-in-aid has been provided for contractual manpower, equipments, medicines, construction of building, training etc.

Rehabilitation Units at CHCs falling under identified districts : There is provision for dedicated health clinics for the elderly persons twice a week. A rehabilitation unit is being set up at all the CHCs falling under identified districts.The grant-in-aid has been provided for manpower, equipments, training. The rehabilitation worker is supposed to provide physiotherapy to the needy elderly persons.

Activity at PHCs under identified districts: Weekly geriatric clinics are arranged at the identified PHCs by a trained Medical Officer. For diseases needing further investigation and treatment, persons will be referred to the first referral unit i.e. the Community Health Centre or District Hospital as per need. One-time grant is given to PHCs for procurement of equipment.

Activity at Sub-centre under districts: The ANMs/Male Health Workers posted in sub-centre will make domiciliary visits to the elderly persons in area under their jurisdiction. She/he will arrange suitable calipers and supportive devices from the PHC and provide the same to the elderly disabled persons to make them ambulatory. Also, there will be a provision for treatment of minor ailments and rehabilitation equipment at the identified sub centers.

The tertiary component of the programme has been renamed as "Rashtriya Varishth Jan Swasthya Yojana" (RVJSY).

NATIONAL PROGRAMME FOR PREVENTION AND CONTROL OF CANCER, DIABETES, CARDIOVASCULAR DISEASES AND STROKE (NPCDCS)

India is experiencing a rapid health transition with large and rising burden of chronic non-communicable diseases (NCDs) especially cardiovascular disease, diabetes mellitus, cancer, stroke, and chronic lung diseases. It is estimated that in 2016 NCDs accounted for 60 per cent of deaths. Considering the fact that NCDs are surpassing the burden of communicable diseases in India and the existing health system is mainly focussed on communicable diseases, need for National Programme on Prevention and Control of Diabetes, Cardiovascular Diseases and Stroke was envisaged. Later on this programme was integrated with National Cancer Control Programme, and National Programme for Prevention and Control of Cancer, Diabetes, Cardiovascular Diseases and Stroke (NPCDCS) came into existence. During the 11th Five Year Plan period, 100 identified districts in 21 states have been covered under the programme. During 12th Five Year Plan, the programme has covered all the districts of the country in a phased manner *(7)*.

A. Diabetes, Cardiovascular Disease and Stroke (DCS) Component under NPCDCS

The programme focuses on the health promotion, capacity building including human resource development, early diagnosis and management of these diseases with integration with the primary health care system.

The major objectives of the programme are as follows *(7)* :

- Prevent and control common NCDs through behaviour and lifestyle changes.
- Provide early diagnosis and management of common NCDs.
- Build capacity at various levels of health care for prevention, diagnosis and treatment of common NCDs.
- Train human resource within the public health set-up *viz* doctors, paramedics and nursing staff to cope with the increasing burden of NCDs, and
- Establish and develop capacity for palliative & rehabilitative care.

The programme is to be implemented in 20,000 sub-centres and 700 community health centres (CHCs) in 100 districts across 21 States/UTs and the strategies include promoting healthy lifestyle through massive health education and mass media efforts at country level, opportunistic screening of persons above the age of 30 years, establishment of Non-Communicable Disease (NCD) Clinic at Community Health Centre (CHC) and District level, development of trained manpower and strengthening of tertiary level health facilities. For long-term sustainability of the programme, service delivery will be through existing public health infrastructure and systems. The various approaches such as mass media, community education and interpersonal communication will be used for behavioural change focusing on the following messages :

- Increased intake of healthy foods
- Increased physical activity
- Avoidance of tobacco and alcohol
- Stress management.

Activities at Sub-Centre

Health promotion for behaviour and lifestyle change will be carried out by organizing various camps, interpersonal communications, posters, banners, etc. Opportunistic screening of population above 30 years will be carried out using BP measurement and blood glucose by strip method. The suspected cases of diabetes and hypertension will be referred to CHCs of higher health facility for further diagnosis and management. For screening of diabetes, glucometer optium xceed, optium test strips and auto disabled lancets are being procured at central level and provided to the concerned states as per their requirements from time to time.

Activities at CHC

NCD clinic at CHC shall do the diagnosis by required investigations/test like blood sugar measurement, lipid profile, ultrasound, X-ray and ECG etc., management and stabilization of common CVD, diabetes and stroke cases (out-patient as well as in-patients). One of the nurses appointed under the programme shall undertake home visits for bedridden cases, supervise the work of health workers and attend monthly clinics being held in the villages on a random basis. Complicated cases of diabetes, high blood pressure etc. shall be referred from CHC to the district hospital for further investigations and management.

Activities at district hospital

NCD clinic at district hospital shall screen persons above the age of 30 years for diabetes, hypertension, cardiovascular diseases etc. to identify individuals who are at a high-risk of developing diabetes, hypertension and CVDs warranting further investigation/action. Detailed investigation will be done in respect of persons those who are at high-risk of developing NCDs on screening and those who are referred from CHCs. They shall provide regular management and annual assessment of persons suffering from cancer, diabetes and hypertension. People with established cardiovascular diseases shall also be managed at district hospital. They shall provide home based palliative care for chronic, debilitating and progressive patients. Apart from clinical services, district hospital shall be involved in promotion of healthy lifestyle through health education and counselling to the patients and their attendants.

Urban health check-up scheme for diabetes and high blood pressure

The scheme has the following objectives :

1. To screen urban slum population for diabetes and high blood pressure.
2. To create database for prevalence of diabetes and high blood pressure in urban slums.
3. To sensitize the urban slum population about healthy lifestyle.

The blood sugar and blood pressure will be checked for all ≥ 30 years and all pregnant women of all age.

The NCD cells at the centre, state and district will implement and monitor the National Programme for Prevention and Control of Cancer, Diabetes, CVD and Stroke (NPCDCS) in various states. The national NCD cell has been established at the centre.

Achievements under the programme

As on 31st March 2021, the programme is under implementation in all 36 states/UTs. The facilities available are as shown in Table 17.

TABLE 17

Comparative progress in achievements 2014–2021

Facilities	As on 31st March, 2014	As on 31st March, 2021
State NCD Cells	21	36
District NCD Cells	96	684
District NCD Clinics	95	640
District CCU facilities	51	194
District Day Care Centres	38	239
CHC NCD Clinics	204	5148

Source : *(6)*

New initiatives under the programme

1. Intervention for prevention and control of Rheumatic Heart Disease under NPCDCS and Rashtriya Bal Swasthya Karyakram (RBSK).
2. Integration of AYUSH with NPCDCS.
3. Integration of RNTCP with NPCDCS to articulate a national strategy for management of TB and diabetes comorbidities in India.

Guidelines for referral and treatment *(66)*

Government of India has developed operational guidelines (2016) for prevention, screening and control of common non-communicable diseases. The guidelines for referral, treatment and for ensuring the continuity of care are as follows :

1. Those with a systolic blood pressure of over 140 and a diastolic blood pressure of over 90 mm of Hg, or random blood sugar of 140 mg/dl and above would be referred to a medical officer, at the nearest facility, for confirmation, conducting relevant laboratory investigations and initiation of treatment.
2. Those who are found positive for cancer/precancerous lesions will be referred by ANM/Staff Nurse in specified screening sites to the appropriate PHC/CHC/District Hospital for confirmation and treatment by trained specialist, as per the operational frame work developed for cancer screening and management.
3. Once the diagnosis of Hypertension/diabetes is established, the patient must receive at least a month's supply of drugs from the PHC. Once the condition is stable, the state could also decide to provide the patient with a three-month supply, with the ANM/ASHA visiting the patient each month for ensuring compliance, checking on diet and life style modification, and measuring the blood pressure/blood glucose. Alternatively, a three-month drug supply could be stocked with the ANM at sub-centre, to be given each month. Either way, sufficient drug supplies need to be made available at the PHC.
4. The patient will need to go to the PHC for the first follow up at the end of the first three months after diagnosis, and sooner if required. An annual specialist consultation at the nearest nodal CHC with NCD clinic, is also recommended, based on the decision of the MO at the PHC.
5. For those individuals who are already on treatment under the care of a private practitioner, they could be offered the choice of taking drugs from the public health system, after appropriate confirmation. However, these individuals would be visited regularly by the frontline workers, monitored for compliance with treatment/ lifestyle changes and recorded in the health card.
6. Community Follow up of these individuals would be by the ASHA making visits to enable positive behaviour modifications, treatment compliance, and encouraging patients to go the sub-centre for regular check-up of BP/ blood glucose. Some states have also provided the ASHA with BP apparatus and glucometers to undertake regular examinations at the village level. The ASHA will prioritize those households where there are treatment defaulters or those who experience complications. The aim is to minimize treatment defaulters and to achieve hypertension and glycaemic control at an individual and population level. The ANM would also conduct regular home visits.

WHO has developed a comprehensive global monitoring framework for prevention and control of NCDs (2013–2020), which was endorsed by World Health Assembly in May 2013. This includes nine voluntary targets to monitor the progress made in the implementation of the programme. India is committed to implementation of the action plan and take necessary steps to meet the objectives. The indicators and targets are as shown in Table 18 *(67)*.

TABLE 18
Indicators and targets for NCD prevention and control in India

Framework element	Targets		
	Outcome	2020	2025
Premature mortality from NCDs	Relative reduction in overall mortality from cardiovascular disease, cancer, diabetes, or chronic respiratory disease	10%	25%
Alcohol use	Relative reduction in alcohol use	5%	10%
Obesity and diabetes	Halt the rise of obesity and diabetes prevalence	No mid-term target set	Halt the rise in obesity and diabetes prevalence
Physical inactivity	Relative reduction in prevalence of insufficient physical activity	5%	10%
Raised blood pressure	Relative reduction in prevalence of raised blood pressure	10%	25%
Salt/sodium intake	Relative reduction in mean population intake of salt, with aim of achieving recommended level of less than 5 gms per day	20%	30%
Tobacco use	Relative reduction in prevalence of current tobacco use	15%	30%
Drug therapy to prevent heart attacks and strokes	Eligible people receiving drug therapy and counselling (including glycaemic control) to prevent heart attacks and strokes	30%	50%
Essential NCD medicines and basic technologies to treat major NCDs	Availability and affordability of quality, safe and efficacious essential NCD medicines including generics, and basic technologies in both public and private facilities	60%	80%
Household indoor air pollution	Relative reduction in household use of solid fuels as a primary source of energy for cooking	25%	50%

Source : *(67)*

B. Cancer component under NPCDCS

Cancer is an important public health problem in India, with nearly 10 lakh new cases occurring every year in the country. It is estimated that there are 2.8 million cases of cancer in the country at any given point of time. With the objectives of prevention, early diagnosis and treatment, the national cancer control programme was launched in 1975–76. In view of the magnitude of the problem and gaps in the availability of cancer treatment facilities across the country, the programme was revised in 1984–85 and subsequently in December 2004. During 2010, the programme was integrated with National Programme on Prevention and Control of Diabetes, Cardiovascular Disease and Stroke. The objectives of the programme are :

a. Primary prevention of cancers by health education;
b. Secondary prevention i.e. early detection and diagnosis of common cancer such as cancer of cervix, mouth, breast and tobacco related cancer by screening/self examination method; and
c. Tertiary prevention i.e. strengthening of the existing institutions of comprehensive therapy including palliative care.

The schemes under the revised programme are :

1. Regional Cancer Centre Scheme

The existing regional cancer centres are being further strengthened to act as referral centres for complicated and difficult cases at the tertiary level. One time assistance of Rs. 3 crores during the plan period is provided to Regional Cancer Centres except TMH, Mumbai and IRCH (AIIMS) for strengthening and to the CNCI, Kolkata on the approved pattern of funding.

2. Oncology Wing Development Scheme

This scheme had been initiated to fill up the geographic gaps in the availability of cancer treatment facilities in the country. Central assistance is provided for purchase of equipment, which include a cobalt unit besides other equipment. A part of the grant can be used for the civil work but the manpower is to be provided by the concerned state government/institution. The quantum of central assistance is Rs. 3 crores per institution under the scheme.

3. Decentralized NGO scheme

This scheme is meant for IEC activities and early detection of cancer. The scheme is operated by the nodal agencies and the NGOs are given financial assistance for undertaking health education and early detection activities of cancer.

4. IEC activities at central level

IEC activities at the central level are to be initiated in order to give wider publicity about the Anti-Tobacco Legislation for discouraging consumption of cigarettes and other tobacco related products, and for creating awareness among masses about the ill effects of consumption of tobacco and tobacco related products. Under this scheme wider publicity would also be given about the rules being formulated for implementation of various provisions of the anti–tobacco legislation. November 7th is observed as National Cancer Awareness Day in the country.

5. Research and training

Training programmes, monitoring and research activities will be organized at the central level under this scheme. Following training manuals have been developed under the NCCP for capacity building in cancer control at district level :

a. Manual for health professionals
b. Manual for cytology
c. Manual for palliative care
d. Manual for tobacco cessation

Cancer services under national programme for prevention and control of cancer, diabetes, CVD and stroke *(46)* :

1. Common diagnostic services, basic surgery, chemotherapy and palliative care for cancer cases is being made available at 100 district hospitals.
2. Each district is being supported with Rs. 1.66 crores per annum for the following :
   - Chemotherapy drugs are provided for 100 patients at each district hospital.
   - Day care chemotherapy facilities is being established at 100 district hospitals.
   - Facility for laboratory investigations including mammography is being provided at 100 district hospitals and if not available, this can be outsourced at government rates.
3. Home based palliative care is being provided for chronic, debilitating and progressive cancer patients at 100 districts.
4. Support is being provided for contractual manpower through 1 Medical Oncologist, 1 Cytopathologist, 1 Cytopathology technician, 2 Nurses for day care.
5. State Cancer Institutes will provide comprehensive cancer diagnosis, treatment and care services. SCI will be apex institution in the state for cancer treatment activities.
6. 45 centres were to be strengthened as Tertiary Cancer Centres (TCCs) to provide comprehensive cancer care services at a cost of Rs. 6.00 crore each during 2011–12.

NATIONAL TOBACCO CONTROL PROGRAMME

A comprehensive tobacco control legislation titled "The Cigarettes and other Tobacco Products (Prohibition of Advertisement and Regulation of Trade and Commerce, Production, Supply and Distribution) Act, 2003" was passed by the parliament in April, 2003 and notified in Gazette of India on 25th Feb, 2004. The important provisons of the Act are :

a. Prohibition of smoking in public places;
b. Prohibition of direct and indirect advertisement of cigarette and other products;
c. Prohibition of sale of cigarette and other tobacco products to a person below the age of 18 years,
d. Prohibition of sale of tobacco products near the educational institutions;
e. Mandatory depiction of statutory warnings (including pictorial warnings) on tobacco packs; and
f. Mandatory depiction of tar and nicotine contents alongwith maximum permissible limits on tobacco packs.

The rules related to prohibition of smoking in public places came into force from the 2nd October, 2008. As per rules, it is mandatory to display smoke free signages at all public places. Labelling and packaging rules mandating the depiction of specified health warnings on all tobacco product packs came into force from 31st May, 2009.

On account of sustained efforts on the part of Ministry of Health and Family Welfare, 34 States/UTs have issued orders for implementation of the Food Safety Regulations banning manufacture, sale and storage of gutka and pan masala containing tobacco or nicotine in the year 2014–15. Besides several states/UTs have banned all forms of smokeless tobacco products such as chewing tobacco, zarda, khaini and other flavoured and processed tobacco irrespective of name and form *(45)*.

On 24th September 2015, Government of India notified that the rules on "tobacco pack pictorial warnings" would come into effect from 1st April 2016. These rules mandate display of pictorial health warnings on 85 per cent of the principle display area of tobacco product pack on both sides (60 per cent of the picture and 25 per cent of the text).

National Tobacco Control Programme *(3)* : In order to facilitate the implementation of the Tobacco Control Laws, to bring about greater awareness about the harmful effects of tobacco, and to fulfill the obligations under the WHO–Framework convention on tobacco control, Govt. of India has launched a new National Tobacco Control Programme in the 11th Five Year Plan. Pilot phase was launched in 16 districts covering 9 states in 2007–08. It now covers 108 districts in 31 states in the country. The main components of the programme are :

1. Public awareness/mass media campaigns for awareness building and for behavioural change;
2. Establishment of tobacco product testing laboratories, to build regulatory capacity, as required under COTPA, 2003;
3. Mainstreaming the programme components as a part of the health delivery mechanism under the NRHM framework;
4. Mainstream research and training on alternate crops and livelihood, with other nodal ministries;
5. Monitoring and evaluation, including surveillance, e.g. adult tobacco survey;
6. Dedicated tobacco control cells for effective implementation and monitoring of anti–tobacco initiatives;
7. Training of health and social workers, NGOs school teachers etc;
8. School programme; and
9. Provision of tobacco cessation facilities.

NATIONAL MENTAL HEALTH PROGRAMME

The National Mental Health Programme was launched during 1982 with a view to ensure availability of Mental Health Care Services for all, especially the community at risk and underprivileged section of the population, to encourage application of mental health knowledge in general health care and social development. A National Advisory Group on mental health was constituted under the Chairmanship of the Secretary, Ministry of Health and Family Welfare for the effective implementation of the National Health Programme. Eleven institutions have been identified for imparting training in basic knowledge and skills in the field of mental health to the primary health care physicians and para-medical personnel. At present this programme covers 517 districts in 36 states.

The aims of the NMHP are : (a) Prevention and treatment of mental and neurological disorders and their associated disabilities; (b) Use of mental health technology to improve general health services; and (c) Application of mental health principles in total national development to improve quality of life *(68)*.

The objectives of the programme are :

1. To ensure availability and accessibility of minimum mental health care for all in the foreseeable future, particularly to the most vulnerable and underprivileged sections of population.
2. To encourage application of mental health knowledge in general health care and in the social development.

3. To promote community participation in the mental health services development, and to stimulate efforts towards self-help in the community.

The programme strategies are :

1. Integration of mental health with primary health care through the NMHP;
2. Provision of tertiary care institutions for treatment of mental disorders;
3. Eradicating stigmatization of mentally ill patients and protecting their rights through regulatory institutions like the Central Mental Health Authority, and State Mental Health Authority.

District Mental Health Programme components are : (a) Training programmes of all workers in the mental health team at the identified nodal institute in the state; (b) Public education in mental health to increase awareness and to reduce stigma; (c) For early detection and treatment, the OPD and indoor services are provided; and (d) Providing valuable data and experience at the level of community to the state and centre for future planning, improvement in service and research.

District Mental Health Programme has now incorporated promotive and preventive activities for positive mental health which includes :

- *School mental health services :* Life skills education in schools, counselling services.
- *College counselling services :* Through trained teachers/ councellors.
- *Work place stress management :* Formal & Informal sectors, including farmers, women etc.
- *Suicide prevention services :* Counselling center at district level, sensitization workshops, IEC, help lines etc.

The National Human Rights Commission also monitors the conditions in the mental hospitals along with the government of India, and the states are acting on the recommendations of the joint studies conducted to ensure quality in delivery of mental care.

Thrust areas *(46)*

1. District mental health programme in an enlarged and more effective form covering the entire country.
2. Streamlining/modernization of mental hospitals in order to modify their present custodial role.
3. Upgrading department of psychiatry in medical colleges and enhancing the psychiatric content of the medical curriculum at the undergraduate as well as postgraduate level.
4. Strengthening the central and state mental health authorities with a permanent secretariat. Appointment of medical officers at state headquarters in order to make the monitoring role more effective.
5. Research and training in the field of community mental health, substance abuse and child adolescent psychiatric clinics.

The Mental Healthcare Act, 2017 *(7)*

The United Nations convention on the rights of persons with disabilities was ratified by the Government of India thus making it obligatory on the Government to align the policies and laws of the country with the convention. There was an increasing realization that persons with mental illness constitute a vulnerable section of society and are subject to discrimination in our society.

The Mental Healthcare Bill, 2013 was introduced in the Parliament in order to protect and promote the rights of persons with mental illness during the delivery of health care in institutions and in the community and to ensure health care, treatment and rehabilitation of persons with mental illness, is provided in the least restrictive environment possible. Further, to regulate the public and private mental health sectors within rights framework, to achieve the greatest public health good and to promote principles of equity, efficiency and active participation of all stakeholders in decision making. Suicide has been decriminalized under the Act. The bill received assent of the Hon'ble President of India on 07.04.2017. The Ministry has constituted a committee of experts for formulating rules and regulations under the Act.

INTEGRATED DISEASE SURVEILLANCE PROJECT

Integrated disease surveillance project is a decentralized state based surveillance system in the country. This project is intended to detect early warning signals of impending outbreaks and help initiate an effective response in a timely manner in urban and rural areas. It will also provide essential data to monitor progress of ongoing disease control programme and help allocate health resources more efficiently. The project was launched in Nov. 2004. It was a 5 year project up to March 2010. The project was restructured and extended up to March 2012. It continues in the 12th Five Year Plan with domestic budget as integrated Disease Surveillance Programme under National Health Mission for all states.

A Central Surveillance Unit (CSU) established and integrated in the National Centre for Disease Control, Delhi, State Surveillance Units (SSU) at all State/UT head quarters and District Surveillance Units (DSU) at all districts in the country have been established. IT network connecting 776 sites in states/district head quarters and premier institutes has been established with the help of National Information Centre and ISRO (Indian Space Research Organization) for data entry, training, video conferencing and outbreak discussions.

Under the project weekly disease surveillance data on epidemic prone diseases are being collected from reporting units such as sub-centres, PHCs, CHCs, hospitals including government and private sector hospitals and medical colleges. The data are being collected on 'S' syndromic; 'P' probable; and 'L' laboratory formats using standard case definitions. Presently more than 90 per cent districts report such weekly data through e-mail/portals. The weekly data are analysed by SSU/DSU for disease trends. Whenever there is rising trend of illness, it is investigated by the Rapid Response Team to diagnose and control the outbreak. It is a multi speciality team of an epidemiologist, a clinician, a microbiologist and other specialists as per requirement.

The surveillance is needed to recognize cases or cluster of cases to initiate interventions to prevent transmission of disease or reduce morbidity and mortality; access the public health impact of health events or determine and measure trends; demonstrate the need for public health intervention programmes and resources and allocate resources during public health planning; monitor effectiveness of prevention and control measures; identify high-risk groups or geographical areas to target interventions and guide analytic studies; and develop hypothesis that lead to analytic studies about risk factors for disease causation, propagation and progression *(69)*.

In this project, different types of integration are proposed. These include : (a) Sharing of surveillance information of disease control programmes; (b) Developing effective partnership with health and non-health sectors in surveillance; (c) Including non-communicable and communicable diseases in the surveillance system; (d) Effective partnership of private sector and NGOs in surveillance activities; and (e) Bringing academic institutions and medical colleges into the primary public health activity of disease surveillance.

The important information in disease surveillance are – who gets the disease, how many get the disease, where did they get the disease, why did they get the disease, and what needs to be done as public health response.

The components of the surveillance activity are :

(a) Collection of data

(b) Compilation of data

(c) Analysis and interpretation

(d) Follow-up action

(e) Feedback.

The prerequisite of the effective surveillance are – use of standard case definition, ensure regularity of reports and the action on reports.

The classification of surveillance in IDSP is as follows :

a. *Syndromic diagnosis* – diagnosis is made on the basis of clinical pattern by paramedical personnel and members of the community;

b. *Presumptive diagnosis* – diagnosis made on typical history and clinical examination by medical officer; and

c. *Confirmed diagnosis* – clinical diagnosis by a medical officer and or positive laboratory identification.

Syndromes under surveillance (69) :

The paramedical health staff will undertake disease surveillance based on broad categories of presentation. The following clinical syndromes will be under surveillance in IDSP :

1. Fever:
   a. Less than 7 days duration without any localizing signs
   b. With rash
   c. With altered sensorium or convulsions
   d. Bleeding from skin or mucus membrane
   e. Fever more than 7 days with or without localizing signs
2. Cough more than 3 weeks duration
3. Acute flaccid paralysis
4. Diarrhoea
5. Jaundice, and
6. Unusual events causing death or hospitalization.

These syndromes are intended to pick up all priority diseases listed under regular surveillance at the level of the community under the Integrated Disease Surveillance Project.

Fever with or without localizing signs	Malaria, Typhoid, JE, Dengue, Measles
Cough more than 3 weeks	Tuberculosis
Acute flaccid paralysis	Polio
Diarrhoea	Cholera
Jaundice	Hepatitis, Laptospirosis, Dengue, Malaria, Yellow fever
Unusual syndromes	Anthrax, Plague, Emerging epidemics

The core conditions under surveillance in IDSP are as follows *(71)* :

(i) Regular Surveillance:

Vector borne disease	: Malaria
Water borne disease	: Acute diarrhoeal disease (cholera)
	: Typhoid
Respiratory diseases	: Tuberculosis
Vaccine preventable diseases	: Measles
Diseases under eradication	: Polio
Other conditions	: Road traffic accidents (Link-up with police computers)
Other international commitments	: Plague
Unusual clinical syndromes (causing death/ hospitalization)	: Meningoencephalitis / Respiratory distress, Haemorrhagic fevers, other undiagnosed conditions

(ii) Sentinel Surveillance:

Sexually transmitted diseases / blood borne	: HIV / HBV, HCV
Other conditions	: Water quality monitoring
	: Outdoor air quality (Large urban centres)

(iii) Regular periodic surveys:

NCD risk factors	: Anthropometry, Physical activity, Blood pressure, Tobacco, Nutrition etc.

(iv) Additional state priorities:

Each state may identify upto five additional conditions for surveillance.

Outbreak

In epidemiology, an outbreak is a sudden increase in occurrence of a disease in a particular time and place. A single case of a communicable disease long absent from a population, or caused by an agent (e.g. bacterium or virus) not previously recognized in that community or area, or emergence of a previously unknown disease, may also constitute an outbreak and should be reported and investigated.

Warning signs of an impending outbreak are as follows *(70)*:

- Clustering of cases or deaths in time and/or space
- Unusual increase in number of cases or deaths
- Even a single case of measles, AFP, cholera, plague, dengue or JE
- Acute febrile illness of unknown aetiology
- Occurrence of two or more epidemiologically linked cases of meningitis, measles

- Unusual isolate
- Shifting in age distribution of cases
- Sudden increase/high vector density
- Natural disasters

Summary of outbreak syndromes and trigger events for investigation *(70)* :

Syndrome	Trigger event
Acute watery stools	– A single case of severe dehydration/death in a patient > 5 years of age with diarrhoea.
	– More than 10 houses having at least one case of loose stools irrespective of age, per village or an urban ward.
Fever < 7 days duration	
(a) Only fever	5 cases in 1000 population.
(b) With rash (Measles / Dengue)	Two similar cases in a village (1000 population).
(c) Altered consciousness	Two cases of fever with altered consciousness in the village/1000 population.
(d) Fever with bleeding	Two cases of fever with bleeding in a village or 1000 population.
Fever with convulsions	Two cases of fever with convulsions in a village or 1000 population.
Fever more than 7 days	More than 2 cases in a village or 1000 population.
Jaundice	More than 2 cases in a village or in 1000 population.
Unusual event	More than 2 deaths or hospitalization.

The reporting units for disease surveillance are :

	Public Health Sector	Private Health Sector
Rural	CHCs, District hospitals	Sentinel private practitioners, and Sentinel hospitals.
Urban	Urban hospitals, ESI / Railway / Medical college hospitals.	Sentinel private nursing homes, sentinel hospitals, Medical colleges, Private and NGO laboratories

1. Sub-centre–health worker/ANM reports all patients fulfilling the clinical syndrome from PHC, private clinic, hospital etc.
2. PHC/CHC medical officers report as probable cases of interest, where this cannot be confirmed by laboratory tests at the peripheral reporting units, and as confirmed when the laboratory information is available as in case of blood smear +ve malaria and sputum AFB +ve tuberculosis.
3. Sentinel private practitioners, district hospitals, municipal hospitals, medical colleges, sentinel hospitals, NGOs – medical officers report as probable cases of interest.

AYUSHMAN BHARAT PROGRAMME

In February 2018, the Govt. of India announced two major initiatives in health sector, with aim to cover preventive and health promotive interventions at primary, secondary and tertiary care system. They are as follows *(72)*:

1. *Health and Wellness Centre:* The National Health Policy, 2017 has envisioned Health and Wellness Centres as the foundation of India's health system. Under this 1.5 lakh centres will bring health care system closer to homes of people. The health centres will provide comprehensive health care, including maternal and child health services, Communicable Diseases services, and services related to Non-Communicable Diseases. To begin with, the common NCDs such as hypertension, diabetes and 3 common cancers of oral, breast and cervix. It is also envisaged to incrementally add primary healthcare services for mental health, ENT, opthalmology, oral health, geriatric and palliative health care and trauma care, as well as health promotion and wellness activities like Yoga. A few States/UTs have already started rolling out these additional packages of services in a phased manner. The centres will also provide free essential drugs and diagnostic services.
2. The second component is the Ayushman Bharat – Pradhan Mantri Jan Arogya Yojana (AB-PMJAY) which provides health coverage upto Rs. 5.00 lakh per family per year to about 10.74 crore poor and vulnerable families identified on the basis of Socio Economic Caste Census data.

The first Health and Wellness Centre was inaugurated on 14th April 2018 in Bijapur district of Chhattisgarh. So far, 77,786 centres are operational in the country as on 16th Sep. 2021.

Primary healthcare team at the Sub Health Centre level AB-HWCs is headed by Community Health Officer (CHO) who is a BSc/GNM Nurse or an Ayurveda Practitioner trained in primary care and public health skills, and certified in a six months certificate programme in community health. Other members of the team being multi-purpose workers (Male and Female) and Accredited Social Health Activists (ASHAs).

The training programme is being carried out with support from IGNOU and state specific Public/Health Universities. 282 IGNOU Programme Study Centres (PSCs) have been notified so far, and another 111 PSCs have been notified under the state specific certificate programme in the state of Maharashtra, Tamil Nadu, Gujarat and West Bengal, taking the total of programme study centres to 393 across the country.

Since the screening, prevention and management of chronic illnesses including NCDs, TB and Leprosy have been introduced at AB-HWCs, training and skill upgradation of the primary health team in all the functional AB-HWCs on NCDs and use of IT application is being done.

To promote wellness and healthy lifestyle, orientation of the public on wellness activities for lifestyle modification like increased physical activity (cyclathons and marathons), eating RIGHT and SAFE, cessation of tobacco and drugs, meditation, laughter clubs, open gyms, etc. is being done. Beside these, Yoga sessions are being conducted at these centres on regular basis. Through annual health calendar, planned activities at these centres on the health condition of the day are resulting in increased awareness and preventive measures to be adopted by the public.

The telemedicine guidelines have also been provided to the States to initiate specialist consultations from the PHCs to the Hub Hospitals and the pilot of the application is being conducted in Andhra Pradesh, Tamil Nadu and Maharashtra.

Expanded service packages planned to be provided at functional AB-HWCs are as follows :

1. Care in pregnancy and child birth.
2. Neonatal and infant health care services.
3. Childhood and adolescent health care services.
4. Family planning, contraceptive services and other reproductive health care services.
5. Management of communicable diseases : National Health programmes.
6. General out-patient care for acute simple illnesses and minor ailments.
7. Screening, prevention, control and management of non-communicable diseases and chronic communicable diseases like tuberculosis and leprosy.
8. Basic oral health care.
9. Screening and basic management of mental health ailments.
10. Care for common ophthalmic and ENT problem.
11. Elderly and palliative health care services.
12. Emergency medical services including burns and trauma.

Expected outcome (6)

- Increasing the trust of people on the service provision by public healthcare facilities through health system strengthening and improvement.
- Availability of assured healthcare services to ensure continuum of care.
- Reduction in out of pocket expenditure of the common people.
- Increased awareness among the people about preventive and promotive healthcare.
- Benefits of healthy lifestyle including Yoga, and eat right & eat safe etc.
- Enabling environment to increase the health seeking behaviour of the poor people.

For further details please refer to chapter 9 for school health programme and chapter 10 for Health and Wellness Centres.

NATIONAL PROGRAMME FOR PREVENTION AND MANAGEMENT OF TRAUMA AND BURN INJURIES (NPPMTBI)

A. Trauma Care component *(6)* :

In India, road traffic crashes are one of the major causes of disability, morbidity and mortality. As per the Road Accident Report for 2019, a total number of 4,49,002 accidents took place in the country during the calendar year 2019 leading to 1,51,113 deaths and 4,51,361 injuries.

The programme for trauma care started during 9th and 10th Five Year Plans as "Pilot Project for Strengthening Emergency Facilities along the Highways". During the 11th FYP, the programme was approved as "Assistance for Capacity Building for Developing Trauma Care Facilities in Government Hospitals on National Highways" for developing a network of trauma care facilities (TCFs) in the Government Hospitals along the Golden Quadrilateral highway corridor as well as North-South & East-West Corridors wherein 116 TCFs were approved in 17 States on these corridors on 100% Central assistance. The scheme was further extended during 12th FYP as "Capacity Building for Developing Trauma Care Facilities in Govt. Hospitals on National Highways" wherein 80 Hospitals/Medical Colleges were approved for financial assistance in addition to other interventions. The scheme is being extended since then.

Objectives of the programme are as follows :

- To establish a network of Trauma Care Facilities on National/State Highways in order to reduce the incidence of preventable deaths and disabilities due to road traffic accidents by observing golden hour principle.
- To develop Surveillance, Trauma Registry and Capacity Building Centre for collection, compilation, analysis and dissemination of information for policy formulation and preventive interventions.
- To improve the awareness about trauma care among the general masses and vulnerable groups by developing and disseminating IEC material.

B. Burn Injuries component *(6)* :

India has one of the largest burdens of burns with an estimated 7,000,000 burn injuries per year, and an estimated 1.4 lakh deaths and 2.4 lakh disabilities, making burn injuries the second largest group of injuries after road accidents. These figures translate to a mortality rate of over 8.3/100,000 population, disfigurement and permanent disability in 250,000 people annually, and a loss of 5 million disability-adjusted life years (DALYs).

This high incidence has been attributed to illiteracy, poverty, and low safety consciousness in the population. The epidemiology of mortality after burns is unique in India; most burn injuries are in young adults and deaths are more common in women than men, contrasting trends observed in other low-and middle-income countries. Burns survivors are also known to be financially distressed, vocationally challenged and socially excluded. Death and disability due to burn injury are preventable to a great extent provided timely and appropriate treatment is provided by trained healthcare professionals.

Keeping in view the magnitude of the problem, a pilot programme on burn care was initiated in the year 2010 by Ministry of Health & Family Welfare in the name of "Pilot Programme for Prevention of Burn Injuries" (PPPBI). This was initiated in three Medical Colleges and six Districts Hospitals. The goal of PPPBI was to ensure prevention of Burn Injuries, provide timely and adequate treatment in case of burn injuries, so as to reduce mortality, complications and ensuing disabilities and to provide effective rehabilitative interventions if disability has set in.

The pilot project continued as full-fledged programme for tertiary care level during the 12th Five Year Plan period. The financial assistance towards District Hospital component was undertaken under National Health Mission (NHM). The scheme is being extended since then.

NATIONAL GUINEAWORM ERADICATION PROGRAMME

India launched its National Guineaworm Eradication Programme in 1984 with technical assistance from WHO. From the very beginning the programme was integrated into the national health system at village level. With well defined strategies, an efficient information and evaluation system, intersectoral coordination at all levels and close collaboration with WHO and UNICEF, India was able to significantly reduce the disease in affected areas. The country has reported zero cases since August 1996. In February 2000, the International Commission for the Certification of Dracunculiasis Eradication recommended that India be certified free of dracunculiasis transmission *(71)*.

The following activities are continuing as per recommendations of International Certification Team of International Commission for Certification of Dracunculiasis Eradication, Geneva :

a. Health education activities with special emphasis on school children and women in rural areas;
b. Rumour registration and rumour investigation;
c. Maintenance of guinea-worm disease on list of notifiable disease and continuation of surveillance in previously infected areas; and
d. Careful supervision of the functioning of hand pumps and other sources of safe drinking water, and provision of additional units, wherever necessary.

YAWS ERADICATION PROGRAMME *(9)*

The disease has been reported in India from the tribal communities living in hilly forest and difficult to reach areas in 49 districts of 10 states, namely Andhra Pradesh, Assam, Chhattisgarh, Gujarat, Jharkhand, Madhya Pradesh, Maharashtra, Orissa, Tamil Nadu and Uttar Pradesh. National Institute of Communicable Diseases is the nodal agency for planning, guidance, coordination, monitoring and evaluation of the programme. The programme is implemented by the State Health Directorates of Yaws endemic states utilizing existing health care delivery system with the coordination and collaboration of department of tribal welfare and other related institutions.

The number of reported cases has come down from more than 3,500 to Nil during the period from 1996 to 2004, since then no new case has been reported.

NATIONAL PROGRAMME FOR CONTROL AND TREATMENT OF OCCUPATIONAL DISEASES

Government of India launched a scheme called "National Programme for Control and Treatment of Occupational Diseases" in 1998–99. The National Institute of Occupational Health, Ahmedabad (ICMR) has been identified as the nodal agency for this programme.

The following research projects have been proposed by the government *(73)* :

1. Prevention, control and treatment of silicosis and silico-tuberculosis in agate industry;
2. Occupational health problems of tobacco harvesters and their prevention;
3. Hazardous process and chemicals, database generation, documentation, and information dissemination;
4. Capacity building to promote research, education, and training at National Institute of Occupational Disease;
5. Health Risk Assessment and development of intervention programme in cottage industries with high risk of silicosis; and
6. Prevention and control of occupational health hazards among salt workers in the remote desert areas of Gujarat and Western Rajasthan.

NUTRITIONAL PROGRAMME

Please refer to chapter 11, for details.

NATIONAL FAMILY WELFARE PROGRAMME

See chapter 8 for details.

NATIONAL WATER SUPPLY AND SANITATION PROGRAMME

The National Water Supply and Sanitation Programme was initiated in 1954 with the object of providing safe water supply and adequate drainage facilities for the entire urban and rural population of the country. In 1972 a special programme known as the **Accelerated Rural Water Supply Programme** was started as a supplement to the national water supply and sanitation programme. Inspite of increased financial outlay during the successive Five Year Plans, only a small dent was made on the overall problem. During the Fifth Plan, rural water supply was included in the Minimum Needs Programme of the State Plans. The Central Government is supporting the efforts of the States in identifying problem villages through assistance under Accelerated Rural Water Supply Programme. A *"problem village"* has been defined as one where no source of safe water is available within a distance of 1.6 km, or where water is available at a depth of more than 15 metres, or where water source has excess salinity, iron, fluorides and other toxic elements, or where water is exposed to the risk of cholera.

The stipulated norm of water supply is 40 litres of safe water per capita per day, and at least one hand pump/spot-source for every 250 persons. Information, education and communication is an integral part of rural sanitation programme to adopt proper environmental sanitation practices including disposal of garbage, refuse and waste water, and to convert all existing dry latrines into low cost sanitary latrines. The priority is to evolve financially viable sewerage systems in big cities and important pilgrimage and tourist centres and recycling of treated effluents for horticulture, irrigation and other non-domestic purposes *(74)*.

The programme was subsequently renamed as the Rajiv Gandhi National Drinking Water Mission in 1991. In 1999–2000, Sector Reform Project was started to involve the community in planning, implementation and management of drinking water schemes which was in 2002 scaled up as the Swajaldhara Programme.

Swajaldhara (75)

Swajaldhara was launched on 25th December 2002. Swajaldhara has certain fundamental reform principles, which need to be adhered to by the state governments and the implementing agencies. Swajaldhara is a community led participatory programme, which aims at providing safe drinking water in rural areas, with full ownership of the community, building awareness among the village community on the management of drinking water projects, including better hygiene practices and encouraging water conservation practices along with rainwater harvesting.

Swajaldhara has two components : Swajaldhara I (First Dhara) is for a gram panchayat or a group of panchayats (at block / tahsil level) and Swajaldhara II (Second Dhara) has district as the project area. District water and sanitation mission sanctions swajaldhara I. The panchayats and communities have the power to plan, implement, operate, maintain and manage all water supply and sanitation schemes. There is an integrated service delivery mechanism, taking up conservation measures through rain water harvesting and ground water recharge systems for sustained drinking water supply and shifting the role of government from direct service delivery to that of planning, policy formulation, monitoring and evaluation and partial financial support. On completion of the project, gram panchayat or village water and sanitation committee manages the project.

The programme was revised from 1st April 2009 and named as National Rural Drinking Water Programme *(60)*. It is now a component of Bharat Nirman which focuses on the creation of rural infrastructure.

Bharat Nirman

Bharat Nirman was launched by the Government of India in 2005 as a programme to build rural infrastructure. While phase-I was implemented in the period of 2005–06 to 2008–09, the phase-II was implemented from 2009–10 to 2011–12. At the beginning of phase-I period, priority was given to cover water quality problem and other contaminants, e.g., arsenic and fluoride affected habitations followed by iron, salinity, nitrate.

New initiatives in 12th Five Year Plan

1. In order to raise coverage of piped water supply, toilet coverage and strengthening of institutions and systems in rural drinking water and rural sanitation sectors the Ministry has proposed a Rural Water Supply and Sanitation Project for low income states;
2. Enhancement of service levels for rural water supply from the norm of 40 lpcd to 55 lpcd for designing of system. The target being at least 50 per cent of rural population in the country to have access to water within their household premises or within 100 metres radius, with at least 30 per cent having individual household connections, as against 13 per cent today *(76)*.

Rural Sanitation Programme *(76)*

Nirmal Bharat Abhiyan (NBA)

In 2012, a paradigm shift was made in the Total Sanitation Campaign, by launching the Nirmal Bharat Abhiyan, in the 12th Five Year Plan. The objective of NBA is to achieve sustainable behavioural change with provision of sanitary facilities in entire communities in a phased manner, saturation mode with "Nirmal Grams" as outcomes.

Swachh Bharat Mission

Swachh Bharat Abhiyan or Swachh Bharat Mission is a national campaign by the government of India to clean streets, roads and infrastructure of the country. The campaign was officially launched by Prime Minister of India on 2nd Oct, 2014, at Rajghat, New Delhi. It aims to eradicate open defecation by year 2019, by constructing 12 million toilets in rural India. Mission has two sub-missions, namely, Swachh Bharat Mission Urban, and Swachh Bharat Mission Gramin.

Swachh Bharat Mission Gramin (SBM-G) (77)

The Mission in rural India will mean improving the level of cleanliness in rural areas through solid and liquid waste management and making gram panchayats free of open defecation, clean and sanitized. The programme includes the key components of earlier sanitation schemes.

The key objectives of the programme are as follows:

(a) Bring about an improvement in the general quality of life in the rural areas, by promoting cleanliness, hygiene and eliminating open defecation;

(b) Accelerate sanitation coverage in rural area to achieve the vision of Swachh Bharat by 2nd October 2019;

(c) Motivate Communities and Panchayati Raj Institutions to adopt sustainable sanitation practices and facilities through awareness creation and health education;

(d) Encourage cost effective and appropriate technologies for ecologically safe and sustainable sanitation; and

(e) Develop wherever required, community managed sanitation systems focusing on scientific solid & liquid waste management systems for overall cleanliness in the rural areas.

The key components of SBM-G include, start up activities including preparation of state plan; construction of household toilets; construction of community sanitary complexes; and capacity building of functionaries etc. Under the programme, construction of toilets in government schools and anganwadi centres will be done by the Ministry of Human Resource Development and Ministry of Women and Child Development respectively. Rural School sanitation focusing on separate toilets for girls and boys is a major intervention which shall be implemented under the programmes of the Department of School Education.

A duly completed household sanitary toilet shall comprise of toilet unit including a substructure which is sanitary (that safely confines human faeces and eliminates the need of human handling before it is fully decomposed), a super structure, with water facility and hand wash unit for cleaning and hand washing. The Mission aims that all rural families have access to toilets. Incentives for construction of household toilets will be available for below poverty line households, and above poverty line households restricted to SCs/STs, small and marginal farmers, landless labourers, physically handicapped and women headed families.

Swachh Bharat Mission–Urban (78)

Swachh Bharat Mission–Urban (SBM-U) is being implemented by Ministry of Urban Development. The main objectives of the mission are as follows:

1. Elimination of open defecation;
2. Eradication of manual scavenging;
3. Modern and scientific municipal solid waste management;
4. To effect behavioural change regarding healthy sanitation practices;
5. Generate awareness about sanitation and its linkage with public health;
6. Capacity augmentation for ULB's; and
7. To create an enabling environment for private sector participation in Capex (capital expenditure) and Opex (operation and maintenance).

Mission components

The Mission has the following components:

1. Household toilets, including conversion of insanitary latrines into pour-flush latrines;
2. Community toilets;
3. Public toilets;
4. Solid waste management;
5. IEC & public awareness; and
6. Capacity building and administrative & office expenses.

By Public Toilets, it is implied that these are to be provided for the floating population/ general public in places such as markets, train station, tourist places, near office complexes, or other public areas where there are considerable number of people passing by.

By Community Toilets, it is implied that a shared facility provided by and for a group of residents or an entire settlement. Community toilet blocks are used primarily in low-income and/or informal settlements / slums, where space and/or land are constraints in providing a household toilet, These are for a more or less fixed user group.

All statutory towns will be covered under the mission. The special focus group under the mission are as follows:

i. All manual scavengers in urban areas are identified, insanitary toilets linked to their employment are upgraded to sanitary toilets, and the manual scavengers are adequately rehabilitated;
ii. In their efforts to streamline and formalize SWM systems it shall be the endeavor of ULBs that the informal sector workers in waste management (rag pickers) are given priority to upgrade their work conditions and are enumerated and integrated into the formal system of SWM in cities;
iii. All temporary accommodation for migrants and the homeless in urban areas have adequate provision for toilets either on the premises or linked to a public/ community toilet;
iv. Mandating that construction labour in urban areas have access to temporary toilets at all sites in urban areas, buildings, parks and roads where construction / maintenance work is taking place or where construction labour is temporarily housed; and
v. Priority shall be accorded pro-actively to cover households with vulnerable sections such as pensioners, girl children, pregnant and lactating mothers.

Household toilet component of SBM-Urban

SBM (Urban) aims to ensure that –

(a) No households engage in the practice of open defecation;
(b) No new insanitary toilets are constructed during the mission period; and
(c) Pit latrines are converted to sanitary latrines.

The target group for construction of household units of toilets, thus, is:

(i) 80% of urban households engaging in open defecation;
(ii) All households with insanitary latrines; and
(iii) All households with single-pit latrines.

These will be targeted under this component for the construction of household toilets or individual household latrines during the mission period. The remaining 20% of households practicing open defecation will be catered by community toilets, due to constraints of space.

Household toilets constructed under SBM (Urban) will have two main structures – the toilet superstructure (including the pan and water closet), and the sub- structure, either an on-site treatment system or a connection to existing underground sewerage system.

Solid waste management component of SBM–Urban

Municipal Solid Waste Management (MSWM) refers to a systematic process that comprises of waste segregation and storage at source, primary collection, secondary storage, transportation, secondary segregation, resource recovery, processing, treatment, and final disposal of solid waste.

PRADHAN MANTRI AWAS YOJNA (URBAN)

Ministry of Housing and Urban Affair (MOHUA) launched the Pradhan Mantri Awas Yojna-Urban (PMAY-U) on 25th June, 2015, as a flagship mission of Government of India. It addresses urban housing shortage among the Economically Weaker Section (EWS)/Low Income Group (LIG) category including slum dwellers by ensuring a pucca house to eligible urban households. An eligible beneficiary family will comprise of a husband, wife, unmarried sons and /or unmarried daughters. The beneficiary family should not own a Pakka House (an all whether dwelling unit) either in his/ her name or in the name of any member of his/her family in any part of India. An adult earning member (irrespective of marital status) can be treated as separate household.

PMAY-U adopts a demand driven approach wherein the housing shortage is decided based on demand assessment by States/Union territories (UTs). All houses built or acquired or purchased under the mission have basic amenities like kitchen, water supply, electricity and toilet. The mission promotes woman empowerment by providing the ownership of houses in the name of female members or in joint name. Preference is also given to women (with overriding preference to widows, single woman) persons belonging to Scheduled Caste/Scheduled Tribes/Other Backward Classes, Minorities, Persons with disability and Transgender *(80)*.

MINIMUM NEEDS PROGRAMME

The Minimum Needs Programme (MNP) was introduced in the first year of the Fifth Five Year Plan (1974–78). The objective of the programme is to provide certain basic minimum needs and thereby improve the living standards of the people. It is the expression of the commitment of the government for the "social and economic development of the community particularly the underprivileged and underserved population". The programme includes the following components :

a. Rural Health
b. Rural Water Supply
c. Rural Electrification
d. Elementary Education
e. Adult Education
f. Nutrition
g. Environmental improvement of Urban Slums
h. Houses for landless labourers

There are two basic principles which are to be observed in the implementation of MNP : (a) the facilities under MNP are to be first provided to those areas which are at present underserved so as to remove disparities between different areas; (b) the facilities under MNP should be provided as a package to an area through intersectoral area projects, to have a greater impact.

In the field of **rural health**, the objectives to be achieved by the end of the Eighth Five Year Plan, under the minimum needs programme were : one PHC for 30,000 population in plains and 20,000 population in tribal and hilly areas; one sub-centre for a population of 5,000 people in the plains and for 3000 in tribal and hilly areas, and one community health centre (rural hospital) for a population of one lakh or one C.D. Block by the year 2000. The establishment of PHCs, sub-centres, upgradation of PHCs, and construction of buildings thereof are all included in the State sector of the minimum needs programme.

In the field of **nutrition,** the objectives are: (a) to extend nutrition support to 11 million eligible persons; (b) to expand "special nutrition programme" to all the ICDS projects; and (c) to consolidate the mid-day meal programme and link it to health, potable water and sanitation.

20-POINT PROGRAMME

In addition to the Five Year Plans and Programmes, in 1975, the Govt. of India initiated a special activity. This was the 20-Point programme – described as an **agenda** for national action to promote social justice and economic growth.

On August 20, 1986, and again in 2006, the existing 20-Point Programme was restructured. Its objectives are spelt out by the Government as "eradication of poverty, raising productivity, reducing inequalities, removing social and economic disparities and improving the quality of life".

The 20 points of twenty point programme 2006 are as follows *(79)*:

1. Poverty eradication
2. Power to people
3. Support to farmers
4. Labour welfare
5. Food security
6. Housing for all
7. Clean drinking water
8. Health for all
9. Education for all
10. Welfare of scheduled castes, scheduled tribes, minorities and OBCs
11. Women welfare
12. Child welfare
13. Youth development
14. Improvement of slums
15. Environment protection and afforestation
16. Social security
17. Rural roads
18. Energization of rural area
19. Development of backward areas
20. IT enabled E-Governance

The restructured 20–Point Programme constitutes the Charter for the country's socio-economic development. It has been described as "the cutting edge of the plan for the poor".

References

1. Govt. of India (2014), *Annual Report 2013-14,* Ministry of Health and Family Welfare, New Delhi.
2. Govt. of India (2012), *Strategic Action Plan for Malaria Control in India 2012-2017,* Scaling up malaria control interventions with a focus on high burden areas, Directorate of National Vector Borne Disease Control Programme, DGHS, Ministry of Health and Family Welfare, New Delhi.
3. Govt. of India (2010), *Annual Report 2009-2010,* DGHS, Ministry of Health and Family Welfare, New Delhi.
4. Govt. of India (2016), *Operational Manual for Malaria Elimination in India 2016 (Version 1),* Directorate of NVBDCP, Ministry of Health and Family Welfare, New Delhi.
5. Govt. of India (2016), *National Framework for Malaria Elimination in India (2016–2030),* Directorate of NVBDCP, Ministry of Health and Family Welfare, New Delhi.
6. Govt. of India (2022), *Annual Report 2021–2022,* Ministry of Health and Family Welfare, New Delhi.
7. Govt. of India (2018), *Annual Report 2017–2018,* Ministry of Health and Family Welfare, New Delhi.
8. Govt. of India (2014), *Press Information Bureau, 2nd Sept. 2014,* Ministry of Health and Family Welfare, New Delhi.
9. Govt. of India (2006), *Annual Report 2005-06,* Ministry of Health and Family Welfare, New Delhi.
10. Rao, C.K. (1987). *Ind. J. Lep.,* 59 (2) 203.
11. Govt. of India (2020), *Annual Report 2019–2020,* Ministry of Health and Family Welfare, New Delhi.
12. Govt. of India (2012), *Disability Prevention and Medical Rehabilitation, Guidelines for Primary,secondary and tertiary level care,* NLEP, DGHS, Ministry of Health and Family Welfare, New Delhi.
13. Govt. of India (2014), *Programme Implementation Plan (PIP) for 12th Plan Period (2012–13 to 2016–17),* Central Leprosy Division, DGHS, Ministry of Health and Family Planning, New Delhi.
14. National Leprosy Eradication Programmme (2017), *Annual Report for year 2016–2017.*
15. Govt. of India (2021), *Nation Wide Implementation of Disease Eradication Programme,* Press release page, 7th Dec. 2021.
16. *Indian Journal of Leprosy,* vol. 78, No. 1, Jan-March 2006.
17. Govt. of India (2012), *TB India 2012,* RNTCP Status Report, Ministry of Health and Family Welfare, New Delhi.
18. Govt. of India (2020), *Training Module (1–4) for programme managers and medical officers,* NTEP.
19. Govt. of India (2014), *T.B. India 2014,* RNTCP Annual Status Report, Central TB Division, DGHS, Ministry of Health and Family Welfare, New Delhi.
20. Govt. of India (2012), *Notification dated 7th May 2012 regarding TB cases,* Ministry of Health and Family Welfare, New Delhi.
21. Govt. of India (2021), *Guidelines for Progrmmatic Management of Drug Resistant Tuberculosis in India,* March 2021, Central TB Division, Ministry of Health and Family Welfare, New Delhi.
22. RNTCP (2017), *Guidelines on Programmatic Management of Drug Resistant Tuberculosis in India,* Ministry of Health and Family Welfare, New Delhi.
23. Govt. of India (2016), *Technical and Operational Guidelines for Tuberculosis Control in India 2016, RNTPC,* Ministry of Health and Family Welfare, New Delhi.

23A. Govt. of India (2007), *NACP III, To Halt and Reverse the HIV Epidemic in India,* NACO, Ministry of Health and Family Welfare, New Delhi.

24. Govt. of India (2022), *India TB Report 2022,* Central TB Division, Ministry of Health and Family Welfare, New Delhi.
25. Govt. of India (2013), *T.B. India 2013,* RNTCP Annual Status Report, Central TB Division, DGHS, Ministry of Health and Family Welfare, New Delhi.
26. RNTCP (2018), *TB India 2018,* Ministry of Health and Family Welfare, New Delhi.
27. Govt. of India (2013), *National AIDS Control Programme Phase-IV (2012–2017),* Strategy Document, Dept of AIDS Control, Ministry of Health and Family Welfare, New Delhi.
28. NACO (2017), *National Strategic Plan for HIV/AIDS and STI 2017–2024,* Paving way for an AIDS Free India, Dec.1.2017.
29. Govt. of India (2006), *National AIDS Control Programme Phase III (2007-12),* Strategy and Implementation Plan, NACO, Ministry of Health and Family Welfare, New Delhi.

30. Govt. of India (2008), *HIV Sentinel Surveillance Round 2008*, National Action Plan Sept 2008 - June 2009, NACO, Ministry of Health and Family Welfare, New Delhi.
31. NACO (2017), *HIV Sentinary Surveillance 2016–2017*, Technical Brief.
32. NACO (2014), *Annual Report 2013–2014*, Department of AIDS Control, Ministry of Health and Family Welfare, New Delhi.
33. Govt. of India (2013), *National Framework for Joint HIV/TB Collaborative Activities, Nov. 2013*, Central TB Division and NACO, Ministry of Health and Family Welfare, New Delhi.
34. Govt. of India (2021), *National Guidelines for HIV Care and Treatment 2021*, NACO, Ministry of Health and Family Welfare, New Delhi.
35. NACO Website, *National AIDS Prevention and Control Policy*.
36. Govt. of India (2007), *Operational Guidelines for Programme Managers and Service Providers for Strengthening STI/RTI Services*, NACO, Ministry of Health and Family Welfare, New Delhi.
37. Govt. of India (2004), *National Programme for Control of Blindness in India*, Ministry of Health and Family Welfare, New Delhi.
38. WHO (2013), *Universal Eye Health, A Global Action Plan* 2014–2019.
39. Allan, D. (1987). *World Health, Jan-Feb*, 1987, p. 9.
40. Grant, J.P. (1987). *World Health, Jan-Feb*, 1987, p. 10.
41. Govt. of India (2017), *Immunization Handbook for Medical Officers*, Ministry of Health and Family Welfare, New Delhi.
42. Govt. of India (2005), *Health Information 2005*, Ministry of Health and Family Welfare, New Delhi.
43. Govt. of India (1987). *Centre Calling*, Nov. 1987.
44. Govt. of India (2011), *National Health Profile 2011*, DGHS, Ministry of Health and Family Welfare, New Delhi.
45. Govt. of India (2016), *Annual Report 2015–2016*, Ministry of Health and Family Welfare, New Delhi.
46. Govt. of India (2012), *Annual Report 2011-2012*, Ministry of Health and Family Welfare, New Delhi.
47. Govt. of India (2011), *Immunization Hand Book for Health Workers*, Ministry of Health and Family Welfare, New Delhi.
48. Govt. of India (2014), *India Newborn Action Plan (INAP), Sept. 2014*, Ministry of Health and Family Welfare, New Delhi.
49. Govt. of India (2015), Press Release, Ministry of Health and Family Welfare, New Delhi, 24th July 2015, *Achievements under the National Rural Health Mission*.
50. Govt. of India (2013), *Guidelines for Preparing NUHM Programme Implementation Plan (PIP) for 2013–14*, July 2013, Urban Health Division, Department of Health and Family Welfare, New Delhi.
51. Govt. of India (2013), *National Urban Health Mission*, Framework for Implementation, May 2013, Ministry of Health and Family Welfare, New Delhi.
52. Govt. of India (2013), *For Healthy Mother and Child, A Strategic Approach to Reproductive, Maternal, Newborn, Child and Adolescent Health (RMNCH+A) in India*, January 2013, Ministry of Health and Family Welfare, New Delhi.
53. Govt. of India (1997), *Reproductive and Child Health Programme*, Schemes for Implementation October 1997, Department of Family Welfare, Ministry of Health and Family Welfare, New Delhi.
54. Govt. of India (2000), *Annual Report 1999-2000*, Ministry of Health and Family Welfare, New Delhi.
55. Govt. of India (2004), *Annual Report 2003-2004*, Ministry of Health and Family Welfare, New Delhi.
56. Govt. of India (2004), *Guidelines for Operationalising First Referral Units*, Maternal Division, Ministry of Health and Family Welfare, New Delhi.
57. Govt. of India (2018), *Guidelines for community based events (CBE), Poshan Abhiyan*, Ministry of Women and Child Development, New Delhi.
58. Govt. of India (2011), *Operational Guidelines on Facility Based Management of children with Severe Acute Malnutrition*, Ministry of Health and Family Welfare, New Delhi.
59. Govt. of India (2011), *Facility Based Newborn Care Operational Guide*, Guidelines for Planning and Implementation, Ministry of Health and Family Welfare, New Delhi.
60. Govt. of India (2014), *Home Based Newborn Care, Revised Operational Guidelines*, Ministry of Health and Family Welfare, New Delhi.
61. WHO (2006), *Working Together for Health*, The World Health Report, 2006.
62. Govt. of India (2013), *Operational Guidelines, Rashtriya Bal Swasthya Karyakram (RBSK), Child Health Screening and early intervention service under NRHM*, Feb. 2013, Ministry of Health and Family Welfare, New Delhi.
63. S. Menon et al (2006), Health Programme Series 10, *Reproductive and Child Health Programme : Flagship Programme of National Rural Health Mission, 2006*.
64. USAID (2013), MCHIP (2014), *India's Reproductive Maternal, Newborn, Child and Adolescent (RMNCH+A) Strategy*, July 2014.
65. Govt. of India (2021), *Reference Manual for Integrated RMNCAH+N Counselling*, Ministry of Health and Family Welfare, New Delhi.
66. Govt. of India (2016), *Operational Guidelines- Prevention, Screening and Control of Common Non-Communicable Diseases: Hypertension, Diabetes, and Common Cancers (Oral, Breast, Cervix) (Part of Comprehensive Primary Health Care)*, Ministry of Health and Family Welfare, New Delhi.
67. Govt. of India (2013), *National Action Plan and Monitoring Framework for Prevention and Control of Non-communicable Diseases (NCDs) in India, Developed through the WHO- Government of India, 2012– 2013 Biennial Workplan*, Ministry of Health and Family Welfare, New Delhi.
68. *National Institute of Health and Family Welfare, website*, Legislations, National Mental Health Programme.
69. Govt. of India (2005), *Integrated Disease Surveillance Project*, Training Manual for state and District Surveillance Officers, Ministry of Health and Family Welfare, New Delhi.
70. Govt. of India, *Training Manual for State and District Surveillance Officers*, Integrated Disease Surveillance Project, Module-8.
71. WHO (2000), *Weekly Epidemiological Record*, No.22, 2nd June 2000.
72. Ministry of Finance Press release 2018.
73. *National Institute of Health and Family Welfare, website*, Legislations, National Programme for Control and Treatment of Occupational Diseases.
74. Bookhive's, *8th Five Year Plan (1992-97)* by E. Chandran, Issues of Current Interest, Series No. 4.
75. Swajaldhara, *Deptt of drinking water supply, Ministry of Rural Development*, GOI, website http://ddws.nic.in / swajaldhara / html / faq.htm.
76. Govt. of India (2014), *Annual Report 2013–14*, Ministry of Drinking Water and Sanitation, New Delhi.
77. Govt. of India (2014), *Swachh Bharat Mission (Gramin) Guidelines*, Ministry of Drinking Water and Sanitation, New Delhi.
78. Govt. of India (2014), *Guidelines for Swachh Bharat Mission*, Ministry of Urban Development, New Delhi.
79. Govt. of India (2016), *Twenty Point Programme-2006*, Progress Report for the period of April 2016-June 2016.
80. Govt. of India (2022), *Years of Pradhan Mantri Awas Yojana-Urban, 2015–2022*, Ministry of Housing and Urban Affairs, New Delhi.

8 Demography and Family Planning

"Delay the first, postpone the second and prevent the third"

Demography, as understood today, is the scientific study of human population. It focuses its attention on three readily observable human phenomena : (a) *changes* in population size (growth or decline); (b) the *composition* of the population; and (c) the *distribution* of population in space. It deals with five "demographic processes", namely fertility, mortality, marriage, migration and social mobility. These five processes are continuously at work within a population determining size, composition and distribution.

Community medicine is vitally concerned with population, because health in the group depends upon the dynamic relationship between the numbers of people, the space which they occupy and the skill that they have acquired in providing for their needs. The main sources of demographic statistics in India are population censuses, National Sample Surveys, registration of vital events, and adhoc demographic studies.

Demographic cycle

The history of world population since 1650 suggests that there is a demographic cycle of 5 stages through which a nation passes:

(1) FIRST STAGE (High stationary)

This stage is characterized by a high birth rate and a high death rate which cancel each other and the population remains stationary. India was in this stage till 1920.

(2) SECOND STAGE (Early expanding)

The death rate begins to decline, while the birth rate remains unchanged. Many countries in South Asia and Africa are in this phase. Birth rates have increased in some of these countries possibly as a result of improved health conditions and shortening periods of breast-feeding *(1)*.

(3) THIRD STAGE (Late expanding)

The death rate declines still further, and the birth rate tends to fall. The population continues to grow because births exceed deaths. India has entered this phase. In a number of developing countries (e.g., China, Singapore) birth rates have declined rapidly.

(4) FOURTH STAGE (Low stationary)

This stage is characterized by a low birth and low death rate with the result that the population becomes stationary. Zero population growth has already been recorded in Austria during 1980–85. Growth rates as little as 0.1 were recorded in UK, Denmark, Sweden and Belgium during 1980–85. In short, most industrialized countries have undergone a demographic transition shifting from a high birth and high death rates to low birth and low death rates.

(5) FIFTH STAGE : (Declining)

The population begins to decline because birth rate is lower than the death rate. Some East European countries, notably Germany and Hungary are experiencing this stage.

WORLD POPULATION TRENDS

At the beginning of the Christian era, nearly 2,000 years ago, world population was estimated to be around 250 million. Subsequent estimates of the world population, and rates of increase are given in Table 1.

TABLE 1
World population

Year	Population (million)	Average annual growth rate (per cent)
1750	791	–
1800	978	0.4
1850	1,262	0.5
1900	1,650	0.6
1950	2,526	1.1
1960	3,037	1.79
1970	3,696	1.92
1975	4,066	1.89
1980	4,432	1.72
1987	5,000	1.63
1991	5,385	1.7
1998	5,884	1.6
2000	6,054	1.4
2003	6,313	1.1
2007	6,655	1.4
2008	6,734	1.2
2010	6,908	1.23
2014	7,238	1.2
2016	7,418	1.2
2018	7,621	1.2
2019	7,715	1.1
2022	7,948	1.23

It required all the human history up to the year 1800 for the world population to reach one billion. The second billion came in 130 years (around 1930), the third billion in 30 years (around 1960), the fourth billion in 15 years (in 1974), the fifth billion in 12 years (in 1987), and the sixth billion in 12 years (1999). The 7th billion came by 31st Oct. 2011 (after 15 years). It is projected to reach 8 billion on 15th Nov. 2022.

About three fourths of the world's population lives in the developing countries. The population of the ten most populous countries of the world and their relative share is shown in Fig. 1. Although, in terms of population USA ranks

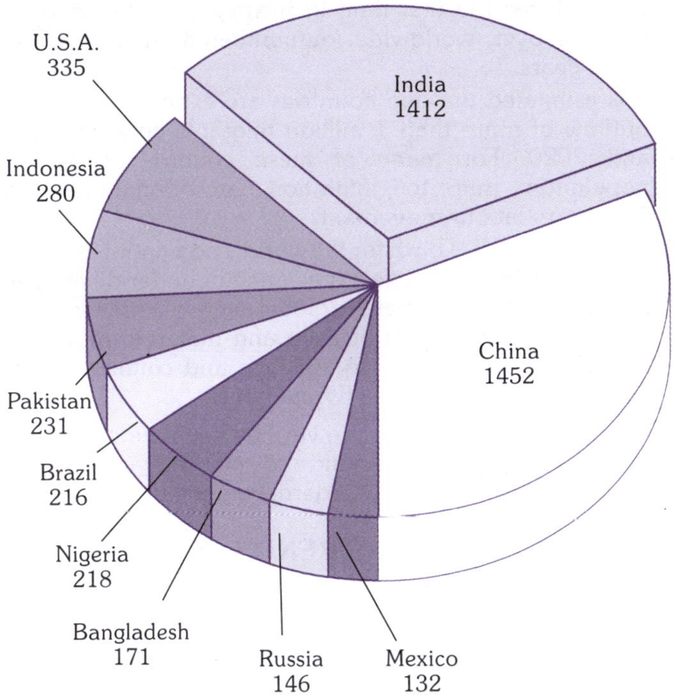

FIG. 1

Ten most populated countries of the world (mid-2022)

Source : *(2)*

third in the world after India, there is a yawning gap of 1076 million between the population of these two countries. The United Nations has estimated that world's population is growing at an annual rate of 1.1 per cent in the year 2022.

Three countries of SEAR, i.e. India (1412 million), Indonesia (280 million), and Bangladesh (171 million) are among the most populous ten countries of the world. At present India's population is second to that of China. According to UN projections, India's population will reach 1.53 billion by the year 2050, and will be the highest population country in the world. The trend of population increase in South East Asia Region countries is as shown in Table 2.

TABLE 2

Trends in increase of population of SEAR countries (in million)

Country	1991	Nov. 2022
India	843.9	1,412.0
Bangladesh	118	171.8
Bhutan	1.5	0.84
Indonesia	187.7	273.1
Maldives	0.221	0.523
Myanmar	42.5	54.32
Nepal	19.6	30.7
Sri Lanka	17.4	21.85
Thailand	56.4	71.73

Source : *(2)*

Birth and death rates

The glaring contrasts in birth and death rates in selected countries are as shown in Table 3.

TABLE 3

Birth and death rates in selected developed and developing countries in mid-2022

Country	Birth rate	Death rate
India	18.7	7.20
Bangladesh	18.6	5.50
Pakistan	21.6	7.00
Sri Lanka	14.8	6.60
Thailand	11.0	7.60
Myanmar	17.7	8.20
Nepal	19.1	6.40
China	12.1	7.10
Japan	8.0	10.40
Singapore	8.7	4.40
UK	12.0	9.40
USA	12.4	8.70

Source : *(2)*

The world's birth rate fell below 30 for the first time around 1975 and had declined to about 17.6 during mid-2022 *(3)*. In most of the world the decline reflected falling birth rates and a global trend towards smaller families. The outstanding examples are Singapore and Thailand. In Singapore, in 50 years, the birth rate fell from 23 per thousand in 1970 to 4.4 in 2022; and in Thailand from 37 per thousand to 7.6 during the same period.

TABLE 4

Reduction in the birth and death rates in selected countries, 1990 – mid-2022

Country	Birth rate		Death rate	
	1990	2022	1990	mid-2022
Bangladesh	35	18.6	10	5.5
Nepal	38	19.1	13	6.4
India	31	18.7	11	7.2
Sri Lanka	21	14.8	7	6.6
Thailand	19	11.0	8	7.6
Singapore	18	8.7	5	4.4
China	23	12.1	8	10.4
Pakistan	40	21.6	11	7.0

Source : *(2)*

In all these countries, key factors in fertility decline included changes in government attitudes towards growth, the spread of education, increased availability of contraception and the extension of services offered through family planning programmes, as well as the marked change in marriage patterns.

Death rates have also declined worldwide over the last decades. The global death rate declined from 11.0 (between 1975–1980) to 7.678 per thousand population during 2022, a reduction of 30.2 per cent. The decline in the death rate of the South-East Asia Region has been more marked, from 14.1 to 7.0 per 1000 population.

In countries with a relative young population, crude death rates are mainly affected by infant and child mortality. With improvement in maternal and child health services, successful implementation of the expanded programme on immunization, diarrhoeal disease and acute respiratory infection control programmes, as well as with the control of other infectious diseases, there has been marked reduction in infant and child mortality rates, which are reflected in the declining crude death rates.

Growth rates

When the crude death rate is substracted from the crude birth rate, the net residual is the current annual growth rate, exclusive of migration. The relation between the growth rate and population increase is as shown in Table 5.

TABLE 5

Relation between growth rate and population

Rating	Annual rate of growth %	Number of years required for the population to double in size
Stationary population	No growth	
Slow growth	Less than 0.5	More than 139
Moderate growth	0.5 to 1.0	139–70
Rapid growth	1.0 to 1.5	70–47
Very rapid growth	1.5 to 2.0	47–35
"Explosive" growth	2.0 to 2.5	35–28
-----"-----	2.5 to 3.0	28–23
-----"-----	3.0 to 3.5	23–20
-----"-----	3.5 to 4.0	20–18

Source : *(4)*

It is said that population growth rates, like railway trains, are subject to momentum. They start slowly and gain momentum. Once in motion, it takes time to bring the momentum under control. In case of the train the control factors are mass and inertia; in population, they are age distribution, marriage customs and numerous cultural, social and economic factors.

The world population growth rate was at, or near to its peak, around 1970, when the human population grew by an estimated 1.92 per cent. The most recent data shows a slight decline since then to 1.1 per cent in mid 2022.

The growth rate is not uniform in the world. There are many countries in the world (e.g., European countries) where the growth rate is less than 0.3 per cent per year. In developing countries, the growth rates are excessive – it is around 2.6 per cent in Africa, 1.0 per cent in Latin America, 0.3 per cent in Europe and industrialized countries, and 0.9 per cent in Asia. A population growing at 0.5 per cent per year will double in about 140 years, a population growing at 3 per cent per year will double in about 20–25 years (Table 5). These differences in growth rates are largely the result of fertility and mortality patterns. The salient features of population growth at a glance are as follows *(5)*:

1. The world's population continues to grow, albeit at a slower pace than at any time since 1950, owing to reduced levels of fertility. From an estimated 7.7 billion people worldwide in 2019 to around 8.5 billion in 2030, 9.7 billion in 2050 and 10.9 billion in 2100.
2. Countries of Sub-Saharan Africa could account for more than half of the growth of the world's population between 2019 and 2050.
3. More than half of the projected increase in global population will be concentrated in just nine countries: The Democratic Republic of the Congo, Egypt, Ethiopia, India, Indonesia, Nigeria, Pakistan, United Republic of Tanzania, and the USA. India is projected to surpass China as world's most populous country around 2027.
4. In most of Sub-Saharan Africa, as well as in parts of Asia, Latin America and Caribbean, recent reductions of fertility means that the population at working ages (25–64 years) is growing faster than in other age groups, providing an opportunity for accelerated economic growth known as the "demographic dividend".
5. In 2018, for the first time in history, persons aged 65 years or over, worldwide, outnumbered children under age 5 years.
6. It is estimated that ten countries are experiencing a net outflow of more than 1 million migrants between 2010 and 2020. For many of these countries losses of population due to migration are dominated by temporary labour movements.
7. Life expectancy at birth for the world's population reached 72.6 years in 2019. Life expectancy in under developed countries is 7.4 years behind global average, due largely to persistently high levels of child and maternal mortality, and in some countries, to violence and conflict, or the continuing impact of the HIV epidemic.

The rampant population growth has been viewed as the greatest obstacle to the economic and social advancement of the majority of people in the underdeveloped world.

DEMOGRAPHIC TRENDS IN INDIA

Demographic indicators

Demographic characteristics provide an overview of its population size, composition, territorial distribution, changes therein and the components of changes such as nativity, mortality and social mobility. Demographic indicators have been divided into two parts–population statistics and vital statistics.

Population statistics include indicators that measure the population size, sex ratio, density and dependency ratio.

Vital statistics include indicators such as birth rate, death rate, natural growth rate, life expectancy at birth, mortality and fertility rates.

These indicators help in identifying areas that need policy and programmed interventions, setting near and far-term goals and deciding priorities, besides understanding them in an integrated structure.

With a population of 1,412 million in the year mid 2022, India is the second most populous country in the world, next only to China, whereas seventh in land area. With only 2.4 per cent of the world's land area, India is supporting about 17.5 per cent of the world's population. The population of India since 1901, averaged annual exponential growth rate (%), and the decadal growth of population (%) was as shown in Table 6.

TABLE 6

Population of India, 1901–2011 (As per census)

Year	Total population (in million)	Average annual exponential growth rate (%)	Decadal growth rate (%)
1901	238.4	–	–
1911	252.1	0.56	0.75
1921	251.3	(–) 0.03	(–) 0.31
1931	279.0	1.04	11.00
1941	318.7	1.33	14.22
1951	361.1	1.25	13.31
1961	439.2	1.96	21.64
1971	548.2	2.20	24.80
1981	683.3	2.22	24.66
1991	846.4	2.16	23.87
2001	1,028.6	1.7	21.52
2011	1,210.1	1.64	17.64

Source : *(6)*

India's population has been steadily increasing since 1921. The year 1921 is called the "big divide" because the absolute number of people added to the population during each decade has been on the increase since 1921 (Table 6). India's population is currently increasing at the rate of 16 million each year.

India's population numbered 238 million in 1901, doubled in 60 years to 439 million (1961); doubled again, this time in only 30 years to reach 846 million by 1991. It crossed 1 billion mark on 11 May 2000, and is projected to reach 1.53 billion by the year 2050. This will then make India the most populous country in the world, surpassing China.

With the division of some states the rank of most populous states have changed. Table 7 shows the ten most populous states in the country by rank. It is seen that Uttar Pradesh comes first with about 231.425 million people, Maharashtra comes second with 128.711 million people and Bihar comes third with 108.377 million people. These ten states account for about 71 per cent of the total population of India *(7)*.

TABLE 7
Ranking of most populous states by projected population size 2020

Rank	State	Population 2020 (000)	Per cent to total population of India 2020
1.	Uttar Pradesh	231,425	16.7
2.	Maharashtra	128,711	9.0
3.	Bihar	108,377	7.8
4.	Andhra Pradesh	90,949	6.5
5.	Madhya Pradesh	82,134	5.9
6.	Rajasthan	76,759	5.5
7.	Tamil Nadu	70,617	5.0
8.	Gujarat	65,532	4.7
9.	Karnataka	64,410	4.6
10.	Odisha	43,732	3.1

Source : *(8)*

It has been estimated that with current trends, the population in India will increase from 1.210 billion to 1.4 billion during the period 2011 to 2026. There is a substantial difference in total fertility rate in between and within states. At one end of spectrum are southern states like Kerala, Tamil Nadu, Karnataka and Andhra Pradesh with total fertility rate at or below replacement levels. At the other end are high fertility states like Uttar Pradesh, Chhattisgarh, Uttarakhand, Rajasthan, Jharkhand, Bihar, Madhya Pradesh and Orissa, with an estimated total fertility rate of more than 2.2.

The Government of India has categorized states according to total fertility rate (TFR) level into very high-focus (more than or equal to 3.0), high-focus (more than 2.1 and less than 3.0) and non-high focus (less than or equal to 2.1) categories. The states categorized as very high-focus and high focus are as follows *(9)*:

TFR 2.2-3.0	–	Assam–2.3, Dadra & Nagar Haveli–2.3, Mizoram–2.3, Chhattisgarh–2.5, Jharkhand–2.6, Manipur–2.6, Rajasthan–2.7, Nagaland–2.7, Madhya Pradesh–2.8
TFR more than or equal to 3.0	–	Bihar–3.3, Uttar Pradesh–3.1 and Meghalaya–3.0

It is matter of concern that these states will delay the attainment of replacement level of fertility in India. These high fertility states are anticipated to contribute about 50 per cent to the nation-wide increase in population. Demographic outcomes in these states will determine the timing and size of population at which India achieves population stabilization.

Age and sex composition

The age–sex composition of India's population is as shown in Table 8. In the age group 0–14 years male population is about 1.1 per cent more than female, whereas in the age group 60+, percentage of female population is 0.6 per cent more than male population. The proportion of population in the age group 0–14 years is higher in rural areas (26.5 per cent) than in urban areas (21.5 per cent), for both male and female population *(10)*.

The proportion of population below 14 years of age is showing decline, whereas the proportion of elderly in the country is increasing. This trend is to continue in the time to come. The increase in the elderly population will impose a greater burden on the already outstretched health services in the country.

TABLE 8
Per cent distribution of estimated population by age and sex, India (2020)

Age group	Population percentage		
	Total	Males	Females
0–4	7.5	7.7	7.4
5–9	8.3	8.4	8.1
10–14	9.0	9.2	8.9
15–19	10.2	10.4	9.9
20–24	11.2	11.0	11.4
25–29	10.5	10.4	10.7
30–34	8.8	8.8	8.7
35–39	7.4	7.4	7.5
40–44	6.2	6.2	6.2
45–49	5.2	5.2	5.3
50–54	4.2	4.2	4.1
55–59	3.4	3.3	3.5
60–64	2.9	2.9	3.0
65–69	2.1	2.1	2.2
70–74	1.4	1.4	1.5
75–79	0.9	0.8	0.9
80–84	0.5	0.4	0.5
85+	0.3	0.2	0.3
Total	100.0	100.0	100.0

Note : * Total may not add upto 100 due to rounding off.

Source : *(10)*

Population pyramid

Population pyramid is also known as "Age and Sex" pyramid. It is a graphical representation of the age and sex of a population. It shows the distribution of ages across a population divided down the center between male and female members of the population. The graphic starts from the youngest at the bottom to oldest at the top. It is called a pyramid because when a population is growing (there are more babies being born then there are people dying) the graphic forms the shape of a triangle. A population pyramid can be used to compare difference between male and female population of an area. They also show the number of dependents and general structure of the population at any given time *(11)*.

Fig. 2 shows age and sex pyramid of India and Switzerland. The pyramid is typical of developing countries, with a broad base and a tapering top.

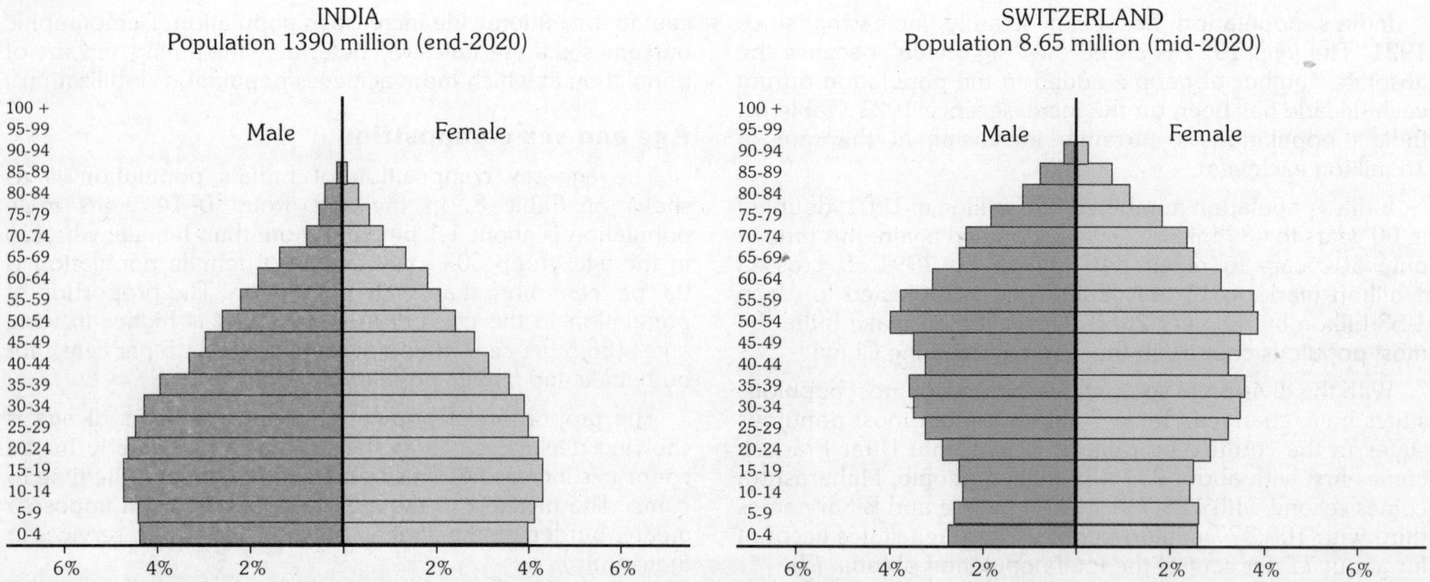

FIG. 2

Percentage distribution by age of the population of India and of the population of Switzerland.

Sex ratio

Sex ratio is defined as "the number of females per 1000 males". One of the basic demographic characteristics of the population is the sex composition. In any study of population, analysis of the sex composition plays a vital role. The sex composition of the population is affected by the differentials in mortality conditions of males and females, sex selective migration and sex ratio at birth. "Female deficit syndrome" is considered adverse because of social implications. A low sex ratio indicates strong male–child preference and consequent gender inequities, neglect of the girl child resulting in higher mortality at younger age, female infanticide, female foeticide, higher maternal mortality and male bias in enumeration of population. Easy availability of the sex determination tests and abortion services may also be proving to be catalyst in the process, which may be further stimulated by preconception sex selection facilities.

The trends in the sex ratio in the country from 1901 onwards are as shown in Table 9.

TABLE 9

Sex ratio in India

Year	Females per 1000 males
1901	972
1911	964
1921	955
1931	950
1941	945
1951	946
1961	941
1971	930
1981	934
1991	927
2001	933
2011	940

Source : *(6)*

The sex ratio in India has been generally adverse to women, i.e., the number of women per 1,000 men has generally been less than 1,000. Apart from being adverse to women, the sex ratio has also declined over the decades.

Sex ratio at birth : The sex ratio at birth for the country for the period 2018–20 (3-years average) has been estimated at 907. At National level, it is 907 in rural areas and 910 in urban areas. Among the bigger States/UTs, the sex ratio at birth varies from 974 in Kerala to 844 in Uttarakhand. In the rural areas, the highest and the lowest sex ratio at birth are in the States of Kerala (973) and Uttarakhand (853) respectively. The sex ratio at birth in urban areas varies from 975 in Kerala to 821 in Uttarakhand. Table 10 shows the variation in sex ratio at birth by residence among bigger States/UTs in the country.

TABLE 10

Sex Ratio (female per 1000 male) at birth by residence, India and bigger states/UTs, 2018–2020

Bigger states	Total	Rural	Urban
Andhra Pradesh	926	930	919
Assam	923	923	930
Bihar	895	894	897
Chhattisgarh	958	970	910
Delhi	860	972	857
Gujarat	877	882	869
Haryana	870	868	874
Himachal Pradesh	950	952	920
Jammu & Kashmir	921	918	930
Jharkhand	914	915	910
Karnataka	916	942	871
Kerala	974	973	975
Madhya Pradesh	919	908	960
Maharashtra	876	881	870
Odisha	925	928	907
Punjab	897	874	932
Rajasthan	911	914	901
Tamil Nadu	917	902	930
Telangana	892	903	875
Uttar Pradesh	905	890	960
Uttaranchal	844	853	821
West Bengal	936	941	920
India	907	907	910

Source : *(10)*

Child sex ratio (0–6 years) : Census 2011 marks a considerable fall in child sex ratio in the age group of 0–6 years and has reached an all time low of 914 since 1961. The fall has been 13 points from 927 to 914 for the country during 2001 to 2011. In rural areas, the fall has been significant – 15 points from 934 to 919 and in urban areas it has been 4 points from 906 to 902 over the decade *(6)*.

Dependency ratio

The proportion of persons above 65 years of age and children below 15 years of age are considered to be dependant on the economically productive age group (15–64 years). The ratio of the combined age groups 0–14 years plus 65 years and above to the 15–65 years age group is referred to as the total dependency ratio. It is also referred to as the **societal dependency ratio** and reflects the need for a society to provide for their younger and older population groups. The dependency ratio can be subdivided into **young age dependency ratio** (0–14 years); and **old age dependency ratio** (65 years and more). These ratios are, however, relatively crude, since they do not take into consideration elderly or young persons who are employed or working age persons who are unemployed. It is given by the formula :

$$\text{Total dependency ratio} = \frac{\text{Children 0–14 years age + Population more than 65 years of age}}{\text{Population of 15 to 64 years}} \times 100$$

For India, the dependency ratio for the year mid-2020 is calculated as :

% of population in 0–14 years age group – 26.2 per cent
% of population above 65 years of age – 6.6 per cent
% of population in 15–64 years age group – 67.3 per cent

$$\text{Total dependency ratio} = \frac{26.2 + 6.6}{67.3} \times 100$$

$$= 48.736 \text{ per cent}$$

The young age dependency ratio is 38.3 per cent, and old age dependency ratio is 9.8 per cent for the year mid 2020 *(12)*.

For international comparison, the child, old and total dependency ratios are used to study the dependency burden of the population. The total dependency ratio tends to decrease in the earlier stages of development when rapid decline in fertility reduces the child population more than the increase in the older persons, but subsequently the increase in older persons far out-weighs the decline in the child population. There is a shift from child dependency to old age dependency, as fertility declines and life expectancy increases.

The rapid decline in dependency ratios, especially the child dependency ratio, has been identified to be a key factor underlying rapid economic development. The term *"demographic bonus"* connotes the period when the dependency ratio in a population declines because of decline in fertility, until it starts to rise again because of increasing longevity. This period depends on the pace of decline in fertility level of a population. If the switch to small families is fast, the demographic bonus can give a considerable push to development. If investment in health care and education for skill development are made during this period, maximum advantage is taken of the demographic transition with high economic growth rates *(13)*.

The term *"demographic burden"* is used to connote the increase in the total dependency ratio during any period of time, mostly caused by increased old age dependency ratio. This is an inevitable consequence of demographic transition, and the country has to face this problem sooner or later *(13)*.

Density of population

One of the important indices of population concentration is the density of population. It is the ratio between (total) population and surface (land) area. This ratio can be calculated for any territorial unit for any point in time, depending on the source of the population data *(13)*. In the Indian census, density is defined as the number of persons, living per square kilometre. The trends of the density in the country from 1901 onwards are as shown in Table 11. For the year 2020 the density of population per sq. km. in India was 464.

TABLE 11

Density of population in India 1901–2011

Year	Per sq.km
1901	77
1911	82
1921	81
1931	90
1941	103
1951	117
1961	142
1971	177
1981	216
1991	267
2001	325
2011	382

Source : *(6)*

Urbanization

By definition, urban population is the number of persons residing in urban localities. The definition of urban locality varies from country to country. In Indian context, the urban areas are the "Towns (places with municipal corporation, municipal area committee, town committee, notified area committee or cantonment board); also, all places having 5,000 or more inhabitants, a density of not less than 1,000 persons per square mile or 390 per square kilometre, pronounced urban characteristics and at least three fourths of the adult male population employed in pursuits other than agriculture" *(13)*.

The population in India continues to be predominantly rural with agriculture as the main occupation for the majority of the people.

As per population totals for the year 2019, the urban population stands at 471.828 million (34.5 per cent). Mumbai is the highest populous city with 12.69 million followed by Delhi 10.927 million, Bengaluru comes third with 5.104 million, Kolkata 4.631 million is fourth and Chennai (4.328 million) is fifth. Fig. 3 indicates the level of urbanization in the country *(14)*.

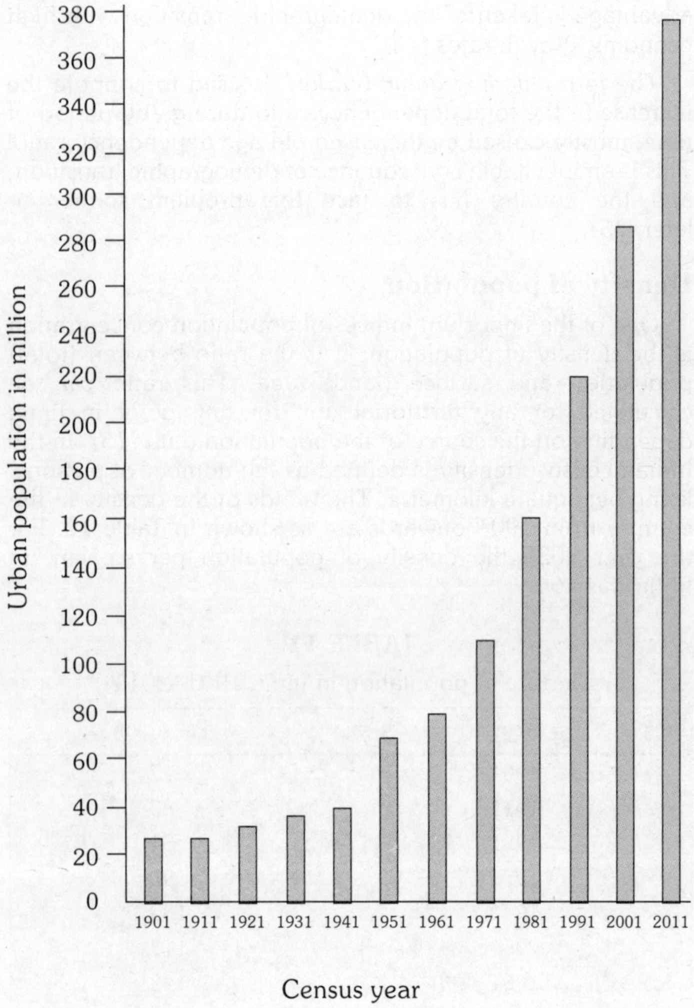

FIG. 3

INDIA – Growth of urban population 1901–2011

The increase in urban population has been attributed both to natural growth (through births) and migration from villages because of employment opportunities, attraction of better living conditions and availability of social services such as education, health, transport, entertainment etc. The continuous migration of people from country side to urban areas in India constitute a social crisis, the ramification of which may eventually impair the quality of life.

The urban-rural scenario in India is as follows *(6)* :

Administrative Units	Census 2011	2020	Increase
No. of States/UTs	35	37	2
No. of Districts	640	741	101
No. of Sub-Districts	5,924	6,553	629
No. of Villages	640,867	664,369	23,502

Family size

While in common parlance, family size refers to the total number of persons in a family, in demography, family size means the **total number of children** a woman has borne at a point in time *(15)*. The completed family size indicates the total number of children borne by a woman during her child-bearing age, which is generally assumed to be between 15 and 45 years. The **total fertility rate** gives the approximate magnitude of the completed family size.

The family size depends upon numerous factors, viz. duration of marriage, education of the couple, the number of live births and living children, preference of male children, desired family size, etc.

The question of family size is undoubtedly important from the demographic point of view. The family planning programme's campaign is currently based on the theme of a "two–child" family norm, with a view to reach the long-term demographic goal of NRR=1. Family planning involves both decision regarding the "desired family size" and the effective limitation of fertility once that size has been reached.

Table 12 shows the total fertility rates (completed family size) in India and selected countries. The decrease in family size does not appear to be due to any reduction in fertility; rather it appears to be due to the result of deliberate family planning.

TABLE 12

Total fertility rates in selected developed and developing countries : 1994 and 2020

Country	1994	2020
India	3.7	1.8
Bangladesh	3.9	2.1
Nepal	4.8	1.9
Sri Lanka	2.3	2.2
Myanmar	3.6	2.2
China	1.9	1.7
Pakistan	5.5	3.6
UK	1.8	1.8
USA	2.0	1.8
Japan	1.5	1.4
Switzerland	1.5	1.5

Source : *(16, 17)*

Literacy and education

In 1948, the Declaration of Human Rights stated that everyone has a right to education. Yet, even today, this right is being denied to millions of children. Education is a crucial element in economic and social development. Without education, development can neither be broad based nor sustained. The benefits that accrue to a country by having a literate population are multidimensional. Spread of literacy is generally associated with modernization, urbanization, industrialization, communication and commerce. It forms an important input in the overall development of individuals enabling them to comprehend their social, political and cultural environment better, and respond to it appropriately. Higher levels of education and literacy lead to a greater awareness and also contribute to improvement of economic conditions, and is a pre-requisite for acquiring various skills and better use of health care facilities.

It was decided in 1991 census to use the term literacy rate for the population relating to seven years age and above. A person is deemed as literate if he or she can read and write with understanding in *any* language. A person who can merely read but cannot write is not considered literate. The same concept has been continued in census 2001 and 2011 also. The literacy rate taking in account the total population in the denominator has now been termed as *"crude literacy rate"*, while the literacy rate calculated taking into account the 7 years and above population in the denominator is called the effective literacy rate. The formula for computing crude literacy rate and effective literacy rate are as follows:

$$\text{Crude literacy rate} = \frac{\text{Number of literate persons} \times 100}{\text{Total population in a given year}}$$

$$\text{Effective literacy rate} = \frac{\text{Number of literate persons aged 7 and above} \times 100}{\text{Population aged 7 and above in a given year}}$$

A significant milestone reached in Census 2011 is that the total number of illiterates has come down from 304.1 million in 2001 to 272.9 million in 2011 showing a decline of 31.1 million. The reverse trend was noted during 1991–2001 period. The decadal increase in the number of literates among males is of 31.9 per cent points and the corresponding increase among females is of 49.1 per cent points *(6)*. These two changes are a clear indication that the gender gap in literacy is shrinking in the country. It will have far reaching consequence on the development of the society. Fig. 4 shows the literacy rates in India after independence.

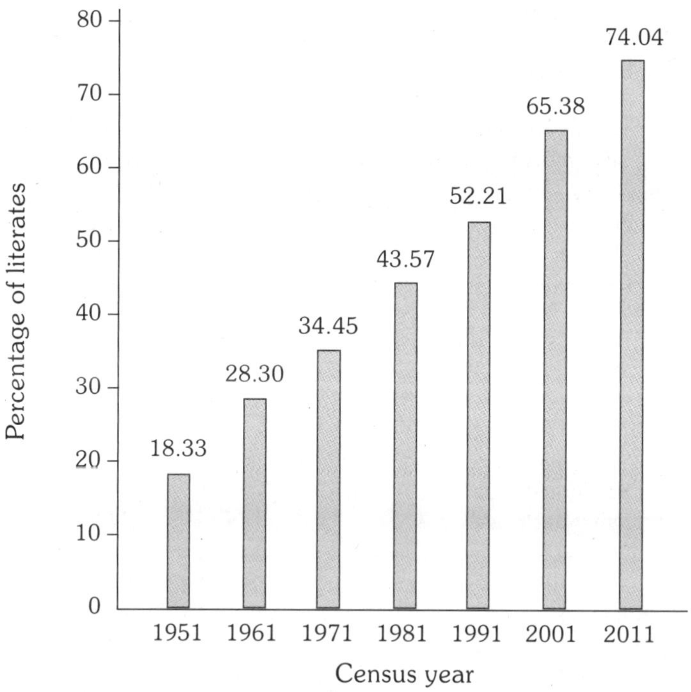

FIG. 4

Literacy rates in India 1951–2011

Source : *(18)*

The national average of literacy rate is misleading as wide variations exist between the states. Table 13 shows the literacy rates in different states in India. The national percentage of literates in the population above 7 years of age is about 74.04 with literate males about 82.14 per cent and females lagging behind with about 65.46 per cent.

Table 13 shows that Kerala continues to occupy the top rank in the country with about 93.91 per cent literates. Mizoram (91.58 per cent, and Lakshadweep (92.28 per cent) closely follow Kerala. On the other end is Bihar and Arunachal Pradesh with literacy rate of only 63.82 and 66.9 per cent respectively. The states which have literacy rates below the national average are Arunachal Pradesh, Andhra Pradesh, Bihar and Jharkhand, Jammu & Kashmir, Uttar Pradesh, Madhya Pradesh, Rajasthan and Odisha etc.

TABLE 13

State-wise literacy rate in India – 2011

State/ Union Territory#	Literacy rate		
	Total	Males	Females
Jammu & Kashmir	68.74	78.26	58.01
Himachal Pradesh	83.78	90.83	76.60
Punjab	76.68	81.48	71.34
Chandigarh#	86.43	90.54	81.38
Uttarakhand	79.63	88.33	70.70
Haryana	76.64	85.38	66.77
NCT of Delhi#	86.34	91.03	80.93
Rajasthan	67.06	80.51	52.66
Uttar Pradesh	69.72	79.24	59.26
Bihar	63.82	73.39	53.33
Sikkim	82.20	87.29	76.43
Arunachal Pradesh	66.95	73.69	59.57
Nagaland	80.11	83.29	76.69
Manipur	79.85	86.49	73.17
Mizoram	91.58	93.72	89.40
Tripura	87.75	92.18	83.15
Meghalaya	75.48	77.17	73.78
Assam	73.18	78.81	67.27
West Bengal	77.08	82.67	71.16
Jharkhand	67.63	78.45	56.21
Odisha	73.45	82.40	64.36
Chhattisgarh	71.04	81.45	60.59
Madhya Pradesh	70.63	80.53	60.02
Gujarat	79.31	87.23	70.73
Daman & Diu#	87.07	91.48	79.59
Dadra & Nagar Haveli#	77.65	86.46	65.93
Maharashtra	82.91	89.82	75.48
Andhra Pradesh	67.66	75.56	59.74
Karnataka	75.60	82.85	68.13
Goa	87.40	92.81	81.84
Lakshadweep#	92.28	96.11	88.25
Kerala	93.91	96.02	91.98
Tamil Nadu	80.33	86.81	73.86
Puducherry#	86.55	92.12	81.22
Andaman & Nicobar Islands#	86.27	90.11	81.84
INDIA	74.04	82.14	65.46

Source : *(6)*

Government of India has made education compulsory up to the age of 14 years in the country. Though considerable progress has been made in expanding primary education, a major concern is high drop out rates in the first few years of schooling.

Life expectancy

Life expectancy – or expectation of life – at a given age is the average number of years which a person of that age may expect to live, according to the mortality pattern prevalent in that country. Demographers consider it as one of the best indicators of a country's level of development and of the overall health status of its population.

Life expectancy at birth has continued to increase globally over the years. For 1950–1955, the combined life expectancy at birth for both sexes was 46.5 years. Five decades later by 2008, it was 69 years – an increase of 22.5 years. The increase has been more marked in less developed regions of the world than in the developed regions *(16)*.

Most countries in the world exhibit a sex differential in mortality favouring women – females live longer than males as shown in Table 14 and 15.

Trends in life expectancy show that people are living longer, and they have a right to a long life in good health, rather than one of pain and disability. Health policy makers thus need to recognize this changing demographic pattern and plan for prevention and control of diseases associated with old age.

Tables 14 and 15 present life expectancy at birth in India and those in selected countries. Japan leads in life expectancy for both males and females, 81 and 87 years respectively for the year 2020.

TABLE 14

Expectation of life at birth, years in India

Year	Males	Females
1901	23.63	23.96
1911	22.59	23.31
1921	19.42	20.91
1931	26.91	26.56
1941	32.09	31.37
1951	32.45	31.66
1961	41.89	40.55
1971	46.40	44.70
1981	54.10	54.70
1991	59.70	60.90
2001	63.90	66.90
2011	64.00	67.00

Source : *(6)*

TABLE 15

Expectation of life at birth, years, in selected countries 2020

Developing countries	2020		Developed countries	2020	
	Male	Female		Male	Female
Nepal	67	70	UK	79	83
Bangladesh	71	74	USA	76	81
Myanmar	64	69	Sweden	81	85
India	68	70	Switzerland	82	85
Sri Lanka	74	80	Russian Federation	68	78
Thailand	73	80	Japan	81	87
Pakistan	67	71	Singapore	81	85

Source : *(19)*

FERTILITY

By fertility is meant the actual bearing of children. Some demographers prefer to use the word natality in place of fertility. A woman's reproductive period is roughly from 15 to 45 years – a period of 30 years. A woman married at 15 and living till 45 with her husband is exposed to the risk of pregnancy for 30 years, and may give birth to 15 children, but this maximum is rarely achieved.

Fertility depends upon several factors. The higher fertility in India is attributed to universality of marriage, lower age at marriage, low level of literacy, poor level of living, limited use of contraceptives and traditional ways of life. National Family Health Survey-5 conducted in India during 2019–2021 provides some detailed information of fertility trends, as shown in Table 16.

TABLE 16

Total fertility rate by selected background characteristics (2019–21)
National Family Health Survey–5

Background characteristics	Total fertility rate
Residence	
Urban	1.63
Rural	2.14
Education	
No education	2.8
<5 years complete	2.30
5-7 years complete	2.21
8-9 years complete	2.12
10-11 years complete	1.88
12 or more years complete	1.78
Religion	
Hindu	1.94
Muslim	2.36
Christian	1.88
Sikh	1.61
Buddhist/Neo-Buddhist	1.39
Jain	1.60
Other	2.15
Caste/tribe	
Scheduled caste	2.08
Scheduled tribe	2.09
Other backward class	2.02
Others	1.78
Don't know	2.54
Wealth index	
Lowest	2.63
Second	2.12
Middle	1.89
Fourth	1.74
Highest	1.57
Total	1.99

Source : *(20)*

Some of the factors which have engaged attention of demographers since long are discussed below.

1. Age at marriage

The age at which a female marries and enters the reproductive period of life has a great impact on her fertility. The Registrar General of India collected data on fertility on a national scale and found that females who marry before the age of 18 gave birth to a larger number of children than those who married after *(21)*. In India some demographers have estimated that if marriages were postponed from the age of 16 to 20–21, the number of births would decrease by 20–30 per cent *(21)*.

Early marriage is a long-established custom in India. As early as 1929, the Sarada Act was enacted forbidding the practice of child marriage. The census data reveals that prior to 1951, the average age at marriage for girls in India was 13 years. There is however, a gradual rise in the age at marriage in the country. The Child Marriage Restraint Act of 1978 raises the legal age at marriage from 15 to 18 years for girls, and from 18 to 21 years for boys. Studies indicate that in many States, the mean age at marriage for girls has already moved upto 20 years in 2006, and many others are very close to this. For the year 2020, the national average for effective marriage is 22.7 years. The exceptions are the rural areas, where a substantial proportion of marriages continue to take place when the girl is around 16 years of age *(10)*.

2. Duration of married life

Studies indicate that 10–25 per cent of all births occur within 1–5 years of married life; 50–55 per cent of all births within 5–15 years of married life. Births after 25 years of married life are very few *(21)*. This suggests that family planning efforts should be concentrated in the first few years of married life in order to achieve tangible results.

3. Spacing of children

Studies have shown that when all births are postponed by one year, in each age group, there was a decline in total fertility. It follows that spacing of children may have a significant impact on the general reduction in the fertility rates.

4. Education

There is an inverse association between fertility and educational status. Education provides knowledge; increased exposure to information and media; builds skill for gainful employment; increases female participation in family decision making; and raises the opportunity costs of women's time. The National Family Health Survey–5 shows that the total fertility rate is 1.02 children higher for illiterate women than for women with at least a high school education (Table 16).

5. Economic status

Operational Research studies support the hypothesis that economic status bears an inverse relationship with fertility. The total number of children born declines with an increase in per capita expenditure of the household. The World Population Conference at Bucharest in fact stressed that economic development is the best contraceptive. It will take care of population growth and bring about reductions in fertility.

6. Caste and religion

Muslims have a higher fertility than Hindus. The National Family Health Survey-5 reported a total fertility rate of 2.36 among Muslims as compared to 1.94 among Hindus. The total fertility rate among Christians was found to be 1.88. Among Hindus, the lower castes seem to have a higher fertility rate than the higher castes *(20)*.

7. Nutrition

There appears to be some relationship between nutritional status and fertility levels. Virtually, all well-fed societies have low fertility, and poorly-fed societies high fertility. The effect of nutrition on fertility is largely indirect.

8. Family planning

Family planning is another important factor in fertility reduction. In a number of developing countries, family planning has been a key factor in declining fertility (Table 4). Family planning programmes can be initiated rapidly and require only limited resources, as compared to other factors.

9. Other factors

Fertility is affected by a number of physical, biological, social and cultural factors such as place of women in society, value of children in society, widow remarriage, breast-feeding, customs and beliefs, industrialization and urbanization, better health conditions, housing, opportunities for women and local community involvement. Attention to these factors requires long-term government programmes and vast sums of money.

FERTILITY RELATED STATISTICS

Fertility may be measured by a number of indicators, as given below. Stillbirths, foetal deaths and abortions, however, are not included in the measurement of fertility in a population *(22)*.

1. Birth Rate

Birth rate is the simplest indicator of fertility and is defined as "the number of live births per 1000 estimated mid-year population, in a given year". It is given by the formula :

$$\text{Birth Rate} = \frac{\text{Number of live births during the year}}{\text{Estimated mid-year population}} \times 1000$$

The birth rate is an unsatisfactory measure of fertility because the total population is not exposed to child bearing. Therefore it does not give a true idea of the fertility of a population.

2. General Fertility Rate (GFR)

It is the "number of live births per 1000 women in the reproductive age-group (15–44 or 49 years) in a given year".

$$\text{GFR} = \frac{\text{Number of live births in an area during the year}}{\text{Mid-year female population age 15–44 (or 49) in the same area in same year}} \times 1000$$

General fertility rate is a better measure of fertility than the crude birth rate because the denominator is restricted to the number of women in the child–bearing age, rather than the whole population. The major weakness of this rate is that not all women in the denominator are exposed to the risk of childbirth.

3. General Marital Fertility Rate (GMFR)

It is the "number of live births per 1000 married women in the reproductive age group (15–44 or 49) in a given year".

$$\text{GMFR} = \frac{\text{Number of live births in a year}}{\text{Mid-year married female population in the age-group 15–49 years}} \times 1000$$

4. Age-specific Fertility Rate (ASFR)

A more precise measure of fertility is age-specific fertility rate, defined as the "number of live births in a year to 1000 women in any specified age-group". The age-specific fertility rates throw light on the fertility pattern. They are also sensitive indicators of family planning achievement.

$$\text{ASFR} = \frac{\text{Number of live births in a particular age group}}{\text{Mid-year female population of the same age-group}} \times 1000$$

5. Age-specific Marital Fertility Rate (ASMFR)

It is the number of live births in a year to 1000 married women in any specified age group.

$$\text{ASMFR} = \frac{\text{Number of live births in a particular age group}}{\text{Mid-year married female population of the same age group}} \times 1000$$

6. Total Fertility Rate (TFR)

Total fertility rate represents the average number of children a woman would have if she were to pass through her reproductive years bearing children at the same rates as the women now in each age group *(23)*. It is computed by summing the age-specific fertility rates for all ages; if 5–year age groups are used, the sum of the rates is multiplied by 5. This measure gives the approximate magnitude of "completed family size".

$$\text{TFR} = \frac{5 \times \sum_{15\text{–}19}^{45\text{–}49} \text{ASFR}}{1000}$$

7. Total Marital Fertility Rate (TMFR)

Average number of children that would be born to a married woman if she experiences the current fertility pattern throughout her reproductive span.

$$\text{TMFR} = \frac{5 \times \sum_{15\text{–}19}^{45\text{–}49} \text{ASMFR}}{1000}$$

8. Gross Reproduction Rate (GRR)

Average number of girls that would be born to a woman if she experiences the current fertility pattern throughout her reproductive span (15–44 or 49 years), assuming no mortality.

$$\text{GRR} = \frac{5 \times \sum_{15\text{-}19}^{45\text{-}49} \text{ASFR for female live births}}{1000}$$

9. Net Reproduction Rate (NRR)

Net Reproduction Rate (NRR) is defined as the number of daughters a newborn girl will bear during her lifetime assuming fixed age-specific fertility and mortality rates *(24)*.

NRR is a demographic indicator. NRR of 1 is equivalent to attaining approximately the 2–child norm. If the NRR is less than 1, then the reproductive performance of the population is said to be below replacement level.

10. Child-woman Ratio

It is the number of children 0–4 years of age per 1000 women of child-bearing age, usually defined as 15–44 or 49 years of age. This ratio is used where birth registration statistics either do not exist or are inadequate. It is estimated through data derived from censuses *(6)*.

11. Pregnancy Rate

It is the ratio of number of pregnancies in a year to married women in the ages 15–44 (or 49) years. The "number of pregnancies" includes all pregnancies, whether these had terminated as live births, stillbirths or abortions or had not yet terminated.

12. Abortion Rate

The annual number of all types of abortions, usually per 1000 women of child-bearing age (usually defined as age 15–44) *(25)*.

13. Abortion Ratio

This is calculated by dividing the number of abortions performed during a particular time period by the number of live births over the same period *(26)*.

14. Marriage Rate

It is the number of marriages in the year per 1000 population :

$$\text{Crude Marriage Rate} = \frac{\text{Number of marriages in the year}}{\text{Mid-year population}} \times 1000$$

Demographers consider this a very unsatisfactory rate, because the denominator is comprised primarily of population that is not eligible to marry. A more sensitive rate is the general marriage rate :

$$\text{General Marriage Rate} = \frac{\text{Number of marriages within one year}}{\text{Number of unmarried persons age 15–49 years}} \times 1000$$

This rate is more accurate when computed for women than for men because more men than women marry at the older ages *(6)*.

Fertility trends

Researches indicate that the level of fertility in India is beginning to decline. The crude birth rate which was about 49 per thousand population during 1901–11 has declined to about 25.0 per thousand population in 2002, and was 20.4 per thousand population in 2016. The rural urban differential has narrowed. However, the crude birth rate has continued to be higher in rural areas as compared to urban areas in the last 3 decades.

The total fertility rate has declined from 3.6 in 1991 to 2.0 in 2020. The TFR in rural areas has declined from 5.4 in 1971 to 2.2 in 2020, whereas the corresponding decline in urban areas has been from 4.1 to 1.6 during the same period. There are considerable inter-state variations in total fertility rate as shown in Fig. 5. In bigger states it varies from 1.4 in West Bengal and Tamil Nadu to 3.0 in Bihar *(7)*.

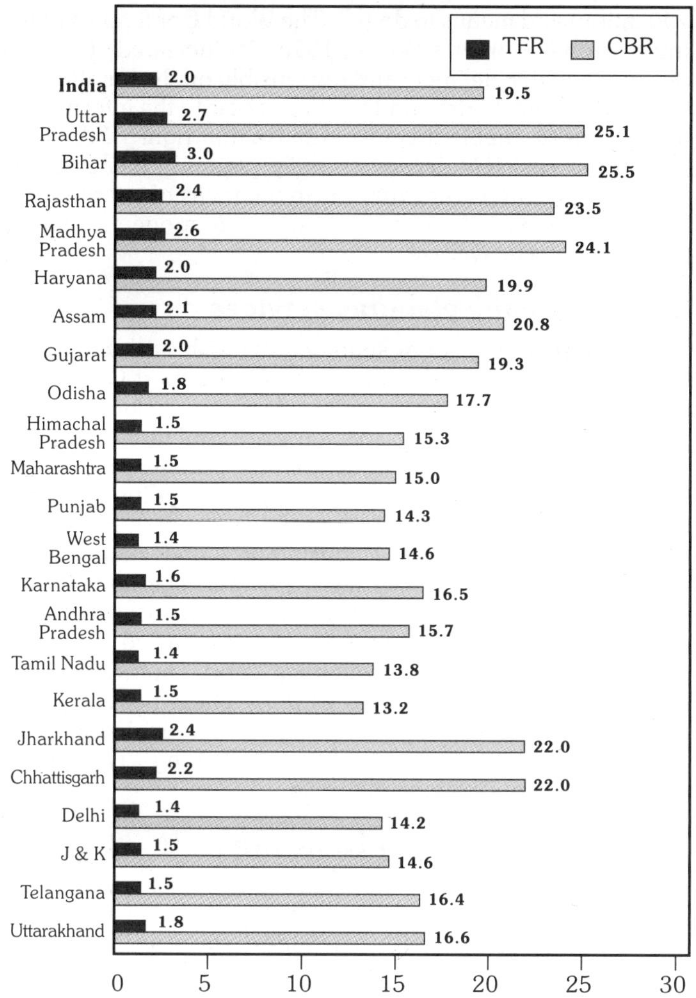

FIG. 5

Crude birth rate (2020) and Total fertility rate (2020) for major states

Source : *(10)*

Recent estimates of the fertility indicators and age-specific fertility rates in India are given in Table 17.

TABLE 17

Fertility indicators of India, 2020

Indicators	Age group	Total	Rural	Urban
Age-specific fertility rate	15–19	11.3	13.2	6.6
	20–24	113.6	128.1	81.8
	25–29	139.6	152.5	115.2
	30–34	84.4	89.4	75.5
	35–39	35.6	38.9	29.5
	40–44	11.7	13.5	8.5
	45–49	4.7	5.2	3.9
Age-specific marital fertility rate	15–19	353.0	361.2	318.2
	20–24	339.1	350.0	306.5
	25–29	199.3	206.2	183.9
	30–34	95.1	98.4	88.8
	35–39	38.1	41.2	32.1
	40–44	12.6	14.5	9.2
	45–49	5.2	5.6	4.4
Crude birth rate		19.5	21.1	16.1
General fertility rate		67.0	73.7	53.7
Total fertility rate		2.0	2.2	1.6
Gross reproduction rate		0.9	1.0	0.8
General marital fertility rate		108.3	118.0	88.5
Total marital fertility rate		5.2	5.4	4.7

Source : *(10)*

Birth and death rates

The birth and death rates are important components of population growth. The birth and death rates in India are shown in Table 18. A look at Table 18 shows that whereas the death rate has considerably declined from 27.4 in 1951 to an estimated 7.2 per thousand population in 2020, the birth rate has declined niggardly from 39.9 in 1951 to an estimated 18.7 per thousand in 2020.

The Fifth Five Year (1974–79) Plan's objective was to reduce the birth rate from 35 per thousand at the beginning of the Plan to 30 per thousand by 1978–79. During 1979–84, the birth rate was stagnating around 33 per thousand with no obvious decline. During 1990, however, the birth rate showed a slight decline, to an estimated 30.2, further declining to 26.4 by the year 1998. The current picture indicates that birth and death rates are both declining in India.

TABLE 18

Birth and death rates in India

Year	Birth rate	Death rate
1941–1950	39.9	27.4
1951–1960	41.7	22.8
1961–1970	41.2	19.0
1971–1980	37.2	15.0
1981	33.9	12.5
1991	29.5	9.8
1995	28.3	9.0
1998	26.8	9.0
1999	26.1	8.7
2002	25.0	8.1
2004	24.1	7.5
2006	23.5	7.5
2008	22.8	7.4
2010	22.1	7.2
2012	21.6	7.0
2015	20.0	7.0
2016	20.4	6.4
2018	20.0	6.2
2022	18.7	7.2

Source : *(7)*

HIGH BIRTH RATE : India like other developing countries is faced with the dilemma of a high birth rate and a declining death rate. This is a vicious circle, not easy to break. The causes of high birth rate are :- (1) *Universality of marriage* : Marriages are universal and sacramental. Everyone, sooner or later (usually sooner) gets married and participates in reproduction. The individual's economic security or emotional maturity are seldom a pre-requisite to marriage. (2) *Early marriage* : Marriages are performed early. Data indicate that about 60 per cent of the girls aged 15–19 years are already married. (3) *Early puberty* : Indian girls attain puberty early, between 12 and 14 years. (4) *Low standard of living* : Where standards of living are low, birth rates are high. (5) *Low level of literacy* : The 2011 census showed that only 74.04 per cent of the population was literate. The female literacy is still lower, especially in the rural areas. (6) *Traditional customs and habits* : Customs dictate that every woman must marry and every man must have a son. Children are considered a gift of God and their birth should not be obstructed. (7) *Absence of family planning habit* : Family planning is of recent origin. It has not yet become part of the marital mores of the people.

DECLINING DEATH RATE : The declining death rate has been attributed to : (1) absence of natural checks, e.g., famines and large scale epidemics, (2) mass control of diseases, e.g., smallpox, plague, cholera, malaria etc., (3) advances in medical science, e.g., extensive use of chemotherapeutics, antibiotics, and insecticides, (4) better health facilities, e.g., establishment of primary health centres and more treatment centres, (5) impact of national health programmes, (6) improvements in food supply, (7) international aid in several directions, and (8) development of social consciousness among the masses.

Demographers opine that further rapid decline in India's death rate may not continue in future. The reason is that most of the "easy" conquest of mortality has been accomplished through the widespread use of vaccines, antibiotics, insecticides, and other life-saving measures. The tasks that remain now are the most difficult ones such as improvements in environmental sanitation and nutrition; and control of non-communicable and genetic diseases.

Growth rate

The population growth rates in India are presented in Table 6. Prior to 1921, the population of India grew at a slow rate. This was due to the operation of natural checks (e.g., famines and epidemics) which took a heavy toll of human life. After 1921, the "great divide", the occurrence of famines and epidemics was effectively controlled through better nutrition and improved health care services, with the result that the death rate declined more steeply than the birth rate. Consequently, there was a net gain in births over deaths, leading to rapid growth in population, which rose from 1.25 per cent in 1951 to 1.96 in 1961, 2.20 in 1971, 2.22 in 1981, 2.16 in 1991, 1.7 in 2001 and 1.64 in 2011 (Table 6).

India is now the second most populous country in the world, adding 17.5 million every year to her 1210 million at the time of 2011 census. However, the most recent data indicates a decline in India's population growth rate. The estimates for the year 2020 is 1.2.

FAMILY PLANNING

Definition

There are several definitions of family planning. An Expert Committee (1971) of the WHO defined family planning as "a way of thinking and living that is adopted voluntarily, upon the basis of knowledge, attitudes and responsible decisions by individuals and couples, in order to promote the health and welfare of the family group and thus contribute effectively to the social development of a country" *(27)*.

Another Expert Committee *(28)* defined and described family planning as follows : "Family planning refers to practices that help individuals or couples to attain certain objectives :

(a) to avoid unwanted births;
(b) to bring about wanted births;
(c) to regulate the intervals between pregnancies;
(d) to control the time at which births occur in relation to the ages of the parent; and
(e) to determine the number of children in the family.

Basic human rights

The United Nations Conference on Human Rights at Tehran in 1968 recognized family planning as a basic human right. The Bucharest Conference *(29)* on the World Population held in August 1974 endorsed the same view and stated in its 'Plan of Action' that "all couples and individuals have the basic human right to decide freely and responsibly the number and spacing of their children and to have the information, education, and means to do so". The World Conference of the International Women's Year in 1975 also declared "the right of women to decide freely and responsibly on the number and spacing of their children and to have access to the information and means to enable them to exercise that right" *(30)*. Thus during the past few decades, family planning has emerged from whispers in private quarters to the focus of international concern as a basic human right, and a component of family health and social welfare.

Scope of family planning services

Family planning is not synonymous with birth control; it is more than mere birth control. A WHO Expert Committee (1970) has stated that family planning includes in its purview:- (1) the proper spacing and limitation of births, (2) advice on sterility, (3) education for parenthood, (4) sex education, (5) screening for pathological conditions related to the reproductive system (e.g., cervical cancer), (6) genetic counselling, (7) premarital consultation and examination, (8) carrying out pregnancy tests, (9) marriage counselling, (10) the preparation of couples for the arrival of their first child, (11) providing services for unmarried mothers, (12) teaching home economics and nutrition, and (13) providing adoption services *(29)*. These activities vary from country to country according to national objectives and policies with regard to family planning. This is the modern concept of family planning.

Health aspects of family planning *(31, 32, 33)*

Family planning and health have a two-way relationship. The principal health outcomes of family planning were listed and discussed by a WHO Scientific Group on the Health Aspects of Family Planning *(31)*. These can be summarized under the following headings.

Women's health

maternal mortality, morbidity of women of child–bearing age, nutritional status (weight changes, haemoglobin level, etc.) preventable complications of pregnancy and abortion.

Foetal health

foetal mortality (early and late foetal death); abnormal development.

Infant and child health

neonatal, infant and pre-school mortality,
health of the infant at birth (birth weight),
vulnerability to diseases.

(a) WOMEN'S HEALTH : Pregnancy can mean serious problems for many women. It may damage the mother's health or even endanger her life. In developing countries, the risk of dying as a result of pregnancy is much greater than in developed countries. The risk increases as the mother grows older and after she has had 3 or 4 children. Family planning by intervening in the reproductive cycle of women, helps them to control the number, interval and timing of pregnancies and births, and thereby reduces maternal mortality and morbidity and improves health. The health impact of family planning occurs primarily through : (i) the avoidance of unwanted pregnancies; (ii) limiting the number of births and proper spacing, and (iii) timing the births, particularly the first and last, in relation to the age of the mother. It is estimated that guaranteeing access to family planning alone could reduce the number of maternal deaths by 25 per cent, and child mortality by 20 per cent *(13)*.

(i) *Unwanted pregnancies* : The essential aim of family planning is to prevent the unwanted pregnancies. An unwanted pregnancy may lead to an induced abortion. From the point of view of health, abortion outside the medical setting (criminal abortion) is one of the most dangerous consequence of unwanted pregnancy. Particular mention must be made of the unmarried mother who faces significantly higher health risks. There is also evidence of higher incidence of mental disturbances among mothers who have had unwanted pregnancies.

(ii) *Limiting the number of births and proper spacing* : Repeated pregnancies increase the risk of maternal mortality and morbidity. These risks rise with each pregnancy beyond the third, and increase significantly with each pregnancy beyond the fifth. The incidence of rupture of the uterus and uterine atony increases with parity as does the incidence of toxaemia, eclampsia and placenta previa. Anaemia is a common problem in mothers with many children and the rate of stillbirths tends to increase significantly with high parity. The somatic consequences of repeated pregnancies may also be exemplified in the clear association between the incidence of cancer of the cervix and high parity. Family planning is the only way to limit the size and control the interval between births with a view to improving the health of the mother.

(iii) *Timing of births* : Generally mothers face greater risk of dying below the age of 20 and above the age of 30–35. In many countries, complications of pregnancy and delivery show the same pattern of risk, with the highest rate below 20 and over 35 years of age.

(b) FOETAL HEALTH : A number of congenital anomalies (e.g., Down's syndrome) are associated with advancing maternal age. Such congenital anomalies can be avoided by timing the births in relation to the mother's age. Further, the "quality" of population can be improved only by avoiding completely unwanted births. In the present state of our knowledge, it is very difficult to weigh the overall genetic effects of family planning.

(c) CHILD HEALTH : Issues relating to family planning are highly relevant to paediatrics. It would seem that family size and birth spacing, if practised by all, will yield substantial child health benefits. These are : (a) *Child mortality* : It is well known that child mortality increases when pregnancies occur in rapid succession. A birth interval of 2 to 3 years is considered desirable to reduce child mortality. Family planning is, therefore, an important means of ensuring the survival of all children in a family. (b) *Child growth, development and nutrition* : Birth spacing and family size are important factors in child growth and development. The child is likely to receive his full share of love and care, including nutrition he needs, when the family size is small and births are properly spaced. Family planning, in other words, is effective prevention against malnutrition. (c) *Infectious diseases* : Children living in large-sized families have an increase in infection, especially infectious gastroenteritis, respiratory and skin infections.

The welfare concept

Family planning is associated with numerous misconceptions – one of them is its strong association in the minds of people with sterilization. Others equate it with birth control. The recognition of its welfare concept came only a decade and half after its inception, when it was named Family Welfare Programme.

The concept of welfare is very comprehensive and is basically related to quality of life. The Family Welfare Programme aims at achieving a higher end – that is, to improve the quality of life of the people.

Small-family norm

Small differences in the family size will make big differences in the birth rate. The difference of only one child per family over a decade will have a tremendous impact on the population growth.

The objective of the Family Welfare Programme in India is that people should adopt the "small family norm" to stabilize the country's population at the level of some 1,533 million by the year 2050 AD. Symbolized by the inverted red triangle, the programme initially adopted the model of the 3–child family. In the 1970s, the slogan was the famous *Do Ya Teen Bas*. In view of the seriousness of the situation, the 1980s campaign has advocated the 2–child norm. The current emphasis is on three themes : "Sons or Daughters – two will do"; "Second child after 3 years", and "Universal Immunization".

A significant achievement of the Family Welfare Programme in India has been the decline in the fertility rate from 6.4 in the 1950s to 2.2 in 2018. The national target was to achieve a Net Reproduction Rate of '1' by the year 2006, which is equivalent to attaining approximately the 2–child norm, which could not be attained. All efforts are being made through mass communication that the concept of small family norm is accepted, adopted and woven into lifestyle of the people.

Eligible couples

An "eligible couple" refers to a currently married couple wherein the wife is in the reproductive age, which is generally assumed to lie between the ages of 15 and 45. There will be at least 150 to 180 such couples per 1000 population in India. These couples are in need of family planning services. About 20 per cent of eligible couples are found in the age group 15–24 years. On an average 2.5 million couples are joining the reproductive group every year. The "Eligible Couple Register" is a basic document for organizing family planning work. It is regularly updated by each functionary of the family planning programme for the area falling within his jurisdiction.

Target couples

In order to pin-point the couples who are a priority group within the broad definition of "eligible couples", the term "target couple" was coined. Hitherto, the term target couple was applied to couples who have had 2–3 living children, and family planning was largely directed to such couples. The definition of a target couple has been gradually enlarged to include families with one child or even newly married couples *(34)* with a view to develop acceptance of the idea of family planning from the earliest possible stage. In effect, the term target couple has lost its original meaning. The term eligible couple is now more widely used and has come to stay.

Couple protection rate (CPR)

Couple protection rate (CPR) is an indicator of the prevalence of contraceptive practice in the community. It is defined as the per cent of eligible couples effectively protected against childbirth by one or the other approved methods of family planning, viz. sterilization, IUD, condom or oral pills. Sterilization accounts for over 60 per cent of effectively protected couples *(35)*. Demographers are of the view that the demographic goal of NRR=1 can be achieved only if the CPR exceeds 60 per cent.

Couple protection rate is based on the observation that 50 to 60 per cent of births in a year are of birth order 3 or more. Thus attaining a 60 per cent CPR will be equivalent to cutting off almost all third or higher order births, leaving 2 or less surviving children per couple *(35)*. Therefore, in India, the previous National Population Policy was to attain a CPR of 42 per cent by 1990 (end of Seventh Five Year Plan), and 60 per cent by the year 2000. In short CPR is a dominant factor in the reduction of net reproduction rate.

NATIONAL POPULATION POLICY 2000

Population policy in general refers to policies intended to decrease the birth rate or growth rate. Statement of goals, objectives and targets are inherent in the population policy.

In April 1976 India formed its first – "National Population Policy". It called for an increase in the legal minimum age of marriage from 15 to 18 for females, and from 18 to 21 years for males. However, for the most part, the 1976 statement became irrelevant and the policy was modified in 1977. New policy statement reiterated the importance of the small family norm without compulsion and changed the programme title to "family welfare programme". The National Health Policy approved by the parliament in 1983 had set the long-term demographic goals of achieving a Net Reproductive Rate (NRR) of one by the year 2000 (which was not achieved).

"National Population Policy 2000" is the latest in this series. It reaffirms the commitment of the government towards target free approach in administering family planning services. It gives informed choice to the people to voluntarily avail the reproductive health care services.

The new NPP 2000 is more than just a matter of fertility and mortality rates. It deals with women education; empowering women for improved health and nutrition; child survival and health; the unmet needs for family welfare services; health care for the under-served population groups like urban slums, tribal community, hill area population and displaced and migrant population; adolescent's health and education; increased participation of men in planned parenthood; and collaboration with NGOs.

The objective of NPP 2000 is to bring the TFR to replacement level by 2010. The long term objective is to achieve requirements of suitable economic growth, social development and environment protection.

The National Socio-Demographic Goals to be achieved by the year 2010 were as follows *(36)*:

(1) Address the unmet needs for basic reproductive and child health services, supplies and infrastructure.
(2) Make school education upto the age 14 free and compulsory, and reduce drop-outs at primary and secondary school levels to below 20 per cent for both boys and girls.
(3) Reduce infant mortality rate to below 30 per 1000 live births.
(4) Reduce maternal mortality ratio to below 100 per 100,000 live births.
(5) Achieve universal immunization of children against all vaccine preventable diseases.
(6) Promote delayed marriage for girls, not earlier than age 18 and preferably after 20 years of age.
(7) Achieve 80 per cent institutional deliveries and 100 per cent deliveries by trained persons.
(8) Achieve universal access to information/counselling, and services for fertility regulation and contraception with a wide basket of choices.
(9) Achieve 100 per cent registration of births, deaths, marriage and pregnancy.
(10) Contain the spread of Acquired Immunodeficiency Syndrome (AIDS), and promote greater integration between the management of reproductive tract infections (RTI) and sexually transmitted infections (STI) and the National AIDS Control Organization.
(11) Prevent and control communicable diseases.
(12) Integrate Indian Systems of Medicine (ISM) in the provision of reproductive and child health services, and in reaching out to households.
(13) Promote vigorously the small family norm to achieve replacement levels of TFR.
(14) Bring about convergence in implementation of related social sector programmes so that family welfare becomes a people centred programme.

If the NPP 2000 was fully implemented, it was anticipated that in the year 2010 the population may be 1107 million instead of 1162 million projected by the Technical Group of Population Projections. However, the provisional population (1210 million) in 2011 is higher by about 110 million compared to the target set for the year 2010. Efforts at population stabilization will be effective only if an integrated package of essential services is directed at village and household levels. Inadequacies in the existing health infrastructure have led to a unmet need of 28 per cent of contraception services and obvious gap in coverage and outreach. The NPP 2000 is to be largely implemented and managed at panchayat and nagar palika levels in coordination with the concerned state/UT administration.

CONTRACEPTIVE METHODS
(Fertility Regulating Methods)

Contraceptive methods are, by definition, preventive methods to help women avoid unwanted pregnancies. They include all temporary and permanent measures to prevent pregnancy resulting from coitus.

The last few years have witnessed a contraceptive revolution, that is, man trying to interfere with the ovulation cycle.

It is now generally recognized that there can never be an ideal contraceptive – that is, contraceptive that is safe, effective, acceptable, inexpensive, reversible, simple to administer, independent of coitus, long-lasting enough to obviate frequent administration and requiring little or no medical supervision. Further, a method which may be quite suitable for one group may be unsuitable for another because of different cultural patterns, religious beliefs and socio-economic milieu. As there is no single method likely to meet the social, cultural, aesthetic and service needs of all individuals and communities, the search for an "ideal contraceptive" has been given up. The present approach in family planning programmes is to provide a "cafeteria choice" that is to offer all methods from which an individual can choose according to his needs and wishes and to promote family planning as a way of life.

The term conventional contraceptives is used to denote those methods that require action at the time of sexual intercourse, e.g., condoms, spermicides, etc. Each contraceptive method has its unique advantages and disadvantages. The success of any contraceptive method depends not only on its effectiveness in preventing pregnancy but on the rate of continuation of its proper use.

The contraceptive methods may be broadly grouped into two classes – spacing methods and terminal methods, as shown below :

I. Spacing methods

1. Barrier methods
   (a) Physical methods
   (b) Chemical methods
   (c) Combined methods
2. Intra-uterine devices
3. Hormonal methods
4. Post-conceptional methods
5. Miscellaneous.

II. Terminal methods

1 Male sterilization
2 Female sterilization.

BARRIER METHODS

A variety of barrier or "occlusive" methods, suitable for both men and women are available. The aim of these methods is to prevent live sperm from meeting the ovum. Barrier methods have increased in popularity quite recently because of certain contraceptive and non-contraceptive advantages. The main contraceptive advantage is the absence of side-effects associated with the "pill" and IUD. The non-contraceptive advantages include some protection from sexually transmitted diseases, a reduction in the incidence of pelvic inflammatory disease and possibly some protection from the risk of cervical cancer *(37)*. Barrier methods require a high degree of motivation on the part of the user. In general they are less effective than either the pill or the loop. They are only effective if they are used consistently and carefully.

a. PHYSICAL METHODS

1. Condom *(38, 39)*

Condom is the most widely known and used barrier device by the males around the world. In India, it is better known by its trade name NIRODH, a sanskrit word, meaning prevention. Condom is receiving new attention today as an effective, simple "spacing" method of contraception, without side effects. In addition to preventing pregnancy, condom protects both men and women from sexually transmitted diseases.

The condom is fitted on the erect penis before intercourse. The air must be expelled from the teat end to make room for the ejaculate. The condom must be held carefully when withdrawing it from the vagina to avoid spilling seminal fluid into the vagina after intercourse. A new condom should be used for each sexual act.

Condom prevents the semen from being deposited in vagina. The effectiveness of a condom may be increased by using it in conjunction with a spermicidal jelly inserted into the vagina before intercourse. The spermicide serves as additional protection in the unlikely event that the condom should slip off or tear.

Condoms can be a highly effective method of contraception, if they are used correctly at every coitus. Failure rates for the condom vary enormously. Surveys have reported pregnancy rates varying from 2–3 per 100 women–years to more than 14 in typical users *(40)*. Most failures are due to incorrect use.

The ADVANTAGES of condom are : (a) they are easily available (b) safe and inexpensive (c) easy to use; do not require medical supervision (d) no side effects (e) light, compact and disposable, and (f) provides protection not only against pregnancy but also against STD. The DISADVANTAGES are : (a) it may slip off or tear during coitus due to incorrect use, and (b) interferes with sex sensation locally about which some complain while others get used to it. The main limitation of condoms is that many men do not use them regularly or carefully, even when the risk of unwanted pregnancy or sexually transmitted disease is high.

Condoms are manufactured in India by the Hindusthan Latex in Trivandrum, London Rubber Industries in Chennai and others. Besides commercial outlets, condoms are supplied under social marketing programme.

Female condom

The female condom is a pouch made of polyurethane, which lines the vagina. An internal ring in the close end of the pouch covers the cervix and an external ring remains outside the vagina. It is prelubricated with silicon, and a spermicide need not be used. It is an effective barrier to STD infection. However, high cost and acceptability are major problems. The failure rates during the first year use vary from 5 per 100 women-years pregnancy rate to about 21 in typical users *(41)*.

2. Diaphragm

The diaphragm is a vaginal barrier. It was invented by a German physician in 1882. Also known as "Dutch cap", the diaphragm is a shallow cup made of synthetic rubber or plastic material. It ranges in diameter from 5–10 cm (2–4 inches). It has a flexible rim made of spring or metal. It is important that a woman be fitted with a diaphragm of the proper size. It is held in position partly by the spring tension and partly by the vaginal muscle tone. This means, for successful use, the vaginal tone must be reasonable. Otherwise, in the case of a severe degree of cystocele, the rim may slip down.

The diaphragm is inserted before sexual intercourse and must remain in place for not less than 6 hours after sexual intercourse. A spermicidal jelly is always used along with the diaphragm. The diaphragm holds the spermicide over the cervix. Side-effects are practically nil. Failure rate for the diaphragm with spermicide vary between 6 to 12 per 100 women–years *(40)*.

ADVANTAGES : The primary advantage of the diaphragm is the almost total absence of risks and medical contraindications. DISADVANTAGES : Initially a physician or other trained person will be needed to demonstrate the technique of inserting the diaphragm into the vagina and to ensure a proper fit. After delivery, it can be used only after involution of the uterus is completed. Practice at insertion, privacy for this to be carried out and facilities for washing and storing the diaphragm precludes its use in most Indian families, particularly in the rural areas. Therefore, the extent of its use has never been great.

If the diaphragm is left in the vagina for an extended period, there is a remote possibility of a toxic shock syndrome, which is a state of peripheral shock requiring resuscitation *(42)*.

Variations of the diaphragm include the cervical cap, vault cap and the vimule cap. These devices are not recommended in the National Family Welfare Programme.

3. Vaginal sponge

Another barrier device employed for hundreds of years is the sponge soaked in vinegar or olive oil, but it is only recently one has been commercially marketed in USA under the trade name **TODAY** for the sole purpose of preventing conception. It is a small polyurethane foam sponge measuring 5 cm × 2.5 cm, saturated with the spermicide, nonoxynol–9. The sponge is far less effective than the diaphragm, but it is better than nothing *(43)*. The failure rate in parous women is between 20 to 40 per 100 women-years and in nulliparous women about 9 to 20 per 100 women-years *(41)*.

b. CHEMICAL METHODS

In the 1960s, before the advent of IUDs and oral contraceptives, spermicides (vaginal chemical contraceptives) were used widely. They comprise four categories *(44)*:

a) Foams : foam tablets, foam aerosols
b) Creams, jellies and pastes – squeezed from a tube
c) Suppositories – inserted manually, and
d) Soluble films – C-film inserted manually.

The spermicides contain a base into which a spermicide is incorporated. The commonly used modern spermicides are "surface-active agents" which attach themselves to spermatozoa and inhibit oxygen uptake and kill sperms *(45)*.

The main drawbacks of spermicides are : (a) they have a high failure rate (b) they must be used almost immediately before intercourse and repeated before each sex act (c) they must be introduced into those regions of the vagina where sperms are likely to be deposited, and (d) they may cause mild burning or irritation, besides messiness. The spermicide should be free from potential systemic toxicity. It should not have an inflammatory or carcinogenic effect on the vaginal skin or cervix. No spermicide which is safe to use has yet been found to be really effective in preventing pregnancy when used alone *(44)*. Therefore, spermicides are not recommended by professional advisers. They are best used in conjunction with barrier methods. Recently there has been some concern about possible teratogenic effects on foetuses, following their use. However, this risk is yet to be confirmed *(42)*.

INTRA-UTERINE DEVICES

Types of IUD

There are two basic types of IUD : **non-medicated** and **medicated**. Both are usually made of polyethylene or other polymers; in addition, the medicated or bioactive IUDs release either metal ions (copper) or hormones (progestogens).

The non-medicated or inert IUDs are often referred to as **first generation IUDs**. The copper IUDs comprise the **second** and the hormone-releasing IUDs the **third** generation IUDs. The medicated IUDs were developed to reduce the incidence of side-effects and to increase the contraceptive effectiveness. However, they are more expensive and must be changed after a certain time to maintain their effectiveness *(46)*. Fig. 6 shows different types of IUDs currently in use.

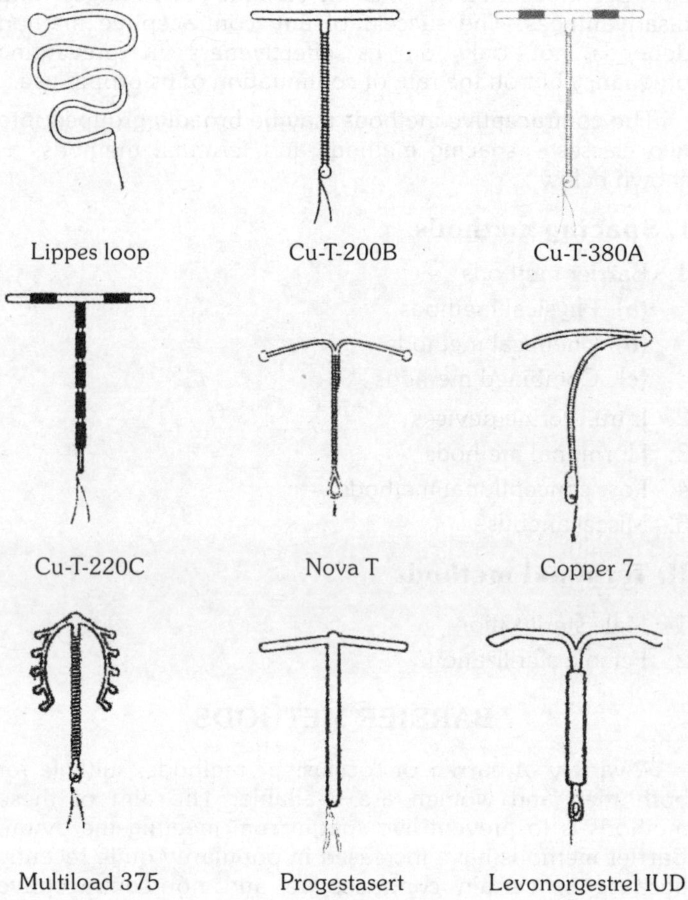

FIG. 6
Types of IUDs

FIRST GENERATION IUDs

The first generation IUDs comprise the inert or non-medicated devices, usually made of polyethylene, or other polymers. They appeared in different shapes and sizes – loops, spirals, coils, rings, and bows. Of all the models, the Lippes Loop is the best known and commonly used device in the developing countries.

Lippes Loop

Lippes Loop is double–"S" shaped device made of polyethylene, a plastic material that is non-toxic, non-tissue reactive and extremely durable. It contains a small amount of barium sulphate to allow X-ray observation. The Loop has attached threads or "tail" made of fine nylon, which project into the vagina after insertion. The tail can be easily felt and is a reassurance to the user that the Loop is in its place. The tail also makes it easy to remove the Loop when desired.

The Lippes Loop exists in four sizes A,B,C, and D, the latter being the largest. A larger sized device usually has a greater anti-fertility effect and a lower expulsion rate but a higher removal rate because of side-effects such as pain and bleeding. The larger Loops (C and D) are more suitable for multiparous women.

SECOND GENERATION IUDs

It occurred to a number of research workers that the ideal IUD can never be developed simply as a result of obtaining changes in the usual shape or size *(43)*. A new approach was tried in the 1970s by adding copper to the IUD. It was found that metallic copper had a strong anti-fertility effect *(47)*. The addition of copper has made it possible to develop smaller devices which are easier to fit, even in nulliparous women. A number of copper bearing devices are now commercially available :

Earlier devices :

- Copper-7
- Copper T-200

Newer devices :

- Variants of the T device
  - (i) Cu-T 220 C
  - (ii) Cu-T 380 A or Ag
- Nova T
- Multiload devices
  - (i) ML-Cu-250
  - (ii) ML-Cu-375

The numbers included in the names of the devices refer to the surface area (in sq. mm) of the copper on the device. Nova T and Cu-T 380 Ag are distinguished by a silver core over which the copper wire is wrapped.

The newer copper devices are significantly more effective in preventing pregnancy than the earlier copper ones or the inert IUDs. The newer copper IUDs – Multiload devices and variants of the T device – offer the further advantage of having an effective life of at least 5 years. They can be left in place safely for the time, unless specific medical or personal reasons call for earlier removal.

Advantages of copper devices

- Low expulsion rate
- Lower incidence of side-effects, e.g., pain and bleeding
- easier to fit even in nulliparous women
- better tolerated by nullipara
- increased contraceptive effectiveness
- effective as post-coital contraceptives, if inserted within 3–5 days of unprotected intercourse

THIRD GENERATION IUDs

A third generation of IUDs based on still another principle, i.e., release of a hormone have become available on a limited scale. The most widely used hormonal device is **progestasert**, which is a T-shaped device filled with 38 mg of progesterone, the natural hormone. The hormone is released slowly in the uterus at the rate of 65 mcg daily. It has a direct local effect on the uterine lining, on the cervial mucus and possibly on the sperms. Because the hormone supply is gradually depleted, regular replacement of the device is necessary.

Another hormonal device LNG-20 (Mirena) is a T-shaped IUD releasing 20 mcg of **levonorgestrel** (a potent synthetic steroid); it has a low pregnancy rate (0.2 per 100 women) and less number of ectopic pregnancies *(41)*. Long-term clinical experience with levonorgestrel releasing IUD has shown to be associated with lower menstrual blood loss and fewer days of bleeding than the copper devices. The levonorgestrel releasing IUD has an effective life of 10 years *(41)*. The hormonal devices would be particularly valuable for women in developing countries in whom excess blood loss caused by inert devices have been shown to result in significant anaemia. But these devices are more expensive, to be introduced on a wide scale.

Mechanism of action of IUDs

At present, the most widely accepted view is that the IUD causes a foreign body reaction in the uterus causing cellular and biochemical changes in the endometrium and uterine fluids, and it is believed that these changes impair the viability of the gamete and thus reduce its chances of fertilization, rather than its implantation.

Medicated IUDs produce other local effects that may contribute to their contraceptive action. Copper seems to enhance the cellular response in the endometrium *(48)*. It also affects the enzymes in the uterus. By altering the biochemical composition of cervial mucus, copper ions may affect sperm motility, capacitation and survival *(48)*.

Hormone-releasing devices increase the viscosity of the cervical mucus and thereby prevent sperm from entering the cervix. They also maintain high levels of progesterone in the endometrium and thus, relatively low levels of oestrogen, thereby sustaining an endometrium unfavourable to implantation *(48)*.

Effectiveness

The IUD is one of the most effective reversible contraceptive methods. The "theoretical effectiveness" of IUD is less than that of oral and injectable hormonal contraceptives. But since IUDs have longer continuation rates than the hormonal pills or injections, the overall effectiveness of IUDs and oral contraceptives are about the same in family planning programmes *(49)*.

Table 19 shows the rates of pregnancy, expulsion and removal of some of the IUDs. It can be seen from Table 19 that copper devices are more effective than the Lippes Loop in preventing pregnancy, with fewer expulsions. Studies have shown that the effectiveness of copper devices is directly related to the amount of copper surface area (usually this is 200 or 220 sq. mm.)

TABLE 19

First year clinical trial experience in parous women

Device	Pregnancy rate (%)	Explusion rate (%)	Removal rate (%)
Lippes Loop	3	12-20	12-15
Cu-7	2-3	6	11
TCu-200	3	8	11
TCu-380A	0.5-0.8	5	14
Progesterone IUD	1.3-1.6	2.7	9.3
Levonorgestrel IUD	0.2	6	17

Source : *(41)*

Change of IUD

Inert IUDs such as Lippes Loop may be left in place as long as required, if there are no side-effects. Copper devices cannot be used indefinitely because copper corrodes and mineral deposits build up on the copper affecting the release of copper ions. They have to be replaced periodically. The same applies to the hormone-releasing devices. This is an inherent disadvantage of medicated devices when they are used in large national family planning programmes.

The Cu-T 380A is approved for use for 10 years. However, the Cu-T 380A has been demonstrated to maintain its efficacy over at least 12 years of use. The Cu-T-200 is approved for 4 years and the Nova T for 5 years. The progesterone-releasing IUD must be replaced every year because the reservoir of progesterone is depleted in 12–18 months. The levonorgestrel IUD can be used for at least 7 years, and probably 10 years. The progesterone IUD has a slightly higher failure rate, but the levonorgestrel device that releases 15–20 μg levonorgestrel per day is as effective as the new copper IUDs *(41)*.

Advantages

The IUD has many advantages : (a) simplicity, i.e., no complex procedures are involved in insertion; no hospitalization is required (b) insertion takes only a few minutes (c) once inserted IUD stays in place as long as required (d) inexpensive (e) contraceptive effect is reversible by removal of IUD (f) virtually free of systemic metabolic side-effects associated with hormonal pills (g) highest continuation rate, and (h) there is no need for the continual motivation required to take a pill daily or to use a barrier method consistently; only a single act of motivation is required. However, as with most contraceptive methods, the IUD can produce side-effects such as heavy menstruation and/or pain.

Contraindications

ABSOLUTE : (a) suspected pregnancy (b) pelvic inflammatory disease (c) vaginal bleeding of undiagnosed aetiology (d) cancer of the cervix, uterus or adnexia and other pelvic tumours (e) previous ectopic pregnancy *(50)*.

RELATIVE : (a) anaemia (b) menorrhagia (c) history of PID since last pregnancy (d) purulent cervical discharge (e) distortions of the uterine cavity due to congenital malformations, fibroids (f) unmotivated person *(46)*.

The ideal IUD candidate

The Planned Parenthood Federation of America (PPFA) has described the ideal IUD candidate as a woman :

- who has borne at least one child
- has no history of pelvic disease
- has normal menstrual periods
- is willing to check the IUD tail
- has access to follow-up and treatment of potential problems, and
- is in a monogamous relationship.

The federation does not, however, rule out women who do not conform to this profile *(51)*.

An important finding that has recently emerged is that the IUD is not a method of first choice for nulliparous women. They have more problems with IUD such as expulsions, low abdominal pain and pelvic infection, than other women. IUDs such as copper-T, which are smaller and more pliable are better suited to the small uterus of the nulliparous women, if they cannot use or accept alternative methods of contraception.

In 1985, the American College of Obstetricians and Gynaecologists stated that IUDs are "not recommended for women who have not had children or who have multiple partners, because of the risk of PID and possible infertility" *(51)*.

Timing of insertion

Although the loop can be inserted at almost anytime during a woman's reproductive years (except during pregnancy), the most propitious time for loop insertion is during menstruation or within 10 days of the beginning of a menstrual period *(43)*. During this period, insertion is technically easy because the diameter of the cervical canal is greater at this time than during the secretory phase. The uterus is relaxed and myometrial contractions which might tend to cause expulsion are at a minimum *(45)*. In addition, the risk that a woman is pregnant is remote at this time.

The IUD insertion can also be taken up during the first week after delivery before the woman leaves the hospital ("immediate postpartum insertion"). Special care is required with insertions during the first week after delivery because of the greater risk of perforation during this time. Furthermore, immediate postpartum insertion is associated with a high expulsion rate. A convenient time for loop insertion is 6–8 weeks after delivery ("post-puerperal insertion"). Post-puerperal insertion of an IUD has several advantages. It can be combined with the follow-up examination of the women and her child. IUD insertion can also be taken up immediately after a legally induced first trimester abortion. But IUD insertion immediately after a second trimester abortion is not recommended *(46)*. Since there is a risk of infection, most physicians still do not approve of an IUD insertion after an illegal abortion *(46)*.

Follow-up

An important aspect of IUD insertion is follow-up which is sadly neglected. The objectives of the follow-up examination are : (a) to provide motivation and emotional support for the woman (b) to confirm the presence of the IUD, and (c) diagnose and treat any side-effect or complication *(51)*. The IUD wearer should be examined after her first menstrual period, for the chances of loop expulsion are high during this period; and again after the third menstrual period to evaluate the problems of pain and bleeding; and thereafter at six-month or one-year intervals depending upon the facilities and the convenience of the patient.

The IUD wearer should be given the following instructions : (a) she should regularly check the threads or "tail" to be sure that the IUD is in the uterus; if she fails to locate the threads, she must consult the doctor (b) she should visit the clinic whenever she experiences any side-effects such as fever, pelvic pain and bleeding, and (c) if she misses a period, she must consult the doctor.

SIDE-EFFECTS AND COMPLICATIONS

1. Bleeding

The commonest complaint of women fitted with an IUD (inert or medicated) is increased vaginal bleeding. It accounts for 10–20 per cent of all IUD removals *(51)*. The bleeding may take one or more of the following forms : greater volume of blood loss during menstruation, longer menstrual periods or mid-cycle bleeding *(48)*. From the woman's point of view, irregular bleeding constitutes a source of personal inconvenience; from a medical point of view, the concern is iron-deficiency anaemia. Usually bleeding or spotting between periods settles within 1–2 months *(49)*. The patient who is experiencing the bleeding episodes should receive iron tablets (ferrous sulphate 200 mg, three times daily).

Studies have shown that the greatest blood loss is caused by the larger non-medicated devices. Copper devices seem to cause less average blood loss. Menstrual blood loss is consistently lower when hormone-releasing devices are used *(46)*.

If the bleeding is heavy or persistent or if the patient develops anaemia despite the iron supplement, the IUD should be removed. Since there is often a direct relationship between the bleeding and the size and configuration of the IUD *(50)*, a change of IUD from the Lippes Loop to one of copper devices is advised. In most women, removal of the device is rapidly followed by a return to the normal menstrual pattern. If an abnormal pattern persists, a full gynaecological examination is required to ensure that there is no pelvic pathology *(46)*.

2. Pain

Pain is the second major side-effect leading to IUD removal. WHO estimates that 15–40 per cent of IUD removals appear to be for pain only *(46)*. Pain may be experienced during IUD insertion and for a few days thereafter, as well as during menstruation *(51)*. It may manifest itself in low backache, cramps in the lower abdomen and occasionally pain down the thighs. These symptoms usually disappear by the third month *(49)*.

If during insertion, the pain is particularly severe, it is possible that the device may have been incorrectly placed in the uterus or there is a disparity in size between the device and the uterine cavity. Severe pain can also indicate a uterine perforation *(46)*. Pain could also be due to infection. Pain is more commonly observed in nullipara and those who have not had a child for a number of years *(52, 53)*.

Slight pain during insertion can be controlled by analgesics such as aspirin and codein. If pain is intolerable, the IUD should be removed. In place of a Lippes Loop, a copper device can be tried. If the woman decides not to have an IUD, another method of contraception should be prescribed.

3. Pelvic infection

Pelvic inflammatory disease (PID) is a collective term that includes acute, subacute and chronic conditions of the ovaries, tubes, uterus, connective tissue and pelvic peritoneum and is usually the result of infection *(50)*. Studies suggest that IUD users are about 2 to 8 times more likely to develop PID than non-contraceptors *(54)*. Risk associated with IUD use is greater among women who have a number of sexual partners *(55)* possibly because of greater potential for exposure to STDs. The greater risk of PID with IUD use may be due to introduction of bacteria into the uterus during IUD insertion. Recent work has focused on PID as being caused by organisms ascending the IUD tail from the lower genital tract to uterus and tubes *(56)*. The organisms include Gardnerella, Anaerobic streptococci, Bacteroides, Coliform bacilli and Actinomyces. The risk of PID appears to be the highest in the first few months after IUD insertion.

The clinical manifestations of PID are vaginal discharge, pelvic pain and tenderness, abnormal bleeding, chills and fever. In many cases, the infection may be asymptomatic or low grade. Even one or two episodes of PID can cause infertility permanently blocking the fallopian tubes. Therefore, young women should be fully counselled on the risks of PID before choosing an IUD.

When PID is diagnosed, it should be treated promptly with broad–spectrum antibiotics. Most clinicians recommend removing IUD if infection does not respond to antibiotics within 24–48 hours *(48)*. The risk of PID calls for proper selection of cases for IUD insertion, better sterilization and insertion techniques, and modified devices without tails.

4. Uterine perforation

Many workers have reported uterine perforation by the IUD *(57)*. The reported incidence ranges from 1:150 to 1 : 9000 insertions *(57)*, depending upon the time of insertion, design of the IUD, technique of insertion and operator's experience. In the hands of trained physicians, it should not be higher than 0.3 per cent *(58)*. The device may migrate into the peritoneal cavity causing serious complications such as intestinal obstruction. Copper devices produce an intense tissue reaction leading to peritoneal adhesions. Perforations occur more frequently when insertions are performed between 48 hours and 6 weeks postpartum. Interestingly, the perforation may be completely asymptomatic and discovered only when searching for a missing IUD. The conclusive diagnosis of perforation is usually made by a pelvic X-ray. Evidence suggests that any IUD that has perforated the uterus should be removed because the risks of intra-abdominal inflammatory response leading to adhesions or perforation of organs within the abdominal cavity outweigh the risks associated with removal *(51)*.

5. Pregnancy

Considering all IUDs together, the actual use failure rate in the first year is approximately 3 per cent *(41)*. It differs, in different types of IUDs. About 50 per cent of uterine pregnancies occurring with the device *in situ* end in a spontaneous abortion *(51)*. Removal of the IUD in early pregnancy has been found to reduce this abortion rate by half. In women who continue the pregnancy with the device *in situ*, a 4–fold increase in the occurrence of premature births compared with other women has been reported *(46)*.

The earlier teaching that pregnancy with an IUD *in situ* is not unsafe is no longer accepted. Pregnancy with an IUD should be regarded as a potential medical complication with the dangers of infection and spontaneous abortion. The options left open are *(45)* :

(a) If the woman requests an induced abortion, this is legally available.

(b) If the woman wishes to continue with the pregnancy and the threads are visible, the device should be removed by gently pulling the threads.

(c) If the woman wishes to continue with the pregnancy and the threads are not visible, there should be careful examination for possible complications. If there are any signs of intrauterine infection and sepsis, evacuation of the uterus under broad–spectrum antibiotic cover is mandatory.

If the woman becomes pregnant with the IUD, she should be advised that only 25 per cent of pregnancies will have a successful outcome if the IUD is left in place.

6. Ectopic pregnancy

The possibility of ectopic pregnancy must be considered when an IUD user becomes pregnant. The ectopic pregnancy rate per 1000 women year in levonorgestrel IUD and Cu-T 380A is about 0.2 as compared to non-contraceptive users, where it is about 3–4.5. With progesteron IUD it is higher–about 6.8, because its action is limited to a local effect on endometrium. With levonorgestrel IUD the chances of ectopic pregnancy are less, because it is associated with a partial suppression of gonadotrophins with subsequent disruption of normal follicular growth and inhibition of ovulation in significant number of cycles *(41)*.

Women using IUDs should be taught to recognize the symptoms of ectopic pregnancy – lower abdominal pain, dark and scanty vaginal bleeding or amenorrhoea. Women at high risk of ectopic pregnancy – because of previous PID, tubal pregnancy or other ectopic pregnancy – should not use an IUD if other methods are feasible *(51)*.

7. Expulsion

Expulsion rates vary between 12–20 per cent (Table 19). Expulsion can be partial or complete. Partial expulsion is diagnosed on speculum examination by observing the stem of the IUD protruding through the cervix. Clinical skill, timing of insertion and the age and parity of the user all influence the likelihood of expulsion.

An expulsion usually occurs during the first few weeks following insertion or during menstruation. Expulsion is most common among young women, nulliparous women and women who have a postpartum insertion. Expulsion rates are somewhat lower for copper than for inert devices. As many as 20 per cent of all expulsions go undetected. In general, expulsion in itself is not a serious problem, but if expulsion is unnoticed, pregnancy may occur.

8. Fertility after removal

Fertility does not seem to be impaired after removal of a device provided there has been no episode of PID, whilst the device was *in situ (48)*. Over 70 per cent of previous IUD users conceive within one year of stopping use *(51)*. It is now established that PID is a threat to woman's fertility. There is no meaningful data available on the long-term use of IUD on subsequent fertility *(46)*.

9. Cancer and teratogenesis

There is no evidence to date that IUD use increases cancer risks. Nor is there any evidence of developmental abnormality or congenital malformations among the offspring of either former users of IUDs or those who conceive with an IUD *in situ (46)*.

10. Mortality

Mortality associated with IUD use is extremely rare and has been estimated to be one death per 100,000 woman–years of use, the deaths usually following complications such as septic spontaneous abortion or ectopic pregnancy *(46)*. In fact, IUD is safer than oral contraceptives in this regard, particularly in older or high-risk patients *(46)*.

Of all the available spacing methods of contraception, IUDs are among the most effective, with an average pregnancy rate after one year of about 3–5 per 100 typical users *(51)*. In comparison with other methods, the IUD is a relatively inexpensive form of contraception, because of its long life. Unlike use of barrier methods, IUD use is independent of the time of intercourse. IUDs have a relatively high continuation rates. Inert devices, as well as those with copper lack the systemic metabolic effects associated with oral pills. Women who cannot tolerate the adverse effects of oral pills may find the IUD an acceptable alternative. It does not interfere with lactation. However, because of expulsion and possible side-effects like menstrual irregularities, IUDs should preferably be used in settings where follow-up facilities are available. Evidence to date shows that for a fully informed woman, the IUD can provide a satisfactory, highly effective, relatively low-risk method of contraception.

HORMONAL CONTRACEPTIVES

Hormonal contraceptives when properly used are the most effective spacing methods of contraception. Oral contraceptives of the combined type are almost 100 per cent effective in preventing pregnancy. They provide the best means of ensuring spacing between one childbirth and another. More than 65 million in the world are estimated to be taking the "pill" of which about 9.52 million are estimated to be in India.

Gonadal steroids

To physicians in general medicine, the term "steroid" refers to adrenocortical hormones, while to those in gynaecology, it implies gonadal steroids, i.e., oestrogens and progestogens.

a. *Synthetic oestrogens* : Two synthetic oestrogens are used in oral contraceptives. These are *ethinylestradiol* and *mestranol*. Both are effective. In fact, mestranol is inactive until converted into ethinylestradiol in the liver *(59)*.

b. *Synthetic progestogens* : These are classified into three groups – pregnanes, oestranes and gonanes. (i) *Pregnanes* : These include megestrol, chlormadinone and medroxy–progesterone acetate. The pregnane progestogens are now not recommended in oral contraceptives because of doubts raised by the occurrence of breast tumours in beagle dogs. (ii) *Oestrones* : These are also known as 19-nortestosterones, e.g., norethisterone, norethisterone acetate, lynestrenol, ethynodiol diacetate and norethynodrel. These are all metabolized to norethisterone before becoming active. For some women, oestranes are more acceptable than gonanes. (iii) *Gonanes* : The most favoured gonane is levonorgestrel *(59)*.

Classification

Hormonal contraceptives currently in use and/or under study may be classified as follows :

A. Oral pills
1. Combined pill
2. Progestogen only pill (POP)
3. Post-coital pill
4. Once–a–month (long–acting) pill
5. Male pill

B. Depot (slow release) formulations
1. Injectables
2. Subcutaneous implants
3. Vaginal rings

A. ORAL PILLS

1. Combined pill

The combined pill is one of the major spacing methods of contraception. The "original pill" which entered into the market in the early 1960s contained 100–200 mcg of a synthetic oestrogen and 10 mg of a progestogen. Since then, a number of improvements have been made to reduce the undesirable side-effects of the pill by reducing the dose of both the oestrogen and progestogen. At the present time, most formulations of the combined pill contain no more than 30–35 mcg of a synthetic oestrogen, and 0.5 to 1.0 mg of a progestogen. The debate continues about the minimum effective dose of the progestogen in the pill which will produce the least metabolic disturbances.

The pill is given orally for 21 consecutive days beginning on the 5th day of the menstrual cycle (for a few preparations

20 or 22 days are advised), followed by a break of 7 days during which period menstruation occurs. When the bleeding occurs, this is considered the first day of the next cycle. The bleeding which occurs is not like normal menstruation, but is an episode of uterine bleeding from an incompletely formed endometrium caused by the withdrawal of exogenous hormones. Therefore it is called "withdrawal bleeding" rather than menstruation. Further, the loss of blood which occurs is about half that occurring in a woman having ovulatory cycle. If bleeding does not occur, the woman is instructed to start the second cycle one week after the preceding one. Ordinarily, the woman "menstruates" after the second course of pill intake.

The pill should be taken everyday at a fixed time, preferably before going to bed at night. The first course should be started strictly on the 5th day of the menstrual period, as any deviation in this respect may not prevent pregnancy. If the user forgets to take a pill, she should take it as soon as she remembers, and that she should take the next day's pill at the usual time.

Types of pills

The Department of Family Welfare, in the Ministry of Health and Family Welfare, Government of India has made available 2 types of low-dose oral pills under the brand names of MALA-N and MALA-D. It contains Levonorgestrel 0.15 mg and Ethinyl estradiol 0.03 mg. Mala-D in a package of 28 pills (21 of oral contraceptive pills and 7 brown film coated 60 mg ferrous fumarate tablets) is made available to the consumer under social marketing at a price of Rs. 3 per packet. Mala-N is supplied free of cost through all PHCs, urban family welfare centres, etc. Some of the combined pills are as shown in Table 20.

TABLE 20
Some combination oral contraceptives

Name	Progestin	(mg)
(A) *With EE 0.02 mg*		
Loestrin 1/20	Norethisterone acetate	1.00
Femilon	Desogestrel	0.15
(B) *With EE 0.03 mg*		
Eugynon 30	Levonorgestrel	0.25
Microgynon, Ovral L Triquilar (Varying E E and levonorgestrel) Primovlar 30, Mala D,	Levonorgestrel	0.15
Choice	Norgestrel	0.30
Novelon	Desogestrel	0.15
Yasmin	Drospirenone	3.00
(C) *With EE 0.05 mg and less progestogenic*		
Eugynon 50, Duoluton, Ovral G	Norgestrel	0.50
Ovral, Primovlar 50	Levonorgestrel	0.25
Minovlar Ed, Orlest	Norethisterone acetate	1.00
Orthonovin 1/50	Norethisterone	1.00
(D) *With EE 0.05 mg and more progestogenic*		
Orgalutin	Lynestrenol	2.50
Norlestrin 2.5/50	Norethisterone acetate	2.50
Gynovlar 21	-Do-	3.00
Anovlar 21	-Do-	4.00

2. Progestogen-only pill (POP)

This pill is commonly referred to as "minipill" or "micropill". It contains only progestogen, which is given in small doses throughout the cycle. The commonly used progestogens are norethisterone and levonorgestrel.

The progestogen-only pills never gained widespread use because of poor cycle control and an increased pregnancy rate *(60)*. However, they have a definite place in modern-day contraception. They could be prescribed to older women for whom the combined pill is contraindicated because of cardiovascular risks. They may also be considered in young women with risk factors for neoplasia *(61)*. The evidence that the progestogens may lower the high-density lipoproteins may be of some concern.

3. Post-coital contraception

Post-coital (or "morning after") contraception is recommended within 72 hours of an unprotected intercourse. Two methods are available :

(a) *IUD* : The simplest technique is to insert an IUD, if acceptable, especially a copper device within 5 days.

(b) *Hormonal* : More often a hormonal method may be preferable. In India Levonorgestrel 0.75 mg tablet is approved for emergency contraception. It is used as one tablet of 0.75 mg within 72 hours of unprotected sex and the 2nd tablet after 12 hours of 1st dose.

or

Two oral contraceptive pills containing 50 mcg of ethinyl estradiol within 72 hours after intercourse, and the same dose after 12 hours.

or

Four oral contraceptive pills containing 30 or 35 mcg of ethinyl estradiol within 72 hours and 4 tablets after 12 hours.

or

Mifepristone 10 mg once within 72 hours.

Post-coital contraception is advocated as an emergency method; for example, after unprotected intercourse, rape or contraceptive failure. Opinion is divided about the effect on foetus, should the method fail. Although the failure rate for post-coital contraception is less than 1 per cent, some experts think a woman should not use the hormonal method unless she intends to have an abortion, if the method fails. There is no evidence that foetal abnormalities will occur. But some doubts remain *(62)*.

4. Once–a–month (long-acting) pill

Experiments with once–a–month oral pill in which quinestrol, a long-acting oestrogen is given in combination with a short-acting progestogen, have been disappointing *(63)*. The pregnancy rate is too high to be acceptable. In addition, bleeding tends to be irregular.

5. Male pill

The search for a male contraceptive began in 1950 *(64)*. Research is following 4 main lines of approach : (a) preventing spermatogenesis (b) interfering with sperm storage and maturation (c) preventing sperm transport in the vas, and (d) affecting constituents of the seminal fluid. Most of the research is concentrated on interference with spermatogenesis. An ideal male contraceptive would decrease sperm count while leaving testosterone at normal levels. But hormones that suppress sperm production tend to lower testosterone and affect potency and libido.

A male pill made of gossypol – a derivative of cotton-seed oil, has been very much in the news. It is effective in producing azoospermia or severe oligospermia, but as many as 10 per cent of men may be permanently azoospermic after taking it for 6 months. Further gossypol could be toxic. Animal studies show a narrow margin between effective and toxic doses. At present it does not seem that gossypol will ever be widely used as a male contraceptive *(65)*.

MODE OF ACTION OF ORAL PILLS

The mechanism of action of the combined oral pill is to prevent the release of the ovum from the ovary. This is achieved by blocking the pituitary secretion of gonadotropin that is necessary for ovulation to occur. Progestogen–only preparations render the cervical mucus thick and scanty and thereby inhibit sperm penetration. Progestogens also inhibit tubal motility and delay the transport of the sperm and of the ovum to the uterine cavity *(63)*.

EFFECTIVENESS

Taken according to the prescribed regimen, oral contraceptives of the combined type are almost 100 per cent effective in preventing pregnancy *(50)*. Some women do not take the pill regularly, so the actual rate is lower. In developed countries, the annual pregnancy rate is less than 1 per cent but in many other countries, the pregnancy rate is considerably higher *(63)*.

Under clinical trial conditions, the effectiveness of progestogen–only pills is almost as good as that of the combination products. However, in large family planning programmes, the effectiveness and continuation rates are usually lower than in clinical trials. The effectiveness may also be affected by certain drugs such as rifampicin, phenobarbital and ampicillin *(63)*.

RISKS AND BENEFITS

a. Adverse effects

1. Cardiovascular effects

Data from the earlier case control studies *(66, 67)* and the Oral Contraceptive Study of the RCGP *(68)* and the Oxford Study in UK *(68, 69)* provided conclusive evidence that the use of the combined pill was associated with an excess mortality. Women who had used the pill were reported to have a 40 per cent higher death rate than women who had never taken the pill. Virtually, all the excess mortality was due to cardiovascular causes, that is myocardial infarction, cerebral thrombosis and venous thrombosis, with or without pulmonary embolus *(70, 71)*. The risk increased substantially with age and cigarette smoking. The evidence was convincing that the cardiovascular complications were positively associated with the oestrogen content of the pill.

The above findings led to the progressive reduction of the oestrogen content to the minimum levels necessary to maintain contraceptive effect. In spite of this reduction, it became clear by 1980 that some of the untoward vascular effects (e.g., hypertension) persisted, in addition to metabolic effects which are attributed to the progestogen content of the pill. It became clear that progestogen levels must also be minimal to avoid the complications of pill use.

2. Carcinogenesis

A review prepared by WHO *(72)* concluded that there was no clear evidence of a relationship, either positive or negative between the use of combined pill and the risk of any form of cancer. However, the WHO Multicentre case-control study on the possible association between the use of hormonal contraceptives and neoplasia indicated a trend towards increased risk of cervical cancer with increasing duration of use of oral contraceptives; this finding is being further explored *(73)*.

3. Metabolic effects

A great deal of attention has been focused recently on the metabolic effects induced by oral contraceptives. These have included the elevation of blood pressure, the alteration in serum lipids with a particular effect on decreasing high-density lipoproteins, blood clotting and the ability to modify carbohydrate metabolism with the resultant elevations of blood glucose and plasma insulin *(74)*. These effects are positively related to the dose of the progestogen component *(75)*. Family planning specialists have voiced a growing concern that the adverse effects associated with oral contraceptives could be a potential long–range problem for the users in that they may accelerate atherogenesis and result in clinical problems such as myocardial infarction and stroke.

4. Other adverse effects

(i) *Liver disorders* : The use of the pill may lead to hepatocellular adenoma and gall bladder disease. Cholestatic jaundice can occur in some pill users. (ii) *Lactation* : Preparations containing a relatively high amount of oestrogen adversely affect the quantity and constituents of breast milk *(73)*, and less frequently cause premature cessation of lactation. In a WHO study *(73)* users of the combined pill experienced a 42 per cent decline in milk volume after 18 weeks, compared with a decline of 12 per cent for users of progestogen-only minipills and 0.16 per cent for controls using non-hormonal preparations. Women taking oral contraceptives, no matter what type, excrete small quantities of hormones in their breast milk, but little is known about the long-term impact, if any, on the child *(71)*. (iii) *Subsequent fertility*: In general, oral contraceptive use seems to be followed by a slight delay in conception *(76)*. The proportion of women becoming pregnant within 2 months of discontinuing the pill may range from 15–35 per cent *(77)*. It is not known whether the prolonged use of the pill beyond 5–10 years affects subsequent fertility. (iv) *Ectopic pregnancies* : These are more likely to occur in women taking progestogen-only pills, but not in those taking combined pills. (v) *Foetal development* : Several reports have suggested that oral pills taken inadvertently during (or even just before) pregnancy might increase the incidence of birth defects of the foetus, but this is not yet substantiated *(78)*.

5. Common unwanted effects

(i) *Breast tenderness* : Breast tenderness, fullness and discomfort have been observed in women taking oral pills. Breast engorgement and fullness are said to be dependent on progestogen; pain and tenderness are attributed to oestrogen. (ii) *Weight gain* : About 25 per cent of users complain of weight gain. It is usually less than 2 kg, and occurs during the first 6 months of use. This is attributed to water retention, in which case restriction of salt intake is usually effective. (iii) *Headache and migraine* : Migraine may be aggravated or triggered by the pill. Women, whose migraine requires treatment with vasoconstrictors such as ergotamine, should not take oral pills. (iv) *Bleeding disturbances* : A small minority of women using oral contraceptives may complain of break-through bleeding or spotting in the early cycles. A few women may not have a withdrawal bleeding at the end of a cycle. Women should be forewarned of these possibilities.

b. Beneficial effects

The single most significant benefit of the pill is its almost 100 per cent effectiveness in preventing pregnancy and thereby removing anxiety about the risk of unplanned pregnancy. Apart from this, the pill has a number of non-contraceptive health benefits *(79)*. Both the Royal College of General Practitioners' and the Oxford Family Planning Association's long-term prospective studies of pill use in Britain have shown that using the pill may give protection against at least 6 diseases: benign breast disorders including fibrocystic disease and fibroadenoma, ovarian cysts, iron–deficiency anaemia, pelvic inflammatory disease, ectopic pregnancy and ovarian cancer.

Contraindications

(a) *Absolute* : Cancer of the breast and genitals; liver disease, previous or present history of thromboembolism; cardiac abnormalities; congenital hyperlipidaemia; undiagnosed abnormal uterine bleeding.

(b) *Special problems requiring medical surveillance* : Age over 40 years; smoking and age over 35 years; mild hypertension; chronic renal disease; epilepsy; migraine; nursing mothers in the first 6 months; diabetes mellitus; gall bladder disease; history of infrequent bleeding, amenorrhoea, etc. *(63)*.

Duration of use

The pill should be used primarily for spacing pregnancies in younger women. Those over 35 years should go in for other forms of contraception. Beyond 40 years of age, the pill is not to be prescribed or continued because of the sharp increase in the risk of cardiovascular complications (*63*).

Medical supervision *(80)*

Women taking oral contraceptives should be advised annual medical examinations. An examination before prescribing oral pills is required (a) to identify those with contraindications, and (b) those with special problems that require medical intervention or supervision. A check-list (Table 21) has been developed for screening women who can be given oral pills by the health workers.

TABLE 21

Check-list for prescription of oral contraceptives

Check the following by history and examination	Yes	No
Above 40 years of age	....	....
Above 35 years of age and a heavy smoker	....	....
Seizures	....	....
Severe pain in the calves or thighs	....	....
Symptomatic varicose veins in the legs	....	....
Severe chest pains	....	....
Unusual shortness of breath after examination	....	....
Severe headaches and/or visual disturbances	....	....
Lactating (yes = for less than 6 months)	....	....
Intermenstrual bleeding and/ or bleeding after sexual intercourse	...	....
Amenorrhoea	....	....
Abnormally yellow skin, eyes	....	....
Blood pressure (yes = above 140 mm Hg systolic and/or 90 mm Hg diastolic)	....	....
Mass in the breast	....	....
Swollen legs (oedema)	....	....
Instructions : If all the above are negative, the woman may be given oral contraceptives. If any are positive, she must first be seen by a doctor.		

Source : *(71)*

B. DEPOT FORMULATIONS

The need for depot formulations which are highly effective, reversible, long-acting and oestrogen-free for spacing pregnancies in which a single administration suffices for several months or years cannot be stressed. The injectable contraceptives, subdermal implants and vaginal rings come in this category.

1. Injectable contraceptives

There are two types of injectable contraceptives. Progestogen–only injectables and the newer once–a–month combined injectables. The formulation and injection schedules of injectable contraceptives are as shown in Table 22.

A. PROGESTOGEN–ONLY INJECTABLES

Thus far, only two injectable hormonal contraceptives – both based on progestogen – have been found suitable. They offer more reliable protection against unwanted pregnancies than the older barrier techniques. These are :

a. DMPA (Depot-medroxyprogesterone acetate)

b. NET-EN (Norethisterone enantate)

c. DMPA-SC

a. DMPA *(81)*

Depot-medroxyprogesterone acetate (DMPA or Depo-provera) has been in use since 1960s. The standard dose is an intramuscular injection of 150 mg every 3 months. It

TABLE 22
Formulations and injection schedules of injectable contraceptives

Common trade names	Formulation	Injection type and schedule
Progestin - Only Injectables		
Depo-Provera®, Megestron®, Contracep®, Depo-Prodasone®	Depot medroxyprogesterone acetate (DMPA) 150 mg	One intramuscular (IM) injection every 3 months
depo-subQ provera 104® (DMPA-SC)	DMPA 104 mg	One subcutaneous injection every 3 months
Noristerat®, Norigest®, Doryxas®	Norethisterone enanthate (NET-EN) 200 mg	One IM injection every 2 months
Combined Injectable (progestin + estrogen)[1]		
Cyclofem®, Ciclofeminina®, Lunelle®[2]	Medroxyprogesterone acetate 25 mg + Estradiol cypionate 5 mg (MPA/E_2C)	One IM injection every month
Mesigyna®, Norigynon®	NET-EN 50 mg + Estradiol valerate 5 mg (NET-EN/E_2V)	One IM injection every month
Deladroxale®, Perlutal®, Topasel®, Patectro®, Deproxone®, Nomagest®	Dihydroxyprogesterone (algestone) acetophenide 150 mg + Estradiol enanthate 10 mg	One IM injection every month
Anafertin®, Yectames®	Dihydroxyprogesterone (algestone) acetophenide 75 mg + Estradiol enanthate 5 mg	One IM injection every month
Chinese Injectable No. 1®	17α-hydroxyprogesterone caproate 250 mg + Estradiol valerate 5 mg	One IM injection every month, except 2 injections in first month

[1] Also called monthly injectables.
[2] The U.S. Food and Drug Administration approved Lunelle, but it is currently not available in the United States.

Source : *(81)*

gives protection from pregnancy in 99 per cent of women for at least 3 months. It exerts its contraceptive effect primarily by suppression of ovulation. However, it also has an indirect effect on the endometrium and direct action on the fallopian tubes and on the production of cervical mucus, all of which may play a role in reducing fertility. DMPA has been found to be a safe, effective and acceptable contraceptive which requires a minimum of motivation or none at all. Another advantage is that it does not affect lactation. Therefore in the experience of several countries, DMPA has proved acceptable during the postpartum period as a means of spacing pregnancies. However, the side-effects of DMPA (viz. weight increase, irregular menstrual bleeding and prolonged infertility after its use) are disadvantages limiting the age groups for which the drug could regularly be used. As now practiced in a number of countries, this contraceptive should find good use among multiparae of age over 35 years who have already completed their families.

b. NET-EN

Norethisterone enantate (NET-EN) has been in use as a contraceptive since 1966. However, it has been less extensively used than DMPA. It is given intramuscularly in a dose of 200 mg every 60 days. Contraceptive action appears to include inhibition of ovulation, and progestogenic effects on cervical mucus. A slightly higher (0.4) pregnancy rate (failure rate) has been reported as compared to DMPA.

Administration

The initial injection of both DMPA and NET-EN should be given during the first 5 days of the menstrual period. This timing is very important to rule out the possibility of pregnancy. Both are given by deep intramuscular injection into the gluteus maximus. The injection site should never be massaged following injections. *(82)*. Although compliance with regular injection intervals should be encouraged, both DMPA and Net-EN may be given two weeks early or two weeks late *(83)*.

c. DMPA-SC 104 mg *(81)*

A new lower-dose formulation of DMPA, *depo-subQ provera 104* (also called DMPA-SC), is injected under the skin rather than in the muscle. It contains 104 mg of DMPA rather than the 150 mg in the intramuscular formulation. Like the intramuscular formulation, DMPA-SC is given at 3-month intervals.

DMPA-SC is just as effective as the formulation injected into the muscle, and the patterns of bleeding changes and amount of weight gain are similar.

Injections of DMPA-SC are given in the upper thigh or abdomen. DMPA-SC should not be injected intramuscularly, and the intramuscular formulation should not be injected subcutaneously. The intramuscular formulation cannot be diluted to make the lower-dose subcutaneous formulation.

Side-effects

Both DMPA and NET-EN have similar side effects, the most common being disruption of the normal menstrual cycle, manifested by episodes of unpredictable bleeding, at times prolonged and at other times excessive. In addition, many women using DMPA or NET-EN may become amenorrhoeic. The unpredictable bleeding may be very inconvenient to the user; and amenorrhoea can be alarming, causing anxiety. Studies showed that women discontinuing DMPA became pregnant some 5.5 months (average) after the treatment period. At 2 years, more than 90 per cent of previous users became pregnant *(82)*. A study is in progress in India to examine the return of fertility among women who discontinued NET-EN. The potential long-term effects of DMPA and NET-EN are not yet known.

Contraindications

These include cancer of the breast; all genital cancers; undiagnosed abnormal uterine bleeding; and a suspected malignancy. Women usually should not start using a progestin-only injectable if they have high blood pressure (systolic ≥ 160 mm Hg or diastolic ≥ 100), certain conditions of the heart, blood vessels, or liver including history of stroke or heart attack and current deep vein thrombosis. Also, a woman breast-feeding a baby less than 6 weeks old should not use progestin-only injectables *(81)*.

The particular advantage of DMPA and NET-EN is that they are highly effective, long-lasting and reversible contraceptives. Check-lists have been developed for auxiliaries primarily for the screening of women who can be given injectable contraceptives without being examined by the physician; they can also be utilized in follow-up visits.

B. COMBINED INJECTABLE CONTRACEPTIVES

These injectables contain a progestogen and an oestrogen. They are given at monthly intervals, plus or minus three days. Combined injectable contraceptives act mainly by suppression of ovulation. The cervical mucus is affected, mainly by progestogen, and becomes an obstacle to sperm penetration. Changes are also produced in endometrium which makes it unfavourable for implantation if fertilization occurs, which is extremely unlikely.

In clinical trials, Cyclofem/Cycloprovera and Mesigyna have both been found to be highly effective with 12 month failure rates of 0.2 per cent or less for Cyclofem/Cycloprovera and 0.4 per cent for Mesigyna. The side-effects are similar to progestogen only injectables, but are much less. Data on return to ovulation and fertility are limited.

The contraindications are confirmed or suspected pregnancy; past or present evidence of thromboembolic disorders; cerebrovascular or coronary artery disease; focal migraine; malignancy of the breast; and diabetes with vascular complications. Combined injectables are not suitable for women who are fully breast feeding until 6 months postpartum. It is less suitable for women with risk factors for oestrogen.

2. Subdermal implants

The Population Council, New York has developed a subdermal implant known as **Norplant** for long-term contraception. It consists of 6 silastic (silicone rubber) capsules containing 35 mg (each) of levonorgestrel *(84)*. More recent devices comprise fabrication of levonorgestrel into 2 small rods, **Norplant (R)-2**, which are comparatively easier to insert and remove. The silastic capsules or rods are implanted beneath the skin of the forearm or upper arm. Effective contraception is provided for over 5 years. The contraceptive effect of Norplant is reversible on removal of capsules. A large multicentre trial conducted by International Committee for Contraception Research (ICCR) reported a 3–year pregnancy rate of 0.7. The main disadvantages, however, appear to be irregularities of menstrual bleeding and surgical procedures necessary to insert and remove implants.

3. Vaginal rings

Vaginal rings containing levonorgestrel have been found to be effective. The hormone is slowly absorbed through the vaginal mucosa, permitting most of it to bypass the digestive system and liver, and allowing a potentially lower dose. The ring is worn in the vagina for 3 weeks of the cycle and removed for the fourth *(85)*.

4. Centchroman non-hormonal pill (Chhaya) :

Centchroman is commonly known as weekly pill as for the first three months it is taken biweekly and from 4th month onwards, once weekly. It can be initiated anytime during the menstrual cycle if it is reasonably certain that the woman is not pregnant.

However, the following timing of initiation can be opted by the women to start the package after proper screening by health-care provider :

- on first day of period
- on the day of abortion itself
- within 4 weeks after childbirth, whether breastfeeding or not

To start with, take one pill at the correct time (mentioned above) and take another pill three days later (2 pills in a week). Then the schedule of these 2 pills per week to be followed for three months. From fourth month onwards, only one pill per week to be taken (the first pill day to be repeated every week) This weekly regime to be continued, regardless of menstrual cycle, till protection from pregnancy is needed *(86)*.

POST-CONCEPTIONAL METHODS

(Termination of pregnancy)

Menstrual regulation

A relatively simple method of birth control is "menstrual regulation". It consists of aspiration of the uterine contents 6 to 14 days of a missed period, but before most pregnancy tests can accurately determine whether or not a woman is pregnant *(45)*. Cervical dilatation is indicated only in nullipara or in apprehensive subjects. No after-care is necessary as a rule.

The immediate complications are uterine perforation and trauma. Late complications (after 6 weeks) include a tendency to abortion or premature labour, infertility, menstrual disorders, increase in ectopic pregnancies and Rh-immunization *(87)*.

Some regard menstrual regulation as very early abortion, others view it as a treatment for delayed periods. Menstrual regulation differs from abortion in 3 respects *(88)* : (a) the lack of certainty if a pregnancy is being terminated. Microscopic examination of the aspirated material can confirm pregnancy *post facto*, but it is not obligatory (b) the lack of legal restrictions, and (c) the increased safety of the early procedure.

Menstrual induction

This is based on disturbing the normal progesterone–prostaglandin balance by intrauterine application of 1–5 mg solution (or 2.5–5 mg pellet) of prostaglandin F2. Within a few minutes of the prostaglandin impact, performed under sedation, the uterus responds with a sustained contraction lasting about 7 minutes, followed by cyclic contractions continuing for 3–4 hours. The bleeding starts and continues for 7–8 days *(87)*.

Oral abortifacient

Mifepristone (RU 486) in combination with misoprostol is 95 per cent successful in terminating pregnancies of upto 9 week's duration with minimum complications. The commonly used regimen is mifepristone 200 mg orally on day 1, followed by misoprostol 800 mcg vaginally either immediately or within 6–8 hours. Commercially it comes as MTP kit having combipack tablets of mifepristone 200 mg one tablet and misoprostol 200 mcg 4 tablets (800 mcg).

The other regimen is a dose of mifepristone 600 mg on day one, followed by 400 mcg orally of misoprostol on day three.

The patient should return for a follow-up visit approximately 14 days after the administration of mifepristone to confirm by clinical examination or ultra-sonographic scan that a complete termination of pregnancy has occurred. Patients who have an ongoing pregnancy at this visit have a risk of foetal malformation resulting from the treatment. Surgical termination is recommended to manage medical abortion treatment failures.

Contraindications

Administration of mifepristone and misoprostol is contraindicated in following conditions : (1) History of allergy or known hypersensitivity to mifepristone, misoprostol or other prostaglandin; (2) Confirmed or suspected ectopic pregnancy or undiagnosed adnexal mass; (3) IUD in place; (4) Chronic adrenal failure; (5) Haemorrhagic disorder or concurrent anticoagulant therapy; (6) Inherited porphyria; and (7) If a patient does not have adequate access to medical facilities equipped to provide emergency treatment of incomplete abortion and blood transfusion.

ABORTION

Abortion is theoretically defined as termination of pregnancy before the foetus becomes viable (capable of living independently). This has been fixed administratively at 28 weeks, when the foetus weighs approximately 1000 g. Abortion is sought by women for a variety of reasons including birth control. In fact, in some countries (e.g., Hungary) the legal abortions exceed live births.

Abortions are usually categorized as spontaneous and induced. Spontaneous abortions occur once in every 15 pregnancies *(89)*. They may be considered "Nature's method of birth control". Induced abortions, on the other hand, are deliberately induced – they may be legal or illegal. Illegal abortions are hazardous; they are usually the last resort of women determined to end their pregnancies at the risk of their own lives.

Abortion hazards

On an average, 73 million induced (safe and unsafe) abortions take place worldwide each year. About 61 per cent of all unintended pregnancies and 29 per cent of all pregnancies, end in induced abortion *(90)*. The rate of abortion was higher in developing regions than in developed world. About 45 per cent unsafe abortions were estimated to have taken place worldwide each year, almost all in developing world. Among these, 8 million were carried out in the least safe or dangerous conditions. Over half of all estimated unsafe abortions globally were in Asia. 3 out of 4 abortions that occurred in Africa and Latin America were unsafe. Each year between 4.7 per cent to 13.2 per cent of maternal deaths can be attributed to unsafe abortion. Around 7 million women are hospitalized every year in developing countries as a result of unsafe abortion.

Abortions are safe if they are done with a method recommended by WHO that is appropriate to the pregnancy duration and if the person providing abortion is trained. Unsafe abortion occurs when a pregnancy is terminated either by a person lacking the necessary skills or in an environment that does not conform to minimal medical standards, or both. The people, skills and medical standards considered safe in the provision of induced abortion are different for medical abortion (which is performed by drugs alone and/or surgical abortion) and that which is performed with a manual or electric aspirator. In developed regions it is estimated that 30 women die for every 100,000 unsafe abortions. This number rises to 220 deaths, per 100,000 unsafe abortions in developing regions and 520 deaths in sub-Saharan Africa *(91)*.

In India an ICMR study documented that the rates of safe (legal) and unsafe (illegal) abortion were 6.1 and 13.5 per 1000 pregnancies respectively. It is evident that perhaps two thirds of all abortions take place outside authorized health service by unauthorized and often unskilled persons *(92)*.

The EARLY COMPLICATIONS of abortion include haemorrhage, shock, sepsis; uterine perforation, cervical injury, thromboembolism and anaesthetic and psychiatric complications. The LATE SEQUELAE include infertility, ectopic gestation, increased risk of spontaneous abortion and reduced birth weight.

Data indicates that the seventh and eighth week of gestation is the optimal time for termination of pregnancy *(93)*. Studies indicate that the risk of death is 7 times higher for women who wait until the second trimester to terminate pregnancy. The Indian Law (MTP Act, 1971) allowed abortion only upto 20 weeks of pregnancy. In the year 2020 the MTP Bill was amended, to increase the duration of pregnancy upto 24 weeks.

Legalization of abortion

During the last 25 years there have been gradual liberalization of abortion laws throughout the world. Until 1971, abortions in India were governed exclusively by the Indian Penal Code 1860 and the Code of Criminal Procedure 1898, and were considered a crime except when performed to save the life of a pregnant woman. The Medical Termination of Pregnancy Act was passed by the Indian Parliament in 1971 and came into force from April 1, 1972 (except in Jammu and Kashmir, where it came into effect from November 1, 1976). Implementing rules and regulations initially written in 1971 were revised again in 1992 *(94)*. The Medical Termination of Pregnancy Act is a health care measure which helps to reduce maternal morbidity and mortality resulting from illegal abortions. It also affords an opportunity for motivating such women to adopt some form of contraception.

THE MEDICAL TERMINATION OF PREGNANCY ACT 1971

The Medical Termination of Pregnancy Act, 1971 lays down :

1. The conditions under which a pregnancy can be terminated.
2. The person or persons who can perform such terminations, and
3. The place where such terminations can be performed.

1. The conditions under which a pregnancy can be terminated under the MTP Act. 1971 :

There are 5 conditions that have been identified in the Act :

a. *Medical* – where continuation of the pregnancy might endanger the mother's life or cause grave injury to her physical or mental health.
b. *Eugenic* – where there is substantial risk of the child being born with serious handicaps due to physical or mental abnormalities.

c. *Humanitarian* – where pregnancy is the result of rape.

d. *Socio-economic* – where actual or reasonably foreseeable environments (whether social or economic) could lead to risk of injury to the health of the mother, and

e. *Failure of contraceptive devices* – The anguish caused by an unwanted pregnancy resulting from a failure of any contraceptive device or method can be presumed to constitute a grave mental injury to the health of the mother. This condition is a unique feature of the Indian law and virtually allows abortion on request, in view of the difficulty of proving that a pregnancy was not caused by failure of contraception.

The written consent of the guardian is necessary before performing abortion in women under 18 years of age, and in lunatics even if they are older than 18 years.

2. The person or persons who can perform abortion

The Act provides safeguards to the mother by authorizing only a Registered Medical Practitioner having experience in gynaecology and obstetrics to perform abortion where the length of pregnancy does not exceed 12 weeks. However, where the pregnancy exceeds 12 weeks and is not more than 20 weeks, the opinion of two Registered Medical Practitioners is necessary to terminate the pregnancy.

3. Where abortion can be done

The Act stipulates that no termination of pregnancy shall be made at any place other than a hospital established or maintained by Government or a place approved for the purpose of this Act by Government.

Abortion services are provided in hospitals in strict confidence. The name of the abortion seeker is kept confidential, since abortion has been treated statutorily as a personal matter.

MTP RULES (1975)

Rules and Regulations framed initially were altered in October 1975 to eliminate time-consuming procedures involved in MTP and to make services more readily available. These changes have occurred in 3 administrative areas *(95, 96)*.

1. Approval by Board

Under the new rules, the Chief Medical Officer of the district is empowered to certify that a doctor has the necessary training in gynaecology and obstetrics to do abortions. The procedure of doctors applying to Certification Boards was removed.

2. Qualification required to do abortion

The new rules allow for registered medical practitioners to qualify through on the spot training :

> "If he has assisted a RMP in the performance of 25 cases of medical termination of pregnancy in an approved institution".

The doctor may also qualify to do MTPs under the new rules if he has one or more of the following qualifications which are similar to the old rules :

(a) 6 months housemanship in obstetrics and gynaecology.

(b) a postgraduate qualification in OBG.

(c) 3 years of practice in OBG for those doctors registered before the 1971 MTP Act was passed.

(d) 1 year of practice in OBG for those doctors registered on or after the date of commencement of the Act.

3. The place where abortion is performed

Under the new rules, non-governmental institutions may also take up abortions provided they obtain a licence from the Chief Medical Officer of the district, thus eliminating the requirement of private clinics obtaining a Board licence.

Impact of liberalization of abortion

Although abortion has been greatly liberalized, the annual number of legal abortions are about 6.1 per 1000 pregnancies, whereas the illegal abortions performed in the country are about 13.5 per 1000 pregnancies. In other words, illegal abortions are still rife although it is now more than 45 years since MTP Act was promulgated.

An amendment to the MTP Act in the year 2003 includes decentralization of power for approval of places as MTP centres, from state to district level with the aim of enlarging the network of safe MTP centres, and MTP service providers. The strategy at the community level is : (a) spread awareness regarding safe MTP in the community and the availability of services thereof ; (b) Enhance access to confidential counselling for safe MTP; train ANMs, AWWs, and link workers/ASHAs to provide such counselling; and (c) Promote post-abortion care through ANMs, AWWs, link workers/ASHAs while maintaining confidentiality. At the facility level the strategy is : (1) To provide manual Vaccum Aspiration facility at all CHCs and at least 50 per cent of PHCs that are being strengthened for 24 hour deliveries; (2) Provide comprehensive and high quality MTP services at all FRUs; and (3) Encourage private and NGO sectors to establish quality MTP services *(98)*.

According to the new Oct. 2022 ruling of Supreme Court, Rule 3B allows abortion between 20 and 24 weeks of pregnancy if there is a change in marital status during pregnancy including widowhood or divorce. The Supreme Court declared that rule 3B must also extend to unmarried women who experience a change in their relationship (even if not married) status, whether due to separation from, desertion by or death of their partners *(97)*.

Repeated abortion is not conducive to the health of the mother. It has to be ensured that abortion does not replace the traditional methods of birth control. The numerous abortion hazards which are inherent should serve as a warning that abortions under the best of circumstances can never be as safe as efficient contraception.

MISCELLANEOUS

1. Abstinence

The only method of birth control which is completely effective is complete sexual abstinence. It is sound in theory; in practice, an oversimplification. It amounts to repression of a natural force and is liable to manifest itself in other directions such as temperamental changes and even nervous breakdown. Therefore, it can hardly be considered as a method of contraception to be advocated to the masses.

2. Coitus interruptus

This is the oldest method of voluntary fertility control.

It involves no cost or appliances. It continues to be a widely practised method. The male withdraws before ejaculation, and thereby tries to prevent deposition of semen into the vagina. Some couples are able to practise this method successfully, while others find it difficult to manage. The chief drawback of this method is that the precoital secretion of the male may contain sperm, and even a drop of semen is sufficient to cause pregnancy. Further, the slightest mistake in timing the withdrawal may lead to the deposition of a certain amount of semen. Therefore, the failure rate with this method may be as high as 25 per cent.

Hitherto, the alleged side-effects (e.g., pelvic congestion, vaginismus, anxiety neurosis) were highly magnified. Today, expert opinion is changing in this respect. If the couple prefers it, there should be no objection to its use. It is better than using no family planning method at all. It is conceded that coitus interruptus along with abstinence and abortion played a major role in reducing birth rates in the developed world during the 18th and 19th centuries *(45)*.

3. Safe period (rhythm method)

This is also known as the *"calendar method"* first described by Ogino in 1930. The method is based on the fact that ovulation occurs from 12 to 16 days before the onset of menstruation (see Fig. 7). The days on which conception is likely to occur are calculated as follows :

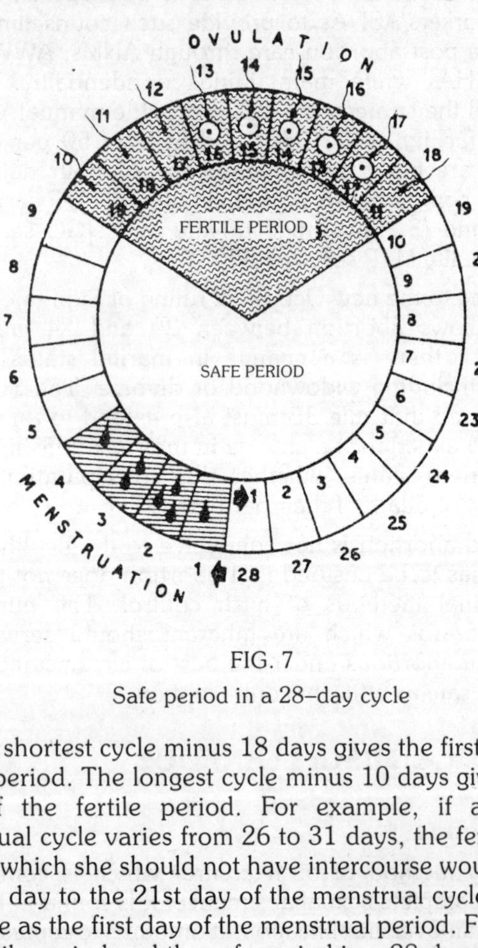

FIG. 7
Safe period in a 28–day cycle

The shortest cycle minus 18 days gives the first day of the fertile period. The longest cycle minus 10 days gives the last day of the fertile period. For example, if a woman's menstrual cycle varies from 26 to 31 days, the fertile period during which she should not have intercourse would be from the 8th day to the 21st day of the menstrual cycle, counting day one as the first day of the menstrual period. Fig. 7 shows the fertile period and the safe period in a 28-day cycle.

However, where such calculations are not possible, the couple can be advised to avoid intercourse from the 8th to the 22nd day of the menstrual cycle, counting from the first day of the menstrual period *(94)*.

The drawbacks of the calendar method are : (a) a woman's menstrual cycles are not always regular. If the cycles are irregular, it is difficult to predict the safe period (b) it is only possible for this method to be used by educated and responsible couples with a high degree of motivation and cooperation (c) compulsory abstinence of sexual intercourse for nearly one half of every month – what may be called "programmed sex" (d) this method is not applicable during the postnatal period, and (e) a high failure rate of 9 per 100 woman–years *(40)*. The failures are due to wrong calculations, inability to follow calculations, irregular use and "taking chances".

Two medical complications have been reported to result from the use of safe period; ectopic pregnancies and embryonic abnormalities. Ectopic pregnancies may follow conception late in the menstrual cycle and displacement of the ovum; embryonic abnormalities may result from conception involving either an over-aged sperm or over-aged ovum. If this is correct, the safe period may not be an absolutely safe period *(99)*.

4. Natural family planning methods

The term "natural family planning" is applied to three methods: (a) basal body temperature (BBT) method (b) cervical mucus method, and (c) symptothermic method. The principle is the same as in the calendar method, but here the woman employs self-recognition of certain physiological signs and symptoms associated with ovulation as an aid to ascertain when the fertile period begins. For avoiding pregnancy, couples abstain from sexual intercourse during the fertile phase of the menstrual cycle; they totally desist from using drugs and contraceptive devices. This is the essence of natural family planning.

(a) Basal body temperature method (BBT)

The BBT method depends upon the identification of a specific physiological event – the rise of BBT at the time of ovulation, as a result of an increase in the production of progesterone. The rise of temperature is very small, 0.3 to 0.5 degree C. When no ovulation occurs (e.g., as after menarche, during lactation) the body temperature does not rise. The temperature is measured preferably before getting out of bed in the morning. The BBT method is reliable if intercourse is restricted to the post-ovulatory infertile period, commencing 3 days after the ovulatory temperature rise and continuing up to the beginning of menstruation. The major drawback of this method is that abstinence is necessary for the entire pre-ovulatory period. Therefore, few couples now use the temperature method alone *(100)*.

(b) Cervical mucus method

This is also known as *"billings method"* or *"ovulation method"*. This method is based on the observation of changes in the characteristics of cervical mucus. At the time of ovulation, cervical mucus becomes watery clear resembling raw egg white, smooth, slippery and profuse. After ovulation, under the influence of progesterone, the mucus thickens and lessens in quantity. It is recommended that the woman uses a tissue paper to wipe the inside of vagina to assess the quantity and characteristics of mucus. To practice this method the woman should be able to distinguish between different types of mucus. This method requires a high degree of motivation than most other methods. The appeal and appropriateness of this method in developing countries such as India, especially among lay people, is dubious.

(c) Symptothermic method

This method combines the temperature, cervical mucus and calendar techniques for identifying the fertile period. If the woman cannot clearly interpret one sign, she can "double check" her interpretation with another. Therefore, this method is more effective than the "Billings method".

To sum up, natural family planning demands discipline and understanding of sexuality. It is not meant for everybody. The educational component is more important with this approach than with other methods. The opinion of the Advisory Group to WHO's Special Programme of Research in Human Reproduction is that the current natural family planning methods have very little application particularly in developing countries *(101)*.

5. Breast-feeding

Field and laboratory investigations have confirmed the traditional belief that lactation prolongs postpartum amenorrhoea and provides some degree of protection against pregnancy *(102)*. No more than 5–10 per cent of women conceive during lactational amenorrhoea, and even this risk exists only during the month preceding the resumption of menstruation *(103)*. However, once menstruation returns, continued lactation no longer offers any protection against pregnancy *(104)*. By and large, by 6 months after childbirth, about 20–50 per cent of women are menstruating and are in need of contraception *(105)*.

6. Birth control vaccine

Several immunological approaches for men and women are being investigated. The most advanced research involves immunization with a vaccine prepared from beta sub-unit of human chorionic gonadotropin (hCG), a hormone produced in early pregnancy. Immunization with hCG would block continuation of the pregnancy. Antibodies appeared in about 4–6 weeks and reached maximum after about 5 months and slowly declined reaching zero levels after a period ranging from 6–11 months. The immunity can be boosted by a second injection. Two types of pregnancy vaccines employing variants of the beta sub-unit of hCG are now about to go into clinical trial *(51)*. Research on birth control vaccines continues. The uncertainties are great *(85)*.

TERMINAL METHODS

(Sterilization)

Voluntary sterilization is a well-established contraceptive procedure for couples desiring no more children. Currently female sterilizations account for about 85 per cent and male sterilizations for 10–15 per cent of all sterilizations in India (*106*), in spite of the fact that male sterilization is simpler, safer and cheaper than female sterilization.

Sterilization offers many advantages over other contraceptive methods – it is a one-time method; it does not require sustained motivation of the user for its effectiveness; provides the most effective protection against pregnancy; the risk of complications is small if the procedure is performed according to accepted medical standards; and it is most cost-effective. It has been estimated that each procedure averts 1.5 to 2.5 births per woman *(107)*.

Guidelines for sterilization

Sterilization services are provided free of charge in Government institutions. Guidelines have been issued from time to time by the Government covering various aspects of sterilization. These are *(108, 109)*:

a. The age of the husband should not ordinarily be less than 25 years nor should it be over 50 years.

b. The age of the wife should not be less than 20 years or more than 45 years.

c. The motivated couple must have 2 living children at the time of operation.

d. If the couple has 3 or more living children, the lower limit of age of the husband or wife may be relaxed at the discretion of the operating surgeon, and

e. It is sufficient if the acceptor declares having obtained the consent of his/her spouse to undergo sterilization operation without outside pressure, inducement or coercion, and that he/she knows that for all practical purposes, the operation is irreversible, and also that the spouse has not been sterilized earlier.

Male sterilization *(110, 111)*

Male sterilization or vasectomy being a comparatively simple operation can be performed even in primary health centres by trained doctors under local anaesthesia. When carried out under strict aseptic technique, it should have no risk of mortality. In vasectomy, it is customary to remove a piece of vas at least 1 cm after clamping. The ends are ligated and then folded back on themselves and sutured into position, so that the cut ends face away from each other. This will reduce the risk of recanalization at a later date. It is important to stress that the acceptor is not immediately sterile after the operation, usually until approximately 30 ejaculations have taken place *(45)*. During this intermediate period, another method of contraception must be used. If properly performed, vasectomies are almost 100 per cent effective.

Following vasectomy, sperm production and hormone output are not affected. The sperm produced are destroyed intraluminally by phagocytosis. This is a normal process in the male genital tract, but the rate of destruction is greatly increased after vasectomy. Vasectomy is a simpler, faster and less expensive operation than tubectomy in terms of instruments, hospitalization and doctor's training. Cost-wise, the ratio is about 5 vasectomies to one tubal ligation.

COMPLICATIONS

The very few complications that may arise are :

(a) *Operative* : The early complications include pain, scrotal haematoma and local infection. Wound infection is reported to occur in about 3 per cent of patients. Good haemostasis and administration of antibiotics will reduce the risk of these complications.

(b) *Sperm granules* : Caused by accumulation of sperm, these are a common and troublesome local complication of vasectomy. They appear in 10–14 days after the operation. The most frequent symptoms are pain and swelling. Clinically the mass is hard and the average size approximately 7 mm. Sperm granules may provide a medium through which re-anastomosis of the severed vas can occur. The sperm granules eventually subside. It has been reported that using metal clips to close the vas may reduce or eliminate this problem.

(c) *Spontaneous recanalization* : Most epithelial tubes will recanalize after damage, and the vas is no exception. The incidence of recanalization is variously placed between 0 to 6 per cent. Its occurrence is serious. Therefore, the surgeon should explain the possibility of this complication to every acceptor prior to the operation, and have written consent acknowledging this fact. In a study, the wives of 6 out of 14,047 men who had vasectomies in the UK became pregnant between 16 months and 3 years later *(112)*. Therefore, the patient should be urged to report for a regular follow-up, may be up to 3 years.

(d) *Autoimmune response* : Vasectomy is said to cause an autoimmune response to sperm. Blocking of the vas causes reabsorption of spermatozoa and subsequent development of antibodies against sperm in the blood. Normally 2 per cent of fertile men have circulating antibodies against their own sperm. In men who have had vasectomies, the figure can be as high as 54 per cent. There is no reason to believe that such antibodies are harmful to physical health. It is likely that the circulating antibodies can cause a reduction in subsequent fertility despite successful reanastomosis of the vas *(44)*.

(e) *Psychological* : Some men may complain of diminution of sexual vigour, impotence, headache, fatigue, etc. Such adverse psychological effects are seen in men who have undergone vasectomy under emotional pressure. That is why it is important to explain to each acceptor the basis of the operation and give him sufficient time to make up his mind voluntarily and seriously to have the operation done.

Causes of failure *(111)*

The failure rate of vasectomy is generally low, 0.15 per 100 person–years. The most common cause of failure is due to the mistaken identification of the vas. That is, instead of the vas, some other structure in the spermatic cord such as thrombosed vein or thickened lymphatic has been taken. Histological confirmation has, therefore, been recommended on all vasectomy specimens by some authors in developed countries. In developing countries, histological confirmation is ruled out because of lack of facilities for such an examination. A simpler method has been recommended, that is, microscopic examination of a smear prepared by gentle squeezing of the vas on a glass slide and staining with Wright's stain. The vas can be identified by the presence of columnar epithelial cells that line the lumen of the vas. In some cases, failure may be due to spontaneous recanalisation of vas. Sometimes there may be more than one vas on one side. Pregnancy could also result from sexual intercourse before the disappearance of sperms from the reproductive tract.

Post-operative advice

To ensure normal healing of the wound and to ensure the success of the operation, the patient should be given the following advice :

1. The patient should be told that he is not sterile immediately after the operation; at least 30 ejaculations may be necessary before the seminal examination is negative *(45)*.
2. To use contraceptives until aspermia has been established.
3. To avoid taking bath for at least 24 hours after the operation.
4. To wear a T-bandage or scrotal support *(langot)* for 15 days : and to keep the site clean and dry.
5. To avoid cycling or lifting heavy weights for 15 days; there is, however, no need for complete bed rest.
6. To have the stitches removed on the 5th day after the operation.

No scalpel vasectomy

No scalpel vasectomy is a new technique that is safe, convenient and acceptable to males. This new method is now being canvassed for men as a special project, on a voluntary basis under the family welfare programme. Under the project, medical personnel all over the country are to be trained. Availability of this new technique at the peripheral level will increase the acceptance of male sterilization in the country. The project is being funded by the UNFPA *(98)*.

Female sterilization

Female sterilization can be done as an interval procedure, postpartum or at the time of abortion. Two procedures have become most common, namely laparoscopy and minilaparotomy.

(a) Laparoscopy

This is a technique of female sterilization through abdominal approach with a specialized instrument called "laparoscope". The abdomen is inflated with gas (carbon dioxide, nitrous oxide or air) and the instrument is introduced into the abdominal cavity to visualize the tubes. Once the tubes are accessible, the Falope rings (or clips) are applied to occlude the tubes. This operation should be undertaken only in those centres where specialist obstetrician–gynaecologists are available. The short operating time, shorter stay in hospital and a small scar are some of the attractive features of this operation.

Patient selection : Laparoscopy is not advisable for postpartum patients for 6 weeks following delivery; however, it can be done as a concurrent procedure to MTP. Haemoglobin per cent should not be less than 8. There should be no associated medical disorders such as heart disease, respiratory disease, diabetes and hypertension. It is recommended that the patient be kept in hospital for a minimum of 48 hours after the operation.

The cases are required to be followed-up by health workers (F) LHVs in their respective areas once between 7–10 days after the operation, and once again between 12 and 18 months after the operation.

Complications : Although complications are uncommon, when they do occur they may be of a serious nature requiring experienced surgical intervention. Puncture of large blood vessels and other potential complications have been reported as major hazards of laparoscopy.

(b) Minilap operation

Minilaparotomy is a modification of abdominal tubectomy. It is a much simpler procedure requiring a smaller abdominal incision of only 2.5 to 3 cm conducted under local anaesthesia. The minilap/Pomeroy technique is considered a revolutionary procedure for female sterilization. It is also found to be a suitable procedure at the primary health centre level and in mass campaigns. It has the advantage over other methods with regard to safety, efficiency and ease in dealing with complications. Minilap operation is suitable for postpartum tubal sterilization.

Evaluation of contraceptive methods

Contraceptive efficacy is generally assessed by measuring the number of unplanned pregnancies that occur during a specified period of exposure and use of a contraceptive method. The two methods that have been used to measure contraceptive efficacy are the Pearl index and life-table analysis.

The **Pearl index** is defined as the number of "failures per 100 woman-years of exposure (HWY)." This rate is given by the formula :

$$\text{Failure rate per HWY} = \frac{\text{Total accidental pregnancies}}{\text{Total months of exposure}} \times 1200$$

In applying the above formula, the total accidental pregnancies shown in the numerator must include every known conception, whatever its outcome, whether this had terminated as live births, still-births or abortions or had not yet terminated. The factor 1200 is the number of months in 100 years. The total months of exposure in the denominator is obtained by deducting from the period under review of 10 months for a full-term pregnancy, and 4 months for an abortion *(99)*.

A failure rate of 10 per HWY would mean that in the lifetime of the average woman about one-fourth or 2.5 accidental pregnancies would result, since the average fertile period of a woman is about 25 years *(99)*.

In designing and interpreting a use–effectiveness trial, a minimum of 600 months of exposure is usually considered necessary before any firm conclusion can be reached *(99)*.

With most methods of contraception, failure rates decline with duration of use. The Pearl index is usually based on a specific exposure (usually one year) and, therefore, fails to accurately compare methods at various durations of exposure. This limitation is overcome by using the method of life-table analysis.

Life-table analysis : Life-table analysis calculates a failure rate for each month of use. A cumulative failure rate can then compare methods for any specific length of exposure. Women who leave a study for any reason other than unintended pregnancy are removed from the analysis, contributing their exposure until the time of the exit.

Element of success in family planning programme

The main strategy of family planning programme is to offer to client easy access to a wide range of affordable contraceptive method through multiple service delivery channels in a good quality, reliable fashion. The key points are as follows : (1) *Make services accessible :* Offering services through a variety of delivery points makes methods available to more potential users; (2) *Make services affordable :* Partnerships between public and private-sector services encourage clients to pay what they can, while public programmes serve the poor for free or for low fees; (3) *Offer client-centered care :* Planning and providing services with the clients in mind help to make sure their needs are met and their preferences are honoured; (4) *Rely on evidence-based technical guidance :* Up-to-date service delivery guidelines, tools, and job aids can help translate research findings into better practice; (5) *Communicate effectively :* Communication grounded in behaviour theory and sensitive to local norms motivates clients to seek services and helps them make good family planning choices; (6) *Assure contraceptive security :* A strong logistics system and a long-term plan for contraceptive security ensure that a variety of methods, and the supplies and equipment to provide them, are always available; (7) *Work for supportive policies :* Showing how family planning contributes to development goals makes the case for continued support for family planning programme; (8) *Coordinate :* When governments, donor agencies, and implementing partners work together, they streamline efforts and avoid duplication; (9) *Build a high-performing staff :* Programme can keep workers motivated and on the job by creating a good working environment, matching skills with tasks, and rewarding a job well done; (10) *Secure adequate budget, use it well :* Spending wisely, doing more with less, and finding ways to recover costs can help ensure financial sustainability; (11) *Base decisions on evidence :* Research, monitoring, and evaluation yield important information to guide decision-making, and they need not be expensive; (12) *Lead strongly, manage well :* Strong leadership helps programmes navigate change. Good management solves operational problems; and (13) *Integrate services appropriately :* Programmes can address a wider range of health needs by integrating services where appropriate and offering referrals where it is not.

Unmet need for family planning *(113)*

Many women who are sexually active would prefer to avoid becoming pregnant, but nevertheless are not using any method of contraception (including use by their partner). These women are considered to have an "unmet need" for family planning. The concept is usually applied to married women. However, it can apply to sexually active fecund women and perhaps to men, but its measurement has been limited to married women only. Unmet need can be a powerful concept for family planning. It poses a challenge to family planning programme – to reach and serve millions of women whose reproductive attitude resembles those of contraceptive user – but who are, for some reason or combination of reasons, not using contraceptives.

Among the most common reason for unmet need are inconvenient or unsatisfactory services, lack of information, fears about contraceptive side-effects and opposition from husband or relatives. Unmet need is defined on the basis of women's response to survey questions.

According to the National Family Health Survey-5, the unmet need for family planning is highest (28.0 per cent) among women between 15 to 24 years of age and is almost entirely for spacing the births rather than for limiting the births. The unmet need for contraception among women aged 30 years and above are mostly for limiting the births.

Unmet need for family planning is higher in rural areas than in urban areas. It also varies by women's education (within range of 11–17 per cent) and religion (hindu and christian women have a lower unmet need than muslim women). Table 23 shows some of the characteristics of unmet need for family planning in India *(20)*.

TABLE 23
Percentage of currently married women with unmet need for family planning in India by selected background characteristics (NFHS–5, 2019–2021)

Background characteristics	Unmet need for family planning		
	For spacing	For limiting	Total
1. Age			
15–19	15.6	2.2	17.8
20–24	12.4	4.9	17.3
25–29	6.2	7.0	13.2
30–34	2.5	6.6	9.1
35–39	0.9	5.5	6.3
40–44	0.3	4.7	5.0
45–49	0.2	3.3	3.4
2. Residence			
Urban	3.5	4.9	8.4
Rural	4.3	5.6	9.9
3. Schooling			
No schooling	2.0	5.3	7.3
<5 years complete	2.4	4.9	7.2
5–7 years complete	2.9	5.4	8.3
8–9 years complete	4.7	5.5	10.3
10–11 years complete	4.8	5.1	9.9
12 or more years complete	6.9	5.6	12.5
4. Religion			
Hindu	3.9	5.2	9.0
Muslim	5.0	6.8	11.8
Christian	5.5	4.8	10.4
Sikh	3.5	6.0	9.5
Buddhist/Neo-Buddhist	3.9	4.3	8.2
Jain	4.8	2.7	7.5
Other	4.5	6.1	10.7
5. Caste/tribe			
Scheduled caste	4.0	5.2	9.2
Scheduled tribe	4.5	4.7	9.2
Other backward class	4.2	5.4	9.6
Other	3.7	5.7	9.4
Don't know	5.0	6.9	12.0
6. Wealth index			
Lowest	4.5	6.9	11.4
Second	4.1	5.6	9.7
Middle	3.9	4.8	8.6
Fourth	4.0	5.0	9.0
Highest	3.7	4.8	8.6
Total	4.0	5.4	9.4

Source : *(20)*

"Demand satisfied" by modern contraceptives

'Demand satisfied' calculates the need satisfied by modern methods out of total demand in the community (includes the cohort using modern contraceptives and traditional methods, and having unmet need for contraception). India's 'demand satisfied' shows an increase from 72 per cent in NFHS-4 to 74.2 per cent in NFHS-5 and modern contraceptive usage. 12 states show 'demand satisfied' of more than 75 per cent.

The National Family Health Survey–5 results show that although current use of contraception has increased, and the extent of unmet need has declined in most of the states in India, there is a need for considerable improvement in the coverage and quality of family planning services, especially in the states of Uttar Pradesh, Bihar, Assam and Jharkhand etc.

Contraception and adolescence *(114)*

Adolescence is the period between puberty and the end of physiological maturation, which occurs between ages 15–19 years. Pregnancy in adolescence constitutes about 11 per cent of all pregnancies in most developing countries and in some developed countries such as the USA. For the year 2014, WHO puts the global adolescent birth rate at 49 per 1000 girls of that age, country rates range from one to 229 births per 1000 girls. This indicates a marked decrease since 1990 *(115)*. These are often "at risk" pregnancies. Many are undesired, and occur in unmarried adolescents who then resort to legal or illegal abortion, performed under unsatisfactory medical conditions. This has serious health and even life-threatening consequences for these young women – the ensuing mortality and morbidity (especially secondary sterility) are quite considerable.

Prevention of undesired pregnancies and of sexually transmitted diseases in young people through educational programmes dealing with responsible sexual behaviour is a major public health challenge. Adolescents are ambivalent about family planning : to request contraception is to "reveal" one's sexuality. For this reason, adolescent girls sometimes choose the risk of an undesired pregnancy and of an abortion.

BARRIER METHODS : Condoms make barrier method worthwhile, because they protect those adolescents, with occasional different sexual partners, against STD and AIDS. However, condoms must be properly used, and it depends on the man's behaviour. Young men seem to be increasingly aware of the importance of safeguarding their own health and that of their partners. Cervical caps and diaphragms, on the other hand, are inappropriate for adolescents since they require foreseeing of intercourse and complicated manipulations, to which young people are loath.

HORMONAL CONTRACEPTION : Hormonal methods are perfectly suitable for adolescents, who generally do not suffer from such problems as cardiovascular contraindications. In fact, these are probably the most adequate methods, since they are completely reversible, and in no way modify the future fertility of these young women. In developed countries, pills are usually preferred, but trimestrial or monthly injections are also appropriate. Implants, with their five year term, cover too long a period for certain adolescents.

IUD : IUD are theoretically contraindicated, because of the risk of pelvic infection and of secondary sterility. However, an adolescent is better protected by an IUD than by illegal repeated abortions. This method has the advantage of being discrete and avoiding demanding routines.

OTHER METHODS : Periodic abstinence is not easy when cycles are irregular and intercourse is unforeseen, and with new partners. In certain countries, however, they are practically the only method taught, for religious reasons, and poor protection is preferable to no protection at all. Similarly, withdrawal is not very suitable method, since young men are usually not very skillful.

Spermicides are not contraindicated, but have two disadvantages – they are costly, and are not effective against STD and AIDS.

A major chunk of the world population is under 25 years age group. An extremely large number of young people will, therefore, be entering their reproductive years at that time. The demographic future of the world will depend on them, on how well informed they are, and on their sense of responsibilities.

DELIVERY SYSTEM

Since family planning is essentially a component of the health care system, the primary responsibility for the delivery of services rests with the Government through its health care system at the Centre and in the States.

At the Centre

The Family Welfare Programme is a centrally sponsored scheme, and the states receive 100 per cent assistance from the central government. Since the entire cost is virtually borne by the central government, the central government controls the planning, and financial management of the programme (e.g., establishment of clinics, pattern of staffing, expenditure); training, research and evaluation, and most important, the formulation of an overall policy for the programme. The current policy is to promote family planning on the basis of voluntary and informed acceptance with full community participation. The emphasis is on a 2–child family. Recently there have been two major changes in the approach to delivery of family planning services : first, a greater emphasis on spacing methods, side by side with terminal methods, and secondly to take the services to every door–step and motivate families to adopt the small family norm.

The administrative apparatus consists of a separate Department of Family Welfare, which was created in 1966 in the Central Ministry of Health and Family Welfare. The Secretary to the Government of India in the Ministry of Health and Family Welfare is in over all charge of the Department of Family Welfare. He is assisted by a **Special Secretary** and Joint Secretaries. The special secretary supervises the programme implementation and coordinates the various activities. There is now an **Advisor** (Mass Media and Communication) – an officer of the rank of an Additional Secretary. The National Institute of Health and Family Welfare acts as an apex technical institute for promoting health and family welfare in the country through education, training services, research and evaluation. There is a Central Family Welfare Council consisting of all the State Health Ministers to review the implementation of the programme. A Population Advisory Council headed by the Union Health Minister, Members of Parliament, and persons from the fields related to population control was set up in 1982. This body acts like a "think tank" to analyze the implementation of the programme and advise the government suitably. A cabinet sub-committee headed by the Prime Minister has also been formed for periodic review of the progress of the family welfare programme. Family planning is no longer viewed as the sole responsibility of the Health Ministry, but will devolve on all ministries connected with human resources and development. This is an important breakthrough in current thinking.

At the state level

Under the Indian constitution, the state governments are responsible for the administration and implementation of the Family Welfare Programme. Since most of the crucial policy decisions are made by the central government, the pattern of organization and many features of the delivery system are fairly well-standardized in the States.

The organizational set-up at the State level consists of a State Family Welfare Bureau, which is part of the State Health and Family Welfare Directorate. At present, 25 State Family Welfare Bureaus are functioning in the country.

In 1979, the offices of the Family Welfare and National Malaria Eradication Programme were merged into one office and named as Regional Office for Health and Family Welfare. These regional offices have been set up to maintain liaison with state governments and give technical assistance to them in connection with the implementation of the Family Welfare Programme and other important health programmes. To co-ordinate the family welfare activities between the state governments and the central government, one Family Welfare Cell has been sanctioned for each State.

At the district level

At the district level, the set-up consists of a District Family Welfare Bureau consisting of 3 divisions – an administrative division headed by the District Family Welfare Officer; mass education and media division, in charge of District Mass Education and Media Officer, and an evaluation division, in charge of a Statistical Officer. These are supported by 1,083 Urban Family welfare centres and 871 Urban Health Posts. Presently there are 4 types of Urban Health Posts–type A for areas with population less than 5,000, type B for areas with population between 5,000–10,000, type C for population between 10,000–25,000, and type D for areas with population between 25,000–50,000. If the population is more than 50,000, then it is to be divided into sectors of 50,000 population and Health Posts provided. Type A, B and C Health Posts are attached to a hospital for providing referral and supervisory services. Type D Health Post is attached to a hospital for sterilization, MTP and referral *(115)*. Only type D health post have a post of medical officer.

The 10 city family welfare bureaus are entrusted with the responsibility of coordination, monitoring and supervision etc. of the family welfare services provided by various institutions in the city.

Presently there are three types of Urban Family Welfare Centres. Type I is for population between 10,000–25,000, type II is for population between 25,000–50,000, and type III is for above 50,000 population *(115)*. These are manned by 2 para-medical staff in type I and II centres and by 6 persons including medical officer in type III centres.

The Urban family welfare centres and health posts provide comprehensive integrated services of MCH and family planning. The staff pattern is different for different types of health posts and urban family welfare centres.

At the community health centre

Community health centre is established and maintained by the state governments. Presently it is manned by four medical specialists i.e. surgeon, physician, gynaecologist and paediatrician, supported by 21 paramedical and other staff. It has 30 in-door beds with one OT, X-ray, labour room and laboratory facilities and serves as a referral centre for four PHCs. According to Indian Public Health Standards, the community health centre is to be manned by 6 medical specialists including an anaesthetist and an eye surgeon supported by 24 paramedical and other staff with inclusion of two nurse midwives. It provides, apart from other emergency obstetric care, full range of family planning services including laproscopic services and safe abortion services. At present as of March 2021, 5,481 community health centres are functional in the country.

At the primary health centre

Since more than 65 per cent of India's population lives in the rural areas an adequate network of service centres has been extended to the rural areas. A Rural Family Welfare Centre with a medical officer and supporting staff forms an integral part of the primary health centre. A total of 5,435 Rural Family Welfare Centres were established in the country at all block level PHCs sanctioned upto 1.4.1980. Most of the states have integrated these centres into their primary health care system and after this date family planning services are being provided through integrated facilities at PHCs. As of March 2021, 25,140 primary health centres were functioning in the country. Each centre is supported by sub-centres. The total number of sub-centres functioning are 1,56,101.

When fully staffed (by 3 medical officers including one lady doctor and supporting personnel) the PHC is expected to provide fairly comprehensive "essential health care" including family planning care. The medical officers are usually trained to provide MTP and sterilization services. The programme of insertion of copper-T IUDs has been intensified. It is intended that laparoscopic services which have become very popular will be made more widely available at the PHC.

The sub-centres are to provide the main thrust of the programme. Each sub-centre is staffed by one male and one female health worker. They are responsible for providing rudimentary health and MCH care; family planning motivation, supplies and services in spacing methods.

Various studies conducted have highlighted that the existing infrastructure is not being optimally utilized because of its inadequacy to provide proper services. To improve matters **popular committees** have been set up at all levels by some states to involve people in the programme and in exercising vigilance over the work of various functionaries.

At the village level

Two schemes are being implemented at the village level to improve the outreach of services and increase local participation: **(a) The Village Health Guides** : An innovative approach has been the creation of a band of village Health Guides (mostly women), one for each village or a population of 1000. They are made responsible for spreading knowledge and information to the eligible couples and providing them with supplies of Nirodh and oral pills. About 3.23 lakh health guides are in position. **(b) Trained dais :** The national target is to provide one trained dai per 1000 population. They conduct safe deliveries in rural areas. They also act as family planning counsellors and motivators, supplementing the delivery system. **(c) ASHA :** 9.39 lakh ASHAs have been selected so far and have been provided with drug kits. At present the village health guides in some states only, trained dais and ASHAs are the lynchpins of the family planning delivery system in India.

Family planning has a significant role in mitigating the impact of high population growth by helping women achieve desired family size and avoid unintended and mistimed pregnancies. Past few years have seen a paradigm shift in family planning programme. Studies show that if the current unmet need for family planning could be fulfilled over the next 5 years, 35,000 maternal deaths and 1.2 million infant deaths can be averted. The focus of the programme is now towards meeting the unmet need of contraception and increasing the use of modern contraceptive use, thereby help in averting unintended and mistimed pregnancies, achieve desired family size, and promote the health of the mother and child.

Currently the family planning methods in India can be broadly classified in two categories – spacing methods, and limiting permanent methods.

(A) *Spacing methods :* These are reversible methods which can be adopted and discontinued as per an individual's choice,

- (a) Oral contraceptives pills (combined oral contraceptive pill (Mala N), Centchroman (Chhaya)
- (b) Condoms
- (c) Intrauterine contraceptive devices (IUCD 380A – effective for 10 years, IUCD 375 – effective for 5 years)
- (d) Contraceptive injectable MPA (Antara programme)

(B) *Permanent method :* These methods are irreversible in nature

- (a) Female sterilization
  - i. Minilap
  - ii. Laparoscopic
- (b) Male sterilization
  - i. Conventional
  - ii. Non scalpel vasectomy (no incision no stitches)

(C) Emergency contraceptive pills

During the year 2020–2021 the number of acceptors by different methods was as follows *(116)*:

Sterilization	....	26.8 lakh
Total IUCD	....	54.72 lakh
Post-partum IUCD	....	27.43 lakh
Injectable MPA	....	18.81 lakh
Centchroman	....	57.11 lakh
Post-abortion IUCD	....	80,165

Performance of social marketing programme in the sale of contraceptives was :

Condoms	....	459.51 million
Oral pills	....	159.19 million cycles
Saheli	....	77.52 lakh tablets

New initiatives *(117)*

1. *Home Delivery of Contraceptives (HDC)*
   - a. A new scheme has been launched to utilize the services of ASHA to deliver contraceptives at the doorstep of beneficiaries. The scheme was launched in 233 pilot districts of 17 States on 11th July 2011 and is now expanded to the entire country from 17th December 2012.
   - b. ASHA is charging a nominal amount from beneficiaries for her effort to deliver contraceptives at doorstep i.e. Rs. 1 for a pack of 3 condoms. Rs.1 for a cycle of OCPs and Rs. 2 for a pack of one tablet of ECP.

2. *Ensuring spacing at birth (ESB)*

   a. Under a new scheme launched by the Government of India, services of ASHAs to be utilized for counselling newly married couples to ensure spacing of 2 years after marriage and couples with 1 child to have spacing of 3 years after the birth of 1st child. The scheme is operational in 18 States (EAG, North-Eastern and Gujarat and Haryana). ASHA would be paid following incentives under the scheme :

   – Rs. 500/- to ASHA for delaying first child birth by 2 years after marriage.

   – Rs. 500/- to ASHA for ensuring spacing of 3 years after the birth of 1st child.

   – Rs.1000/- in case the couple opts for a permanent limiting method upto 2 children only.

   b. Ministry of Health & Family Welfare has introduced short term IUCD (5 years effectively), Cu IUCD 375 under the National Family Planning programme. Training of State level trainers has already been completed and process is underway to train service providers upto the sub-centre level.

   c. A new method of IUCD insertion (post-partum IUCD insertion) has been introduced by the Government.

   d. Promoting Post-partum Family Planning services at district hospitals by providing for placement of dedicated Family Planning Counsellors and training of personnel.

3. *Pregnancy Testing Kits*

   Nischay-Home based pregnancy test kits (PTKs) was launched under NRHM in 2008 across the country. The PTKs are being made available at sub-centres and to the ASHAs to facilitate the early detection and decision making for the outcomes of pregnancy.

4. *Mission Parivar Vikas (MPV)*

   A programme launched in 146 high total fertility rate districts to accelerate the use and awareness of family planning methods. States and districts fact sheet highlight the current indicators and trends in these districts and will act as baseline and roadmap for future work in these districts, A five pronged strategy has been developed under the mission parivar vikas, which comprise of *(9)*:

   a. Delivering assured services;

   b. Building additional capacity/human resources development for enhanced service delivery;

   c. Ensuring commodity security;

   d. Implementing new promotional schemes; and

   e. Creating an enabling environment.

5. *New contraceptive launch (9)*

The new contraceptive injectable MPA under "Antara programme" and oral contraceptive pill centchroman "chhaya" have been added to the existing contraceptive basket of choice thus providing the users with new options.

The public sector provides a wide range of contraceptive services for limiting and spacing of births at various levels of health system as described in Table 24.

Government of India is promoting "Fixed Day Static Services" (FDS) approach in sterilization services within the

TABLE 24

Family planning services in public health sector

Family planning method	Service provider	Service location	Service strategy and promotional schemes
Spacing Methods			
IUCD 380 A/IUCD 375	Trained & certified ANMs, LHVs, SNs and Doctors	Sub-centre & higher levels	• On demand • Camp approach • Revised Compensation Scheme
Oral contraceptive pills (OCPs)	Trained ASHAs, ANMs, LHVs, SNs and Doctors	At door step (in pilot districts), Village level Sub-centre & higher levels	• On demand • Village Health Nutrition Days
Condoms	Trained ASHAs, ANMs, LHVs, SNs and Doctors	At door step (in pilot districts), Village level Sub-centre & higher levels	• On demand • Village Health Nutrition Days
Injectable contraceptive MPA	Trained doctors, SNs and ANMs	Medical colleges and district hospitals (in MPV districts at all levels upto sub-centres)	
Limiting Methods			
Minilap	Trained & certified MBBS Doctors & Specialist Doctors	PHC & higher levels	• Fixed Day Static Approach • Camp approach • Revised Compensation Scheme
Laparoscopic sterilization	Trained & certified Specialist Doctors (OBG & General Surgeons)	Usually CHC & higher levels	• National Family Planning Insurance Scheme
NSV (No Scalpel Vasectomy)	Trained & certified MBBS Doctors & Specialist Doctors	PHC & higher levels	
Emergency Contraception			
Emergency contraceptive pills (ECPs)	Trained ASHAs, ANMs, LHVs, SNs and Doctors	At door step (in pilot districts) Village level, Sub-centre & higher levels	• On demand • Village Health Nutrition Days

ANM : Auxiliary Nurse Midwife; LHV : Lady Health Visitor; SN : Staff Nurse; ASHA : Accredited Social Health Activist.

Source : *(9)*

public health system with the aim of increasing access to sterilization services. States are being provided technical and financial support for the development of human resources and upgradation of health facilities for the functioning of FDS. In the states with high unmet need for limiting methods, sterilization camps will continue till the time FDS is implemented effectively. The frequency of sterilization services at different health facilities at FDS is as follows *(98)* :

District hospital – twice a week
Sub-district hospital – weekly
CHC/Block PHC – fortnightly
24x7 PHC/PHC – monthly

Community Needs Assessment Approach *(118)*

Till recently, the achievements of family welfare programme were assessed on the basis of the targets given from the centre for individual contraceptives. This led to a situation where the achievement of the contraceptive targets had become the ends by themselves. Over the years it became apparent that there were many drawbacks in the top down target approach in which types and quantity of contraceptive need to be canvassed was decided by the higher authorities. Firstly, the user preference was not reflected in the targets. If the contraceptive required in accordance with the user was not available, the targets were not likely to be achieved. There was no authentic system of feedback regarding which type of contraceptive was to be promoted in a particular area or among a particular age group. Secondly, the quality of the services became secondary. For example, if in an attempt to fulfil targets for the number of IUD insertions, the quality of care is compromised (especially while screening women for pre-existing reproductive tract infections and sexually transmitted diseases before IUD insertion) the acceptability of IUD programme would receive a serious setback and discontinuation rate will be high. Thirdly, people may be tempted to resort to false reporting to claim fulfilment of the target. In other words, contraceptive targets and cash incentives resulted in the inflation of performance statistics and deterioration in the quality of services.

Government of India deliberated objectively on the utility of retaining the practice of targets at national and state levels. In the year 1995–96, one district in each of 18 states (including a pilot project in Kerala and Tamil Nadu) were made target free. Later on the practice of fixing up of targets for individual contraceptive method was given up from April 1996. This does not mean a licence to do no work. The population goals remain the same as before. Health workers are expected to consult families and local community in the beginning of the year in order to assess their needs and preference and then work-out for themselves the programme and workload for the coming year. The requirement for each village needs to be worked out to arrive at the workload for the ANM, this becomes the target for the ANM for the year. The workload of different ANMs under one PHC when added up would determine the workload for the PHC. Similarly requirements at the district level would be worked out by adding up the requirements at all the PHCs.

Later on it was found that due to complex calculations required the health workers were unable to fix the performance norms for themselves. Therefore, it was decided to modify and rename the target free manual as *Community Needs Assessment Approach Manual*.

Involvement of private sector

The family planning programme, to be successful, will have to be extended beyond the government delivery system to include the private sector. Grants-in-aid are provided to voluntary organizations and industrial organizations for running family welfare centres and postpartum centres. The scheme for involvement of private medical practitioners in the family welfare programme has been extended to practitioners of integrated medicine. Government has also created nation-wide retail outlets for selling subsidized condoms.

Incentives

The use of incentives and disincentives to encourage couples to practise family planning has become a common strategy in many developing countries. Financial compensation of individuals undergoing sterilization was first introduced in 1966; over the years, it has been gradually increased. The acceptors now receive a one-time payment as shown in Table 25 *(9)*:

National Family Planning Indemnity Scheme (NFPIS)

With effect from, 01.04.2013, it has been decided that States/UTs would process and make payment of claims to accepters of sterilization in the event of death/failures/complications/indemnity cover to doctors/health facilities. The States/UTs would make suitable budget provisions for implementation of the scheme through their respective State/UT Programme Implementation Plans (PIPs) under the National Rural Health Mission (NRHM) and the scheme is renamed as "Family Planning Indemnity Scheme".

	Claims arising out of sterilization operation	Amount (Rs.)
A	Death at hospital/within seven days of discharge	2,00,000
B	Death following sterilization (8th-30th day from discharge)	50,000
C	Expense for treatment of medical complications	25,000
D	Failure of Sterilization	30,000
E	Doctors/facilities covered for litigations upto 4 cases per year including defence cost	2,00,000 (per case)

State government employees, who undergo sterilization after two or three children are eligible for a special increment (two increments after 2 children and one after 3 children). Central government employees get one increment after sterilization. It is under the scheme introduced in Dec. 1979 to promote small family norm, provided the employee is below 50 years of age and his spouse below 45 years. They get special leave (14 days for women and 7 days for men). No maternity leave is allowed after 3 children.

The State Governments have been requested to : issue Green Cards to individual acceptors of terminal methods after two children as a mark of recognition and for priority attention in schemes where preferential treatment was feasible. Cash awards have been instituted for the best performing states, the amount of which will be spent on promoting family welfare activities *(119)*.

TABLE 25

Compensation scheme in public facilities and private accredited facilities

Compensation scheme in public facilities *(Amount in Rs.)*

States	Type of operation	Acceptor	ASHA/Health Worker	Others	Total
11 High focus states (Uttar Pradesh, Bihar, Madhya Pradesh, Rajasthan, Chhattisgarh, Jharkhand, Odisha, Uttarakhand, Assam, Haryana, Gujarat)	Vasectomy	2000	300	400	2700
	Tubectomy	1400	200	400	2000
	Post-partum sterilization	2200	300	500	3000
Mission Parivar Vikas Districts	Vasectomy	3000	400	600	4000
	Tubectomy	2000	300	500	2800
	Tubectomy (PPS)	3000	400	600	4000
	Vasectomy (COT)	3000	400	1600	5000
	Tubectomy (COT)	2000	300	2200	4500
Other High focus states (North-East States, J&K, Himachal Pradesh)	Vasectomy	1100	200	200	1500
	Tubectomy	600	150	250	1000
Non-high focus states	Vasectomy	1100	200	200	1500
	Tubectomy (BPL+SC/ST only)	600	150	250	1000
	Tubectomy (APL)	250	150	250	650

Compensation scheme in private accredited facilities *(Amount in Rs.)*

States	Type of operation	Facility	Others/Acceptor	Total
11 High focus states (Uttar Pradesh, Bihar, Madhya Pradesh, Rajasthan, Chhattisgarh, Jharkhand, Odisha, Uttrakhand, Assam, Haryana, Gujarat)	Vasectomy (All)	2000	1000	3000
	Tubectomy (All)	2000	1000	3000
Mission Parivar Vikas Districts	Vasectomy (All)	2500	1000	3500
	Tubectomy (All)	2500	1000	3500
	Post Partum Sterilization (PPS)	3000	1000	4000
Other High focus states (North-East States, J&K, Himachal Pradesh)	Vasectomy (All)	1300	200	1500
	Tubectomy (All)	1350	150	1500
Non-high focus states	Vasectomy (All)	1300	200	1500
	Tubectomy (All)	1350	150	1500

Source: *(9)*

Family welfare linked health insurance scheme *(98)*

Government of India has introduced a family planning insurance scheme for acceptors of sterilization and indemnity cover for doctors performing sterilization procedures in both government and accredited private/ NGO/corporate health facilities. The insurance scheme will be operated by the ICICI.

Compensation in the event of death :

In the event of death following sterilization (inclusive of death during process of sterilization operation) in hospital or within 7 days from the date of discharge from the hospital, the compensation available as stated above.

All the doctors and health facilities rendering family planning services, conducting such operations shall stand indemnified against claims arising out of failure of sterilization, death or medical complications resulting therefrom up to a maximum amount of Rs 2 lacs per doctor/ health facility per case. The cover would also include the legal costs and actual modality of defending the prosecuted doctor/ health facility in court, which would be borne by the insurance company within certain limits *(120)*.

Postpartum Programme *(121)*

An All India Hospital Postpartum Programme (AIHPP) was introduced in 1969. It is a hospital-based, maternity centred approach to family planning. The primary objective of the postpartum programme is to improve the health of the mother and children through MCH and Family Welfare programme which includes antenatal, neonatal, and postnatal services; immunization services to children and mothers; and prophylaxis against anaemia and blindness. The programme is based on the following rationale :

a. That women who have recently delivered are of proven fertility, and are at risk to become pregnant again rapidly
b. At the time of delivery and during the lying-in period, they are generally more receptive to adopt one or the other family planning method.

The postpartum programme offers necessary facilities to such women. It has proved to be an efficient way of delivering family planning services. The programme now covers 550 medical institutions at national, state and district levels inclusive of 100 medical colleges and 2 post-graduate institutions. A scheme of PAP smear test facilities has been sanctioned for all medical colleges.

With a view to provide MCH and family welfare services in rural and semi-urban areas, as well as to improve the health of mothers and children, the postpartum programme has been extended to sub-divisional and sub-district hospitals. 1,012 such centres are functioning in the country *(122)*.

Population education

Population education has been defined as "an educational programme which provides for a study of the population situation in the community, nation and world with the purpose of developing in the students rational and responsible attitudes and behaviour towards that situation" *(121)*. The content of population education programme is influenced by the specific national situation as well as by political and educational goals *(123)*.

In the Indian context, the concept of population education is designed to bring home to the students, both at school and university level the consequences of uncontrolled population growth; the benefits of a small family norm; the economics, sociology and statistics of population growth, its distribution and its relation to the levels of living.

SOCIOLOGY OF FAMILY PLANNING

The institution of family is as old as man himself. It is the basic social cell. The need for its discipline has only recently dawned because of changing economic, social and cultural patterns in the world – and above all, because of concern of what might be called "quality of life" criteria. Sociologists and economists have shown that it will be difficult to raise the living standards of the people while population growth continues unchecked. The gains of the five year developmental plans are being absorbed by the rapidly growing population for basic consumption, e.g., food, shelter, clothing, education and medical care.

Attitude surveys have shown that awareness of family planning is very widespread and over 60 per cent people have attitudes favourable to restricting or spacing births *(29)*. People are generally in favour of family planning, and there is no organized opposition to it. In spite of this, the rate of contraceptive use by couples in the developing countries is very low. This is the crux of the family planning problem. Studies have shown that the population problem is complicated by deep-rooted religious and other beliefs, attitudes and practices favouring larger families (e.g., strong preference for male children). The common beliefs are – that children are the gift of God; the number of children is determined by God; children are a poor man's wealth; children are an asset to which parents can look forward in periods of dependency caused by old age or misfortune, etc. Most of these beliefs stem from ignorance and lack of communication.

The problem of family planning is, therefore, essentially the problem of social change. Contraceptive technology is no short cut to the problem. What is more important is to stimulate social changes affecting fertility such as raising the age of marriage, increasing the status of women, education and employment opportunities, old age security, compulsory education of children, accelerating economic changes designed to increase the per capita income, etc. It is now axiomatic that economic development is the best contraceptive. The experience of all countries which have had a successful population control show that the best motivation is economic, a desire to improve standard of living. The solution to the problem is one of mass education and communication, so that people may understand the benefits of a small family.

VOLUNTARY ORGANIZATIONS

Voluntary organizations have played a major role in population control programmes since the beginning. They are involved in every possible way so as to complement governmental efforts to promote Family Welfare Programme. Apart from educational and motivational efforts, their activities include running of Family Welfare Centres, post-partum centres, ANM training schools, population research centres and other innovative projects.

Some of the well-known voluntary agencies in India are the Family Planning Association of India, the Family Planning Foundation and the Population Council of India. Others include the Indian Red Cross, the Indian Medical Association, Rotary Clubs, Lions Clubs, Citizens Forum, Christian Missionaries and Private Hospitals.

At the international level, the International Planned Parenthood Federation is the world's largest private voluntary organization supporting family planning services in developing countries. It is an international federation of independent Family Planning Associations with headquarters in London. Others with long experience in this field include the United Nations Fund for Population Activities (UNFPA), the US Agency for International Development (USAID), the Population Council, Ford Foundation, the Pathfinder Fund and World Bank besides WHO and UNICEF. The international agencies are assisting in funding family planning research, services, training and information programmes designed to reduce the family size.

NATIONAL FAMILY WELFARE PROGRAMME

India launched a nation-wide family planning programme in 1952, making it the first country in the world to do so, though records show that birth control clinics have been functioning in the country since 1930. The early beginnings of the programme were modest with the establishment of a few clinics and distribution of educational material, training and research. During the Third Five Year Plan (1961–66), family planning was declared as "the very centre of planned development". The emphasis was shifted from the purely "clinic approach" to the more vigorous "extension education approach" for motivating the people for acceptance of the "small family norm". The introduction of the Lippes Loop in 1965 necessitated a major structural reorganization of the programme, leading to the creation of a separate Department of Family Planning in 1966 in the Ministry of Health. During the years 1966–1969, the programme took firmer roots. The family planning infrastructure (e.g., primary health centres, sub-centres, urban family planning centres, district and State bureaus) was strengthened. During the Fourth Five Year Plan (1969–74), the Government of India gave "top priority" to the programme. The Programme was made an integral part of MCH activities of PHCs and their sub-centres. In 1970, an All India Hospital Postpartum Programme and in 1972, the Medical Termination of Pregnancy (MTP) Act were introduced. During the Fifth Five Year Plan (1975–80) there have been major changes. In April 1976, the country framed its first "National Population Policy". The disastrous forcible sterilization campaign of 1976 led to the Congress defeat in the 1977 election. In June 1977, the new (Janata) Government that came into power formulated a new population policy, ruling out compulsion and coercion for all times to come. The Ministry of Family Planning was renamed "Family Welfare".

Although the performance of the programme was low during 1977–78, it was a good year in as much as the programme moved into new healthier directions. The 42nd Amendment of the Constitution has made "Population control and Family Planning" a concurrent subject, and this provision has been made effective from January 1977. The acceptance of the programme is now purely on voluntary basis. The launching of the Rural Health Scheme in 1977 and the involvement of the local people (e.g., Health Guides, trained Dais, Opinion leaders) in the family welfare programme at the grass-root level were aimed at accelerating the pace of progress of the programme. India was a signatory to the Alma Ata Declaration in 1978. The acceptance of the primary health care approach to the achievement of HFA/2000 AD led to the formulation of a National Health Policy in 1982. The National Health Policy was approved by the Parliament in 1983. It laid down the long-term demographic goal of NRR=1 by the year 2000 – which implies a 2-child family norm – through the attainment of a birth rate of 21 and a death rate of 9 per thousand population, and a couple protection rate of 60 per cent by the year 2000. The Sixth and Seventh Five Year Plans were accordingly set to achieve these goals. The National Health Policy also called for restructuring the health care delivery system to achieve HFA/2000 AD, and family planning has been accorded a central place in health development.

The Universal Immunization Programme aimed at reduction in mortality and morbidity among infants and younger children due to vaccine preventable diseases was started in the year 1985–86. The oral rehydration therapy was also started in view of the fact that diarrhoea was a leading cause of death among children. Various other programmes under MCH were also implemented during the Seventh Five Year Plan. The objective of all these programmes were convergent and aimed at improving the health of the mothers and young children, and to provide them facilities for prevention and treatment of major diseases. During 1992 these programmes were integrated under Child Survival and Safe Motherhood (CSSM) Programme.

The process of integration of related programmes initiated was taken a step further during 1994 when the International Conference on Population and Development in Cairo recommended implementation of Unified Reproductive and Child Health Programme (RCH). It is obviously sensible that integrated RCH programme would help in reducing cost of inputs to some extent because overlapping of expenditure would no longer be necessary and outcome will be better. Accordingly, during Ninth Five Year Plan the RCH Programme integrates all the related programmes of the Eighth Five Year Plan. The concept of RCH is to provide need based, client oriented, demand driven, high quality integrated services.

The Government of India evolved a more detailed and comprehensive National Population Policy 2000 (see page 568) to promote family welfare.

In the year 2005 Govt. of India launched National Rural Health Mission, initially for seven years (2005–2012) which was extended for 5 years up to 2017. Then came National Urban Health Plan and merging both these plans as National Health Mission. In the year 2013, RMNCH+A strategy was launched which was based on a continuum of care approach and defines integrated packages of services for different stages of life. In the year 2014, India Newborn Action Plan (INAP) came with the goal to attain single digit neonatal mortality rate by 2030 and single digit stillbirth rate by 2030. In the year 2017, National Health Policy was launched.

Table 26 shows the achievements of the Health and Family Welfare Programme.

TABLE 26

Achievements of Health & Family Welfare Programme

Parameter	2015	2017	2018
Crude Birth Rate (Per 1000 Population)	20.8	20.2	20.0
Crude Death Rate (Per 1000 Population)	6.5	6.3	6.2
Total Fertility Rate (Per women)	2.3	2.2	2.2
Maternal Mortality Ratio (Per 100,000 live births)	130 (2014–16)	122 (2015–17)	113 (2016–18)
Neo-natal Mortality Rate (Per 1000 live births)	25	23	23
Under Five Mortality Rate (Per 1000 live births)	43	37	36
Expectation of life at Birth	69.0 (2013–17)	69.4 (2014–18) Mid-year 2016	

Source : *(116)*

EVALUATION OF FAMILY PLANNING

Evaluation is defined as a "process of making judgements about selected objectives and events by comparing them with specified value standards for the purpose of deciding alternative course of action". The purpose of evaluation is to improve the design and delivery of family planning services.

Five types of evaluation have been defined by a WHO Expert Committee in 1975 *(32)* on evaluation of family planning in health services :

1. *Evaluation of need*

That is, health, demographic and socio-economic needs for family planning. For example, the current status of maternal mortality in a given area is an indicator of the need for family planning.

2. *Evaluation of plans*

That is, an assessment of the feasibility and adequacy of programme plans.

3. *Evaluation of performance*

(a) *Services* : Clinic services, mobile services, post-partum services, contraceptive distribution, follow up services, education and motivation activities;

(b) *Response* : Number of new acceptors, characteristics of acceptors;

(c) *Cost analysis; and*

(d) *Other activities* : Administration, manpower, data system, etc.

4. *Evaluation of effects*

Changes in knowledge, attitudes, motivation and behaviour.

5. Evaluation of impact

A WHO Study Group in 1976 *(125)* proposed the following indices for evaluating the impact : (a) Family size (number of living children (b) desired number of additional children (c) birth interval (d) age of the mother at birth of first child and last child (e) birth order, and (f) number of abortions. To this may be added, changes in birth rate and growth rate.

Evaluation is a technical activity that requires trained personnel, statistical facilities and adequate flow of data and information.

The Family Welfare Programme in India has come a long way and holds forth the promise that in the not very distant future it may be accepted as a way of life by most people. Although birth control continues to occupy the same important position in the programme as it used to be in the earlier days the programme now aims at achieving a higher end – and that is, to improve, in conjunction with other development programmes, the quality of life of the people (*124*).

References

1. International Planned Parenthood Federation (1981). *People* 8 (2) 26.
2. Macrotrends.net, *World Population 1950–2022*.
3. World Population review 2022, *2022 World Population by country*.
4. Bogue, D.N. (1969). *Principles of Demography,* John Wiley.
5. UNO (2019), *World Population Prospects,* 2019, Highlights.
6. Govt. of India (2012). *Census 2011,* Provisional Population Report, Office of the Registrar General and Census Commissioner India, Ministry of Home Affairs, March 31st, 2011.
7. Govt. of India (2019). *Sample Registration System Statistical Report 2018,* Office of the Registrar General and Census Commissioner India, Ministry of Home Affairs, New Delhi.
8. Govt. of India (2020), *Population projections for India and States 2011–2036,* Report of the Technical Group on Population Projections, July, 2020.
9. Govt. of India (2020), *Annual Report, 2019–20,* Ministry of Health and Family welfare, New Delhi.
10. Govt. of India (2022), *SRS Report for year 2020,* Ministry of Home Affairs, New Delhi.
11. *Population Pyramid, National Geographic Society,* 2020.
12. WHO (2020), *State of World's Population, 2020,* Against my WILL defying the practice that harm women and girls and undermine equality.
13. WHO (2008). *Health Situation in the South-East Asia Region 2001-2007.*
14. India Demographic's, *Population of India, 2020*.
15. Bhende, Asha A and Kanitkar, T. (1985). *Principles of Population Studies,* Himalaya Publ. House, Mumbai.
16. UNICEF (2009). *State of the World's Children 2009,* Special Edition.
17. UNO (2020), *Countries in the world by population,* 2020.
18. Govt. of India (2011). *Census of India 2011,* Provisional Population Totals, Paper – 1 of 2011.
19. Population Reference Bureau (2020), *Population Data Sheet*.
20. *National Family Health Survey NFHS 5 India 2019–21,* International Institute for Population Sciences, Mumbai, India MEASURE DHS + ORC & MACRO.
21. Agarwala, S.N. (1977). *India's Population Problems,* 2nd Ed., Tata Mc Graw Hill.
22. Last, J.M. (1983). *A Dictionary of Epidemiology,* Oxford Medical Publications.
23. The John Hopkins University (1985). *Population Reports,* M.8, Sept–Oct. 85, Baltimore, Maryland.
24. World Bank (1987). *World Development Report,* 1987, Oxford University Press, New Delhi.
25. John M. Last (2001). *A Dictionary of Epidemiology,* 4th ed.
26. *International Family Planning Perspectives* (1983). 9 (3) 84, New York, USA.
27. WHO (1971). *Techn. Rep. Ser.,* No. 483.
28. WHO (1971). *Tech. Rep. Ser.,* No. 476.
29. Department of Medical and Public Affairs. The George Washington University Medical Centre, Washington DC (1974). *Population Reports,* No.1974.
30. United Nations (1975). *World Conference of the International Women's Year : World Plan of Action,* Document E/Cof.66/5, 1975, UN Secretariat.
31. WHO (1970). *Techn. Rep. Ser.,* No.442.
32. WHO (1975). *Techn. Rep. Ser.,* No.569.
33. Siegel, E. et al (1974). *Am. J. Obs & Gyn,* 118 : 995.
34. Mukerji, S. (1987). *J. Family Welfare,* 33 (3) 14.
35. Mohan, M. (1985). *J. Family Welfare,* 31 (3) 3–12.
36. Govt. of India (2000). *National Population Policy* 2000, Ministry of Health and Family Welfare, New Delhi
37. Skrine, R. (1984). *The Practitioner,* 229 : 441–446.
38. Dalsimer, I. et al, eds (1973). *Barrier Methods,* Population Report Series H : I.
39. Sherris, J.D. ed (1982). *Barrier Methods,* Population Report Series H:6.
40. WHO, USAID (1997). *The Essentials of Contraceptive Technology,* Population Information programme. Ed. by Robert A. Hatcher et al.
41. Leon Speroff and Philip D. Darney, *A Clinical Guide for Contraception,* 3rd Ed.
42. Hofmann, A.D. (1984). *Bull WHO,* 2 (2) 331–344.
43. Clive Wood (1975). *Contraception Explained,* Geneva, WHO.
44. Belsky Raymond, ed (1975). *Barrier Methods,* George Washington University Medical Centre (Population Report Series B : 3), Washington, DC.
45. Hawkins, D.F. and Elder M.G. (1979). *Human Fertility Control : Theory and Practice,* Butterworth, London.
46. WHO (1983). *Offset Publication,* No.75.
47. Zipper, J.A. et al (1969). *Am. J. OBG,* 105 : 1275.
48. Gray, R.H. et al (1980). *Manual for the Provision of IUDs,* WHO, Geneva.
49. Liskin, L. ed (1982). *Intra–Uterine Devices,* The John Hopkins University (Population Report Series B : 4).
50. WHO (1971). *Techn. Rep. Ser.,* No.473.
51. Hutchings, J.E. et al (1985). *International Family Planning Perspectives,* 11 (3) 77–85.
52. WHO (1966). *Techn. Rep. Ser.,* No.322.
53. WHO (1968). *Techn. Rep. Ser.,* No.397.
54. Vassey, M. et al (1982). *Lancet,* 1 : 841.
55. Eschenbach, D.A. et al (1977). *Am. J. OBG,* 128 (8) 838.
56. Sparks, R.A. et al (1981). *Brit. Med. J.,* 282 : 1189–91.
57. Padma Rao, K. (1972). *J. OBG of India,* 22 : 268.
58. Snowden R. et al (1977). *The IUD,* A Practice Guide Croom Helm, London.
59. V. Wynn, et al (1979). *Lancet,* 1 : 1045.
60. Spellacy, W.N. (1982). *Am. J. OBG,* 142 : 717.
61. McEwan, J. (1985). *The Practitioner,* 229 : 415–423.
62. *People* (1983). 10 (3) 30.
63. WHO (1982). *Offset Publication,* No.64.
64. Ericsson, R. (1974). *Control of Male Fertility,* Harper and Row, Hagerstown.
65. Royal College of General practitioners (1974). *Oral Contraceptives and Health,* London, Pitman Medical.
66. Inman, W.H.W. and Vessey, M.P. (1968). *Brit. Med.* J. 2 : 193.
67. Mann, J.I. and Inman, WHW (1975). 2 : 245.
68. Vassey, M. et al (1976). *Jr. Biosocial Science,* 8 : 373.
69. Vassey, M. and Mann J.I. (1978). *Br. Med. Bull,* 34 : 157.
70. Stradel, B.V. (1981). *New Eng. J. Med.,* 305 : 612–618.
71. Kols, A. et al (1982). *Oral Contraceptives,* The Johns Hopkins University (Population–Report Series A : 6).
72. WHO (1978). *Techn. Rep. Ser.,* No.619.
73. WHO (1974). *The Work of WHO,* 1982–83.
74. Knopp, R.H. et al (1982). *Am. J. OBG,* 142 : 725.
75. Kay, C.R. (1982). *Am. J. OBG,* 142 : 762–765.
76. Hull, M.G.R. et al (1981). *Lancet,* 1 : 1329.
77. WHO (1981). *Techn. Rep. Ser.,* No. 657.
78. Ambani, L.M. et al (1977). *Fertility and Sterility,* 28 : 791.
79. Mishall, D.R. (1982). *Am.J.OBG,* 142 : 809.

80. Any Questions (1970). *Brit. Med. J.*, 1 : 354.
81. Info Reports (2007). *Injectable Contraceptives : Tool for Providers,* Jan-Feb, 2007, Johns Hopkins Bloomberg, Info Project centre for communication programme.
82. WHO (1982). *Offset Publication* No.65.
83. *IPPF Medical Bulletin (1996)*. Vol. 30, Number 2, April 1996.
84. Fathalla, M. (1981). *People,* 8 (4) 12.
85. WHO (1978). *The Work of WHO 1976–77,* Biennial Report.
86. Govt. of India (2021). *Reference Manual for Integrated RMNCAH+N Counselling,* Ministry of Health and Family Welfare, New Delhi.
87. Robinson, P. (1975). *An Aid to the Teaching of Human Reproduction, Family Planning and Population Dynamics,* WHO, SEARO, New Delhi.
88. International Planned Parenthood Federation (1974). *IPPF Medical Bulletin,* Feb 1974.
89. Vlugt, T. et al (1973). *Pregnancy Termination,* The George Washington University (Population Report Series F : 3).
90. WHO (2021). *Fact Sheet on Abortion,* 25th Nov. 2021.
91. WHO (2018). *Preventing unsafe abortions,* 19th Feb. 2018.
92. Govt. of India (2012). *Annual Report 2011–2012,* Ministry of Health and Family Welfare, New Delhi.
93. WHO (1980). *The Work of WHO 1978–79.*
94. Govt. of India (1978). *Manual for Health Worker, Female,* Vol I, Ministry of Health & Family welfare, New Delhi.
95. Grewal, S. (1976). *J. Indian M.A.,* 66 : 269.
96. Cook, R.J. (1976). *IFPP Bulletin,* April 1966.
97. A New direction for Abortion Law in India, Courts have promises to keep, 3rd Oct. 2022.
98. Govt. of India (2010). *Annual Report 2009-2010,* Ministry of Health and Family Welfare, New Delhi.
99. Peel, John and Potts Malcom (1970). *Textbook of Contraceptive Practice,* Cambridge University Press.
100. *People* (1981). 8 (4) 20.
101. *People* (1982). 9 (2) 47.
102. *Population Reports* (J) (1981). 24 : 525.
103. Jain, A.K. et al (1981). *Stud. Family Plan,* 12 : 79.
104. *ICMR Bulletin*, Dec. 1983.
105. *People* (1982). 9 (2) 41.
106. Govt. of India (1984). *Year Book–Family Welfare Programme in India, 1983–84,* Ministry of Health, New Delhi.
107. Bhiwandiwala, P. (1981). *People* 8 (4) 14.
108. Govt. of India (1978). *Central Calling,* March 1978. Dept. of Family Welfare.
109. Govt. of India (1978). *Central Calling,* Aug. 78, Dept. of Family Welfare.
110. Elstein, M. (1970). *The Practitioner,* 205 : 30.
111. Kanti Giri (1976). *Bibliography on Human Reproduction, Family Planning and Population Dynamics,* WHO, SEARO New Delhi.
112. Philip, T. et al (1984). *Brit. Med. J.* 289 : 77Ä9.
113. France Donnay (1991). *Children in the Tropics,* Controlling Fertility, 1991 No.193–194.
114. P&P (1997). *Population Report,* Meeting Unmet Needs; New Strategies, No. 43, Series J, June 1997.
115. WHO (2014). *Adolescent : Health Risks and Solutions,* Fact Sheet No. 345, May 2014.
116. Govt. of India (2022). *Annual Report 2021–2022,* Ministry of Heatlh and Family Welfare, New Delhi.
117. Govt. of India (2014). *Annual Report 2013–14,* Ministry of Health and Family Welfare, New Delhi.
118. Govt. of India (1985). *Annual Report,* 1984–85, Ministry of Health and Family Welfare, New Delhi.
119. Veena Soni (1983). *International Family Planning Perspectives,* 9 (2) 35.
120. Govt. of India (2006). *Annual Report 2005–06,* DGHS, Ministry of Health and Family Welfare, New Delhi.
121. UNESCO. Regional Office for Education in Asia (1979). *Regional Workshop on Population and Family Education,* Final Report, Sept/ Oct 1970, Bangkok, Thailand.
122. Govt. of India (2002). *Bulletin on Rural Health Statistics in India,* March 2002, Issued by Rural Health Division, DGHS, New Delhi.
123. Sherris, J.D. (1982). *Population Education in the Schools,* The Johns Hopkins University, Maryland (Population Rep.Ser. M : 6).
124. Govt. of India (2004). *Annual Report 2003–2004*, Ministry of Health and Family Welfare, New Delhi.
125. WHO (1976). *Techn. Rep. Ser.,* No. 587.

9 Preventive Medicine in Obstetrics, Paediatrics and Geriatrics

"The test of any civilization is the measure of consideration and care which it gives to its weaker members"

In any community, mothers and children constitute a priority group. In sheer numbers, they comprise approximately 71.14 per cent of the population of the developing countries. In India, women of the child-bearing age (15 to 44 years) constitute 52.4 per cent of total female population, and children under 15 years of age about 26.5 per cent of the total population. Together they constitute nearly 57.5 per cent of the total population. By virtue of their numbers, mothers and children are the major consumers of health services, of whatever form.

Mothers and children not only constitute a large group, but they are also a "vulnerable" or special-risk group. The risk is connected with child-bearing in the case of women; and growth, development and survival in the case of infants and children. Whereas 50 per cent of all deaths in the developed world are occurring among people over 70, the same proportion of deaths are occurring among children during the first five years of life in the developing world. Global observations show that in developed regions maternal mortality ratio averages at 12 per 100,000 live births; in developing regions the figure is 232 for the same number of live births *(1)*. From commonly accepted indices, it is evident that infant, child and maternal mortality rates are high in many developing countries. Further, much of the sickness and deaths among mothers and children is largely preventable. By improving the health of mothers and children, we contribute to the health of the general population. These considerations have led to the formulation of special health services for mothers and children all over the world.

The problems affecting the health of mother and child are multifactorial. Despite current efforts, the health of mother and child still constitutes one of the most serious health problems affecting the community, particularly in the developing countries. The present strategy is to provide mother and child health services as an integrated package of "essential health care", also known as **primary health care** which is based on the principles of equity, intersectoral coordination and community participation. The primary health care approach combines all elements in the local community necessary to make a positive impact on the health status of the population, including the health of mothers and children.

Mother and child – one unit

Mother and child must be considered as one unit. It is because: (1) during the antenatal period, the foetus is part of the mother. The period of development of foetus in mother is about 280 days. During this period, the foetus obtains all the building materials and oxygen from the mother's blood; (2) child health is closely related to maternal health. A healthy mother brings forth a healthy baby; there is less chance for a premature birth, stillbirth or abortion; (3) certain diseases and conditions of the mother during pregnancy (e.g., syphilis, german measles, drug intake) are likely to have their effects upon the foetus; (4) after birth, the child is dependant upon the mother. At least up to the age of 6 to 9 months, the child is completely dependant on the mother for feeding. The mental and social development of the child is also dependant upon the mother. If the mother dies, the child's growth and development are affected (maternal deprivation syndrome); (5) in the care cycle of women, there are few occasions when service to the child is not simultaneously called for. For instance, postpartum care is inseparable from neonatal care and family planning advice; and (6) the mother is also the first teacher of the child. It is for these reasons, the mother and child are treated as one unit.

Obstetrics, Paediatrics and Preventive and Social Medicine

In the past, maternal and child health services were rather fragmented, and provided piecemeal "personal health services" by different agencies, in different ways and in separate clinics. The current trend in many countries is to provide integrated MCH and family planning services as compact family welfare service. This implies a close relationship of maternity health to child health, of maternal and child health to the health of the family; and of family health to the general health of the community. In providing these services, specialists in obstetrics and child health (paediatrics) have joined hands, and are now looking beyond the four walls of hospitals into the community to meet the health needs of mothers and children aimed at positive health. In the process, they have linked themselves to preventive and social medicine, and as a result, terms such as "social obstetrics", "preventive paediatrics" and "social paediatrics" have come into vogue.

OBSTETRICS

Obstetrics is largely preventive medicine. The aim of obstetrics and preventive medicine is the same, viz. to ensure that throughout pregnancy and puerperium, the mother will have good health and that every pregnancy may culminate in a healthy mother and a healthy baby. The age-old concept that obstetrics is only antenatal, intranatal and postnatal care, and is thus concerned mainly with technical skills, is now considered as a very narrow concept, and is being replaced by the concept of **community obstetrics** which combines obstetrical concerns with concepts of primary health care.

SOCIAL OBSTETRICS

The concept of **social obstetrics** has gained currency in recent years. It may be defined as the study of the interplay of social and environmental factors and human reproduction going back to the preconceptional or even premarital period. The social and environmental factors which influence human reproduction are a legion, viz. age at marriage, child bearing, child spacing, family size fertility patterns, level of education, economic status, customs and beliefs, role of women in society, etc. A study of these factors is an important aspect of social obstetrics. The social obstetric problems in India, differ from the social obstetric problems in the developed countries, because of various differing social, economic, cultural and other factors. While accepting the influence of environmental and social factors on human reproduction, social obstetrics has yet another dimension, that is the influence of these factors on the organization, delivery and utilization of obstetric services by the community. In other words, social obstetrics is concerned with the delivery of comprehensive maternity and child health care services including family planning so that they can be brought within the reach of the total community *(2)*.

Preventive paediatrics

Paediatrics which is synonymous with child health is that branch of medical science that deals with the care of children from conception to adolescence, in health and disease. Paediatrics is one of the first clinical subjects to link itself to preventive medicine. Like obstetrics, paediatrics has a large component of preventive and social medicine. There is no other discipline so comprehensive as paediatrics that teaches the value of preventive medicine. Recent years have witnessed further specialization within the broad field of paediatrics viz. preventive paediatrics, social paediatrics, neonatology, perinatology, developmental paediatrics, paediatric surgery; paediatric neurology, and so on.

Preventive paediatrics comprises efforts to avert rather than cure disease and disabilities. It has been broadly divided into *antenatal paediatrics* and *postnatal paediatrics*. The aims of preventive paediatrics and preventive medicine are the same: prevention of disease and promotion of physical, mental and social well-being of children so that each child may achieve the genetic potential with which he/she is born. To achieve these aims, hospitals for children have adopted the strategy of "primary health care" to improve child health care through such activities as growth monitoring, oral rehydration, nutritional surveillance, promotion of breast-feeding, immunization, community feeding, regular health check-ups, etc. Primary health care with its potential for vastly increased coverage through an integrated system of service delivery is increasingly looked upon as the best solution to reach millions of children, especially those who are most in need of preventive and curative services.

Social paediatrics

The challenge of the time is to study child health in relation to community, to social values and to social policy. This has given rise to the concept of social paediatrics. Social paediatrics has been defined as "the application of the principles of social medicine to paediatrics to obtain a more complete understanding of the problems of children in order to prevent and treat disease and promote their adequate growth and development, through an organized health structure *(3)*". Social paediatrics, like social obstetrics, covers a wide responsibility. It is concerned not only with the social factors which influence child health but also with the influence of these factors on the organization, delivery and utilization of child health care services. In other words, social paediatrics is concerned with the delivery of comprehensive and continuous child health care services and to bring these services within the reach of the total community. Social paediatrics also covers the various social welfare measures – local, national and international – aimed to meet the total health needs of a child.

Preventive and social medicine, with its involvement in total community care, and expertise in epidemiology and in the methodology of collection and utilization of data relating to the community and the environment, makes an indispensable contribution to social obstetrics and social paediatrics in the :

1. collection and interpretation of community statistics, delineating groups "at risk" for special care;
2. correlation of vital statistics (e.g., maternal and infant morbidity and mortality rates, perinatal and child mortality rates) with social and biological characteristics such as birth weight, parity, age, stature, employment etc. in the elucidation of aetiological relationships;
3. study of cultural patterns, beliefs and practices relating to childbearing and childrearing, knowledge of which might be useful in promoting acceptance and utilization of obstetric and paediatric services by the community;
4. to determine priorities and contribute to the planning of MCH services and programmes; and
5. for evaluating whether MCH services and programmes are accomplishing their objectives in terms of their effectiveness and efficiency.

Hitherto, obstetrics, paediatrics and preventive and social medicine were operating in watertight compartments. The emergence of social paediatrics, social obstetrics and their association with preventive and social medicine are certainly new developments in contemporary medicine. In some Universities, a chair of social paediatrics has also been established. The increasing coming together of these disciplines augurs well for the provision of comprehensive mother and child health care and family planning services as a compact family welfare service.

Maternity cycle

The stages in maternity cycle are :

(i) Fertilization;
(ii) Antenatal or prenatal period;
(iii) Intranatal period;
(iv) Postnatal period; and
(v) Inter-conceptional period.

Fertilization takes place in the outer part of the fallopian tube. Segmentation of the fertilized ovum begins at once and proceeds at a rapid rate. The fertilized ovum reaches the uterus in 8 to 10 days. Cell division proceeds at a rapid rate. By a process of cell division and differentiation, all the organs and tissues of the body are formed. The periods of growth have been divided as follows :

1. Prenatal period :
   (a) Ovum – 0 to 14 days
   (b) Embryo – 14 days to 9 weeks
   (c) Foetus – 9th week to birth
2. Premature infant – from 28 to 37 weeks
3. Birth, full term – average 280 days.

MCH problems

MCH problems cover a broad spectrum. At one extreme, the most advanced countries are concerned with problems such as perinatal problems, congenital malformations, genetic and certain behavioural problems. At the other extreme, in developing countries, the primary concern is reduction of maternal and child mortality and morbidity, spacing of pregnancies, limitation of family size, prevention of communicable diseases, improvement of nutrition and promoting acceptance of health practices. Currently, the main health problems affecting the health of the mother and the child in India, as in other developing countries, revolve round the triad of *malnutrition, infection* and the consequences of *unregulated fertility (4)*. Associated with these problems is the scarcity of health and other social services in vast areas of the country together with poor socio-economic conditions.

1. MALNUTRITION

Malnutrition is like an iceberg; most people in the developing countries live under the burden of malnutrition. Pregnant women, nursing mothers and children are particularly vulnerable to the effects of malnutrition. The adverse effects of maternal malnutrition have been well documented–maternal depletion, low birth weight, anaemia, toxemias of pregnancy, postpartum haemorrhage, all leading to high mortality and morbidity. The effects of malnutrition are also frequently more serious during the formative years of life. Previously it was thought that malnutrition was largely concentrated in school age children, and in toddlers. Now it is realized that the *intrauterine period* of life is a very important period from the nutritional standpoint. Infants born with adequate birth weight have relatively low mortality even under poor environmental conditions. The next critical period of childhood is the *period of weaning*. Severe malnutrition coincides with the age at which babies are usually weaned. Susceptibility to infection and severity of illness are significantly less in well nourished, than in malnourished children. Nutrition protection and promotion is, therefore, an essential activity of MCH care.

Measures to improve the nutritional status of mothers and children may be broadly divided into *direct* and *indirect* nutrition interventions *(4)*. *Direct interventions* cover a wide range of activities, viz. supplementary feeding programmes, distribution of iron and folic acid tablets, fortification and enrichment of foods, nutrition education, etc. *Indirect nutrition* interventions have still wider ramifications because they are not specifically related to nutrition. These include measures such as control of communicable diseases through immunization, improvement of environmental sanitation, provision of clean drinking water, family planning, food hygiene, education and primary health care. Nutritional surveillance is becoming increasingly important for identifying subclinical malnutrition, as it tends to be overlooked in both the mother and the child. The primary health worker (community worker) can play a vital role in improving the nutritional status of mothers and children.

2. INFECTION

Maternal infections may cause a variety of adverse effects such as foetal growth retardation, low birth weight, embryopathy, abortion and puerperal sepsis. In industrial societies, the risk of the mother acquiring infections during pregnancy is relatively low, but in underdeveloped areas, the mother is exposed to significantly higher risks. Many women are infected with HIV, hepatitis B, cytomegalo viruses, herpes simplex virus or toxoplasma during pregnancy. Furthermore, about 2 to 10 per cent pregnant women suffer from asymptomatic bacteriuria.

As far as the baby is concerned, infection may begin with labour and delivery and increase as the child grows older. Children may be ill with debilitating diarrhoeal, respiratory and skin infections for as much as a *third of their first year of life*. In some regions, the situation is further aggravated by such chronic infections as malaria and tuberculosis. The occurrence of multiple and frequent infections may precipitate in the children a severe protein-energy malnutrition and anaemia. When the child becomes ill, traditions, beliefs and taboos enter into play; the indirect effect of infections may be more important than the direct one in traditional societies.

Prevention and treatment of infections in mother and children is a major and important part of normal MCH care activity. It is now widely recognized that children in developing areas need to be immunized against nine infections – tuberculosis, diphtheria, whooping cough, tetanus, hepatitis B, haemophilus influenza type B, Japanese encephalitis in endemic states, measles and polio. Many countries, including India, have adopted the WHO Expanded Programme on Immunization as part of everyday MCH care. Tetanus toxoid application during pregnancy has also been taken up. Education of mothers in medical measures such as oral rehydration in diarrhoea and febrile diseases. In addition, a good knowledge and practice of personal hygiene and appropriate sanitation measures, particularly in and around the home, are essential pre-requisites for the control of the most common infections and parasitic diseases.

3. UNCONTROLLED REPRODUCTION

The health hazards for the mother and the child resulting from unregulated fertility have been well recognized – increased prevalence of low birth weight babies, severe anaemia, abortion, antepartum haemorrhage and a high maternal and perinatal mortality, which have shown a sharp rise after the 4th pregnancy. Statistics have shown that in almost every country in the world, a high birth rate is associated with a high infant mortality rate and under-five death rate (Table 1).

TABLE 1

Selected rates by country for crude birth rates, infant mortality rates and under-five mortality rates (mid 2020)

Country	Crude birth rate per 1000 population (mid 2020)	IMR per 1000 live births (mid 2020)	Under–five mortality rate per 1000 live births (2020)
India	17	28	33
Pakistan	27	54	65
Bangladesh	18	24	29
Thailand	10	7	9
Sri Lanka	15	6	7
China	9	5	7
Switzerland	10	4	4
UK	10	4	4
USA	11	5	6
Singapore	9	2	2
Japan	7	2	2

Source : *(5, 6)*

Because family planning has a striking impact on the health of the mother and the child, a number of countries have integrated family planning in the MCH care activities. The introduction of new types of IUD; easier and safer techniques of pregnancy termination and female sterilization; oral pills and long-acting injectable medroxyprogesterone acetate (MPA) have contributed a good deal in the utilization of family planning services. In some countries, MCH programmes are extending their scope to include family-life education in schools. There is also an increasing acceptance of the role of traditional midwives and community health workers, with suitable training for the extension of family planning services to remote rural areas.

Maternal and child health

The term "maternal and child health" refers to the promotive, preventive, curative and rehabilitative health care for mothers and children. It includes the sub-areas of maternal health, child health, family planning, school health, handicapped children, adolescence, and health aspects of care of children in special settings such as day care *(4)*.

The specific objectives of MCH are (a) reduction of maternal, perinatal, infant and childhood mortality and morbidity; (b) promotion of reproductive health; and (c) promotion of the physical and psychological development of the child and adolescent within the family. The ultimate objective of MCH services is lifelong health *(4)*.

Pregnancy detection

The simple way to confirm pregnancy in the first trimester is to conduct a urine examination using a pregnancy test kit. The kit detects pregnancy on the basis of presence of human chorionic gonadotrophin hormone in the urine. The test is performed soon after a missed period and is simple to perform. The pregnancy test should be offered to any women who is in reproductive age group and comes with a history of amenorrhoea or symptoms of pregnancy. The Government of India has made "Nischay" pregnancy test kit available across the country. Other test kits are also available in the market. The kit is provided to ASHA or other link workers and the women should be advised appropriately on the result of the test *(7)*.

ANTENATAL CARE

Antenatal care (ANC) can be defined as the care provided by skilled health-care professionals to pregnant women and pregnant adolescent girls in order to ensure the best health conditions for both mother and baby during pregnancy. The components of ANC include: risk identification; prevention and management of pregnancy-related or concurrent diseases; health education and health promotion *(8)*. ANC reduces maternal and perinatal morbidity and mortality both directly, through detections, and indirectly, through the identification of women and girls at increased risk of developing complications during labour and delivery, thus ensuring referral to an appropriate level of care *(8)*.

Ideally this care should begin soon after conception and continue throughout pregnancy. In some countries, notification of pregnancy is required to bring the mother in the prevention care cycle as early as possible.

Objectives

The objectives of antenatal care are :

(1) To promote, protect and maintain the health of the mother during pregnancy;

(2) To detect "high-risk" cases and give them special attention;

(3) To foresee complications and prevent them;

(4) To remove anxiety and dread associated with delivery;

(5) To reduce maternal and infant mortality and morbidity;

(6) To teach the mother elements of child care, nutrition, personal hygiene, and environmental sanitation;

(7) To sensitize the mother to the need for family planning, including advice to cases seeking medical termination of pregnancy; and

(8) To attend to the under-fives accompanying the mother.

The above objectives are achieved by the following programme of health care services :

(1) Antenatal visits

Ideally the mother should attend the antenatal clinic once a month during the first 7 months; twice a month, during the next month; and thereafter, once a week, if everything is normal. A high proportion of mothers in India are from lower socio-economic group, and many of them are working women. Attendance at the antenatal clinic may mean loss of daily wages. Consequently, it is difficult for them to attend the antenatal clinic so often. In these cases, a minimum of 4 visits covering the entire period of pregnancy should be the target, as shown below :

The suggested schedule is as follows *(7)* :

1st visit – within 12 weeks, preferably as soon as the pregnancy is suspected, for registration of pregnancy and first antenatal check-up.

2nd visit – between 14 and 26 weeks.

3rd visit – between 28 and 34 weeks.

4th visit – between 36 weeks and term.

It is advisable for the woman to visit medical officer at the PHC for an antenatal check-up during the period of 28–34 weeks (3rd visit). Besides this, she may be advised to avail investigation facilities at the nearest PHC/CHC/FRU.

Registration of pregnancy within 12 weeks is the primary responsibility of the ANM. Opportunities such as Village Health Nutrition Day should be availed to ensure early registration of pregnancy and antenatal check-up.

Early pregnancy detection is important for the following reasons *(7)* :

1. It facilitates proper planning and allows for adequate care to be provided during pregnancy for both the mother and the foetus.
2. Record the date of last menstrual period and calculate the expected date of delivery.
3. The health status of the mother can be assessed and any medical illness that she might be suffering from can be detected. Also to obtain and record the baseline information on blood pressure, weight, haemoglobin etc.
4. It helps in timely detection of complications at an early stage and helps to manage them appropriately by referral as and where required.
5. It also helps to confirm if the pregnancy is wanted and if not, then refer the women at the earliest to a 24 hours PHC or FRU that provides safe abortion services. The health personnel should be alert to the possibility of sex selective abortion as such abortions are illegal.

6. Early detection of pregnancy and provision of care from the initial stage facilitates a good interpersonal relationship between the care giver and the pregnant woman.

Estimation of number of pregnancies in a specified area and pregnancy tracking *(7)*

To ensure complete registration, it is essential that the ANM should know the estimated number of pregnancies to be registered annually in her area. Calculating the expected number of annual pregnancies in the area will help her judge how good her pregnancy registration is. In case the number of pregnancies registered is less than that of the estimated pregnancies, she needs to track down the pregnancies she has missed, with the help of ASHAs and AWWs. Estimating the number of pregnancies will also help her judge whether she has an adequate stock of the supplies required to provide routine ANC (such as TT injections, IFA tablets and ANC record forms) and tackle any complications that arise during this period.

The number of expected pregnancies per year :

The ANM must know the population size and birth rate of the area under her jurisdiction. The expected number of live births may be calculated as shown below :

$$\text{Expected no. of live births (Y)/year} = \frac{\text{Birth rate (per 1000 population)} \times \text{population of the area}}{1000}$$

As some pregnancies may not result in a live birth (i.e. abortions and stillbirths may occur), the expected number of live births would be an under-estimation of the total number of pregnancies. Hence, a correction factor of 10% is required, i.e. add 10% to the figure obtained above.

So, the total number of expected pregnancies

(Z) = Y + 10% of Y

As a thumb rule, in any given month, approximately half the number of pregnancies estimated above should be in records.

Example of estimation of the number of pregnancies annually

Birth rate	= 25/1000 population
Population under the sub-centre	= 5000
Therefore, expected number of live births	= (25×5000)/1000 = 125 births
Correction factor (pregnancy wastage)	= 10% of 125 = say 13
Therefore, total no. of expected pregnancies in a year	= 125 + 13 = 138

In any month, the ANM should have about 69 pregnancies registered with her.

If the number of women registered is less than expected, the ANM should approach community leaders and key people to ensure that the pregnant women are registered and come for ANC. ASHA and link worker should visit every house in the area and ensure that all pregnant women are registered. Some women may be receiving ANC from the private sector. Ensure that their names together with the names of the facilities where they are registered are mentioned in the antenatal register.

The ANM must keep track of all pregnant women in her area. In case a registered women does not turn-up for her ANC check-up, ANM must follow her and counsel her for the regular ANC check-up. An antenatal check-up after a missed appointment should include all the components of the missed visit(s) as well as those that correspond to the present visit. For example, the woman should be given her TT injection and supply of IFA tablets, her weight and blood pressure should be checked besides being screened for complications.

A policy decision has been taken for a name-based tracking system whereby pregnant women and children can be tracked for their ANCs and immunization along with a feedback system for the ANM, ASHA etc. This has been done to ensure that all pregnant women receive their ANCs and PNCs, and children receive full immunization. This will also help in tracking and ensuring ANC/PNC for missed/left out cases.

PREVENTIVE SERVICES FOR MOTHERS (ANTENATAL CHECK-UP)

The first visit, irrespective of when it occurs, should include the following components :

I. **History-taking**

During the first visit, a detailed history of the woman needs to be taken to : (1) Confirm the pregnancy (first visit only); (2) Identify whether there were complications during any previous pregnancy/confinement that may have a bearing on the present one; (3) Identify any current medical/ surgical or obstetric condition(s) that may complicate the present pregnancy; (4) Record the date of 1st day of last menstrual period and calculate the expected date of delivery by adding 9 months and 7 days to the 1st day of last menstrual period; (5) Record symptoms indicating complications, e.g. fever, persisting vomiting, abnormal vaginal discharge or bleeding, palpitation, easy fatigability, breathlessness at rest or on mild exertion, generalized swelling in the body, severe headache and blurring of vision, burning in passing urine, decreased or absent foetal movements etc; (6) History of any current systemic illness, e.g., hypertension, diabetes, heart disease, tuberculosis, renal disease, epilepsy, asthma, jaundice, malaria, reproductive tract infection, STD, HIV/AIDS etc. Record family history of hypertension, diabetes, tuberculosis, and thalassaemia. Family history of twins or congenital malformation; and (7) History of drug allergies and habit forming drugs.

II. **Physical examination**

1. *Pallor* : Presence of pallor indicates anaemia. The woman should be examined for pallor at each visit. Examine woman's conjunctiva, nails, tongue, oral mucosa and palms. Pallor should be co-related with haemoglobin estimation.
2. *Pulse* : The normal pulse rate is 60 to 90 beats per minute. If the pulse rate is persistently low or high, with or without other symptoms, the woman needs medical attention.
3. *Respiratory rate* : It is important to check the respiratory rate, especially if the woman complaints of breathlessness. Normal respiratory rate is 18–20 breaths per minute.
4. *Oedema* : Oedema (swelling), which appears in the evening and disappears in the morning after a full night's sleep, could be a normal manifestation of pregnancy. Any oedema of the face, hands, abdominal wall and vulva is abnormal. Oedema can be suspected if a woman

complains of abnormal tightening of any rings on her fingers. She must be referred immediately for further investigations. If there is oedema in association with high blood pressure, heart disease, anaemia or proteinuria, the woman should be referred to the medical officer.

5. *Blood pressure :* Measure the woman's blood pressure at every visit. This is important to rule out hypertensive disorders of pregnancy. Hypertension is diagnosed when two consecutive readings taken four hours or more apart show the systolic blood pressure to be 140 mmHg or more and/or the diastolic blood pressure to be 90 mmHg or more. High blood pressure during pregnancy may signify Pregnancy-Induced Hypertension (PIH) and/or chronic hypertension. If the woman has high blood pressure, check her urine for the presence of albumin. The presence of albumin (+2) together with high blood pressure is sufficient to categorize her as having pre-eclampsia. Refer her to the MO immediately. If the diastolic blood pressure of the woman is above 110 mmHg, it is a danger sign that points towards imminent eclampsia. The urine albumin should be estimated at the earliest. If it is strongly positive, the woman should be referred to the FRU IMMEDIATELY. If the woman has high blood pressure but no urine albumin, she should be referred to the MO at 24×7 PHC. A woman with PIH, pre-eclampsia or imminent eclampsia requires hospitalization and supervised treatment at a 24-hour PHC/FRU.
6. *Weight :* A pregnant woman's weight should be taken at each visit. The weight taken during the first visit/ registration should be treated as the baseline weight. Normally, a woman should gain 9–11 kg during her pregnancy. Ideally after the first trimester, a pregnant woman gains around 2 kg every month. If the diet is not adequate, i.e. if the woman is taking less than the required amount of calories, she might gain only 5–6 kg during her pregnancy. An inadequate dietary intake can be suspected if the woman gains less than 2 kg per month. She needs to be put on food supplementation. The help of the AWW should be taken in this matter, especially for those categories of women who need it the most. Low weight gain usually leads to Intrauterine Growth Retardation and results in the birth of a baby with a low birth weight. Excessive weight gain (more than 3 kg in a month) should raise suspicion of pre-eclampsia, twins (multiple pregnancy) or diabetes. Take the woman's blood pressure and test her urine for proteinuria and sugar. If the blood pressure is high and the urine is positive for protein or sugar, refer her to medical officer.
7. *Breast examination :* Observe the size and shape of the nipples for the presence of inverted or flat nipples.

III. Abdominal examination

Examine the abdomen to monitor the progress of the pregnancy and foetal growth. The abdominal examination includes the following :

1. *Measurement of fundal height :* Enlargement of the uterus and the height of the uterine fundus is as shown in Fig. 1.
   a. 12 weeks – Uterine fundus just palpable per abdomen.
   b. 20 weeks – Fundus flat at the lower border of umbelicus.
   c. 36 weeks – Fundus felt at the level of xiphisternum.

   The duration of pregnancy should always be expressed in terms of completed weeks. In the first half of pregnancy the size of the uterus is of the greatest value in confirming the calculated duration of pregnancy.
2. *Foetal heart sounds :* The foetal heart sounds can be heard after 6th month. The rate varies between 120 to 140 per minute. They are usually best heard in the midline; after the 28th week, their location may change because of the position and lie of the foetus.
3. *Foetal movements :* Foetal movements can be felt by the examiner after 18–22nd week by gently palpating the abdomen.
4. *Foetal parts :* These can be felt about the 22nd week. After the 28th week, it is possible to distinguish the head, back and limbs.
5. *Multiple pregnancy :* This must be suspected if the uterus is larger than the estimated gestational age or palpation of multiple foetal parts.
6. *Foetal lie and presentation :* Relevant only after 32 weeks of pregnancy.
7. Inspection of abdominal scar or any other relevant abdominal findings.

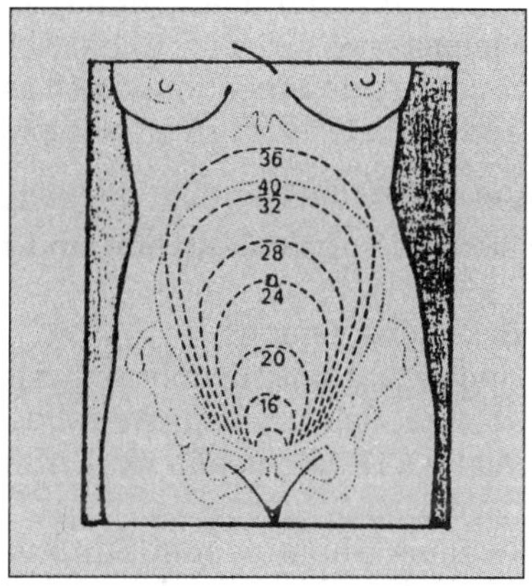

FIG. 1

Uterine fundal height at various stages of pregnancy (numbers indicate weeks of pregnancy)

IV. Assessment of gestational age *(9)*

Measurement of gestational age has changed over the time. As the dominant effect of gestational age on survival and long-term impairment has become apparent over the last 30 years, perinatal epidemiology has shifted from measuring birth weight alone to focusing on gestational age. The most accurate "gold standard" for assessment is routine early ultrasound assessment together with foetal measurements ideally in the first trimester. Gestational age assessment based on the date of last menstrual period (LMP) was previously the most widespread method used and remains the only available method in many settings. Many countries now use "best obstetric estimate", combining ultrasound and LMP as an approach to estimate gestational age. It can have a large impact on the number of preterm births reported.

Any method using ultrasound requires skilled technicians, equipment and for maximum accuracy, first trimester antenatal clinic attendance. These are not common in low-income settings, where majority of preterm births occur. Alternative approaches to LMP in these settings include fundal height, clinical assessment of the newborn after birth or birth weight as a surrogate.

V. **Laboratory investigations**

The following laboratory investigations are carried out at the facilities indicated below :

a. At the sub-centre :
- Pregnancy detection test.
- Haemoglobin examination.
- Urine test for presence of albumin and sugar.
- Rapid malaria test.

b. At the PHC/CHC/FRU :
- Blood group, including Rh factor.
- VDRL/RPR.
- HIV testing.
- Rapid malaria test (if unavailable at SC).
- Blood sugar testing.
- HBsAg for hepatitis B infection.

Essential components of every antenatal check-up :

1. Take the patient's history.
2. Conduct a physical examination–measure the weight, blood pressure and respiratory rate and check for pallor and oedema.
3. Conduct abdominal palpation for foetal growth, foetal lie and auscultation of foetal heart sound according to the stage of pregnancy.
4. Carry out laboratory investigations, such as haemoglobin estimation and urine tests for sugar and proteins.

Interventions and counselling

1. Iron and folic acid supplementation and medication as needed.
2. Immunization against tetanus.
3. Group or individual instruction on nutrition, family planning, self care, delivery and parenthood.
4. Home visiting by a female health worker/trained dai.
5. Referral services, where necessary.
6. Inform the woman about Janani Suraksha Yojana and other incentives offered by the government.

RISK APPROACH (10)

The central purpose of antenatal care is to identify "high risk" cases (as early as possible) from a large group of antenatal mothers and arrange for them skilled care, while continuing to provide appropriate care for all mothers. These cases comprise the following :

1. Elderly primi (30 years and over).
2. Short statured primi (140 cm and below).
3. Malpresentations, viz breech, transverse lie, etc.
4. Antepartum haemorrhage, threatened abortion.
5. Pre-eclampsia and eclampsia.
6. Anaemia.
7. Twins, hydramnios.
8. Previous still-birth, intrauterine death, manual removal of placenta.
9. Elderly grandmultiparas.
10. Prolonged pregnancy (14 days–after expected date of delivery).
11. History of previous caesarean or instrumental delivery.
12. Pregnancy associated with general diseases, viz. cardiovascular disease, kidney disease, diabetes, tuberculosis, liver disease, malaria, convulsions, asthma, HIV, RTI, STI, etc.
13. Treatment for infertility.
14. Three or more spontaneous consecutive abortions.

The "risk approach" is a managerial tool for improved MCH care. Its purpose is to provide better services for all, but with special attention to those who need them most. Inherent in this approach is maximum utilization of all resources, including some human resources that are not conventionally involved in such care – traditional birth attendants, community health workers, women's groups, for example. The risk strategy is expected to have far–reaching effects on the whole organization of MCH/FP services and lead to improvements in both the coverage and quality of health care, at all levels, particularly at primary health care level.

MAINTENANCE OF RECORDS

A Mother and Child Protection Card should be duly completed for every woman registered. It contains a registration number, identifying data, previous health history and main health events etc. The case record should be handed over to the woman. She should be instructed to bring the record with her during all subsequent check-ups/visits and also to carry it along with her at time of delivery. This card has been developed jointly by the Ministry of Health and Family Welfare (MOHFW) and Ministry of Women and Child Development (MOWCD) to ensure uniformity in record keeping. This will also help the service provider to know the details of previous ANCs/PNCs both for routine and emergency care. The information contained in the card should also be recorded in the antenatal register as per the Health Management Information System (HMIS) format.

HOME VISITS

Home visiting is the backbone of all MCH services. Even if the expectant mother is attending the antenatal clinic regularly, it is suggested that she must be paid at least one home visit by the Health Worker Female or Public Health Nurse. More visits are required if the delivery is planned at home. The mother is generally relaxed at home. The home visit will win her confidence. The home visit will provide an opportunity to observe the environmental and social conditions at home and also an opportunity to give prenatal advice.

(2) Prenatal advice

A major component of antenatal care is antenatal or prenatal advice. The mother is more receptive to advice concerning herself and her baby at this time than at other times. The "talking points" should cover not only the specific problems of pregnancy and child-birth but overflow into family and child health care.

(i) *DIET :* Reproduction costs energy. A pregnancy in total duration consumes about 60,000 kcal, over and above normal metabolic requirements. Lactation demands about 550 kcal a day. Further, child survival is correlated with birth weight. And birth weight is correlated to the weight gain of the mother during pregnancy. On an average, a normal healthy woman gains about 9–11 kg of weight during pregnancy. Several studies have indicated that weight gain of poor Indian women averaged 6.5 kg during pregnancy *(11)*. Thus pregnancy imposes the need for considerable extra calorie and nutrient requirements. If maternal stores of iron are poor (as may happen after repeated pregnancies) and if enough iron is not available to the mother during pregnancy, it is possible that foetus may lay down insufficient iron stores. Such a baby may show a normal haemoglobin at birth, but will lack the stores of iron necessary for rapid growth and increase in blood volume and muscle mass in the first year of life. Stresses in the form of malaria and other childhood infections will make the deficiency more acute, and many infants become severely anaemic during early months of life. A balanced and adequate diet is therefore, of utmost importance during pregnancy and lactation to meet the increased needs of the mother, and to prevent "nutritional stress".

(ii) *PERSONAL HYGIENE* : Of equal importance is advice regarding personal hygiene. (a) *Personal cleanliness* : The need to bathe every day and to wear clean clothes should be explained. The hair should also be kept clean and tidy. (b) *Rest and sleep* : 8 hours sleep, and at least 2 hours rest after mid-day meals should be advised. (c) *Bowels*: Constipation should be avoided by regular intake of green leafy vegetables, fruits and extra fluids. Purgatives like castor oil should be avoided to relieve constipation. (d) *Exercise*: Light household work is advised, but manual physical labour during late pregnancy may adversely affect the foetus. (e) *Smoking*: Smoking should be cut down to a minimum. Expectant mothers who smoke heavily produce babies much smaller than the average – it is because nicotine has a vasoconstrictor influence in the uterus and induces a degree of placental insufficiency. The adverse effects of smoking range from low birth-weight to an increased risk of perinatal death of the infant *(12)*. Women who smoke during pregnancy give birth to babies which on an average weigh 170g less at term than the babies of non-smokers. The perinatal mortality amongst babies whose mothers smoked during pregnancy is between 10–40 per cent higher than in non-smokers. (f) *Alcohol* : Evidence is mounting that alcohol can cause a range of fertility problems in women. Moderate to heavy drinkers who became pregnant have greater risk of pregnancy loss *(13)*, and if they do not abort, their children may have various physical and mental problems *(14)*. Heavy drinking has been associated with a fetal syndrome (FAS) which includes intrauterine growth retardation and developmental delay. More recently, it has been shown that the consumption of even moderate amount of alcohol during pregnancy is associated with an increased risk of spontaneous abortion *(15)*. (g) *Dental care*: Advice should also be given about oral hygiene. (h) *Sexual intercourse*: This should be restricted especially during the last trimester.

(iii) *DRUGS* : The use of drugs that are not absolutely essential should be discouraged. Certain drugs taken by the mother during pregnancy may affect the foetus adversely and cause foetal malformations. The classical example is thalidomide, a hypnotic drug, which caused deformed hands and feet of the babies born. The drug proved most serious when taken between 4 to 8 weeks of pregnancy. Other examples are LSD which is known to cause chromosomal damage, streptomycin which may cause 8th nerve damage and deafness in the foetus, iodide-containing preparations which may cause congenital goitre in the foetus *(16)*. Corticosteroids may impair foetal growth, sex hormones may produce virilism, tetracyclines may affect the growth of bones and enamel formation of teeth. Anaesthetic agents including pethidine administered during labour can have depressant effect on the baby and delay the onset of effective respiration. Later still in the puerperium, if the mother is breast-feeding, there are certain drugs which are excreted in breast milk. A great deal of caution is required in the drug-intake by pregnant women *(17)*.

(iv) *RADIATION* : Exposure to radiation is a positive danger to the developing foetus. The most common source of radiation is abdominal X-ray during pregnancy. Case cohort studies have shown that mortality rates from leukaemia and other neoplasms were significantly greater among children exposed to intrauterine X-ray. This is in addition to congenital malformations such as microcephaly. The X-ray examination in pregnancy should be carried out only for definite indications, X-ray dosage kept to minimum. Furthermore, in all women of child-bearing age among whom there is a possibility of pregnancy, elective X-ray should be avoided in the two weeks preceeding the menstrual period.

(v) *WARNING SIGNS* : The mother should be given clear-cut instructions that she should report immediately in case of the following warning signals : (a) swelling of the feet (b) fits (c) headache (d) blurring of the vision (e) bleeding or discharge per vagina, and (f) any other unusual symptoms.

(vi) *CHILD CARE* : The art of child care has to be learnt. Special classes are held for mothers attending antenatal clinics. Mother-craft education consists of nutrition education, advice on hygiene and childrearing, cooking demonstrations, family planning education, family budgeting, etc.

(3) Specific health protection

(i) *ANAEMIA* : According to NFHS IV, about 50 per cent of pregnant women in India are anaemic. The major aetiological factors being iron and folic acid deficiencies. It is well known that anaemia per se is associated with high incidence of premature births, postpartum haemorrhage, puerperal sepsis and thromboembolic phenomena in the mother. The Government of India has initiated a programme in which 100 mg of elemental iron and 500 mcg of folic acid are being distributed daily for 100 days to pregnant women through antenatal clinics, primary health centres and their subcentres.

(ii) *OTHER NUTRITIONAL DEFICIENCIES* : The mother should be protected against other nutritional deficiencies that may occur, particularly protein, vitamin and mineral especially vit A and iodine deficiency. In some MCH Centres fresh milk is supplied free of cost to all expectant mothers; where this is not possible, skimmed milk should be given. Capsules of vitamin A and D are also supplied free of cost.

(iii) *ASYMPTOMATIC BACTERIURIA (ASB)*: Urinary tract infection during pregnancy are associated with risks to both mother and foetus. It includes pyelonephritis preterm birth, low birth weight and increased perinatal mortality. Because of physiological changes during pregnancy, the pregnant woman is more prone to urinary tract infection. Midstream urine culture is the recommended method for diagnosis of ASB. If culture facility is not available on-site, midstream urine gram-staining is recommended for the diagnosis *(8)*. The patient should be appropriately treated for ASB.

(iv) *GESTATIONAL DIABETES*: Hyperglycaemia first detected at any time during pregnancy should be classified as either gestational diabetes mellitus or diabetes mellitus in pregnancy according to WHO criteria. Gestational diabetes is high blood sugar that develops during pregnancy and usually disappears after giving birth. It can occur at any stage of pregnancy but is more common in the second half. Having gestational diabetes also means that the woman is at increased risk of developing type 2 diabetes in the future. At the first antenatal visit, family history of diabetes should be recorded to determine if the woman is more at risk of gestational diabetes *(8)*. The general symptoms are excessive thirst and hunger, frequent urination, drowsiness or fatigue, dry itchy skin, blurring of vision, slow healing of wounds. The second pregnancy may be associated with type 2 diabetes. Hyperglycaemia during pregnancy can harm mother and the foetus, increasing risk of high blood pressure, preeclampsia, miscarriage or stillbirth, birth defects and big baby (birth weight more than 4.5 kg).

(v) *TOXEMIAS OF PREGNANCY* : The presence of albumine in urine and an increase in blood pressure indicates toxemias of pregnancy. Their early detection and management are indicated. Efficient antenatal care minimizes the risk of toxemias of pregnancy.

(vi) *TETANUS* : If the mother was not immunized earlier, 2 doses of adsorbed tetanus toxoid should be given – the first dose at 16–20 weeks and the second dose at 20–24 weeks of pregnancy. The minimum interval between the 2 doses should be one month. No pregnant woman should be denied even one dose of tetanus toxoid, if she is seen late in pregnancy. For a woman who has been immunized earlier, one booster dose will be sufficient. When such a booster has been given, it will provide necessary cover for subsequent pregnancies, during the next 5 years. It is advised not to inject tetanus toxoid at every successive pregnancy because of the risk of hyperimmunization and side-effects.

(vii) *SYPHILIS* : Syphilis is an important preventable cause of pregnancy wastage in some countries. Pregnancies in women with primary and secondary syphilis often end in spontaneous abortion, stillbirth, perinatal death, or the birth of a child with congenital syphilis. Syphilitic infection in the pregnant woman is transmissible to the foetus. Neurological damage with mental retardation is one of the most serious consequences of congenital syphilis. When the mother is suffering from syphilis, infection of the foetus does not occur before the 4th month of pregnancy; it is most likely to occur after the 6th month by which time the Langhan's cell layer has completely atrophied *(18)*. Infection of the foetus is most likely to occur when the mother is suffering from primary or secondary stages of syphilis than late syphilis.

It is routine procedure in antenatal clinics to test blood for syphilis at the first visit. Since the mother can subsequently get infected with syphilis, the ideal procedure would be to test blood for syphilis both early and late in pregnancy. Congenital syphilis is easily preventable. Ten daily injections of procaine penicillin (600,000 units) are almost always adequate *(18)*.

(viii) *GERMAN MEASLES* : Maternal viraemia associated with the rubella infection during pregnancy may result in infection of placenta and foetus. Only a limited number of foetal cells become infected. The growth rate of infected cell is reduced, resulting in fewer number of cells in affected organ at birth. The infection may lead to deranged and hypoplastic organ development, resulting in structural anomalies in the newborn. The timing of infection determines the extent of teratogenic effect. In general, the earlier in pregnancy infection occurs, the greater the damage to the foetus. Infection during first trimester of pregnancy results in abnormalities in infant in about 85 per cent of cases, but detectable defects are found in about 16 per cent of infants who acquired infection during second trimester. Birth defects are uncommon if maternal infection occurs after 20 weeks of gestation *(19)*.

Ideally we should prevent infection during pregnancy by preventing and controlling the disease in the general population. Currently this is being attempted by vaccination of all school-aged children with rubella vaccine, and including the rubella vaccine in the routine immunization schedule. Supplementing the community control of infection is the vaccination of all women of childbearing age who are sero-negative. Before vaccinating, it is advisable that pregnancy be ruled out and effective contraception be maintained for 8 weeks after vaccination because of the possible risk to the foetus from the virus.

(ix) *Rh STATUS* : The foetal red cells may enter the maternal circulation in a number of different circumstances, during labour, caesarean section, therapeutic abortion, external cephalic version, and apparently spontaneously in the late pregnancy. The intrusion of these cells, if the mother is Rh-negative and the child is Rh-positive, provokes an immune response in her so that she forms antibodies to Rh which can cross the placenta and produce foetal haemolysis. The same response may be produced to a greater degree by a transfusion of Rh-positive blood. In a pregnant woman, isoimmunization mainly occurs during labour, so that the first child although Rh-positive, is unaffected except where the mother has been already sensitized. In the second or subsequent pregnancies, if the child is Rh-positive, the mother will react to the smallest intrusion of foetal cells by producing antibodies to destroy foetal blood cells causing haemolytic disease in the foetus. Clinically haemolytic disease takes the form of *hydrops foetalis, icterus gravis neonatorum* (of which kernicterus is often a sequel) and congenital haemolytic anaemia.

It is a routine procedure in antenatal clinics to test blood for Rhesus type in early pregnancy. If the woman is Rh-negative and the husband is Rh-positive, she is kept under surveillance for determination of Rh-antibody levels during antenatal care. The blood should be further examined at 28 weeks and 34–36 weeks of gestation for antibodies. Rh anti-D immunoglobulin should be given at 28 weeks of gestation so that sensitization during the first pregnancy can be prevented. If the baby is Rh-positive, the Rh anti D immunoglobulin is given again within 72 hours of delivery. It should also be given after abortion. Post maturity should be avoided. Whenever there is evidence of haemolytic process in foetus-in-utero, the mother should be shifted to an equipped centre specialized to deal with Rh problems. The incidence of haemolytic disease due to Rh factor in India is estimated to be approximately one for every 400 to 500 live births.

(x) *HIV INFECTION* : HIV may pass from an infected mother to her foetus, through the placenta or to her infant during delivery or by breast-feeding. About one-third of the children of HIV–positive mothers get infected through this route. The risk of transmission is higher if the mother is newly infected or if she has already developed AIDS. Voluntary prenatal testing for HIV infection should be done as early in pregnancy as possible for pregnant women who are at great risk (if they or their partner has a number of sexual partners; has a sexually transmitted disease; uses illicit injectable drugs etc.). Universal confidential voluntary screening of pregnant women in high-prevalence areas may allow infected women to choose therapeutic abortion, make an informed decision on breast-feeding, or receive appropriate care. Screening should not be used as a substitute for primary prevention through community-wide education on safe sexual practice, making condoms readily available and preventing parenteral transmission *(20)*.

(xi) *HEPATITIS B INFECTION* : Spread of infection from HBV carrier mothers to their babies appears to be a factor for the high prevalence of HBV infection in some regions. The mechanism of perinatal infection is uncertain. Most infections appear to occur at birth. Transmission of the virus to the baby after delivery is likely if both surface antigen and e antigen are positive. Vertical transmission can be blocked by immediate post-delivery administration of B immunoglobulin and hepatitis B vaccine. Please refer to page 254 for details.

(xii) *PRENATAL GENETIC SCREENING* : Prenatal genetic screening includes screening for chromosomal abnormalities associated with serious birth defects, screening for direct evidence of congenital structural anomalies, and screening for haemoglobinopathies and other inherited conditions detectable by biochemical assay. Universal genetic screening is generally not recommended. Screening for chromosomal abnormalities and for direct evidence of structural anomalies is performed in pregnancy in order to make the option of therapeutic abortion available when severe defects are detected. Typical examples are screening for trisomy 21 (Down's syndrome) and severe neural tube defects. Women aged 35 years and above, and those who already have an afflicted child are at higher risk.

(4) Mental preparation

Antenatal care does not mean only palpation, blood and urine examination and pelvic measurements. These are no doubt important aspects of antenatal care. Mental preparation is as important as physical or material preparation. Sufficient time and opportunity must be given to the expectant mothers to have a free and frank talk on all aspects of pregnancy and delivery. This will go a long way in removing her fears about confinement. The "mothercraft" classes at the MCH Centres help a great deal in achieving this objective.

(5) Family planning

Family planning is related to every phase of the maternity cycle. The mother is psychologically more receptive to advice on family planning than at other times. Educational and motivational efforts must be initiated during the antenatal period. If the mother has had 2 or more children, she should be motivated for puerperal sterilization. In this connection, the All India Postpartum Programme services are available to all expectant mothers in India.

(6) Paediatric component

It is suggested that a paediatrician should be in attendance at all antenatal clinics to pay attention to the under-fives accompanying the mothers.

INTRANATAL CARE

Childbirth is a normal physiological process, but complications may arise. Septicaemia may result from unskilled and septic manipulations, and *tetanus neonatorum* from the use of unsterilized instruments. The need for effective intranatal care is therefore indispensable, even if the delivery is going to be a normal one. The emphasis is on the cleanliness. It entails – clean hands and fingernails, a clean surface for delivery, clean cord care i.e., clean blade for cutting the cord and clean tie for the cord, no application on cord stump, and keeping birth canal clean by avoiding harmful practices. Hospitals and health centres should be equipped for delivery with midwifery kits, a regular supply of sterile gloves and drapes, towels, cleaning materials, soap and antiseptic solution, as well as equipment for sterilizing instruments and supplies. There are delivery kits available with the items needed for basic hygiene for delivery at home, where a midwife with a midwifery kit is not likely to be present. The aims of good intranatal care are :

(i) thorough asepsis;
(ii) delivery with minimum injury to the infant and mother;
(iii) readiness to deal with complications such as prolonged labour, antepartum haemorrhage, convulsions, malpresentations, prolapse of the cord, etc.; and
(iv) Care of the baby at delivery – resuscitation, care of the cord, care of the eyes, etc.

Domiciliary care

Mothers with normal obstetric history may be advised to have their confinement in their own homes, provided the home conditions are satisfactory. In such cases, the delivery may be conducted by the Health Worker Female or trained dai. This is known as "domiciliary midwifery service."

The advantages of the domiciliary midwifery service are : (1) the mother delivers in the familiar surroundings of her home and this may tend to remove the fear associated with delivery in a hospital; (2) the chances for cross infection are generally fewer at home than in the nursery/hospital; and (3) the mother is able to keep an eye upon her children and domestic affairs; this may tend to ease her mental tension.

Domiciliary midwifery is also not without disadvantages : (1) the mother may have less medical and nursing supervision than in the hospital; (2) the mother may have less rest; (3) she may resume her domestic duties too soon; and (4) her diet may be neglected. Strictly speaking, many homes in India are unsuitable for even a normal delivery. The argument that childbirth is a natural event and should take place at home does not guarantee that everything will be normal.

Since 72.2 per cent of India's population live in rural areas, most deliveries will have to take place in the home with the aid of Female Health Workers or trained dais. Domiciliary out–reach is a major component of intranatal health care : The Female Health Worker, who is a pivot of domiciliary care, should be adequately trained to recognize the 'danger signals' during labour and seek immediate help in transferring the mother to the nearest Primary Health Centre or Hospital. The danger signals are :

(1) sluggish pains or no pains after rupture of membranes;
(2) good pains for an hour after rupture of membranes, but no progress;
(3) prolapse of the cord or hand;
(4) meconium-stained liquor or a slow irregular or excessively fast foetal heart;
(5) excessive 'show' or bleeding during labour;
(6) collapse during labour;
(7) a placenta not separated within half an hour after delivery;
(8) post-partum haemorrhage or collapse; and
(9) a temperature of 38 deg C or over during labour.

There should be a close liaison between domiciliary and institutional delivery services.

Institutional care

About one per cent of deliveries tend to be abnormal, and four per cent "difficult", requiring the services of a doctor. Institutional care is recommended for all 'high-risk" cases, and where home conditions are unsuitable.

The mother is allowed to rest in bed on the first day after delivery. From the next day, she is allowed to be up and about. The current practice is to discharge the woman after 48 hours lying-in period after a normal delivery.

Rooming-in

Keeping the baby's crib by the side of the mother's bed is called "rooming-in". This arrangement gives an opportunity for the mother to know her baby. Mothers interested in breast feeding usually find there is a better chance for success with rooming-in. Rooming-in also allays the fear in the mother's mind that the baby is not misplaced in the central nursery. It also builds up her self-confidence.

POSTNATAL CARE

Care of the mother (and the newborn) after delivery is known as postnatal or postpartal care. Broadly this care falls into two areas: care of the mother which is primarily the responsibility of the obstetrician; and care of the newborn, which is the combined responsibility of the obstetrician and paediatrician. This combined area of responsibility is also known as perinatology.

Care of the mother

The objectives of postpartal care are :

(1) To prevent complications of the postpartal period;
(2) To provide care for the rapid restoration of the mother to optimum health;
(3) To check adequacy of breast-feeding;
(4) To provide family planning services; and
(5) To provide basic health education to mother/family.

Complications of the postpartal period

Certain complications may arise during the postpartal period which should be recognized early and dealt with promptly. These are (1) *Puerperal sepsis* : This is infection of the genital tract within 3 weeks after delivery. This is accompanied by rise in temperature and pulse rate, foul–smelling lochia, pain and tenderness in lower abdomen, etc. Puerperal sepsis can be prevented by attention to asepsis, before and after delivery. This is particularly important in domiciliary midwifery service. (2) *Thrombophlebitis* : This is an infection of the veins of the legs, frequently associated with varicose veins. The leg may become tender, pale and swollen. (3) *Secondary haemorrhage* : Bleeding from vagina anytime from 6 hours after delivery to the end of the puerperium (6 weeks) is called secondary haemorrhage, and may be due to retained placenta or membranes. (4) *Others* : Urinary tract infection and mastitis, etc. It is extremely important to look for these complications in the postpartal period and prevent or treat them promptly.

Restoration of mother to optimum health

The second objective of postpartal care is to provide care whereby, the woman can recuperate physically and emotionally from her experience of delivery. The broad areas of this care fall into three divisions :

PHYSICAL

(1) *Postnatal examinations* : Soon after delivery, the health check-ups must be frequent, i.e., twice a day during the first 3 days, and subsequently once a day till the umbilical cord drops off. At each of these examinations, the FHW checks temperature, pulse and respiration, examines the breasts, checks progress of normal involution of uterus, examines lochia for any abnormality, checks urine and bowels and advises on perineal toilet including care of the stitches, if any. The immediate postnatal complications, viz. puerperal sepsis, thrombophlebitis, secondary haemorrhage should be kept in mind. At the end of 6 weeks, an examination is necessary to check-up involution of uterus which should be complete by then. Further visits should be done once a month during the first 6 months, and thereafter once in 2 or 3 months till the end of one year. In rural areas only limited postnatal care is possible. Efforts should be made by the FHWs to give at least 3 to 6 postnatal visits. The common conditions found on examination during the late postnatal period are subinvolution of uterus, retroverted uterus, prolapse of uterus and cervicitis. Postnatal examination offers an opportunity to detect and correct these defects.

(2) *Anaemia* : Routine haemoglobin examination should be done during postnatal visits, and when anaemia is discovered, it should be treated. In some cases, it may be necessary to continue treatment for a year or more.

(3) *Nutrition* : Though a malnourished mother is able to secrete as much breast milk as a well nourished one, she does it at the cost of her own health. The nutritional needs of the mother must be adequately met. Often the family budget is limited; the mother should be shown the means how she can eat better with less money.

(4) *Postnatal exercises* : Postnatal exercises are necessary to bring the stretched abdominal and pelvic muscles back to normal as quickly as possible. Gradual resumption of normal house-hold duties may be enough to restore one's figure.

PSYCHOLOGICAL : The next big area of postnatal care involves a consideration of the psychological factors peculiar to the recently delivered woman. One of the psychological problems is fear which is generally borne of ignorance. Other problems are timidity and insecurity regarding the baby. If a woman is to endure cheerfully the emotional stresses of childbirth, she requires the support and companionship of her husband. Fear and insecurity may be eliminated by proper prenatal instruction. The postpartum psychosis is perhaps precipitated by birth; and it is rather uncommon.

SOCIAL : It has been said that the most important thing a woman can do is to have a baby. This is only part of the truth. The really important thing is to nurture and raise the child in a wholesome family atmosphere. She, with her husband, must develop her own methods.

Breast-feeding

Postnatal care offers an excellent opportunity to find out how the mother is getting along with her baby, particularly with regard to feeding. For many children, breast milk provides the main source of nourishment in the first year of life. In some societies, lactation continues to make an important contribution to the child's nutrition for 18 months or longer. In the world's more affluent societies, breast–feeding appears to have become a lost art and the feeding bottle has usurped the breast. When the standard of environmental sanitation is poor and education low, the content of the feeding bottle is likely to be as nutritionally poor as it is bacteriologically dangerous. It is therefore very important to advise the mothers to avoid the feeding bottle.

A great asset in India is that an average Indian mother, although poor in nutritional status, has a remarkable ability to breast-feed her infant for prolonged periods, sometimes extending to nearly 2 years and beyond. Longitudinal and cross-sectional studies indicate that poor Indian women secrete as much as 400 to 600 ml of milk per day during the first year (Table 2). No other food is required to be given until 6 months after birth. At the age of 6 months, breast milk should be supplemented by additional foods rich in protein and other nutrients (e.g., animal milk, soft-cooked mashed vegetables, etc.). These are called supplementary foods which should be introduced very gradually in small amounts.

TABLE 2

Output of breast milk at different stages of lactation

Months of lactation	Number examined	Per day mean–output of breast milk (ml)
0–2	20	530
3–4	18	640
5–6	14	730
7–8	14	660
9–10	17	600
11–12	30	525
13–15	11	515
16–18	29	440
19–24	14	400
25–36	12	425
37–38	4	345

Family planning

It has already been stressed that family planning is related to every phase of maternity cycle. Every attempt should be made to motivate mothers when they attend postnatal clinics or during postnatal contacts to adopt a suitable method for spacing the next birth or for limiting the family size as the case may be. Postpartum sterilization is generally recommended on the 2nd day after delivery. Although lactation confers some protection against conception, it cannot be depended upon; contraceptives have to be supplied immediately postpartum. To ask the mother to come at the time of her first menstruation may be too late. A contraceptive must therefore be used, that will not affect lactation in the early postpartum period. In this connection, IUD and conventional (non–hormonal) contraceptives are the choices during the first 6 months following delivery. In general, combined or sequential oral "pills" should be avoided in a lactating mother as they do suppress lactation. Fortunately, evidence is accumulating that progestogens alone have little or no effect on lactation. The injection of medroxy-progesterone acetate (MPA) after delivery has been found to be successful in ensuring spacing of pregnancy without suppressing lactation; however, because of its side-effects (e.g., irregular uterine bleeding, prolonged infertility) some countries have limited its use to multiparae at ages 35 and over, or who have already completed their families. MPA is not recommended for general use.

Basic health education

Health education during the postnatal period should cover the following broad areas : (a) hygiene – personal and environmental; (b) feeding for mother and infant; (c) pregnancy spacing; (d) importance of health check-up; and (e) birth registration.

CARE OF CHILDREN

This section focuses on children in the age group 0–14 years. This is the most important age group in all societies, not because they constitute about 40 per cent of the total population, but because there is a renewed awareness that the determinants of chronic disease in later life and health behaviour are laid down at this stage *(21)*. Family influences and education are of the highest importance, and these experiences ultimately influence patterns of their future life-styles, occupational skills, and even political attitudes and leadership. The childhood period is also a vital period because of the so called socialization process, that is, transmission of attitudes, customs and behaviour. In addition, of course, they are vulnerable to disease, death and disability owing to their age, sex, place of living, socio-economic class and a host of other variables. Certain specific biological and psychological needs must be met to ensure the survival and healthy development of the child and future adult.

It is customary to divide the childhood into the following age-periods :

1. Infancy (upto 1 year of age) :
   a. Neonatal period (first 28 days of life).
   b. Post neonatal period (28th day to 1 year).
2. Pre-school age (1–4 years).
3. School age (5–14 years).

Antenatal paediatrics

Fifty years ago, the main purpose of antenatal care was the prevention of maternal mortality. With the fall in the maternal mortality to about 0.2 per 1000 live births, attention has shifted to the child – first to decrease perinatal mortality, secondly to prevent perinatal morbidity; and more recently to the "foetus at risk". This has given rise to the concept of antenatal paediatrics. Recent technical developments such as amniocentesis, ultrasonography, fetoscopy and chorion biopsy have contributed significantly to the diagnosis of congenital abnormalities and inborn errors of metabolism *(22, 23)*. This knowledge has led to the recognition that causation and possible prevention may lie in intra-uterine life. The emphasis has greatly changed in the care of the child with the prevention of disorders (e.g., low birth weight, foetal disorders and neonatal asphyxia) assuming greater importance.

Antenatal care should, appropriately, begin even before the mother conceives and enters the maternity cycle; this care comprising such measures as genetic counselling for prospective parents; limitation and proper spacing of births with intervals of 2–3 years; delaying a young woman's first pregnancy until she is physically and socially mature enough to cope with it; ensuring adequate maternal nutrition; protection of the unborn against intrauterine infections and other adverse influences. In a developing country such as India, all this may not be possible, but certainly some elements, such as improvement of maternal nutrition, family planning and counselling could go a long way in ensuring maternal and foetal health.

INFANCY

Infants (0–1 year) constitute about 2.92 per cent of the total population in India. Of the 136 million children born each year in the world, 90 per cent are in the third world. Although the chances of survival of these newborns has improved by 50 per cent in the last 20 years, the first few hours, days and months of their lives are still an obstacle race. From the time of birth, 20–30 per cent of babies are under-weight. That makes them vulnerable to infection and disease. About 40 per cent of total infant mortality occurs in the first month of life. Then comes the weaning period, when one out of four surviving children receives neither the quality nor the quantity of food needed to replace the substances provided by mother's milk. The result is that more and more children in developing countries reach adulthood with their health already largely impaired. An infant mortality rate of

58 per thousand, as compared to 5 per thousand in the developed countries, places India in the unenviable position of being among the less developed in the world. Many low-cost measures are available for saving life of millions of children, like immunization, breast feeding, birth spacing, growth monitoring, improved weaning, oral rehydration. Attention is focused on these elements of child health care in developing countries.

NEONATAL CARE

A flow chart of the optimum care of the newborn is as shown in Fig. 2. This aspect of family health services has been termed neonatology. This branch of medicine is, perhaps, more than any other, dependant on teamwork in which disciplines of obstetrics and gynaecology, paediatrics, preventive and social medicine, community health services and nursing have an important part to play, if any impact is to be made on the vast problems of perinatal and neonatal mortality and morbidity. The paediatrician has a key role as a coordinator and guide for the whole team.

Early neonatal care

The first week of life is the most crucial period in the life of an infant. In India, 61.3 per cent of all infant deaths occur within the first month of life. Of these, more than half may die during the first week of birth. This is because the new born has to adapt itself rapidly and successfully to an alien external environment. The risk of death is the greatest during the first 24–48 hours after birth. The problem is more acute in rural areas where expert obstetric care is scarce, and the home environmental conditions in which the baby is born, are usually unsatisfactory.

The objective of early neonatal care is to assist the newborn in the process of adoption to an alien environment, which involves :

(i) establishment and maintenance of cardio–respiratory functions;
(ii) maintenance of body temperature;
(iii) avoidance of infection;
(iv) establishment of satisfactory feeding regimen; and
(v) early detection and treatment of congenital and acquired disorders, especially infections.

Congenital infections caused by toxoplasmosis, rubella, human (alpha) herpes-virus 1 or 2, human (beta) herpes virus, and syphilis (TORCHES synonyms) is associated with high mortality rate in the neonates *(24)*.

Immediate care

1. CLEARING THE AIRWAY

Establishment and maintenance of cardio-respiratory functions (e.g., breathing) is the most important thing the moment the baby is born, and everything else is secondary. To help establish breathing, the airways should be cleared of mucus and other secretions. Positioning the baby with his head low may help in the drainage of secretions. This process can be assisted by gentle suction to remove mucus and amniotic fluid. Resuscitation becomes necessary if natural breathing fails to establish within a minute, as in the case of babies who have already been subject to hypoxia during labour. In these cases, resuscitation may require more active measures such as suction, application of oxygen mask, intubation and assisted respiration. All labour wards should be equipped with resuscitation equipment including oxygen. If the heart has stopped beating for 5 minutes, the baby is probably dead.

2. APGAR SCORE

The Apgar score is taken at 1 minute and again at 5 minutes after birth. Today it is considered as negligence to omit Apgar scoring of a newborn infant, especially low birth weight babies *(25)*. It requires immediate and careful observation of the heart rate, respiration, muscle tone, reflex response and colour of the infant. Each sign is given a score of 0, 1 or 2 (Table 3). It provides an immediate estimate of the physical condition of the baby. A perfect score should be 9 or 10; 0–3 indicates that the baby is severely depressed and 4–6 moderately depressed. A score below 5 needs prompt action. Infants with low Apgar scores at 5 minutes of age are subject to a high-risk of complications and death during the neonatal period *(25)*.

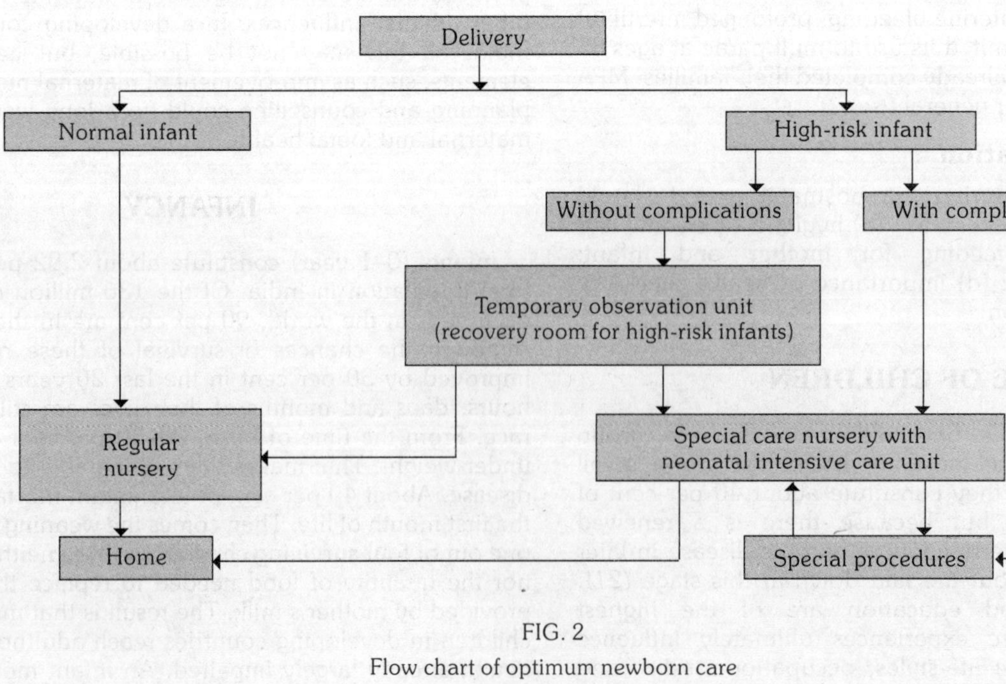

FIG. 2
Flow chart of optimum newborn care

TABLE 3

Apgar score

Sign	Score		
	0	1	2
Heart rate	Absent	Slow (below 100)	Over 100
Respiratory effort	Absent	Slow Irregular	Good crying
Muscle tone	Flaccid	Some flexion of extremities	Active movements
Reflex response	No response	Grimace	Cry
Colour	Blue, pale	Body pink Extremities blue	Completely pink
Total score = 10	Severe depression 0–3	Mild depression 4–6	No depression 7–10

3. CARE OF THE CORD

In the case of the normal infant, the umbilical cord should be cut and tied when it has stopped pulsating. The advantage is that the baby derives about 10 ml of extra blood, if the cord is cut after pulsation ceases. This is particularly important in India, where anaemia is frequent. Care must be taken to prevent tetanus of the newborn by using properly sterilized instruments and cord ties. It is essential to apply an antiseptic preparation on the cord stump and the skin around the base. The cord should be kept as dry as possible. It dries and shrivels up and separates by aseptic necrosis in 5–8 days.

4. CARE OF THE EYES

Before the eyes are open, the lid margins of the newborn should be cleaned with sterile wet swabs, one for each eye from inner to outer side. Instil a drop of freshly prepared silver nitrate solution (1 per cent) to prevent gonococcal conjunctivitis, alternatively, a single application of tetracycline 1 per cent ointment can be given. Any discharge from the eye of an infant is pathological and calls for immediate treatment.

Ophthalmia Neonatorum : A variety of organisms are implicated – *N. gonorrhoea, C. trachomatis* (commonest), staphylococcus, streptococcus, Candida spp, etc. The most serious cause of conjunctivitis of the newborn is infection with *N. gonococcus* as it can rapidly cause blindness. *C. trachomatis* is also an important cause of neonatal conjunctivitis. Since gonococcal ophthalmia neonatorum has become much less frequent than conjunctivitis due to other acquired organisms, application of topical neomycin might be more useful *(26)*.

As a preventive measure, specific maternal genital tract infection should be treated effectively prior to, or during pregnancy, and specific care should be taken while conducting face or breech delivery.

5. CARE OF THE SKIN

A newborn baby is wet from amniotic fluid and can easily become cold. Drying the baby with clean cloth to remove vernix, meconium and blood clots is done by the nursing staff. The baby is then wrapped in dry, clean cloth from head to foot to prevent heat loss. First bath is given after temperature stabilization, preferably after a week.

6. MAINTENANCE OF BODY TEMPERATURE

The normal body temperature of a newborn is between 36.5 to 37.5°C. A newborn baby is projected out of warm womb of the mother into an environment which may be 10 to 20°C cooler especially in winter months in India.

A newborn has little thermal control and can lose body heat quickly. Immediately after birth; most of the heat loss occurs through evaporation of the amniotic fluid from the body of the wet child. As much as 75 per cent of the heat loss can occur from the head. It is important that immediately after birth the child is quickly dried with a clean cloth and wrapped in warm cloth and given to the mother for skin-to-skin contact and breast-feeding. Practices such as separating the baby from the mother for the first 12–24 hours of life are harmful. Pre-term and low birth weight babies lose heat more easily through their thin skin as they have less sub-cutaneous fat for insulation. Putting the newborn on a cold surface such as metallic tray, rubber sheeting or weighing scale should be avoided, and the child should be kept away from cold walls, open windows and from draught *(27)*.

7. BREAST-FEEDING

Breast-feeding should be initiated within an hour of birth instead of waiting several hours as is often customary. Although there is little milk at that time, it helps to establish feeding and a close mother–child relationship, known as "bonding".

The first milk which is called "colostrum" is the most suitable food for the baby during this early period because it contains a high concentration of protein and other nutrient the body needs; it is also rich in anti-infective factors which protect the baby against respiratory infections and diarrhoeal diseases. Supplementary feeds are not necessary. The regular milk comes on the third to sixth day after birth. The baby should be allowed to breast-feed whenever it wants. Feeding the baby on demand helps the baby to gain weight. It is very important to advise mother to avoid feeding bottles.

Neonatal examinations

a. FIRST EXAMINATION

The first examination is made soon after birth, and preferably in the delivery room. This examination is (a) to ascertain that the baby has not suffered injuries during the birth process; (b) to detect malformations especially those requiring urgent treatment; and (c) to assess maturity.

The following abnormalities found on examination should be immediately attended to : (a) cyanosis of the lips and skin; (b) any difficulty in breathing; (c) imperforated anus; (d) persistent vomiting; (e) signs of cerebral irritation such as twitchings, convulsions, neck rigidity, bulging of anterior fontanel, and (g) temperature instability.

b. SECOND EXAMINATION

The second examination should be made preferably by a paediatrician within 24 hours after birth. This examination should form the first stage of a continual process of health care surveillance. It is a detailed systematic examination from head to foot, conducted in good light. The following protocol will be found useful for such an examination *(28)*.

1. Body size:
   Body weight; crown–heel length; head and thoracic perimeters.
2. Body temperature.

3. Skin :
   Observe for cyanosis of lips and skin; jaundice; pallor; generalized erythema; vesicular and bullous lesions.
4. Cardio-respiratory activities :
   Cardiac murmurs; absence of femoral pulse; central cyanosis, a respiratory rate of over 60 per minute; thoracic cage retraction on inspiration.
5. Neuro-behavioural activity :
   (i) Posture : neck retraction; frog-like posture; hyper-extension of all limbs; hyperflexion of all limbs; asymmetrical posture (ii) Muscle tone : tendon reflexes; cry; movements.
6. Head and face :
   Hydrocephalus; large fontanelles; prominent scalp vein (i) Eyes : cataract; coloboma; conjunctivitis (ii) Ears : dysmorphism; accessary auricles; pre-auricular pits (iii) Mouth and lips : Hare lip; cleft palate.
7. Abdomen :
   Signs of distension; abnormal masses; imperforate anus.
8. Limbs and joints :
   Deformities of joints; congenital dislocation of the hips; extra digits.
9. Spine :
   Neural tube defects
10. External genitalia :
    Male : Hypospadius; undescended testis; hydrocele; Female : fused labia; enlarged clitoris.

The infected newborn *(27)*

Neonatal infection is particularly frequent in Africa. It is the main cause of neonatal mortality in many developing countries. Contributing factors are related to the environment (traditional practices, poor hygiene), the course of pregnancy (premature rupture of membranes) and constitutional fragility (prematurity, small–for–date, dysmaturity). Transplacental contamination is one of the important cause of infection in new-borns. Early detection of newborns at risk of transplacental infection is important, so that close monitoring and preventive action may be implemented.

NEONATAL TETANUS : It can be prevented by vaccination of pregnant women and sero-vaccination of newborns in case of at-risk delivery. These measures have proved effective in those countries where they are systematically applied.

CONGENITAL SYPHILIS : The frequency of congenital syphilis is on rise in some large African cities. Diagnosis is essentially based on the evidence of syphilis in the mother, since clinical signs of congenital syphilis often do not occur at once. In case of doubt and if there is risk of inadequate subsequent medical surveillance of the baby, treatment with 2.4 to 4.8 million I.U. of Benzathine Penicillin may be recommended.

NEWBORN WITH A HBV-POSITIVE MOTHER : Chronic carriers of hepatitis virus are extremely frequent in some countries. Babies may be infected at birth when the mother is a carrier of this virus. The risk of transmission is somewhere around 20 per cent when the mother has the HBs antigen only, and around 90 per cent when she also has the HBe antigen. Transmission occurs through the blood and the genital secretions and therefore affects the newborn during the immediate perinatal period and throughout infancy. It is not a contraindication of breast-feeding.

If the newborn is infected, there is a risk that he/she will become a chronic carrier, and tend to develop active chronic hepatitis, cirrhosis or primary cancer of liver during adulthood. 50 per cent of severe cases of infantile hepatitis before age one year are the outcome of untreated perinatal transmission.

It is possible to prevent perinatal transmission by seroprophylaxis combined with vaccination – an intra-muscular injection of 0.5 ml of hepatitis B immunoglobulin along with hepatitis B vaccine within 24 hours of birth. The vaccine must be repeated at 6, 10 and 14 weeks of age.

This prophylaxis has proved effective. The real problem is to detect mothers who are chronic carriers of the HBs antigen, and the high cost of prevention.

NEWBORN WITH A HIV-POSITIVE MOTHER : The rapidity of the propagation of HIV infection is a source of great concern. About 30 per cent babies born to HIV-positive mothers get infected. Transmission of infection mostly occurs at the end of the pregnancy, and it is not influenced by the type of delivery. The virus has been isolated in breast-milk. Although there is probably a risk of transmission of infection through breast-milk, prohibiting breast-feeding is debatable, as it is so essential for the survival of newborn in developing countries. The risk of transmission depends on the severity of the mother's case. It is higher from mothers with AIDS, but may also occur from seropositive cases. The infection can be prevented by giving ART. Please refer to page 402 for details. The question of whether to perform BCG vaccination arises – it is contraindicated in infected children, and therefore, should not be performed in the offspring of HIV positive mothers until it is determined whether the baby is infected or not. This is only feasible at the end of several months when the maternal antibodies are completely eliminated *(27)*.

MEASURING THE BABY

Measurements of birth-weight, length (height) and head circumference are the simplest and one of the reliable means by which the health and maturity of a baby is evaluated.

1. Birth-weight

The birth-weight should be taken preferably within the first hour of life, before significant post-natal weight loss has occurred *(29)*. The naked baby should be placed on a clean towel on the scale pan. In home delivery, weight is taken by placing the baby in a sling bag using a salter weighing scale. The child is weighed to the nearest 100 g according to the standard method for weight measurement.

The average birth-weight of infants is lower in many developing countries than it is in developed countries. There are reasons to believe that this difference is not of genetic origin but is due largely to maternal malnutrition.

2. Length (height)

This need not be taken immediately if the baby's condition gives rise to any anxiety, but should be recorded within the first 3 days. Length can be taken most accurately with a measuring board (infantometer) with a fixed head piece on which the infant lies supine with its legs fully extended and the feet flexed at right angles to the lower legs. Two people are needed to hold the baby correctly. The sliding board is moved firmly against the feet before the reading is taken. Length is taken to the nearest 0.1 cm.

3. Head circumference

This measurement may change slightly during the first 3 days owing to moulding during labour. It is taken with a tape measure at the maximum circumference of the head in the occipito-frontal diameter.

The purpose of taking these measurements are :

(i) to assess the baby's size against known standards for the population;
(ii) to compare the size with estimated period of gestation; and
(iii) to provide a baseline against which subsequent progress can be measured.

Anthropometric measurements may be classified as *(30)* :

(a) Weight : kg
(b) Length : total height, sitting height, heel knee-length
(c) Perimeters : head, chest, abdomen, arm, calf
(d) Diameters : biacromial, bicristal, biepicondylar, bistyloid, bicondylar
(e) Skinfold thickness : triceps, biceps, superiliac subscapular.

NEONATAL SCREENING

The object of screening newborns is primarily to detect infants with treatable genetic, developmental and other abnormalities, and secondarily, to provide their parents with genetic counselling. The Apgar score and routine clinical examinations are simple screening tests which should be carried out on all newborn infants. 10 to 15 ml of cord blood should be collected at birth and saved in the refrigerator for 7 days for typing, coombs' testing and other tests if needed. Recent years have witnessed development of numerous tests for screening congenital metabolic disorders, inherited haemoglobinopathies and red blood cell disorders. Since these diseases are rare, general screening of the population for them is neither justified nor technically possible. However, only a few tests qualify for a screening programme. The most common disorders which are screened are discussed below.

(a) *Phenylketonuria (PKU)* : PKU is a rare (incidence 1 in 10,000–20,000 births) disorder of amino acid metabolism. This is an autosomal recessive trait in babies who are homozygous with a deficiency in the enzyme phenylalanine hydrozylase (PAH) which normally converts phenylalanine to tyrosin. The deficiency results in raised serum phenylalanine concentrations causing mental retardation and tendency to seizures if the child does not receive low phenylalanine diet. Mass screening of blood phenylalanine in neonates is performed in many countries by the Guthrie test. It is possible to test for all three types of metabolic error, namely PKU, galactosaemia and maple syrup urine disease by taking blood from the 6–10 days old baby by heel prick and collecting 3 or 4 separate drops of it on thick absorbent filter paper. The treatment of PKU consists of a diet free of phenylalanine. Careful dietary management in affected children results in normal physical and mental development. (b) *Neonatal hypothyroidism* : This is the most common disorder that is screened. Congenital hypothyroidism leads to serious sequelae, including severe mental retardation, which can be prevented if medical treatment is given within the first 1–2 months of life. The test involves measuring the radioimmunoassays of the thyroid hormone T4 or the thyroid-stimulating hormone (TSH). By examining the cord blood of newborns, potential victims of IDD could be identified and proper prevention can be taken at such an early stage of life. (c) *Coombs' test* : This is done routinely on infants of all Rh-negative mothers. (d) *Sickle cell or other haemoglobinopathies* : Agar-gel electrophoresis is done on infants whose mothers have sickle cell or other haemoglobinopathies, e.g., thalassaemia, G6PD. (e) *Congenital dislocation of hip* : The test consists of manipulating the hip of the child from the adducted to abducted position while the thigh is flexed. A positive or abnormal result is indicated by a click or snap being produced during the test. The test is carried out on all babies at 6–14 days after birth, and at monthly intervals until the child is 4 months old. Diagnosis within a week or two of birth means that treatment can be completed before the infant could normally have reached the stage of standing. Failure to diagnose the condition will expose the child to a whole series of difficult operations in later life *(20)*.

The requirements for effective screening for inborn errors are discussed in detail in chapter 4.

Identification of "at-risk" infants

The number of infants (and children 1–5 years of age) in a community, or attending a child health clinic, may be so large that it may not be possible to give sufficient time and attention to all of them. It is therefore necessary to identify particularly those "at-risk" and give them special intensive care, because it is these "at-risk" babies that contribute so largely to perinatal, neonatal and infant mortality. The basic criteria for identifying these babies include :

1. birth weight less than 2.5 kg;
2. twins;
3. birth order 5 and more;
4. artificial feeding;
5. weight below 70 per cent of the expected weight (i.e., II and III degrees of malnutrition);
6. failure to gain weight during three successive months;
7. children with PEM, diarrhoea; and
8. working mother/one parent.

Late neonatal care

The remaining three weeks of the neonatal period carry the common and serious hazards of infection and failure of satisfactory nutrition. Diarrhoea and pneumonia take a heavy toll of life in infants exposed to an unsatisfactory environment. The case fatality rate of what would normally be trivial episodes can increase dramatically when elementary care is not given.

LOW BIRTH WEIGHT

The birth weight of an infant is the single most important determinant of its chances of survival, healthy growth and development.

There are two main groups of low birth weight babies – (a) those born prematurely (short gestation); and (b) those with foetal growth retardation. In countries where the population of low birth weight infants is less, short gestation period is the major cause. In countries where the proportion is high (e.g. India), the majority of cases can be attributed to foetal growth retardation.

By international agreement low birth weight has been defined as a birth weight of less than 2.5 kg (upto and including 2499 g), the measurement being taken preferably within the first hour of life, before significant postnatal weight loss has occurred *(30)*. Apart from birth weight, babies can also be classified into 3 groups according to gestational age, using the word "preterm", "term" and "postterm", as follows *(29)* :

a. *Preterm* : Babies born before the end of 37 weeks gestation (less than 259 days).
b. *Term* : Babies born from 37 completed weeks to less than 42 completed weeks (259 to 293 days) of gestation.
c. *Postterm* : Babies born at 42 completed weeks or any time thereafter (294 days and over) of gestation.

A LBW infant then, is any infant with a birth weight of less than 2.5 kg regardless of gestational age. It includes two kinds of infants :

PRETERM BABIES (9)

Preterm is defined as babies born alive before 37 weeks of pregnancy are completed. There are sub-categories of preterm birth, based on gestational age :

- extremely preterm (<28 weeks)
- very preterm (28 to <32 weeks)
- moderate to late preterm (32 to 37 weeks).

These are babies born too early. Their intrauterine growth may be normal. That is, their weight, length and development may be within normal limits for the duration of gestation. Given good neonatal care, these babies may catch up growth and by 2 to 3 years of age will be of normal size and performance.

INCIDENCE

More than 1 in 10 of the world's babies born in 2015 were born prematurely, making an estimated 15 million preterm births (defined as before 37 weeks of gestation) of which more than 1 million died as a result of their prematurity. Prematurity is now the second-leading cause of death in children under 5 years, and the single most important cause of death in the critical first month of life. For the babies who survive, many face a lifetime of significant disability.

Preterm births is a global problem. More than 60 per cent of preterm births occur in Africa and South Asia. In the lower income countries, on average, 12 per cent babies are born too early compared to 9 per cent in higher-income countries. Within countries, poorer families are at higher risk. The 10 countries with the greatest number of preterm births in 2015 are : (1) India 3519100; (2) China 1172300; (3) Nigeria 773600; (4) Pakistan 748100; (5) Indonesia 675700; (6) USA 517400; (7) Bangladesh 424100; (8) Philippines 348900; (9) DPR of the Congo 341400; and (10) Brazil 279300 *(31)*.

The 10 countries with the highest rates of preterm birth per 100 live births is; (1) Malawi 18.1; (2) Comoros 16.7; (3) Congo 16.7; (4) Zimbabwe 16.6; (5) Equatorial Guinea 16.5; (6) Mozambique 16.4; (7) Gabon 16.3; (8) Pakistan 15.8; (9) Indonesia 15.5; and (10) Mauritania 15.4 *(31)*.

There is a dramatic difference in survival of premature babies depending on where they are born. More than 90 per cent of extremely preterm babies (less than 28 weeks) born in low-income countries die within the first few days of life; yet less than 10 per cent of extremely preterm babies die in high income countries.

Causes of preterm births *(9)*

Preterm birth is a syndrome with a variety of causes which can be classified into two broad subtypes: (1) spontaneous preterm birth (spontaneous onset of labor or following prelabor premature rupture of membranes (pPROM) and (2) provider-initiated preterm birth (defined as induction of labor or elective caesarean birth before 37 completed weeks of gestation for maternal or fetal indications (both "urgent" or "discretionary"), or other non-medical reasons.

Spontaneous preterm birth is a multi-factorial process, resulting from the interplay of factors causing the uterus to change from quiescence to active contractions and to birth before 37 completed weeks of gestation. The precursors to spontaneous preterm birth vary by gestational age, social and environmental factors, but the cause of spontaneous preterm labor remains unidentified in upto half of all cases. Maternal history of preterm birth is a strong risk factor and most likely driven by the interaction of genetic, epigenetic and environmental risk factors.

Elevated risk of preterm birth also demands increased attention to maternal health, including the antenatal diagnosis and management of NCDs and other conditions known to increase the risk of preterm birth. Premature babies, in turn, are at greater risk of developing NCDs, like hypertension and diabetes, and other significant health condition later in life, creating an intergenerational cycle of risk. The link between prematurity and an increased risk of NCDs takes on an added public health importance when considering the reported increase in the rates of both worldwide. Table 4 summarizes the types of preterm births and the risk factors involved.

TABLE 4

Types of preterm birth and risk factors involved

Type:	Risk Factors:	Examples:
Spontaneous preterm birth:	Age at pregnancy and pregnancy spacing	Adolescent pregnancy, advanced maternal age, or short inter-pregnancy interval
	Multiple pregnancy	Increased rates of twin and higher order pregnancies with assisted reproduction
	Infection	Urinary tract infections, malaria, HIV, syphilis, bacterial vaginosis.
	Underlying maternal chronic medical conditions	Diabetes, hypertension, anaemia, asthma, thyroid disease
	Nutritional	Undernutrition, obesity, micronutrient deficiencies
	Lifestyle/ work related	Smoking, excess alcohol consumption, recreational drug use, excess physical work/activity
	Maternal psychological health	Depression, violence against women
	Genetic and other	Genetic risk, e.g., family history, Cervical incompetence
Provider-initiated preterm birth:	Medical induction or caesarean birth for: obstetric indication, Foetal indication Other-Not medically indicated	There is an overlap for indicated provider-initiated preterm birth with the risk factors for spontaneous preterm birth.

Source : *(9)*

SMALL–FOR–DATE (SFD) BABIES :

Also known as small for gestational age babies. These may be born at term or preterm. They weigh less than the 10th percentile for the gestational age. These babies are clearly the result of retarded intrauterine foetal growth.

Computation : The percentage of LBW babies is computed as :

$$\frac{\text{Live-born babies with birth weight less than 2.5 Kg}}{\text{Total number of live births}} \times 100$$

The factors associated with intrauterine growth retardation are multiple and interrelated to mother, the placenta or to the foetus. The maternal factors include malnutrition, severe anaemia, heavy physical work during pregnancy, hypertension, malaria, toxaemia, smoking, low economic status, short maternal stature, very young age, high parity and close birth spacing, low education status etc. *(32)*. The placental causes include placental insufficiency and placental abnormalities. The foetal causes include foetal abnormalities, intrauterine infections, chromosomal abnormality and multiple gestation.

SFD babies have a high risk of dying not only during the neonatal period but during their infancy, thus significantly raising the rate of infant and perinatal mortality and contribute greatly to immediate and long term health problems. Most of them become victims of protein-energy malnutrition and infections.

In the developing countries, adverse prenatal and post-natal development of the child is associated with 3 interrelated conditions : malnutrition, infection and unregulated fertility which are often due to poor socio-economic and environmental conditions.

IMPORTANCE

LBW is one of the most serious challenges in maternal and child health in both developed and developing countries. Its public health significance may be ascribed to numerous factors – its high incidence; its association with mental retardation and a high risk of perinatal and infant mortality and morbidity (half of all perinatal and one-third of all infant deaths are due to LBW); human wastage and suffering; the very high cost of special care and intensive care units and its association with socio-economic underdevelopment *(33)*.

LBW is the single most important factor determining the survival chances of the child. Many of them die during their first year. The infant mortality rate is about 20 times greater for all LBW babies than for other babies. The lower the birth weight, the lower is the survival chance. Many of them become victims of protein–energy malnutrition and infection. LBW is thus an important guide to the level of care needed by individual babies. LBW also reflects inadequate nutrition and ill-health of the mother. There is a strong and significant positive correlation between maternal nutritional status and the length of pregnancy and birth weight. A high percentage of LBW therefore points to deficient health status of pregnant women, inadequate prenatal care and the need for improved care of the newborn.

As premature babies are born before their bodies and organ systems have completely matured, they may need help breathing, eating, fighting infection and staying warm. Very premature babies who are born before 28 weeks, are especially vulnerable. Many of their organs may not be ready for life outside the mother's uterus and may be too immature to function well.

Some of the problems premature babies may experience include *(34)* :

- Temperature instability – inability to stay warm due to low body fat
- Respiratory problems;
  - hyaline membrane disease/respiratory distress syndrome – a condition in which the airsacs cannot stay open due to lack of surfactant in the lung
  - chronic lung disease/bronchopulmonary dysplasia-long-term respiratory problems caused by injury to the lung tissue
  - air leaking out of the normal lung spaces into other tissues
  - incomplete lung development
  - apnea (stopping breathing) – occurs in about half of babies born at or before 30 weeks
- Cardiovascular
  - patent ductus arteriosus (PDA) – a heart condition that causes blood to divert away from the lungs
  - too low or too high blood pressure
  - low heart rate – often occurs with apnea
- Blood and metabolic;
  - anaemia – may require blood transfusion
  - jaundice – due to immaturity of liver and gastrointestinal function
  - too low or too high levels of minerals and other substances in the blood such as calcium and glucose (sugar)
- Gastrointestinal;
  - difficulty feeding – many are unable to coordinate suck and swallow before 35 weeks gestation
  - poor digestion
  - necrotizing enterocolitis (NEC) – a serious disease of the intestine common in premature babies
- Neurologic;
  - intraventricular haemorrhage – bleeding in the brain
  - periventricular leukomalacia – softening of tissues of the brain around the ventricles (the spaces in the brain containing cerebrospinal fluid).
  - poor muscle tone
  - seizures – may be due to bleeding in the brain
  - retinopathy of prematurity – abnormal growth of the blood vessels in a baby's eye
- Infections – premature infants are more susceptible to infection and may require antibiotics

PREVENTION

Experts opine that the rates of LBW babies could be reduced to not more than 10 per cent in all parts of the world *(35)*. It is clear from the multiplicity of causes that there is no universal solution. Interventions have to be cause–specific. Main attention has been given in recent years to ways and means of preventing LBW through good prenatal care and intervention programmes, rather than "treatment" of LBW babies born later.

DIRECT INTERVENTION MEASURES

The incidence of LBW can be reduced if pregnant women "at risk" are identified and steps are taken to reduce the risk. For this approach the women need to be identified early in pregnancy. To achieve this goal, the mothers health card –

which is simple and can be used by primary health care worker – has been found very useful. The risk factors are : mother's malnutrition, heavy work load, diseases and infections and high blood pressure. Added to malnutrition, too many and too frequent pregnancies contribute to the continued depletion of her body. Both malnutrition and morbidity due to infections during pregnancy are amenable to correction or can be prevented. Some of the direct interventions are as follows :

(i) *Increasing food intake* : Studies have shown that even a relatively small dietary improvement in the malnourished pregnant mother, even during the last trimester, can result in a significant improvement in the birth weight of an infant. In Southern India, treatment of anaemic mothers led to an increase in birth weight of offspring. Direct intervention covers a wide range of activities, viz. supplementary feeding, distribution of iron and folic acid tablets, fortification and enrichment of foods, etc.; (ii) *Controlling infections* : Many maternal infections go unrecognized. They should be diagnosed and treated (e.g., malaria, urinary tract infection, infections due to cytomegalovirus, toxoplasmosis, rubella and syphilitic infection) or otherwise prevented. These infections can affect foetal growth in several ways; and (iii) *Early detection and treatment of medical disorders* : These include hypertension, toxemias, and diabetes.

INDIRECT INTERVENTION

Family planning, avoidance of excessive smoking, improved sanitation measures, and measures aimed at improving the health and nutrition of young girls, each have a role to play. These measures can be expected to be more effective and to have lasting effects only if, at the same time there are improvements in the socio-economic and environmental conditions and in the distribution of health and social services especially in the under-served areas. Government support could be provided through such measures as maternity leave with full wages and child benefits.

Fig. 3 summarizes the integrated services delivery package for maternal and newborn care.

TREATMENT

From the point of view of treatment, LBW babies can be divided in to 2 groups : (a) those under 2 kg and (b) those between 2–2.5 kg. The first group requires first class modern

Clinical

REPRODUCTIVE CARE:
- Family planning.
- STIs, HIV and immunizations.
- Care after pregnancy loss.

CHILDBIRTH CARE:
- Skilled care and immediate newborn care (hygiene, warmth, breast-feeding) and resuscitation.
- Antenatal steroids, antibiotics for pPROM.
- PMTCT of HIV.
- Emergency obstetric care if needed.

EMERGENCY NEWBORN CARE:
- Extra care of preterm babies, including Kangaoroo Mother Care.
- Emergency care of sick newborns (context-specific e.g. CPAP, surfactant).

EMERGENCY CHILD CARE:
- Hospital care of childhood illness, including HIV care.

Outreach/outpatient

REPRODUCTIVE HEALTH CARE:
- Family planning, including birth spacing.
- Prevention and management of STIs and HIV.
- Nutritional counselling.

ANTENATAL CARE:
- 4-visit focused ANC package.
- IPTp and bednets for malaria.
- Prevention and management of STIs and HIV.
- Calcium supplementation.
- Diagnosis and treatment of maternal chronic conditions.

POSTNATAL CARE:
- Promotion of healthy behaviours, e.g. hygiene, breastfeeding, warmth.
- Early detection of and referral for illness.
- Extra care of at-risk mothers and babies.
- Prevention of mother-to child transmission of HIV.

CHILD HEALTH CARE:
- Immunizations, nutrition, e.g. Vit A. supplementation and growth monitoring.
- IPTi and bednets for malaria.
- Care of children with HIV, including cotrimoxazole.
- First level assessment and care of childhood illness (IMCI).
- Diagnosis and treatment of prematurity associated disability.

Family/community

- Adolescent and pre-pregnancy nutrition.
- Gender violence.
- Education.
- Prevention of STIs and HIV.
- Optimize prepregnancy maternal conditions.

Counselling and preparation for newborn care, breast-feeding, birth and emergency preparedness.

Where skilled care is not available, consider clean birth and immediate newborn care (hygiene, warmth and immediate breast-feeding).

Healthy home care including:
- Promoting preventive care, including newborn care (hygiene, warmth), nutrition (exclusive breast-feeding, complementary feeding) and family planning for women.
- Seeking curative services for women, babies and children, including oral rehydration salts for prevention of diarrhoea, and where referral is not available, consider case management for pneumonia, malaria and neonatal sepsis.

INTERSECTORAL Improved living and working conditions including housing, water and sanitation, and nutrition; education and empowerment, especially of girls; folic acid fortification; safe and healthy work environment for women and pregnant women.

Pre-pregnancy → Pregnancy → Birth → Newborn/Postnatal → Childhood

FIG. 3

Integrated service delivery packages for maternal, newborn and child health

Source : *(9)*

neonatal care (which is hardly available globally) in an intensive care unit until the weight reaches that of the second group. The second group may need an intensive care unit for a day or two.

KANGAROO MOTHER CARE

Kangaroo mother care for low birth-weight babies was introduced in Colombia in 1979 by Drs. Hector Martinez and Edzar Rey as a response to, inter alia, high infection and mortality rates due to overcrowding in hospitals. It has since been adopted across the developing world and has become essential element in the continuum of neonatal care. The four components of kangaroo mother care are all essential for ensuring the best care option, especially for low birth-weight babies. They include skin-to-skin positioning of a baby on the mother's chest; adequate nutrition through breast-feeding; ambulatory care as a result of earlier discharge from hospital; and support for the mother and her family in caring for the baby *(36)*.

The intensive care comprises of:- (a) *Incubatory* care: that is, adjustment of temperature, humidity and oxygen supply. There is increasing evidence that low levels of oxygen in a baby's blood stream (hypoxia) can produce cerebral palsy. Therefore, continuous monitoring of the level of oxygen in baby's blood stream is now carried out in the best incubatory care units. If the oxygen is excessive, it may lead to retrolental fibroplasia; (b) *Feeding* : Breast-feeding is rarely possible – the baby cannot suck. However, breast milk should be used if available. Feeding is often by nasal catheter; and (c) *Prevention of infection* : Infection presents the greatest hazard. Death may occur within a few hours following respiratory infection. Prevention of infection is therefore, one of the most important functions of an intensive care unit.

The leading causes of death in low birth weight babies are :

a. atelectasis;
b. malformation;
c. pulmonary haemorrhage;
d. intracranial bleeding, secondary to anoxia or birth trauma; and
e. pneumonia and other infections.

Facility based newborn care services like newborn care corner, newborn stablization unit and special newborn care unit have improved the management of low birth weight babies. Some of these units are linked to obstetric units capable of monitoring the foetus. The development of perinatal intensive care units has been associated with a decline in neonatal mortality.

FEEDING OF INFANTS

A detailed discussion of the feeding of infants is outside the scope of this book. However, a brief mention may be made of some of the important aspects of the problem.

(1) Breast-feeding

Under any circumstances, breast milk is the ideal food for the infant. No other food is required by the baby until 6 months after birth. Under normal conditions, Indian mothers secrete 450 to 600 ml of milk daily with 1.1 gm protein per 100 ml. The energy value of human milk is 70 kcals per 100 ml.

A child who is breast-fed has greater chances of survival than a child artificially fed. Prolonged breast feeding does protect the infant from early malnutrition and some infections. The data suggests that infant mortality rates in developing countries are 5–10 times higher among children who have not been breast-fed or who have been breast-fed for less than 6 months. Despite the marked advantages of breast-feeding, its popularity has declined significantly in many parts of the world.

Advantages of breast-feeding

Among the advantages of breast milk are the following : (1) it is safe, clean, hygienic, cheap and available to the infant at correct temperature; (2) it fully meets the nutritional requirements of the infant in the first few months of life; (3) it contains antimicrobial factors such as macrophages, lymphocytes, secretory IgA, anti-streptococcal factor, lysozyme and lactoferrin which provide considerable protection not only against diarrhoeal diseases and necrotizing enterocolitis, but also against respiratory infections in the first months of life; (4) it is easily digested and utilized by both the normal and premature babies; (5) it promotes "bonding" between the mother and infant; (6) sucking is good for the baby – it helps in the development of jaws and teeth; (7) it protects babies from the tendency to obesity; (8) it prevents malnutrition and reduces infant mortality; (9) it provides several biochemical advantages such as prevention of neonatal hypocalcaemia and hypomagnesemia *(37)*; (10) it helps parents to space their children by prolonging the period of infertility; and (11) special fatty acids in breast milk lead to increased intelligence quotients and better visual acuity. A breast-fed baby is likely to have an IQ of around 8 points higher than a non-breast fed baby *(38)*.

Early initiation of breast-feeding lowers the mother's risk of postpartum haemorrhage and anaemia, boosts mother's immune system, delays next pregnancy and reduces the insulin of diabetic mothers. It protects mothers from ovarion and breast cancers and osteoporosis *(38)*.

It is neither necessary nor desirable to train a baby to "feed by the clock". It should be explained to the mother, however, that intervals between feeds are necessary for herself and for the baby, though they may vary between 1 to 4 hours, according to the baby's needs, size, strength of sucking and the mother's milk supply.

(2) Artificial feeding

The main indications for artificial feeding are failure of breast milk, prolonged illness or death of the mother. It is crucial for the baby to be fed "breast-milk substitutes" – e.g., dried whole milk powder, fresh milk from a cow or other animal, or commercial formulae.

PRINCIPLES OF ARTIFICIAL FEEDING

In planning an artificial feed, the nutritional needs of infants should be kept in view. These include :

1. Infants require an average of 100 kcal of energy per kg of body weight per day, i.e., about 150 ml of milk per kg of body weight each day;
2. The estimated protein requirement is about 2 g/kg of body weight during the first 6 months; it declines to about 1.5 g/kg by the end of one year. This works out to 13–14 g protein daily during the first year of life. In terms of calories, 8 to 10 per cent of calories are given as protein;
3. The carbohydrate requirement is about 10 g/kg of body weight daily;
4. After 4 months of age, undiluted boiled and cooled milk should be given;

5. Infants need feeding at frequent intervals about 6–8 times a day; older babies 5 times a day; and
6. During illness (e.g., fevers) the calorie need is increased, and it should be met.

(a) *DRIED MILK* : The safest milk is undoubtedly dried whole milk, which is scientifically prepared for infant feeding. It is free from bacteria; there is little danger from flies; it does not become sour and is simple to reconstitute. It is usually fortified with vitamins. But it is expensive and, therefore, beyond the reach of many Indian families.

(b) *COW'S MILK* : A cheaper alternative which is well within the reach of many Indian families is cow's milk, which in fact is widely used for infant feeding. Most health workers give very conflicting advice on the use of cow's milk for infant feeding. A small minority of over-enthusiastic paediatricians recommend undiluted cow's milk right from the birth, forgetting the fact that human milk is made for the human baby and cow's milk for the calf. Both cannot be equated. Most authorities in India and abroad including the World Health Organization have persistently recommended dilution of cow's milk during the first 2 months in order to reduce the solute load on neonatal kidneys. The Government of India in the Ministry of Health and Family Welfare in the "Manual for Health Worker (Female) Vol. I (1978) have also recommended dilution of cow's milk during the first two months. A suggested schedule for infant feeding with cow's milk is given in Table 5.

TABLE 5

Quantities per feeding – assuming five feedings per day

	Infant's weight (kg)			
	3	4	5	6
Cow's milk (ml)	70	100	150	180
Water (ml)	20	20	0	0
Sugar (g)	5	10	10	10
kcal	64	103	135	153
Protein (g)	2.1	3.0	4.5	5.4

- Place milk, water, and sugar in pan
- bring to boil, then cool
- pour into feeding utensil

Source : *(39)*

Artificial feeding is a hazardous procedure in poor homes because of the dangers of contamination and over-dilution of the feed.

The composition of cow's milk and human milk is given in Table 6.

Table 6 shows that cow's milk and human milk are dissimilar in many respects. The differences may be seen as great as the difference between "brain" and "brawn", (a) *PROTEIN* : One of the striking difference is the low protein content of human milk; this is about 3 times less than in cow's milk and lower than in most mammals. The proteins in human breast milk and in cow's milk are completely different. Human milk contains more cystine, essential for the prematures, and less methionine than cow's milk. It is rich in taurine, indispensable for infants, but which they, unlike adults, are unable to synthesize. Breast milk is almost completely digested and utilized for growth, whereas much of cow's milk protein is excreted by the infant undigested producing whitish curdy stool. Breast milk contains other proteins whose functions are not nutritive, but anti-infective, e.g., IgG, lysozyme, living cells, etc. Human milk is virtually a

TABLE 6

Comparison between breast milk during the 1st month of lactation and unprocessed cow milk

Constituent	Breast milk grammes per litre	Cow milk grammes per litre
PROTEINS :	11	33
– Casein	4	28
– Soluble proteins	7	5
Lactalbumin	3.5	1.5 to 1.8
Beta-lactaglobulin	0	3.7
Lactotransferrin	1 to 2	0.2 to 0.5
Immunoglobulin	1 to 2	0.5
Lysozyme	0.5	Traces
NON-PROTEIN : NITROGENOUS SUBSTANCES	0.32	0.32
LIPIDS :	35	35
– Linoleic acid	3.5	1
CARBOHYDRATES :	70	50
– Lactose	62	50
– Nitrogenous oligosaccharides	8	0
MINERALS :	2	8
– Ca (Calcium)	0.33	1
– P (Phosphorus)	0.15	1
– Fe (Iron)	0.4 to 1.5 mg	0.3 to 0.5 mg
VITAMINS :		
– C	60 mg	20 mg
– D	50 IU	25 IU
ENERGY :	640–720 kcal 2670–3000 kJ	650 kcal 2717 kJ

Source : *(40)*

"living" fluid. (b) *FATS* : Mother's milk is especially rich in fats, which represents between 35–50 per cent of total energy value. There are two main ways in which the fats of human milk differ from those of other milks – first, levels of essential polyunsaturated fatty acids, especially linoleic acid and alpha–linolenic acid are higher in human milk than in cow's milk; secondly, the fats of human milk are easier for the baby to digest and absorb than are those of cow's milk. With cow's milk, unabsorbed fatty acids tend to bind with calcium and prevent it from being absorbed. Although there is less calcium in human milk than in cow's milk, it is much better absorbed, (c) *CARBOHYDRATES* : Human milk contains more lactose than most other milks. It may be specially useful for the growing brain. In the intestine, lactose helps the "right" kind of bacteria (i.e., *Lactobacillus bifidus*) to grow. Lactobacillus and lactose help to keep the intestinal contents acidic, which inhibits the growth of harmful bacteria. Lactose plays an important role in maintaining low electrolyte concentration. (d) *VITAMINS AND MINERALS* : If the mother takes adequate amount of vitamins, there is no reason why the child should have a vitamin supplement. The earlier teaching that human milk was deficient in vitamin D is no longer accepted. Vitamin D is present in human milk in water–soluble form. Human milk contains more vitamin A and vitamin C than cow's milk. Another factor which was supposed to be deficient in human milk was iron, but again recent work has shown that iron contained in human milk has a high level of bio-availability, thanks to complex phenomena (the action of lactoferrin, acidity of the digestive track, presence of appropriate proportions of zinc and copper). The coefficient of uptake of the iron in breast milk may be as high as 70 per cent, whereas it is only 30 per cent for cow's milk and infant formulas *(40)*, and no iron supplement is necessary for the baby reared on human milk. Human milk is richer in copper, selenium and cobalt than cow's milk. It contains less sodium than cow's milk and does not put any unnecessary strain on the infant's kidneys. The calcium/ phosphorus ratio is high, so that the uptake of calcium is better than cow's milk. The high phosphorus content of cow's milk causes this mineral to be assimilated to the detriment of calcium. It has the added disadvantage of combining with certain fatty acids to form non-soluble calcium soaps.

WEANING : Weaning is not sudden withdrawal of child from the breast. It is a gradual process starting around the age of 6 months, because the mother's milk alone is not sufficient to sustain growth beyond 6 months. It should be supplemented by suitable foods rich in protein and other nutrients. These are called "supplementary foods". These are usually cow's milk, fruit juice, soft cooked rice, suji, dhal and vegetables. The weaning period is the most crucial period in child development, for during the weaning process children are particularly exposed to the deleterious synergistic interaction of malnutrition and infection. Weaning, if not done properly, is often followed by diarrhoea and months of growth failure leading to kwashiorkor, marasmus and immunodeficiency marked by recurrent and persistent infections which may be fatal. A knowledge of weaning foods and practices is an important aspect of preventive and social paediatrics. At the age of one year, the child should receive solid foods consisting of cereals, pulses, vegetables and fruits. There is now enough evidence to show that children can be properly weaned by local foods of a kind usually consumed by the older children and adults in their families. Efforts should therefore be made to design and promote the use of adequate home-made weaning foods.

Baby friendly hospitals initiatives (2018)

Since 1993 WHO's efforts to improve infant and young child nutrition have focused on promoting breast feeding. It has been calculated that breast feeding could prevent deaths of at least one million children a year. A "baby-friendly hospital initiative" (BFHI), created and promoted by WHO and UNICEF, has proved highly successful in encouraging proper infant feeding practices, starting at birth *(41)*. BFHI is supported by the major professional medical and nursing bodies in India. The implementation guidelines have been revised recently in the year 2018. The ten steps summarize a package of policies and procedures that facilities providing maternity and newborn services should implement to support breastfeeding. The steps are : (1a) Comply fully with the international code of marketing of breast-milk substitutes and relevant World Health Assembly resolutions; (1b) Have a written infant feeding policy that is routinely communicated to staff and parents; (1c) Establish ongoing monitoring and data-management system; (2) Ensure that staff have sufficient knowledge, competence and skills to support breastfeeding; (3) Discuss the importance and management of breastfeeding with pregnant women and their families; (4) Facilitate immediate and uninterrupted skin to skin contact and support mothers to initiate breastfeeding as soon as possible after birth; (5) Support mothers to initiate and maintain breastfeeding and manage common difficulties; (6) Do not provide breastfed newborns any food or fluids other than breast milk, unless medically indicated; (7) Enable mothers and their infants to remain together and to practice rooming-in 24 hours a day; (8) Support mothers to recognize and respond to their infant's cues for feeding; (9) Counsell mothers on the use and risk of feeding bottles, teats and pacifiers; and (10) Coordinate discharge so that parents and their infants have timely access to ongoing support and care *(42)*. The "Baby friendly" hospitals in India are also expected to adopt and practice guidelines on other interventions critical for child survival including antenatal care, clean delivery practices, essential newborn care, immunization and ORT *(43)*.

National guidelines on infant and young child feeding

In view of the vulnerability of young infant to the risk of breast milk substiutes, the Government of India enacted the Infant Milk Substitutes, Feeding Bottles and Infant Food (Regulation of Production, Supply and Distribution) Act 1992. It came into force on 1st Aug. 1993. It prohibits the promotion of infant food, infant milk substitutes and feeding bottles as Government of India is committed to promote breast-feeding.

The new norms of infant and young child feeding i.e., exclusive breast-feeding for the first 6 months (replacing the 4–6 months age range of earlier guidelines), introduction of complementary foods at 6 months while continuing breast-feeding upto the age of 2 years or beyond; replaces the previous policy. The infant milk substitutes, feeding bottles and infant foods (Regulation of Production, Supply and Distribution) Amendment Act 2003, was passed and came into action since 1st January 2004 *(38)*. Goals set to be achieved by the year 2007 were :

1. Intensify nutrition and health education to improve infant and child feeding and caring practices so as to (a) bring down the prevalence of under-weight children under three years from the current level of 47 per cent to 40 per cent; (b) reduce prevalence of severe undernutrition in children in the 0–6 years age group by 50 per cent;
2. Enhance early institution of breast feeding (colostrum feeding) from the current level of 15.8 per cent to 50 per cent;
3. Enhance the exclusive breast-feeding rate for the first six months from the current rate of 55.2 per cent (for 0–3 months) to 80 per cent; and
4. Enhance the complementary feeding rate at six months from the current level of 33.5 per cent to 75 per cent.

GROWTH AND DEVELOPMENT

1. Definition

A phenomenon peculiar to the paediatric age group is growth and development. The term growth refers to increase in the physical size of the body, and development to increase in skills and functions. Growth and development are considered together because the child grows and develops as a whole. Growth and development include not only physical aspect, but also intellectual, emotional and social aspects. Normal growth and development take place only if there is optimal nutrition, if there is freedom from recurrent episodes of infections, and if there is freedom from adverse genetic and environmental influences. MCH care is concerned with the process of growth and development, which is the foundation of human life. It is the nature of this process of physical and psychological growth and development of the child which is crucial for health or ill-health, for life or death.

Determinants of growth and development

It is beyond the scope of this book to delve into the subject of growth and development which indeed is a vast one, except to make a passing reference to some of the more important factors influencing it. Briefly these are : (1) *GENETIC INHERITANCE* : Genetic factors influence growth and development, especially height and weight, mental and social development and personality. (2) *NUTRITION* : Nutrition influences growth and development before as well as after birth. In fact, retardation of growth rate is an indication of malnutrition. When the diet is improved the child begins to grow in height and weight. (3) *AGE* : Growth rate is maximum during foetal life, during the first year of life and then again at puberty. At other periods, growth is slower. (4) *SEX* : At about the age of 10 to 11 years, female children show a sudden increase in height and weight. This growth spurt corresponds to puberty. In male children, the growth spurt occurs a little later, i.e., between 12 and 13 years. (5) *PHYSICAL SURROUNDINGS* : Sunshine, good housing, lighting and ventilation have their effects on growth and development (6) *PSYCHOLOGICAL FACTORS*: Love, tender care and proper child-parent relationship do affect the social, emotional and intellectual development of children. (7) *INFECTIONS AND PARASITOSIS* : Certain infections of the mother during pregnancy (e.g., rubella, syphilis) affect the intrauterine growth of the foetus. Infections after birth (e.g., diarrhoea, measles) slow down growth and development, especially in the malnourished child. The intestinal parasites (e.g., roundworms) by consuming considerable quantities of nutrients hamper growth and development. (8) *ECONOMIC FACTORS* : The standard of living of the family is an important factor. Children from well-to-do families have better height and weight. The economic factor is connected with the nutrition and living of the people. (9) *OTHER FACTORS*: These comprise the birth order of the child, birth spacing, birth weight in single and multiple pregnancies, education of the parents, etc. In short, a normal childhood implies proper physical, mental and emotional development, and is a prerequisite for a full adult life. The study of normal development and its determinants is the basis for paediatric education.

The process of growth from birth to age 20 may be represented diagrammatically in 3 curves (Fig. 4) which shows the level accomplished (as a percentage of development between birth and maturity). These curves are so drawn that height at age 20 corresponds to 100 on the vertical scale. It will be seen from Fig. 4 that the growth of the brain is spectacular during the pre-school age.

2. Normal growth

CONCEPT OF NORMALITY

When speaking of human growth and development, mention must be made of the difficulty of defining normality. A normal child may be defined as one whose characteristics fall within the range of measurements accepted as normal for the majority of children in the same (or reference) age group. Conventionally, these limits – the limits of normal variation – are assumed to include two standard deviations above and below the mean (i.e., between the 3rd and the 97th centiles). This presupposes the availability of accurate measurement techniques of growth, and a satisfactory set of reference values or standards for comparison.

As far as physical development is concerned, we have measurement techniques. For example, we measure growth in terms of kilograms and centimetres. But very great difficulties are encountered in connection with psychomotor, emotional and social development; most measurement techniques are based on observations such as "milestones of development."

Methods of assessment *(44, 45)*

In children, the parameters of growth generally used are : weight, height (or length in infants), and head and chest circumferences. These characteristics are measured and compared with the reference standards. Three methods are

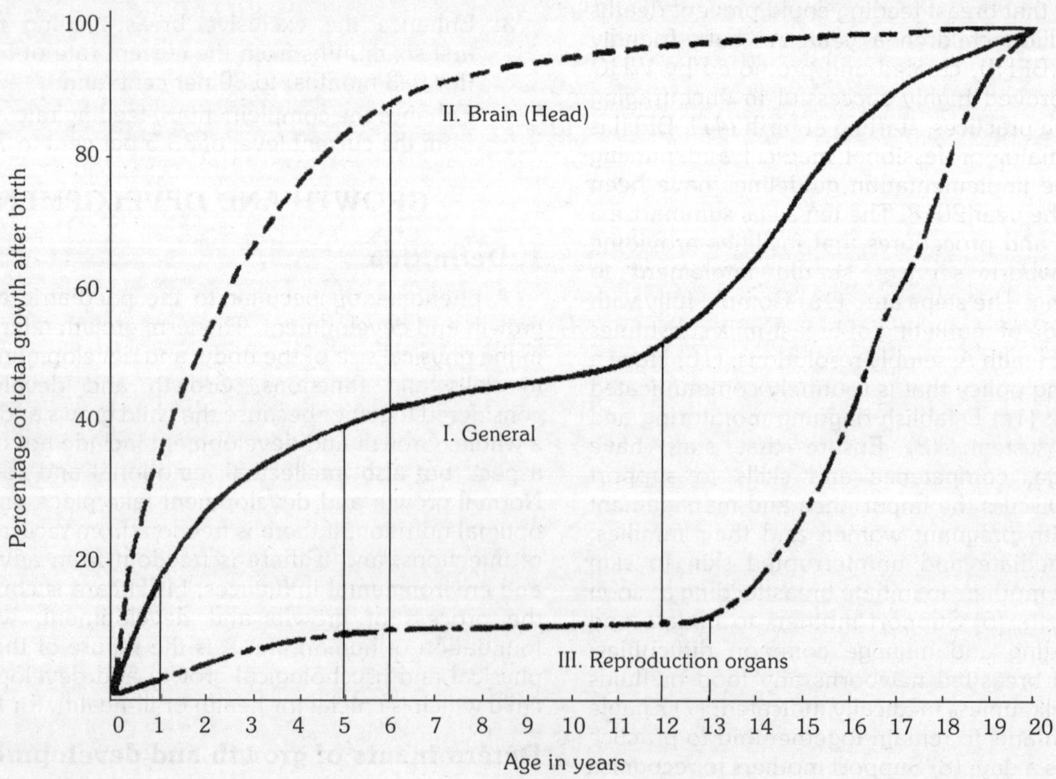

FIG. 4
Growth after birth

generally used for making comparisons : (i) The first method is based on mean (or median) values. The median, rather than mean is used where possible because of the skewed distribution of most anthropometric measurements. A variation of 2 standard deviations from either side of the mean (or median) is considered as within normal limits; (ii) The second method is by means of percentile or (centiles). Percentiles are easier to understand than standard deviations. Percentiles refer to the percentage of individuals falling below a particular level. By definition 3 per cent of children are below the 3rd percentile, and a further 3 per cent are above the 97th percentile. The remaining 94 per cent of individuals who fall between these two lines (i.e. between 3rd and 97th percentiles) should therefore be regarded as being within the range of "normal." However, the 6 per cent of the children outside this range may not necessarily be "abnormal", particularly if their growth is parallel with their centile lines. A measurement outside 3 standard deviation (above 99th and below 1st centile) is more likely to indicate a significant degree of abnormality; and (iii) Thirdly, it is also possible to assess the growth of a child by such indices as weight for length, and weight for height. These are age-independent indices.

The assessment of growth may be longitudinal or cross-sectional. Longitudinal assessment of growth entails measuring the same child at regular intervals. This provides valuable data about a child's progress. Cross-sectional studies are also essential to compare a child's growth with that of his peers. Cross-sectional comparisons involve large number of children of the same age. These children are measured and the range of their measurements (e.g., weight, height) is plotted, usually on percentile charts.

Reference values

For national and international comparisons and for monitoring, reference or "standard" values of growth are essential. The well known reference standards are : *(i) Harvard (or Boston) standards (46)* : These are based on observations made on children in Boston from 1930 to 1956. They have been carefully compiled longitudinally on a large series of children, mostly from North European origin. They became widely used throughout the world; *(ii) WHO reference values (47, 48)* : The Harvard values were replaced by WHO reference values for weight and height. These values were based on extensive cross-sectional data assembled by the United States National Centre for Health Statistics (NCHS) which were considered the best available for international use. The WHO reference values are used for children upto 5 years of age since the influence of ethnic or genetic factors on young children at this age period is considered insignificant, given the similar socio-economic environment; and *(iii) Indian standards (49)* : The Indian Council of Medical Research (ICMR) undertook a nationwide cross-sectional study during the year 1956 and 1965 to establish the much needed reference standards of growth and development of Indian children, for the country as a whole, as well as for each of the states in the country. As the Indian data are based on measurements of children belonging to the lower socio-economic groups which form the majority of Indian communities, the values cannot be considered as representing standard values *(50)*.

The use of local standards of reference is not recommended unless these are based on well-nourished and healthy samples of local population. Further, local standards do not permit international comparisons *(51)*. It was the opinion of WHO that countries or regions might eventually develop their own reference standards; in the interim, the WHO reference value should provide an effective substitute *(47)*.

Reference versus standard values

A distinction must be made between reference values and standard values. If the values are derived from a population racially different from the population under study, such values should be considered as reference values only and not as standard values *(52)*. That is, reference values cannot be used as standard values applicable to a population racially different. For example, it would be absurd to apply the Harvard standards of growth to Pigmies and Eskimos who are racially different *(51)*.

Surveillance of growth and development

Surveillance of growth and development is a specific function of the mother and child health services. It is an important component of the routine anticipatory care of children. The main purpose of growth surveillance is to identify those children who are not growing normally. Surveillance also reflects the effectiveness of other components of child care such as nutrition, sanitation and control of infection. Surveillance of growth and development covers the following aspects :

PHYSICAL GROWTH

1. Weight-for-age

Measurement of weight and rate of gain in weight are the best single parameters for assessing physical growth. A single weight record only indicates the child's size at the moment; it does not give any information about whether a child's weight is increasing, stationary or declining. This is because, normal variation in weight at a given age is wide. What is important is careful repeated measurement at intervals, ideally monthly, from birth to 1 year, every two months during the second year and every 3 months thereafter upto 5 years of age, since this age group is at greatest risk from growth faltering. By comparing the measurements with reference standards of weight of children of the same age (Table 7), the trend of growth becomes obvious. This is best done on growth chart. Serial weighing is also useful to interpret the progress of growth when the age of the child is not known. Thus, without the aid of a growth chart, it is virtually impossible to detect changes in the rate of growth, such as sudden loss of weight or halt in gain. Each baby should have its own growth chart.

A baby should gain at least 500 gram wt. per month in the first three months of life. That is the minimum. The children who gain less weight are malnourished. It is usual for babies to gain about 1 kg a month, especially in the first 3 months. Healthy babies, on an average double their birth weight by 5 months, and treble it by the end of first year and quadruple by the age of two. During the first year, weight increases by about 7 kg. After that the increase in weight is not so fast – only about 2.5 kg during the second year and from then until puberty by about 2 kg per year. The weight and height gain patterns in India are as shown in Table 8.

In different parts of India, the average birth weight is between 2.7 and 2.9 kg *(54)*. The Indian infant manages to grow well upto the age of 3–4 months, even at the expense of its malnourished mother. Thereafter, the growth falters due to lack of supplementary feeding *(55)*. However, Indian children from well-to-do families display growth patterns as good as their counterparts in the Western world *(49)*.

TABLE 7

2006 – WHO standards of weight for age of boys and girls upto the age of 5 years (kg)

Age (months)	Boys			Girls		
	– 2SD	Median	+ 2SD	–2SD	Median	+2SD
0	2.5	3.3	4.4	2.4	3.2	4.2
4	5.6	7.0	8.7	5.0	6.4	8.2
8	6.9	8.6	10.7	6.3	7.9	10.2
12	7.7	9.6	12.0	7.0	8.9	11.5
16	8.4	10.5	13.1	7.7	9.8	12.6
20	9.1	11.3	14.2	8.2	10.4	13.5
24	9.7	12.2	15.3	9.0	11.5	14.8
28	10.2	12.9	16.3	9.7	12.3	16.0
32	10.8	13.7	17.4	10.3	13.1	17.1
36	11.3	14.3	18.3	10.8	13.9	18.1
40	11.8	15.0	19.3	11.3	14.6	19.2
44	12.2	15.7	20.2	11.8	15.3	20.4
48	12.7	16.3	21.2	12.3	16.1	21.5
52	13.2	17.0	22.2	12.8	16.8	22.6
56	13.6	17.7	23.2	13.3	17.5	23.8
60	14.1	18.3	24.2	13.7	18.2	24.9

Source : *(53)*

TABLE 8

Average weight and height increase during the first 5 years

Age	Increments
	Weight increments per week
0 – 3 months	200 g
4 – 6 months	150 g
7 – 9 months	100 g
10 – 12 months	50 – 75 g
	Weight increments per year
1 – 2 years	2.5 kg
3 – 5 years	2.0 kg
	Length increments per year
1st year	25 cm
2nd year	12 cm
3rd year	9 cm
4th year	7 cm
5th year	6 cm

Source : *(52)*

Weight-for-age is often used to classify malnutrition and determine its prevalence. Jelliffe suggested that 80 per cent of the median weight-for-age of the reference be the cut-off point below which children could be considered malnourished.

2. Height (length)-for-age

Height should be taken in a standing position without foot wear. If the height machine is not available, the measuring scale fixed to the wall can be employed. This arrangement is suitable for children 2 years and above. The measuring scale should be capable of measuring to an accuracy of 0.1 cm *(48)*. A very great effort should be made to measure children accurately. Errors in the measurement of a young child may lead to significant errors in the classification of the nutritional status. The WHO standards (2006) for height-for-age are as shown in Table 9.

The length of a baby at birth is about 50 cm. It increases by about 25 cm during first year, and by another 12 cm during the second year. During growth spurt, boys add something like 20 cm in their height, and girls gain about 16 cm. The spurt is followed by a rapid slowing of growth. Indian girls reach 98 per cent of their final height on an average by the age of 16.5 years, and boys reach the same stage by the age of 17.75 years. With the exception of a few ethnic groups, there is evidence showing that all children have a similar growth potential.

Height is a stable measurement of growth as opposed to body weight. Whereas weight reflects only the present health status of the child, height indicates the events in the past also. The use of growth (height) centile chart is particularly valuable in studying the trend of height curve.

Low height for age : This is also known as nutritional stunting or dwarfing. It reflects past or chronic malnutrition. The cut-off point commonly taken for the diagnosis of stunting is 90 per cent of the United States NCHS height-for-age values *(56)*. Waterlow recorded the use of 2SD below the median reference as the cut-off point.

3. Weight-for-height

Height and weight are interrelated. Weight in relation to height is now considered more important than weight alone. It helps to determine whether a child is within range of "normal" weight for his height. For example, a child on the 75th centile of both his height and weight is neither overweight nor under-weight, but a child on the 75th centile of his weight chart and the 25th centile of his height chart is clearly overweight.

Low weight for height : This is also known as nutritional wasting or emaciation (acute malnutrition). It is associated with an increased risk of mortality and morbidity *(56)*. A child who is less than 70 per cent of the expected weight-for-height is classed as severely wasted.

The WHO has compiled reference value for children giving weight according to height. For details see reference 53.

Weight records

Weight records are generally kept by all infant clinics; the aim is the prevention of underfeeding, and in the developing world, the weight chart is an important tool in the prevention of malnutrition.

TABLE 9

2006 – WHO standards for length/height-for-age of boys and girls upto the age of 5 years (cm)

Age (months)	Boys			Girls		
	– 2SD	Median	+ 2SD	–2SD	Median	+2SD
0	46.1	49.9	53.7	45.4	49.1	52.9
4	59.7	63.9	68.0	57.8	62.1	66.4
8	66.2	70.6	75.0	64.0	68.7	73.5
12	71.0	75.7	80.5	68.9	74.0	79.2
16	75.0	80.2	85.4	73.0	78.6	84.2
20	77.7	83.2	88.8	76.7	82.7	88.7
24	81.7	87.8	93.9	80.0	86.4	92.9
28	83.8	90.4	97.0	82.2	89.1	96.0
32	86.4	93.4	100.4	84.9	92.2	99.4
36	88.7	96.1	103.5	87.4	95.1	102.7
40	90.9	98.6	106.4	89.8	97.7	105.7
44	93.0	101.0	109.1	92.0	100.3	108.6
48	94.9	103.3	111.7	94.1	102.7	111.3
52	96.9	105.6	114.2	96.1	105.0	114.0
56	98.8	107.8	116.7	98.1	107.3	116.5
60	100.7	110.0	119.2	99.9	109.4	118.9

Source : *(53)*

4. Head and chest circumference

At birth the head circumference is about 34 cm. It is about 2 cm more than the chest circumference. By 6 to 9 months, the two measurements become equal, after which the chest circumference overtakes the head circumference. In severely malnourished children, this overtaking may be delayed by 3 to 4 years due to poor development of the thoracic cage. In a ICMR study *(49)*, the crossing over of chest and head circumference did not take place until the age of two years and six months. This has been attributed to growth retardation in poor Indian children.

Besides increase in height and weight, the term "growth" also includes various physiological events which occur at predictable periods such as, dentition, ossification of bones and secondary sexual characteristics.

BEHAVIOURAL DEVELOPMENT

A closely related development is behavioural development. It is assessed in four fields :

1. Motor development;
2. Personal-social development;
3. Adaptive development; and
4. Language development.

The developmental landmarks or milestones of development provide an estimate of the time when the child can be expected to attain certain skills or points in development. Since the milestones are averages, each child is bound to differ from the other. For instance, some children sit up and speak earlier than others. Table 10 shows some of the normal developmental milestones and ages at which these are reached in the Indian context. When a child takes longer time to cross these milestones, the possibility of his being mentally handicapped should not be overlooked.

The behavioural development of the child is a complex affair. The work of ethnologists and sociologists show how quickly the child's behaviour conform to the models adult society offers them. For proper behaviour development, the child must be assured emotional and moral stability, that is, a home where he will find bonds of affection, regular discipline and parents who accept him and provide him with

TABLE 10

Milestones of development

The 'milestones' given here are approximations and to assess any individual child, all types of growth development and behaviour must be taken into account.

Age	Motor development	Language development	Adaptive development	Socio-personal development
6-8 weeks	–	–	–	Looks at mother and smiles
3 months	Holds head erect	–	–	–
4-5 months	–	listening	begins to reach out for objects	recognizes mother
6-8 months	sits without support	experimenting with noises	transfers objects hand to hand	enjoys hide and seek
9-10 months	crawling	increasing range of sounds	releases objects	suspicious of strangers
10-11 months	stands with support	first words		
12-14 months	walks wide base		builds	
18-21 months	walks narrow base beginning to run	joining words	beginning to explore	
24 months	runs	short sentences		dry by day

models of balanced conduct. Many children will not find themselves in ideal conditions. They consequently have trouble with behaviour, speech, sleep and appetite and these problems will have to be anticipated, diagnosed and treated.

THE GROWTH CHART

The growth or "road-to-health" chart (first designed by David Morley and later modified by WHO) is a visible display of the child's physical growth and development. It is designed primarily for the longitudinal follow-up (growth monitoring) of a child, so that changes over time can be interpreted.

It is important to note that in the weight-for-age chart, the height of the child is not taken into consideration. This is because weight is the most sensitive measure of growth, and any deviation from "normal" can be detected easily by comparison with **reference curves**. A child can lose weight, but not height. In short, the growth chart offers a simple and inexpensive way of monitoring weight gain, and in fact child health over time.

1. WHO child growth standards, 2006 *(53)*

In 1993 the WHO undertook a comprehensive review of the uses and interpretation of anthropometric references. The review concluded that the NCHS growth references, which had been recommended for international use since the late 1970s, did not adequately represent early childhood growth and that new growth curves were necessary. A Multicentre Growth Referenece Study (MGRS) was undertaken between 1997 and 2003 in Brazil, Ghana, India, Norway, Oman and USA and primary growth data and related information were gathered from 9,440 healthy breast-fed infants and young children (0 to 60 months boys and girls) from widely diverse ethnic background and cultural settings. In addition their mothers followed health practices such as breast feeding their children, and not smoking during and after pregnancy.

The new standards were generated for boys and girls aged 0–60 months – percentile and Z-score curves for length/height-for-age, weight-for-age, weight-for-length, weight-for-height and BMI-for-age. The last standard is an addition of the set of indicators previously available as part of the NCHS/WHO reference.

As expected, there are notable differences with the NCHO/WHO reference that vary by age, sex, anthropometric measure and specific percentile or Z-score curve. Differences are particularly important in infancy. Stunting will be greater throughout childhood when assessed using the new WHO standards compared to the NCHS/ WHO reference. The growth pattern of breast-fed infant will result in a substantial increase in rates of underweight during the first half of infancy and a decrease thereafter. For wasting, the main difference is during infancy when wasting rate will be substantially higher using the new WHO standards. With respect to overweight, use of the new standards will result in a greater prevalence that will vary by age, sex and nutritional status of the index population.

The new WHO standards depict normal early childhood growth under optimal environmental conditions and can be used to assess children everywhere, regardless of ethnicity, socio-economic status and type of feeding.

Fig. 5 and 6 show the comparison of WHO with NCHS weight-for-age reference curve from birth to 5 years of age for boys and girls respectively *(53)*.

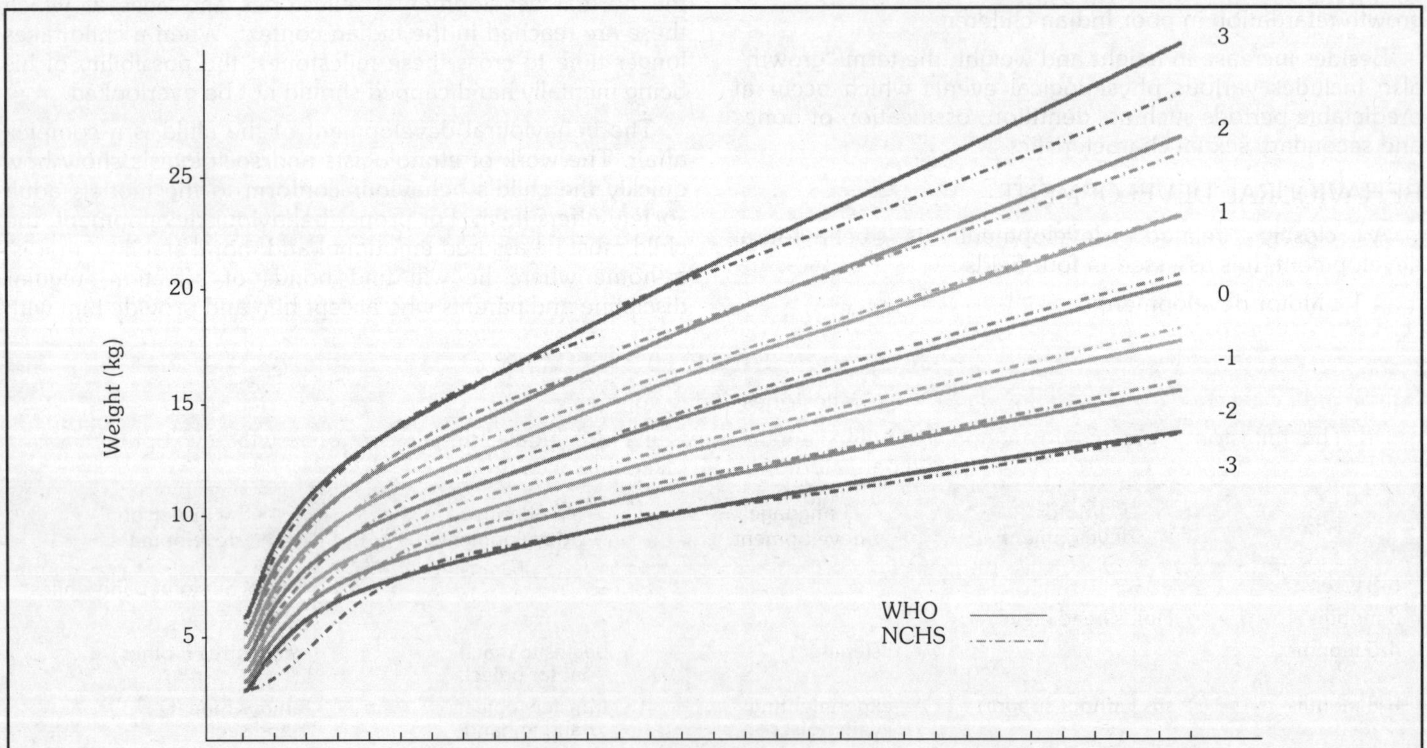

FIG. 5

Comparison of WHO with NCHS weight-for-age Z-scores for boys

Source : *(53)*

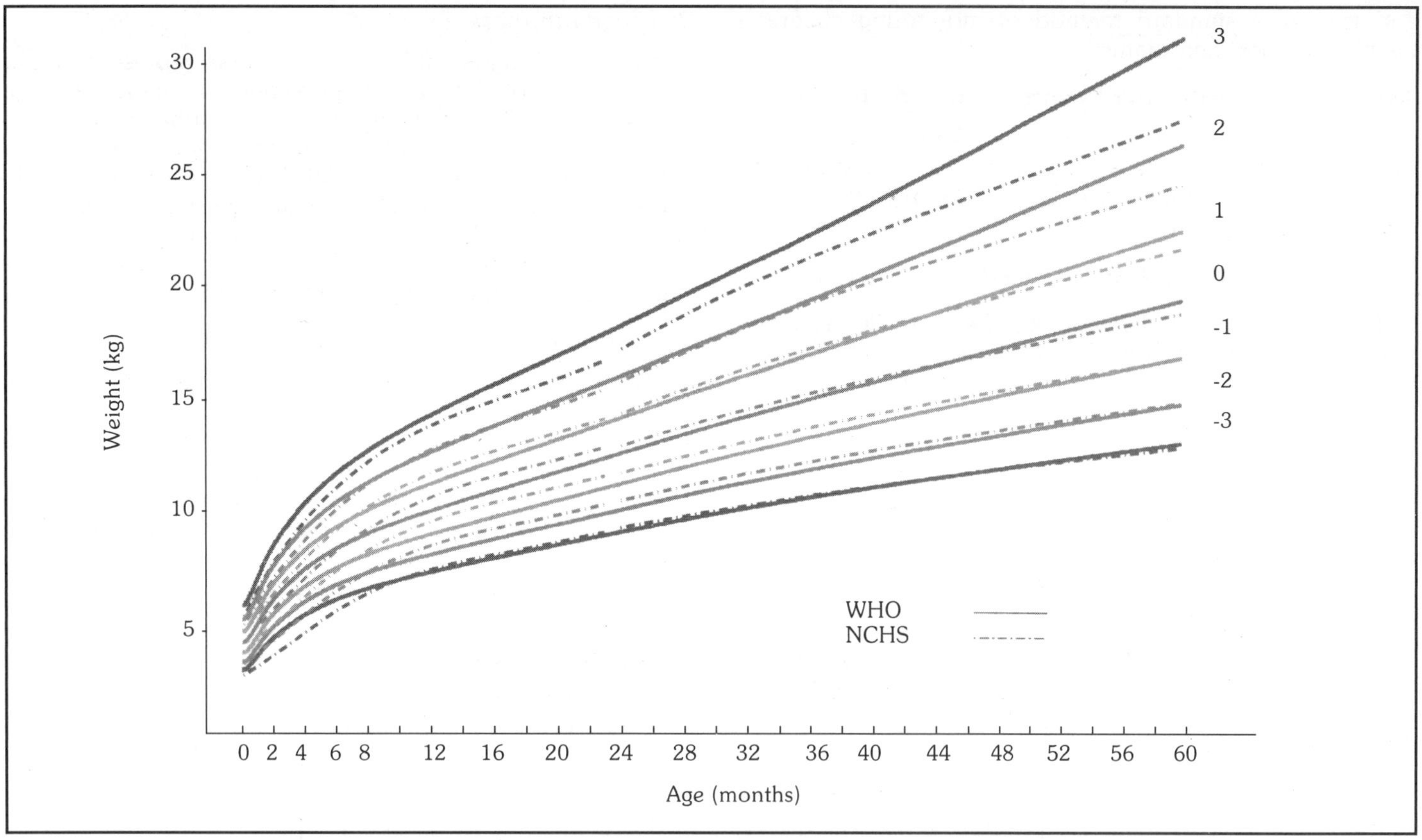

FIG. 6

Comparison of WHO with NCHS weight-for-age Z-scores for girls

Source : *(53)*

2. Growth chart used in India

India has adopted the new WHO Child Growth Standards (2006) in February 2009, for monitoring the young child growth and development within the National Rural Health Mission and the ICDS. The same standards will be used for research too in future.

These standards are available for both boys and girls below 5 years of age. With these new standards the child care workers will know when the nutrition and care needs of the child is being compromised and it will enable them to take timely corrective action at different levels.

A joint "Mother and Child Protection Card" has been developed, as shown in Fig. 7 and 8, which provides space for recording the family identification and registration, birth record, pregnancy record, institutional identification, care during pregnancy, preparation for delivery, registration under Janani Suraksha Yojana, details about immunization procedures, breast-feeding and introduction of supplementary food, milestones of the baby, birth spacing and reasons for special care. The chart is easily understood by the health workers and the mother, with a visual record of the health and nutritional status of the child. It is kept by the mother and brought to the health centre at each visit.

The growth chart shows normal zone of weight for age, undernutrition (below –2SD) and severely underweight zone (below –3SD). In some states like Maharashtra, the growth chart contains normal weight for age zone and undernutrition zone of grade one, second, third and fourth. It is the direction of growth that is more important than the position of dots on the line. The importance of the direction of growth is illustrated at the left hand, upper corner of the chart. Flattening or falling of the child's weight curve signals growth failure, which is the earliest sign of the protein-energy malnutrition and may precede clinical signs by weeks and months. Such a child needs special care. The objective in child care is to keep the child in normal zone.

Uses of growth chart

A growth chart has many potential uses :

1. for **growth monitoring** which is of great value in child health care;
2. **diagnostic tool:** for identifying "high-risk" children. For example, malnutrition can be detected long before signs and symptoms of it become apparent;
3. **planning and policy making:** by grading malnutrition, it provides an objective basis for planning and policy making in relation to child health care at the local and central levels;
4. **educational tool:** because of its visual character, the mother can be educated in the care of her own child and encourage her to participate more actively in growth monitoring;
5. **tool for action:** it helps the health worker on the type of intervention that is needed; it will help to make referrals easier;
6. **evaluation:** it provides a good method to evaluate the effectiveness of corrective measures and the impact of a programme or of special interventions for improving child growth and development; and
7. **tool for teaching:** it can also be used for teaching, for example, the importance of adequate feeding; the deleterious effects of diarrhoea.

The growth chart has been described as a passport to child health care *(57)*. It has won international recognition and is now a standard method of monitoring children's health and nutritional status.

Alternative methods of growth monitoring

Growth charting is only one method of growth monitoring. There are other indicators such as height-for-age, weight-for-height, and arm circumference. The last two are independent of age and are particularly useful when age is not known.

CARE OF THE PRE-SCHOOL CHILD

Children between 1–4 years of age are generally called pre-school age children or toddlers. In the history of health services of many developing countries, their social and health needs were realized rather late. Today, more than ever before, the pre-school age child has become a focus for organized medical–social welfare activities, and their death rate is considered a significant indicator of the social situation in a country.

The pre-school age is distinguished by the following characteristics :

1. Large numbers

Pre-school age children (1–4 years) represent about 9.7 per cent of the general population in India. A large majority of these children live in rural and tribal areas and in urban slums. By virtue of their numbers, they are entitled to a large share of health and social services. Further, children are the human resources of the future. Their development is in the interest of the total national development; therefore, they need special attention. Unfortunately, pre-school age children are comparatively less attended to.

2. Mortality

The pre-school age (1–4 years) mortality in India is 2.3 per cent of all deaths. This high mortality which is largely due to infection and malnutrition is characteristic of this age group in underprivileged areas. Malnutrition was shown to be an underlying cause in 3.4 per cent of all deaths in young children and associated cause in no less than 46 per cent *(40)*.

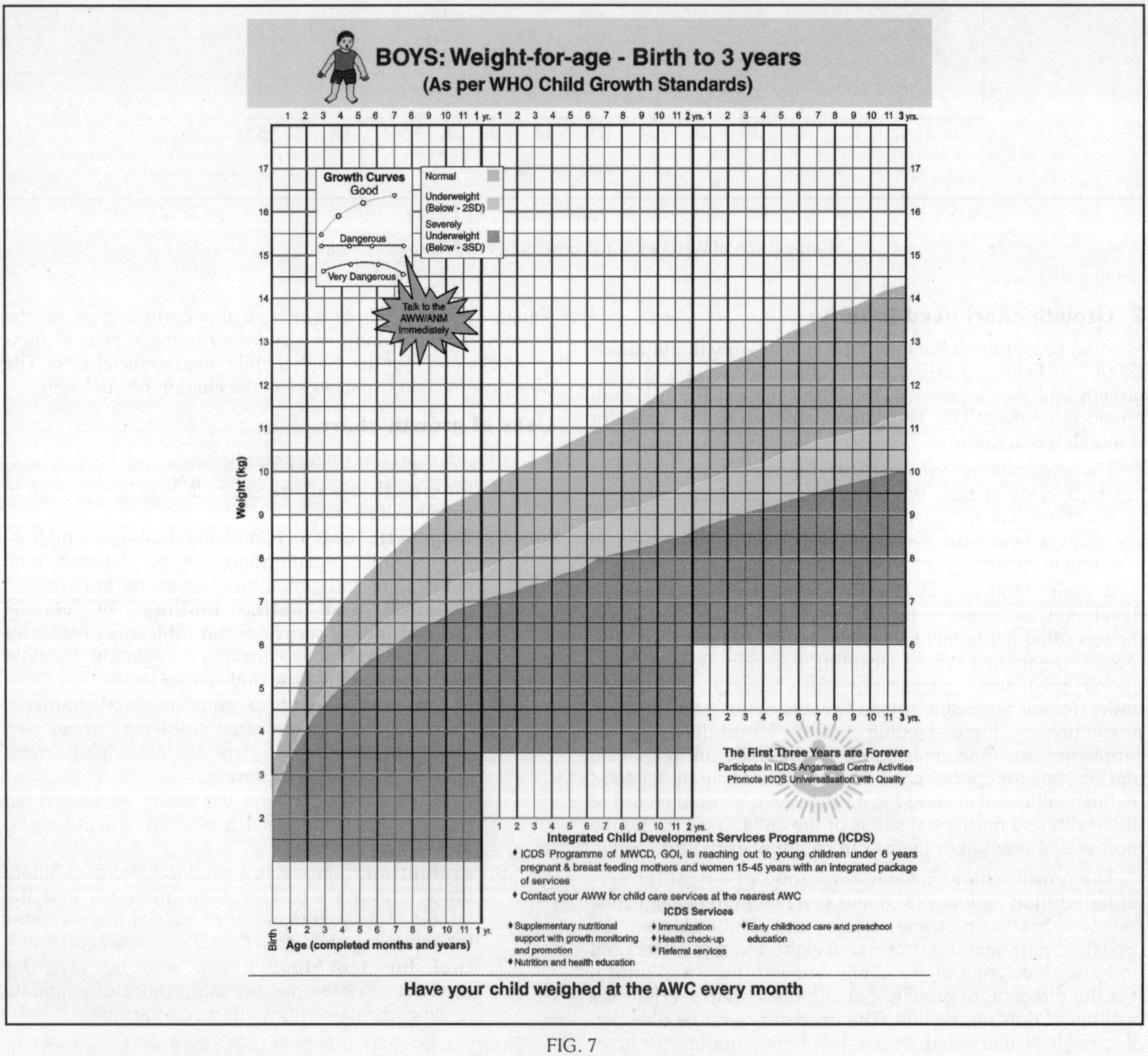

FIG. 7

ICDS growth chart for boys

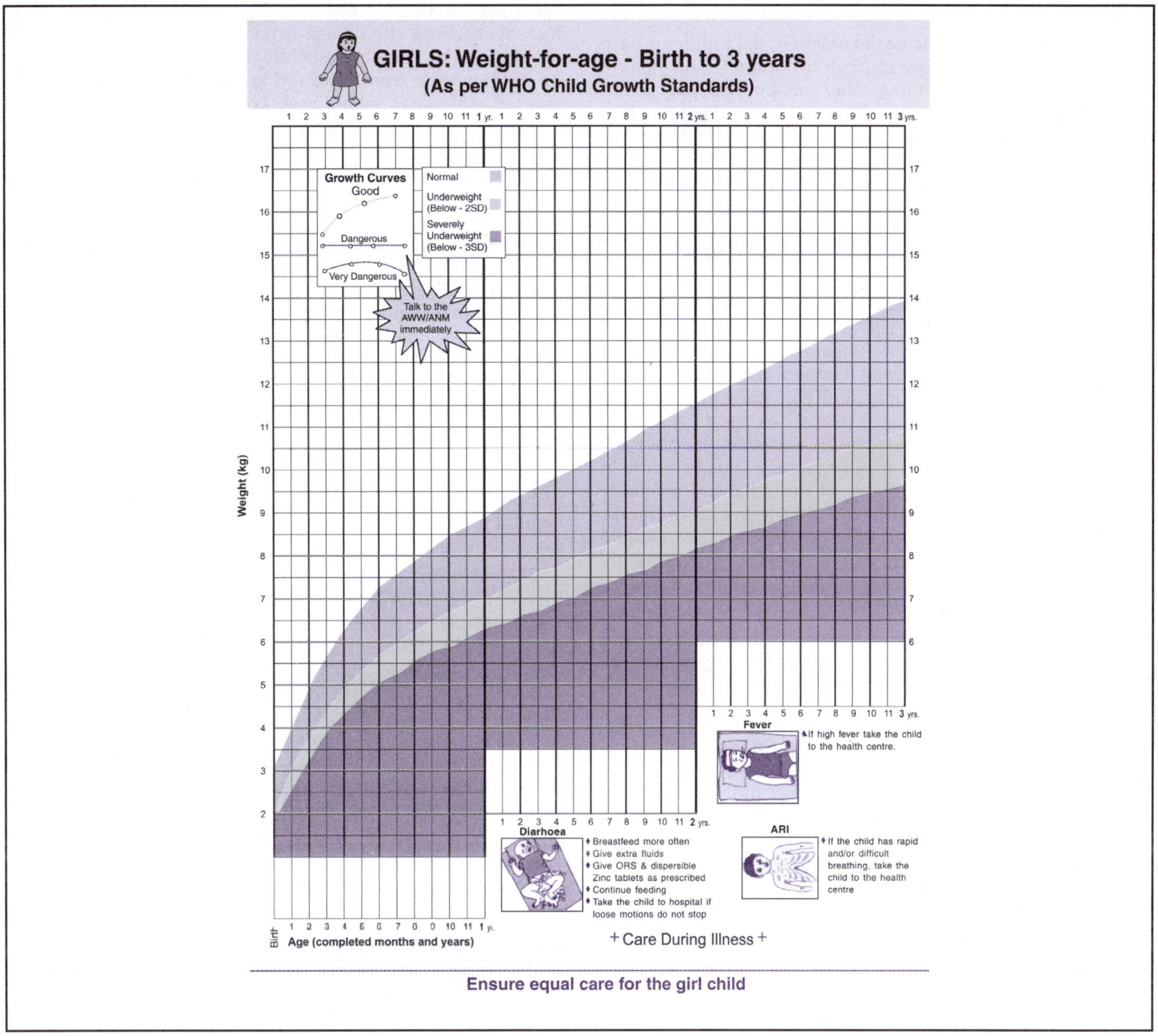

FIG. 8

ICDS growth chart for girls

3. Morbidity

The data on the extent of morbidity of pre-school children are scarce. Some hospital records and a few surveys suggest that children in this age group are usually victims of PEM accompanied by retarded growth and development. Surveys indicate that the main morbidity problems are malnutrition and infections. The prevalence of severe protein-energy malnutrition ranged between 5–6 per cent, and mild protein energy malnutrition about 40 per cent. PEM is often associated with other nutritional deficiency such as anaemia, xerophthalmia, etc. Diarrhoea, diphtheria, tetanus, whooping cough, measles and other eruptive fevers, skin and eye infections, and intestinal parasitic infestations are usually common under the existing environmental conditions. Atleast 5 per cent of the pre-school age children belonging to poor socio-economic groups show signs of vitamin A deficiency. Accidents are also becoming frequent, especially burns and trauma from home accidents, and to an increasing degree, traffic accidents. Some childhood diseases and conditions do not kill their victims, but cause serious disability (e.g., blindness, paralysis); and some diseases become manifest later in life (e.g., heart disease and mental retardation). In many developing countries, periods of illness take up 25–30 per cent of the child's life and each represents either loss of weight or failure to gain weight. These episodes are well documented by several authors *(55)*.

4. Growth and development

The importance of the first 5 or 6 years of life of a child for its growth and development is well known. Any adverse influences operating on children during this period (e.g., malnutrition and infection) may result in severe limitations in their development, some of which at least are irreversible. The concept of vulnerability calls for preventive care and special actions to meet the biological and psychological needs inherent in the process of human growth and development *(33)*.

5. Accessibility

While the infant may be easily reached, the toddler is hard to reach, and it is therefore difficult to look after his health. Special inputs are needed (e.g., day care centres, play group centres, children's clubs) to reach the toddler and to bring him into the orbit of health care. Operations research all over the world has demonstrated that parents are unlikely to travel more than 5–8 kms to obtain medical care. For the toddler who needs to be carried, the distance may be reduced even further.

6. Prevention in childhood of health problems in adult life

Results of research indicate how events in early life (e.g. child's diet, infections) affect its health when it becomes an adult, and how many conditions can be prevented through early action, for example, dental diseases in adulthood. Early treatment of streptococcal infection can prevent rheumatic heart disease. Longitudinal studies suggest that the foundations of obesity, hypertension, cardiovascular diseases, and certain mental disorders may be laid in early life. Some of the chronic orthopaedic ailments of the adult are probably connected with anomalies in the development or minor uncorrected infirmities of the infant (e.g. talipes, congenital dislocation of the hip). Many of the measures subsequently undertaken to treat these disorders often do not fully succeed.

Since young children are "vulnerable" to social and health hazards which can retard or arrest their physical and mental development during these critical years, they deserve special attention by the administration, general population and the family.

CHILD HEALTH PROBLEMS

The problems facing the health worker in the developing world are vast and are nowhere more evident than in the field of childcare. The main health problems encountered in the child population comprise the following :

1. low birth weight;
2. malnutrition;
3. infections and parasitosis;
4. accidents and poisoning; and
5. behavioural problems.

1. Low birth weight

This has been discussed in detail earlier.

2. Malnutrition

Malnutrition is the most widespread condition affecting the health of children. Scarcity of suitable foods, lack of purchasing power of the family as well as traditional beliefs and taboos about what the baby should eat, often lead to an insufficient balanced diet, resulting in malnutrition. It is estimated that no less than 45 per cent of the children who died before the age of 5 years were found to have malnutrition as underlying factor and 80 per cent of newborn mortality occurs in babies who are of low birth weight *(55)*. During 2020, more than 22 per cent of the world's children under the age of 5 years were stunted and 6.7 per cent were having wasting for their age. The proportion ranged from 0.7 per cent of children in the Regions of Americas to 14.1 per cent in the countries of South East Asia Region *(59)*. In India, the National Family Health Survey (NFHS-5) 2019–21 included survey of the nutritional status of young children. Both chronic and acute undernutrition were found to be high. The prevalence of undernutrition is almost same among girls and boys, although, girls are slightly less well nourished than boys on all three measures. The prevalence of stunting increases with a child's age from 6–8 months through 6–23 months, and it decreases slightly thereafter. Over 44 per cent of children who were reported to be very small at birth are stunted, compared with 35 per cent of children who were of average size or larger. Children born to thin mothers (BMI less than 18.5 kg/m^2) are more likely to be stunted, wasted, and underweight than children born to mothers with a normal BMI, stunting is higher in rural areas (37 per cent) than in urban areas (30 per cent). 46 per cent of children born to mothers with no schooling are stunted, compared to 26 per cent of children born to mothers with 12 or more years of schooling. The corresponding proportion of underweight children are 42 and 23 per cent respectively. The prevalence of stunting decreases steadily with an increase in wealth quintiles, from 46 per cent of children in households in the lowest wealth quintile to 23 per cent of children in households in the highest wealth quintile. Prevalence of stunting in children under five years age is highest in Meghalaya (47 per cent), followed by Bihar (43 per cent), Uttar Pradesh and Jharkhand (40 per cent each), and it is lowest in Puducherry (20 per cent) and Sikkim (22 per cent). Bihar has the highest level of underweight children (41 per cent). Maharashtra has the highest level of wasting (26 per cent) *(58)*.

Malnutrition makes the child more susceptible to infection, recovery is slower and mortality is higher. Undernourished children do not grow to their full potential of physical and mental abilities. Malnutrition in infancy and childhood leads to stunted growth. It also manifests by clinical signs of micronutrient and vitamin deficiencies. Prevention and appropriate treatment of diarrhoea, measles and other infections in infancy and early childhood are important to reduce malnutrition rates as infection and malnutrition often make vicious cycle. Exclusive breast-feeding in first 6 months of life is very important.

Specific nutritional deficiencies

(a) Protein-energy malnutrition

Protein-energy malnutrition (PEM) has been identified as a major health and nutrition problem in India. It occurs particularly in weaklings and children in the first years of life. It is characterized by low birth weight if the mother is malnourished, poor growth in children and high level of mortality in children between 12 and 24 months, and is estimated to be an underlying cause in 30 per cent of deaths among children under age 5.

As many as 27 per cent of the children in the low income countries have low height for their age i.e. stunting, and 17 per cent children have low weight for height. The rate of low height for age reflects the cumulative effects of undernutrition and infections since birth or even before birth; high rates are often suggestive of bad environmental conditions and/or early malnutrition. On the other hand, a greater frequency of low weight for height, often reflects current severe undernutrition or disease. The scenario in India is discussed in detail under the heading malnutrition.

(b) Micronutrient malnutrition

Micronutrient malnutrition refers to a group of conditions caused by deficiency of essential vitamins and minerals such as vitamin A, calcium, iodine, iron and zinc. It is estimated that about 2 billion people are affected by this type of malnutrition. Vitamin A deficiency is still the most common cause of preventable childhood blindness worldwide; iodine deficiency causes goitre, cretinism and brain damage; and anaemia results from insufficient iron intake.

Nutritional anaemia : It affects all age groups, including pre-school children, school children and elders. Even mild anaemia reduces resistance to fatigue. It has a profound effect on psychological and physical behaviour. Overall, 67 per cent of children are having same degree of anaemia, 29 per cent of children have mild anaemia, 36 per cent have moderate anaemia, and 2 percent have severe anaemia *(58)*.

Vitamin A deficiency and nutritional blindness : Young children are at greater risk of developing xerophthalmia, partly because their vitamin A requirements are proportionately greater than those of any other group and partly because they suffer most from infections. The result is that severe, blinding corneal destruction is most frequently seen in children between the age of six months and six years. Vitamin A deficiency is in fact, the single most frequent cause of blindness among pre-school children in developing countries. Some 20 per cent children with this deficiency are at increased risk of death from common infections, and around 2 per cent are blinded or suffer serious sight impairment.

Iodine deficiency : Iodine deficiency disorders pose a public health problem as about 1.5 billion people are living in environments lacking this mineral. As a result at least 30,000 babies are stillborn each year and over 120,000 are born mentally retarded, physically stunted, deaf–mute or paralysed. Even when children are born otherwise healthy, lack of iodine may still cause mental dullness and apathy.

Nutritional deficiencies not only lead to severe illnesses, entailing long and costly treatment, but also influence physical development, psychic behaviour and susceptibility to infection.

3. Infectious and parasitic diseases

Young children fall an easy prey to infectious diseases. The leading childhood diseases are : diarrhoea, respiratory infections, measles, pertussis, polio, neonatal tetanus, tuberculosis, and diphtheria. It is known that a child may get affected several times in a year; the incidence increases with the aggravation of a state of malnutrition. Of about 4 million deaths a year from acute respiratory infections in the developing world, a quarter are linked to malnutrition, and a further quarter associated with complications of measles, pertussis, malaria and HIV/AIDS. During 2018, about 8 per cent of under-five mortality worldwide was due to diarrhoeal diseases, about 12 per cent due to ARI, about 2 per cent deaths were due to measles and about 5 per cent due to malaria. In India, during the year 2020, 1,991 cases of diphtheria, 12,081 cases of measles, 11,985 cases of pertussis, and 162 cases of neonatal tetanus were reported *(60)*. The actual figures may be several times higher since there is considerable under-reporting. This is so, for example, in the case of eruptive fevers, malaria, intestinal parasites such as ascariasis, hookworm, giardiasis and amoebiasis etc. which are common because of poor environmental sanitation and paucity of potable drinking water. The prevention and treatment of children's illnesses may interrupt the transmission of infection in the community.

These few facts, which are merely examples and could be multiplied, show that the prevention and treatment of infections and parasitosis of children are bound to have important long-term consequences.

4. Accidents and poisoning

In the developed world, accidents and poisoning have become a relatively more important child health problem. There is every reason to believe that accidents among children are frequent in the developing countries also, especially burns and trauma as a result of home accidents and, to an increasing degree, traffic accidents. Children and young adolescents are particularly vulnerable to domestic accidents – including falls, burns, poisoning and drowning.

5. Behavioural problems

Behavioural disturbances are notable child health problem, the importance of which is increasingly recognized in most countries. Children abandoned by their families present severe social and health problems. Over 60,000 children are abandoned each year in India *(61)*.

6. Other factors affecting the health of children

a. Maternal health

A major determinant of child health is the health of his/ her mother. Child health is adversely affected (the risk begin to appear even before birth) if the mother is malnourished, if she is under 18 years (too young) or over 35 (too old), if her last child was born less than 2 years ago (too close), if she has already more than 4 births (too many) and if she is deprived of basic pregnancy care. A healthy mother brings forth a healthy baby, with better chances of survival.

b. Family

In pre-school years, the child is very much an organic part of the immediate family. Whatever happens to him or her affects the other members of the family, and vice versa. Therefore, "child health" has to be "family health". It depends upon the family's physical and social environment, which includes its lifestyle, customs, culture, traditional habits, and the childbearing and childrearing practices are greatly influenced by this. The family and social environment has a considerable influence on the development of speech, personality and the intellectual potentials of the small child. Other factors are the family size, the family relationships, and family stability. Infancy and early childhood is the time when the child contracts common contagious illness from contact with others (elder brothers and sisters, playmates, schoolmates). Data shows that the number of episodes of infectious diarrhoea increases with the size of the family. Studies also show an increase in the prevalence of malnutrition in families with more than 4 children. In short, fewer children would mean better nutrition, better health care, less morbidity and lower infant mortality.

c. Socio-economic circumstances

The socio-economic situation in which the family is placed is a very important factor in child health. In every region of the world, the physical and intellectual development of children varies with the family's socio-economic level. Under-privileged children of the same age are smaller, lighter and less advanced in psychomotor and intellectual performance, compared to children of privileged group. A detailed analysis of socio-economic factors shows the part played by the parents' education, profession and income, their housing, the urban or rural, industrialized or non-industrialized nature of the population.

Poverty, illiteracy (especially mothers' illiteracy) and sickness create a vicious circle spanning from one generation to the next, and from which it is difficult for the individual to escape. The differences in health between rich and poor, which can be observed in all age-groups are particularly striking among children.

d. Environment

After the first week of a child's life, the environmental factors play a very great role as determinants of infant and childhood morbidity and mortality. Tetanus infection of the newborn may take a heavy toll of the newborn in the first few weeks of life. Diarrhoea, pneumonia and other infections – bacterial, viral and parasitic – are extremely common in children exposed to insanitary and hostile environment. The stages at which these infections occur vary according to the ecological conditions, home and family hygiene, local epidemiological conditions and the extent to which they come into contact with earth, water and above all with adults and other children. An insufficient supply of safe water, inadequate disposal of human excreta and other waste, an abundance of insects and other disease carriers are among the environmental factors continuously menacing family health.

Another important factor which influences child development is environmental stimulations. Children also develop skills if they are given the opportunity. Stimulation, particularly the interaction with people who take interest and talk to them helps children to develop. Other sources of environmental stimulation are the radio, TV and illustrated magazines.

e. Social support and health care

Other factors affecting the health status of children include community and social support measures, ranging from creches and day care facilities to organized health care systems.

RIGHTS OF THE WOMEN AND CHILDREN

Women and children are the most vulnerable section of the society. It is, therefore, vital to improve their health and well-being in order to achieve complete development of overall human resources.

One of the core function assigned to the WHO in its Constitution of 1948 was to "promote maternal and child health and welfare". By the 1950s, national health plans and policy documents from development agencies invariably stressed that mothers and children were vulnerable groups and, therefore, priority "targets" for public health action. The notion of mother and children as vulnerable group was also central to the primary health care movement launched at Alma-Ata in 1978. The plight of mothers and children soon came to be seen as much more than a problem of biological vulnerability. The 1987 Call to Action for Safe Motherhood explicitly framed it as "deeply rooted in the adverse social, cultural and economic environment of the society, and specially the environment that societies create for women". Women's relative lack of decision-making power and their unequal access to employment, finances, education, basic health care and other resources are considered to be the root causes of their ill-health, and that of their children. The unfairness of this situation has made it obvious that the health of mothers and children is an issue of rights, entitlements and day to day struggle to secure these entitlements. The milestones in this establishment of the rights of women and children are as shown in Fig. 9 *(62)*.

1948 The Universal Declaration of Human Rights states that "motherhood and childhood are entitled to special care and assistance".

1952 The General Conference of the International Labour Organization adopts the Maternity Protection Convention.

1959 The Declaration of the Rights of the Child.

1966 The International Covenant on Economic, Social and Cultural Rights recognizes the right to the highest attainable standard of physical and mental health.

1981 The Convention on the Elimination of All Forms of Discrimination Against Women enjoins States parties to ensure appropriate maternal health services.

1989 The Convention on the Rights of the Child guarantees children's right to health. States commit themselves to ensuring appropriate maternal health services.

1990 At the United Nations World Summit on Children governments declare their "joint commitment... to give every child a better future", and recognize the link between women's rights and children's well-being.

1993 The United Nations Human Rights Committee expresses concern over high rates of maternal mortality.

1994 1995 The United Nations International Conference on Population and Development and the United Nations Fourth World Conference on Women affirm women's right of access to appropriate health care services in pregnancy and childbirth.

1996 The United Nations Human Rights Committee rules that, when abortion gives rise to a criminal penalty even if a woman is pregnant as a result of rape, a woman' right to be free from inhuman and degrading treatment might be violated.

2000 The United Nations Committee on Economic, Social and Cultural Rights states that measures are required to "Improve child and maternal health, sexual and reproductive health services".

2003 The United Nations Committee on the Rights of the Child states that adolescent girls should have access to information on the impact of early marriage and early pregnancy and have access to health services sensitive to their needs and rights.

The United Nations Committee on the Rights of the Child adopts its General Comment on HIV/AIDS and that on the Rights of the Child.

2003 The United Nations Commission on Human Rights, states that sexual and reproductive health are integral elements of the right to health.

2004 The United Nations Committee Against Torture calls for an end to the extraction of confession for prosecution purposes from women seeking emergency medical care as a result of illegal abortion. The United Nations Special Rapporteur on the Right to Health reports that all forms of sexual violence are inconsistent with the right to health.

2004 The United Nations Sub-Commission on the Promotion and Protection of Human Rights adopts a resolution on "harmful traditional practices affecting the health of women and the girl child".

FIG. 9
Milestones in the establishment of the rights of women and children

RIGHTS OF THE CHILD

One of the most encouraging signs of our times is the awakening of the public to the needs and rights of children. The needs of children and our duties towards them are enshrined in our Constitution; the relevant articles are :

a. Article 24 prohibits employment of children below the age of 14 in factories;
b. Article 39 prevents abuse of children of tender age; and
c. Article 45 provides for free and compulsory education for all children until they complete the age of 14 years.

In the country's Five Year Plans, special attention has been given to the welfare of children particularly the weaker sections. Various schemes have been introduced and implemented to achieve this goal. However, despite constitutional provisions, organized efforts for stepping up child welfare services did not take place until 1959.

UN DECLARATION OF THE RIGHTS OF THE CHILD

The year 1959 ushered in a new era in child welfare. To meet the special needs of the child, the General Assembly of the United Nations adopted on 20th November 1959, the Declaration of the Rights of the Child. India was a signatory to this Declaration. The Rights of the Child are :

1. Right to develop in an atmosphere of affection and security and, wherever possible, in the care and under the responsibility of his/her parents;
2. Right to enjoy the benefits of social security, including nutrition, housing and medical care;
3. Right to free education;
4. Right to full opportunity for play and recreation;
5. Right to a name and nationality;
6. Right to special care, if handicapped;
7. Right to be among the first to receive protection and relief in times of disaster;
8. Right to learn to be a useful member of society and to develop in a healthy and normal manner and in conditions of freedom and dignity;
9. Right to be brought up in a spirit of understanding, tolerance, friendship among people, peace and universal brotherhood; and
10. Right to enjoy these rights, regardless of race, colour, sex, religion, national or social origin.

UNIVERSAL CHILDREN'S DAY

November 14 is observed as Universal Children's Day. It was started by the International Union for Child Welfare and the UNICEF. In 1954, the UN General Assembly passed a formal resolution establishing Universal Children's Day and assigned to UNICEF the responsibility for promoting this annual day.

A non-governmental organization (Defence for Children International, Geneva) was set up in 1979 (during the International Year of the Child) to ensure ongoing, systematic international action specially directed towards promoting and protecting the Rights of the Child.

The 1990 World Summit for children agreed on a series of specific social goals for improving the lives of the children including measurable progress against malnutrition, preventable diseases and illiteracy. The vital vulnerable years of childhood should be given a first call on society's concerns and capacities. A child has only one chance to develop normally, and the protection of that one chance, therefore, demands the kind of commitment that will not be superseded by other priorities. The following are the goals that have been accepted by almost all nations.

Social goals for the year 2000 *(63)*

The end-of-century goals agreed to by the nations following the 1990 World Summit for children were :

1. A one-third reduction in 1990 under-five death rates (or to 70 per 1000 live births, whichever is less);
2. A halving of 1990 maternal mortality rates;
3. A halving of 1990 rates of malnutrition among the world's under-five (to include the elimination of micronutrient deficiencies, support for breast-feeding by all maternity units, and a reduction in the incidence of low birth weight to less than 10 per cent;
4. Achievement of 90 per cent immunization among under-ones, eradication of polio, elimination of neonatal tetanus, a 90 per cent reduction in measles cases and a 95 per cent reduction in measles deaths (compared to pre-immunization level);
5. A halving of child deaths caused by diarrhoeal disease;
6. A one-third reduction of child deaths from acute respiratory infections;
7. Basic education for all children and completion of primary education by at least 80 per cent girls as well as boys;
8. Clean water and safe sanitation for all communities;
9. Acceptance in all countries of the Convention on the Rights of Child, including improved protection for children in especially difficult circumstances; and
10. Universal access to high quality family planning information and services in order to prevent pregnancies that are too early, too closely spaced, too late or too many.

NATIONAL POLICY FOR CHILDREN

Keeping in view the constitutional provisions and the United Nations Declaration of the Rights of the Child, the Government of India adopted a National Policy for Children in August 1974. The Policy declares :

> *"It shall be the policy of the State to provide adequate services to children, both before and after birth and through the period of growth, to ensure their full physical, mental and social development. The State shall progressively increase the scope of such services so that, within a reasonable time, all children in the country enjoy optimum conditions for their balanced growth".*

According to the Declaration, the development of children has been considered an integral part of national development. The Policy recognizes children as the "nation's supremely important asset" and declares that the nation is responsible for their "nurture and solicitude". It further spells out various measures to be adopted and priorities to be assigned to children's programmes with a focus on areas like child health, child nutrition and welfare of the handicapped and destitute children.

A high level National Children's Board with the Prime Minister as Chairman was established. It provides a forum where problems relating to child welfare and their purposeful development into useful members of society are evolved, reviewed and coordinated into an effective programme *(64)*.

Following the enunciation of the National Policy for Children, a number of programmes were introduced by the Government of India, viz. The ICDS Scheme, programmes of supplementary feeding, nutrition education and production of nutritious food, constitution of the "National Children's Fund" under the Charitable Endowments Act, 1980, institution of National Awards for Child Welfare, Welfare of the Handicapped *(65)*.

Review of existing policies and legislations *(66)*

The Constitution of India follows the principle of protective discrimination and thereby commits itself to safeguard the rights of children through policies, laws and action. These commitments are reflected through the national polices which are as follows :

1. *National Policy for Children, 1974* provides the conceptual basis for an integrated approach to address the whole child and commits the State to provide adequate services to children, both before and after birth and through the period of growth, to ensure their full physical, mental and social development.
2. *National Policy on Education, 1986* and its *National Plan of Action*, which has a full section on early childhood care and education. It clearly recognizes the holistic nature of child development, and that ECCE is the crucial foundation for human resource development and cumulative lifelong learning. It is viewed as a feeder and support programme for universal elementary education – especially for first generation learners, and an important support service for working mothers and girls.
3. *The National Children's Fund* was created during the international year of the child in 1979 under the Charitable Endowment Fund Act, 1890. The fund provides financial assistance to voluntary agencies for implementing programmes for the welfare of children including rehabilitation of destitute children.
4. *National Health Policy, 2002* accords primacy to preventive and first line curative care at primary health level, and emphasizes convergence, and strategies to change care behaviours in families and communities.
5. *National Charter for Children, 2003* intends to secure for every child its inherent right to be a child and enjoy a healthy and happy childhood, to address the root causes that negate the healthy growth and development of children, and to awaken the conscience of the community in the wider societal context to protect children from all forms of abuse, while strengthening the family, society and the nation.

   The national charter for children affirms India's commitment to the child. However, it does not declare India's acceptance of children's entitlements as their rights. The national policy for children, 1974 still stands as the official policy commitment to children of India. With India's accession to the UNCRC and its two optional protocols rights based framework has been accepted as the guiding frame for policy measures and programming for children. This is clearly reflected in the national plan of action for children, 2005.
6. *Commission for the Protection of Child Rights Act, 2005* provides for the constitution of a national commission and state commissions for protection of child rights and children's courts for providing speedy trial of offences against children or of violation of child rights and for matters connected therewith or incidental thereto.
7. *National Plan of Action for Children, 2005* articulates clearly the rights, perspective, and agenda for the development of children. It provides a robust framework within which to promote the development and protection of children. The guiding principles of the NPAC are :

   a. To regard the child as an asset and a person with human rights;
   b. To address issues of discriminiation emanating from biases of gender, class, caste, race, religion and legal status in order to ensure equality;
   c. To accord utmost priority to the most disadvantaged, poorest of the poor and the least served child in all policy and programme interventions; and
   d. To recognize the diverse stages and settings of childhood, and address the needs of each, providing all children the entitlements that fulfill their rights and meet their needs in each situation.

   Time targets in the NPAC 2005 extend to 2012, the end-year of the Eleventh Plan. The NPAC 2005 has identified 12 key priority areas for the highest and most sustained attention in terms of outreach, programme interventions and resource allocations. These are :

   – Reducing infant mortality rate.
   – Reducing maternal mortality rate.
   – Reducing malnutrition among children.
   – Achieving 100% civil registration of births.
   – Universalization of early childhood care and development and quality education for all children achieving 100% access and retention in schools, including pre-schools.
   – Complete abolition of female foeticide, female infanticide and child marriage and ensuring the survival, development and protection of the girl child.
   – Improving water and sanitation coverage in both rural and urban areas.
   – Addressing and upholding the rights of children in difficult circumstances.
   – Securing for all children all legal and social protection, from all kinds of abuse, exploitation and neglect.
   – Complete abolition of child labour with the aim of progressively eliminating all forms of economic exploitation of children.
   – Monitoring, review, and reform of policies, programmes and laws to ensure protection of children's interest and rights.
   – Ensuring child participation and choice in matters and decisions affecting their lives.

   A new alienation of children from their rights has arisen with the plight of children affected by HIV/AIDS. Since the finalization of the NPAC the issues of these children have also been accepted as key priorities by MWCD and therefore found a place in the Eleventh Plan among critical concerns that need to be addressed.
8. *Integrated Child Protection Scheme (ICPS) (67, 68)*

   During the year 2009-10, the Ministry of Women and Child Development launched a new centrally sponsored scheme called "Integrated Child Protection Scheme" (ICPS) with a view to create a safe and secure environment in the country for the comprehensive development of children who are in need of care and protection, children in conflict and in contact with law (either as a victim or as a witness or due to any other circumstances), children of migrant families, children of prisoners, prostitutes, working children, street children, trafficked or sexually exploited children, child drug abusers, child beggars etc.

The objectives of the scheme are : (1) Improve access to and quality of child protection services; (2) Raise public awareness about child rights; (3) Clearly articulated responsibilities and accountability for child protection; (4) Establish structures at all government levels for delivery of statutory and support services to children in difficult circumstances; and (5) Setting-up of an evidence based monitoring and evaluation system.

The services provided under ICPS are as follows :

(1) Emergency outreach service through 'Child line', dedicated number is 1098. It is a 24-hour toll free telephone service available to all children in distress.
(2) Open shelters for children in need, in urban and semi-urban areas.
(3) Family based non-institutional care through sponsorship, foster-care, adoption, cradle baby centres and after-care.
(4) Institutional services through shelter homes, children homes, observation homes, special homes, and specialized services for children with special needs.
(5) Web-enabled child protection management system including website for missing children.
(6) General grant-in-aid for need based interventions.

9. *National Policy for Children 2013 (NPC) (69)*

The National Policy for Children 2013 is a long term sustainable, multi-sectoral, and integrated approach for the development and protection of children i.e. 0–18 years age group. Survival, health, nutrition, development, education, protection and participation are the key priorities of the policy. It reiterates the State's commitment to ensure equitable access to essential, preventive, promotive, curative and rehabilitative health care for all children. Towards this goal, NPC envisages that state shall take measures to :

- Improve maternal health care (pre-natal, natal, post-natal);
- Provide universal access to services for informed choices related to births and spacing;
- Address key causes of child mortality through appropriate interventions including access to safe drinking water and sanitation;
- To improve new born and child care practices;
- To protect children from water borne, blood borne, vector borne, communicable and other childhood diseases by providing universal and affordable access to appropriate services;
- Prevent disabilities, physical and mental through timely measures to take pre-natal, natal, peri-natal and post-natal care of mother and child;
- Ensure availability of services, support and provisions for nutritive attainment in a life cycle approach with focus on infant and young child feeding (IYCF) practices and on the health and nutrition needs of adolescent girls and other vulnerable groups;
- Prevent HIV infections at birth and ensure proper treatment to infected children; and
- Provide the adolescents access to information regarding ill effects of alcohol and substance use, and support for the choice of healthy life style.

The state commits to allocate the required financial, material and human resources for the implementation of NPC 2013. The Ministry of Women & Child Development is the nodal ministry for implementation of NPC.

10. *Protection of Children from Sexual Offences (POCSO) Act, 2012*

In order to effectively address the heinous crime of sexual abuse and sexual exploitation of children through less ambiguous and more stringent legal provisions, the Ministry of Women and Child Development introduced the Protection of Children from Sexual Offences (POCSO) Act, 2012.

The Act defines a child as any person below 18 years of age and regards the best interest and well-being of a child as being of paramount importance at every stage, to ensure a healthy physical, emotional, intellectual and social development of the child. It defines different forms of sexual abuse, including penetrative and non-penetrative assault, as well as sexual harassment and pornography, and deems a sexual assault to be "aggravated" under certain circumstances, such as when abused child is mentally ill or when the abuse is committed by a person in a position of trust or authority vis-a-vis the child, like a family member, police officer, teacher or doctor. People who traffic children for sexual purpose are also punishable under the provisions relating to abetment in the said Act *(70)*.

An ordinance providing the death penalty for rapist of girls below 12 years of age "The Criminal Law Amendment Ordinance, 2018" was promulgated. The salient features of the Ordinance are:

a. Minimum punishment for rape made 10 years;
b. Minimum punishment of 20 years to a person committing rape on a girl aged below 16 years;
c. Minimum punishment of 20 years rigorous imprisonment and maximum death penalty / life imprisonment for committing rape on a girl aged below 12 years,
d. Police officer committing rape anywhere shall be awarded rigorous imprisonment of minimum 10 years;
e. Investigation of rape cases to be completed within 2 months;
f. Appeals in rape cases to be disposed within 6 months; and
g. No anticipatory bail can be granted to a person accused of rape of girl of age less than 16 years.

The POCSO Act 2012 was further amended in the year 2019 with insertion of the following clause :

Under the Act, a person is guilty of using a child for pornographic purposes if he uses a child in any form of media for the purpose of sexual gratification. The Act also penalises persons who use children for pornographic purposes resulting in sexual assault. The Bill defines child pornography as any visual depiction of sexually explicit conduct involving a child including photograph, video, digital or computer generated image indistinguishable from an actual child. The punishment is minimum 5 years in Jail. The Act penalises storage of pornographic material for commercial purposes with a punishment of upto three years, or a fine or both *(71)*.

The POCSO amendment Bill 2020 proposes that child offenders between 15 and 18 years of age should be covered under the ambit of the POCSO Act 2012 and be given the same punishment as is given to adults *(72)*.

The growing vulnerability of children in urban settlements, including those caught in the shifting frame of migratory and transient labour are also now in the MWCD portfolio. Their distress and the difficult circumstances of their childhoods merit special measures of development and protection.

11. *National Plan of Action for Children, 2016*

The Government of India adopted a new National Plan of Action for Children (NPAC) 2016 which is based on the principles embedded in earlier Action Plan. The Action Plan has four key priority areas: survival, health and nutrition; education and development; protection and participation. The NPAC seeks to ensure convergence of ongoing programmes and initiation of new programmes so as to focus on objectives through well-defined strategies and activities to achieve desired level of outcome for children.

Goals and targets set by Government of India for child health under various national and international commitments are as follows *(66)* :

CHILD HEALTH GOALS/TARGETS

Common Minimum Programme	To raise public spending on health to at least 2-3% of GDP over the next five years and focus on primary health care ...special attention will be paid to the poorer sections in the matter of health care.
Twelfth Five Year Plan 2012–17	– Reduction of infant mortality rates to 25 per thousand live births by 2017. – To raise the sex ratio for age group 0–6 from 914 to 950 by 2017. Prevention and reduction of under-nutrition in children under 3 years to half of NFHS-3 (2005–06) levels.
National Plan of Action for Children, 2005	– To reduce infant mortality rate to below 30 per 1000 live births by 2010. – To reduce child mortality rate to below 31 per 1000 live births by 2010. – To reduce neonatal mortality rate to below 18 per 1000 live births by 2010. – To explore possibilities of covering all children with plan for health insurance.
Millennium Development Goals (MDG)	– Reduce by two-thirds, between 1990 and 2015, the under-five mortality rate (Goal 4). – Reduce by three-quarters, between 1990 and 2015, the maternal mortality rate. – Combat HIV/AIDS, malaria and other diseases.
National Health Policy, 2017	– Reduce under five mortality to 23 per 1000 live births by 2025. – Reduce infant mortality rate to 28 by 2019. – Reduce neo-natal mortality to 16 and stillbirth rate to "single digit" by 2025. – Increase life expectancy at birth from 67.5 to 70 years by 2025. – Reduce prevalence of blindness to 0.25/1000 by 2025, and reduce disease burden by one third from current level. – Achieve global target of HIV/AIDS of 90–90–90 by 2020. – Achieve and maintain a cure rate of > 85% in new sputum positive patients of TB and reach elimination level by 2025. – Achieve and maintain elimination status of leprosy by 2018, Kala-azar by 2017 and lymphatic filariasis in endemic pockets by 2017. – Antenatal coverage and skilled birth attendance at birth above 90 per cent by 2025. – More than 90 per cent full immunization by one year of age by 2025. – Reduction of 40 per cent in prevalence of stunting of under-five children by 2025. – Access to safe water and sanitation to all by 2020.
NITI Aayog Three Year Action Agenda 2017-18 to 2019-20	– Reduce infant mortality rate to 30/1000 live births by 2020. – Reduce under 5 mortality rate to 38/1000 live births by 2020. – Reduce incidence of TB to 130/100,000 by 2020. – Eliminate Kala-azar and lymphatic filariasis.
Global Strategy for Women's, Children's and Adolescent Health (2016–2030) with 2030 Sustainable Development Agenda	– By 2030, end all forms of malnutrition (stunting and wasting in children under 5 years of age). – By 2030, end preventable deaths of newborns and children under 5 years of age, with all countries aiming to reduce neonatal mortality to atleast as low as 12 per 1000 live births and under five mortality to at least as low as 25 per 1000 live births.

DELIVERING THE MCH SERVICES

MCH (mother and child health) is not a new speciality. It is a method of delivering health care to special group in the population which is especially vulnerable to disease, disability or death. These groups (i.e., children under the age 5 years and women in the reproductive age group (15–44 years) comprise about 32.4 per cent of the total population in India.

The MCH services encompass the curative, preventive and social aspects of obstetrics, paediatrics, family welfare, nutrition, child development and health education. The **specific objectives** of MCH are :

1. reduction of morbidity and mortality rates for mothers and children;
2. promotion of reproductive health; and
3. promotion of the physical and psychological development of the child within the family.

Through concern with child development and the health education of parents and children, the ultimate objective of MCH services is life-long health.

Sub-areas

The components of MCH include the following sub-areas:

a. maternal health
b. family planning
c. child health

d. school health
e. handicapped children
f. care of the children in special settings such as day care centres.

The content of MCH care will vary according to the demographic, social and economic patterns. Factors such as urbanization, rural migration, changing patterns of women's work and status have far-reaching effects on childbearing and child-rearing. It is now generally accepted that the MCH services should always be flexible and based on, and adapted to the local needs and resources of the community it serves; they should be moulded to the local traditions, cultures and other environmental characteristics and cannot be modelled on patterns copied from other countries. Health care, social legislation and social support measures also will have to be adapted to these changing needs and problems of the community.

MCH care is now conceived of as all activities which promote health and prevent or solve health problems of mother and children, irrespective of whether they are curative, diagnostic, preventive or rehabilitative, and whether they are carried out in health centres or in the home by primary health care workers, traditional dais, or highly trained specialists.

Recent trends in MCH care

Maternal and child care was traditionally designed and provided in the form of vertical programmes with "standard" technical content based on models from a few developed countries. Applied in different socio-economic situations, such vertical programmes have been unable to provide more than minimum coverage because of their cost, and they have scarcely been of a kind to solve the priority problems of the majority of mothers and children. The emergence of some new concepts is now changing the organization and management of MCH care in increasing number of countries. These are discussed below :

1. Integration of care

Conventional MCH services tended to be fragmented into antenatal care, postnatal care, infant care, family planning etc. The various components were dealt with separately by different staff or departments. This approach has changed over the years. The trend now is an "integrated" approach. This integration is based on the fact that it is inconvenient for the mother to go to one place to receive care for herself, to another for care for her children, and yet another for family planning services.

An integrated approach implies that all those involved in maternity care from the obstetrician down to the local dai, must work as a team. Obstetric and paediatric units should be closely linked so that there can be regular contact between obstetricians, paediatricians, community physicians, health and social workers so that services for the care of the mother and the child in the hospital and community be planned and reviewed including teaching and research. This approach helps to promote continuity of care as well as improves efficiency and effectiveness of MCH care.

2. Risk approach

A promising means of improving the coverage and efficiency of MCH care and family planning is the "risk approach". This is a managerial tool for better use of scarce resources. It is based on the early detection of mothers and children with high-risk factors. All mothers and children with high risk factors are given additional and more skilled care including hospitalization, while at the same time essential care is provided for the rest of the mothers and children so that every one gets care appropriate to their need.

It is also possible to assess the "degrees" of risk of each factor, by scoring according to their (a) *magnitude* – i.e., extent and severity; (b) *treatability* – responsiveness to treatment and control; (c) *cost-effect* – in terms of alleviating human suffering; and (d) *community attitude* – social concern. Such an approach when applied on a community-wide basis enables the determination of priority activities, within the MCH programme based on the "degrees" of risk.

Application of the risk approach to the problems of mothers and children is a departure from past or traditional practices to promote the health of mothers and children.

3. Manpower changes

The special category of "maternal and child health worker" (e.g., auxiliary-nurse-midwives, health visitors) at the peripheral level is gradually being phased out. A wide range of workers are now considered necessary for maternal and child health work. They include :

(i) *Professionals :* Specialists
(ii) *Field workers :* Multi-purpose workers, Health Guides, dais (traditional birth attendants), Bal Sevikas, Anganwadi workers, extension workers, ASHA etc
(iii) *Voluntary workers :* Members of women's organizations

Taking for example, the local dais in the past were not generally recognized by the national health authorities, who thought that their services were inimical to the safety of the mother and child. The current trend is to assist them perform safe deliveries through training and supervision. In India, where 70 per cent of population lives in rural areas, there are not enough obstetricians to attend to all deliveries. Therefore, a trained dai or midwife is absolutely essential in every village. The same thing can be said about paediatrics. It is now recognized that obstetric and paediatric services can only be improved by cooperation and liaison with these practitioners.

4. Primary health care

Primary health care is now recognized as a way of making essential health care available to all. It has all the elements necessary to make a positive impact on the health of mothers and children – i.e., MCH care, family planning, control of infections, education about health problems and how to prevent them, and measures to ensure nutritious food – all closely related. Primary health care emphasizes family oriented care and support, and community self-reliance in health matters. MCH care is an indispensable priority element of primary health care in every country.

Targets for MCH Services

From time to time Government of India has suggested MCH goals with quantifiable time bound targets for achievement. Table 11 shows the MCH indicators with their goal period and the current level of achievement.

Organization of MCH/FP services

The mother and child health, and family planning services were integrated in the Fourth Five Year Plan for better effectiveness. They both are now an integral part of primary health care, which places emphasis on community participation and intersectoral coordination. The National Health Policy 2002 and National Population Policy 2000 has provided the necessary directives for reorienting and

TABLE 11

MCH goals and current level of achievement (India)

Indicator	Current level	Goals and target period		
		Three Year Action Agenda of Niti Ayog (2018-19-20)	National Health Policy 2017	Sustainable Development Goals (2030)
A. Family Planning Indicators				
Crude birth rate	19.5 (2020)	–	21	–
Total fertility rate	2.0 (2020)	2.1	2.1 by 2025	–
Couple protection rate (%)	67.0 (2015–19)	–	Meet all needs	–
B. Mortality indicators per 1000				
Infant mortality	28 (2020)	30	< 28 by 2019	–
Neonatal mortality	20 (2020)	–	16 by 2025	< 12
Maternal mortality per 100,000	97 (2018–2020)	120	100 by 2020	70
Under-5 mortality	32 (2020)	38	23 by 2025	≤ 25
C. Services (% coverage)				
Infants immunized (2020)		–	> 90 by 2025	
– $Measles_2$	81	–	–	
– DPT_3	85	–	–	
– $Polio_3$	85	–	–	
– BCG	85	–	–	
– $HepB_3$	85	–	–	
– Hib_3	85	–	–	
– Rotavirus	82	–	–	
– PCV_3	90	–	–	
Pregnant women TT	90	–	–	
Antenatal care coverage %	(2015–2020)	–	100	
at least once	79.0			
at least four times	51.0		90	
Institutional deliveries	88.6 (2019–2021)	–	80	
Deliveries by trained personnel	81.0 (2013–2018)	–	100	
D. Prevalence of low-birth-weight babies	28 (2011–2016)	–	–	

Source : *(73, 74)*

restructuring the health services, based on primary health care approach with short and long-term goals.

The infrastructure in rural areas is based on the complex of community health centres, primary health centres and their subcentres. They provide preventive and promotive health care services. Since deliveries by trained health personnels are crucial in reducing maternal and infant mortality in rural areas, the government of India undertook a scheme to train local dais to conduct safe deliveries. These dais are now available in most villages. Mention must be made of ICDS (Integrated Child Development Services) projects which are functioning all over the country providing a package of basic health services (eg. supplementary nutrition, immunization, health check-up, referral, nutrition and health education, and non-formal education services) to mother and children.

Maternal health care was a part of family welfare programme from its inception. Interventions were introduced on vertical schemes, but family planning remained a separate intervention. In 1992, the Child Survival and Safe Motherhood Programme integrated all the schemes for better compliance. More recently, Reproductive and Child Health Programme was launched in 1997, which integrated family planning, Child Survival and Safe Motherhood Programme, Preventive management of STD/RTI, AIDS, and a client approach to health care. This programme has entered into phase II, with reorientation to make it consistant with the requirement of the National Rural Health Mission.

In urban areas, the general trend is towards institutional delivery. In larger cities, almost 90 per cent of deliveries take place in maternity hospitals and maternity homes. Some of the institutions are under the auspices of the Municipal Corporations and voluntary organizations. The services of obstetricians are available at district hospitals, which are the apical hospitals for MCH care at the district level. For specialized care of children, paediatric units have been established in several district hospitals.

Table 12 shows the evolution of maternal and child health programmes in India.

TABLE 12

Evolution of maternal and child health programmes in India

Year	Milestones
1952	Family Planning programme adopted by Government of India (GOI)
1961	Department of Family Planning created in Ministry of Health
1971	Medical Termination of Pregnancy Act (MTP Act), 1971
1977	Renaming of Family Planning to Family Welfare
1978	Expanded Programme on Immunization (EPI)
1985	Universal Immunization Programme (UIP) + National Oral Rehydration Therapy (ORT) Programme
1992	Child Survival and Safe Motherhood Programme (CSSM)
1996	Target-free approach
1997	Reproductive and Child Health Programme-1 (RCH-1)
2005	Reproductive and Child Health Programme-2 (RCH-2)
2005	National Rural Health Mission
2013	RMNCH+A Strategy
2013	National Health Mission
2014	India Newborn Action Plan (INAP)
2021	NMNCAH+N Strategy

Source : *(75)*

INDICATORS OF MCH CARE

Maternal and child health status is assessed through measurements of mortality, morbidity, growth and development. In many countries, mortality rates are still the only source of information. Morbidity data are scarce and poorly standardized. In recent years, attention has been paid to systematizing the collection, interpretation and dissemination of data on growth and development. The commonly used mortality indicators of MCH care are :

1. Maternal mortality ratio
2. Mortality in infancy and childhood
   a. Perinatal mortality rate
   b. Neonatal mortality rate
   c. Post-neonatal mortality rate
   d. Infant mortality rate
   e. 1–4 year mortality rate
   f. Under-5 mortality rate
   g. Child survival rate.

MATERNAL MORTALITY RATIO

According to WHO, a maternal death is defined as "the death of a woman while pregnant or within 42 days of termination of pregnancy, irrespective of the duration and site of pregnancy, from any cause related to or aggravated by the pregnancy or its management but not from unintentional or incidental causes" *(1)*.

This definition allows identification of a maternal death, based on the cause of the death being identified as either a direct or indirect maternal cause. It is calculated as :

$$= \frac{\text{Total no. of female deaths due to complications of pregnancy, childbirth or within 42 days of delivery from "puerperal causes" in an area during a given year}}{\text{Total no. of live births in the same area and year}} \times 1000 \text{ (or } 100{,}000)$$

Direct obstetric deaths (or direct maternal deaths) : those resulting from obstetric complications of the pregnant state (pregnancy, labour and puerperium), from interventions, omissions, incorrect treatment, or from a chain of events resulting from any of the above. Deaths due to obstetric haemorrhage or hypertensive disorders in pregnancy, for example, or those due to complications of anaesthesia or caesarean section are classified as direct maternal deaths *(1)*.

Indirect obstetric deaths (or indirect maternal deaths) : those resulting from previous existing disease or disease that developed during pregnancy and which was not due to direct obstetric causes, but which was aggravated by physiological effects of pregnancy. For example, deaths due to aggravation (by pregnancy) of an existing cardiac or renal disease are considered indirect maternal deaths.

The maternal mortality rate, the direct obstetric rate and the indirect obstetric rate are fine measures of the quality of maternity services.

Late maternal death : It is "the death of a woman from direct or indirect obstetric causes, after more than 42 days but less than one year after termination of pregnancy" *(1)*. Like maternal deaths, late maternal deaths also include both direct and indirect maternal/obstetric deaths. Complications of pregnancy or childbirth can lead to death beyond the six-week (42 day) postpartum period, and the increased availability of modern life-sustaining procedures and technologies enables more women to survive adverse outcomes of pregnancy and delivery, and also delays some deaths beyond that postpartum period. Specific codes for "late maternal deaths", are included in the ICD-10 (096 and 097) to capture these delayed maternal deaths, which may not be categorized as maternal deaths in civil registration and vital statistics systems despite being caused by pregnancy-related events.

Maternal deaths and late maternal deaths are combined in the 11th revision of the ICD under the new grouping of "comprehensive maternal deaths".

Pregnancy-related death (also known as death occurring during pregnancy, childbirth and puerperium) : is defined as "The death of a woman while pregnant or within 42 days of termination of pregnancy, irrespective of the cause of death (obstetric and non-obstetric)"; this definition includes unintentional/accidental and incidental causes. This definition allows measurement of deaths that occur during pregnancy, childbirth and puerperium while acknowledging that such measurements do not strictly conform to the standard "maternal death" concept in settings where accurate information about causes of death based on medical certification is unavailable *(1)*.

The number of maternal deaths in a population (during a specified time period, usually one calendar year) reflects two factors: (i) the risk of mortality associated with a single pregnancy or a single birth (whether live birth or stillbirth); and (ii) the fertility level (i.e. the number of pregnancies or births that are experienced by women of reproductive age, i.e. age 15–49 years).

Maternal mortality ratio (MMR) : is defined as the number of maternal deaths during a given time period per 100,000 live births during the same time period; thus, it quantifies the risk of maternal death relative to the number of live births, and essentially captures the first factor mentioned above *(1)*.

Maternal mortality rate (MMRate) : is defined and calculated as the number of maternal deaths divided by person-years lived by women of reproductive age in a population. The MMRate captures both the risk of maternal death per pregnancy or per birth (whether live birth or stillbirth), and the level of fertility in the population (i.e. both factors mentioned above) *(1)*.

Adult lifetime risk of maternal death : for women in the population, is defined as the probability that a 15 year-old girl (in the year of the estimate) will eventually die from a maternal cause. This indicator takes into account competing causes of death *(1)*.

The proportion of maternal deaths of women of reproductive age (PM) : The number of maternal deaths in a given time period divided by the total deaths, among women aged 15–49 years.

The 43rd World Assembly in 1990 adopted the recommendation that countries consider the inclusion on death certificates of questions regarding current pregnancy and pregnancy within one year preceding death in order to improve the quality of maternal mortality data and provide alternative methods of collecting data on deaths during pregnancy or related to it, as well as to encourage the recording of deaths from obstetric causes occurring more than 42 days following termination of pregnancy.

Approaches for measuring maternal mortality (1)

In the absence of complete and accurate civil registration systems, MMR estimates are based upon a variety of methods :

(1) Civil registration systems : This approach involves routine registration of births and deaths. Ideally, maternal mortality statistics should be obtained through civil registration data.

(2) Household survey : Where civil registration data are not available, household survey provides an alternative.

(3) Sisterhood methods : Sisterhood methods obtain information by interviewing a representative sample of respondents about the survival of all their adult sisters (to determine the number of ever married sisters, how many are alive, how many are dead, and how many died during pregnancy, delivery, or within six weeks of pregnancy.

(4) Reproductive-age mortality studies (RAMOS) : This approach involves identifying and investigating the causes of all deaths of women of reproductive age in a defined area/population by using multiple sources of data.

(5) Verbal autopsy : This approach is used to assign cause of death through interview with family or community members, where medical certification of cause of death is not available. Records of births and deaths are collected periodically among small populations, under demographic surveillance systems maintained by the research institutions in developing countries.

(6) Census : A national census, with the addition of a limited number of questions, could produce estimates of maternal mortality; this approach eliminates sampling errors and hence allows a more detailed breakdown of the results, including time trends, geographic subdivisions and social strata.

Incidence

WORLD SCENARIO

The methodology employed by the Maternal Mortality Estimation Inter-Agency Group to estimate 1990–2015 maternal mortality ratio followed an improved approach referred to as Bayesian maternal mortality estimation model or BMat model. These results supersede all previously published estimates for the years within that time period and differences with previously published estimates should not be interpreted as representing time trends *(1)*.

An estimated 295,000 maternal deaths occurred globally in 2017, yielding an overall MMR of 211 (199–243) maternal deaths per 100,000 live births. The global adult life-time risk of maternal mortality (i.e. the probability that a 15 years old woman will die eventually from a maternal cause) is approximately 1 in 190 for the year 2017. For the purpose of categorization, MMR is considered to be high if it is 300–499, very high if it is 500–999, and extremely high if it is $\geq$ 1000 maternal deaths per 100,000 live births *(1)*.

MMR in the world's least developed countries is high, estimated at 415 maternal deaths per 100,000 live births which is more than 40 times higher than MMR in Europe (10), and almost 60 times higher than in Australia and New Zealand *(7)*. The lifetime risk of maternal death in least developed countries is 1 in 56, Sub Saharan Africa is the only Region with very high MMR for 2017, estimated at 542 with life time risk of maternal death at 1 in 37. Three countries namely, South Sudan (1150), Chad (1140) and Sierra Leone (1120) fall under extremely high MMR in 2017. Nigeria (67000) and India (35000) had the highest estimated number of maternal deaths accounting for approximately 35 per cent of estimated global maternal deaths *(1)*.

Between 2000 and 2017, the sub-region of South Asia achieved the greatest percentage reduction in MMR, i.e. from 384 to 157 (59 per cent). Central Asia (52 per cent), Eastern Asia (50 per cent), Europe (53 per cent), and Northern Africa (54 per cent) halved their MMR during that period.

A woman is most vulnerable at the post-partum period. About 50–70 per cent maternal deaths occur in the postpartum period of which 45 per cent deaths occur in the first 24 hours after delivery and more than two-thirds during the first week. Between 11–17 per cent of maternal deaths occur during child birth itself *(76)*.

Maternal mortality ratios strongly reflect the overall effectiveness of health systems, which in many low-income developing countries suffer from weak administrative, technical and logistical capacity, inadequate financial investment and a lack of skilled health personnel. Scaling up key interventions – for example, increasing the number of births attended by skilled health personnel, providing access to emergency obstetric care when necessary and providing post-natal care for mothers and babies – could sharply reduce both maternal and neonatal deaths. Enhancing women's access to family planning, adequate nutrition, improved water and sanitation facilities and affordable basic health care protection from abuse, violence, discrimination, empowerment of women, greater involvement of men in maternal and child care, would lower mortality rates further still. These are not impossible, impractical actions, but proven, cost-effective provisions that women of reproductive age have a right to expect.

The low status of women in the society coupled with their low literacy levels prevent the women from taking antenatal care even if services are available. Most deliveries take place at home without the services of the trained midwifery personnel. There is an inverse relationship between lifetime risk of maternal death and the availability of the trained health worker during pregnancy and at the time of delivery.

It is a tragic situation as these deaths are not caused by disease but occurred during or after a natural process. It is one of the leading cause of death for women of reproductive age in many parts of the world. Most maternal deaths and pregnancy complications can be prevented if pregnant women have access to good-quality antenatal, natal and postnatal care, and if certain harmful birth practices are avoided. Estimates of antenatal care coverage, deliveries conducted by skilled personnel, lifetime risk of maternal death and maternal mortality ratio in some developing and developed countries are shown in Table 13.

Maternal health, however, goes beyond the survival of pregnant women and mothers. For every woman who dies from causes related to pregnancy or childbirth, it is estimated that there are 20 others who suffer pregnancy-related illness or experience other severe consequences. The number is striking: An estimated 10 million women annually who survive their pregnancies experience such adverse outcomes.

Causes

Maternal deaths mostly occur from the third trimester to the first week after birth (with the exception of deaths due to complications of abortion). Studies show that mortality risks for mothers are particularly elevated within the first two days after birth. Most maternal deaths are related to obstetric complications – including postpartum haemorrhage, infections, eclampsia and prolonged or obstructed labour – and complications of abortion. Most of these direct causes of maternal mortality can be readily addressed if skilled health

TABLE 13

Maternal mortality ratio, deliveries conducted by skilled personnel, antenatal care coverage and lifetime risk of maternal deaths in some developing and developed countries.

Country	Antenatal care coverage (%) (2013–2018)		Deliveries conducted by skilled personnel (%) (2012–2021)	Lifetime risk maternal death (one in) (2017)	Maternal mortality ratio (per 100,000 live births) (2020)
	At least once	At least four times			
India	79	51	81	290	97 (2018–2020)
Bangladesh	64	31	59	250	173
Bhutan	98	85	96	250	183
Indonesia	98	77	95	240	177
Myanmar	81	59	60	190	195
Nepal	84	69	77	186	220
Thailand	99	90	99	1,900	37
Sri Lanka	99	93	100	1,300	36
Pakistan	86	51	71	140	188
China	100	81	100	2,100	29
Japan	100	100	100	16,700	5
Singapore	100	100	100	9,900	8
UK	–	–	99	8,400	7
USA	–	97	99	3,000	19
World	87	59	84	190	211

Source : *(59)*

personnel are on hand and key drugs, equipment and referral facilities are available.

About 80 per cent of maternal deaths are due to direct causes i.e. obstetric complications of pregnancy, labour and puerperium to interventions or incorrect treatment. As shown in Fig. 10 the single most common cause-accounting for a quarter of all maternal deaths – is obstetric haemorrhage, generally occurring postpartum which can lead to death very rapidly in the absence of prompt life-saving care.

Puerperal infections, often the consequence of poor hygiene during delivery, or untreated reproductive tract infections account for about 15% of maternal mortality. Such infections can be easily prevented. Hypertensive disorders of pregnancy, particularly eclampsia (convulsions), result in about 13% of all maternal deaths. They can be prevented through careful monitoring during pregnancy and

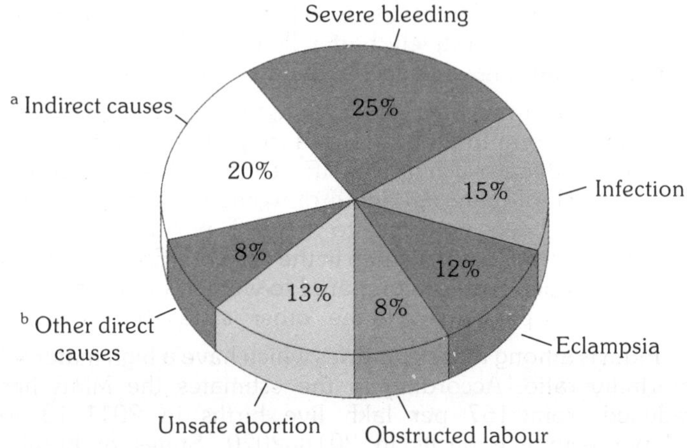

[a] Indirect causes including for example: anaemia, malaria, heart diseases

[b] Other direct causes including, for example : ectopic pregnancy, embolism, anaesthesia-related

FIG. 10
Causes of maternal deaths worldwide

treatment with relatively simple anticonvulsant drugs in cases of eclampsia.

Of the estimated 210 million pregnancies that occur every year, about 42 million end in induced abortion, of which only approximately 60 per cent are carried out under safe conditions. More than 20 million induced abortions each year are performed by people lacking the necessary skills or in an environment lacking the minimal medical standards, or both.

Around 8% of maternal deaths occur as a result of prolonged or obstructed labour. Other direct causes include ectopic pregnancies, embolism and deaths related to interventions. Around 20 per cent of maternal deaths are due to indirect causes, that is, the result of pre-existing diseases or disease that developed during pregnancy, which are not due to direct obstetric cause but are aggravated by the physiological effect of pregnancy. One of the most significant is anaemia, which can cause death. Maternal anaemia affects about half of all pregnant women. Pregnant adolescents are more prone to anaemia than older women, and they often receive less care. Infectious diseases such as malaria, and intestinal parasites can exacerbate anaemia, as can poor quality diet – all of which heighten vulnerability to maternal death. Severe anaemia contributes to the risk of death in cases of haemorrhage. Other important causes of indirect death are hepatitis, cardiovascular diseases, diseases of the endocrine and metabolic system and infections such as tuberculosis, malaria and increasingly HIV/AIDS *(77)*. Each year, approximately 50 million women living in malaria-endemic countries throughout the world become pregnant. Around 10,000 of these women die as a result of malaria *(78)*.

Social correlates

A number of social factors influence maternal mortality. The important ones are : (a) *Women's age* : The optimal child-bearing years are between the ages of 20 and 30 years. The further away from this age range, the greater the risks of a woman dying from pregnancy and childbirth.

(b) *Birth interval* : Short birth intervals are associated with an increased risk of maternal mortality. (c) *Parity*: High parity contributes to high maternal mortality.

Not only are these three variables interrelated, but there are also other factors which are involved, e.g., economic circumstances, cultural practices and beliefs, nutritional status, environmental conditions and violence against women. The social factors often precede the medical causes and make pregnancy and child-birth a risky venture.

Global Strategy for Women's, Children's and Adolescent's Health 2016–2030

The Global Strategy for Women's, Children's and Adolescent's Health, 2016–2030 was launched in the year 2015 with a vision to have by the year 2030, a "world in which every woman, child and adolescent in every setting realize their rights to physical and mental health and well-being, has social and economic opportunities, and is able to participate fully in shaping prosperous and sustainable society" *(79)*. The strategy is a road map for the post-2015 agenda as described by the Sustainable Development Goals and seeks to end all preventable deaths of women, children and adolescents and create an environment in which these groups not only survive, but thrive, and see their environments, health and wellbeing transformed. The global strategy goals of SURVIVE, THRIVE and TRANSFORM and the targets to be achieved by 2030 are as follows *(79)*:

SURVIVE

End preventable deaths

- Reduce global maternal mortality to less than 70 per 100,000 live births
- Reduce newborn mortality to at least as low as 12 per 1000 live births in every country
- Reduce under-5 mortality to at least as low as 25 per 1000 live births in every country
- End epidemics of HIV, tuberculosis, malaria, neglected tropical diseases and other communicable diseases
- Reduce by one third premature mortality from non-communicable diseases and promote mental health and well-being

THRIVE

Ensure health and well-being

- End all forms of malnutrition, and address the nutritional needs of adolescent girls, pregnant and lactating women and children
- Ensure universal access to sexual and reproductive health-care services (including for family planning) and rights
- Ensure that all girls and boys have access to good quality early childhood development
- Substantially reduce pollution-related deaths and illnesses
- Achieve universal health coverage including financial risk protection and access to quality essential services, medicines and vaccines

TRANSFORM

Expand enabling environment

- Eradicate extreme poverty
- Ensure that all girls and boys complete free, equitable and good quality primary and secondary education
- Eliminate all harmful practices and all discrimination and violence against women and girls
- Achieve universal and equitable access to safe and affordable drinking water, and to adequate sanitation and hygiene
- Enhance scientific research, upgrade technological capabilities and encourage innovation
- Provide legal identity for all, including birth registration
- Enhance the global partnership for sustainable development.

INDIA

Despite significant improvements in maternal health over the last decade or so, which is evident in the reductions in maternal mortality in the country, an estimated 44,000 mothers continue to die every year due to causes related to pregnancy, childbirth and the post-partum period. The major medical causes of these deaths are haemorrhage, sepsis, abortion, hypertensive disorders, obstructed labor and other causes including anaemia. A host of socio-economic-cultural determinants like illiteracy, low socio-economic status, early age of marriage, low level of women's empowerment, traditional preference for home deliveries and other factors contribute to the delays leading to these deaths.

From year 2000 onwards, SRS (Sample Registration System) included a new method called the "RHIME" or Representative, Re-sampled, Routine Household Interview of Mortality with Medical Evaluation. This is an enhanced form of *"verbal autopsy"* which is the key feature of a prospective study of 1 million deaths within the SRS. RHIME include random re-sampling of field-work by an independent team for maintaining quality of data. For comparability with WHO estimates for India and for other countries, the WHO's "Global Burden of Disease" categorization of maternal deaths have been used, which includes various categories with their ICD-10 codes such as : haemorrhage, sepsis, hypertensive disorder, obstructed labour, abortion, and other conditions.

The SRS report has been grouped into three categories; (a) EAG states of Bihar and Jharkhand, Madhya Pradesh and Chhattisgarh, Odisha, Rajasthan, Uttar Pradesh and Uttaranchal and Assam. These states have high mortality indicators; (b) This category includes southern states of Andhra Pradesh, Karnataka, Kerala and Tamil Nadu. These states have comparatively better health indicators; (c) The remaining states have been classified as others *(80)*.

Table 14 shows live births, maternal deaths, maternal mortality ratio in India by states during 2018–2020, special survey of deaths using RHIME. During this period the life time risk of maternal death of women in the age group 15–49 has been reported to be 0.3 per cent. This is substantially higher for women in the category EAG states and Assam (0.5 per cent) as compared to women in the category southern (0.1 per cent) or in the "other" states (0.2 per cent).

India is among those countries which have a high maternal mortality ratio. According to the estimates the MMR has reduced from 167 per lakh live births in 2011–13 to 97 per lakh live births in 2018–2020. States of Kerala, Maharashtra, Andhra Pradesh, Gujarat, Tamil Nadu, Karnataka, Telangana, Haryana and Jharkhand have already achieved the goal of a MMR of 100 per lakh live births. In EAG and Assam category of states, MMR is about 137 per lakh live births, with Assam on top (195) and Madhya Pradesh (173), Uttar Pradesh (167), Chhattisgarh (137), Odisha (119),

TABLE 14

Maternal Mortality Ratio (MMR), 95% Confidence Interval (CI), Maternal Mortality Rate and lifetime risk; India, EAG and Assam, South and other states, 2018–2020

India and major states	MMR	95% CI	Maternal mortality rate	Lifetime risk
India Total	97	(88–106)	6.0	0.21%
Assam	195	(117–272)	12.1	0.42%
Bihar	118	(78–157)	11.2	0.39%
Jharkhand	56	(10–101)	4.2	0.15%
Madhya Pradesh	173	(126–220)	15.3	0.53%
Chhattisgarh	137	(54–219)	9.9	0.35%
Odisha	119	(71–167)	7.3	0.25%
Rajasthan	113	(71–155)	9.6	0.33%
Uttar Pradesh	167	(126–207)	14.3	0.50%
Uttarakhand	103	(52–154)	6.3	0.22%
EAG and Assam Subtotal	137	(121–154)	11	0.38%
Andhra Pradesh	45	(13–78)	2.4	0.08%
Telangana	43	(4–83)	2.3	0.08%
Karnataka	69	(35–103)	3.5	0.12%
Kerala	19	(0–42)	0.9	0.03%
Tamil Nadu	54	(24–85)	2.7	0.09%
South Subtotal	49	(35–64)	2	0.09%
Gujarat	57	(28–86)	3.9	0.14%
Haryana	110	(58–162)	8.0	0.28%
Maharashtra	33	(10–56)	1.8	0.06%
Punjab	105	(40–170)	5.4	0.19%
West Bengal	103	(64–143)	5.0	0.18%
Other states	77	(55–98)	3.9	0.14%
Other Subtotal	76	(63–89)	4	0.15%

Source : *(80)*

Rajasthan (113) closely following. Assam, Madhya Pradesh and Rajasthan have shown an acceleration in reduction in last three years *(80)*.

The age distribution of maternal and non-maternal deaths from the 2018–2020 Special Survey of Deaths are given in Table 15. It shows that more than two-thirds of the maternal deaths are of women in age group 20–34 years. In contrast, non-maternal deaths are more evenly distributed over the reproductive age span of 15–49 years.

TABLE 15

Age distribution of maternal and non-maternal deaths, India, 2018–2020

Age groups	Maternal deaths		Non-maternal deaths	
	Proportion	95% CI	Proportion	95% CI
15–19	6%	(4–8)	9%	(8–9)
20–24	32%	(27–36)	11%	(11–12)
25–29	30%	(25–34)	12%	(12–13)
30–34	20%	(16–24)	13%	(12–14)
35–39	8%	(6–11)	14%	(13–15)
40–44	3%	(1–4)	18%	(17–19)
45–49	2%	(1–3)	22%	(21–23)
15–49	**100%**		**100%**	

(Figures may not add to 100 due to round-off)

Source : *(80)*

Causes

The major causes of maternal mortality according to the 2001–2003 SRS survey are haemorrhage (38 per cent), sepsis (11 per cent), hypertension (5 per cent), obstructed labour (5 per cent), abortion (8 per cent) and other conditions (34 per cent). Anaemia (19 per cent) is not only the leading cause of death but also an aggravating factor in haemorrhage, sepsis and toxaemia. Illegal abortions are also one of the leading causes of maternal death. That this should continue despite MTP facilities points to the need for wider dissemination of information about these facilities. Induced abortions also point to a large unmet need for contraceptives, as with each pregnancy the woman faces increased risk of death. The percentage distribution of causes of maternal deaths during the year 2001–2003 are as shown in Fig. 11.

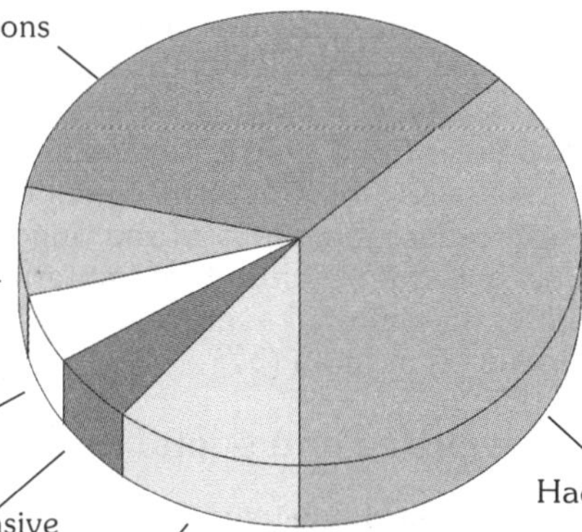

FIG. 11

Major causes of maternal deaths in India (2003)

(Figures may not add to 100 due to round-off)

Source : *(81)*

The determinants of maternal mortality in India are as listed in Table 16.

TABLE 16

Determinants of maternal mortality in India

Medical causes	Social factors
Obstetric causes: Toxaemias of pregnancy; Haemorrhage; Infection; Obstructed labour; Unsafe abortion	Age at child birth; Parity; Too close pregnancies; Family size; Malnutrition; Poverty; Illiteracy; Ignorance and prejudices; Lack of maternity services
Non-obstetric causes: Anaemia; Associated diseases, e.g., cardiac, renal, hepatic metabolic and infectious; Malignancy; Accidents	Shortage of health manpower; Delivery by untrained dais; Poor environmental sanitation; Poor communications and transport facilities; Social customs, etc.

Newer approaches such as "risk approach" and primary health care are steps in the right direction to reduce maternal mortality and morbidity. Despite best antenatal care, some women may develop complications without warning signs and require emergency care. Essential obstetric care and establishment of first referral units (FRUs) for emergency obstetric care is, therefore, a high priority under the safe motherhood component of Reproductive and Child Health Programme. Janani Suraksha Yojna, Janani Shishu Suraksha Karyakram, establishment of MCH wings and mother and child traking system; and RMNCH+A and more recently RMNCAH+N are key strategies to accelerate the pace of decline of MMR. Equally important is an attack on social and cultural factors (e.g., ignorance, low levels of female literacy, prejudices inherent in the socio-cultural milieu, low levels of nutrition and poor environmental sanitation). It calls for socio-economic development of the community through active community involvement.

National maternal health care indicators

The estimates of maternal mortality can only be used as a rough indicator of maternal health situation in any given country. Hence indicators such as antenatal check-up, institutional delivery and delivery by trained personnel etc. are used to assess the maternal health status. These indicators also reflect the status of the ongoing programme interventions and the situation of maternal health *(60)*. Table 17 shows the national average of key indicators as per NFHS-5 conducted in India *(57)*.

Preventive and social measures

High maternal mortality reflects not only in inadequacy of health care services for mothers, but also a low standard of living and socio-economic status of the community. In the world as a whole, the problem of maternal mortality is principally one of applying existing obstetric knowledge through antenatal, intranatal and postnatal services rather than developing new skills. Any attempt to lower MMR must take into consideration the following measures :

1. Early registration of pregnancy;
2. At least four antenatal check-ups;
3. Dietary supplementation, including correction of anaemia;
4. Prevention of infection and haemorrhage during puerperium;
5. Prevention of complications, e.g., eclampsia, malpresentations, ruptured uterus;
6. Treatment of medical conditions, e.g., hypertension, diabetes, tuberculosis, etc;
7. Anti-malaria and tetanus prophylaxis;
8. Clean delivery practice;
9. In India, a large number of maternal deaths could be prevented with the help of trained village level health workers;
10. Institutional deliveries for women with bad obstetric history and risk factors;
11. Promotion of family planning – to control the number of children to not more than two, and spacing of births;
12. Identification of every maternal death, and searching for its cause; and
13. Safe abortion services.

TABLE 17

National average of key indicators (per cent) in India 2019–2021

Indicators	NFHS-5 (2019–2021)		
Maternal and Child Health	Urban	Rural	Total
Maternity Care (for last birth in the 5 years before the survey)			
Mothers who had antenatal check-up in the first trimester (%)	75.5	67.9	70.0
Mothers who had at least 4 antenatal care visits (%)	68.1	54.2	58.1
Mothers whose last birth was protected against neonatal tetanus (%)	92.7	91.7	92.0
Mothers who consumed iron folic acid for 100 days or more when they were pregnant (%)	54.0	40.2	44.1
Mothers who consumed iron folic acid for 180 days or more when they were pregnant (%)	34.4	22.7	26.0
Registered pregnancies for which the mother received Mother and Child Protection (MCP) card (%)	94.9	96.3	95.9
Mothers who received postnatal care from a doctor/nurse/LHV/ANM/midwife/other health personnel within 2 days of delivery (%)	84.6	75.4	78.0
Average out of pocket expenditure per delivery in public health facility (Rs.)	3,385	2,770	2,916
Children born at home who were taken to a health facility for check-up within 24 hours of birth (%)	3.8	4.3	4.2
Children who received postnatal care from a doctor/nurse/LHV/ANM/midwife/other health personnel within 2 days of birth (%)	85.7	76.5	79.1
Delivery Care (for births in the 5 years before the survey)			
Institutional births (%)	93.8	86.7	88.6
Institutional births in public facility (%)	52.6	65.3	61.9
Home births that were conducted by skilled health personnel (%)	2.1	3.7	3.2
Births attended by skilled health personnel (%)	94.0	87.8	89.4
Births delivered by caesarean section (%)	32.3	17.6	21.5
Births in private health facility that were delivered by caesarean section (%)	49.3	46.0	47.4
Births in a public health facility that were delivered by caesarean section (%)	22.7	11.9	14.3

Source : *(58)*

MORTALITY IN INFANCY AND CHILDHOOD

Mortality rates are good indicators to measure the level of health and health care in different countries. They also help in assessing the overall socio-economic development of a country and correlate well with certain economic variables such as GNP. Medical and social progress have substantially reduced mortality in childhood.

It has become customary to consider mortality in and around infancy in a number of time periods convenient from both the analytical and programmatic point of view as under :

a. perinatal period
b. early neonatal period
c. late neonatal period
d. neonatal period
e. post neonatal period

These are as illustrated in Fig. 12.

FOETAL DEATH : Foetal death is death prior to the complete expulsion or extraction from its mother of a product of conception, irrespective of the duration of pregnancy; the death is indicated by the fact that after such separation the foetus does not breathe or show any other evidence of life, such as beating of the heart, pulsation of the umbilical cord, or definite movement of voluntary muscles *(82)*. Defined variously as death after the 20th or 28th week of gestation (the definition of length of gestation varies between countries).

Some observers have expressed the view that vital statistical reports are less reliable on foetal deaths occurring at 20–27 weeks than on those occurring after 28 completed weeks, and have preferred to analyze the data separately for the two intervals. Stillbirths are seldom reported in developing countries.

Because of the above difficulties WHO has recommended that within any country the term "stillbirth" be applied to a foetus born dead, and weighing over 500 g – the birth weight most frequently associated with a gestation period of 22 weeks. But for international comparison, however, they suggested a boundary of 1000 g or more, which is more frequently associated with a gestation period of 28 weeks.

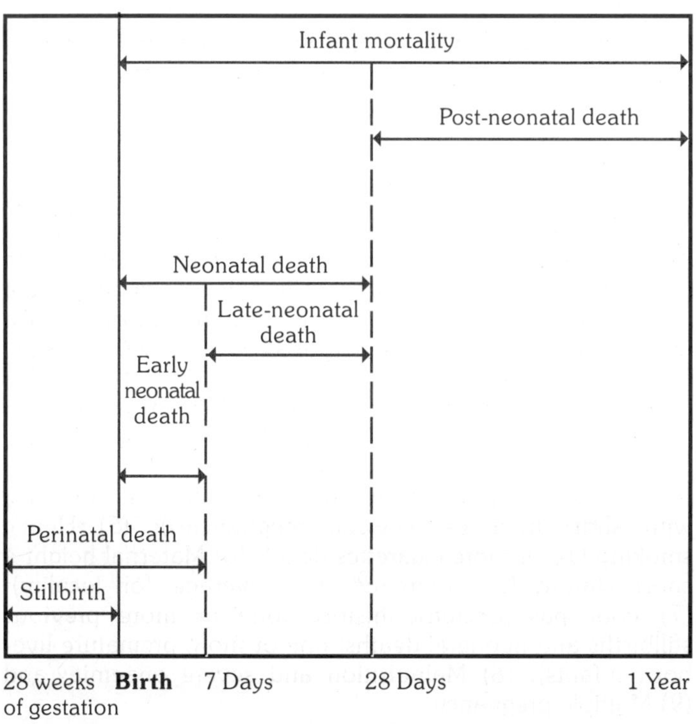

FIG. 12
Mortality in and around infancy

STILLBIRTH RATE

The most widespread use of the term is, "death of a foetus weighing 1000 g (this is equivalent to 28 weeks of gestation) or more" occurring during one year in every 1000 total births (live births plus stillbirths). Stillbirth rate is given by the formula :

$$\text{Stillbirth rate} = \frac{\text{Foetal deaths weighing over 1000 g at birth during the year}}{\text{Total live + stillbirths weighing over 1000 g at birth during the year}} \times 1000$$

It is a frequent occurrence in the developing countries. Its prevention involves the detection and treatment of infectious pathology in the course of pregnancy as well as of high blood pressure and its complications, Rh incompatibility, diabetes and premature rupture of the membrane. Some causes are difficult or impossible to eliminate, such as multiple pregnancies, cord anomalies, foetal malformations, placenta anomalies.

Approximately 1.9 million babies were stillborn in the year 2019 worldwide, the rate was 14 per 1000 total births. The rate varies between 22 per 1000 total births in least developed countries to 3 in Western European countries *(74)*. In India, the SRS estimates for the year 2020 for the whole country was about 3 per 1000 total births (4 for the rural and 3 for the urban areas). Among the bigger states, the highest level of stillbirths has been estimated for Odisha (10). Table 18 shows the statewise break-up of stillbirth rate.

TABLE 18
Perinatal mortality rates and stillbirth rates by residence, India and bigger states, 2020

India and bigger states/UTs	Perinatal mortality rate Total	Rural	Urban	Stillbirth rate Total	Rural	Urban
India	18	21	12	3	4	3
Andhra Pradesh	14	16	9	1	1	3
Assam	17	18	8	3	3	2
Bihar	17	18	12	1	1	1
Chhattisgarh	26	26	24	6	6	6
Delhi	6	8	6	0	0	0
Gujarat	15	18	11	4	4	3
Haryana	21	23	17	7	6	7
Himachal Pradesh*	13	14	10	4	4	4
Jammu & Kashmir	11	11	10	3	2	4
Jharkhand	15	16	10	2	2	2
Karnataka	14	17	9	3	4	2
Kerala	8	6	10	4	4	4
Madhya Pradesh	28	30	20	5	6	4
Maharashtra	11	14	6	3	4	1
Odisha	30	32	20	10	10	6
Punjab	12	11	13	3	3	4
Rajasthan	20	21	16	4	4	5
Tamil Nadu	8	11	5	2	3	1
Telangana	13	14	11	2	1	4
Uttar Pradesh	24	27	15	4	4	2
Uttarakhand	18	17	20	6	6	6
West Bengal	15	15	11	4	5	4

*(Based on three year period 2018–20)
Source : *(73)*

The estimates provided by Lancet Stillbirth Series for India is 22 per 1000 live births for the year 2009. This estimate is being used as a target-setting excercise by India Newborn Action Plan (launched in June 2014). With the current level of average annual rate of reduction, which is less than 1 per cent, India is expected to reach SBR of 19 per 1000 live births by 2030 *(83)*.

PERINATAL MORTALITY RATE

As currently defined, the term "perinatal mortality" includes both late foetal deaths (stillbirths) and early neonatal deaths. The Eighth Revision of the International Classification of Diseases (ICD) defined the "perinatal period" as lasting from the 28th week of gestation to the seventh day after birth. The Tenth Revision (1993) of ICD added that :

i) Babies chosen for inclusion in perinatal statistics (this means late foetal deaths, live births and early neonatal deaths) should be those above a minimum birth weight, i.e., 1000 g at birth (A birth weight of 1000 g is considered equivalent to gestational age of 28 weeks);

ii) if the birth weight is not available, a gestation period of at least 28 weeks should be used; and

iii) where (i) and (ii) are not available, body length (crown to heel) of at least 35 cm should be used. But the preferred criterion is birth weight.

The Conference for the Tenth Revision (ICD-10) made no changes to these definitions.

DEFINITIONS *(84)*

The WHO's definition, more appropriate in nations with well established vital records of stillbirths is as follows :

$$\text{PMR} = \frac{\text{Late foetal deaths (28 weeks gestation and more)} + \text{early neonatal deaths (first week) in one year}}{\text{Live births + late foetal deaths (28 weeks gestation and more) in the same year}} \times 1000$$

The WHO's definition, more appropriate in nations with less well established vital records, is :

$$\text{Perinatal mortality rate} = \frac{\text{Late foetal deaths (28 weeks + of gestation)} + \text{postnatal deaths (first week) in a year}}{\text{Live births in a year}} \times 1000$$

There is a difference in denominator of the perinatal mortality rate defined by the WHO and industrially developed nations. This makes international comparisons difficult.

International comparisons

For international comparisons, the WHO Expert Committee on the Prevention of Perinatal Mortality and Morbidity (1970) recommended a more precise formulation : "Late foetal and early neonatal deaths weighing over 1000 g at birth, expressed as a ratio per 1000 live births weighing over 1000 g at birth". It is calculated as :

$$\text{Perinatal mortality rate} = \frac{\text{Late foetal and early neonatal deaths weighing over 1000 g at birth}}{\text{Total live births weighing over 1000 g at birth}} \times 1000$$

Why perinatal mortality rate ?

With the decline of infant mortality rate to low levels in many developed countries, perinatal mortality rate has assumed greater significance as a yardstick of obstetric and paediatric care before and around the time of birth.

First, two types of death rate i.e., stillbirths and deaths under the first week of life are combined in perinatal mortality rate because the factors responsible for these two types of deaths are often similar, being those operating before and around the time of birth. *Secondly*, a proportion of deaths which occur after birth are incorrectly registered as stillbirths, thereby inflating the stillbirth rate and lowering the neonatal death rate. The perinatal mortality rate, being a combination of stillbirths and early neonatal deaths, is not influenced by this error, by removing from consideration the dividing line between a stillbirth and a live birth with death shortly after birth.

Although perinatal period occupies less than 0.5 per cent (less than 168 hours) of the average life span, there are more deaths within this period than during the next 30–40 years of life in many developing countries *(85)*. The value of perinatal mortality rate is that it gives a good indication of the extent of pregnancy wastage as well as the quality and quantity of health care available to the mother and the newborn. It reflects the results of maternity care more clearly than the neonatal death rate.

Incidence

Perinatal mortality is a problem of serious dimensions in all countries. It now accounts for about 90 per cent of all foetal and infant mortality in the developed countries. In India, stillbirths are seldom registered. Consequently, most studies on perinatal mortality in this country are hospital-based. The SRS estimates for perinatal mortality rate in India for the year 2020 was about 18 per 1000 live births and stillbirths, with about 21 for rural areas and 12 for the urban areas. The statewise perinatal mortality rate is shown in Table 18.

In developed countries, perinatal mortality rates have gradually declined during the past decades due to improved obstetric and perinatal technologies.

Social and biological variables

A number of social and biological factors are known to be associated with perinatal mortality. The degree to which these factors influence perinatal mortality varies from country to country. Many of these factors also endanger the life of the mother, causing high maternal mortality. An appreciation of these factors (at-risk factors) will certainly make the greatest impact on reducing perinatal mortality. The overall risk is increased in the following categories : (1) Low socio-economic status; (2) High maternal age (35 years or more); (3) Low maternal age (under 16 years); (4) High parity (fifth and subsequent pregnancies, especially with short intervals between pregnancies); (5) Heavy smoking (10 or more cigarettes daily); (6) Maternal height – short stature (as compared with average for locality); (7) Poor past obstetric history (one or more previous stillbirths and neonatal deaths, one or more premature live-born infants); (8) Malnutrition and severe anaemia; and (9) Multiple pregnancy.

For further details see page 648 under "factors affecting infant mortality".

Causes of perinatal mortality

About two-thirds of all perinatal deaths occur among infants with less than 2500 g birth weight. The causes involve one or more complications in the mother during pregnancy or labour, in the placenta or in the foetus or neonate.

Main causes : The main causes of death are intrauterine and birth asphyxia, low birth weight, birth trauma, and intrauterine or neonatal infections. The various causes of perinatal mortality may be grouped as below :

(a) Antenatal causes

(1) Maternal diseases : hypertension, cardiovascular diseases, diabetes, tuberculosis, anaemia
(2) Pelvic diseases : uterine myomas, endometriosis, ovarian tumours
(3) Anatomical defects : uterine anomalies, incompetent cervix
(4) Endocrine imbalance and inadequate uterine preparation
(5) Blood incompatibilities
(6) Malnutrition
(7) Toxaemias of pregnancy
(8) Antepartum haemorrhages
(9) Congenital defects
(10) Advanced maternal age

(b) Intranatal causes

(1) Birth injuries
(2) Asphyxia
(3) Prolonged effort time
(4) Obstetric complications

(c) Postnatal causes

(1) Prematurity
(2) Respiratory distress syndrome
(3) Respiratory and alimentary infections
(4) Congenital anomalies

(d) Unknown causes

In some cases; the causes are not clinically ascertainable.

Interventions for the reduction of perinatal mortality

Measures to reduce perinatal mortality rates are essential to accelerate the declining trend in neonatal and infant mortality rates. For further details, refer to Table 21.

International certificate of perinatal death

For international comparability, the 9th (1975) Revision of International Classification of Diseases (ICD-9) recommended a special certificate of cause of perinatal death. The ICD has also a list of 100 causes (the "P" list) for tabulation of perinatal morbidity and mortality *(28)*.

Prevention of perinatal mortality

See page 650 under Preventive & Social Measures.

NEONATAL MORTALITY RATE

Neonatal deaths are deaths occurring during the neonatal period, commencing at birth and ending 28 completed days after birth. Neonatal mortality rate is the number of neonatal deaths in a given year per 1000 live births in that year.

The neonatal mortality rate is tabulated as :

$$= \frac{\text{Number of deaths of children under 28 days of age in a year}}{\text{Total live births in the same year}} \times 1000$$

Causes of neonatal mortality

The main causes of neonatal death globally are as shown in Fig 13.

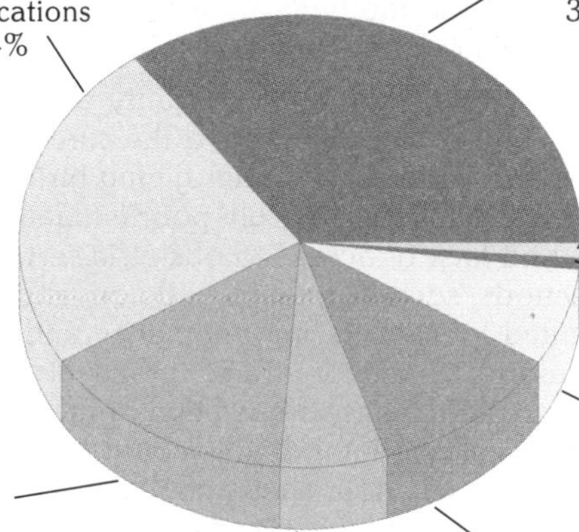

FIG. 13
Global distribution of neonatal deaths by cause, 2018

Source : *(86)*

No woman should die giving life. Nor should any mother endure pregnancy and childbirth, only to go through the agony of having her child born dead or watching the baby die minutes after birth. Yet for countless women around the world this scenario remains a tragic reality. The first 28 days of life – the neonatal period, is the most vulnerable time for a child's survival. In order to continue to accelerate progress in under-five mortality, focussing on newborns is critical.

Neonatal mortality is a measure of intensity with which "endogenous factors" (e.g., low birth weight, birth injuries) affect infant life. The neonatal mortality is directly related to the birth weight and gestational age. Intrapartum related complications, low birth weight and preterm birth is a causal factor in 60 per cent of neonate deaths.

Prematurity and congenital anomalies account for about 60 per cent of newborn deaths, and these often occur in the first week of life. A further quarter of neonatal deaths are attributable to asphyxia – also mainly in the first week of life. In the late neonatal period, that is, after the first week, deaths attributable to infection (including diarrhoea and tetanus) predominate. The importance of tetanus as a cause of neonatal death, however, has diminished sharply due to intensified immunization efforts.

Neonatal mortality rates of babies born to mothers with no education are nearly twice as high as those of babies born to mothers with secondary education or higher. The family's wealth and rural/urban residence also remain powerful determinant of inequities in neonatal mortality. Ending child marriage, reducing adolescent pregnancy and extending birth intervals are crucial to reducing the risk of newborn mortality.

Direct causes of newborn death vary from region to region. In general, the proportions of deaths attributed to prematurity and congenital disorders increase as the neonatal mortality rate decreases, while the proportions caused by infections, asphyxia, diarrhoea and tetanus decline as care improves. Patterns of low birth weight vary considerably between countries. Babies with a low birth weight are especially vulnerable to the hazards of the first hours and days of life, particularly if they are premature. Majority of low-birth-weight babies are not actually premature but have suffered from *in utero* growth restriction, usually because of the mother's poor health. These babies too are at increased risk of death.

The main causes of neonatal mortality are intrinsically linked to the health of the mother and the care she receives before, during and immediately after giving birth. Asphyxia and birth injuries usually result from poorly managed labour and delivery, and lack of access to obstetric services. Many neonatal infections, such as tetanus and congenital syphilis, can be prevented by care during pregnancy and childbirth. Inadequate calorie or micronutrient intake also results in poorer pregnancy outcomes. It has been argued that nearly three quarters of all neonatal deaths could be prevented if women were adequately nourished and received appropriate care during pregnancy, childbirth and in the postnatal period.

However, neonatal mortality is the most difficult part of infant mortality to alter, because of the endogenous factors which are not sensitive to improvements in environmental conditions. Neonatal mortality is greater in boys throughout the world, because newborn boys are biologically more fragile than girls.

Incidence

About 2.5 million newborns died before they are 4 weeks old and half of them died in their first 24 hours in the year 2020. 98 per cent of these deaths occur in developing countries.

The global number of neonatal deaths declined from 5.0 million in 1990 to 2.4 million in 2019 – 6,700 deaths every day in 2020, compared to 14,000 in 1990. Neonatal deaths accounted for about 47 per cent of all under-five deaths in 2020, increasing from 40 per cent in 1990 due to faster global decline in mortality among children aged 1–59 months, than in their first month of life. Based on a recent systematic review, about a third of all neonatal deaths occur on the day of birth and close to three quarters die in the first week of life. These findings suggest that focusing on the critical period before and immediately following birth is essential to saving more newborn lives *(6)*.

The mortality rate comparison for children under 19 years of age is as shown in Fig. 14.

In 2020, the neonatal mortality rate was estimated to be at 17 deaths per 1000 live births globally. The probability of dying after the first month, in post-neonatal period was 11 per 1000, and probability of dying after reaching 1 year of age and before reaching 5 years of age was at 10 per 1000 live births.

The burden of neonatal mortality is uneven across regions. Some countries have relatively high neonatal mortality given their level of under-five mortality. Most of these countries are in Southern Asia. Sub-Saharan Africa had the highest neonatal mortality rate in 2020, at 27 deaths per 1000 live births, followed by Central and Southern Asia with 23 deaths per 1000 live births. A child born in

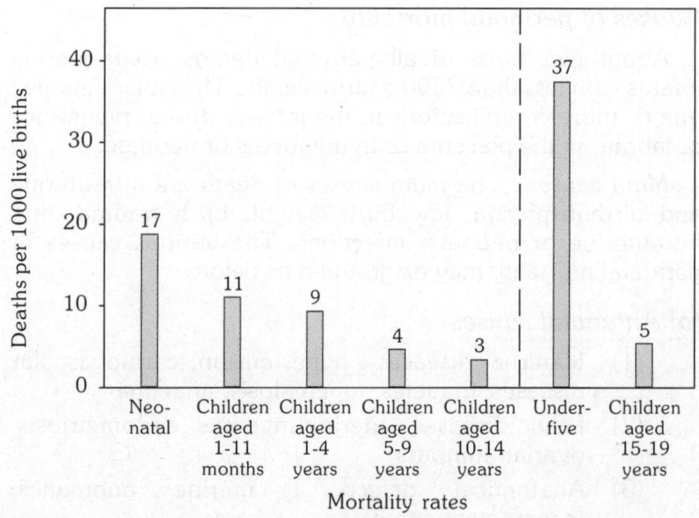

FIG. 14
Global mortality rates by age, 2020

Source : *(6)*

Sub-Saharan Africa is 11 times more likely to die in the first month than a child born in high-income country *(6)*.

India

In India the SRS estimates for the year 2020 was about 15 per 1000 live births, in early-neonatal period (0–7 days), with about 17 for rural areas and 9 for urban areas. Table 19 shows the early neonatal mortality rate and percentage share of early neonatal mortality to infant deaths in the country and the major states. Among the bigger states,

TABLE 19

Early neonatal mortality rates and percentage share of early neonatal deaths to infant deaths by residence, India and bigger states/UTs, 2020

India and bigger states/UTs	Early neonatal mortality rate			Percentage of early neonatal deaths to infant deaths		
	Total	Rural	Urban	Total	Rural	Urban
India	15	17	9	53.3	54.7	46.8
Andhra Pradesh	13	15	6	52.6	57.9	35.1
Assam	14	15	6	39.6	39.6	38.1
Bihar	16	17	12	59.5	60.9	47.4
Chhattisgarh	20	20	18	51.9	50.5	59.5
Delhi	6	8	6	49.0	40.0	49.4
Gujarat	11	14	8	50.5	51.5	48.1
Haryana	14	17	10	51.4	54.4	43.7
Himachal Pradesh*	10	10	6	54.9	55.6	41.3
Jammu & Kashmir	8	8	6	47.3	48.3	42.9
Jharkhand	13	15	8	53.6	56.4	39.3
Karnataka	11	13	6	55.5	61.8	40.8
Kerala	4	2	6	60.7	48.9	66.7
Madhya Pradesh	23	25	16	52.8	52.5	54.6
Maharashtra	8	11	5	50.8	54.1	43.1
Odisha	21	22	14	58.1	58.8	52.3
Punjab	9	9	9	46.8	44.6	50.3
Rajasthan	16	18	11	50.4	50.6	49.0
Tamil Nadu	6	9	4	50.0	56.6	41.1
Telangana	10	13	7	48.4	51.3	41.8
Uttar Pradesh	21	23	13	54.8	56.5	45.9
Uttarakhand	13	12	15	51.7	48.1	62.1
West Bengal	10	11	8	54.2	56.9	44.7

*(Based on three year period 2018–2020)

Source : *(73)*

Kerala (4), Madhya Pradesh (23), and Odisha (21) are the two extremes. The percentage of early neonatal deaths to the total infant deaths during the year 2020, at the national level, has been 53.3, and it varied from 54.7 in rural areas to 46.8 in urban areas. In most of the states rural proportion is relatively higher than the urban proportion. Among the bigger states, the percentage for total varied from 39.6 in Assam to 60.7 in Kerala.

Table 20 shows the neonatal mortality rate in the country and the percentage of neonatal deaths to infant deaths for the year 2020, both at the national and state levels. At the national level, the neonatal mortality rate was 20 and ranged from 12 in urban areas to 23 in rural areas. Among the bigger states neonatal mortality ranges from 31 in Madhya Pradesh to 4 in Kerala. The percentage of neonatal deaths to total infant deaths was 71.9 per cent at the national level and varied from 62.4 per cent in urban areas to 74.1 per cent in rural areas. Among the bigger states Bihar (77.7) registered the highest percentage of neonatal deaths to infant deaths, and the lowest was in Assam (53.0).

TABLE 20

Neonatal mortality rates and percentage share of neonatal deaths to infant deaths by residence, India and bigger states, 2020

India and bigger states/UTs	Neonatal mortality rate			Percentage of neonatal deaths to infant deaths		
	Total	Rural	Urban	Total	Rural	Urban
India	20	23	12	71.9	74.1	62.4
Andhra Pradesh	17	21	8	70.3	77.7	45.4
Assam	19	20	10	53.0	52.6	61.7
Bihar	21	22	17	77.7	79.0	66.6
Chhattisgarh	26	28	20	68.8	69.3	65.9
Delhi	9	12	9	71.3	60.0	71.8
Gujarat	16	20	9	68.7	73.6	56.8
Haryana	19	22	15	68.6	70.3	64.2
Himachal Pradesh*	13	13	10	72.7	73.0	66.5
Jammu & Kashmir	12	12	10	71.1	70.5	73.9
Jharkhand	17	19	11	68.8	71.8	53.2
Karnataka	14	18	8	74.7	85.0	50.5
Kerala	4	3	6	66.4	66.0	66.7
Madhya Pradesh	31	34	19	70.8	71.8	64.8
Maharashtra	11	15	6	70.2	75.3	58.3
Odisha	28	29	20	77.6	78.2	72.1
Punjab	12	12	12	65.7	63.7	69.0
Rajasthan	23	26	14	71.5	73.6	60.7
Tamil Nadu	9	12	6	70.5	78.6	59.6
Telangana	15	17	13	71.8	68.7	79.0
Uttar Pradesh	28	31	18	74.1	76.1	63.8
Uttarakhand	17	17	18	71.0	70.1	73.8
West Bengal	14	15	11	72.9	76.1	61.5

*(Based on three year period 2018–2020)

Source : *(73)*

CAUSES OF NEONATAL DEATHS IN INDIA

The major causes of neonatal deaths are shown in Fig. 15.

It is estimated that 40 per cent of all stillbirths and neonatal deaths take place during labour and the day of birth, and about 75 per cent of total neonatal deaths occur within the first week of life. Notably half of all the maternal deaths also take place in this period *(83)*.

India accounts for 40 per cent of the global burden of low birth weight babies with 7.5 million babies (or about 30 per cent of the country's total annual live births) being born with a birth weight less than 2500 grams. Of these 7.5 million babies, about 60 per cent are born at term after foetal growth retardation, while the remaining 40 per cent are born preterm, constituting one fourth of global burden of preterm births. Preterm babies in addition to being at a higher risk of neonatal mortality, are at an increased risk of post-neonatal mortality, stunting, and long-term neuro-developmental impairment during childhood *(83)*.

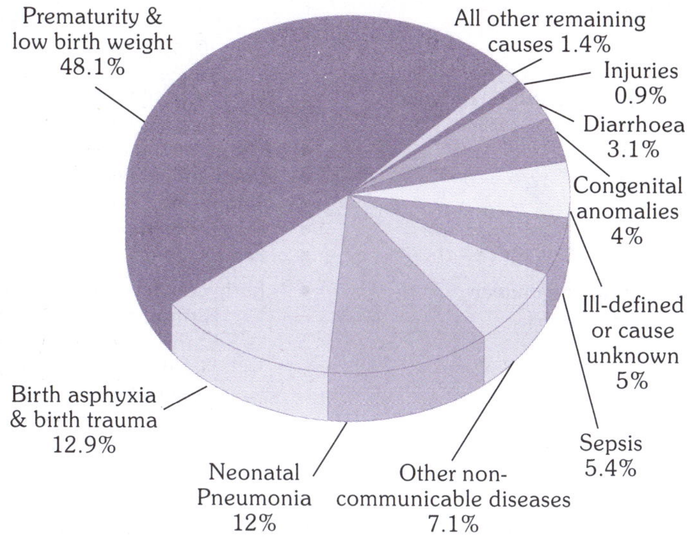

FIG. 15

Causes of neonatal deaths in India, 2017

Source : *(87)*

Interventions for the reduction of neonatal mortality

Measures to reduce neonatal mortality rates and to improve newborn health are enumerated in Table 21.

POST-NEONATAL MORTALITY RATE

Deaths occurring from 28 days of life to under one year are called "post-neonatal deaths". The post-neonatal death rate is defined as : "the ratio of post-neonatal deaths in a given year to the total number of live births in the same year; usually expressed as a rate per 1000" *(88)*.

The post-neonatal mortality rate is tabulated as :

$$= \frac{\text{Number of deaths of children between 28 days and one year of age in a given year}}{\text{Total live births in the same year}} \times 1000$$

Whereas neonatal mortality is dominated by endogenous factors, post-neonatal mortality is dominated by exogenous (e.g., environmental and social) factors. Diarrhoea and respiratory infections are the main causes of death during the post-neonatal period. Malnutrition is an additional factor, reinforcing the adverse effects of the infections. In the developed countries, the main cause of post-neonatal mortality is congenital anomalies. Studies show that post-neonatal mortality increases steadily with birth order, and that infants born into already large families run a higher risk of death from infectious diseases.

In some areas of South East Asia (including India), during the post-neonatal period girls die more frequently than boys. This is attributed to neglect of the female children in terms of nutrition and health care.

The SRS estimates for post-neonatal mortality rate in

TABLE 21

Priority areas to improve newborn health

Before and during pregnancy	• Delayed child-bearing. • Well-timed, well-spaced and wanted pregnancies • Well-nourished and healthy mother • Pregnancy free of drug abuse, tobacco and alcohol • Tetanus and rubella immunization • Prevention of mother-to-child transmission of HIV • Female education
During preganancy	• Early contact with health systems including : – Birth and emergency preparedness – Early detection and treatment of maternal complications – Monitoring of foetal well-being and timely interventions for foetal complications – Tetanus immunization – Prevention and treatment of anaemia – Prevention and treatment of infections (malaria, hookworm, syphilis and other STIs) – Voluntary HIV counselling and testing, and prevention of mother-to-child transmission of HIV • Good diet • Prevention of violence against women
During and soon after delivery	• Safe and clean delivery by skilled attendant • Early detection and prompt management of delivery and foetal complications • Emergency obstetric care for maternal and foetal conditions • Newborn resuscitation • Newborn care ensuring warmth and cleanliness • Newborn cord, eye and skin care • Early initiation of exclusive breast-feeding • Early detection and treatment of complications of the newborn • Special care for infants born too early or too small and/or complications • Prevention and control of infections • Prevention of mother-to-child transmission of HIV • Information and counselling on home care, danger signs and care seeking
During the first month of life	• Early post-natal contact • Protection, promotion and support of exclusive breast feeding • Prompt detection and management of diseases in newborn infant • Immunization • Protection of girl child

Source : *(89)*

India for the year 2020 was about 8 per 1000 live births for the whole country, and 8 for rural areas and 7 for the urban areas. The state-wise break-up is shown in Table 22.

TABLE 22

SRS estimates of post neonatal mortality in India, 2020

State	Post-neonatal mortality rate		
	Total	Urban	Rural
Andhra Pradesh	7	10	6
Assam	17	6	18
Bihar	6	8	6
Chhattisgarh	12	11	12
Gujarat	7	7	7
Haryana	9	8	9
Himachal Pradesh	5	5	5
Jharkhand	8	10	7
Karnataka	5	8	3
Kerala	2	3	1
Madhya Pradesh	13	10	13
Maharashtra	5	4	5
Odisha	8	8	8
Punjab	6	5	7
Rajasthan	9	9	9
Tamil Nadu	4	4	3
Telangana	6	4	8
Uttar Pradesh	10	10	10
Uttarakahand	7	6	7
West Bengal	5	7	5
India	8	7	8

Source : *(73)*

INFANT MORTALITY RATE

Infant mortality rate (IMR) is defined as "the ratio of infant deaths registered in a given year to the total number of live births registered in the same year; usually expressed as a rate per 1000 live births" *(90)*. It is given by the formula :

$$\text{IMR} = \frac{\text{Number of deaths of children less than 1 year of age in a year}}{\text{Number of live births in the same year}} \times 1000$$

IMR is universally regarded not only as a most important indicator of the health status of a community but also of the level of living of people in general, and effectiveness of MCH services in particular. Infant mortality is given a separate treatment by demographers because : (a) infant mortality is the largest single age–category of mortality; (b) deaths at this age are due to a peculiar set of diseases and conditions to which the adult population is less exposed or less vulnerable; (c) infant mortality is affected rather quickly and directly by specific health programmes and hence may change more rapidly than the general death rate.

International comparisons

During the past decades, there has been a steady decline in infant mortality (Table 23)

TABLE 23
Infant mortality rate in selected countries (1990–2020)

Country	1990	2020
India	88	28
Sri Lanka	18	6
Bangladesh	100	24
Pakistan	106	54
Thailand	30	7
Myanmar	78	35
China	42	5
Nepal	99	24
New Zealand	9	4
USA	9	5
UK	8	4
Japan	5	2
World	63	27

1990 is the baseline for MDGs

Source : *(6)*

There are wide variations between countries or regions in the levels of infant mortality. The world average of IMR for 2020 has been estimated at about 27 per 1000 live births. However, IMR varies from 4 per 1000 live births in the developed countries to 46 per 1000 live births in the least developed countries. The average in the South Asian countries was 35 per 1000 live births. Although infant mortality declined significantly, the drop was greatest for the developed countries and lowest for least developed countries. The developed world had a much greater reduction in infant mortality compared to child mortality, while in the developing world the situation was reverse *(6)*.

The IMRs in industrialized countries were around 200 or even more, some 150 years ago. Even at the beginning of the 20th century. USA, UK, Japan, France, etc, had rates above 140 per 1000 live births. Within 50 years (1950) a spectacular fall in the rate was observed in all developed countries. By 1980s, most developed countries achieved IMR rates below 10 per 1000 live births. Demographers opine that in most developed countries, further decline in IMRs would be difficult to achieve without some revolutionary advances in perinatology. Any further reduction in infant mortality in developed countries will depend upon preventing one of its principal causes, namely, congenital abnormalities.

In general, the infant mortality rates reflect the socio-economic development of a country. Deaths during the first four weeks are largely preventable by good health care. Much of the variations between developed and developing world in death among newborn can be explained by differences in antenatal care – about half of all pregnant women in the least developed countries have no antenatal care, and 7 out of 10 babies are born without the help of a trained birth attendant. The other major factors being malnutrition and high parity of the mother, low birth weight of the baby, and congenital anomalies.

The decline in infant mortality has been attributed to : (a) improved obstetric and perinatal care, e.g., availability of oxygen, foetal monitoring during labour, improved techniques for the induction of labour (b) improvement in the quality of life, that is, economic and social progress (c) better control of communicable diseases, e.g., immunization and oral rehydration (d) advances in chemotherapy, antibiotics and insecticides (e) better nutrition, e.g., emphasis on breast feeding, and (f) family planning, e.g., birth spacing.

In the industrial world, the dominant factor in the decline of infant mortality was economic and social progress (i.e., quality of life), with medical services playing secondary role. On the other hand, in most of the developing countries, this pattern has been almost turned upside down. That is, medical services (e.g., mass control of disease, immunization, antibiotics and insecticides) have made the major impact, with social and economic progress taking the supporting role. Therefore, infant mortality rates are reluctant to fall below 100 per 1000 live births in many developing countries. It is now conceded that only socio-economic development can re-accelerate the progress and lead to further significant fall in infant deaths.

Infant mortality in India

India is still among high infant mortality rate countries (28 in the year 2020). IMR has declined slowly from 204 during 1911–15, to 129 per 1000 live births in 1970 and remained static at around 127 for many years, and then declined a bit once again to 114 in 1980 and coming down to 28 in the year 2020. Despite this significant decline, the rates are high as compared to developed countries (Table 23) which are now mostly in the range of 3–7 per 1000 live births.

India is a vast country with widely differing populations. The all-India rate masks variations that exist among sub-groups of the population. An examination of state-wise IMR for the year 2020 shows a vast regional variation, with Madhya Pradesh having IMR of 43 and Kerala as low as 6 per thousand live births during the year 2020. Among the larger States Kerala, Maharashtra, Punjab, Tamil Nadu, West Bengal, Andhra Pradesh, Haryana, Karnataka, Gujarat, Himachal pradesh, Bihar, and Jharkhand have achieved IMR below the national average of 28. Within each state there is rural urban variation. A critical infant mortality belt runs through Odisha, Madhya Pradesh, Assam, Chhattisgarh, Uttar Pradesh, and Rajasthan; all these states have infant mortality rates above the national average.

Table 24 shows infant mortality rates in major states of India.

TABLE 24
Infant mortality rates in major states of India (2020)

India and major states/UTs	Total	Rural	Urban
Andhra Pradesh	24	26	18
Assam	36	39	17
Bihar	27	27	25
Chhattisgarh	38	40	31
Delhi	12	20	12
Gujarat	23	27	17
Haryana	28	31	23
Himachal Pradesh*	17	18	15
Jammu & Kashmir	17	18	13
Jharkhand	25	26	21
Karnataka	19	21	16
Kerala	6	4	9
Madhya Pradesh	43	47	30
Maharashtra	16	20	11
Odisha	36	37	28
Punjab	18	19	17
Rajasthan	32	35	23
Tamil Nadu	13	15	10
Telangana	21	24	17
Uttar Pradesh	38	40	28
Uttarakhand	24	25	24
West Bengal	19	19	17
India	28	31	19

Source : *(73)*

There is plenty of evidence to show that better control of infant mortality is related to a wider spread of literacy (particularly female literacy) and primary health care. Also, the states with the highest infant mortality are also the states with the highest fertility. Table 25 illustrates the impact of the above variables on infant mortality.

TABLE 25

IMR, female literacy rate and birth rate in major Indian States

State	IMR per 1000 live births (2020)	Female literacy rate (2011)	Birth rate per 1000 population (2020)
Andhra Pradesh	24	59.74	15.7
Assam	36	67.27	20.8
Bihar	27	53.33	25.5
Chhattisgarh	38	60.59	22.0
Gujarat	23	70.73	19.3
Haryana	28	66.77	19.9
Himachal Pradesh	17	76.60	15.3
Jharkhand	25	56.21	22.0
Karnataka	19	63.13	16.5
Kerala	6	91.98	13.2
Madhya Pradesh	43	60.20	24.1
Maharashtra	16	70.48	15.0
Odisha	36	64.36	17.7
Punjab	18	71.34	14.3
Rajasthan	32	52.66	23.5
Tamil Nadu	13	73.86	13.8
Telangana	21	–	16.4
Uttar Pradesh	38	59.26	25.1
Uttarakhand	24	–	16.6
West Bengal	19	71.16	14.6

Source : *(73, 91, 92)*

Table 25 shows that Kerala has managed to surpass all the Indian states in certain important measures of social development. It has the lowest infant mortality rate, the lowest birth rate and the highest literacy rate.

Mortality pattern

(a) *Age* : Deaths in the age–group 0–1 year account for 10.5 per cent of the total deaths in the country. About 71.7 per cent of infant deaths occur within the first month (neonatal period) of life. Of these, 54.6 per cent may die during the first week of birth *(73)*. The risk of death is the greatest during the first 24–48 hours after birth. The problem is more acute in rural areas where expert obstetric care is scarce. (b) *Sex* : Whereas in all developed countries, male death rates are higher than female deaths, in India, after the age of one month (post-neonatal period) female deaths are invariably higher than male deaths. Social scientists have attributed this phenomenon to social factors unfavourable to females in India *(93)*.

Medical causes of infant mortality

The causes of infant mortality are multifactorial. The medical causes are shown in Table 26 under two subdivisions – neonatal and post-neonatal mortality.

TABLE 26

Causes of infant mortality

Neonatal mortality (0–4 weeks)	Post-neonatal mortality (1–12 months)
1. Low birth weight and prematurity 2. Birth injury and difficult labour 3. Sepsis 4. Congenital anomalies 5. Haemolytic diseases of newborn 6. Conditions of placenta and cord 7. Diarrhoeal diseases 8. Acute respiratory infections 9. Tetanus	1. Diarrhoeal diseases 2. Acute respiratory infections 3. Other communicable diseases 4. Malnutrition 5. Congenital anomalies 6. Accidents

The principal causes of infant mortality in India are low birth weight (57%), respiratory infections (17%), diarrhoeal diseases (4%), congenital malformations (5%) and cord infection (2%), birth injury (3%) and unclassified about (18%) *(62)*. Neonatal deaths make a major contribution to infant mortality. Whereas in developing countries, the high infant mortality is mainly due to low birth weight, and the combined effects of infection (e.g., diarrhoea, respiratory infections) and malnutrition, in developed countries, it is mainly due to congenital anomalies, anoxia and hypoxia.

Factors affecting infant mortality

Infant mortality is due to the interaction of several factors in combination. They may be classified as biological, economic and social factors.

1. BIOLOGICAL FACTORS

(a) *Birth weight*

Birth weight is a major determinant of infant and perinatal mortality and morbidity. Babies of low birth weight (under 2.5 kg) and high birth weight (over 4 kg) are at special risk. Virtually, all infants weighing less than 1000 g at birth succumb. One major cause of low birth weight is poor maternal nutrition – not only during pregnancy, but even before that. It has been observed that the mother who was adequately nourished during her own growing-up years has an excellent chance of delivering a normal size baby even if she has taken an inadequate diet during her pregnancy. An increase in birth weight would lower the perinatal and neonatal mortality.

(b) *Age of the mother*

There is a definite relationship between the age of the mother and the fate of the child. Infant mortality rates are greater when the mother is either very young (below the age of 19 years) or relatively older (over 30 years). Very young mothers also tend to be poorer and less educated *(94)*.

(c) *Birth order*

The live births are classified according to their order of rank. The highest mortality is found among first born, and the lowest among those born second. The risk of infant mortality escalates after the third birth. The fate of the 5th and later children is always worse than the fate of the 3rd child. Infant mortality from nutritional deficiencies are 3–4 times higher for infants born with fifth or higher birth order compared to the first three. These deaths occur mostly in post-neonatal period.

(d) *Birth spacing*

Repeated pregnancies exert a great influence on infant mortality. They cause malnutrition and anaemia in the mother, again predispose to low birth weight, which results in higher infant death. The mother who becomes pregnant again too early and whose youngest baby is displaced from the breast, and prematurely weaned – that baby is more prone to develop (a) protein energy malnutrition (b) diarrhoea and dehydration, both of which cause an increased mortality in infants and young children. The Khanna Study in India showed that IMR was highest for infants born after an interval of one year, lower for those born after an interval of 2–3 years, and lowest for those born after an interval of 4 years *(95)*. A WHO study in rural India also showed similar findings *(96)*. Evidence from the World Fertility Survey – the largest survey into human behaviour ever undertaken – suggests that the risks to life for babies born within a year of each other is 2–4 times higher than for babies born more than 2 years apart. Wider spacing of births curtails infant mortality, and is considered as important part of health care as immunization *(97)*.

(e) *Multiple births*

Infants born in multiple births face a greater risk of death than do those in single births due in large part to the greater frequency of low birth weight among the former.

(f) *Family size*

Studies show the infant mortality increases with family size. The number of episodes of infectious diarrhoea, prevalence of malnutrition, and severe respiratory infections have been found to increase with family size. Besides the frequency of disease, the duration of illness is also affected by the family size. It was found that the duration of illness is much longer in families with 3 or more children. Deprivation of maternal care is also found in large families. Fewer children would mean better maternal care, a better share of family resources, less morbidity and greatly decreased infant mortality.

(g) *High fertility*

Fertility is one of the most important factors that influence infant mortality. High fertility and high infant mortality go together.

(2) ECONOMIC FACTORS

One of the most important variables affecting infant mortality rates, both directly and indirectly, is socio-economic status. The availability and quality of health care and the nature of the child's environment are closely related to socio-economic status. Statistics reveal that infant mortality rates are highest in the slums and lowest in the richer residential localities. Major improvements in health status and a decrease in infant mortality require continuing socio-economic development, including provision of health services.

(3) CULTURAL AND SOCIAL FACTORS

(a) *Breast-feeding*

Infant health is related to breast feeding because of the nutritional content and natural immunizing agents contained in breast milk, at least for fully breast-fed infants. Early weaning and bottle-fed infants living under poor hygienic conditions are more prone to die than the breast-fed infants living under similar conditions.

(b) *Religion and caste*

The differences are attributed to socio-cultural patterns of living, involving age-old habits, customs, traditions affecting cleanliness, eating, clothing, child care and almost every detail of daily living.

(c) *Early marriages*

The baby of teen-age mother has the highest risk for neonatal and post-neonatal mortality.

(d) *Sex of the child*

In most parts of India, female infants receive far less attention than males. This is especially the case, where there are already several female children. In many families, the birth of a female child is unwelcome. Statistics show that female infant mortality is higher than the male infant mortality. But when the total infant mortality is split into neonatal and postneonatal deaths, the picture gets reversed, i.e., neonatal death rate is higher for males than for female infants; post-neonatal death rate is higher for female infants than male infants *(93)*.

(e) *Quality of mothering*

The art of child care has to be learnt. Even in conditions of extreme poverty, children could reasonably survive if they had an efficient mother. It is the "quality of mothering" that helps to reduce infant mortality.

(f) *Maternal education*

Illiteracy is the greatest barrier to any improvement in the health conditions. Mother's education level, even within the same socio-economic class is a key determinant of their children's health. There is extensive evidence (e.g. Kerala experience) that maternal education plays a major role in the decline of infant and child mortality, presumably reflecting personal health behaviour, care and access to and use of health services. Women with schooling tend to marry later, delay child-bearing and are more likely to practice family planning. They generally have fewer children with wider spacing between births.

(g) *Quality of health care*

Another likely factor affecting infant mortality in contemporary India is inadequate prenatal care and infrequent attendance at delivery.

The percentage of deliveries attended by untrained persons or relatives is very high in rural India. Shortage of trained personnel like dais, midwives and health visitors is another determinant of high infant mortality in India. According to estimates only 47 per cent of the deliveries are attended by trained birth attendants.

(h) *Broken families*

Infant mortality tends to be high where the mother or father has died or separated.

(i) *Illegitimacy*

Illegitimacy is also an important factor contributing to high infant mortality rate. A child born out of wedlock is generally unwanted both by the mother as well as society. Consequently such a child does not receive the care in terms of nutrition and medical care that it needs.

(j) *Brutal habits and customs*

Certain age-old customs and beliefs greatly influence infant mortality rate. These include depriving the baby of the first milk or colostrum, frequent purgation, branding the skin, application of cowdung to the cut end of umbilical cord, faulty feeding practices and early weaning.

(k) *The indigenous dai*

The untrained midwife is greatly responsible for the high infant mortality in India. She is usually an illiterate person devoid of all knowledge of rules of hygiene. Her unhygienic delivery practice is an important cause of high infant mortality.

(l) *Bad environmental sanitation*

Infants are highly susceptible to bad environmental sanitation. Lack of safe water supply, poor housing conditions, bad drainage, overcrowding, and insect breeding, all increase the risk of infant mortality.

The fourth National Family Health Survey conducted in India during 2019–2021 provides vast information on factors associated with mortality in infancy and childhood.

Preventive and social measures

There is no single specific health programme or a single set of action that can reduce IMR. Since the aetiology of infant and perinatal mortality is multifactorial, nothing less than a multipronged approach will reduce infant and perinatal mortality. Under ideal conditions of Social Welfare, no baby should die, except possibly the few who are born with serious handicaps such as congenital abnormalities or disorders originating in uterine life. The measures needed to achieve reduction of infant mortality comprise the following :

1. *Prenatal nutrition*

The risk of death begins to appear even before birth, if the mother is malnourished. Therefore, the very first need is to improve the state of maternal nutrition. There is mounting evidence that the addition of even a small amount of extra food by way of supplementation to the mother's basic diet goes a long way in improving the birth weight of babies. In a controlled study in India, poor women were fed an additional 500 kcals and 10 g of protein during the last 4 weeks of pregnancy. Their infants' birth weights were on an average 300 g above those infants born to the control group *(98, 99)*. This points to the need for food supplementation programmes during pregnancy. ICDS (Integrated Child Development Services) in India is active in this field.

2. *Prevention of infection*

The major causes of sickness and death of children in India are infectious diseases, many of which are preventable by immunization, as for example, neonatal tetanus. A large number of cases of EPI targeted diseases are reported each year. The Universal Immunization Programme launched in 1985 aims at providing protection to all the expectant mothers and children against 9 vaccine preventable diseases, and thereby ensure greater child survival.

3. *Breast-feeding*

The most effective measure for lowering infant mortality is to promote breast-feeding, which is a safeguard against gastrointestinal and respiratory infections and PEM.

4. *Growth monitoring*

It is a low cost technology available for reducing infant mortality. All infants should be weighed periodically (at least once a month) and their growth charts maintained. These charts help to identify children at risk of malnutrition early. Babies who do not thrive or show growth failure are given special health care to pull them on to the road-to-health. Thus systematic use of growth chart will help to promote health in children.

5. *Family planning*

Family limitation and spacing of births contribute substantially to lowering of infant mortality rate. The risk of death is greatly enhanced if the last child was born less than 2 years ago, and if the mother already has four or more children. Smaller sibship and longer spacing between pregnancies are associated in all societies with improved infant and child survival.

6. *Sanitation*

For infants and young children, the risk of dying is very closely related to the environment in which they live. Exposure to infections through contaminated food and polluted water, lack of elementary hygiene, flies and poor housing pose hazards which the young cannot escape. This is why infant mortality rate is universally recognized not only as a most important indicator of the health status of the children, but also of the level of social environment.

7. *Provision of primary health care*

(a) All those involved in maternity care, from the obstetrician down to the local dai should collaborate and work together as a team, (b) Prenatal care must be improved with a view to detecting mothers with "high-risk factors", and those with prenatal conditions associated with high-risk (e.g., toxaemia of pregnancy, antipartum haemorrhage, diabetes mellitus) are hospitalized and treated. (c) "Special care baby units" must be provided for all babies weighing less than 2000 g. (d) Proper referral services.

8. *Socio-economic development*

Since the causes of infant and perinatal mortality are also social, there is no getting away from the fact that the ultimate solution for lowering IMR and PMR lies in socio-economic development. This must include spread of education (especially female literacy), improvement of nutritional standards, provision of safe water and basic sanitation, improvement of housing conditions, the growth of agriculture and industry and the availability of commerce and communication; in short, it implies allround health and social development of the community.

9. *Education*

Education of females as a driving force for better health has been extensively studied and documented. Educated women generally do not have early pregnancies, are able to space their pregnancies, have better access to information related to personal hygiene and care of their children, and make better use of health care services. Higher literacy rate among women is associated with low fertility and low maternal mortality, as well as low infant mortality. A study during 1991 in the Indian State of Tamil Nadu, with a population of more than 60 million, showed that a mid-day meal programme for school children together with improvement of health care for women and their babies raised retention levels in school, reduced child mortality, increased immunization rates and led to dramatic fall in infant deaths from 90 per 1000 live births in 1984 to 57 in 1991. This in turn seems to have reduced the fertility level to 2.5 children per women in 1991 *(40)*, and Tamil Nadu has now achieved zero population growth.

1–4 YEAR MORTALITY RATE

(Child death rate)

Child death rate is the number of deaths of children aged 1–4 years per 1000 children in the same age group in a given year. It thus excludes infant mortality. The rate is computed by the formula :

$$= \frac{\text{No.of deaths of children aged 1–4 years during a year}}{\text{Total no. of children aged 1–4 years at the middle of the year}} \times 1000$$

The child death rate is a more refined indicator of the social situation in a country than infant mortality rate. It reflects the adverse environmental health hazards (e.g., malnutrition, poor hygiene, infections and accidents), including economic, educational and cultural characteristics of the family. Mortality in this age group no longer depends on perinatal hazards and other endogenous factors, which often cause loss of life during the first year of life.

In the age group 1–4 years, the second year is the period when the young child runs the highest risk of dying. In the developing countries, death in the second year of life commonly accounts for 50 per cent of all deaths between 1–4 years of age. After the second year, death rates decline progressively. The infectious diseases of childhood such as measles, whooping cough, diphtheria, diarrhoea and acute respiratory infections affect mostly this age group, and can lead to high case–fatality rate in malnourished children.

Mortality rate at ages 1–4 years is about 30 in some developing countries whereas it is less than one in developed countries. The contrast is glaring. While on an average, the IMR is 10–20 times higher in developing countries than in the developed countries, the average mortality rate between the age 1–4 years is 30–50 times higher.

In India, for the year 2020, 1–4 years age crude death rate was estimated to be 1.0 per cent of total deaths. Like infant mortality, 1–4 year age mortality also shows wide state-wise variations as shown in Table 27. The states reporting rates higher than the national average are Madhya Pradesh 2.0, Rajasthan 1.9, Himachal Pradesh 1.7, Uttar Pradesh 1.4, and Haryana with 1.2 *(73)*. Tamil Nadu recorded the lowest with 0.2 per cent followed by Gujarat with 0.3 per cent.

TABLE 27

SRS estimates for child death (1-4 years) and under-five mortality in major states of India, 2020

State	Child death (1–4 years) crude death rate	Under-five mortality rate (per 1000 live births)		
		Total	Rural	Urban
Andhra Pradesh	0.7	27	29	21
Assam	0.9	40	42	19
Bihar	0.8	30	31	27
Chhattisgarh	0.8	41	43	31
Delhi	0.6	14	20	14
Gujarat	0.3	24	28	17
Haryana	1.2	33	37	25
Himachal Pradesh*	1.7	24	24	18
Jammu & Kashmir	0.2	17	18	14
Jharkhand	0.4	27	28	22
Karnataka	0.6	21	23	18
Kerala	0.5	8	5	12
Madhya Pradesh	2.0	51	56	33
Maharashtra	0.6	18	23	12
Odisha	0.9	39	40	31
Punjab	0.9	22	24	18
Rajasthan	1.9	40	43	27
Tamil Nadu	0.2	13	16	11
Telangana	0.4	23	25	19
Uttar Pradesh	1.4	43	46	32
Uttarakhand	0.4	26	26	26
West Bengal	0.8	22	22	20
India	1.0	32	36	21

*(Based on three year period 2018–2020)

Source : *(73)*

Leading causes of death

The leading causes of death in the 1–4 years age group are as shown in Table 28.

TABLE 28

Leading causes of death in 1–4 years age group

Developing countries	Developed countries
Diarrhoeal diseases Respiratory infections Malnutrition Infectious diseases (e.g., measles, whooping cough) Other febrile diseases Accidents and injuries	Accidents Congenital anomalies Malignant neoplasms Influenza Pneumonia

The leading causes of death in 1–4 years age group in developing countries are diarrhoeal diseases and respiratory infections, closely followed by other communicable diseases such as whooping cough and measles. When combined with malnutrition these diseases have high case fatality rates. In the developed countries deaths from infectious diseases are quite rare, while accidents are the leading cause of death from the age of one year. Four groups of home accidents have been identified – (a) falls from unprotected stairs, and balconies (b) suffocation (c) burns and scalds (d) poisoning. Almost all accidents are preventable. The factors such as congenital anomalies and neoplasms are not easy to prevent or to cure. These conditions also affect children in developing countries, but their relative importance is overshadowed by infections.

UNDER-5 MORTALITY RATE

(Child mortality rate)

UNICEF defines this as the "annual number of deaths of children age under 5 years, expressed as a rate per 1000 live births." More specifically, it measures the probability of dying between birth and exactly 5 years of age. UNICEF considers this as the best single indicator of social development and well-being rather than GNP per capita, as the former reflects income, nutrition, health care and basic education etc *(100)*. The rate is calculated by the formula :

$$\text{Child mortality rate} = \frac{\text{Number of deaths of children less than 5 years of age in a given year}}{\text{Number of live births in the same year}} \times 1000$$

Around the world, remarkable progress in child survival has been made and millions of children have better survival chances than in 1990. The under-5 mortality rate fell to 33 deaths per 1000 live births in 2020, from 126 in 1990 – a 73.8 per cent reduction. This is equivalent to 1 in 11 children dying before reaching age 5 years in 1990, compared to 1 in 26 in 2020. In most of the SDG regions, the under-5 mortality rate was reduced by at least half since 1990. The total number of under-5 deaths dropped to 5.0 million in 2020 from 12.6 million in 1990. On average, 14,520 children died every day in 2018, as compared to 34,000 in 1990 *(86)*.

Despite progress over the past 2 decades, millions of newborns and children die every year, mostly from preventable or treatable causes such as infectious diseases and injuries. These deaths reflect the limited access of children and communities to basic medical treatment of infectious diseases, adequate nutrition, health interventions such as vaccination, clean water and sanitation. Children face wide-spread regional and income disparities in their chances of survival. Sub-Saharan Africa continues to be the region with the highest under-five mortality rate in the world – 74 deaths per 1000 live births in 2020. This translates to 1 child in 13 dying before his fifth birthday - 14 times higher than the average ratio of 1 in 185 in high income countries and 20 times higher than the ratio of 1 in 263 in the region of Australia and New Zealand. In 2020, about 26 per cent under-five mortality occurred in Southern Asia. About 38 per cent of all deaths occur in least developed countries. The number of countries with gender disparities in child mortality continues to decline. On an average, boys are expected to have a higher probability of dying before reaching age 5 years than girls. The estimated under-5 mortality rate in 2020 was 41 deaths per 1000 lives birth for boys and 35 deaths per 1000 live births for girls. In 2020, an estimated 2.7 million boys and 2.3 million girls under 5 years of age died *(6)*.

A recent analysis showed that children in the poorest households are nearly twice likely to die before the age of 5 as those from the richest. The risk of death in rural areas is 1.5 times higher than for children in the urban areas and within urban areas children from poorer household tend to have higher mortality rates. Children of mothers who lack any education are 2.6 times more likely to die before reaching 5 years age. Poor air quality is another risk factor for child mortality *(101)*.

Table 29 shows child mortality rate in some selected developed and developing countries.

TABLE 29

Under-5 mortality rate in some selected countries during 1990 and mid 2020

(Per 1000 live births)

Country	1990	2020
India	126	33.0
Sri Lanka	21	7.0
Thailand	37	9.0
Nepal	142	28.0
China	54	7.0
Bangladesh	144	29.0
Pakistan	139	65.0
UK	9	4.0
USA	11	6.0
Japan	6	2.0
Singapore	8	2.0
World	90	37.0

Source : *(6)*

Causes of under five deaths

Understanding the causes of child mortality provides important public health insights. Of the 5.3 million deaths in children under-5, that occurred in 2018, almost 40% were caused by infectious diseases and conditions such as pneumonia, diarrhoea, malaria, meningitis, tetanus, HIV and measles. Around 47% of all under-five deaths occurred in the neonatal period (within the first 28 days of life), the majority from preterm birth complications and intrapartum-related complications (complications during delivery). Globally, more than half of the under-five deaths are attributable to undernutrition *(102)*.

Worldwide, the leading causes of death among children under-5 years include pneumonia (12% of all under-five deaths), preterm birth complications (16%), diarrhoea (8%), intrapartum-related complications (11%), malaria (5%), and neonatal sepsis (7.0%), meningitis (2.1%), tetanus (0.1%), measles (2%), injury (6%) and others (12%). Cross-country comparisons show a wide variation among countries in the proportions of under-five deaths attributable to specific causes. Such variations indicate that optimal programmatic approaches for child survival will differ from country to country. Fig. 16 shows the causes of death of children under-five in 2018.

Summarizing data across regions and countries masks substantial differences in the distribution of causes of death. Approximately 90% of all malaria and HIV/AIDS deaths in children, more than 50% of measles deaths and about 40% of pneumonia and diarrhoeal deaths are in the African Region. On the other hand, deaths from injuries and non-communicable diseases other than congenital anomalies, account for 20–30% of under-five deaths in the region of the Americas and in the European and Western Pacific Regions *(103)*.

The steady improvement in under-five survival is explained by a combination of advances. They include developments in science and technology (for example, oral rehydration salts that treat diarrhoeal dehydration and insecticide-treated mosquito nets for malaria prevention), improved health-seeking behaviours (such as women's increasing use of antenatal care and skilled providers for care around the time of birth), improved sanitation and improved coverage of effective interventions to prevent or treat the most important causes of child mortality. Each one

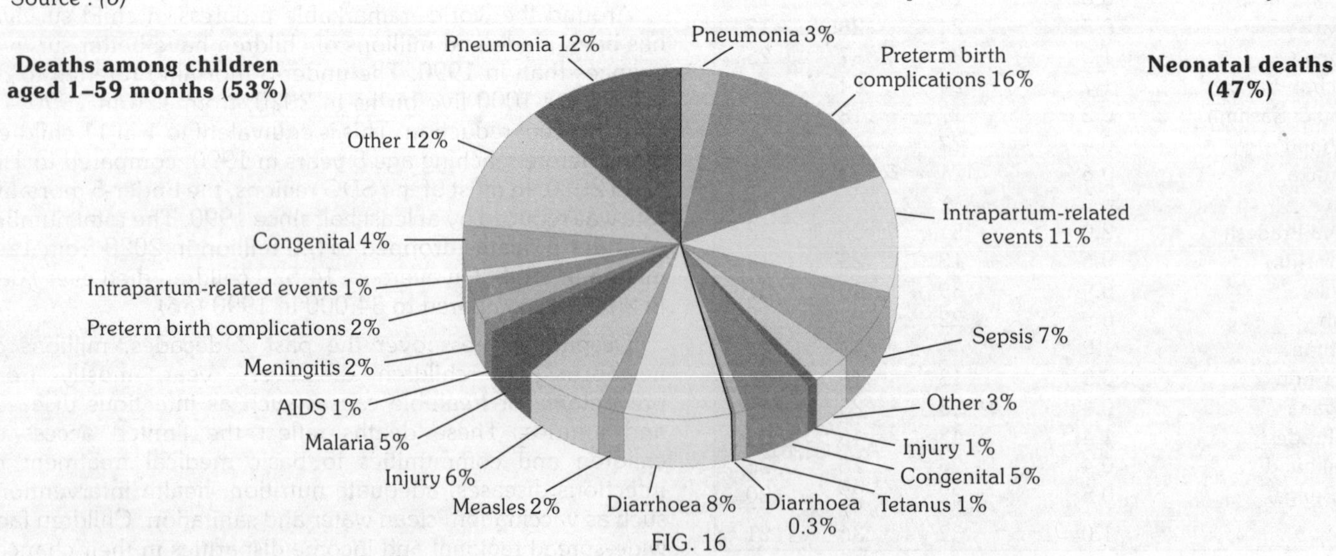

FIG. 16

Global distribution of deaths among children under-5 by cause, 2018

Source : *(86)*

of these advances is due to the political will of committed governments and the expansion of innovative partnerships involving civil society and the public and private sectors. Taken together, these efforts are reducing the number of young lives claimed by the leading causes of under-five mortality: pneumonia, diarrhoea, malaria, measles and AIDS. As a result 3 million fewer children died from these five diseases in 2015 than in the year 2000 *(103)*.

The Expanded Programme on Immunization started in 1974 and widened range of vaccines routinely provided, from smallpox, BCG and DPT to include polio and measles and more recently hepatitis B, Hib, Rota virus vaccine and JE vaccine. It set-out to increase coverage in line with the international commitment to achieve the universal child immunization goal of 80 per cent coverage in every country.

As mortality from diarrhoeal diseases and vaccine preventable diseases decreased, pneumonia came to the forefront as a cause of death, and in the 1980s programmes were developed around simplified diagnostic and treatment techniques. In the meantime, promotion of breast-feeding continued, backed by international initiative and countries widely implemented the Baby-Friendly Hospitals initiative.

The Integrated Management of Childhood Illness (IMCI) strategy addresses the principal causes of child mortality i.e. diarrhoeal disease, acute respiratory infection, measles, malaria and underlying malnutrition. Several countries like India have added neonatal care in the national adaptations. It combines effective interventions for preventing death and for improving healthy growth and development, e.g., oral rehydration therapy for diarrhoea; antibiotics for sepsis, pneumonia and ear infection, antimalarials and insecticide-treated bed-nets; vitamin A, treatment of anaemia, promotion of breast-feeding and complementary feeding for healthy nutrition and for recovery from illness; and immunization. Some countries have included guidelines to treat children with HIV/AIDS, others for dengue fever, wheezing or sore throat, or for the follow-up of healthy children.

More recently, Every Newborn Action Plan proposes five strategic objectives for achieving two clear and measurable targets : (1) Ending preventable newborn deaths – By 2035, all countries reach a national target of 10 or fewer newborn deaths per 1000 live births and continue to reduce death and disability; and (2) Ending preventable stillbirths – By 2035, all countries reach the target of 10 or fewer stillbirths per 1000 total births and continue to narrow gaps in equity. Developed under WHO and UNICEF, the ENAP recommends the integrated delivery of high-impact interventions across the full continuum of maternal and newborn care, including care during labour, newborn care during the first week of life and care of small and sick newborns. Fig. 17 shows the package of interventions.

Child mortality rate in India

Each year about 27 million children are born in India. Around 10 per cent of them do not survive to 5 years of age. In absolute figures, India contributes to 25 per cent of the over 5.3 million under-five deaths occurring worldwide every year. Nearly 62 per cent of the under-five deaths occur in neonatal period, 20 per cent takes place on the day of birth, and 49 per cent within the first 7 days *(86)*. The mortality rates for children below age 5 years for the year 2020, by residence are shown in Table 27. At the national level the mortality rate was estimated at 27 per 1000 live births, and the rate varies from 8 in Kerala to 51 in Madhya Pradesh. The rate for rural areas is about 36 and for urban areas 21. The mortality rate in female children in India is higher than the male children *(73)*.

Among children who die before their fifth birthday, almost one-third die of infectious causes nearly all of which are preventable. The estimates of the cause of death for the year 2016 are shown in Fig. 18.

Focus of the Every Newborn Action Plan
The time around birth results in the majority of maternal and newborn deaths and stillbirths as well as human capital loss. These packages have the highest impact yet some of the lowest coverage of equitable and quality care across the continuum.

	Adolescence and before pregnancy	Pregnancy	Labour and birth	Postnatal	Child
Referral and tertiary level facility	Reproductive health, including family planning	Management of pregnancy complications	Skilled care at birth	Essential newborn care Emergency care of small and sick newborns	Hospital care of childhood illness
First and secondary level facility	Reproductive health, including family planning	Pregnancy care	Skilled care at birth Basic emergency obstetric and newborn care	Essential newborn care Postnatal visits Care of small and sick newborns	Prevention and management of childhood illness
Community	Adolescent and pre-conception health care and nutrition Gender violence prevention	Counselling and birth preparedness	Home birth with skilled care and clean practices	Essential newborn care Postnatal home visits for mothers and newborns	Ongoing care for the child at home

Intersectoral : Improved living and working conditions, including housing, water and sanitation, and nutrition, education and empowerment, especially of girls, folic acid fortification; safe and healthy work environments for women and pregnant women

Labour, birth and first week

FIG. 17

Packages of interventions in the continuum of care

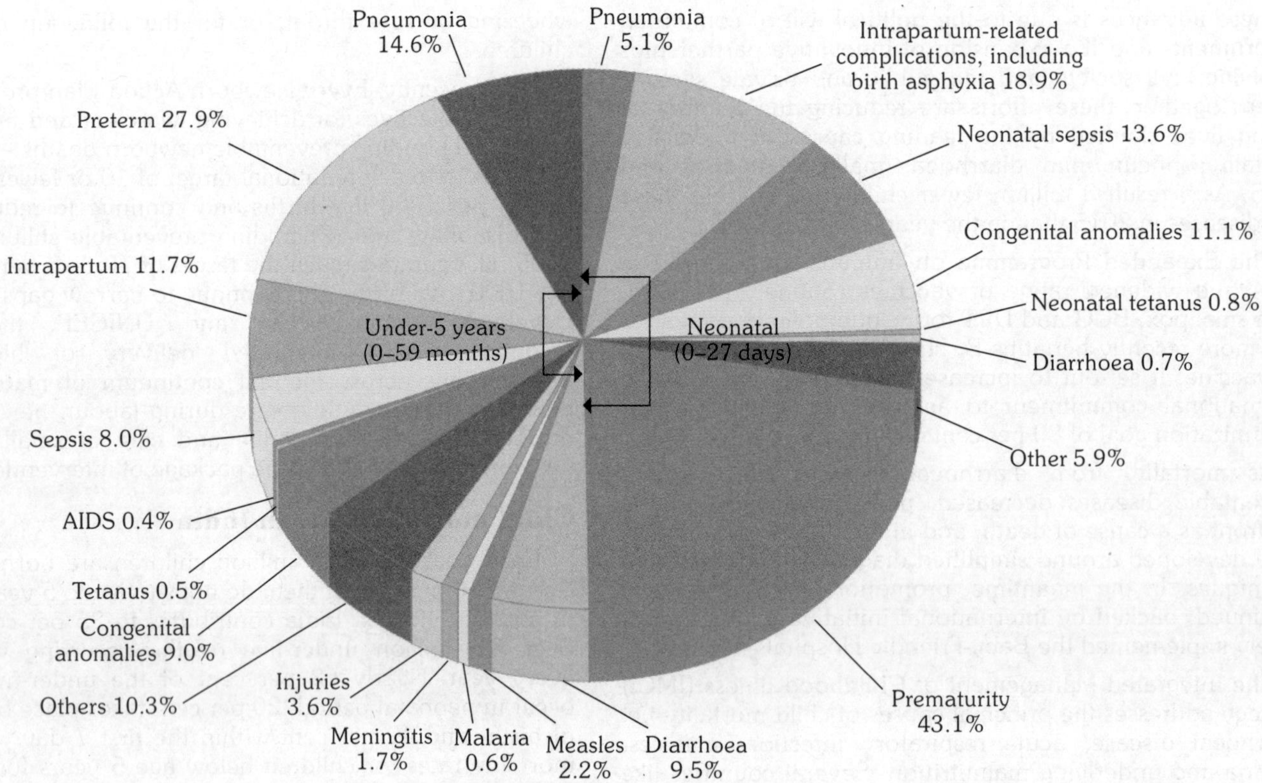

FIG. 18

Causes of death among children under 5 years, India, 2016

Source : *(102)*

Preterm birth has emerged as the leading cause of neonatal death, underlying the need for rapid scale-up of maternal health interventions in order to improve neonatal health outcomes.

Social determinants for maternal and child mortality include marriage and childbirth at a very young age, less spacing between births and low literacy level among women, in particular those belonging to the urban poor and rural settings, and socially-disadvantaged groups (such as scheduled caste and tribes). Access to and use of contraceptives, particularly modern, non-permanent contraceptives, and access to safe abortion services are also factors that influence maternal health and child survival. The TFR for those women who have no education is higher compared to those who are literate. Furthermore, there is a gradual decline of TFR with the increase in the level of education. Low level of education is itself linked to the low status of women, and associated risks such as violence against women, emotional and physical abuse and malnutrition *(104)*.

A large number of maternal and child deaths are attributable to the 'three delays' : (1) the delay in deciding to seek care, (2) the delay in reaching the appropriate health facility, and (3) the delay in receiving quality care once inside an institution. The delay in deciding to seek care can occur due to inadequate resources, poor access to high-quality health care and lack of awareness of the importance of maternal and newborn health care at the household level. The unavailability of basic reproductive health services, including contraceptives, pre and postnatal care and emergency obstetric and neonatal care, as well as delays in seeking institutional care and the poor quality of care provided in the health facility can potentially contribute to child deaths *(104)*.

The reproductive, maternal, neonatal and child health packages that are currently being implemented under the NRHM address the most common causes of maternal and child deaths. However, the coverage of key interventions, such as antenatal care, deliveries by skilled birth attendants, and use of oral rehydration solution (ORS) for the management of childhood diarrhoea during the NRHM period has been slow and of variable quality across states.

To pursue the goals of NPP, the Government of India constituted a National Technical Committee on Child Health in June 2000. New initiatives taken on the basis of this are *(64)* :

- Launch of Immunization Strengthening Project;
- Organization of RCH camps, health "melas" and RCH outreach scheme to reach disadvantageous segments of the population;
- Launch of Hepatitis B vaccine in the immunization programme;
- Operationalization of newborn care facilities in identified weak districts;
- Operations research by ICMR for provision of home-based neonatal care through community-level providers;
- Policy for exclusive breast-feeding upto 6 months of age;
- Preparation and approval of concept note on development of community based mid-wives;
- Implementation of Dai training to provide key messages for newborn health in 166 districts; and
- Adaptation of IMCI to incorporate newborn issues and development of IMNCI.

The Government of India established an IMCI Adaptation Committee that has led the development of Integrated

Management of Newborn and Childhood Illnesses (IMNCI). Separate tools and guidelines have been produced that focus on newborn issues; these are used to train field staff and for supervision and monitoring purposes.

In the year 2013, RMNCH+A strategy and in the year 2014, India Newborn Action Plan were launched in view to reduce the mortality rates in children. Newer vaccines were introduced in the national immunization schedule. Please refer to chapter 7 for details.

The Global Strategy for Women's, Children's and Adolescent's Health (2016–2030) and the 2030 agenda for Sustainable Development have three overarching objectives – Survive, Thrive and Transform. The SDGs contain ambitious targets for child mortality with SDG 3.2 seeking to end preventable deaths of newborns and children under 5 year. These include national targets of a U5MR of no more than 25 per 1000 live births and neonatal mortality rate to no more than 12 per 1000 live births *(105)*. Target 4.2, which calls for efforts to ensure that all girls and boys have access to quality early childhood development, care and pre-primary education; which is likely to have an impact on child mortality, while also improving children's chances of long and rewarding lives *(105)*.

CHILD SURVIVAL INDEX

The basic measure of infant and child survival is the Under-5 mortality (number of deaths under the age of 5 years, per 1000 live births). A child survival rate per 1000 births can be simply calculated by subtracting the Under-5 mortality rate from 1000. Dividing this figure by ten shows the percentage of those who survive to the age of 5 years *(106)*.

$$\text{Child survival rate} = \frac{1000 - \text{under-5 mortality rate}}{10}$$

The following table (Table 30) shows the child survival rates of some countries.

TABLE 30

Child survival rates of some countries during 1990 and 2020

Country	1990	2020
India	87.4	96.7
Sri Lanka	97.9	99.3
Bangladesh	85.6	97.1
Nepal	85.8	97.2
Pakistan	86.1	93.5
China	94.6	99.3
UK	99.1	99.6
USA	98.4	99.4
Japan	99.4	99.8
Singapore	99.2	99.8

The difference in the survival rates of children in developed and developing countries is a grim pointer to the Third World's need for preventive services. Through breast-feeding, adequate nutrition, clean water, immunization programmes, oral rehydration therapy and birth spacing, a virtual revolution in child survival could be achieved. The impact would be dramatic in humanitarian and fertility terms.

INTEGRATED MANAGEMENT OF CHILDHOOD ILLNESS (IMCI)

The notion of integration has a long history. Integration is supposed to tackle the need for complementarity of different independent services and administrative structures, so as to better achieve common goals. In 1950s, the goals were defined in terms of outcome, in 1960s of process and in the 1990s of economic impact. Integration has different meanings at different levels. At the patient level it means case management. At the point of delivery it means that multiple interventions are provided through one delivery channel, e.g., where vaccination is used as an opportunity to provide vitamin A to the child, boosting efficiency and coverage. At the system level integration means bringing together management and support function of different sub-programmes and ensuring complimentarity between different levels of care. IMCI is now the only child health strategy that aims for improved integration at these three levels simultaneously. More than just adding more programmes to a single delivery channel, it has sought to transform the way the health system looks at the child care.

Most sick children present with signs and symptoms related to more than one conditions. This overlap means that a single diagnosis may not be possible or appropriate, and that treatment may be complicated by the need to combine therapy for several conditions. Surveys of the management of sick children at these facilities reveal that many children are not properly assessed and treated and that their parents are poorly advised. Providing quality care to sick children in these conditions is a serious challenge. In response to these challenge, WHO and UNICEF developed a strategy known as IMCI. The strategy combines improved management of childhood illness with aspects of nutrition, immunization, and other important disease prevention and health promotion elements. The objectives are to reduce deaths and the frequency and severity of illness and disability and to contribute to improved growth and development.

The strategy includes three main components :

(1) Improvements in the case-management skills of health staff through the provision of locally adapted guidelines on IMCI and through activities to promote their use;

(2) Improvements in the health system required for effective management of childhood illness; and

(3) Improvements in family and community practices.

The core of the IMCI strategy is integrated case management of the most common childhood problems, with a focus on the most important causes of death i.e. diarrhoea, ARI, malaria, measles and malnutrition. A guided process of adaptation ensures that the guidelines, and the learning materials that go with them, reflect the epidemiology within a country and are tailored to fit the needs, resources and capacity of a country's health system.

The clinical guidelines, which are based on expert clinical opinion and research results, are designed for the management of sick children aged 1 week up to 5 years. They promote evidence-based assessment and management, using a syndromic approach that supports the rational, effective and affordable use of drugs. They include methods for assessing signs that indicate severe disease; assessing a child's nutrition, immunization, and feeding; teaching parents how to care for a child at home; counselling parents to solve feeding problems; and advising parents about when to return to a health facility.The guidelines also include recommendations for checking the parent's understanding of the advice given and for showing them how to administer the first dose of treatment.

When assessing a sick child, a combination of individual signs leads to one or more classifications, rather than to a diagnosis. IMCI classifications are action oriented and allow a health care provider to determine if a child should be urgently referred to another health facility, if the child can be treated at the first-level facility (e.g. with oral antibiotic, antimalarial, ORS, etc.) or if the child can be safely managed at home.

The complete IMCI case management process involves the following elements *(107)* :

a. Assess a child by checking first for danger signs (or possible bacterial infection in a young infant), asking questions about common conditions, examining the child, and checking nutrition and immunization status. Assessment includes checking the child for other health problems.

b. Classify a child's illnesses using a colour-coded triage system. Because many children have more than one condition, each illness is classified according to whether it requires :
   - urgent pre-referral treatment and referral (pink), or
   - specific medical treatment and advice (yellow), or
   - simple advice on home management (green).

c. After classifying all conditions, **identify** specific treatments for the child. If a child requires urgent referral, give essential treatment before the patient is transferred. If a child needs treatment at home, develop an integrated treatment plan for the child and give the first dose of drugs in the clinic. If a child should be immunized, give immunization.

d. Provide practical **treatment** instructions, including teaching the caretaker how to give oral drugs, how to feed and give fluids during illness, and how to treat local infections at home. Ask the caretaker to return for follow-up on a specific date, and teach her how to recognize signs that indicate the child should return immediately to the health facility.

e. Assess feeding, including assessment of breast-feeding practices, and **counsel** to solve any feeding problems found. Then counsel the mother about her own health.

f. When a child is brought back to the clinic as requested, **give follow-up care and,** if necessary, reassess the child for new problems.

The IMCI guidelines address most, but not all, of the major reasons a sick child is brought to a clinic. A child returning with chronic problems or less common illnesses may require special care. The guidelines do not describe the management of trauma or other acute emergencies due to accidents or injuries.

Although AIDS is not addressed specifically, the case management guidelines address the most common reasons children with HIV seek care : diarrhoea and respiratory infections. When a child, who is believed to have HIV, presents with any of these common illnesses, he or she can be treated the same way as any child presenting with an illness. If a child's illness does not respond to the standard treatments described or if a child becomes severely malnourished, or returns to the clinic repeatedly, the child is referred to a hospital for special care.

Case management can only be effective to the extent that families bring their sick children to a trained health worker for care in a timely way. If a family waits to bring a child to a clinic until the child is extremely sick, or takes the child to an untrained provider, the child is more likely to die from the illness. Therefore, teaching families when to seek care for a sick child is an important part of the case management process.

The case management process is presented on two different sets of charts : one for children age 2 months up to five years, and one for children age 1 week up to 2 months. Annexure 'A' at the end of this chapter shows the flowchart about the IMNCI guidelines for the management of various conditions of childhood.

The Indian version of IMCI is known as IMNCI (Integrated Management of Neonatal and Childhood Illness) as it includes the first 7 days of age in the programme. Please refer to page 528 chapter 7 for further details.

CONGENITAL MALFORMATIONS

Definitions

Congenital disorders are defined as "those diseases that are substantially determined before or during birth and which are in principle recognizable in early life" *(110)*. Some are obvious at birth like, cleft palate; some are obvious in early life like congenital dislocation of hip which may escape detection until walking should commence; and some may not become apparent until much later in life, like patent ductus arteriosus which may escape diagnosis until school age or even later. Internal defects, when they are not lethal, may go unrecognized. In addition to the list of late diagnoses are a host of inborn errors of metabolism like PKU, Tay-Sachs disease, galactosaemia, and mental retardation. Some defects are classified as major which may require surgical intervention, and some are classified as minor that have no functional implications like skin tags in front of the ear. Thus a broad definition of **congenital malformation** includes not only anatomical defects but also molecular and cellular abnormalities present at birth *(108)*. A WHO document in 1972, however, held that the term **congenital malformation** should be confined to structural defects at birth, and the term **congenital anomaly** being used to include all biochemical, structural and functional disorders present at birth *(88)*. Thus the basic difficulty in the study of congenital defects is the actual definition of the term without which comparisons between studies are difficult to make.

Incidence

Congenital anomalies (also referred as birth defects) affect approximately 1 in 33 infants and result in approximately 3.2 million birth defect-related disabilities every year. An estimated 270,000 newborns die during the first 28 days of life every year from congenital anomalies. Congenital anomalies may result in long-term disability, which may have significant impacts on individuals, families, health-care systems and societies. The most common serious congenital disorders are heart defect, neural tube defects and Down's syndrome. Congenital anomalies may have a genetic, infectious or environmental origin; although in most of the cases it is difficult to identify their cause *(109)*.

Causes

The aetiology of most congenital anomalies is poorly understood; both genetic and environmental factors have been implicated. They include :

1. GENETIC FACTORS : The congenital disorders with genetic aetiology are : (a) *Chromosomal abnormalities :* The chromosome is either missing or in excess. The examples include Down's syndrome, Klinefelter's syndrome and Turner's syndrome. (b) *Inborn errors of metabolism :* These include PKU, Tay-Sachs disease and galactosaemia (c) *Others :* Other genetically inherited disorders, presumably due to single gene defects, are much more common than conditions with demonstrable chromosomal abnormalities. Single gene disorders may be dominant (e.g., Huntington's chorea), recessive (e.g., thalassaemia, sickle cell disease) or sex-linked disorders (e.g., haemophilia) (d) *Those with probable or possible genetic aetiology :* This applies to congenital dislocation of hip, club foot and neural tube defects.

2. ENVIRONMENTAL FACTORS : These include intra–uterine Infections (e.g., rubella, cytomegalovirus, toxoplasmosis, syphilis), Drugs (e.g., thalidomide, stilboestrol, anti-convulsants, tobacco, high dose of vitamin A during early pregnancy, alcohol, anaesthetics, etc.), Maternal diseases complicated by pregnancy (e.g., diabetes, cardiac failure), Irradiation, and Dietary factors (e.g., folic acid deficiency).

Risk factors

The factors significantly associated with the occurrence of congenital malformations are : (a) *Maternal age :* Advanced maternal age at conception is a recognized risk factor. The overall risk of giving birth to an infant with Down's syndrome is 1 : 800. The risk rises sharply with age; it is 1 : 67 for those aged 40–45. (b) *Consanguinity :* In consanguineous marriages (e.g., first-cousin and uncle-niece marriages), there is a relatively high incidence of mental retardation and congenital malformations.

Prenatal diagnosis

It is now possible to detect certain congenital anomalies *in utero* using the following techniques : (a) **Alpha fetoprotein** : Neural tube defects can be detected by measurement of a specific protein of foetal origin, called alpha fetoprotein in maternal blood and in amniotic fluid during pregnancy. (b) **Ultrasound** : This can be used to visualize the foetus and detect many abnormalities of the foetus. (c) **Amniocentesis :** This test is possible only in the second trimester (i.e., after the completion of 12 weeks). It can detect many abnormalities (e.g., Down's syndrome, Neural tube defects). (d) **Chorionic villus sampling** : This new technique allows prenatal diagnosis at 9 to 11 weeks of pregnancy. By this test, the chromosome status can be easily determined. Prenatal diagnosis of congenital abnormalities offers the parents the option of therapeutic abortion.

PREVENTION OF CONGENITAL DEFORMITIES

There are 3 main approaches to the reduction of congenital abnormalities: *(111)*. (1) By discouraging further reproduction after the birth of a malformed child; after such a birth, the frequency of malformations in subsequent pregnancies is increased by about 10 times; (2) The avoidance of pregnancy in circumstances where malformations are likely to occur, e.g., advanced maternal age and Down's syndrome; (3) the identification and removal of teratogens such as certain drugs (e.g., thalidomide, steroid hormones, folate antagonists, anti-convulsants); infective agents (e.g., rubella, cytomegalovirus, herpes simplex virus, varicella zoster virus, *Toxoplasma gondii*); and physical agents such as X-rays and irradiation, alcohol and pesticides. Immunization against rubella is now routine in many countries which is bound to lead to some reduction in congenital abnormalities. A largely untapped preventive measure is the avoidance of drugs in pregnancy except where they are absolutely necessary *(112)*.

Congenital malformations may be regarded as one form of reproductive failure. The most unfavourable environmental and genetic factors result in sterility, and the favourable factors lead to normal reproduction. Between these extremes there may be abortions, stillbirths, premature births or neonatal deaths. Malformation represent a relative reproductive "success" when compared with sterility or early abortion *(103)*. Penrose (1961) stressed that major advances in the prevention of malformations must be achieved by attention to environmental factors rather than by attempting to improve heredity. It is more within reach than genetic control *(104)*.

SCHOOL HEALTH SERVICE

School health is an important branch of community health. According to modern concepts, school health service is an economical and powerful means of raising community health, and more important, in future generations. The school health service is a personal health service. It has developed during the past 70 years from the narrower concept of medical examination of children to the present-day broader concept of comprehensive care of the health and well-being of children throughout the school years.

Historical development

The beginning of School Health Service in India dates back to 1909, when for the first time medical examination of school children was carried out in Baroda city. The Bhore Committee (1946) *(115)* reported that School Health Services were practically non-existent in India, and where they existed, they were in an under-developed state. In 1953, the Secondary Education Committee emphasized the need for medical examination of pupils and school feeding programmes. In 1960, the Government of India constituted a School Health Committee to assess the standards of health and nutrition of school children and suggest ways and means to improve them. The Committee submitted its report in 1961, which contains many useful recommendations *(116)*. During the Five Year Plans, many State Governments have provided for school health, and school feeding programmes. In spite of these efforts to improve school health, it must be stated that in India, as in other developing countries, the school health services provided are hardly more than a token service because of shortage of resources and insufficient facilities.

HEALTH PROBLEMS OF THE SCHOOL CHILD

Any discussion of a school health service must be based on the local health problems of the school child, the culture of the community and the available resources in terms of money, material and manpower. While the health problems of school children vary from one place to another, surveys carried out in India indicate that the main emphasis will fall in the following categories : (1) malnutrition; (2) infectious diseases; (3) intestinal parasites; (4) diseases of skin, eye and ear; and (5) dental caries.

OBJECTIVES OF SCHOOL HEALTH SERVICE

The objectives of the programme of a school health service are as follows *(117, 118)* :

1. the promotion of positive health;
2. the prevention of diseases;
3. early diagnosis, treatment and follow-up of defects;
4. awakening health consciousness in children; and
5. the provision of healthful environment.

Aspects of School Health Service

The tasks of a school health service are manifold, and vary according to local priorities. Where resources are plentiful, special school health services may be developed. Some aspects of a school health service are as follows :

1. Health appraisal of school children and school personnel.
2. Remedial measures and follow-up.
3. Prevention of communicable diseases.
4. Healthful school environment.
5. Nutritional services.
6. First-aid and emergency care.
7. Mental health.
8. Dental health.
9. Eye health.
10. Health education.
11. Education of handicapped children.
12. Proper maintenance and use of school health records.

1. Health appraisal

The health appraisal should cover not only the students but also the teachers and other school personnel. Health appraisal consists of periodic medical examinations and observation of children by the class teacher. (a) *Periodic Medical Examination* : The school health committee (1961) in India recommended medical examination of children at the time of entry and thereafter every 4 years *(116)*. In big cities, where facilities for medical examination are available, this could be more frequent. The initial examination should be thorough and unhastened and should include a careful history and physical examination of the child, with tests for vision, hearing and speech. A routine examination of blood and urine should be carried out. Clinical examination for nutritional deficiency, and examination of faeces for intestinal parasitosis are particularly important in India. Tuberculin testing or mass screening should not be withheld. The parents should be persuaded to be present at these examinations. The teacher should help in the medical inspection by recording the medical history, regular (quarterly) recording of height and weight, annual testing of vision, and preparing children for the medical examination by helping them understand the "how" and "why" of health appraisal. (b) *School Personnel* : Medical examination should be given to teachers and other school personnel as they form part of the environment to which the child is exposed. (c) *Daily Morning Inspection* : The teacher is in a unique position to carry out the "daily inspection", as he is familiar with the children and can detect changes in the child's appearance or behaviour that suggest illness or improper growth and development. The following clues will help the school teacher in suspecting children who need medical attention : (1) unusually flushed face (2) any rash or spots (3) symptoms of acute cold (4) coughing and sneezing (5) sore throat (6) rigid neck (7) nausea and vomiting (8) red or watery eyes (9) headache (10) chills or fever (11) listlessness or sleepiness (12) disinclination to play (13) diarrhoea (14) pains in the body (15) skin conditions like scabies and ringworm (16) pediculosis *(119)*. Children showing any such signs or symptoms should be referred to the school medical officer. Teacher observation of school children is of particular importance in India because of the limited number of trained personnel for school health work. For this work, the teachers should be adequately trained during Teacher Training Courses and subsequently by short In-service Training Courses.

2. Remedial measures and follow-up

Medical examinations are not an end in themselves; they should be followed by appropriate treatment and follow-up. Special clinics should be conducted exclusively for school children at the primary health centres in the rural areas, and in one of the selected schools or dispensaries for a group of about 5,000 children in the urban areas *(118)*. The clinic days and time should be intimated to all the concerned schools. Considering the high prevalence of dental, eye, ear, nose and throat defects in the school children in India, special clinics should be secured or provided for the exclusive use of school children for examination and treatment of such defects. In the big cities, the required number of specialists should be employed in the School Health Service. There should be provision for beds in the existing referral hospitals for the children to be admitted for investigation and treatment as and when required.

3. Prevention of communicable diseases

Communicable diseases control through immunization is the most emphasized school health service function. A well planned immunization programme should be drawn up against the common communicable diseases.

A record of all immunizations should be maintained as part of the school health records. When the child leaves school, the health record should accompany him.

4. Healthful school environment

The school building, site and equipment are part of the environment in which the child grows and develops. A healthful school environment therefore is necessary for the best emotional, social and personal health of the pupils. Schools should also serve as demonstration centres of good sanitation to the community. The following minimum standards for sanitation of the school and its environs have been suggested in India *(117, 118, 120)*.

(1) *Location* : The school should normally be centrally situated with proper approach roads and at a fair distance from busy places and roads, cinema houses, factories, railway tracks and market places. The school premises should be properly fenced and kept free from all hazards. (2) *Site* : The site should be on suitable high land, and not subject to inundation or dampness and can be properly drained. The School Health Committee (1961) had recommended that 10 acres of land be provided for higher elementary schools and 5 acres for primary schools with an additional one acre of land per 100 students. In congested areas, the nearest public park or playground should be made available to the students. (3) *Structure* : Nursery and secondary schools, as far as possible, be single storied. Exterior walls should have a minimum thickness of 10 inches and should be heat resistant. (4) *Classroom* : Verandhas should be attached to classrooms. No classroom should accommodate more than 40 students. Per capita

space for students in a classroom should not be less than 10 sq. ft. (5) *Furniture* : Furniture should suit the age group of students. It is desirable to provide single desks and chairs. Desks should be of "minus" type. Chairs should be provided with proper back-rests, with facilities for desk-work. (6) *Doors and windows*: The windows should be broad with the bottom sill, at a height of 2'–6" from the floor level; combined door and window area should be at least 25 per cent of the floor space; windows should be placed on different walls for cross-ventilation; the ventilators should not be less than 2 per cent of the floor area. (7) *Colour* : Inside colour of the classroom should be white and should be periodically white-washed. (8) *Lighting* : Classrooms should have sufficient natural light, preferably from the left, and should not be from the front. (9) *Water supply* : There should be an independent source of safe and potable water supply, which should be continuous, and distributed from the taps. (10) *Eating facilities* : Vendors other than those approved by the school authorities should not be allowed inside school premises; there should be a separate room provided for mid-day meals. (11) *Lavatory* : Privies and urinals should be provided – one urinal for 60 students and one latrine for 100 students. Arrangements should be separately made for boys and girls.

5. Nutritional services

A child who is physically weak will be mentally weak, and cannot be expected to take full advantage of schooling. The diet of the school child should, therefore receive first attention. The diet should contain all the nutrients in proper proportion, adequate for the maintenance of optimum health. Studies in India have shown that nutritional disorders are widely prevalent among school children, particularly deficiencies relating to proteins; vitamins A, C, thiamine and riboflavin, calcium and iron.

Mid-day School Meal : In order to combat malnutrition and improve the health of school children, it is now an accepted procedure in all advanced countries to provide a good nourishing meal to school children. The School Health Committee (1961) recommended that school children should be assured of at least one nourishing meal *(121)*. Those who can afford it may bring their lunch packets from home, and during lunch hours take their meals in school. Otherwise, schools should have some arrangement for providing mid-day meals through their own cafeteria on a 'no profit no loss' basis. In view of the limited finances in India, it is recommended that the school meal should provide at least one-third of the daily calorie requirement and about half of daily protein requirement of the child.

Applied Nutrition Programme : UNICEF is assisting in the implementation of the Applied Nutrition Programme in the form of implements, seeds, manure and water supply equipment. Wherever land is available, the facilities provided by the UNICEF should be utilized in developing school gardens. The produce may be utilized in the school feeding programmes as well as for nutrition education.

Specific Nutrients : Advances in the knowledge of nutrition have revealed that specific nutrients may be necessary for the prevention of some nutrient disorders. Dental caries, endemic goitre, nightblindness, protein malnutrition, anaemias and a host of other nutrient disorders are eminently preventable. Use of specific nutrients is indicated where such nutrient disorders are problems in a community.

6. First-aid and emergency care

The responsibility of giving first-aid and emergency care to pupils who become sick or injured on school premises rests with the teacher and therefore all teachers should receive adequate training during "Teacher Training Programmes" or "In-service Training programmes" to prepare them to carry out this obligation. The emergencies commonly met within schools are – (a) accidents leading to minor or serious injuries, and (b) medical emergencies such as gastroenteritis, colic, epileptic fits, fainting, etc. In every school a fully equipped First-Aid-Post should be provided as per regulations of St. John Ambulance Association of India.

7. Mental health

The mental health of the child affects his physical health and the learning process. Juvenile delinquency, maladjustment and drug addiction are becoming problems among school children. The school is the most strategic place for shaping the child's behaviour and promoting mental health. The school teacher has both a positive and preventive role – he should be concerned with helping all children attain mental health, so that they may develop into mature, responsible and well adjusted adults. The school routine should be so planned that there is enough relaxation between periods of intense work, and every effort should be made to relieve the tedium of the class room. No distinction should be made between race, religion, caste or community; between the rich and poor; and between the clever and the dull. It is now increasingly realized that there is a great need for vocational counsellors and psychologists in schools for guiding the children into careers for which they are suited.

8. Dental health

Children frequently suffer from dental diseases and defects. Dental caries and periodontal diseases are the two common dental diseases in India. A school health programme should have provision for dental examination, at least once a year. In the developed countries, dental hygienists are employed in schools to assist the school dentist with the examination of the teeth. They make preliminary inspection of the teeth and do prophylactic cleansing which is of great value in preventing gum troubles and in improving personal appearance. They take part in the teaching of dental hygiene as they work with the children.

9. Eye health services

Schools should be responsible for the early detection of refractive errors, treatment of squint and amblyopia, and detection and treatment of eye infections such as trachoma. Administration of vitamin A to children at risk, has shown gratifying results. In other words, basic eye health services should be provided in schools.

10. Health education

The most important element of the school health programme is health education. The goal of health education should be to bring about desirable changes in health knowledge, in attitudes and in practice, and not merely to teach the children a set of rules of hygiene.

Health education in schools should cover the following areas: (1) *Personal hygiene* : Health education programme in schools should be lively, practical and based on everyday needs and interests of children. The need for hygiene of skin, hair, teeth and clothing should be impressed upon them. Attention to posture is also important. Children often adopt bad postures while sitting and standing. Such tendencies, should be observed and corrected. It is increasingly recognized that the major degenerative diseases of adults have their origin in poor health habits formed early in life. Cigarette smoking is an example of a public health problem that should be tackled in schools. (2) *Environmental Health* : Encouraging young people to take part in health activities and keep their environment clean is an important function of school health services. Visits to observe community health programmes, and even better participation in community action programmes (e.g., vaccination, fly control campaigns, construction of sanitary wells and latrines) are excellent opportunities for health education. (3) *Family life* : Family life education is being increasingly recognized as a priority in both developed and developing countries. The school health service is concerned not only with the development of healthy lives but also with healthy attitudes towards human reproduction.

Health education in schools is a function of the school teacher. The health officer and the public health nurse/ health worker/health assistant may furnish teaching materials and advice, but the teacher is the key person in the presentation of the material to the children. To do this important work, the teacher should be well versed in health education techniques, and sincerely interested in the welfare of the pupils. Children take back to their parents the health instructions they receive in schools, and even more important, when they become adults they apply this knowledge to their own families. In developing countries, where ill-health is a major problem, "every school child is a health worker".

11. Education of handicapped children

The ultimate goal is to assist the handicapped child and his family so that the child will be able to reach his maximum potential, to lead as normal a life as possible, to become as independent as possible, and to become a productive and self-supporting member of the society. The resources for managing handicapped child vary from country to country. It requires the cooperation of health, welfare, social and educational agencies.

12. School health records

A cumulative health record of each student should be maintained. Such records should contain (a) Identifying data – name, date of birth, parent's name and address, etc. (b) past health history (c) record of findings of physical examination and screening tests and record of services provided. The purpose of maintaining school health records is to have cumulative information on the health aspects of school children in order to give continuing intelligent health supervision. These records will also be useful in analysing and evaluating school health programmes and providing a useful link between the home, school and the community.

School health programme under Ayushman Bharat

The programme has been developed based on the learning and experiences from a variety of global and national school based interventions. Two teachers, preferably one male and one female, in every school, designated as "Health and Wellness Ambassadors" will be trained to transact heath promotion and disease prevention information in the form of interesting activities for one hour every week. These health promotion messages will also have bearing on improving health practices in the country as students will act as "Health and Wellness Messengers" in the society *(122)*.

Activities in school

Weekly

- Classroom transactions by health and wellness ambassadors
- Administration of IFA tablets

Fortnightly/Monthly

- Thematic school assembly
- Question box responses

Quarterly

- Thematic AHDs
- Parent teacher meetings

Bi-annual

- Administration of albendazole tablet (National deworming day)

The Health and Wellness Ambassadors will facilitate linkages with other ongoing school based programmes like WIFS, NDD, MHS and RBSK; and coordinate referral of students requiring any support or treatment to the Adolescent Friendly Health Centres and Health & Wellness Clinics. For any greater information that the students require, they may also be referred to the Adolescent friendly health resource centres at the district level.

School health promotion activities

The health promotion activities will be given a special focus. Age appropriate health education for the students will be taken up to influence behaviour and enhance skills. The framework developed pays special attention to physical, psycho-social and mental aspects based on the developmental stages of the child. The broad components are :

Age appropriate health promotion		
Primary school	*Middle school*	*High school*
• Health, growth and development • Personal safety • Nutrition and physical activity • Hygiene practices • Prevention of diseases like malaria, dengue, TB, worms infestation, diarrhoea and vaccine preventable diseases	• Puberty and related changes • Eye care, oral hygiene • Nutrition • Bullying prevention • Meditation and yoga • Internet safety and media literacy • Prevention of substance abuse • HIV/AIDS • Mental health	• Prevention of substance abuse • Sexual & reproductive health • Violence prevention • Unintentional injury • Road safety • Nutrition • Meditation and Yoga

Health screening *(122)*

Rashtriya Bal Swasthya Karyakram (RBSK) is an important initiative aiming at early identification and early intervention for children from birth to 18 years to cover 4 'D's viz. Defects at birth, Deficiencies, Diseases, Development delays including disability. The 0–6 years age group, will be specifically managed at District Early Intervention Center (DEIC) level while for 6–18 years age group, management of conditions will be done through existing public health facilities. DEIC will act as referral linkage for both the age groups. Once the child is screened and referred from school, it would be ensured that the necessary treatment/intervention is delivered at zero cost to the family.

Provision of services *(122)*

Weekly iron folic acid supplementation through 6–19 years of age will follow the existing guidelines in the schools. These services will continue to be delivered through school teachers.

Age groups	6–10 years	10–19 years
Intervention/ dose	Tablets of 45 mg elemental iron and 400 mcg of folic acid	Tablets of 100 mg elemental iron and 500 mcg of folic acid
Regime	Weekly, throughout the period 6–10 years of age	Weekly, throughout the period 10–19 years of age
Service delivery	Through teachers	Through teachers

Deworming : To combat parasitic worm infections, Government of India has declared 10th August and 10th February as fixed days to provide Albendazole tablets for deworming school-age children. During NDD, Albendazole 400mg chewable tablets will be administered to children at government, government-aided, and private schools. This will continue to follow the current NDD guidelines.

Menstrual hygiene management : Sanitary napkins may be provided in the schools for adolescent girls as per MHS guidelines.

Health screening : Under RBSK, identification of 30 diseases including malnutrition and anaemia with appropriate referrals. Identification of children with refractive errors may be done and spectacles provided.

Physical and mental fitness : Classes on yoga and meditation through Health & Wellness Ambassadors may be promoted on the lines of 'International Yoga Day' to inculcate the habits of yoga and meditation among children since their childhood.

Research : Provisions may be made for research and studies on health, wellness and nutrition for children to assess the impact of the programme.

Other preventive services in the form of regular age appropriate vaccination of children through local health staff are being considered.

Electronic health records

It is envisaged to develop an electronic health record for each student. Student Health Card will include health screening and service access data for each student. Under the RBSK, the screening and referral records of all the school children will be digitalized .The relevant information related to school health activities will be added to existing electronic records maintained under RBSK.

Upgrading skills in emergency care

A child spends a considerable part of the day in school, which makes it the responsibility of the school to ensure the safety of all children in every possible way during their stay at school. Thus students and teachers should know the basis of first aid and should be able to respond to emergencies. There should be a first aid box available in each school. The teachers and students will be made aware of the various services available in each school to emergencies like the ambulance, fire brigade, police, closest health facility etc. Sessions of the basic first aid will be taken up and linkage with local disaster response team will be made, to build the capacity of school teachers and children to respond to emergencies.

School health administration

The health of the school child is the responsibility of the parents, teachers, health administrators and the community. The success or efficiency of school health service depends largely on effective coordination between the participating agencies. There is no uniform pattern of school health administration, both here and abroad. In England, school health service is part of the Education service of the country. In India, school health service is administered by different departments in different States – these are usually the departments of Health and Education. The School Health Committee set up by the Government of India, in 1960 recommended that school health service should be an integral part of the general health services. The general health services in India are administered largely through the primary health centres in the rural areas, where the bulk of India's population lives. School health service is, therefore, an important function of the primary health centres.

(a) Primary health centres

The primary health centres are charged with the responsibility of administering school health service within their jurisdiction. It requires a whole-time, medical officer to cover 5,000 to 6,000 children a year. The School Health Committee (1961) has, therefore, recommended that the staff of the primary health centres should be augmented by additional staff to carry out effectively the school health programme.

(b) School Health Committees

The School Health Committee (1961) in India recommended the formation of school health committees at the village level, block level, district level, state level and national level. These Committees should mobilize community resources and make the school health programme continuous and self-supporting. The National School Health Council will be an advisory and coordinating body.

HANDICAPPED CHILDREN

Definitions

"Handicap" may be defined as "reduction in a person's capacity to fulfil a social role as a consequence of an impairment, inadequate training for the role, or other circumstances. Applied to children, the term usually refers to the presence of an impairment or other circumstances that are likely to interfere with normal growth and development or with the capacity to learn" *(123)*.

International Classification of Impairments, Disabilities and Handicaps (ICIDH) : First published by WHO in 1980, this is an attempt to produce a systematic taxonomy of the consequences of injury and disease. In the year 2001, International Classification of Functioning, Disability and Health (ICF, WHO 2001) was published.

An *impairment* is defined as "any loss or abnormality of psychological, physiological, or anatomical structure or function". Impairments are disturbances at the level of the organ and include defects, loss of limb, organ or other body structure and defects or loss of mental function.

A *disability* is defined as "any restriction or lack (resulting from an impairment) of ability to perform an activity in a manner or within the range considered normal for a human being". The term disability reflects the consequences of impairment in terms of functional performance and activity by the individual; disability thus represents disturbances at the level of the person.

A *handicap* is defined as a disadvantage for a given individual, resulting from an impairment or a disability, that limits or prevents the fulfilment of a role that is normal (depending on age, sex, and social and cultural practice) for that individual. The term handicap thus reflects interaction with and adaptation to the individual's surroundings.

Handicap may be intrinsic or extrinsic. For example, blindness is an intrinsic handicap, and loss of parents is an extrinsic handicap. One handicap can give rise to further handicaps and the terms "primary" and "secondary" are used to denote this relationship. Blindness is a primary handicap; it can lead to poverty, which will be secondary handicap.

Extent of the problem

Nearly 83 million of the world's population are estimated to be mentally retarded, with 41 million having long-term or permanent disability. It ranks fourth in the list of leading causes of disability. Hearing loss (41 decibels and above) over the age of 3 is estimated to affect 42 million people, ranking 3rd in the list. Disability resulting from poliomyelitis has affected about 10 million people *(41)*. It is difficult to state how many people are mentally retarded in India as the census estimates do not cover mental handicap. About 16.15 million persons (1.9 per cent of the population) suffer from some or the other physical disability in the country. About 3 per cent child population in 1–14 years age group is affected by developmental delays *(124)*.

Classification

It is usual to classify handicapped children into the following groups :

1. Physically handicapped
2. Mentally handicapped
3. Socially handicapped.

1. Physically handicapped children

This category includes children who are blind, deaf and mute; those with hare-lip, cleft palate, talipes; and the "crippled" – e.g., resulting from polio, cerebral palsy, congenital heart disease, road accidents, burns, injuries, etc. These conditions fall into three broad causative groups : (a) birth defects (b) infections, and (c) accidents. These are all preventable to a large extent through adequate prenatal, natal, postnatal services, and genetic counselling.

2. Mentally handicapped children

Mental handicap is the present term used for mental retardation. It is a condition of sub-average intellectual function combined with deficits in adaptive behaviour. Terms which were previously used such as idiot, moron and imbecile are now discarded. At least 2 per cent of India's population is said to be suffering from some kind of mental disability *(125)*.

Causes

Mental handicap has many causes. These may be genetic, or environmental and include prenatal as well as postnatal causes. The possible and earliest time to recognize the problem of mental retardation is to look for any delayed milestones and development.

The known causative factors include the following : (a) *Genetic conditions* : Down's syndrome, Klinefelter syndrome, PKU, Tay-Sach disease, galactosaemia, microcephaly, congenital hypothyroidism involving both single and multiple gene action and chromosomal abnormalities. (b) *Antenatal factors* : These comprise neural tube defects, Rh incompatibility, certain infections (e.g., rubella, cytomegalovirus, toxoplasmosis, syphilis), drugs and irradiation. (c) Perinatal *factors* : These include birth injuries, hypoxia and cerebral palsy. (d) *Postnatal factors* : Head injuries, accidents, encephalitis, physical and chemical agents such as lead and mercury poisoning may result in mental retardation. (e) *Miscellaneous* : Maternal malnutrition, protein-energy malnutrition, iodine deficiency (endemic goitre), consanguineous marriages, pregnancy after the age of 40 (late marriages) are all known to be associated with mental retardation.

Categories of mental retardation

Psychologists have used the concept of IQ to classify the degree of mental retardation. The IQ scores rest on the assumption that intelligence distribution in the general public follow the normal or Gaussian curve, with a mean of 100. The half of the general population achieve scores above 100, and one half below. The lower 3 per cent or so of the population achieve scores of 70 or less. They are usually considered to be mentally retarded. The WHO gave the following classification of mental retardation :

Mild mental retardation	....	IQ	50–70
Moderate mental retardation	....	IQ	35–49
Severe mental retardation	....	IQ	20–34
Profound mental retardation	....	IQ	under 20

Children scoring above 70 are no longer described as mentally handicapped. The number of mild cases far exceed the severe and profound cases. English statistics which have been widely quoted suggest that, among 100 mentally handicapped persons, the following proportion will be found : 70 mild, 20 moderate and 5 severe cases. In other words, a very great majority of cases of mental handicap are of the mild type and potentially capable of being taught to make a fairly adequate social adaptation in appropriate circumstances *(126)*.

Severe mental retardation is uncommon. The great majority of severely handicapped children remain more or less dependant throughout life. Mental retardation often involves psychiatric disturbances. It has been stressed that the IQ range suggested must not be applied too rigidly. IQ level is not necessarily constant during the individual's life span.

3. Socially handicapped children

A "socially handicapped child" may be defined as a child whose opportunities for a healthy personality development and a full unfolding of potentialities are hampered by certain elements in his social environment such as parental inadequacy, environmental deprivation (i.e. lack of stimulation of learning process), and emotional disturbances. Such children would include children who are orphaned either due to death or loss of parents; neglected and destitute children; those who are exploited or victimized; and, delinquent children. It may be pointed out that a child who is physically or mentally handicapped also meets with social handicaps to the extent to which he is subject to social rejection or misunderstanding and cannot make use of the normal value of social fulfilment.

More recently, WHO has come out with International classification of functioning disability and health (IFC).

International Classification of Functioning, Disability and Health (ICF) *(69)*

Like ICD-10, ICF is a core classification in the WHO-FIC, where ICD-10 provides users an aetiologic framework for classification of disease, disorder and other health conditions, ICF classifies functioning and disability associated with health conditions. ICD-10 and ICF are complementary classifications and WHO encourages users to use both systems together to create a broader and more meaningful picture of health of individuals and populations.

Developed by WHO, ICF represents a revision of the International Classification of Impairment, Disability and Handicaps (ICIDH). The focus of ICIDH was consequences of disease whereas focus of ICF is "components of health". ICF is a classification of health and health related domain that describe body function and structure, activities and participation. Since an individual's functioning and disability occur in a context, ICF is a tool for measuring functioning in society, no matter what the reason for one's impairment.

The model of ICF

Two major model of disability have been proposed. The *medical* model views disability as a feature of the person, directly caused by disease, trauma or other health conditions; which requires medical care provided in the form of individual treatment by professionals. The *social model* of disability, on the other hand, sees disability as a socially-created problem and not at all an attribute of an individual. On the social model, disability demands a political response, since the problem created by an unaccomodating physical environment brought about by attitude and other features of the social environment.

Components of ICF

The ICF framework consists of two parts:

a. Functioning and disability
b. Contextual factors

a. Functioning and disability includes :
   - *Body function and structure* – describes actual anatomy and physiology/psychology of human body.
   - *Activity and participation* – describes the person's functional status, including communication, mobility, interpersonal interactions, self-care, learning, applying knowledge, etc.

b. Contextual factors includes :
   - *Environmental factors* – factors that are not within the person's control, such as family, work, government agencies, laws, and cultural beliefs.
   - *Personal factors* – include race, gender, age, educational level, coping styles, etc.

ICF is used by persons with disability and professionals alike to evaluate health care settings that deal with chronic illness and disability, such as rehabilitation centres, nursing homes, psychiatry institutions and common services.

The overall organization of the classification of ICF

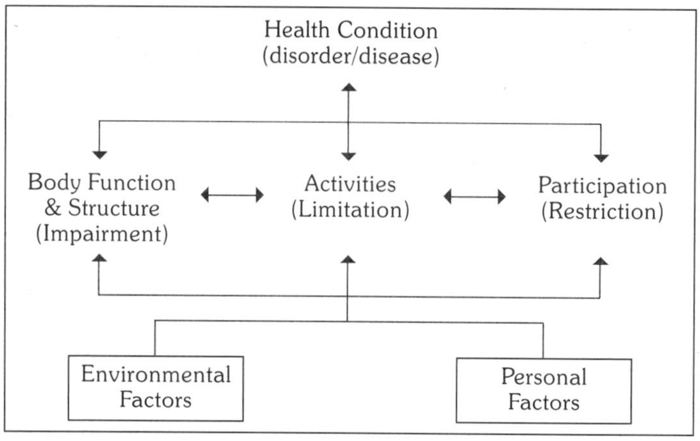

Source : *(69)*

Approaches to prevention

One of the objectives of Mother and Child Health Services is the prevention of handicapping conditions, and the early management of illness to prevent crippling sequelae.

1. Primary prevention

The ideal is to prevent the handicap from occurring through the application of preventive measures during preconceptional, prenatal and intranatal periods and during infancy, childhood and adolescence. The approaches in primary prevention include (a) *Genetic counselling* : The optimum maternal age for producing normal babies is between 20 and 30 years. After the age of 30 or 35 years, there is a greater chance of producing a genetically abnormal child, especially one with Down's syndrome. The mother should be advised accordingly. In some communities consanguineous marriages are common. The incidence of such marriage should be reduced through educational efforts. (b) *At-risk approach* : People "at-risk" of transmitting inherited diseases (e.g., chromosomal or sex–linked diseases) should be identified. They should be offered all the investigations currently available and should have competent advice about future risks. (c) *Immunization* : In India, the main cause of disability is poliomyelitis which is preventable by immunization *(127)*. Immunization against other diseases such as rubella should also be considered. (d) *Nutrition* : Proper nutrition of the expectant mother is important for the welfare of the unborn child, especially to reduce the incidence of prematurity which is associated with mental handicaps. (e) *Others* : These include health care of mothers and children through prenatal, natal and postnatal periods; avoidance of infectious diseases, potentially teratogenic drugs, X-rays and smoking; special care of high risk women especially during labour, and accident prevention. The Medical Termination of Pregnancy Act of 1971 allows abortion of the foetus which may be seriously handicapped. In short, the obstetrician has a major role to play in reducing the frequency of handicaps in the population.

2. Secondary prevention

The broad objective for all children whatever their condition or problem is to bring them as close to normality as possible – physically, mentally and socially. This will involve : (a) *Early diagnosis of handicap* : Parents themselves have the responsibility to bring the child to paediatrician and seek advice. Investigation of the child requires full history, assessment of the degree of handicap and perhaps special investigations including the natural potentialities of the child. This should be done through MCH and School Health Services and such other agencies. (b) *Treatment* : Handicapped children need specialized treatment facilities such as physiotherapy, (the deformities are corrected, the weakened muscles are given exercise as in polio, infrared rays, diathermy etc.); occupational therapy (the child is taught, according to his ability and taste, things like music, painting, weaving, woodwork, pottery, basket making etc.); speech therapy (the child is trained to talk normally); and prosthetics (provision of artificial limbs, hearing aids and other equipment). The modern term for this branch of medicine is "Physical Medicine and Rehabilitation". The purpose of treatment is to improve the physical condition of the patient. (c) *Training and education* : the handicapped child is trained for an independent living. This is called "vocational guidance". He is trained to "work with what is left", so that he is not a burden on others. In India, there are over 150 schools and institutions for the handicapped. The following are some of the important ones : (1) Occupational Therapy School, Mumbai; (2) Physical Therapy School, Mumbai; (3) Occupational Therapy School, Nagpur; (4) All India Institute of Physical Medicine and Rehabilitation, Mumbai; (5) Institute of Physical Medicine and Rehabilitation, Christian Medical College, Vellore; and (6) Occupational Therapy College, New Delhi. Beside these, there are schools for the blind, deaf, and special hospitals and wards for crippled children. Institutional care of the handicapped children is being replaced by various social support measures and services, enabling families to assume a larger share of rehabilitation within the family cycle *(33)*.

The mentally handicapped children can be helped to reach their optimal capacity through attention to the following : (a) they should get love and warmth, patience and tolerance, besides discipline (b) their natural potentials should be identified, and the child must be helped to develop in that direction in all possible manner.

The mentally handicapped require attention from diverse disciplines such as medicine, psychology, education, rehabilitation and social welfare. Taking into account the gravity of the problem, the Ministry of Social Welfare, Govt. of India, has set-up the National Institute for Mentally Handicapped (NIMH) in 1984 at Secunderabad. It has Regional Branches at Mumbai, New Delhi and Kolkata. The NIMH serves as an apex organization for developing appropriate models for care for the mentally handicapped *(125)*.

Apart from NIMH, 3 other premier National Institutes are working in specific disabilities : (a) Ali Yavar Jung National Institute for the Hearing Handicapped, Mumbai with Regional branches at New Delhi, Kolkata and Secunderabad; (b) National Institute for the visually Handicapped, Dehradun with Regional branch at Chennai; (c) National Institute for the Orthopaedically Handicapped, Kolkata. Apart from developing models for care and services, these institutions conduct research, promote human resource development, crises management, education, placement and employment, development and supply of appropriate aids and appliances, and documentation and dissemination of information *(124)*.

In India, the Ministry of Social Welfare operates through five major schemes of assistance to voluntary organizations providing services to disabled persons. These are : (a) Assistance to voluntary organizations for the disabled : Assistance upto 90 per cent in urban and 95 per cent in rural areas is given to NGOs for education, training and rehabilitation of the disabled; for rehabilitation of people recovering from mental illness; emphasis on vocational guidance and training; liaison with nearest psychiatrist centre or hospital; provision for Half-way Homes. (b) Assistance for aids and appliances : Aids and appliances upto Rs 3,600 are provided to people with disabilities free, if the monthly income is up to Rs 1,200, and at 50 per cent cost if the monthly income is between Rs 1,201 to 2,500. (c) Assistance to voluntary organizations for rehabilitation of leprosy-cured persons : Assistance to voluntary organizations working for leprosy-cured persons is given upto 90 per cent for public education and awareness, early intervention, educational and vocational training, economic rehabilitation and social integration. (d) Development in the field of cerebral palsy and mental retardation : For manpower training of professionals and also for developing organizational infrastructure such as class room/library/hostel in the field of cerebral palsy and mental retardation. (e) Assistance to voluntary organization for establishment of special schools : For setting up special schools NGOs receive grants upto 90 per cent. Preference is given for opening schools in new districts and upgradation of existing schools.

On 26th August 1995, Ministry of Social Welfare, Govt. of India introduced a comprehensive Bill in the Parliament known as "Persons with disabilities (equal opportunities, protection of right and full participation) Bill 1995". It deals with preventive and promotional aspects of rehabilitation.

The Rights of Persons with Disabilities Bill - 2016

The Lok Sabha has passed "The Rights of Persons with Disabilities Bill-2016". The Bill replaced the existing PWD Act, 1995, which was enacted 21 years back. The Rajya Sabha has already passed the Bill on 14.12.2016. The salient features of the Bill are *(128)*:

Disability has been defined based on an evolving and dynamic concept. The types of disabilities have been increased from existing 7 to 21 and the Central Government will have the power to add more types of disabilities. The 21 disabilities are given below:

1. Blindness
2. Low-vision
3. Leprosy cured persons
4. Hearing impairment (deaf and hard of hearing)
5. Locomotors disability
6. Dwarfism
7. Intellectual disability
8. Mental Illness
9. Autism spectrum disorder
10. Cerebral palsy
11. Muscular dystrophy
12. Chronic neurological conditions
13. Specific learning disabilities
14. Multiple sclerosis

15. Speech and language disability
16. Thalassemia
17. Haemophilia
18. Sickle cell disease
19. Multiple disabilities including deaf blindness
20. Acid attack victim
21. Parkinson's disease

Speech and language disability and specific learning disability have been added for the first time. Acid attack victims have been included. Dwarfism, muscular dystrophy have been indicated as separate class of specified disability. The new categories of disabilities also include three blood disorders, thalassemia, hemophilia and sickle cell disease. In addition, the government has been authorized to notify any other category of specified disability. Responsibility has been cast upon the appropriate governments to take effective measures to ensure that the persons with disabilities enjoy their rights equally as others.

In considering the management of the socially handicapped child, we must remember that such children are normal in their needs and development. Their needs should be identified and met. The children Act, 1960 provides for the "care, protection, maintenance, welfare, training, education and rehabilitation" of the socially handicapped children.

Lastly, we need to strengthen the family. The family is the most effective bulwark to prevent children from becoming socially handicapped. There were times when the handicapped child was considered a liability to the parents and to the society. All over the world, there is an awakening that handicapped children can and must be helped to make their lives as happy and useful as possible.

BEHAVIOUR PROBLEMS

The behaviour problems in children may be classified as below :

(a) *Problems antisocial in nature :* Stealing, lying, gambling, cruelty, sexual offences, destructiveness.

(b) *Habit disorders :* Thumb sucking, nail-biting, bed-wetting, masturbation.

(c) *Personality disorders :* Jealousy, temper-tantrums, timidity, shyness, day-dreaming, fears and anxieties, unsociability, hysterical manifestations.

(d) *Psychosomatic complaints :* Tremors, headache, asthma, depression, delusion, hallucinations.

(e) *Educational difficulties :* Backwardness in studies, school phobia, school failures, etc.

Some of the behaviour disorders are due to mental deficiency; some are due to organic disease and some due to failure in adjustment to external environment. The answer to these problems lies in improvement of living conditions, better social environment and education.

JUVENILE DELINQUENCY

The Children Act, 1960 in India defines delinquent as "a child who has committed an offence". Juvenile means a boy who has not attained the age of 16 years and a girl who has not attained the age of 18 years. In a broad sense, delinquency is not merely "juvenile crime". It embraces all deviations from normal youthful behaviour and includes the incorrigible, ungovernable, habitually disobedient and those who desert their homes and mix with immoral people, those with behaviour problems and indulge in antisocial practices.

INCIDENCE : In the United States it is reported that 2 per cent of children between 7 and 17 years attend juvenile courts. Comparable statistics are not available in India to denote the size of the problem, but it is agreed that juvenile delinquency is on the increase in India during the past few decades, due to changes in the cultural pattern of the people, urbanization and industrialization. The highest incidence is found in children aged 15 and above. The incidence among boys is 4 to 5 times more than among girls.

CAUSES : (1) *Biological causes* : Certain biological causes such as hereditary defects, feeble-mindedness, physical defects and glandular imbalance may be at the bottom of juvenile delinquency. Recent studies indicate that chromosome anomaly might be associated with a tendency for delinquency and crime. A survey of criminal patients in Scotland and elsewhere demonstrated such a link – some of the patients showing an extra Y chromosome. The XYY men suffer from severe disturbance of the whole personality *(129)*. (2) *Social causes* : Among the social causes may be mentioned broken homes, e.g., death of parents, separation of parents, step mothers and disturbed home conditions, e.g., poverty, alcoholism, parental neglect, ignorance about child care, too many children, etc. (3) *Other causes* : Absence of recreation facilities, cheap recreation, sex-thrillers, urbanization and industrialization, cinemas and television, slum-dwelling, etc.

PREVENTIVE MEASURES : (1) *Improvement of family life* : A well adjusted family can stem the tide of delinquency. Parents should be prepared for parenthood. The needs of children should be appreciated and met. (2) *Schooling* : The school comes next to home in the community in ordering the behaviour of children. There should be a healthy teacher–pupil relationship. The school teacher can play an important part by detecting early signs of maladjustment. (3) *Social welfare services* : These comprise recreation facilities, parent-counselling, child guidance, educational facilities and adequate general health services.

Children in difficult circumstances *(66)*

In a globalized economy, the increased vulnerability of some children due to their identity, and/or their socio-economic and geo-political circumstances calls for more focused attention as well as coordination of social and economic policies and monitoring of child impact. Besides being victims of globalization, these children may be barred from benefits meant for all children simply because they belong to a group or community with difficulties of access. These barriers must be overcome.

Over the years, some children have been categorized as children in difficult circumstances and these categorizations include :

- Homeless children (pavement dwellers, displaced/evicted, etc.).
- Orphaned or abandoned children.
- Children whose parents cannot or are not able to take care of them.
- Children separated from parents.
- Migrant and refugee children.
- Street children.
- Working children.
- Trafficked children.

- Children in bondage.
- Children in prostitution.
- Children of sex workers/prostitutes/sexual minorities.
- Children of prisoners.
- Children affected by conflict.
- Children affected by natural disasters.
- Children affected by HIV/AIDS.
- Children suffering from terminal diseases.
- The girl child.
- Children with disabilities and related special needs.
- Children belonging to the ethnic and religious minorities, and other minority communities, and those belonging to the Scheduled Castes and Scheduled Tribes.
- Children in institutional care, be it in state-run institutions or religious and other charitable institutions.
- Children in conflict with law (those who commit crimes).
- Children who are victims of crime.

For the first time in the history of planning for children, India has adopted a clear understanding and definition of the child in the NPAC 2005. The NPAC definition of the child as a person upto the age of 18 years and its clear declaration that 'all rights apply to all age-groups, including before birth' reiterates the 1974 National Policy mandate that the State takes responsibility for children 'both before and after birth,' and the child's interests are to receive paramount attention. This national reaffirmation must set the frame for future planning and intervention to secure the well-being of all children of the country and provide them a caring and protective environment.

Battered baby syndrome

It has been defined as "a clinical condition in young children, usually under 3 years of age who have received non-accidental wholly inexcusable violence or injury, on one or more occasions, including minimal as well as severe fatal trauma, for what is often the most trivial provocation, by the hand of an adult in a position of trust, generally a parent, guardian or foster parent. In addition to physical injury, there may be deprivation of nutrition, care and affection in circumstances which indicate that such deprivation is not accidental".

Battered baby syndrome has been found in all strata of society. Its incidence is not known. So far as sequelae are concerned, the most worrying is the risk of mental and neurological complications. Thus it has been tentatively suggested that 10–15 per cent of cases of cerebral palsy and almost double that proportion of the new mentally retarded children each year may be the result of the battered baby syndrome.

Girl child and gender bias *(66)*

Gender biases pose a specific threat to girl children across the social and economic strata. For a girl child, life is a constant fight for survival, growth and development from the time she is conceived till she attains 18 years. The life chart of a girl child and the many life threatening problems she might face are as follows :

Years	Problems faced
Before birth to 1 year	– Being unwanted, risk of prenatal detection. – Foeticide and infanticide. – Infant mortality. – Discrimination in breast-feeding and infant food. – Neglect of health (immunization).
1 to 5 years	– Discrimination in access to food. – Poorer health attention and poorer access to health care; high risk of nutritional anaemia. – Discrimination in overall treatment, parental care; expression of value and worth. – Vitamin and micro-nutrient deficiencies. – Early definition and imposition of 'suitable' roles; limits on permitted learning and play activities. – Child marriages in some areas of country. – Household/near-home sexual abuse. – If enrolled in school, less time for learning. – Assignment of domestic duties, minor small domestic chores.
6 to 11 years	– Malnutrition and anaemia. – Health problems like diarrhoea. – Iodine and Vitamin A deficiency. – Low school enrolment, school drop outs. – Vulnerable to trafficking, child labour, child marriage. – Abuse, exploitation and violence. – Increasing domestic duties/workload. – Looking after siblings. – Restrictions on mobility, play.
12 to 18 years	– Poor health, poor health attention. – High risk/high levels of anaemia. – Frequent illness due to malnutrition and micro-nutrient deficiency. – Child marriage. – High-risk/incidence of early child-bearing related morbidity/mortality. – Becoming a 'child-mother', health risks and burden of childcare. – Denied information, mobility, access to services. – Low literacy/learning level. – Early and frequent pregnancy coupled with abortions. – Marital and domestic violence. – Dowry harassment, desertion, polygamy, divorce. – Child labour, trafficking. – STDs and HIV/AIDS. – Unpaid and unrecognized work, and drudgery. – No voice either in home or society.

It is evident from the text above that age-specific and setting-specific interventions have to be put in place for appropriate and effective response to the above problems, highlighting the inter-sectoral nature of actions required.

Protecting girl children in India will not be easy. The nation cannot any longer afford the cost of hoping that society will change its mindset on its own, in a situation where pervasive negative attitudes towards women are being reflected on girl children, to the extent of denying them life itself.

The well-being of daughters in the community must become the subject of government monitoring (with NGO assistance if appropriate), covering every age and stage of childhood. Such vigilance must apply to all stages of a girl child's childhood. Panchayats, gram sabhas and local self-government bodies should be brought into this benevolent surveillance.

The specific goals for girls in the National Plan of Action for Children 2005

- Assurance of equality of status for girl child as an individual and a citizen in her own right through promotion of special opportunities for her growth and development.
- To ensure survival, development and protection of the girl child and to create an environment wherein she lives a life of dignity with full opportunity for choice and development.
- To stop sex selection, female foeticide and infanticide.
- To eliminate child marriages.
- To ensure the girl child's security and protect her from abuse, exploitation, victimization and all other forms of violence.
- To protect the girl child from deprivation and neglect and to ensure to the girl child an equal share of care and resources in the home and community, and equal access to services.
- To take measures to protect girl children from any treatment which undermines their self-esteem, and causes their exclusion from social mainstream and also to break down persistent gender stereotype.
- To eliminate all obstacles that prevent girls from full enjoyment of human rights and fundamental freedom including equal rights in succesion and inheritance.
- To ensure equal opportunity for free and compulsory elementary education to all girls.
- Health and nutrition.

Child abuse

The WHO defines child abuse and child maltreatment as "all forms of physical and/or emotional ill-treatment, sexual abuse, neglect or negligent treatment or commercial or other exploitation resulting in actual or potential harm to the childs health, survival, development or dignity in the context of a relationship of responsibility, trust or power". The Center for Disease Control and Prevention (CDC) uses the term child maltreatment to refer to both acts – commission (abuse), or acts of omission (neglect) *(130)*. These public health problems include all types of abuse and neglect under the age of 18 years by a parent, caregiver or another person in a custodial role (such as clergy, a coach, a teacher) that result in harm to the child. There are four types of abuse and neglect *(131)*:

a. *Physical abuse* – It is the intentional use of physical force that can result in physical harm. Examples include hitting, kicking, shaking, burning or other show of force against a child;
b. *Sexual abuse* – It involves pressuring or forcing a child to engage in a sexual act. It includes behaviours such as fondling, penetration and exposing a child to other sexual activities;
c. *Emotional abuse* – It refers to behaviours that harm a child's self-worth or emotional well-being. Examples include name calling, shaming, rejection, withholding love and threatening; and
d. *Neglect* – It is failure to meet a child's basic physical and emotional needs. These needs include housing, food, clothing, education and access to medical care.

Child abuse and neglect are common. At least 1 in 7 children have experienced child abuse and/or neglect in the past year. Children living in poverty experience more abuse and neglect. Rates are 5 times higher for children in families with low socio economic status. The consequences of physical battering – death, blindness, mental and emotional retardation, stunting of growth – are only one part of the whole picture of child abuse. Some contributory factors of child abuse are poverty, alcohol and other drug abuse, loneliness, immaturity and a host of other factors. Many causes are embedded in the family and in its function of child rearing.

The adverse effects of child-abuse are summarized in Fig. 19.

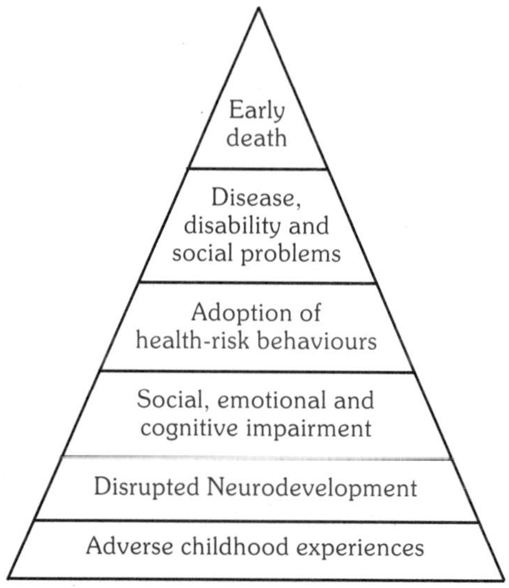

FIG. 19

Impact of adverse childhood experiences

Source : *(131)*

The strategies and approaches to prevent child abuse can be summarized as :

a. Strengthen economic support to the family;
b. Change social norms to support parents and positive parenting;
c. Provide quality care and education early in life;
d. Enhance parenting skills to promote healthy child development;
e. Intervene to lessen harms and prevent future risk; and
f. Child protection.

Studies carried out throughout the past two decades have shown that the provision of supportive home visitors, either public health nurse or trained lay people, to families who are at risk of using violence against children can prevent the abuse from happening. However, we have not yet reached a similar level of confidence about our ability to prevent the sexual abuse of children, which is also a worldwide phenomenon.

Street children

The UN defines street children as "boys and girls for whom the street has become their home and/or source of livelihood and who are inadequately protected or supervised by responsible adults".

The issue of street children is considered to be an urban problem. There are three major categories of street children :

1. Children who live on street with their families and often work on street. They may be from migrated families or temporarily migrated and are likely to go back to their home;
2. Children who live on the street by themselves or in groups and have remote access or contacts with their families in the village; and
3. Children who have no ties to their families such as orphans, refugees or runaways.

According to UNICEF street children fall under two categories: "on the street" and "of the street". Children of the street are homeless who live and sleep on the streets in the urban areas. They are on their own and do not have parental supervision or care though some do live with other homeless adults. Children on the street earn a livelihood from street such as street urchins and beggars. They return home at night to have contact with their families. The distinction is important one because children of the street lack emotional and psychological support of a family.

A large number of children without any family support, particularly in the megacities of the developing world are at high-risk of malnutrition, tuberculosis, STDs including HIV, parasite and worm infestation and skin diseases. Both sexes are highly vulnerable to drug abuse, prostitution and criminal exploitation.

Most street children describe major losses in their lives. Many have lost family members through diseases, natural or man-made disasters, or may be by-product of war and riots.

Although poverty and rapid urbanization are major contributing factors to the problem, many claim that physical and sexual abuse were the reason for their leaving home.

During the year 2003, global estimates placed their number at as many as 100 million. There may be 40 million in Latin America, 25 million in Asia and 10 million in Africa, with about 25 million in other areas including the developed world. In 1993 WHO launched an innovative project to study links between street children and substance abuse. The study noted regular use of alcohol and other drugs by a major proportion of street children. Often the lives of street children are intimately entwined with the illicit drug industry. Street children are used in the production and marketing of cocain and the trafficking of cannabis and heroin *(40)*.

There are particular problems in the provision of health and welfare services to street children with regard not only to health care but also to housing, educational opportunities and employment. The rehabilitation of these children should be taken up by the government and non-government voluntary agencies.

The "Integrated Programme for Street Children" without homes and families was launched to prevent destitution of children and provide facilities for their withdrawal from life on the streets. During 2008–09 the scheme was merged to Integrated Child Protection Scheme. Under the scheme NGOs are given financial support to run 24 hour shelters and provide food, clothing, non-formal education, recreation, counselling, guidance and referral services for children. The other components of the scheme include enrolment in schools, vocational training, occupational placement, mobilizing preventive health services and reducing incidence of drug substance abuse, HIV/AIDS etc. *(67)*.

Refugee and displaced children *(132)*

At the end of 2004, roughly 48 per cent of all refugees worldwide were children.

During the same year, the total number of people displaced within their own countries by conflict or human rights violations amounted to roughly 25 million.

Refugee and internally displaced children face many risks, given the violence and uncertainty surrounding both their flight and their lives in the country and/or place of asylum. They may become separated from their families, lose their homes and find themselves living in poor conditions that jeopardize their health and education.

Displacement complicates birth registration and the issuance of travel documents, thereby compromising displaced persons' right to an identity. Both refugees and internally displaced people may have been forced to leave their homes without proper documentation, making it difficult to establish their identities. They may, therefore, be unable to prove their right to receive basic social services, such as education or health care, or to work in a different part of the country.

The loss of family protection, and inadequate resources to address the needs and challenges that refugee and internally displaced children face, can leave them at significant risk of recruitment by armed groups and forces, abuse and sexual exploitation. Girls are especially at risk of abduction, trafficking and sexual violence, including rape used as a weapon of war.

Orphaned children are much more vulnerable to protection violations. The death of a parent, in situations where no adequate alternative care systems are in place, opens up a protection gap. Children living on their own are at much greater risk of abuse and exploitation. Assessments by the International Labour Organization (ILO) have found that orphaned children are much more likely than non-orphans to be working in commercial agriculture, as street vendors, in domestic service and in the sex trade.

Primary responsibility for both refugee and displaced children lies with national governments. However, the Office of the United Nations High Commissioner for Refugees (UNHCR) has a mandate to assist and protect refugees, while the International Committee of the Red Cross (ICRC) has a mandate to assist internally displaced people if displacement is a result of armed conflict and internal violence.

Child labour and child exploitation

A sizeable number of growing children of poor socio-economic class especially in rural areas are known to be inducted as child labour. Studies have shown that labour at very young ages can have dire consequences on the child's development, both physical and mental. Child labourers always had lower growth and health status compared to their non-working counterparts, besides exposure to occupational hazards at a very young stage in their lives. The Declaration of the Rights of the Child and our own Constitution has laid down that childhood and youth should be protected against exploitation. In 1973, the ILO passed a convention establishing 15 as the minimum work age for most sectors while permitting light work from age 13, provided that such work was unlikely to harm child's health, morals and safety or prejudice his school attendance *(133)*.

The facts and figures of child labour are summarized as *(134)*:

1. Worldwide 218 million children between 5 and 17 years are in employment. Among them, 152 million are victims of child labour, almost half of them, about 73 million work in hazardous conditions;
2. In absolute terms, almost half of child labour (72.1 million) is in Africa; 62.1 million in the Asia and the Pacific; 10.7 million in the Americas; 1.2 million in the Arab States and 5.5 million in Europe and Central Asia;
3. In terms of prevalence, 1 in 5 children in Africa (19.6%) are in child labour, whilst prevalence in other regions is between 3% and 7%; 2.9% in the Arab States (1 in 35 children); 4.1% in Europe and Central Asia (1 in 25); 5.3% in the Americas (1 in 19) and 7.4% in Asia and the Pacific region (1 in 14);
4. Almost half of all 152 million children victims of child labour are aged 5–11 years;
5. Hazardous child labour is most prevalent among the 15–17 years old. Nevertheless up to a fourth of all hazardous child labour (19 million) is done by children less than 12 years old;
6. Among 152 million children in child labour, about 88 million are boys and 64 million are girls;
7. 58% of all children in child labour and 62% of all children in hazardous work are boys. Boys appear to face a greater risk of child labour than girls, but this may also be a reflection of an under-reporting of girls' work, particularly in domestic child labour; and
8. Child labour is concentrated primarily in agriculture (71%) , which includes fishing, forestry, livestock herding and aquaculture, and comprises both subsistence and commercial farming; 17% in service; and 12% in the industrial sector, including mining.

According to ILO, forced child labour is present in all regions and kinds of economy. For the most part, there is neither official data on the incidence of forced labour nor a widespread awareness among society at large that forced labour is a problem. Children in domestic service are the most invisible child labourers. Their work is performed within individual homes, removed from public scrutiny and their conditions of life and labour are entirely dependant on the whims of their employers. The number of children involved in domestic service around the world is unquantifiable because of the hidden nature of the work, but it certainly runs into millions. Many of these children are girls, and in many countries domestic service is seen as the only avenue of employment for a young girl, though in some places, such as Nepal and South Africa, boys are more likely to be domestic workers than girls. Children exploited in domestic service are generally paid little or nothing over and above food and lodging. In addition, children in domestic service are especially susceptible to physical and psychological harm. Many are forced to undertake tasks that are completely inappropriate for their age and physical strength. Another form of forced labour is debt bondage, whatever the origin of the debt, it leaves children under complete control of a money lender in a state little distinguishable from slavery.

India fosters the largest number of child labour in the world. In 2014, about 82.2 lakh child labour population was estimated in India. Child labour contributes about 20 per cent of India's GNP. Child workers work for 12 hours at an average every day *(134)*. Jammu and Kashmir has the highest percentage of child labour, where children are mainly engaged in carpet weaving industry. The other fields where child labour is used is in agriculture, plantations, mining, building construction, beedi-making, garbage picking, cashew descalding and processing, cloth printing, dyeing and weaving etc.

In India, various items of health and social legislation have been enacted to protect the health, safety and welfare of working children below the age of 15 years.

The Child Labour (Prohibition and Regulation) Act, 1986

Except in the process of family-based work or recognized school-based activities, children are not permitted to work in occupations concerned with :

- Passenger, goods mail transport by railways.
- Carpet weaving.
- Cinder picking, cleaning of ash-pits.
- Cement manufacturing.
- Building construction operations.
- Cloth printing.
- Dyeing, weaving.
- Manufacturing of matches, explosives, fire-works.
- Beedi making.
- Mica cutting, splitting.
- Abattoirs.
- Wool cleaning.
- Printing.
- Cashew descalding and processing.
- Soldering process in electronic industries.

Child labour is rooted in poverty, unemployment and lack of education. A great deal of effort is needed to eliminate these basic causes. It is felt that instead of proliferating the laws relating to children, all the statutory provisions of the various Acts relating to children should be grouped in one comprehensive code of children. It is not feasible to abolish child labour entirely in the present context, but it is expedient to protect such children against abuse, exploitation and health hazards, and regulate the conditions of work in occupations where child labour is permitted.

Child trafficking *(132)*

Child trafficking is the recruitment, transportation,

transfer, harbouring or receipt of a child for the purpose of exploitation. A child trafficker is anyone who contributes to an element of the trafficking process with the intent to exploit the child. This included those who play only a part in the entire process, such as recruiters, intermediaries, document providers, transporters, corrupt officials, service providers and unscrupulous employers. Girls are trafficked disproportionately for commercial sexual exploitation and child domestic labour. The ILO 2005 Global Report estimates that Asia has the highest number of child trafficking victims followed by industrialized countries, Latin America and Caribbean, the Middle East Countries *(135)*.

"Poverty-plus" at source, transit and destination : Poverty alone does not guarantee that a child will be trafficked, usually it is poverty plus one or many other risk factors that make a child vulnerable to trafficking. These could be at the individual, household, community or institutional level. Some common causes of vulnerability include lack of birth registration, discrimination, orphanhood, illness in the family, family abuse, conflict or natural disaster, travelling alone or through a non-registered agency or smuggler, inability to speak the language, unregulated informal economy, weak legal framework and enforcement, corruption and a large youth population with low labour market absorption. Vulnerability is not static, it changes over time, and different risk factors are present in different contexts *(135)*.

Trafficking of children takes many different forms. Some children are forcibly abducted, others are tricked and still others opt to let themselves be trafficked by promise of earnings, but not suspecting the level of exploitation they will suffer at the other end of the recruiting chain. Trafficking always involves journey, whether within the country or across the international border. The relocation takes children away from their families, communities and support network, leaving them isolated and utterly vulnerable to exploitation. Collecting data about these children is very difficult. It is estimated that trafficking affects about 1.2 million children each year.

Though the trafficking of children is a shadowy practice, some dominant regional patterns are identifiable. In West and Central Africa, children are "placed" in a marginal position within other families. This practice is being used to exploit children both within and outside home. Children are also trafficked into plantations and mines, and in those countries affected by conflict, they are directly abducted by militias. In East Asia and Pacific, most trafficking is into child prostitution, though some children are also recruited for industrial and agricultural work. In South Asia, trafficking forms most of immense child labour problem in the sub-continent, often related to debt bondage. In addition, significant number of children are trafficked for other purposes, including into prostitution, carpet and garment factories, construction projects and begging. In Europe, children are mainly trafficked from east to west, reflecting the demand for cheap labour and child prostitution in richer countries of the continent. Children are also used as unskilled labour and in the entertainment sector.

An estimated 8.4 million children work under terrible circumstances and are forced into bondage or other forms of slavery (Fig. 19).

Making children safe requires creating a protective environment for them. The key elements of a protective environment include :

- Strengthening the capacity of families and communities to care for and protect children.
- Government commitment to child protection by providing budgetary support and social welfare policies targeted at the most excluded and invisible children.
- Ratification and implementation of legislation, both national and international, concerning children's rights and protection.
- Prosecution of perpetrators of crimes against children, and avoidance of criminalizing child victims.
- An open discussion by civil society and the media of attitudes, prejudices, beliefs and practices that facilitate or lead to abuses.
- Ensuring that children know their rights, are encouraged to express them and are given vital life skills and information to protect themselves from abuse and exploitation.
- Availability of basic social services to all children without discrimination.
- Monitoring, transparent reporting and oversight of abuses and exploitation.

The key to building the protective environment is the responsibility of members of the society, by ensuring that children are not exploited. While families and the State have the primary responsibility for protecting children, ongoing and sustained efforts by individuals and organizations at all levels, are essential to break patterns of abuse.

UJJAWALA : "Ujjawala", a comprehensive scheme to combat trafficking was launched in India by the Ministry of Women and Child Development on 4th December, 2007 and is being implemented mainly through NGOs. The scheme has five components of prevention, rescue, rehabilitation, reintegration and repatriation of victims trafficked for commercial sexual exploitation. Some of the provisions under the scheme are *(67)* :

(1) Formation of community vigilance groups, adolescents groups, awareness creation and preparation of IEC material, organizing workshops;

(2) Safe withdrawal of victims from the place of exploitation;

(3) Rehabilitation of victims by providing them safe shelter, basic amenities, medical care, legal aid, vocational training and employment;

(4) Re-integration of victims into society; and

(5) Provide support to cross-border victims for their safe repatriation to the country of origin.

Preventing Violence Against Children *(136)*

Globally, it is estimated that one out of two children aged 2–17 years suffer some form of violence each year. Worldwide, close to 300 million children aged 2–4 years regularly experience violent discipline by their caregivers. A third of students aged 11–15 years worldwide have been bullied by their peers in the past month, and 120 million girls are estimated to have suffered some form of forced sexual contact before the age of 20 years. Emotional violence affects one in three children and worldwide one in four children lives with a mother who is the victim of intimate partner violence. An estimated 40,150 children worldwide were victims of homicide in the year 2017. The global homicide rate for 0–17 years old was 1.7 per 100,000 population, and the rate for boys of 2.4 per 100,000 was over twice than in girls (1.1 per 100,000 population). The COVID-19 pandemic and societies response to it has had a dramatic impact on the prevalence of violence against children and is likely to have long-lasting negative consequences.

Over their lifetime, children exposed to violence are at increased risk of mental illness and anxiety disorders; high risk behaviours like alcohol and drug abuse, smoking and unsafe sex; chronic diseases such as cancers, diabetes and heart disease; infectious diseases like HIV; and social problems including educational underattainment, further involvement in violence and crime. The economic costs of these consequences are enormous.

The elimination of violence against children is called for in several targets of the 2030 Agenda for Sustainable Development Goals, specially in Target 16.2 : "end abuse, exploitation, trafficking and all forms of violence and torture of children". It focusses on interpersonal violence which accounts for most acts of violence against children, and includes child maltreatment, bullying and other types of youth violence and intimate person violence. The governments can monitor their progress towards reaching the SDG over course of 2020–2030, through the lens of Seven INSPIRE evidence-based strategies for ending violence against children.

INSPIRE: Seven strategies for ending violence against children *(136)*

INSPIRE is a set of seven evidence-based strategies for countries and communities working to eliminate violence against children. Launched in 2016, INSPIRE serves as a technical package and handbook for selecting, implementing and monitoring effective policies, programmes and services to prevent and respond to violence against children.

INSPIRE is an acronym, with each letter representing a strategy : I for the implementation and enforcement of laws; N for norms and values; S for safe environments; P for parent and caregiver support; I for income and economic strengthening; R for response and support services; and E for education and life skills. There are also two cross-cutting activities (multisectoral action and coordination, and monitoring and evaluation) that connects the seven strategies and monitor the extent of their implementation and impact on the problem.

The strategies and approaches of INSPIRE for preventing and responding to violence against children are as follows :

Strategy	Approach
Implementation and enforcement of laws	– Laws banning violent punishment of children by parents, teachers or other caregivers – Laws criminalizing sexual abuse and exploitation of children – Laws that prevent alcohol misuse – Laws limiting youth access to firearms and other weapons
Norms and values	– Changing adherence to restrictive and harmful gender and social norms – Community mobilization programmes – Bystander interventions
Safe environments	– Reducing violence by addressing "hotspots" – Interrupting the spread of violence – Improving the built environment
Parent and caregiver support	– Delivered through home visits – Delivered in groups in community settings – Delivered through comprehensive programmes
Income and economic strengthening	– Cash transfers – Group saving and loans combined with gender equity training – Micro-finance combined with gender norm training
Response and support services	– Counselling and therapeutic approaches – Screening combined with interventions – Treatment programmes for juvenile offenders in the criminal justice system – Foster care interventions involving social welfare services
Education and life skills	– Increase enrolment in pre-school, primary and secondary schools – Establish a safe and enabling school environment – Improve children's knowledge about sexual abuse and how to protect themselves against it – Life and social skills training – Adolescent intimate partner violence prevention programmes

The COVID-19 pandemic and violence against children *(136)*

The COVID-19 pandemic and societies response to it affects all aspects of our lives. School closures have impacted some 1.5 billon children. Movement restrictions, loss of income, isolation, and overcrowding have heightened levels of stress and anxiety in parents, caregivers and children, and cut families and individuals off from their usual sources of support.

These consequences have altered the prevalence and patterns of interpersonal violence. Decreases in homicides and violence-related injuries receiving emergency medical treatment (which mostly involve older adolescents and adult males) have been reported, particularly where lockdowns were accompanied by bans on alcohol sales. Spikes in calls to helplines about child abuse and intimate partner violence have been observed, alongside declines in the number of child abuse cases referred to child protection services. An increase in potential or actual online harms, including sexual exploitation and cyber-bullying resulting from increased internet use by children, has also been identified. The economic devastation wrought by COVID-19 and the response to it may take years to overcome, and could exacerbate economic inequalities, poverty, unemployment, and household financial insecurity.

Child marriage

Early marriage is a long-established custom in India. As early as 1929, the Sharda Act was enacted forbidding the practice of child marriages. In spite of the spread of literacy and legislations prohibiting early marriages, child marriages are still in vogue in the countryside particularly in Rajasthan, Madhya Pradesh and Uttar Pradesh, where substantial proportion of marriages take place when the girl is around 15 years of age *(137)*. The census data reveal that prior to 1951, the average age at marriage for girls in India was 13 years. There is however a gradual rise in the age at marriage in the country. The Child Marriage Restraint Act of 1978 raises the legal age of marriage from 15 to 18 years for girls; and from 18 to 21 years for boys. Studies indicate that in many states, the mean age at marriage for girls has already moved into 19 years and 24 years for the boys. The Prohibition of Child Marriage Act, 2006 (PCMA) was enacted repealing the Child Marriage Restraint Act of 1929 in order to prohibit child marriage rather than only restraining them. PCMA has been enforced with effect from 1st November, 2007. It makes child marriage an offence and makes provision for punishment for those conducting / abetting /promoting / permitting the marriage *(67)*.

The age at which the girl marries and enters the reproduction period of life has a great impact on her fertility. Girls who marry before the age of 18 give birth to larger number of children than those who married late. It is estimated that if the marriages were postponed from the age of 16 to 20–21, the number of births would decrease by 20–30 per cent.

Child guidance clinic

The first child guidance clinic was started in Chicago in 1909 and ever since, they have grown in number and complexity throughout the world. Originally intended to deal with problems of juvenile delinquency, child guidance clinics deal with all children or adolescents who for one reason or other, are not fully adjusted to their environment. The object of child guidance is to prevent children from the possibility of becoming neurotics and psychotics in later life.

Team work : Child guidance is a team work job – the team comprising of a psychiatrist, clinical psychologist, educational, psychologist, psychiatric social workers, public health nurses, paediatrician, speech therapist, occupational therapist and a neurologist. The psychiatrist is the central figure and is helped by the others in arriving at a correct diagnosis and formulating the line of treatment.

Services : The paediatrician takes care of the physical health of the child. The core of therapy is psychotherapy in order to restore positive feelings of security in the child. To achieve this, many methods are employed, e.g., play therapy, counselling, suggestions, change in the physical environment, easing of parental tensions, reconstruction of parental attitudes, etc. The child guidance clinics operate on the premise that if sound foundations of mental health are laid in childhood and adolescence, the same will continue into adulthood.

Child placement

(1) ORPHANAGES : Children who have no home or who for some reason could not be cared for by their parents are placed in orphanages. Scientific studies of human behaviour have revealed that mass care of infants and children in large institutions is undesirable. In such institutions, there is little opportunity for the child to experience the warmth and intimacy of family life, to develop emotional security and to participate in activities that would help him to become an adequate citizen. (2) FOSTER HOMES : Fostering is an arrangement whereby a child lives, usually on a temporary basis, with an extended or unrelated family member. Such an arrangement ensures that the birth parents do not lose any of their parental rights or responsibilities. This arrangement cater to children who are not legally free for adoption, and whose parents are unable to care for them due to illness, death or desertion by one parent, or any other crisis. The aim is to eventually re-unite the child with his/her own family, when the family circumstances improve *(66)*. (3) ADOPTION : In addition to the more or less temporary placement of children in foster or boarding homes, children are legally adopted. Legal adoption confers upon the child and adoptive parents, rights and responsibilities similar to that of natural parents. The laws of adoption vary from country to country; the relevant law in India is the "Hindu Adoptions and Maintenance Act, 1956". (4) BORSTALS : Boys over 16 years who are too difficult to be handled in a certified school or have misbehaved there, are sent to a Borstal. This institution falls in a category between a certified school and an adult prison. A Borstal sentence which is usually for three years, is regarded as a method of training and reformation. There are about six Borstals for boys in India but none for girls. Borstals do not come under the Children Act but are governed by the State Inspector General of Prisons *(138)*. (5) REMAND HOMES : In the remand home, the child is placed under the care of doctors, psychiatrists and other trained personnel. Every effort is made to improve the mental and physical wellbeing of the child. Elementary schooling is given, various arts and crafts are taught, games are played and other recreational activities are arranged.

THE CHILDREN ACT, 1960

The Children Act, 1960 in India (amended in 1977) provides for the care, maintenance, welfare, training, education and rehabilitation of the delinquent child. It covers the neglected and destitute, socially handicapped, uncontrollable, victimized and delinquent children. In Article 39 (f) the Constitution of India provides that "the state shall in particular direct its policy towards securing that childhood and youth are protected against moral and material abandonment."

JUVENILE JUSTICE ACT 1986

With the implementation of the Juvenile Justice Act, 1986, all Children's Acts applicable in different parts of the country have been repealed. The new Act, apart from rectifying the inadequacies of Children's Act, provides a comprehensive scheme for care, protection, treatment, development and rehabilitation of delinquent juveniles. The new Act has come into force from 2nd Oct 1987. Some of the special features of the Act are :

a. It provides a uniform legal framework for juvenile justice in the country so as to ensure that no child under any circumstances is put in jail or police lock-up;
b. It envisages specialized approach towards prevention

and treatment of juvenile delinquency in keeping with the developmental needs of children;

c. It establishes norms and standards for administration of juvenile justice in terms of investigation, care, treatment and rehabilitation; and

d. It lays down appropriate linkages and coordination between the formal system of juvenile justice and voluntary organizations. It specifically defines the roles and responsibilities of both.

Juvenile Justice Act 2000 *(66)*

Juvenile Justice (Care and Protection of Children) Act, 2000 (now Amendment Act 2006) is an Act to consolidate and amend the law relating to juveniles in conflict with law and children in need of care and protection, by providing for proper care, protection and treatment by catering to their development needs, and by adopting a child-friendly approach in the adjudication and disposition of matters in the best interest of children and for their ultimate rehabilitation. The Act defines a juvenile/child as a person who has not completed the age of 18 years. It has two separate chapters – one for juveniles in conflict with law and the other for children in need of care and protection. It also contains an exclusive chapter concerning rehabilitation and social reintegration of children. The Act defines Juvenile in conflict with law as a child who is alleged to have committed an offence and Children in need of care and protection broadly as children who are neglected, abused, abandoned, victim of any armed conflict or natural calamity amongst others. Offences committed against a child as listed in the Act, are cognizable and punishable under the provisions of this Act.

In order to implement its provisions and procedure, the Act provides for :

- Juvenile Justice Boards
- Child Welfare Committees
- Institutional care through children's homes, observation homes, shelter homes, special homes and aftercare organizations
- Non-institutional care through Adoption, Foster Care, Sponsorship Act and After Care
- Special Juvenile Police Units
- Juvenile Justice Fund
- Central/State/District Advisory Boards
- Selection Committee
- Inspection Committee.

Juvenile Justice (Care and Protection of Children) Act 2015

Juvenile Justice (Care and Protection of Children) Act 2015 came into force from January 15, 2016. The Act allows children aged 16 to 18 years and in conflict with law to be tried as adults in cases of heinous offences. When pronounced guilty, such children can be detained in a place of safety until they reach the age of 21 years. If still not found to have reformed by 21, they can be sent to jails housing adults.

SOCIAL WELFARE PROGRAMMES

The various social welfare programmes for women and children in India may be broadly categorized under six heads : (1) programmes for the welfare of women; (2) programmes for the welfare of children; (3) composite programmes (both for women and children); (4)schemes for the maladjusted groups; (5) schemes for the physically handicapped persons; and (6) programmes for the welfare of backward classes.

CHILD WELFARE

Child welfare covers the entire spectrum of needs of children who by reason of handicap – social, economic, physical or mental – are unable to avail of services provided by the community *(139)*. Child welfare programmes thus seek to provide supportive services to the families of these children because one of the important responsibility of the society and state is to assist the family in its natural obligations for the welfare of the children.

Child welfare services in their various facets are preventive, promotive, developmental and rehabilitative in nature. The problem is gigantic, and the resources available are only supplementary in nature and are designed to meet certain needs of the most deprived and vulnerable among country's child population. Attention is generally focussed on 3 categories of children in the poverty groups : children of working mothers; destitute children, and handicapped children *(139)*.

CHILD WELFARE AGENCIES

The important child welfare agencies in India are : (1) Indian Council for Child Welfare (ICCW); (2) Central Social Welfare Board; (3) Kasturba Gandhi Memorial Trust; and (4) the Indian Red Cross Society. These agencies have got branches all over the country. They get financial aid from the government to organize child welfare services in the country. The following are some of their activities. (a) DAY CARE SERVICES : This is for children of working mothers. Nursery schools, BALWADIS and creches are set up to help the children of working mothers. Day care centres are mainly for infants and toddlers. (b) HOLIDAY HOMES : These are organized for children in the age group 12 to 16 years at hill stations and sea-side resorts. The children spend their holidays in a useful manner. (c) RECREATION FACILITIES : These comprise organization of play centres, public parks, children's libraries, BAL BHAVANS, children's films, national museums, hobby classes, etc. Besides the national agencies, the following international agencies are interested in child welfare : UNICEF, WHO, International Union for Child Welfare, CARE and FAO of the United Nations.

INTEGRATED CHILD DEVELOPMENT SERVICES (ICDS)

Currently, the most important scheme in the field of child welfare is the ICDS scheme. The blue print for the scheme was prepared by the Department of Social Welfare in 1975. Considering the magnitude of the task, it was decided to take up on an experimental basis 33 projects in the year 1975–76 in 4 urban, 19 rural and 10 tribal areas spread over 22 states and the Union Territory of Delhi. The projects were sanctioned in October 1975. The Government of India decided to expand the project to cover 100 areas by 1978–79. Two major evaluations were conducted in 1978 and 1982. The positive results of these evaluations formed the basis for the governments decision to accelerate the expansion of ICDS in 1982.

Prior to 2005–06, providing supplementary nutrition was the responsibility of the states and administrative cost was provided by the central government. Government of India has modified the cost sharing pattern under ICDS by giving aid of 60 per cent of the financial expenditure to the states/UTs. In North-East states and Himalayan states the share is 90:10 and in Union Territories without legislation it is 100% central share.

The population norms for setting up of Angan Wadi Centres (AWC) and Mini-AWC have been revised to cover all habitations by SC/ST/minorities. The revised norms are as follows :

For AWCs in rural/urban projects

1 AWC for 400–800 population

2 AWCs for 800–1600 population

3 AWCs for 1600–2400 population

Thereafter, one AWC for multiples of 800 population. For Mini-AWC, the norm is one mini-AWC for 150 to 400 population.

Anganwadi on demand – where a settlement has atleast 40 children under 6 years but no anganwadi centre.

For tribal/reverine/desert/hilly and other difficult areas

1 AWC for 300–800 population

1 Mini-AWC for 150–300 population.

The ICDS seeks to lay a solid foundation for the development of the nation's human resource by providing an integrated package of early childhood services. These consist of – (1) supplementary nutrition; (2) immunization (3) health check-up; (4) medical referral services; (5) nutrition and health education for women; and (6) non-formal education of children up to the age of 6 years, and pregnant and nursing mothers in rural, urban, slums and tribal areas. ICDS scheme is designed both as a preventive and development effort. The services of immunization, health check-up and referral services are provided through public health infrastructure i.e., sub-centres, PHC and CHC. The services are provided concurrently.

Objectives *(140)*

The objectives of the ICDS scheme are :

(a) to improve the nutritional and health status of children in the age group 0–6 years;

(b) to lay the foundations for proper psychological, physical and social development of the child ;

(c) to reduce mortality and, morbidity, malnutrition and school drop-out;

(d) to achieve an effective coordination of policy and implementation among the various departments working for the promotion of child development; and

(e) to enhance the capability of the mother and nutritional needs of the child through proper nutrition and health education.

To achieve the above objectives the ICDS aims at providing the following package of services.

Beneficiary	Services
Pregnant women	Heath check-up Immunization against tetanus Supplementary nutrition Nutrition and health education
Nursing mothers	Health check-up Supplementary nutrition Nutrition and health education
Other women 15–45 years	Nutrition and Health education
Children less than 3 years	Supplementary nutrition Immunization Health check-up Referral services
Children in age group 3–6 years	Supplementary nutrition Immunization, Health check-up Referral services Non-formal education
Adolescent girls 11–18 years	Supplementary nutrition Nutrition and health education

The strategy adopted in ICDS is one of simultaneous delivery of early childhood services. While the health component forms a major component, ICDS is much more than a mere health programme for delivery of social services input for development.

Delivery of services

1. Supplementary nutrition

Supplementary nutrition is given to children below 6 years, and nursing and expectant mothers from low income group. The type of food depends upon local availability, type of beneficiary, location of the project etc. The aim is to supplement nutritional intake as follows *(141)* :

a. each child 6–72 months of age to get 500 calories and 12–15 grams of protein (financial norm of Rs 8.00 per child per day);

b. Severely malnourished child 6–72 months to get 800 calories and 20–25 grams protein (financial norm of Rs 12.00 per child per day); and

c. Each pregnant and nursing woman to get 600 calories and 18–20 grams of protein (financial norm of Rs 9.50 per beneficiary per day.

Under the revised nutritional and feeding norms for supplementary nutrition, state governments/UTs have been mandated to provide more than one meal to the children who come to AWCs, which include providing a morning snack in the form of milk/banana/egg/seasonal fruit/micro-nutrient fortified food followed by a hot cooked meal. For children below 3 years of age, and pregnant and lactating mothers, "take home ration" is to be provided. All are eligible for availing of the services of ICDS, below poverty line is not a criteria for registration of beneficiaries. The scheme is universal.

Supplementary nutrition is given 300 days in a year *(140)*. Adequate funds for supplementary nutrition is provided in the State Plan under Minimum Needs Programme. Children are weighed every month. Nutrition education and health education is given to mothers of children suffering from 1st degree of malnutrition. Supplementary nutrition (therapeutic food) is given to children suffering from 2nd and 3rd degree malnutrition. Children suffering from 4th degree malnutrition are recommended hospitalization.

2. Nutrition and health education

Nutrition education and health education is given to all women in the age group 15–45 years, giving priority to nursing and expectant mothers. It is imparted by specially organized courses in village during home visits by anganwadi workers.

3. Immunization

Immunization of children against 9 vaccine preventable diseases is being done, while for expectant mothers, immunization against tetanus is recommended.

4. Health check-up

This includes (a) antenatal care of expectant mothers; (b) postnatal care of nursing mother and care of newborn infants; (c) care of children under 6 years of age. Besides immunization, expectant mothers are given iron and folic acid tablets along with protein supplements. A minimum of 3 physical examinations are done. High risk mothers are referred to appropriate institutions for special care.

The health care of children under 6 years of age consists of :

1. Record of weight and height of children at periodical intervals;
2. Watch over milestones;
3. Immunization;
4. General check-up every 3-6 months to detect disease, malnutrition etc.;
5. Treatment for disease like diarrhoea, dysentery, respiratory tract infections etc. which are widely prevalent;
6. Deworming;
7. Prophylaxis against vitamin A deficiency and anaemia; and
8. Referral of serious cases to hospital has also been provided for.

Health records : Health records of the children, antenatal care and delivery card etc. are maintained. A card containing the health record of the child is given to the mother.

5. Non-formal pre-school education

Children between the ages 3–6 years are imparted non-formal pre-school education in an anganwadi in each village with about 1000 population. The objective is to provide opportunities to develop desirable attitude, values and behaviour pattern among children. Locally produced inexpensive toys and material are used in organizing play and creative activity.

Schemes for adolescent girls (67)

At present, there are two schemes for adolescent girls viz. "Kishori Shakti Yojana" and "Nutrition Programme for Adolescent Girls".

Kishori Shakti Yojana is being implemented using the infrastructure of ICDS. The scheme targets adolescent girls in the age group of 11 to 18 years and addresses their needs of self development, nutrition and health status, literacy and numerical skills, vocational skills etc.

Nutrition Programme for Adolescent Girls was approved in the year 2009–10, on a pilot project basis. The project is being implemented in 51 identified districts from the major states. Undernourished adolescent girls in the age group of 11 to 19 years (with body weight less than 30 kg in the age group of 11 to 15 years and 35 kg in the age group of 15 to 19 years) are covered under the scheme. 6 kg of free food grain is provided to each beneficiary per month. The programme is being implemented through the administrative set-up of ICDS scheme at the state, district, block and Anganwadi Centre level.

Poshan Abhiyan *(140)*

Government of India has launched "Poshan Abhiyan" on 18th December 2017 for a period of three years commencing from 2017–18, in all 36 states/UTs. The goals are to achieve improvement in nutritional status of children from 0–6 years, adolescent girls, pregnant women and lactating mothers with fixed targets. It ensures convergence of various programmes i,e anganwadi services, Pradhan Mantri Matru Vandana Yojana; schemes for adolescent girls of Ministry of Women and Child Development; Janani Suraksha Yojana; National Health Mission of Ministry of Health and Family Welfare; Swachh Bharat Mission of Ministry of Jal Shakti etc.

The objectives and targets are as follows *(140)* :

	Objective	Target
1.	Prevent and reduce stunting in children (0–6 years)	By 6 per cent (2 per cent/ year)
2.	Prevent and reduce under nutrition and underweight prevalence in children (0–6 years)	By 6 per cent (2 per cent/ year)
3.	Reduce the prevalence of anaemia among children (6–59 months)	By 9 per cent (3 per cent/ year)
4.	Reduce the prevalence of anaemia among girls and women in the age group (15–49 years)	By 9 per cent (3 per cent/ year)
5.	Reduce low birth weight (LBW)	By 6 per cent (2 per cent/ year)

The Abhiyan aims to reduce malnutrition in the country through a life cycle approach.

Two more schemes are being implemented at the ICDS level. They are (a) Rajiv Gandhi Scheme for Empowerment of Adolescent Girls – "SABLA" for the age group 11 to 18 years to improve their nutritional and health status; and (b) Indira Gandhi Matritva Sahyog Yojana (IGMSY), under which conditional cash transfer will be made to pregnant and lactating mothers in order to improve their nutritional and health status *(67)*.

At the end of 2019, about 7,075 ICDS projects and 13.77 lakh Anganwadi Centres/Mini-Anganwadi Centres were functional in the country. About 305.09 lakh children are pre-school education beneficiaries and 836.25 lakh supplementary nutrition beneficiaries are children and pregnant and lactating mothers.

Administration

The administrative unit of an ICDS project is the "community development block" in rural areas, the "tribal development block" in tribal areas and a group of slums in urban areas. In selection of project areas preference was given to areas predominantly inhabited by backward tribes, backward areas, draught prone areas and areas in which nutritional deficiencies are rampant. The rural/urban project has a population of 100,000 and a tribal project about 35,000 population. The number of villages in the rural project may be 100 while in tribal areas, it may be only about 50, taking into account the difficult terrain in which the tribal projects are located. The focal point for the delivery of integrated early childhood services under the ICDS scheme is the trained local woman known as Anganwadi worker (AWW). Other functionaries in the ICDS are the Child Development Project Officer (CDPO), who is in charge of 4 Supervisors (Mukhya Sevika) and 100 AWWs. Each Supervisor is responsible for 20–25 anganwadis and acts as mentor to AWWs; assists in record keeping, visits of health personnel and organizing community visits; and provides on-the-job training to AWWs. Anganwadi worker is the multipurpose agent, selected from the community. AWW provides direct link to children and mother; assists CDPO in survey of community and beneficiaries; organizes non-formal education sessions; provides health and nutrition education to mothers; assists PHC staff in providing health services; maintains records of immunization, feeding and pre-school attendance; liaises with block administrator, local school, health staff and community, and works for other community based activities, e.g., family planning.

The Government of India is committed to child development as a policy priority and is steadily expanding ICDS programme with the ultimate aim of reaching every child. The impact of the programme on the lives of children is evident in several crucial indicators : increased birth weight, reduced incidence of malnutrition, increased immunization coverage, and a reduced infant and child mortality rate in areas covered by the ICDS *(121)*.

Health of adolescents

The term "adolescence" has been defined as including those aged between 10 and 19, and "youth" as those between 15 and 24; "young people" is a term that covers both age groups, i.e. those between the ages of 10 and 24. True adolescence, however, being the period of physical, psychological and social maturing from childhood to adulthood, may fall within either age range. The development that takes place in adolescence is generally uneven, in that physical maturity may well be achieved in advance of psychological or social maturity; in most societies, in fact, reproductive capability is now established at an earlier age than in the past.

The importance of the health of adolescents has started to receive increasing recognition, particularly in developing countries where four out of five of the world's young people live, and where more than half the population is under the age of 25. These young men and women are, or will become, the parents of the next generation. They must be given every opportunity to develop to their full potential as healthy individuals.

Because adolescents are less vulnerable to disease than the very young and the very old, health problems specific to their age group have been given little prominence until now. Moreover, in societies where girls in particular have traditionally married at an early age, adolescence has been regarded merely as a brief interlude between puberty and marriage. As the average age of menarche has fallen, and with an increasing trend towards late marriage, however, this period has been extended and traditional attitude has begun to change. At the same time, the influence of the family has declined, urbanization and migration have become more common, and young people have been increasingly exposed to the mass media – all factors that contribute to major changes in social and sexual behaviour.

High rate of mortality and morbidity has always been associated with pregnancy and childbirth in pubertal and adolescent girls. This problem is now compounded by the dramatic rise in the number of pregnancies, both wanted and unwanted, among adolescents, who are also having more abortions and contracting sexually transmitted diseases more often. There appears also to be an increase in the number of abandoned and abused children born to adolescent mothers. As long as these problems are allowed to persist, much of the energy, creativity and idealism of youth will be lost to society. However, the problems are preventable, and efforts to eliminate them must involve the young people themselves, contributing in ways appropriate to their particular cultures.

Society today demands more of young people than ever before. With the decline of the extended family greater autonomy is expected of them, especially in the raising of children; increasing urbanization and industrialization means that economic independence is achieved only through more education and training. Early parenthood, particularly for girls, may limit or preclude social and educational development and the ability to achieve full status in society and is associated with greater morbidity and mortality. The World Fertility Survey observed an inverse relationship between fertility and the education of women: women with no education have, on average, twice as many children as those with seven or more years of schooling. Corollaries of this finding are the increased earning power of educated women, their improved status within the family, and the greater control they are able to exercise over their own lives.

A more universal consequence of early and more frequent childbearing is the increase in population size and growth rate. Where girls marry at 15, the age gap between successive generations may be less than 20 years; this gap may widen to as much as 30 years where the age at marriage is 25. The sexual behaviour and reproductive patterns of young people are highly susceptible to social influences and related to their own sense of psychological well-being.

Although an adolescent girl is likely to give birth and rear her children within the context of an extended family, the risks she and her children run of illness, injury and death are far greater than those for a mature woman in her twenties. The chances of anaemia, developing during pregnancy, and of retarded fetal growth; premature birth and complications during labour are all significantly higher for the adolescent mother, as are the risks of her own death during pregnancy or child-birth.

Formal education of girls generally ends with marriage, and from then on their social status may well depend on fecundity. An adolescent girl who proves to be infertile (or whose husband is infertile) runs the risk of being rejected by both husband and family and thus of losing what little status she has. The second major set of problems of reproductive health in adolescence results from the profound socio-economic changes taking place in most developing countries. The average age of menarche has fallen, there is a trend towards later marriage, and young people are often less directly supervised than was the case in the past – all of which have the effect of increasing the opportunities for sexual encounter. Since the subject of adolescent sexuality remains taboo in most societies, there is widespread ignorance among young people of the risks associated with unprotected sexual activity. Sources of information and contraceptive advice are rarely available or accessible to them. In addition, impulsive sexual behaviour and non-use of contraceptives are sometimes exacerbated by alcohol and drug abuse.

A number of major approaches to reducing problems by modification of the contributing factors will serve to promote good health among the young and thus to improve health and social development of their communities. These approaches include the following :

1. Informing, educating and sensitizing key groups in society to individual health and social development needs.
2. Advocating appropriate policy, legislation and programmes for promoting adolescent reproductive health.
3. Using appropriate and innovative research to improve knowledge of, and disseminate information about, the factors that influence and determine young people's sexual, contraceptive and reproductive decisions and behaviour.
4. Modifying, extending and evaluating services specially designed to meet young people's needs.
5. Mobilizing the energy, creativity and idealism of young people in promoting health and developing appropriate activities in their communities.
6. Facilitating action to extend education opportunities for girls.

PREVENTIVE MEDICINE AND GERIATRICS

Ageing is a natural process. In the words of Seneca; "Old age is an incurable disease", but more recently, Sir James Sterling Ross commented : "You do not heal old age. You protect it; you promote it; you extend it" *(142)*. These are in fact the basic principles of preventive medicine. Old age should be regarded as a normal, inevitable biological phenomenon. The study of the physical and psychological changes which are incident to old age is called gerontology. The care of the aged is called clinical gerontology or geriatrics. Another aspect of gerontology is social gerontology which was born on the one hand out of the instincts of humanitarian and social attitudes and on the other out of the problems set by the increasing number of old people. Experimental gerontology is concerned with research into the basic biological problems of ageing, into its physiology, biochemistry, pathology and psychology. The fields of studies range from studies of populations through individuals, organs, systems, tissues and cells, down to the molecular level. GERIATRIC GYNAECOLOGY : With the lengthening span of life a new chapter in gynaecology – geriatric gynaecology – is fast opening up. More patients are coming for repair of prolapse of varying degrees, non-specific vaginitis, ovarian tumours, psychic aberrations and sexual problems. There is ample scope for research into the degenerative and other diseases of old age; their treatment in hospital and general practice; and finally into preventive geriatrics and the epidemiology of conditions affecting the aged.

Size of the problem

Discoveries in medical science and improved social conditions during past few decades have increased the life span of man. The expectation of life at birth in developed countries is over 80 years. The age structure of the population in the developed countries has so evolved that the numbers of old people is continually on the increase. These trends are appearing in all countries where medical and social services are well developed and the standard of living is high.

In the year 2019, there were an estimated 694 million old persons in the world, of which 540 million were living in developing countries *(5)*. Italy and Japan have the highest proportion of older persons (about 24 per cent and 16 per cent respectively in the year 2019). By 2025, the number of elderly people is expected to rise more than 1.2 billion with about 840 million of these in low-income countries. In India, although the percentage of aged persons to the total population is low in comparison to the developed countries, nevertheless, the absolute size of aged population is considerable. For the year 2019 the estimates are : 9.3 per cent of total population were above the age of 65 years. This profound shift in the share of older Indians, brings with it a variety of social, economic and healthcare policy challenges *(143)*.

Health problems of the aged

(1) PROBLEMS DUE TO THE AGEING PROCESS

No one knows when old age begins. The "biological age" of a person is not identical with his "chronological age". It is said that nobody grows old merely by living a certain number of years. Years wrinkle the skin, but worry, doubt, fear, anxiety and self-distrust wrinkle the soul. While ageing merely stands for growing old, senescence is an expression used for the deterioration in the vitality or the lowering of the biological efficiency that accompanies ageing. With the passage of time, certain changes take place in an organism. These changes are, for the most part deleterious and eventually lead to the death of the organism. Our knowledge about the ageing process is incomplete. We do not know much about the disabilities incident to the ageing process. However the following are some of the disabilities considered as incident to it; (a) senile cataract, (b) glaucoma, (c) nerve deafness, (d) osteoporosis affecting mobility, (e) emphysema, (f) failure of special senses, (g) changes in mental outlook. This list is not exhaustive; we need to know a lot more about the disabilities incident to the ageing process.

(2) PROBLEMS ASSOCIATED WITH LONG-TERM ILLNESS

Certain chronic diseases are more frequent among the older people than in the younger people. These are : (a) DEGENERATIVE DISEASES OF HEART AND BLOOD VESSELS : Of particular importance after the age of 40, are the degenerative diseases of the heart and blood vessels. The inner walls of arteries break down, and a lipoid material is deposited. This in time is replaced by calcium which leads to narrowing of blood vessels or atherosclerosis. This leads to diminished blood supply, thrombus formation, rupture of blood vessels and high blood pressure. No single factor has been identified as the cause of atherosclerosis. Diet, heredity, overweight, nervous and emotional strain have all been implicated. Cardiovascular diseases are the major causes of death in the developed countries. A reduction of body weight and modification of the habits of life are needed to decrease the strain on heart and blood vessels. By these, it is possible to lead a longer and more useful life. (b) CANCER : The danger of cancer looms large past middle life. In the developed countries, cancer is a leading cause of death. The incidence of cancer rises rapidly after the age of 40. Cancer of the prostate is common after the age of 65. (c) ACCIDENTS : Accidents are a health problem in the elderly. The bones become fragile due to a certain amount of decalcification as a result of which they break easily. Accidents are more common in the home than outside. Fracture neck of femur is a very common geriatric problem. (d) DIABETES : Diabetes is a long-term illness due to faulty carbohydrate metabolism. It is a leading cause of death as the population grows older. About 75 per cent of the diabetics are over 50 years of age. (e) DISEASES OF LOCOMOTOR SYSTEM : A wide range of articular and non-articular disorders affect the aged – fibrositis, myositis, neuritis, gout, rheumatoid arthritis, osteoarthritis, spondylitis of spine, etc. These conditions cause more discomfort and disability than any other chronic disease in the elderly. (f) RESPIRATORY ILLNESSES : In the upper decades of life, respiratory diseases such as chronic bronchitis, asthma, emphysema are of major importance. (g) GENITOURINARY SYSTEM : Enlargement of the prostate, dysuria, nocturia, frequent and urgency of micturition are the common complaints.

(3) PSYCHOLOGICAL PROBLEMS

(1) MENTAL CHANGES : Impaired memory, rigidity of outlook and dislike of change are some of the mental changes in the aged. Reduced income leads to a fall in the living standards of the elderly; it does have mental and social consequences. (2) SEXUAL ADJUSTMENT : Between 40 and 50, there is cessation of reproduction by women and diminution of sexual activity on the part of men. During this phase, physical and emotional disturbances may occur. Irritability, jealousy and despondency are very frequent. (3) EMOTIONAL DISORDERS : Emotional disorders result from social maladjustment. The degree of adaptation to the fact of ageing is crucial to a man's happiness in this phase of life. Failure to adapt can result in bitterness, inner withdrawal, depression, weariness of life, and even suicide.

Lifestyle and healthy ageing

People can do a great deal to influence their individual risk of developing many of the diseases of later life by paying careful attention to lifestyle factors. By adopting a healthier lifestyle, the risk of a whole range of diseases can be reduced. These factors are : (a) DIET AND NUTRITION : A good diet reduces the chances of developing the diseases of old age. As countries rapidly develop economically, diets and lifestyles change considerably and overnutrition replaces undernutrition. One of the problem is excessive fat intake. Saturated fats and trans-fatty acids, have been linked to raised cholesterol levels in the blood, leading to increased risk of cardiovascular disease. People should eat healthy diet since very early age to avoid or delay diseases. The diet should be balanced with less saturated fats and oils; should contain lots of fruits and vegetables; salt and sugar should be less; include plenty of calcium rich food; eat high fibre diet; (b) EXERCISE : Exercise helps maintain good health, as it helps to control weight, improves emotional well-being and relieves stress, improves blood circulation, increases flexibility, lowers blood pressure, increases energy levels, improves balance and thus reduces the dangers of falls, lowers blood sugar levels thus helps in diabetes, improves bone density and thus helps prevent osteoporosis; (c) WEIGHT : Overweight and obesity have become major problem worldwide and it contributes to many diseases of later life. Obesity is an important factor in heart disease, stroke, hypertension, diabetes, arthritis (especially in the knees), and breast cancer; (d) SMOKING : It is estimated that 22 per cent of men and 18 per cent of women aged 65 to 74 years in developed countries are smokers *(144)*. Though this figure is lower than among younger adults, older people have usually smoked for longer, have been and continue to be heavy smokers, and are likely to have chronic diseases, with smoking causing further deterioration. Former smokers live longer than continuing smokers; smoking cessation at the age of 50 years reduces the risk of dying within the next 15 years by 50 per cent. For some, but not for all former smokers, the risk of developing smoking-related diseases reverts to that of lifelong non-smokers *(144)*; (e) ALCOHOL : Drinking beyond a specified amount contributes to a number of later life diseases. Research suggests that sensitivity to the effect of alcohol increases with age. Older people achieve a higher blood alcohol concentration, than younger people after consuming an equal amount of alcohol. This is largely as a result of the age-related decrease in the amount of body water which dilutes alcohol. While younger people are likely to develop tolerance to increasing amount of alcohol, older people have a decreased ability to develop this tolerance *(144)*. Drinking is linked to liver diseases, stomach ulcers, gout, depression, osteoporosis, heart disease, breast cancer, diabetes and hypertension *(143)*; and (f) SOCIAL ACTIVITIES : People who become socially isolated – who rarely go out, do not join in the community activities, have few friends or do not see much of their family – are less healthy. Getting out and keeping involved with others creates a sense of belonging. Mixing with other people of similar age, at similar stage of life or perhaps with similar health concerns, can help people realize that they are not alone. The support gained from others can be important in recovering from illness. Simply knowing that others care, helps *(143)*.

Health status of the aged in India

A few hospital based studies have been made in India on the health status of the aged persons, but such studies provide only a partial view of the spectrum of illness in the aged. The overall data on aged are scarce. The main causes of illness are arthritis, cataract, bronchitis, avitaminosis, ear diseases, hypertension, diabetes, rheumatism, helminthic infestations, accidents, etc.

The government of India announced a *National Policy on older persons* in January 1999. This policy identifies principal areas of intervention as financial security, health care, nutrition, shelter, education, welfare, protection of life and property of older citizens. The policy provides for a broad framework for collaboration and cooperation, both within as well as between governmental and non-governmental agencies. An important thrust in the policy is on active and productive involvement of older persons, and not just their care. A national council for older persons (NCOP) was constituted to operationalize the policy. An integrated programme for older persons has been formulated by revising the earlier scheme of assistance to voluntary organizations for programmes relating to the welfare of the aged. The objective is to promote a society for all ages, to empower and improve the quality of life of older persons.

The programme for the first time recognizes formation of self-help groups, association of older persons for advancement of their rights and utilization of their experience and services. 234 Old age homes, 398 day care centres and 40 mobile medical units are operational. Scheme of assistance to Panchayat Raj Institutions / Voluntary Organizations / Self Help Groups, for construction of old age homes has also been revised to encourage Multi Service Centres for older persons.

As a part of National Social Assistance Programme, old age pension is being provided to more than 4 million destitute elderly all over the country. The amount of pension varies from state to state – from Rs 75 per month in Assam to Rs 300 per month in West Bengal and Rajasthan *(144)*. An Old Age Social and Income Security (OASIS) project was launched to comprehensively examine policy questions, connected with Old Age Income Security. Travel related concessions / facilities are provided to the older people by Indian Railways, Indian Airlines and State Transport Corporations. Health care is being provided to the older persons through Bhavishya Arogya Mediclaim, and Rural Group Life Insurance Schemes. Income Tax Concessions are also available to the elderly citizens.

On 19th Nov. 2007, the Indira Gandhi National Old Age Pension Scheme was launched to provide monthly pension to people over 65 years and living below poverty line. The scheme is to cover about 1.57 crore people, the central government is to provide a monthly pension of Rs. 200 to each beneficiary and the state governments are expected to contribute an equal amount.

In India, *HelpAge India* is the largest voluntary organization working for the cause and care of the disadvantaged older people. In the 26 years since its inception, it has made an impact on the lives of nearly 6 million senior citizens, through 3,084 projects. HelpAge India supports the following programmes to make life easier for older people : (a) Free cataract operations; (b) Mobile medicare units; (c) Income generation and micro-credit; (d) Old-age homes and day-care centres; (e) Adopt-a-Gran (grand parent); and (f) Disaster mitigation.

Implication of the ageing population in terms of preventive and social medicine

The ageing population is both a medical and sociological problem. It makes a greater demand on the health services of a community. In rapidly greying world, healthy ageing is vital for countries. It is a prerequisite for economic growth. The predicted explosion of non-communicable diseases like cardiovascular diseases, cancer, and depression in the ever increasing number of older persons globally, will result in enormous human and social costs unless preventive action is taken.

The alteration of the age pyramid, however, poses significant new challenges for governments, societies, and families in the 21st century. Ageing developing countries are slated to face a heavy double burden of infectious and non-communicable diseases, yet they often lack significant resources, including comprehensive ageing policies, to cope. Industrialized countries, on the otherhand, were fortunate enough to become affluent before they became old *(144)*.

The modern philosophy is that the old must continue to take their share in the responsibilities and in the enjoyment of the privileges, which are an essential feature of remaining an active member of the community. The community must assist the aged to fight the triple evils of poverty, loneliness and ill-health.

Potential for disease prevention in the elderly

For older individuals, a great proportion of the disease burden derives from existing conditions, whether this burden is measured by prevalence rates, indicators of morbidity, disability, mortality, or by health and long term care utilization. In addition, older people with disability, resulting from chronic diseases, appear at high risk of acute illness and injuries. The evidence arrayed of the role of existing and often immutable disease argues for the importance of secondary and tertiary prevention, in combination with primary screening or prevention for this population *(145)*.

Among older individuals, categories of conditions, occurrences, and illnesses exist in a variety of combinations, and risk factors as well as disease sequelae often overlap. Examples of conditions potentially amenable to prevention in older persons are outlined in Table 31.

Many factors that contribute to decrements of ageing and the burden of illness are potentially responsive to preventive interventions. In view of this evidence, the design of preventive strategies appropriate to this population becomes crucial for the utility of preventive care, both in reducing risk and maintaining functional independence.

Much care is bestowed upon the old people in Western societies by providing Social Welfare measures such as national assistance, supplementary pensions, home services, home care services, meals on wheels services, old folk's homes, sitters-up service and provision of services of health visitors. By providing these services, the State ensures that the years of retirement of those who have worked hard in its service shall be free from anxiety, want and boredom.

TABLE 31

Areas potentially amenable to preventive health care in the elderly

Primary	Secondary	Tertiary
Health habits	Screening for	Rehabilitation
-smoking	- hypertension	- physical deficits
-alcohol abuse	- diabetes	- cognitive deficits
-obesity	- periodontal disease	- functional deficits
-nutrition	- dental caries	
-physical activity	- sensory impairment	
-sleep	- medication side-effects	Caretaker support
Coronary heart disease risk factors	- colo-rectal cancer breast cancer, cervical cancer prostatic cancer	Introduction of support necessary to prevent loss of autonomy
Immunization -influenza	- nutritionally-induced anaemias	
-pneumovax	- depression, stress	
-tetanus	- urinary incontinence	
	- podiatric problems	
Injury prevention Iatrogenesis prevention	- fall risk - tuberculosis (high-risk)	
Osteoporosis prevention	- syphilis (high-risk) - stroke prevention - myocardial infarction	

Source : *(145)*

ANNEXURE A *(146)*

PRINCIPLES OF THE INTEGRATED CLINICAL CASE MANAGEMENT

IMCI clinical guidelines are based on the following principles :

1. **Examining all sick children aged up to five years** of age for general danger signs and all young infants for signs of **very severe disease**. These signs **indicate** severe illness and the need for immediate referral or admission to hospital.
2. The children and infants are then **assessed for main symptoms :**
   - In older children the main symptoms include :
     - Cough or difficulty in breathing
     - Diarrhoea,
     - Fever, and
     - Ear infection.
   - In young infants, the main symptoms include :
     - Local bacterial infection,
     - Diarrhoea, and
     - Jaundice.
3. Then in addition, all sick children are **routinely checked** for :
   - Nutritional and immunization status,
   - HIV status in high HIV settings, and
   - Other potential problems.
4. Only a **limited number of clinical signs** are used, selected on the basis of their sensitivity and specificity to detect disease through classification.

A combination of individual signs leads to a **child's classification** within one or more symptom groups rather than a diagnosis. The classification of illness is based on a colour-coded triage system :

- **"PINK"** indicates urgent hospital referral or admission.
- **"YELLOW"** indicates initiation of specific outpatient treatment.
- **"GREEN"** indicates supportive home care.

5. IMCI management procedures use a **limited number of essential drugs** and encourage active participation of caregivers in the treatment of their children.
6. An essential component of IMCI is the **counselling of caregivers** regarding home care :
   - Appropriate feeding and fluids,
   - When to return to the clinic immediately, and
   - When to return for follow-up.

SICK YOUNG INFANT AGE UPTO 2 MONTHS
ASSESS AND CLASSIFY THE SICK YOUNG INFANT

ASSESS	CLASSIFY	IDENTIFY TREATMENT
DO A RAPID APPRAISAL OF ALL WAITING INFANTS **ASK THE MOTHER WHAT THE YOUNG INFANT'S PROBLEMS ARE** • Determine if this is an initial or follow-up visit for this problem. – If follow-up visit, use the follow-up instructions. – If initial visit, assess the child as follows:	USE ALL BOXES THAT MATCH THE INFANT'S SYMPTOMS AND PROBLEMS TO CLASSIFY THE ILLNESS	

CHECK FOR VERY SEVERE DISEASE AND LOCAL BACTERIAL INFECTION

ASK :

- Is the infant having difficulty in feeding ?
- Has the infant had convulsions (fits) ?

LOOK, LISTEN, FEEL :

- Count the breaths in one minute. Repeat the count if more than 60 breaths per minute.
- Look for severe chest indrawing.

(YOUNG INFANT MUST BE CALM)

- Measure axillary temperature.
- Look at the umbilicus. Is it red or draining pus ?
- Look for skin pustules.
- Look at the young infant's movements.
  If infant is sleeping, ask the mother to wake him/her.
  – Does the infant move on his/her own ?
  If the young infant is not moving, gently stimulate him/her.
  – Does the infant not move at all ?

Classify ALL YOUNG INFANTS

Signs	Classify	Treatment
Any one of the following signs: • Not feeding well, or • Convulsions, or • Fast breathing (60 breaths per minute or more), or • Severe chest indrawing, or • Fever (37.5°C* or above), or • Low body temperature (less than 35.5°C*) or • Movement only when stimulated or no movement at all.	***Pink :*** VERY SEVERE DISEASE	➢ **Give first dose of intramuscular antibiotics.** ➢ **Treat to prevent low blood sugar.** ➢ **Refer *URGENTLY* to hospital**** ➢ **Advise the mother how to keep the infant warm on the way to the hospital.**
• Umbilicus red or draining pus. • Skin pustules.	***Yellow :*** LOCAL BACTERIAL INFECTION	➢ **Give an appropriate oral antibiotic.** ➢ Teach the mother to treat local infections at home. ➢ Advise mother to give home care for the young infant. ➢ Follow-up in 2 days.
• None of the signs of very severe disease or local bacterial infection.	***Green :*** SEVERE DISEASE OR LOCAL INFECTION UNLIKELY	➢ Advise mother to give home care.

* These thresholds are based on axillary temperature. The thresholds for rectal temperature readings are approximately 0.5° C higher.

** If referral is not possible, manage the sick young as described in the national referral care guidelines or WHO Pocket Book for hospital care for children.

CHECK FOR JAUNDICE

If jaundice present, ASK :	***LOOK, AND FEEL :***	*Classify JAUNDICE*	Signs	Classification	Treatment
• When did the jaundice appear first ?	• Look for jaundice (yellow eyes or skin) • Look at the young infant's palms and soles. Are they yellow ?		• Any jaundice if age less than 24 hours or • Yellow palms and soles at any age.	***Pink :*** SEVERE JAUNDICE	➢ **Treat to prevent low blood sugar.** ➢ **Refer *URGENTLY* to hospital.** ➢ **Advise the mother how to keep the infant warm on the way to the hospital.**
			• Jaundice appearing after 24 hours of age and • Palms and soles not yellow.	***Yellow :*** JAUNDICE	➢ Advise the mother to give home care for the young infant. ➢ Advise the mother to return immediately if palms and soles appear yellow. ➢ If the young infant is older than 14 days, refer to a hospital for assessment. ➢ Follow-up in 1 day.
			• No jaundice	***Green :*** NO JAUNDICE	➢ Advise the mother to give home care for the young infant.

THEN ASK: Does the young infant have diarrhoea* ?

IF YES, LOOK AND FEEL:	Classify DIARRHOEA *For DEHYDRATION*	Signs	Classification	Treatment
• Look at the young infant's general condition : Infant's movements – Does the infant move on his/her own ? – Does the infant move when stimulated but then stops ? – Does the infant not move at all ? – Is the infant restless and irritable ? • Look for sunken eyes. • Pinch the skin of the abdomen. Does it go back: – Very slowly (longer than 2 seconds) ? – or slowly ?		**Two of the following signs:** • Movement only when stimulated or no movement at all. • Sunken eyes. • Skin pinch goes back very slowly.	***Pink :*** SEVERE DEHYDRATION	➢ **If infant has no other severe classification :** – Give fluid for severe dehydration (Plan C) OR ***If infant also has another severe classification :*** – **Refer *URGENTLY* to hospital with mother giving frequent sips of ORS on the way.** – **Advise the mother to continue breast-feeding.**
		Two of the following signs: • Restless and irritable. • Sunken eyes. • Skin pinch goes back slowly.	***Yellow :*** SOME DEHYDRATION	➢ Give fluid and breast milk for some dehydration (Plan B) ➢ ***If infant has any severe classification :*** ***– Refer urgently to hospital with mother giving frequent sips of ORS on the way.*** ***– Advise the mother to continue breast-feeding.*** ➢ Advice the mother when to return immediately. ➢ Follow-up in 2 days if not improving.
		Not enough signs to classify as some or severe dehydration.	***Green :*** NO DEHYDRATION	➢ Give fluids to treat diarrhoea at home and continue breast feeding (Plan A). ➢ Advise the mother when to return immediately. ➢ Follow-up in 2 days if not improving.

Details of Plan A, B, C on page 688, 689

* **What is diarrhoea in a young infant ?**
A young infant has diarrhoea if the stools have changed from usual pattern and are many and watery (more water than faecal matter). The normally frequent or semi-solid stools of a breastfed baby are not diarrhoea.

THEN CHECK FOR FEEDING PROBLEM OR LOW WEIGHT FOR AGE

If an infant has no indications to refer urgently to hospital :

ASK :

- Is the infant breastfed ? If yes, how many times in 24 hours ?
- Does the infant usually receive any other drinks ? If yes, how often ?
- If yes, what do you use to feed the infant ?

LOOK, LISTEN, FEEL :

- Determine weight for age.
- Look for ulcers or white patches in the mouth (thrush).

Classify FEEDING

ASSESS BREAST-FEEDING :

- **Has the infant breastfed in the previous hour ?**
  If the infant has not fed in the previous hour, ask the mother to put her infant to the breast. Observe the breastfeed for 4 minutes.
  (If the infant was fed during the last hour, ask the mother if she can wait and tell you when the infant is willing to feed again.)
  - Is the infant well attached ?
    not well attached good attachment
- **TO CHECK ATTACHMENT, LOOK FOR :**
  - Chin touching breast
  - Mouth wide open
  - Lower lip turned outwards
  - More areola visible above than below the mouth.

  (All of these signs should be present if the attachment is good)
- Is the infant suckling effectively (that is, slow deep sucks, sometimes pausing) ?
  not suckling effectively suckling effectively
  Clear a blocked nose if it interferes with breastfeeding.

Signs	Classify	Treatment
• Not well attached to breast, or • Not suckling effectively, or • Less than 8 breastfeeds in 24 hours, or • Receives other foods or drinks, or • Low weight for age, or • Thrush (ulcers or white patches in mouth).	***Yellow :*** FEEDING PROBLEM OR LOW WEIGHT	➢ If not well attached or not suckling effectively, teach correct positioning and attachment. – If not able to attach well immediately, teach the mother to express breast milk and feed by a cup. ➢ If breastfeeding less than 8 times in 24 hours, advise to increase frequency of feeding. Advice the mother to breastfeed as often and as long as the infant wants, day and night. ➢ If receiving other foods or drinks, counsel the mother about breastfeeding more, reducing other drinks, and using a cup. ➢ If not breastfeeding at all*: – Refer for breastfeeding counselling and possible relactation*. – Advice about correctly preparing breast-milk substitutes and using a cup. ➢ Advice the mother how to feed and keep the low weight infant warm at home. ➢ If thrush, teach the mother to treat thrush at home. ➢ Advise the mother to give home care for the young infant. ➢ Follow-up any feeding problem or thrush in 2 days. ➢ Follow-up low weight for age in 14 days.
• Not low weight for age and no other signs of inadequate feeding.	***Green :*** NO FEEDING PROBLEM	➢ Advise mother to give home care for the young infant. ➢ Praise the mother for feeding the infant well.

* Unless not breastfeeding because the mother is HIV positive.

SICK CHILD AGE 2 MONTHS UPTO 5 YEARS
ASSESS AND CLASSIFY THE SICK CHILD

ASSESS	CLASSIFY	IDENTIFY TREATMENT
ASK THE MOTHER WHAT THE CHILD'S PROBLEMS ARE • Determine if this is an initial or follow-up visit for this problem. – If follow-up visit, use the follow-up instructions on *TREAT THE CHILD* chart. – If initial visit, assess the child as follows :	USE ALL BOXES THAT MATCH THE CHILD'S SYMPTOMS AND PROBLEMS TO CLASSIFY THE ILLNESS	

CHECK FOR GENERAL DANGER SIGNS

ASK :
- Is the child able to drink or breastfeed ?
- Does the child vomit everything ?
- Has the child had convulsions ?

LOOK :
- See if the child is lethargic or unconscious.
- Is the child convulsing now ?

URGENT Attention

Signs	Classify	Identify treatment
• Any general danger sign.	*Pink :* VERY SEVERE DESEASE	➢ **Give diazepam if convulsing now.** ➢ **Quickly complete the assessment.** ➢ **Give any pre-referral treatment immediately.** ➢ **Treat to prevent low blood sugar.** ➢ **Keep the child warm.** ➢ **Refer URGENTLY.**

A child with any general danger sign needs *URGENT* attention; complete the assessment and any pre-referral treatment immediately so referral is not delayed.

THEN ASK ABOUT MAIN SYMPTOMS :

Does the child have cough or difficult breathing ?

IF YES, ASK :
- For how long ?

LOOK, LISTEN, FEEL :* (CHILD MUST BE CALM)
- Count the breaths in one minute.
- Look for chest indrawing.
- Look and listen for stridor.
- Look and listen for wheezing.

If wheezing with either fast breathing or chest indrawing :
Give a trial of rapid acting inhaled bronchodilator for up to three times 15–20 minutes apart. Count the breaths and look for chest indrawing again, and then classify.

If the child is :	*Fast breathing is :*
2 months up to 12 months	50 breaths per minute or more.
12 months up to 5 years	40 breaths per minute or more.

Classify COUGH or DIFFICULT BREATHING

Signs	Classify	Identify treatment
• Any general danger sign or • Stridor in calm child.	*Pink :* SEVERE PNEUMONIA OR VERY SEVERE DISEASE	➢ **Give first dose of an appropriate antibiotic.** ➢ **Refer URGENTLY to hospital.****
• Chest indrawing. • Fast breathing.	*Yellow :* PNEUMONIA	➢ **Give oral Amoxicillin for 5 days***.** ➢ If wheezing (or disappeared after rapidly acting bronchodilator) give an inhaled bronchodilator for 5 days****. ➢ If chest indrawing in HIV exposed/ infected child, give first dose of amoxicillin and refer. ➢ Soothe the throat and relieve the cough with a safe remedy. ➢ If coughing for more than 14 days or recurrent wheeze, refer for possible TB or asthma assessment. ➢ Advise mother when to return immediately. ➢ Follow-up in 3 days.
• No signs of pneumonia or very severe disease.	*Green :* COUGH OR COLD	➢ If wheezing (or disappeared after rapidly acting bronchodilator) give an inhaled bronchodilator for 5 days****. ➢ Soothe the throat and relieve the cough with a safe remedy. ➢ If coughing for more than 14 days or recurrent wheezing, refer for possible TB or asthma assessment. ➢ Advise mother when to return immediately. ➢ Follow-up in 5 days if not improving.

* If pulse oximeter is available, determine oxygen saturation and refer if < 90%.

** If referral is not possible, manage the child as described in the pneumonia section of the national referral guidelines or as in WHO Pocket Book for hospital care for children.

*** Oral Amoxicillin for 3 days could be used in patients with fast breathing but no chest indrawing in low HIV settings.

**** In settings where inhaled bronchodilator is not available, oral salbutamol may be tried but not recommended for treatment of severe acute wheeze.

DOES THE CHILD HAVE DIARRHOEA ?

IF YES ASK :

- For how long ?
- Is there blood in the stool ?

LOOK AND FEEL:

- Look at the child's general condition. Is the child :
  - Lethargic or unconscious ?
  - Restless and irritable ?
- Look for sunken eyes.
- Offer the child fluid. Is the child :
  - Not able to drink or drinking poorly ?
  - Drinking eagerly, thirsty ?
- Pinch the skin of the abdomen. Does it go back:
  - Very slowly (longer than 2 seconds) ?
  - Slowly ?

Classify DIARRHOEA

	Signs	Classify	Treatment
For DEHYDRATION	Two of the following signs : • Lethargic or unconscious. • Sunken eyes. • Not able to drink or drinking poorly. • Skin pinch goes back very slowly.	***Pink :*** SEVERE DEHYDRATION	➢ If child has no other severe classification : – Give fluid for severe dehydration (Plan C). **If child also has another severe classification :** **– Refer URGENTLY to hospital with mother giving frequent sips of ORS on the way.** **– Advise the mother to continue breastfeeding.** **➢ If child is 2 years or older and there is cholera in your area, give antibiotic for cholera.**
	Two of the following signs : • Restless, irritable. • Sunken eyes. • Drinks eagerly, thirsty. • Skin pinch goes back slowly.	***Yellow :*** SOME DEHYDRATION	➢ Give fluid, zinc supplements, and food for some dehydration (Plan B). **➢ If child also has a severe classification :** **– Refer URGENTLY to hospital with mother giving frequent sips of ORS on the way.** **– Advise the mother to continue breastfeeding.** ➢ Advise mother when to return immediately. ➢ Follow-up in 5 days if not improving.
	Not enough signs to classify as some or severe dehydration.	***Green:*** NO DEHYDRATION	➢ Give fluid, zinc supplements, and food to treat diarrhoea at home (Plan A). ➢ Advise mother when to return immediately. ➢ Follow-up in 5 days if not improving.
and if diarrhoea 14 days or more	• Dehydration present.	***Pink :*** SEVERE PERSISTENT DIARRHOEA	➢ Treat dehydration before referral unless the child has another severe classification. ➢ Refer to hospital.
	• No Dehydration.	***Yellow :*** PERSISTENT DIARRHOEA	➢ Advise the mother on feeding a child who has PERSISTENT DIARRHOEA. ➢ Give multivitamins and minerals (including zinc) for 14 days. ➢ Follow-up in 5 days.
and if blood in stool	• Blood in the stool.	***Yellow :*** DYSENTERY	**➢ Give ciprofloxacin for 3 days.** ➢ Follow-up in 3 days.

DOES THE CHILD HAVE FEVER ?

(by history or feels hot or temperature 37.5°C* or above)

IF YES:

- Decide Malaria Risk : High or Low

THEN ASK:

- For how long ?
- If more than 7 days, has fever been present every day ?
- Has the child had measles within the last 3 months ?

LOOK AND FEEL :

- Look or feel for stiff neck.
- Look for runny nose.
- Look for any bacterial cause of fever**.
- Look for signs of MEASLES.
  - Generalized rash and
  - One of these : cough, runny nose, or red eyes.

Do a malaria test :***
If NO severe classification

- In all fever cases if High malaria risk.
- In Low malaria risk if no obvious cause of fever present.

Classify FEVER

High or Low Malaria Risk

Signs	Classify as	Treatment
• Any general danger sign or • Stiff neck.	***Pink :*** VERY SEVERE FEBRILE DISEASE	➢ **Give first dose of artesunate or quinine for severe malaria.** ➢ **Give first dose of an appropriate antibiotic.** ➢ **Treat the child to prevent low blood sugar.** ➢ **Give one dose of paracetamol in clinic for high fever (temp. 38.5°C or above).** ➢ **Refer URGENTLY to hospital.**
• Malaria test POSITIVE	***Yellow:*** MALARIA	➢ **Give recommended first line oral antimalarial.** ➢ **Give one dose of paracetamol in clinic for high fever (temp. 38.5°C or above).** ➢ Give appropriate antibiotic treatment for an identified bacterial cause of fever. ➢ Advise mother when to return immediately. ➢ Follow-up in 3 days if fever persists. ➢ If fever is present every day for more than 7 days, refer for assessment.
• Malaria test NEGATIVE • Other cause of fever PRESENT	***Green:*** FEVER NO MALARIA	➢ **Give one dose of paracetamol in clinic for high fever (temp. 38.5°C or above).** ➢ Give appropriate antibiotic treatment for an identified bacterial cause of fever. ➢ Advise mother when to return immediately. ➢ Follow-up in 3 days if fever persists. ➢ If fever is present every day for more than 7 days, refer for assessment.

No Malaria Risk and No Travel to Malaria Risk Area

Signs	Classify as	Treatment
• Any general danger sign or • Stiff neck.	***Pink:*** VERY SEVERE FEBRILE DISEASE	➢ **Give first dose of an appropriate antibiotic.** ➢ **Treat the child to prevent low blood sugar.** ➢ **Give one dose of paracetamol in clinic for high fever (temp. 38.5°C or above).** ➢ **Refer URGENTLY to hospital.**
• No general danger signs. • No stiff neck.	***Green:*** FEVER	➢ **Give one dose of paracetamol in clinic for high fever (temp. 38.5°C or above).** ➢ Give appropriate antibiotic treatment for any identified bacterial cause of fever. ➢ Advise mother when to return immediately. ➢ Follow-up in 2 days if fever persists. ➢ If fever is present every day for more than 7 days, refer for assessment.

If the child has measles now or within the last 3 months :

- Look for mouth ulcers. Are they deep and extensive ?
- Look for pus draining from the eye.
- Look for clouding of the cornea.

If MEASLES Now or within last 3 months, Classify

Signs	Classify as	Treatment
• Any general danger sign or • Clouding of cornea or • Deep or extensive mouth ulcers.	***Pink:*** SEVERE COMPLICATED MEASLES****	➢ **Give Vitamin A treatment.** ➢ **Give first dose of an appropriate antibiotic.** ➢ **If clouding of the cornea or pus draining from the eye, apply tetracycline eye ointment.** ➢ **Refer URGENTLY to hospital.**
• Pus draining from the eye or • Mouth ulcers.	***Yellow:*** MEASLES WITH EYE OR MOUTH COMPLI-CATIONS****	➢ **Give Vitamin A treatment.** ➢ **If pus draining from the eye, treat eye infection with tetracycline eye ointment.** ➢ If mouth ulcers, treat with gentian violet. ➢ Follow-up in 3 days.
• Measles now or within the last 3 months.	***Green:*** MEASLES	➢ **Give Vitamin A treatment.**

* These temperatures are based on axillary temperature. Rectal temperature readings are approximately 0.5°C higher.

** Look for local tenderness; oral sores; refusal to use a limb; hot tender swelling; red tender skin or boils; lower abdominal pain or pain on passing urine in older children.

*** If no malaria test available : High malaria risk - classify as MALARIA; Low malaria risk AND NO obvious cause of fever - classify as MALARIA.

**** Other important complications of measles - pneumonia, stridor, diarrhoea, ear infection, and acute malnutrition - are classified in other tables.

DOES THE CHILD HAVE AN EAR PROBLEM ?

IF YES, ASK :
- Is there ear pain ?
- Is there ear discharge ? If yes, for how long ?

LOOK AND FEEL :
- Look for pus draining from the ear.
- Feel for tender swelling behind the ear.

Classify EAR PROBLEM

Signs	Classify as	Treatment
• Tender swelling behind the ear.	***Pink :*** MASTOIDITIS	➢ **Give first dose of an appropriate antibiotic.** ➢ **Give first dose of paracetamol for pain relief.** ➢ **Refer URGENTLY to hospital.**
• Pus is seen draining from the ear and discharge is reported for less than 14 days, or • Ear pain.	***Yellow :*** ACUTE EAR INFECTION	➢ **Give an antibiotic for 5 days.** ➢ **Give paracetamol for pain relief.** ➢ Dry the ear by wicking. ➢ Follow-up in 5 days.
• Pus is seen draining from the ear and discharge is reported for 14 days or more.	***Yellow :*** CHRONIC EAR INFECTION	➢ Dry the ear by wicking. ➢ Treat with topical quinolone eardrops for 14 days. ➢ Follow-up in 5 days.
• No ear pain, and No pus seen draining from the ear.	***Green :*** NO EAR INFECTION	No treatment.

THEN CHECK FOR ACUTE MALNUTRITION

CHECK FOR ACUTE MALNUTRITION
LOOK AND FEEL :

Look for signs of acute malnutrition
- Look for oedema of both feet.
- Determine WFH/L* — z-score.
- Measure MUAC** — mm in a child 6 months or older.

If WFH/L less than –3 z-scores or MUAC less than 115 mm, then :

- Check for any medical complication present :
  - Any general danger signs
  - Any severe classification
  - Pneumonia with chest indrawing
- If no medical complications present :
  - Child is 6 months or older, offer RUTF*** to eat. Is the child :
    Not able to finish RUTF portion ?
    Able to finish RUTF portion ?
  - Child is less than 6 months, assess breastfeeding :
    Does the child have a breastfeeding problem ?

Classify NUTRITIONAL STATUS

Signs	Classify as	Treatment
• Oedema of both feet or • WFH/L less than –3 z-scores, or MUAC less than 115 mm AND any one of the following: – Medical compli-cation present, or – Not able to finish RUTF, or – Breast-feeding problem	***Pink :*** COMPLICATED SEVERE ACUTE MALNUTRITION	➢ **Give first dose appropriate antibiotic.** ➢ **Treat the child to prevent low blood sugar.** ➢ **Keep the child warm.** ➢ **Refer URGENTLY to hospital.**
• WFH/L less than –3 z-scores, or • MUAC less than 115 mm AND • Able to finish RUTF.	***Yellow :*** UNCOMPLI-CATED SEVERE ACUTE MALNUTRITION	➢ **Give oral antibiotics for 5 days.** ➢ Give ready-to-use therapeutic food for a child aged 6 months or more. ➢ Counsel the mother on how to feed the child. ➢ Assess for possible TB infection. ➢ Advise mother when to return immediately. ➢ Follow-up in 7 days.
• WFH/L between –3 and –2 z-scores or • MUAC 115 up to 125 mm.	***Yellow :*** MODERATE ACUTE MALNUTRITION	➢ Assess the child's feeding and counsel the mother on the feeding recommendations. ➢ If feeding problem, follow up in 7 days. ➢ Assess for possible TB infection ➢ Advise mother when to return immediately. ➢ Follow-up in 30 days.
• WFH/L-2 z-scores or more or • MUAC 125 mm or more.	***Green :*** NO ACUTE MALNUTRITION	➢ If child is less than 2 years old, assess the child's feeding and counsel the mother on feeding according to the feeding recommendations. ➢ If feeding problem, follow-up 7 days.

* WFH/L is Weight-for-Height or Weight-for-Length determined by using the WHO growth standards charts.
** MUAC is Mid-Upper Arm Circumference measured using MUAC tape in all children 6 months or older.
*** RUTF is Ready-to-Use Therapeutic Food for conducting the appetite test and feeding children with severe acute malnutrition.

THEN CHECK FOR ANAEMIA

Check for anaemia
- Look for palmar pallor. Is it :
  - Severe palmar pallor* ?
  - Some palmar pallor ?

Classify ANAEMIA

Signs	Classification	Treatment
• Severe palmar pallor	***Pink :*** SEVERE ANAEMIA	➢ **Refer URGENTLY to hospital.**
• Some palmar pallor	***Yellow :*** ANAEMIA	➢ **Give iron.**** ➢ Give mebendazole if child is 1 year or older and has not had a dose in the previous 6 months. ➢ Advise mother when to return immediately. ➢ Follow-up in 14 days.
• No palmar pallor	***Green :*** NO ANAEMIA	➢ – If child is less than 2 years old, assess the child's feeding and counsel the mother according to the feeding recommendations. – If feeding problem, follow-up in 5 days.

* Assess for sickle cell anaemia if common in your area.
** If child has severe acute malnutrition and is receiving RUTF. DO NOT give iron because there is already adequate amount of iron in RUTF.

THEN CHECK THE CHILD'S IMMUNIZATION*, PROPHYLACTIC VITAMIN A & IRON-FOLIC ACID SUPPLEMENTATION STATUS

IMMUNIZATION SCHEDULE :

Please refer to page 136 for national immunization schedule.

PROPHYLACTIC VITAMIN A

Give a single dose of vitamin A :

100,000 IU at 9 months with measles immunization.

200,000 IU at 16-18 months with DPT Booster.

200,000 IU at 24 months.

200,000 IU at 30 months.

200,000 IU at 36 months.

PROPHYLACTIC IFA

Give 20 mg elemental iron + 100 mcg folic acid (one tablet of Paediatric IFA or 5 ml of IFA syrup or 1 ml of IFA drops) for a total of 100 days in a year after the child has recovered from acute illness if :

➢ The child 6 months of age or older, and

➢ Has not received Paediatric IFA tablet syrup/drops for 100 days in last one year.

* A child who needs to be immunized should be advised to go for immunization the day vaccines are available at AW/SC/PHC.

ASSESS OTHER PROBLEMS

MAKE SURE CHILD WITH ANY GENERAL DANGER SIGN IS REFERRED after first dose of an appropriate antibiotic and other urgent treatments.

Exception : Rehydration of the child according to Plan C may resolve danger signs so that referral is no longer needed.

GIVE EXTRA FLUID FOR DIARRHOEA AND CONTINUE FEEDING

PLAN A: TREAT DIARRHOEA AT HOME

Counsel the mother on the 4 rules of home treatment:

1. Give extra fluid;
2. Give zinc supplements (age 2 months up to 5 years);
3. Continue feeding; and
4. When to return.

1. ***GIVE EXTRA FLUID* (as much as the child will take)**
   - **Tell the mother :**
     - Breastfeed frequently and for longer at each feed.
     - If the child is exclusively breastfed, give ORS or clean water in addition to breast milk.
     - If the child is not exclusively breastfed, give one or more of the following: ORS solution, food-based fluids (such as soup, rice water, and yoghurt drinks), or clean water.
   - **It is especially important to give ORS at home when :**
     - the child has been treated with Plan B or Plan C during this visit.
     - the child cannot return to a clinic if the diarrhoea gets worse.
   - **Teach the mother how to mix and give ORS. Give the mother 2 packets of ORS to use at home.**
   - **Show the mother how much fluid to give in addition to the usual fluid intake :**

Up to 2 years	50 to 100 ml after each loose stool
2 years or more	100 to 200 ml after each loose stool

   Tell the mother to:
   - Give frequent small sips from a cup.
   - If the child vomits, wait 10 minutes. Then continue, but more slowly.
   - Continue giving extra fluid until the diarrhoea stops.

2. ***GIVE ZINC* (age 2 months up to 5 years)**
   - **Tell the mother how much zinc to give (20 mg tab) :**

2 months up to 6 months	½ tablet daily for 14 days
6 months or more	1 tablet daily for 14 days

   - **Show the mother how to give zinc supplements :**
     - Infants - dissolve tablet in a small amount of expressed breast milk, ORS or clean water in a cup.
     - Older children - tablets can be chewed or dissolved in a small amount of water.

3. ***CONTINUE FEEDING*** (exclusive breastfeeding if age less than 6 months).
4. ***WHEN TO RETURN***

PLAN B: TREAT SOME DEHYDRATION WITH ORS

In the clinic, give recommended amount of ORS over 4-hours period

- **Determine amount of ORS to give during first 4 hours**

WEIGHT	<6 kg	6 -<10 kg	10-<12 kg	12-19 kg
AGE*	Up to 4 months	4 months up to 12 months	12 months up to 2 years	2 years up to 5 years
In ml	200–450	450–800	800–960	960–1600

* *Use the child's age only when you do not know the weight. The approximate amount of ORS required (in ml) can also be calculated by multiplying the child's weight (in kg) times 75.*
- If the child wants more ORS than shown, give more.
- For infants under 6 months who are not breastfed, also give 100-200 ml clean water during this period if you use standard ORS. This is not needed if you use new low osmolarity ORS.

- **Show the mother how to give ORS solution :**
  - Give frequent small sips from a cup.
  - If the child vomits, wait 10 minutes. Then continue, but more slowly.
  - Continue breastfeeding whenever the child wants.
- **After 4 hours :**
  - Reassess the child and classify the child for dehydration.
  - Select the appropriate plan to continue treatment.
  - Begin feeding the child in clinic.
- **If the mother must leave before completing treatment :**
  - Show her how to prepare ORS solution at home.
  - Show her how much ORS to give to finish 4-hours treatment at home.
  - Give her enough ORS packets to complete rehydration. Also give her 2 packets as recommended in **Plan A**.
  - Explain the 4 Rules of Home Treatment:
    1. GIVE EXTRA FLUID;
    2. GIVE ZINC (age 2 months up to 5 years);
    3. CONTINUE FEEDING (exclusive breastfeeding if age less than 6 months); and
    4. WHEN TO RETURN.

GIVE EXTRA FLUID FOR DIARRHOEA AND CONTINUE FEEDING

PLAN C: TREAT SEVERE DEHYDRATION QUICKLY

Follow the arrows. If answer is "YES", go across. If "NO", go down.

START HERE

Can you give intravenous (IV) fluid immediately? YES →

- **Start IV fluid immediately.** If the child can drink, give ORS by mouth while the drip is set up. Give 100 ml/kg Ringer's Lactate Solution (or, if not available, normal saline), divided as follows :

Age	First give 30 ml/kg in :	Then give 70 ml/kg in :
Infants (under 12 months)	1 hour *	5 hours
Children (12 months upto 5 years)	30 minutes *	2½ hours

** Repeat once if radial pulse is still very weak or not detectable.*

- Re-assess the child every 1–2 hours. If hydration status is not improving, give the IV drip more rapidly.
- Also give ORS (about 5 ml/kg/hour) as soon as the child can drink : usually after 3–4 hours (infants) or 1–2 hours (children).
- Re-assess an infant after 6 hours and a child after 3 hours. Classify dehydration. Then choose the appropriate plan (A, B or C) to continue treatment.

NO ↓

If IV treatment available nereby (within 30 minutes)? YES →

- Refer UNGENTLY to the hospital for IV treatment.
- If the child can drink, provide the mother with ORS solution and show her how to give frequent sips during the trip or give ORS by naso-gastric tube.

NO ↓

Are you trained to use a naso-gastric (NG) tube for rehydration? YES →

NO ↓

Can the child drink? YES →

- Start rehydration by tube (or mouth) with ORS solution : give 20 ml/kg/hour for 6 hours (total of 120 ml/kg)
- Re-assess the child every 1–2 hours while waiting for transfer :
  - If there is repeated vomiting or increasing abdominal distension, give the fluid more slowly.
  - If hydration status is not improving after 3 hours, send the child for IV therapy.
- After 6 hours, reassess the child. Classify dehydration. Then choose the appropriate plan (A, B or C) to continue treatment.

NO ↓

Refer URGENTLY to the hospital for IV or NG treatment

NOTE :

- If the child is not referred to hospital, observe the child at least 6 hours after rehydration to be sure the mother can maintain hydration giving the child ORS solution by mouth.

References

1. WHO (2019). *Trends in Maternal Mortality : 1990 to 2017,* Estimates by WHO etc.
2. Menon, M.K.K. (1975). *J.Obs & Gynae. of India,* XXXV, 113.
3. WHO (1969). *Report of Training Courses on Organization of MCH Field Practice Programmes in Medical Colleges,* SEA/MCH/56 Dec. 1969, New Delhi.
4. WHO (1976). *Techn. Rep. Ser.,* No. 600.
5. data.wordbank.org. (2022). *Birth rate of the countries.*
6. UNICEF (2021), *Level and Trends in Child Mortality,* Report 2021.
7. Govt. of India (2010). *Guidelines for Antenatal Care and Skilled Attendance at Birth by ANM/LHV/SNS,* Ministry of Health and Family Welfare, New Delhi.
8. WHO (2017), *WHO recommendations on antenatal care for a positive pregnancy experience.*
9. WHO (2012). Save the Children etc. *Born Too Soon, The Global Action Report on Preterm Birth, 2012.*
10. WHO (1978). *Risk Approach for MCH Care,* WHO Offset Publication No.39.
11. ICMR (1977). *ICMR Bulletin,* Dec. 1977.
12. Editorial (1973). *Brit.Med.J. 1,* 370.
13. Klina, J. et al (1980). *Lancet,* 2 : 176–180.
14. Davis, R.P. et al (1981). Pregnancy and alcohol, *Current Problems in Obst and Gynaecology 4 (6) 2–48,* Feb 1981.
15. Harlops, Shiono, PH (1980). *Lancet 2* : 173–6.
16. Carswell, F. et al (1970). *Lancet,* 1, 1241.
17. Noble, I.M. (1974). *The Practitioner,* 212, 657.
18. King, A and Nicol, C. (1969). *Venereal Diseases,* 2nd Ed., Bailliere Tindal and Cassel.
19. Jawetz, Melnik, and Adelberg's *Medical Microbiology (2019)*, 28th ed., A Lange Publication.
20. Paula A. Braveman and E. Tarimo, WHO (1994). *Screening in Primary Health Care,* Setting priorities with limited resources.
21. Rodrek, C.H. and Nicolaides, K.H. eds. (1984). *Prenatal Diagnosis,* Recordings of the 11th Study Group (RCOG).
22. Ferguson – Smith, M.A. ed. (1983). *Br. Med. Bull. Early prenatal diagnosis Vol.* 39 No.4.
23. WHO (1986). *Tech. Rept.* Sr.No.736.
24. WHO (1980). *Guide to the Care of the LBW Infants,* SEARO, Ref Publ. Sr.No. 10 New Delhi.
25. Mallinson, H. et al (1985). *Lancet 1* : 351.
26. Govt. of India (1994). CSSM review, *A newsletter on the Child Survival and Safe Motherhood Programme,* August 1994, No.20.

27. Christine HURAUX-RENDU (1991). *Children in the Tropics,* Early Detection of Transplacental Infections in Maternity Units, 1991 – No 190/191.
28. WHO (1993). *International Classification of Diseases, Tenth Revision,* Vol. 2.
29. WHO (2014). *Fact Sheet, Preterm birth,* No. 363, Nov. 2014.
30. WHO (1978). *WHO Chronicle,* 32 : 231.
31. WHO (2018), *Fact sheet, Preterm birth,* 19th Feb. 2018.
32. Harfouche, J.K. (1979). *Bull WHO,* 57 (3) 387–403.
33. WHO (1980). *Towards a better future* : MCH.
34. Boston Children Hospital, *Contact the Vision of Newborn Medicine, Prematurity - Symptoms and Causes.*
35. UNICEF (2009). *State of World's Children, 2009,* Maternal and Newborn Health.
36. Medical Annual. (1976). p. 130.
37. Govt. of India (2004). *National Guidelines on Infant and Young Child Feeding (2004),* Dept. of Women and Child Development, Govt. of India.
38. Helsing, E. and King F.S. (1984). *Breast feeding in Practice, Oxford University Press,* New Delhi.
39. Anne-Marie Masse-Raimbault, *Children in the Tropics (1992). Feeding Babies : From Breast Milk To The Family Dish,* No.202–203.
40. WHO (1995). Bridging the gaps, *The World Health Report 1995,* Report of the Director General .
41. Govt. of India (1993). *CSSM review,* A news letter on the Child Survival and Safe Motherhood Programme, July 1993, No.7.
42. WHO (2018). *Baby Friendly Hospital Initiative 2018,* Implementation, guidance to protect, promote and support breast-feeding in health facilities.
43. Brooks, G.D. (1982). *Growth Assessment in Childhood and Adolescence,* Oxford.
44. Tanner, J.M. (1978). In : *Textbook of Paediatrics, Forfav, J.O., Arneil G.C., eds,* 3rd Ed. Churchil Livingston.
45. Stuart, H.C. and Stevenson, S.S. (1959). In : *Nelson, W.E. ed "Textbook of Paediatrics" 7th Ed.,* Saunders.
46. WHO (1978). *A Growth Chart for International Use in MCH care.*
47. WHO (1983). *Measuring Changes in Nutritional Status.*
48. ICMR (1984). *Growth and Development of Indian Infants,* TRS No.18
49. ICMR (1976). *ICMR Bull* 6 (3) 1.
50. Gueri, M. et al (1980). *Bull WHO,* 58 (5) 773–777.
51. Govt. of India (1995). *CSSM review,* A newsletter on Child Survival and Safe Motherhood Programme Jan.1995, No.25.
52. ICMR (1983). *ICMR Bull., Oct,* Vol 13, No 10.
53. WHO (2006). *WHO Child Growth Standards,* Length/height–for–age, weight–for–age, weight–for–length, weight–for height and body mass index–for age, Methods and development.
54. Nutrition News (1979). *Nutrition,* April 1979 P–2–10.
55. WHO (1985). *Tech.Rep.Sr.,* 724, P–142.
56. Morley, David (1973). *Paediatric Priorities in the Developing World,* Butterworths.
57. Govt. of India (2017), *National Family Health Survey-4, 2015–2016,* Ministry of Health and Family Welfare, New Delhi.
58. Govt. of India (2022), *National Family Health Survey-5, 2019–2021,* Ministry of Health and Family Welfare, New Delhi.
59. WHO (2022), *World Health Statistics, 2022.*
60. Govt. of India (2021). *National Health Profile 2021,* Central Bureau of Health Intelligence, Ministry of Health & Family Welfare, New Delhi.
61. *International Business times, 4th June 2013.*
62. WHO (2005). *World Health Report 2005,* Make every mother and child count, Report of the Director General WHO.
63. UNICEF (1995). *The State of the World's Children* 1995.
64. WHO (2005). *Improving Maternal, Newborn and Child Health in the South-East Asia Region,* New Delhi.
65. Govt. of India (1982). *Swasth Hind, 22:297,* Central Health Education Bureau.
66. Govt. of India (2012). *Working Group on Development of Children for the Eleventh Five Year Plan (2007-2012),* A Report, Ministry of Women and Child Development, New Delhi.
67. Govt. of India (2010). *Annual Report 2009-10,* Ministry of Women and Child Development, New Delhi.
68. Govt. of India (2010). *The Integrated Child Protection Scheme;* Ministry of Women and Child Development, New Delhi.
69. Govt. of India (2015). *Manual in Health Statistics in India,* Central Statistics Office, Ministry of Statistics and Programme Implementation, New Delhi.
70. Govt. of India (2017), *National Commission for Protection of Child Rights, Protection of Children from Sexual Offence Act (POCSO) 2012.*
71. Govt. of India (2019), *The Gazette of India,* Ministry of Law and Justice, No. 25 of 2019, 5th Aug. 2019.
72. *Bill No. IV of 2020, as introduced in Rajya Sabha,* 7th Feb. 2020.
73. Govt. of India (2022). *Sample Registration System Statistical Report 2022,* Office of Registrar, General of India.
74. UNICEF (2021), *State of World's Children, 2021.*
75. WHO, UNICEF, World Bank (2012). *Trends in Maternal Mortality : 1990–2010.*
76. WHO, UNICEF, World Bank (2010). *Trends in Maternal Mortality; 1990-2008,* Estimates Developed by WHO, UNICEF, UNFPA and The World Bank.
77. WHO (1998). *World Health Report 1998,* Life in the 21st century, A vision for all, Report of the Director General, WHO.
78. WHO (2005). *Regional Health Forum,* Vol. 9, No. 1, 2005.
79. Every Women Every Child (2016), *Operational Framework for the Global Strategy for Women's, Children's and Adolescent's Health,* 2016–2030.
80. Govt. of India (2022). *Special Bulletin on Maternal Mortality in India 2018–2020,* SRS, Nov. 2022, Office of Registrar General of India.
81. Govt. of India (2013). *Annual Report 2012–13,* Ministry of Health and Family Welfare, New Delhi.
82. WHO (1975). *International Classification of Diseases,* 9th Revision.
83. Govt. of India (2014). *INAP-India Newborn Action Plan,* Sept. 2014, Ministry of Health and Family Welfare, New Delhi.
84. John M. Last (2001). *A Dictionary of Epidemiology,* Fourth Ed., Oxford University Press.
85. Meredith Davis, J.B. (1983). *Community Health, Preventive Medicine and Social Services,* 5th ed., Bailliere Tindall.
86. UNICEF, WHO (2019), *Levels and trends of child mortality,* 2019 Report.
87. Govt. of India (2020), *Annual Report 2019–2020,* Ministry of Health and Family Welfare, New Delhi.
88. Hogarh, J. (1978). *Glossary of Health Care Terminology,* WHO, Copenhagen.
89. WHO (2004). *Strategic Directions to Improve Newborn Health in the South-East Asia Region,* New Delhi.
90. Govt. of India (2008). *Sample Registration System. Statistical Report 2007,* Report No. 2 of 2008, Ministry of Home Affairs, New Delhi.
91. Govt. of India (2022). *Sample Registration System. Statistical Report 2020,* Ministry of Home Affairs, New Delhi.
92. Govt. of India (2011). *Census 2011,* Office of the Registrar General and Census Commissioner India, Ministry of Home Affairs, New Delhi.
93. WHO (1993). *Implementation of the Global Strategy for Health for All by the year 2000,* Second evaluation, Eighth report on the World Health Situation, Vol.4, South-East Asia Region.
94. WHO (1986). *Tech. Rept. Sr.,*731.
95. Wyon, J.B. and Gordan, J.E. (1962). *Research in Family Planning.*
96. Omran, A.R., and Stanley, C.C. et al (1976). *Family Function Pattern and Health,* Geneva.
97. Govt of India (1984). *Swasth Hind* March – April.
98. Iyangar, L. (1972). *In Proceedings of the 9th International Congress of Nutrition,* Mexico, Karger, Basal P 48–53.
99. Mora, J.O., et al (1979). *Am.J.Cli Nutrition* 32 : 455–462.
100. WHO (1992). *Global Health Situations and Projections, Estimates,* Division of Epidemiological Surveillance and Health Situation and Trend Assessment.
101. UNICEF (2018), *Levels and trends in child mortality,* Report 2018.
102. UNICEF (2018), *Child mortality estimates, country, global and regional specific estimates,* 18th sept. 2018.
103. UNICEF (2014). *Committing to Child Survival, A Promise Renewed Progress Report, 2014.*
104. Govt. of India (2013). *A Strategic Approach to Reproductive, Maternal, Newborn, Child and Adolescent Health (RMNCH+A) in India for Healthy Mother and Child,* January 2013, Ministry of Health and Family Welfare, New Delhi.
105. WHO (2015). *From MDGs - Millennium Development Goals to SDGs- Sustainable Development Goals.*

106. UNICEF (1987). *The State of the World's Children 1987.*
107. WHO, UNICEF (2005). *Handbook IMCI, Integrated Management of Childhood Illness,* 2005.
108. WHO (1968). *Techn. Rep. Ser.,* No.400.
109. WHO (2012), *Congenital Anomalies,* Fact Sheet No. 370, Oct. 2012.
110. Bhende, Asha A. and Tara Kanitkar (1985). *Principles of Population Studies,* 3rd ed., Himalaya Publishing House, Mumbai.
111. Editorial (1976). *Brit. Med. Bull,* 32,1.
112. Editorial (1976). *Brit. Med. J.,* 1, 676.
113. Nelson, W.E. (1964). *Textbook of Paediatrics,* Saunders.
114. Penrose, L.S. (1961). *Recent Advances in Human Genetics,* Churchill, London.
115. Govt. of India (1946). *Report of the Health Survey and Development Committee,* Govt. of India Press, Shimla.
116. Govt. of India (1961). *Report of the School Health Committee, part I,* Central Health Education Bureau, New Delhi.
117. Central Health Education Bureau (1965). *Report of Seminar on School Health Services,* New Delhi.
118. Idem (1965). *Report of Workshop for the Development of Criteria for Health Aspects of a School Programme,* New Delhi.
119. Turner, C.E. et al (1957). *School Health and Health Education,* C.V. Mosby.
120. Govt. of India (1955). *Model Public Health Act,* Ministry of Health, New Delhi.
121. UNICEF (1984). *Nanoy S. Sadka,* ICDS Integrated Programme in India.
122. Govt. of India (2018), *Operational Guidelines on school Health Programme under Ayushman Bharat,* April 2018, Ministry of Health and Family Welfare, and Ministry of Human Resource & Development, New Delhi.
123. John M. Last (1995). *A Dictionary of Epidemiology,* Oxford University Press.
124. *Times of India,* Dated 4th Dec. 1995.
125. *Social Welfare,* Oct 1985, PÄ28.
126. WHO *Tech. Rept. Sr.,* Mentally Handicapped.
127. WHO (1985). *SEARO* MCH Paper No.5 New Delhi.
128. Indian Express.com.
129. Koller, P.C. (1968). *Chromosomes and Genes,* Oilver & Boyd.
130. WHO (2017), *World Report on Violence and Health,* Child abuse and neglect by parents and other care givers, 2017.
131. CDC (2017), *Fact sheet, Preventing child abuse and neglect,* 2017.
132. UNICEF (2006). *State of World's Children,* 2006.
133. WHO (1981). *World Health,* Nov 1981, P–19.
134. ILO (2017), *Global estimates of child labour, results and trends,* 2012–2016, Geneva 2017.
135. ILO (2010), *Child Trafficking Essentials,* ILO International Programme on the Elimination of Child Labour.
136. UNICEF, WHO (2020), *Global Status Report on Preventing Violence against Children,* 2020.
137. Chanda, A. (1970). *Illustrated Weekly of India,* March 1, 1970.
138. *Social Welfare* (1983). May/June Vol XI No.2–3.
139. Govt. of India (1978). *National Plan of Action for International Year for the Children 1979,* Ministry of Education and Social Welfare, New Delhi.
140. Govt. of India (2020), *Annual Report 2019–20,* Ministry of Women and Child Development, New Delhi.
141. Govt. of India (2015). *Annual Report 2014–2015,* Ministry of Women and Child Development, New Delhi.
142. Weir, J.H. (1967). *Roy.Soc.Hlth.Jr.,* 87, 144.
143. Population Reference Bureau USA, (2012).
144. Health Action (2004). *Eldercare,* Feb. 2004, Vol. 17, No. 2.
145. German, P.S., Fried, L.P. (1989). *Annual Review of Public Health,* Vol.10, 1989, P. 325.
146. WHO (2014). *Integrated Management of Childhood Illness – CHART BOOKLET.*

10 Health Care of the Community

"The needs of the many must prevail over those of the few"

Health has been declared a fundamental human right. This implies that the State has a responsibility for the health of its people. National governments all over the world are striving to expand and improve their health care services. The current criticism against health care services is that they are (a) predominantly urban-oriented (b) mostly curative in nature, and (c) accessible mainly to a small part of the population. The present concern in both developed and developing countries is not only to reach the whole population with adequate health care services, but also to secure an acceptable level of Health for All, through the application of primary health care programmes.

Concept of health care

Since health is influenced by a number of factors such as adequate food, housing, basic sanitation, healthy lifestyles, protection against environmental hazards and communicable diseases, the frontiers of health extend beyond the narrow limits of medical care. It is thus clear that "health care" implies more than "medical care". It embraces a multitude of "services provided to individuals or communities by agents of the health services or professions, for the purpose of promoting, maintaining, monitoring, or restoring health"*(1)*.

The term "medical care" is not synonymous with "health care". It refers chiefly to those personal services that are provided directly by physicians or rendered as the result of physicians's instructions. It ranges from domiciliary care to resident hospital care. Medical care is a subset of health care system.

Health care is a public right, and it is the responsibility of governments to provide this care to all people in equal measure. These principles have been recognized by nearly all governments of the world and enshrined in their respective constitutions. In India, health care is completely or largely a governmental function.

Health system

Health services are designed to meet the health needs of the community through the use of available knowledge and resources. It is not possible to define a fixed role for health services when the socio-economic pattern of one country differs so much from another. The health services are delivered by the "health system", which constitutes the management sector and involves organisational matters.

Two major themes have emerged in recent years in the delivery of health services : (a) First, that health services should be organised to meet the needs of entire populations and not merely selected groups. Health services should cover the full range of preventive, curative and rehabilitation services. Health services are now seen as part of the basic social services of a country *(2)*; (b) Secondly, it is now fully realised that the best way to provide health care to the vast majority of underserved rural people and urban poor is to develop effective "primary health care" services supported by an appropriate referral system. The social policy throughout the world was to build up health systems based on primary health care, towards the policy objective of Health for All by 2000 A.D.

Community participation is now recognized as a major component in the approach to the whole system of health care – treatment, promotion and prevention. The stress is on the provision of these services to the people – representing a shift from medical care to health care and from urban population to rural population.

Levels of health care

It is customary to describe health care service at 3 levels, viz. primary, secondary and tertiary care levels. These levels represent different types of care involving varying degrees of complexity.

1. Primary care level

It is the first level of contact of individuals, the family and community with the national health system, where "primary health care".("essential" health care) is provided. As a level of care, it is close to the people, where most of their health problems can be dealt with and resolved. It is at this level that health care will be most effective within the context of the area's needs and limitations *(3)*.

In the Indian context, primary health care is provided by the complex of primary health centres and their subcentres through the agency of multipurpose health workers, ANM, ASHA, Anganwadi worker, village health guides and trained dais. Besides providing primary health care, the village "health teams" bridge the cultural and communication gap between the rural people and organised health sector. Since India opted for "Health for All" by 2000 AD, the primary health care system has been reorganized and strengthened to make the primary health care delivery system more effective.

2. Secondary care level

The next higher level of care is the secondary (intermediate) health care level. At this level more complex problems are dealt with. In India, this kind of care is generally provided in district hospitals and community health centres which also serve as the first referral level *(4)*.

3. Tertiary care level

The tertiary level is a more specialized level than secondary care level and requires specific facilities and attention of highly specialized health workers *(5)*. This care is provided by the regional or central level institutions, e.g., Medical College Hospitals, All India Institutes, Regional Hospitals, Specialized Hospitals and other Apex Institutions.

A fundamental and necessary function of health care system is to provide a sound **referral system**. It must be a two-way exchange of information and returning patients to those who referred them for follow-up care *(6)*. It will ensure continuity of care and inspire confidence of the consumer in the system. For a large majority of developing countries (including India) this aspect of the health system remains very weak.

Changing concepts

With political independence, there was a national commitment to improve health in developing countries. Against this background different approaches to providing health care came into existence. These are :

1. Comprehensive health care

The term "comprehensive health care" was first used by the Bhore Committee in 1946. By comprehensive services, the Bhore committee meant provision of integrated preventive, curative and promotional health services from "womb to tomb" to every individual residing in a defined geographic area. The Bhore Committee defined comprehensive health care as having the following criteria :

(a) provide adequate preventive, curative and promotive health services;
(b) be as close to the beneficiaries as possible;
(c) has the widest cooperation between the people, the service and the profession;
(d) is available to all irrespective of their ability to pay;
(e) look after specifically the vulnerable and weaker sections of the community; and
(f) create and maintain a healthy environment both in homes as well as working places.

The Bhore Committee suggested that comprehensive health care should replace the policy of providing more medical care. This concept formed the basis of national health planning in India and led to the establishment of a network of primary health centres and subcentres.

The Government of India, during the successive 5 year plans has built up a vast infrastructure of rural health services based on primary health centres and subcentres. However, experience during the past 60 years has indicated that the primary health centres were not able to effectively cover the whole population under their jurisdiction, and their sphere of service did not extend beyond a 2–5 km radius. These facilities often did not enjoy the confidence of the people because they were understaffed and poorly supplied with medicines and equipment; as a result, there was growing dissatisfaction with the delivery of health services.

2. Basic health services

In 1965, the term "basic health services" was used by UNICEF/WHO in their joint health policy *(7)*. They defined the term as follows "A basic health service is understood to be a network of coordinated, peripheral and intermediate health units capable of performing effectively a selected group of functions essential to the health of an area and assuring the availability of competent professional and auxiliary personnel to perform these functions."

The change in terminology from comprehensive to basic health services did not affect materially the quality or content of health services. The handicaps or drawbacks of the basic health services are those shared by the comprehensive health care services, viz., lack of community participation, lack of intersectoral coordination and dissociation from the socio-economic aspects of health.

3. Primary health care

A new approach to health care came into existence in 1978, following an international conference at Alma-Ata (USSR). This is known as "primary health care". It has all the hallmarks of a primary health care delivery, first proposed by the Bhore Committee in 1946 and now espoused worldwide by international agencies and national governments *(8)*.

Before Alma-Ata, primary health care was regarded as synonymous with "basic health services", "first contact care", "easily accessible care", "services provided by generalists", etc. The Alma-Ata international conference gave primary health care a wider meaning. The Alma-Ata Conference defined primary health care as follows *(9)* :–

> *"Primary health care is essential health care made universally accessible to individuals and acceptable to them, through their full participation and at a cost the community and country can afford".*

The primary health care is equally valid for all countries from the most to the least developed, although it takes varying forms in each of them. The concept of primary health care has been accepted by all countries as the key to the attainment of Health for All by 2000 AD. It has also been accepted as an integral part of the country's health system.

Elements of primary health care

Although specific services provided will vary in different countries and communities, the Alma-Ata Declaration has outlined 8 essential components of primary health care *(9)*.

1. education concerning prevailing health problems and the methods of preventing and controlling them;
2. promotion of food supply and proper nutrition;
3. an adequate supply of safe water and basic sanitation;
4. maternal and child health care, including family planning;
5. immunization against major infectious diseases;
6. prevention and control of locally endemic diseases;
7. appropriate treatment of common diseases and injuries; and
8. provision of essential drugs.

Principles of primary health care

1. Equitable distribution

The first key principle in the primary health care strategy is equity or equitable distribution of health services, i.e., health services must be shared equally by all people irrespective of their ability to pay, and all (rich or poor, urban or rural) must have access to health services. At present, health services are mainly concentrated in the major towns and cities resulting in inequality of care to the people in rural areas. The worst hit are the needy and vulnerable groups of the population in rural areas and urban slums. This has been termed as social injustice. The failure to reach the majority of the people is usually due to inaccessibility. Primary health care aims to redress this imbalance by shifting the centre of gravity of the health care system from cities (where three-quarters of the health budget is spent) to the rural areas (where three-quarters of the people live), and bring these services as near people's homes as possible.

2. Community participation

Notwithstanding the overall responsibility of the Central and State Governments, the involvement of individuals, families, and communities in promotion of their own health and welfare, is an essential ingredient of primary health care. Countries are now conscious of the fact that universal coverage by primary health care cannot be achieved without the involvement of the local community. There must be a continuing effort to secure meaningful involvement of the community in the planning, implementation and maintenance of health services, besides maximum reliance on local resources such as manpower, money and materials. In short, primary health care must be built on the principle of community participation (or involvement).

One approach that has been tried successfully in India is the use of village health guides and trained dais. They are selected by the local community and trained locally in the delivery of primary health care to the community they belong, free of charge. By overcoming cultural and communication barriers, they provide primary health care in ways that are acceptable to the community. It is now considered that ASHA and Anganwadi workers are an essential feature of primary health care in India. These concepts are revolutionary. They have been greatly influenced by experience in China where community participation in the form of **bare-foot doctors** took place on an unprecedented scale.

3. Intersectoral coordination

There is an increasing realization of the fact that the components of primary health care cannot be provided by the health sector alone. The Declaration of Alma-Ata states that "primary health care involves in addition to the health sector, all related sectors and aspects of national and community development, in particular agriculture, animal husbandry, food, industry, education, housing, public works, communication and others sectors" *(9)*. To achieve such cooperation, countries may have to review their administrative system, reallocate their resources and introduce suitable legislation to ensure that coordination can take place. This requires strong political will to translate values into action. An important element of intersectoral approach is planning – planning with other sectors to avoid unnecessary duplication of activities.

4. Appropriate technology

Appropriate technology has been defined as "technology that is scientifically sound, adaptable to local needs, and acceptable to those who apply it and those for whom it is used, and that can be maintained by the people themselves in keeping with the principle of self reliance with the resources the community and country can afford" *(10)*. The term "appropriate" is emphasized because in some countries, large, luxurious hospitals that are totally inappropriate to the local needs, are built, which absorb a major part of the national health budget, effectively blocking any improvement in general health services. This also applies to using costly equipment, procedures and techniques when cheaper, scientifically valid and acceptable ones are available, viz, oral rehydration fluid, standpipes which are socially acceptable, and financially more feasible than house-to-house connections, etc.

It will be seen from the above discussion that primary care is qualitatively a different approach to deal with the health problems of a community. Unlike the previous approaches (e.g, basic health services, integrated health care, vertical health services) which depended upon taking health services to the doors of the people, primary health care approach starts with the people themselves. This approach signifies a new dynamism in health care and has been described as Health by the people, placing people's health in people's hands *(11)*. The ends of the primary health care approach are the same as those of earlier approaches (i.e., attainment of an acceptable level of health by every individual), but the means adopted are different *(12)*, that is, more equitable distribution and nation-wide coverage, more intersectoral coordination and more community involvement in health related matters. In short, primary health care goes beyond the conventional health services. It forms part of the larger concept of Human Resources and Development.

HEALTH FOR ALL

In 1977, it was decided in the World Health Assembly to launch a movement known as "Health for All by the year 2000". The fundamental principle of HFA strategy is equity, that is, an equal health status for people and countries, ensured by an equitable distribution of health resources. The Member countries of WHO at the 30th World Health Assembly defined Health for All as :

> *"attainment of a level of health that will enable every individual to lead a socially and economically productive life."*

In 1978, the Alma-Ata International conference on Primary Health Care reaffirmed Health for All as the major social goal of governments, and stated that the best approach to achieve the goal of HFA is by providing primary health care, especially to the vast majority of underserved rural people and urban poor. It was envisaged that by the year 2000, at least essential health care should be accessible to all individuals and families in an acceptable and affordable way, with their full participation.

The Alma-Ata Conference called on all governments to formulate national policies, strategies and plans of action to launch and sustain primary health care as part of a national health system. It is left to each country to develop its norms and indicators for providing primary health care according to its own circumstances.

In 1981, a global strategy for HFA was evolved by WHO *(13)*. The global strategy provides a global framework that is broad enough to apply to all Member States and flexible enough to be adapted to national and regional variations of conditions and requirements. This was followed by individual countries developing their own strategies for achieving HFA, and synthesis of national strategies for developing regional strategies.

The WHO has established 12 global indicators *(13)* as the

basic point of reference for assessing the progress towards HFA, as for example, a minimum life expectancy of 60 years and maximum IMR of 50 per 1000 live births.

National strategy for HFA/2000

As a signatory to the Alma-Ata Declaration in 1978, the Government of India was committed to taking steps to provide HFA to its citizens by 2000 AD. In pursuance of this objective various attempts were made to evolve suitable strategies and approaches. In this connection two important reports appeared : (i) Report of the Study Group on "Health for All – an alternative strategy", sponsored by ICSSR and ICMR, and (ii) Report of the Working Group on "Health for All by 2000 AD" sponsored by the Ministry of Health and Family Welfare, Government of India *(14, 15)*. Both the groups considered in great detail the various issues involved in providing primary health care in the Indian context. These reports formed the basis of the National Health Policy formulated by the Ministry of Health and Family Welfare, Government of India in 1983 *(16)* which committed the Government and people of India to the achievement of HFA.

The National Health Policy echoes the WHO call for HFA and the Alma-Ata Declaration. It had laid down specific goals in respect of the various health indicators by different dates such as 1990 and 2000 AD. Foremost among the goals to be achieved by 2000 AD were :

(1) Reduction of infant mortality from the level of 125 (1978) to below 60.
(2) To raise the expectation of life at birth from the level of 52 years to 64.
(3) To reduce the crude death rate from the level of 14 per 1000 population to 9 per 1000.
(4) To reduce the crude birth rate from the level of 33 per 1000 population to 21.
(5) To achieve a net reproduction rate of one.
(6) To provide potable water to the entire rural population.

THE MILLENNIUM DEVELOPMENT GOALS

During September 2000, representatives from 189 countries met at the Millennium Summit in New York, to adopt the United Nations Millennium Declaration. The goals in the area of development and poverty eradication are now widely referred to as **"Millennium Development Goals"** (MDGs). The MDGs placed health at the heart of development and represent commitments by governments throughout the world to do more to reduce poverty and hunger and to tackle ill-health; gender inequality; lack of education; access to clean water; and environmental degradation. They were an integral part of the road map towards the implementation of the UN Millennium Declaration. Three of the 8 goals, 8 of the 18 targets required to achieve them, and 18 of the 48 indicators of progress, were health related. They assist in the development of national policies focussing on poor, and help track the performance of health programmes and systems. Although, the MDGs do not cover the whole range of public health domains, a broad interpretation of the goals provides an opportunity to tackle important cross cutting issues and key constraints to health and development. Governments had set a date of 2015 by which they would meet the MDGs, i.e. eradicate extreme poverty and hunger; achieve universal primary education; promote gender equality; improve maternal health; combat HIV/AIDS, malaria and other communicable diseases; ensure environmental sustainability; and develop a global partnership for development *(17,18,19)*. For details, please refer to chapter 2.

THE SUSTAINABLE DEVELOPMENT GOALS

On 25th September 2015, the UN General Assembly adopted a new development agenda "Transforming our world : the 2030 agenda for sustainable development". The 17 goals of the new development agenda integrates all three dimentions of sustainable development (economic, social and environmental) around the theme of people, planet, prosperity, peace and partnership. The SDGs aim to be universal, integrated and interrelated in nature. For details, please refer to chapter 14.

HEALTH CARE DELIVERY

The challenge that exists today in many countries is to reach the whole population with adequate health care services and to ensure their utilization. The "large hospital" which was chosen hitherto for the delivery of health services has failed in the sense that it serves only a small part of the population, that too, living within a small radius of the building and the services rendered are mostly curative in nature. Therefore, it has been aptly said that these large hospitals are more ivory towers of diseases than centres for the delivery of comprehensive health care services. Rising costs in the maintenance of these large hospitals and their failure to meet the total health needs of the community have led many countries to seek 'alternative' models of health care delivery with a view to provide health care services that are reasonably inexpensive, and have the basic essentials required by rural population.

THE MODEL

A number of models have been developed for the delivery of health care services *(20)*. One of the simplest models is shown in Fig. 1.

In actual practice the model is more detailed and complex. The INPUTS are the health status or health problems of the community; they represent the health needs and health demands of the community. Since resources are always limited to meet the many health needs, priorities have to be set. This envisages proper planning so that resources are not wasted. An account of the health planning has already been given in the preceding chapter. The HEALTH CARE SERVICES are designed to meet the health needs of the community through the use of available knowledge and resources. The services provided should be comprehensive and community-based. The resources must be distributed according to the needs of the community. The HEALTH CARE SYSTEM is intended to deliver the health care services; in other words, it constitutes the management sector, and involves organisational matters. The final outcome or the OUTPUT is the changed health status or improved health status of the community which is expressed in terms of lives saved, deaths averted, diseases prevented, cases treated, expectation of life prolonged, etc. Models such as these are being employed for improving health care services. A discussion of the application of the model (Fig. 1) in the Indian context is given in the following pages.

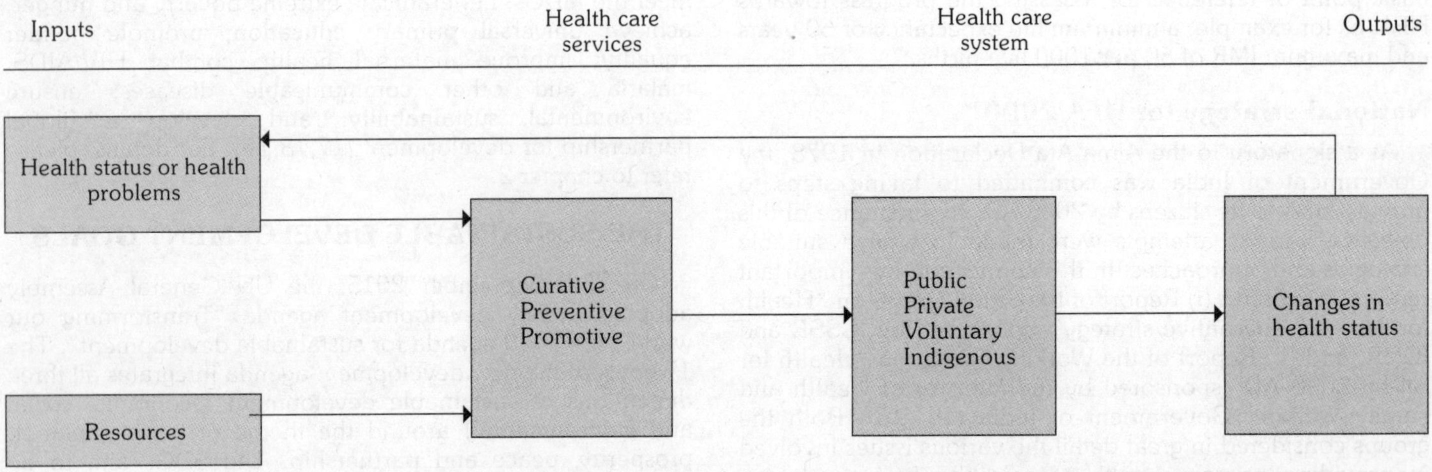

FIG. 1
Model of health care system

HEALTH STATUS AND HEALTH PROBLEMS

An assesment of the health status and health problems is the first requisite for any planned effort to develop health care services. This is also known as Community Diagnosis. The data required for analyzing the health situation and for defining the health problems comprise the following :

1. Morbidity and mortality statistics.
2. Demographic conditions of the population.
3. Environmental conditions which have a bearing on health.
4. Socio-economic factors which have a direct effect on health.
5. Cultural background, attitudes, beliefs, and practices which affect health.
6. Medical and health services available.
7. Other services available.

An analysis of the health situation in the light of the above data will bring out the health problems and health needs of the community. These problems are then ranked according to priority or urgency for allocation of resources. A brief description of current demographic and mortality profile and the health problems of India is given in the following pages.

1. Demographic profile

A major concern today is population explosion. The demographic profile is characterised by:

a. large population base;
b. high fertility both in terms of birth rate and family size;
c. low or declining mortality;
d. "young" population (about 26.2 per cent of the population) is below the age of 15 years;
e. the proportion of illiterate population is close to 34.62 per cent: this explains why the decline in birth rate has been so slow; and
f. dependency ratio of 48.73 per cent for the year 2020; that is, every economically productive member has to support almost one dependant.

Table 1 summarizes the most recent demographic information available.

TABLE 1
India: Demographic profile

Total population (2022)	1,412 million
Crude birth rate (2022)	18.7
Crude death rate (2022)	7.2
Annual growth rate % (2022)	1.3
Population doubling time (at current growth rate)	30 years
Population rural % (2020)	65.0
Adult literacy rate % (2011)	74.04
Density of population per sq.km (2020)	464
Sex ratio female per 1000 male (2018–20)	907
Population below 15 years % (2020)	26.2
Population above 65 years % (2020)	6.6
Average family size (2020)	1.8
Age at marriage, female (2020)	22.7 years
Annual per capita GNP (at current prices 2018–19)	Rs. 126,521

Source : *(21, 22, 23)*

2. Mortality profile

During the last few decades, there has been a notable improvement in the health status of the population. The death rate has steadily declined from 21 (1965) to 7.2 (2022). The life expectancy at birth has gone up considerably since 1951, recording an estimated 67 years for males and 70 years for females during 2020. The mortality rates for a number of infectious and communicable diseases have also registered a decline (e.g., cholera, tuberculosis, malaria).

However, a deeper study reveals distressing situation. India's health standards are still low compared to those in developed countries. While in the world as a whole, the IMR for the year 2019 is about 28 per 1000 live births, and in the developed countries as low as 5, in India it is as high as 28. Our life expectancy of about 67 years lags behind by almost 12–15 years compared to that in developed countries where it is currently between 71 and 80 years.

The current urban death rate (during 2022) was 5.1 and the rural death rate 6.4 per 1000 of population. There were also considerable interstate variations in death rate, as for example, during 2020 the death rate in Chhattisgarh was highest, about 7.9 as compared to the national average of 7.3, and 3.6 in Delhi. Among the states, Kerala had the lowest IMR of 6 per 1000 live births and Madhya Pradesh had the highest IMR of 43 per 1000 live births *(24)*.

Table 2 shows that the death rate is the highest in the age group 0–4 years. This is as a result of malnutrition and infection. 15 to 25 per cent of total deaths are attributed to infectious and parasitic diseases.

TABLE 2
Child (Under 5 years) and infant mortality indicators, India 2020

Indicators	Total	Rural	Urban
Child mortality rate	3.2	36	21
Infant mortality rate	28	31	19
Neo-natal mortality rate	20	23	12
Early neo-natal mortality rate	15	17	9
Late neo-natal mortality rate	5	6	3
Post neo-natal mortality rate	8	8	7
Peri-natal mortality rate	18	21	12
Still birth rate	3	1	3

Source : *(22)*

Health problems

The HEALTH PROBLEMS of India may be conveniently grouped under the following heads:

1. Communicable disease problems;
2. Non-communicable disease problems;
3. Nutritional problems;
4. Environmental sanitation problems;
5. Medical care problems; and
6. Population problems.

1. Communicable disease problems

Communicable diseases continue to be a major problem in India. Diseases considered to be of great importance today are : (a) **Malaria :** Malaria continues to be a major health problem in India. Although total malaria cases has declined compared to previous years, the proportion of *P. falciparum* has increased. Malaria cases have increased in North-East states, Madhya Pradesh, Chhattisgarh, Jharkhand, Orissa, Andhra Pradesh, Maharashtra etc. During 2021 there were 0.16 million cases of malaria (which included 63.1% cases of *Pf* malaria) and 73 deaths. (b) **Tuberculosis :** Tuberculosis remains a public health problem, with India accounting for one-fifth of the world incidence. Every year about 2.2 million persons develop tuberculosis, of which about 0.62 million are new smear positive highly infectious cases and about 0.24 million people die of TB every year. The emergence of HIV-TB co-infection and multidrug resistant TB has increased the severity and magnitude of the disease. In March 2006 RNTCP has achieved nation-wide coverage. (c) **Diarrhoeal diseases :** Diarrhoeal diseases constitute one of the major causes of morbidity and mortality, specially in children below 5 years of age. They are responsible for about 7.2 million cases of diarrhoea each year. Outbreaks of diarrhoeal diseases (including cholera) continue to occur in India due to poor environmental conditions. (d) **ARI :** Acute repiratory diseases are one of the major causes of mortality and morbidity in children below 5 years of age. During 2020, 23.67 million episodes of ARI were reported with 5,160 deaths. (e) **COVID-19 :** India had its share of COVID-19 cases during the pandemic, as of 20th Sept. 2022, India reported 44.52 million cases with 528 million deaths due to COVID-19. Large scale vaccination drive is going on in the country. (f) **Leprosy :** Leprosy is another important public health problem in India. During the year 2020–2021, total of 65,147 new cases were detected, out of which child cases were 9.49% and deformity grade II and above was 4.14%. 51.48 per cent of these cases are estimated to be multibacillary. All the States and Union Territories report cases of leprosy. However, there are considerable variations not only between one State and another, but also between one district and another. With the prevalence rate of about 0.68 per 10,000 population, India has achieved the goal of leprosy elimination at national level. (g) **Filaria :** The problem of filaria remains endemic in about 272 districts in 16 States and 4 UTs. The population at risk is over 670 million. To achieve elimination of LF, the Govt. of India has launched nationwide Annual Mass Drug Administration (MDA) with annual single recommended dose of diethylcarbamazine citrate tablets in addition to scaling up home based foot care and hydrocele operations. In 2014, 250 endemic districts implemented MDA targeting a population of about 554 million. (h) **AIDS :** The problem of AIDS is stable. It is estimated that by the end of year 2021 there were about 2.4 million HIV positive cases in the country. (i) **Others :** Kala-azar, meningitis, viral hepatitis, Japanese encephalitis, dengue fever, enteric fever and helminthic infestations are among the other important communicable disease problems in India. The tragedy is that most of these diseases can be either easily prevented or treated with minimum input of resources. In fact most of the developed countries of the world have overcome many of these problems by such measures as manipulation of environment, practice of preventive medicine and improvement of standards of living.

2. Non-communicable diseases (NCDs)

India is experiencing a rapid epidemiological transition with a large and rising burden of chronic diseases, which were estimated to account for 63 per cent of all deaths in 2016. NCDs, especially diabetes mellitus, CVDs, cancer, stroke, and chronic lung diseases have emerged as major public health problems due to an ageing population and environmentally driven changes in behaviour.

Cancer has become an important public health problem in India with an estimated 1.1 million cases occurring every year. At any point of time, it is estimated that there are nearly 3.9 million cases in the country. In India, tobacco related cancers account for about half the total cancers among men and 20% among women. About one million tobacco related deaths occur each year, making tobacco related health issues a major public health concern. In India, more then 12 million people are blind. Cataract (62.6 per cent) is the main cause of blindness followed by Refractive Error (19.70 per cent). There has been a significant increase in proportion of cataract surgeries with Intra Ocular Lens (IOL) implantation from <5 per cent in 1994 to 95 per cent in 2016–17. Oral Health Care has not been given sufficient importance in our country. Most of the district hospitals have a post of dental surgeon but they lack equipment, machinery, and material. Even where the equipment exists, the maintenance is poor, hence service delivery is affected.

3. Nutritional problems

From the nutritional point of view, the Indian society is a dual society, consisting of a small group of well fed and a very large group of undernourished. The high income groups are showing diseases of affluence which one finds in developed countries.

The specific nutritional problems in the country are : (a) **Protein-energy malnutrition :** Insufficiency of food – the so-called "food gap"– appears to be the chief cause of PEM, which is a major health problem particularly in the first years of life. The great majority of cases of PEM, nearly 80 per cent are mild and moderate cases. The incidence of severe cases is 1 to 2 per cent in preschool age children. The problem exists in all the States and the nutritional marasmus is more frequent than kwashiorkor. (b) **Nutritional anaemia :** India has probably the highest prevalence of nutritional anaemia in women and children. About one-half of non-pregnant women and young children are estimated to suffer from anaemia. 52.2 per cent of pregnant women are anaemic. 19 per cent of maternal deaths are attributed to anaemia. According to NFHS-5, about 52.2 per cent women are anaemic of which 45.5 per cent are in urban areas and 54.3 per cent in rural areas. The survey also shows that the incidence of anaemia in children aged 6-59 months is 67.1 per cent with 64.2 per cent in urban areas and 68.7 per cent in rural areas. By far the most frequent cause of anaemia is iron deficiency, and less frequently folate and vitamin B_{12} deficiency. (c) **Low birth weight :** This is a major public health problem in India. About 28 per cent of babies born are of low birth weight (less than 2.5 kg). Maternal malnutrition and anaemia are mainly responsible for this condition. (d) **Xerophthalmia (nutritional blindness) :** About 0.04 per cent of total blindness in India is attributed to nutritional deficiency of vitamin A. Keratomalacia has been the major cause of nutritional blindness in children usually between 1–3 years of age. Subclinical deficiency of vitamin A is also widespread and is associated with increased morbidity and mortality from respiratory and gastro-intestinal infections. (e) **Iodine deficiency disorders :** Goitre and other iodine deficiency disorders (IDD) have been known to be highly endemic in sub-Himalayan regions. Reassessment of the magnitude of the problem by the Indian Council of Medical Research showed that the problem is not restricted to the "goitre belt" as was thought earlier, but is extremely prevalent in other parts of India as well. It has been found that out of 324 districts surveyed in 29 states and all UTs, 263 districts are endemic i.e. where the prevalence of IDD is more than 10 per cent. It is also estimated that more than 71 million people are suffering from goitre and other IDD *(25)*. (f) **Others :** Other nutritional problems of importance are lathyrism and endemic fluorosis in certain parts of the country. To these must be added the widespread adulteration of foodstuffs.

4. Environmental sanitation

The most difficult problem to tackle in this country is perhaps the environmental sanitation problem, which is multifaceted and multifactorial. The twin problems of environmental sanitation are lack of safe water in many areas of the country and sanitary way of excreta disposal. Besides these, there has been a growing concern about the impact of "new" problems resulting from population explosion, urbanization and industrialization leading to hazards to human health in the air, in water and in the food chain. As of year 2017 safe water is available to 97 per cent of the urban and 93 per cent of the rural population; and adequate facilities for waste disposal to 63 per cent of the urban and 28 per cent of the rural population. The problem is gigantic.

5. Medical care problems

India has a national health policy. The existing hospital-based, disease-oriented health care model has provided health benefits mainly to the urban elite. Approximately 80 per cent of health facilities are concentrated in urban areas. Even in urban areas, there is an uneven distribution of doctors. With large migrations occurring from rural to urban areas, urban health problems have been aggravated and include overcrowding in hospitals, inadequate staffing and scarcity of certain essential drugs and medicines. The rural areas where nearly 65 per cent of the population live, do not enjoy the benefits of the modern curative and preventive health services. Many villages rely on indigenous systems of medicine. Thus the major medical care problem in India is inequable distribution of available health resources between urban and rural areas, and lack of penetration of health services to the social periphery. The primary health care approach, which lays stress on equity, intersectoral coordination and community participation seek to redress these imbalances.

6. Population problem

The population problem is one of the biggest problem facing the country, with its inevitable consequences on all aspects of development, especially employment, education, housing, health care, sanitation and environment. The country's population has already reached one billion mark by the turn of the century.

Currently, the country's growth rate is 1.3 per cent. This calls for the "two child family norm". The population size and structure represent the most important single factor in health and manpower planning in India today where the law of diminishing returns, among other factors, plays an important role in the economic development of the country.

RESOURCES

Resources are needed to meet the vast health needs of a community. No nation, however rich, has enough resources to meet all the needs for all health care. Therefore an assessment of the available resources, their proper allocation and efficient utilization are important considerations for providing efficient health care services. The basic resources for providing health care are :

(i) Health manpower;
(ii) Money and material; and
(iii) Time.

Health manpower

The term "health manpower" includes both professional and auxiliary health personnel who are needed to provide the health care. An auxiliary is defined by WHO as "technical worker in a certain field with less than full professional training". Health manpower requirements of a country are based on (i) health needs and demands of the population; and (ii) desired outputs. The health needs in turn are based on the health situation and health problems and aspirations of the people.

Health manpower planning is an important aspect of community health planning. It is based on a series of accepted ratios such as doctor-population ratio, nurse-population ratio, bed-population ratio, etc. They are given in Table 3. The country is producing annually, on an average

31,298 allopathic doctors; 9,865 Ayurvedic graduates; 1525 Unani graduates; 320 Siddha graduates and 12785 Homoeopathic graduates *(26)*.

TABLE 3

Suggested norms for health personnel

Category of personnel	Norms suggested
1. Nurses	1 per 5,000 population
2. Health workers female and male	1 per 5,000 population in plain area and 3,000 population in tribal and hilly areas.
3. Trained dai	One for each village
4. Health assistants (male and female)	1 per 30,000 population in plain area and 20,000 population in tribal and hilly areas. Provides supportive supervision to 6 health workers (male / female).
5. Pharmacists	1 per 10,000 population
6. Lab. technicians	1 per 10,000 population
7. ASHA	1 per 1,000 population

Source : *(25)*

Although the averages are satisfactory on a national basis, they vary widely within the country. There is also maldistribution of health manpower between rural and urban areas. Studies in India have shown that there is a concentration of doctors (upto 73.6 per cent) in urban areas where only 26.4 per cent of population live. This maldistribution is attributed to absence of amenities in rural areas, lack of job satisfaction, professional isolation, lack of rural experience and inability to adjust to rural life.

The national averages of doctor-population ratio, population-bed ratio and nurse to doctor ratio in some countries are shown in Table 4.

TABLE 4

Health manpower in some countries 2010–2018

Country	Doctors per 10000 population	Beds per 10000 population	Nurses and Midwives per 10000 population
India	7.8	7.0	20.9
Bangladesh	5.6	8.0	2.2
Sri Lanka	9.6	36.0	16.4
Thailand	8.1	21.0	20.8
Myanmar	8.6	9.0	10.0

Source : *(27)*

Health manpower requirements are subject to change, both qualitatively and quantitatively, as new programmes, projects and philosophies are introduced into the health care system. For example, there has been a change from unipurpose to multipurpose strategy. Then came the goal of Health for All. In addition, national health programmes such as tuberculosis control, leprosy eradication and control of blindness needed more trained workers and technicians. Thus during the past decade many new categories of health manpower have been introduced. They include village health guides, multipurpose workers, technicians, ophthalmic assistants, etc. Table 5 gives the total health manpower current stock under the "rural health scheme".

TABLE 5

Health man-power in India as on March 2021

Category			In position
Health worker female/ANM at sub-centre		rural	187,557
Health worker male at sub-centre		rural	52,978
PHC		rural	27,263
Health Assistant PHC		rural	12,428
Health Assistant PHC		urban	8,058
Allopathic Doctors at PHC		rural	31,716
Ayush Doctors at PHC		rural	8,709
Ayush Doctors at CHC			514
CHC (rural)	General duty doctor		17,012
	Surgeon		923
	Gynaecologist		1,433
	Physician		975
	Paediatrician		1,074
	Anaesthetist		805
	Eye surgeon		289
Total specialists			4405
Radiographer	CHC	rural	2,418
Pharmacist	PHC	rural	19,574
	CHC	rural	8,963
Lab. Technician	PHC	rural	14,498
	CHC	rural	8,225
Staff nurse	PHC	rural	34,420
	CHC	rural	44,624
	CHC	urban	6,905

Source : *(28)*

Money and material

Money is an important resource for providing health services. Scarcity of money affects all parts of the health delivery system. In most developed countries, average government expenditure for health is about 18 per cent of GNP. In developing countries it is less than 1 per cent of the GNP and it seldom exceeds 2 per cent of the GNP. This translates into an average of a few dollars per person per year in the underdeveloped countries as compared to several hundred dollars in developed ones. To make matters worse, much of the spending is for services that reach only a small fraction of the population. At present India is spending about 3 per cent of GNP on health and family welfare development.

Since money and material are always scarce resources they must be put to the most effective use, with an eye on maximum output of results for investment. Since deaths from preventable diseases such as whooping cough, measles, tuberculosis, tetanus, diphtheria, acute respiratory infection, diarrhoea, malaria and malnutrition frequently occur in developing countries, the case is strong for investing resources on preventing these diseases. Management techniques such as cost-effectiveness and cost-benefit analysis are now being used for allocation of resources in the field of community health.

Time

"Time is money", someone said. It is an important dimension of health care services. Administrative delays in sanctioning health projects imply loss of time. Proper use of man-hours is also an important time factor. To summarize, resources are needed to meet the many health needs of a community. But resources are desperately short in the health sector in all poor countries. What is important is to employ suitable strategies to get the best out of limited resources.

HEALTH CARE SERVICES

The purpose of health care services is to improve the health status of the population. The goals to be achieved have been fixed in terms of mortality and morbidity reduction, increase in expectation of life, decrease in population growth rate, improvements in nutritional status, provision of basic sanitation, health manpower requirements and resources development and certain other parameters such as food production, literacy rate, reduced levels of poverty, etc.

The scope of health services varies widely from country to country and influenced by general and ever changing national, state and local health problems, needs and attitudes as well as the available resources to provide these services.

There is now broad agreement that health services should be (a) comprehensive (b) accessible (c) acceptable (d) provide scope for community participation, and (e) available at a cost the community and country can afford. These are the essential ingredients of primary health care which forms an integral part of the country's health system, of which it is the central function and main agent for delivering health care *(9)*.

HEALTH CARE SYSTEMS

The health care system is intended to deliver the health care services. It constitutes the management sector and involves organisational matters. It operates in the context of the socioeconomic and political framework of the country. In India, it is represented by five major sectors or agencies which differ from each other by the health technology applied and by the source of funds for operation. These are :

1. PUBLIC HEALTH SECTOR
   - (a) Primary Health Care
     - Primary health centres
     - Sub- centres
   - (b) Hospitals/Health Centres
     - Community health centres
     - Rural hospitals
     - District hospital/health centre
     - Specialist hospitals
     - Teaching hospitals
   - (c) Health Insurance Schemes
     - Employees State Insurance
     - Central Government Health Scheme
   - (d) Other agencies
     - Defence services
     - Railways
2. PRIVATE SECTOR
   - (a) Private hospitals, polyclinics, Nursing homes, and dispensaries
   - (b) General practitioners and clinics
3. INDIGENOUS SYSTEMS OF MEDICINE
   - Ayurveda and Siddha
   - Unani and Tibbi
   - Homoeopathy
   - Unregistered practitioners
4. VOLUNTARY HEALTH AGENCIES
5. NATIONAL HEALTH PROGRAMMES

PRIMARY HEALTH CARE IN INDIA

In 1977, the Government of India launched a Rural Health Scheme, based on the principle of "placing people's health in people's hands". It is a three tier system of health care delivery in rural areas based on the recommendation of the Shrivastav Committee in 1975. Close on the heels of these recommendations an International conference at Alma-Ata in 1978, set the goal of an acceptable level of Health for All the people of the world by the year 2000 through primary health care approach. As a signatory to the Alma-Ata Declaration, the Government of India was committed to achieving the goal of Health for All through primary health care approach which seeks to provide universal comprehensive health care at a cost which is affordable.

Keeping in view the WHO goal of "Health for All" by 2000 AD, the Government of India evolved a National Health Policy based on primary health care approach. It was approved by Parliament in 1983. The National Health Policy laid down a plan of action for reorienting and shaping the existing rural health infrastructure with specific goals to be achieved by 1985, 1990 and 1995 within the framework of the Sixth (1980–85) and Seventh (1985–90) Five Year Plans and the new 20 point Programme. Steps were taken to implement the National Health Policy objectives towards achieving Health for All by the year 2000. During the last decade further development of rural health infrastructure took place in view to implement National Health Policy 2002 and 2017, National Population Policy 2000 and more recently National Rural Health Mission, National Urban Health Mission and Health and Wellness Centres with formulation of Indian Public Health Standards.

VILLAGE LEVEL

One of the basic tenets of primary health care is universal coverage and equitable distribution of health resources. That is, health care must penetrate into the farthest reaches of rural areas, and that everyone should have access to it. To implement this policy at the village level, the following schemes are in operation :

a. ASHA Scheme;
b. ICDS Scheme; and
c. Training of Local Dais.

a. ASHA

ASHA must be resident of the village – a woman (married/widow/divorced) preferably in the age group of 25 to 45 years with formal education upto eight class, having communication skill and leadership qualities. Adequate representation from the disadvantaged population group will ensure to serve such groups better. The general norm of selection is one ASHA for 1000 population. In tribal, hilly and desert areas the norm could be relaxed to one ASHA per habitation.

Role and responsibilities of ASHA

ASHA will be a health activist in the community who will create awareness on health. Her responsibilities will be as follows *(29)* :

1. ASHA will take steps to create awareness and provide

information to the community on determinants of health such as nutrition, basic sanitation and hygienic practices, healthy living and working conditions, information on existing health services, and the need for timely utilization of health and family welfare services.

2. She will counsel women on birth preparedness, importance of safe delivery, breast-feeding and complementary feeding, immunization, contraception and prevention of common infections including reproductive tract infection/sexually transmitted infection and care of the young child.
3. ASHA will mobilize the community and facilitate them in accessing health and health related services available at the anganwadi/subcentre/primary health centres, such as immunization, antenatal check-up, postnatal check-up, supplementary nutrition, sanitation and other services being provided by the government.
4. She will work with the village health and sanitation committee of the gram panchayat to develop a comprehensive village health plan.
5. She will arrange escort/accompany pregnant women and children requiring treatment/admission to the nearest pre-identified health facility i.e. primary health centre/community health centre/First Referral Unit.
6. ASHA will provide primary medical care for minor ailments such as diarrhoea, fevers, and first-aid for minor injuries. She will be a provider of directly observed treatment short-course (DOTS) under revised national tuberculosis control programme.
7. She will also act as a depot holder for essential provisions being made available to every habitation like oral rehydration therapy, iron folic acid tablet, chloroquine, disposable delivery kits, oral pills and condoms etc. A drug kit will be provided to each ASHA. Contents of the kit will be based on the recommendations of the expert/technical advisory group set up by the government of India, and include both AYUSH and allopathic formulations.
8. Her role as a provider can be enhanced subsequently. States can explore the possibility of graded training to her for providing newborn care and management of a range of common ailments, particularly childhood illnesses.
9. She will inform about the births and deaths in her village and any unusual health problems/disease outbreaks in the community to the sub-centre/primary health centre.
10. She will promote construction of household toilets under total sanitation campaign.

Role and integration with Anganwadi *(29)*

Anganwadi worker will guide ASHA in performing following activities : (a) Organizing Health Day once/twice a month. On health day, the women, adolescent girls and children from the village will be mobilized for orientation on health related issues such as importance of nutritious food, personal hygiene, care during pregnancy, importance of antenatal check-up and institutional delivery, home remedies for minor ailment and importance of immunization etc. AWWs will inform ANM to participate and guide organizing the Health Days at anganwadi centre; (b) AWWs and ANMs will act as resource persons for the training of ASHA; (c) IEC activity through display of posters, folk dances etc. on these days can be undertaken to sensitize the beneficiaries on health related issues; (d) Anganwadi worker will be depot holder for drug kits and will be issuing it to ASHA. The replacement of the consumed drugs can also be done through AWW; (e) AWW will update the list of eligible couples and also the children less than one year of age in the village with the help of ASHA; and (f) ASHA will support the AWW in mobilizing pregnant and lactating women and infants for nutrition supplement. She would also take initiative for bringing the beneficiaries from the village on specific days of immunization, health check-ups/health days etc. to anganwadi centres.

Role and integration with ANM *(29)*

Auxiliary Nurse Midwife (ANM) will guide ASHA in performing following activities : (a) She will hold weekly/ fortnightly meeting with ASHA and discuss the activities undertaken during the week/fortnight. She will guide her in case ASHA had encountered any problem during the performance of her activity; (b) AWWs and ANMs will act as resource persons for the training of ASHA; (c) ANMs will inform ASHA regarding date and time of the outreach session and will also guide her for bringing the beneficiary to the outreach session; (d) ANM will participate and guide in organizing the Health Days at anganwadi centre; (e) She will take help of ASHA in updating eligible couple register of the village concerned; (f) She will utilize ASHA in motivating the pregnant women for coming to sub-centre for initial check-ups. She will also help ANMs in bringing married couples to sub-centres for adopting family planning; (g) ANM will guide ASHA in motivating pregnant women for taking full course of iron and folic acid tablets and tetanus toxoid injections etc.; (h) ANMs will orient ASHA on the dose schedule and side effects of oral pills; (i) ANMs will educate ASHA on danger signs of pregnancy and labour so that she can timely identify and help beneficiary in getting further treatment; and (j) ANMs will inform ASHA on date, time and place for initial and periodic training schedule. She will also ensure that during the training ASHA gets the compensation for performance and also TA/DA for attending the training.

b. Anganwadi worker

Angan literally means a courtyard. Under the ICDS (Integrated Child Development Services) Scheme, there is an anganwadi worker for a population of 400–800. There are about 100 such workers in each ICDS Project. As of date over 7,067 ICDS blocks are functioning in the country. The anganwadi worker is selected from the community she is expected to serve. She undergoes training in various aspects of health, nutrition, and child development for 4 months. She is a part-time worker and is paid an honorarium of Rs. 1500 per month for the services rendered, which include health check-up including maintenance of growth chart, immunization, supplementary nutrition, health education, non-formal pre-school education and referral services. The beneficiaries are especially nursing mothers, pregnant women, other women (15–45 years), children below the age of 6 years and adolescent girls *(30)*. Along with Village Health Guides, the anganwadi workers are the community's primary link with the health services and all other services for young children.

c. Local dais *(31)*

A scheme for training of Dais was initiated during 2001–02. The scheme was implemented in 156 districts in 18 states/UTs of the country. The districts selected were on the basis of the safe delivery rate being less than 30 per cent. The scheme was extended to all the districts of EAG states. The aim was to train at least one Dai in every village with the objective of making deliveries safe.

INDIAN PUBLIC HEALTH STANDARDS AT PRIMARY HEALTH CARE LEVEL (2022)

Focus on urban health came during RCH-I and continued in RCH-II as part of NRHM. Since the last revision of the Indian Public Health Standards in 2012, a number of new initiatives, interventions and programmes have been introduced in the public health system of India. The introduction of comprehensive primary health care through upgraded sub-centres and PHCs (now known as Health and Wellness Centres), and similarly, in urban areas, Urban Health and Wellness Centres, speciality UPHCs (polyclinics), are some of the new additions, with special focus on people living in listed and unlisted slums, homeless, rag-pickers, migrants and other vulnerable population. Since then, some key policy shifts have been proposed under the National Health Policy (2017) for public health care delivery system in the following areas *(32)* :

- *Clinical care* – from stand-alone curative to a preventive, promotive and rehabilitative approach for achieving comprehensive wellness in health.
- *Primary care* – from selective care to assured comprehensive care with linkages to referral hospitals.
- *Drugs, diagnostics, and emergency services* – from user fees and cost recovery to assured free drugs, diagnostic and emergency services to all in public hospitals.
- *Infrastructure and human resource development* – from normative approach to targeted approach to reach under-served areas with "time to care approach".
- *Urban health* – from token interventions to on-scale assured interventions to organize Primary Health Care delivery and referral support for urban poor. Collaboration with other sectors to address wider determinants of urban health is advocated.
- *National health programmes* – integration with health systems for programme effectiveness and in turn contributing to strengthening of health systems for efficiency.

In the public health sector, the sub health centre (SHC) and urban health and wellness centre (UHWC) are the most peripheral and first point of contact between the primary health care system and the community in rural and urban areas respectively. These health facilities act as an interface with the community at the grass-root level, providing all the comprehensive primary health care services.

Revised IPHS guidelines 2022 also define the components specific to urban health facilities to set benchmarks to achieve the goal of universal health coverage.

The 2022 IPHS guidelines have been framed for :

- Sub-District Hospitals (SDH) & District Hospitals (DH),
- Community Health Centres (CHC) – rural and urban,
- Health and Wellness Centre – Primary Health Centres (PHC) – rural and urban, including Multispeciality UPHC (Polyclinics) in urban areas,
- Health and Wellness Centre – Sub Health Centre (SHC) – rural and urban.

The 2022 revised guidelines emphasize on the services to be delivered at each level of facility. Service delivery defined for each level of health facility will be the basis for developing other health system strengthening components viz. infrastructure, human resources, drugs, diagnostics/ equipment, quality improvement, monitoring/supervision, governance, and leadership.

The 2022 IPHS norms supports government health facilities to attain a minimum acceptable functional standard (indicated as 'essential') while striving and aspiring for improvement (indicated as 'desirable') so as to accelerate India's progress towards achievement of Universal Health Coverage (UHC) and Sustainable Development Goal - 3 (SDG-3) in alignment with the National Health Policy 2017.

In comparison with the IPHS guidelines of 2012, the revised IPHS 2022 guidelines classify the HWCs as :

1. Health and Wellness Centres - Primary Health Centre:
   a. HWC-PHC in rural areas
   b. HWC- UPHC in urban areas
2. Health and Wellness Centres - Sub Health Centre:
   a. Health and Wellness Centre - Sub Health Centre in rural areas
   b. Urban Health & Wellness Centre in urban areas

Depending on the services provided at a particular facility, it may be deemed as a primary or secondary care service provider facility :

- Health and Wellness Centres (HWC-SHC, UHWCs and PHCs), in both rural and urban areas will provide primary care services.
- Multispeciality polyclinics nearer to the community will provide ambulatory specialist services, particularly in urban areas.
- Community Health Centres in rural areas can be either FRU or non- FRU, depending on the range of services provided. In urban areas, CHCs will provide services at par with FRU.
- District and Sub-District Hospitals will provide secondary care services.

Implementation of all national programmes at individual facilities must be in line with the latest GoI/state guidelines developed for that programme. All Rural and Urban-HWCs should have a National Identification Number (NIN-Id) and register on the AB-HWC portal.

A Citizen's Charter should be prominently displayed near the entrance of the facility. This should provide information about the various services being offered, timings, responsibilities of patients and providers, details of referral vehicles and facilities, the number of free drugs and diagnostics being provided and other citizen friendly information. Patient's rights should be ensured, and they should also be made aware of their responsibilities (e.g., to keep the facility clean and avoid spitting in corners, avoiding over-crowding by attendants, respecting visiting hours, not causing any harm to public property or indulging in violence against healthcare professionals, etc.). A sample of citizen's charter for the level of HWC-PHC is shown below *(33)*.

CITIZEN'S CHARTER *(33)*

Name of the state

*Name & type of facility (HWC-PHC/HWC-UPHC/24*7 - UPHC*)

Contact No. (facility In charge)

(This facility is IPHS & KAYAKALP/NQAS/LaQshya* Certified)

Mission statement & Objective :

The NHM envisages achievement of universal access to equitable, affordable & quality healthcare services as per IPHS for all with respect, dignity & without any discrimination.

General Information :

No. of General Beds

Staff

No of GDMO ....

No of Nursing staff ....

No of Paramedical staff ....

Any other *

Services Available			
Services (as per Type of PHC)		Days	Timings
OPD services including special services		Mon- Sat (except on public holidays)	8:00 am to 2:00pm
Key services available during OPD			
General OPD			
Antenatal Care (ANC)			
Immunization			
Emergency Services		24×7	
Minor O.T./Dressing		24×7	
Dental Clinic*			
AYUSH* OPD			
Yoga Day Wellness activities			
Fixed day clinics			
NCD Clinics			
Geriatric Clinic			
Disability & Palliative Clinic			
Mental Health Clinic (Screening)*			
Eye Optometry (Screening)*			
ENT Clinic (Screening)*			
DOTS Centre			
Adolescent clinic			
Laboratory	Routine Lab	Mon- Sat	00:00-00:00
	Referral Lab	24×7 *(Hub and spoke, if any)*	
Pharmacy		Mon- Sat	00:00-00:00
Ambulance Service		24×7	
Administrative Office Services		Mon-Sat	00:00- 00:00
Medico-Legal Services*			

Out bench Services :

Services	Venue	Day/Date	Time
Village Health & Nutrition days (VHNDs)/UHNDs			
Mobile Medical Units (MMU) visits			
RBSK Team Visit			
Population based screening			
Any Other*			

Support Services : (In House /Linked)

- Equipment sterilization services
- Laundry services
- Dietary services
- Security services

Other Basic Amenities

- Stretcher & wheelchair
- Separate queue for senior citizens*
- Disabled & elderly-friendly facilities
- Potable water
- Washroom facility
- Waiting areas
- Generic drug store*

Free Entitlements:

- Free drugs as per the Essential Drug List (EDL)
- Free diagnostic as per Free Diagnostic Initiative (FDI) guidelines
- 24x7 Ambulance services (including drop back service)
- Dietary Services
- Services under various schemes like.
- Pradhan Mantri Jan Arogya Yojana(PM-JAY)
- Pradhan Mantri Surakshit Matritava Abhiyan (PMSMA)
- Janani Suraksha Yojana (JSY)
- Janani Shishu Suraksha Karyakram (JSSK)
- Mission Indradhanush
- Direct Observed Treatment Short course(DOTS)

Paid Services *(if applicable)*

- The user fee for the payable services is displayed in respective services areas. Do not pay any extra money to anybody.

Note : This is a suggestive draft for HWC(PHC/UPHC).The states can add or delete as per the services available at the facility

(Continued on page 704)

(Continued on page 703)

CITIZEN'S CHARTER

Financial Benefits :

Schemes	Benefits	
Janani Suraksha Yojana (JSY)		
Compensation for family planning procedures * Tubectomy * NSV * IUCD * Indemnity Scheme		
National TB Elimination Programme (NTEP)		

Expanded range of comprehensive services packages being implemented :

- Care in pregnancy and childbirth
- Neonatal & infant health care services
- Childhood and adolescent health care services
- Family planning, contraceptive services & other Reproductive Health care services
- Management of communicable disease including National Health Programmes
- Management of Common Communicable Disease & Outpatient care for acute simple illnesses and minor ailments.
- Screening, Prevention, Control & Management of Non-Communicable disease
- Care for Common Ophthalmic & ENT problems
- Basic Oral Health Care
- Elderly & Palliative health care services
- Emergency Medical Services
- Screening & Basic Management of Mental Health ailments

* *(State specific programme to be entered)*

Referral Services :

Toll free Number

Details of nearest CHC ....

Details of nearest FRU ....

Details of nearest District Hospital ....

Details of nearest Tertiary care Hospital ....

Tele-consultation services :

- Tele-medicine, Tele- radiology
- Tele-conferencing- ECHO ZOOM

Patient Rights :

- Right to informed consent prior to specific treatment, tests and digitalization of medical records
- Right to confidentiality and privacy during treatment.
- Right to be treated with respect and dignity without any discrimination
- Timely release of dead body commensurate to legal Protocols.
- Right to emergency care and grievance redressed

Patient Responsibilities :

- Respect dignity of doctors & other hospital staff
- Never resort to violence
- Please refrain from causing any damage to public property
- Please do not cause inconvenience to other patient and staff
- Maintain queues & respect others particularly the elderly, disabled, women & children
- Please do not spit on the floor/walls/inside the campus
- Please cooperate to keep the facility clean and tidy. Use the dustbin
- Hospital is a no smoking zone and smoking is a punishable offence
- Please register your experience through Mera Aspataal

Visitors policy :

Visiting time : Morning : Evening :

- Only one person allowed to visit at a time *(Maintain about pass system)
- Respect visiting hours

Complaints & Grievance :

- Any Patient /Attendant can register their grievance through Grievance redressed (GR) Helpdesk/Calling toll free number (...) online GR, web portal (www...)
- Every Grievance will be duly acknowledged with an SMS & registration number for status tracking
- We aim to settle your genuine complaints within (7) days of its receipt
- Suggestions /complaints may also be put in the complaint boxes provided at every department
- Contact details of the RTI officer are displayed below

Grievance & Redressal :

- Toll free number
- Designated officer: (with mobile number & Email)
- Complaint Box

Funds :

- RKS details
- United fund detail - Rs............... /-

Note : The details of the nodal person can be displayed based on the program requirement * Marked patients can be edited according to the condition/services provided in the respective facilities "a" indicate amount as applicable.

The healthcare services to be provided at these Centres include health promotion, early identification, ensuring treatment adherence, follow-up care, ensuring continuity of care by appropriate referrals, optimal home and community follow-up, disease surveillance, and health promotion and prevention for the expanded range of CPHC services. The twelve packages envisaged under CPHC are *(32)* :

1. Care in Pregnancy and Childbirth.
2. Neonatal and Infant Health Care Services
3. Childhood and Adolescent Health Care Services.
4. Family Planning, Contraceptive Services and other Reproductive Health Care Services
5. Management of Communicable Diseases : National Health Programme
6. Management of Common communicable diseases and outpatient care for acute simple illness and minor ailments
7. Screening, Prevention, Control and Management of Non-communicable Diseases
8. Care for Common Ophthalmic and ENT Problems
9. Basic Oral Health Care
10. Elderly and Palliative Health Care Services
11. Emergency Medical Services including Burns and Trauma
12. Screening and Basic Management of Mental Health Ailments

In addition to providing clinical services, HWCs are also to be utilized as a platform for teleconsultation and expanding the range of diagnostics.

Indian Public Health Standards for Health and Wellness Centre - Sub Health Centre (2022)

The population norms for HWC-SHC and UHWC are as follows :

a. *HWC-SHC (rural)* : In rural areas, one Sub Health Centre is established for every 5000 population in plain areas and 3000 population in hilly/tribal/desert areas.

b. *UHWC (urban)* : In urban areas one Urban-HWC per 15,000–20,000 population caters predominantly to poor and vulnerable populations, residing in slums or other such pockets.

Manpower recommended under IPHS are as follows :

HR at HWC-SHC

Human Resource required	Required Numbers
Community Health Officer (CHO)	1
Multipurpose Health Worker	1 Male +1 Female

Sanitation and security services can be hired/outsourced

There should be one ASHA per 1000 population or one ASHA per habitation in tribal, hilly and desert areas, and should be attached with the HWC as part of the entire team.

Manpower at UHWC:

The Urban-HWC is to be staffed with a Medical Officer, a Staff Nurse/Pharmacist, Male-MPW and one support staff. Staff Nurses will also be supporting the doctors while examining the patients particularly the female patients to ensure their privacy and dignity. Ideally, the ANM and ASHA are responsible for the catchment area of a UPHC. Wherever available, they will be drawn from HWC-UPHC / UCHC for respective Urban-HWC while their salaries can continue to be drawn from their linked HWC-UPHC. In case where ANM, ASHA are not available, the state may engage new ASHA, ANM for Urban-HWCs depending on the local needs and resources available.

The services provided at HWC-SHC and UHWC are discussed in detail at page 706 to 712.

Indian Public Health Standards for Health and Wellness Centre - Primary Health Centre *(33)*

In comparison with the IPHS guidelines of 2012, the revised IPHS 2022 guidelines classify the rural and urban PHC as :

a. *HWC-PHCs* : Ideally, for rural areas, the states should aspire to make all PHCs functional as 24×7 facilities. However, there is a need to prioritize PHCs conducting deliveries to function as 24×7 HWC-PHCs. All other PHCs should continue to provide routine care along with preventive and promotive health interventions and function as PHCs-HWCs.

b. *Urban HWC-PHCs* : In urban areas, assured round-the-clock emergency and secondary care services are readily available, owing to the presence of higher level health care facilities. Thus primary health centres are expected to provide routine OPD care along with preventive and promotive health interventions and function as UPHCs-HWCs. However, the UPHCs with indoor beds already conducting deliveries can continue to function as 24×7 UPHCs-HWCs.

c. *Specialist UPHC/Polyclinic (Urban)* : "Multispeciality UPHC/Polyclinics" in urban areas should be established with the aim to further reduce morbidity and mortality by providing specialist services on ambulatory/day care basis, closer to the urban community. Such poly clinic services would be limited to outpatient care.

The population norms for HWC-PHC are as follows :

Population norm for HWC-PHC

Type of PHC facility	Plain (population)	Hilly and Tribal areas (population)
Rural PHC	30,000	20,000
Urban PHC	50,000	-
Polyclinic	2.5 lakh–3 lakh	-

Human resources for health

Human Resource for Health	PHC		UPHC		Polyclinic		24×7 PHC		24×7 UPHC	
	E	D	E	D	E	D	E	D	E	D
MO MBBS	1	1	2	-	2	-	2	1	2	1
MO AYUSH	-	1	-	-	-	-	-	1	-	-
MO Dental	-	1	-	1	1	-	-	1	-	1
*Specialist for Medicine, Obstetrics & Gynecology, Pediatrics, Ophthalmology, Dermatology and Psychiatry on rotation basis	-	-	-	-	1	-	-	-	-	-
Staff Nurses	2	1	1	1	2	-	7	-	7	-
Pharmacist	1	-	1	-	1	1	1	1	1	1
Medical Laboratory Technologist/Lab Technician	1	-	1	-	1	-	2	1	2	1
Optometrist/Ophthalmic Assistant/Vision Technician	-	1	-	-	1	-	-	1	-	1
Health Worker (Female)/ANM	1	-	5	-	5	-	1	-	5	-
Health Worker/ Health Assistant (Male)	1	-	-	-	-	-	1	-	-	-
Health Assistant (Female)/ Lady Health Visitor	1	-	1	-	1	-	1	-	1	-
Health Educator/Counsellor	-	1	-	1	1	-	-	1	-	1
Dental Assistant	-	1	-	1	-	1	-	1	-	1
Cold chain/Vaccine logistic Assistant	-	1	-	1	-	1	1	-	1	-
Physiotherapist	-	-	-	-	1	-	-	1	-	1
Public Health Manager	-	-	1	-	1	-	-	-	1	-
Dresser	1	-	1	-	-	-	1	-	1	-
LDC-1/Accountant	1	-	1	-	1	-	1	-	1	-
Data Entry Operator	1	-	1	-	1	-	1	-	1	-
Sanitation staff	1	-	1	-	2	-	4	-	4	-

Source : *(33)*

The recommended service delivery framework *(32)*

S. No.	Health care services	Care at community level	Care at the Health and Wellness Centres-Sub Health Centres/ Urban Health and Wellness Centres	Care at the referral site** (PHC and upwards)
1.	Care in pregnancy and childbirth	• Early diagnosis of pregnancy • Ensuring four antenatal care checks • Counselling regarding care during pregnancy including information about nutritional requirements • Identifying of high-risk pregnancies and follow up • Enabling access to take home ration from Anganwadi Centre • Follow up to ensure compliance to IFA in normal and anemic cases • Facilitating institutional delivery and supporting birth planning • Post- partum care visits • Identifying high risk pregnancies, child births and post-partum cases and facilitating timely referrals	• Early registration of pregnancy and issuing ID number and Mother and Child Protection (MCP) Card. • Antenatal check-up including screening for hypertension, diabetes, anemia. Immunization for pregnant women-Td, IFA and Calcium supplementation • Identifying high risk pregnancies, postpartum cases for regular follow up, timely referral for institutional births and complication management. • Screening, referral and follow up care in cases of gestational diabetes, and syphilis during pregnancy • Normal vaginal delivery in specified delivery sites as per state context -where CHO or MPW (F) is trained as skill birth attendant. • Provide first aid treatment and referral for obstetric emergencies, e.g., eclampsia, PPH, sepsis, and prompt referral.	• Antenatal and postnatal care of high-risk cases • Blood grouping and Rh typing and blood cross matching • Linkage with nearest ICTC/ PPTCT Centre for voluntary testing for HIV and PPTCT services • Normal vaginal delivery and assisted vaginal delivery • Surgical interventions like caesarean section, • Management of all complications including ante-partum and post-partum haemorrhage, eclampsia, puerperal sepsis, obstructed labour, retained placenta, shock, severe anaemia, breast abscess. • Blood transfusion facilities

S. No.	Health care services	Care at community level	Care at the Health and Wellness Centres-Sub Health Centres/ Urban Health and Wellness Centres	Care at the referral site** (PHC and upwards)
2.	Neonatal and infant Health	• Home based new-born care through 7 visits in case of home delivery and 6 visits in case of institutional delivery • Identification and care of high-risk new-born – low birth weight/ preterm new-born and sick new-born (with referral as required), • Counselling and support for early breast feeding, improved weaning practices. • Iron supplementation • Adoption of safe and hygiene WASH practices • Growth Monitoring • Counselling for early childhood growth and development. • Identification of birth asphyxia, sepsis and referral after initial management • Identification of congenital anomalies and appropriate referral • Family /community education for prevention of infections and keeping the baby warm • Identification of ARI/Diarrhoea-identification, initiation of treatment- ORS and timely referral as required • Mobilization and follow up for immunization services	• Identification and management of high-risk new-born - low birth weight/preterm/ sick new-born and sepsis (with referral as required), • Management of birth asphyxia • Identification, appropriate referral and follow up of congenital anomalies • Management of ARI/Diarrhoea and other common illness and referral of severe cases. • Screening, referral and follow up for disabilities and developmental delays • Complete immunization • Vitamin A supplementation • Identification and follow up, referral and reporting of Adverse Events Following Immunization (AEFI).	• Care for low-birth-weight new-borns (<2500gms) • Treatment of asphyxia and neonatal sepsis, • Treatment of severe ARI and Diarrhoea/Dehydration cases • Vitamin K for premature babies • Management of all emergency and complication cases.
3.	Childhood and Adolescent health care services including immunization	• Growth Monitoring, IYCF continued and enable access to food supplementation- all linked to ICDS • Detection of SAM, referral and follow up care for SAM • Prevention of Anaemia, iron supplementation and deworming • Prevention of diarrhoea/ARI, prompt and appropriate treatment of diarrhoea/ ARI with referral where needed • Pre-school and School Child Health: Biannual Screening, School Health Records, eye care, de-worming • Screening of children under national program to cover 4'D's Viz. Defect at birth, Deficiencies, Diseases, Development delay including disability **Adolescent Health** Counselling on - Improving nutrition • Sexual and reproductive health • Enhancing mental health / Promoting favourable attitudes for preventing injuries and violence, prevent substance misuse • Promote healthy lifestyle • Personal hygiene- oral hygiene and menstrual hygiene • Peer counselling and life skills education • Prevention of anaemia, identification and management, with referral if needed • Provision of IFA under National Program for Iron Supplementation	• Complete immunization • Detection and treatment of Anaemia and other deficiencies in children and adolescents • Identification and management of vaccine preventable diseases in children such as Diphtheria, Pertussis and Measles • Early detection of growth abnormalities, delays in development and disability and referral • Prompt Management of ARI, acute diarrhoea and fever with referral as needed • Management (with timely referral as needed) of ear, eye and throat problems, skin infections, worm infestations, febrile seizure, poisoning, injuries/accidents, insect and animal bites **Adolescent Health** • Detection of SAM, referral and follow up care for SAM. • Adolescent health-counselling • Detection for cases of substance abuse, referral and follow up • Detection and treatment of Anaemia and other deficiencies in adolescents • Detection and referral for growth abnormality and disabilities, with referral as required	• NRC Services • Management of SAM children, severe anaemia or persistent malnutrition • Severe diarrhoea and ARI management • Management of all ear, eye and throat problems, skin infections, worm infestations, febrile seizure, poisoning, injuries/accidents, insect and animal bites • Diagnosis and treatment for disability, deficiencies and development delays • Surgeries for any congenital anomalies like cleft lips and cleft palates, club foot etc. **Adolescent Health** • Screening for hormonal imbalances and treatment with referral if required • Management of growth abnormality and disabilities, with referral as required • Management including rehabilitation and counselling services in cases of substance abuse • Counselling at Adolescent Friendly Health Clinics (AFHC)

S. No.	Health care services	Care at community level	Care at the Health and Wellness Centres-Sub Health Centres/ Urban Health and Wellness Centres	Care at the referral site** (PHC and upwards)
4.	Family planning, contraceptive services and other reproductive care services	• Counselling for creating awareness against early marriage and delaying early pregnancy • Identification and registration of eligible couples • Motivating for family planning (Delaying first child and spacing between 2 children) • Provision of condom, oral contraceptive pills and emergency contraceptive pills • Follow up with contraceptive users • Other reproductive care services • Counselling and facilitation of safe abortion services • Post abortion contraceptive counselling • Follow up for any complication after abortion and appropriate referral if needed • Education and mobilizing of community for action on violence against women • Counselling on prevention of RTI/STI • Identification and referral of RTI/STI cases • Follow up and support PLHA (People living with HIV/AIDS) groups • Ensure regular treatment and follow of diagnosed cases	• Insertion of IUCD • Removal of IUCD • Provision of condoms, oral contraceptive pills and emergency contraceptive pills • Provision of Injectable Contraceptives in MPV districts • Counselling and facilitation for safe abortion services • Medical methods of abortion (up to 7 weeks of pregnancy) on fix days at the HWC by PHC MO • Post abortion contraceptive counselling • Follow up for any complication after abortion and appropriate referral if needed • First aid for GBV related injuries – link to referral centre and legal support centre • Identification and management of RTIs/STIs • Identification, management (with referral as needed) in cases of dysmenorrhea, vaginal discharge, mastitis, breast lump, pelvic pain, pelvic organ prolapse	• Insertion of IUCD and Post-Partum IUCD • Removal of IUCD • Male sterilization including Non-scalpel Vasectomy • Female sterilization (Mini- Lap and Laparoscopic Tubectomy) • Management of all complications • Provision of Injectable Contraceptives • Medical methods of abortion (up to 7 weeks of pregnancy) with referral linkages MVA up to 8 weeks • Referral linkages with higher centre for cases beyond 8 weeks of pregnancy up to 20 weeks • Treatment of incomplete/ Inevitable/ Spontaneous Abortions • Second trimester MTP as per MTP Act and Guidelines • Management of all post abortion complications • Management of survivors of sexual violence as per medico legal protocols. • Management of GBV related injuries and facilitating linkage to legal support centre • Management of hormonal and menstrual disorders and cases of dysmenorrhea, vaginal discharge, mastitis, breast lump, pelvic pain, pelvic organ prolapse • Provision of diagnostic tests services such as (VDRL, HIV) • Management of RTIs/STIs • PPTCT at district level
5.	Management of communicable diseases and General Outpatient care for acute simple illness and minor ailments	• Symptomatic care for fevers, URIs, LRIs, body aches and headaches, with referral as needed • Identify and refer in case of skin infections and abscesses • Preventive action and primary care for waterborne disease, like diarrhoea, (cholera, other enteritis) and dysentery, typhoid, hepatitis (A and E) • Creating awareness about prevention, early identification and referral in cases of helminthiasis and rabies • Preventive and promotive measures to address Musculoskeletal disorders- mainly osteoporosis, arthritis and referral or follow up as indicated • Providing symptomatic care for aches and pains – joint pain, back pain etc	• Identification and management of common fevers, ARIs, diarrhoea, and skin infections. (Scabies and abscess) • Identification and management (with referral as needed) in cases of cholera, dysentery, typhoid, hepatitis and helminthiasis • Management of common aches, joint pains, and common skin conditions, (rash/urticaria)	• Diagnosis and management of all complicated cases (requiring admission) of fevers, gastroenteritis, skin infections, typhoid, rabies, helminthiasis, patitis acute • Specialist consultation for diagnostics and management of Musculoskeletal disorders, e.g.- arthritis.
6.	Management of Communicable diseases : National Health Programmes (Tuberculosis, Leprosy, Hepatitis, HIV-AIDS, Malaria, Kala-azar, Filariasis and Other vector borne diseases)	• Community awareness for prevention and control measures • Screening, Identification, prompt presumptive treatment initiation and referral as appropriate and specified for that level of care • Ensure compliance with follow up medication compliance	• Diagnosis, (or sample collection) treatment (as appropriate for that level of care) and follow up care for vector borne diseases – Malaria, Dengue, Chikungunya, Filaria, Kala Azar, Japanese Encephalitis, TB and Leprosy • Provision of DOTS for TB and MDT for leprosy	• Confirmatory diagnosis and initiation of treatment • Management of Complications, • Rehabilitative surgery in case of leprosy

S. No.	Health care services	Care at community level	Care at the Health and Wellness Centres-Sub Health Centres/ Urban Health and Wellness Centres	Care at the referral site** (PHC and upwards)
		• Mass drug administration in case of filariasis and facilitate immunization for Japanese encephalitis • Collection of blood slides in case of fever outbreak in malaria prone areas • Provision of DOTS/ensuring treatment adherence as per protocols in cases of TB	• HIV screening, appropriate referral and support for HIV treatment. • Referral of complicated cases	
7.	Prevention, Screening and Management of Non-Communicable diseases	• Population empanelment, support screening for universal screening for population - age 30 years and above for Hypertension, Diabetes, and three common cancers – Oral, Breast and Cervical Cancer • Health promotion activities – to promote healthy lifestyle and address risk factors • Early detection and referral for - Respiratory disorders – COPD, Epilepsy, Cancer, Diabetes, Hypertension and occupational diseases (Pneumoconiosis, dermatitis, lead poisoning) and Fluorosis • Mobilization activities at village level and schools for primary and secondary prevention • Treatment compliance and follow up for positive cases	• Screening and treatment compliance for Hypertension and Diabetes, with referral if needed • Screening and follow up care for occupational diseases (Pneumoconiosis, dermatitis, lead poisoning); fluorosis; respiratory disorders (COPD and asthma) and epilepsy • Cancer – screening for oral, breast and cervical cancer and referral for suspected cases of other cancers • Confirmation and referral for deaddiction – tobacco/ alcohol/ substance abuse • Treatment compliance and follow up for all diagnosed cases • Linking with specialists and undertaking two-way referral for complication	• Diagnosis, treatment and management of complications of Hypertension and Diabetes • Diagnosis, treatment and follow up of cancers (esp. Cervical, Breast, Oral) • Diagnosis and management of occupational diseases such as Silicosis, Fluorosis and respiratory disorders (COPD and asthma) and epilepsy
8.	Screening and Basic management of Mental health ailments	• Healthy life style tips-balanced diet, exercise, stress management. • Screening using CIDT tool for mental illness • Community awareness about mental disorders (Psychosis, Depression, Neurosis, Dementia, Mental Retardation, Autism, Epilepsy and Substance Abuse related disorders) • Patient Health Questionnaires 2 to be included in CBAC form. • Identification and referral to the HWC/ PHC for diagnosis • Ensure treatment compliance and follow up of patients with Severe Mental Disorders • Support home-based care by regular home visits to patients of Severe Mental Disorders • Facilitate access to support groups, day care centres and higher education/ vocational skills	• Awareness and stigma reduction activities at individual level & psychoeducation for all groups of MNG conditions • Promotion of mental health through family enrichment programme • Detection and referral of patients with severe mental disorders • Confirmation and referral to deaddiction Centres • Dispense follow up medication as prescribed by the Medical Officer at PHC/ CHC or by the Psychiatrist at DH. • Counselling and follow up of patients with Severe Mental Disorders • Suicide risk assessment, suicide management by gatekeepers, referrals, and follow-up for suicidal ideation and behaviour. • Formulation of comprehensive plan for persons with Dementia. • Establish linkages with NGOs, Government departments, PRIs, ULBs to facilitate access to entitlements and referral linkages with faith healers and referral and integrated coordination with other programmes. • Management of Violence related concerns	• Awareness and stigma reduction activities at individual level • Diagnosis and Treatment of mental illness • Suicide risk assessment, suicide management, referral, follow up and emergency management of poisoning • Emergency care for seizures • Provision of out -patient and in-patient services • Counselling services to patients (and family if available)
9.	Care for Common Ophthalmic and ENT problems	• Community based services, Counselling and support for care seeking for blindness, other eye and ENT disorders	• Awareness about common ophthalmic & ENT problems and illness through IEC • Screening for visual acuity, blindness, cataract and for refractive errors	• Advocacy for ENT services. • Management of all Acute and chronic eyes, ear, nose and throat problems • Surgical care for ear, nose, throat and eye

S. No.	Health care services	Care at community level	Care at the Health and Wellness Centres-Sub Health Centres/ Urban Health and Wellness Centres	Care at the referral site** (PHC and upwards)
		• Health Promotion through appropriate IEC with special emphasis on prevention of ophthalmic and ENT problems. • Community screening for congenital disorders and referral and early identification of ENT related problems like sign of hearing loss in infants, children and adults. • Screening for blindness and refractive errors and ENT problems • AWC based screening for children from 6 to 18 year through RBSK. • Recognizing and treating acute suppurative otitis media and other common ENT problems	• Identification and treatment of common eye problems – conjunctivitis, acute red eye, trachoma; spring catarrh, xeropthalmia as per the STG • Management of common colds, Acute Suppurative Otitis Media, injuries, pharyngitis, laryngitis, rhinitis, URI, sinusitis, epistaxis • Early detection of hearing impairment and deafness with referral • Diagnosis and treatment services for common diseases like otomycosis, otitis externa, ear discharge etc. • First aid for injuries/ stabilization and then referral. • Removal of Foreign Body. (Eye, Ear, Nose and throat) • Identification and referral of thyroid swelling, discharging ear, blocked nose, hoarseness and dysphagia	• Management of Cataract, Glaucoma, Diabetic retinopathy and Corneal ulcers and of referral cases from HWC-SHCs/ UHWCs. • Diagnosis and management of blindness, hearing and speech impairment • Management including nasal packing, tracheostomy, foreign body removal etc. • Offering support services to hearing aid users e.g., day to day care such as change of batteries, Do's & Don'ts while handling the aid etc. • Counselling and referral of patients with complications and which require surgical treatment.
10.	Basic oral health care	• Providing awareness about oral health & hygiene, and health care seeking practices through IEC and planned interactive sessions in home visits, community meetings of the VHSNC, MAS and VHNDS/ UHNDs and nutritional days in rural and urban area. • Create awareness, early detection and referral for fluorosis, and other common oral problems like caries, gingivitis and tooth loss etc. • Creating awareness about ill effects of Substance Abuse like tobacco, beetle and areca nut, smoking, reverse smoking and alcohol • Co-ordinate various Oral Health Care training programs to school teachers, volunteers and other self- Help groups for imparting preventive and promotive oral health education. • Participate and coordinate the outreach activities. • Symptomatic care for tooth ache and first aid for tooth trauma, with referrals • Mobilization for screening of oral cancer on screening day	• Providing awareness about oral health & hygiene, and health care seeking practices through IEC and planned interactive sessions. • Screening and early identification of common dental problems like gingivitis, periodontitis, malocclusion, dental caries, dental fluorosis and oral cancers, with referral • Oral health education about dental caries, periodontal diseases, malocclusion and oral cancers • Co-ordinate various Oral Health Care training programs to school teachers, volunteers and other self- Help groups for imparting preventive and promotive oral health education. • Management of conditions like apthous ulcers, candidiasis and glossitis, with referral for underlying disease • Participate and coordinate the outreach activities of PHC. • Symptomatic care for tooth ache and first aid for tooth trauma, with referral • Counselling for tobacco cessation and referral to Tobacco Cessation Centres. • Maintain records of all the identified oral diseases reporting in the OPD in a standardized recording format.	• Providing awareness to OPD patients about oral health & hygiene, and health care seeking practices through IEC and planned interactive sessions Diagnosis and management of oral cancer • Monitoring and ensuring quality care and smooth functioning of oral health services at HWCs. • Record keeping and maintenance of registries. • Conduct various Oral Health Care training programs to schoolteachers, volunteers and other Self- Help Groups. **Assured Services :** • Management of malocclusion, trauma cases, Tooth abscess, caries • Topical application of fluoride for caries prevention.
11.	Elderly and palliative health care service	• Identification of high-risk groups • Support to family in palliative care • Home visits for care to home bound/ bedridden elderly, disabled elderly persons • Support family in identifying behavioural changes in elderly and providing care • Linkage with other support groups and day care Centres etc. operational in the area.	• Home based care must be supported by a home visit by health care professional trained in palliative care and by linkages to day-to-day Centres and hospices to manage situations that are difficult to handle at home. • The CHO will be provided with a "Palliative- Care Kit". • Arrange for suitable supportive devices from higher Centres to the elderly /disabled persons to make them ambulatory.	• Provide awareness by sensitizing care givers, on prevention of fall, malnutrition and neglect of care, social security schemes, social entitlements etc. • OPD : Diagnosis, treatment and referral for complications. • Drugs & Consumables : Essential Drugs including Narcotics should be made available at PHC level. • Home care and End or Life Care. • Referral for those requiring secondary level of palliative care.

S. No.	Health care services	Care at community level	Care at the Health and Wellness Centres-Sub Health Centres/ Urban Health and Wellness Centres	Care at the referral site** (PHC and upwards)
		• Community mobilization on promotional, preventive and rehabilitative aspects of elderly. • Community awareness on various social security schemes for elderly • Identify and report elderly abuse cases, and provide family counselling	• Palliative care team should provide out of hours care to those who require end of life care. • Referral for diseases needing further investigation and treatment, to PHC/CHC/DH • CHOs to undertake Comprehensive Geriatric Assessment twice in a year for cognitive decline, limited mobility, malnutrition, visual impairment, hearing loss, and depressive symptoms. • Develop elderly self-help groups named Sanjeevani & ensure involvement of active and mobile elderly in various activities like awareness generation, assessment of fit elders. • Undertake monthly visit to bedbound elderly. • Ensure mobile elderly & restricted mobile elderly attend yoga/ activity sessions at HWCs. • Promote healthy behaviours. • Promote inter-generational bonding and involvement of elderly, ASHA & MPW to identify volunteers from youth groups. • Management of common geriatric ailments; counselling, supportive treatment • Pain Management and provision of palliative care with support of ASHA. • VHSNCs/JAS/MAS/RWA will ensure availability of benefits from various governments and non-governmental programs schemes to the eligible patients caregivers.	• Rehabilitation through physiotherapy and counselling • Identify care givers and empower them to take care of bed bound elderly. • Ensure continuous psychosocial support to family members and other informal care givers of care dependent elderly patients. • Impart training to care givers. • Provide dietary advice like oral supplemental nutrition etc. for undernourished elderly. • Advanced Comprehensive Geriatric Assessment. • Provision of diagnostics, equipment, consumables, medicines and services for Elderly leveraging other National Health Programmes. • Referral of elderly patients requiring secondary & tertiary care to higher Centre.
12.	Emergency Medical Services, including for Trauma and Burns	• Providing awareness to the community for handling emergencies in health. • First aid for trauma including management of minor injuries, fractures, animal bites and poisoning	• Providing awareness to the community for handling emergencies in health. • Stabilization care with Triaging based on ABCD criteria and first aid before referral in cases of – poisoning, trauma, minor injury, burns, respiratory arrest and cardiac arrest, fractures, shock, chocking, fits, drowning, animal bites and haemorrhage, infections (abscess and cellulitis), acute gastrointestinal conditions and acute genito urinary condition • Identify and refer cases for surgical correction – lumps and bumps (cysts/ lipoma/ hemangioma/ganglion); anorectal problems, hemorrhoids, rectal prolapse, hernia, hydrocele, varicocele, epidymo-orchitis, lymphedema, varicose veins, genital ulcers, bed ulcers, lower urinary tract symptoms (Phimosis, paraphimosis), and atrophic vaginitis. • Facilitate referral and basic management with communication to higher Centre. • Administer Td if not immunized.	• Triage and management of trauma cases • Management of poisoning, • Management of simple fractures and poly trauma • Basic surgery and surgical emergencies (Hernia, Hydrocele, Appendicitis, Haemorrhoids, Fistula, and stitching of injuries) etc. • Handling of all emergencies like animal bite, Congestive Heart Failure, Left Ventricular Failure, acute respiratory conditions, burns, shock, acute dehydration etc.

S. No.	Health care services	Care at community level	Care at the Health and Wellness Centres-Sub Health Centres/ Urban Health and Wellness Centres	Care at the referral site** (PHC and upwards)
13.	Linkages with Outreach Public Health surveillance, VHNDs, UHND and special outreach.	• The PRIs/ULBs and frontline workers shall be oriented on identification and reporting of any abnormal morbidity and mortality in human beings and animals. • VHNDs, UHNDs, AWCs and other community level facility platform can be identified for organizing VHND. • Community linkages with existing SHGs and Galli/Mohalla committees may also be utilized for the purpose. • The PRIs, ULBs and community should be oriented to participate in VHNDs and UHNDs for availing specific services being organized. • While attending physical distancing and infection prevention protocols needs to be adhered. • Collaboration with Urban Local bodies to strengthen the outreach and preventive and promotive functions including public health actions and surveillance.	• Capacity building/sensitization/ • Orientation of community/PRIs ULBs, frontline workers on public health issues, challenges and importance of timely reporting. • Facilitate testing of samples and timely submission of designated public health surveillance forms. • Planning for emergency preparedness and disaster management • Capacity building of PRIs/ULBs/ frontline workers as first responders during emergency. • Screening of early childhood diseases, through an active School Health Programme. • Identification of site for VHND/UHND. • Service delivery through VHND/UHND as per the GoI guidelines. • Need- based special outreach in urban areas.	• To support HWCs in their designated activities in public health importance including emergency preparedness and disaster management plan. • Timely management of all the referred cases.
14.	Services to be given by MO at UHWCs.	• In addition to the above the Medical Officer at UHWCs will also manage the clinical cases by proper diagnosis, treatment and follow up of patients. • He/she will supervise all the staff members working under UHWC, guide them, monitor their performance to ensure services are available to the community seamlessly.		

Please refer to Government of India publication "Indian Public Health Standards – Community Health Centre" 2022, Vol.-II, Ministry of Health and Family Welfare, New Delhi, for details about the types of Community Health Centres, human resources and services available in each type of community health centre.

JOB DESCRIPTION OF MEMBERS OF THE HEALTH TEAM

1. Medical Officer, PHC

1. He is the captain of the health team at the primary health centre. He devotes the morning hours attending to patients in the out-door; in the afternoon he supervises the field work.
2. His tour programme is so designed as to cover all the basic health services including family planning.
3. He will plan and implement UIP as per guidelines and ensure maximum possible coverage of the population in the PHC. He will ensure proper storage of vaccine and maintenance of cold chain equipment. He will ensure adequate supplies of vaccine and miscellaneous items required for the effective implementation of UIP.
4. He will ensure proper implementation of IMNCI as per guidelines.
5. He will visit schools in the PHC area at regular intervals and arrange for medical check up and immunization.
6. He will organize and conduct tubectomy and vasectomy camps.
7. Organize training of all health personnel like ASHA, anganwadi worker, Dais etc.
8. He ensures that national health programmes are being implemented in his area properly.
9. He visits each subcentre regularly on fixed days and hours and provides guidance, supervision and leadership to the health team.
10. He spends one day in each month organising staff meetings at the primary health centre to discuss the problems and review the progress of health activities.
11. The success of a primary health centre depends largely on the team leadership which the medical officer is able to provide. The medical officer must be the planner, the promoter, the director, the supervisor, the coordinator as well as the evaluator.

Second Medical Officer

The second medical officer performs identical duties.

2. Health worker Male and Female

Under The Multipurpose Worker Scheme, one health worker female and one health worker male are posted at each sub-centre and are expected to cover a population of 5000 (3000 in tribal and hilly areas). However, health worker female limits her activities among 350–500 families.

A. HEALTH WORKER FEMALE (ANM)

She will carry out the following functions :

1. Maternal and Child Health :

1.1 Register and provide care to pregnant women throughout the period of pregnancy.

1.2 Ensure that every pregnant woman makes at least 4 (four) visits for antenatal check-up according to suggested schedule.

1.3 Test urine of pregnant women for albumin and sugar. Estimate haemoglobin level.

1.4 Refer all pregnant women to PHC for RPR test for syphilis.

1.5 Refer cases of abnormal pregnancy and cases with medical and gynaecological problems to Health Assistant Female (LHV) or the Primary Health Centre.

1.6 Conduct deliveries in her area when called for.

1.7 Supervise deliveries conducted by Dais and assist them whenever called in.

1.8 Refer cases of difficult labour and newborns with abnormalities, help them to get institutional care and provide follow-up to the patients referred to or discharged from hospital.

1.9 ANM will identify the beneficiaries, complete necessary formalities and obtain necessary approvals of the competent authority before disbursement to the beneficiaries under Janani Suraksha Yojana (JSY), and by 7th of each month will submit accounts of the previous month in the prescribed format to be designed by the State. ANM will prepare a monthly work schedule in the meeting of all accredited workers to be held on every 3rd Friday of every month, which is mandatory. The guideline under JSY is to be followed.

1.10 Tracking of all pregnancies by name for scheduled ANC/PNC services.

1.11 Make post-natal home visits on 0, 3, 7 and 42nd day for deliveries at home and sub-centre and on 3,7, and 42nd day for institutional delivery. Post-natal visits are to be made for each delivery happened in her area and she should render advice regarding care of the mother and care and feeding of the newborn.

1.12 In case of low birth weight baby, a total of six post natal visits are to be made on 0, 3, 7, 14, 21 and 28th day to screen for congenital abnormalities, assess the neonate for danger signs of sickness etc. as per IMNCI guidelines and appropriate referral.

1.13 Initiation of early breast-feeding within one hour of birth, exclusive breast-feeding for 6 months and timely weaning at 6 months as per infant and young child feeding guidelines.

1.14 Assess the growth and development of the infants and under 5 children and make timely referral.

1.15 Provide treatment for all cases of diarrhoea, acute respiratory infections (pneumonia) and other minor ailments and refer cases of severe dehydration, respiratory distress, infections, severe acute malnutrition and other serious conditions as per IMNCI guidelines/national guidelines.

1.16 Educate mothers individually and in groups in better family health including maternal and child health, family planning, nutrition, immunization, control of communicable diseases, personal and environmental hygiene.

1.17 Assist Medical Officer and Health Assistant (Female) in conducting antenatal and postnatal clinics at the sub-centre.

2. Family Planning :

2.1 Utilize the information from the eligible couple and child register for the family planning programme. She will be responsible for maintaining eligible couple registers and updating at all times.

2.2 Distribute conventional contraceptives and oral contraceptives to the couples, provide facilities and to help prospective acceptors in getting family planning services, if necessary, by accompanying them or arranging for the Dai/ ASHA to accompany them to hospital.

2.3 Provide follow-up services to female family planning acceptors, identify side effects, give treatment on the spot for side effects and minor complaints and refer those cases that need attention by the physician to the PHC/Hospital.

2.4 Establish female depot holders, and provide a continuous supply of conventional contraceptives to the depot holders.

2.5 Build rapport with acceptors, village leaders, ASHA, Dais and others and utilize them for promoting Family Welfare Programme.

2.6 Identify women leaders and help the Health Assistant (Female) to train them.

2.7 Participate in Mahila Mandal meetings and utilize such gatherings for educating women in Family Welfare Programme.

3. Medical Termination of Pregnancy :

3.1 Identify the women requiring help for medical termination of pregnancy and refer them to nearest approved institution.

3.2 Educate the community of the consequences of septic abortion and inform them about the availability of services for medical termination of pregnancy.

4. Nutrition :

4.1 Identify cases of malnutrition among infants and young children (birth to five years), give the necessary treatment and advice and refer serious cases to the Primary Health Centre.

4.2 Distribute Iron and Folic Acid tablets as prescribed to pregnant women, nursing mothers, and young children (up to five years) as per the guidelines.

4.3 Administer Vitamin A solution to children as per the guidelines.

5. Universal Programme on Immunization (UIP) :

5.1 Immunize pregnant women with tetanus toxoid.

5.2 Administer pentavalent vaccine, DPT vaccine, oral poliomyelitis vaccine, IPV, measles vaccine, hepatitis B vaccine and BCG vaccine to all infants and children, as per immunization schedule.

5.3 Ensure injection safety, safe disposal and record, report and manage minor & serious Adverse Events Following Immunization (AEFI). Submit monthly UIP reports, weekly surveillance reports (AFP, measles under IDSP). Serious AEFI and outbreak should be reported immediately.

5.4 ANM is responsible for cold chain maintenance for vaccines during fixed and outreach sessions.

5.5 Manage waste generated during immunization as per GOI/CPCB guidelines.

5.6 Preparing work plan, estimating beneficiaries and logistics, preparing due list of expected beneficiaries in coordination with anganwadi worker and ASHA/mobilizer on the session day and ensure their vaccination through adequate mobilization.

5.7 Maintain tracking bag/tickler box at each sub-centre, file updated counterfoils and utilize them for follow up.

5.8 Tracking of dropouts and left outs, records/ reports (including MCH register and immunization card counterfoils), surveillance/ reporting Vaccine Associated Paralytic Poliomyelitis (VAPP) and AEFI incidents in catchment area.

5.9. Indent order of vaccines and logistics should be weekly, based on the due beneficiary list. HW/ alternate vaccinator should receive the required quantity of vaccine and logistics on the day of immunization and supply to the session site.

5.10 Work plan indicating village, place, date & time of organizing proposed session, including the names of ASHA and AWW must be displayed at each sub-centre.

5.11 Posters/paintings on key messages, immunization schedule, positioning during vaccine administration, Safe injection practices, VVM, AEFI awareness, use of hub cutters.

5.12 Village-wise dropout list for display at sub-centre.

5.13 Norm for due beneficiaries : 3 per session.

6. Dai Training : List Dais in her area and involve them in promoting family welfare; and help the Health Assistant (Female) / LHV in the training programme of Dais.

7. Communicable Diseases :

7.1 Notify the M.O. PHC immediately about any abnormal increase in cases of diarrhoea/ dysentery, fever with rigors, fever with rash, fever with jaundice acute flaccid paralysis in a child < 15 years (AFP), minor or serious AEFIs, or fever with unconsciousness which she comes across during her home visits, take the necessary measures to prevent their spread, and inform the Health Worker (male) to enable him to take further action.

7.2 If she comes across a case of fever during her home visits, she will take blood smear, administer radical treatment if the person is positive for malaria and inform Health Worker (male) for further action.

7.3 Identify cases of skin patches, especially if accompanied by loss of sensation, which she comes across during her home visits and bring them to the notice of the Health Worker (male)/ MO (PHC).

7.4 Assist the Health Worker (male) in maintaining a record of cases in her area, who are under treatment for malaria, tuberculosis and leprosy, and check whether they are taking regular treatment, motivate defaulters to take regular treatment and bring these cases to the notice of the Health Worker (male) or Health Assistant (male).

7.5 Give oral rehydration solution to all cases of diarrhoea/dysentery/vomiting.

Identify and refer all cases of blindness including suspected cases of cataract to M.O., PHC.

7.6 Education, counselling, referral, follow-up of cases STI/RTI, HIV/AIDS.

7.7 Where Filaria is endemic :

- Identification of cases of lymphoedema/ elephantiasis and hydrocele and their referrals to PHC/CHC for appropriate management.
- Training of patients with lymphoedema/ elephantiasis about care of feet and home based management remedies.
- Identification and training of drug distributors for mass drug distribution of DEC + albendazole on National Filaria Day.

8. Non Communicable Diseases : IEC for prevention and detection of non communicable diseases.

9. Vital Events : Record and report to the health authority of vital events including births and deaths, particularly of mothers and infants; and maintenance of all the relevant records concerning mothers, children and eligible couples in the area.

10. Record Keeping : (1) Register (a) pregnant women at earliest contact; (b) infants zero to one year of age; (c) under 5 years and adolescents; and (d) women aged 15 to 44 years; (2) Maintain the prenatal and maternity records and child care records; (3) Prepare the eligible couple and child register and maintaining it up-to-date; (4) Maintain the records as regards contraceptive distribution, IUD insertion, couples sterilized, clinics held at the sub-centre and supplies received and issued; (5) Prepare and submit the prescribed weekly/monthly reports in time to the Health Assistant (Female); and (6) While maintaining

passive surveillance register for malaria cases, she will record no. of fever cases, no. of blood slides prepared, no. of malaria positive cases reported, and no. of cases given radical treatment.

11. Treatment of minor ailments :

11.1 Provide treatment for minor ailments, provide first-aid for accidents and emergencies and refer cases beyond her competence to the Primary Health Centre/Community Health Centre or nearest hospital.

11.2 Provide treatment as per Indian System of Medicine (ISM), as needed, at the local level.

12. Team Activities :

12.1 Attend and participate in staff meetings at Primary Health Centre/Community Development Block or both.

12.2 Coordinate her activities with the Health Worker (male) and other health workers including the Health volunteers/ASHA and Dais.

12.3 Coordinate with the PRI and Village Health and Sanitation Committee.

12.4 Meet the Health Assistant (Female) each week and seek her advice and guidance whenever necessary.

12.5 Maintain the cleanliness of the sub-centre.

12.6 Dispose medical waste as per the guidelines.

12.7 Participate as a member of the team in camps and campaigns.

B. HEALTH WORKER MALE (HWM) *(34)*

I. National health programmes

His duties pertaining to different national health programmes are as follows:

A. National vector borne disease control programme

I. Malaria

1. Surveillance activities.
2. He shall collect thick and thin blood smears on one glass slide from case having fever or giving history of fever.
3. He shall contact the ASHAs and other FTDs, if any, during his fortnightly visit to the village and collect blood smears already taken by the ASHA, FTD and replenish both drugs and glass-slides and Rapid Diagnostic Kits (RDKs) and look into the account of consumption of anti malarial drugs and use of RDKs.
4. He shall dispatch blood smears along with MF-2 to the PHC Laboratory twice a week, or as instructed by the Medical Officer PHC.
5. He shall see the results obtained by the use of RDKs and verify the radical treatment administered by the ASHA, FTD, if any, during his visit.
6. He shall administer radical treatment to the positive cases as per drug schedule prescribed, and as per instructions issued by the Medical Officer PHC, and take laid down action if toxic manifestations are observed in a patient receiving radical treatment with primaquine.
7. He shall contact the ASHA and FTD and inform the spray dates, and make request to motivate the community and prepare them for accepting the spray operations.
8. Assist the Health Supervisor (Male)/ Health Assistant (Male) in supervising spraying operations and training of field spraying staff.

II. Kala-azar endemic areas : (1) From each family, he will enquire about presence of any fever case of more than 15 days duration; whether any guest of the house had fever/Kala-azar; or any family member of the house/ guest who had fever of more than 15 days duration left the village; (2) He will guide the suspected cases to the nearest PHC/CHC for diagnosis and treatment. He will keep a record of such cases and make sure that they take complete treatment; and (3) Health education about Kala-azar disease.

III. Japanese encephalitis (JE) endemic areas : From each family he will enquire about any fever case with symptoms of encephalitis and guide the suspected cases to the nearest PHC/CHC for diagnosis and treatment by the medical officer. He will keep the record of all the cases of JE in his area for follow-up.

IV. Filaria endemic areas : (1) Identification of cases of lymphoedema/elephantiasis and hydrocele and their referrals to PHC/CHC for appropriate management; (2) Train patients with lymphoedema/elephantiasis about care of feet and home based management remedies; and (3) Identification and training of drug distributors including ASHA for mass drug distribution of DEC + albendazole on National Filaria Day.

B. Leprosy eradication programme

1. Identify cases of skin patches, especially if accompanied by loss of sensation and refer these cases to M.O., PHC for further investigations diagnosis.
2. Check whether all cases of leprosy are taking regular treatment. Motivate defaulter to take regular treatment.
3. Maintain patient records.

C. Revised national tuberculosis control programme

(1) Identify persons especially 15 years and above, with prolonged cough or spitting of blood, and take sputum smears from these individuals. Refer cases to the M.O.PHC for further investigations; (2) Check whether all cases of tuberculosis are taking regular treatment. Motivate defaulters to take regular treatment; and (3) Assist the ASHA and similar village health volunteers to carry-out DOTS activities, and to motivate the TB patients in taking regular treatment.

D. National blindness control programme :

Identify and refer all cases of blindness including suspected cases of cataract to M.O., PHC.

E. Expanded programme on immunization :

(1) Administer DPT vaccine, oral poliomyelitis vaccine, measles vaccine and BCG vaccine to all infants and children and administer tetanus toxoid to all pregnant women in his area in collaboration with health worker (female); and (2) Assist the Health Assistant Male in the school immunization programme.

F. Reproductive and child health programme (RCH)

(1) Utilize the information from the eligible couple and child register for the family planning programme and spread the message of family planning to the couples;

(2) Distribute conventional contraceptives and oral contraceptives to the couples and help prospective acceptors of sterilization in obtaining the services; (3) Provide follow-up services to male family Planning acceptors, and refer those cases that need attention by the physician to PHC/Hospital; (4) Build rapport with satisfied acceptors, village leaders, ASHA, Dais and others and utilize them for promoting family welfare Programme; (5) Educate the community on the availability of service for Medical Termination of Pregnancy; (6) Report any outbreak of diarrhoea disease; (7) Measures such as chlorination of drinking water to be carried out; (8) Proper sanitation to be maintained; (9) Encourage use of latrines; and (10) Identify and refer cases of genital sore or urethral discharge or non-itchy rash over the body to medical officer.

II. Communicable diseases

(1) Identify cases of diarrhoea/dysentery, fever with rash jaundice, encephalitis, diphtheria, whooping cough, tetanus, and acute eye infections and notify the Health Assistant Male and M.O. PHC immediately about these cases; (2) Give Oral Rehydration solution to all cases of diarrhoea/dysentery/vomiting; (3) Educate the community about the importance of control and preventive measures against communicable diseases and about the importance of taking regular and complete treatment; and (4) Counselling about HIV and STD.

III. Environmental sanitation

(1) Chlorinate public water sources including wells at regular intervals; and (2) Educate community on (a) the method of disposal of liquid wastes; (b) the method of disposal of solid wastes; (c) home sanitation; (d) advantage and use of sanitary type of latrines; and (e) construction and use of smokeless chulhas.

IV. Nutrition

Identify cases of low birth weight and malnutrition among infants and young children (0–5 years) in his area, give the necessary treatment and advice or refer them to the anganwadi for supplementary feeding and refer serious cases to the PHC.

V. Vital events

Record births and deaths occurring in his area, and educate the community on the importance of registration of births and deaths.

VI. Record Keeping

(1) Survey all the facilities in his area and prepare/maintain maps and charts for the village; (2) Prepare, maintain and utilize family and village records; (3) Assist the Health Worker (Female)/ANM to prepare and maintain the eligible couple as well as maternal & child health register; (4) Maintain a record of cases in his area, who are under treatment for tuberculosis and leprosy; (5) Prepare and submit the prescribed monthly reports in time to the Health Supervisor (Male); and (6) While maintaining passive surveillance register for malaria cases, he will record: no. of fever cases, no. of blood slides prepared, no. of malaria positive cases reported, and no. of cases given radical treatment.

3A. Job responsibilities of Health Assistant (Female)

Under the multipurpose workers scheme, a health assistant (female) is expected to cover a population of 30,000 (20,000 in tribal and hilly areas) in which there are six sub-centres, each with one health worker (female).

The health assistant (female) will carry out the following functions :

1. Supervision and guidance : (1) Supervise and guide the health worker (female) in the delivery of health care services to the community; (2) Strengthen the knowledge and skills of the health worker (female); (3) Visit each sub-centre at least once a week on a fixed day to observe and guide the health worker (female) in her day-to-day activities; (4) Assess periodically the progress of work of the health worker (female), and submit an assessment report to the medical officer of the primary health centre; and (5) Carry out supervisory home visits in the area of the health worker (female).
2. Team work : (1) Help the health worker to work as part of the health team; (2) Co-ordinate her activities with those of the health assistant (male) and other health personnel including the *dais*; (3) Co-ordinate the health activities in her area with the activities of workers of other departments and agencies, and attend meetings at block level; (4) Conduct regular staff meetings with the health workers in coordination with the health assistant (male); (5) Attend staff meetings at the primary health centre; (6) Assist the medical officers of the primary health centre in the organization of the different health services in the area; and (7) Participate as a member of the health team in mass camps and campaigns in health programmes.
3. Supplies, equipment and maintenance of sub-centre : (1) In collaboration with the health assistant (male), check at regular intervals the stores at the sub-centre and help in the procurement of supplies and equipment; (2) Check that the drugs at the sub-centre are properly stored and the equipment is well maintained; (3) Ensure that the health worker (female) maintains her general kit and midwifery kit in the proper way; and (4) Ensure that the sub-centre is kept clean.
4. Records and reports : (1) Scrutinize the maintenance of records by the health worker (female) and guide her in their proper maintenance; (2) Maintain the prescribed records and prepare the necessary reports; and (3) Review reports received from the health workers (female), consolidate them, and submit periodical reports to the medical officer of the primary health centre.
5. Where Kala-azar is endemic, her additional duties are: (1) She should check minimum of 10% of the house in a village to verify that the health worker (female) really visited those houses and carried her job of identifying suspected Kala-azar cases and ensuring complete treatment has been done properly; (2) She will carry with her the proper record forms, diary and guidelines for identifying suspected Kala-azar cases; and she will be responsible along with Health Assistant (Male) for ensuring complete treatment of Kala-azar patients in her area; (3) She will be responsible along with health assistant (male) for ensuring complete coverage during the spray activities and search operation; and (4) She will also undertake health education activities

particularly through interpersonal communication, arrange group meetings with leaders and organizing and conducting training of community leaders with the assistance of health team.

6. Where lymphatic filariasis is endemic, her specific duties are: (1) She should check minimum of 10% of the houses in a village to verify that the health worker (female) really visited those houses and carried her job properly; (2) She will be responsible along with Health Assistant (male) for ensuring compliance of drug more than 80% during mass drug administration; and (3) She will also undertake health education activities particularly through interpersonal communication, arrange group meetings with leaders and organizing and conducting training of community leaders with the assistance of health team.
7. Where Japanese Encephalitis is endemic, her specific duties are: (1) She should check along with minimum of 10% of the houses in a village to verify that the health worker (female) really visited those houses and carried her job properly. Her job of identifying suspected JE cases and ensuring complete treatment has been done properly; (2) She will carry with her proper record form and guidelines for identifying suspected JE cases; (3) She will be responsible for ensuring complete treatment of JE patients in her area; (4) She will be responsible along with health assistant male for ensuring complete coverage during the spray activities and search operation; and (5) She will undertake health education activities about the disease particularly through interpersonal communication.
8. Training : Organize and conduct training for *dais*/ASHA with the assistance of the health worker (female).
9. Maternal and child health : (1) Conduct weekly MCH clinics at each sub-centre with the assistance of the health worker (female); (2) Respond to calls from the health worker (female) and trained *dais*, and from the health worker (male) and render necessary help; and (3) Conduct deliveries when required at PHC level and provide domiciliary and midwifery services.
10. Family welfare and medical termination of pregnancy : (1) Conduct weekly family welfare clinics (alongwith the MCH clinics) at each sub-centre with the assistance of the health worker (female); (2) Personally motivate resistant cases for family planning; (3) Provide information on the availability of services for medical termination of pregnancy and refer suitable cases to the approved institutions; (4) Guide the health worker (female) in establishing female depot holders for the distribution of conventional contraceptives and train the depot holders with the assistance of the health worker (female); (5) Through spot checking, she will ensure that health worker (female) maintains up-to-date eligible couple register; (6) Provide IUD services and their follow-up; and (7) Assist medical officer PHC in organizing family planning camps.
11. Nutrition :

    (1) Identify cases of malnutrition among infants and young children (zero to five years), give the necessary treatment and advice and refer serious cases to the primary health centre/community health centre; (2) Ensure that iron and folic acid tablets; and vitamin A solution are distributed to the beneficiaries; and (3) Educate the expectant mother regarding breast feeding.
12. Immunization : (1) Supervise the immunization of all pregnant women and children (0–5) years; and (2) She will guide the health worker (female) to procure supplies, organize immunization camps, provide guidance for maintaining cold chain, storage of vaccine and health education about immunization programme.
13. Acute respiratory infection : (1) Ensure early diagnosis of pneumonia cases; (2) Provide suitable treatment to mild/moderate cases of ARI; and (3) Ensure early referral in doubtful/severe cases.
14. School health : Help medical officer in school health services.
15. Primary medical care : (1) Provide treatment for minor ailments, provide first-aid for accidents and emergencies, and refer cases beyond her competence to the primary health centre or nearest hospital; and (2) Attend to cases referred by the health workers and refer cases beyond her competence to the primary health centre or nearest hospital.
16. Health education : (1) Carry out educational activities for MCH, family planning, nutrition, control of blindness, dental care and immunization with the assistance of the health worker (female); (2) Arrange group meetings with leaders and involve them in spreading the message for various health programmes; (3) Organize and conduct training of woman leaders with the assistance of health worker (female); and (4) Organize and utilize *mahila mandals*, teachers, ICDS personel and other women in the community in the family welfare programmes.

3B. Specific Job functions of Health Assistant (Male) *(35)*

Under the Multipurpose workers scheme a Health Assistant Male is expected to cover a population of 30,000 (20,000 in tribal and hilly areas) in which there are six sub-centres, each with the health worker male. He will carry out following duties:

1. Supervise and guidance : (1) Supervise and guide the Health Worker Male, in the delivery of health care service to the community; (2) Strengthen the knowledge and skills of the Health Worker Male; (3) Help the Health Worker Male in improving his skills in working in the community; (4) Help and guide the Health Worker Male in planning and organizing in programmes of activities; (5) Visit each Health Worker Male at least once a week on a fixed day to observe and guide him in his day to day activities; (6) Assess monthly the progress of work of the Health Worker Male and submit with assessment report to the medical officer of the primary helth centre; and (7) Carry out supervisory home visits in the area of the Health Worker Male.
2. Team Work : (1) Help the health workers to work as part of the health team; (2) Coordinate his activities with those of the Health Assistant Female and other health personnel including the Dais and Health Guide; (3) Coordinate the health activities in his area with the activities of workers of other departments and agencies and attend meetings; (4) Conduct staff meetings fortnightly with the health workers in coordination with

the Health Assistant Female at one of the sub-centres by rotation; (5) Attend staff meetings at the primary health centre; (6) Assist the medical officer of the primary health centre in the organization of the different health services; (7) Participate as a member of the health team in mass camps and campaigns in health programmes; (8) Assist the medical officer of the primary health centre in conducting training programmes for various categories of health personnel; and (9) Facilitate and participate in the activities of village health & nutrition day.

3. Supplies, equipment and maintenance of sub-centres : (1) In collaboration with the Health Assistant Female, check at regular intervals the stores at the sub-centres and ensure timely placement of supplies and equipment; (2) Check that the drugs at the sub-centre are properly stored and that the equipment is well maintained; and (3) Ensure that the Health Worker Male maintains his general kit in proper way.

4. Records and reports : (1) Scrutinize the maintenance of records by the Health Worker Male and guide him in their proper maintenance; and (2) Review records received from the Health Worker Male, consolidate them and submit reports to the medical officer of the primary health centre.

5. Malaria :

   (1) He will supervise the work of Health Worker Male during concurrent visits and will check whether the worker is performing his duty as laid down in the schedule; (2) He should check minimum of 100 of the houses in a village to verify the work of the Health Worker Male; (3) He will carry with him a kit for collection of blood smears during his visit to the field and collect thick and thin smears from any fever case he comes across.; (4) He will be responsible for prompt radical treatment to positive cases in his area. He will plan, execute and supervise the administration of radical treatment in consultation with PHC medical officer; and (5) Supervise the spraying of insecticides during local spraying along with the Health Worker Male.

6. Where Kala-Azar is endemic additional duties are:

   (1) He will supervise the work of Health Worker Female during concurrent visit and will check whether the worker is performing her duties; (2) He should check minimum of 10% of the house in a village to verify that the Health Worker Male really visited those houses and carried his job properly. His job of identifying suspected Kala-Azar cases and ensuring complete treatment has been done properly; (3) He will carry with him the proper record forms, diary and guidelines for identifying suspected Kala-Azar cases; (4) He will be responsible for ensuring complete coverage treatment of Kala-Azar patients in his area; (5) He will be responsible for ensuring complete coverage during the spray activities and search operation; and (6) He will also undertake health education activities particularly through interpersonal communication, arranging group meetings with leaders and organizing and conducting training of community leaders with the assistance of health team.

7. Where Japanese Encephalitis is endemic his specific duties are as below :

   (1) He will supervise the work of Health Worker Female during concurrent visit and will check whether the worker is performing her duties; (2) He should check minimum of 10% of the house in a village to verify that the Health Worker Male really visited those houses and carried his job properly. His job of identifying suspected encephalitis cases and ensuring motivation of community has been done properly; (3) He will carry with him the proper record forms , diary and guidelines for identifying suspected encephalitis cases; and (4) He will also undertake health education activities particularly through interpersonal communication, arranging group meetings with leaders and organizing and conduction training of community leaders with the assistance of health team.

8. Where Lymphatic Filariasis is endemic, his specific duties are as follows :

   (1) He will supervise the work of Health Worker Male and volunteers during concurrent visit and will check whether the worker is performing his duties; (2) He should check minimum 10% of the houses in a village to verify that the health worker (male) really visited those houses and carried his job properly; (3) He will carry with him the proper record forms, diary and guidelines for Mass Drug Administration (MDA) and drug distribution; (4) He will be responsible for ensuring coverage and compliance of drug above 80% during MDA; and (5) He will also undertake health education activities particularly through interpersonal communication, arranging group meetings with leaders and organizing and conducting training of community leaders with the assistance of health team.

9. Communicable diseases :

   9.1 Be alert to the sudden outbreak of epidemics of diseases such as diarrhoea/dysentery, fever with rash, jaundice, enecephalitis, diphtheria, whooping cough or tetanus, acute eye infections and take all possible remedial measures.

   9.2 Take the necessary control measures when any notifiable disease is reported to him. Carry out the destruction of stray dogs with the help of the Health Worker Male.

10. Leprosy :

    Ensure that all cases of Leprosy take regular and complete treatment and inform the Medical Officer PHC about any defaulters to treatment.

11. Tuberculosis :

    Ensure that all cases of tuberculosis take regular and complete treatment and inform the M.O. PHC about any defaulters to treatment.

12. Environmental sanitation

    Help the community in the construction of :

    (a) safe water source; (b) soakage pits; (c) kitchen garden; (d) manure pits; (e) compost pits; (f) Sanitary latrines; and (g) smokeless chulhas and supervise their construction. Supervise the chlorination of water source including wells.

13. Expanded programme on immunization :

    13.1 Conduct immunization of all school going children with the help of the Health Worker Male.

    13.2 Supervise the immunization of all children from one to five years.

14. Family planning : (1) Personally motivate resistant cases for family planning; (2) Guide the Health Worker Male in establishing male depot holders with the assistance of the Health Worker Male and supervise the functioning; (3) Assist M.O.PHC in organization of Family Planning camps and drives; (4) Provide information on the availability of services for medical termination of pregnancy and refer suitable cases to the approved institutions; and (5) Ensure follow-up of all cases of vasectomy, tubectomy, IUD and other Family Planning acceptors.
15. Nutrition : Ensure that all cases of malnutrition among infants and young children (0–5 years) are given the necessary treatment and advice and refer serious cases to the PHC and ensure that Iron and Folic Acid and Vitamin A are distributed to the beneficiaries as prescribed.
16. Control of blindness : All cases of blindness including suspected cases of cataract be referred to Medical Officer of Primary Health Centre.

4. Accredited Social Health Activist (ASHA)

The job responsibility of ASHA, and the integration of her role with anganwadi and ANM are described in detail on page 700.

HEALTH INSURANCE

Rashtriya Swasthya Bima Yojana (RSBY) *(40)*

Rashtriya Swasthya Bima Yojana (RSBY) was a centrally sponsored scheme to provide health insurance cover of Rupees 30,000/- per family per annum on family floater basis (maximum 5 members per family) to Below Poverty Line (BPL) families and 11 other categories of Unorganized Workers i.e MGNREGA Workers, Construction Workers, Domestic workers, Sanitation Workers, Mine Workers, licensed Railway Porters, Street Vendors, Beedi Workers, Rickshaw Pullers, Rag Pickers, and Auto/Taxi drivers. The Scheme was launched by Ministry of Labour and employment in 2008 and transferred to Ministry of Health & Family Welfare on "as is where is" basis with effect from 01.04.2015.

Each family enrolled in the scheme was entitled to hospitalization benefits of up to INR 30,000 per annum in Government as well as empanelled private hospitals. 1516 treatment packages were covered under RSBY. A network of more than eight thousand hospitals was developed by empanelling 4860 private hospitals and 3677 public hospitals under RSBY scheme. Before the launch of Pradhan Mantri Jan Arogya Yojana (PMJAY), around 2.75 crore families were covered under the scheme. With the launch of PMJAY on 23.09.2018, RSBY was subsumed in it.

Ayushman Bharat – Pradhan Mantri Jan Arogya Yojana (AB-PMJAY) *(40)*

The Ayushman Bharat – Pradhan Mantri Jan Arogya Yojana (AB PM-JAY) is the flagship scheme of Government of India that provides a health cover of up to Rs. 5 Lakhs per family per year, for secondary and tertiary hospitalizations to over 10.74 Crore poor and vulnerable families (approximately 50 Crore people). Launched on 23rd September 2018, PM-JAY has been designed to provide financial risk protection against catastrophic health expenditure that impoverishes an estimated 6 Crore people every year.

The number of individual beneficiaries verified under AB PM-JAY stands at nearly 16 Crores. Over 21,800 hospitals have been empanelled under the scheme till date. This has facilitated over 1.82 Crore hospitalizations, saving beneficiaries over Rs. 22,500 Crore in out of pocket medical expenditure.

Benefits

- Health cover of up to Rs. 5,00,000 per family per year, for secondary and tertiary care hospitalization;
- Cashless access to hospitalization services;
- No cap on family size, age or gender;
- All pre-existing conditions are covered;
- Benefits are portable across the country in all empanelled hospitals;
- 1685 procedures covering treatment, food, drugs and supplies, and diagnostics services; and
- PM-JAY covers cost of hospitalization, treatment, up to 3 days of pre-hospitalization and 15 days of post hospitalization follow-up care.

For further details refer to chapter 7.

Employees State Insurance Scheme

The ESI scheme, introduced by an Act of Parliament in 1948, is a unique piece of social legislation in India. It has introduced for the first time in India the principle of contribution by the employer and employee. The Act provides for medical care in cash and kind, benefits in the contingency of sickness, maternity, employment injury, and pension for dependents on the death of worker because of employment injury. The Act covers employees drawing wages not exceeding Rs. 21,000 per month (see chapter 18 for details).

Central Government Health Scheme

The Central Government Health Scheme (previously known as Contributory Health Service Scheme) for the Central Government employees was first introduced in New Delhi in 1954 to provide comprehensive medical care to Central Government employees. The scheme is based on the principle of cooperative effort by the employee and the employer, to the mutual advantage of both.

The facilities under the scheme include : (a) out-patient care through a network of dispensaries; (b) supply of necessary drugs; (c) laboratory and X-ray investigations (d) domiciliary visits; (e) hospitalization facilities at Government as well as private hospitals recognized for the purpose; (f) specialist consultation; (g) paediatric services including immunization; (h) antenatal, natal and postnatal services; (i) emergency treatment; (j) supply of optical and dental aids at reasonable rate; and (k) family welfare services.

The scope of the scheme has been gradually extended over the years to cover cities outside Delhi as well as other sectors of population such as the employees of the autonomous organizations, retired Central Govt. servants, widows receiving family pension, Members of Parliament, Ex-Governors and retired Judges. The Scheme now covers besides Delhi, the cities of Mumbai, Allahabad, Meerut, Kanpur, Patna, Kolkata, Nagpur, Chennai, Hyderabad, Bangalore, Jaipur, Pune, Lucknow, Ahmedabad, Bhubaneswar, and Jabalpur.

The scheme which started with 16 allopathic dispensaries in 1954 covering 2.3 lakh beneficiaries. Over the time, the scheme has spread to 72 cities. It serves nearly 12.83 lakh primary cardholders and about 37.49 lakh beneficiaries.

CGHS has 4 hospitals in Delhi and 417 CGHS Wellness Centres and Units (329 Allopathic and 88 AYUSH) in the country at different locations / cities and providing medical care to its members in Allopathic, Homeopathic, Ayurvedic, Unani and siddha systems of medicine. CGHS has empanelled 1403 Hospitals (including Eye Care and Dental Clinics) and 272 Diagnostic Centres in different CGHS Cities *(40)*.

The Employees State Insurance Scheme and the Central Government Health Scheme cover two large groups of wage -earners in the country. They are well-organized health insurance schemes, and are providing reasonable medical care plus some essential preventive and promotive health services. Experience in other countries has shown that health insurance is a logical step towards nationalization of health services.

OTHER AGENCIES

Defence Medical Services

Defence services have their own organization for medical care to defence personnel under the banner "Armed Forces Medical Services". The services provided are integrated and comprehensive embracing preventive, promotive and curative services.

Health Care of Railway Employees

The Railways provide comprehensive health care services through the agency of Railway Hospitals, Health Units and clinics. Environmental sanitation is taken care of by Health Inspectors in big stations. A chief Health Inspector supervises the division's work. Heath check-up of employees is provided at the time of entry into service, and thereafter at yearly intervals. There are lady medical officers, health visitors and midwives who look after the MCH and School Health Services. Specialists' services are also available at the Divisional Hospitals.

PRIVATE AGENCIES

In a mixed economy such as India, private practice of medicine provides a large share of the health services available. There has been a rapid expansion in the number of qualified allopathic physicians from about 50,000 at the time of Independence to about 7.67 lakhs in 2005 and the doctor-population ratio for the country as a whole was 1 : 1428. The general practitioners constitute 70 per cent of the medical profession. Most of them tend to congregate in urban areas. They provide mainly curative services. Their services are available to those who can pay. The private sector of the health care services is not organized. Some statutory bodies like the Medical Council of India and the Indian Medical Association regulate some of the functions and activities of the large body of private registered medical practitioners.

INDIGENOUS SYSTEMS OF MEDICINE

The practitioners of indigenous systems of medicine (e.g., Ayurveda, Siddha, Homoeopathy, etc.) provide the bulk of medical care to the rural people. Ayurvedic physicians alone are estimated to be about 7.73 lakhs *(36)*. Studies indicate that nearly 90 per cent of Ayurvedic physicians serve the rural areas. Most of them are local residents and remain very close to the people socially and culturally. In recent years there has been considerable state patronage to foster these systems of medicine. Many ayurvedic dispensaries are state-run. The Govt. of India has established a National Institute of Ayurveda in Jaipur and a National Institute of Homoeopathy in Kolkata. A Central Council of Indian Medicine was established in 1971 to prescribe minimum standards of education in Indian medicine. The Govt. of India is studying the question of how indigenous systems of medicine could best be utilized for more effective or total health coverage.

VOLUNTARY HEALTH AGENCIES

The voluntary health agencies occupy an important place in community health programmes. "A voluntary health agency may be defined as an organisation that is administered by an autonomous board which holds meetings, collects funds for its support chiefly from private sources and expends money, whether with or without paid workers, in conducting a programme directed primarily to furthering the public health by providing health services or health education, or by advancing research or legislation for health, or by a combination of these activities" *(37)*. The one country where voluntary health agencies have developed and flourished to an enormous extent is the United States. Even in 1945, it was estimated that there were more than 20,000 voluntary agencies in the United States. The voluntary health agencies have been compared to "motor trucks" which can penetrate the by-ways, and the official agencies to "Railway Trunk Lines" which must run on tracks established by law *(38)*.

FUNCTIONS

The types of service rendered by voluntary health agencies have been classified as : (a) SUPPLEMENTING THE WORK OF GOVERNMENT AGENCIES : It is well known that government agencies cannot provide complete service because they operate under financial and statutory restrictions. The voluntary health agencies can help strengthen the work of government agencies by lending personnel, or by contributing funds for special equipment, supplies or services. (b) PIONEERING : The voluntary health agencies are in a position to explore ways and means of doing new things. Research is one form of pioneering. When the efforts succeed and bear fruit, the government agencies can step in and take over the project for the benefit of the larger numbers. The family planning programme in India is an example of pioneering by the voluntary agencies which first spearheaded the movement, in the face of much opposition. When the importance of family planning was realised, the government accepted family planning as a national policy. (c) EDUCATION : There is unlimited scope for health education in India. The government agencies cannot cope with the problem, unless it is supplemented by voluntary effort on the part of the people. (d) DEMONSTRATION : By putting up demonstrations and experimental projects, the voluntary health agencies have advanced the cause of public health. The demonstration of bore hole latrines by the Rockefeller Foundation to solve the problem of hookworm in India is a case in point. The bore-hole latrine and its modifications have since become an essential part of the environmental sanitation programme in India. (e) GUARDING THE WORK OF GOVERNMENT AGENCIES : By setting a good example the voluntary health agencies can always guide and criticise the work of government agencies. (f) ADVANCING HEALTH LEGISLATION : The voluntary agencies can also mobilise public opinion and advance legislation on health matters for the benefit of the whole community.

VOLUNTARY HEALTH AGENCIES IN INDIA *(39)*

1. INDIAN RED CROSS SOCIETY : The Indian Red Cross Society was established in 1920. It has a network of over 400 branches all over India. It has been executing programmes for the promotion of health, prevention of disease and mitigation of suffering among the people. Its activities are : (a) RELIEF WORK : When disaster strikes any part of the country in the shape of earth-quakes, floods, drought, epidemics, etc., the Red Cross Society immediately mobilises all its resources and goes to the rescue of the affected people. (b) MILK AND MEDICAL SUPPLIES : A number of hospitals, dispensaries, maternity and child welfare centres, schools and orphanges receive assistance from the society every year. The assistance given consists mainly of milk powder, medicines, vitamins and other supplies. (c) ARMED FORCES : The care of the sick and the wounded among the members of the forces is one of the primary obligations of the Red Cross. The Society runs a well-equipped hospital, 'the Red Cross Home' in Bangalore – the only one of its kind in India and the Far East – for permanently disabled ex-servicemen. (d) MATERNAL AND CHILD WELFARE SERVICES : There are a large number of maternity and child welfare centres all over India, either directly administered by or are affiliated to the Red Cross. There is a bureau of Maternity and Child Welfare, which provides technical advice and financial aid to schemes for establishing model maternity and child welfare centres. (e) FAMILY PLANNING : Several States in India are running family planning clinics under the auspices of the Indian Red Cross. (f) BLOOD BANK AND FIRST AID : Some of the State branches have started blood banks. The St. John Ambulance Association in India which is part of the Red Cross has trained several lakh men and women in first aid, home nursing and allied subjects.

2. HIND KUSHT NIVARAN SANGH : The Hind Kusht Nivaran Sangh was founded in 1950 with its headquarters in New Delhi. Its precursor was the Indian Council of the British Empire Leprosy Relief Association (B.E.L.R.A.) which was renamed as LEPRA in 1950. The programme of work of the Sangh includes rendering of financial assistance to various leprosy homes and clinics, health education through publications and posters, training of medical workers and physiotherapists, conducting research and field investigations, organising All-India Leprosy Workers Conferences and publication of 'Leprosy in India', a quarterly journal. The Sangh has branches all over India and works in close cooperation with the Government and other voluntary agencies.

3. INDIAN COUNCIL FOR CHILD WELFARE : Indian Council for Child Welfare was established in 1952. It is affiliated with the International Union for Child Welfare. Since its formation, the I.C.C.W. has built up a network of State Councils and district councils all over the country. The services of I.C.C.W. are devoted to secure for India's children those "opportunities and facilities, by law and other means" which are necessary to enable them to develop physically, mentally, morally, spiritually and socially in a healthy and normal manner and in conditions of freedom and dignity.

4. TUBERCULOSIS ASSOCIATION OF INDIA : The Tuberculosis Association of India was formed in 1939. It has branches in all the States in India. The activities of this Association comprise organising a T.B. Seal campaign every year to raise funds, training of doctors, health visitors and social workers in antituberculosis work, promotion of health education and promotion of consultations and conferences. The following institutions are under the management of the Association : The New Delhi Tuberculosis Centre, the Lady Linlithgow Sanatorium at Kasauli, the King Edward VII Sanatorium at Dharampur and the Tuberculosis Hospital at Mehrauli.

5. BHARAT SEVAK SAMAJ : The Bharat Sevak Samaj which is a non-political and non-official organization was formed in 1952. One of the prime objectives of the Bharat Sevak Samaj (B.S.S.) is to help people to achieve health by their own actions and efforts. The B.S.S. has branches in all the States and in nearly all the districts. Improvement of sanitation in villages is one of the important activities of the B.S.S.

6. CENTRAL SOCIAL WELFARE BOARD : The Central Social Welfare Board is an autonomous organization under the general administrative control of the Ministry of Education. It was set up by the Government of India in August 1953. The functions of the Board are :– (1) surveying the needs and requirements of voluntary welfare organizations in the country (2) promoting and setting up of social welfare organizations on a voluntary basis (3) rendering of financial aid to deserving existing organizations and institutions. The Board initiated, in 1968, "Family and Child Welfare Services" in rural areas for the welfare of women and children. The activities of these projects comprise teaching of craft, social education, literacy classes, maternity aid for women, distribution of milk, balwadis, and organisation of play centres for children. The Board has also started a scheme of Industrial Cooperatives to help the lower-middle class women in urban areas supplement their family income by doing paid work.

7. THE KASTURBA MEMORIAL FUND : Created in commemoration of Kasturba Gandhi, after her death in 1944, the Fund was raised with the main object of improving the lot of women, especially in the villages, through gram-sevikas. The trust has nearly a crore of rupees and is actively engaged in various welfare projects in the country.

8. FAMILY PLANNING ASSOCIATION OF INDIA : The Family Planning Association was formed in 1949 with its headquarters at Mumbai. It has done pioneering work in propagating family planning in India. The Association has branches all over the country. These branches are running family planning clinics with grants-in-aid from the Government. The Association has trained several hundred doctors, health visitors and social workers. One of the activities of the Headquarters is to answer enquiries on family planning by correspondence or by personal interviews.

9. ALL INDIA WOMEN'S CONFERENCE : It is the only women's voluntary welfare organisation in the country. Established in 1926, it has now branches all over the country. Most of the branches are running M.C.H. Clinics, Medical centres, and adult education centres, milk centres and family planning clinics.

10. THE ALL-INDIA BLIND RELIEF SOCIETY : The All-India Blind Relief Society was established in 1946 with a view to coordinate different institutions working for the blind. It organises eye relief camps and other measures for the relief of the blind.

11. PROFESSIONAL BODIES : The Indian Medical Association, All India Licentiates Association, All India Dental Association, The Trained Nurses Association of India

are all voluntary agencies of men and women who are qualified in their respective specialities and possess registerable qualifications. These professional bodies conduct annual conferences, publish journals, arrange scientific sessions and exhibitions, foster research, set up standards of professional education and organise relief camps during periods of natural calamities.

12. INTERNATIONAL AGENCIES : The Rockefeller Foundation, Ford Foundation, and CARE (Cooperative for Assistance & Relief Everywhere) are examples of voluntary international health agencies.

HEALTH PROGRAMMES IN INDIA

Since India became free, several measures have been undertaken by the National Government to improve the health of the people. Prominent among these measures are the NATIONAL HEALTH PROGRAMMES, which have been launched by the Central Government for the control/eradication of communicable diseases, improvement of environmental sanitation, nutrition, control of population and rural health. Various international agencies like WHO, UNICEF, UNFPA, World Bank, as also a number of foreign agencies like SIDA, DANIDA, NORAD and USAID have been providing technical and material assistance in the implementation of these programmes. A brief account of these programmes which are currently in operation is given in chapter 7.

References

1. Last J.M. ed (1993). *A Dictionary of Epidemiology,* Oxford University Press. New York.
2. WHO (1971). *Techn Rep Ser.,* 472.
3. WHO (1984). *Public Health Paper,* No. 80.
4. WHO (1987). *Seventh Rep. World Health Situation*. Vol. 1.
5. WHO (1987). *Techn Rep. Ser.,* No. 746.
6. WHO (1984). *Glossary of Terms,* HFA Series 1-8.
7. UNICEF//WHO (1975). *Joint Committee on Health Policy.*
8. Ashish Bose (1984). *In : Practising Health for All, David Morley et al (eds),* Oxford University Press.
9. WHO (1978). *Alma Ata 1978 : Primary Health Care,* HFA Sr. No. 1.
10. Brelet, C. (1985). *World Health,* June 1985, p. 21.
11. Newell, K.W. (1975). *Health by the People,* WHO Geneva.
12. Banerjee, D. (1980). *In : Proceedings of the Primary Health Care Programmes,* ICMR, New Delhi.
13. WHO (1981). *Global Strategy for Health for All by the Year 2000,* HFA Ser. No. 3.
14. ICSSR and ICMR (1980). *Health for All – An Alternative Strategy,* Indian Institute of Education, Pune.
15. Govt. of India (1981). *Report of the Working Group on Health for All by 2000 AD,* Ministry of Health and Family Welfare, New Delhi.
16. Govt. of India (1983). *Statement on National Health Policy.*
17. WHO (2003). *The World Health Report 2003 : Shaping the Future.*
18. UNDP (2003). *Human Development Report 2003,* Millennium Development Goals : A Compact among nations to end human poverty.
19. UNICEF (2004). *The State of World's Children 2004.*
20. Govt. of India (1998). *Year Book 1996-1997,* Family Welfare Programme in India, Ministry of Health and Family Welfare, New Delhi.
21. *Macrotrends.net, world population 1950–2022.*
22. Govt. of India (2022). *Sample Registration System, Statistical Report 2020,* Office of the RGI.
23. Govt. of India (2011). *Census of India 2011,* Registrar General and Census Commissioner, New Delhi, India.
24. Govt. of India (2022). *SRS Bulletin, May 2022,* Office of the RGI.
25. Govt.of India (2008). *Annual Report 2007-08,* Ministry of Health and Family Welfare, New Delhi.
26. Govt. of India (2007). *Eleventh Five Year Plan, 2007-2012,* Vol. II, Planning Commission, Govt. of India.
27. UNDP (2019). *Human Development Report, 2019.*
28. Govt. of India (2016–17). *Bulletin on Rural Health Statistics in India,* March 2017, DGHS, New Delhi.
29. Govt. of India (2005). *National Rural Health Mission, Accredited Social Health Activist (ASHA), Guidelines,* Ministry of Health and Family Welfare, New Delhi.
30. WHO (1985). Notes for the Practising Midwife, *SEARO, Regional Health Paper* No. 5.
31. Govt. of India (2002). *Bulletin on Rural Health statistics in India,* June 2002, Rural Health Division, DGHS, Ministry of Health and Family Welfare, New Delhi.
32. Govt. of India (2022). *Indian Public Health Standards – Health and Wellness Centre – Sub Health Centre,* 2022 Volume-IV, Ministry of Health and Family Welfare, New Delhi.
33. Govt. of India (2022). *Indian Public Health Standards – Health and Wellness Centre – Primary Health Centre,* 2022, Ministry of Health and Family Welfare, New Delhi.
34. Govt. of India (2012). *Indian Public Health Standards for sub-centre,* Ministry of Health and Family Welfare, New Delhi.
35. Govt. of India (2012). *Indian Public Health Standards for Primary Health Centre,* Ministry of Health and Family Welfare, New Delhi.
36. Govt. of India (2006). *Health Information of India 2005,* Ministry of Health and Family Welfare, New Delhi.
37. Gunn, S.M. and Platt, P.S. (1945). *Voluntary Health Agenies,* The Ronald Press, New York.
38. Leavell, H. and Clark, E.G. (1958). *Preventive Medicine for the Doctor in his Community,* Mc Graw Hill.
39. Govt. of India (1961). *Voluntary Health Organizations and India's Health Programmes,* Central Health Education Bureau, New Delhi.
40. Govt. of India (2021). *National Health Profile, 2021,* Ministry of Health and Family Welfare, New Delhi.

11 Nutrition and Health

"What people eat is not calories but food, and consideration of fads, flavours and variations of appetite can make nonsense of the dietician's theories"

Nutrition may be defined as the science of food and its relationship to health. It is concerned primarily with the part played by nutrients in body growth, development and maintenance *(1)*. The word *Nutrient* or "food factor" is used for specific dietary constituents such as proteins, vitamins and minerals. *Dietetics* is the practical application of the principles of nutrition; it includes the planning of meals for the well and the sick. Good nutrition means "maintaining a nutritional status that enables us to grow well and enjoy good health" *(2)*. The subject of nutrition is very extensive. Since our concern is with community aspects of nutrition, the subject will be dealt with in five sections : dietary constituents, nutritional requirements, assessment of nutritional status, nutritional problems in public health and nutritional programmes in India.

Changing concepts

Through centuries, food has been recognized as important for human beings, in health and disease. The history of man to a large extent has been a struggle to obtain food. Until the turn of the nineteenth century the science of nutrition had a limited range. Protein, carbohydrate and fat had been recognized early in the 19th century as energy-yielding foods and much attention was paid to their metabolism and contribution to energy requirements *(3)*. The discovery of vitamins "rediscovered" the science of nutrition. Between the two World Wars, research on protein gained momentum. By about 1950, all the presently known vitamins and essential amino acids had been discovered. Nutrition gained recognition as a scientific discipline, with roots in physiology and biochemistry. In fact nutrition was regarded as a branch of physiology and taught as such to medical students.

Great advances have been made during the past 50 years in knowledge of nutrition and in the practical application of that knowledge. Specific nutritional diseases were identified and technologies developed to control them, as for example, protein energy malnutrition, endemic goitre, nutritional anaemia, nutritional blindness and diarrhoeal diseases.

While attention was concentrated on nutritional deficiency diseases during the first decades of the century, the science of nutrition was extending its influence into other fields – agriculture, animal husbandry, economics and sociology. This led to "green revolution" and "white revolution" in India and increased food production. However, studies of the diets and state of nutrition of people in India showed that poorer sections of the population continued to suffer from malnutrition despite increased food production. One result was that for the first time the problem of nutrition began to attract international attention *(3)* as a cause of social problems. International activities in the field of nutrition initiated by the League of Nations, later continued by FAO, WHO and UNICEF form a striking part of the story.

Significant advances have been made during the past two decades. The association of nutrition with infection, immunity, fertility, maternal and child health and family health have engaged scientific attention. More recently, a great deal of interest has been focussed on the role of dietary factors in the pathogenesis of non-communicable diseases such as coronary heart disease, diabetes and cancer.

It has been said that most nutrition scientists are far more familiar with rats than with humans. Of greater significance during recent years is that the science of nutrition has moved out of the laboratory and linked itself to epidemiology. This association has given birth to newer concepts in nutrition such as epidemiological assessment of nutritional status of communities, nutritional and dietary surveys, nutritional surveillance, nutritional and growth monitoring, nutritional rehabilitation, nutritional indicators and nutritional interventions all parts of what is broadly known as **nutritional epidemiology.** Epidemiological methods are now increasingly used not only in the elucidation of disease aetiology and identification of risk factors of disease, but also in the planning and evaluation of nutritional programmes. With these newer concepts and newer approaches, nutritional science has become more dynamic.

Another concept that has emerged in recent years is that nutrition is the cornerstone of socio-economic development, and that nutritional problems are not just medical problems but are "multifactorial" with roots in many other sectors of development such as education, demography, agriculture and rural development. It has become apparent that lasting improvement in the health and nutritional status of people can be brought about only through a successful attack on the basic problems of poverty and injustice. The old concept that the health sector alone is responsible for all nutritional ills of the community has faded away. It is now realized that a broad intersectoral and integrated approach of sectors of development is needed to tackle today's nutritional problems.

In the global campaign of Health for All, promotion of proper nutrition is one of the eight elements of primary health care *(4)*. Nutritional indicators *(5)* have been developed to monitor "Health for All". Greater emphasis is now placed on integrating nutrition into primary health care systems whenever possible, and formulation of **national dietary goals** to promote health and nutritional status of families and communities.

CLASSIFICATION OF FOODS

There are many ways of classifying foods :

1. *Classification by origin :*
   1) Foods of animal origin
   2) Foods of vegetable origin.
2. *Classification by chemical composition :*
   1) Proteins 2) Fats
   3) Carbohydrates 4) Vitamins
   5) Minerals.
3. *Classification by predominant function :*
   1) *Body-building foods,* e.g., milk, meat, poultry, fish, eggs, pulses, nuts, and oil seeds etc.
   2) *Energy-giving foods,* e.g., cereals, sugars, roots and tubers, fats and oils.
   3) *Protective foods,* e.g., vegetables, fruits, milk.
4. *Classification by nutritive value :*
   1) Cereals and millets
   2) Pulses (legumes)
   3) Vegetables
   4) Nuts and oilseeds
   5) Fruits
   6) Animal foods
   7) Fats and oils
   8) Sugar and jaggery
   9) Condiments and spices
   10) Miscellaneous foods.

NUTRIENTS

Nutrients are organic and inorganic complexes contained in food. There are about 50 different nutrients which are normally supplied through the foods we eat. Each nutrient has specific functions in the body. Most natural foods contain more than one nutrient. These may be divided into :

(i) Macronutrients : These are proteins, fats and carbohydrates which are often called "proximate principles" because they form the main bulk of food. In the Indian dietary, they contribute to the total energy intake in the following proportions.

Proteins	....	10 to 15 per cent
Fats	....	15 to 30 per cent
Carbohydrates	....	50 to 80 per cent

(ii) Micronutrients : These are vitamins and minerals. They are called micronutrients because they are required in small amounts which may vary from a fraction of a milligram to several grams. A short review of basic facts about these nutrients is given below.

PROTEINS

The word "protein" by derivation means that which is of first importance. Indeed they are of the greatest importance in human nutrition. Proteins are complex organic nitrogenous compounds. They are composed of carbon, hydrogen, oxygen, nitrogen and sulphur in varying amounts. Some proteins also contain phosphorus and iron and occasionally other elements. Proteins differ from carbohydrates and fats in that they contain nitrogen, this usually amounts to about 16 per cent. Proteins constitute about 20 per cent of the body weight in an adult.

Essential amino acids

Proteins are made up of smaller units, called amino acids. Some 20 amino acids are stated to be needed by the human body, of which 9 are called "essential" because the body cannot synthesize them in amounts corresponding to its needs, and therefore, they must be obtained from dietary proteins. They are : leucine, isoleucine, lysine, methionine, phenylalanine, threonine, valine, tryptophan and histidine. Evidence is now accumulating that histidine is essential even for adults *(6)*. Non-essential amino acids include arginine, asparagine, serine, glutamic acid, proline and glycine. Both essential and non-essential amino acids are needed for synthesis of tissue proteins, the former must be supplied through diet, whereas the latter can be synthesized by the body provided other building blocks are present.

Some of the essential amino acids have important biological functions, e.g., formation of niacin from tryptophan; the action of methionine as a donor of methyl groups for the synthesis of choline, folates and nucleic acids. There is evidence that cystine and tyrosine are essential for premature babies *(7)*. New tissues cannot be formed unless all the essential amino acids (EAA) are present in the diet.

A protein is said to be "biologically complete" if it contains all the EAA in amounts corresponding to human needs. When one or more of the EAA are lacking, the protein is said to be "biologically incomplete". The quality of dietary protein is closely related to its pattern of amino acids. From the nutritional standpoint, animal proteins are rated superior to vegetable proteins because they are "biologically complete". For example milk and egg proteins have a pattern of amino acids considered most suitable for humans.

Functions

Proteins are needed by the body for (a) body building, – this component is small compared with the maintenance component, except in the very young child and infant; (b) repair and maintenance of body tissues; (c) maintenance of osmotic pressure; and (d) synthesis of certain substances like antibodies, plasma proteins, haemoglobin, enzymes, hormones and coagulation factors. Proteins are connected with the immune mechanism of the body. The cell mediated immune response and the bactericidal activity of leucocyte have been found to be lowered in severe forms of protein energy malnutrition. Proteins can also supply energy (4 kcal per one gram) when the calorie intake is inadequate, but this is not their primary function. It is considered wasteful if proteins were used for such a purpose.

Sources

Humans obtain protein from two main dietary sources; *(a) ANIMAL SOURCES :* Proteins of animal origin are found in milk, meat, eggs, cheese, fish and fowl. These proteins contain all the essential amino acids (EAA) in adequate amounts. Egg proteins are considered to be the best among food proteins because of their high biological value and digestibility. They are used in nutrition studies as a "reference protein". *(b) VEGETABLE SOURCES :* Vegetable proteins are found in pulses (legumes), cereals, beans, nuts, oil-seed cakes, etc. They are poor in EAA. In developing countries such as India, cereals and pulses are the main sources of dietary protein because they are cheap, easily available and consumed in bulk. Protein content of some foods are as given in Table 1.

TABLE 1
Protein contents of some foods

Food	Protein (g. per 100 g. of food)
Animal foods :	
Milk	3.2-4.3
Meat	18.0-26.0
Egg	13.0
Fish	15.0-23.0
Plant foods :	
Cereals	6.0-13.0
Pulses	21.0-28.0
Vegetables	1-4
Fruits	1-3
Nuts	4.5-29.0
Soyabean	43.2
Others :	
Oils and fats	nil
Sugar and jaggery	nil

Supplementary action of proteins

Man derives protein not from a single source, but from a variety of food sources, animal and vegetable. Cereal proteins are deficient in lysine and threonine; and pulse proteins in methionine. These are known as "limiting" amino acids. When two or more of vegetarian foods are eaten together (as for example, rice–dal combination in India) their proteins supplement one another and provide a protein comparable to animal protein in respect of EAA. Thus with proper planning, it is possible for a vegetarian to obtain a high grade protein, at low cost, from mixed diets of cereals, pulses and vegetables. This is known as supplementary action of proteins, and is the basis of counselling people to eat mixed diets.

Protein metabolism

There are three features of protein metabolism : (a) since proteins are not stored in the human body in the way that energy is stored in adipose tissue, they have to be replaced every day; (b) the body proteins are constantly being broken down into their constituent amino acids and then reused for protein synthesis. The rates of turnover vary from tissue to tissue. The reutilization of amino acids is a major contributory factor to the economy of protein metabolism *(6)*. The overall rate of turnover in adult man is equivalent to replacement between 1–2 per cent of body protein each day *(7)*; (c) it is not only the amount of protein that is maintained constant, but also the pattern of specific protein in body. For maximum utilization of dietary proteins, the calorie intake should be adequate.

Evaluation of proteins

A knowledge of the amino acid content of protein is not sufficient for the evaluation of protein quality. Information is also required about the digestibility and suitability to meet the protein needs of the body. The parameters used for such an evaluation include the estimation of the biological value, digestibility coefficient, protein efficiency ratio and net protein utilization *(8)*. The net protein utilization (NPU) is considered of more practical value because it is the product of biological value and digestibility coefficient divided by 100. In exact terms, it is the "proportion of ingested protein that is retained in the body under specified conditions for the maintenance and/or growth of the tissues". In other words, growth is an important yardstick for ascertaining the essentiality of a nutrient.

Assessment of protein nutrition status

A battery of tests have been suggested to assess the state of protein nutrition. These include : arm muscle circumference, the creatinine – height index, serum albumin and transferrin, total body nitrogen, etc.

At the present time the best measure of the state of protein nutrition is probably serum albumin concentration. It should be more than 3.5 g/dl, a level of 3.5 g/dl is considered mild degree of malnutrition; a level of 3.0 g/dl severe malnutrition. Serum albumin and transferrin assess the ability of the liver to synthesize proteins.

Protein requirements

It is customary to express protein requirements in terms of body weight. The Indian Council of Medical Research in 2020 *(11)* recommended 0.83 g protein/kg body weight per day as a safe intake for an Indian adult, assuming a median obligatory nitrogen loss of 48 mg/kg body weight. Daily allowances recommended by the ICMR for various population groups are as given in Table 28.

FATS

Fats are solid at 20 deg. C; they are called "oils" if they are liquid at that temperature. Fats and oils are concentrated sources of energy. They are classified as :

(a) *Simple lipids,* e.g., triglycerides
(b) *Compound lipids,* e.g., phospholipids
(c) *Derived lipids,* e.g., cholesterol

The human body can synthesize triglycerides and cholesterol endogenously. Most of the body fat (99 per cent) in the adipose tissue is in the form of triglycerides. In normal human subjects, adipose tissue constitutes between 10 to 15 per cent of body weight. The accumulation of one kilogram of adipose tissue corresponds to 7,700 kcal of energy *(10)*.

Fatty acids

Fats yield fatty acids and glycerol on hydrolysis. Fatty acids are divided into **saturated** fatty acids such as lauric, palmitic and stearic acids, and **unsaturated** fatty acids which are further divided into monounsaturated (MUFA) (e.g., oleic acid) and poly-unsaturated fatty acids (PUFA) (e.g., linoleic acid and α-linolenic acid). Table 2 shows the fatty acid content of different fats.

The poly-unsaturated fatty acids are mostly found in vegetable oils, and the saturated fatty acids mainly in animal fats. However, there are exceptions, as for example, coconut and palm oils, although vegetable oils, have an extremely high percentage of saturated fatty acids. On the other hand, fish oils, although they are not vegetable oils, contain poly and mono-unsaturated fatty acids.

Essential fatty acids

Essential fatty acids are those that cannot be synthesized by humans. They can be derived only from food. The most important essential fatty acid (EFA) is ***linoleic acid,*** which serves as a basis for the production of other essential fatty acids (e.g., linolenic and arachidonic acids). Not all polyunsaturated fatty acids are essential fatty acids.

TABLE 2

Approximate fatty acid composition of dietary fats and oils consumed in India (% of total fatty acids)

Fats/oils	SFAs	MUFAs	LA	ALA
High (medium chain) SFAs				
Coconut	92	6	2	–
Palm kernel	83	15	2	–
Butter/Ghee	68	29	2	1
High SFAs & MUFAs				
Palmolein	39	46	11	<0.5
High MUFAs & Moderate LA				
Groundnut	19	41	32	<0.5
Rice bran	17	43	38	1
Sesame	16	41	42	<0.5
High LA				
Cottonseed	24	29	48	1
Corn	12	35	50	1
Safflower	9	13	75	–
Sunflower	12	22	62	–
LA & ALA				
Soyabean	14	24	53	7
Canola	6	60	22	10
Mustard/rapeseed	4	65	15	14
Flax-seed	10	21	16	53
High TFAs				
Vanaspati	61	34	5	–

SFA – Saturated fatty acids; MUFA – Mono-unsaturated fatty acids; LA – Linoleic acid; ALA – alpha-linolenic acid; TFA – trans-fatty acids.

Source : *(11)*

Linoleic acid is abundantly found in vegetable oils. The dietary sources of EFA are as shown in Table 3.

TABLE 3

Dietary sources of EFA

Essential fatty acids	Dietary source	Per cent content
Linoleic acid	Safflower oil	73
	Corn oil	57
	Sunflower oil	56
	Soyabean oil	51
	Sesame oil	40
	Groundnut oil	39
	Mustard oil	15
	Palm oil	9
	Coconut oil	2
Arachidonic acid	Meat, eggs	0.5–0.3
	Milk (fat)	0.4–0.6
Linolenic acid	Soyabean oil	7
	Leafy greens	Varied
Eicosapentaenoic acid	Fish oil	10

Source : *(12)*

Sources

The dietary sources of fats may be classified as :

(a) ANIMAL FATS : The major sources of animal fats are ghee, butter, milk, cheese, eggs, and fat of meat and fish. Animal fats with few exceptions like cod liver oil and sardine oil are mostly saturated fats.

(b) VEGETABLE FATS : Some plants store fat in their seeds, e.g., groundnut, mustard, sesame, coconut, etc. They are sources of vegetable oils.

(c) OTHER SOURCES : Small quantities of fat (invisible fat) are found in most other foods such as cereals, pulses, nuts and vegetables. For example, rice carries 3 per cent of fat, wheat 3 per cent, jowar 4 per cent and bajra 6.5 per cent. Large cereal consumption, as in India, provides considerable amounts of "invisible fat". Moreover, the body can convert carbohydrate into fat.

Visible and invisible fats

"Visible" fats are those that are separated from their natural source, e.g., ghee (butter) from milk, cooking oils from oil-bearing seeds and nuts. It is easy to estimate their intake in the daily diet. "Invisible" fats are those which are not visible to the naked eye. They are present in almost every article of food, e.g., cereals, pulses, nuts, milk, eggs, etc. It is difficult to estimate their intake. In fact, the major contribution to total fat intake is from invisible sources rather than visible sources as cereals and pulses constitute the bulk of Indian diet.

Edible plant foods have a low content of fat and saturated fatty acids but they are good source of mono-unsaturated fatty acids and poly-unsaturated fatty acids. In most cereals, millets, pulses and legumes, fat content ranges between 1.5 to 3 per cent. In cereals, millets and most oil seeds, linoleic acid is the major fatty acid whereas pulses, legumes, green leafy vegetables and some oil seeds (e.g. soyabean, rapeseed/mustard and flaxseed) and fenugreek are good sources of both linoleic acid and alpha-linolenic acid. Animal foods like butter, ghee, whole milk cream, fatty cheese and fatty meats provide cholesterol and high amount of saturated fatty acids, and are natural source of trans-fatty acids. Lean meats have a fairly high content of long chain poly-unsaturated fatty acids (PUFA). Poultry meat contains less fat and cholesterol and have high amount of PUFA including long chain PUFA. Egg has high cholesterol but are good source of linoleic acid, alpha-linolenic acid and docosahexaenoic acid (DHA). Fish has less fat, saturated fatty acids and cholesterol but are good source of PUFAs. The total quantity of invisible fat and its fatty acid composition depends on the kind of diet consumed *(9)*.

Vegetable oil used in cooking is the major type of visible fat consumed; vanaspati and ghee are the other sources. India has a wide range of edible vegetable oils (groundnut, rapeseed/mustard, soyabean, sunflower, sesame, safflower, ricebran, cottonseed and linseed). In India, the type of vegetable oil consumed varies from one part of the country to the other. Vanaspati (PHVO) promoted as vegetable ghee is used as a substitute for ghee and is used in preparing commercially fried, processed, ready to eat, packaged, frozen, pre-mixed foods and street foods. In recent years, there is change in choice of cooking oils in the urban population. The daily intake of visible fat in rural India is about the same as reported about 25 years back *(9)*.

Functions

Fats have always been equated with calories. They are high energy foods, providing as much as 9 kcal for every gram. By supplying energy, fats spare proteins from being used for energy. Besides providing energy, fats serve as vehicles for fat-soluble vitamins. Fats in the body support viscera such as heart, kidney and intestine; and fat beneath the skin provides insulation against cold. Without fat, food is limited in palatability.

It is only recently that the "non-calorie" roles of fats have been discovered. For example vegetable fats are rich sources of essential fatty acids which are needed by the body for growth, for structural integrity of the cell membrane and decreased platelet adhesiveness. Diets rich in EFA have been reported to reduce serum cholesterol and low-density lipoproteins *(13)*. Poly-unsaturated fatty acids are precursors of prostaglandin – a group of compounds, now recognized as "local hormones"; they play a major role in controlling many of the physiological functions of the body such as vascular haemostasis, kidney function, acid secretion in stomach, gastro-intestinal motility, lung physiology and reproduction. Cholesterol is essential as a component of membranes and nervous tissue and is a precursor for the synthesis of steroid hormones and bile acids. Thus fats and oils are useful to the body in several ways.

Hydrogenation

When vegetable oils are hydrogenated under conditions of optimum temperature and pressure in the presence of a catalyst, the liquid oils are converted into semi-solid and solid fat. The resulting hydrogenated fat is known as "vanaspati" or vegetable ghee, which is a popular cooking medium in India.

During the process of hydrogenation, unsaturated fatty acids are converted into saturated acids and the EFA content is drastically reduced. The main advantage of vanaspati is its ghee-like consistency and its keeping quality even in hot humid climates. Since vanaspati is lacking in fat-soluble vitamins, it is fortified with vitamins A and D by government regulation to the extent of 2500 IU of vitamin A and 175 IU of vitamin D per 100 grams.

Trans-fatty acids

Trans-fatty acids are geometrical isomers of Cis-unsaturated fatty acids that adapt a saturated fatty acid like configuration. Partial hydrogenation, the process used to increase shelf-life of poly-unsaturated fatty acids (PUFAs) create trans fatty acids and also removes the critical double bonds in essential fatty acids. Metabolic studies have demonstrated that trans-fatty acids render the plasma lipid profile even more atherogenic than saturated fatty acids, by not only elevating LDL cholesterol but also by decreasing HDL cholesterol. Several large cohort studies have found that intake of trans-fatty acids increases the risk of coronary heart disease *(14)*. It takes years for trans fatty acids to be flushed from the body. Deep fried fast foods, cake mixes, cereals and energy bars, chips and crackers and whipped toppings, packaged cookies and candy, packaged doughnuts, pies and cakes are major sources of trans-fatty acids. It is better to look for "partially hydrogenated oil" on the label of any packaged food.

Refined oils

Refining is usually done by treatment with steam, alkali, etc. Refining and deodourization of raw oils is done mainly to remove the free fatty acids and rancid materials which may be present in them. Refining does not bring about any change in the unsaturated fatty acid content of the oil. It only improves the quality and taste of oils. Refined oils are costly.

Fats and disease

(a) OBESITY : A diet, rich in fat, can pose a threat to human health by encouraging obesity. In fat people, adipose tissue may increase upto 30 per cent. *(b) PHRENODERMA* : Deficiency of essential fatty acids in the diet is associated with rough and dry skin, a condition known as phrenoderma or "toad skin". This condition is reported in Kerala, Karnataka and Gujarat *(15)*. It is characterized by horny papular eruptions on the posterior and lateral aspects of limbs and on the back and buttocks. Phrenoderma can be cured rapidly by the administration of linseed or safflower oil which are rich in EFA, along with vitamins of the B-complex group. *(c) CORONARY HEART DISEASE* : High fat intake (i.e., dietary fat representing 40 per cent or over of the energy supply and containing a high proportion of saturated fats) has been identified as a major risk factor for CHD *(16)*. Epidemiological studies indicate that LDL and VLDL fractions are atherogenic and HDL exerts a protective effect against the development of artherosclerosis. There is evidence indicating an inverse relationship between EFA intake and CHD mortality. *(d) CANCER* : In recent years, there has been some evidence that diets high in fat increase the risk of colon cancer and breast cancer *(17)*. *(e) OTHERS* : The skin lesions of kwashiorkor and those induced by EFA deficiency are similar. The possible association between the skin lesions of kwashiorkor and EFA deficiency has attracted attention *(18)*.

The WHO/FAO Expert Group on diet, nutrition and prevention of chronic diseases endorse that qualitative composition of fats in the diet has a significant role to play in modifying risk factors of CVD and set the following ranges for population nutrient goals (% of Energy) : total fat, 15–30 (at least 20%E (energy) is consistent with good health); Saturated fatty acids less than 10 per cent; PUFAs 6–10 per cent; n-6 about 5–8 per cent; n-3 about 1–2 per cent; Trans-fatty acids less than 1 per cent; MUFAs by difference, and cholesterol less than 300 mg a day *(9)*.

The FAO/WHO expert consultation on fats and fatty acids in human nutrition held in November 2008 in Geneva, Switzerland, reviewed the scientific evidence on nutrient intake values for total fat and fatty acids for different life stages. It also assessed the risks to adequate growth, development and maintenance of health and provided recommendations for infants, children, adults and for women during pregnancy and lactation. Some of their conclusions and recommendations are as follows :

(a) There is convincing evidence on the following :

Energy balance is critical to maintain healthy body weight and ensure optimal nutrient intakes, regardless of macronutrient distribution of energy as % total fat and % total carbohydrates.

Saturated fatty acids (SFAs) :

(1) Replacing SFAs with PUFAs decreases LDL cholesterol concentration and the total/HDL cholesterol ratio. A similar but lesser effect is achieved by replacing these SFAs with MUFAs.

(2) Replacing SFAs with carbohydrates decreases both LDL and HDL cholesterol concentration but does not change the total/HDL cholesterol ratio.

(3) Replacing SFAs with trans-fatty acids (TFAs) decreases HDL cholesterol and increases the total/HDL cholesterol ratio.

(4) Considering the data from epidemiological studies on morbidity and mortality due to coronary heart disease (CHD) and controlled clinical trials (using CHD events and death), it was also agreed that replacing SFAs with PUFAs decrease the risk of CHD.

MUFAs (Monounsaturated fatty acids)

(1) Replacing carbohydrates with MUFAs increases HDL cholesterol concentrations.

(2) Replacing SFA with MUFA reduces LDL cholesterol concentration and total/HDL cholesterol ratio.

PUFAs (Polyunsaturated fatty acids)

Linoleic acid (LA) and alpha-linolenic acid (ALA) are indispensable since they cannot be synthesized by humans. Minimum intake levels for essential fatty acids to prevent deficiency symptoms are estimated to be 2.5% E LA plus 0.5% E ALA.

Trans-fatty acids (TFAs)

TFAs from commercial partially hydrogenated vegetable oils (PHVO) increase CHD risk factors and CHD events to a greater extent than what was thought earlier.

(b) Based on epidemiologic studies and randomized controlled trials of CHD events, 6% has been fixed as the minimum recommended consumption level of total PUFAs for lowering LDL and total cholesterol concentrations, increasing HDL cholesterol concentrations and decreasing the risk of CHD events.

(c) Whilst ALA may have individual properties in their own right, there is evidence that the n-3 long chain PUFAs may contribute to the prevention of CHD and possibly other degenerative diseases of ageing.

(d) Based on both the scientific evidence and conceptual limitations, there is no compelling scientific rationale for recommending a specific ratio of n-6 to n-3 fatty acids or LA to ALA, especially if intakes of n-6 and n-3 fats lie within the recommendations established.

(e) In promoting the removal of TFA, which are predominantly a by-product of industrial processing (partial hydrogenation) usually in the form of PHVO, particular attention must be given to what would be their replacement; this is a challenge for the food industry.

Choice of cooking oils *(9)*

Taking into account the contribution of various fatty acids from all foods (visible fats and invisible fats), the complete dependence on just one vegetable oil does not ensure the recommended intake of fatty acids for optimal health. To achieve intake of individual fatty acids, the type of visible fats and correct combination of vegetable oils to be used are as follows :

1. Use correct combination/blend of 2 or more vegetable oils (1:1)
   (a) Oil containing LA + oil containing both LA and ALA
   Groundnut/Sesame/Rice bran/Cottonseed + Mustard/Rapeseed
   Groundnut/Sesame/Rice bran/Cottonseed + Canola
   Groundnut/Sesame/Rice bran/Cottonseed + Soyabean
   Palmolein + Soyabean
   Safflower/Sunflower + Palm oil/Palmolein + Mustard/Rapeseed.
   (b) Oil containing high LA + oil containing moderate or low LA
   Sunflower/Safflower + Palmolein/Palm oil/Olive
   Safflower/Sunflower + Groundnut/Sesame/Ricebran/Cottonseed.
2. Limit use of butter/ghee.
3. Avoid use of PHVO as medium for cooking/frying.
4. Replacements for PHVO

Frying : oils which have higher thermal stability – palm oil/palmolein, sesame, ricebran, cottonseed - single/blends (home/commercial)

Fat requirements

Recommendations for dietary fats for Indians have been revised taking into account the recent FAO and WHO recommendations for : (1) total fat, individual fatty acids and health promoting non-glyceride components; (2) source of dietary fats in Indians; and (3) availability of fat. The recommendations are directed towards meeting the requirements of optimal foetal and infant growth and development, maternal health and for combating chronic energy deficiency in children and adults, and diet related non-communicable diseases in adults.

Taking into account the unfavourable effect of low fat-high carbohydrate diets and the energy requirement set on the basis of age, physiological status and physical activity, the minimum intakes of visible fat for Indian adults have been based on the sedentary, moderate and heavy physical activity and set at 25, 30 and 40 g/d for adult man, and 20, 25 and 30 g/d for adult women as against a single level recommendation earlier *(11)*. The minimum level of total fat should be 20 per cent of energy. To furnish 20 per cent of total energy, diet of pregnant and lactating mothers should contain at least 30 grams of visible fat *(11)*. For further details see Table 27.

CARBOHYDRATES

The third major component of food is carbohydrate, which is the main source of energy, providing 4 kcals per gram. Carbohydrate is also essential for the oxidation of fats and for the synthesis of certain non-essential amino acids. There are three main sources of carbohydrates, viz., starches, sugar and cellulose. ***Starch*** is basic to the human diet. It is found in abundance in cereals, roots and tubers. ***Sugars*** comprise monosaccharides (glucose, fructose and galactose) and disaccharides (sucrose, lactose and maltose). These free sugars are highly water soluble and easily assimilated. Free sugars along with starches constitute a key source of energy. ***Cellulose*** which is the indigestible component of carbohydrate with scarcely any nutritive value, contributes to dietary fibre.

The carbohydrate reserve (glycogen) of a human adult is about 500 g. This reserve is rapidly exhausted when a man is fasting. If the dietary carbohydrates do not meet the energy needs of the body, protein and glycerol from dietary and endogenous sources are used by the body to maintain glucose haemostasis.

Glycaemic index *(9)*

Glycaemic index of a food is defined by the area under the two-hour blood glucose response curve (AUC) following the ingestion of a fixed portion of test carbohydrate (usually 50 g) as a proportion (%) of the AUC of the standard (either glucose or white bread).

Some foods containing different fractions of soluble and insoluble fibres favour slow release of sugar into small intestine and its absorption into blood (reduced peak and prolonged rate). They are therefore termed low glycaemic index foods as compared to high glycaemic foods with readily digestible and absorbable sugar. The concept has practical utility in management of diabetes and control of obesity.The classification of foods according to GI is as follows :

Classification	GI range	Examples
Low GI	55 or less	most fruit and vegetables (except potatoes, watermelon and sweet corn), whole grains, pasta foods, beans, lentils
Medium GI	56-69	sucrose, basmati rice, brown rice
High GI	70 or more	corn flakes, baked potato, some white rice varieties (e.g. jasmine), white bread, candy bar and syrupy foods.

GI - Glycaemic index

DIETARY FIBRE

By definition "Dietary fibre is the remnants of the edible part of plants and analogous carbohydrates that are resistant to digestion and absorption in the human small intestine with complete or partial fermentation in the human large intestine". It includes polysaccharides, oligosaccharides, lignin and associated plant substances. Dietary fibre exhibits one or more of either laxation (faecal bulking and softening; increased frequency; and or regularity), blood cholesterol attenuation, and or blood glucose attenuation. Organic acids (butyric acid) and polyols (sorbitol) are also considered as part of fibre. Animal foods do not contain any fibre.

Type and sources

Dietary fibres have been characterized by its source, e.g., cereal, vegetable and fruits or its solubility in water – soluble (partly or fully) or insoluble. Both characters of solubility are essential for health promotion. Digestibility of fibre is determined by physiochemical and structural properties of the dietary component and the process used. When exposed to longer duration of degradative conditions in large intestine, more fibre is digested. It forms the substance for fermentation by intestinal microbes. It is through this mechanism that part of energy from resistant starch is rendered available. Apart from the energy yielding reactions during digestion, at different pH, the action of enzymes on dietary fibres promotes interaction between nutrients. It also changes the pattern of microbes colonizing the colon and thus the metabolic products of such fermentation over the time. Vegetarians may have different digestion pattern than that of the non-vegetarians and thus derive different health benefits. This knowledge of probiotics characterized by helpful microbes and prebiotics (substrates promoting the colonization of probiotic strains) has opened up new areas for research *(9)*.

Original estimates of fibre covered all that was insoluble in boiling water or in dilute acid and alkali conditions. It was reported as 'crude fibre', which may include all structural fibre, cellulose, lignin and haemicellulose. It is related to digestibility and has the property of holding water and swelling properties of the diet. It adds to the bulk of the food, favours satiety, increases transit time of the food in the gut and is an active substrate in the large intestine for release of important functional components like organic acids and nutraceuticals. Mostly complex carbohydrates, such as polysaccharides i.e. cellulose, haemicellulose, pectin and a variety of gums, mucilages form the fibre.

Dietary fibre is known to be associated with reduced incidence of coronary heart disease. The mechanism of its action is attributed to its binding to bile salts and preventing its reabsorption and thus reducing cholesterol level in circulation. The fibre, particularly the gum and pectin, when ingested with a diet, are reported to reduce post-prandial glucose level in blood. Recent studies have shown that gum present in fenugreek seeds, which contains 40 per cent gum, is most effective in reducing blood glucose and cholesterol levels as compared to other gums.

Fibre have no metabolic effects. However, too much of fibre can decrease the absorption of valuable micronutrients. There is conflicting evidence as to whether fibre tends to bind some vitamins and minerals like calcium, magnesium, iron and zinc, and reduce their bio-availability. People who eat well-balanced diet obtain enough roughage. Considering the qualitative and quantitative decrease in fibre content of diet over the past many decades, an increase in dietary fibre, particularly from cereals emerge as a recommendation. Intake in excess of 60 g of fibre over a day can reduce the nutrient absorption and cause bowel irritation *(9)*. A daily intake of about 30 grams of dietary fibre per 2000 kcal is desirable. The estimates of dietary fibre intake in different income segments reported from western India are : rural – 39 grams per day for men and 30 g/day for women; tribal – 19 g/day for men and 15 g/day for women; industrial – 41 g/day for men and 31 g/day for women; high income group – 31 g/day for men and 21 g/day for women; middle income group – 43 g/day for men and 22 g/day for women; and low income group – 24 g/day for men and 20 g/day for women *(11)*. The actual quantity of fibre intake depends upon the nature of cereals, pulses, whole grain, vegetables and millets used. The total fibre content of common foods are as shown in Table 4.

TABLE 4

Different dietary fibre fractions in selected Indian foods

Food Group	Food Name	Dietary Fibre (g/100 g)		
		Total	Insoluble	Soluble
Cereals and millets	Bajra	11.49	9.14	2.34
	Jowar	10.22	8.49	1.73
	Ragi	11.18	9.51	1.67
	Rice, raw, milled	2.81	1.99	0.82
	Wheat, whole	11.23	9.63	1.60
Grain legumes	Bengal gram, whole	25.22	22.70	2.52
	Green gram, whole	17.04	14.59	2.44
	Rajmah, red	16.57	13.86	2.70
	Soya bean, brown	21.55	16.56	5.00
Green leafy vegetables	Amaranth leaves, green	4.41	3.21	1.20
	Colocasia leaves, green	5.60	4.32	1.29
	Drumstick leaves	8.21	6.12	2.10
	Tamarind leaves, tender	10.70	9.34	1.36
Other vegetables	Brinjal	3.98	2.84	1.14
	Drumstick	6.83	5.60	1.23
	Ladies finger	4.08	2.80	1.28
Fruits	Apple, big	2.59	1.43	1.16
	Pine apple	3.46	2.88	0.59
	Sapota	9.60	8.46	1.14
Roots and tubers	Carrot, orange	4.18	2.81	1.37
	Potato, brown skin	1.71	1.13	0.58
	Tapioca	4.61	3.85	0.76
Condiments and spices	Chillies, red	31.15	26.55	4.60
	Fenugreek seeds	47.55	27.63	19.92
	Pepper, black	33.16	30.61	2.54
Nuts and oil seeds	Almond	13.06	10.55	2.52
	Gingelly seeds, black	17.16	13.57	3.59
	Mustard seeds	14.10	10.63	3.47
Mushrooms	Button mushroom, fresh	3.11	2.76	0.35
	Shiitake mushroom, fresh	3.02	2.03	0.99
	Oyster mushroom, dried	39.12	35.64	3.48

Source : *(11)*

VITAMINS

Vitamins are a class of organic compounds categorized as essential nutrients. They are required by the body in very small amounts. They fall in the category of micronutrients. Vitamins do not yield energy but enable the body to use other nutrients. Since the body is generally unable to synthesize them (at least in sufficient amounts) they must be provided by food. A well balanced diet supplies in most instances the vitamin needs of a healthy person.

Vitamins are divided into two groups : (a) fat soluble vitamins, viz., vitamins A, D, E and K; and (b) water soluble vitamins, viz., vitamins of the B-group and vitamin C. Each vitamin has a specific function to perform and deficiency of any particular vitamin may lead to specific deficiency diseases. For some vitamins (e.g., vitamin E), no deficiency disease is yet known. The minimum intake for the maintenance of health in respect of many of the vitamins has been determined, but the optimum intake remains somewhat speculative.

VITAMIN A

"Vitamin A" covers both a pre-formed vitamin, retinol, and a pro-vitamin, beta carotene, some of which is converted to retinol in the intestinal mucosa *(17)*. The international units (IU) originally established for vitamin A and provitamin were discarded in 1954 and 1956 respectively *(18)*. In 1960, the term "retinol" was introduced for vitamin A – 1 alcohol (which is available in crystalline form), but most workers prefer the older term vitamin A and the international unit. The international unit (IU) of vitamin A is equivalent to 0.3 microgram of retinol (or 0.55 microgram of retinol palmitate).

Some food composition tables give separate values for retinol and beta-carotene. To convert these into a single value, the term "retinol equivalent" (RE) has been conventionally adopted. The conversion can be done in the following way.

1 mcg of retinol = 1 RE
1 mcg of β-carotene = 0.167 mcg of RE
1 mcg of other carotenoids = 0.084 mcg of RE
1 RE = 3.333 IU of Vitamin A

Functions

Vitamin A participates in many bodily functions : (a) it is indispensable for normal vision. It contributes to the production of retinal pigments which are needed for vision in dim light. (b) it is necessary for maintaining the integrity and the normal functioning of glandular and epithelial tissue which lines intestinal, respiratory and urinary tracts as well as the skin and eyes. (c) it supports growth especially skeletal growth. (d) it is anti-infective; there is increased susceptibility to infection and lowered immune response in vitamin A deficiency, and (e) it may protect against some epithelial cancers such as bronchial cancers, but the data are not fully consistent *(19)*. However, the role of vitamin A at the molecular level is not yet known.

Sources

Vitamin A is widely distributed in animal and plant foods – in animal foods as preformed vitamin A (retinol), and in plant foods as provitamins (carotenes).

(a) ANIMAL FOODS : Foods rich in retinol are liver, eggs, butter, cheese, whole milk, fish and meat. Fish liver oils are the richest natural sources of retinol (Table 5), but they are generally used as nutritional supplements rather than as food sources.

(b) PLANT FOODS : The cheapest source of vitamin A is green leafy vegetables such as spinach and amaranth which are found in great abundance in nature throughout the year. The darker the green leaves, the higher its carotene content. Vitamin A also occurs in most green and yellow fruits and vegetables (e.g., papaya, mango, pumpkin) and in some roots (e.g., carrots). The most important carotenoid is beta-carotene which has the highest vitamin A activity. Carotenes are converted to vitamin A in the small intestine. This action is poorly accomplished in malnourished children and those suffering from diarrhoea.

(c) FORTIFIED FOODS : Foods fortified with vitamin A (e.g., vanaspati, margarine, milk) can be an important source. Vitamin A content of selected foods is as given in Table 5.

TABLE 5
Retinol content of selected foods

Retinol equivalents (RE) (mcg/100 g)			
Halibut liver oil	900,000	Carrot	1,167
Cod liver oil	18,000	Spinach	607
Liver, Ox	16,500	Amaranth	515
Butter	825	Green leaves	300
Margarine	900	Mango, ripe	313
Cheese	350	Papaya	118
Egg	140	Orange	25
Milk, Cow	38	Tomato	84
Fish	40		

Source : *(20)*

The liver has an enormous capacity for storing vitamin A, mostly in the form of retinol palmitate. Under normal conditions, a well-fed person has sufficient vitamin A reserves to meet his needs for 6 to 9 months or more. Free retinol is highly active but toxic and is therefore transported in the blood stream in combination with retinol-binding protein, which is produced by the liver. In severe protein deficiency, decreased production of retinol-binding protein prevents mobilization of liver retinol reserves.

Deficiency

The signs of vitamin A deficiency are predominantly ocular. They include nightblindness, conjunctival xerosis, Bitot's spots, corneal xerosis and keratomalacia. The term "xerophthalmia" (dry eye) comprises all the ocular manifestations of vitamin A deficiency ranging from nightblindness to keratomalacia, Given below is a short description of the ocular manifestations.

(a) Nightblindness

Lack of vitamin A, first causes nightblindness or inability to see in dim light. The mother herself can detect this condition when her child cannot see in late evenings or find her in a darkened room. Nightblindness is due to impairment in dark adaptation. Unless vitamin A intake is increased, the condition may get worse, especially when children also suffer from diarrhoea and other infections.

(b) Conjunctival xerosis

This is the first clinical sign of vitamin A deficiency. The conjuctiva becomes dry and non-wettable. Instead of looking smooth and shiny, it appears muddy and wrinkled. It has been well described as "emerging like sand banks at receding tide" when the child ceases to cry *(21)*.

(c) Bitot's spots

Bitot's spots are triangular, pearly-white or yellowish, foamy spots on the bulbar conjunctiva on either side of the cornea. They are frequently bilateral. Bitot's spots in young children usually indicate vitamin A deficiency. In older individuals, these spots are often inactive sequelae of earlier disease.

(d) Corneal xerosis

This stage is particularly serious. The cornea appears dull, dry and non-wettable and eventually opaque. It does not have a moist appearance. In more severe deficiency there may be corneal ulceration. The ulcer may heal leaving a corneal scar which can affect vision.

(e) Keratomalacia

Keratomalacia or liquefaction of the cornea is a grave medical emergency. The cornea (a part or the whole) may become soft and may burst open. The process is a rapid one. If the eye collapses, vision is lost.

EXTRA-OCULAR MANIFESTATIONS

These comprise follicular hyperkeratosis, anorexia and growth retardation which have long been recognized. They are non-specific and difficult to quantify. Recent studies seem to indicate that even mild vitamin A deficiency causes an increase in morbidity and mortality due to respiratory and intestinal infection *(22)*. Deficiency of vitamin A has recently been linked to child mortality *(23)*.

Treatment

Vitamin A deficiency should be treated urgently. Nearly all of the early stages of xerophthalmia can be reversed by administration of a massive dose (200,000 IU or 110 mg of retinol palmitate) orally on two successive days *(24)*. All children with corneal ulcers should receive vitamin A whether or not a deficiency is suspected.

Prevention

Prevention and/or control takes two forms – (a) improvement of people's diet so as to ensure a regular and adequate intake of foods rich in vitamin A, and (b) reducing the frequency and severity of contributory factors, e.g., PEM, respiratory tract infections, diarrhoea and measles. Both are long term measures involving intensive nutrition education of the public and community participation.

Since vitamin A can be stored in the body for 6 to 9 months and liberated slowly, a short term, simple technology had been evolved by the National Institute of Nutrition at Hyderabad (India) for community based intervention against nutritional blindness, which has subsequently been adopted by other countries *(25)*. The strategy is to administer a single massive dose of 200,000 IU of vitamin A in oil (retinol palmitate) orally every 6 months to preschool children (1 year to 6 years), and half that dose (100,000 IU) to children between 6 months and one year of age *(24)*. In this way, the child would be, as it were "immunized" against xerophthalmia. The protection afforded by six-monthly dosing seems very adequate as measured by clinical signs of deficiency *(26)*.

Assessment of vitamin A deficiency

The formulation of an effective intervention programme for prevention of vitamin A deficiency (VAD) begins with the characterization of the problem. This is done by population surveys employing both clinical and biochemical criteria. These surveys (prevalence surveys) are done on preschool children (6 months to 6 years) who are at special risk. The criteria recommended by WHO *(18)* are as given in Table 6. The presence of any one of the criteria should be considered as evidence of a xerophthalmia problem in the community.

TABLE 6

Prevalence criteria for determining the xerophthalmia problem

Criteria	Prevalence in population at risk (6 months to 6 years)
Nightblindness	more than 1 per cent
Bitot's spots	more than 0.5 per cent
Corneal xerosis/corneal ulceration/keratomalacia	more than 0.01 per cent
Corneal scar	more than 0.05 per cent
Serum retinol (less than 10 mcg/dl)	more than 5 per cent

Source : *(18)*

Recommended allowances

The present committee revised the carotene conversion ratio to account for tissue conversion, and general conversion factor of 6:1 is recommended for all carotenoids except β-cryptoxanthine and α-carotene where a CF of 12:1 is recommended.The detailed recommendations are as given in Table 28.

Toxicity

An excess intake of retinol causes nausea, vomiting, anorexia and sleep disorders followed by skin desquamation and then an enlarged liver and papillar oedema. High intakes of carotene may colour plasma and skin, but do not appear to be dangerous *(19, 27)*. The teratogenic effects of massive doses of vitamin A is the most recent focus of interest *(28)*.

VITAMIN D

The nutritionally important forms of Vitamin D in man are Calciferol (Vitamin D_2) and Cholecalciferol (Vitamin D_3). Calciferol may be derived by irradiation of the plant sterol, ergosterol. Cholecalciferol is the naturally occurring (preformed) vitamin D which is found in animal fats and fish liver oils. It is also derived from exposure to UV rays of the sunlight which convert the cholesterol in the skin to vitamin D. Vitamin D is stored largely in the fat depots.

Vitamin D : Kidney hormone

Major advances have been made in recent years in our understanding of the metabolism of vitamin D in the body *(29)*. It is now known that vitamin D, by itself, is metabolically inactive unless it undergoes endogenous transformation into several active metabolites (e.g., 25 HCC; 1 : 25 DHCC) first in the liver and later in the kidney. These metabolites are bound to specific transport proteins and are carried to the target tissues – bone and intestine. It has been proposed that vitamin D should be regarded as a kidney hormone *(30)* because it does not meet the classic definition of a vitamin, that is, a substance which must be obtained by dietary means because of a lack of capacity in the human body to synthesize it. In fact, vitamin D_3 is not a dietary requirement at all in conditions of adequate sunlight. It can be synthesized in the body in adequate amounts by simple exposure to sunlight even for 5 minutes per day.

Functions

The functions of vitamin D are as summarized in Table 7.

TABLE 7
Functions of vitamin D and its metabolites

Intestine	Promotes intestinal absorption of calcium and phosphorus
Bone	Stimulates normal mineralization, enhances bone reabsorption, affects collagen maturation.
Kidney	Increases tubular reabsorption of phosphate, Variable effect on reabsorption of calcium
Other	Permits normal growth.

Source : *(31)*

Sources

Vitamin D is unique because it is derived both from sunlight and foods. (a) **Sunlight :** Vitamin D is synthesized by the body by the action of UV rays of sunlight on 7-dehydrocholesterol, which is stored in large abundance in the skin. Exposure to UV rays is critical; these can be filtered off by air pollution. Dark-skinned races such as Negros, also suffer from this disadvantage because black skin can filter off up to 95 per cent of UV rays. (b) **Foods :** Vitamin D occurs only in foods of animal origin. Liver, egg yolk, butter and cheese, and some species of fish contain useful amounts. Fish liver oils, although not considered to be a food, are the richest source of vitamin D. Human milk has been shown to contain considerable amounts of water-soluble vitamin D sulphate *(31)*. Other sources of vitamin D are foods artificially fortified with vitamin D, such as milk, margarine, vanaspati and infant foods. Dietary sources of vitamin D are as given in Table 8.

TABLE 8
Dietary sources of vitamin D

	μg/per 100g		μg/per 100g
Butter	0.5–1.5	Shark liver oil	30–100
Eggs	1.25–1.5	Cod liver oil	200–750
Milk, whole	0.1	Halibut liver oil	500–10,000
Fish fat	5–30		

Deficiency

(1) *Rickets* : Vitamin D deficiency leads to *rickets,* which is usually observed in young children between the age of six months and two years. There is reduced calcification of growing bones. The disease is characterized by growth failure, bone deformity, muscular hypotonia, tetany and convulsions due to hypocalcaemia. There is an elevated concentration of alkaline phosphate in the serum. The bony deformities include curved legs, deformed pelvis, pigeon chest, Harrison's sulcus, rickety rosary, kyphoscoliosis, etc. The milestones of development such as walking and teething are delayed. (2) *Osteomalacia :* In adults, vitamin D deficiency may result in osteomalacia which occurs mainly in women, especially during pregnancy and lactation when requirements of vitamin D are increased.

Both rickets and osteomalacia were frequently reported in India, although they do not appear to be a problem of public health importance. In the world as a whole, their prevalence has declined as a result of changes in social customs (e.g., purdah system), and the expansion of mother and child health services leading to better care and feeding of infants and children *(3)*. In the developing countries today, rickets as a menace to child health is overshadowed by the prevalence of protein-energy-malnutrition.

Prevention

Prevention measures include (a) educating parents to expose their children regularly to sunshine; (b) periodic dosing (prophylaxis) of young children with vitamin D; and (c) vitamin D fortification of foods, especially milk. Some industrialized countries still carry out the last measure. Periodic dosing and education appear to be the most practical approaches in developing countries.

Fraser *(32)* urges caution concerning oral supplementation, because orally administered vitamin D appears to bypass the protective mechanism that prevent excessive $25(OH)D_3$ formation. The margin of safety with oral vitamin D between the nutrient requirement and toxic intake is narrow.

Vitamin D is stored in the body in fatty tissues and in the liver. An excessive intake is harmful and may result in anorexia, nausea, vomiting, thirst, and drowsiness. The patient may lapse into coma, while cardiac arrhythmias and renal failure may occur. The effects are due to hypercalcaemia induced by increased intestinal absorption and mobilization of calcium from bone. Recent literature contains warning against the administration of amounts of vitamin D that greatly exceed accepted requirement levels. This warning applies to pregnant women also since manifestations of hypercalcaemia may develop *in utero (4)*.

Daily requirements

The expert committee of ICMR emphasizes importance of outdoor physical activities as a means of achieving adequate vitamin D status in a tropical country like India. However, under minimal exposure to sunlight, particularly in certain urban groups, like 1–2 year old children, a specific recommendation of a daily supplement of 600 IU is suggested *(11)*.

VITAMIN E
(Tocopherol)

Vitamin E is the generic name for a group of closely related and naturally occurring fat soluble compounds, the **tocopherols**. Of these alpha-tocopherol is biologically the most potent. Vitamin E is widely distributed in foods. By far the richest sources are vegetable oils, cotton-seed, sunflower seed, egg yolk and butter. Foods rich in polyunsaturated fatty acids are also rich in vitamin E. The usual plasma level of vitamin E in adults is between 0.8 and 1.4 mg per 100 ml *(31)*. While there is no doubt that man requires tocopherol in his diet, there is no clear indication of dietary deficiency. The role of vitamin E at the molecular level is little understood. The current estimate of vitamin E requirement is about 0.8 mg/g of essential fatty acids. This roughly works out to 7.5–10 mg tocopherol per day depending on the edible oil used *(11)*.

Recently the cytotoxic effect of vitamin E on human lymphocytes *in vitro* at high concentrations has been reported. This being so, caution should be exercised against the mega-dose consumption of vitamin E in clinical practice.

VITAMIN K

Vitamin K occurs in at least two major forms – vitamin K_1 and vitamin K_2. Vitamin K_1 is found mainly in fresh green vegetables particularly dark green ones, and in some fruits. Cow's milk is a richer source (60 mcg/L) of vitamin K than human milk (15 mcg/L). Vitamin K_2 is synthesized by the intestinal bacteria, which usually provides an adequate supply in man. Long-term administration of antibiotic doses for more than a week may temporarily suppress the normal intestinal flora, (a source of vitamin K_2) and may cause a deficiency of vitamin K. Vitamin K is stored in the liver.

The role of vitamin K is to stimulate the production and/ or the release of certain coagulation factors. In vitamin K deficiency, the prothrombin content of blood is markedly decreased and the blood clotting time is considerably prolonged.

The vitamin K requirement of man is met by a combination of dietary intake and microbial synthesis in the gut. The daily requirement for man appears to be about 0.03 mg/kg for the adult. Newborn infants tend to be deficient in vitamin K due to minimal stores of prothrombin at birth and lack of an established intestinal flora. Soon after birth, all infants or those at increased risk should receive a single intramuscular dose of a vitamin K preparation (0.1–0.2 mg of menadione sodium bisulphite or 0.5 mg of vitamin K_1) by way of prophylaxis *(33)*.

B GROUP OF VITAMINS
THIAMINE (B_1)

Thiamine (vitamin B_1) is a water-soluble vitamin. It is essential for the utilization of carbohydrates. Thiamine pyrophosphate (TPP), the coenzyme of cocarboxylase plays a part in activating transketolase, an enzyme involved in the direct oxidative pathway for glucose. In thiamine deficiency, there is accumulation of pyruvic and lactic acids in the tissues and body fluids.

Sources

Thiamine occurs in all natural foods, although in small amounts. Important sources are : whole grain cereals, wheat, gram, yeast, pulses, oilseeds and nuts, especially groundnut. Meat, fish, eggs, vegetables and fruits contain smaller amounts. Milk is an important source of thiamine for infants, provided the thiamine status of their mothers is satisfactory. The main source of thiamine in the diet of Indian people is cereals (rice and wheat) which contribute from 60–85 per cent of the total supply. The thiamine content of selected food stuff is given in Table 9.

TABLE 9

Dietary sources of thiamine

Foods of vegetable origin	mg/100 g	Foods of animal origin	mg/100 g
Wheat (whole)	0.45	Milk, cow's	0.05
Rice, raw homepounded	0.21	Egg hen's	0.10
Rice, milled	0.06	Mutton	0.18
Bengal gram dhal	0.48	Liver, sheep	0.36
Almonds	0.24		
Gingelly seeds	1.01		
Groundnut	0.90		

Source : *(34)*

Thiamine losses

Thiamine is readily lost from rice during the process of milling. Being a water-soluble vitamin, further losses take place during washing and cooking of rice. This is the basis for advising people to eschew highly polished rice and eat parboiled or under-milled rice (see page 741). Much of thiamine in fruits and vegetables is generally lost during prolonged storage *(35)*. Thiamine is also destroyed in toast and in cereals cooked with baking soda. The occurrence or absence of beriberi is determined by the local customs and cultural practices concerning the processing and cooking of rice and other foodstuffs.

Deficiency

The two principal deficiency diseases are beriberi and Wernick's encephalopathy. Beriberi may occur in three main forms : (a) the **dry** form characterized by nerve involvement (peripheral neuritis); (b) the **wet** form characterized by heart involvement (cardiac beriberi); and (c) **infantile** beriberi, seen in infants between 2 and 4 months of age. The affected baby is usually breast-fed by a thiamine-deficient mother who commonly shows signs of peripheral neuropathy. Wernick's encephalopathy (seen often in alcoholics) is characterized by ophthalmoplegia, polyneuritis, ataxia and mental deterioration. It occurs occasionally in people who fast.

A few short decades ago, frank cases of beriberi used to be frequently seen in the coastal districts of Andhra Pradesh where people eat highly polished rice. Investigations by the ICMR showed that such cases are now rarely encountered because of improved socio-economic conditions and diversification in the diet consumed now *(36)*.

Prevention

Beriberi can be eliminated by educating people to eat well-balanced, mixed diets containing thiamine-rich foods (e.g., parboiled and undermilled rice) and to stop all alcohol. Direct supplementation of high-risk groups (e.g., lactating mothers) is another approach. Beriberi tends to disappear as economic conditions improve and diets become more varied *(10)*. The disease, as has been shown, is not completely vanquished but the knowledge and resources needed to bring about its disappearance are available *(3)*.

Recommended allowances

The body content of thiamine is placed at 30 mg, and if more than this is given it is merely lost in the urine *(19)*. Patients on regular haemodialysis should routinely be given supplements of thiamine. Thiamine should also be given prophylactically to people with persistent vomiting or prolonged gastric aspiration and those who go on long fasts. For further details see Table 28.

RIBOFLAVIN (B_2)

Riboflavin (Vitamin B_2) is a member of the B-group vitamins. It has a fundamental role in cellular oxidation. It plays an important role in maintaining the integrity of mucocutaneous structure. It is a co-factor in a number of enzymes involved with energy metabolism. It is also involved in antioxidant activity, being a co-factor for the enzymes like glutathione reductace and is required for the metabolism of other vitamins like vitamin B6, niacin and vitamin K *(9)*.

Sources

Its richest natural sources are milk, eggs, liver, kidney and green leafy vegetables. Meat and fish contain small amounts. Cereals (whether whole or milled) and pulses are relatively poor sources but because of the bulk in which they are consumed, they contribute much of the riboflavin to Indian diets. Germination increases the riboflavin content of pulses and cereals. The riboflavin content of some common foods is given in Table 10.

TABLE 10
Dietary sources of riboflavin

Foods of animal origin	mg/100 g	Foods of vegetable origin	mg/100 g
Liver, sheep	1.70	Whole cereals	0.10–0.16
Milk, cow's	0.19	Milled cereals	0.03–0.08
Egg, hen	0.40	Pulses	0.21–0.32
Meat	0.14	Leafy vegetables	0.15–0.30

Source : *(34)*

Deficiency

The most common lesion associated with riboflavin deficiency is angular stomatitis, which occurs frequently in malnourished children and its prevalence is used as an index of the state of nutrition of groups of children *(3)*. Other clinical signs suggestive (but not specific) include cheilosis, glossitis, nasolabial dyssebacia, etc. Hyporiboflavinosis, even when severe, seldom incapacitates the individual, but it may have subtle functional effects such as impaired neuromotor function, wound healing and perhaps increased susceptibility to cataract *(37)*. Riboflavin deficiency almost always occurs in association with deficiencies of other B-complex vitamins such as pyridoxine; it is usually a part of a multiple deficiency syndrome.

Requirement

There are no real body stores of riboflavin. Daily requirement is 1.96 mg per 1000 kcal of energy intake *(11)*. For further details see Table 28.

NIACIN (B_3)

Niacin or nicotinic acid (B_3) is essential for the metabolism of carbohydrate, fat and protein. It is also essential for the normal functioning of the skin, intestinal and nervous systems. This vitamin differs from the other vitamins of the B-complex group in that an essential amino acid, tryptophan serves as its precursor. Another characteristic of niacin is that it is not excreted in urine as such, but is metabolized to at least 2 major methylated derivatives : N-methyl-nicotinamide and N-methyl pyridones.

Sources

Foods rich in niacin and/or tryptophan are liver, kidney meat, poultry, fish, legumes and groundnut. Milk is a poor source of niacin but its proteins are rich in tryptophan which is converted in the body into niacin (about 60 mg of tryptophan is required to result in 1 mg of niacin). In many cereals, especially maize, niacin occurs in "bound" form unavailable to the consumer.

Deficiency

Niacin deficiency results in pellagra. The disease is characterized by three D's – diarrhoea, dermatitis and dementia. In addition glossitis and stomatitis usually occur. The dermatitis is bilaterally symmetrical and is found only on those surfaces of the body exposed to sunlight, such as back of the hands, lower legs, face and neck. Mental changes may also occur which include depression, irritability and delirium.

Once a formidable and widespread deficiency disease among malnourished population subsisting mainly on maize diets, pellagra has declined in all parts of the world. It is still prevalent in some parts of Western Asia and Southern Africa where people subsist on maize and little else *(38)*. While pellagra is historically a disease of the maize-eating population, it was reported in India in the Telangana area of Andhra Pradesh in some segments of the population eating another cereal – that is jowar (Sorghum vulgare), these people consuming very little of milk or other foods of animal origin. Studies by Gopalan and others *(39)* have shown that amino acid imbalance caused by an excess of leucine is the cause of pellagra in both jowar and maize eaters. Excess of leucine appears to interfere in the conversion of tryptophan to niacin.

Prevention

Pellagra is a preventable disease. A good mixed diet containing milk and/or meat is universally regarded as an essential part of prevention and treatment. Avoidance of total dependence on maize or sorghum is an important preventive measure. Pellagra is a disease of poverty. Given modern knowledge and opportunities for economic, agricultural and social development, there is every reason to hope that this disease could be eliminated *(3)*.

Requirement

The recommended daily allowance is 12 mg per day of energy intake *(11)*. For further details see Table 28.

PYRIDOXINE (B_6)

Pyridoxine (vitamin B_6) exists in three forms : pyridoxine, pyridoxal and pyridoxamine. It plays an important role in the metabolism of amino acids, fats and carbohydrate. It is widely distributed in foods, e.g., milk, liver, meat, egg yolk, fish, whole grain cereals, legumes and vegetables. Pyridoxine deficiency is associated with peripheral neuritis. Riboflavin deficiency impairs the optimal utilization of pyridoxine. INH, an antituberculosis drug is a recognized antagonist, and patients receiving INH are provided with a supplement of pyridoxine (10 mg/day).

The requirements of adults vary directly with protein intake. Adults may need 2 mg/day; during pregnancy and lactation, 2.5 mg/day. Balanced diets usually contain pyridoxine, therefore deficiency is rare. For further details see Table 28.

PANTOTHENIC ACID (B_5)

There is a long standing evidence for a relation between pantothenic acid and adrenal cortical function. Work indicates a more specific role for pantothenic acid in the biosynthesis of corticosteroids *(7)*. Human blood normally contains 18 to 35 mg of pantothenic acid per 100 ml, mostly present in the cells as coenzyme A. The daily requirement is set at 5 mg *(31)*. All foods contribute to dietary intake. About 3 mg are excreted daily in urine.

FOLATE

The recommended name is folate, alternative name is folacin and the usual pharmaceutical preparation is folic acid *(19)*.

Folic acid occurs in food in two forms : free folates and bound folates. The total folates represent both the groups. In man, free folate is rapidly absorbed, primarily from the proximal part of small intestine. The availability of bound folate is uncertain. Folic acid plays a role in the synthesis of the nucleic acids (which constitute the chromosomes). It is also needed for the normal development of blood cells in the marrow.

Sources

The name comes from the latin folia (leaf) but foods such as liver, meat, dairy products, eggs, milk, fruits and cereals are as good dietary sources as leafy vegetables. Overcooking destroys much of folic acid and thus contributes to folate deficiency in man. Folate deficiency has been reported in babies given milk foods subjected to heat sterilization.

Deficiency

Folate deficiency may occur simply from a poor diet. It is commonly found in pregnancy and lactation *(40)* where requirements are increased. It results in megaloblastic anaemia, glossitis, cheilosis and gastrointestinal disturbances such as diarrhoea, distension and flatulence. Severe folate deficiency may cause infertility or even sterility. There is also evidence that the administration of folic acid antagonists (e.g., alcohol, pyrimethamine, and cotrimoxazole) in early pregnancy may produce abortions or congenital malformations.

The laboratory diagnosis of folate deficiency is based on measurement of serum and red cell folate concentrations, usually by microbiological assay *(41)*.

Requirement

Body stores of folate are not large, about 5–10 mg, and therefore, folate deficiency can develop quickly. Folic acid requirements are greatest in conditions where there is rapid cell multiplication, such as during growth in young children and during pregnancy *(41)*. Folic acid supplementation during pregnancy has been found to increase the birth weight of infants and decrease the incidence of low birth weight babies. Intake values recommended by ICMR (2020) are given in Table 28.

VITAMIN B_{12}

Vitamin B_{12} is complex organo-metallic compound with a cobalt atom. The preparation which is therapeutically used is cyanocobalmin, which is relatively cheap. Vitamin B_{12} cooperates with folate in the synthesis of DNA, so deficiency of either leads to megaloblastosis. Vitamin B_{12} has a separate biochemical role, unrelated to folate, in synthesis of fatty acids in myelin *(19)*. The physiological mechanism for its absorption requires intrinsic factor from the stomach, and the complex is absorbed only at a special site in the terminal ileum.

Sources

Good sources are liver, kidney, meat, fish, eggs, milk and cheese. Vitamin B_{12} is not found in foods of vegetable origin. It is also synthesized by bacteria in colon. Unlike folic acid, vitamin B_{12} is relatively heat stable. Liver is the main storage site of vitamin B_{12}. About 2 mg are stored in liver, and another 2 mg elsewhere in the body. These stores are sufficient to tide over any deficiency for one to three years. Because of these reserves, deficiency of vitamin B_{12} appears to be rare.

Deficiency

Vitamin B_{12} deficiency is associated with megaloblastic anaemia (pernicious anaemia), demyelinating neurological lesions in the spinal cord and infertility (in animal species); which is rarely seen in India. While clinical deficiency of B_{12} is not manifested, sub-clinical deficiency is reported to exist in India. Reports indicate that there exist more than 30 per cent deficiency in adults and children in the country. It is not surprising that blood levels of vitamin B_{12} are low, since a large proportion of population depends on plant food for nutrients *(9)*.

Requirement

Intake values recommended by ICMR (2020) are as below *(11)*. Detailed requirements are as shown in Table 28.

		Per day
a) Normal adults	....	2.2 mcg
b) Pregnancy	....	+0.25 mcg
c) Lactation	....	+1.0 mcg
d) Infants & children	....	1.2 mcg

VITAMIN C

Vitamin C (ascorbic acid) is a water-soluble vitamin. It is the most sensitive of all vitamins to heat. Man, monkey and guinea pig are perhaps the only species known to require vitamin C in their diet.

Functions

Vitamin C is a potent antioxidant and has an important role to play in tissue oxidation. It is needed for the formation of collagen, which accounts for 25 per cent of total body protein *(7)*. Collagen provides a supporting matrix for the blood vessels and connective tissue, and for bones and cartilage. That explains why in vitamin C deficiency this support fails, with the result that local haemorrhages occur and the bones fracture easily. Vitamin C, by reducing ferric iron to ferrous iron, facilitates the absorption of iron from vegetable foods. It inhibits nitrosamine formation by the intestinal mucosa. Other claims such as prevention of common cold and protection against infections are not substantiated.

Sources

The main dietary sources of vitamin C are fresh fruits and green leafy vegetables. Traces of vitamin C occur in fresh meat and fish but scarcely in cereals. Germinating pulses contain good amounts. Roots and tubers contain small amounts. Amla or the Indian gooseberry is one of the richest sources of vitamin C both in the fresh as well as in the dry condition. Guavas are another cheap but rich source of this vitamin. The dietary sources of vitamin C are as given in Table 11.

TABLE 11

Dietary sources of vitamin C

		mg/100 g			mg/100 g
Fruits :			Vegetables :		
Amla	..	600	Cabbage	..	124
Guava	..	212	Amaranth	..	99
Lime	..	63	Cauliflower	..	56
Orange	..	30	Spinach	..	28
Tomato	..	27	Brinjal	..	12
Germinated pulses :			Potatoes	..	17
Bengal gram	..	16	Raddish	..	15

Source : *(34)*

Deficiency

Deficiency of vitamin C results in scurvy, the signs of which are swollen and bleeding gums, subcutaneous bruising or bleeding into the skin or joints, delayed wound healing, anaemia and weakness. Scurvy which was once an important deficiency disease is no longer a disease of world importance *(3)*.

Requirement

The estimated requirement for vitamin C is 40 mg per day for adults. The normal body when fully saturated contains about 5 g of vitamin C. Daily intakes recommended by the ICMR *(11)* are as given in Table 28.

MINERALS

More than 50 chemical elements are found in the human body, which are required for growth, repair and regulation of vital body functions. These can be divided into three major groups : (a) MAJOR MINERALS : These include calcium, phosphorus, sodium, potassium and magnesium; (b) TRACE ELEMENTS : These are elements required by the body in quantities of less than a few milligrams per day, e.g. iron, iodine, fluorine, zinc, copper cobalt, chromium, manganese, molybdenum, selenium, nickel, tin, silicon and vanadium *(41)*. Many more have been added to the list in the last few years; and (c) TRACE CONTAMINANTS WITH NO KNOWN FUNCTION : These include lead, mercury, barium, boron, and aluminium.

Only a few mineral elements (e.g., calcium, phosphorus, potassium, sodium, iron, fluorine, iodine) are associated with clearly recognizable clinical situations in man. For none of the other elements do we know with any certainty for their metabolic roles, and much less the clinical effects of dietary insufficiency *(42)*. The bio-availability of minerals such as iron and zinc may be low in a total vegetarian diet because of the presence of substances such as phytic acid. Besides, large amounts of dietary fibre may interfere with proper absorption. Man is not likely to suffer from trace element deficiencies as long as he is omnivorous. Surveys have shown that mineral deficiencies are no greater among vegetarians than among non-vegetarians. In fact, man's need for trace elements has not yet been precisely determined. Trace elements should not be used as dietary supplements, since excessive amounts can have injurious effects.

CALCIUM

Calcium is a major mineral element of the body. It constitutes 1.5–2 per cent of the body weight of an adult human. An average adult body contains about 1200 g of calcium of which over 98 per cent is found in the bones. The amount of calcium in the blood is usually about 10 mg/dl. The developing foetus requires about 30 g of calcium. There is a dynamic equilibrium between the calcium in the blood and that in the skeleton; this equilibrium is maintained by the interaction of vitamin D, parathyroid hormone, and probably calcitonin.

Functions

Ionized calcium in the plasma has many vital functions including formation of bones and teeth, coagulation of blood, contraction of muscles, cardiac action, milk production, relay of electrical and chemical messages that arrive at a cell's surface membrane to the biochemical machinery within the cell, keeping the membranes of cells intact and in the metabolism of enzymes and hormones. It also plays a crucial role in the transformation of light to electrical impulses in the retina. In short, the calcium ion controls many life processes ranging from muscle contraction to cell division.

Sources

Calcium is readily available from many sources. By far the best natural sources are milk and milk products, (e.g., cheese, curd, skimmed milk and butter milk), eggs and fish. A litre of cow's milk provides about 1200 mg of calcium, and human milk about 300 mg. Calcium occurs in milk as calcium caseinate which is readily assimilated by the body. The cheapest dietary sources are green leafy vegetables, cereals and millets. The limiting factor in the complete absorption of calcium from green leafy vegetables (e.g., spinach, amaranth) is the presence of oxalic acid with which calcium forms an insoluble compound, calcium oxalate which interferes with the absorption of calcium. Most cereals are generous providers of calcium, and the millet "ragi" is particularly rich in calcium. Rice is very deficient in calcium *(43)*. The bioavailability of calcium from cereals is poor because of the presence of phytic acid which forms an insoluble compound with calcium, calcium phytate. An additional source of calcium is drinking water which may provide up to 200 mg/day. Some fruits (e.g. Sitaphal) contain good amounts of calcium.

Absorption

Overall, about 20–30 per cent of dietary calcium is normally absorbed. Absorption of calcium is enhanced by vitamin D and decreased by the presence of phytates, oxalates and fatty acids in the diet. Calcium absorption is regulated to some extent by the body's needs.

Deficiency

No clear-cut disease due to calcium deficiency has ever been observed, even under conditions of low intake *(44)*. It has been established that if the intake of vitamin D is adequate, the problems of rickets and osteomalacia do not arise even with low calcium intake. On the other hand, no deleterious effects have been observed in man as a result of prolonged intakes of large amounts of dietary calcium, neither have any benefits been demonstrated.

Requirement

A daily intake of 1,000 mg of calcium has been suggested for adults which is 1.5 times higher than earlier recommendation *(11)*. The physiological requirements are higher in children, expectant and nursing mothers. Intake values recommended by ICMR *(11)* are as given in Table 28.

PHOSPHORUS

Phosphorus is essential for the formation of bones and teeth. It plays an important part in all metabolisms. An adult human body contains about 400–700 g of phosphorus as phosphates, most of this occurs in bones and teeth. Phosphorus is widely distributed in foodstuffs; its deficiency rarely occurs. A large part of phosphorus present in vegetable foods occurs in combination with phytin and is available to the body only to the extent of 40–60 per cent. Phosphorus requirements have not been specifically considered by FAO/WHO Committees, but other groups of experts have suggested that phosphorus intake should be at least equal to calcium intakes in most age groups, except in infancy where the ratio suggested is 1:1.5 *(9)*.

SODIUM

Sodium is found in all body fluids. The adult human body contains about 100 g of sodium ion. Sodium occurs in many foods, and is also added to food during cooking in the form of sodium chloride. Sodium is lost from the body through urine and sweat; that which is passed out in urine is regulated by the kidney but that which is lost by sweating is not controlled. Depletion of sodium chloride causes muscular cramps. The requirement of sodium chloride depends upon climate, occupation and physical activity. Adult requirement is about 5 g per day. A strong relationship between hypertension and dietary salt intake has been observed and intake of more than 10 g of salt per day is considered to have definitive tendency to raise blood pressure *(9)*.

POTASSIUM

The adult human body contains about 250 g of potassium. Potassium occurs widely in foodstuffs, so there is little likelihood of its deficiency. Potassium is vasoactive, increases blood flow and sustains metabolic needs of the tissue. Potassium is released by endothelial cells. Potassium supplements lower blood pressure, although the response is slow. Much of the information regarding potassium and blood pressure is in relation to dietary sodium. High dietary sodium, low dietary potassium have been implicated in the aetiology of hypertension as evidenced by epidemiological clinical studies *(9)*.

The ideal desirable sodium : potassium ratio in the diet is 1:1 (in mmol).

MAGNESIUM

Magnesium is a constituent of bones, and is present in all body cells. Human adult body contains about 25 g of magnesium of which about half is found in the skeleton. It appears that magnesium is essential for the normal metabolism of calcium and potassium *(45)*. Magnesium deficiency may occur in chronic alcoholics, cirrhosis of liver, toxemias of pregnancy, protein-energy malnutrition and malabsorption syndrome *(46)*. The principal clinical features attributed to magnesium deficiency are irritability, tetany, hyper-reflexia and occasionally hypo-reflexia. Requirements are estimated to be about 440 mg/day for adults *(11)*. For details see Table 28.

IRON

Iron is of great importance in human nutrition. The adult human body contains between 3–4 g of iron, of which about 60–70 per cent is present in the blood (Hb iron) as circulating iron, and the rest (1 to 1.5 g) as storage iron. Each gram of haemoglobin contains about 3.34 mg of iron.

Functions

Iron is necessary for many functions in the body including formation of haemoglobin, brain development and function, regulation of body temperature, muscle activity, and catecholamine metabolism. Lack of iron directly affects the immune system; it diminishes the number of T-cells and the production of antibodies. Besides haemoglobin, iron is a component of myoglobin, the cytochromes, catalase and certain enzyme systems. Iron is essential for binding oxygen to the blood cells. The central function of iron is "oxygen transport", and cell respiration.

Sources

There are two forms of iron, haem-iron and non-haem iron. Haem-iron is better absorbed than non-haem iron. Foods rich in **haem-iron** are liver, meat, poultry and fish. They are not only important sources of readily available iron but they also promote the absorption of non-haem iron in plant foods eaten at the same time *(47)*. The iron content of milk is low in all mammalian species. Iron content of breast milk averages less than 0.2 mg/dl, and it is well utilized. Foods containing **non-haem** iron are those of vegetable origin, e.g., cereals, green leafy vegetables, legumes, nuts, oilseeds, jaggery and dried fruits. They are important sources of iron in the diets of a large majority of Indian people. The bioavailability of non-haem iron is poor owing to the presence of phytates, oxalates, carbonates, phosphates and dietary fibre which interfere with iron absorption. Other foods which inhibit iron absorption are milk, eggs and tea *(48)*. The Indian diet which is predominantly vegetarian contains large amounts of these inhibitors, e.g., phytates in bran, phosphates in egg yolk, tannin in tea and oxalates in vegetables. In some areas, significant amounts of iron may be derived from cooking in iron vessels.

Absorption

Iron is mostly absorbed from duodenum and upper small intestine in the ferrous state, according to body needs. The rate of iron absorption is influenced by a great many factors like iron reserves of the subjects, the presence of inhibitors (e.g., phosphates), and promoters (e.g., ascorbic acid and ascorbic acid-rich foods) of iron absorption, and disorders of duodenum and jejunum (e.g., coeliac disease, tropical sprue). Iron absorption is greater when there is an increased demand for iron, as for example during pregnancy. Iron absorption from habitual Indian diets is less than 5 per cent, the bioavailability being poor.

The absorbed iron is transported as plasma ferritin and stored in liver, spleen, bone marrow and kidney. The characteristic feature of iron metabolism is conservation. When red cells are broken down, the liberated iron is reutilized in the formation of new red cells.

Iron losses

The total daily iron loss of an adult is probably 1 mg, and about 12.5 mg per 28 days cycle in menstruating women. Major routes of iron loss are : (a) through **haemorrhage**, that is, wherever blood is lost, iron is lost, the causes of which may be physiological (e.g., menstruation, childbirth) or pathological (e.g., hookworms, malaria, haemorrhoids, peptic ulcer); (b) **basal losses**, such as excretion through urine, sweat and bile, and desquamated surface cells. The widespread use of IUDs in the family planning programme is an additional cause of iron loss. IUDs have been shown to increase the average monthly blood loss by between 35 and 146 per cent depending upon the type of the device *(49, 50)*. Hormonal contraceptives, on the other hand, decrease menstrual blood loss by about 50 per cent *(51)*.

Iron deficiency

Three stages of iron deficiency have been described : (a) First stage characterized by decreased storage of iron without any other detectable abnormalities. (b) An intermediate stage of "latent iron deficiency", that is, iron stores are exhausted, but anaemia has not occurred as yet. Its recognition depends upon measurement of serum ferritin levels. The percentage saturation of transferrin falls from a normal value of 30 per cent to less than 15 per cent. This stage is the most widely prevalent stage in India. (c) The third stage is that of overt iron deficiency when there is a decrease in the concentration of circulating haemoglobin due to impaired haemoglobin synthesis *(49)*.

The end result of iron deficiency is nutritional anaemia which is not a disease entity. It is rather a syndrome caused by malnutrition in its widest sense *(51)*. Besides anaemia, there may be other functional disturbances such as impaired cell-mediated immunity, reduced resistance to infection, increased morbidity and mortality and diminished work performance.

Diagnosis of anaemia

A WHO Expert Group *(52)* proposed that "anaemia or deficiency should be considered to exist" when haemoglobin is below the following levels (see Table 12).

TABLE 12

Cut-off points for the diagnosis of anaemia

	g/dl (Venous blood)	MCHC (per cent)
Adult males	13	34
Adult females, non-pregnant	12	34
Adult females, pregnant	11	34
Children, 6 months to 6 years	11	34
Children, 6 to 14 years	12	34

At all ages the normal MCHC should be 34; values below that indicate that red cells are hypochromic, which occurs in iron deficiency anaemia. A haemoglobin level of 10 to 11 g/dl has been defined as early anaemia; a level below 10 g/dl as marked anaemia *(53)*.

EVALUATION OF IRON STATUS

Evaluation of iron status is based on the following parameters :

(a) *Haemoglobin concentration* : Values below those given in Table 13 indicate anaemia. Haemoglobin concentration is a relatively insensitive index of nutrient depletion. Its value is less in population groups in which anaemia is not severe. This is because anaemia is a late manifestation of iron deficiency which can frequently occur without the manifestation of anaemia *(52)*.

(b) *Serum iron concentration* : This is a more useful index than haemoglobin concentration. The normal range is 0.80 to 1.80 mg/L; values below 0.50 mg/L indicate probable iron deficiency *(54)*.

(c) *Serum ferritin* : The single most sensitive tool for evaluating the iron status is by measurement of serum ferritin. It reflects the size of iron stores in the body. It is the most useful indicator of iron status in a population where the prevalence of iron deficiency is not high. Values below 10 mcg/L probably indicate an absence of stored iron *(19)*.

(d) *Serum transferrin saturation* : This should be above 16 per cent. Normal value is 30 per cent.

Iron requirements

Because of the recycling of iron, only a small amount of iron is needed by the body. In general, iron requirements are greater when there is rapid expansion of tissue and red cell mass, as for example during pregnancy, childhood & adolescence. The recommended dietary intakes of iron are as given in Table 28.

IODINE

Iodine is an essential micronutrient. It is required for the synthesis of the thyroid hormones, thyroxine (T_4) and triiodothyronine (T_3) containing respectively 4 and 3 atoms of iodine. Iodine is essential in minute amounts for the normal growth and development and well-being of all humans. The adult human body contains about 50 mg of iodine, and the blood level is about 8–12 micrograms/dl *(31)*.

Sources

The best sources of iodine are sea foods (e.g., sea fish, sea salt) and cod liver oil. Smaller amounts occur in other foods, e.g., milk, meat, vegetables, cereals, etc. The iodine content of fresh water is small and very variable, about 1–50 micrograms/L *(31)*.

About 90 per cent of iodine comes from foods eaten; the remainder from drinking water. The iodine content of the soil determines its presence in both water and locally grown foods. The deficiency is geochemical in nature.

Goitrogens

"Goitrogens", are chemical substances leading to the development of goitre. They interfere with iodine utilization by the thyroid gland. They may occur in food and water. The brassica group of vegetables (e.g., cabbage, cauliflower) may contain goitrogens. Most important among the dietary goitrogens are probably cyanoglycosides and the thiocyanates.

Deficiency

The most obvious consequence of iodine deficiency is goitre but recent studies have indicated that there is a much wider spectrum of disorders, some of them so severe as to be disabling. They include : (a) hypothyroidism (b) retarded physical development and impaired mental function (c) increased rate of spontaneous abortion and stillbirth (d) neurological cretinism, including deaf-mutism; and

(e) myxoedematous cretinism, including dwarfism and severe mental retardation. To express this state of affairs more accurately, the term "endemic goitre", is now replaced by the term **Iodine Deficiency Disorders** (IDD) to refer to all the effects of iodine deficiency on human growth and development which can be prevented by correction of iodine deficiency *(55, 56, 57)*. The spectrum of IDD is as shown in Table 13.

TABLE 13

The spectrum of iodine-deficiency disorders in approximate order of increasing severity

Disorders	Levels of severity
Goitre	– Grade I – Grade II – Grade III – Multinodular
Hypothyroidism	– Varying combinations of clinical signs (depending on age of onset, duration and severity)
Subnormal intelligence Delayed motor milestones Mental deficiency Hearing defects Speech defects	Variable severity
Strabismus (squint) Nystagmus	– Unilateral – Bilateral
Spasticity (extrapyramidal) Neuromuscular weakness	– Muscle weakness in legs, arms, trunk – Spastic diplegia – Spastic quadriplegia
Endemic cretinism	– Hypothyroid cretinism – Neurological cretinism
Intrauterine death (spontaneous abortion, miscarriage)	

It can be seen from Table 15 that the problem of IDD is of far greater magnitude than one of goitre and cretinism. It is a national problem with grave socio-economic consequences. Adequate technology exists for the successful prevention of iodine deficiency disorders.

Requirement

The daily requirement of iodine for adults is placed at 150 micrograms. The recommendations of WHO of 250 mcg per day for iodine during pregnancy have also been adopted. This amount is normally supplied by well-balanced diet and drinking water except in regions where food and water are deficient in iodine. Table 28 shows the requirements for different age groups.

Epidemiological assessment of iodine deficiency

This is necessary before initiating an iodization programme, and for surveillance of goitre control programmes. The following indicators are useful in this regard *(58)* :

- prevalence of goitre;
- prevalence of cretinism;
- urinary iodine excretion;
- measurement of thyroid function by determination of serum levels of thyroxine (T_4) and pituitary thyrotropic hormone (TSH); and
- prevalence of neonatal hypothyroidism.

Since the objective of goitre control programme is to increase iodine intake, indices of urinary excretion are particularly recommended for use in surveillance. Neonatal hypothyroidism has been found to be a sensitive indicator of environmental iodine deficiency. Serum T_4 level is a more sensitive indicator of thyroid insufficiency than T_3.

FLUORINE

Fluorine is the most abundant element in nature. Being so highly reactive, it is never found in its elemental gaseous form, but only in combined form. About 96 per cent of the fluoride in the body is found in bones and teeth. Fluorine is essential for the normal mineralization of bones and formation of dental enamel.

Sources

The principal sources of fluorine available to man are : (a) **Drinking water** : The major source of fluorine to man is drinking water. In most parts of India, the fluoride content of drinking water is about 0.5 mg/L, but in fluorosis-endemic areas, it may be as high as 3 to 12 mg/L *(59)*. (b) **Foods** : Fluorides occur in traces in many foods, but some foods such as sea fish, cheese and tea are reported to be rich in fluorides *(38)*.

Deficiency/excess

Fluorine is often called a two-edged sword. Prolonged ingestion of fluorides through drinking water in excess of the daily requirement is associated with dental and skeletal fluorosis; and inadequate intake with dental caries. The use of fluoride is recognized as the most effective means available for the prevention of dental caries.

Requirements

The recommended level of fluorides in drinking water in India is accepted as 0.5 to 0.8 mg per litre *(60, 61)*. In temperate countries where the water intake is low, the optimum level of fluorides in drinking water is accepted as 1 to 2 mg per litre *(62)*.

OTHER TRACE ELEMENTS

Zinc

Zinc is a component of more than 300 enzymes. It is active in the metabolism of glucides and proteins, and is required for the synthesis of insulin by the pancreas and for the immunity function. Zinc is present in small amounts in all tissues. Zinc-plasma level is about 96μg per 100 ml for healthy adults, and 89 μg per 100 ml for healthy children *(63)*. The average adult body contains 1.4 to 2.3 g of zinc *(64)*. Zinc deficiency has been reported to result in growth failure and sexual infantilism in adolescents, and in loss of taste and delayed wound healing *(10)*. There are also reports of low circulating zinc levels in clinical disorders such as liver disease, pernicious anaemia, thalassaemia and myocardial infarction. Zinc deficiency is common in children from developing countries due to lack of intake of animal food, high dietary phytate content, inadequate food intake and increased faecal losses during diarrhoea. Zinc supplementation in combination with oral rehydration therapy has been shown to significantly reduce the duration and severity of acute and persistent diarrhoea and to increase survival in a number of randomized control trials. Adequate zinc intake is essential for maintaining the integrity of immune system. Zinc affects multiple aspects of the immune system, from the barrier of the skin to gene regulation within lymphocytes. Severe maternal zinc deficiency has been associated with spontaneous abortion and congenital malformations like anencephaly. Milder forms of zinc deficiency has been associated with low birth weight, intrauterine growth retardation and preterm delivery. Several studies have indicated that zinc supplementation may reduce the incidence of clinical attacks of malaria in children. Zinc plays an important role as antioxidant agent *(65)*. These reports suggest that zinc deficiency may not be uncommon in man *(63)*. Zinc is widely distributed in foodstuffs, both animal and vegetable – but the bioavailability of zinc in vegetable foods is low. Animal foods such as meat, milk and fish are dependable sources. Suggested daily intake for adults is 17 mg per day for men, 13.2 mg per day for women, 10 mg per day for children and 5 mg for infants. Refer to Table 28 for details. Growing children and pregnant and lactating women need more. Most human diets provide these amounts.

Copper

The amount of copper in an adult body is estimated to be between 100–150 mg. Copper is widely distributed in nature. Even poor diets provide enough copper for human needs. Deficiency or excess of this element is very rare. Hypocupremia occurs in patients with nephrosis, Wilson's disease and protein-energy malnutrition and in infants fed for long periods exclusively on cow's milk. Neutropenia is the best documented abnormality of copper deficiency. Hypercupremia may reflect excessive intake which may result from eating food prepared in copper cooking vessels, or it may be associated with several acute and chronic infections (leukaemia, Hodgkin's disease, severe anaemia, haemochromatosis, myocardial infarction and hyperthyroidism *(66)*. Estimated copper requirement for adults is about 2.0 mg per day.

Cobalt

The only established function of cobalt in the human is as a part of the vitamin B_{12} molecule, which must be ingested preformed. There is no evidence as yet of cobalt deficiency in man *(10)*. Recently cobalt deficiency and cobalt iodine ratio in the soil have shown to produce goitre in humans. It is suggested that cobalt may be necessary for the first stage of hormone production. i.e., capture of iodine by the gland *(67)*. Cobalt may interact with iodine and affect its utilization *(10)*.

Chromium

Total body content of chromium is small, less then 6 mg. Current interest in chromium is based on the occurrence of unusual glucose tolerance curves that are responsive to chromium *(41)*. Thus there is suggestive evidence that chromium plays a role in relation to carbohydrate and insulin function *(10)*.

Selenium

Little attention had been given earlier to selenium in human nutrition. The first report that selenium deficiency may occur in man appeared in 1961, and a similar report in 1967. Selenium administration to children with kwashiorkor resulted in significant weight increase. Studies indicate that human selenium deficiency may occur in protein-energy malnutrition *(66)*. Selenium deficiency especially when combined with vitamin E deficiency, reduces antibody production *(68)*. 40 µg/day is recommended intake of selenium *(11)*.

Molybdenum

Excess absorption of molybdenum has been shown to produce bony deformities. On the other hand, deficiency of molybdenum is associated with mouth and oesophageal cancer *(67)*.

Dietary antioxidants *(9)*

Antioxidants are substances which are both nutrients, viz. vitamins E, C, β-carotene, selenium, and non-nutrients, viz. plant phenols, flavonoids, coumarins, benzyl isothiocyanates, caffeic, ferulic, gallic and ellagic acids, some enzymes like superoxide dismutase and catalase superoxides mutase. These antioxidants reduce the adverse effects of reactive oxygen species (ROS) and nitrogen species which are generated during physiological or pathological conditions and result in oxidant damage. Literature is replete with evidence that ageing and several diet/nutrient related chronic disorders are due to chronic exposure to ROS. It is well established that vegetables, fruits, legumes, spices, beverages such as tea and wine, and cereals are excellent sources of AO, however scientific evidence for their protective role is available only for vegetables and fruits in several chronic disorders. None of the randomized clinical trials conducted so far with nutrient AO supplements has demonstrated a significant benefit in community trials barring one or two major trials in high-risk populations.

Experimental studies have amply indicated that both pro-oxidant and AO have a fundamental role in pathogenesis of diseases. Reactive oxygen species (ROS) damage the bio-molecules such as DNA, protein, carbohydrates and lipids, and affect the enzyme processes and genetic machinery. The oxidation products of bio-molecules accumulate with age. ROS can be derived from an enviornmental source also. There are several endogenous and exogenous sources of ROS, which play an important role in diseases such as cardiovascular, cancer, cataract, diabetes, neuro-degenerative disorders and age-related masculopathy. Chronic infections aggravate the damage. Further, research in this field has highlighted the mechanistic details about the role of antioxidants in mitigating the damage.

Free radicals produced during tissue metabolism and their consequent damage are reduced by nutrient antioxidants. The antioxidants, particularly vitamin E, C, co-enzyme Q and glutathione seem to work in concert by recycling each other.

In healthy subjects, the dietary antioxidants from a balanced diet with adequate fruits and vegetables ranging from 500–600 gm/d will probably be enough to take care of oxidant damage and repair cellular and tissue defects. However, certain groups of populations like pre-mature infants, smokers, alcoholics, and those exposed to environmental pollutants including carcinogens, individuals with chronic infections as well as those engaged in strenous physical activity and geriatric population, are at high-risk of oxidant damage.

At present the amount of antioxidants to be consumed daily to protect against risk factors cannot be quantitatively fixed *(9)*.

NUTRITIONAL PROFILES OF PRINCIPAL FOODS

When planning balanced diets, it is important to know what foods are available according to origin, approximate chemical composition, predominant function and how to combine them to increase nutritive value. Since each food has a different nutritional profile, an intake of different types of foods is desired to achieve optimum health.

1. Cereals and millets

CEREALS

Cereals (e.g., rice, wheat) constitute the bulk of the daily diet. Rice is the staple food of more than half the human race. Next to rice, wheat is the most important cereal. Maize ranks next to rice and wheat in world consumption. Maize is also used as food for cattle and poultry because it is rich in fat, besides being cheaper than rice or wheat.

Cereals are the main sources of energy (carbohydrates). They also contribute significant quantities of proteins (6 to 12 per cent), minerals and B-group vitamins. The yellow variety of maize contains significant amounts of carotene. In terms of energy, cereals provide about 350 kcal per 100 grams. Considering the large amounts in which they are consumed, cereals contribute 70 to 80 per cent of the total energy intake, and more than 50 per cent of protein intake in typical Indian diets.

Cereal proteins are poor in nutritive quality, being deficient in the essential amino acid, lysine. The proteins of maize are still poorer, being deficient in lysine and tryptophan (a precursor of niacin). However, if cereals are eaten with pulses, as is common in the traditional Indian diets, cereal and pulse proteins complement each other and provide a more balanced and "complete" protein intake. Some strains of maize contain an excess of leucine which interferes with the conversion of tryptophan into niacin; this aggravates the pellagragenic action of maize.

Table 14 gives the nutritive value of some common cereals.

TABLE 14

Nutritive value of cereals (values per 100 g.)

		Raw rice milled	Wheat whole	Maize dry
Protein	(g)	6.8	11.81	11.1
Fat	(g)	0.5	1.5	3.6
Carbohydrate	(g)	78.2	71.2	66.2
Thiamine	(mg)	0.06	0.45	0.42
Niacin	(mg)	1.9	5.0	1.8
Riboflavin	(mg)	0.06	0.17	0.1
Minerals	(g)	0.6	1.5	1.5
Energy	(kcal)	345	346	342

Source : *(34)*

Rice

Rice is the staple food of more than half the human race. The rice grain consists of 3 parts – the germ (embryo), the inner endosperm, and the outer pericarp and aleurone grain layer. The endosperm is composed mostly of starch; the outer pericarp aleurone layer and germ contain most of the essential nutrients. The protein content of rice varies from 6–9 per cent. Rice proteins are richer in lysine than the other cereal proteins, and for this reason, rice protein is considered to be of better quality. Rice is a good source of B group vitamins, especially thiamine. It is devoid of vitamins A, D and C. In regard to minerals rice is a poor source of calcium and iron (Table15).

TABLE 15

Effect of milling on rice

	Protein (g)%	Calcium (g)%	Phosphorus (g)%	Iron (mg)%	Vit.B (mg)%	Niacin (mg)%
Raw, husked rice	7.7	0.015	0.368	4.0	0.40	3.5
Raw, undermilled or home pounded rice (about 7% polishings removed)	7.2	0.013	0.146	2.2	0.22	2.2
Raw milled rice (about 14% polishings removed)	7.0	0.010	0.110	2.0	0.11	1.0

Effect of milling

The milling process deprives the rice grain of its valuable nutritive elements (thiamine, riboflavin, protein). The losses may be upto 15 per cent of protein, 75 per cent of thiamine and 60 per cent of riboflavin and niacin *(69)*. The resulting white or polished rice, although attractive in appearance, is poor in nutritive value. People subsisting mainly on white or polished rice are prone to beriberi, the best known deficiency disease of rice eaters. Nutrition workers therefore advocate under-milled or "parboiled" rice in place of white rice.

Washing and cooking

The rice grain is subjected to further loss of essential nutrients during the process of washing and cooking. Washing in large quantities of water would remove upto 60 per cent of the water-soluble vitamins and minerals. The practice of cooking rice in large quantities of water and draining away the excess of water at the end of cooking leads to further loss of B-group vitamins. Thus the combined effect of washing and cooking may affect seriously the nutritive value of rice. It is therefore best to cook rice in just enough water (about 2 measure of water for 1 measure of rice).

Parboiling

Parboiling (partial cooking in steam) is an ancient Indian technique of preserving the nutritive quality of rice. There are many techniques of parboiling. The technique recommended by the Central Food Technological

Research Institute, Mysore *(8)* is known as the **hot soaking process**.

The process starts with soaking the paddy (unhusked rice) in hot water at 65 to 70 deg. C for 3 to 4 hours, which swells the grain. This is followed by draining of water and steaming the soaked paddy in the same container for 5 to 10 minutes. The paddy is then dried and later homepounded or milled.

During the steaming process, a greater part of the vitamins and minerals present in the outer aleurone layer of the rice grain are driven into the inner endosperm. With subsequent milling, even to a high degree, the nutrients are not removed. During the drying process, the germ gets attached more firmly to the grain. In addition, the heat used in drying hardens the rice grain. It results in the grain becoming more resistant to insect invasion and more suitable for storage than raw rice. The starch also gets gelatinized which improves the keeping quality of rice *(8)*. The serious disadvantage of parboiling is the development of a peculiar smell or "off flavour" which some consumers do not relish. Modern methods of parboiling rice have been developed by which the finished product does not give any bad odour.

Wheat

Next to rice, wheat is the most important cereal. The nutritive composition of wheat is given in Table 14. The protein content of wheat varies from 9 to 16 per cent, the limiting amino acids are lysine and threonine. The wheat grain is much less subjected to loss of essential nutrients during processing than rice. In India, the bulk of wheat is consumed as whole grain wheat flour or atta. Maida or white flour which represents 70 per cent extraction of wheat is poorer from the nutrition standpoint. The whiter the flour the greater the loss of vitamins and minerals. Thus whole grain wheat flour is richer source of vitamin B than refined white flour.

Maize

Maize (Corn, *bhutta*) ranks next to rice and wheat in world consumption, and in certain areas it is the principal source of proteins and energy both. It is also used as a food for cattle and poultry. The yellow variety of maize contains significant amount of carotenoid pigments. Maize is fairly rich in fat (Table 16). The proteins of maize are deficient in tryptophan and lysine; and some strains contain an excess of leucine. Studies indicate that excess of leucine interferes in the conversion of tryptophan into niacin, and thus aggravates the pellagragenic action of maize. Maize is also used in the manufacture of breakfast foods such as cornflakes. Maize flour or corn flour is widely used in the preparation of custards and table desserts. The incorporation of opaque-2 gene into maize has greatly improved the quality of its protein.

MILLETS

The term "millet" is used for smaller grains which are ground and eaten without having the outer layer removed; they are jowar (sorghum), bajra (pearl millet), ragi, kodo and a few others known as "minor millets" or pseudocereals *(70)*. The nutritive value of millets is as shown in Table 16.

TABLE 16

Nutritive value of millets (values per 100 g)

		Jowar	Bajra	Ragi
Protein	(g)	10.4	11.6	7.3
Fat	(g)	1.9	5.0	1.3
Carbohydrate	(g)	72.6	67.5	72.0
Minerals	(g)	1.6	2.3	2.7
Calcium	(mg)	25.0	42.0	344.0
Iron	(mg)	4.1	8	3.9
Thiamine	(mg)	0.3	0.3	0.2
Riboflavin	(mg)	1.3	0.25	0.18
Niacin	(mg)	3.1	2.3	2.3
Energy	(kcal)	349	361	328

Source : *(34)*

Jowar (sorghum)

Jowar is also known as kaffir corn or Milo. It is a major crop grown in India next only to wheat and rice. For several population groups, it is a staple diet. The protein content of jowar varies from 9 to 14 per cent, and the proteins are limiting in lysine and threonine. Certain varieties of jowar have a high leucine content and consumption of these varieties is associated with pellagra. This disorder is often seen in the Telangana and Marathwada regions where jowar is predominantly consumed.

Bajra (pearl millet)

Bajra is grown extensively in the dry belts of northern and peninsular India, viz. Rajasthan, Gujarat and Maharashtra, where it forms the staple food of large sections of the population. The protein content varies from 10 to 14 per cent; the proteins are deficient in lysine and threonine. Bajra contains significant amounts of B-group vitamins and minerals such as calcium and iron.

Ragi

Ragi is a popular millet in Andhra Pradesh and Karnataka. It is the cheapest among millets. Ragi flour is cooked and eaten as porridge. Ragi is rich in calcium (see Table 16).

2. Pulses (legumes)

Pulses comprise a variety of grams, also known as dhals. Most commonly eaten pulses are bengal gram (chana), red gram (tuvar or arhar), green gram (mung) and black gram (urd). Others include lentils (masur), peas and beans including soyabean. Khesari dhal *(lathyrus sativus)*, is consumed in parts of Madhya Pradesh, Uttar Pradesh and Bihar, excessive consumption of which is associated with lathyrism.

Pulses contain 20 to 25 per cent of proteins, which is double that found in wheat and three times that found in rice. In fact, pulses contain more protein than eggs, fish or flesh foods. But in regard to quality, pulse proteins are inferior to animal proteins. Pulse proteins are poor in methionine and to a lesser extent in cysteine. On the other hand they are rich in lysine. Soyabean is exceptionally rich in protein, containing up to 40 per cent. In addition, pulses are rich in minerals and B-group vitamins such as riboflavin and thiamine. In the dry state, pulses do not contain vitamin C. Germinating pulses, however, contain higher concentration of vitamins, especially vitamin C and B vitamins. Fermentation also modifies the nutritive value of pulses in that the vitamin content particularly that of riboflavin, thiamine and niacin is enhanced.

Although pulses are called "poor man's meat", they are eaten by the rich and poor alike in India. They give variety to the diet and make the food more palatable. Table 17 gives the nutritive value of some common pulses.

TABLE 17
Nutritive value of pulses (values per 100 g)

Pulses	Energy (kcal)	Proteins g	Fat g	Calcium mg	Iron mg	Thiamine mg	Riboflavin mg	Niacin mg	Vit-C mg
Bengal gram	360	17.1	5.3	202	4.6	0.30	0.15	2.9	3
Black gram	347	24.0	1.4	154	3.8	0.42	0.20	2.0	0
Red gram	335	22.3	1.7	73	2.7	0.45	0.19	2.9	0
Soyabean	432	43.2	19.5	240	10.4	0.73	0.39	3.2	0
Green gram	348	24.5	1.2	75	3.9	0.47	0.21	2.4	0
Peas dry	315	19.7	1.1	75	7.05	0.47	0.19	3.4	0
Horse gram	321	22.0	0.5	287	6.77	0.42	0.2	1.5	1

Source : *(34)*

Anti-nutritional factors : In the raw state, pulses have some anti-nutritional factors such as phytates and tannins which adversely affect the availability of some nutrients to the body. However, most of the anti-nutritional factors are destroyed by heat. Presence of high amounts of certain sugars known as oligosaccharides is known to be associated with flatulence *(71)*.

Soyabean

Soyabean is the richest among pulses. It contains about 40 per cent of protein, 20 per cent of fat and 4 per cent of minerals. The proteins of soyabean are of relatively high nutritive value. The limiting amino acid is methionine. Soyabean can be cooked and eaten as dhal. It can be tried in other forms like mixing its powder with atta for chappatis, soyabean milk and curd and in baby foods. Soyabean is yet to become popular in India despite many years of publicity.

3. Vegetables

Vegetables are classed as "protective foods"; their value resides in their high vitamin and mineral content. Some vegetables (e.g., green peas, beans) are also good sources of protein. Vegetables usually have a large water content, low energy and protein content and varying amounts of "dietary fibre". Vegetables are divided into three groups "green leaves"; "roots and tubers"; and "others".

a. Green leaves

The term "green leaves" designates a number of indigenous leafy vegetables consumed by the people. They include palak (spinach), amaranth, cabbage, fenugreek (methi) etc. The darker the green leaves, the greater their nutritive value. With the possible exception of vitamin B_{12}, green leaves are rich sources of carotenes, calcium, iron and vitamin C. They are also fairly good sources of riboflavin, folic acid and many other micronutrients. In addition, leaf proteins (2 to 4 per cent) are good sources of lysine, although deficient in sulphur – containing amino acids. The bioavailability of calcium and iron from greens is rather poor because of the presence of high amounts of oxalates. Leafy vegetables are high in water content and dietary fibre. Because of their low calorific value (25 to 50 kcal per 100 g) and large bulk, they have an important place in the dietaries of obese people who wish to cut down their calorie intake. The recommended daily intake of green leafy vegetables is about 40 g for an adult.

b. Roots and tubers

Included in this group are potato, sweet potato, tapioca, yam, carrots, onion, radish and colocasia. They vary widely in composition, some are good sources of carbohydrates such as potatoes and tapioca. In general roots and tubers are poor in protein, minerals and vitamins. Carrots are exceptionally high in beta-carotene. In times of cereal shortage, potatoes, sweet potatoes, and tapioca can serve as subsidiary foods for limited periods. But bulk and low protein make them unsuitable as staple foods for longer periods, unless supplemented by foods richer in protein. The recommended daily intake of roots and tubers is 50 to 60 g for an adult.

c. Other vegetables

There is a wide range of "other" vegetables such as brinjal, tomatoes, cauliflower, etc. They bring variety to the diet. Many of them are fairly good sources of minerals and vitamins. Some vegetables like cluster beans, drumsticks and green mango contain fair amounts of iron. The daily recommended intake is 60 to 70 grams.

4. Nuts and oilseeds

Included in this group are groundnut (Peanut), cashewnut, coconut, walnut, almonds, pistachio, mustard seeds, sesame seeds, cotton seeds, sunflower seeds, maize germ and many others from which cooking oils are extracted.

Nuts and oilseeds contain good amount of fat and good quality protein in a relatively small bulk. Regarding the fat content, walnuts contain 64.5 per cent, almonds 58.7 per cent, cashewnuts 46.9 per cent and groundnut 40 per cent. Peanut (groundnut) butter is a very valued article of the diet. Regarding protein content, groundnut tops the list with 26.7 per cent. Being of vegetable origin, their protein is not equal to that of meat or eggs in quality. Nuts are good sources of vitamins of the B-group. They contribute minerals such as calcium, phosphorus, and iron. Among the commonly used nuts, cashewnuts and almonds are good sources of iron, but pistachio is the richest containing 14 mg of iron per 100 g.

Most of the vegetable oils are rich in essential fatty acids. After oil extraction in the case of some, the residue (oilseed cake) can be formulated into acceptable foods rich in protein. For example, groundnut flour is used in the manufacture of Indian Multipurpose Food, balahar and balanced malt food. Due partly to their high fat content and partly to their high cellulose content, nuts are not easily digestible. However nuts eaten in a mixed diet are an extremely valuable source of protein. Peanuts for human consumption should be thoroughly dried and properly stored to avoid the growth of *Aspergillus flavus* which produces "aflatoxin".

5. Fruits

Fruits are protective foods. They are invaluable in human nutrition because they are good sources of vitamins and minerals. One special feature which distinguishes fruits from other foods is that they can be eaten raw and fresh. This makes the vitamins and minerals present in fruit easily available.

Nutritive value

(1) *Vitamins* : Fruits are prized for their vitamins. Most fruits contain significant amounts of ascorbic acid. The orange, guava and the Indian gooseberry (amla) are particularly rich in ascorbic acid. One medium sized orange can provide enough juice to meet the daily requirement of ascorbic acid of an adult. Apart from ascorbic acid, several fruits contain good amounts of carotene. The papaya and mango are excellent sources of carotene. (2) *Minerals* : Fruits are good sources of minerals especially sodium and potassium. Some fruits like sitaphal (custard apple) are rich in calcium. Dried fruits like raisins, dates and apricots are good sources of calcium and iron. Fruits also contain a great variety of organic acids which are responsible for the sourness of unripe fruits. The intake of fruits leads to an alkaline urine. (3) *Carbohydrates* : Fruits in general have a low energy value but some fruits like banana and mango contain good amounts of carbohydrate and can act as good source of energy. Pectin, a kind of sugar, present in fruits like guavas is helpful in the preparation of fruit jellies. The fruit sugars are easily digestible and completely absorbed. The more ripe a fruit is, the higher its sugar content. (4) *Cellulose* : Fruits contain cellulose which assists in normal bowel movements.

Nutrition experts recommend a daily intake of 85 grams or more of fresh fruit for maintenance of good health. Fruits are costly and it may not be within the reach of all to afford them daily. If green leafy vegetables are included in the daily diet, the need for fruit as an essential item in the diet is much reduced. The aim in nutrition education should be to promote the intake of seasonal fruits which are cheaper and easily available. The costly fruits are not necessarily the best in respect of nutrients. The food values of some common fruits are as given in Table 18.

TABLE 18
Nutritive value of some common fruits
(per 100 g of edible portion)

Name	Calories	Calcium (mg)	Iron (mg)	Carotene (µg)	Vit. C (mg)
Fresh fruits :					
Banana	104	10	0.5	124	7
Grapes	71	20	1.5	0	1
Guava	51	10	0.27	0	212
Mango	74	14	1.3	2,210	16
Orange	48	26	0.32	2,240	68
Papaya	32	17	0.5	2,740	57
Sitaphal	104	17	4.31	0	37
Amla	58	50	1.2	9	600
Dry fruits :					
Dates	317	120	7.3	44	3
Raisins	308	87	7.7	2.4	1
Almonds	655	230	5.09	0	0
Cashew nut	596	50	5.81	0	0
Ground nut	567	90	2.5	37	0

Source : *(34)*

6. Animal foods

Foods of animal origin include meat, poultry, fish, eggs, milk and dairy products. They provide high quality protein (containing all the essential amino acids) and good amounts of fat, besides some vitamins and minerals. Vitamin B_{12} is one of the rare nutrients found only in animal foods. Since they are expensive, animal foods are consumed in small amounts in most developing countries. Even small amounts of animal foods add considerably to the nutritive value of the diet. Among animal foods, cow's milk and hen's egg are perhaps nature's two most "nearly perfect" foods.

Milk

Milk is the best and most complete of all foods. It is secreted by the animals to serve as the sole and wholesome food for their suckling young ones. It is a fine blend of all the nutrients necessary for growth and development of the young ones. Thus milk is a good source of proteins, fats, sugars, vitamins and minerals.

(i) *Proteins* : The chief protein of milk is casein; it occurs in combination with calcium as calcium caseinate. The other proteins are lactalbumin and lactoglobulin. Animal milks contain nearly three times as much protein as human milk. Milk proteins contain all the essential amino acids. Human milk proteins contain greater amounts of tryptophan and sulphur–containing amino acids (especially cysteine) than the animal milk proteins. (ii) *Fat* : The fat content of milk varies from 3.4 per cent in human milk to 8.8 per cent in buffalo milk. Human milk contains a higher percentage of linoleic acid and oleic acid than animal milks. Milk fat is a good source of retinol and vitamin D. (iii) *Sugar* : The carbohydrate in all milks is lactose or milk sugar. It is found nowhere else in nature. It is less sweet than cane sugar and is readily fermented by lactic acid bacilli. Human milk contains more sugar than animal milks. (iv) *Minerals* : Milk contains almost all known minerals needed by the body such as calcium, phosphorus, sodium, potassium, magnesium, cobalt, copper, iodine, etc. Milk is particularly rich in calcium; it is however a poor source of iron. (v) *Vitamins* : Milk is a good source of all vitamins except vitamin C.

Human and animal milks are as compared in Table 19, which illustrates that milk is to a great extent species-specific.

TABLE 19
Nutritive value of milks compared
(value per 100 grams)

		Buffalo	Cow	Goat	Human
Fat	(g)	6.5	4.1	4.5	3.4
Protein	(g)	4.3	3.2	3.3	1.1
Lactose	(g)	5.1	4.4	4.6	7.4
Calcium	(mg)	210	120	170	28
Iron	(mg)	0.2	0.2	0.3	0.4-0.5
Vitamin C	(mg)	1	2	1	3
Minerals	(g)	0.8	0.8	0.8	0.1
Water	(g)	81.0	87	86.8	88
Energy	(kcal)	117	67	72	65

Source : *(34)*

Milk products

Milk is consumed in a variety of forms – as whole milk, butter, ghee, cheese, dried and condensed milk, khoa, ice cream, etc. Milk from which fat has been removed, is known as "skimmed milk". It is devoid of fat and fat soluble vitamins, but a good source of milk protein (35 per cent) and calcium.

Toned milk

The term "toned" is an Indian coinage. It is a blend of

natural milk and "made-up" milk. It contains 1 part of water, 1 part of natural milk and 1/8 part of skim milk powder. The mixture is stirred, pasteurized and supplied in bottles. Toned milk has a composition nearly equivalent to cow's milk. It is cheaper and yet a wholesome product.

Vegetable milk

Milk prepared from certain vegetable foods (viz. groundnut, soyabean) is termed "vegetable milk". It may be used as a substitute for animal milk. The Central Food Technological Research Institute, Mysore has perfected techniques for the preparation of vegetable milk *(72)*.

Egg

Egg contains all the nutrients except carbohydrate and vitamin C. About 12 per cent of egg is made of shell, 58 per cent of egg white, and 30 per cent of egg yolk. An egg weighing 60 grams contains 6 g of protein, 6 g of fat, 30 mg of calcium and 1.5 mg of iron, and supplies about 70 kcal of energy. Egg proteins have all the nine essential amino acids needed by the body in right proportions. Nutritionists consider egg protein as the best among food proteins. In fact, egg protein is the standard against which the quality of other proteins is compared. Except for vitamin C, egg contains all the fat-soluble and water-soluble vitamins in appreciable amounts. Important minerals such as calcium, phosphorus, iron, zinc and other trace elements are present in the egg. Barring milk, no other food can supply such a diverse range of nutrients. Net protein utilization (NPU) which combines in a single value the biological value and digestibility, is 100 for egg compared to 80 for meat and 75 for milk. Raw egg white is not assimilated by the intestinal mucosa, therefore it must be cooked before consumption. Boiling destroys 'avidin', a substance which prevents the body from obtaining biotin, one of the B-complex vitamins. Boiled egg is therefore nutritionally superior to raw egg. In recent years the cholesterol content of egg (250 mg/egg) has generated a sense of fear because of the risk of CHD. A reduction in intake of eggs is advised for those at risk of CHD. This should not distract others from eating eggs. Eggs or no eggs, cholesterol is formed in the body endogenously and is controlled by what is known as feedback mechanism.

Fish

Fish is nutritious food rich in proteins (15 to 25 per cent) with a good biological value and a satisfactory amino acid balance. The fat of fish is rich in unsaturated fatty acids and A and D vitamins. Fish liver oils are the richest source of vitamins A and D. Fish bones when eaten are an excellent source of calcium, phosphorus and fluorides. Fish are less rich in iron (0.7 to 3 mg per 100 g) than meat. Fresh water fish do not contain iodine, but sea fish do. Of all the sea foods, oysters and lobsters are the richest in iodine. There is practically no carbohydrate in fish. The fish proteins are easily digested. The nutritive value of diet is greatly enhanced by inclusion of fish.

Meat

The term "meat" is applied to the flesh of cattle, sheep and goats. Meats contain 15 to 20 per cent of protein, which is less than that found in pulses, but meat proteins are a good source of essential amino acids. Iron contained in meat (2 to 4 mg per 100 g) is more easily absorbed than iron in plants and this is another major quality of meat. In addition, meat contains varying amounts of fat, which is composed of non-essential saturated fat. The energy provided by meat depends upon its fat content. Besides iron, meat provides minerals such as zinc and B-vitamins. It is poor in calcium (10 to 25 mg per 100 g) but rich in phosphorus. Liver is extremely rich in many nutrients.

Table 20 shows the nutritive value of meat, fish and eggs.

TABLE 20
Nutritive value of Meat, Fish and Eggs (g/100 g)

	Proteins	Fat	Minerals
Meat, Goat	21.4	3.6	1.1
Fish	19.5	2.4	1.5
Egg. hen*	13.3	13.3	1.0
Liver goat	20.0	3.0	1.3

* Two large eggs without shell weigh about 100 g.

7. Fats and oils

Good cooking demands liberal use of oils and fats. Fats which are liquid at room temperature are called oils. Fats and oils are good sources of energy and fat-soluble vitamins. Fats of animal origin are poor sources of essential fatty acids. Those of vegetable origin are rich in poly-unsaturated fatty acids, excepting coconut and palm oils. The vegetable oils contain no vitamin A and D, except for red palm oil which is extremely rich in carotene. During the past 25 years, there has been a great increase in manufacture of vanaspati (hydrogenated fat) under various trade names. Margarine is made from vegetable oils and is fortified with vitamin A and D.

8. Sugar and jaggery

These are carbohydrate foods. Sugar is produced from sugarcane in India, and from sugar beet elsewhere. Refined sugar is pure sucrose and contains no other nutrients. Jaggery is prepared from sugarcane in India and is consumed in place of sugar. It contains useful amounts of carotene and iron derived from cooking pans. Honey consists of about 75 per cent sugars, mostly fructose and glucose.

9. Condiments and spices

These include asafoetida, cardamom, chillies, garlic, cloves, ginger, mustard, pepper, tamarind, turmeric, etc. They are mainly used to enhance the palatability of foods and stimulate appetite. The essential oils present in them have carminative properties and may aid in digestion. Excessive consumption of condiments is associated with peptic ulcer.

10. Miscellaneous

Beverages : Diet includes beverages, and especially water which is essential to life. Beverages include drinks which are appreciated for their flavour or their stimulating properties. They may be classified as follows :

(i) Coffee, tea, cocoa.
(ii) Soft drinks : aerated water, lemonade, pepsi cola, fruit juices, etc.
(iii) Alcoholic beverages : wine, beer, whisky and traditional preparations. Alcoholic beverages are rich in calories.

Coffee, tea and cocoa

(a) *Coffee* : Coffee contains caffeine (0.6 to 2.0 per cent), volatile oils (caffeol) and tannic acid. Caffeine is a stimulant of the nervous system. When coffee seeds are roasted, tannin is destroyed, proteins are coagulated and the pleasant aroma is liberated.

(b) *Tea* : There are two main varieties of tea – the green and the black varieties. Green tea which is more astringent than the black variety is popular in China, Japan and Assam. The chemical composition of tea is as follows : (i) *caffeine* : 2 to 6 per cent; (ii) *tannic acid* : 6 to 12 per cent; (iii) *theophylline* : traces; and (iv) *essential volatile oils:* 5 per cent. Tea is prepared by adding leaves to boiling water. When milk is added; the casein of milk combines with tannin and forms a harmless complex.

(c) *Cocoa* : Cocoa is obtained from cocoa beans. It is rich in fat, and contains theobromine which has stimulating properties. The composition of a cup of tea, coffee and cocoa containing the usual amount of sugar is given in Table 21. The nutritive value of a cup of tea or coffee is really due to its milk and sugar content.

TABLE 21
The chemical composition of coffee, tea and cocoa
(values per cup of 150 ml)

		Coffee	Tea	Cocoa
Protein	(g)	1.8	0.9	7.2
Fat	(g)	2.2	1.1	8.8
Carbohydrate	(g)	17.8	16.4	26.2
kcal		98.0	79.0	213.0

Soft drinks

Some are carbonated (e.g., soda water incorporating carbon dioxide under high pressure) and others non-carbonated such as fruit juices. The principal ingredients of soft drinks are carbon dioxide, sugars, acids such as citric acid or tartaric acid, colouring and flavouring agents. Fruit beverages comprise fruit juices, squashes and cordials. Fruit squashes and cordials are diluted with water before consumption.

Alcoholic beverages

These are beer, whisky, rum, gin, arrack, etc. The alcoholic content of these beverages varies widely from 5 to 6 per cent in beers to 40 to 45 per cent in whisky, rum, gin and brandy. Alcohol supplies about 7 kcal per gram.

b. Vinegar

Natural vinegar is made from fermentation of fruits, malt and molasses. It contains a minimum of 3.7 per cent acetic acid. Synthetic vinegar should not be harmful if it is free from lead, copper, arsenic or mineral acids. Synthetic vinegar should be distinctly labelled "SYNTHETIC" according to Prevention of Food Adulteration Act rules.

NUTRITIONAL REQUIREMENTS

Basic concepts

The science of human nutrition is mainly concerned with defining the nutritional requirements for the promotion, protection and maintenance of health in all groups of the population. Such knowledge is necessary in order to assess the nutritional adequacy of diets for growth of infants, children and adolescents, and for maintenance of health in adults of both sexes and during pregnancy and lactation in women *(83)*. In this context, a variety of terms have been used to define the amount of nutrients needed by the body such as : *optimum requirements, minimum requirements, recommended intakes* or *allowances,* and *safe level of intake.* Of these, the term "recommended dietary intake or allowance" (RDA) has been widely accepted *(1)*.

Recommended dietary allowance (RDA) : The average daily dietary nutrient intake level sufficient to meet the nutrient requirement of nearly all (97–98 per cent) healthy individuals in a particular life stage and gender group *(11)*.

Adequate intake : A recommended average daily intake level based on observed or experimentally determined approximations or estimates of nutrient intake by a group (or groups) of apparently healthy people, that are assumed to be adequate – used when an RDA cannot be determined. In the Indian context, this is referred to as "acceptable intake" *(11)*.

Tolerable upper intake level (TUL) : The highest average daily nutrient intake level that is likely to pose no risk of adverse health effects for almost all individuals in the general population. As intake increases above the TUL, the potential risk of adverse effect increases *(9)*.

Estimated average requirement (EAR) : The average daily nutrient intake level estimated to meet the requirement of half of the healthy individuals in a particular life stage and gender group *(11)*.

The RDA is derived from (a) the individual variability; and (b) the nutrient bioavailability from the habitual diet.

Individual variability : Definition of RDA takes into account the variability that exist in the requirement of a given nutrient between individuals in a given population group. The distribution of nutrient requirement in a population group is considered normal when the RDA corresponds to a requirement, which covers most of the individuals (97.5 per cent) in a given population. This corresponds to mean + 2 SD. This is termed as a safe level of nutrient; the chances of individual having requirements above the RDA is only 2.5 per cent. This principle is used in case of all nutrients except energy. In case of energy, intakes either in excess or below the actual requirement of energy are not safe. In respect to other nutrients, the RDA is 25 per cent (+ 2 SD) higher than the mean requirement, 12.5 per cent being considered as the extent of individual variability in the requirement of all those nutrients *(9)*.

Bioavailability : Bioavailability of a given nutrient from a diet, i.e., the release of the nutrient from the food, its absorption in the intestine and bioresponse have to be taken into account. It is the level of the nutrient that should be present in the diet to meet the requirement. The bio-availability factor is quite important in calcium, protein and trace elements like iron and zinc. In case of iron, the amount present in the diet is to be 20–30 times higher than the actual iron requirement to account for the low bioavailability of iron from a given diet, particularly a cereal-based diet.

RDA presents the level of the nutrient to be consumed daily to meet all the requirements of most of the individuals in a given population. However, it must be recognized that the RDA is not meant to be used as a standard to determine whether or not a given individual requirement has been met, since it is a level above the requirement of most individuals in a given population. RDA value of a nutrient is valid only when all other dietary nutrient intakes are satisfactory.

REFERENCE BODY WEIGHTS *(9)*

Age, gender and body weight largely determine the nutritional requirement of an individual. Body weights and heights of children reflect their state of health, nutrition and growth rate, while weight and heights of adults represent what can be attained by an individual with normal growth. Anthropometric measurements of infants and children of well-to-do families having access to good health care and no nutritional constraints are usually treated as reference values. The purpose of recommending nutrient requirements is to help attaining these anthropometric reference standards.

WHO standard weights and heights of infants and pre-school children

World Health Organization has recently published multi-centre growth reference standards for 0–60 month boys and girls, based on studies carried out among predominantly exclusively breast-fed children in six countries viz., USA, Brazil, Ghana, Norway, Oman and India. The median weights of infants and pre-school children (1–3 years) can be taken as reference values for Indian children.

Reference Indian adult man and woman

"Reference man" is aged between 19–39 years and weighs 65 kg with a height of 1.77 metre and a BMI of 20.75; is free from disease and physically fit for active work. On each working day, he is engaged in 8 hours of occupation which usually involves moderate activity; while when not at work he spends 8 hours in bed, 4-6 hours in sitting and moving about, 2 hours in walking and in active recreation or household duties.

"Reference woman" is aged between 19–39 years, non-pregnant non-lactating (NPNL) and weighs 55 kg with a height of 1.62 metre and a BMI of 20.95, is free from disease and physically fit for active work. On each working day she is engaged in 8 hours of occupation, which usually involves moderate activity, while when not at work she spends 8 hours in bed, 4–6 hours in sitting and moving about, 2 hours in walking and in active recreation or household duties.

Infants

The average of birth weight and body weight at 6 months is used for computing the reference body weight for infants 0–6 months of age. For 6–12 months, an average of body weight at 6 months and at 12 months is taken for computation.

Children

For children 1–3 years of age, an average of body weight at 18 months, 30 months, 42 months of WHO median weight is taken (as mentioned above).

The reference body weight for children of 4–6 years are obtained by averaging the body weight of 4+, 5+ and 6+ years. Similarly for other age groups also the reference body weights were obtained from the 95th centile value of body weights of rural India.

Adults

The average of values for age category of 18–19, 20–24, and 25–29 years was used for computing the reference weights for adult man and woman.

The summary of reference body weights for population in specified age groups is as shown in Table 22.

TABLE 22

Reference body weights for Indian population in specified age groups

Age Group	Category	Body weights (kg)
Men	>18 years	65.0
Women	>18 years	55.0
Infants	0–6 months	5.8
	6–12 months	8.5
Children	1–3 years	11.7
	4–6 years	18.3
	7–9 years	25.3
Boys	10–12 years	34.9
Girls	10–12 years	36.4
Boys	13–15 years	50.5
Girls	13–15 years	49.6
Boys	16–18 years	64.4
Girls	16–18 years	55.7

Source : *(11)*

ENERGY

Energy is a prime requisite for body function and growth. When a child's intake of food falls below a standard reference, growth slows, and if low levels of intake persist, adult stature will be reduced. Similarly, if adults fail to meet their food requirements they lose weight. This may lead to reduced ability to work, to resist infection, and weakened will to enjoy the normal satisfaction of life. This underlines the need for an adequate intake of food which is the source of all energy.

Measurement of energy

The energy value of foods has long been expressed in terms of the kilocalorie (kcal). The kilocalorie is generally expressed as "Calorie"– written with a capital "C" *(74)*. This has been replaced by the "joule" expressed as J, which has been accepted internationally. These units are defined as follows :

Joule, a physical unit of energy, is defined as the energy required to move 1 kg of mass by 1 metre by a force of 1 Newton acting on it (One Newton is the force needed to accelerate one kg mass by 1 metre per sec^2).

Kilocalorie (kcal) is defined as the heat required to raise the temperature of one kg of water by 1°C from 14.5°C to 15.5°C. The unit kcal is still popularly used.

The relationship between the two units of energy is as follows :

1 kcal = 4.184 KJ (Kilo Joule)
1 KJ = 0.239 kcal
1000 kcal = 4184 KJ = 4.18 MJ (Mega Joule)
1 MJ = 239 kcal

Reference man and woman

Energy intake recommendations are formulated for a "reference man" and a "reference woman" whose profiles are described, and then necessary adjustments are made for subjects who deviate from the standard reference. This procedure was first devised by the FAO Committee on calorie requirements in 1950 *(75)* and has been in use ever since.

Energy requirements

The energy requirement of an individual is defined as that level of energy intake from food that balances energy expenditure, when the individual has a body size and composition and level of physical activity, consistent with long-term good health, also allowing for maintenance of economically essential and socially desirable activity. In children and pregnant and lactating women, it includes the energy needs associated with the deposition of tissues or secretion of milk at rates consistent with good health *(9)*. The two standard deviation value is not added to the average requirement. This is because the energy intake and expenditure of an individual are finely balanced, and any surplus energy consumption will be stored as fat and a continuous excess of intake will lead to obesity *(9)*. Adults and even growing children are known to adapt either intake to suit their output, or output to suit intake over a very wide range. We do not have a proper understanding of the lower limit of adaption.

Factors affecting energy requirements

Energy requirements vary from one person to another depending upon inter-related variables acting in a complex way, such as age, sex, working condition, body composition, physical activity, physiological state etc. All these factors lead to differences in food intake.

Currently, it is recommended that energy requirement must be assessed in terms of energy expenditure rather than in terms of energy intake. It is a logical approach, where one can specify the energy requirements in terms of energy output for productive work and leisure activity of adults and tissue deposition in infants, children and during pregnancy and milk secretion during lactation. This does imply that there is a need to specify an appropriate body weight of individual as well as the quantum of physical activity that is considered 'desirable' for the same individual *(11)*.

There are three important terms while defining energy expenditure using physical activity estimations. These are – Physical Activity Ratio (PAR), Physical Activity Level (PAL) and Total Energy Expenditure (TEE). The physical activity ratio (PAR) is expressed as the ratio of the energy cost of an individual activity per minute to the cost of the basal metabolic rate (BMR) per minute.

$$\text{Physical Activity Ratio (PAR)} = \frac{\text{Energy cost of an activity per minute}}{\text{Energy cost of basal metabolism per minute}}$$

The PAR is unit-less, and the distinct advantage of expressing energy expenditure of an activity in terms of PAR values relates to its use for both sexes, at all ages and at all body sizes. This is because these covariates appear in both the numerator and denominator and cancel out *(11)*.

Table 23 shows the energy requirement as proposed by ICMR 2020, for various age groups.

Vulnerable groups

(a) *Pregnant and lactating mothers :* The energy requirements of women are increased by pregnancy

TABLE 23

Energy requirement (kcal/d) as proposed by ICMR 2020

Age group	Category	ICMR 2020	ICMR 2010	Difference
Adult Men	Sedentary work	2110	2320	–210
	Moderate work	2710	2730	–20
	Heavy work	3470	3490	–20
Adult Women	Sedentary work	1660	1900	–240
	Moderate work	2130	2230	–100
	Heavy work	2720	2850	–130
	Pregnant	+ 350	+ 350	–
	Lactating (0–6 m)	+600	+600	–
	Lactating (7–12 m)	+520	+520	–
Infants	0–6 months	550	520	+30
	6–12 months	670	670	–
Children	1–3 y	1010	1060	-50
	4–6 y	1360	1350	+10
	7–9 y	1700	1690	+10
Boys	10–12 y	2220	2190	+30
Girls	10–12 y	2060	2010	+50
Boys	13–15 y	2860	2750	+110
Girls	13–15 y	2400	2330	+70
Boys	16–18 y	3320	3020	+300
Girls	16–18 y	2500	2440	+60

Source : *(11)*

(+350 kcal daily throughout pregnancy) and lactation (+600 kcal daily during the first 6 months, and +520 kcals daily during the next 6 months) over and above their normal requirements. This is to provide for the extra energy needs associated with the deposition of tissues or the secretion of milk at rates consistent with good health *(11)*.

(b) *Children :* Because of their rapid growth rate, young children require proportionately more energy for each kilogram of body weight than adults (see Table 23).

A problem that arises is in recommending intakes in communities where a large number of children are underweight because of malnutrition. In order to provide for "catch-up growth" during childhood, intakes should be based on age rather than weight where practical *(77)*. The ICMR standards are based on age, and not on body weight (except during the first year of life).

Children above the age of 13 years need as much energy as adults. This is because they show a good deal of physical activity, almost equal to hard work by adults. This is also the age when puberty sets in and there is a spurt in growth and an increase in metabolic rate. This fact should be borne in mind when planning dietaries for children.

(c) *Adults :* The energy requirements decrease with age because of a fall in BMR and a decrease in physical activity in most persons. In general, there is a 2 per cent decline of resting metabolism for each decade for adults *(31)*. The FAO/WHO committee suggested that after the age of 40 years, requirements should be reduced by 5 per cent per each decade until the age of 60, and by 10 per cent for each decade thereafter *(76)*.

Source of energy

The main source of energy in Indian diets, which are predominantly plant food based, are carbohydrate, fat, protein and dietary fibre. They supply energy at the following rates :

Protein	–	4 kcal/g
Fat	–	9 kcal/g
Carbohydrate	–	4 kcal/g
Dietary fibre	–	2 kcal/g

Dietary fibre forms an indigestible and important component of plant food and was never earlier considered as source of energy. These dietary fibres (soluble and insoluble) undergo fermentation in the colon and yield short chain fatty acids, such as butyric, propionic and acetic acids which are utilized as a source of energy by the colon cells and by the liver. Hence they are known to yield energy from fermentable fibre and no energy from non-fermentable fibre. In conventional foods, 70 per cent of fibre is fermentable. In general, energy conversion factor for fibre is taken as 2.0 kcal/g. Hitherto, dietary fibre was not determined directly as a source of energy and there is a need to recalculate energy yield of various foods on the basis of their revised content of carbohydrates, proteins, fat and dietary fibre *(9)*.

The main source of energy in diets is carbohydrates derived largely from cereals. These cereals constitute about 80 per cent of our diet and provide 50–80 per cent of daily energy intake. However, energy contribution from diets varies very widely. Those belonging to low income group have only 5 per cent fat in their diet, whereas affluent families derive as high as 30 per cent of their dietary energy from fat. Most families derive 10–12 per cent of energy from proteins *(9)*.

Nutritional individuality

In normal individuals at all ages and of both sexes, there is a large variation in energy intake but the reasons for this wide range of nutritional requirements are not known. The concept of nutritional individuality needs to be stressed, and its neglect may result in the over-feeding of some whose needs happen to be less than the "average standard requirement" *(78)*.

PROTEIN

Protein requirements vary from individual to individual. Apart from age, sex and other physiological variables, factors like infection, worm infestation, emotional disturbances and stress situations can affect a person's protein requirement.

Assessment of protein

(a) *PROTEIN QUALITY*

The quality of a protein is assessed by comparison to the "reference protein" which is usually egg protein. Two methods of assessment of protein quality needs mention :

(i) Amino acid score : It is a measure of the concentration of each essential amino acid in the test protein expressed as a percentage of that amino acid in the reference protein.

$$\text{Amino acid score} = \frac{\text{mg of amino acid per g of test protein}}{\text{mg of the same amino acid per g of reference protein.}} \times 100$$

The amino acid (or chemical) score is somewhere between 50 and 60 for starches, and 70 and 80 for animal foods *(69)*.

(ii) Net protein utilization (NPU) : It is a product of digestibility coefficient and biological value divided by 100 *(8)*. The NPU gives a more complete expression of protein quality than the amino acid score. It is a biological method that requires special laboratory facilities.

$$\text{NPU} = \frac{\text{Nitrogen retained by the body}}{\text{Nitrogen intake}} \times 100$$

In calculating protein quality, 1 gram of N is assumed to be equivalent to 6.25 g of protein.

The protein requirement varies with the NPU of dietary protein. If the NPU is low, the protein requirement is high and vice versa. The NPU of the protein of Indian diets varies between 50 and 80.

(b) *PROTEIN QUANTITY*

The protein content of many Indian foods has been determined and published in food composition tables. One way of evaluating foods as source of protein is to determine what per cent of their energy value is supplied by their protein content. This is known as **Protein–Energy Ratio** (PE ratio or percentage).

$$\text{PE per cent} = \frac{\text{Energy from protein}}{\text{Total energy in diet}} \times 100$$

This concept is useful because in many population groups adequate diet is not consumed to meet energy needs, resulting in energy deficits. The ratio of protein requirement, expressed as the ratio of protein calories to the energy requirement is as given in Table 24.

TABLE 24

Protein-energy ratio for different age groups (2020)

Group	Protein requirement g/kg/d[a]	Energy requirement kcal/kg/d	PE ratio of requirement
Pre-school children[b] 1–5 years[b]	0.95	79	4.8
School children 6–10 years	0.91	68	5.4
Adolescents[b] 11–17 years (Boys)	0.88	56	6.3
11–17 years (Girls)	0.86	51	6.7
Adults			
Men (Sedentary)	0.83	32	10.4
Women (Sedentary)	0.83	30	11.1
Men (Moderate active)	0.83	39	8.5
Women (Moderate active)	0.83	37	9.0

PE Ratio = Protein Energy ratio; these values refer to the requirement

a Safe requirement of high-quality protein

b Assuming moderately active children and adolescents

Source : *(11)*

The protein-energy percentage value of some commonly used foods is as shown in Table 25.

TABLE 25

Relative protein value of some foods : per cent of total energy supplied by protein

Food	Nutrients per 100 g		Energy from proteins	
	kcal	Protein (g)	Actual (kcal)	PE%
Fish	100	20.0	80	80
Milk (cow)	67	3.2	13	20
Dhal	350	21.0	84	24
Rice	350	7.0	28	8
Potato	100	1.6	6	6
Banana	100	1.0	4	4
Tapioca	160	0.7	3	2

If the PE is less than 4 per cent, the subject will be unable to eat enough to satisfy protein requirements. It is recommended that protein should account for approximately 10–12 per cent of the total daily energy intake.

Dietary intakes

It is customary to express requirement in terms of grams per kg of body weight. This principle applies to all age groups, although absolute additions in units of grams of protein per day are made for pregnancy and lactation.

The ICMR Expert Group *(11)* suggested an intake of 0.88 gram of protein per kg of body weight for adult males and females, assuming a NPU of 65 for the dietary protein. Table 28 gives the protein intakes for individuals of different ages and physiological states.

Vulnerable groups

The protein requirements of women are increased during pregnancy. For 10 kg gestational weight gain the requirement increases by 1, 9.5 and 22 g/day in 1st, 2nd and 3rd trimesters respectively; and during lactation by about 13 g per day (during 0 to 6 months), over and above their normal requirements.

Young children (0 to 6 years) require proportionately more protein for each kilogram of body weight than adults. They are more vulnerable to malnutrition.

The ICMR Expert Group *(11)* has made recommendations for the elderly. It seems reasonable to assume that the requirement of the aged are not less than that for young adults, as shown in Table 31.

All estimates of protein requirement are valid only when the energy requirements are fully met. If the total energy intake is inadequate some dietary protein will be diverted to provide energy. It is now accepted that there are no body protein stores which can be filled up by a high protein intake.

At present there is no evidence that higher intakes of protein confer greater benefit, although the possibility cannot be ruled out. Most people, if they can, apparently choose to eat more protein than the physiological requirement. The question remains whether high protein intakes, far from being beneficial, may actually be harmful *(7)*.

Amino acid requirements

The protein intake must also satisfy the need for essential amino acids. The 2007 WHO Expert Committee Report on Energy and Protein Requirements gives current estimates of amino acid requirements (in mg/kg per day) for adults. These are reproduced in Table 26.

TABLE 26

Essential amino acid (EAA) requirements : Adult

Amino acid	FAO/WHO/UNU 2007	
	mg/kg/d	mg/g protein
Histidine	10	15
Isoleucine	20	30
Leucine	39	59
Lysine	30	45
Methionine	10	16
Cysteine	4	6
Methionine + Cysteine	15	22
Threonine	15	23
Phenylalanine + Tyrosine	25	38
Tryptophan	4	6
Valine	26	39
Total EAA	184	277
Total protein	0.66 g/kg/d	
Safe level of protein (Mean + 1.96 × SD)	0.83 g/kg/d	

Source : *(11)*

New tissues cannot be formed unless all the essential amino acids are present in the diet. The requirement of EAA decreases sharply as one advances in age. The quality of the diet is far more critical for the infant than for the adult.

FAT

The daily requirement of fat is not known with certainty. During infancy, fats contribute to a little over 50 per cent of the total energy intake. This scales down to about 20 per cent in adulthood. The ICMR Expert Group (2020) has recommended an intake of 20 per cent of the total energy intake as fat, of which at least 50 per cent of fat intake should consist of vegetable oils rich in essential fatty acids. The requirement of essential fatty acids ranges from 3 per cent energy intake to 5.7 per cent of energy intake in young children.

Suggested levels of fat intake are as given in Table 27.

TABLE 27

Recommendations for dietary fat intake for Indians (2020)

Age/Gender/ Physiological groups	Physical activity	Minimum level of Total fat (% E)	Fat from foods other than visible fats, % E	Visible fat	
				%E	g/p/d
Adult Man	Sedentary				25
	Moderate	20	10	10	30
	Heavy				40
	Sedentary				20
	Moderate	20	10	10	25
	Heavy				30
Adult Woman	Pregnant women				30
		20	10	10	
	Lactating women				30
Infants	0 - 6 months	40-60	Human milk		
	7-24 months	35	10	25	25
Children	3-6 years				25
	7-9 years				30
Boys	10-12 years				35
	13-15 years	25	10	15	45
	16-17 years				50
Girls	10-12 years				35
	13-15 years				40
	16-17 years				35

Source : *(11)*

CARBOHYDRATE

The recommended intake of carbohydrate in balanced diets is placed so as to contribute between 50 to 80 per cent of total energy intake. Most Indian diets contain amounts more than this, providing as much as 90 per cent of total energy intake in some cases, which makes the diet imbalanced. This needs to be corrected through nutrition education.

The recommended dietary allowances for energy, protein, fat and minerals is summarized in Table 28.

OTHER RECOMMENDED INTAKES

The recommended daily allowances of nutrients for Indians are as summarized in Table 28; Table 29 shows acceptable macronutrients distribution range; Table 30 shows summary of recommended intake of some of the minerals and trace elements; Table 31 shows the daily nutrients recommendation for the elderly and Table 32 shows Tolerable Upper Limit (TUL) for nutrients.

All nutritional requirements are interrelated. For example, there is a close interrelationship between the energy and protein requirements, between requirements for phosphorus, calcium and vitamin D, between fats and vitamins, and between carbohydrates and vitamins.

It has been said that food is not only a collection of nutrients open to statistical or dietary study, but also simultaneously a system of communication, a protocol for customs, situations and behaviour.

BALANCED DIET

A diet may be defined as the kinds of food on which a person or group lives. A balanced diet is defined as one which contains a variety of foods in such quantities and proportions that the need for energy, amino acids, vitamins, minerals, fats, carbohydrate and other nutrients is adequately met for maintaining health, vitality and general well-being and also makes a small provision for extra nutrients to withstand short duration of leanness *(69)*. A balanced diet has become an accepted means to safeguard a population from nutritional deficiencies *(79)*.

In constructing balanced diet, the following principles should be borne in mind : (a) First and foremost, the daily requirement of protein should be met. This amounts to 10–15 per cent of the daily energy intake. (b) Next comes the fat requirement, which should be limited to 15–30 per cent of the daily energy intake (c) Carbohydrates rich in natural fibre should constitute the remaining food energy. The requirements of micronutrients (Table 28, 29, 30 and 31) should be met.

TABLE 28

Summary of RDA for Indians – 2020

Age Group	Category of work	Body Wt (kg)	Protein (g/d)	Dietary Fibre* (g/d)	Cal-cium (mg/d)	Magn-esium (mg/d)	Iron (mg/d)	Zinc (mg/d)	Iodine (µg/day)	Thia-mine (mg/d)	Ribo-flavin (mg/d)	Niacin (mg/d)	Vit B6 (mg/d)	Folate (µg/d)	Vit B12 (µg/d)	Vit C (mg/d)	Vit A (µg/d)	Vit D (IU/d)
	Sedentary			32						1.4	2.0	14	1.9					
Men	Moderate	65	54.0	41	1000	440	19	17	150	1.8	2.5	18	2.4	300	2.2	80	1000	600
	Heavy			52						2.3	3.2	23	3.1					
	Sedentary			25						1.4	1.9	11	1.9					
	Moderate	55	46.0	32	1000	370	29	13	150	1.7	2.4	14	1.9	220	2.2	65	840	600
	Heavy			41						2.2	3.1	18	2.4					
Women	Pregnant woman	55 + 10	+9.5 (2nd trimester) +22.0 (3rd trimester)	–	1000	440	27	14.5	250	2.0	2.7	+2.5	2.3	570	+0.25	+15	900	600
	Lactation 0–6m		+17.0							2.1	3.0	+5	+0.26	330				
				–	1200	400	23	14	280						+1.0	+50	950	600
	7–12m		+13.0							2.1	2.9	+5	+0.17	330				
Infants	0–6 m*	5.8	8.0	–	300	30	–	–	100	0.2	0.4	2	0.1	25	1.2	20	350	400
	6–12m	8.5	10.5	–	300	75	3	2.5	130	0.4	0.6	5	0.6	85	1.2	30	350	400
	1–3 y	12.9	12.5	15	500	90	8	3.3	90	0.7	1.1	7	0.9	120	1.2	30	390	
Children	4–6 y	18.3	16.0	20	550	125	11	4.5	120	0.9	1.3	9	1.2	135	1.2	35	510	600
	7–9 y	25.3	23.0	26	650	175	15	5.9	120	1.1	1.6	11	1.5	170	2.2	45	630	
Boys	10–12 y	34.9	32.0	33	850	240	16	8.5	150	1.5	2.1	15	2.0	220	2.2	55	770	600
Girls	10–12 y	36.4	33.0	31	850	250	28	8.5	150	1.4	1.9	14	1.9	225	2.2	50	790	600
Boys	13–15 y	50.5	45.0	43	1000	345	22	14.3	150	1.9	2.7	19	2.6	285	2.2	70	930	600
Girls	13–15 y	49.6	43.0	36	1000	340	30	12.8	150	1.6	2.2	16	2.2	245	2.2	65	890	600
Boys	16–18 y	64.4	55.0	50	1050	440	26	17.6	150	2.2	3.1	22	3.0	340	2.2	85	1000	600
Girls	16–18 y	55.7	46.0	38	1050	380	32	14.2	150	1.7	2.3	17	2.3	270	2.2	70	860	600

* Adequate Intake (AI)

Source : *(11)*

TABLE 29

Acceptable macronutrients distribution range (AMDR) by age and physiological groups as per cent of energy (%E)

Nutrients	Age group			
	1–2 years	3–18 years	Adults	Pregnant and lactating women
Protein (PE ratio)*	5–15	5–15	5–15	5–15
Total Fat	30–40	25–35	15–35	20–35
n-6 PUFA#	4–10	4–10	4–10	4–10
n-3-PUFA	0.5–1	0.5–1	0.5–1	0.5–1
Carbohydrate	40–60	45–65	45–65	45–65

* Depends on protein quality and total energy intake

\# n-6 to n-3 ratio should be between 5–10:1

Note : For good health, adults should consume minimum of 100 to 130 g of carbohydrates and atleast 20 g fats (food sources)

Source : *(11)*

TABLE 30

Summary of recommended intakes for other minerals and trace elements

S.No.	Minerals/ Trace Element	Recommended intake (per day)
1	Phosphorous	1000 mg/day
2	Sodium	2000 mg/day
3	Potassium	3500 mg/day
4	Copper	2 mg/day
5	Manganese	4 mg/day
6	Chromium	50 µg/day
7	Selenium	40 µg/day

Source : *(11)*

TABLE 31

Daily Nutrient recommendations for the elderly in India – 2020

Nutrients		Energy (Kcal)*	Dietary Fibre	Protein (gr)	Vit-A (µg)	Thiamin B_1(mg)	Riboflavin B_2(mg)	Niacin (mg)	Vit-C (mg)	Vit-B_6 (mg)	Folate (µg)	Vit-B_{12} (µg)	Vit-D (IU)	Calcium (mg)	Magnesium (mg)	Iron (mg)	Zinc (mg)	Iodine (µg)
Men ≥60 Yrs	EAR	1700	-	42.9	460	1.2	1.6	12	65	1.6	250	2.0	400	800	370	11	14	95
	RDA	-	32	54.0	1000	1.4	2.0	14	80	1.9	300	2.2	800	1200	440	19	17	150
Women ≥60 Yrs	EAR	1500	-	36.3	390	1.1	1.6	9	55	1.6	180	2.0	400	800	310	11	11	95
	RDA	-	25	45.7	840	1.4	1.9	11	65	1.9	200	2.2	800	1200	370	19	13.2	150

*: There is no RDA for Energy. The EAR is equivalent to the Estimated Energy Requirements (EER)

Source : *(11)*

TABLE 32

Tolerable Upper Limit (TUL) for Nutrients – 2020

Age Group	Category of work	Protein (PE ratio)	Calcium (mg/d)	Magnesium* (mg/d)	Iron (mg/d)	Zinc (mg/d)	Iodine (µg/day)	Niacin (mg/d)	Vit. B_6 (mg/ d)	Folate (µg/d)	Vit. C (mg/d)	Vit. A (µg/d)	Vit. D (IU/d)
Men	Sedentary												
	Moderate	<40%	2500	350	45	40	1100			1000	2000	3000	
	Heavy							35	100				4000
	Sedentary												
	Moderate	<40%	2500	350	45	40	1100			1000	2000	3000	
	Heavy												
Women	Pregnant woman	<30%	2500	350	45	40	1100	–	–	1000	2000	3000	4000
	Lactation 0–6 months 7–12 months	<40%	2500	350	45	40	1100	–	–	1000	2000	3000	4000
Infants	0–6 months	<15%	–	–	40	4	–	–	–	–	–	600	1000
	6–12 months	<15%	–	–	40	5	–	–	–	–	–	600	1500
Children	1–3 years	<15%	1500	65	40	7	200			–	350	600	2500
	4–6 years	<15%	2500	110	40	12	300	–	–	–	550	900	3000
	7–9 years	<15%	2500	110	40	12	400			300	800	900	3000
Boys	10–12 years	<15%	3000	350	40	23	600	–	–	600–800 (9–17y)	1050	1700	4000
Girls	10–12 years	<15%	3000	350	40	23	600	–	–	–	1300	1700	4000
Boys	13–15 years	<15%	3000	350	45	34	900	–	–	–	1550	2800	4000
Girls	13–15 years	<15%	3000	350	45	34	900	–	–	–	1800	2800	4000
Boys	16–18 years	<15%	3000	350	45	34	1100	–	–	–	1950	2800	4000
Girls	16–18 years	<15%	3000	350	45	34	1100	–	–	–	2000	2800	4000

The TUL is the maximum level of habitual intake from all sources of a nutrient or related substance judged to be unlikely to lead to adverse health effects in humans

*Note: TUL values are only for non-dietary pharmacological doses.

Source : *(11)*

The dietary pattern varies widely in different parts of the world. It is generally developed around the kinds of food produced (or imported) depending upon the climatic conditions of the region, economic capacity, region, customs, taboos, tastes and habits of the people. Balanced diets formulated by the Indian Council of Medical Research are given in Annexure II at the end of this chapter.

A nutritional education guide "The Food Guide Pyramid" emphasizes foods from the five major food groups shown in the three lower sections of the Pyramid (Fig. 1). Each of these food groups provides some, but not all, of the nutrients required. Foods in one group can't replace those in another. No one of these major food groups is more important than another – for good health, one needs them all.

DIETARY GOALS

All countries should develop a national nutrition and food policy setting out "dietary goals" for achievement *(72)*. The dietary goals **("prudent diet")** recommended by the various Expert Committees of WHO *(16, 79)* are as below :

(a) dietary fat should be limited to approximately 15–30 per cent of total daily intake;

(b) saturated fats should contribute no more than 10 per cent of the total energy intake; unsaturated vegetable oils should be substituted for the remaining fat requirement;

(c) excessive consumption of refined carbohydrate should be avoided; some amount of carbohydrate rich in natural fibre should be taken;

(d) sources rich in energy such as fats and alcohol should be restricted;

(e) salt intake should be reduced to an average of not more than 5 g. per day; (salt intake is more in tropical countries. In India it averages 15 g. per day);

(f) protein should account for approximately 10–15 per cent of the daily intake; and

(g) junk foods such as colas, ketchups and other foods that supply empty calories should be reduced.

There may be conditions under which the above recommendations for daily food intake do not apply. For example, diet should be adapted to the special needs of growth, pregnancy, lactation, physical activity, and medical disorders (e.g., diabetes).

NUTRITIONAL PROBLEMS IN PUBLIC HEALTH

There are many nutritional problems which affect vast segments of our population. The major ones which deserve special mention are highlighted :

1. Low birth weight

Low birth weight (i.e., birth weight less than 2500 g) is a major public health problem in many developing countries. According to Rapid Survey Report on Children 2014, about 18.6 per cent of babies born in India are LBW *(81)* as compared to 4 per cent in some developed countries. In countries where the proportion of LBW is high, the majority are suffering from foetal growth retardation. In countries where the proportion of LBW infants is low, most of them are preterm. Although we do not know all the causes of LBW, maternal malnutrition and anaemia appear to be significant risk factors in its occurrence. Among the other causes of LBW are hard physical labour during pregnancy, and illnesses

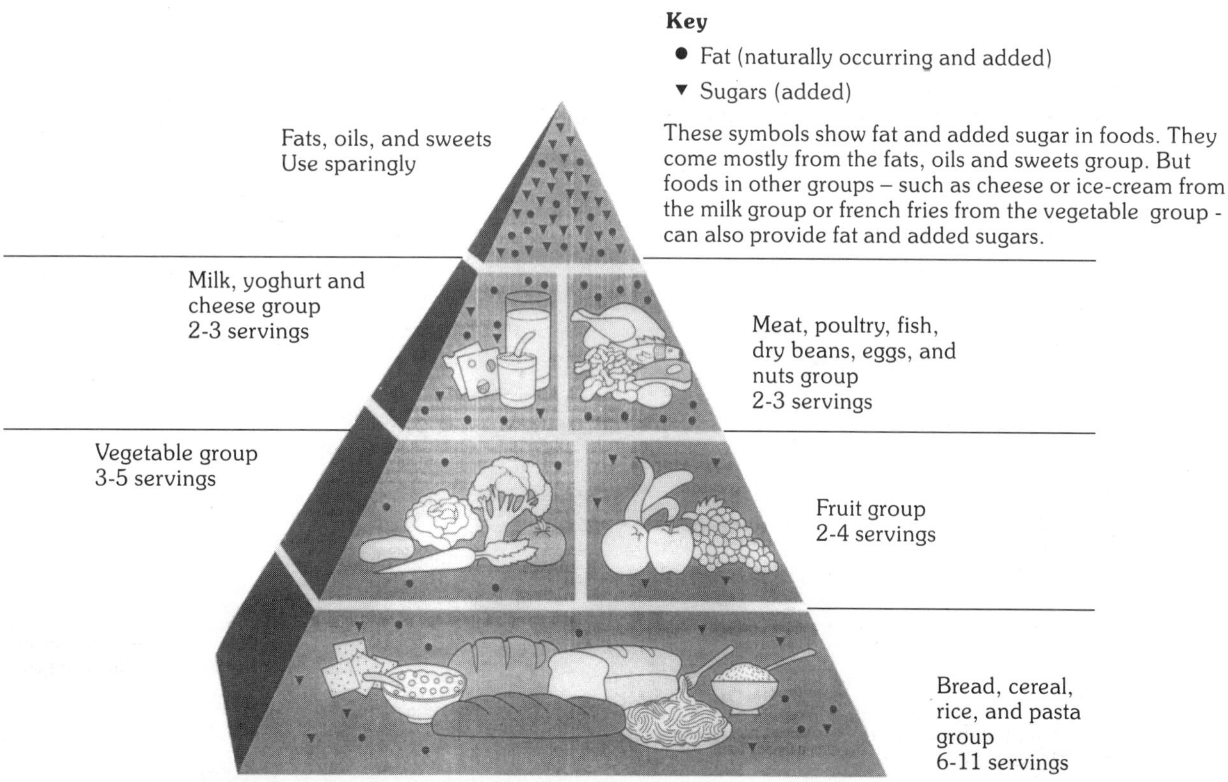

FIG. 1

The food guide pyramid

Source : *(80)*

especially infections. Short maternal stature, very young age, high parity, smoking, close birth intervals are all associated factors. All these factors are interrelated *(82)*.

Since the problem is multifactorial, there is no universal solution. Interventions have to be cause-specific. This matter has already been discussed in Chapter 11.

2. Under nutrition

Undernutrition is identified as a major health and nutrition problem in India. It is not only an important cause of childhood morbidity and mortality, but leads also to permanent impairment of physical and possibly, of mental growth of those who survive *(9)*.

The nutrition problem frequently encountered, particularly among the rural poor and urban slums in India are protein-energy malnutrition and micronutrient deficiencies. The term undernutrition encompasses stunting (chronic malnutrition), wasting (acute malnutrition) and underweight.

Persistent undernutrition through the growing phase of childhood leads to short stature in adults. About 16.2 per cent of adult men and 18.7 per cent women have Body Mass Index (BMI) below 18.5, which indicates chronic energy deficiency. In case of tribal adults 40 per cent of men and 49 per cent of women are below 18.5 BMI *(84)*.

Children are more vulnerable to the effects of undernutrition. According to NFHS-5, about 18.5 per cent of children are born with low birth weight, 32.1 per cent are underweight (weight for age < 5 years of age), 35.5 per cent are stunted (height for age <5 years), 19.3 per cent are wasted (weight for hight) and <1 per cent children under 5 years are having kwashiorkor/Marasmus.

In the 1970s, it was widely held that PEM was due to protein deficiency. Over the years, the concept of "protein gap" has given place to the concept of "food gap". That is, PEM is primarily due to (a) an inadequate intake of food (food gap) both in quantity and quality, and (b) infections, notably diarrhoea, respiratory infections, measles and intestinal worms which increase requirements for calories, protein and other nutrients, while decreasing their absorption and utilization. It is a vicious circle – infection contributing to malnutrition and malnutrition contributing to infection, both acting synergistically (Fig. 2).

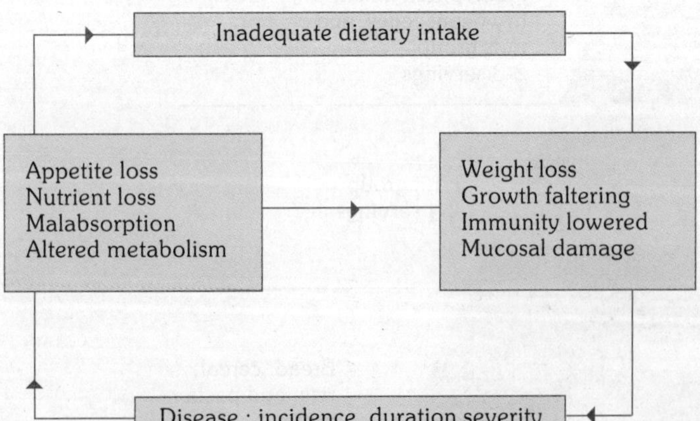

FIG. 2
Malnutrition/Infection cycle

Source : *(68)*

There are numerous other contributory factors in the web of causation, viz. poor environmental conditions, large family size, poor maternal health, failure of lactation, premature termination of breast-feeding, and adverse cultural practices relating to child rearing and weaning such as the use of over-diluted cow's milk and discarding cooking water from cereals and delayed supplementary feeding *(83)*.

Malnutrition is self-perpetuating. A child's nutritional status at any point of time depends on his or her past nutritional history, which may particularly account for the present status. To some extent, this nutritional history is linked to the mother's health and nutritional status. This in turn has been influenced by her living conditions and nutritional history during her own childhood (Fig. 3).

Measurement of Undernutrition

In children, undernutrition is synonymous with growth failure – undernourished children are shorter and lighter than they should be for their age/height. To get a measure of malnutrition in a population, young children are weighed and/or their height is measured and the results compared to those of a 'reference population' known to have grown well. Measuring weight and height is the most common way of assessing malnutrition in a given population. Such use of measurements of dimensions of the human body is known as anthropometry.

Anthropometry is a widely used, inexpensive and non-invasive measure of the general nutrirional status of an individual or a population group. The three commonly used anthropometric indices are :

- Weight-for-Age (WFA).
- Length-for-Age or Height-For-Age (HFA).
- Weight-for-Length or Weight-for-Height (WFH).

Types of Undernutrition *(73)*

The three indices – weight-for-age, height/length-for-age, weight-for-height/length are used to identify three nutrition conditions : underweight, stunting and wasting, respectively.

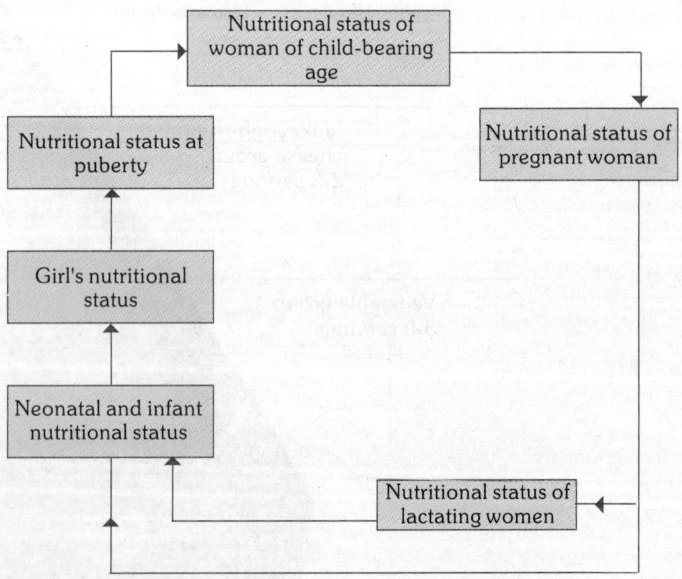

FIG. 3
Influence of each generation's nutritional status on the following generation.

Source : *(68)*

Each of the three nutrition indicators is expressed in standard deviation units (Z-scores) from the median of the reference population based on which undernutrition may be further classified as moderate or severe.

Underweight

Underweight, based on weight-for-age, is a composite measure of stunting and wasting, and is recommended as the indicator to assess changes in the magnitude of malnutrition over time. This condition can result from either chronic or acute malnutrition, or both. Underweight is often used as a basic indicator of the status of a population's health as weight is easy to measure. Evidence has shown that the mortality risk of children who are even mildly underweight is increased, and severely underweight children are at even greater risk.

An underweight child has a weight-for-age Z-score that is at least two standard deviations (–2SD) below the median in the World Health Organization (WHO) Child Growth Standards.

Stunting

Failure to achieve expected height/length as compared to healthy, well-nourished children of the same age is a sign of stunting. Stunting is an indicator of linear growth retardation that results from failure to receive adequate nutrition over a long period or recurrent adequate nutrition over a long period or recurrent infections. It may be exacerbated by recurrent and chronic illness. It is an indicator of past growth failure. It is associated with a number of long-term factors including chronic insufficient nutrient intake, frequent infection, sustained inappropriate feeding practices and poverty. Stunting often results in delayed psycho-social and cognitive development and poor school performance.

A stunted child has a height-for-age Z-score that is at least two standard deviations (–2SD) below the median for the WHO Child Growth Standards.

Wasting

Wasting represents a recent failure to receive adequate nutrition and may be affected by recent episodes of diarrhoea and other acute illnesses. Wasting indicates current or acute malnutrition resulting from failure to gain weight or actual weight loss. Causes include inadequate food intake, incorrect feeding practices, disease, and infection or, more frequently, a combination of these factors. Wasting in individual children and population groups can change rapidly and shows marked seasonal patterns associated with changes in food availability or disease prevalence to which it is very sensitive.

A wasted child has a weight-for-height Z-score that is at least two standard deviations (–2SD) below the median for the WHO Child Growth Standards.

Severe Acute Malnutrition (SAM)

Severe acute malnutrition is defined by very low weight-for-height/length (Z-score below –3SD of the median WHO child growth standards), a mid-upper arm circumference <115 mm, or by the presence of nutritional oedema.

SAM increases signficantly the risk of death in children under five years of age. It can be an indirect cause of child death by increasing the case fatality rate in children suffering from common illnesses such as diarrhoea and pneumonia. Children who are severely wasted are 9 times likely to die than well-nourished children.

Kwashiorkor and Marasmus

Kwashiorkor and marasmus are the two different forms of protein and energy malnutrition. The main cause of this form of malnutrition is inadequate protein intake and low concentration of essential amino acids. Kwashiorkor is a severe form of undernutrition, which develops in individuals on diets with a low protein/energy ratio. The main symptoms of Kwashiorkor are oedema, wasting, liver enlargement, hypoalbuminaemia, steatosis and the possible depigmentation of skin and hair.

Marasmus is the other form of malnutrition, which is caused by inadequate intake of both protein and energy. It is a form of severe cachexia with weight loss as a result of wasting in infancy and childhood. The main symptoms of marasmus are severe wasting, with little or no oedema, minimal subcutaneous fat, severe muscle wasting and non-normal serum albumin levels.

Early detection of PEM

The first indicator of PEM is under-weight for age. The most practical method to detect this, which can be employed even by field health workers, is to maintain growth charts. These charts indicate at a glance whether the child is gaining or losing weight.

Arm circumference : Arm circumference yields a relatively reliable estimation of the body's muscle mass, the reduction of which is one of the most striking mechanisms by which the body adjusts to inadequate energy intakes. Arm circumference cannot be used before the age of one year; between ages one and five years, it hardly varies. An arm circumference exceeding 13.5 cm is a sign of a satisfactory nutritional status, between 12.5 and 13.5 cm it indicates mild–moderate malnutrition and below 12.5 cm, severe malnutrition *(68)*.

Preventive measures

There is no simple solution to the problem of PEM. Many types of actions are necessary. The following is adapted from the 8th FAO/WHO Expert Committee on Nutrition *(1)* for the prevention of PEM in the community :

(a) *Health promotion :*

1. Measures directed to pregnant and lactating women (education, distribution of supplements);
2. Promotion of breast-feeding;
3. Development of low cost weaning foods : the child should be made to eat more food at frequent intervals;
4. Measures to improve family diet;
5. Nutrition education – Promotion of correct feeding practices;
6. Home economics;
7. Family planning and spacing of births; and
8. Family environment.

(b) *Specific protection :*

1. The child's diet must contain protein and energy rich foods. Milk, eggs, fresh fruits should be given if possible;
2. Immunization; and
3. Food fortification.

(c) *Early diagnosis and treatment :*

1. Periodic surveillance;
2. Early diagnosis of any lag in growth;
3. Early diagnosis and treatment of infections and diarrhoea;
4. Development of programmes for early rehydration of children with diarrhoea;
5. Development of supplementary feeding programmes during epidemics; and
6. Deworming of heavily infested children.

(d) *Rehabilitation :*

1. Nutritional rehabilitation services;
2. Hospital treatment; and
3. Follow-up care.

3. Xerophthalmia

Xerophthalmia (dry eye) refers to all the ocular manifestations of vitamin A deficiency in man. It is the most widespread and serious nutritional disorder leading to blindness *(85)* particularly in South-East Asia.

Xerophthalmia is most common in children aged 1–3 years, and is often related to weaning. The younger the child, the more severe the disease. It is often associated with PEM. Mortality is often high in this age group *(21)*. The victims belong to the poorest families. Associated risk factors include ignorance, faulty feeding practices and infections particularly diarrhoea and measles which often precipitate xerophthalmia. In some countries, "epidemics" of xerophthalmia have occurred in association with food donation programmes involving skimmed milk, which is totally devoid of vitamin A *(86)*.

The States badly affected are the southern and eastern States of India notably Andhra, Tamil Nadu, Karnataka, Bihar and West Bengal. These are predominantly rice-eating States and rice is devoid of carotene. The North Indian States have relatively few cases of xerophthalmia *(87)*.

Prevention and control

Prevention and control of xerophthalmia must be an integral part of primary health care. An overall strategy can be defined, according to WHO, in terms of short-term, medium-term and long-term action *(24)*.

(a) *Short-term action :* A short-term preventive approach that has already demonstrated its efficacy is the administration of large doses of vitamin A orally, in recommended doses to vulnerable groups, on a periodic basis. This can be organized quickly and with a minimum of infrastructure.

(b) *Medium-term action :* An approach widely used to promote regular and adequate intake of vitamin A is **fortification** of certain foods with vitamin A. Addition of vitamin A to *dalda* in India is a typical example. Many other foods have also been considered for vitamin A fortification, viz. sugar, salt, tea, margarine and dried skimmed milk. Fortifying an appropriate food with vitamin A is a complex process. The greatest challenge to successful fortification programmes is choosing a food that is likely to be consumed in sufficient quantities by groups at risk *(88)*.

(c) *Long-term action :* These are measures aimed at reduction or elimination of factors contributing to ocular disease, e.g., persuading people in general, and mothers in particular, to consume generously dark green leafy vegetables or other vitamin A rich foods; promotion of breast-feeding for as long as possible; improvements in environmental health such as ensuring safe and adequate water supply and construction and maintenance of sanitary latrines to safeguard against diarrhoea; immunization against infectious diseases such as measles, prompt treatment of diarrhoea and other associated infections; better feeding of infants and young children; improved health services for mothers and children; social and health education. All these are components of primary health care.

Vitamin A deficiency in India (VAD) *(89)*

VAD has been recognized as a major controllable public health and nutritional problem in India. An estimated 5.7 per cent children in India suffer from eye signs of VAD. Recent evidence suggests that even mild VAD probably increases morbidity and mortality in children, emphasizing the public health importance of this disorder. VAD is one of the major deficiencies among lower income strata population in India.

Though the prevalence of severe forms of VAD such as corneal ulcers/softening of cornea i.e. keratomalacia has in general become rare, Bitot spots were present in varying magnitudes in different parts of the country as reported by National Nutritional Monitoring Bureau in 2005–06. The prevalence was higher than WHO cut-off level of 0.8–1.0 per cent, indicating the public health significance of the problem of VAD *(84)*. There is huge inter-state variation in the prevalence of VAD among children. It is also a matter of concern that only 21 per cent of children of age 12 to 35 months receive a vitamin A dose. Less than 10 per cent coverage was reported in Nagaland, Uttar Pradesh reported 7.3 per cent coverage. Only states such as Tamil Nadu (37.2 per cent), Goa (37.3 per cent), Kerala (38.2 per cent) and West Bengal (41.2 per cent) have better coverage, though it is still low.

In India, in 1970 a national programme for prevention of nutritional blindness was initiated to fight this deficiency. The beneficiaries of this programme were pre-school children (1–5 years). The programme was modified in 1992 to cover children in age group of nine months to three years only. Since Tenth Five Year Plan vitamin A supplementation exists as an integral component of RCH programme which is now a part of NRHM. The guidelines issued in November 2006 cover children upto 5 years of age.

The programme focusses on *(90)*: (a) Promoting consumption of vitamin A rich foods by pregnant and lactating women and by children under-five years of age and appropriate breast-feeding; (b) Administration of massive dose of vitamin A up to five years. First dose of 100,000 IU with measles vaccination at nine months and subsequent doses of 200,000 IU each, every six months up to the age 5 years; (c) For sick children – all children with xerophthalmia to be treated at health facilities; all children suffering from measles to be given one dose of vitamin A if they have not received it in the previous one month; all cases of severe malnutrition to be given one additional dose of vitamin A *(90)*.

4. Nutritional anaemia

Nutritional anaemia is a disease syndrome caused by malnutrition in its widest sense *(54)*. It has been defined by

WHO as "a condition in which the haemoglobin content of blood is lower than normal as a result of a deficiency of one or more essential nutrients, regardless of the cause of such deficiency" *(52)*. Anaemia is established if the haemoglobin is below the cut-off points recommended by WHO (Table 12). By far the most frequent cause of nutritional anaemia is iron deficiency, and less frequently folate or vitamin B_{12} *(49)*.

The problem

WORLD

Nutritional anaemia is a worldwide problem with the highest prevalence in developing countries. It is found especially among women of child-bearing age, young children and during pregnancy and lactation. It is estimated to affect nearly two-thirds of pregnant and one-half of non-pregnant women in developing countries *(91)*. The populations of developed countries are not by any means completely free of anaemia, and a significant percentage of women of child-bearing age (estimated between 4 and 12 per cent) suffer from anaemia *(92)*.

INDIA

Iron deficiency anaemia is the most widespread micronutrient deficiency affecting all age groups irrespective of gender, cast, creed and religion. In India, this silent emergency is rampant among women belonging to reproductive age group (15–49 years), children (6–35 months) and low socio-economic strata of the population. For details about anaemia in under 5 years children refer to chapter 9.

As per National Family Health Survey-5 (2019–2021), the prevalence of anaemia in women in 15–49 years age group is about 57 per cent and in men it is much less, about 25.1 per cent. For women it is highest in West Bengal (71.4%) followed by Assam (65.9%), J & Kashmir (65.9%). In Union territories it is highest in Ladakh (92.8%) and lowest in Lakshadweep (25.8%). In case of men, it is highest in Assam (36%) and J & Kashmir (36.7%). In Ladakh it is 75.6 per cent *(92A)*.

Prevalence of anaemia in adolescent girls is very high (72.6%) in India, with prevalence of severe anaemia among them much higher (21.1%) than that in preschool children (2.1%). In adolescent girls, educational or economic status does not seem to make much of a difference in terms of prevalence of anaemia. Prevention, detection, or management of anaemia in adolescent girls has till now not received much attention. In view of the high prevalence of moderate and severe anaemia in this group and the fact that many of them get married early, conceive, and face the problems associated with anaemia in pregnancy, it is imperative to screen them for anaemia and treat them.

Iron deficiency can arise either due to inadequate intake or poor bioavailability of dietary iron or due to excessive losses of iron from the body. Although most habitual diets contain seemingly adequate amounts of iron, only a small amount (less than 5 per cent) is absorbed *(94)*. This poor bio-availability is considered to be a major reason for the widespread iron deficiency *(93)*. Women lose a considerable amount of iron especially during menstruation. Some of the other factors leading to anaemia are malaria and hookworm infestations. In addition mothers who have born children at close intervals become anaemic due to the additional demands of the rapid pregnancies and the loss of blood in each delivery.

Megaloblastic anaemia is not encounterd frequently in general population, but it occurs occasionally in pregnant women from poor income groups. It is possible that the widespread iron deficiency (microcytic anaemia) could mask megaloblastic anaemia. In a recent study, sub-clinical folate deficiency was found to be about 30 per cent in pregnant women from rural North India. A high level of sub-clinical folate deficiency was also reported in semi-urban school children. There are some sporadic reports indicating its prevalence in adults *(9)*.

Detrimental effects

The detrimental effects of anaemia can be seen in three important areas *(49)* : (a) *Pregnancy :* Anaemia increases the risk of maternal and foetal mortality and morbidity. In India, 19 per cent of maternal deaths were found to be due to anaemia *(54)*. Conditions such as abortions, premature births, postpartum haemorrhage and low birth weight were especially associated with low haemoglobin levels in pregnancy. (b) *Infection :* Anaemia can be caused or aggravated by parasitic diseases, e.g., malaria, intestinal parasites. Further, iron deficiency may impair cellular responses and immune functions and increase susceptibility to infection (c) *Work capacity :* Anaemia (even when mild) causes a significant impairment of maximal work capacity. The more severe the anaemia, the greater the reduction in work performance, and thereby productivity. This has great significance on the economy of the country.

Interventions

An estimation of haemoglobin should be done to assess the degree of anaemia. If the anaemia is "Severe", less than 10 g/dl high doses of iron or blood transfusion may be necessary. If haemoglobin is between 10–12 g/dl, the other interventions are :

(1) Iron and folic acid supplementation

In order to prevent nutritional anaemia among mothers and children, the Government of India sponsored a National Nutritional Anaemia Prophylaxis Programme during the Fourth Five Year Plan. The Programme is based on daily supplementation with iron and folic acid tablets to prevent mild and moderate cases of anaemia. The beneficiaries are "at risk" groups viz., pregnant women, lactating mothers and children under 12 years.

Eligibility criteria (95) : These are determined by the haemoglobin levels of the patients. If the haemoglobin is between 10 and 12, daily supplement with iron and folic acid tablets is advised; if it is less than 10 g, the patient is referred to the nearest primary health centre.

Dosage : (a) MOTHERS : One tablet of iron and folic acid containing 100 mg of elemental iron (300 mg of ferrous sulphate) and 0.5 mg of folic acid should be given daily. The daily administration should be continued until 2 to 3 months after haemoglobin level has returned to normal so that iron stores are replenished. It is necessary that estimation of haemoglobin is repeated at 3–4 month intervals. The exact period of supplementation will depend upon the progress of the beneficiary. (b) CHILDREN : If anaemia is suspected, a screening test for anaemia may be done on infants at 6 months, and 1 and 2 years of age. One tablet of iron and folic acid containing 20 mg of elemental iron (60 mg of ferrous sulphate) and 0.1 mg of folic acid should be given daily for 100 days. For children 6–60 months, ferrous sulphate and folic acid is to be provided in a liquid formulation. For safety sake, the liquid formulation should be dispensesd in bottles so designed that only 1 ml can be dispensed each time. School children, 6 to 10 year old and adolescents are also to be included in the national programme. Children 6-10 years of age are to be provided 30 mg. elemental iron and 250 mcg. folic acid per day for 100 days. Adolescents are given the same dosage and duration as adults *(90)*.

(2) Iron fortification

The WHO experts *(49)* did not recommend iron fortification strategy for control of anaemia in regions where its prevalence is high. However, studies in India at the National Institute of Nutrition, Hyderabad showed that simple addition of ferric ortho-phosphate or ferrous sulphate with sodium bisulphate was enough to fortify salt with iron *(96)*. When consumed over a period of 12–18 months, iron fortified salt was found to reduce prevalence of anaemia significantly. Fortification of salt with iron has been accepted by the Government of India as a public health approach to reduce prevalence of anaemia. Commercial production of iron fortified salt was started in 1985 *(96)*.

Iron fortification has many advantages over iron supplementation. As salt is a universally consumed dietary item, all segments of the population stand to benefit. No special delivery systems are required *(53)*.

(3) Other strategies

There are other strategies such as changing dietary habits, control of parasites and nutrition education. These are longterm measures applicable to situations where the prevalence and severity of anaemia are lower. Cost and time involved to meet the desired goals through these strategies are disproportionately high *(53)*.

5. Iodine deficiency disorders (IDD)

Iodine deficiency is yet another major nutrition problem in India. Previously, iodine deficiency was equated with goitre. In recent years, it has become increasingly clear that iodine deficiency leads to a much wider spectrum of disorders commencing with the intrauterine life and extending through childhood to adult life with serious health and social implications. Table 16 presents the iodine deficiency disorders in approximate order of increasing severity. The social impact of iodine deficiency arises not so much from goitre as from the effect on the central nervous system *(56)*.

The problem

Whereas goitre has ceased to be a major problem in many developed countries (although not eradicated) it continues to be a serious health problem in many Third World Countries. For example iodine deficiency is a health problem of considerable magnitude in India and the neighbouring countries of Bangladesh, Bhutan, Myanmar, Indonesia, Nepal, Sri Lanka and Thailand. More people are affected and levels of severity are higher in South-East Asia than anywhere else in the world *(97)*.

It has always been thought in India that goitre and cretinism were only found to a significant extent in the "Himalaya goitre belt" which is the world's biggest goitre belt. It stretches from Kashmir to the Naga Hills in the east, extending about 2,400 km and affecting the northern States of Jammu and Kashmir, Himachal Pradesh, Punjab, Haryana, Delhi, Uttar Pradesh, Bihar, West Bengal, Sikkim, Assam, Arunachal Pradesh, Nagaland, Mizoram, Meghalaya, Tripura and Manipur. In recent years renewed surveys outside the conventional goitre belt have identified endemic foci of iodine deficiency and the associated IDD in parts of Madhya Pradesh, Gujarat, Maharashtra, Andhra Pradesh, Kerala, Karnataka and Tamil Nadu. More and more new areas are being identified. Even areas near the sea coast like Bharuch district in Gujarat and Ernakulam district in Kerala are found goitre-affected. In short, no State in India can be said to be entirely free from goitre.

The magnitude of the problem in India is far greater than what had been estimated in 1960s, when it was estimated that about 9 million persons were affected by goitre. Results of sample surveys conducted in 325 districts covering all the states/UTs have revealed that 263 districts are endemic where the prevalence of IDD is more than 10 per cent. It is estimated that more than 71 million persons are suffering from goitre and other iodine deficiency disorders in the country *(98)*.

National Iodine deficiency disorders control programme

There are four essential components of National Iodine Deficiency Disorder control programme. These are iodized salt, monitoring and surveillance, manpower training and mass communication. Please refer to page 494 for details.

Hazards of iodization

A mild increase in incidence of thyrotoxicosis has now been described following iodized salt programmes. An increase in lymphocytic thyroiditis (Hashimoto's disease) has also been claimed. The risk of iodism or iodide goitre however seems to be very small *(58)*.

6. Endemic fluorosis

In many parts of the world where drinking water contains excessive amounts of fluorine (3–5 mg/L), endemic fluorosis has been observed. Endemic fluorosis has been reported to be an important health problem in certain parts of the country, e.g., Andhra Pradesh (Nellore, Nalgonda and Prakasam districts), Punjab, Haryana, Karnataka, Kerala and Tamil Nadu *(60)*. The toxic manifestation of fluorosis comprise the following :

(a) *Dental fluorosis :* Fluorosis of dental enamel occurs when excess fluoride is ingested during the years of tooth calcification – essentially during the first 7 years of life *(99)*. It is characterized by "mottling" of dental enamel, which has been reported at levels above 1.5 mg/L intake *(100)*. The teeth lose their shiny appearance and chalk-white patches develop on them. This is the early sign of dental fluorosis. Later the white patches become yellow and sometimes brown or black. In severe cases, loss of enamel gives the teeth a corroded appearance. Mottling is best seen on the incisors of the upper jaw. It is almost entirely confined to the permanent teeth and develops only during the period of formation *(61)*.

(b) *Skeletal fluorosis :* This is associated with lifetime daily intake of 3.0 to 6.0 mg/L or more *(100)*. There is heavy fluoride deposition in the skeleton. When a concentration of 10 mg/L is exceeded, crippling fluorosis can ensue *(101)*. It leads to permanent disability.

(c) *Genu valgum* : A new form of fluorosis characterized by genu valgum and osteoporosis of the lower limbs has been reported in some districts of Andhra Pradesh and Tamil Nadu *(102)*. The syndrome was observed among people whose staple was sorghum *(jowar)*. Further studies showed that diets based on sorghum promoted a higher retention of ingested fluoride than do diets based on rice *(15)*.

Intervention

(a) *Changing the water source* : One solution to the problem is to find a new source of drinking water with a lower fluoride content (0.5 to 0.8 mg/L) if that is possible. Running surface water contains lower quantities of fluorides than ground water sources such as wells. (b) *Chemical treatment* : If the above is not possible, the water can be chemically defluoridated in a water treatment plant, even though such treatment is moderately expensive *(99)*. The National Environmental Engineering Research Institute, Nagpur developed a technique for removing fluoride by chemical treatment. It is called **Nalgonda technique** for defluoridation of water *(103)*. It involves the addition of two chemicals (viz. lime and alum) in sequence followed by flocculation, sedimentation and filtration. (c) *Other measures* : Fluoride supplements should not be prescribed for children who drink fluoridated water. The use of fluoride toothpaste in areas of endemic fluorosis is not recommended for children upto 6 years of age *(99)*.

7. Lathyrism

Lathyrism is a paralyzing disease of humans and animals. In the humans it is referred to as **neurolathyrism** because it affects the nervous system, and in animals as **osteolathyrism** (odoratism) because the pathological changes occur in the bones resulting in skeletal deformities *(8)*. Neurolathyrism is a crippling disease of the nervous system characterized by gradually developing spastic paralysis of lower limbs, occurring mostly in adults consuming the pulse, Lathyrus sativus in large quantities.

The problem

Neurolathyrism is prevalent in parts of Madhya Pradesh, Uttar Pradesh, Bihar and Orissa. It has also been reported in Maharashtra, West Bengal, Rajasthan, Assam and Gujarat where the pulse is grown. The magnitude of the problem can be assessed from the fact that at one time in Rewa and Satna districts of Madhya Pradesh alone, there were 25,000 and 32,000 cases respectively. According to reports, there are no fresh outbreaks of the disease in endemic areas. This is attributed to the shifting trends in agronomical practices in the region *(104)*. Lathyrism has also been reported to occur in Spain and Algeria where *Lathyrus* is eaten *(8)*.

The pulse

Lathyrus sativus is commonly known as "Khesari dhal". It is known by local names such as Teora dhal, Lak dhal, Batra, Gharas, Matra etc. *(106)*. The seeds of lathyrus have a characteristic triangular shape and grey colour. When dehusked the pulse looks similar to red gram dhal or bengal gram dhal. Like other pulses, lathyrus is a good source of protein, but for its toxin which affects the nerves. It is eaten mostly by the poor agricultural labourer because it is relatively cheap. Studies have shown that diets containing over 30% of this dhal if taken over a period of 2–6 months will result in neurolathyrism.

The toxin

The toxin present in lathyrus seeds has been identified as Beta oxalyl amino alanine (BOAA). It has been isolated in crystalline form and is water soluble; this property has been made use of in removing the toxin from the pulse by soaking it in hot water and rejecting the soak water. Studies indicate that there is a blood-brain barrier to this toxin. In order to overcome this barrier, the pulse must be eaten in large amounts over a period of time for 2 months or more. Besides BOAA several other toxins have also been reported *(105)*.

The disease

The disease affects mainly young men between the age of 15 to 45 years and manifests itself in stages : (a) *Latent stage* : The individual is apparently healthy, but when subjected to physical stress exhibits ungainly gait. Neurological examination shows characteristic physical signs. This stage is considered important from the preventive aspect, since at this stage, if the pulse is withdrawn from the diet, it will result in complete remission of the disease. (b) *No-stick stage* : the patient walks with short jerky steps without the aid of a stick. A large number of patients are found in this stage. (c) *One-stick stage* : The patient walks with a crossed gait with a tendency to walk on toes. Muscular stiffness makes it necessary to use a stick to maintain balance. (d) *Two-stick stage* : the symptoms are more severe. Due to excessive bending of knees and crossed legs, the patient needs two crutches for support. The gait is slow and clumsy and the patient gets tired easily after walking a short distance. (e) *Crawler stage* : Finally the erect posture becomes impossible as the knee joints cannot support the weight of the body. There is atrophy of the thigh and leg muscles. The patient is reduced to crawling by throwing his weight on his hands *(104)*.

Interventions

The possible interventions for the prevention and/or control of lathyrism are :

(a) *Vitamin C prophylaxis* : Although this condition is believed to be irreversible, in certain instances the damages could be repaired by the daily administration of 500–1000 mg of ascorbic acid for a week or so. The damage could also be prevented by generous provision of ascorbic acid in the lathyrogenic diet, as demonstrated in guinea pigs and monkeys.

(b) *Banning the crop* : This is an extreme step not feasible for immediate implementation. The Prevention of Food Adulteration Act in India has banned *lathyrus* in all forms – whole, split or flour. But the ban is not operative where it is needed, viz. Madhya Pradesh, Bihar, Orissa and Gujarat where the pulse is widely grown.

If however, it is not possible to avoid consuming khesari dhal, it is desirable that the proportion of the *dhal* should never form more than a quarter of the total amount of cereals and pulses eaten per day.

(c) Removal of toxin

(1) *Steeping method* : Since the toxins are water soluble, they can be removed by soaking the pulse in hot water. This method can be practised at home. A large quantity of water is boiled and the pulse is soaked in hot water for 2 hours;

after which the soaked water is drained off completely. The pulse is washed again with clean water, then drained off and dried in the sun. The pulse is then used for consumption. The drawback with this method is that it entails loss of vitamins and minerals.

(2) *Parboiling* : An improved method of detoxicating the pulse is "parboiling" as is done in the case of parboiled rice. This technique is suitable for large scale operation. Simple soaking in lime water overnight followed by boiling is credited to destroy the toxin. This treatment also destroys trypsin inhibitiors. Lime is easily available as it is used with betel leaves.

(c) *Education* : The public must be educated on the dangers of consuming this pulse and the need for removing its toxin before consumption.

(d) *Genetic approach* : Certain strains of *lathyrus* contain very low levels of toxin (0.1%). The selective propagation and cultivation of such strains may be the most effective way to eradicate lathyrism without any drastic change in the food habits of the people. Low toxin varieties can be obtained from the Indian Agricultural Research Institute, New Delhi.

(e) *Socio-economic changes* : In the final analysis, it is only socio-economic changes or overall development that can root out lathyrism.

NUTRITIONAL FACTORS IN SELECTED DISEASES

1. Cardiovascular disease

It is now generally agreed that diet governs many situations favouring the onset of "heart disease", particularly coronary heart disease. Of all the factors associated with CHD (e.g., plasma cholesterol, high blood pressure, cigarette smoking, lack of physical activity) plasma cholesterol has a very high statistical significance with the incidence of CHD. The risk of CHD appears to increase as the plasma cholesterol concentration rises *(106)*. Various studies have supported the role of elevated blood levels of cholesterol and low density lipoproteins (LDL) in the development of atherosclerosis. Geographical studies have shown that there is no population in whom CHD is common that does not have a relatively high mean level of plasma total cholesterol (TC) in adults *(16)*. These observations have been reinforced by metabolic studies. In addition trials of the effect of dietary changes on CHD have suggested that altering the fatty acid composition of the diet in favour of greater intake of polyunsaturated fatty acids (PUFA) and less intake of saturated fats, while restricting the intake of fat calories to less than 30 per cent of the total calories, may lower the risk that CHD will subsequently develop *(107)*. The evidence of association is now so strong for cholesterol and CHD that the WHO Expert committee (1982) considered its effect to be "causal" in populations although this cannot be claimed yet for individuals *(16)*. The WHO Expert Committee *(16)* concludes that there is a well established triangular relationship between habitual diet, blood cholesterol levels and CHD. The current report of the expert group of the ICMR (2010) on Nutrient Requirement and Recommended Dietary Allowances for Indians endorses the views.

Cholesterol

Cholesterol occurs in all foods of animal origin. Part of it is synthesized in the body. The plasma cholesterol is determined by (a) the amount absorbed from food (b) the amount synthesized in the body (c) the rate of catabolism and excretion in the bile (d) intestinal reabsorption of bile acids, and (e) the equilibrium between plasma and tissues. The extent to which cholesterol intake influences total cholesterol levels is highly variable.

Lipoproteins

Cholesterol is carried in plasma lipoproteins. Lipoproteins are divided into four major classes – chylomicrons, very low-density lipoproteins (VLDLs), low-density lipoproteins (LDLs) and high-density lipoproteins (HDLs). The total serum cholesterol is the sum of the cholesterol in 3 lipoprotein fractions, viz. VLDL, LDL, and HDL cholesterol. Most of the serum cholesterol (close to 50 per cent) is in LDL. Whereas LDL is dominated by its cholesterol content, VLDL is dominated by its triglyceride content.

LDL has been shown to function in the delivery of cholesterol to body cells. Excessive level of LDL thus leads to the accumulation of cholesterol in tissue cells particularly the smooth muscle cells of the vascular system. It is thus involved in the arteriosclerotic process. In contrast, HDL functions in the removal of cholesterol from cells. This mechanism underlines its protective effect in CHD. From long-term observations it became quite clear that HDL levels, the higher they are, the more protective they seem to be against CHD.

Fatty acids

In populations where the plasma cholesterol is high, there is also generally a high consumption of saturated fats. Clinical studies on selected volunteers under well-defined conditions have clearly demonstrated that a high intake of saturated fatty acids over several weeks or months causes an increase in plasma cholesterol. The cholesterol-raising effect is mainly produced by C_{12}, C_{14} and C_{16} acids; stearic acid and fatty acids with less than 12 carbon atoms have a smaller effect on plasma cholesterol. The mechanisms by which these saturated fatty acids act (possibly on cholesterol synthesis) is not fully known.

Dietary unsaturated fatty acids with two or more double bonds have been shown to lower plasma cholesterol. The mechanism of reduction of serum cholesterol by polyunsaturated fatty acids is not clear but includes reduced synthesis of VLDL. The proposition has often been made that a low HDL/LDL ratio favours the development of atheroma, thus favouring the onset of CHD *(108)*.

Polyunsaturated fatty acids (e.g., linoleic and arachidonic acids) have an additional role, that is, to inhibit platelet aggregation and thus prevent thrombus formation. Recent research indicates that arachidonic acid metabolizes in the vascular endothelium to form two important metabolites, namely prostacyclin and thromboxane (Fig. 4). These two compounds have opposing effects on the cardiovascular system. Whereas thromboxane induces platelet aggregation, prostacyclin inhibits the same and prevents intravascular thrombus formation. Prostacyclin was found also to relax coronary blood vessels, thus opposing the action of thromboxane. It has been suggested that generation of

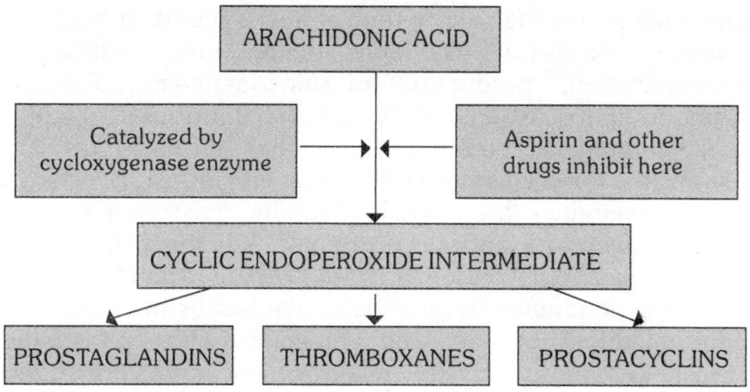

FIG. 4

Steps in the conversion of arachidonic acid to prostaglandins, etc.

prostacyclin is the biochemical mechanism underlying the well-known ability of blood vessels to resist platelet aggregation. Linoleic acid which is the main precursor of arachidonic acid is therefore regarded as the body's best bulwark against CHD. In short, essential fatty acids have in the last decade come to be regarded as of major importance in clinical nutrition.

It has been shown that cholesterol in blood can be reduced by controlling the amount and type of fat in the diet. However, several populations, particularly in Africa and in the South Pacific have intakes of fat similar to those observed in Western countries, but the average plasma cholesterol level remains below 200 mg/dl, and coronary heart disease is rare. It has been argued that this discrepancy may be due to a "favourable" intrinsic (possibly genetic) mechanism for lipid handling, when receiving a diet shown experimentally to raise total cholesterol. This illustrates an important interplay between dietary and genetic determinants of individual blood cholesterol levels *(16)*.

Evidence is emerging that ischaemic myocardium may not metabolise all fatty acids equally, and that the accumulation of some of these in the myocardium may be more closely associated with sudden cardiac death *(108)*.

Triglycerides

In a very large proportion of individuals with a raised cholesterol level, the blood concentration of triglycerides (TG) is also markedly increased. Some workers have indeed claimed that correlation between TG and CHD is as good as that between total serum cholesterol and CHD. It has been shown that TG levels act as a significant independent risk factor for CHD *(100)*. Both cholesterol and TG are associated with specific proteins in the plasma to form lipoproteins.

The most important determinant of TG level is the activity of the enzyme, lipoprotein lipase in the endothelial lining of the capillaries and in a variety of tissues. This enzyme removes TG particularly from the very low density lipoproteins (VLDL) and converts these to the lipoproteins of higher density. In certain genetically determined diseases, this enzyme may be absent. A reduction in its activity or a reduced capacity to deal with increased levels of TG may be important in more common diseases such as diabetes where high concentrations of TG are often observed.

Carbohydrate

Coronary heart disease rates are lowest in populations eating high carbohydrate diets. Support for the hypothesis that consumption of complex carbohydrates may decrease the risk of CHD comes from historical trends of food consumption patterns and mortality rates in US. It is generally recognized that such mortality rates were quite low until about 1920. After 1920 there was a steady increase in the mortality rate until 1968 when a decline began *(107)*. The principal nutritional change that has occurred since the early 1920 has been a decrease in the consumption of dietary carbohydrate. Further support comes from feeding studies. A decrease in serum cholesterol was observed during the vegetable feeding period. Neither high carbohydrates nor high sucrose feeding has induced atherosclerosis in animals, An inverse association of fibre intake with the risk of CHD has also been observed *(109)*.

Salt

There are good and consistent correlations between dietary sodium intake and the incidence of hypertension. Thus the highest incidence of hypertension is found in north Japan where the sodium intake is above 400 mmol/day, while primitive societies ingesting less than 60 mmol/day have virtually no hypertension. Susceptible individuals in primitive populations who change from low to high intake of sodium have been found to develop hypertension. Hypertension can be successfully treated with a drastically low sodium diet (less than 10 mmol/day *(108)*.

2. Diabetes

In a diabetic, there is impaired metabolism of glucose in the body, which leads to excess of glucose in blood and urine. Insulin helps in checking and maintaining the level of glucose in blood. Insulin deficiency leads to accelerated utilization of energy reserves from fat stores. The fatty acids are oxidized by liver to ketone bodies. Excess of ketone bodies leads to their accumulation in urine. This condition is known as ketoacidosis and can result in diabetic coma. Due to insulin deficiency excess of fatty acids are converted to triglycerides. In diabetes these accumulate in the blood. Insulin is also important for synthesis of proteins and deficiency of insulin leads to muscle wasting.

Studies in England showed that diabetics ate an average 1000 kcal per day more than non-diabetics. It was also found that most diabetics were in non-manual occupations than non-diabetics. And the diet of diabetics did not appear to differ in any marked way from that of non-diabetics, except in quantity. There is no sound evidence that any specific dietary factor is diabetogenic.

It has been suggested that deficiencies of trace elements such as chromium, copper and zinc may play a role in the pathogenesis of diabetes mellitus, but clinical evidence is lacking *(110)*.

Malnutrition-related diabetes mellitus has recently attracted attention. Protein deficiency may be involved in the pathogenesis of some forms of diabetes. Excessive consumption of alcohol can increase the risk of diabetes by damaging the pancreas and liver and by promoting obesity.

3. Obesity

In richer countries and in some developing countries, obesity is a health problem. The connection between severe obesity and premature death from diabetes, hypertension and CHD is well established *(111)*. The basic cause of obesity is overnutrition. A diet containing more energy than needed may lead to prolonged postprandial hyperlipidaemia and to deposition of triglycerides in adipose tissue resulting in obesity *(108)*.

It is known that a relative insulin resistance takes place in obesity in peripheral tissues, mainly adipose tissues, while the insulin secretion is normal or increased. The demonstrated reduction in the sensitivity to insulin of the large adipocyte can be attributed to the decreased affinity of the insulin receptors or to a reduction in their number in the cell membrane. Through a feedback mechanism the insulin secretion is stepped up, thus leading to a state of hyperinsulinism.

From a practical point of view all hypotheses concerning the genesis of obesity could be put down to over-nutrition, to a hyper-energy food intake. This is a sound basis for preventive and therapeutic recommendations *(112)*.

4. Cancer

It is postulated that 80 per cent of cancers may be due to environmental factors, and it is possible that some dietetic factors may be involved. Existing knowledge is reviewed briefly as below:

(a) *Dietary fat*

Population surveys have shown a strong positive correlation between cancer colon and dietary intake of fat *(113)*. It has been suggested that the high fat intake accounts for the high incidence of colon cancer in Western communities. In Japan, recent increases in fat consumption have been associated with striking increase in rates of colon cancer *(114)*. Dietary fat is believed to increase the secretion of bile acids in the bowel which are then metabolized by bacterial flora into carcinogen or co-carcinogens *(115)*. However, no known carcinogen has yet been identified from faeces and the evidence is thus incomplete.

A positive correlation between per capita consumption of dietary fat and breast cancer rates has also been noted. A reduction in dietary fat may alter the risk of breast cancer *(116)*, perhaps by increasing oestrogen production or prolactin release *(117)*.

(b) *Dietary fibre*

Several studies indicate that the risk of colon cancer is inversely related to the consumption of dietary fibre, which may protect against intestinal carcinogens or precursors by dilutional or other effects *(108)*. Although the available epidemiological data are not entirely consistent, the weight of evidence generally supports the hypothesis that fibre protects against colon cancer *(114)*.

(c) *Micronutrients*

Micronutrients may also have a protective influence, since cancers of the lung and several other sites have been associated with a low intake of vitamin A *(115)*. The risk of stomach cancer has been related to a deficiency of vitamin C, which may act by inhibiting the formation of carcinogenic nitrosamines in the stomach *(119)*. Trace elements (e.g., selenium) have also been implicated in the aetiology of cancer *(114)*.

(d) *Food additives and contaminants*

Food additives and contaminants (e.g., preservatives, artificial colours, artificial sweeteners, pesticides, flavours, anti-oxidants) have always been under suspicion as possible carcinogens in their long-term effects. Food processing involves exposure to high temperature, oxidation, polymerization, production of nitrosamines, polycyclic aromatic hydrocarbons, etc which are injurious to health. It is thought in some quarters that nitrosamines are responsible for certain types of gastric carcinoma. Saccharin and cyclamate are weak bladder carcinogens or co-carcinogens in laboratory animals, but the risk in man is very small if present at all *(120)*. Aflatoxin is a carcinogenic metabolite. Coffee intake has been associated with bladder cancer and recently with pancreatic cancer *(121)* but causal relationships have not been established. The mutagenic properties of food additives are under constant surveillance.

(e) *Alcohol*

Heavy drinking increases the risk of liver cancer. It is estimated that alcohol contributes to about 3 per cent of all cancer deaths *(122)*. Some recent studies have suggested that beer consumption may be related to cancer rectum, but the association has not been confirmed *(115)*.

The above review indicates that much evidence has accumulated to indicate that nutrition has an influence on cancer incidence and mortality. There is in this field a remarkable dearth of facts and an abundance of speculation.

ASSESSMENT OF NUTRITIONAL STATUS

The nutritional status of an individual is often the result of many interrelated factors. It is influenced by the adequacy of food intake both in terms of quantity and quality and also by the physical health of the individual *(123)*. The nutritional status of a community is the sum of the nutritional status of the individuals who form that community. The main objective of a "comprehensive" nutritional survey is to obtain precise information on the prevalence and geographic distribution of nutritional problems of a given community, and identification of individuals or population groups "at risk" or in greatest need of assistance. In the absence of this information, problems cannot be defined and policies formulated. The purpose of nutritional assessment is to develop a health care programme that meets the needs defined by that assessment, including evaluation of the effectiveness of such programmes *(58)*.

In nutritional surveys, it is not necessary to examine all the persons in a given community. Examination of a random and representative sample of the population covering all ages and both sexes in different socio-economic groups is sufficient to be able to draw valid conclusions. All surveys should be planned with the aid of expert statistical advice. Decisions of many kinds have to be made in advance : duration of survey; type of survey whether cross-sectional or longitudinal; standardization of measurement techniques and survey instruments, etc. Opportunity might be taken of conducting, perhaps on a sub-sample, an intensive investigation of nutritional status.

Assessment methods

The assessment of the nutritional status involves various techniques. Proper evaluation demands a many angled approach, covering all the different stages in the natural history of nutritional diseases, including prepathogenesis stage as shown in Fig. 5 *(124)*.

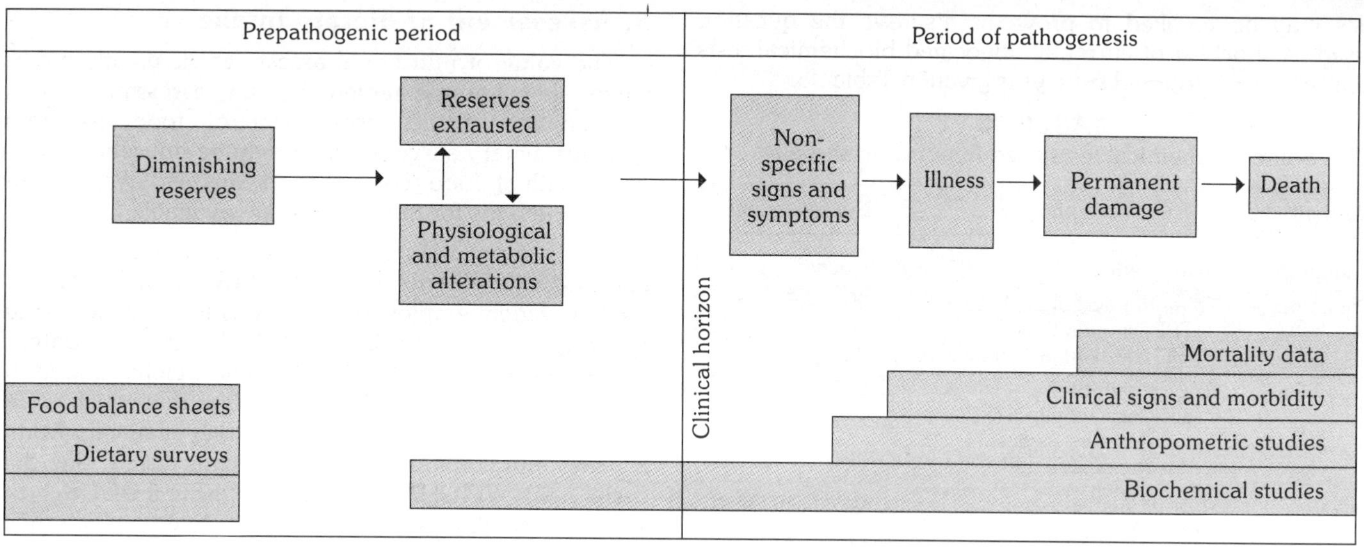

FIG. 5
Methods of nutritional assessment and their relationship to the natural history of disease

The assessment methods include the following :

1. Clinical examination;
2. Anthropometry;
3. Biochemical evaluation;
4. Functional assessment;
5. Assessment of dietary intake;
6. Vital and health statistics; and
7. Ecological studies.

The different methods used for the appraisal of nutritional status are not mutually exclusive; on the contrary, they are complimentary.

1. Clinical examination

Clinical examination is an essential feature of all nutritional surveys since their ultimate objective is to assess levels of health of individuals or of population groups in relation to the food they consume. It is also the simplest and the most practical method of ascertaining the nutritional status of a group of individuals. There are a number of physical signs, some specific and many non-specific, known to be associated with states of malnutrition. When two or more clinical signs characteristic of a deficiency disease are present simultaneously, their diagnostic significance is greatly enhanced. A WHO Expert Committee *(125)* classified signs used in nutritional surveys into three categories as those :

(a) *not related to nutrition,* e.g., alopecia, pyorrhoea, pterygium;
(b) *that need further investigation,* e.g., malar pigmentation, corneal vascularization, geographic tongue; and
(c) *known to be of value,* e.g., angular stomatitis, Bitot's spots, calf tenderness, absence of knee or ankle jerks (beri-beri), enlargement of the thyroid gland (endemic goitre), etc.

However, clinical signs have the following drawbacks : (a) malnutrition cannot be quantified on the basis of clinical signs (b) many deficiencies are unaccompanied by physical signs and (c) lack of specificity and subjective nature of most of the physical signs. To minimize subjective and objective errors in clinical examination, standard survey forms or schedules have been devised covering all areas of the body. A specimen nutrition assessment schedule is given at the end of this chapter (Annexure I).

2. Anthropometry

Anthropometric measurements such as height, weight, skinfold thickness and arm circumference are valuable indicators of nutritional status. In young children, additional measurements such as head and chest circumference are made. If anthropometric measurements are recorded over a period of time, they reflect the patterns of growth and development, and how individuals deviate from the average at various ages in body size, build and nutritional status. Anthropometric data can be collected by non-medical personnel, given sufficient training. This subject is discussed in detail in Chapter 11.

3. Laboratory and biochemical assessment

(a) LABORATORY TESTS : (i) *Haemoglobin estimation :* It is the most important laboratory test that is carried out in nutrition surveys. Haemoglobin level is a useful index of the overall state of nutrition irrespective of its significance in anaemia. An RBC count and a haematocrit determination are also valuable. (ii) *Stools and urine :* Stools should be examined for intestinal parasites. History of parasitic infestation, chronic dysentery and diarrhoea provides useful background information about the nutritional status of persons. Urine should also be examined for albumin and sugar.

(b) BIOCHEMICAL TESTS : With increasing knowledge of the metabolic functions of vitamins and minerals, assessment of nutritional status by clinical signs has given way to more precise biochemical tests which may be applied to measure individual **nutrient** concentration in body fluids (e.g., serum retinol, serum iron) or detection of abnormal amounts of **metabolites** in urine (e.g., urinary iodine) frequently after a loading dose, or measurement of **enzymes** in which the vitamin is a known co-factor (for example in riboflavin deficiency) to help establish malnutrition in its preclinical stages.

Biochemical tests are time consuming and expensive. They cannot be applied on a large scale, as for example in the nutritional assessment of a whole community. They are often carried out on a subsample of the population. Most biochemical tests reveal only current nutritional status; they are useful to quantify mild deficiencies. If the clinical examination has raised a question, then the biochemical tests may be invoked to prove or disprove the question raised. A short list of currently advocated biochemical tests applicable in nutritional surveys is given in Table 33.

TABLE 33
Some biochemical tests used in nutrition surveys

Nutrient	Method	Normal value
Vitamin A	Serum retinol	20 mcg/dl
Thiamine	Thiamine pyrophosphate (TPP) stimulation of RBC transketolase activity	1.00–1.23 (ratio)
Riboflavin	RBC glutathione reductase activity stimulated by flavine adenine dinucleotide	1.0–1.2 (ratio)
Niacin	Urine N-methyl nicotinamide	(not very reliable)
Folate	Serum folate	6.0 mcg/ml
	Red cell folate	160 mcg/ml
Vitamin B_{12}	Serum vitamin B_{12} concentration	160 mg/L
Vitamin C	Leucocyte ascorbic acid	15 mcg/10^8 cells
Vitamin K	Prothrombin time	11–16 seconds
Protein	Serum albumin (g/L)	35
	Transferrin (g/L)	20
	Thyroid-binding pre-albumin (mg/L)	250

Source : *(126)*

4. Functional indicators

Static indices of nutritional status (biochemical indicators) will continue to play an important role as they are well established and familiar to practitioners and public health workers. Functional indices of nutritional status are emerging as an important class of diagnostic tools. Some of these are given in Table 34.

TABLE 34
Functional indices of nutritional status

System	Nutrients
1. *Structural integrity*	
Erythrocyte fragility	Vit.E,Se
Capillary fragility	Vit.C
Tensile strength	Cu
2. *Host defence*	
Leucocyte chemotaxis	P/E, Zn
Leucocyte phagocytic capacity	P/E, Fe
Leucocyte bactericidal capacity	P/E, Fe, Se
T-cell blastogenesis	P/E, Zn
Delayed cutaneous hypersensitivity	P/E, Zn
3. *Haemostasis*	
Prothrombin time	Vit.K
4. *Reproduction*	
Sperm count	Energy, Zn
5. *Nerve function*	
Nerve conduction	P/E, Vit B_1, B_{12}
Dark adaptation	Vit A, Zn
EEG	P/E
6. *Work capacity*	
Heart rate	P/E, Fe
Vasopressor response	Vit.C

Source : *(127)*

5. Assessment of dietary intake

The value of nutritional assessment is greatly enhanced when it is supplemented by an assessment of food consumption. Direct assessment of food consumption involves dietary surveys which may be household inquiries or individual food consumption surveys. Well organized survey methods for this purpose are available *(128, 129)*.

A diet survey may be carried out by one of the following methods : (i) WEIGHMENT OF RAW FOODS : This is the method widely employed in India as it is practicable and if properly carried out is considered fairly accurate. The survey team visits the households, and weighs all food that is going to be cooked and eaten as well as that which is wasted or discarded. The duration of the survey may vary from 1 to 21 days, but commonly 7 days which is called "one dietary cycle". (ii) WEIGHMENT OF COOKED FOODS : Foods should preferably be analyzed in the state in which they are normally consumed, but this method is not easily acceptable among people. (iii) ORAL QUESTIONNAIRE METHOD : This is useful in carrying out a diet survey of a large number of people in a short time. Inquiries are made retrospectively about the nature and quantity of foods eaten during the previous 24 or 48 hours. If properly carried out, oral questionnaire method can give reliable results. A diet survey may also include collection of data relating to dietary habits and practices.

The data that is collected have to be translated into (a) mean intake (grams) of food in terms of cereals, pulses, vegetables, fruits, milk, meat, fish and eggs, and (b) the mean intake of nutrients per adult man value or "consumption unit". This exercise requires the use of suitable tables of food composition. An excellent guide for carrying out this analysis is the Indian Council of Medical Research (ICMR) publication : "Nutritive Value of Indian Foods" *(43)*.

A diet survey provides information about dietary intake patterns, specific foods consumed and estimated nutrient intakes. It indicates relative dietary inadequacies as judged by present standards. Not only will such information be valuable for planning health education activities, but it will also allow an assessment to be made of the extent and nature of changes needed in the agriculture and food production industries.

6. Vital statistics

An analysis of vital statistics – mortality and morbidity data – will identify groups at high risk and indicate the extent of risk to the community. Mortality in the age group 1 to 4 years is particularly related to malnutrition. In developing countries, it may be as much as 20 times that in countries such as Australia, Denmark or France. The other rates commonly used for this purpose are : infant mortality rate, second-year mortality rate, rate of low birth-weight babies and life expectancy. These rates are influenced by nutritional status and may thus be indices of nutritional status. Mortality data, however, do not provide a satisfactory picture of the nutritional status of a population *(130)*.

Data on morbidity (e.g., hospital data or data from community health and morbidity surveys) particularly in relation to protein energy malnutrition, anaemia, xerophthalmia and other vitamin deficiencies, endemic goitre, diarrhoea, measles and parasitic infestations can be of value in providing additional information contributing to the nutritional status of the community.

7. Assessment of ecological factors

Malnutrition is the end result of many interacting ecological factors. In any nutrition survey it is necessary to collect ecological information of the given community in order to make the nutrition assessment complete. A study of the ecological factors comprise the following : (a) FOOD BALANCE SHEET : This is an indirect method of assessing food consumption, in which supplies are related to census population to derive levels of food consumption in terms of per capita supply availability. The estimate refers to the country as a whole, and so conceals differences which may exist between regions, and among economic, age and sex groups. The great advantage of this method is that it is cheaper and probably simpler than any method of direct assessment. Used intelligently, this method does give an indication of the general pattern of food consumption in the country. (b) SOCIO-ECONOMIC FACTORS : Food consumption patterns are likely to vary among various socio-economic groups. Family size, occupation, income, education, customs, cultural patterns in relation to feeding practices of children and mothers, all influence food consumption patterns. (c) HEALTH AND EDUCATIONAL SERVICES : Primary health care services, feeding and immunization programmes should also be taken into consideration. (d) CONDITIONING INFLUENCES : These include parasitic, bacterial and viral infections which precipitate malnutrition. It is necessary to make an "ecological diagnosis" of the various factors influencing nutrition in the community before it is possible to put into effect measures for the prevention and control of malnutrition.

NUTRITIONAL SURVEILLANCE

The concept of nutritional surveillance is derived from disease surveillance. Nutritional surveillance has been defined as "Keeping watch over nutrition, in order to make decisions that will lead to improvement in nutrition in population" *(131)*. Three distinct objectives have been defined for surveillance systems : (a) to aid long-term planning in health and development, (b) to provide input for programme management and evaluation, and (c) to give timely warning and intervention to prevent short-term food consumption crises *(131, 132)*.

Nutritional surveillance and growth monitoring

Nutritional surveillance should not be confused with growth monitoring. The differences are shown in Table 35.

Growth monitoring is oriented to the individual child, and is a dynamic measure of its health from month to month. It focuses on normal nutrition and the means to promote continued growth and good health. It requires enrolment of the infant at an early stage, preferably before 6 months. Regular monthly participation is crucial to detect early onset of growth faltering.

Nutritional surveillance, on the other hand, can be carried out on a representative sample of children in the community. It gives a reliable idea of the overall nutritional condition of village (or area) A – whether it is good or bad, is better or worse than that of village B or C (and so requires supplies and personnel), and whether it is improving or deteriorating with time. It can help to diagnose malnutrition and assess the impact of occurrence like drought or measures designed to alleviate malnutrition in the community at large.

TABLE 35

Comparison of growth monitoring and nutritional surveillance

Factor	Growth monitoring	Nutritional surveillance
Strategy	Preservation of normal growth	Detection of undernutrition
Approach	Educational, motivational	Diagnostic–interventional
Enrolment	All infants	Representative sample
Age	Start before 6 months and continue monthly	Representative ages at longer intervals
Number	Small groups, preferably between 10 and 20	Any size group; 50 to 100 most efficient
Weigher/Recorder	Mothers guided by worker	Trained worker
Weight card	Simple, emphasis growth	Precise, nutritional status
Nutritional emphasis	Maintaining good nutrition	Detect malnutrition
Response	Early home intervention based on local knowledge	Nutritional rehabilitation often with supplements
Response time	Brief, resumption of normal growth	Long, regain of good nutrition in community
Interventions	Primary health care; oral rehydration therapy; vaccines; vitamin A; deworming; contraceptives; chloroquine; other treatment	Food supplements of community-wide response, such as food subsidy
Referral	Health system for check-up and possible brief food supplements	Malnutrition rehabilitation, often in special centre

Source : *(133)*

Nutritional status indicators

Indicators that are considered useful for the surveillance of nutritional status are given in Table 36. There is an increasing trend to use nutritional indicators to measure quality of life, specially as a means of evaluating both development programmes and health programmes. Many of the indicators used in nutritional surveillance are the same as the socio-economic and health status indicators recommended for monitoring progress in health.

TABLE 36

Concise list of indicators of nutritional status

Phenomenon	Indicator
Maternal Nutrition	birth weight
Infant and preschool child nutrition	proportion being breast fed and proportion on weaning foods, by age in months, mortality rates in children aged 1,2,3 and 4 years, with emphasis on 2 year olds If age known : height for age weight for age If age unknown : weight for height arm circumference clinical signs and syndromes
School child nutrition	height for age, and weight for height at 7 years or school admission clinical signs

Source : *(132)*

SOCIAL ASPECTS OF NUTRITION

Food means not only proteins, fats, minerals, vitamins and other nutrients – but much more; it is part of security and civilization. Nations and civilizations are linked together not only by *ideas*, but also by *bread*. Hunger and malnutrition are problems everywhere and have harassed mankind and threatened peace throughout history. It is no wonder that the growing incidence of hunger and malnutrition should have come to the forefront of international concern.

Problem of malnutrition

Malnutrition has been defined as "a pathological state resulting from a relative or absolute deficiency or excess of one or more essential nutrients". It comprises four forms – undernutrition, overnutrition, imbalance and the specific deficiency *(134)*. (1) *Undernutrition :* This is the condition which results when insufficient food is eaten over an extended period of time. In extreme cases, it is called starvation. (2) *Overnutrition :* This is the pathological state resulting from the consumption of excessive quantity of food over an extended period of time. The high incidence of obesity, atheroma and diabetes in western societies is attributed to overnutrition. (3) *Imbalance :* It is the pathological state resulting from a disproportion among essential nutrients with or without the absolute deficiency of any nutrient. (4) *Specific deficiency :* It is the pathological state resulting from a relative or absolute lack of an individual nutrient.

On a global scale the five principal nutritional deficiency diseases that are being accorded the highest priority action are wasting, stunting, xerophthalmia, nutritional anaemias and endemic goitre. These diseases represent the tip of the "iceberg" of malnutrition; a much larger population are affected by "hidden" malnutrition which is not easy to diagnose.

The effects of malnutrition on the community are both direct and indirect. The direct effects are the occurrence of frank and subclinical nutrition deficiency diseases such as kwashiorkor, marasmus, vitamin and mineral deficiency diseases. The indirect effects are a high morbidity and mortality among young children (nearly 50 per cent of total deaths in the developing countries occur among children under-5 years of age as compared to less than 5 per cent in developed countries), retarded physical and mental growth and development (which may be permanent), lowered vitality of the people leading to lowered productivity and reduced life expectancy. Malnutrition predisposes to infection and infection to malnutrition; and the morbidity arising therefrom as a result of complications from such infectious diseases as tuberculosis and gastroenteritis is not inconsiderable. The high rate of maternal mortality, stillbirth and low birth-weight are all associated with malnutrition.

In the more developed countries of the world nutritional problems are somewhat different. Overnutrition is encountered much more frequently than undernutrition. The health hazards from overnutrition are a high incidence of obesity, diabetes, hypertension, cardiovascular and renal diseases, disorders of liver and gall bladder. From this brief review, it is obvious that the consequences of malnutrition are ominous.

Ecology of malnutrition

Malnutrition is a man-made disease. It is a disease of human societies. It begins quite commonly in the womb and ends in the grave. The great advantage of looking at malnutrition as a problem in human ecology is that it allows for variety of approaches towards prevention. Jelliffe (1966) *(134)* listed the ecological factors related to malnutrition as follows : conditioning influences, cultural influences, socio-economic factors, food production and health and other services.

(1) CONDITIONING INFLUENCES : Infectious diseases are an important conditioning factor responsible for malnutrition, particularly in small children. Diarrhoea, intestinal parasites, measles, whooping cough, malaria, tuberculosis all contribute to malnutrition. In fact it is a vicious circle – infection contributing to malnutrition, and malnutrition causing an otherwise minor childhood ailments to become killers. It has been shown that where environmental conditions are poor, small children may suffer from some infection or the other for almost half of their first three years of life. The interrelationship between malnutrition and infection has been well documented.

(2) CULTURAL INFLUENCES : Lack of food is not the only cause of malnutrition. Too often there is starvation in the midst of plenty. People choose poor diets when good ones are available because of cultural influences which vary widely from country to country, and from region to region. These may be stated as follows : (a) *Food habits, customs, beliefs, traditions and attitudes :* Food habits are among the oldest and most deeply entrenched aspects of any culture. They have deep psychological roots and are associated with love, affection, warmth, self image and social prestige. The family plays an important role in shaping the food habits, and these habits are passed from one generation to another. Rice is the staple cereal in the eastern and southern States of India and wheat is the staple cereal in the northern States. During the second World War, when wheat was made available in place of rice in South India people refused to buy wheat because it was not their staple cereal. The story is told of a Philippine student who died of beriberi after writing an essay explaining how the disease could be prevented. The crux of the problem is that many customs and beliefs apply

most often to vulnerable groups, i.e. infants, toddlers, expectant and lactating women. Papaya is avoided during pregnancy because it is believed to cause abortion. In Gujarat, valuable foods such as dhals, leaf greens, rice and fruits are avoided by the nursing mother. There is a widespread belief that if a pregnant woman eats more, her baby will be big and delivery difficult. Certain foods are "forbidden" as being harmful for the child. Then there are certain beliefs about hot and cold foods, light and heavy foods. (b) *Religion :* Religion has a powerful influence on the food habits of the people. Hindus do not eat beef, and Muslims pork. Some orthodox Hindus do not eat meat, fish, eggs and certain vegetables like onion. These are known as food taboos which prevent people from consuming nutritious foods even when these are easily available. (c) *Food fads :* In the selection of foods, personal likes and dislikes play an important part. These are called "food-fads". The food fads may stand in the way of correcting nutritional deficiencies. (d) *Cooking practices :* Draining away the rice water at the end of cooking, prolonged boiling in open pans, peeling of vegetables, all influence the nutritive value of foods. (e) *Child rearing practices :* These vary widely from region to region and influence the nutritional status of infants and children. Examples of this situation are premature curtailment of breast feeding, the adoption of bottle feeding and adoption of commercially produced refined foods. (f) *Miscellaneous :* In some communities, men eat first and women eat last and poorly. Consequently, the health of women in these societies may be adversely affected. Chronic alcoholism is another factor which may lead to serious malnutrition.

(3) SOCIO-ECONOMIC FACTORS : Malnutrition is largely the by-product of poverty, ignorance, insufficient education, lack of knowledge regarding the nutritive value of foods, inadequate sanitary environment, large family size, etc. These factors bear most directly on the quality of life and are the true determinants of malnutrition in society. The speed with which populations are growing in many developing countries is another important factor to reckon with. It has made the solution of the malnutrition problem more difficult. In short, the causes of malnutrition are built into the very nature of society, in the socio-economic and political structures, both nationally and internationally *(135)*.

(4) FOOD PRODUCTION : Increased food production should lead to increased food consumption. The average Indian has 0.6 hectare of land surface compared to 5.8 hectare per head in the developed countries. The per capita arable land for an average Indian is only 0.3 hectare *(136)*. Yields per hectare are only about one-fourth of those achieved in the industrialized countries. Given the best technology known at present, most developing countries could increase their food production several fold. But increased food production will not solve the basic problem of hunger and malnutrition in much of the developing world. Scarcity of food, as a factor responsible for malnutrition, may be true at the family level; but it is not true on a global basis, nor is it true for most of the countries where malnutrition is still a serious problem. It is a problem of uneven distribution between the countries and within the countries. It is said that there will be very little malnutrition in India today if all the food available can be equitably distributed in accordance with physiological needs *(137)*.

(5) HEALTH AND OTHER SERVICES : The health sector can, if properly organized and given adequate resources can combat malnutrition. Some of the remedial actions that can be taken up by the health sector are : (1) *Nutritional surveillance :* Nutritional surveillance implies the continuous monitoring in a community or area of factors or conditions which indicate, relate to, or impinge on the nutritional status of individuals or groups of people (WHO, 1976) *(138)*. The first task is to identify the groups and individuals affected – through clinical examination and simple body measurements of persons attending health centres and hospitals. A further step is to carry out surveys in the villages. The data will give a more realistic picture of the nutritional status of the community. (2) *Nutritional rehabilitation :* Immediate measures are required as soon as the malnourished subjects are located. Children suffering from severe PEM with complications need urgent care, may be in a hospital. Less severely affected children can be treated on a domiciliary basis or in special nutrition rehabilitation centres. These centres should be linked with health centres. (3) *Nutrition supplementation :* The target groups are mothers and children. Supplementary feeding is normally regarded as a stop-gap measure for the rehabilitation of malnourished children. (4) *Health education :* It is opined that by appropriate educational action, about 50 per cent of nutritional problems can be solved. Health education programmes in nutrition is often a weak component. Its reinforcement is a key element in all health services development.

Preventive and social measures

Since malnutrition is the outcome of several factors, the problem can be solved only by taking action simultaneously at various levels – family, community, national and international levels. It requires a coordinated approach of many disciplines – nutrition, food technology, health administration, health education, marketing, etc. In short, it calls for a comprehensive programme of social development of the entire country.

ACTION AT THE FAMILY LEVEL

The principal target of nutritional improvement in the community is the family, and the instrument for combating malnutrition at the family level is nutrition education. The housewife is the "manager" to the consumption of foods in the family. In some families, the husband determines what foods will reach the table. Both the husband and the wife need to be educated on the selection of right kinds of local foods and in the planning of nutritionally adequate diets within the limits of their purchasing power. Harmful food taboos and dietary prejudices can be identified and corrected. Since food expenditure often amounts to 50–70 per cent of family budgets, nutrition education programmes should be a good investment *(139)*. The promotion of breast-feeding and improvement in infant and child feeding practices are the two areas where nutrition education can have a considerable effect. Action is also needed to counter misleading commercial advertising with regard to baby foods. Attention should also be focused on the nutritional needs of expectant and nursing mothers and children in the family. The shortage of protective foods can be met to some extent by planning a kitchen garden or keeping poultry. Adequate nutrition can be obtained in most countries with a combination of locally available and acceptable foods. Other related activities at the family level are the "package" of mother and child health, family planning and immunization services. The community health workers and the multipurpose workers are the kind of people in key positions to impart nutrition education to the families in their respective areas.

ACTION AT THE COMMUNITY LEVEL

Action at the community level should commence with the analysis of the nutrition problem in terms of (a) the extent, distribution and types of nutritional deficiencies; (b) the population groups at risk, and (c) the dietary and non-dietary factors contributing to malnutrition. To obtain this information, diet and nutrition surveys in carefully chosen representative population samples will have to be carried out using standardized methodologies which will permit comparisons in time and space. Having obtained information about the magnitude of the nutrition problem in the community, the next important step will be to plan realistic and feasible approaches to the control of the problem based on local resources. In many developing countries such as India, it is usual to start with direct intervention measures such as supplementary feeding programmes, midday school meals, vitamin A prophylaxis programme, but these will only provide palliative, partial or temporary solutions. The real permanent solution can only come from fundamental measures that will correct the basic causes of malnutrition. This implies, first of all, increasing the availability of foods both in quantity and quality, but – much more important – making sure that the people suffering or at risk of malnutrition can obtain these foods. The Applied Nutrition Programme is an attempt at production of various types of protective foods by the community for the community. The Integrated Child Development Services (ICDS) Programme makes a concerted and coordinated effort to deliver a basic minimum package consisting of supplementary nutrition, immunization, health check-ups, health and nutrition education for the mothers and non-formal education for the preschool age children. The target groups are children up to six years, pregnant and lactating women, and other women in the age group 15 to 44 years. Significant improvements in the overall living conditions of the people is also called for at the community level. This includes such measures as health education, improvement of water supply, control of infectious diseases. In brief, a broad socio-economic development of the entire community is called for.

ACTION AT THE NATIONAL LEVEL

The burden of improving the nutritional status of the people, by and large, is the responsibility of the State. The ninth Report of the Joint FAO/WHO Expert Committee on Nutrition (1976) *(138)* suggested several new approaches and strategies for action at the national level. Some of the strategies and approaches undertaken at the national level in India are : (1) *Rural development :* The nutritional uplift of people, especially in a country like India, can come about only as part and parcel of an overall socio-economic development of rural areas where 72 per cent of people live. Even an impressive increase in total food production will not solve the problem of undernutrition if the income levels of vast sections of the people continue to be so low that they cannot afford to buy the foods they need. It is therefore necessary to raise the living standards and purchasing power of the people. This implies a broad–based programme of rural development. (2) *Increasing agricultural production :* The food production potential is still greatly under-utilized. It must keep pace with population growth. This implies application of modern farming practices, the expansion of cultivated areas, the use of fertilisers, better seeds, and so on. Increased food production is meaningless if not accompanied by an effective food distribution system. This implies marketing, land tenure and food price policies. Irrigation projects undertaken to increase food production could be counter-productive if parallel measures aimed at prevention of mosquito–breeding and other vector control measures are not built into the programmes. (3) *Stabilization of population :* The population policy in India is related to food and nutrition policy. The accent now is on birth spacing and a small family norm. (4) *Nutrition intervention programmes :* Several nutritional problems of developing countries today can be mitigated, if not entirely solved by short-term programmes. The prevention and control of endemic goitre through iodized common salt; the control of anaemia through distribution of iron and folic acid tablets to pregnant and nursing mothers, or possibly through fortification of common foods with iron; the control of nutritional blindness through periodic administration of massive oral doses of vitamin A to children at risk; supplementary feeding programmes for preschool children are examples of such measures. These programmes have a direct impact on the health and nutritional status of particular segments of the population. These programmes alleviate the situation as a temporary measure : (5) *Nutrition related health activities :* Several programmes within the field of health, seemingly unrelated to nutrition, may have a profound impact on the nutritional status. The National Malaria Eradication Programme, by opening up vast tracts of land for cultivation, has made an outstanding contribution to health and nutrition. Since malnutrition is closely related to infection, all programmes of immunization and improvement of environmental sanitation will inevitably have a beneficial effect on nutrition. Programmes of family planning could make a major contribution to the improvement of nutritional status of mothers and children. All these programmes may be considered as alternative approaches to improving the nutritional status of the people. The FAO/WHO Expert Committee on Nutrition (1976) stressed that food and nutrition planning must be an integral part of the overall socio-economic development.

ACTION AT THE INTERNATIONAL LEVEL

Food and nutrition are global problems, just as health and sickness; and both are interrelated. There is considerable scope for international cooperation in solving the problems of malnutrition. International cooperation can play an important role in mitigating the effects of acute emergencies caused by floods and droughts. The establishment of the multilateral *World Food Programme* in 1963 to stimulate and promote economic and social development as a means of providing enough safe food to those in need and to come to the aid of victims of emergency is an example of international cooperation. Several international agencies such as the FAO, UNICEF, WHO, World Bank, UNDP, and CARE are working in close collaboration helping the national governments in different parts of the world in their battle against malnutrition.

FOOD SURVEILLANCE

Food surveillance is essential for the protection and maintenance of community health. Broadly it implies the monitoring of food safety/food hygiene. The WHO *(140)* has defined food safety/food hygiene as "all conditions and measures that are necessary during the production, processing, storage, distribution and preparation of food to ensure that it is safe, sound, wholesome and fit for human consumption." The Declaration of Alma-Ata considered food safety as an essential component of primary health care.

The importance of surveillance of foodborne diseases has been underlined in the WHO Sixth General Programme of Work for the period 1978–1983. The most important international programme carrying out activities in the field of food hygiene is the Joint FAO/WHO Food Standard Programme *(141)*.

FOOD HYGIENE

Food is a potential source of infection and is liable to contamination by microorganisms, at any point during its journey from the producer to the consumer. Food hygiene, in its widest sense, implies hygiene in the production, handling, distribution and serving of all types of food *(142)*. The primary aim of food hygiene is to prevent food poisoning and other food-borne illnesses. Food hygiene can be grouped under the following headings.

MILK HYGIENE

Source of Infection

Milk is an efficient vehicle for a great variety of disease agents. The sources of infection or contamination of milk may be (1) the dairy animal (2) human handler or (3) the environment, e.g., contaminated vessels, polluted water, flies, dust, etc. *(143)*.

Milkborne diseases

A Joint FAO/WHO Expert Committee (1970) on Milk Hygiene classified milkborne diseases as under *(144)*.

(1) Infections of animals that can be transmitted to man:

Primary importance :

- Tuberculosis
- Brucellosis
- Streptococcal infections
- Staphylococcal enterotoxin poisoning
- Salmonellosis
- Q fever

Lesser importance :

- Cow-pox
- Foot and mouth disease
- Anthrax
- Leptospirosis
- Tick-borne encephalitis

(2) Infections primary to man that can be transmitted through milk :

- Typhoid and paratyphoid fevers
- Shigellosis
- Cholera
- Enteropathogenic Escherichia coli (EEC)
- Non-diarrhoeal diseases
  - (a) Streptococcal infections
  - (b) Staphylococcal food poisoning
  - (c) Diphtheria
  - (d) Tuberculosis
  - (e) Enteroviruses
  - (f) Viral hepatitis

Clean and safe milk

The safety and keeping quality of milk are related to its microbial content. The first essential in the production of clean and safe milk, therefore, is a healthy and clean animal. Milk from a healthy udder contains only a few organisms, and these are relatively unimportant. Secondly, the premises where the animal is housed and milked should be sanitary. The milk vessels must be sterile and kept covered. The water supply must be bacteriologically safe. Milk handler must be free from communicable diseases, and before milking they must wash their hands and arms. Where possible, milking machines must be used. Milk should be cooled immediately to below 10 deg.C after it is drawn to retard bacterial growth. In the production of good quality milk, cleanliness of all containers and equipment in which milk is handled is very important.

Methylene blue reduction test : It is an indirect method for detection of microorganisms in milk. The test is carried out on the milk accepted for pasteurization. It is based on the observation that bacteriae growing in milk bring about a decrease in the colour imparted to milk. In conducting the test, definite quantities of methylene blue are added to 10 ml of milk and the sample is held at a uniform temperature of 37 deg C until the blue colour has disappeared. The milk which remains blue the longest is considered to be of the best quality and a scale of grading different milk samples, on the basis of the time required to reduce a definite quantity of methylene blue has been worked out. The test thus serves as confirmation of heavy contamination and compared with direct counts of bacteriae, it saves time and money.

Pasteurization of milk

Pasteurization may be defined as the heating of milk to such temperatures and for such periods of time as are required to destroy any pathogens that may be present while causing minimal changes in the composition, flavour and nutritive value (WHO, 1970) *(144)*. There are several methods of pasteurization. Three are widely used : (1) *Holder (Vat) method :* In this process, milk is kept at 63–66 deg C for at least 30 minutes, and then quickly cooled to 5 deg C. Vat method is recommended for small and rural communities. In larger cities, it is going out of use. (2) *HTST method :* Also known as "High Temperature and Short Time Method". Milk is rapidly heated to a temperature of nearly 72 deg C, is held at that temperature for not less than 15 seconds, and is then rapidly cooled to 4 deg C. This is now the most widely used method. Very large quantities of milk per hour can be pasteurized by this method. (3) *UHT Method :* Also known as "ultra-high temperature method." Milk is rapidly heated usually in 2 stages (the second stage usually being under pressure) to 125 deg C for a few seconds only. It is then rapidly cooled and bottled as quickly as possible.

Pasteurization is a preventive measure of public health importance and corresponds in all respects to the modern principles of supplying safe milk. Pasteurization kills nearly 90 per cent of the bacteria in milk including the more heat-resistant tubercle bacillus and the Q fever organisms. But it will not kill thermoduric bacteria nor the bacterial spores. Therefore, despite pasteurization, with subsequent rise in temperature, the bacteria are bound to multiply. In order to check the growth of microorganisms, pasteurized milk is rapidly cooled to 4 deg C. It should be kept cold until it reaches the consumer. Hygienically produced pasteurized milk has a keeping quality of not more than 8 to 12 hours at 18 deg C.

Tests of pasteurized milk

(1) *Phosphatase test :* This test is widely used to check the efficiency of pasteurization. The test is based on the fact that raw milk contains an enzyme called phosphatase which is destroyed on heating at a temperature which corresponds closely with the standard time and temperature required for pasteurization. At 60 deg C for 30 minutes phosphatase is completely destroyed. Consequently, the test is used to detect inadequate pasteurization or the addition of raw milk. (2) *Standard plate count :* The bacteriological quality of pasteurized milk is determined by the standard plate count. Most countries in the West enforce a limit of 30,000 bacterial count per ml of pasteurized milk. (3) *Coliform count :* Coliform organisms are usually completely destroyed by pasteurization, and therefore, their presence in pasteurized milk is an indication either of improper pasteurization or post-pasteurization contamination. The standard in most countries is that coliforms be absent in 1 ml of milk.

MEAT HYGIENE

The term "meat" includes various tissues of animal origin. The diseases which may be transmitted by eating unwholesome meat are: (1) TAPEWORM INFESTATIONS : Taenia solium, T. saginata, *Trichinella spiralis and Fasciola hepatica*. (2) BACTERIAL INFECTIONS : anthrax, actinomycosis, tuberculosis and food poisoning.

Meat inspection

Animals intended for slaughter are subjected to proper ante mortem and post mortem inspection by qualified veterinary staff. The principal causes of antemortem rejection of animals are emaciation, exhaustion, pregnancy, sheeppox, footrot, actinomycosis, brucellosis, febrile conditions, diarrhoea and other diseases of an infectious nature rendering meat unfit for human consumption. The main causes of the post mortem rejection are cysticercus bovis, liver fluke, abscesses, sarcocystis, hydatidosis, septicaemia, parasitic and nodular infections of liver and lungs, tuberculosis, cysticercus cellulosae, etc. *(145)*. The characteristics of good meat are that it should be neither pale pink nor a deep purple tint, firm and elastic to touch, should not be slimy and have an agreeable odour.

Slaughter houses

Slaughter houses are the places where animals, whose flesh is intended for human consumption, are killed. The hygiene of the slaughter house is of paramount importance to prevent the contamination of meat during the process of dressing. The following minimum standards for slaughter houses have been suggested under the Model Public Health Act (1955) in India *(146)*. (1) *Location :* Preferably away from residential areas. (2) *Structure :* Floors and walls upto 3 feet should be impervious and easy to clean. (3) *Disposal of wastes :* Blood, offal, etc. should not be discharged into public sewers but should be collected separately. (4) *Water supply :* should be independent, adequate and continuous. (5) *Examination of animals :* Ante mortem and post mortem examination to be arranged. Animals or meat found unfit for human consumption should be destroyed or denatured. (6) *Storage of meat :* Meat should be stored in fly-proof and rat-proof rooms; for overnight storage, the temperature of the room shall be maintained below 5 deg C. (7) *Transportation of meat :* Meat shall be transported in fly-proof covered vans. (8) *Miscellaneous :* Animals other than those to be slaughtered should not be allowed inside the shed.

FISH

Fish deteriorates or loses its freshness because of autolysis which sets in after death and because of the bacteria with which they become infected. Stale fish should be condemned. The signs of fresh fish are : (1) it is in a state of stiffness or rigor mortis, (2) the gills are bright red, and (3) the eyes are clear and prominent.

Fish is the intermediate host of the tape worm, *Dibothriocephalus latus*. This cestode is communicable to man, but is very rarely encountered. Sewage, bacteria and viruses (e.g., the virus of hepatitis type A) may be concentrated in shellfish such as oysters, and fish may carry *Vibrio parahaemolyticus, Salmonella spp., Clostridium botulinum* type E, and other organisms *(147)*. Consumption of certain fish may sometimes give rise to 'fish poisoning'.

TINNED FISH : When called upon to inspect tinned fish (or meat or any food), the following points should be noted : the tin must be new and clean without leakages or rusting; there should be no evidence of having been tampered with such as sealed openings; on opening the tin, the contents should not be blown out which indicates decomposition.

EGG

Although the majority of freshly laid eggs are sterile inside, the shells become contaminated by faecal matter from the hen. Microorganisms including pathogenic Salmonella can penetrate a cracked shell and enter the egg *(147)*.

FRUITS AND VEGETABLES

Fruits and vegetables constitute another important source for the spread of pathogenic organisms, protozoans and helminths. These infections are a serious menace to public health where sewage is used for growing vegetables. The vegetables which are consumed raw in the form of salads pose a problem in food sanitation. People should be educated to wash the vegetables before eating them raw. Vegetables which are cooked are free from this danger.

Sanitation of eating places

Sanitation of eating establishments is a challenging problem in food sanitation. The following minimum standards have been suggested for Restaurants and Eating Houses in India under the Model Public Health Act (1955) *(146)*. (1) *Location :* Shall not be near any accumulation of filth or open drain, stable, manure pit and other sources of nuisances. (2) *Floors :* To be higher than the adjoining land, made with impervious material and easy to keep clean. (3) *Rooms :* (a) Rooms where meals are served shall not be less than 100 sq. feet and shall provide accommodation for a maximum of 10 persons. (b) Walls up to 3 feet should be smooth, corners to be rounded; should be impervious and easily washable. (c) Lighting and ventilation – ample natural lighting facilities aided by artificial lighting with good circulation of air are necessary. (4) *Kitchen :* (a) Floor space minimum 60 sq. ft. (b) Window opening to be 25 per cent of floor area. (c) Floor to be impervious, smooth, easy to keep clean and non-slippery. (d) Doors and windows to be rat-proof, fly-proof, and of the self-closing type. (e) Ventilators 2 per cent of the floor area in addition to smoke pipes. (5) *Storage of cooked food :* Separate room to be provided. For long storage, control of temperature is necessary. (6) *Storage of uncooked foodstuffs :* Perishable and non-perishable articles to be kept separately, in rat-proof and vermin-proof space; for storage of perishable articles temperature control should be adopted. (7) *Furniture* : Should be reasonably strong and easy to keep clean and dry. (8) *Disposal of refuse* : To be collected in covered, impervious bins and disposed off twice a day. (9) *Water supply* : To be an independent source, adequate, continuous and safe. (10) *Washing facilities* : To be provided. Cleaning of utensils and crockery to be done in hot water and followed by disinfection.

Food handlers

Food sanitation rests directly upon the state of personal hygiene and habits of the personnel working in the food establishments. Proper handling of foods, utensils and dishes together with emphasis upon the necessity for good personal hygiene are of great importance. The infections which are likely to be transmitted by the food handlers are diarrhoeas, dysenteries, typhoid and paratyphoid fevers, enteroviruses, viral hepatitis, protozoal cysts, eggs of helminths, streptococcal and staphylococcal infections, and salmonellosis.

The first essential is to have complete medical examination carried out of all food handlers at the time of employment. Any person with a history of typhoid fever, diphtheria, chronic dysentery, tuberculosis or any other communicable disease should not be employed. Persons with wounds, otitis media or skin infections should not be permitted to handle food or utensils. The day to day health appraisal of the food handlers is also equally important; those who are ill should be excluded from food handling. It is also important that any illness which occurs in a food handler's family should at once be notified.

Education of food handlers in matters of personal hygiene, food handling, utensils, dish washing, and insect and rodent control is the best means of promoting food hygiene. Many of the food handlers have little educational background. Certain aspects of personal hygiene are therefore required to be continually impressed upon them: (a) *Hands* : The hands should be clean at all times. Hands should be scrubbed and washed with soap immediately after visiting a lavatory and as often as necessary at other times. Finger nails should be kept trimmed and free from dirt. (b) *Hair* : Head coverings should be provided, particularly in the case of females to prevent loose hair entering the food-stuffs. (c) *Overalls* : Clean white overalls should be worn by all food handlers. (d) *Habits* : Coughing and sneezing in the vicinity of food, licking the fingers before picking up an article of food, smoking on food premises are to be avoided.

FOOD-BORNE DISEASES

The term "food-borne disease" is defined as : "A disease, usually either infectious or toxic in nature, caused by agents that enter the body through the ingestion of food." With the increase in urbanization, industrialization, tourism and mass catering systems, food-borne diseases are on the increase throughout the world. Food-borne diseases may be classified as :

A. Food-borne intoxications

1. Due to naturally occurring toxins in some foods *(148)* :
   a. Lathyrism (beta oxalyl amino-alanine)
   b. Endemic ascitis (Pyrrolizidine alkaloids).
2. Due to toxins produced by certain bacteria *(128, 149)* :
   a. Botulism
   b. Staphyloccus poisons
3. Due to toxins produced by some fungi *(147, 150)* :
   a. Aflatoxin
   b. Ergot
   c. Fusarium toxins
4. Food-borne chemical poisoning *(151, 152)* :
   a. Heavy metals, e.g., mercury (usually in fish), cadmium (in certain shellfish) and lead (in canned food)
   b. Oils, petroleum derivatives and solvents (e.g., Tricresyl phosphate or TCP)
   c. Migrant chemicals from package materials
   d. Asbestos
   e. Pesticide residues (DDT, BHC)

B. Food-borne infections

Group	Examples of illness in each group
(1) Bacterial diseases	Typhoid fever, Paratyphoid fever, Salmonellosis, Staphylococcal intoxication, *C.perfringens* illness, Botulism, B.cereus Food Poisoning, *E.coli* diarrhoea, Non-cholera vibrio illness, V.parahaemolyticus infection, Streptococcal infection, Shigellosis Brucellosis.
(2) Viral diseases	hepatitis A and E, Norovirus Gastroenteritis, Rotavirus.
(3) Parasites	Taeniasis Hydatidosis, Trichinosis, Ascariasis, Amoebiasis, Oxyuriasis.

FOOD TOXICANTS

1. Neurolathyrism

The cause of neurolathyrism is a toxin, Beta oxalyl amino alanine (BOAA) which is found in the seeds of the pulse, *L.sativus* (Khesari dhal). Neurolathyrism is a public health problem in certain parts of the country where this pulse is eaten (see page 734).

2. Aflatoxins *(153, 154)*

Aflatoxins are a group of mycotoxins produced by certain fungi, *Aspergillus flavus* and *A parasiticus*. These fungi infest foodgrains such as groundnut, maize, parboiled rice, sorghum, wheat, rice, cotton seed and tapioca under conditions of improper storage, and produce aflatoxins of which B_1 and G_1 are the most potent hepatotoxins, in addition to being carcinogenic. The most important factors affecting the formation of the toxin are moisture and temperature. Moisture levels above 16 per cent and temperatures ranging from 11 to 37°C favour toxin formation. Aflatoxicosis is quite a public health problem in India. The latest report (1975) of 400 cases of aflatoxin poisoning including 100 deaths from Banswada and Panchmahal districts of Rajasthan and Gujarat respectively highlight the problem in India. Aflatoxin B_1 has also been detected in samples of breast milk and urine collected from children suffering from infantile cirrhosis, Attempts are also being made to relate aflatoxin with human liver cirrhosis.

Control and preventive measures : A crucial factor in the prevention of fungal contamination of foodgrains is to ensure their proper storage after drying, Moisture content should be kept below 10 per cent. If the food is contaminated, it must not be consumed. It is also essential to educate the local population on the health hazards of consuming contaminated foodgrains.

3. Ergot *(155, 156)*

Unlike Aspergillus, ergot is not a storage fungus, but a field fungus. Foodgrains such as bajra, rye, sorghum, and wheat have a tendency to get infested during the flowering stages by the ergot fungus *(Claviceps purpurea).* Fungus grows as a blackish mass and the seeds become black and irregular and are harvested along with food grains. Consumption of ergot infested grain leads to ergotism. Sporadic outbreaks of ergot poisoning in human population have been reported from time to time in areas where bajra is consumed as a staple. The symptoms are acute but rarely fatal and include nausea, repeated vomiting, giddiness and drowsiness extending sometimes for periods upto 24 to 48 hours after the ingestion of ergoty grain. In chronic cases, painful cramps in limbs and peripheral gangrene due to vasoconstriction of capillaries have been reported. However, the long-term effects of consuming small amounts of the toxin are not known. A disquieting feature is that the recently introduced high-yielding varieties of bajra are more susceptible to infestation. Ergot-infested grains can be easily removed by floating them in 20 per cent salt water. They can also be removed by hand-picking or air floatation. The upper safe limit for the ergot alkaloids has been estimated to be 0.05 mg per 100 grams of the food material.

4. Epidemic dropsy *(157, 142)*

From time to time, outbreaks of "epidemic dropsy" are reported in India. The cause of epidemic dropsy was not known until 1926, when Sarkar ascribed it to the contamination of mustard oil with argemone oil. Lal and Roy (1937) and Chopra et.al., (1939) gave experimental proof of the cause of epidemic dropsy. Mukherji *et.al.*, (1941) isolated a toxic alkaloid, *sanguinarine* from argemone oil and found out its chemical formula. This toxic substance interferes with the oxidation of pyruvic acid which accumulates in the blood.

The symptoms of epidemic dropsy consist of sudden, non-inflammatory, bilateral swelling of legs, often associated with diarrhoea. Dyspnea, cardiac failure and death may follow. Some patients may develop glaucoma. The disease may occur at all ages except breast-fed infants. The mortality varies from 5–50 per cent.

The contamination of mustard or other oils with argemone oil may be accidental or deliberate. Seeds of *Argemone mexicana* (prickly poppy) closely resemble mustard seeds. The plant grows wild in India. It has prickly leaves and bright yellow flowers. Crops of mustard are gathered during March, and during this period, the seeds of argemone also mature and are likely to be harvested along with mustard seeds. Sometimes unscrupulous dealers mix argemone oil with mustard or other oils.

Argemone oil is orange in colour with an acrid odour. The following tests may be applied for the detection of argemone oil : (1) *Nitric acid test :* A simple test is to add nitric acid to the sample of oil in a test tube. The tube is shaken and the development of a brown to orange-red colour shows the presence of argemone oil. The nitric acid test is positive only when the level of argemone oil is about 0.25 per cent *(158)*. (2) *Paper chromatography test :* This is the most sensitive test yet devised. It can detect argemone oil up to 0.0001 per cent in all edible oils and fats.

The accidental contamination of mustard seeds can be prevented at the source by removing the argemone weeds growing among oil-seed crops. Unscrupulous dealers may be dealt with by the strict enforcement of the Prevention of Food Adulteration Act.

5. Endemic ascites *(159, 160)*

In Kusmi Block of Sarguja district in Madhya Pradesh, during 1973 and again during 1976, an outbreak of rapidly developing ascites and jaundice was reported among the Nagesia tribals. Both the sexes and all the age groups, except infants, were affected. The overall mortality was 40 per cent.

Studies conducted by the National Institute of Nutrition, Hyderabad showed that the local population subsist on the millet *Panicum miliare* (known locally as Gondhli) which gets contaminated with weed seeds of Crotalaria (locally known as *Jhunjhunia*). On chemical analysis. *Jhunjhunia seeds* were found to contain *pyrrolizidine alkaloids* which are *hepatotoxins.*

The preventive measures comprise educating the people in the affected areas about the disease, deweeding of the Jhunjhunia plants which grow along with the staple, and simple sieving of the millet at the household level to remove the seeds of *Jhunjhunia* which are considerably smaller than those of the millet.

6. Fusarium toxins *(161)*

Fusarium species of field fungi are known to contaminate food crops and pose health hazards to livestock and man. The problem of fusarium contamination of sorghum is believed to be on the increase. Rice is also known to be a good substrate for fusarium. Work is now in progress at the National Institute of Nutrition to isolate, and identify the toxic metabolites produced by *fusarium incamatum.*

Food additives

The concept of adding "non-food" substances to food products is not new. Pickling is an ancient culinary practice aimed at preserving food articles such as mango, lime, etc for fairly long periods by the addition of salt and spices. Modern science of food technology has revolutionized food processing with the introduction of chemical additives to increase the shelf-life of food, improve its taste, and to change its texture or colour. Majority of the processed foods such as bread, biscuits, cakes, sweets, confectionary, jams, jellies, soft drinks, ice creams, ketchup and refined oils contain food additives.

Food additives are defined as non-nutritious substances which are added intentionally to food, generally in small quantity, to improve its appearance, flavour, texture or storage properties *(162)*. This definition also includes animal food adjuncts which may result in residues in human food and components of packing materials which may find their way into food *(163)*.

Food additives may be classified into two categories : Additives of the **first category** include colouring agents (e.g., saffron, turmeric), flavouring agents (e.g., vanilla essence), sweeteners (e.g., saccharin), preservatives (e.g., sorbic acid, sodium benzoate), acidity imparting agents (e.g., citric acid, acetic acid), etc *(164)*. These agents are generally considered safe for human consumption. Additives of the **second category** are, strictly speaking, contaminants incidental through packing, processing steps, farming practices (insecticides) or other environmental conditions *(165)*. Uncontrolled or indiscriminate use of food additives may pose health hazards among consumers. For example, certain preservatives such as nitrites and nitrates can lead to the production of toxic substances, e.g., nitrosamines that have been implicated in cancer aetiology.

The use of food additives is subjected to government regulations throughout the world. In India two regulations (viz. the Prevention of Food Adulteration Act and the Fruit Products Order) govern the rules and regulations of food additives *(165)*. Any food that contains food additives that are not permitted is considered to be adulterated; if the permissible limit exceeds then also the food is considered adulterated. The nature and quantity of the additive shall be clearly printed on the label to be affixed to the container. Whenever, any extraneous colouring matter has been added to any article of food, the words "Artificially Coloured" shall be written on the label. At the international level, in 1963, a joint FAO/WHO programme on food standards was established, with the FAO/WHO Codex Alimentarius Commission as its principal organ. Protection of the health of consumers is the primary aim of the Commission. The ultimate effects of food additives on man is an important problem of public health and is therefore of great concern to the public and the health administrators.

Food fortification

Fortification of food is a public health measure aimed at reinforcing the usual dietary intake of nutrients with additional supplies to prevent/control some nutritional disorders. WHO *(1)* has defined "food fortification" as "the process whereby nutrients are added to foods (in relatively small quantities) to maintain or improve the quality of the diet of a group, a community, or a population."

Programmes of demonstrated effectiveness of fortification of food or water are : fluoridation of water as a preventive of dental caries; iodization of salt for combating the problem of endemic goitre, and food fortification (e.g., vanaspati, milk) with vitamins A and D. Technology has also been developed for the twin fortification of salt with iodine and iron.

In order to qualify as suitable for fortification, the vehicle and the nutrient must fulfil certain criteria *(25)* :

(a) the vehicle fortified must be consumed consistently as part of the regular daily diet by the relevant sections of the population or total population;

(b) the amount of nutrient added must provide an effective supplement for low consumers of the vehicle, without contributing a hazardous excess to high consumers;

(c) the addition of the nutrient should not cause it to undergo any noticeable change in taste, smell, appearance, or consistency; and

(d) the cost of fortification must not raise the price of the food beyond the reach of the population in greatest need.

Finally, an adequate system of surveillance and control is indispensable for the effectiveness of food fortification. Food fortification is a long-term measure for mitigating specific problems of malnutrition in the community.

Adulteration of foods

Adulteration of foods is an age-old problem. It consists of a large number of practices, e.g., mixing, substitution, concealing the quality, putting up decomposed foods for sale, misbranding or giving false labels and addition of toxicants. Adulteration results in two disadvantages for the consumer : first, he is paying more money for a foodstuff of lower quality; secondly, some forms of adulteration are injurious to health, even resulting in death, as for example, adulteration of mustard oil with argemone oil causing epidemic dropsy or adulteration of edible oils with tricresyl phosphate (TCP) resulting in paralysis and death.

Food adulteration practices vary from one part of the country to another, and from time to time. Our knowledge about the current practices of food adulteration is by no means complete. Table 37 shows the types of adulteration seen in India *(166)*.

TABLE 37

Adulteration of foods

Food material	Common adulterants
Cereals such as wheat, rice	Mud, grits, soapstone bits
Dals	Coal-tar dyes, khesari dal
Haldi (Turmeric) powder	Lead chromate powder
Dhania powder	Starch, cow dung or horse dung powder
Black pepper	Dried seeds of papaya
Chilli powder	Saw dust, brick powder
Tea dust/leaves	Blackgram husk, tamarind seeds powder, saw dust, used tea dust
Coffee powder	Date husk, tamarind husk, Chicory
Asafoetida (Hing)	Sand, grit, resins, gums
Mustard seeds	Seeds of prickly poppy-Argemone
Edible oils	Mineral oils, argemone oil
Butter	Starch, animal fat
Ice-cream	Cellulose, starch, non-permitted colours
Sweetmeats	Non-permitted colours
Fresh green peas in packing	Green dye
Milk	Extraction of fat, addition of starch and water
Ghee	Vanaspati

Source : *(166)*

Prevention of Food Adulteration Act, 1954

Enacted by the Indian Parliament in 1954, with the objective of ensuring pure and wholesome food to the consumers and to protect them from fraudulent and deceptive trade practices, the Prevention of Food Adulteration (PFA) Act was amended in 1964, 1976 and lately in 1986 to make the Act more stringent. A minimum imprisonment of 6 months with a minimum fine of Rs.1,000 is envisaged under the Act for cases of proven adulteration, whereas for the cases of adulteration which may render the food injurious to cause death or such harm which may amount to grievous hurt (within the meaning of section 320 of I.P.C.) the punishment may go upto life imprisonment and a fine which shall not be less than Rs.5,000. With the amendment in 1986, the consumer and the voluntary organizations have been empowered under the Act to take samples of food.

Rules are framed which are revised from time to time by an expert body called the "Central Committee for Food standards" which is constituted by the Central Government under the provisions of the Act. Any food that does not conform to the minimum standards is said to be adulterated. Although it is a Central Act, its implementation is largely carried out by the State Governments and local bodies in their respective areas. However, the Centre plays a vital role in proper coordination, monitoring and surveillance of the programme throughout the country. A chain of food laboratories and four regional appellate Central Food Laboratories (Kolkata, Mysore, Ghaziabad and Pune) whose report is considered to be final have been established.

Training being an important component of the programme for prevention of food adulteration, the Directorate General of Health Services organizes in-service training programme for different functionaries responsible for implementation of the PFA Act. Food inspectors, analysts and the senior officers concerned with the implementation of the Act in States are provided training.

Food adulteration is a social evil. The general public, traders, and Food Inspectors are all responsible for perpetuating this evil – the public, because of lack of awareness of the dangers of adulteration and their general disinterest; the traders, for their greed for money, and Food Inspectors who find food adulteration a fertile ground to make easy money. Unless the public rises up against the traders and unscrupulous food inspectors, this evil cannot be curbed. It is here the voluntary agencies and consumer guidance societies can play a vital role.

Food Safety and Standards Act, 2006 was enacted with the objective to consolidate the laws relating to food and for laying down science based standards for articles of food as well as to regulate their manufacture, storage, distribution, sale and import to ensure availability of safe and wholesome food for human consumption and for matters connected therewith or incidental thereto. The Food Safety and Standards Authority of India (FSSAI) was established in the year 2008 *(174)*. FSS Act 2006 is being implemented by all states/UT governments *(174)*.

Food standards

(a) CODEX ALIMENTARIUS : The Codex Alimentarius Commission, which is the principal organ of the joint FAO/WHO Food Standards Programme formulates food standards for international market. The food standards in India are based on the standards of the codex alimentarius. (b) PFA STANDARDS : Under the Prevention of Food Adulteration Act (1954) standards have been established which are revised from time to time by the "Central Committee for Food Standards". The purpose of the PFA standards is to obtain a minimum level of quality of foodstuffs attainable under Indian conditions. (c) THE AGMARK STANDARDS : These standards are set by the Directorate of Marketing and Inspection of the Government of India. The Agmark gives the consumer an assurance of quality in accordance with the standards laid down. (d) BUREAU OF INDIAN STANDARDS : The ISI mark on any article of food is a guarantee of good quality in accordance with the standards prescribed by the Bureau of Indian Standards for that commodity. The Agmark and ISI standards are not mandatory; they are purely voluntary. They express degrees of excellence above PFA standards.

National Nutrition Policy 1993 *(167)*

In spite of the significant improvement in food production and advancement in science since independence, under-nutrition continues to be a widespread problem in India. In the year 1993, Govt. of India announced National Nutrition Policy 1993. As nutrition is a multi-sectoral issue, it needs to be tackled at various levels through direct nutrition interventions for specifically vulnerable groups as well as through various development policy instruments which will create conditions for improved nutrition. The strategy consists of the following :

A. Direct intervention – Short-term

1. Nutrition interventions for specially vulnerable groups.
   a. Expanding the Safety Net – The universal immunization programme, oral rehydration therapy and the integrated child development services have a considerable impact on child survival and extreme forms of malnutrition.
   b. Improving growth monitoring between age group 0 to 3 years, with closer involvement of the mothers.
   c. Reaching the adolescent girls through ICDS so as to make them ready for safe motherhood.
   d. Ensuring better coverage of expectant women in order to reduce the incidence of low birth weight babies.
2. Fortification of essential foods.
3. Popularization of low cost nutritious food.
4. Control of micro-nutrient deficiencies among vulnerable groups.

B. Indirect Policy Instruments : Long-term institutional and structural changes

1. Food security – In order to ensure aggregate food security, a per capita availability of 215/kg/person/year of food grain needs to be attained.
2. Improvement of dietary pattern through production and demonstration.
3. Improving the purchasing power of the urban and rural poor and improving the public food distribution system.
4. Land reforms.
5. Health and family welfare.
6. Basic health and nutrition knowledge.
7. Prevention of food adulteration.
8. Nutrition surveillance.
9. Monitoring of nutrition programmes.
10. Research into various aspects of nutrition, both on the consumption side and the supply side.
11. Equal remuneration for women.
12. Communication through established media for the implementation of nutrition policy.
13. Minimum wage administration.
14. Community participation.
15. Education and literacy particularly that of women.
16. Improvement of the status of women.

Anaemia Mukt Bharat Strategy *(175)*

The Anaemia Mukt Bharat Strategy is a universal strategy and will focus on the following six interventions :

1. Prophylactic iron and folic acid supplementation.
2. Deworming.
3. Intensified year-round behaviour change communication campaign (solid body, smart mind) focussing on four key behaviours – (a) improving compliance to iron folic acid supplementation and deworming; (b) appropriate infant and young child feeding practices; (c) increase in intake of iron-rich food through diet diversity/quantity/ frequency and/or fortified foods with focus on harnessing locally available resources; and (d) ensuring delayed cord clamping after delivery (by 3 minutes) in health facilities.
4. Testing and treatment of anaemia, using digital methods and point of care treatment, with special focus on pregnant women and school-going adolescents.
5. Mandatory provision of iron and folic acid fortified foods in government-funded public health programmes.
6. Intensifying awareness, screening and treatment of non-nutritional causes of anaemia in endemic pockets, with special focus on malaria, haemoglobinopathies and fluorosis.

The Anaemia Mukt Bharat Strategy will be implemented in all villages, blocks, and districts of all the states/UTs of India through existing delivery platforms as envisaged in the National Iron Plus Initiative (NIPI) and Weekly Iron Folic Acid Supplementation (WIFS) programme *(175)*.

COMMUNITY NUTRITION PROGRAMMES

The Government of India have initiated several large-scale supplementary feeding programmes, and programmes aimed at overcoming specific deficiency diseases through various Ministries to combat malnutrition. They are as shown in Table 38.

TABLE 38
Nutrition programmes in India

Programme	Ministry
1. Vitamin A prophylaxis programme	Ministry of Health and Family Welfare
2. Prophylaxis against nutritional anaemia	Ministry of Health and Family Welfare
3. Iodine deficiency disorders control programme	Ministry of Health and Family Welfare
4. Special nutrition programme	Ministry of Social Welfare
5. Balwadi nutrition programme	Ministry of Social Welfare
6. ICDS programme	Ministry of Social Welfare
7. Mid-day meal programme	Ministry of Education
8. Mid-day meal scheme	Ministry of Human Resources Development

1. Vitamin A prophylaxis programme

One of the components of the National Programme for Control of Blindness is to administer a single massive dose of an oily preparation of vitamin A containing 200,000 IU (110 mg of retinol palmitate) orally to all pre-school children in the community every 6 months through peripheral health workers. This programme was launched by the Ministry of Health and Family Welfare in 1970 on the basis of technology developed at the National Institute of Nutrition at Hyderabad. An evaluation of the programme has revealed a significant reduction in vitamin A deficiency in children (see page 705, 706 for details).

2. Prophylaxis against nutritional anaemia

In view of its public health importance, a national programme for the prevention of nutritional anaemia was launched by the Govt. of India during the fourth Five Year Plan. The programme consists of distribution of iron and folic acid (folifer) tablets to pregnant women and young children (1–12 years). Mother and Child Health (MCH) Centres in urban areas, primary health centres in rural areas and ICDS projects are engaged in the implementation of this programme. The technology for the control of anaemia through iron fortification of common salt has also been developed at the National Institute of Nutrition at Hyderabad (see page 732 for more details).

3. Control of iodine deficiency disorders

The National Goitre Control Programme was launched by the Government of India in 1962 in the conventional goitre belt in the Himalayan region with the objective of identification of the goitre endemic areas to supply iodized salt in place of common salt and to assess the impact of goitre control measures over a period of time.

Surveys, however, indicated that the problem of goitre and iodine deficiency disorders was more widespread than it was thought earlier, with nearly 145 million people estimated to be living in known goitre endemic areas of the country. As a result, a major national programme – the IDD Control Programme – was mounted in 1986 with the objective to replace the entire edible salt by iodide salt, in a phased manner by 1992 (see page 494, 733 for more details).

4. Special nutrition programme

This programme was started in 1970 for the nutritional benefit of children below 6 years of age, pregnant and nursing mothers and is in operation in urban slums, tribal areas and backward rural areas. The supplementary food supplies about 300 kcal and 10–12 grams of protein per child per day. The beneficiary mothers receive daily 500 kcal and 25 grams of protein. This supplement is provided to them for about 300 days in a year. This programme was originally launched as a Central programme and was transferred to the State sector in the fifth Five Year Plan as part of the Minimum Needs Programme *(168)*. The main aim of the Special Nutrition Programme is to improve the nutritional status of the target groups. This programme is gradually being merged into the ICDS programme.

5. Balwadi nutrition programme

This programme was started in 1970 for the benefit of children in the age group 3–6 years in rural areas. It is under the overall charge of the Department of Social Welfare. Four national level organizations including the Indian Council of Child Welfare are given grants to implement the programme. Voluntary organizations which receive the funds are actively involved in the day-to-day management. The programme is implemented through ***Balwadis*** which also provide pre-primary education to these children. The food supplement provides 300 kcal and 10 grams of protein per child per day. Balwadis are being phased out because of universalization of ICDS.

6. ICDS programme

Integrated Child Development Services (ICDS) programme was started in 1975 in pursuance of the National Policy for Children. There is a strong nutrition component in this programme in the form of supplementary nutrition, vitamin A prophylaxis and iron and folic acid distribution. The beneficiaries are preschool children below 6 years, and adolescent girls 11 to 18 years, pregnant and lactating mothers. The States and Union Territories are encouraged to undertake additional ICDS projects on the Central pattern to cover more beneficiaries *(168)*.

The workers at the village level who deliver the services are called ***Anganwadi workers.*** Each Anganwadi unit covers a population of about 400 to 800 and mini anganwadi centre about 150 to 400. A network of Mahila Mandals has been built up in ICDS Project areas to help Anganwadi workers in providing health and nutrition services. The work of Anganwadis is supervised by *Mukhyasevikas.* Field supervision is done by the Child Development Project Officer (CDPO).

7. Mid-day meal programme

The mid-day meal programme (MDMP) is also known as School Lunch Programme. This programme has been in operation since 1961 throughout the country. The major objective of the programme is to attract more children for admission to schools and retain them so that literacy improvement of children could be brought about *(167)*.

In formulating mid-day meals for school children, the following broad principles should be kept in mind *(169)*.

(a) the meal should be a *supplement* and not a substitute to the home diet;
(b) the meal should supply at least one-third of the total energy requirement, and half of the protein need;
(c) the cost of the meal should be reasonably low;
(d) the meal should be such that it can be prepared easily in schools; no complicated cooking process should be involved;
(e) as far as possible, locally available foods should be used; this will reduce the cost of the meal; and
(f) the menu should be frequently changed to avoid monotony.

MODEL MENU

A model menu for a mid-day school meal is given in Table 39.

TABLE 39
A mid-day school meal

Foodstuffs	g/day/child
Cereals and millets	75
Pulses	30
Oils and fats	8
Leafy vegetables	30
Non-leafy vegetables	30

The National Institute of Nutrition, Hyderabad has prepared model recipes for the preparation of school meals suitable for North and South Indians. Copies of these publications can be had gratis on request. The National Institute of Nutrition is of the view that the minimum number of feeding days in a year should be 250 to have the desired impact on the children *(170)*.

School feeding should not be considered as an end in itself. The important goals to be accomplished are : reorientation of eating habits; incorporating nutrition education into the curriculum; encouraging the use of local commodities; improving school attendance as well as educational performance of the pupils. Since the number to be fed are in millions, the problem is one of balance between the resources and the number to be fed.

The mid-day meal programme became part of the Minimum Needs Programme in the Fifth Five Year Plan *(168)*.

8. Mid-day meal scheme *(171)*

Mid-day meal scheme now known as PM Poshan Scheme is also known as National Programme of Nutritional Support to Primary Education. It was launched as a centrally sponsored scheme on 15th August 1995 and revised in 2004. Its objective being universalization of primary education by increasing enrolment, retention and attendance and simultaneously impacting on nutrition of students in primary classes. It was implemented in 2,408 blocks in the first year and covered the whole country in a phased manner by 1997–98. The programme originally covered children of primary stage (classes I to V) in government, local body and government aided schools and was extended in Oct. 2002, to cover children studying in Education Guarantee Scheme and Alternative and Innovative Education Centres also.

The central assistance provided to states under the programme is by way of free supply of food grain from nearest Food Corporation of India godown at the rate of 100 g. per student per day and subsidy for transport of food grain. To achieve the objective, a cooked mid-day meal with minimum 300 Calories and 8 to 12 grammes of protein content will be provided to all the children in class I to V.

Some suggesstions for preparation of nutritious and economical mid-day meals are as under :

- Foodgrains must be stored in a place away from moisture, in air tight containers/bins to avoid infestation.
- Use whole wheat or broken wheat (dalia) for preparing mid-day meals.
- Rice should preferably be parboiled or unpolished.
- 'Single Dish Meals' using broken wheat or rice and incorporating some amount of a pulse or soyabeans, a seasonal vegetable/green leafy vegetable, and some amount of edible oil will save both time and fuel besides being nutritious. Broken wheat pulao, leafy khicheri, upma, dal-vegetable bhaat are some examples of single dish meals.
- Cereal pulse combination is necessary to have good quality protein. The cereal pulse ratio could range from 3:1 to 5:1.
- Sprouted pulses have more nutrients and should be incorporated in single dish meals.
- Leafy vegetables when added to any preparation should be thoroughly washed before cutting and should not be subjected to washing after cutting.
- Soaking of rice, dal, bengal gram etc. reduces cooking time. Wash the grains thoroughly and soak in just sufficient amount of water required for cooking.
- Rice water if left after cooking should be mixed with dal if these are cooked separately and should never be thrown away.
- Fermentation improves nutritive value. Preparation of idli, dosa, dhokla etc. may be encouraged.

- Cooking must be done with the lid on to avoid loss of nutrients.
- Over cooking should be avoided.
- Reheating of oil used for frying is harmful and should be avoided.
- Leafy tops of carrots, radish, turnips etc. should not be thrown but utilized in preparing mid-day meals.
- Only "iodized salt" should be used for cooking mid-day meals.

Monitoring and evaluation of nutrition programmes

Good preventive medicine demands effective planning, monitoring and evaluation of health programmes. An important advance in this field is the development of the **randomized controlled trial** for the evaluation of the effectiveness and efficiency of health care programmes.

Criticism is often voiced that nutrition programmes are not based on good intentions. It is considered unethical to launch a major nutritional programme (or for that matter any other health programme) without a built-in-provision for monitoring, evaluation and feedback.

Since health and nutrition of the young child is indivisible from the health and nutrition of the family as a whole, there is now increasing recognition that it is only through an improvement of the family diet as a whole, that the diet of the young child in the poor family can be improved *(172)*. Secondly, a question is raised : How long will a country be able to feed its children who may number 100 million or more without any socio-economic improvements? An eminent nutrition scientist in India has said : "In the long run, we can hope to improve the nutritional status of our children only through improvement in the economic conditions of the community to a level at which families can afford balanced diets. Organized State-sponsored feeding programmes cannot be the permanent answer to the problem" *(84)*.

ANNEXURE–1

Nutrition Assessment Schedule

Serial No.	Date :
Name :	Age :
Address :	Sex :
District :	Village :

CLINICAL :

(1)	*General appearance*	:	Normal built/Thin built/Sickly.
(2)	*Hair*	:	Normal/lack of lustre/dyspigmented/thin and sparse/easily pluckable/flag sign.
(3)	*Face*	:	Diffuse depigmentation/naso-labial dyssebacea/moon face.
(4)	*Eyes*	:	Conjunctiva - normal/dry on exposure for 1/2 min/dry and wrinkled/bitot's spots/ brown pigmentation/angular conjunctivitis/pale conjunctiva Cornea - normal/dryness/hazy or opaque.
(5)	*Lips*	:	Normal/angular stomatitis/cheilosis.
(6)	*Tongue*	:	Normal/pale and flabby/red and raw/fissured/geographic.
(7)	*Teeth*	:	Mottled enamel/caries/attrition.
(8)	*Gums*	:	Normal/spongy/ bleeding.
(9)	*Glands*	:	Thyroid enlargement/parotid enlargement.
(10)	*Skin*	:	Normal/dry and scaly/follicular hyperkeratosis/petechiae/pellagrous dermatosis/flanky paint dermatosis/scrotal and vulval dermatosis.
(11)	*Nails*	:	Koilonychia.
(12)	*Oedema*	:	Independent parts.
(13)	*Rachitic changes*	:	Knock-knees or bow legs/epiphyseal enlargement/beading of the ribs/pigeon chest.
(14)	*Internal systems*	:	Hepatomegaly/psychomotor change/mental confusion/sensory loss/muscle wasting/ motor weakness/loss of position sense/loss of vibration sense/loss of ankle and knee jerks/calf tenderness/cardiac enlargement/tachycardia.

ANTHROPOMETRIC :

Weight (kg) :	Head circumference (cm) :
Height (cm) :	Chest circumference (cm) :
Mid-upper-arm circumference (cm) :	Skinfold :

LABORATORY :

(1) Haemoglobin : (specify method).

(2) Stool : negative/ascariasis/ancylostomiasis/giardiasis/amoebiasis/strongyloides/others (state).

(3) Blood smear : negative/M.T./B.T./Filaria.

Investigator

ANNEXURE–2

BALANCED DIETS

(The quantities are given in grams)

Food Item	Adult man			Adult woman			Children		Boys	Girls
	Seden-tary	Moderate work	Heavy work	Seden-tary	Moderate work	Heavy work	1-3 years	4-6 years	10-12 years	10-12 years
Cereals	460	520	670	410	440	575	175	270	420	380
Pulses	40	50	60	40	45	50	35	35	45	45
Leafy vegetables	40	40	40	100	100	50	40	50	50	50
Other vegetables	60	70	80	40	40	100	20	30	50	50
Roots and tubers	50	60	80	50	50	60	10	20	30	30
Milk	150	200	250	100	150	200	300	250	250	250
Oil and Fat	40	45	65	20	25	40	15	25	40	35
Sugar or Jaggery	30	35	55	20	20	40	30	40	45	45

Source : *(138)*

ANNEXURE–3

Suggested substitution for non-vegetarians

Food item which can be deleted from non-vegetarian diets	Substitution that can be suggested for deleted item or items
50% of pulses (20-30 g)	1. One egg or 30 g of meat or fish 2. Additional 5 g of fat or oil
100% of pulses (40-60 g)	1. Two eggs or 50 g of meat or fish 2. One egg plus 30 g meat 10 g of fat or oil

Source : *(138)*

ANNEXURE–4

Low cost Indian vegetarian high protein diet for an adult woman during 2nd and 3rd trimester of pregnancy (10 kg GWG)

Food group composition[a]	2nd trimester Amount (g/d)	Digestible protein content[b] (g/d)	3rd trimester Amount (g/d)	Protein content[b]
Cereals & Millets	325	24	260	20
Pulses (legumes)	65	11	80	14
Green leafy vegetables (GLVs)	250		250	
Other vegetables	100	9	100	9
Roots & tubers	50		30	
Fruits	50		50	
Milk and milk products	300	9	750	23
Fats & oils	30		22	
Sugar & Jaggery	20		5	
Energy (kcal)	2019		2031	
Protein (g)[b]	54		65	
PE Ratio (%)	11		13	

a Cereals and millets are presumed to be in the ratio 40:40:20 for rice: wheat: millets (Ragi/Bajra/Jowar). For calculation purpose, nutritive values for all three millets are averaged. Spinach, french beans, potato and guava represents green leafy vegetables, other vegetables, roots and tubers and fruits respectively. Source of nutritive values of foods: IFCT, 2017.

b Represents digestible protein content of the diet. Protein contents of each food group (except for GLVs, roots and tubers, fruits) are corrected for true faecal digestibility values

Source : *(11)*

ANNEXURE–5

Exercise and physical activity

Individuals over the age of 20 years should undertake a minimum of 30 minutes of physical activity of moderate intensity (such as walking 5–6 km/hr) on most, if not all days of the week. Greater health benefits can be obtained by engaging in physical activity of longer duration or more vigorous intensity (such as jogging, running, cycling and swimming).

Sedentary people embarking on a physical activity programme should undertake a moderate intensity activity of short duration to start with and gradually increase the duration or intensity. Other day-to-day activities like walking, housework, gardening, will be beneficial not only in weight reduction but also for lowering of blood pressure and serum triglycerides. This also elevates HDL (good) cholesterol in blood. Simple modification in lifestyle like deliberately climbing up the stairs instead of using the lift and walking for short distance instead of using a vehicle could also immensely help in increasing our physical activity.

Exercise programme should include 'warm up' and 'cool down' periods each lasting for 5 minutes. During exercise, the intensity of exercise should ensure 60–70% increase in heart rate.

Previously inactive men over the age of 40 years, women over the age of 50 years and people at high risk for chronic diseases like heart disease and diabetes should first consult a physician before engaging in a programme of vigorous physical activity such as running and swimming.

Computation of energy expenditure of adult Indian population using factorial approach

Main daily activities	Duration (h)	Major lifestyles, energy expenditure (PAR values)		
		Sedentary	Moderate active	Heavy or vigorously active
Sleep	8	1.0	1.0	1.0
Occupational activity	8	1.3	2.5	4.1
Non-occupational activity	8	1.9	1.9	1.9
Mean		1.41	1.80	2.33
Non-occupational activity				
Personal care	1	1.6	1.6	1.6
Eating	1	1.2	1.2	1.2
Commuting to work by bus or by vehicle or by walk	1	2.0	2.0	2.0
General household or other activities	2	2.0	2.0	2.0
Walking at various speeds without load	1	3.4	3.4	3.4
Light leisure activity	2	1.4	1.4	1.4
Mean non-occupational activity	8	1.9	1.9	1.9
Men : body wt. (65kg), BMR (1506kcal)	–	2123	2711	3509
Women : body wt. (55kg), BMR (1184 kcal)	–	1670	2131	2759

Source : *(11)*

ANNEXURE–6

Approximate calorific value of some cooked preparations

Preparation	Quantity for one serving	Calories (kcal)
1. Cereal :		
Rice	1 cup	170
Phulka	1 No.	80
Paratha	1 No.	150
Puri	1 No.	100
Bread	2 slices	170
Poha	1 cup	270
Upma	1 cup	270
Idli	2 Nos.	150
Dosa	1 No.	125
Khichidi	1 cup	200
Wheat porridge	1 cup	220
Semolina porridge	1 cup	220
Cereal flakes with milk (corn/wheat/rice)	1 cup	220
2. Pulse :		
Plain dhal	1/2 cup	100
Sambar	1 cup	110
3. Vegetable :		
With gravy	1 cup	170
Dry	1 cup	150
4. Non-Vegetarian :		
Boiled egg	1 No.	90
Omelette	1 No.	160
Fried egg	1 No.	160
Mutton curry	3/4 cup	260
Chicken curry	3/4 cup	240
Fish fried	2 big pieces	220
Fish cutlet	2 Nos.	190
Prawn curry	3/4 cup	220
Keema kofta curry	3/4 cup (6 small koftas)	240
5. Savoury snacks :		
Bajji or pakora	8 Nos.	280
Besan ka pura	1 No.	220
Chat (Dahi-pakori)	5 pieces	220
Cheese balls	2 Nos.	250
Dahi vada	2 Nos.	180
Vada	2 Nos.	140
Masala vada	2 Nos.	150
Masala dosa	1 No.	200
Pea-kachori	2 Nos.	380
Potato bonda	2 Nos.	200
Sago vada	2 Nos.	210
Samosa	1 No.	200
Sandwich (butter - 2 tsp)	2 Nos.	200
Vegetable puff	1 No.	170
Pizza (Cheese and tomato)	1 slice	200
6. Chutneys :		
Coconut/ground/til	2 tbsp	120
Tomato	1 tbsp	10
Tamarind (with jaggery)	1 tbsp	60
7. Sweets and desserts :		
Besan barfi	2 pieces	400
Chikki	2 pieces	290
Fruit cake	1 piece	270
Rice puttu	1/2 cup	280
Sandesh	2 Nos.	140
Double ka meetha	1/2 cup	280
Halwa (kesari)	1/2 cup	320
Jelly/Jam	1 tsp	20
Custard (caramel)	1/2 cup	160
Srikhand	1/2 cup	380
Milk chocolate	25 g	140
Ice-cream	1/2 cup	200
8. Beverages :		
Tea (2 tsp sugar+ 50 ml. toned milk)	1 cup	75
Coffee (2 tsp sugar+ 10 ml toned milk)	1 cup	110
Cow's milk (2 tsp sugar)	1 cup	180
Buffalo's milk (2 tsp sugar)	1 cup	320
Lassi (2 tsp sugar)	1 glass (200 ml)	110
Squash	1 glass (200 ml)	75
Syrups (Sherbat)	1 glass (200 ml)	200
Cold drinks	1 bottle (200 ml)	150
Fresh lime juice	1 glass (200 ml)	60

	Serving	Calories
Nuts :		
Almonds	10 Nos.	85
Cashewnuts	10 Nos.	95
Coconut (fresh)	1/4	130
Coconut (dry)	1/4	140
Peanuts	50 Nos.	90
Fresh fruits :		
Apple	1 medium	65
Banana	1 medium	90
Grapes	30 Nos.	70
Guava	1 medium	50
Jackfruit	4 pieces	90
Mango	1 medium	180
Mosambi/orange	1 medium	40
Papaya	1 piece	80
Pineapple	1 piece	50
Sapota	1 medium	80
Custard apple	1 medium	130
Watermelon/muskmelon	1 slice	15
Salads :		
Beetroot	1 medium	30
Carrot	1 medium	20
Cucumber	1 medium	15
Onion	1 medium	25
Radish	1 medium	10
Tomato	1 medium	10

Source : *(173)*

ANNEXURE–7

Ranges of population nutrient intake goals

Dietary factor	Goal (% of total energy, unless otherwise stated)
Total fat	15-30%
Saturated fatty acids	<10%
Polyunsaturated fatty acids (PUFAs)	6-10%
n-6 Polyunsaturated fatty acids (PUFAs)	5-8%
n-3 Polyunsaturated fatty acids (PUFAs)	1-2%
Trans fatty acids	<1%
Monounsaturated fatty acids (MUFAs)	By difference[a]
Total carbohydrate	55-75%[b]
Free sugars[c]	<10%
Protein	10-15%[d]
Cholesterol	<300 mg per day
Sodium chloride (sodium)[e]	<5 g per day (<2 g per day)
Fruits and vegetables	≥ 400 g per day
Total dietary fibre	From foods
Non-starch polysaccharides (NSP)	From foods

a This is calculated as : total fat – (saturated fatty acids + polyunsaturated fatty acids + trans-fatty acids).

b The percentage of total energy available after taking into account that counsumed as protein and fat, hence the wide range.

c The term "free sugars" refers to all monosaccharides and disaccharides added to foods by the manufacturer, cook or consumer, plus sugars naturally present in honey, syrups and fruit juices.

d The suggested range should be seen in the light of the Joint WHO/FAO/UNU Expert Consultation on Protein and Amino Acid Requirements in Human Nutrition, held in Geneva from 9 to 16 April 2002.

e Salt should be iodized appropriately. The need to adjust salt iodization, depending on observed sodium intake and surveillance of iodine status of the population, should be recognized.

Source : *(13)*

References

1. WHO (1971). *Techn. Rep. Ser.*, No. 477.
2. WHO (1988).*World Health* May 1988.
3. Aykroyd, W.R. (1970). *Conquest of Deficiency Diseases,* FFHC Basic Study, No. 24, Geneva, WHO.
4. WHO/UNICEF (1978). *Primary Health Care* HFA Sr.No. 1.
5. WHO (1981). *Health for All,* Sr.No. 4.
6. WHO (1985). *Techn. Rep. Ser.*, No. 724.
7. ARC/MRC (1974). Report : *Food and Nutrition Research,* London, HMSO.
8. Swaminathan, M. (1977). *Handbook of Food and Nutrition,* Ganesh & Co., Madras.
9. ICMR (2010). *Nutrient Requirement and Recommended Dietary Allowances for Indians,* A Report of the Expert Group of the ICMR.
10. Beaton, G.H. (1976). *Nutrition in Preventive Medicine* P. 482. WHO Monograph Sr.No. 62.
11. ICMR (2020), *Recommended Dietary Allowances and Estimated Average Requirements, Nutritional Requirements for Indians - 2020.*
12. National Institute of Nutrition (1983). *Nutrition News,* March, 1983.
13. Rivers, J.P.H. and Frankel, T.L. (1981). *Br. Med. Bull.*, 37 (1) 59.
14. WHO (2003). *Tech. Rep. Ser.*, No. 916.
15. National Institute of Nutrition (1976). *Annual Report,* 1975.
16. WHO (1982). *Techn. Rep. Ser.*, No. 678.
17. Willet, W.C. and MacMahon, B (1984). *Diet and Cancer: An Overview,* N.Eng.J.Med., 310 (11) 697.
18. WHO (1982). *Techn. Rep. Ser.*, No. 672.
19. Truswell, A.S. (1985). *Br. Med. J. 291* : 1033.
20. N I N Hyderabad (1988). *Nutrition,* Oct. 1988.
21. Somer, A. (1978). *Field guide to detection and control of xerophthalmia,* Geneva, WHO.
22. Demaeyer, E M (1986). *Children in the Tropics* No. 165.
23. Hussaini, G et al (1983). *Lancet 2* : 585.
24. WHO (1984). *Strategies for the Prevention of Blindness in National Programmes,* Geneva, WHO.
25. WHO (1973). *WHO Chr.* 27 (1) 28.
26. West, K.P. and Sommer, A (1987). *Food and Nutrition* Bull 9 70.
27. *Lancet* (1985). 1 : 319.
28. *Med. Dig.* 1988 : 6 (9) P 32.
29. DeLuca, H.F. (1979). *Vitamin D Metabolism and Function,* New York, Springer–Verlag.
30. Kodicek (1974). *Lancet, 1* : 325.
31. McLaren, D.S. (1981). *Nutrition and Its Disorders,* 3rd ed., Edinburgh, Churchill Livingstone.
32. Fraser, D.R. (1981). *Brit. Med. Bull.*, 37 : 37.
33. Vaughan, V.C. et al (1979). Nelson : *Textbook of Pediatrics,* Philadelphia, Saunders.
34. Gopalan, C. et al (1989). *Nutritive Value of Indian Foods,* National Institute of Nutrition, Hyderabad.
35. WHO (1967). *Techn. Rep. Ser.*, No. 362.
36. Pandit, C.G. et al (1960). *Nutrition in India,* New Delhi, ICMR.
37. Bamji, M.S. (1989). *Nutrition News* 10 (2) March 1989.
38. Passmore, R et al (1974). *Handbook on Human Nutritional Requirements,* Geneva, WHO.
39. Krishnaswamy, K. and Gopalan, C. (1971). *Lancet, 2* : 1167.
40. Layrisse, M. et al (1976). In :*Nutrition in Preventive Medicine,* WHO Monograph No. 62.
41. WHO (1973). *Techn. Rep. Ser.*, No. 532.
42. Golden, M.H.N. (1981). *Br. Med. Bull.*, 37 : 31.
43. ICMR (1980). *Nutritive Value of Indian Foods,* National Institute of Nutrition, Hyderabad.
44. WHO/FAO (1962). *Techn. Rep. Sr.*, No. 230.
45. Havard , C. W. H. (1970). *The Medical Annual,* John Wright & Sons.
46. Kundu, S. C. (1970). *J. Indian M. A.*, 55, 25.
47. Layrisse, H.H. et al (1976). *WHO Monograph* 62.
48. WHO (1975). *Techn. Rep. Ser.*, No. 580.
49. Hefnawi, F.et al (1974). *Contraception,* 9; 133.
50. Guilleband, J. et al (1976). *Lancet,* 1 : 387.
51. Royston, E. (1982). *WHO Statis Q.* 14 35 :52.
52. WHO (1968). *Techn. Rep. Ser.* No. 405.
53. Sood, S.K. and U. Rusia (1986). *Ann of Nat Acad of Med Sci.*,India, 22 (4) 235.
54. WHO (1982). *Wld Hlth Statis Qrly,* 35 : 52.
55. Editorial (1983). *Lancet,* 2 : 1121.
56. Hetzel, B.S. (1983). *Lancet, 2* : 1126.
57. WHO (1985). *IDD in SE Asia,* SEARO Reg.Health Paper No.10 New Delhi.
58. Hetzel, B.S. (1985). In :*Oxford Textbook of Public Health,* Vol 4, p. 28.
59. Gopalan, C. (1974). *Ann Indian Acad Med.Sci.*, 10 :1.
60. Jolly, S.S. et al (1969). *Ind. J. Med. Res.*, 57 : 1333.
61. Jolly, S.S. (1970). *J. Assoc. Phy. of India,* 18 : 459.
62. WHO (1970). *WHO Chr.* 24 (6) 271.
63. Halsted, J. (1970). *Lancet,* 1,322.
64. Swaminathan, M. (1974). *Essentials of Food and Nutrition.* Ganesh & Co., Madras 17.
65. CIMS, *Role of Zinc in Health and Disease.*
66. Standstead, H. H. et al (1970). *Med. Cli. N. Amer.* 54, 1509.
67. J. Indian M. A. (1976). *Current Medical Literature,* 66, P. 248.
68. Jean – Gerard Pelletier (1993), *Children in the Tropics,* Severe Malnutrition : A Global Approach, 1993 – No.208–209.
69. Chauliac, M. (1984). *Children in the Tropics* No.147–148 P. 26.
70. Narsinga Rao, B.S. (1986). *Nutrition,* 20 (1) 14.
71. Deosthale, Y.G. (1983). *Nutrition,* July 1983.
72. Swaminathan, M. (1983). *Human Nutrition and Diet,* The Banglore Printing and Publishing Co.Ltd. Bangalore.
73. Govt. of India (2011), *Operational Guidelines on Facility Based Management of Children with Severe Acute Malnutrition,* Ministry of Health and Family Welfare, New Delhi.
74. *Taber's Cyclopedic Medical Dictionary* 17th Edn, 1993, Vol.2 Page 2222.

75. FAO (1950). *Nutritional Studies* No. 5.
76. WHO (1973). *Techn. Rep. Ser.*, No. 522.
77. WHO (1979). *The Health Aspects of Food and Nutrition, Manila.*
78. Falkner, F. ed (1980). *Prevention in Childhood of Health Problems in adult life,* WHO.
79. WHO (1986). *Techn. Rep. Ser.*, No. 732.
80. Lawrence M. Tierney et al, *Current Medical Diagnosis and Treatment,* 43rd Ed., A Lange Medical Books Publication.
81. Public Health Foundation of India (2015), *India Health Report : Nutrition 2015.*
82. WHO (2012). Save the Children etc. (2012). *Born Too Soon,* The Global Action Report on Preterm Birth, 2012.
83. Shah, P. M. (1974). *Early Detection and Prevention of Protein–Calorie Malnutrition,* Popular Prakashan, Bombay.
84. National Institute of Nutrition Hyderabad (2011). *Dietry Guidelines for Indians - A manual.*
85. Editorial (1982). *Lancet 2* : 28–29.
86. John Bland (1979). *World Health,* Aug–Sept. 1979.
87. WHO (1976). *Techn. Rep. Ser.*, 590.
88. Central Health Education Bureau (1986). *Swasth Hind,* 30 (3–4) 85. Ministry of Health and Family Welfare, Govt. of India, New Delhi.
89. Govt. of India (2008). *Eleventh Five Year Plan (2007-2012),* Vol II, Planning Commission, New Delhi.
90. Govt. of India (2008). *Annual Report 2007-08,* Ministry of Health and Family Welfare, New Delhi.
91. WHO (1982). *The Work of WHO,* 1980–81, Biennial Report.
92. WHO (1980). *Sixth Report World Health Situation,* Vol I.
92A. Govt. of India (2022), *National Family Health Survey-5, 2019–2021,* Ministry of Health and Family Welfare, New Delhi.
93. Srikantia, S.G. (1983). *Proceed.Nut.Society of India* No.28, P. 7.
94. Narsinga Rao, B.S. (1978). *Ind. J. Med. Res.* No. 58.
95. Govt.of India (1978). *Manual for Health Worker (F),* Vol I. Ministry of Health and Family Welfare, New Delhi.
96. N.I.N., Hyderabad (1989). *Nutrition,* Jan. 1989.
97. Clugston, G.A. and K. Bagchi (1986). *World Health Forum,* 7 (1) 33
98. Govt. of India (2010). *Annual Report 2009-2010,* Ministry of Health and Family Welfare, New Delhi.
99. WHO (1984). *Techn. Rep. Ser.*, 713.
100. WHO (1984). *Guidelines for Drinking Water Quality,* Vol 1 P 55 Geneva WHO.
101. WHO (1970). *Fluorides and Human Health* Geneva, WHO Monograph S No. 59.
102. Krishnamachary, K.A.V.R. (1976). *Ind. J. Med. Res.*, 64 : 284.
103. Nawlakha, W.G. et al (1975). *Ind. J. Env. Hlth.* 17 : 26.
104. Mohan Ram M and I Gopalan (1981). *Nutritional Disabilities,* ICMR, National Institute of Nutrition, Hyderabad.
105. Ramachandran, L.K. (1978). *Science Reporter, Feb.1978,* Council of Scientific and Industrial Research, New Delhi.
106. The pooling project Research Group (1978). *J.Chr.Dis.*, 31 : 201.
107. Kushi, L.H. et al (1985). *N. Eng. J. Med.*, 312 : 811.
108. Oliver, M.F. (1981). *Br. Med. Bull.* 37 (1) 49–58.
109. Morris, J.N. et al (1977). *Brit. Med. J.*, 2 : 1307–1314.
110. WHO (1985). *Techn. Rep. Ser.*, No. 727.
111. WHO (1984). *Techn. Rep. Ser.*, 706, P. 44.
112. Tasher, T. (1986). *Food and Nutrition Bulletin,* 8 (13) 12.
113. Jain, M. et al (1980). *Int. J. Cancer,* 26 : 757–68.
114. Willet, W.C. and B. MacMahon (1984). *N. Eng. J. Med.*, 310 (11) 697.
115. Fraumenti, J.F. (1982). *Ann. Rev. Pub Health* 3 : 85–100.
116. Miller, A.B. et al (1978). *Am. J. Epid,* 107 : 499–509.
117. Wynder, E.L. and Hill, P. (1977). *Lancet, 2* : 840–841.
118. Burkitt, D.P. (1971). *Cancer,* 28 : 3–13.
119. Weisburger, J.H. et al (1980). *Prev. Med.*, 9 : 352–61.
120. Hoover, R.N. and Strasser, P.H. (1980). *Lancet, 1* : 837–40.
121. MacMohan, B. et al (1981). *N. Eng. J. Med.*, 304 : 630–33.
122. Rothma, K.J. (1980). *Prev. Med.*, 9 : 174–79.
123. WHO (1978). *Bull WHO* 56 (4) 519.
124. Behar, M. (1976). In : *Nutrition in Preventive Medicine,* WHO Monograph Ser.No. 62.
125. WHO (1963). *Techn. Rep. Ser.*, No. 258.
126. James W.P.T. (1982). *Medicine International,* 1 (15) 663.
127. Solomons, N.W. and Allen, L.H. (1983). *Nutrition Review,* 41 (2) 33–50.
128. Bourne, G.H. ed (1971). *World Review of Nutrition and Dietetics,* Vol 13, pp 106–164, Karger Basel.
129. Taskar, A.D. et al (1967). *Ind. J. Med. Res.*, 55 : 90.
130. Bengoa, J.M. (1974). *WHO Chronicle,* 28 : 3–7.
131. Mason, J.B. et al (1984). *Nutritional Surveillance,* Geneva, WHO.
132. WHO (1976). *Techn. Rep. Ser.*, No. 593.
133. WHO (1984). *World Health,* Oct. 1984, p. 8.
134. Jelliffe, D.B. (1966). *The Assessment of the Nutritional Status of the Community,* WHO Monograph Sr. No. 53.
135. WHO (1963). *World Health,* May 1977.
136. Sukhatma, P.V. et al (1972). In : *Proceedings of the First Asian Congress of Nutrition.* National Institute of Nutrition, Hyderabad.
137. Gopalan, C. (1977). *Swasth Hind,* 21, 335.
138. ICMR (1990). *Recommended Dietary Intakes for Indians,* New Delhi.
139. WHO (1976). *Proc. Nutrition Society,* 20, 1–5 National Institute of Nutrition, Hyderabad.
140. WHO (1984). *Techn. Rep. Ser.*, No. 705.
141. WHO (1978). *Wkly. Epi. Rec.*,53, 37–44.
142. Stewart, S. (1975). *Sanitary Officers Practice; Food Inspection,* Butterworth, London.
143. WHO (1962). *Milk Hygiene,*Monograph Ser. No. 48.
144. WHO (1970). *Techn. Rep. Ser.*, No. 453.
145. Parulekar, V. P.P. (1968). *National Seminar on Zoonoses in India,* National Institute of Communicable Diseases, Delhi.
146. Govt. of India (1955). *Model Public Health Act,*Ministry of Health.
147. WHO (1972). *Hazards of the Human Environment,* Geneva, WHO.
148. Morton, L.D. (1977). *Proce. Nutr. Soc.* 36 : 101.
149. WHO (1976). *Techn. Rep. Ser.*, No. 598.
150. Rodricks, J.V. (1976). *Food Nutrition* (FAO) 2 :9.
151. WHO (1977). *Techn. Rep. Ser.*, No. 612.
152. Elton, G.A.H. (1977). *Proc. Nutr. Soc.* 36 : 113.
153. Nagarajan, V. (1970). *A Decade of Progress,* 1961–1970, National Institute of Nutrition, Hyderabad.
154. Krishnamachari, K.A.V.R. et al (1975). *Indian J.Med.Res.*, 63, 1036.
155. Bhatt, R.V. et al (1976). *Indian J. Medical Res.* 64, 1629.
156. Krishnamachary, K.A.V.R. et al (1976). *Ibid,* 64, 1624.
157. Lal R.B. and Roy, S.C. (1937). Ibid, 25, 163.
158. Garrow, J.S. (1968). *The Practitioner,* 201, 283.
159. National Institute of Nutrition, Hyderabad (1977). *Ann.Rep.*1976.
160. National Institute of Nutrition, Hyderabad (1977). *Nutrition,* April, 1977.
161. National Institute of Nutrition, Hyderabad (1976). *Annual Report,* 1975.
162. WHO/FAO (1955). *Techn. Rep. Ser.*, No. 97.
163. WHO (1989). *Techn. Rep. Ser.*, No. 776.
164. Bhat, R. (1977). *Nutrition,* July 1977, Hyderabad.
165. Thankamma Jacob (1976). *Food Adulteration,* MacMillan, Delhi.
166. Ramadasmurthy, V. and M. Mohanram (1984). *Your Nutrition and Health,* N.I.N., Hyderabad.
167. Govt. of India (1993). *National Nutrition Policy 1993,* Ministry of Human Resource Development, New Delhi.
168. Planning Commission, Govt. of India (1985). *Seventh Five Year Plan,* 1985–90. Vol II, Delhi.
169. Swaminathan, M.C. (1970). *Nutrition* Oct. 1970 NIN.
170. Govt.of India, Planning Commission (1972). *Report of the Committee on Preschool Children Feeding Programmes.*
171. Guidelines of Revised National Programme of Nutritional Support to Education, 2004, http://education.nic.in/mdm/mdm2004.asp
172. Gopalan, C. (1980). *Nutrition and Health Care,* Nutrition Foundation of India, Spl, Publ. No. 1.
173. *Dietary Guidelines for Indians,* National Institute of Nutrition, ICMR Hyd. 1998.
174. Govt. of India (2020), *Annual Report 2019–20,* Ministry of Health and Family Welfare, New Delhi.
175. Govt. of India (2017), *Nourishing India, National Nutrition Strategy,* Niti Aayog.

12 Medicine and Social Sciences

"The secret of national health lies in the homes of the people"

The term "social sciences" refers to a composite of several disciplines. These disciplines are anthropology, economics, political science, psychology, sociology etc. In general, these disciplines contribute to our understanding of society and human behaviour. The social sciences relevant to medicine are psychology and sociology. They should be considered like anatomy and physiology, the basic sciences of medicine.

Social context of medicine

Health cannot be isolated from its social context. The last few decades have shown that social and economic factors have as much influence on health as medical interventions. All these factors have a direct bearing on the incidence, course and outcome of a wide variety of communicable and non-communicable diseases as well as on many other health problems besetting the world today. They also have an important effect on the provision of health care to all strata of society *(1)*. Poverty, malnutrition, poor sanitation, lack of education, inadequate housing, unemployment, poor working conditions, cultural and behavioural factors all predispose to ill-health. Today more than ever before, there has been an increasing recognition that successful application of medicine to individuals and groups involves more than mere scientific or biological knowledge; it involves an understanding of the behaviour of individuals and groups who live together and also share certain values of life. Man is a social animal. The patient is no longer considered as one who is under strict laboratory control, but an individual with personal idiosyncrasies, erratic habits, customs and beliefs reacting on his body and mind. It has been aptly said that even a person with a broken leg may present complex social and personal factors which may influence his recovery. Thus there has been a shift from the earlier concept of visualizing disease in terms of a specific germ to the involvement of "multiple factors" in the causation of disease. Good doctors are being identified as those who treat people, and bad ones as those who treat cases. As a result of this new outlook, concepts of sociology are increasingly being used in the study of disease in human societies.

How much effect social changes might have on health of the people is shown in Fig. 1.

It suggests that health is influenced by four sets of variables – individual predispositions, ecological predispositions, current circumstances, and opportunities. These variables are in turn influenced by the major sources of social changes : economic, political, educational and other systems. The health status of the people can feed back into and influence factors relating to social structure which may in turn influence the predisposing variables, and therefore health *(2)*.

Medicine and the social sciences are concerned, in their own special way, with human behaviour. Specialists in community health, clinical medicine, epidemiology are all seeking the cooperation and help of social scientists in understanding problems such as the social component of health and disease, "illness behaviour" of people, efficient use of medical care and the study of medical institutions. A brief sketch of the current interest of these disciplines in social science is given below :

1. COMMUNITY HEALTH

Community health workers are often faced with the problem of why people who need a particular service are least likely to use it or fail to secure the total benefit which is expected. A case in point is immunization against communicable diseases. Although, there is a wide range of prophylactic vaccines, immunization has not gained universal acceptance. The family planning programme in India is a recent example of a health service of which people are not making use to the extent desired. Similarly, health programmes relating to mother and child health care services, improvement of water supplies, installation of sanitary latrines, improvement of dietary patterns and infant rearing practices have all proved abortive or only partially successful. The resistance of the people is felt not only in the field of community health, but in fact even in fields designed to improve their general standard of living. The central question in community health is : Why do people behave as they do ? This is the basic problem which the social scientists are studying in India, and are often asked to explain this failure of health measures. In the western countries, social scientists are working on problems of mental health, hospital organization, social class difference in disease, rehabilitation, and professional roles and relationships. In industries, the social scientists are invited to look into the relationships between members of a team who are concerned with doing a job in order to improve the overall performance of the work team. In short, the social scientists are stepping in increasing numbers into the field of community health. The theme common to community health and social sciences is human behaviour. Many community health problems in essence are social problems, and vice versa.

2. CLINICAL MEDICINE

During the past half century, the scientific content of medicine has increased enormously. The acute

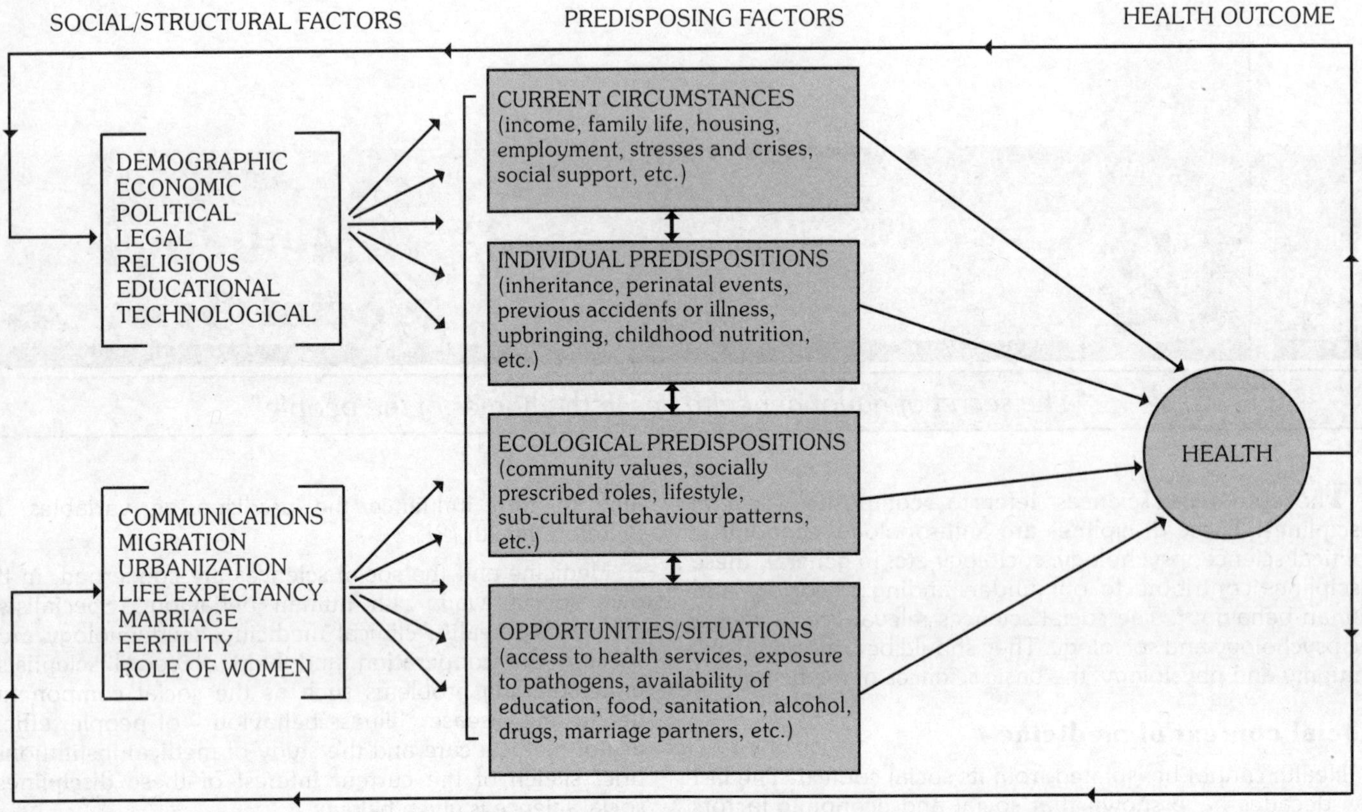

FIG. 1
Social factors influencing the health of people

Source : *(2)*

communicable diseases have been brought under control, and good medical care is available to more people than ever before. This has brought to a sharp focus, the so-called "modern diseases" such as cardiovascular disease, cancer, diabetes and mental illness. These diseases have defied "cure" and prevention, and are currently the major causes of morbidity and mortality in developed societies. The clinicians also tend to believe that "psychophysiological stress reactions" are involved in cases of rheumatoid arthritis, obesity, ulceration of intestine, skin diseases, constipation, diarrhoea and epilepsy. It has become apparent that control of these diseases involves not merely medical care but basic changes in the behaviour and habits of the patients, which is a field of specialization of social scientists. The social scientists are asked to investigate the life situations of the patients with a view to discover linkages between specific life situations and specific types and cases of illness.

The clinicians have also shown interest in what is known as "illness behaviour" of patients, i.e., why different people react in different ways to the same disease process or regimen of treatment. It is not known why some people (whether by reason of education, religion, social class difference or occupational status) make light of symptoms and some respond in an exaggerated manner, to the slightest pain or discomfort. This is an important area of medical sociology. The doctor-patient relationship, patient care management, hospital organization, collusion of medical treatment and cultural practices are all current interests of medical sociology.

Criticism is often voiced that the present medical sciences (e.g., anatomy, physiology, microbiology, pathology) are insufficient to train the physician to cope with the socio-cultural aspects of medicine. It is recognized that the physician needs two kinds of knowledge – medical knowledge and social knowledge, so that he could more effectively serve the patient and the community. Hence is the current interest in social sciences.

3. EPIDEMIOLOGY

Epidemiologists have also forged a close alliance with social scientists in studying the distribution of health and disease in human population, and of factors that cause the distribution. Disease is studied in relationship to factors such as social status, income, occupation, housing, overcrowding, social customs, habits and behaviour. Examples can be found in researches into the ecology of coronary heart disease, duodenal ulcer, schizophrenia, mental subnormality, suicide, accidents, and several other conditions.

To sum up, social scientists are studying a great many things of considerable interest to medicine and public health. They have "given fruitful attention to the growing place of medicine and medical practice in the social system, and to different attitudes and values which various segments of the population have towards health, illness and medical care. They have made noteworthy advances in mapping out the social organization of health personnel; the social structure and functioning of hospitals have been studied to advantage, as have the social roles played by patients and health personnel as they interact in different settings. They have paid particular attention to the situation of health personnel who are professionals, and to the social processes through which these persons acquire the outlook, standards and competence considered necessary for providing satisfactory professional services. They have also undertaken investigations which relate various social and psychological factors to different kinds of diseases in patients as well as to the course of certain diseases" *(3)*.

SOCIAL AND BEHAVIOURAL SCIENCES

Medicine and social sciences are concerned in their own special way with human behaviour. The term 'social sciences' is applied to those disciplines which are committed to the scientific examination of human behaviour. These are economics, political science, sociology, social psychology and social anthropology. The term 'behavioural sciences' is applied to the last three, i.e., sociology, social psychology and social anthropology, because they deal directly with human behaviour. Each of these disciplines, while sharing the major goals of social sciences, i.e., the scientific examination of human behaviour deals with specific aspects of public health in the study of man.

(a) ECONOMICS

The field of economics has a very close relationship with sociology. It is the parent discipline from which sociology has emerged. Economics deals with human relationships in the specific context of production, distribution, consumption and ownership of scarce resources, goods and services. Sociology and economics overlap in many senses; both are concerned with interdependence in human relations.

(b) POLITICAL SCIENCE

Historically economics and political science tended to be a single discipline. As a separate discipline, political science is concerned with the study of the system of laws and institutions which constitute government of whole societies.

(c) SOCIOLOGY

Sociology deals with the study of human relationships and of human behaviour for a better understanding of the pattern of human life. It is also concerned with the effects on the individual of the ways in which other individuals think and act.

(d) SOCIAL PSYCHOLOGY

This discipline sprang from psychology. It is concerned with the psychology of individuals living in human society or groups. The emphasis is on understanding the basis of perception, thought, opinion, attitudes, general motivation and learning in individuals and how these vary in human societies and groups. In other words, it deals with the effect of social environment on persons, their attitudes and motivations.

(e) ANTHROPOLOGY

The word 'anthropology' is derived from the root words, anthropos meaning man and *logos* meaning science. It is the study of the physical, social and cultural history of man. The study of human evolution, racial differences, inheritance of bodily traits, growth and decay of the human organism is called *physical anthropology*. The study of the development and various types of social life is called *social anthropology*. The study of the total way of life of contemporary primitive man, his ways of thinking, feeling and action is called *cultural anthropology (4)*. Of all the sciences, which study various aspects of man, anthropology is one which comes nearest to being a total study of man. *Medical anthropology*, deals with the cultural component in the ecology of health and disease.

SOCIOLOGY

Sociology is derived from the Latin socio, meaning society and the Greek *logos,* meaning science. The word *'society'* is derived from the root words *socius,* meaning individual and *societa,* meaning group. Society is a group of individuals who have organized themselves and follow a given way of life, and sociology is the study of individuals as well as groups in a society. Sociology can be viewed from two angles : (a) First, it can be seen as the *study of relationships between human beings,* and how these relationships change or vary in different parts of the world and at different times. The unit of study can be a small group (e.g., family) consisting of parents and children, or the study can extend beyond the family or small groups into the complex society where a greater number of people interact and interdepend in terms of economics, political power, general organization and ways of living. (b) The other part of sociology is concerned with the *study of human behaviour.* Human behaviour is determined not merely by biological and physical environmental factors but also by social factors. Every form of human behaviour has a social component. Sociologists are interested in the study of the social determinants of human behaviour. In the final analysis it may be stated that the aim of sociology is to search for the pattern of relationships between people in order to pave the way for the betterment of individuals in relation to society *(5)*.

SPECIALIZATION WITHIN SOCIOLOGY

Sociology has grown rapidly since World War II resulting in an increase in specialization within the general field of sociology. Some of the major fields of specialization are : medical sociology, urban sociology, rural sociology, industrial sociology, sociology of religion, sociology of education, criminology, hospital sociology, and demography.

MEDICAL SOCIOLOGY

Medical sociology is a specialization within the field of sociology. Its main interest is in the study of health, health behaviour and medical institutions. As a specialized field, it was first proposed by Charles McIntire in 1894 *(6)*. It is defined as "professional endeavour devoted to social epidemiology, the study of cultural factors and social relations in connection with illness, and the social principles in medical organization and treatment" *(6)*.

Broadly speaking medical sociology includes studies of the medical profession, of the relationship of medicine to public, and of the social factors in the aetiology, prevalence, incidence and interpretation of disease.

CONCEPTS IN SOCIOLOGY

Such terms as society, social structure, social institutions, role, socialization, social control mechanisms, customs, culture, acculturation, social problems, social pathology and social survey are frequently used by all sociologists and form part of the necessary equipment by means of which they organize their thinking, do research and communicate the results of research *(7)*. Some of these concepts have also crept into medical terminology and are being increasingly used in epidemiological studies. A brief account of these concepts is given below.

SOCIETY

Human beings everywhere are members of a group or groups. A man who can live without society, said Aristotle, is either a beast or God. A group of people may or may not form a society. For example, a group of people coming together temporarily for a while to witness a hockey match do not constitute a society; they are merely a crowd. But if the same group of people settle down and organize themselves, then they form a society. Thus, society may be defined in simple terms as an organization of member agents. The outstanding feature of society is a *system* – a system of social relationships between individuals. The importance of society lies in the fact that it controls and regulates the behaviour of the individual both by law and customs. It can exert pressure on the individual to conform to its norms. In short, society is a vast network of relationships and compulsions that propel, direct and constrain man's individual efforts. The character of society is dynamic; it changes over time and place. Public health is an integral part of the social system. It is influenced by society, and society by public health. In many places it is the social organization that has made it possible to translate into practice the scientific concepts and achievements. As a result, the mortality rates have been brought to low levels and the life expectancy at birth has soared to very high levels.

COMMUNITY

Various definitions of community are given in dictionaries and other publications. Some imply homogenity, e.g., "The people living in a particular place or region and usually linked by common interests" *(8)*; or "A group of individuals and families living together in a defined geographic area, usually comprising a village, town or city" *(8)*.

The definition accepted by WHO Expert Committee is – "A community is a social group determined by geographical boundaries and/or common values and interests". Its members know and interact with each other. It functions within a particular social structure and exhibits and creates certain norms, values, and social institutions. The individual belongs to the broader society through his family and community *(8)*.

SOCIAL STRUCTURE

Social structure refers to the pattern of inter-relations between persons. Every society has a social structure – a complex of major institutions, groups, power structure and status hierarchy. The study of social structure is comparable to the study of anatomy and that of social organization to that of physiology.

SOCIAL INSTITUTIONS

A social institution is an organized complex pattern of behaviour in which a number of persons participate in order to further group interest. The family, the school, the church, the club, the hospital, political parties, professional associations and the panchayats are all social institutions. Within each institution, the rights and duties of the members are defined.

ROLE

In a society, individuals are allocated roles as people in a drama. Sociologists have classified roles into ascribed and achieved, according to whether a particular role is "given" by virtue of sex, age, and birth status or "acquired" by virtue of education or otherwise. In a single day, a man may play a role of husband, father, employee, friend, son, brother, committee chairman, guest, neighbour. The playing of these roles enables him to cooperate with others in many situations according to well-defined roles *(9)*. When a person falls ill, he assumes what is known as a "Sick role". In this role he is expected to decrease or relinquish his normal duties, seek medical aid, and carry out the orders given by the physician.

SOCIALISM

Socialism, to put it briefly, is the general term for any economic doctrine that favours the use of property and resources of the country for the public welfare. It is a system of production and distribution based on *social ownership* for raising the living standard of the working class, as opposed to capitalism which is based on *private ownership* of the means of production and aims at maximum private profit at the expense of the working masses. While the motto of capitalism is 'all for each' and 'each for each', that of socialism is 'all for all' and 'each for all'. These are two extremes. Ever since Louis Blanc set forth the socialist principle "from each according to his abilities, to each according to his needs", socialism has undergone many changes and taken varied shades.

SOCIALIZATION

Every society has its beliefs, customs, traditions and prejudices. A man acquires these in his everyday social interaction with the people of the society. This is called "socialization" or the process by which an individual gradually acquires culture and becomes a member of a social group. Children going to school is an instance of socialization. The internship training programme of doctors is another instance; it gives them an opportunity to learn how to become acceptable to the public at large as doctors.

SOCIAL CONTROL MECHANISMS

In every society there are rules, formal and informal, for the maintenance of relationships of authority and subordination. The laws and enactments of Parliament are social control mechanisms. In the field of health, there are various Acts, some central and others state or local which help to maintain the standards of health. Even in small organizations, there are sets of formal rules and regulations which control the behaviour of individuals to perform different roles. Besides formal rules, sometimes, informal social pressures are brought to bear upon individuals to help construct "norms" of behaviour. The informal social pressure may be exerted by powerful groups, individuals or friends. These mechanisms work largely through reward and punishment. For example, in India, the government is offering a small financial reward to those who undergo sterilization operation. It is a sort of informal social pressure to further the programme of family planning in India. The social control mechanisms vary from group to group. A study of these mechanisms may be helpful to the community health worker in carrying out the health programmes.

CUSTOMS

The mere existence of a society, the mere plurality of individuals gives rise to customs from which no single member of the community can escape. The 'highly developed' societies of the modern world are just as replete with social customs as the 'primitive societies' of the past. These customs are quite numerous and quite as powerful. Customs are technically divided into "folkways" and 'mores'. The folkways are the right ways of doing things in what is regarded as the less vital areas of human conduct. The more stringent customs are called "mores". The public takes an active part in their enforcement. Laws are generally customs-inspired. The starting point of all customs is convention. Convention is the practice promoted by convenience of the society or the individual.

CULTURE

The word "culture" is widely used in sociology. It is the central concept around which cultural anthropology has grown. Culture is defined as "learned behaviour which has been socially acquired". Culture is the product of human societies, and man is largely a product of his cultural environment. Culture is transmitted from one generation to another through learning processes, formal and informal. Culture plays an important role in human societies. It lays down norms of behaviour and provides mechanisms which secure for an individual his personal and social survival *(4)*. In general, it is widely held, that culture stands for the customs, beliefs, laws, religion and moral precepts, arts and other capabilities and skills acquired by man as a member of the society.

Cultural factors in health and disease have engaged the attention of medical scientists and sociologists. Every culture has its own customs, some of which have a profound influence on the incidence of disease. In developed countries, for example, cancer of the lung from smoking and cirrhosis of liver from drinking are the result of the abuse of widely proclaimed social habits. In India, chewing pan is associated with oral cancer. It is now fairly established that cultural factors are deeply involved in matters of personal hygiene, nutrition, immunization, seeking early medical care, family planning, child rearing, disposal of refuse and excreta, outlook on health and disease – in short, the whole way of life.

ACCULTURATION

Acculturation means "culture contact." When there is contact between two people with different types of culture, there is diffusion of culture both ways. There are various ways by which culture contact takes place *(10)* : (1) trade and commerce; (2) industrialization; (3) propagation of religion; (4) education; and (5) conquest. The British brought their culture into India through conquest. An Indian is said to be the next best Englishman. It is because of culture contact, which has both good and bad aspects. The introduction of scientific medicine is through culture contact. The changes in food habits of people is brought about through culture contact; many orthodox brahmins in India today eat meat. The widespread use of tobacco all over the world is because of culture contact. The radio, the television, the cinema have been important factors in shaping the cultural-behaviour patterns of people.

STANDARD OF LIVING

The term "standard of living" refers to the usual scale of our expenditure, the goods we consume and the services we enjoy. It includes food, dress, house, amusements and in short the mode of living.

The standard of living in a country depends upon : (1) the level of national income; (2) the total amount of goods and services a country is able to produce; (3) the size of the population; (4) the level of education; (5) general price level; and (6) the distribution of national income.

There are vast inequalities in the standard of living of the people in different countries of the world. The extent of differences in the level of living can be known through the comparison of *per capita income* on which the standard of living of people primarily depends.

DYNAMICS OF SOCIAL CHANGE

The interaction between social factors and health issues is complex and sometimes unpredictable. For example, in Western Europe during the nineteenth century, increase in income and wealth, resulting from the Industrial Revolution, was accompanied by decrease in both – birth and death rates. Many authors have in fact argued that increased income was the main cause of these changes *(2)*. The situation in the developing world has varied and differs from the so-called "demographic transition" in Europe. In many parts of Asia, and to a certain extent in Latin America, death rates, particularly among infants, have declined steadily in the past decade and birth rates have declined rather dramatically. Yet the increase in income has been very modest. In Africa, on the whole, death rates, particularly of infants, remain high, birth rates are not declining, the benefits of increased income are not yet apparent, and concern over population growth is just emerging. The relationship between wealth, birth, and death rates observed in the development of West European countries, is thus obviously not universal *(2)*.

A typical feature of traditional societies is a sense of continuity and immutability in patterns of social life. Transitional societies may be better able to cope with change, and modern societies are perhaps best adapted to assimilate rapid changes. A major difference between traditional and modern societies is that, in the former, young people can be fairly sure that their lives will be substantially similar to their parent's, while, in the latter, young people can be fairly sure that their lives will be substantially different from their parent's, and that their children's lives will be different from their own. In transitional societies, young people may simultaneously be involved in two cultures : the traditional one in which their parents grew up and which they still value, and the modern one which may be portrayed in the mass media. A similar clash of cultures may occur in the lives of young people whose families have migrated to another country or from a rural to an urban area *(2)*.

SOCIAL STRESS

A major source of stress, particularly in transitional societies, is the conflict generated by new opportunities and frustrations arising from societal changes. These stress-inducing conditions include : the wave of migration from rural to urban areas and the consequent diminution in the traditional family support system; a greater exposure through mass media to ideas that had been previously culturally alien; tourism; changes in the technological needs of society requiring skills that are different from those of the previous generation and for which the training or education available may be inadequate and the encouragement by commercial interests of economic aspirations that are often unrealistic *(2)*. The pressure is mostly felt where young people have little control over their own destinies, where rapid population expansion means greater competition in the younger age groups, and where resources are inadequate to meet their needs.

It is well understood that the causation of physical and psychological disorders is multifactorial. The experience of stress, particularly in the absence of a social support system or when there is a discrepancy between the actual and perceived demands of a stressful situation, may contribute to further disorders *(2)*. Psychological stress and inadequate coping ability has been implicated as a contributory factor in virtually all diseases *(2)*. In particular, there are direct links between stress and hypertension and coronary heart disease.

SOCIAL PROBLEMS

In a community, there are both individual and social problems. Individual problems become social problems when they affect a large number of people amounting to a threat to the welfare or safety of the whole group. But all individual problems are not social problems. Poverty, crime and disease are the common social problems. Many public health problems are social problems and vice versa. Alcoholism, sexually transmitted diseases, mental illness and narcotic addiction are both, public health and social problems. Such social problems as housing, divorce, population growth, increased number of old people have public health implications calling for a combined sociological and public health action.

SOCIAL PATHOLOGY

The term "social pathology" is given a restricted interpretation linking it to poverty, crime, delinquency and vagrancy. In the modern context, the term is also used to describe the relation between disease and social conditions. The social pathology of accidents, diabetes, cardiovascular disease, cancer, chronic bronchitis have all been subject of recent investigations in medical literature. Social pathology is uncovered by "social surveys".

SOCIAL SURVEYS

Social surveys disclose social pathology. Social surveys have played an important part, in the development of public health. It was such a survey by Chadwick that led to the foundation of the General Board of Health in 1848 in Great Britain. There is a strong kinship between epidemiological survey and social survey. When the objective of the research is to study the role of social factors in the aetiology of disease, the two merge into what is known as "social epidemiology". Large scale social epidemiological studies have investigated the relationship of social factors to heart disease, cancer and arthritis *(11)*.

CASE STUDY

Case study is a method of exploring and analyzing the life of a social unit – be that unit a person, a family, an institution, culture group, or even an entire community. Its aim is to determine the factors that account for the complex behaviour patterns of the unit and the relationships of the unit to its surrounding milieu. The case study differs from the survey in the respect that it attempts to collect a large amount of information from a small number of units whereas a survey collects a relatively small amount of information from a large number of units. Thus the case study can yield valuable data about the unit studied than is possible from survey data. A combination of survey and case study could, for example, provide more information about a population of interest than either method could do alone. A case study also has its limitations, i.e., a single instance may or may not be representative of a larger population.

FIELD STUDY

Whereas surveys are concerned with the breadth of knowledge (systematic collection of data from population or samples of population through personal interviews or other data-gathering devices), field studies are concerned with depth of knowledge; they involve observation of people *in situ*.

COMMUNICATION

The term "communication" refers to a social process – the flow of information, the circulation of knowledge and ideas, and the propagation of thoughts. The role of communication in community health is to help motivate people to accept ideas; the ultimate aim of communication is to bring about changes in behaviour. The *mass media* (e.g., song and drama, radio talks, posters) are extensively used as vehicles of dissemination of information.

SOCIAL DEFENCE

A new concept has come into vogue in recent times – the concept of social defence. It covers the entire gamut of preventive, therapeutic and rehabilitative services for the protection of society from antisocial, criminal or deviant conduct of man. Included in this are measures relating to the prevention and control of juvenile delinquency, eradication of beggary, social and moral hygiene programmes, welfare of prisoners, prison reforms, elimination of prostitution, control of alcoholism, drug addiction, gambling and suicides *(12)*. Many States in India have enacted the Children Act for the prevention and control of juvenile delinquency. Under the Suppression of Immoral Traffic in Women and Girls Act, services are being provided for the elimination of prostitution in society. Social defence is a system developed to defend society against criminality not merely by treating and defending the offended, but also by creating such conditions in the community which are conducive for a healthy and wholesome growth of human life. The Government of India renamed the Central Bureau of Correctional Services as National Institute of Social Defence in 1975. This Institute is under the Department of Social Welfare.

PSYCHOLOGY

Psychology is defined as "the study of human behaviour – of how people behave and why they behave in just the way they do". It is concerned with the individual, his personality and behaviour. A knowledge of psychology is essential to know others better; to differentiate between the normal and abnormal, to understand attitudes, beliefs, learning and memory processes; and to help promote mental health in individuals and families.

Scope of psychology

Psychology is vast in its scope, as indicated by the numerous branches of psychology, e.g., normal psychology, abnormal psychology, educational psychology, social psychology, child psychology, applied psychology, psychoanalysis, etc. Medical psychology deals with patients suffering from disorders of the mind. Persons trained in medicine and psychology are called psychiatrists. Thus psychology includes every aspect of human life and every type of human relation.

DYNAMICS OF BEHAVIOUR

The theme common to community medicine and psychology is human behaviour i.e., manner of acting or of conducting one self. The main concern of psychology is to study human behaviour. Human behaviour is the result of physical and mental factors (body and mind) interacting in complicated ways. Behaviour is "the total reactions (of an individual) accessible to external observation. Thought and understanding are implicit behaviour which are observable not directly. but solely by inference from other observable behaviours."

The broad categories of factors that may influence individual and community health behaviour include :

knowledge, beliefs, values, attitudes, skills, finance, materials, time, and the influence of family members, friends, co-workers, opinion leaders, and even health workers themselves. Serious consideration must also be given to the community or social context in which a given type of behaviour occurs. Pervasive issues such as norms, male/female roles, ethnic discrimination, poverty, unemployment, and educational opportunities may limit the ability of some of the sections of the community to behave in a healthy manner *(13)*.

Cultural and social factors provide a setting for individuals. However, behavioural decisions may also be made that are other than those predicted on the basis of these factors. Psychological factors relating to public health programmes may be considered under the heading of health, illness and treatment behaviours.

Health behaviour

Health behaviour refers to those activities people undertake to avoid disease and to detect asymptomatic infections through appropriate screening tests. For instance, sexually transmitted diseases can be prevented by avoiding sexual exposure with infectious sexual partners. Other health behaviours that might reduce the risks of infection include the use of condoms, of bactericidal products immediately before and after sexual exposure, and the appropriate use of antimicrobial agents with proper supervision *(13)*. In addition the risks of transmission can be reduced by assisting in the detection of infection in sexual partners before they have further unprotected sexual exposure with other susceptible partners. People with good health habits (e.g., daily brushing of teeth, non-smoking) are less likely to develop sexually transmitted diseases than persons with poor health habits *(13)*.

Illness behaviour

Illness behaviour refers to how people react to symptoms. Generally, people who detect symptoms will wait to see if the symptoms persist or worsen. If the symptoms continue, the affected person may ask a friend or acquaintance for advice, before seeking medical help.

Treatment behaviour

Treatment behaviour refers to those activities used to cure diseases and restore health. It is important for patients to take medication as directed, return for tests for cure, and cooperate in efforts to identify untreated cases. Research has not shown that any particular group or personality type is more compliant than any other.

All forms of behaviour are responses to stimuli. For example, a child sees a dog rushing towards him, and starts running away. The sight of a dog rushing towards him is the stimulus and running away is the response. To understand behaviour, we must find out the cause for stimulus. The goal of psychology is to find relations that exist between stimuli and responses.

RESPONSES

The various responses may be classified as follows :

i) *Physical responses* : habits, skills;

ii) *Organic responses* : emotions, feelings, tension; and

iii) *Intellectual responses* : perceptions, thinking, reasoning.

CAUSES

All behaviour is caused, and the causes are very complex. They include :

i) *Environmental stimuli*

The environmental stimuli (e.g., sight, smell, touch, etc.) reach the cerebral cortex through nerve impulses. The information received is assembled and evaluated. By another set of impulses, the cerebral cortex "orders" the behaviour of the individual. This is known as **conscious behaviour.** It is the behaviour determined by the standards or expectations of the society, e.g., professional behaviour of doctors with patients. This accounts for the variation in a person's behaviour in different situations.

ii) *Emotions and feelings*

Behaviour is also dependant on our feelings and emotions. These stimuli arise from within the body. When we say a person is blind with rage or paralysed with fear, we mean that he is a victim or captive to his own emotions. Emotions thus affect our behaviour. The seat of primary emotions (e.g., anger, joy, hunger) is the thalamus in the brain. It is under the control of cerebral cortex. When the influence of cerebral cortex is removed, as for example, when an injury to cerebral cortex occurs, the person's behaviour may be affected.

iii) *Needs*

An individual's behaviour is also influenced by his needs. The terms – needs, wants, desires and urges are used synonymously.

iv) *Motivation*

Motivation is an inner force which drives an individual to a certain action. It also determines human behaviour. Without motivation, behavioural changes cannot take place.

v) *Intellectual perception*

A person's intellectual perception, thinking and reasoning can influence his behaviour in a given situation. That is why each individual behaves in ways which make sense to him.

Making adjustments

Behaviour is also described as an **adjustment** to meet the needs of a given situation. For example, when a person does not succeed in something there are several ways he or she can react:

- losing temper and complaining to every one;
- isolating oneself or simply avoiding facing others;
- making excuses for the failure; and
- accepting failure with good grace and making amends by changing his behaviour or otherwise.

This adjustment is both active and passive. That is why some people blow hot and cold to suit their physical and social environment.

Unconscious behaviour

There is also behaviour of which the individual is not conscious. For example, if ten people witness an accident, we get ten conflicting reports of the accident. This is because of certain forces (e.g., perceptions, prejudices, and notions) which colour the incident, over which the individual has no control. Another example is that some people forget important things because they are unpleasant and remain happily unconscious about them.

EMOTIONS

An emotion is a strong feeling of the whole organism. Emotions motivate human behaviour. An emotional experience is characterized by both external and internal changes in the human being. The "external" changes are those which are apparent and easily seen by others such as changes in facial expression, changes in posture. By studying the facial expression we can find out if a person is angry, happy, depressed or elevated. The "internal" changes brought about by emotions are psychological such as rapid pulse, respiration, increased blood pressure, tension and pain. Usually these changes are temporary, and subside when the individual returns to the "normal".

Some of the major emotions are :

Fear	Jealousy	Sympathy
Anger	Moodiness	Pity
Love	Joy	Lust
Hate	Sorrow	Grief

Scientists have proved that emotions can be a major barrier to communication. Man is indeed a slave to his emotions. The doctor should be able to understand the emotions of the patient. Once the emotional barriers are broken down, a mutual trust between the patient and the doctor develops, and the patient will begin to talk more freely about himself. This is the basis of doctor–patient relationship. The desirable qualities in a doctor are cheerfulness and an even temperament. Moodiness, emotional instability and getting easily upset are undesirable qualities.

Some specific emotions

(1) FEAR : Fear is the most common emotion of man. It may produce excitement or depression; flight or fight. Some of the common fears of man are – fear of the dark, fear of dogs, fear of snakes, fear of ghosts, fear of sickness, fear of death, etc. When the fear becomes exaggerated or unnecessary, it is called **phobia**. Such fears are common in patients with mental disorders; (2) ANGER : Anger or rage is another basic emotion of man. It is a reaction of the offensive type. Anger is a destructive force. If it is not controlled, it may impel a person even to commit murder; (3) ANXIETY : Anxiety may manifest in such symptoms as rapid pulse and breathing, flushing, tremors, sweating, dry mouth, nausea, diarrhoea, raised blood pressure, etc. Patients admitted to hospitals are anxious. Anxiety leads to tension, and tension to pain. The doctor must understand the patient's anxiety and give him reassurance. A kind word from the doctor or nurse works like a magic and gives the patient considerable relief from mental anxiety; and (4) LOVE : Love is a feeling of attachment to some person. It is a basic emotion of man.

Role of emotions in health and disease

Emotional states determine human behaviour. Anger can cause a person to be rude and sarcastic. Disorders of emotion interfere with human efficiency – lack of concentration, lack of appetite, increased risk of accidents, lack of sleep, palpitation, etc. Emotional disorders in children may appear in the form of temper tantrums, abdominal pain, spasms, tics, and anti-social behaviour such as aggressiveness.

Psychosocial illness : There are a group of diseases known as "psychosocial diseases" (mind acting on body), e.g., essential hypertension, peptic ulcer, asthma, ulcerative colitis which are attributed to disturbed emotional states.

Control of emotions

A well-adjusted and mentally healthy person is one who is able to keep his emotions under control. One should not be carried away by one's emotions. Children should be shown love and appreciation so that they may grow into emotional maturity. For adults, a happy family life is basic for emotional adjustment. Patients who are anxious need reassurance and their fears must be allayed. The following tips may be useful in controlling one's emotions : (i) cultivate hobbies, good habits of reading and recreation; (ii) adopt a philosophy of life to enable you to avoid mental conflicts; (iii) try to understand your own limitations; and (iv) develop a sense of humour. A study of psychology helps us to understand the basis of emotions and the need to keep emotions under control.

MOTIVATION

Motivation is a key word in psychology. It is an inner force which drives an individual to a certain action. It also determines human behaviour. Motivation may be positive (the carrot) or negative (the stick). Without motivation, behavioural changes cannot be expected to take place. Positive motivation is often more successful than negative motivation. Motivation is not manipulation. A motivated person acts willingly and knowingly. The terms motives, needs, wants, desires and urges are all used synonymously; these terms are interrelated and interdependent.

Kinds of needs and urges

It is difficult to define human needs. There are many kinds of needs and urges : (a) *Biological needs :* These are survival needs. A hungry man needs food, a thirsty man water, a sick man medicine. There are other needs such as sleep, rest, recreation and fresh air. The doctor should be aware of these needs in the day-to-day care of the patients; (b) *Social needs :* The need for company, the need for love and affection, the need for recognition, the need for education are all social needs. Some of these needs are met by the family, and some by the community; (c) *Economic needs :* Economic security, that is security from want, is one which everyone desires; and (d) *Ego-integrative needs :* The desire for prestige, power and self-respect come in this category.

Motivation is contagious; it spreads from one motivated person to another. We make use of motives and incentives in community health work. Motivation of eligible couples for a small family norm is an important activity in the National Family Welfare Programme. Motivation is required to enlist people's participation in community health work.

INCENTIVES

Incentives are among the factors that stimulate motivation and encourage specific behaviours. Incentives can be either intrinsic or extrinsic, material or psychological, self determined or selected by others. An intrinsic incentive is the benefit that comes from solving one's own problems. Extrinsic incentives are rewards that do not relate directly to the goal towards which the desired behaviour is aimed, for example, financial compensation of individuals undergoing sterilization operation for family planning. Material incentives are tangible goods or services; psychological incentives include the satisfaction, self-esteem, or enhanced capabilities gained through a proposed course of action *(13)*.

LEGISLATION

Legislation can serve as an important tool to support, promote and sustain activities at the community level. Laws should satisfy requirements and, at the same time be compatible with the political, cultural, social, and economic situation of the country. This is essential because laws may antagonize the population and make the community uncooperative.

OBSERVATION

Treatment involves lot of correct observation of the patient's condition. Observation involves two mental activities – perception and attention. Hippocrates, the Father of Medicine, laid the foundation of modern medicine by accurate observation of signs and symptoms. By observing an apple fall, Newton formulated the theory of gravitation. By observation penicillin was discovered. Observation is a psychological skill. It consists of the noting of the phenomena of life as they occur. It requires correct use of the senses of seeing, hearing, touch, smell, movements etc. A doctor should cultivate the habit of correct observation. Correct observation leads to correct thinking, reasoning and learning.

Observation promotes attention. To observe more carefully is called attention. A moving object attracts more attention than a static object, a large object attracts more attention than a small object, an uncommon object attracts more attention than, a common one, a bright colour attracts more attention than a dull colour. In attention, certain adjustments of sense organs are involved such as turning the head, converging the eyes, In other words, attention means closer observation. Attention is not a fixed state or power of the mind. We constantly change our attention from one object to another according to the demands of the situation. Concentration, i.e., the focusing of consciousness on a particular object to the exclusion of all other objects has been defined as sustained attention.

Errors in perception

The word perception implies observation, recognition and discrimination. Perception takes place with the help of sensory organs. Thus we have visual perception, auditory perception, olfactory perception, and muscular perception. The disorders of perception are : (1) *Imperception :* That is, inability to recognize. This may be due to damage to the sense organs, e.g., anaesthesia; (2) *Illusion :* An illusion is a false perception. Mistaking a rope for a snake, a tree for an animal are called illusions. Illusions occur in mental diseases. Illusions may be auditory or visual; and (3) *Hallucination :* Hallucination is an imaginary perception. It is a gross error of perception. Seeing objects that do not exist, hearing sounds that are false, seeing objects moving in a room are called hallucinations. Hallucinations occur in mental disorders.

ATTITUDES

Attitudes are acquired characteristics of an individual. They are more or less permanent ways of behaving. An attitude includes three components : (a) a cognitive or knowledge element; (b) an affective or feeling element; and (c) a tendency to action. An attitude has been defined as a relatively enduring organization of beliefs around an object, subject or concept which pre-disposes one to respond in some preferential manner.

Attitudes are not learnt from textbooks, they are acquired by social interaction, e.g., attitude towards persons, things, situations and issues (e.g., government policies, programmes and administrative measures). It has been truly said that attitudes are caught, and not taught. Once formed, attitudes are difficult to change. The responsibility to develop healthy attitudes devolves upon parents, teachers, religious leaders and elders. Our success or failure in life depends upon our attitudes. Social psychology is largely a study of attitudes. In recent years, attitude surveys and attitude measurements have been widely used by psychologists and health professionals.

OPINIONS AND BELIEFS

Opinions are views held by people on a point of dispute. They are based on evidence available at the time. Opinions by definition are temporary, provisional. They can be looked on as beliefs for the time being. Beliefs, on the other hand are permanent, stable, almost unchanging. These are usually derived from our parents, grand-parents, and other people we respect. We accept beliefs, without trying to prove that they are true. Every community has its own beliefs. As beliefs are held strongly, they are often difficult to change. They can be harmful, helpful or neutral. It is thus easier to give up one's opinions when faced with the facts; attitudes and beliefs do not succumb so easily.

INTERESTS

Numerous interests come into play in a communication situation. Most significant are our own interests – of security, pleasure, and self-esteem. Then come the interests of the various groups we are associated with : primary and secondary, as well as the reference groups whose values and norms we aspire to promote. Our communities, castes, language groups, peer groups, and other religious, social, political and professional groups so dear to us are vital to our interests. One must not overlook the social, regional and national interests that shape our selection of communications, and also the way we perceive them *(14)*.

LEARNING

Learning is any relative permanent change in behaviour that occurs as a result of practice or experience. It means acquiring something new – new knowledge, new techniques, new skills, new fears and new experiences.

Learning is necessary for man's survival and for human progress. It includes not only acquiring knowledge but also skills and formation of habits, and development of perception. Learning depends largely upon intelligence. Learning also depends upon motivation, and motivation depends on the need students feel to learn. Learning is a continuous process. It is both conscious and unconscious.

Conditions affecting learning

(1) *Intelligence :* Learning depends upon the intelligence or mental faculty of an individual. It involves the activity of sensory adjustment and motor mechanisms of the body. The mental faculty is related to heredity, nutrition and IQ. Children with low IQ are poor learners; they may not learn at all. (2) *Age* : The curve of learning reaches its peak between 22 and 25 years of age. After the age of 30, there is a sharp decline. It has been appropriately said : You cannot

teach "an old dog a new trick". (3) *Learning situation :* Physical facilities for learning, viz, institutions, teachers, textbooks, audio-visual aids promote learning. (4) *Motivation :* In order to learn effectively, there must be adequate motivation. The powerful motives are encouragement, praise, reward and success. These stimulate learning. (5) *Mental health :* Worries, anxieties, and fears interfere with learning.

Types of learning

There are 3 types of learning :

(1) **Cognitive** learning (knowledge);

(2) **Affective** learning (attitudes); and

(3) **Psychomotor** learning (skills).

Psychologists have experimented a good deal with animals and man to find out how learning takes place. They have proposed a number of theories : (1) *Learning by conditioned reflex :* It is well known that when dogs see food, they begin to salivate; this is an inborn reflex. Pavlov, the Russian physiologist discovered that if a bell was rung when the dogs were fed, eventually, salivation could be induced by the ringing of the bell alone. This is called conditioned reflex. The psychologists proposed that learning takes place partly by the mechanism. (2) *Trial and error :* The lower animals such as apes and cats learn by trial and error method. We also learn a good deal by this method. A child tries and tries again using a number of approaches until accidentally the ideal approaches, becomes obvious. This method of learning is very slow, laborious and primitive. (3) *Learning by observation and imitation :* We learn a good deal by observation and imitation. A child copies or imitates gestures, facial expressions and movements such as walking. He learns language by observation and imitation. Observation is an important element in medical examination. Observation promotes attention, discrimination and recognition. It was by observation, Hippocrates, Father of Medicine, separated medicine from magic. Part of the doctor's and nurse's education has always been to observe the patient's condition, and to make decisions based on these observations. (4) *Learning by doing :* In this type of learning there is coordination of muscular responses with sensory impulses. Nursing skills (e.g., bed making, applying bandages, giving bath) are learnt by doing. Learning to type-write or learning a new game or a musical instrument are all examples of learning by doing. (5) *Learning by remembering :* We also learn by memorizing – remembering dates, events, memorising a poem, remembering faces, etc. (6) *Learning by insight :* When we are faced with a problem, we solve it by insight or mental exploration. When the doctor makes a diagnosis, some amount of insight is involved. It appears that human beings learn by a combination of methods. (7) *Demonstration :* Here a procedure is carried out step by step, slowly and accurately before an audience, the demonstrator ascertaining that the audience understands how to perform it. The demonstration involves the audience in discussion, when possible. (8) *Field experience :* It involves a series of activities for diagnosing problems, planning procedures to solve them and implementing and evaluating these programmes. It provides opportunities to acquire with number of skills. (9) *Problem solving :* It is closely related to field experience in that the problems are identified and plans to solve them are made, but if the time is short, the plans may be executed by another group of trainees or by the service staff.

Learning is measured by student's performance. There are many ways of measuring student's learning viz., multiple choice questions, essay writing, project work, practical examination, oral examination, etc. Usually a combination of different methods is used.

HABITS

Habit is an accustomed way of doing things, example in the field of health is washing one's hands before handling food. It is usual way of action or an act performed without thinking. Habits are said to have 3 characteristics : (a) they are acquired through repetition (b) they are automatic, and (c) they can be performed only under similar circumstances. Habits accumulated through generations emerge as customs; and customs in turn create habits. Habits once formed persist and influence human behaviour.

Habit formation

Habits are formed. They are of many kinds, e.g., habits relating to food, sleep, work, smoking, intake of drugs and alcohol, etc. There are both good and bad habits. Good habits promote health; bad habits (e.g., drug dependance) may ruin health. Therefore, cultivation of good habits is desirable. The principles involved in habit formation are :

(1) Habit formation should begin early in childhood, when the child has not yet formed any habits, and is receptive to all influences;

(2) Habits are formed by frequent repetition;

(3) It takes time to form habits; they cannot be formed overnight;

(4) There should be a strong emotional stimulus to form habits (e.g., taking a vow, reward, recognition, etc.); and

(5) Good habits kill bad habits. The best way to break bad habits is to cultivate good habits.

Habits build up human personality. Man should not become a slave to his habits, he should remain a master. It is the job of the psychologist to find out how good habits can be developed, and bad ones eliminated.

FRUSTRATIONS AND CONFLICTS

Frustrations

All people have needs – biological, social, economic, which they try to satisfy. When they are unable to meet their needs and desires, they feel frustrated.

The sources of frustration may be external – e.g., unemployment, failures and defeats, or, internal – e.g., lack of health, lack of intellectual ability, etc.

Sometimes, frustration may rouse the individual to higher and bigger effort to overcome failures. The individual may bypass the frustration conditions by changing his goals in life. Frustration, if it is allowed to continue, may damage one's personality. It may generate feelings of anger, dejection, hostility, withdrawal or even attempts at suicide. That is why some people take to drugs and alcohol to escape frustration.

Conflicts

A conflict is like a tug of war between two or more courses of action or between opposing ideas. The person is required to act one way or the other, often generating painful emotions as for example in choosing a life partner or a job. He has to weigh the pros and cons of the situation to be able to make a correct decision. It is essential for a person's mental health that conflicts should be resolved as quickly as possible, within a reasonable period of time, before emotional disturbances occur.

DEFENCE MECHANISMS

When an individual is faced with problems, difficulties or failures, he employs certain ways or devices to achieve health, happiness or success. These are called **defence mechanisms**. Psychologists have identified a number of such defence mechanisms, which include the following :

1. Rationalization

Instead of accepting failure and correcting himself, the individual tries to make excuses and justifies his behaviour. It is like the proverbial fox declaring that the grapes were sour, when it could not reach them. This is called rationalization. It is a face-saving device.

2. Projection

Sometimes the individual blames others for his mistakes or failures. It is just like the student saying that he could not score good marks in the examination because, his teacher did not like him.

3. Compensation

Many people make use of compensation to enhance their self-esteem and prestige. The familiar example is that the student who is not good in his studies may distinguish himself in sports or dramatics, music or other activities.

4. Escape mechanism

Some individuals adopt what is known as an "escape mechanism" to overcome failure or defeat. Some students pretend illness and do not appear for examinations. This is an escape phenomenon. Then there are others who take to alcohol or drugs trying to solve their problems. This is also an escape phenomenon.

5. Displacement

An office clerk badly snubbed by his superior takes it out on his wife and children on reaching home. This is like a rebound phenomenon. It is trying to escape from one situation and fixing blame on another situation.

6. Regression

Some people resort to childhood practices (e.g., weeping when something goes wrong) as a mode of adjustment.

The above list of "defence mechanisms" serves to illustrate the various modes of adjustments the individual adopts to escape from realities. He is either too keen to hide his faults, or run away from his troubles and problems. A mentally healthy person will not use defence mechanisms for achieving success or happiness.

PERSONALITY

The term "personality" is a key word in psychology. It implies certain *physical* and *mental* traits which are characteristic of a given individual; these traits determine to some extent, the individual's behaviour or adjustments to his surroundings. The terms personality and human behaviour are inter-related. Psychology, in its broader concept, implies study of human personality. It is important to bear in mind that the personality of the doctor affects very much the well-being of the patient.

Components of personality

There are at least 4 components of human personality :

(1) PHYSICAL : These are the physical traits or features of an individual namely height, weight, colour, facial expression, physical health, etc. To the layman, a good personality means an impressive, symmetrical and healthy body; (2) EMOTIONAL : A person's emotions also go into the make-up of his personality. Emotions are the feelings we have – fear, anger, love, jealousy, guilt, worries. These feelings affect an individual's personality; (3) INTELLIGENCE : Personality also implies intellectual ability. An intelligent person will have a forceful personality. A person with sub-normal intelligence is described as a "dull" person; and (4) BEHAVIOUR : Behaviour is a reflection of one's personality. It is partly dependent upon our feelings and partly on the expectations of the society. Behaviour is described in such terms as gentle, kind, affectionate, balanced, submissive and aggressive. When we assess human personality, all these components must be taken into consideration.

Personality traits

A trait is described as tendency to behave in a consistent manner in variable situations. Human personality is a bundle of traits. The basic personality traits are established by the age of 6 years. Some traits, we cultivate (e.g., good manners); some, we may conceal (e.g., kindliness); and some, we modify depending upon the society in which we are placed (e.g., sense of humour). The following are some of the personality traits :

- Cheerfulness
- Good manners
- Sportsmanship
- Honesty
- Kindliness
- Loyalty
- Reliability
- Sense of humour
- Tactfulness
- Willing to help others.

The personality traits we look for in a doctor are kindliness, honesty, patience, tolerance, perseverance, consciousness, thoroughness and initiative. It is possible to cultivate these traits.

The Swiss Psychiatrist, Carl Jung (1875–1961) divided personalities into 2 types – **extrovert** and **introvert**. The extrovert is a person who is thought to be dashing, practical, active, showing-off and easily mixes with people. An introvert is a person who is reserved, shy and generally keeps to himself. Most people exhibit characteristics of both.

Development of personality

Human life consists of definite stages of growth, and each stage is marked by distinctive psychology. (1) INFANCY : The first one year of life is called infancy. The infant is hardly a social creature. There is rapid physical and mental growth. The infant is totally dependent on the mother. By the end of first year, the infant is able to stand up for a short while and tries to walk with a little support. He enjoys simple tricks and games. (2) PRE-SCHOOL CHILD: This stage is marked by considerable growth of brain. The child feeds himself, speaks, loves his home, fears dark, loves stories and wants to assume responsibility. He begins to mix with other small children. (3) SCHOOL-AGE : The school-age period ranges from 5 to 15 years. The school going child is active all the time. By the age of 8, the mental powers are fully developed. The brain of the child at the age of 8 years is almost of the same size as an adult. The child begins to reason. There is a gradual detachment from the family, and greater attachment to his playmates and friends. He begins to form groups. The period of childhood terminates with the onset of puberty, which is about 11 years in the case of girls and 13 in the case of boys. (4) ADOLESCENCE : Adolescence or "teenage" is a turbulent period in one's life. This is a period of rosy dreams, adventure, love and romance. The teenager strives for independence. He dislikes parental authority. He becomes fully aware of social values and norms. There is rapid physical growth. (5) ADULTS : The person is mature and more balanced. The physical and mental characteristics are fully developed. It is difficult to draw a line when adolescence ceases, and adulthood begins. (6) OLD AGE : It is difficult to say when old age begins. It is a gradual process marked by decline in physical powers and acuity of sense organs. Old age is marked by certain psychological changes such as impaired memory, rigidity of outlook, irritability, bitterness, inner withdrawal and social maladjustment.

Character and will

The concept of personality also involves assumptions about character and will of the person. Will indicates determination and character implies moral worth. Personality and character are not identical; both are different. Man's character may be good at one time and bad at another time, though his personality remains the same. There is no acceptable definition of character.

THINKING

Man is called a thinking animal. Thinking includes perception, memory, imagination and reasoning. It is an active mental process. Imaginative thinking is a mental process, it involves thinking in the absence of original sensory stimuli. Day-dreaming and thinking about our future plans are examples of imaginative thinking. The highest form of thinking is said to be creative thinking , e.g., an artist painting a picture. Creative thinking is said to be responsible for new inventions, new views of life and new discoveries. The anatomical basis of thinking is cerebral cortex. In fact, the purpose of education is to teach people to think, and not merely to memorize facts and figures.

Problem solving

An aspect of thinking is problem solving. It is regarded as the highest stage in human learning. Some problems in life are relatively simple; there are others which are more difficult and complex calling for thinking and reasoning. REASONING requires intelligence. There are several steps in the reasoning process – collection of information on the subject, the arrangement of data carefully, observation of the implications, drawing conclusions and testing the conclusions. An intelligent person reasons well. Reasoning is not always fool-proof. Fallacies may also occur.

INTELLIGENCE

Intelligence is an important aspect of personality. It has not been satisfactorily defined as yet. The widely accepted definition is that it is the ability to see meaningful relationships between things. It includes perceiving, knowing, reasoning and remembering. Psychologists believe that intelligence results from an interplay between hereditary and environmental factors. Some psychologists emphasize genetic factors as having major significance while others emphasize environmental factors.

There is considerable relationship between a person's degree of intelligence and range of activities, the level of achievement and the depth of understanding possible to him. As psychologists observed the differences between animals and human beings, and the differences between organisms of the same species, they were impressed by the fact that there are variations in the case and adequacy with which adjustments to new situations occur. It was out of such observations that the concept of intelligence arose.

Mental age

The first tests of intelligence were devised by Binet and Simon (1896). They developed the concept of *mental age.* That is, a child who could do the five-year tests but who could not go on to the six-year level, was credited with mental age of five years. The concept of mental age indicated the level of intelligence achieved, but it gave no indication of the brightness or dullness of the individual concerned. Terman revised these tests, defining intelligence as the capacity to use abstract ideas for solving problems. Gessel indicated four sectors of intellectual development for consideration : (a) motor ability (b) adoptive behaviour (c) language development and (d) personal-social behaviour.

Intelligence Quotient

This is an improvement over the concept of mental age. It is obtained by dividing the mental age by chronological age, and multiplying by 100.

$$IQ = \frac{\text{Mental age}}{\text{Chronological age}} \times 100$$

When the mental age is the same as chronological age, the IQ is 100. The higher the IQ, the more brilliant the child. 80 per cent of people have an IQ of or near 100. On the other hand, say for example, if a child is 10 years of age and his mental age level is that of 5 years, the IQ is 50.

Levels of Intelligence		IQ Range
Idiot	.....	0–24
Imbecile	.....	25–49
Moron	.....	50–69
Borderline	.....	70–79
Low normal	.....	80–89
Normal	.....	90–109
Superior	.....	110–119
Very superior	.....	120–139
Near genius	.....	140 and over

The current interpretation is that the IQ is the measurement of the quality and potential of intelligence. The higher the IQ the more *"brilliant"* the child is and is more capable of higher performance at school age.

ADULT INTELLIGENCE

The components of adult intelligence have been analyzed by many specialists. Thurstone *(15)*, for instance, defines them as :

(1) space : the ability to perceive objects.
(2) number : familiarity with elementary arithmetic.
(3) verbal comprehension : the ability to reason from verbal concepts.
(4) facility of expression : the ability to employ the appropriate words.
(5) memory : the ability to retain words and ideas.

(6) induction : the ability to discover principles.
(7) deduction : the ability to use those principles to solve concrete problems.
(8) flexibility and quickness of thought.

Intelligence tests

Intelligence tests can be classified under the categories of group tests and individual tests. These two kinds of tests have been constructed mostly to meet practical necessities. Naturally, if large numbers of subjects are to be tested, it would be more convenient to test them in large group to save time and trouble. But under particular situations, such as in a guidance clinic, each individual could be tested separately and would need to be tested separately. To suit these different requirements, we now have both group tests and individual tests. In a group test, all the subjects must start at one time and finish at the same time just as in an examination. Here, the time factor is constant. One's intelligence is measured in terms of the amount of work successfully completed within the given time. Individual tests on the other hand need not necessarily depend on a constant time factor. Time tests can also be used for individuals. Strictly speaking, all tests of intelligence are measures of *performance*. However, the term *performance* is customarily applied to tests which call for a minimal understanding and use of language. These tests provide a measure of fundamental psychological process, such as reasoning and seeing relationship, without at the same time depending upon particular cultural or educational opportunities. They enable us to measure the intelligence of individuals : – (1) who are too young to have learned a language, (2) who are illiterate through lack of educational opportunity or feeble-mindedness, and (3) who speak only a foreign tongue.

As the child grows older, his intelligence undergoes a gradual increase. There is an improvement with age in his versatility of adjustment – in the readiness with which he gathers information and acquires new skills which enable him to adjust to the changing circumstances of his environment. When a normally healthy school child, whose educational opportunities have been average, is tested year after year, his IQ remains fairly constant. Changes in educational opportunities lead to fluctuations in IQ. There are cases on record, too, where the IQ rose considerably after glandular therapy.

The chief values of discovering a child's IQ are that : (1) those of low IQ can be taken aside for special education in line with their capacity to acquire intelligent behaviour; (2) those of very high capacity can be selected for education in keeping with their capacity; (3) intelligence tests as an aid in the determination of the right time to enter school; (4) the use of intelligence test in maintaining the adjustment of a pupil to his work; (5) the selection of applicants for college and professional school; (6) the use of intelligence test in educational guidance; and (7) the use of intelligence test to the therapist *(16)*.

Measurement of disability

There have been many attempts to measure or record in standardized form the aspects of behaviour, psychological functions and social performance. One of the most important is Wing's Comprehensive Handicaps, Behaviour and Skills Schedule (HBS) which has been used in epidemiological studies to assess the total child population in terms of detailed scales of specific abilities and disabilities. Results from these surveys have raised important questions about ethnic differences in disability profiles, individual programme planning, defining new syndromes of disability and the possibilities of new parameters for classification. The HBS is essentially a research tool, but Wing has developed from it a small practical schedule for use in service contexts using what had emerged as the most important aspect of mobility, communication and social interaction. The resulting Disability Assessment Schedule (DAS) is being used in several communities as a source of high quality routine data for total population *(17)*.

SOCIAL PSYCHOLOGY

Social psychology is an important branch of psychology. It is defined *as the science of behaviour of the individual in society*. That is, it studies the behaviour of the individual in group, crowd, mob, audience and other social situations. It also studies the *attitudes* of the individuals towards cultural and social values.

Group behaviour

Man is a social being. From birth till death, he is associated with people. He is born in particular culture which is made up of customs, laws, ideals, art, literature, crafts, science, technology and institutions. All these act on the individual and influence his social behaviour. Group behaviour is also known as social behaviour.

Social interaction

(a) *Inter-personal relationships :* The individual learns many things from his parents, teachers and friends. This is known as person-to-person interaction.

(b) *Inter-group relationships :* The individual is a member of a group, of a family and of a community. He has to follow the traditions of the group. For example, in many communities in India the person is not permitted to marry outside his caste. This is the result of person-to-group interaction.

The individual, through social interaction and social learning acquires patterns of behaviour prevalent in his society, and is accepted as a member of that community. This process of adaptation is known as socialization. Social interaction converts the biological organism into human, social and moral.

As a result of social interaction, the individual acquires attitudes towards persons, things, situations and issues. Social attitudes are shared by others in the community, e.g., attitude to prohibition, family planning, child marriage, etc. In any democratic society, people's attitudes are a matter of vital importance to the State.

Group morale

Every group has leaders. They are responsible for the solidarity of the group behaviour and the morale of the people in the group.

Groups work together. They have definite programmes and objectives. Often their members think, feel and act together. Many community problems can be solved by group effort. We can approach the group through group discussions. The problem is one of how to make these group activities happy and satisfying experiences for those who participate in them.

SOCIOLOGY

Sociology is the science of society. It deals with the study of relationship between human beings, it also deals directly with the study of human behaviour. Whereas the unit of study of psychology is the *individual*, the unit of study of sociology is the *group*. Sociology studies man in the context of society and as a part of it.

Medical sociology is a specialization within the field of sociology. Its main interest is in the study of health, health behaviour and medical institutions. Illness is viewed not only as a medical problem but also as a psychological and social problem. The problems presented by patients are not always purely medical but also psycho-social. Diseases such as tuberculosis, leprosy, sexually transmitted diseases have a big social component in their aetiology. Medical scientists are increasingly turning their attention to the study of social, behavioural and cultural factors of illness. A social approach to disease treatment is also emphasized. The doctor needs to have a fuller appreciation of biological, behavioural and social sciences. A successful doctor must possess a knowledge of the community and the factors which affect the health of the community.

THE INDIVIDUAL

Rights of the Individual

During the 19th Century, the rights of man received some small recognition. In 1946 the subject of human rights again received attention. In 1948, the General Assembly of the United Nations adopted the Universal Declaration of Human Rights. The declaration consists of 30 Articles, and recognizes that all human beings are born free and equal in dignity and rights. The Right to better living conditions, and the Right to Health and Medical Service are vital articles. In 1959, the General Assembly of the United Nations also adopted. "The Declaration of the Rights of the Child''. The Universal Declaration of Human rights speaks of the right to health in the following terms :

> Everyone has the right to a standard of living adequate for the health and well-being of himself and of his family, including food, clothing, housing, and medical care and necessary social services, and the right to security in the event of unemployment, sickness, disability, widow-hood, old age or other lack of livelihood in circumstances beyond his control.
>
> Motherhood and childhood are entitled to special care and assistance. All children, whether born in or out of wedlock, shall enjoy the same social protection.

The Constitution of the World Health Organization expressed itself as follows :

> The enjoyment of the highest attainable standard of health is one of the fundamental rights of every human being without distinction of race, religion, political belief, economic or social condition.

Most countries of the world have accepted the idea of the right to health.

The Constitution of India guarantees 7 broad categories of fundamental rights :

(1) the right to equality;
(2) the right to freedom of speech and expression;
(3) the right against exploitation;
(4) the right to freedom of practice and propagation of religion;
(5) the right of minorities to conserve their culture;
(6) the right to property; and
(7) the right to constitutional remedies for the enforcement of fundamental rights.

Responsibility for health

Although health is now recognized as a fundamental right of every human being, it has to be earned by individual effort. It cannot be given by one person to another.

The responsibility for health rests not only on the individual but also upon the community or State. There are certain responsibilities which the individual must accept or exercise in order to achieve optimum health. These are responsibilities regarding personal health, e.g., diet, care of teeth, skin, recreation, exercise, cultivation of healthful habits, immunization, reporting early when falling sick, optimum utilization of available health services, etc.

In all civilized societies, the Government or State assumes responsibility to safeguard or promote the health and welfare of its citizens. Russia was the first country to give its citizens a constitutional right to all health services. There is provision for health in the Constitution of India. The Directive principles of State policy of the Constitution of India states :

The State shall, in particular, direct the policy towards securing –

> That the health and strength of workers, men and women and the tender age of children are not abused and that citizens are not forced by economic necessity to enter a vocation unsuited to their age or strength.
>
> That children and youth are protected against exploitation and against moral and material abandonment.
>
> The State shall, within the limits of its economic capacity and development, make effective provision for securing the right to work, to education and to public assistance in case of unemployment, old age, sickness and disablement, and in other cases of undeserved want.
>
> The State shall, make provision for securing just and humane conditions of work and maternity relief.
>
> The State shall regard the raising of the level of nutrition and standard of living of its people and the improvement of public health as among its primary duties.

SOCIAL ORGANIZATION

Society is a group of individuals drawn together by a common bond of nearness and who act together in general for the achievement of certain common goals. The individual needs the group – not necessarily a particular group or always the same group or the same group for all needs. Different groups are needed for different purposes; these groups comprise social organization.

The social groups to which people belong are the family, the kinship and caste, religion, village, town or city and the state. Besides these, there are certain functional groups such as the panchayat, the club and various associations. Cutting across these groups, there are groups based on social status.

1. THE FAMILY

The family is the basic unit in all societies. It is the most powerful example of social cohesion. A detailed discussion of the nature and functions of the family is given in the following pages.

2. RELIGION AND CASTE

The caste system in India is an example of a "closed class", i.e., there is no mobility or shifting from one class to another, and the members remain throughout life time wherein they are born. Each caste is governed by certain rules and sanctions relating to endogamy, food taboos, ritual purity, etc. Each caste group within a village is expected to give certain standardized services to the families of other castes. For example, a carpenter repairs tools, a barber (nai) cuts hair, a potter supplies earthenware vessels. In the towns and cities and industrial areas, the caste system, although existing, is not rigid : there is considerable inter-communication and interpersonal relationships not strictly based on caste hierarchy.

3. TEMPORARY SOCIAL GROUPS

(1) *The Crowd* : When a group of people come together temporarily, for a short period, motivated by a common interest or curiosity (e.g., to witness a football match), it is known as a crowd. The crowd lacks internal organization and leadership. When the interest is over, the crowd disperses. (2) *The Mob* : The mob is essentially a crowd, but has a leader who forces the members into action. There may be a symbol in the shape of a flag or slogan. The mob is more emotional than a crowd. Like the crowd, it is unstable and without internal organization. When the purpose of the mob is achieved, the group disperses. (3) *The Herd* : This is also a crowd with a leader. Here the members of the group have to follow the orders of the leader without question, e.g., the tourist group under a guide.

4. PERMANENT SPATIAL GROUPS

(1) *The Band* : It is the most elementary community of a few families living together. Here the group has organized itself and follows a pattern of life e.g., gypsies in India. (2) *The Village* : The village is a small collection of people permanently settled down in a locality with their homes and cultural equipments. From time immemorial, the village has constituted a basic unit in India. According to the 2011 census, there were 6,40,867 villages in India. The average population of a village is estimated to be 550. This is the general picture, although there are variations. In Kerala for example, houses are not in clusters. It has been stated that the villages in India are like "little republics having nearly everything they want within themselves; and almost independent of foreign relations; they seem to last where nothing else lasts". The survival of the villages and in fact Indian culture, during periods of foreign dependence, has been due to the continuity of village organization. Castes, religion, rituals, kinship, marriages and economy are some of the important aspects of the Indian villages. (3) *The Towns and Cities* : From a sociological point of view, a city or town may be defined as a relatively large, dense and permanent settlement of socially heterogeneous individuals. The community is subdivided into smaller groups on the basis of wealth and social class. Because of their size, primary contact among all its inhabitants is difficult. The 2011 census enumerated 7,935 towns and cities in India. When the population exceeds 100,000 it is called a city; on this basis, there were only 107 cities in India at the time of 1961 census. (4) *The State* : The state is an ecological social group based on territory. It is more stabilized and formalized. It is heterogeneous in nature. The Indian Union is a large State.

5. GOVERNMENT AND POLITICAL ORGANIZATION

Some form of government is detectable even among primitive societies. Government is an association of which law is the institutional activity. There is no society which lacks government. It is the supreme agent authorized to regulate the balanced social life in the interests of the public. To understand the organization of medical services in any country, it is essential to know its social and administrative organization.

The various types of government in different countries of the modern world are as follows : (1) *Democracy* : This is government of the people, by the people and for the people. India and USA have this form of government. (2) *Autocracy* : The ruler is absolute in his power, as in Jordan and Ethiopia (3) *Monarchy* : The head of the State is a monarch as found in UK, and Nepal, (4) *Socialistic* : The production and wealth are owned and controlled by the State. Examples are China and Poland. (5) *Oligarchy* : The country is ruled by a family group e.g., Thailand, Cambodia, Saudi Arabia.

In Capitalist countries, medical service is given to the population by various agencies in various ways. State medicine, insurance medicine, charity medicine and private medicine exist side by side. Medicine has developed into a trade – a service that is purchased by the patient and sold by the physician under a competitive system. In socialist countries, medicine, like education, is not a trade; it is a public function of society. All health activities are directed and controlled by central bodies, medical service is free and therefore available to all. It is, in other words, socialized medicine.

THE FAMILY

The family is a primary unit in all societies. It is a group of biologically related individuals living together and eating from a common kitchen. The term family differs from household in that all the members of a *household* may not be blood relations, e.g., servants. As a biological unit, the family members share a pool of genes : as a social unit, they share a common physical and social environment. As a cultural unit, the family reflects the culture of the wider society of which it forms a part and determines the behaviour and attitudes of its members. The family is also an epidemiological unit, and a unit for providing social services as well as comprehensive medical care. The family therefore has engaged the attention of sociologists, anthropologists, demographers, epidemiologists, medical scientists, and in fact all those who are concerned with family welfare.

The word, family, which is used in popular term, has made a good deal of confusion among the professionals. It is used in very many different senses. To avoid confusion, social scientists have used the term : (1) *Family of origin* or the family into which one is born, and (2) *Family of procreation* or the family which one sets up after marriage.

Family life cycle

Families are not constant; they are ever changing. A normal family-cycle is generally conceived as having six phases (Table 1).

TABLE 1

Basic model of nuclear family life cycle

Phases of family life cycle		Events characterizing	
No.	Description	Beginning of phase	End of phase
I.	Formation	Marriage	Birth of 1st child
II.	Extension	Birth of 1st child	Birth of last child
III.	Complete extension	Birth of last child	1st child leaves home
IV.	Contraction	1st child leaves home	Last child leaves home of parents
V.	Completed contraction	Last child has left home of parents	1st spouse dies
VI.	Dissolution	1st spouse dies	Death of survivor (extinction)

Source : *(18)*

Such a model, however, tends to apply only to areas of low mortality and requires amendment in high mortality situations to reflect the early death of children and even the death of the mother before any of the children are old enough to leave home. Moreover, "leaving home" is essentially an American and European phenomenon that has little relevance in many developing countries in Africa and Asia. A number of variations and exceptions, then, to the typical life-cycle such as the early death of children or one spouse, divorce, childlessness, etc., need to be taken into account.

Family cycle and stress

Structure

Each family experiences its own dynamics of formation, growth, maturation, and dissolution. Crises confronted may be divided into those that are transitional in the family life cycle (e.g., birth of first child or loss of spouse) or nontransitional (e.g., acts of war, uprooting, mental disorders, etc.). Family sociologists have studied effects of sudden shifts in economic status, migration, uprooting, disasters, physical change or incapacity of a family member, and impact of crises at various stages of the family life-cycle. It has been suggested that stress and health hazards are likely to increase when environmental changes occur at critical developmental periods such as, adolescence, first pregnancy, menopause, and retirement. The ability to cope in given situation depends, in part, on perception of threat, motivation and readiness to respond creatively, available emotional and social supports, and cultural provisions. Compared with other social organizations, the average family has distinct disadvantages. Its age composition is heavily weighted by dependents and is of uncertain sex distribution. No other institution is so exposed to crises and stress yet so potentially capable of resolving frustration and releasing tension *(19)*.

Childhood

As noted by number of observers, the literature on delinquency, psychiatric conditions, mental disorders, and other childhood disorders has produced considerable knowledge on insecurity, and incompetence, and on the damage done by marital discord, prenatal rejection, and institutional rearing. Much less is known about conditions facilitating normal development or why some children with a variety of unfortunate disadvantages still manage to develop a healthy personality, emotional security and social competence. Concern with childhood mental disorders is especially appropriate in developing countries, where children under 15 years of age account for about 40 per cent of the population compared to about 25 per cent in developed countries. Poverty and low socio-economic status appear to be associated with a greater incidence of mental disorder *(19)*.

Adolescence

While the age of puberty and physical maturation does not vary greatly throughout the world, adolescence as a stage of physiological growth is more closely associated with economic development, social and cultural values, and historical traditions. The age at which this development phase occurs may differ between countries within the same geographic region. Few nations really have adequate information on drug abuse, the sequelae of inappropriate sex behaviour, alcoholism, and related difficulties.

Parenthood

In modern society, preparation for parenthood is a complex and changing task. Parental skills do not necessarily come easily and naturally. In part, parents behave the way they do because of their own childhood experiences. Persons reared in unhappy, discordant, or disrupted homes are more likely to marry in their teens, to have out–of–wedlock children and to experience unhappy marriages and difficulties in child rearing *(19)*. Such links between childhood experiences and subsequent parental behaviour are not inevitable. There appears to be considerable capacity for modification of parental behaviour, as shown most frequently in the differential treatment of the second child. The stereotype roles of parenthood are losing their validity amidst cultural changes. There appears to be greater social sensitivity too, for example, parent-child communication when one parent dies, the death of an infant in the family, early childhood intervention, single parent families headed by women, and the relationship of family circumstances to wider social environment.

Ageing

India's population ages 60 and older is projected to increase dramatically from 8 per cent in 2010 to 19 per cent in 2050. By mid-century, this age group is expected to encompass 323 million people, a number greater than the total U.S. population in 2012. This profound shift in the share of older Indians, taking place in the context of changing family relationships and severely limited old-age income support, brings with it a variety of social, economic, and health care policy challenges. The ageing of India's population will lead to increases in the prevalence of chronic conditions such as diabetes and hypertension. By one measure, nearly one-half (45 per cent) of India's disease burden is projected to be borne by older adults in 2030, when the population age groups with high levels of chronic conditions will represent a much greater share of the total population *(19A)*. Similar increase in the population of older persons can be anticipated in other regions of the world.

Types of families

Family units throughout the world are not the same. Industrialization, urbanization, democratization and acculturation have affected the family structure and life. Social scientists have described three main types of families.

1. NUCLEAR FAMILY

The *nuclear* or *elementary* family is universal in all human societies. It consists of the married couple and their children while they are still regarded as dependents. They tend to occupy the same dwelling space. In the nuclear family, the husband usually plays a dominant role in the household. The absence of grandparents, uncles, aunts and near relatives places a greater burden on the nuclear family in terms of responsibilities for child rearing. The husband-wife relationship is likely to be more intimate in the nuclear family than in the joint family. The term "new families" has come recently into vogue; it is applied to those under 10 years duration and consists of parents and children. The concept is important in view of studies relating to family planning *(20)*.

2. JOINT FAMILY

The *joint* or *extended* family is a kind of family grouping which is common in India, Africa, the Far East and the Middle East. It is more common in agricultural areas than in urban areas. The orthodox Hindu family in India is a joint family. As a price for education, urbanization and industrialization, we are losing the joint family system.

The main characteristics of a typical joint family are *(21)* : (1) It consists of a number of married couples and their children who live together in the same household. All the men are related by blood and the women of the household are their wives, unmarried girls and widows of the family kinsmen. (2) All the property is held in common. There is a common family purse to which all the family income goes and from which all the expenditures are met. (3) All the authority is vested in the senior male member of the family. He is the most dominant member and controls the internal and external affairs of the family. The senior female member by virtue of her being the wife of the male head shares his power so far as the women of the family are concerned. (4) The familial relations enjoy primacy over marital relations. Early and arranged marriage is advocated to ward off any threat from marital relationship.

The merit of the joint family system is that it is based on the motto : "union is strength". There is a sharing of responsibilities practically in all matters which gives the family a greater economic and social security. It provides economic and social security to the old, the helpless and the unemployed. It pools its income to help the young through school, to pay for a marriage or begin a commercial venture. It offers many of the services and advantages which an industrial society offers through more impersonal governmental, educational and financial agencies.

3 THREE GENERATION FAMILY

The three generation family is confused with the joint family. It is fairly common in the west. This tends to be a household where there are representatives of three generations. It occurs usually when young couples are unable to find separate housing accommodation and continue to live with their parents and have their own children. Thus, representatives of three generations related to each other by direct descent live together.

Functions of the family

The functions of the family have been stated as follows : (1) *Residence* : One of the major social functions of the family is to provide a clean and decent home to its members. In the west when a man marries he separates from his parents and sets up his own home. In India, it is the prevalent custom among the Hindus that the married couple should reside in the house of the parent. There are two types of residence – patrilocal and matrilocal. In the case of patrilocal residence, the wife goes to the house of the husband; in the matrilocal residence, the husband goes to live in the house of the wife. (2) *Division of labour* : In primitive societies, the roles and functions performed by people in family groups were rather well defined. The male had the sole duty to earn a living and support the family. The female had the total responsibility for the day to day care of children and running of the household. In industrialized and urbanized communities, there is less marked distinction between the functions of men and women. On the other hand, there has been an increasing coming together and sharing of responsibilities by men and women. The young wife in India now-a-days brings to marriage a professional or semi-professional education and she seeks a professional career. This is another new feature of the modern family. The steady enlargement of the freedom of wives, and even children in the family, is leading towards a "communal family" where all its members play a part in its management. (3) *Reproduction and bringing up of children* : This is a very important function of a family. The mother takes absolute care of the infant and children up to a certain age. The father provides for education and teaches the child the social traditions and customs. (4) *Socialization* : The family is a bridge between generations and between parents and children. It is the transfer point of civilization. The cultural patterns relating to eating, cleanliness, dress, speech, language, behaviour, and attitudes are all transmitted through the family. (5) *Economic functions* : The family implies economic partnership for the family and the progeny. The inheritance of the property and the ownership and/or control of certain kinds of property like the farm, shop or dwelling are controlled by the family. Eventually the property is handed down to the children. (6) *Social care* : The family provides social care by (a) giving status in a society to its members, i.e., use of family names where it occurs. Some have a strong feeling of kinship that they belong to a particular family – it denotes some kind of association with someone distinguished in history in that particular society, (b) protecting its members from insult, defamation, etc., (c) regulating marital activities of its members, (d) regulating to a certain extent political, religious and general social activities, (e) regulating sex relations through incest-taboos.

FAMILY IN HEALTH AND DISEASE

Anyone who is concerned with medical practice or community health activities will come to know that family is ultimately the unit with which one has to deal. The family is a group of biologically related individuals. It is a pretty universal picture in all societies. Family performs many functions. There are certain functions which are relevant to health and health behaviour, and are important from the medical-sociology point of view.

1. CHILD REARING

One of the important functions of the family with which medical and community health workers are concerned, is the physical care of the dependent young in order that they may survive to adulthood and perpetuate the family. The way in which child rearing is undertaken differs enormously from society to society, and from time to time, depending upon factors such as capital resources, level of knowledge, state of technology and system of values. It is important to note that patterns of child care (e.g., feeding, nutrition, hygiene, sleep, clothing, discipline, habit training) are passed on from one generation to another. In many societies, child care is socially determined by tradition. The ideas people have about nutrition, exercise, sleep and clothing have a large social component which varies from society to society and from time to time. For instance child care is more permissive in the East starting with the "on demand" schedule at mother's breast : in the West, child care is more rigid and confined to a set of rules. When the community health worker seeks to improve the health of the child, he meets several obstacles. These obstacles are the traditional ways which are supported by appeals to religion and other sanctions. For example, the problem of overcrowding is not merely a question of room space, but in many instances a question of sleeping habits, a part of a pattern of social customs which foster better relations between groups. Once again, variations between societies may be complex and difficult to change.

2. *SOCIALIZATION*

The second responsibility of the family is to socialize the "stream of new-born barbarians." It refers to the process whereby individuals develop qualities essential for functioning effectively in the society in which they live. It is a latent function. By socialization is meant teaching the young the values of society and transmitting information, culture, beliefs, general codes of conduct, by example and precept, in order to make them fit for membership in the wider society of which the family is a part. Organizations such as schools and religious places perform cultural functions for the introduction of the young into adult society. The young are persuaded, given punishments, rewards for good behaviour – all these vary from time to time. In some societies, the young are given freedom to develop into individuals who are freely able to take initiatives.

3. *PERSONALITY FORMATION*

This is even a more latent function. It is an area in which sociology comes closest to psychology. The capacity of an individual to withstand stress and strain and the way in which he interacts with other people is to a large extent determined by his early experience in the family, mainly with the father, mother and siblings who provide the earliest and most immediate component of the child's external environment. The family acts as a "placenta" excluding various influences, modifying others that pass through it and contributes some of its own in laying the foundation of physical, mental and social health of the child.

4. *CARE OF DEPENDANT ADULTS*

(a) *Care of the sick and injured :* In all forms of society, adults may become dependant either through injury, illness or because of basic biological limitation for performing functions normally expected by adults. The attitude of the society in regard to individuals who need care and attention varies considerably. In some societies, there is a great deal of harshness in respect of those who are sufferers. Such individuals are excluded from the full range of benefits. The kind of illness is also of great importance in determining the attitudes of society where the illness arouses fear (e.g., leprosy). However, the family is charged with the responsibility of care of such individuals. The family is expected to provide the front-line care, particularly the mother. Much depends upon her understanding of illness and the extent she believes herself capable of providing nursing care. Studies have shown that the family does more nursing than the hospital, even in highly developed countries *(20)*.

(b) *Care of women during pregnancy and child birth :* From the public health point of view, care of women during periods of recognized dependency, i.e., pregnancy and childbirth is an important function of the family. The attitude of society to pregnancy and child-bearing may have an important bearing on the infant deaths, premature and stillbirths, maternal morbidity and mortality. In many societies today, women are given financial help, maternity leave facilities, diet and nutritional supplements and decreased responsibilities during pregnancy and puerperium.

(c) *Care of the aged and handicapped :* An area of increasing importance, particularly in the western societies, is the care of the aged and infirm. The increased number of such people have created new problems in terms of long term care and specialist facilities. Without the support of the family, no amount of medical care can succeed. In India, the joint family provides for such support.

5. *STABILIZATION OF ADULT PERSONALITY*

The family is like a "shock absorber" to the stress and strains of life. The stress could be injury, illness, births, deaths, tension, emotional upsets, worry, anxiety, economic insecurity and the like. In such situations, the family provides an opportunity, both for adults and children, for release of tension so that the individual can attain mental equilibrium and strive to maintain a stable relationship with other people. The stress of modern living has increased the importance of mental illness as a public health problem. Alcoholism and narcotic addiction are also a reflection of this trend. Certain chronic illnesses such as peptic ulcer, colitis, high blood pressure, rheumatism, skin diseases are accepted as "stress diseases" having a prominent emotional element in their development. Thus the family has an important function in the stabilization of the personality of both adults and children, and in meeting their emotional needs.

6. *FAMILIAL SUSCEPTIBILITY TO DISEASE*

The members of a family share a pool of genes and a common environment and together, these decide their susceptibility to disease *(22)*. Certain diseases such as haemophilia, colour blindness, diabetes and mental illness are known to run through families. Schizophrenia, psychoneurosis and some forms of mental deficiency are also known to have a familial incidence. The family is often the playground also for such communicable diseases as tuberculosis, common cold, scabies, diphtheria, measles, mumps, rubella, chickenpox, dysentery, diarrhoea, and enteric fever. These diseases are known to spread rapidly in families because of the common environment which the family members share.

It is generally agreed that the incidence of congenital malformation is higher among offsprings of consanguineous as compared with non-consanguineous marriages.

7. *BROKEN FAMILY*

A broken family is one where the parents have separated, or where death has occurred of one or both the parents. Dr. John Bowlby brought out clearly the concept of "mental deprivation" as one of the most dangerous pathogenic factors in child development *(23)*. Separation of the child from its father (paternal separation) and separation of the child from both of its parents (dual-parental separation) are important factors in child development. Children who are victims of broken families early in their childhood have been found sometimes to display in later years psychopathic behaviour, immature personality and even retardation of growth, speech and intellect *(22)*. Children from these families may drift away to prostitution, crime and vagrancy.

8. *PROBLEM FAMILIES*

Problem families are those which lag behind the rest of the community. In these families, the standards of life are generally far below the accepted minimum and parents are unable to meet the physical and emotional needs of their children. The home life is utterly unsatisfactory. The underlying factors in most problem families are usually those of personality and of relationship, backwardness, poverty, illness, mental and emotional instability, character defects and marital disharmony. These families are recognized as problems in social pathology *(24)*. Children who are reared in such an environment are victims of prostitution, crime and vagrancy. Problem families may be found in all social classes but are more common in the lower social classes. The health visitor, the health inspector, the midwife, the social worker, the medical officer of health, all can render useful service in rehabilitating such families in a community.

The family therefore plays an important part both in health and disease – in the prevention and treatment of individual illness, in the care of children and dependent adults, and in the stabilization of the personality of both adults and children. In most societies the family is the fulcrum of health services *(25)*. Medical schools are developing teaching programmes in family medicine, because, as Florence Nightingale had said : "the secret of national health lies in the homes of the people".

CULTURAL FACTORS IN HEALTH AND DISEASE

All people, whether rural or urban, have their own beliefs and practices concerning health and disease. It is now widely recognized that cultural factors are deeply involved in all the affairs of man, including health and sickness. Not all customs and beliefs are bad. Some are based on centuries of trial and error and have positive values, while others may be useless or positively harmful. Some of these cultural factors, hallowed by centuries of practice, have stood in the way of implementing health programmes. Where a change of behaviour was involved, the resistance of the people was maximum in accepting new programmes. Information about these factors, i.e., customs, cultural mores, habits, beliefs and superstitions is still woefully lacking. A brief account of the cultural factors relating to health and sickness, as observed in India, is given below :

1. Concept of aetiology and cure

Broadly, the causes of disease, as understood by the majority of rural people, fall into two groups : (a) supernatural and (b) physical.

(a) SUPERNATURAL CAUSES : (1) *Wrath of gods and goddesses :* There are good many people (even among the educated) who believe that certain diseases are due to the wrath of some god or goddess. Chickenpox is an outstanding example, it is known as *Chhoti Mata*. Where the disease is considered to be due to the wrath of gods and goddesses, administration of drugs is considered harmful. Cases are not notified and *pujas* are made to appease the gods (2) *Breach of taboo :* Breach of taboos is believed by some people to be responsible for certain diseases. Venereal diseases are believed by some to be due to illicit sexual intercourse with a woman of low caste, or a woman during menstruation. (3) *Past sins :* Diseases such as leprosy and tuberculosis are believed by some to be due to their past sins. (4) *Evil eye :* A widely held belief throughout the country is the effect of "evil eyes". Children are considered to be most susceptible to the effect of evil eyes. In order to ward off the effects of the evil eye, charms and amulets are prescribed and incantations recited by the exorcist. (5) *Spirit or ghost intrusion :* Some diseases such as hysteria and epilepsy are regarded as due to a spirit or ghost intrusion into the body. The services of an exorcist are sought to drive away the evil spirit or ghost.

(b) PHYSICAL CAUSES : Physical causes are also considered to be responsible for certain diseases. Among these are : (1) *The effects of weather :* Exposure to heat during summer is responsible for an attack of *loo* (heat stroke). The folk remedies consist of application of oil and ghee on the soles of feet and administration of *mango-phool* (prepared by keeping unripe mangoes under hot ashes for a few minutes, and extracting the pulp in cold water) with a pinch of salt. (2) *Water :* Impure water is associated with disease. (3) *Impure blood :* Skin diseases, viz. boils and scabies are considered to be due to impure blood. Eating neem leaves and flowers is considered to purify blood.

2. Environmental sanitation

(a) DISPOSAL OF HUMAN EXCRETA : Large percentage of people in rural areas use open fields for defecation. This practice is time-honoured and is considered harmless. The average Indian villager is averse to the idea of latrines. He considers that latrines are meant for city dwellers, where there are no fields for defecation. He is ignorant that faeces is infectious and pollutes water and soil and promotes fly breeding. Thus the problem of excreta disposal is bound up with numerous beliefs and habits based on ignorance. (b) DISPOSAL OF WASTES : The average villager is not aware that mosquitoes breed in collections of waste water. It is permitted to flow into the streets. The solid waste (refuse) is invariably thrown in front of the houses where it is permitted to accumulate and decompose. Periodically it is removed to the fields and used as manure. The animal dung (cow dung) is allowed to accumulate. It is used sometimes as manure and often times pressed into cakes, sun-dried and used as fuel. (c) WATER SUPPLY : The well occupies a pivotal place in the cultural environment of villages. It is also a common meeting place of men and women of the village, when they go to draw their supply of water. It is a place where people bathe and wash their clothes. It is a place where animals are washed and given a drink. These cultural practices lead to the pollution of well water. Tanks and ponds are used for washing, bathing, ablution and sometimes even as a source of drinking water. Some rivers are considered "holy". People go on pilgrimage to these rivers to have a dip. They not only have a dip but drink the raw water which they consider sacred. Samples of 'holy water' are bottled and carried over long distances for distribution among friends and relatives. Epidemics of cholera and gastroenteritis have been due to these cultural practices. Step-wells are associated with guineaworm disease. (d) HOUSING : Rural houses are practically the same all over the country. They are usually *katcha* and damp, ill-lighted and ill-ventilated. For reasons of security, no windows are provided, and if at all one is provided, it is merely a small hole. Absence of a separate kitchen, latrine, bathroom and drainage are characteristic features of an average rural house. Animal keeping is very common in villages. Infrequently, human beings and animals live under one roof. Houses are generally kept clean inside, regularly white-washed or plastered with mud and cowdung.

3. Food habits

Food habits have deep psychological roots and are associated with love, affection, warmth, self-image and social prestige. The diet of the people is influenced by local conditions (e.g., soil, climate) religious customs and beliefs. Vegetarianism is given a place of honour in Hindu society. Even among vegetarians, the pattern of eating is not the same; some do not take onions and garlic on religious grounds. Muslims abhor pork, and Hindus beef – these food habits have a religious sanction from early days. The concept of hot and cold food is widely prevalent in the country. Foods such as meat, fish, eggs, and jaggery are considered to generate heat in the body; foods such as curd, milk, vegetables and lemon are considered to cool the body. These concepts are encountered by the modern physician when treating disease. Adulteration of milk is a common practice. Although the motive is economic gain, a deep-rooted belief is also responsible for this practice, i.e., if pure milk is boiled, the milk secretion of the donor animal may dry up. Muslims observe fasts during Ramzan and Hindus on several occasions. These fasts are considered important adjuncts to religion. Drinks and drugs are among the food habits of the people. Alcoholic drinks are tabooed by Muslims and high-caste *Hindus. Ganja, bhang* and *charas* are frequently consumed by *sadhus;* these habits are now spreading into the general population, especially the younger generation. Eating and drinking from common utensils is considered as a sign of brotherhood among Muslims. Hindu women often take food left over by their husband. In some societies, men eat first and women last and poorly. Some people do not eat unless they have taken a bath. Thus food is a subject of widespread customs, habits and beliefs, which vary from country to country, and from one region to another.

4. Mother and child health

Mother and child health is surrounded by a wide range of customs and beliefs all over the world. Marriage is universal in Indian society, and the family is incomplete without the birth of a male child. This has obvious implications in the context of the country's population problem and male : female ratio. The various customs in the field of MCH have been classified as good, bad, unimportant and uncertain. (1) *Good :* Customs such as prolonged breast-feeding, oilbath, massage and exposure to sun are good customs. (2) *Bad :* These vary from society to society. For example, some foods (e.g., eggs, meat, fish, milk, leafy vegetables) are forbidden during pregnancy in some parts of the country. In rural areas, deliveries may be conducted by the traditional untrained dai or birth attendant whose methods of conducting delivery may be far from safe. Branding of the skin, administration of opium and drastic purgatives are all bad customs. (3) *Uncertain :* Sometimes, it may be difficult to say whether certain customs are good or bad. The practice of applying *kajal* or black soot mixed with oil to the eye-lids partly for beautification and partly for warding off the effects of "evil eye". Often-times, this custom has been blamed for transmitting trachoma and other eye infections. A knowledge of the local customs and beliefs is therefore very important for improving the health status of mothers and children. This is part of social paediatrics.

5. Personal hygiene

Indians have an immense sense of personal cleanliness, much of which is closely interwoven with ideas of ritual purification. Rituals are "a set or series of acts, usually involving religion or magic, with the sequence established by tradition." (1) *Oral hygiene :* Indians are very particular about oral hygiene. Many people in the countryside use twigs of neem tree as a toothbrush; some use ashes; and some charcoal. The educated and those who have come in contact with urban life use toothbrushes. Eating pan leaves smeared with lime with or without tobacco is a common social custom. (2) *Bathing :* Apart from regular baths of which Indians are very fond, there are baths fixed on special occasions. After childbirth, there may be two or three ceremonial baths, the time for which is fixed upon the advice of the priest. The practice of an oil bath is a good Indian custom. Womenfolk in the countryside use a paste consisting of gram, mustard oil and turmeric powder and rub it on the body before a bath. Thus, bathing is a ritual in India. (3) *Shaving :* This is done by the traditional barber (nai) in the countryside. He does not sterilize the instruments used, as he does not have any idea of micro-organisms. (4) *Smoking :* Smoking hubble-bubble is a social custom in some parts of the country. It can spread tuberculosis. Smoking with the burning end of the cigar in the mouth, which is a common custom among villagers in Andhra Pradesh, is associated with oral cancer. The 1971 Report of the Royal College of Physicians of London *(26)* on the effects of smoking and health provides useful summary of information on the diseases now known to be associated with smoking – cancer of the lung, chronic bronchitis and emphysema, coronary artery occlusion, angina pectoris, cancers of the mouth, pharynx, larynx, and oesophagus, cancer of the bladder and pulmonary tuberculosis. Among patients with peptic ulcer those who smoke have a higher death rate than those who do not. A mother's smoking during pregnancy may retard the growth of the foetus. (5) *Purdah :* Muslims and some high caste Hindu women observe *purdah*. The incidence of tuberculosis is reported to be high amongst those who observe *purdah,* which also deprives them of the beneficial effect of the sunrays. (6) *Sleep :* Many people in the villages sleep on the ground for reasons of poverty, and they are exposed to insect bites. (7) *Wearing shoes :* The transmission of hook-worm disease is associated with bare feet. Many villagers in South India do not wear shoes. (8) *Circumcision :* This is a prevalent custom among Muslims, which has a religious sanction.

6 Sex and marriage

Sexual customs vary among different social, religious and ethnic groups. For certain religious groups menstruation is a time of uncleanness when women are forbidden to pray or have intercourse; orthodox Jews are forbidden to have intercourse for seven days after the menstruation ceases *(27)*. These customs have an important bearing in family planning.

Marriage is a sacred institution. It is the usual social custom in India to perform marriages early. It is considered a sound and desirable practice, because late marriages may create problems in adjustment, especially in joint family systems. Because of the universality of marriage in India problems of unmarried mothers and of illegitimate births are less than in the western countries. The mean age at marriage in India is 24 years in the case of boys and 21 years in the case of girls. There are differences in marriage-age by caste, females of the depressed classes have lower mean age at marriage. Child marriages are fortunately disappearing. Monogamy is the most universal form of marriage.

THE COMMUNITY

"No man is an island". From the time of birth until death, all normal human beings are part of a group, the family or community. The characteristics of a community are :

(1) the community is a contiguous geographic area;

(2) it is composed of people living together;

(3) people cooperate to satisfy their basic needs; and

(4) there are common organizations, e.g., markets, schools, stores, banks, hospitals.

In other words, a community is a network of human relationships. It is a major functioning unit of **society.** It is the place where our home is located; children are educated; sick people are treated and individual basic needs and desires are met.

Structure of society

(1) *Caste:* Indian society is mostly based on caste system. There are further sub-divisions into sub-castes. Each caste is governed by certain rules and regulations relating to food, drink, marriage, social contact and rituals. Castes follow a definite occupation. In urban areas, the caste system is less rigid. The Indian caste system is supported by religion.

(2) *Income :* On the basis of income, people have been grouped into classes – upper, middle and lower classes. People in the upper class enjoy better standards of life.

(3) *Occupation :* Occupation has also been adopted for classifying people. In India, there is no satisfactory occupational class system.

Rural societies

India is a land of villages. There are 6,40,867 villages. Out of every 1,000 population, 690 live in villages (as per 2011 census). The average population of an Indian village is about 550 or 100 families. The villages are self sufficient units for most of the routine requirements of its people. The rural people depend primarily upon agriculture. Caste, religion, ritual, kinship, marriage, and economy are some of the important aspects of Indian village society.

Urban societies

Towns and cities comprise the urban society. They are relatively large, dense and permanent settlements of people. According to the 2011 Census, there were 7,935 towns and cities in India. It has been said that civilization means the city and the city means civilization. The city represents the way of living of man in modern age. The occupational pattern of the urban people is different. They depend less on agriculture. There is an occupational diversity. The social life is impersonal and less intimate. Cities are the melting pots of races, people and cultures. Traditional patterns of belief and behaviour tend to be broken down. New ideas and patterns of behaviour emerge which further spread to villages.

Social mobility

Indian society is rigidly based on caste system. There is little social mobility, i.e., people do not change their caste or religion. In other words, Indian society is a "closed-class" system. There are societies known as the "open class societies" where movement of the social ladder is unrestricted, on the basis of achievement or gaining wealth. Open class societies are therefore more progressive where people according to their ability can go up the social ladder. In closed-class systems, it is difficult to make reforms without meeting resistance of the people.

SOCIAL CLASS

People in a community are differentiated by certain characteristics which they bear. These may be personal characteristics such as age, sex, marital status, place of birth and citizenship; *economic* characteristics such as occupation, type of activity; *cultural* characteristics such as language, religion and caste; and *educational* characteristics such as literacy and level of education. In Indian communities, especially in rural areas, caste is an important basis of social differentiation. The caste groups are hierarchial and carry different degrees of social prestige, which is correlated with a host of other socio-cultural factors.

Although defined differently in different societies and by different investigators, social class is closely bound up with economic status, level of education, way of life, attitudes and expectations, and exposure to different types and degree of stress. More important, it seems to have a direct bearing on the external resources and internal mechanisms available to individuals in attempting to deal with health problems *(1)*.

Social scientists have used *occupation* widely as a means of determining the level of social standing of an individual in a community, because occupation has an enormous importance in all societies for understanding human behaviour. In urbanized and industrialized communities, where there is a substantial division of labour, occupation is a major determinant of : (1) *Economic rewards :* That is income and wealth which can promote or achieve health easier. (2) *Extent of authority :* That is, occupation is an important determinant of authority which the individual has over other people; it spills over into his life itself, his pleasures and other activities, through control of purchasing power. Those who receive higher economic rewards tend to be vested with greater authority. For example, a person who is a judge exercises authority not only in the courts but commands respect from other people. His position enables him to acquire authority. (3) *Extent of obligations :* The extent of obligations demanded of individuals by the rest of the community will be determined by the occupation he holds. One who holds a high place occupationally has greater obligations. (4) *Degree of status :* Closely allied with the occupational role is the degree of status and standing of the individual in the community. For example, medical practitioners in India enjoy a higher status in society than others. The occupation itself will give the person status irrespective of personal characters, age, and experience.

(5) *Values and life styles* : The occupation of an individual very largely will determine many of the values the individual has, the things he feels worth pursuing, his life goals, his life style; his pleasures, friendships and relationships with others. Therefore, occupation is widely used as a measure of social differentiation. In technically advanced countries, occupation tends to range in a hierarchy – those who have high economic rewards have a higher level of prestige than those who are placed low in the social hierarchy.

Occupational classification

The International Standard Classification of Occupation 2008 (ISCO–08) (27A)

The international standard classification of occupation 2008 (ISCO–08) provides a system for classifying and aggregating occupational information obtained by means of statistical censuses and surveys, as well as from administrative records. It is a revision of ISCO–88, which it supersedes. ISCO–08 is a four-level hierarchically structured classification that allows all jobs in the world to be classified into 436 unit groups. These groups form the most detailed level of the classification structure and are aggregated into 130 minor groups, 43 sub-major groups and 10 major groups, based on their similarity in terms of the skill level and skill specialization required for the jobs. They are:

1. Managers
2. Professionals
3. Technicians and associate professionals
4. Clerical support workers
5. Service and sales workers
6. Skilled agricultural, forestry and fishery workers
7. Craft and related trade workers
8. Plant and machine operators and assemblers
9. Elementary occupations
10. Armed forces occupations

Limitations of occupational classification

Occupation is a useful measure of social differentiation particularly in communities highly industrialised and urbanized. We all tend to compare, for example, different social classes in relation to mortality and morbidity. But, there are certain limitations in using social classification based on occupations alone. These may be stated as follows : (1) *Heterogeneous grouping* : Each social class is a heterogeneous grouping of a wide variety of occupations. There is an assumption that these occupations are related to each other, which in fact, is not so. The people in each social class differ not only occupationally, but also in respect of educational status and family background. We have to recognize that categorization into social classes is merely one of convenience. (2) *Occupational mobility* : People sometimes change their occupations. This occupational mobility can lead to discrepancies in using social classes correctly over a period of time. Social classes themselves are subject to change. Certain occupations are promoted in social hierarchy and some demoted. Such changes in social classification may invalidate their comparative use over time. (3) *Women* : There are differences in classifying women alongside men. Some occupations are exclusively occupied by males and some by females. There is also sometimes ambiguity in the nomenclature of occupations occupied by men and women. If a man describes himself as a secretary, it is a highly paid occupation; if a woman describes herself as a secretary, it is usually a position in an office in a low capacity. In spite of these limitations, social classification by occupation is an effective tool for examining various kinds of data related to people. Much research in social medicine in recent years has centred round social class and disease prevalence.

Other measures of social differentiation

There are other measures of social differentiation which may be of greater use or significance than occupation. These are : (1) *Education* : It measures the inculcation of values, knowledge and achievements of the individual. (2) *Income* : Another important way of distinguishing people is by the amount of income or wealth. Here again, there are difficulties because people have great reluctance to talk about their income truthfully. (3) *Purchasing power* : This may be of more important value than occupation in classifying people. (4) *Religion* : This is another important attribute of the individual which may have tremendous bearing on the health of the people. An examination of infant mortality among Christians, Hindus and Muslims in India revealed a low rate for Christians, a high rate for Hindus and highest for Muslims. These differences are attributed to religion which has a bearing on the socio-cultural patterns of living involving age-old habits, customs, and traditions affecting cleanliness, eating, clothing, child care and almost every detail of daily living. (5) *Rural and urban* : There are differences in the health and sickness status of people living in rural and urban areas. Rural and urban people differ in their life-style, opinions and values, which have a bearing on the health and sickness status. To sum up, it may be stated that each of these measures which may be employed for social differentiation have a "snag" too and therefore each must be examined critically and used with discrimination depending upon the subject matter of the enquiry.

Socio-economic status scale

Socio-economic status has been defined as the position that an individual or family occupies with reference to the prevailing average standards of cultural and material possessions, income, and participation in group activity of the community. The social status may be inherited, but in modern society, it is achieved on the basis of occupation, income, type of housing and neighbourhood, membership of certain associations and organizations, material possessions, etc.

There have been many attempts at developing scales for measuring socio-economic status. Hollingshed in USA employed three variables, viz education, occupation and residential address for measuring socio-economic status. Kuppuswamy *(28)* – in India prepared a scale based on education, occupation and income which are the three major variables contributing to socio-economic status in urban areas. Similar scales have also been prepared by Pareek and Kulshrestha *(29)* for use in rural and urban areas. Kuppuswamy's scale is fairly widely known. The modified version of the Kuppuswamy's socio-eonomic status scale for the year 2007 is given in Table 2.The income scale has been recalculated using All India Average Consumer Price Index for the industrial workers for the year 2001 as the new base year *(30, 31)*.

TABLE 2

Kuppuswamy's socio-economic status scale

(A) Education	Score
1. Profession or Honours	7
2. Graduate or postgraduate	6
3. Intermediate or post high school diploma	5
4. High school certificate	4
5. Middle school certificate	3
6. Primary school certificate	2
7. Illiterate	1

(B) Occupation	Score
1. Profession	10
2. Semi-profession	6
3. Clerical, shop-owner, farmer	5
4. Skilled worker	4
5. Semi-skilled worker	3
6. Unskilled worker	2
7. Unemployed	1

(C) Family income per month (in Rs.) original	Score	Modified for 1998	Modified for 2007
1. = 2000	12	= 13,500	= 19,575
2. 1000–1999	10	6750–13499	9788-19,574
3. 750–999	6	5050–6749	7323–9,787
4. 500–749	4	3375–5049	4894–7,322
5. 300–499	3	2025–3374	2936–4,893
6. 101–299	2	676–2024	980–2,935
7. < 100	1	< 675	< 979

Total score	Socio-economic class
26–29	Upper (I)
16–25	Upper-middle (II)
11–15 middle	Lower-middle (III)
5–10 lower	Upper-lower (IV)
<5	Lower (V)

Source : *(30)*

Wealth Index *(32)*

One of the background characteristics used in the National Family Health Survey-III was an index of the economic status of households called the wealth index. The wealth index has been developed and tested in a large number of countries in relation to inequalities in household income, use of health services, and health outcomes. It is an indicator of the level of wealth that is consistent with expenditure and income measures. The economic index was constructed using the following household asset data and housing characteristics : household electrification; type of windows; drinking water source; type of toilet facility; type of flooring; material of exterior walls; type of roofing; cooking fuel; house ownership; number of household members per sleeping room; ownership of a bank or post-office account; and ownership of a mattress, a pressure cooker, a chair, a cot/bed, a table, an electric fan, a radio/transistor, a black and white television, a colour television, a sewing machine, a mobile telephone, any other telephone, a computer, a refrigerator, a watch or clock, a bicycle, a motorcycle or scooter, an animal-drawn cart, a car, a water pump, a thresher, and a tractor.

Each household asset is assigned a weight (factor score) generated through principal components analysis, and the resulting asset scores are standardized in relation to a normal distribution with a mean of zero and standard deviation of one. Each household is then assigned a score for each asset, and the scores were summed for each household; individuals are ranked according to the score of the household in which they reside. The sample is then divided into quintiles i.e., five groups with an equal number of individuals in each. In National Family Health Survey-III, one wealth index has been developed for the whole sample and for the country as a whole. Thus, at the national level, 20 per cent of the household population is in each wealth quintile although this is not necessarily true at the state level. Table 3 shows the wealth quintiles in India for National Family Health Survey-4 according to residence as urban and rural areas and in major states *(32)*.

As shown in Table 3, 45.5 per cent of the population in urban areas is in the highest wealth quintile; in contrast only

TABLE 3

Per cent distribution of the population by wealth quintiles, according to residence and state, India, 2019–21

Residence/state /Union territory	Wealth quintile Lowest	Second	Middle	Fourth	Highest	Total
India	20.0	20.0	20.0	20.0	20.2	100.0
Urban	3.2	7.2	15.5	28.6	45.5	100.0
Rural	27.8	26.0	22.1	16.0	8.1	100.0
North						
Chandigarh	1.1	2.2	5.8	11.5	79.4	100.0
Delhi	0.2	2.6	9.2	20.3	67.7	100.0
Haryana	2.0	8.3	15.8	26.2	47.7	100.0
Himachal Pradesh	3.8	13.4	24.7	29.2	28.9	100.0
Jammu & Kashmir	10.2	16.5	20.8	27.2	25.2	100.0
Ladakh	13.3	30.6	27.0	22.8	6.3	100.0
Punjab	1.1	5.0	11.4	21.9	60.6	100.0
Rajasthan	13.3	20.6	22.5	22.0	21.6	100.0
Uttarakhand	5.9	17.6	20.6	22.3	33.6	100.0
Central						
Chhattisgarh	29.9	24.0	18.6	15.8	11.7	100.0
Madhya Pradesh	31.5	21.4	16.8	15.3	15.1	100.0
Uttar Pradesh	23.9	23.6	18.3	16.4	17.8	100.0
East						
Bihar	42.8	26.1	15.4	10.3	5.4	100.0
Jharkhand	45.9	21.8	14.3	10.6	7.5	100.0
Odisha	35.1	25.2	18.3	12.6	8.7	100.0
West Bengal	32.7	26.1	19.3	14.2	7.7	100.0
Northeast						
Arunachal Pradesh	23.3	31.8	24.8	15.2	4.9	100.0
Assam	38.1	32.0	16.1	9.6	4.1	100.0
Manipur	18.3	32.6	24.1	17.2	7.8	100.0
Meghalaya	31.0	34.9	20.2	9.7	4.2	100.0
Mizoram	6.6	13.2	25.2	30.2	24.8	100.0
Nagaland	27.6	28.6	21.0	15.4	7.4	100.0
Sikkim	2.7	18.9	34.7	31.0	12.8	100.0
Tripura	31.6	33.1	22.3	10.6	2.5	100.0
West						
Dadra & Nagar Haveli and Daman & Diu	12.3	24.4	22.7	23.3	17.3	100.0
Goa	0.5	2.7	9.8	25.7	61.3	100.0
Gujarat	12.2	16.4	19.3	24.7	27.4	100.0
Maharashtra	8.6	15.3	22.1	26.1	27.9	100.0
South						
Andaman & Nicobar Islands	8.0	15.2	25.6	33.3	18.0	100.0
Andhra Pradesh	5.2	19.2	31.2	28.9	15.6	100.0
Karnataka	7.3	18.2	28.4	27.2	19.0	100.0
Kerala	0.8	4.7	17.9	36.5	40.1	100.0
Lakshadweep	0.1	2.0	15.0	46.7	36.2	100.0
Puducherry	2.4	7.2	14.7	30.0	45.7	100.0
Tamil Nadu	4.8	15.2	26.4	29.0	24.6	100.0
Telangana	5.1	17.2	28.1	27.5	22.2	100.0

Source : *(32)*

8.1 per cent of the rural population is in the highest wealth quintile. The distribution of the population across wealth quintiles shows large variations across states, with Chandigarh (79.4 per cent), Punjab (60.6 per cent), Delhi (67.7 per cent) and Goa (61.3 per cent) having over one-half of their populations in the highest quintile and Chhattisgarh, Orissa, Bihar, and Tripura, having less than one-tenth of their populations in the highest quintile. In Jharkhand and Bihar, half of the population falls into the lowest wealth quintile. By contrast, in about half of the states, less than 10 per cent of households are in the lowest wealth quintile.

Social class and health

There are a large number of studies linking social class to incidence of disease. Income, occupation and education which are the major components of most measures of social class are also each generally positively correlated with health status. It adds to the conviction that social class affects health. Individuals in the upper social classes have a longer life expectancy, less mortality and a better health and nutritional status than those in the lower classes. Diseases also have been shown to affect people at various social levels differently. For example, coronary heart disease, hypertension, diabetes all have been shown to have a high incidence in social class I and a gradual decline in incidence in the other social classes. Diseases of skin, eye and ears, diarrhoea and dysentery have also shown a higher incidence in the lower classes, which can be ascribed to the poor state of physical environment in which they live. Social class differences in mental illness have also been reported. Infant mortality, general mortality, maternal mortality are all related to social class. To serve as an illustration (Table 4), the National Family Health Survey-5 (2019–21) conducted in India shows the glaring differences in early childhood mortality rates among the households belonging to various wealth index brackets. Infant mortality rates are high among the lowest wealth index households and is lowest among the highest wealth index households.

TABLE 4

Early childhood mortality rates by wealth index in India (2019–21)

Wealth index	Neonatal mortality rate	Post-neonatal mortality rate	Infant mortality rate	Child mortality rate	Under-5 mortality rate
Lowest	33.8	14.1	48.0	11.6	59.0
Second	29.8	11.1	40.9	7.3	48.0
Middle	23.2	10.4	33.7	5.6	39.1
Fourth	19.9	8.6	28.5	4.3	32.7
Highest	12.2	4.8	17.0	3.2	20.1

Source : *(32)*

Social class differences have also been observed in the family structure, and utilization of medical and health services. Families in the lower classes are bigger in size, women marry early and bear more children. The upper social classes are characterized by small sized families and fewer children. Individuals in the lower social classes have been found to make less use of the hospital facilities, consult the doctors less often and are less likely to utilize preventive health services such as prenatal and postnatal care, general check-ups and immunization services. Social classification therefore provides an important means of studying health and disease phenomena in communities, and has proved an effective tool.

Factors involved in social class differences in health and disease

It is the first concern of those in preventive medicine and those who provide medical care service to know why there are differences in mortality and morbidity from particular diseases in certain social classes. Many factors may be involved, the following are some : (1) *Physical environment :* Differences in mortality and morbidity may be due to differences in physical environment, e.g., housing, safe water, access to clean air, etc. People in the upper social hierarchy enjoy better physical facilities than those in the lower rungs of society. (2) *Differences in services provided :* There are differences in the availability of services for different social groups. So far as general practitioners are concerned, some areas are relatively undoctored as compared to others. On the whole, it seems the undoctored areas are the areas where a substantial proportion of individuals live. (3) *Material resources :* Differences in material resources, e.g., income, wealth and possession of tools which can promote or help achieve better health also intervene in the occurrence of disease or in the maintenance of health status in different social groups. (4) *Genetic endowment :* People in one social class tend to marry in the same social class. The differences in genetic endowment may also influence one's liability to disease. (5) *Educational status :* The educational level varies in different social classes. The ignorant and the illiterate are likely to have much difficulty in pursuing measures which may conduce to good health. (6) *Attitude to disease :* The attitude of people to health and sickness may vary in different social classes, which may account for differences in distribution of disease in the social classes. There are people who regard that illness is a punishment and there are others who regard that illness is due to natural causes. There are people who diagnose illness themselves and there are others who seek early medical aid. The attitudes of people therefore vary in different social classes. The continued differences which show up in many studies of morbidity and mortality and use of medical services are due to the persistence of substantial differences in social class. There is a great field for exploration of value systems, the significance of illness to families in different classes. The aim of preventive medicine should be to reduce the social class differences in health and disease.

HOSPITAL SOCIOLOGY

Hospitals are among the most complex organizations in modern society. There has been in recent years an examination from a sociology point of view of hospitals, of medical personnel and of the utilization of medical services. The modern hospital is a social universe with a multiplicity of goals, profusion of personnel and an extremely fine division of labour. The care of the patient is a master value even for those whose work seldom brings them into direct contact with sick people. The patient is the hospital's client *(33)*. This complex character of the hospital has fascinated the social scientists as a compelling scene for the study of human behaviour.

Social structure of a hospital

A hospital is not a static organization. It is subject to change in structure and function depending upon the changes which occur in the community. The structure and functions of the hospital have changed considerably to what they were 100 years ago. Historically, the hospital was more nearly a place of refuge for the sick and homeless, than a place for medical treatment. It was a charitable institution where one went to die rather than to be cured *(33)*. In contrast, hospitals today are concerned with active medical treatment, mobilizing all that is latest in medical sciences to produce a cure. In the 19th century, hospitals were occupied by poor and old patients. Hospitals today are occupied by all classes of people. The shift in the type of patients occupying hospitals has led to a new doctor-patient relationship. There is an increasing demand for higher academic qualifications which was not typical of the earlier medical organization of the 19th century. This has led to an increasing complexity of specialization within the medical profession and no doctor today can provide single-handedly all the skills and facilities needed for treatment.

The other functions performed by hospitals are *teaching* either medical or nursing personnel and *research* designed to increase medical knowledge in which the patient is of secondary importance. The rural and district hospitals concentrate mainly on patient care. Teaching should take precedence over research in teaching hospitals.

The hospital today is a system of increasing complexity – it is a hotel and a school, a laboratory and a stage set for treatment – employing a large number of medical and paramedical personnel unlike the earlier hospitals in which very few professional groups were involved. At heart the hospital is like a federal system with several departments each enjoying considerable autonomy and discretion in its management of work. The great challenge is one of coordination *(33)*. It requires an administrative machinery to run the hospital smoothly and to avoid conflicts between administrative and professional staff, and between professionals. If a sizable portion of a group is dissatisfied, the system will break down.

The democratic ideal has certainly not yet been achieved in medicine. The structure of the wards, semi-private rooms and private rooms in hospitals is an obvious reflection of class lines. The service of the doctor in his private chamber tends to differ from that given in a public clinic not only in the time spent for case examination but in interpersonal attitudes. The public has come to expect hospitals to give tender, loving care to every patient every day *(34)*.

It is said that each hospital has a "personality" of its own – a tempo of work and an emotional atmosphere peculiar to a given hospital, its traditions, its community of staff and patients. The nature of the staff relationships will influence the staff-patient relationships and consequently the outcome of therapy. It is for this reason there are different atmospheres in different hospitals. Some have a good name, others a bad name.

Medical profession

There has been an examination from a sociological point of view of the medical profession. The medical profession, like any other occupational group is distinguished by certain characteristics. There is a professional body which controls the right to practice. The licence to practice is embodied in the legislation, and is given to those who have reached a level of competence that is considered minimum. In India, the Indian Medical Council Act was passed in 1933 to establish uniform standards of medical education in the country. A revision of the Act was made in 1956, which provides, in addition, for the maintenance of the All India Medical Register. The State Medical Councils control the right to practice and certain standards of practice and personal conduct are imposed upon its members. There is great insistence of maintenance of confidentiality, and right to practise medicine is withdrawn if there is professional misconduct. In other words, the State is regulating the relationship between professional men and their clients. Some of the possible conflicts in the medical profession may stem from the rules and regulations to which they are bound. The abolition of private practice, by Government doctors is an example of recent conflict.

Medical care – an Industry ?

The traditional physician was a self-employed small businessmen, with many of the same problems, goals and attitudes as other small businessmen. His practice was "solo-practice" based on "fee-for-service." Significant changes have taken place in the practice of medicine. The development of new diagnostic and therapeutic techniques require not only large capital investment but also skilled team of personnel. A large number of non-medical personnel are also involved in producing medical care. Society is being increasingly asked to subsidize medical education and medical care. There is a rapid development of insurance and other types of pre-payment. Now it is a national policy in many countries to make the best of known medical care available to all who need it regardless of economic status. Medical profession with its knowledge, experience and dedication is leading the way to developing better systems of health care for all. In economics, an industry is defined simply as a collection of individuals and institutions engaged in the use of similar scarce resources to produce similar goods or services. Sociologically speaking, medical care has the features similar to, big industry *(35)*.

Specialization *(36)*

The vast increase of medical knowledge during the 20th century has contributed to specialization in medicine. There are at present no less than 20 recognized specialities and many more sub-specialities. A specialist is defined as one who learns more about less and less. He is concerned with a particular organ or part of the body as opposed to the traditional general practitioner or "family doctor" who is concerned with the "whole person" or even the family.

Specialization has created problems for the traditional doctor–patient relationships. The specialist does not establish close relationship with the patient. As a consultant, he is less likely to maintain a continuing relationship with the patient. It is difficult for him to give the patient the requisite emotional support and understanding that is needed and which is the essence of a good doctor–patient relationship. Besides, specialization has encouraged jurisdictional disputes between one speciality and another and between specialists and generalist.

In short, specialization divides both doctor and patient; places strain on the traditional doctor–patient relationship; contributes to depersonalization. The social role of medicine with the assistance of the humanities and social sciences is forgotten. Over-specialization can lead to a lopsided development of the health services. Sociologists are paying increasing attention to an examination of the medical value system, the forces behind specialization, and selective factors in medical career choices *(36)*.

Doctor–patient relationship

An important area of medical sociology is doctor–patient relationship in which complex social factors are implicated. The patient comes unbidden to a doctor and enters voluntarily into a contract in which he agrees to follow the doctor's advice. By virtue of his technical superiority, knowledge and skill, the doctor exercises an authoritative role and issues "orders" to his patient. Some individuals may not be prepared to invest the doctor with full authority, this may lead to conflict between the doctor and patient.

Besides technical competence, the doctor must know how to communicate with his patient. In fact, a successful doctor is one who knows how well to communicate with his patient. In this regard, three levels of communication have been described *(37)* : (1) *Communication on an emotional plane :* The doctor must give a sympathetic ear to the complaints made by the patient and his relatives. This is necessary to establish a quick rapport. The reason why folk medicine is successful is because the patient and his relatives feel they can talk more freely to a folk medical practitioner than with the modern physician. The interpersonal relationships between villagers and folk practitioners on one hand, and the villagers and the practitioners of modern medicine on the other hand are considerably different. (2) *Communication on a cultural plane :* Secondly, the doctor should be aware of the general concepts of culture and social organization of the community with which he is dealing. This helps to acquire certain "flexibility" in his dealings with patients. The reason why the indigenous and folk systems of medicine are successful in the rural areas is because they are part of the total way of life of the people; treatment is based mostly on charity, and payment to the physician may be in kind, and the medicines are prepared from ordinary plants common to the region. All these are appealing to the common man. Against this background, the western system of medicine is alien to the cultural patterns of the rural folk. To be successful, the modern doctor should couch his scientific advice in terms which fit an already existing cultural pattern. Then there is a great chance that this advice will be followed. For example, in communities where diseases and medicine are classified as *hot* and *cold,* it might be helpful for the doctor not to challenge this belief openly. A mere statement to a patient that the medicine is "hot" and will help to cure a "cold" disease may make for increased confidence. Anthropologists have therefore stressed the importance of understanding the community as a whole, its general cultural patterns and its social and political structure, and the native concepts of health and disease. (3) *Communication on an intellectual plane :* Practitioners of modern medicine come from well-to-do-families. By their education and training, they tend to be sophisticated. This leaves a wide gap between the intellectual level of the practitioners of modern medicine and the illiterate masses. In other words, there is an enormous "social distance" between the two groups. A successful doctor is one who reduces this distance and is able to communicate with his patient freely and wins his confidence. A most important component of doctor-patient communication is *humour.* It is the best icebreaker for the patient frozen by fear and anxiety.

The doctor who is able to communicate with his patient on these three planes is bound to give maximum psychological satisfaction to his patients. The other qualities which mar the reputation of a doctor are his greed for money, differential treatment between the rich and poor and lack of a sympathetic and friendly attitude. The patient can challenge the doctor's professional adequacy if the doctor does not know how to communicate. Patients who do not behave according to the doctor's expectations are often labelled as "un-cooperative."

Doctor–nurse relationship *(38)*

Medicine and nursing have common goals – the preservation and restoration of health. Yet their roles in achieving these objectives are not identical. The primary role of medicine comprises diagnosis and treatment – the "cure" process. In contrast, the primary role of nursing lies in the "care" process – consisting of caring, helping, comforting and guiding.

In the medical-care team, the physician tends to be autocratic and looks upon the nurse primarily as his helper following his orders and carrying out whatever he chooses to delegate. Because of the authoritarian role of the physician, the role of the nurse in guiding, helping and comforting the patient go largely unrealized. This is more so as technology is advancing, the nurse is asked increasingly to take up tasks instrumental to diagnosis and treatment. In effect, many of the patient's psychosocial needs persist, unidentified and unmet.

Currently, leaders in both the professions are exploring new approaches and roles with a view to provide improved patient care *(36)*.

The sick role

To be ill is more than a medical condition. The sick person has to behave in certain prescribed ways. He comes unbidden to a hospital. As he strips off his clothing, so he strips off his customary identity in the world. He becomes subject to a time schedule and a pattern of activity not of his own making. He becomes passive for most part. He may even become child-like *(33)*. Four aspects of the sick role have been described : (1) the sick person is exempted from his normal social responsibilities depending upon the severity of his illness, (2) he needs to be cared for, (3) sick role is regarded as a misfortune. (4) the sick person is obliged to seek competent medical care, and to cooperate with the doctor in the process of getting well. A typical sick role is temporary, but some patients prefer a prolonged sick role in order to escape everyday responsibilities.

Medical social work

Medical social work had its beginning in England in 1895 when a social worker, known as "Almoner" was appointed at the Royal Free Hospital, London. Later on in the United States, the term was expanded into medical social work. Today, medical social work, has grown into an important field of social work, and an integral part of medicine. Medical social work uses "case work" as its main technique to find out the social background of illness; this information helps the doctor in arriving at a social diagnosis, treating illness and estimating the prognosis. The purpose of medical social work is to help sick people – individual by individual, both through the best use of the patient's capabilities and community resources in matters of personal and social adjustments in the community, including rehabilitation. The person who can best do this type of work is one who had special training in social case work, the medical social worker.

Medical social worker

The medical social worker is a paramedical worker who has been trained in social case work, and in the art of interviewing people. There are many situations, in medical and public health organisations, where medical social workers are being employed, e.g., hospitals, tuberculosis clinics, family planning clinics, cancer control centres, mental health, maternal and child welfare, school and university health services. The medical social worker forms a link between the institution where he is employed and the community. The principal work of the medical social worker is to visit the family and probe into the personal, economic and social causes of illness and collect social history of the patient with a view to supplement the medical history. The medical social worker also tries to secure help to the patient through the community resources. In chronic disabling illnesses like tuberculosis, leprosy and poliomyelitis, the medical social worker helps in the rehabilitation of the patient. The medical social worker is now recognized as an essential professional colleague of the doctor in the analysis and correction of the social and emotional factors and is increasingly relied upon for supplying information that is of fundamental importance in formulating the complete diagnosis and in directing the treatment of many patients. A medical social worker bears the same relationship to the effectiveness of social medicine, as does the nurse to clinical medicine.

From medical ethics to social ethics *(39)*

Since antiquity, the doctor/patient relationship has been governed by systems of medical ethics drawn from the Hippocratic, Chinese, Indian and other traditions. All held that the patient's good transcended other considerations. The physician determined what was the patient's good. Modern codes have added a social dimension, a responsibility for the health – the good of society and humanity in general, and a concern for justice. "Health for all", with its emphasis on social justice, on the equitable allocation of resources and on the responsibility of communities and individuals for their own health, is an expression of this change, and thus represents an ethical as well as a social goal.

The transformation of medical ethics has been stimulated partly by the progress of medical biotechnology and partly by profound social changes, associated with a recognition of human rights and freedoms, and of individual autonomy. Many medical choices can no longer be made purely on the basis of medical science. The emphasis on the social good has confronted lay individuals, whether policy-makers or patients, with ethical decisions and choices, requiring them to share with or often replace the physician or the scientist in determining what is ethically acceptable and good, to balance the patient's interests with those of society.

The explosion of expensive medical technologies, often of limited value to the patient, and the rise in people's expectations, have accentuated the problem of making the best use of limited resources. Policy-makers must set priorities to guide the allocation of resources among health goals and between health and other social goals. They do so under many pressures – social, economic, political, technological and ethical. They are forced to make choices often with tragic consequences. In principle medicine can use the full potential of modern biotechnology – for transplanting organs, for assisting reproduction, for postponing death, for reducing hereditary diseases, even for manipulating the genetic make-up of human beings. In practice the policy-maker by controlling resources and trying to reflect the dominant values of society, determines how much medicine can do, and even which patients may benefit. Thus the good of society and individual good may come into conflict.

For their part, individual patients today exercise autonomy and informed consent in deciding whether or not to accept or continue with treatment, even to continue to live, to become a subject of research, to permit the use of personal health data for study purposes, to be told – or not told – the truth, to permit the use of embryos, to donate organs and to withdraw life-support systems.

Individuals, like communities, are often the subjects of research, such as trials of drugs or vaccines or epidemiological studies. Some living in deprivation or even oppression are liable to exploitation. Researchers have a particular ethical responsibility to safeguard the rights of such people and to observe scrupulously the ethical principles of beneficence, avoidance of harm, and justice.

Consumer Protection Act

Consumer rights have become an important issue. For the first time in India, the Consumer Protection Act 1986 provided consumers a forum for speedy redressal of their grievances against medical services. In the entire health care delivery system the most vital sector is the medical profession. The active participation and dedication of doctors is very important for its survival. Over the centuries the medical profession has been accorded respect by the society. Since last decade or so, increasing commercialization of the profession has eroded this faith.

As far as the professional services are concerned, the evolution of law has followed a set course. Under the general law, a member of a profession is required to show a standard of care which a person of that profession is expected to posses. In developed nations such as USA and UK, patients do not encounter many difficulties, as the courts have developed principles of law which give important rights to patients. In India, people were not going to Civil Courts freely because court fee is very heavy and there is long delay to get final verdict. It may take several years. Parliament has provided an alternative, a quick, efficacious and economic remedy. According to this Act, the decision should be taken within 3 to 6 months. There is no court fee payment and the person can plead his own case. More recently even ESI hospitals have been brought within the ambit of the Consumer Protection Act. COPRA is a piece of comprehensive legislation and recognizes six rights of the consumer, namely : right to safety; right to be informed; right to choose; right to be heard; right to seek redressal; and right to consumer education.

If a patient or the relations of a patient feel that the suffering or death of a patient is because of either negligence by the concerned doctor or the heatlh facility, they can complain to the Medical Council of India or to the Consumer Court. The Medical Council of India, which is a statutory body created to monitor the medical profession has only ethical jurisdiction. The council can only cancel the registration of the concerned doctor temporarily or permanently but cannot punish a doctor or give a compensation.

A complaint against the medical professional can be filed in the consumer court. It should contain all the details of the case, an expert certificate or opinion from the doctor of concerned speciality (stating the complaint is prima facie true and needs further investigation) and the compensation demanded. These courts can only give compensation. The monetary limits of the compensation that can be granted by the consumer courts are as follows : (a) District Consumer Court – up to Rs. 20 lacs; (b) State Commission – Rs. 20 lacs to Rs. 1 crore; and (c) National Commission – above Rs. 1 crore.

Rights of the patient

1. Right to information on healthcare services available to them, diagnosis and treatment;
2. Right to have information about professionals involved in the patient care;
3. Right to safety from errors and malpractice;
4. Right to confidentiality and privacy;
5. Right to have prompt treatment in an emergency;
6. Right to get copies of medical records;
7. Right to informed consent;
8. Right to refuse to participate in human experimentations, and research;
9. Right to be informed about the rules and regulations of the hospital that apply to the patient and the facilities obtainable by the patient;
10. Right to choose and to seek second opinion about the disease and treatment etc.; and
11. Right to complain and have compensation within reasonably short time.

THE ART OF INTERVIEWING *(40)*

Interview is a device for investigation. It is an instrument of research. The chemist carries out research in test tubes; the bacteriologist uses the microscope in his laboratory. In much the same way, the social scientist uses the interview technique in his investigations. Modern medicine has changed its character; it has emerged as a social science in recent years. Social and psychological factors have come to be recognized as dominant factors in the natural history of disease. In order to elicit these factors, it may be necessary to employ the interview technique. It may be said that the interview technique is one of the contributions of social science to modern medicine.

Aims of interview

The major aims of interview are : (1) to secure information through face-to-face association and thereby gain the portrait of the entire personality, broad enough to encompass the social and psychological background (2) to form a hypothesis (3) to collect personal data for quantitative purposes and (4) to collect data from persons who are secondary sources of information.

Kinds of interview

Social scientists have described four kinds of interview : (a) *Direct or structured interview :* A schedule containing a set of predetermined questions is prepared. The researcher gets answers to these questions only. Generally the researcher does not add anything to what has been stated by the subject. He does not even alter the language. (b) *Non-directive or Unstructured interview :* No predetermined questions are asked. The researcher collects information by free discussion. The subject is asked to narrate in his own words his experiences, opinions or reactions about the particular subject under investigation. (c) *Focussed interview :* This type of interview is generally used to study the social and psychological effects of mass communication, e.g., reaction of a film show or radio programme. The researcher tries to focus his attention on a particular aspect of the problem and tries to know the experience, attitude and emotional responses regarding the concrete situation under study. (d) *Repetitive interview :* It is used when it is desired to note the gradual influence of some social or psychological process. A record has also to be maintained to study the change in continued sequence.

Technique of interview

Conducting an interview is both an art and science. Sociologists have described the following steps for conducting an interview *(40)*.

1. ESTABLISHING CONTACT

The first requisite before conducting an interview is to establish contact with the interviewee. Prior appointment regarding the time and place of interview is always desirable. It gives the interviewee a sense of satisfaction and a feeling of importance that his time has been valued.

2. STARTING AN INTERVIEW

The beginning should always be made from a general discussion of the problem. The researcher should create an atmosphere in which the interviewee freely tells his story in his own way. The researcher should let the interviewee do most of the talking, while he should himself listen to it attentively guiding and directing the interviewee about the subject matter wherever necessary. All controversial matters must be carefully avoided.

3. SECURING RAPPORT

A state of rapport must be established between the interviewee and the researcher. In the beginning every interviewee proceeds very cautiously giving only formal information. He may not like to discuss personal matters with a stranger. It therefore requires tact on the part of the researcher to create a friendly atmosphere and gain the confidence of the interviewee. Once rapport is gained and hesitation and shyness are overcome, the interviewee may feel overzealous to tell everything that he knows, and all that he feels without any attempt at secrecy or formality. The research worker must utilize this situation to the fullest advantage, and use it as best as he can. The state of rapport, sometimes may not last long; once the interviewee has relapsed into his former state, it may be very difficult to bring him back to rapport.

4. RECALL

At times, during the course of an interview, the interviewee may be so full of emotion that he drifts away from the main subject, and may even go into silence at the end of the narration. At such times, the researcher should give enough time to the interviewee to recollect and start again. At times, it may be necessary to refresh his memory by pointing out what he had been saying last.

5. PROBE QUESTIONS

When the interviewee, during an interview knowingly or unknowingly side-tracks some important aspect of the problem, the researcher has to be very cautious in catching these slips. Great care should be taken in putting probe questions. They should appear to the interviewee to be born of mere curiosity. If the interviewee has deliberately side-tracked a particular point, a very shrewd effort is needed to make him discuss a point at length, the same should not be doggedly pursued, lest rapport should be lost.

6. ENCOURAGEMENT

During the course of an interview, it is necessary to encourage the interviewee from time to time, by interpolating such complimentary expressions as "what you have said is really very illuminating; I never had such an enlightening discussion; you really have a very unique approach to the problem; I myself had never thought of it from that angle, etc." Great care should be taken that complimentary remarks should sound true appreciations, and not flattery otherwise they will lose all their effect.

7. GUIDING THE INTERVIEW

Sometimes, the interviewee digresses in his narration to less important topics, which he is most eager to relate, and if stopped from continuing the conversation he may get offended. It is the duty of the researcher to guide the subject in the right path without offending him.

8. RECORDING

Recording the statements should be reduced to a minimum during the course of an interview. If recording is continued, the flow of the conversation will slow down and the interview may take the form of questions and answers. Further, the interviewee will be conscious that his statements are being recorded. The researcher should jot down only important points.

9. CLOSING THE INTERVIEW

An interview should not be ended abruptly. The interviewee should not feel, at the close of the interview, that he has divulged many of his secrets to a stranger. The researcher should bring the interview to a natural close, followed by the usual forms of greetings.

10. REPORT

Soon after the interview, the report should be compiled when the mind is still fresh about the narration.

OPERATIONAL RESEARCH

The term 'operational research' was coined during the World War II in connection with the best use of a new invention, the radar. Since the war, the term has spread rapidly in Britain and America and it has come to mean today more than the study of the use of new inventions – the study of the whole systems of services rendered in industry, administration, education and health services *(38)*.

Operational research is defined as the application of scientific methods of investigation to the study of complex human organizations and services. A mathematician working on atomic structure is pursuing pure research; an engineer designing a new plant for an industry is pursuing applied research. In operational research, one is concerned all the time with the activities of a group of people with the purpose of inducing beneficial changes. Thus, operational research is a sociological science, and has an immense social content which distinguishes it from pure or applied research. The main objective of operational research is "to develop new knowledge about institutions, programmes, use of facilities, the people working in these activities and the individuals and communities served by them" in order to secure optimal utilization of resources in men, material and money in the service of the community *(41)*. A new area of operational research is emerging, i.e., "health operational research" *(42)*.

Phases in operational research

The procedure to be adopted in operational research differs according to the nature of the study. The usual procedure adopted generally consists of the following phases.

1. Formulation of the problem.
2. Collection of relevant data, if necessary, by a suitable sample.
3. Analysis of data and formulation of hypothesis.
4. Deriving solutions from the hypothesis or "model".
5. Choosing the optimal solution and forecasting results.
6. Testing of solution, e.g., pilot projects.
7. Implementing the solution in the whole system.

Operational research team

Operational research is a team work job and involves several workers. The composition of the team varies with the type of research. The minimum composition in social medicine applications is probably a public health administrator, an epidemiologist, a statistician, and a social scientist. This is in addition to ancillary workers such as clerks, peons and field workers. The team is headed by a director who is responsible for the whole project.

Operational research in health services *(42)*

Practically everything within the broad field of public health and social medicine – either a whole system or part of it – could be the subject of operational research. Examples of part problems are : optimal size of area and population to be covered by a midwife, or basic health unit; ideal vehicle for local health workers; leaving maximum time for technical personnel to utilize their skills; architectural design of hospitals and health centres; queuing problems in out-patient departments and hospital waiting lists; solutions to integration problems where specialised services have developed on emergency basis outside the general health services; study of bed load and nursing services in teaching and non-teaching hospitals; length of stay in hospitals and length of sickness absence; effectiveness or the extent to which the stated objective of a programme, e.g., malaria eradication, family planning is achieved; quality of medical care services; investigation of outbreaks of epidemic diseases and many others. Whenever social medicine passes from the stage of observation and classification to that of discovering and recommending appropriate action, it is involved in operational research.

SOCIAL PROBLEMS

In a community, there are both individual and social problems. When individual problems affect a large number of people, they become social problems. Some of the present day social problems are alcoholism, drug dependence, STD, vagrancy, juvenile delinquency, prostitution etc. Some of the social problems have medical implication, e.g., venereal diseases. Social problems are solved by social and political action, that is by social welfare programmes, social assistance, social legislation in the community to curb the social evils (e.g., The Prevention of Food Adulteration Act; The Prevention of Immoral Traffic Act; The Medical Termination of Pregnancy Act).

Prostitution

Prostitution is an age-old social evil. It is a social problem in most urban areas, and to a lesser extent in rural areas. Sociologists who have studied prostitution have mentioned the following underlying causes of prostitution. (1) changes in environment (2) breakdown of family relations (3) parenteral quarrels (4) want of affection (5) illegitimate love (6) easy money (7) low I.Q. (8) low moral standards (9) poverty, etc. The Government of India passed an Act in 1956 known as "The Suppression of Immoral Traffic Act in women and girls" which bans prostitution in its commercialized form as an organized means of living. The Act was amended and retitled as "Immoral Traffic (Prevention) Act" in 1986. It covers all persons, whether male or female, who are exploited sexually for commercial purposes.

Delinquency

A delinquent is one who shows deviation from normal behaviour. In other words, he is one who has committed an offence, e.g., theft, sexual offence, murder, burglary, etc. Delinquency is a social problem in many communities. The causes responsible for delinquency are social maladjustment, poverty, disturbed home conditions, alcoholism, drug addiction, and modern ways of living.

The programmes for the prevention and control of juvenile delinquency centre round the implementation of **The Children Act, 1960** which provides a specialized approach towards the care, protection, maintenance, training and rehabilitation of delinquent children. The institutional infrastructure consists of Juvenile/Children's Courts, child welfare boards, remand homes, certified schools, children homes and after-care facilities.

Dowry system

Dowry started as an innocent custom, a symbol of love from parents to their daughter on the eve of her marriage. But it has, in recent years, grown into a social evil with many instances of bride-burning and suicides. These are symptoms of societal corruption.

Under the **Dowry Prohibition (Amendment) Act, 1986** the minimum punishment for taking or abetting the taking of dowry has been raised to 5 years imprisonment and a fine of Rs.15,000. What is required is a sustained effort to go into the root causes of these evils. Well-entrenched social customs cannot be easily erased by an Act of Parliament.

Drug addiction

Drug addiction is defined as a state of periodic or chronic intoxication detrimental to the individual and society produced by the repeated intake of habit-forming drugs.

Drug abuse has reached an alarming proportion in recent years. "Drug culture" is fast making inroads into the lives of young people from all walks of life. The reasons given for drug dependence include the following :

- curiosity and natural tendency to experiment with drugs.
- disturbed home environment : children from broken homes, indifferent parents, lack of communication between parents and children.
- an escape phenomenon from tensions and frustrations in life, e.g., unemployment, failure in examinations.
- impact of disco culture, mobile, TV, internet etc.
- ignorance regarding the habit-forming nature of the drugs.

To call a person a drug addict, the following criteria must be satisfied :

(1) *Psychological dependance* : there is an overpowering desire (compulsion) to take the drug and obtain it by any means.

(2) *Physical dependance* : when the drug is withdrawn, the patient shows "withdrawal symptoms" such as irrational and violent behaviour, nausea, diarrhoea, watering of eyes and nose, etc.

(3) *Development of tolerance* : there is a tendency to increase the dose.

Management

Though drug addiction may be considered as a social problem, the first step in its management is medical care, which includes :

a. identification of drug addicts and their motivation for drug detoxification;
b. detoxification (requires hospitalization);
c. Post-detoxification counselling and follow-up (based on clinic and home visits); and
d. rehabilitation.

Simultaneously with medical treatment, changes in environment (home, school, college, social circle) are important. The patient must effect a complete break with his group, otherwise the chances of relapse are 100 per cent. Psychotherapy has a valuable place in the management of the addict.

Preventive measures include **education** of target groups and the general public through TV, radio, leaflets, and posters to create awareness of the problem. The Government have promulgated an Act called the "Narcotic Drugs and Psychotropic Substances Act" which came into force in 1985 to combat this problem. Refer to Chapter 20 for further details.

Alcohol abuse

Alcoholism is world-wide social and medical problem. Over the past 30 to 40 years, alcohol consumption has increased in quantity and frequency. The age at which people start drinking has also declined. The population groups at great risk are those undergoing rapid socio-economic and cultural changes; they view alcohol as a symbol of prestige and social status.

Consequences : The consequences of alcohol abuse cover a wide spectrum : crime, murder, prostitution, neglect of families, malnutrition, disease (e.g., cirrhosis of liver, alcohol-dependant syndrome, alcoholic psychosis), unemployment, indebtedness, child delinquency, road accidents, loss of friends and self-esteem. In short excessive alcohol results in serious medical, psychological and sociological problems.

Drinking by adults serves as a role model for the young. The identification of risk factors is essential for prevention. As drinking patterns vary considerably, the prevention of alcoholism is not easy. A widespread public education and discussion, and investigation of public attitudes may result in measurable improvement. This should be combined with social welfare and health services. Refer to Chapter 20 for further details.

Unmarried mothers

We do not have accurate statistics regarding unmarried mothers in India. Because of social customs and traditions in India, the problem of unmarried mothers in India must be insignificant. Such mothers have a multiplicity of needs – not only for medical termination of pregnancy and health risks but for understanding, warmth and guidance. In Western societies, where this problem is acute, they have special schools and counselling programmes for teenage mothers.

Handicapped

The handicapped comprise 7 main categories as shown below, during 2011 *(43)*.

	Categories	*Estimated number in India*
(i)	The blind	5.03 million
(ii)	The hearing disability	5.07 million
(iii)	The orthopaedically handicapped	5.43 million
(iv)	Multiple disabilities	2.11 million
(v)	The mentally retarded	1.50 million
(vi)	The mental illness	0.72 million
(vii)	The speech disability	1.99 million
(vii)	Others	4.92 million

The above figures are not static, but ever growing. In all civilized countries, the State looks after the handicapped. The rehabilitation services available for the handicapped in India are as follows : (1) medical care facilities (2) education for the blind, deaf and the orthopaedically handicapped (3) vocational training (4) job placement and sheltered workshops (5) pensions, scholarships and allowances for the education and training of the handicapped.

SOCIAL AGENCIES

Social welfare services have always been an integral part of the socio-cultural tradition of India. Soon after Independence, on the basis of a survey made by the Planning Commission, it was estimated that there were 10,000 voluntary organizations in the field of social welfare. Today the number is much greater. The activities are coordinated and assisted by the Ministry of Social Welfare and Women's Affairs. An autonomous Central Social Welfare Board is the main agency of the Ministry for undertaking and implementing programmes for women through the voluntary sector. Activities include welfare, training, health care, provision of women's hostels, as well as legal aid and support to women being exploited by families or employers. A few of the principal agencies are listed below :

1. All India Women's Conference, 6 Bhagwandas Road, New Delhi–110 001
2. National Association of Rural Women, Room No. 9/104, Jamnagar Hutments Block 11, Mansingh Road, New Delhi–110 001
3. National Council of Women, 12 Circular Road, Patna–800 001
4. India Social Institute, Department of Women's Development, 24 Benson Road, Bangalore–560046
5. Centre of Science for Villages, Magan, Sangrahalaya, Wardha – 442 001
6. Eastern India Women's Association
E Ahmed Building, Lakhtokia, Guwahati.

COMMUNITY SERVICES

Administrative pattern of the country

(1) CENTRE

India is a Union of 29 States and 7 Union territories. Last state Telangana was formed on 2nd June 2014. The Constitution of India came into force on 26 January, 1950. The Union Executive consists of the President, the Vice President, the Prime Minister and the Council of Ministers. Rules of business have been framed under the Constitution.

India is a sovereign Democratic Republic with a Parliamentary form of government. Sovereignty ultimately rests with the people. The Parliament consists of the President, and the two Houses of Parliament – The Rajya Sabha and the Lok Sabha. The Rajya Sabha consists of 250 indirectly elected members, and the Lok Sabha 544 directly elected members. The main functions of Parliament are to make laws for the country, and to make finances available to the Government. The Parliament is assisted by several committees. The term of the Lok Sabha is 5 years.

(2) STATE

The administrative pattern in the States closely resembles that of the Union. The States executive consists of a Governor, and a council of Ministers with a Chief Minister as its head. The Governor who is the head in each state is appointed by the President for a term of 5 years. The State Legislature consists of Vidhan Sabha (Legislative Assembly) and its members are chosen by direct election. In Some States, there is also an Upper House known as Vidhan Parishad or Legislative Council. The powers of the State Legislature have been defined in the Constitution.

The Union territories (e.g. Puducherry, Andaman and Nicobar are administered by the President through an Administrator).

(3) LOCAL GOVERNMENT

(a) *Urban areas* : In big cities, the local Government institution is known as Corporation, and in medium and small towns as Municipal Committee or Council. The Corporations are headed by elected Mayors. The executive power of the Corporation vests in the Commissioner. The Corporation deals with matters concerning public health and sanitation, maintenance of roads, bridges, markets, playgrounds, parks and education. Municipalities are headed by elected Presidents.

(b) *Rural areas* : The rural areas are governed by the system of Panchayati Raj or democratic decentralization.

Democratic decentralization

In democratic societies, the trend is to distribute power as much as possible to the people themselves so that they may be able to manage their own affairs. The Panchayati Raj in India is nothing but democratic decentralization. It is a 3–tier system of local self-government.

Village level	...	*Gram Panchayat*
Block level	...	*Panchayat Samiti*
District level	...	*Zilla Parishad*

Gram Panchayats are elected by Gram Sabhas consisting of the entire adult population of the village. The panchayat consists of 9 to 15 elected members. The Panchayats are responsible for agricultural production, rural industries, medical relief, mother and child health, maintenance of village roads and streets, tanks and sanitation. It is envisaged that the Panchayat institutions will control everything including primary health centres and local schools. The Panchayat Samiti or Janpad Panchayat federates at the Block level, and the Zilla Parishad at the District level. The Panchyat Raj institutions have their own powers of taxation. For the speedy dispensation of Justice, Nyaya (Judicial) Panchyats or village courts have also been established.

LAWS

Laws are rules of the State. They regulate the individual and community behaviour. Some laws come into existence out of the local customs and traditions, e.g., the Hindu marriage Act. There are laws which are enacted by Parliament and State Legislatures. The supreme law of the land is the Constitution which sets out the rights of Government and an individual. Some of the important laws in the field of community health in India are :

(1) The Prevention of Food Adulteration Act. 1954.
(2) The Medical Termination of Pregnancy Act, 1971.
(3) The Employees' State Insurance Act, 1948.
(4) The Indian Factories Act, 1948.
(5) The Central Maternity Benefit Act, 1961.
(6) The Children Act, 1960.
(7) The Central Birth and Death Registration Act, 1969.
(8) The Epidemic Diseases Act, 1897.
(9) Juvenile Justice Act 1986.

COOPERATIVES

Cooperatives are a form of conducting business in society. Profits are distributed after all the costs are paid. The Government has established a system of cooperative societies for helping the farmers to obtain loans for dairy, poultry, and irrigation purposes. There are also other cooperatives such as Consumer Societies in urban and rural areas. There are also District Cooperative Unions and State Cooperative Unions.

EDUCATIONAL SERVICES

Education is one of the fundamental rights of man. The purpose of education is to "socialize" children so that they may imbibe the social values and norms of society and to prepare them as useful citizens. Education in India is primarily a responsibility of the State. The Constitution provides for free and compulsory education up to the age of 14 years. The National Policy on Education aims at achieving this goal, and for an investment of 6 per cent of National Income on education. The literacy rate in India for the year 2011 was 74.04 per cent; male literacy rate 82.14 per cent, female literacy rate 65.46 per cent. Education is fundamental to health and health to education.

The Central Government is concerned with the determination of educational standards, scientific and technical education, and research. The Medical Council of India prescribes standards for medical education in the country. There is a Ministry of Education at the Central and State levels. Education is thus an important community service, and the school is an important community institution.

RECREATION AND CULTURAL ACTIVITIES

India has a great cultural heritage of dance, drama, music and art. There are 3 National Academies for the promotion of art, music and dance. Besides these, there are State Academies for the promotion of art. The All India Radio with its network of stations and the Television are powerful mass media in the country. India also leads the world in the production of films. The documentary films depict the life, art and culture of people in different regions of the country.

ECONOMICS

The word "economics" literally means "house-keeping". It deals with the human relationships in the specific context of production, distribution, consumption, ownership of resources, goods and services. Economics and sociology overlap in many areas.

Natural resources of the country

India is rich in natural resources and man-power (1) *Agriculture :* Agriculture is the main plank of the Indian economy. It accounts for nearly 44 per cent of the National Income, and provides employment to nearly 70 per cent of India's population. (2) *Forestry :* Forests constitute another important basic natural resource of the country. Nearly 19.4 per cent of the total land area of the country is occupied by forests. Forests are a source of timber, bamboo, canes, tendu leaves, gum, resins, tanning materials, rubber, dyes, honey, etc. (3) *Fisheries :* India has a vast sea-coast. The marine products earn foreign exchange. (4) *Minerals :* India is richly endowed with minerals, e.g., bauxite, coal, copper, diamond, gold, iron ore, manganese, mica, nickel, etc. (5) *Man-power :* The greatest natural resource of the country is its man-power. The population of the country is 1,210.1 million (2011). The people of India account for about 16 per cent of the world's population, while occupying only 2.4 per cent of the world's land area.

OCCUPATIONS

One of the first questions we ask a stranger or new acquaintance is "What are you doing ? or "What is your job ?". Occupation is thus a basis of social differentiation. Some occupations are prestigious (e.g., doctors, judges); others (e.g., manual labour) are not. Occupation also reflects the income of the individual, and his standard of living. The occupational structure in India is as shown in Table 5.

TABLE 5

Main workers by industrial categories, 2007

Industry	Total numbers (000)
Primary sector	
Agricultural & allied activities	1,425
Mining & quarrying	1,237
Secondary sector	
Manufacturing	5,837
Electricity, gas & water supply	899
Construction	936
Tertiary sector	
Wholesale and retail Trade, Hotels & Restaurant etc.	588
Transport, storage & communications	2,737
Other services	13,289
Total main workers	27,242

Source : *(44)*

INDUSTRIALIZATION

During the early years of this century, the major industries in India were cotton mill industry, jute industry and coal mining. During recent years, there has been considerable industrial expansion. A number of new industries have come up such as steel, sugar, cement, glass, chemicals, soap, vanaspati, heavy electrical and machine tools, etc.

Industries create new conditions of life and new conditions for adaptation. There is shifting of the population from rural to urban areas. People are removed from the warm intimacy of village life to the isolated and impersonal life in towns and cities. The community health problems arising out of industrialization are water and air pollution, creation of slums; accidents; communicable disease problems such as tuberculosis and sexually transmitted diseases; mental health problems such as delinquency; psychoneurosis and social problems such as alcoholism, drug dependence, prostitution, gambling and crime.

Health problems in industrialized countries have passed through various evolutionary stages, each characterized by different challenges to public health and personal health care. In the initial stage, infectious diseases, malnutrition, and poor housing were combated by socio-economic improvements in combination with public health measures such as the provision of pure water supply and sewage disposal facilities. As scientific advances were made, broader control of acute bacterial and viral diseases were achieved by means of immunization and chemotherapy as well as increased health care for individuals.

The second evolutionary stage has been dominated by chronic diseases, particularly cardiovascular and cerebrovascular diseases and cancer. Scientific and technological progress has produced a wide array of medical interventions for diagnosis and cure, higher levels of specialization in medical practice, and transfer of much of the care previously rendered in doctor's clinic to elaborate and expensive hospitals. The cost of health care has risen dramatically.

There is evidence in some industrialized countries of a third stage, which might be described as social and environmental pathology. Threats to health arise not from intrinsic disorders of bodily structure and function, but from environmental hazards related to urban development and exposure to toxic substances, as well as from changes in social behaviour associated with violence, alcohol, and drug abuse of epidemic proportion. Industrialized countries have passed through these three stages over the course of more than a century. Developing countries, on the other hand, face the challenge of coping with all the three stages simultaneously, with just a fraction of the human and material resources available to their industrialized counterparts. Policies must be closely related to overall socio-economic development if countries with limited resources are to achieve the greatest possible benefits in health *(46)*.

ECONOMIC LEVELS

National Income

An important background influence is the size and strength of a country's economy, which is usually expressed in terms of one of the national aggregates, such as gross national product (GNP) or gross domestic product (GDP). These aggregates measure the total volume of national economic activity at current or constant price. By dividing the GNP or GDP by the total population, one arrives at **per capita** GNP or GDP, which are common general purpose indicators of national wealth. Per capita GNP may thus serve as a general measure of human welfare – that is, of health in a very broad sense. In practice, many health variables are indeed correlated with per capita GNP or GDP. Countries with a high per capita GNP are predominantly industrially developed, while those with a low one are predominantly agricultural, or developing.

Gross National Income (GNI)

Formerly known as GNP or Gross National Product. It is gross income generated from within the country as also net income received from abroad. It is expressed either "at current prices" i.e., at prices prevailing during the period to which the figure refers, or "at constant prices"; i.e., at prices prevailing during a fixed base period in the past, irrespective of the period to which the figures refers. Thus figures 'at constant prices' discount the effect of inflation after the base period and measure the changes in real terms. Figures 'at current prices' are naturally influenced by inflation but are more useful for, say, international comparisons for the same period.

For GNI per capita US $, the national currency is converted to current US Dollars using the Work Bank Atlas Method. This involves using a 3 year average of exchange rates *(45)*.

PER CAPITA INCOME

An index of the standard of living of the people is "per capita income". Per capita income in India is among the lowest in the world. According to recent statistics, the per capita income in India (2012–13) was Rs. 68,748 at current prices.

Gross Domestic Product (GDP)

GDP is gross income generated within a country, i.e., it excludes net income received from abroad.

Net National Product (NNP)

It is the GNP minus the capital we consume (e.g., equipment, machinery, etc.,) in the production process. In other words, NNP is the market value of all final goods and services after providing for depreciation.

Net Domestic Product (NDP)

It is the gross domestic product minus the value of depreciation on fixed assets.

GDP at Market Price

It is GDP at factor cost plus indirect taxes minus subsidies.

NNP at Market Price

It is NNP at factor cost plus indirect taxes minus subsidies.

GNP at Market Price

It is GNP at factor cost plus indirect taxes minus subsidies.

Purchasing Power Parity (PPP)

It is defined as the number of units of a country's currency required to buy the same amount of goods and services in the domestic market as one dollar would buy in the USA. According to the latest calculation of per capita GNI and overall GNP of the World Bank, based on PPP, India's per capita GNP in 2019 has been estimated at $ 6920 (PPP). It is the fourth largest country in terms of GNP (PPP) with about $ 2.5 trillion, preceded by the USA ($ 9.98 trn.), China (about $ 5.4 trn.) and Japan ($ 3.5 trn.) *(44)*.

Gross domestic savings

It is excess of current income over current expenditure.

Poverty

The number of people living in extreme poverty in the world has increased, and was estimated that about

19 per cent of world's population was living below one dollar per day income during the year 2005 *(47)*. Poverty wields its destructive influence at every stage of human life from the moment of conception to the grave. Poverty is the main reason why babies are not vaccinated, clean water and sanitation are not provided, and curative drugs and other treatments are unavailable. It is the main cause of low life expectancy, low birth weight babies, higher maternal mortality, handicap and disability, mental illness, stress, suicide, family disintegration and substance abuse. Table 6 shows the influence of income on health in South-East Asia Region.

TABLE 6

Per capita GNI (PPP), life expectancy at birth and infant mortality rate in SEAR countries (2019)

Country	Per capita GNI PPP US $ (2019)	Life expectancy at birth (2019)	Infant mortality rate (2019)
India	6,920	70.8	28
Bangladesh	5,200	74.3	26
Bhutan	11,230	73.1	24
Indonesia	11,070	71.3	20
Maldives	18,380	79.6	7
Myanmar	5,170	69.1	36
Nepal	3,610	70.9	26
Sri Lanka	13,260	76.9	6
Thailand	18,570	77.7	8

Source : *(51, 52)*

The health consequences of poverty are severe. The poor die younger and suffer more from disability. They are exposed to greater risk from unhealthy conditions at home and at work. Malnutrition and the legacy of past illness mean that they are more likely to fall ill and slower to recover, especially if they have little access to health care. When a family's breadwinner becomes ill, other members of the household may at first cope by working harder themselves and by reducing consumption, even of food. Both adjustments can harm health of the whole family *(48)*.

The poor are forced into occupations that harm their health, lack of access to health care and education, live shorter life and in general lack access to resources and means to improve their lives. These social and economic aspects of poverty are inextricably linked. Addressing these underlying social factors can enable people to escape poverty. Sound economic policies must go hand-in-hand with addressing the social needs of the poor.

Investments to reduce health risks among poor and provision of insurance against catastrophic health care costs are important elements in a strategy for reducing poverty.

Global Hunger Index (GHI) *(50)*

The Global Hunger Index (GHI) is a tool designed to comprehensively measure and track hunger globally, by region and country. It highlights successes and failures in hunger reduction. It is calculated each year by the International Food Policy Research Institute.

GHI combines three equally weighted indicators into one index :

1. *Undernourishment* : the proportion of undernourished people as a percentage of the population (reflecting the share of the population with insufficient calorie intake);
2. *Child underweight* : the proportion of children under the age of five who are underweight (that is, have low weight for their age, reflecting wasting, stunted growth, or both), which is one indicator of child undernutrition; and
3. *Child mortality* : the mortality rate of children under the age of five (partially reflecting the fatal synergy of inadequate food intake and unhealthy environments).

The global hunger index is calculated by the following formula :

$$\text{GHI} = \frac{\text{Proportion of undernourished population (PNU)} + \text{Children under weight (CUW)} + \text{Child mortality in per centage (CM)}}{3}$$

For India the GHI for the year 2014 was :

$$\frac{17.0 + 30.7 + 5.6}{3} = 17.8$$

The calculations result in a 100-point scale on which zero is the best score (no hunger) and 100 the worst, although neither of these extremes is reached in practice. A value of 100 would be reached only if the whole population was undernourished, all children younger than five were underweight, and all children died before their fifth birthday. A value of zero would mean that a country had no undernourished people in the population, no children younger than five who were underweight, and no children who died before their fifth birthday.

Some definitions

1. *Hunger* : distress related to lack of food.
2. *Malnutrition* : an abnormal physiological condition, typically due to eating the wrong amount and/or kinds of foods; encompasses undernutrition and overnutrition.
3. *Undernutrition* : deficiencies in energy, protein, and/or micronutrients.
4. *Micronutrient deficiency (also known as hidden hunger)* : a form of undernutrition that occurs when intake or absorption of vitamins and minerals is too low to sustain good health and development in children and normal physical and mental function in adults. Causes include poor diet, disease, or increased micronutrient needs not met during pregnancy and lactation.
5. *Undernourishment* : chronic calorie deficiency, with consumption of less than 1,800 kilocalories a day, the minimum most people need to live a healthy, productive life.
6. *Overnutrition* : excess intake of energy or micronutrients.

Hidden hunger

Hidden hunger (micronutrient deficiency) is a form of undernutrition that occurs when intake and absorption of vitamins and minerals (such as zinc, iodine, and iron) are too low to sustain good health and development. Factors that contribute to micronutrient deficiencies include poor diet, increased micronutrient needs during certain life stages, such as pregnancy and lactation, and health problems such as diseases, infections, or parasites.

While clinical signs of hidden hunger, such as night blindness due to vitamin A deficiency and goitre from inadequate iodine intake, become visible once deficiencies become severe, the health and development of a much larger share of the population is affected by less obvious "invisible" effects. That is why micronutrient deficiencies are often referred to as hidden hunger.

Hidden hunger afflicts more than 2 billion individuals, or one in three people, globally (FAO 2013). Its effects can be devastating, leading to mental impairment, poor health, low productivity, and even death. Its adverse effects on child health and survival are particularly acute, especially within the first 1,000 days of a child's life, from conception to the age of two, resulting in serious physical and cognitive consequences. Even mild to moderate deficiencies can affect a person's well-being and development. In addition to affecting human health, hidden hunger can curtail socio-economic development, particularly in low and middle income countries.

The nature of the malnutrition burden facing the world is increasingly complex. Developing countries are moving from traditional diets based on minimally processed foods to highly processed, energy-dense, micronutrient-poor foods and drinks, which lead to obesity and diet-related chronic diseases. With this nutrition transition, many developing countries face a phenomenon known as the "triple burden" of malnutrition-undernourishment, micronutrient deficiencies, and obesity. In higher income, more urbanized countries, hidden hunger can co-exist with overweight/ obesity when a person consumes too much dietary energy from macronutrients such as fats and carbohydrates. While it may seem paradoxical, an obese child can suffer from hidden hunger.

The consequences of hidden hunger on the different stages of lifecycle are shown in Fig. 2.

Reproductive health and poverty reduction

Reproductive health has a significant role in poverty reduction and it is expected that successful programmes to promote reproductive health will contribute to the reduction of healthy year of life lost and hence the poverty reduction in equal measure. In addition to reduction of mortality and morbidity, reproductive health programmes address to unmet needs for family planning, relieving the poor of the burden of unwanted pregnancies and large families; they provide much-needed information and services to promote sexual health and responsible behaviour among adolescents and young people; and they promote gender equality and women's empowerment which is necessary for the success of reproductive health interventions. In doing so, these programmes contribute directly to the Millennium Development Goals of United Nations *(49)*. Fig. 3 shows how reproductive health can be used as a tool to poverty reduction.

Poverty is the most obvious problem in India. According to 2011–12 estimate about 22 per cent (270 million) population of the country was living below the "poverty line". The *"poverty line"* is defined as expenditure required for a daily Calorie intake of 2,400 per person in rural areas and 2,100 in urban areas. On the basis of these calculations, for the year 2000, the poverty line for a person was fixed at Rs. 328 per month for rural areas and Rs. 454 for the urban areas *(44)*.

STANDARD OF LIVING

Please see page 787 for details.

SOCIAL SECURITY

Social security is defined as "security that society furnishes through appropriate organization, against certain risks to which its members are exposed". The risks which social security covers in most countries are **sickness, invalidity, maternity, old age and death.** Social security also includes social insurance and social assistance.

Social security for Industrial workers

The social security measures for industrial workers in India are contained in the following legislations :

(1) Workmen's Compensation Act, 1923

(2) Central Maternity Benefit Act, 1961

(3) Employees State Insurance Act, 1948

(4) The Family Pension Scheme, 1971

Some of these Acts have been described elsewhere in the text.

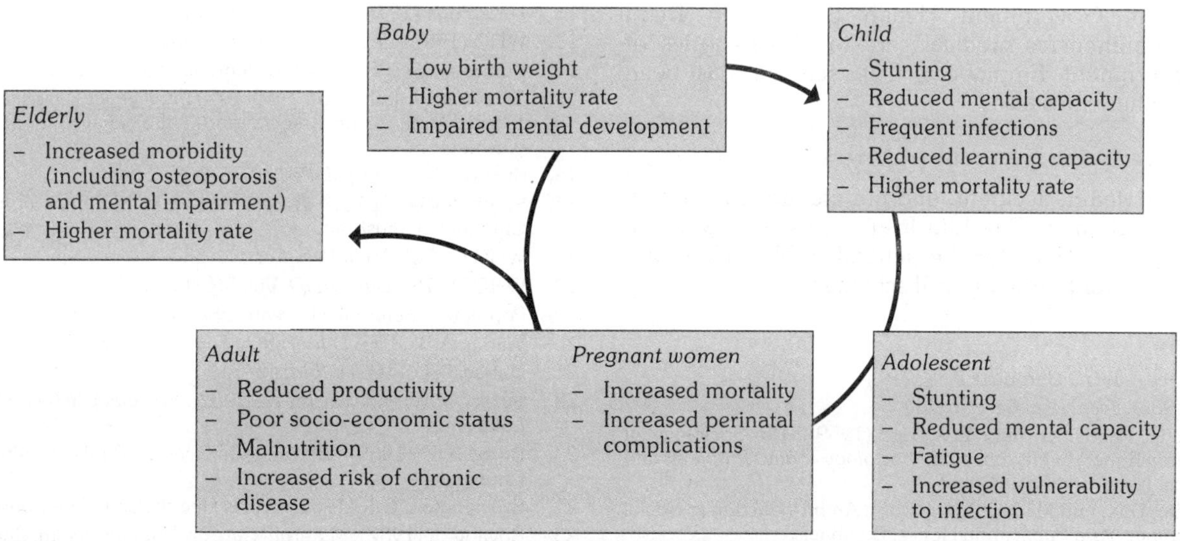

FIG. 2

Consequences of micronutrient deficiencies throughout the lifecycle

Source : *(50)*

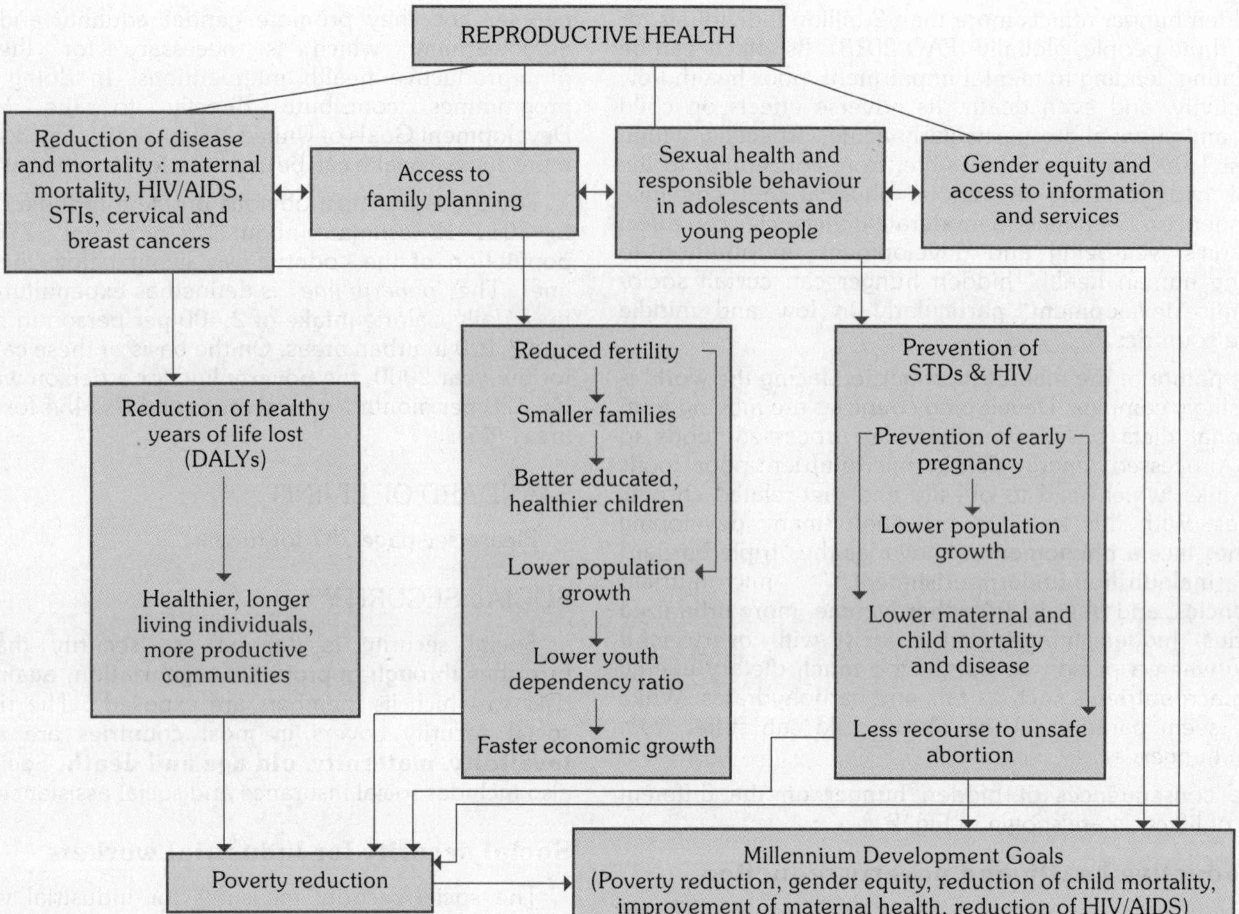

FIG. 3
Reproductive health as a poverty reduction strategy

Source : *(49)*

Social security for civil servants

The employees of the Central and State Government have pension, gratuity, provident fund and family pension schemes.

The Central Government Health Scheme in Delhi provides comprehensive medical care to all categories of Central Government Employees. The scheme has been extended to other cities also.

Social security for general public

The risks of death, accident, and fire etc. are covered by the Insurance schemes. The Life Insurance Corporation of India has many schemes for the general public. There are also public provident fund and ESI schemes.

References

1. WHO (1976). *WHO Chronicle* 3 : 337–9.
2. WHO (1986), *Tech. Rep. Ser.* No. 731.
3. George, G. Reader & Mary E.W.Goss (1959). The Sociology of Medicine in Robert K. Merton, et.al., *Sociology Today : Problems and Prospects,* New York, Basic Books.
4. Majumdar, D.N. and Madan, T.N. (1956). *An Introduction to Social Anthropology,* Asia Publication House, Bombay.
5. Dakshinamurthy, S. (1961). *J. Indian M.A.* 36, 520.
6. Hawkins, Norman G. (1958). *Medical Sociology,* Charles C. Thomas, USA.
7. Bottomore, T.B. (1964). *Sociology – A Guide to Problems and Literature,* Unwin University Books, London.
8. WHO (1974). *Tech. Rep. Ser.* No. 558.
9. Burton, Benedict (1966). *The Eugenics Review,* 58, 71.
10. Basu, M.N. (1967). *Sociology,* The World Press Pvt. Ltd., Calcutta.
11. Suchman, E.A. (1963). *Sociology and the Field of Public Health,* Russel Sage Foundation, New York.
12. Hira Singh (1976). *Social Defence,* 12 (45), 1.
13. WHO (1987). *Tech. Rep. Ser.* No. 755.
14. Kumar, K.J. (1987). *Mass Communication in India.*
15. Thurstone, L.L. (1946). *Theories of Intelligence, Science Monthly,* 5. 175–197, American Association for the Advancement of Science, Washington.
16. Steisel, I.N. (1969). *J. Pediat,* 75, 969.
17. Smith Alwyn (1985). *Recent Advances in Community Medicine,* Churchill Livingstone.
18. WHO (1976). *Tech. Rep. Ser.* No. 587.
19. WHO (1978). *Bull. WHO,* Vol. 56, No.3.

19A. Population Reference Bureau, USA, March 2012.

20. Wadia, A.B. (1967). *Journal of Family Welfare,* 14, 9.
21. Dubey, D.C. (1967). *Ibid,* 42–51.
22. Susser, M.W. and Watson W. (1962). *Sociology in Medicine,* Oxford, London.
23. Burn, J.L. (1959). *Recent Advances in Public Health,* 2nd Ed., Churchill.
24. Brockington, C.F. (1967). *World Health,* Churchill, London.
25. Bowlby, J. (1952). *Maternal Care and Mental Health,* 2nd Ed., WHO Monograph Series No.2 Geneva.
26. Royal College of Physicians, London (1971). *Smoking and Health Now,* Pitman, London.
27. Peel, John and Potts, Malcom (1970). *Textbook of Contraceptive Practice,* Cambridge University Press.

27A. International Labour Office (2012), *International Standard Classification of Occupation (ISCO–08),* structure, group definitions and correspondance tables, Vol. 1.

28. Kappu Swamy, B. (1976). *Manual of Socio-economic Status Scale (Urban),* Manasayan, 32, Netaji Subhash Marg, Delhi–6.

29. Kulshreshtha, S.P. (1975). *Manual for Socio-economic Status Scale,* National Psychological Corporation, Labh Chand Market, Raja Mandi, Agra–2.

30. Kumar, N. et al (2007). *Indian Journal of Paediatrics,* Vol. 74-Dec. 2007, letter to editor.

31. Mishra, D., Singh, H.P. (2003). *Indian Journal of Paediatrics,* Kuppuswamy's socio-economic status scale - A revision, (2003), 70 (3).

32. Govt. of India (2022). *National Family Health Survey-5,* 2019–2021, vol. 1, Ministry of Health and Family Welfare.

33. Willson, Robert, N. (1963). *"The Social Structure of a General Hospital" in Medicine and Society,* The Annuals of the American Academy of Political and Social Science, 346, 67.

34. Roemer, Milton, I (1963). *Ibid,* 44–56.

35. Fuchs, V.R. (1970). *Arch.Intern.Med.,* 125, 154.

36. Menke, W.G. (1970). *Ann.Intern.Med.,* 72, 943.

37. Hasan, K.A. (1967). *The Cultural Frontier of Health in Village India,* Manaktalas, Bombay.

38. Bates, B. (1970). *N. Eng. J. Med.* 283, 129.

39. WHO (1995). The *World Health Report* 1995, Bridging the gaps, Report of the Director–General WHO.

40. Bajpai, S.R. (1960). *Methods of Social Survey and Research,* Kitab Ghar, Kanpur.

41. Bailey, N.T.J. (1962). *"Operational Research" in Society – Problems and Methods of Study,* Eds, Welford, A.T. et. al., Routledge and Kagan Paul, London.

42. WHO (1972). The *Use of Operational Research in Health Services,* Regional Office for Europe, Copenhagen.

43. Govt. of India (2006). *Health Information of India 2005,* Ministry of Health & Family Welfare, New Delhi.

44. Current affairs, December 2016 e Book, *Poverty and Poverty Line in India.*

45. WHO (2003). *Health Situation in South-East Asia, Basic Indicators 2002.*

46. WHO (1984). *Public Health Papers* No.77.

47. WHO (2018). *World Health Statistics,* 2018.

48. World Bank (1993). *World Development Report.*

49. UNPF (2002). *Promoting Reproductive Health as a Poverty Reduction Strategy,* Nov. 2002.

50. *Global Hunger Index (2014).* The Challenge of Hidden Hunger.

51. UNICEF (2019). *The State of World's Children,* 2019.

52. UNICEF (2021). *The State of World's Children,* 2021.

13 Tribal Health in India

Underprivileged, who need more, get less

The term "Scheduled Tribes" first appeared in the constitution of India. Article 366 (25) defined scheduled tribes as "such tribes or tribal communities or parts of or groups within such tribes or tribal communities as are deemed under Article 342 to be Scheduled Tribes for the purpose of this constitution". The list is state/UT specific and a community declared as a scheduled tribe in one state need not be so in another state.

Over 104 million tribal people live in India spread across 705 tribes, and account for 8.6 per cent of the country's population *(1)*. Tribal people have remained marginal-geographically, socio-economically, politically and therefore, health and healthcare in tribal areas remained unsolved problem.

Demographic Profile

The tribal population are largely concentrated in ten states and in 8 North-East states. Nearly 90 per cent of the tribal population live in rural areas. Numerically, Madhya Pradesh has the largest tribal population (15 million), followed by Maharashtra (10 million), Odisha (9 million) and Rajasthan (9 million). However the concentration of tribal population is highest amongst the North-East states. They mostly live in hilly and forested areas.

The population of tribal males is 52.5 million and females is 52.0 million. The total fertility rate is 2.48, which is within reasonable limit and the decline in total fertility rate is comparable to other populations in some major states. The sex ratio in 2011 was 990, which is higher than the national average of 943. The child sex ratio of STs in 0-6 years age group has declined from 972 in 2001 to 957 in 2011 census, but still it is higher than the general population at 914 girls to 1000 boys *(2)*.

Literacy rate : As per census data, literacy rate for STs in India has improved from 47.1 per cent in 2001 to 59 per cent in 2011. The male literacy rate has increased from 59.2 to 68.5 per cent and female literacy rate increased from 34.8 per cent to 49.4 per cent during the same period. Table 1 compares the literacy rate in STs and all India population.

TABLE 1

Literacy rate among STs and all India population

Year	All India			Scheduled Tribes		
	Persons	Males	Females	Persons	Males	Females
1961	28.30	40.40	15.35	8.53	13.83	3.16
1971	34.45	45.96	21.97	11.30	17.63	4.85
1981	43.57	56.38	29.76	16.35	24.52	8.04
1991	52.21	64.13	39.29	29.60	40.65	18.19
2001	64.84	75.26	53.67	47.10	59.17	34.76
2011	73.00	80.90	64.60	59.00	68.50	49.40

Source : *(2)*

Life expectancy

The life expectancy at birth for ST population in India is 63.9 years, as against 67 years for the general population *(1)*.

Reproductive, maternal, newborn, child health and adolescent (RMNCH+A) strategy (1):

No recent estimates for maternal mortality among tribal women are available separately. Early marriage, early child birth, low BMI and high incidence of anaemia are known factors for high maternal mortality. The 68.0 per cent rate of institutional delivery is much lower than the national average of 78.9 per cent. 71.5 per cent deliveries are conducted by skilled health personnel. Coverage of post-natal care remains poor. Only about 37 per cent tribal women reported receiving any postnatal care within 48 hours after home delivery.

As per NFHS-5, the estimated infant mortality rate for scheduled tribe was 41.6, 1–4 year child mortality rate was 9.0, under five mortality rate 50.3, and neonatal mortality rate 28.8 per 1000 live births. The time trend shows a major improvement in the mortality rates.

Immunization coverage of the tribal children remains lower than the total population as shown in Table 2.

The percentage of stunting, wasting and underweight in tribal children has reduced but malnutrition (micro-malnutrition and macro-malnutrition) is still higher than in all population children as shown in Table 2.

The burden of disease in tribal community

Epidemiological transition is taking place in tribal areas also, as in rest of country. The health care needs of the tribal people is much more than RMNCH+A. The tribal population in the country faces a triple burden of diseases. While malnutrition and communicable diseases like malaria and tuberculosis continue to be rampant, rapid urbanization, environmental distress and changing lifestyles have resulted in a rise in the prevalence of non-communicable diseases like cancer, hypertension and diabetes. To add to this is the third burden i.e. of mental illnesses, especially the addictions.

TABLE 2

Comparison of some MCH indicators in ST and all population (2019–2021)

Indicator	ST	All population
A. *Child mortality indicators per 1000*		
Infant mortality rate	41.7	35.2
Neonatal mortality rate	28.8	24.9
Post neonatal mortality rate	12.9	10.3
Under-5 mortality rate	50.3	41.9
Child mortality rate	9.0	6.9
B. *Immunization services*		
Infants fully immunized %	76.8	76.6
No vaccination	4.1	3.6
Measles	86.7	87.9
Pentavalent 1	92.9	93.6
Pentavalent 3	85.9	85.5
Polio 1	92.2	92.4
Polio 3	80.4	80.5
BCG	94.3	95.2
Hep. B1	89.7	91.5
Hep. B3	81.2	88.6
Polio 0 dose	84.5	85.5
Hep. B 0 dose	67.0	67.4
Pregnant women TT	79.0	85.5
C. *Nutritional status*		
Under-5 years children stunted	40.9	35.5
Under-5 years children wasted	23.2	19.3
Under-5 years children underweight	39.5	32.1
D. *Maternal Health*		
Institutional delivery %	68.0	88.6
Deliveries attended by skilled health personnel %	71.5	89.4
Total fertility rate	2.09	1.99
Couple using any contraceptive %	64.4	66.7

ST - Scheduled Tribe

Source : *(3)*

1. Communicable diseases

The tribal population bears a disproportionate burden of communicable diseases. These include tuberculosis, malaria, leprosy, sexually transmitted diseases, AIDS/HIV, skin infections, diarrhoeal diseases, hepatitis etc.

a. Tuberculosis :

The estimated prevalence of pulmonary tuberculosis in tribal community is significantly higher than in the rest of the country, i.e., 703 against 256 per 100,000 population *(1)*. RNTCP provides free diagnosis and treatment to all the patients. The programme has started the newer interventions like active case finding to improve the case detection rate in hard to reach areas. Around 40,000 tribal patients have been diagnosed and treated under RNTCP since 2015 *(4)*. To improve access to tribal and other marginalized groups, there is provision for: (a) Additional TB Units and Designated Microscopy Centres (DMC) in tribal/difficult areas; (b) Compensation for transportation of patient & attendant in tribal areas; (c) Higher rate of salary to contractual staff posted in tribal areas; (d) Enhanced vehicle maintenance and travel allowance in tribal areas; and (e) Provision of TB Health Visitors (TBHVs) for urban areas.

The programme would intensify its case finding activities through systematic active TB screening among clinically and socially vulnerable population in campaign mode. Here the tribal districts of the state are mapped among vulnerable population and door to door case finding efforts are carried out. Phase 1 of the campaign was executed in January, 2017 and the 2nd Phase was implemented in July-August 2017. During this campaign, the programme screened more than 72,000 target tribal population across the country and diagnosed 27 additional TB cases.

The most significant aspect of the project is the deployment of the Mobile TB Diagnostic Van (MTDV) equipped with X-ray facilities and Sputum Microscopy facilities which offer diagnostic services for Tuberculosis at the doorstep of the patient's home in difficult to reach areas of the tribal populations. This project has been initially undertaken in 5 States (Madhya Pradesh, Gujarat, Chhattisgarh, Rajasthan and Jharkhand) in 17 districts. 35 MTDVs have been fabricated for this purpose.

The project covers a total population of approximately 17.65 million. This intervention is expected to improve the 'Standard of Care' among the extremely deprived populations. The efforts are expected to improve early seeking of care, reduction in out of pocket expenditure of individual patients and curbing of individual patients being directed to multiple providers for treatment which results in huge economic burden to patients and their families.

b. Leprosy :

Under the national leprosy eradication programme, state wise disaggregated data of tribal population is collected on monthly basis. During the year 2016–17, out of 1,35,485 new leprosy cases detected, 25,474 (18.90%) were scheduled tribes and 25,449 (18.78%) were scheduled castes.

Facilities for Scheduled Castes and Scheduled Tribes : Leprosy services are uniformly available to all including scheduled castes & scheduled tribes population irrespective of caste and religion. Under the programme, funds are allotted to NGOs, who are encouraged to work in tribal areas for providing services like IEC, prevention of deformity and follow up of cases. Intensified IEC activities have been taken up through various media including the rural media under which population residing in remote, inaccessible and tribal areas is being covered.

c. Malaria and other vector borne diseases

Although tribal communities constitute only about 8% of the national population, they account for about 30% of all cases of malaria, more than 60% of *P. falciparum*, and as much as 50% of the mortality associated with malaria.

Under National Vector Borne Disease Control Programme, services for prevention and control of Malaria, Kala-azar, Filaria, Japanese Encephalitis, Dengue/Dengue Haemorrhagic Fever (DHF) and Chikungunya, are provided to all sections of the community without any discrimination. However, since vector borne diseases are more prevalent in low socio-economic groups, focussed attention is given to areas dominated by the tribal population in North Eastern States and parts of Andhra Pradesh, Chhattisgarh, Gujarat, Jharkhand, Karnataka, Madhya Pradesh, Maharashtra and Odisha. Additional inputs under externally assisted projects from Global fund to North Eastern states and from World Bank to other states, especially for control of Malaria are provided. For Kala-azar elimination in the states of Bihar, Jharkhand and West Bengal, World Bank support is also being provided. In addition, North Eastern states are being provided 100% central assistance for implementation of the programme *(6)*.

2. Non-communicable diseases

The evidence of an early epidemiologic transition in tribal areas and associated increase in the incidence of non-communicable diseases is being observed.

(a) Hypertension:

One out of every four tribal adults suffer from hypertension. Further the prevalence of hypertension increases significantly with age, consumption of tobacco, alcohol and a sedentary lifestyle. Yet two out three tribal adult men and women did not know the signs and symptoms of the ailment. Only 5 per cent men and 9 per cent women suffering from hypertension knew their hypertensive status.

(b) Blindness and visual impairment:

The national programme for control of blindness and visual impairment is a centrally sponsored scheme (60:40 in all states and 90:10 in NE states) with the goal to reduce the prevalence of blindness to 0.3 per cent by 2020. The benefits of the scheme are meant for all including SC/ST population as per the need. The following initiatives have been implemented under NPCBVI, keeping in view the needs of NE states including Sikkim, which are tribal predominant *(6)*:

- Assistance for construction of dedicated eye units in North-Eastern states including Sikkim and other hilly states,
- Appointment of contractual ophthalmic manpower (ophthalmic surgeons, ophthalmic assistants and eye donation counsellors) to meet shortage of ophthalmic manpower in states,
- Assistance for setting up of multipurpose district mobile ophthalmic units for diagnosis and medical management of eye diseases for coverage in difficult areas,
- Besides cataract, assistance for treatment and management of other eye diseases viz. diabetic retinopathy, glaucoma, refractive errors corneal transplantation, vitreo-retinal surgery and childhood blindness, is provided.

3. Genetic disorders

The prevalence of sickle cell disease (anaemia and trait together) and thalassaemia – another genetic disorder – varies between 1–40 per cent in different tribal communities. However, most of the prevalence is due to the heterozygous form of the disease. Sickle cell anaemia, the more serious form, is prevalent in 1 in 86 births among tribal communities in central India *(1)*.

Another genetic disease prevalent in many tribal groups in India is the G6PD deficiency. Among the 14 primitive tribal populations from four different states showing a high frequency of sickle gene, the prevalence of G6PD deficiency varied from 0.7 to 15.6 per cent *(1)*.

4. Mental health and addictions :

Almost 72 per cent of the tribal men in 15–54 years age group use tobacco as compared to 56 per cent non-tribal men and about 50 per cent tribal men consume some form of alcohol *(5)*. Tobacco and alcohol, both are risk factors for non-communicable diseases and cause serious diseases, and increases mortality. They reduce productivity and increase poverty, disrupt family harmony and generate law and order problems.

5. Animal attacks and violence in conflict areas

As tribal areas are often surrounded by forests, animal bites from snakes, dogs and scorpions are common.

Health care infrastructure and tribal development

Tribal development has been a challenge to the planners and policy makers since independence. This is mainly on account of their traditional life styles, remoteness of habitation, dispersed population and displacement. Tribal sub-plan (TSP) strategy now known on Scheduled Tribal Component (STC), was adopted in 5th Five year plan for accelerated development of tribal people. Ministry of Tribal Affairs and Ministry of Health and Family welfare are making efforts through tailored educational, infrastructural and livelihood schemes for the improvement in terms of various indicators relating to literacy, health and socio-economic status etc. However, there is still significant gap in human development indicators between scheduled tribes and all category group *(2)*.

Facilities for scheduled tribes under National Health Mission *(5)*

Health Care Infrastructure

As per the present norms, tribal and hilly areas should have one Health Sub-centre (HSC) per 3,000 population, one Primary Health Centre (PHC) per 20,000 population, and a Community Health Centre (CHC) per 80,000 population. Data on 'required versus shortfall' of sub-centres, PHCs and CHCs in tribal areas of 18 states and three UTs was studied. Data in 18 states showed:

Sub-centres: In seven states no shortfall in number of HSCs against the required number was observed. In the remaining 11 states, a shortfall of 4,996 sub-centres i.e. 27 per cent of the required numbers in these states was noted.

PHCs: No shortfall existed in 11 states. In the remaining seven deficient states a shortfall was noted of 1,023 PHCs which was 40% of the required number in these states.

CHCs: In eight states, there was no shortfall. In the remaining 10 states a shortfall of 209 CHCs was observed. The shortfall accounted for 31% of the required number of CHCs in these states.

Among the UTs an 8% shortfall in Sub-centres and of 1 CHC (against the requirement of 1) was reported from Dadra and Nagar Haveli. No other shortfall was noted at any level. Thus in about half of the states, the health institutions in tribal areas were deficient in number by 27 to 40 per cent as compared to the present norms.

Health Human Resource (HHR)

A huge gap in human resources in health centres in tribal areas is attributed to reasons such as limited scope for professional interaction or growth for the staff, a feeling of social and professional isolation, weak human resource policies, poor working conditions and environment in the government health institutions, limited social infrastructure, etc. Various states have tried different measures to overcome this shortage of doctors, but the problem persists. Several states have introduced a bond for compulsory rural service, but it is flouted by most of the doctors completing MBBS. The medical education and the health departments seem unwilling or unable to enforce the execution of the bond.

The Ministry of Health and Family Welfare (MoHFW) and the Ministry of Tribal Affairs (MoTA), in October 2013, jointly constituted an expert committee on tribal health, under the chairmanship of Dr. Abhay Bang. It had as its members prominent academicians, civil society members and policy makers who have long been working with the tribal people. The expert committee suggests following measures to improve human resources for tribal health *(5)*:

1. Features of tribal society demand that the health care provider, as far as possible, should be a local tribal. The present health workforce pattern is opposite of this.
2. The only way of effecting a vibrant, responsive and accessible health workforce in the tribal areas in a sustained manner, is by ensuring that local tribal people are trained and deployed in the health force.
3. It is important to place the centre of gravity of the workforce not at the top – the specialists and doctors - but closer to the communities.

The ASHA in tribal areas should have an expanded role. Eight type of functions and total 4 hours of work per-day is expected from tribal ASHAs.

Mid-level care providers should be created through bridge courses and placed at the sub-centres.

To attract doctors to work in tribal areas, the total salary of MOs needs to be substantially increased.

To provide doctors dedicated to work in tribal areas, the committee recommended creation of dedicated medical colleges in tribal districts, exclusively for tribal students in the scheduled areas.

References

1. Govt. of India, *Report of the Expert Committee on Tribal Health,* Tribal health in India, Bridging the gap and a roadmap for the future, Executive Summary and Recommendations, Ministry of Health and Family Welfare, New Delhi and Ministry of Tribal Affairs New Delhi.
2. Govt. of India (2018), *Annual Report 2017–2018,* Ministry of Tribal Affairs New Delhi.
3. Govt. of India (2022), *National Family Health Survey-5 Report,* Ministry of Health and Family Welfare, New Delhi.
4. Govt. of India (2018), *Annual Report 2017–2018,* Ministry of Health and Family Welfare, New Delhi.
5. Govt. of India, *Tribal Health in India, Policy Brief,* Report of the Expert Committee on Tribal Health, Bridging the gap and a roadmap for the future, Ministry of Health and Family Welfare, New Delhi and Ministry of Tribal Affairs, New Delhi.
6. Govt. of India (2020), *Annual Report 2019–2020,* Ministry of Health and Family Welfare, New Delhi.

14 Sustainable Development Goals

"Sabka saath, Sabka vikas"

In December 2015, the Millennium Development Goals (MDGs) came to the end of their term, and a post–2015 Agenda, comprising of 17 Sustainable Development Goals (SDGs) took their place. World stood at the threshold of a new era as on 1st January 2016, the SDGs of the 2030 Agenda for Sustainable Development officially came into force. While progress towards the MDGs has been impressive in many ways, much work remains to be done. In health, unprecedented progress has been made in reducing maternal and child mortality and in the fight against infectious diseases; even though several global and country MDG targets were not met. The dramatic progress of MDGs paved the way for more ambitious achievements by 2030. Notable among them are the challenges of acute epidemic diseases, disasters, conflict situations, the newly spreading epidemic of non-communicable diseases, mental health disorders, and large inequalities in all parts of the world. The new goals are unique in that they call for action by all countries to promote prosperity while protecting the planet. They recognize that ending poverty must go hand-in-hand with strategies that build economic growth and addresses a range of social needs including education, health, social protection, raising basic standard of living, job opportunities, while tackling climate changes and environmental protection. The five Ps of the new agenda are people, planet, prosperity, peace and partnership.

The sustainable development has been defined as "development that meets the needs of the present without compromising the ability of future generations to meet their own needs" *(2)*. Implementation of SDGs and the success will rely on countries sustainable development policies, plans and programmes. It will require resource mobilization and financing strategies. All stakeholders : governments, civil societies, the private sector, and others are expected to contribute to the realization of the new agenda.

The 2030 Agenda is designed to benefit all. Universal in scope, the agenda will require a comprehensive, integrated approach to sustain development, as well as collective action at all levels. "Leaving no one behind" will be an overarching theme. The paragraph 26 of the 2030 agenda addresses health as follows :

> *"To promote physical and mental health and well-being, and to extend life expectancy for all, we must achieve universal health coverage and access to quality health care. No one must be left behind. We commit to accelerating the progress made to date in reducing newborn, child and maternal mortality by ending all such preventable deaths before 2030. We are committed to ensuring universal access to sexual and reproductive health-care services, including for family planning, information and education. We will equally accelerate the pace of progress made in fighting malaria, HIV/AIDS, tuberculosis, hepatitis, Ebola and other communicable diseases and epidemics, including by addressing growing anti-microbial resistance and the problem of unattended diseases affecting developing countries. We are committed to the prevention and treatment of non-communicable diseases, including behavioural, developmental and neurological disorders, which constitute a major challenge for sustainable development" (1).*

Health is centrally positioned within the 2030 Agenda, with one comprehensive goal – SDG 3 : Ensure healthy lives and promote well-being for all ages. Goal 3 includes 13 targets covering all major health priorities with four targets on the unfinished and expended millennium development goals, four targets to address non-communicable diseases, mental health, injuries and environmental issues and four "means-of-implementation" targets. The Universal Health Coverage (UHC) is the key to achievement of all targets and development of strong resilient health system. The SDGs are not solely focussed on developing countries. Thus, while some targets and indicators may be more relevant for developing countries, SDG monitoring should in principle cover all.

Even though the 2030 Agenda refers several times to the term "human right(s)" (right to development, self determination, an adequate standard of living, food, water and sanitation, good governance and the rule of law), it does not specifically mention that health is a human right *(1)*.

Table 1 enumerates the 13 targets of goal 3 with their proposed indicators. It shows that millennium development goals on maternal mortality (3.1) child mortality (3.2) and infectious diseases (3.3) have been retained in SDG framework and expanded to include neonatal mortality and more infectious diseases such as hepatitis and waterborne diseases. The target on access to sexual and reproductive health care services (3.7) and access to vaccines and medicines (3.b) are also closely related to MDG targets. Sexual and reproductive rights are addressed under MDG 5 on gender equality. The SDGs include new targets on non-communicable diseases and mental health (3.4), substance abuse (3.5), injuries (3.6), health impact from hazardous

TABLE 1

Sustainable Development Goal 3 : Ensure healthy lives and promote well-being for all at all ages.

Goal and targets from the 2030 Agenda		Indicator	
3.1	By 2030, reduce the global maternal mortality ratio to less than 70 per 100,000 live births.	3.1.1 3.1.2	Maternal deaths per 100,000 live births. Global–217, India–103 (2017–19) Proportion of births attended by skilled health personnel. Global–84, India–89 (2012–2021)
3.2	By 2030, end preventable deaths of newborns and children under 5 years of age, with all countries aiming to reduce neonatal mortality to at least as low as 12 per 1,000 live births and under-5 mortality to at least as low as 25 per 1,000 live births.	3.2.1 3.2.2	Under-5 mortality rate (deaths per 1,000 live births) Global–37, India–33 (2020) Neonatal mortality rate (deaths per 1,000 live births) Global–17, India–20 (2020)
3.3	By 2030, end the epidemics of AIDS, tuberculosis, malaria and neglected tropical diseases and combat hepatitis, water-borne diseases and other communicable diseases.	3.3.1 3.3.2 3.3.3 3.3.4 3.3.5	Number of new HIV infections per 1,000 uninfected population (by age group, sex and key populations). Global–0.19%, India–0.04% (2020) Tuberculosis incidence per 1,000 persons per year. Global–127, India–188 (2020) Malaria incident cases per 1,000 persons at risk, per year. Global–59, India–3.2 (2020) Number of new hepatitis B infections per 100,000 population in a given year. The indicator used is infants receiving three doses of hepatitis B vaccine % Global–83, India–85 (2020) Number of people requiring interventions against neglected tropical diseases. Global–1733.6 million, India–751.7 million (2020)
3.4	By 2030, reduce by one third premature mortality from non-communicable diseases through prevention and treatment and promote mental health and well-being.	3.4.1 3.4.2	Mortality of cardiovasular disease, cancer, diabetes or chronic respiratory disease. Global–17.8%, India–21.9% (2019) Suicide mortality rate. Global–9.2, India–12.7 (2019)
3.5	Strengthen the prevention and treatment of substance abuse, including narcotic drug abuse and harmful use of alcohol.	3.5.1 3.5.2	Coverage of treatment interventions (pharmacological, psychosocial and rehabilitation and aftercare services) for substance use disorders. Harmful use of alcohol, defined according to the national context as alcohol per capita consumption (aged 15 years and older) within a calendar year in litres of pure alcohol. Global–5.8, India–5.6 (2019)
3.6	By 2020, halve the number of global deaths and injuries from road traffic accidents.	3.6.1	Number of road traffic fatal injury deaths within 30 days, per 100,000 population (age-standardized) Global–16.7, India–15.6 (2019)
3.7	By 2030, ensure universal access to sexual and reproductive health-care services, including for family planning, information and education, and the integration of reproductive health into national strategies and programmes.	3.7.1 3.7.2	Percentage of women of reproductive age (aged 15–49) who have their need for family planning satisfied with modern methods. Global–76.7, India–72.8 (2012–2020) Adolescent birth rate (aged 10–14; aged 15–19) per 1,000 women in that age group. Global–42.5, India–12.2 (2012–2020)
3.8	Achieve universal health coverage, including financial risk protection, access to quality essential health-care services and access to safe, effective, quality and affordable essential medicines and vaccines for all.	3.8.1 3.8.2	Coverage of tracer interventions (e.g. child full immunization, antiretroviral therapy, tuberculosis treatment, hypertension treatment, skilled attendant at birth, etc.) Fraction of the population protected against catastrophic/ impoverishing out-of-pocket health expenditure.
3.9	By 2030, substantially reduce the number of deaths and illnesses from hazardous chemicals and air, water and soil pollution and contamination.	3.9.1 3.9.2	Mortality rate attributed to household and ambient air pollution per lac population. Global–114.1, India–184.3 (2016) Mortality rate attributed to hazardous chemicals, water and soil pollution and contamination per lac population. Global–11.7, India–187 (2016)
3.a	Strengthen the implementation of the World Health Organization Framework Convention on Tobacco Control in all countries, as appropriate.	3.a.1	Age-standardized prevalence of current tobacco use among persons aged 15 years and older %. Global—India–male–20.6, female–1.9 (2016)
3.b	Support the research and development of vaccines and medicines for the communicable and non-communicable diseases that primarily affect developing countries, provide access to affordable essential medicines and vaccines, in accordance with the Doha Declaration on the TRIPS Agreement and Public Health, which affirms the right of developing countries to use to the full the provisions in the Agreement on Trade-Related Aspects of Intellectual Property Rights regarding flexibilities to protect public health, and, in particular, provide access to medicines for all.	3.b.1 3.b.2	Proportion of the population with access to affordable medicines and vaccines on a sustainable basis. Total net official development assistance to the medical research and basic health sectors.
3.c	Substantially increase health financing and the recruitment, development, training and retention of the health workforce in developing countries, especially in least developed countries and small island developing states.	3.c.1.	Health worker density and distribution per 10,000 population. Global–25, India–30.2 (2006–13)
3.d	Strengthen the capacity of all countries, in particular developing countries, for early warning, risk reduction and management of national and global health risks.	3.d.1	Percentage of attributes of 13 core capacities that have been attained at a specific point in time. Global–71, India–95 (2010–17)

The indicator shows Global and Indian data.

Source : *(3, 4, 7)*

chemicals, water and soil pollution and contamination (3.9), and the implementation of the WHO framework convention on tobacco control (3.a). Target 3.d addresses reducing and managing national and global health risks, health financing and health work-force issue in least developed countries and small island developing states are addressed by target 3.c. Universal health care (UHC) is also a new target (3.8), which provides an overall framework for the implementation of a broad and ambitious agenda in all countries. UHC is the only target that cuts across all targets of health goal, as well as linked to health-related targets in other goals *(1)*.

Health is linked to many of the non-health goals, reflecting the fact that health affects and in turn is affected by many economic, social and environmental determinants. More than a dozen targets in other goals can be considered health-related and should be given special attention in strategies, policies and plans to achieve the health goal and in monitoring progress. Table 2 shows the targets in other goals linked to health SDG 3.

At the global level the SDGs will be monitored and reviewed using a set of global indicators developed by the Inter Agency and Expert Group on SDG Indicators. The governments will also develop their own national indicators to assist in monitoring progress made on the goals and targets.

Almost all targets of goal 3 can be linked to strategies and global action plans that have been adopted by the World Health Assembly in recent years or are under development. However, there are few gaps, e.g., there is no mention of immunization coverage as a specific target although it is integral to the achievement of at least four targets that are listed. Access to sexual and reproductive health care is included, but sexual and reproductive rights, violence and discrimination against women and girls are dealt with elsewhere (goal 5), older people are mentioned in goal 2. The ageing population as an important implication for health system is absent except indirectly through its impact on non-communicable diseases and mental health.

TABLE 2

Examples of targets in other goals linked to the health SDG 3

Target	Description
1.3	Implement nationally appropriate social protection systems and measures for all, including floors, and by 2030 achieve substantial coverage of the poor and the vulnerable.
2.2	By 2030, end all forms of malnutrition, including achieving, by 2025, the internationally agreed targets on stunting and wasting in children under five years of age, and address the nutritional needs of adolescent girls, pregnant and lactating women and older persons.
4.2	By 2030, ensure that all girls and boys have access to quality early childhood development, care and pre-primary education so that they are ready for primary education.
4.a	Build and upgrade education facilities that are child, disability and gender sensitive and provide safe, non-violent, inclusive and effective learning environments for all.
5.2	Eliminate all forms of violence against all women and girls in the public and private spheres, including trafficking and sexual and other types of exploitation.
5.3	Eliminate all harmful practices, such as child, early and forced marriage and female genital mutilation.
5.6	Ensure universal access to sexual and reproductive health and reproductive rights as agreed in accordance with the Programme of Action of the International Conference on Population and Development and the Beijing Platform for Action and the outcome documents of their review conferences.
6.1	By 2030, achieve universal and equitable access to safe and affordable drinking water to all.
6.2	By 2030, achieve access to adequate and equitable sanitation and hygiene for all and end open defecation, paying special attention to the needs of women and girls and those in vulnerable situations.
6.3	By 2030, improve water quality by reducing pollution, eliminating dumping and minimizing release of hazardous chemicals and materials, halving the proportion of untreated wastewater and substantially increasing recycling and safe reuse globally.
10.4	Adopt policies, especially fiscal, wage and social protection policies, and progressively achieve greater equality.
11.5	By 2030, significantly reduce the number of deaths and the number of people affected and substantially decrease the direct economic losses relative to global gross domestic product caused by disasters, including water-related disasters, with a focus on protecting the poor and people in vulnerable situations.
16.1	Significantly reduce all forms of violence and related death rates everywhere.
16.2	End abuse, exploitation, trafficking and all forms of violence against and torture of children.
16.6	Develop effective accountable and transparent institutions at all levels.
16.9	By 2030, provide legal identity for all, including birth registration.
17.18	By 2020, enhance capacity-building support to developing countries, including for least-developed countries and small island developing states, to increase significantly the availability of high-quality, timely and reliable data disaggregated by income, gender, age, race, ethnicity, migratory status, disability, geographic location and other characteristics relevant in national contexts.

Source : *(1)*

Fig. 1 presents these targets in a way that distinguishes those that have been carried forward and enhanced from the MDGs, those that have been added and those that are means of implementation.

Reproductive, maternal, newborn and child health

Multiple targets in SDG 3 and other goals refer to reproductive, maternal, newborn and child health (RMNCH). These include targets for mortality, service coverage, risk factors and health determinants (Table 3). The global strategy for Women's, Children's and Adolescent's Health, 2016–2030 is fully aligned with the SDG target and is organized around the broad themes of "Survive-Thrive-Transform". It is an example of how a range of health and health-related goals and targets must be addressed to improve health and well-being of women, children and adolescents.

New in the SDGs is the emphasis on youth as a vulnerable population. Though, generally a healthy group, adolescents are exposed to a range of risks and diseases. As many health behaviours established during adolescence have profound effect over rest of the life course, they are a population deserving more concerted attention. Globally, road injuries, HIV/AIDS and self-harm are the leading causes of adolescent death.

Reproductive, maternal, newborn and child health is one of the four categories of the universal health coverage indicators: family planning, antenatal care (four visits or more) with skilled attendance at birth; full child immunization coverage and health-seeking behaviour for suspected child pneumonia. The indicator for SDG target 2.2 on ending all forms of malnutrition are focussed on stunting, wasting and overweight among children under 5 years of age. Children are at greater risk of stunting if they are born in rural areas, poor household or to mothers

TABLE 3

Selected SDG targets and proposed indicators linked to reproductive, maternal, newborn and child health, by type of indicator

Type of Indicator	SDG target	Proposed indicator
Impact	3.1	Maternal mortality
	3.2	Under-five mortality
	3.2	Neonatal mortality
	3.7	Adolescent birth rate
	3.9	Mortality due to unsafe water, sanitation and hygiene; Mortality due to air pollution (household and ambient)
Coverage	3.1	Births attended by skilled health personnel
	3.7	Family planning coverage
	3.8	UHC:RMNCH 3 tracers (family planning, antenatal and delivery care, full immunization coverage, health-seeking behaviour for suspected child pneumonia)
	37 (22)	Model life table systems
Risk factors/ determinants	2.2	Child stunting, child wasting, child overweight
	6.1	Access to safely managed drinking-water source
	6.2	Access to safely managed sanitation
	7.1	Clean household energy
	11.6	Ambient air pollution
	Other	Part of targets in goals on poverty, education, gender etc.

RMNCH - reproductive, maternal, newborn and child health
UHC – Universal health care.

Source : *(2)*

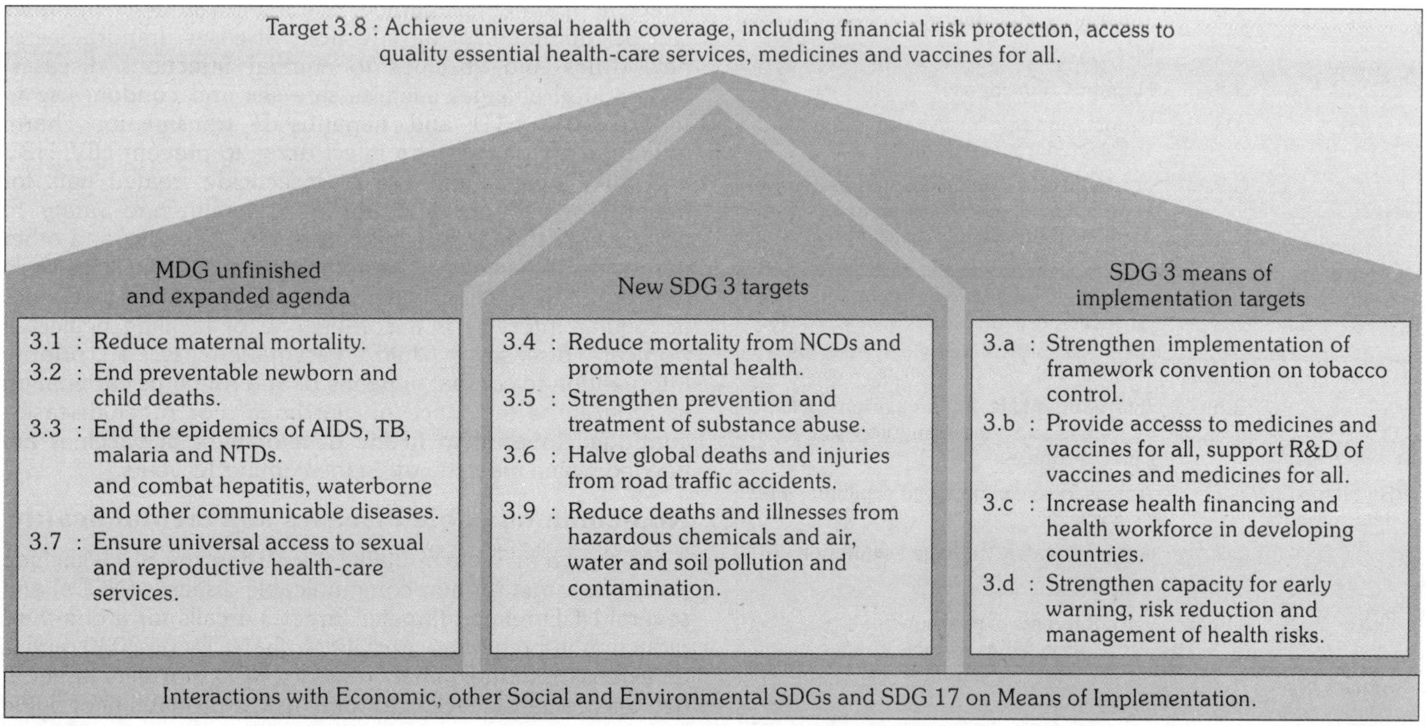

FIG. 1

Framework for the SDG health goal and targets.

Source : *(1)*

denied basic education. Several environmental targets and indicators are also relevant to this group. They include water and sanitation, and air pollution (causes for diarrhoea and pneumonia in under 5 age group).

Infectious diseases

The main target relating to infectious diseases is SDG 3.3, which refers to ending the epidemic of AIDS, tuberculosis, malaria and neglected tropical diseases, and combating hepatitis, water-borne diseases and other communicable diseases. Table 4 shows the selected targets and proposed indicators linked to infectious diseases by type of indicator.

The SDG targets for infectious diseases are very ambitious, but are in line with what a number of disease-specific strategies and World Health Assembly resolutions have already been exploring. For all infectious diseases, the targetted reductions aimed at progressing towards elimination goals in the coming 15 years far outstrip what has been achieved since 2000.

New strategies include *(1)* :

- UNAIDS global strategy fast track: Ending the AIDS epidemic by 2030 and the draft WHO Global Health Sector Strategy on HIV 2016–2021;
- The End TB strategy;
- Global technical strategy for Malaria 2016–2030;
- NTD roadmap, and water sanitation and hygiene for accelerating and sustaining progress on NTDs: A global strategy 2015–2020; and
- Draft global health sector strategy on viral hepatitis 2016–2021.

TABLE 4

Selected SDG targets and proposed indicators linked to infectious diseases, by type of indicator

Type of indicator	SDG target	Proposed indicator
Impact	3.3	HIV incidence
	3.3	Tuberculosis incidence
	3.3	Malaria incidence
	3.3	Hepatitis B incidence
	3.3	People requiring interventions against neglected tropical diseases
	3.9	Mortality due to unsafe water, sanitation and hygiene; mortality due to air pollution (household and ambient)
Coverage/ system	3.8	UHC : infectious diseases tracer (ART coverage, tuberculosis treatment, use of insecticide-treated nets, access to safely managed drinking-water source and sanitaiton)
	3.d	International Health Regulations (IHR) capacity and health emergency preparedness
Risk factors/ determinants	6.1	Access to safely managed drinking-water source
	6.2	Access to safely managed sanitation
	7.1	Clean household energy.
	Other	Part of targets in goals on poverty, education, cities, climate change etc.

Source : *(2)*

The strategies and related documents have proposed a number of more specific targets and indicators for monitoring progress towards the goals, linked to the overall SDG target as shown in Table 5.

TABLE 5

Summary of specific targets in global plans and other international agreements for SDG Target 3.3 on infectious diseases

	Specific plan-main targets 2030
Ending the epidemic of AIDS	Reduce the annual number newly infected with HIV by 90% and the annual number of people dying from AIDS-related causes by 80% (compared with 2010)
Ending the epidemic of TB	90% reduction in TB deaths 80% reduction in TB incidence rate (to less than 20 per 100,000 population) Zero TB-affected families facing catastrophic costs due to TB
Ending the epidemic of malaria	90% reduction in global malaria mortality rate 90% reduction in global malaria case incidence Malaria eliminated from at least 35 countries Re-establishment of malaria prevented in all countries identified as malaria-free
Ending the epidemic of NTDs	90% reduction in the number of people requiring interventions against NTDs
Control hepatitis	95% decline in new cases of chronic HBV infection between 2010 and 2030; 80% reduction in new cases of chronic HCV infection over the same period; 65% reduction in HBV- and HCV-related deaths.
Combat Water-borne diseases	No one practices open defecation (by 2025) Everyone uses a basic drinking-water supply and handwashing facilities at home Everyone uses adequate sanitation when at home (by 2040) All drinking-water supply, sanitation and hygiene services are delivered in progressively affordable, accountable and financially and environmentally sustainable manner

Source : *(1)*

The battle against infectious diseases need to focus on the preventive efforts complemented by rapid diagnosis and effective treatment. A number of common strategic priorities can be identified for all infectious diseases. Importance of new drugs and vaccines to combat infectious diseases; behavioural changes such as safe sex and condom use to reduce HIV, STD and hepatitis B transmission; harm reduction for people who inject drugs to prevent HIV, HBV and HCV acquisition; use of insecticide treated nets for malaria prevention; and improved health-care safety to reduce nosocomial transmission of HIV, hepatitis and other pathogens. Preventive chemotherapy based on large-scale delivery of free, safe, single-dose, quality-assured medicines at regular intervals is a cornerstone of tackling neglected tropical diseases. Child vaccination is a priority intervention to combat hepatitis B, and rotavirus vaccination to reduce the incidence of diarrhoea. For other diseases, continued investment in the development of vaccines are needed which may pay off in the coming 15 years.

Non-communicable diseases and mental health

As shown in Table 6, unlike the MDGs, the SDGs include a specific target for non-communicable diseases (NCDs) and several NCD-related targets. Target 3.4 calls for a one-third reduction in premature mortality from NCDs by 2030, and is an extension of the global voluntary NCD mortality target. It defines premature NCD mortality as the probability of dying from any of the main NCDs between the age 30 and 70 years. Other targets include : Target 3.a on improvements in tobacco control; target 3.5 on substance abuse, including harmful use of alcohol along with mental health; target 3.b on supporting research and development of vaccines and medicines for NCDs that primarily affect developing countries, as well as providing access to affordable essential medicines and vaccines for NCDs; and target 3.9 on deaths and illnesses related to hazardous chemicals, as well as air, water and soil pollution and contamination. Finally 3.8 target addresses universal health care which has implication for a wide range of NCD–related promotion, prevention and treatment interventions *(2)*.

TABLE 6

Selected SDG targets and proposed indicators linked to non-communicable diseases and mental health, by type of indicator

Type of indicator	SDG target	Proposed indicator
Impact	3.4	NCD mortality
	3.4	Suicide mortality
	3.9	Mortality due to air pollution (household and ambient)
Coverage/ risk factors	3.8	UHC: NCDs tracers (hypertension treatment coverage diabetes treatment coverage, cervical cancer screening; tobacco use)
	3.a	Tobacco use
	3.5	Substance abuse (harmful use of alcohol)
Risk factors/ determinants	7.1	Clean household energy
	11.6	Ambient air pollution
	Other	Part of targets in goals on poverty, education, cities, etc.

Source : *(2)*

Lack of awareness and late detection is an issue with all leading NCDs and it is essential to support and develop primary health-care services required for their early detection and management. An integrated approach to NCD care is more effective, e.g., the monitoring of blood pressure status should be integrated with monitoring of blood cholesterol and blood sugar. The prevention of heart attacks and strokes through a "total cardiovascular risk approach" is more cost-effective than treatment based on individual risk factor thresholds only, and should be part of the basic package of UHC.

The SDG targets for NCDs is based on previous UN and WHO declarations that provide strategic directions. In the year 2014 the UN General Assembly adopted Outcome Document on NCDs with national targets for 2025. Of these targets first target is closely linked to SDG target 3.4. The Global Voluntary Indicators are as follows *(1)*:

1. A 25% relative reduction in the risk of premature mortality from CVD, cancer, diabetes or CRD;
2. AT least 10% relative reduction in the harmful use of alcohol;
3. A 10% relative reduction in prevalence of insufficient physical activity;
4. A 30% relative reduction in mean population intake of salt/sodium;
5. A 30% relative reduction in prevalence of current tobacco use;
6. A 25% relative reduction in the prevalence of raised blood pressure;
7. Halt the rise in diabetes and obesity;
8. At least 50% of eligible people receive drug therapy and counselling (including glycaemic control) to prevent heart attacks and strokes; and
9. An 80% availability of the affordable basic technologies and essential medicines, including generics, required to treat major NCDs in both public and private facilities.

Mental disorder occurs in all regions and cultures of the world. The most prevalent being depression and anxiety, which are estimated to affect nearly one in 10 people. At its worst, depression can lead to suicide. Globally, among young adults aged 15–29 years, suicide accounts for 8.5 per cent of all deaths and is second leading cause of death in this group after road traffic injuries *(2)*.

Substance use and substance-use-disorder including the harmful use of alcohol cause a significant public health burden. Worldwide alcohol consumption in 2015 was estimated to be 6.3 litres of pure alcohol per person aged 15 years or older. Tobacco use is a leading risk factor for NCDs and SDG 3.a addresses the implementation of the WHO Framework Convention on Tobacco Control; with tobacco use selected as an indicator of progress. In 2015, over 1.1 billion people used tobacco *(2)*.

Air pollution is a major risk factor for NCDs causing cardiovascular diseases, stroke, chronic obstructive pulmonary disease and lung cancer as well as increasing the risk of acute respiratory infections. In 2012, ambient air pollution (from traffic, industrial sources, waste burning or residential fuel combustion) caused 3 million deaths. Target 11.6 focusses on urban environmental risk and includes an indicator on the annual mean level of the particulate matter such as PM 2.5 and PM10 in cities.

Injuries and violence

Unlike the MDGs, injuries and violence are included in multiple SDGs targets. Road traffic injuries and unintentional injuries are included in the health goal with targets related to violence and disasters as part of other goals as shown in Table 7.

TABLE 7

Selected SDG targets and proposed indicators linked to injuries and violence, by type of indicator

Type of indicator	SDG target	Proposed indicator
Impact	3.6	Deaths due to road traffic injuries
	3.9	Mortality due to unintentional poisoning
	1.5, 11.5, 13.1	Deaths due to disasters
	16.1	Homicide
	16.1	Conflict-related deaths
Coverage/ risk factors/ determinants	5.2	Women and girls subjected to physical; sexual or physiological violence
	16.1	Population subjected to physical, sexual or physiological violence
	Other	Part of targets in goals on peaceful and inclusive societies, cities, poverty, education, etc.

Source : *(2)*

Injuries sustained accidentally or as a result of intentional act of violence, kills more than 5 million people worldwide annually. It accounts for 9 per cent of global mortality. The leading cause of injury deaths is road traffic injury, followed by suicide, fall and interpersonal violence. Other important cause of injuries include drowning, fires and burns, poisoning, war and conflict and natural disasters.

Each year about 1.25 million people die from road traffic injuries and another 20–50 million people sustain non-fatal injuries as a result of road traffic collisions or crashes. Road traffic injuries are among the top 10 causes of deaths globally and the leading cause of death for people in 15–29 years age group. Homicide and collective violence accounts for around 10 per cent of global injury related deaths. Four-fifths of homicide victims are men and 60 per cent of victims are of 15–44 years age group *(1)*.

A proposed indicator for SDG target 16.1 is conflict death per lac population. In 2015, it is provisionally estimated that 1,52,000 people were killed in wars and conflicts, corresponding to about 0.3 per cent of global deaths *(2)*.

New indicators *(3)*

New indicators for SDGs have been added in the year 2020. They are as follows :

- SDG 2.2.3 : In 2016, the global prevalence of anaemia among women of reproductive age was 32.8 per cent (compared with 30.3 per cent in 2012). Applied to the latest UN population estimates, that equated to 615.8 million women with anaemia. The rates of anaemia were highest in the WHO South-East Asia (45.8 per cent), Eastern Mediterranean (39.8 per cent) and African (39.0 per cent) regions.
- SDG 3.b.1 : Human papillomavirus (HPV) is the most common viral infection of the reproductive tract, and can cause cervical cancer. The vaccine targetting 9–14 years-old girls is now offered in 90 countries, but is yet to reach the poorest countries where the risk of cervical cancer is the greatest. Global coverage for a full course of HPV vaccines increased from 3 per cent in 2010 to 12 per cent in 2018.
- SDG 3.b.3 : Based on a sample of 25 countries, surveyed between 2008 and 2019, on an average only 22.4 per cent of health facilities provided an available and affordable (accessible) core set of relevant essential medicines for treatment, prevention and management of acute and chronic, communicable and non-communicable diseases in primary health care settings. A lot of variation in access to medicines is observed between these 25 countries. Specifically, in 28 per cent of countries none of the facilities provided accessible medicines.
- SDG 3.d.2 : By rendering medicines ineffective, antimicrobial resistance undermines the treatment of common infections and increases the risk of spread to others. After the launch of the Global Antimicrobial Resistance Surveillance System (GLASS) in 2016, as of 21st April 2020, a total of 91 countries and territories have been supported to enroll into the system and participate in the annual data call on antimicrobial resistance and consumption. Data on the overall prevalence of antimicrobial resistance pathogens are currently limited, but completeness and representativenes of the data have continuously increased at every GLASS data call. The last data call run in 2019 gathered frequency of antimicrobial resistant pathogens in common acute bacterial infections, including bloodstream infections from 66 countries and territories. Monitoring AMR will help inform control strategies and actions to mitigate impact on the population such as informing the treatment protocols, enhancing Infection Prevention and Control (IPC) and water, sanitation and hygiene (WASH) in health care facilities, increasing the availability of "Access" group antibiotics, as well as continuous improvement of AMR surveillance capacities. Establishing AMR surveillance systems will also build country capacity to monitor and respond to risks from emerging pathogens.
- SDG 6.2.2(b) : Proportion of population using a hand-washing facility with soap and water.

GPW13 indicators

- Number of cases of poliomyelitis caused by wild poliovirus.
- Age-standardized prevalence of raised blood pressure among persons aged 18+ years (defined as systolic blood pressure of >140 mmHg and/or diastolic blood pressure >90 mmHg) and mean systolic blood pressure.
- Prevalence of obesity.

Health system

Health system strengthening is a core focus of the SDGs. This is reflected by the fact that universal health care (UHC) is central to the overall health goal as set out in SDG declaration and is assigned a special target (3.8). In order to move towards the UHC goal, country health system needs to be strengthened as well as adapted to meet the shifting health priorities associated with demographic and epidemiological transition, rapidly developing technologies and changing public expectations. Table 8 shows the targets and indicators linked to health system.

TABLE 8

Selected SDG targets and proposed indicators linked to health systems, by type of indicator

Type of indicator	SDG target	Proposed indicator
Coverage/ financial protection	3.8	UHC index: tracer indicators on service access (hospital access, health workforce density by specific cadres, access to medicines and vaccines, IHR capacities)
	3.8	UHC: financial protection (catastrophic and impoverishing out-of-pocket health spending)
System	3.b	Access to medicines and vaccines
	3.b	Research and development on health issues that primarily affect developing countries, including official development assistance (ODA)
	3.c	Health workforce density and distribution
	3.d	IHR capacity and health emergency preparedness
	17.18	Data disaggregation
	17.19	Coverage of birth and death registration, completion of regular population census.

Source : *(2)*

Access to affordable medicines and vaccines on a sustainable basis is an indicator to SDG target 3.b which focusses on support for research and development and on the affordability of medicines and vaccines for communicable diseases and non-communicable diseases that primarily affect developing countries. A second indicator under SDG target 3.b aims to capture the level of research and development investments.

The transition from MDGs to SDGs cannot be seen solely as exchange of a short list of goals and targets for a longer one. The SDGs are fundamentally different to the MDGs, as is the political context in which they have been developed, and as in which they will be implemented. The MDGs had a consistent and more or less singular purpose. They were about the achievement of improved human development outcome (primarily in terms of poverty, education and health) in developing countries. They were closely associated with aid-spending. The SDGs in the words of declaration are "integrated and indivisible, global in nature and universally applicable". It is relevant to all countries and not just about developing countries.

While MDGs were about limited set of human development targets, the SDGs cover the economic environmental and social pillars of sustainable development with strong focus on equity; expressed more frequently in the phrase "no one will be left behind".

Several health targets follow on from the unfinished MDG agenda and many are derived from World Health Assembly resolutions and related Action Plans *(1)*.

Sustainable development goals and COVID-19

Before the COVID-19 pandemic, the progress in the achievement of SDG remained uneven and were not on track to meet the goals by 2030. Some gains were visible: the share of children and youth out of school had fallen; the incidence of many communicable diseases was in decline; access to safely managed drinking water had improved; and women's representation in leadership roles was increasing. At the same time, the number of people suffering from food insecurity was on the rise, the natural environment continued to deteriorate at an alarming rate, and dramatic levels of inequality persisted in all regions. Change was still not happening at the speed or scale required.

Now, due to COVID-19, an unprecedented health, economic and social crisis is threatening lives and livelihoods, making the achievement of Goals even more challenging. The death toll continues to climb, with almost no country spared. Health systems in many countries have been driven to the brink of collapse. The livelihood of half the global work-force has been severely affected. More than 1.6 billion students are out of school, and tens of millions of people are being pushed back into extreme poverty and hunger, erasing the modest progress made in recent years. It could reverse the progress in reducing maternal and child deaths, COVID-19 has disrrupted childhood immunization efforts globally with potentially deadly consequences. The critical care for the people with non-communicable diseases is affected as many people are not receiving the health services and medicines they need. Same is the case of communicable diseases like tuberculosis, malaria and HIV.

Although the novel coronavirus affects every person and community, it does not do so equally. Instead, it has exposed and exacerbated existing inequalities and injustice. In advanced economies, fatality rates have been highest among marginalized groups. In developing countries, the most vulnerable – including those employed in the informal economy, older people, children, persons with disabilities, indigenous people, migrants and refugees – risk being hit even harder. A large-scale multilateral response is needed to ensure that developing countries have resources they need to protect household and businesses *(5)*.

India and Sustainable Development Goals *(6)*

As the MDGs reached their December 2015 deadline, the new set of Sustainable Development Goals were being adapted by India also. There is now a remarkable convergence of vision underlying the priorities for the proposed SDGs and those of the new government in India. Building on the MDGs, the SDGs propose to end poverty and deprivation in all forms, leaving no one behind, while making development economically, socially and environmentally sustainable. The government of India has also adopted the principle of *Sabka Saath Sabka Vikas* ("together with all, development for all"), with pledge that the first claim on development belong to the poor. The government is calling for improved sanitation, health education, financial inclusion, security and dignity for all, especially women. The priority is improving environmental development with respect to water, air, soil and biosphere by treating challenges of climate change adaptation as an opportunity rather than a problem.

India can progress towards sustainable development in health if health is high on the national and state agenda. This requires high political commitment. India should invest in public health and finish agenda through further improvement in maternal and child health, confronting neglected tropical diseases, eliminating malaria, AIDS and hepatitis and increasing the fight against TB. For all these challenges. the programmes and interventions need to give quality services, with implementation of universal health care. India needs to build robust health system in all aspects and strengthen both the urban and rural components, with primary health care at its centre. More involvement of private health sector is vital. India needs to develop a strong system for monitoring, evaluation and accountability.

The goal of sustainable development cannot be achieved globally without India, and the world will be watching how India will implement its new strategic directives.

References

1. WHO (2015), *Health in 2015 from MDGs (Millennium Development Goals) to SDGs (Sustainable Development Goals)*.
2. WHO (2016), *World Health Statistics, 2016, Monitoring Health for the SDGs*.
3. WHO (2020), *World Health Statistics, 2020, Monitoring Health for the SDGs*.
4. UNICEF (2019), *State of World's Children*, 2019.
5. United Nations (2020), *The Sustainable Development Goals Report – 2020*.
6. UN-India (2015), *India and the MDGs: Towards a Sustainable Future for All*.
7. WHO (2022), *World Health Statistics, 2022, Monitoring Health for the SDGs*.

15 Environment and Health

"The study of disease is really the study of man and his environment"

The term environment implies all the external factors – living and non-living, material and non-material – which surround man. In its modern concept, environment includes not only the water, air and soil that form our environment but also the social and economic conditions under which we live.

For descriptive purpose, environment has been divided into three components, all closely related :

(i) Physical : Water, air, soil, housing, wastes, radiation, etc.
(ii) Biological : Plant and animal life including bacteria, viruses, insects, rodents and animals.
(iii) Social : Customs, culture, habits, income, occupation, religion etc.

The key to man's health lies largely in his environment. In fact, much of man's ill-health can be traced to adverse environmental factors such as water pollution, soil pollution, air pollution, poor housing conditions, presence of animal reservoirs and insect vectors of diseases which pose a constant threat to man's health. Often man is responsible for the pollution of his environment through urbanization, industrialization and other human activities. In 1972 the UN conference on the Human Environment focussed worldwide attention on the environmental hazards that threaten human beings. To facilitate work in this area, WHO has compiled a wide-ranging survey of environmental hazards to human health *(1)*.

The dictionary meaning of the word sanitation is "the science of safe-guarding health." One of the best definitions is that given by the National Sanitation Foundation of the USA, which is as follows : 'Sanitation is a way of life. It is the quality of living that is expressed in the clean home, the clean farm, the clean business, the clean neighbourhood and the clean community. Being a way of life it must come from within the people; it is nourished by knowledge and grows as an obligation and an ideal in human relations'. The term "environmental sanitation" has been defined by WHO as "the control of all those factors in man's physical environment which exercise or may exercise a deleterious effect on his physical development, health and survival".

In the past, sanitation was centred on the sanitary disposal of human excreta. Even now, to many people sanitation still means the construction of latrines. In actual fact, the term sanitation covers the whole field of controlling the environment with a view to prevent disease and promote health. Man has already controlled a number of factors in his environment, e.g., food, water, housing, clothing, sanitation. These controllable factors are those included in the "standard of living". It is the control of these factors that has been responsible for considerable improvement in the health of the people during the past century in the developed countries. However, man's mastery over his environment is not complete. As old problems are being solved, new problems are arising. Air pollution is of growing concern in many urban centres. Industrial growth has given rise to the problem of environmental pollution by industrial wastes. Advances in nuclear technology have produced the problem of radioactive pollution of the environment. The demographic growth and fast urbanization all over the world are bringing profound social and environmental changes. Therefore, the attainment of a healthy environment is becoming more and more complex. The term *environmental sanitation* is now being replaced by environmental health. Proper environmental health now requires the services of the public health qualified doctor, the epidemiologist, the public health engineer, the town planner, the sociologist, the economist, and the health inspector. A purely medical or engineering approach by itself is no longer sufficient; a combined multi-disciplinary programme of action is needed to achieve a healthy environment.

The purpose of environmental health is to create and maintain ecological conditions that will promote health and thus prevent disease. One of the essential public health care element is safe drinking water and sanitation. In 1990, more than 1 billion people in developing world lacked access to safe drinking water and nearly 2 billion people lacked an adequate system for disposing off their excreta *(2)*. Faeces deposited near homes, contaminated drinking water (sometimes caused by poorly designed or maintained sewerage systems), fish from polluted rivers and coastal waters, and agricultural produce, fertilized with human waste are all health hazards. Water quantity is as important as water quality. Washing hands after defecation and before preparing food is of particular importance in reducing disease transmission, but without abundant water in or near home, hygiene becomes difficult or impossible. The lack of water supply and sanitation is the primary reason why diseases transmitted via faeces are so common in developing countries. The most important of these diseases, diarrhoea and intestinal worm infestations, account for 10 per cent of the total burden of disease in developing countries. In addition, an inadequate water supply increases the risk of schistosomiasis, skin and eye infections, and guineaworm disease. Table 1 shows the percentage of population with access to safe water and adequate sanitation in South-East Asia countries.

Two of the changes needed to achieve "Health for All" are concerned with a healthy environment and healthy lifestyle and require initiatives by the individual, the family and the community. Available data from 138 countries show that safely managed drinking water services (that is, located on premises, available when needed and free from

TABLE 1

Population with access to improved drinking water and improved sanitation in South-East Asia countries 2020

Countries	Safe water (%)	Adequate sanitation (%)
India	90	71
Bhutan	97	77
Bangladesh	98	54
Indonesia	92	80
Maldives	100	99
Myanmar	84	74
Nepal	90	77
Sri Lanka	92	94
Thailand	100	99

Source : *(3)*

contamination) was accessible by 74% of the global population in 2020. This translated into 2 billion people still lacking safely managed water services-including 1.2 billion people with only basic services, 282 million with limited services, 367 million using unimproved sources, and 122 million drinking surface water. In the same year, safely managed sanitation services (with excreta safely disposed on-site or treated off-site) were available to only 54% of the global population, leaving 3.6 billion people with insufficient sanitation services. While hand hygiene is one of the first lines of defence against the spread of infectious diseases, 2.3 billion people, or 29% of the global population, lacked a basic handwashing facility with water and soap at home in 2020. For both water and sanitation, safely managed services are enjoyed by a higher proportion of populations in urban areas compared to rural areas *(2)*.

While the available data do not yet allow a global baseline estimate for industrial wastewater generation or treatment, estimates for the generation and treatment of domestic wastewater were available for 128 countries and territories in 2020 (covering 80% of the global population). They show that 44% of household wastewater was discharged without safe treatment *(2)*.

Much of the ill-health in India is due to poor environmental sanitation, that is, unsafe water, polluted soil, unhygienic disposal of human excreta and refuse, poor housing, insects and rodents. Air pollution is also a growing concern in many cities. The high death rate, infant mortality rate, sickness rate and poor standards of health are in fact largely due to defective environmental sanitation. Improvement of environmental sanitation is therefore crucial for the prevention of disease and promotion of health of individuals and communities. Since more than 65 per cent of the population of India live in rural areas, the problem is one of rural sanitation. The first step in any health programme is the elimination through environmental control of those factors which are harmful to health. The environmental factors which are basic and fundamental to individual and community health are discussed in this chapter.

WATER

Much of the ill-health which affects humanity, especially in the developing countries can be traced to lack of safe and wholesome water supply. Water that is easily accessible, adequate in quantity, free from contamination, safe and readily available throughout the year. There can be no state of positive health and well-being without safe water. Water is not only a vital environmental factor to all forms of life, but it has also a great role to play in socio-economic development of human population. Each country should develop its own water resources agency which would collect all pertinent data on water resources, exploitation and hydrogeology. In 1981, the 34th World Health Assembly in a resolution emphasized that safe drinking water is a basic element of "primary health care" which is the key to the attainment of "Health for All by the year 2000 AD". The Millennium Development Goals included safe water and sanitation in the attainable goals. Water is integrated with other PHC components because it is an essential part of health education, food and nutrition, and also MCH.

Safe and wholesome water

Water intended for human consumption should be both safe and wholesome. This has been defined as water that is–

a. free from pathogenic agents;
b. free from harmful chemical substances;
c. pleasant to the taste, i.e., free from colour and odour; and
d. usable for domestic purposes.

Water is said to be *polluted* or *contaminated* when it does not fulfil the above criteria. Water pollution is a growing hazard in many developing countries owing to human activity. Without ample and safe drinking water, we cannot provide health care to the community.

Water requirement

The basic physiological requirements for drinking water have been estimated at about 2 litres per head per day. This is just for survival. But from the standpoint of public health and improvement of the quality of life, water should be provided in adequate volume. It will help to reduce the incidence of many water-related diseases among the people most at risk. The consumption of water, however, depends upon climate conditions, standard of living and habits of the people. A daily supply of 150–200 litres per capita is considered as an adequate supply to meet the needs for all urban domestic purposes. In India 40 litres of water supply per capita per day was the set target to be achieved in rural areas.It must be available close to the people, else they have to spend hours and a lot of energy, going back and forth to obtain it and the water is often polluted in the process.

Uses of water

The uses of water in a community are many, and the requirement in quantity and quality are varied. Conventionally, it has been convenient and economical to provide a single water supply sufficient in quantity to serve all uses and suitable in quality to meet drinking requirements, even though only a small fraction of the total water supply is actually used for drinking.

The uses of water include : (1) Domestic use : on domestic front, water is required for drinking, cooking, washing and bathing, flushing of toilets, gardening etc. (2) Public purposes : cleaning streets, recreational purposes like swimming pools, public fountains and ornamental ponds, fire protection and public parks. (3) Industrial purposes : for processing and cooling; (4) Agricultural purpose : irrigation (5) Power production from hydropower and steam power; (6) Carrying away waste from all manner of establishments and institutions. Water is therefore an essential factor in the economic, social and cultural development of a community. It can eliminate diseases, promote rural development and improve quality of life.

Sources of water supply

Water may be abstracted for use from any one of a number of points in its movement through the hydrological cycle. The safe yield of the source must be sufficient to serve the population expected at the end of the design period, which may be 10 to 50 years in future. The safe yield is generally defined as the yield that is adequate for 95 per cent of the year. The selection of a source requires professional advice. In general, water sources must conform to two criteria : (a) the quantity must be sufficient to meet present and future requirement (b) the quality of water must be acceptable. There are three main sources of water :

1. RAIN
2. SURFACE WATER
   - Impounding reservoirs
   - Rivers and streams
   - Tanks, ponds and lakes
3. GROUND WATER
   - Shallow wells
   - Deep wells
   - Springs

1. Rain

Rain is the prime source of all water. A part of the rain water sinks into the ground to form ground water; part of it evaporates back into the atmosphere, and some runs off to form streams and rivers which flow ultimately into the sea. Some of the water in the soil is taken up by the plants and is evaporated in turn by the leaves. These events are spoken of as "water cycle". *CHARACTERISTICS* : Rain water is the purest water in nature. Physically, it is clear, bright and sparkling. Chemically, it is very soft water containing only traces of dissolved solids (0.0005 per cent). Being soft, it has a corrosive action on lead pipes. Bacteriologically, rain water from clean districts is free from pathogenic agents. *IMPURITIES* : Rain water tends to become impure as it passes through the atmosphere. It picks up suspended impurities from the atmosphere such as dust, soot and microorganisms and gases such as carbon dioxide, nitrogen, oxygen and ammonia. Gaseous sulphur and nitrogen oxides are emitted from power plants that use fossil fuels. These gases react with atmospheric water, forming dilute solution of sulphuric and nitric acid. The precipitation of these acids (acid rain) has begun to have serious impacts on surface water quality and on plants etc. There are very few places in the world like Gibralter which depend upon rain as a source of water supply.

2. Surface water

Surface water originates from rain water. It is the main source of water supply in many areas. Examples of surface water include rivers, tanks, lakes, wadis (water source which are dry, except in rainy season), man-made reservoirs and sea water. Surface water is prone to contamination from human and animal sources. As such it is never safe for human consumption unless subjected to sanitary protection and purification before use.

The vast majority of Indian cities and towns depend upon surface water sources, which are (1) Impounding Reservoirs. (2) Rivers and Streams, and (3) Tanks, Ponds and Lakes. In general, surface water supplies possess a high probability of organic, bacterial and viral contamination.

(1) IMPOUNDING RESERVOIRS

These are artificial lakes constructed usually of earthwork or masonry in which large quantities of surface water is stored. Dams built across rivers and mountain streams also provide large reserves of surface water. The area draining into the reservoir is called "Catchment area". Cities such as Mumbai, Chennai and Nagpur derive their water supply from impounding reservoirs. One disadvantage of storing water for long periods in reservoirs is the growth of algae and other microscopic organisms, which impart bad tastes and odours to water. *CHARACTERISTICS* : Impounding reservoirs usually furnish a fairly good quality of water. The water is usually clear, palatable and ranks next to rain water in purity. If the surrounding hills are covered with peat, the water may acquire a brownish coloration. The water is usually soft and considered to be free of pathogenic organisms. *IMPURITIES* : The upland surface water derives its impurities from the catchment area, the sources being human habitations and animal keeping or grazing. It is therefore very necessary to keep the catchment area free from human or animal intrusion. The general belief that mountain streams are very pure water is often untrue. Even if there is no human habitation or cattle near, there is still a possibility of contamination caused by wild animals.

(2) RIVERS

Many rivers furnish a dependable supply of water. Cities such as Delhi, Kolkata and Allahabad rely on river water for their needs. The chief drawback of river water is that it is always grossly polluted and is quite unfit for drinking without treatment. *CHARACTERISTICS* : River water is turbid during rainy season; it may be clear in other seasons. Clarity of water is no guarantee that the river water is safe for drinking. River water contains dissolved and suspended impurities of all kinds. The bacterial count, including the human intestinal organisms may be very high. *IMPURITIES* : Rivers are described as a direct connection between the alimentary canal of the people living upstream and the mouths of those below. The impurities of river water are derived from surface washings, sewage and sullage water, industrial and trade wastes, and drainage from agricultural areas. The customs and habits of the people like bathing, animal washing and disposal of the dead, all add to the pollution of water. *SELF–PURIFICATION* : Certain amount of self-purification does occur in river water by natural forces of purification such as dilution, sedimentation, aeration, oxidation, sunlight, plant and animal life but these agencies are not sufficient to render the water potable. River water needs purification before it can be used for drinking purposes.

(3) TANKS *(5,6)*

Tanks are large excavations in which surface water is stored. They are an important source of water supply in some Indian villages. Tanks are recipients of contamination of all sorts. They are full of silt and colloidal matter, especially immediately after the rains. The older tanks may be full of aquatic vegetation. Tanks are often used for washing of clothes, cattle, humans, cooking pots; children use it for swimming and there may be regular defecation around the edges which will be washed into the tank at the next rains. Tanks are thus subjected to unlimited possibilities of contamination and are highly dangerous, as a source of drinking water, even at the best of times. But unfortunately, the tank water is drunk without being boiled, disinfected or having undergone treatment of any kind which is responsible for an incalculable number of cases of sickness and death, particularly of children.

Improvement of tanks : A certain amount of natural purification does take place in tank water because of storage, oxidation and other agencies but these are not sufficient to render the water safe. The sanitary quality of tank water may be considerably improved by observing the following : (1) the edges of the tank should be elevated in order to prevent the entry of surface washings; (2) there should be a fence around the tank to prevent access to animals; (3) no one should be permitted to get into the tank directly (note the hazard of guineaworm infestation); (4) there should be an elevated platform from where people can draw water; (5) the weeds should be periodically removed; and (6) the tank should be cleaned at the end of the dry season. Inspite of these precautions, from a practical point of view, it is not possible to prevent pollution of tanks as the people who consume the tank water are often among the poorest in the country and do not have sanitary concepts. Considerable research is now in progress at national and international levels to ensure the village tank as a safe source of drinking water *(5)*. It is believed that the simplest solution consists of subjecting the tank water to some sort of sand filtration. Fig. 1 illustrates how this could be brought about. The addition of chlorine would undoubtedly add to the value of sand filtration.

Sea water

Though this source is plentiful, it has great many limitations. It contains 3.5 per cent of salts in solution. Off-shore waters of the oceans and seas have a salt concentration of 30,000 to 36,000 mg/litre (30–36 g/litre) of dissolved solids including 19,000 mg/litre of chloride, 10,600 mg/litre of sodium and 1,270 mg/litre of magnesium. Desalting and demineralization process involves heavy expenditure. It is adopted in places where sea water is the only source available *(4)*.

3. Ground water

Rain water percolating into ground constitutes ground water. Water used by humans comes mainly from land. It is now realized that there is a limit to ground water in the world. We should withdraw only quantities of water that can be renewed.

Ground water is the cheapest and most practical means of providing water to small communities. Ground water is superior to surface water, because the ground itself provides an effective filtering medium. The advantages of ground water are: (1) it is likely to be free from pathogenic agents; (2) it usually requires no treatment; (3) the supply is likely to be certain even during dry season; and (4) It is less subject to contamination than surface water. The disadvantages are: (1) it is high in mineral content, e.g., salts of calcium and magnesium which render the water hard (2) it requires pumping or some arrangement to lift the water *(7)*. The usual ground water sources are wells and springs. Wells have been classified into shallow and deep wells, dug and tube wells.

WELLS

Traditionally wells are an important source of water supply. Even today, they are an important source of water supply in many communities. Technically, wells are of two kinds – shallow and deep. (1) *Shallow wells :* Shallow wells tap subsoil water i.e. the water from above the first impervious layer in the ground. They yield limited quantities of water, and the water is notoriously liable to pollution unless care is taken in well construction. (ii) *Deep wells :* A deep well is one which taps water from the water-bearing stratum below the first impervious layer in the ground (Fig. 2). Deep wells are usually machine-dug and may be several hundred metres deep. Deep wells furnish the safest water, and are often the most satisfactory sources of water supply.

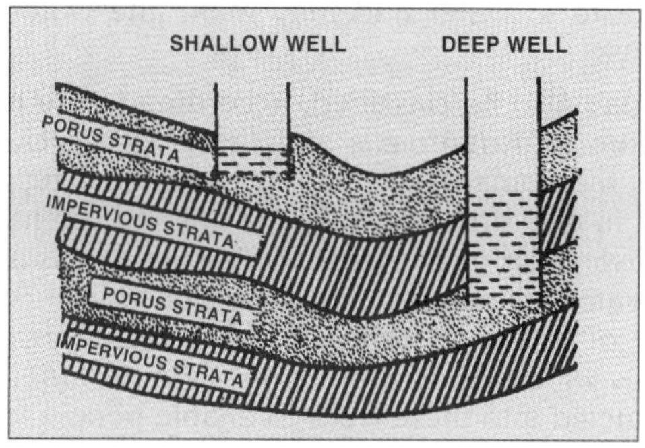

FIG.2
Shallow and deep wells

The points of difference between a shallow well and deep well are set out in Table 2.

Most of the wells in India are of the shallow type. Speaking generally, shallow wells are liable to pollution from neighbouring sources of contamination such as latrines,

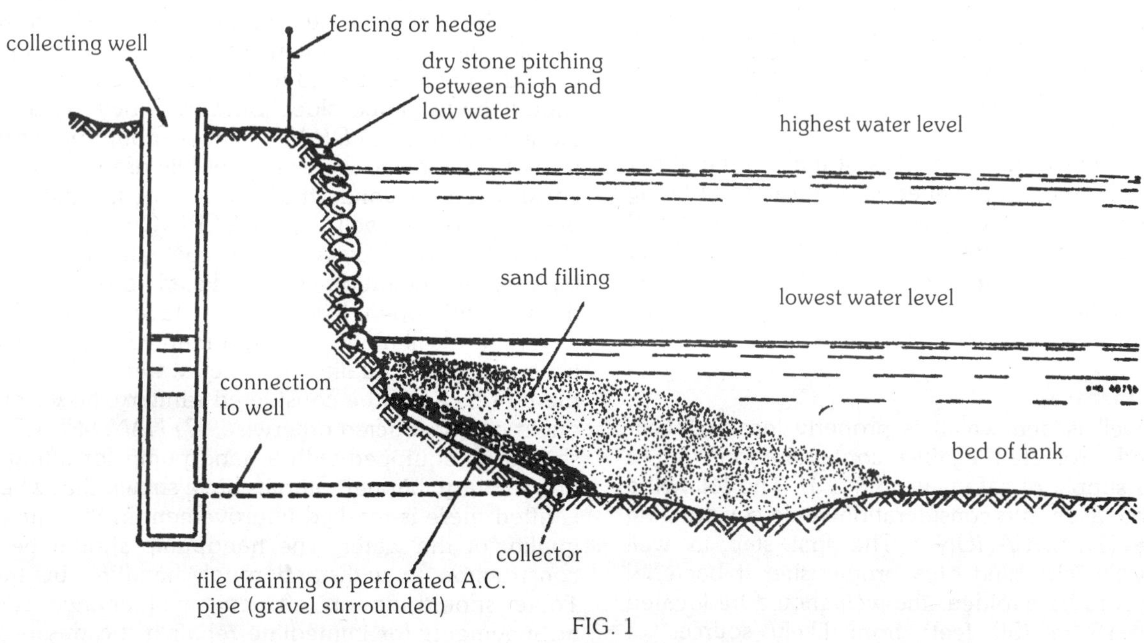

FIG. 1
Slow sand filtration of tank water

TABLE 2

Differences between a shallow well and deep well

	Shallow well	Deep well
1. *Definition*	Taps the water from above the first impervious layer	Taps the water from below the first impervious layer
2. *Chemical quality*	Moderately hard	Much hard
3. *Bacteriological quality*	Often grossly contaminated	Taps purer water
4. *Yield*	Usually goes dry in summer	Provides a source of constant supply

urinals, drains, cesspools, soakage pits and collections of manure. Shallow wells are therefore a health hazard to the community if they are not made sanitary. A deep well can also become a health hazard if it is open, poorly constructed and not protected against contamination. ARTESIAN WELLS are a kind of deep wells in which the water rises above the level of ground water, because it is held under pressure between two impervious strata. Artesian wells are not common in India.

Saline intrusion : Near the sea, there is danger of infiltration of sea water in to deep wells. This gives a brackish taste to water and may make the water unfit for domestic use.

Wells may also be classified, according to the method of construction, into *dug wells* and *tube wells*. DUG WELLS are by far the commonest type in India. Two types of dug wells exist in our rural areas: (a) the unlined katcha well and (b) the masonry or pucca well. The katcha well is a hole dug into the water-bearing stratum. The pucca well is an open well, built of bricks or stones. STEP WELLS are a kind of pucca wells which are becoming obsolete, fortunately. Steps are constructed into these wells to enable people to descend into the well to fetch water or quench their thirst. In these wells, there is considerable personal contact between the user and the water. Some people may even wash their faces, hands and feet which is a common Indian custom. The open dug wells and step wells are a health hazard to the community.

Improvement of dug wells

The unlined katcha wells may be made sanitary by deepening the bottom, installing a hand-pump with screen, and filling the well with coarse sand up to the water level, and with clay above that level. When the material used for filling is completely consolidated a platform and drainage may be constructed.

Masonry well improvement consists of making the upper 10 feet or more of the lining water-tight, raising the lining one foot above the ground, and providing a reinforced concrete slab cover at the top. One or more hand-pumps may be installed for lifting the water. Special attention should be paid to the foundation of the pump to prevent any possible leakage of waste water into the well.

SANITARY WELL

A sanitary well is one which is properly located, well-constructed and protected against contamination with a view to yield a supply of safe water (Fig. 3). The following points should be taken into consideration while constructing sanitary wells: (1) *LOCATION* : The first step in well construction is the choosing of a proper site. If bacterial contamination is to be avoided, the well should be located not less than 15 m (50 feet) from likely sources of contamination. The well should be located at a higher

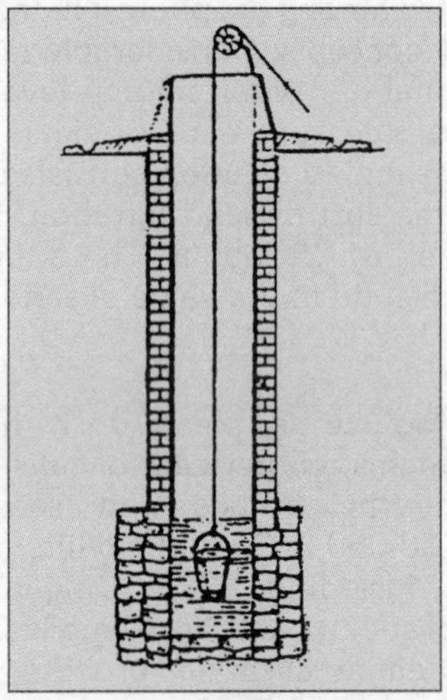

FIG. 3

Sanitary open well

elevation with respect to a possible source of contamination. The distance between the well and the houses of the users should also be considered. If the well is situated far away, people may not use it. It is therefore recommended that the well should be so located that no user will have to carry water for more than 100 m (100 yards) *(7)*. (2) *LINING* : The lining of the well should be built of bricks or stones set in cement up to a depth of at least 6 m (20 feet) so that water enters from the bottom and not from the sides of the well. The lining should be carried 60–90 cm (2–3 feet) above the ground level. (3) *PARAPET WALL* : There should be a parapet wall up to a height of at least 70–75 cms (28 inches) above the ground. (4) *PLATFORM* : There should be a cement-concrete platform round the well extending at least 1 m (3 feet) in all directions. The platform should have gentle slope outwards towards a drain built along its edges. (5) *DRAIN* : There should be a pucca drain to carry off spilled water to a public drain or a soakage pit constructed beyond the "cone of filtration" (area of drainage) of the well. (6) COVERING : The top of the well should be closed by a cement concrete cover because the bulk of the pollution is introduced into the well directly through the open top. Studies have shown that merely covering a well alone caused a marked improvement in the bacteriological quality of the water *(5)*. *Open* wells, therefore, cannot be considered sanitary, however well they might be constructed otherwise. (7) *HAND-PUMP* : The well should be equipped with a hand-pump for lifting the water in a sanitary manner. Studies have shown that when a pump is fitted there is marked improvement in the bacteriological quality of the water. The handpump should be of robust construction to withstand rough handling by the people. There should be an efficient maintenance service and arrangements for immediate repair if the pumps go out of order. (8) *CONSUMER RESPONSIBILITY* : The provision of sanitary wells does not guarantee freedom from water-borne diseases unless the consumers observe certain basic precautions at the individual and family level. Strict cleanliness should be enforced in the vicinity of the well; personal ablutions, washing of clothes and animals, and the dumping of refuse and wastes should be prohibited. Ropes and buckets from individual homes should not be used for drawing a supply from the well. Water from the well should be carried in clean sanitary vessels to individual houses. All this requires health education. (9) *QUALITY* : The physical, chemical and bacteriological quality of water should conform to the acceptable standards of quality of safe and wholesome water.

TUBE WELLS

Tube wells are successful as a source of drinking water in many parts of India. They yield water which is bacteriologically safe, and are also cheap in comparison to other sources of supply. Shallow tube wells or "driven wells" have become the largest individual source of water supply to the rural community. The tube well consists of a pipe (usually galvanized iron) sunk into the water-bearing stratum and fitted with a *strainer* at the bottom, and a hand-pump at the top. A water-tight concrete platform with a drain all round should be provided. The area within 15 m of the tube well should be kept free from pollution with liquid and solid wastes. The hand-pump should be kept in good repair. The life of the tube well is not the same everywhere. It varies from place to place depending upon the type of strainer, quality of underground water and the nature of soil. An average well may last for a period of 5 to 10 years; in some cases, tube wells have given satisfactory service even after 30 years *(8)*. When the tube well is derelict, it is withdrawn and then resunk with a new strainer using as much of the withdrawn pipes as can be recovered. *Deep tube* wells or bored wells are sunk by drilling through successive substrata of gravel or rock until a suitable supply of ground water is located. They may be several hundred feet deep and require complicated mechanical drilling equipment and skilled engineering direction. This type of wells, although costly to construct and to operate, are in many ways the ideal supply. The yield is normally very high and does not depend upon direct rainfall in the immediate vicinity. Chandigarh, the capital of Punjab, derives its entire water supply from tube wells.

SPRINGS

When ground water comes to the surface and flows freely under natural pressure, it is called a "spring". Springs may be of two types – shallow springs and deep springs. Shallow springs dry up quickly during summer months, whereas deep springs do not show seasonal fluctuations in the flow of water. In some geographic areas, springs constitute an important source of water. Springs are simpler to exploit, as no pumping is needed to bring the water to the surface. Springs are exposed to contamination. Well built protective structures are necessary to safeguard water quality.

WATER POLLUTION

Pure uncontaminated water does not occur in nature. It contains impurities of various kinds – natural and man-made. The natural impurities are not essentially dangerous. These comprise dissolved gases (e.g. nitrogen, carbon dioxide, hydrogen sulphide, etc. which may be picked up during rainfall), and dissolved minerals (e.g., salts of calcium, magnesium, sodium, etc.) which are natural constituents of water following its contact with soil; and suspended impurities (e.g., clay, silt, sand and mud), and microscopic organisms. These impurities are derived from the atmosphere, catchment area and the soil.

A more serious aspect of water pollution is that caused by human activity – urbanization and industrialization. The sources of pollution resulting from these are : (a) *sewage*, which contains decomposable organic matter and pathogenic agents (b) *industrial and trade wastes*, which contain toxic agents ranging from metal salts to complex synthetic organic chemicals (c) *agricultural pollutants,* which comprise fertilizers and pesticides, and (d) *physical pollutants,* viz heat (thermal pollution) and radioactive substances *(9)*.

The indicators of pollution include the amount of total suspended solids, biochemical oxygen demand (BOD) at 20 deg. C, concentration of chlorides, nitrogen and phosphorus and absence of dissolved oxygen.

Even if the source of water supply and its treatment are of a high standard, water pollution may still occur as often happens, due to corrosion of pipe lines, leaky joints and cross connections between water supply pipes and sewage drainage pipes. Surveillance has to be exercised at every point in the distribution system to ensure supply of safe water to the consumer.

Water-related diseases

Man's health may be affected by the ingestion of contaminated water either directly or through food; and by the use of contaminated water for purpose of personal hygiene and recreation. The term water-related diseases includes the classical water-borne diseases. Developing countries carry a heavy burden of water-related diseases, the heaviest being the diarrhoeal diseases. Water-related diseases may be classified as follows ;

A. Biological (Water-borne diseases)

1. *Those caused by the presence of an infective agent :*

(a) Viral	: Viral hepatitis A, hepatitis E, poliomyelitis, rotavirus diarrhoea in infants.
(b) Bacterial	: typhoid and paratyphoid fever, bacillary dysentery, *Esch. coli* diarrhoea, cholera.
(c) Protozoal	: amoebiasis, giardiasis
(d) Helminthic	: roundworm, threadworm, hydatid disease.
(e) Leptospiral	: weil's disease

2. *Those due to the presence of an aquatic host :*

(a) Snail	: schistosomiasis
(b) Cyclops	: guineaworm , fish tape worm.

B. Chemical

Chemical pollutants of diverse nature derived from industrial and agricultural wastes are increasingly finding their way into public water supplies. These pollutants include detergent solvents, cyanides, heavy metals, minerals and organic acids, nitrogenous substances, bleaching agents, dyes, pigments, sulphides, ammonia, toxic and biocidal organic compounds of great variety. Chemical pollutants may affect man's health not only directly, but also indirectly by accumulating in aquatic life (e.g. fish) used as human food. The present concern about chemical pollutants in water relates not so much as to their acute toxic effects on human health as to the possible long-term effects of low level exposure, which are often non-specific and difficult to detect. Further, some of the new pollutants are not easily removed by conventional water treatment or purification processes. In many developed countries where water-borne communicable diseases have virtually disappeared, more attention is now being paid to chemical pollution.

In addition to the above, water is associated with the following :

(a) *Dental health :* The presence of fluoride at about 1 mg/litre in drinking water is known to protect against dental caries, but high levels of fluoride cause mottling of the dental enamel;

(b) *Cyanosis in infant :* High nitrate content of water is associated with methaemoglobinaemia. This is a rare occurrence but may occur when surface water from farmland, treated with a fertilizer, gain access to the water supply;

(c) *Cardiovascular diseases :* Hardness of water appears to have a beneficial effect against cardiovascular diseases;

(d) Some diseases are transmitted because of inadequate use of water like shigellosis, trachoma and conjunctivitis, ascariasis, scabies *(10)*; and

(e) Some diseases are related to the disease carrying insects breeding in or near water, like : malaria, filaria, arboviruses, onchocerciasis, African trypanosomiasis *(10)*.

While pollution seems to be an inevitable consequence of modern industrial technology, the problem, now, is to determine the level of pollution that permits economic and social development without presenting hazards to health. The evaluation of the health effects of environmental pollutants is currently being carried out as part of the WHO Environmental Health Criteria Programme.

WATER POLLUTION LAW

In India, water pollution is becoming a serious problem. To protect water from being contaminated, the Indian Parliament in 1974 passed the Water (Prevention and Control of Pollution) Act. The Act seeks to provide legal deterrent against the spread of water pollution. The Act is a comprehensive piece of legislation. It provides for the constitution of Central and State Water Boards and Joint Water Boards endowed with wide powers for controlling pollution.

PURIFICATION OF WATER

Purification of water is of great importance in community medicine. It may be considered under two headings :

1. Purification of water on a large scale.
2. Purification of water on a small scale.

1. PURIFICATION OF WATER ON A LARGE SCALE

The purpose of water treatment is to produce water that is safe and wholesome. The method of treatment to be employed depends upon the nature of raw water, and the desired standards of water quality. For example, ground water (e.g., wells and springs) may need no treatment, other than disinfection. Surface water (e.g., river water) which tends to be turbid and polluted, requires extensive treatment. The components of a typical water purification system comprise one or more of the following measures :

I. Storage
II. Filtration
III. Disinfection

(I) Storage

Water is drawn out from the source and impounded in natural or artificial reservoirs. Storage provides a reserve of water from which further pollution is excluded. As a result of storage, a very considerable amount of purification takes place. This is natural purification, and we may look at it from three points of view : (a) *Physical :* By mere storage, the quality of water improves. About 90 per cent of the suspended impurities settle down in 24 hours by gravity. The water becomes clearer. This allows penetration of light, and reduces the work of the filters, (b) *Chemical :* Certain chemical changes also take place during storage. The aerobic bacteria oxidize the organic matter present in the water with the aid of dissolved oxygen. As a result, the content of free ammonia is reduced and a rise in nitrates occurs. (c) *Biological :* A tremendous drop takes place in bacterial count during storage. The pathogenic organisms gradually die out. It is found that when river water is stored the total bacterial count drops by as much as 90 per cent in the first 5–7 days. This is one of the greatest benefits of storage. The optimum period of storage of river water is considered to be about 10–14 days. If the water is stored for long periods, there is likelihood of development of vegetable growths such as algae which impart a bad smell and colour to water.

(II) Filtration

Filtration is the second stage in the purification of water, and quite an important stage because 98–99 per cent of the bacteria are removed by filtration, apart from other impurities. Two types of filters are in use, the "biological" or "slow sand" filters and the "rapid sand" or "mechanical" filters. A brief description of these filters is given below :

SLOW SAND OR BIOLOGICAL FILTERS *(11)*

Slow sand filters were first used for water treatment in 1804 in Scotland and subsequently in London. During the 19th century their use spread throughout the world. Even today, they are generally accepted as the standard method of water purification.

Elements of a slow sand filter

Fig. 4 shows in diagrammatic form, the various elements of a slow sand filter. Essentially these consists of :

(1) supernatant (raw) water;
(2) a bed of graded sand;
(3) an under-drainage system; and
(4) a system of filter control valves.

(1) Supernatant water

The supernatant water above the sand bed, whose depth varies from 1 to 1.5 metre, serves two important purposes : it provides a constant head of water so as to overcome the resistance of the filter bed and thereby promote the downward flow of water through the sand bed; and secondly, it provides waiting period of some hours (3 to 12 hours, depending upon the filtration velocity) for the raw water to undergo partial purification by sedimentation,

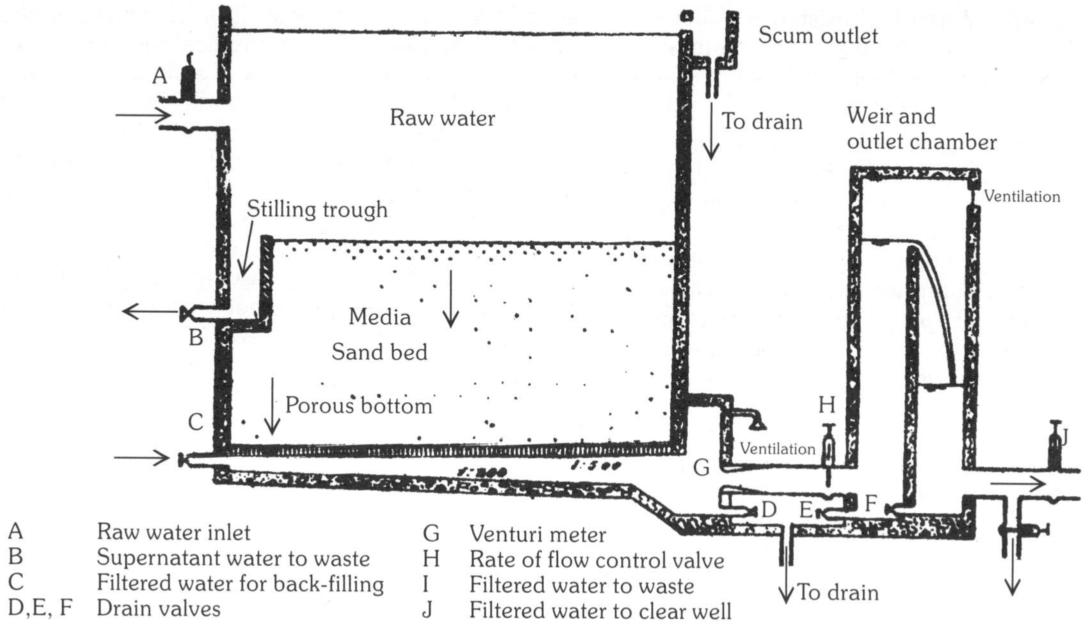

FIG. 4
Slow sand filter

oxidation and particle agglomeration. The level of supernatant water is always kept constant.

(2) Sand bed

The most important part of the filter is the sand bed. The thickness of the sand bed is about 1 metre. The sand grains are carefully chosen so that they are preferably rounded and have an "effective diameter" between 0.2 and 0.3 mm. The sand should be clean and free from clay and organic matter. The sand bed is supported by a layer of graded gravel (Fig. 5), 30–40 cm deep which also prevents the fine grains being carried into the drainage pipes.

The sand bed presents a vast surface area; one cubic metre of filter sand presents some 15,000 sq. metres of surface area. Water percolates through the sand bed very slowly (a process taking two hours or more), and as it does so, it is subjected to a number of purification processes – mechanical straining, sedimentation, adsorption, oxidation and bacterial action, all playing their part. The designed rate of filtration of water normally lies between 0.1 and 0.4 m^3/hour/per square metre of sand bed surface.

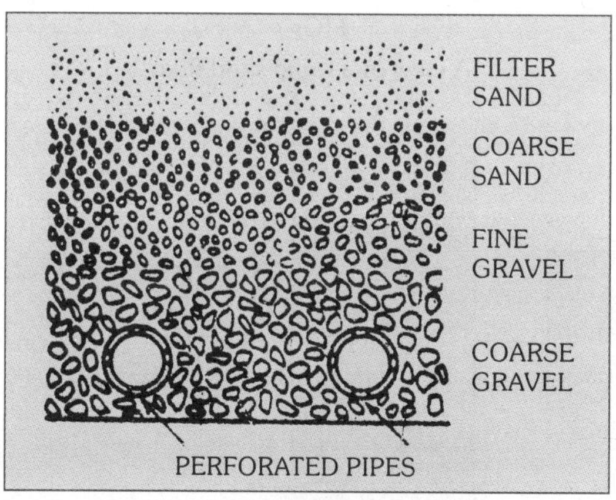

FIG. 5
Section of filter bed

Vital layer : When the filter is newly laid, it acts merely as a mechanical strainer, and cannot truly be considered as "biological". But very soon, the surface of the sand bed gets covered with a slimy growth known as "Schmutzdecke", vital layer, zoogleal layer or biological layer. This layer is slimy and gelatinous and consists of threadlike algae and numerous forms of life including plankton, diatoms and bacteria. The formation of vital layer is known as "ripening" of the filter. It may take several days for the vital layer to form fully, and when fully formed it extends for 2 to 3 cm into the top portion of the sand bed. The vital layer is the "heart" of the slow sand filter. It removes organic matter, holds back bacteria and oxidizes ammonical nitrogen into nitrates and helps in yielding a bacteria-free water. Until the vital layer is fully formed, the first few days filtrate is usually run to waste.

(3) Under-drainage system

At the bottom of the filter bed is the under-drainage system. It consists of porous or perforated pipes which serve the dual purpose of providing an outlet for filtered water, and supporting the filter medium above. Once the filter bed has been laid, the under-drainage system cannot be seen.

Filter box : The first 3 elements (e.g. supernatant water, sand bed and under-drainage system) are contained in the filter box. The filter box is an open box, usually rectangular in shape, from 2.5 to 4 metres deep and is built wholly or partly below ground. The walls may be made of stone, brick or cement. The filter box consists from top to bottom :

Supernatant water	.....	1 to 1.5 metre
Sand bed	.....	1.2 metre
Gravel support	.....	0.30 metre
Filter bottom	.....	0.16 metre

(4) Filter control

The filter is equipped with certain valves and devices which are incorporated in the outlet-pipe system. The purpose of these devices is to maintain a constant rate of filtration. An important component of the regulation system is the "Venturi meter" (Fig. 4) which measures the bed resistance or "loss of head". When the resistance builds up, the operator opens the regulating valve so as to maintain a steady rate of filtration. When the "loss of head" exceeds 1.3 metre it is uneconomical to run the filter.

Filter cleaning : Normally the filter may run for weeks or even months without cleaning. When the bed resistance increases to such an extent that the regulating valve has to be kept fully open, it is time to clean the filter bed, since any further increase in resistance is bound to reduce the filtration rate. At this stage, the supernatant water is drained off, and the sand bed is cleaned by "scraping" off the top portion of the sand layer to a depth of 1 or 2 cm. This operation may be carried out by unskilled labourers using hand tools or by mechanical equipment. After several years of operation, and say 20 or 30 scrapings, the thickness of the sand bed will have reduced to about 0.5 to 0.8 metre. Then the plant is closed down and a new bed is constructed.

The advantages of a slow sand filter are : (1) simple to construct and operate (2) the cost of construction is cheaper than that of rapid sand filters (3) the physical, chemical and bacteriological quality of filtered water is very high. When working ideally, slow sand filters have been shown to reduce total bacterial counts by 99.9 to 99.99 per cent and *E. coli* by 99 to 99.9 per cent.

In recent years, a mistaken idea has grown that biological or slow sand filtration is an old fashioned, outdated method of water treatment which has been completely superseded by rapid sand filtration. This is definitely not the case. Slow sand filtration is still the chosen method of water purification in a number of highly industrialized cities as well as urban areas. In a number of cities in U.S. and Europe, slow sand filters have recently been constructed.

RAPID SAND OR MECHANICAL FILTERS

In 1885, the first rapid sand filters were installed in the USA. Since that time, they have gained considerable popularity especially in highly industrialized countries .

Rapid sand filters are of two types, the gravity type (e.g. Paterson's filter) and the pressure type (e.g. Candy's filter). Both the types are in use. The following steps are involved in the purification of water by rapid sand filters : (Fig. 6).

(1) *Coagulation* : The raw water is first treated with a chemical coagulant such as alum, the dose of which varies from 5 to 40 mg or more per litre, depending upon the turbidity and colour, temperature and the pH value of the water. (2) *Rapid mixing* : The treated water is then subjected to violent agitation in a "mixing chamber" for a few minutes. This allows a quick and thorough dissemination of alum throughout the bulk of the water, which is very necessary. (3) *Flocculation* : The next phase involves a slow and gentle stirring of the treated water in a "flocculation chamber" for about 30 minutes. The mechanical type of flocculator is the most widely used. It consists of a number of paddles which rotate at 2 to 4 rpm. The paddles rotate with the help of motors. This slow and gentle stirring results in the formation of a thick, copious, white flocculant precipitate of aluminium hydroxide. The thicker the precipitate or flock diameter, the greater the settling velocity. (4) *Sedimentation* : The coagulated water is now led into sedimentation tanks where it is detained for periods varying from 2–6 hours when the flocculent precipitate together with impurities and bacteria settle down in the tank. At least 95 per cent of the flocculant precipitate needs to be removed before the water is admitted into the rapid sand filters. The precipitate or sludge which settles at the bottom is removed from time to time without disturbing the operation of the tank. For proper maintenance, the tanks should be cleaned regularly from time to time, otherwise they may become a breeding ground for molluscs and sponges. (5) *Filtration* : The partly clarified water is now subjected to rapid sand filtration.

Filter beds

Each unit of Filter bed has a surface of about 80 to 90 m^2 (about 900 sq. feet). Sand is the filtering medium. The "effective size" of the sand particles is between 0.4–0.7 mm. The depth of the sand bed is usually about 1 metre ($2\frac{1}{2}$ to 3 feet). Below the sand bed is a layer of graded gravel, 30 to 40 cm. ($1-1\frac{1}{2}$ feet) deep. The gravel supports the sand bed and permits the filtered water to move freely towards the under-drains. The depth of the water on the top of the sand bed is 1.0 to 1.5 m (5–6 feet). The under-drains at the bottom of the filter beds collect the filtered water. The rate of filtration is 5–15 m^3/m^2/hour. A view of the rapid sand filter is given in Fig. 7.

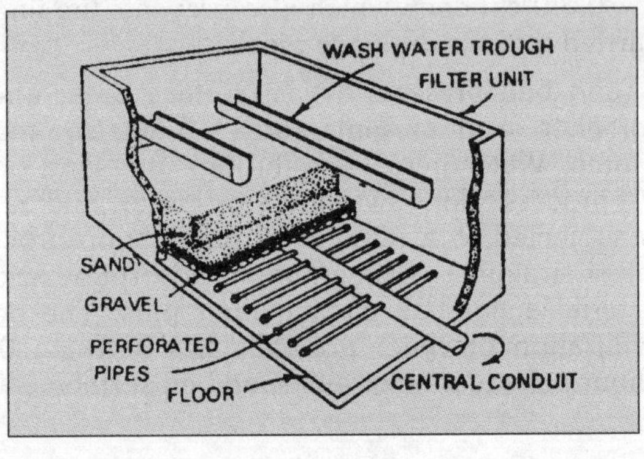

FIG. 7
A view of a rapid sand filter

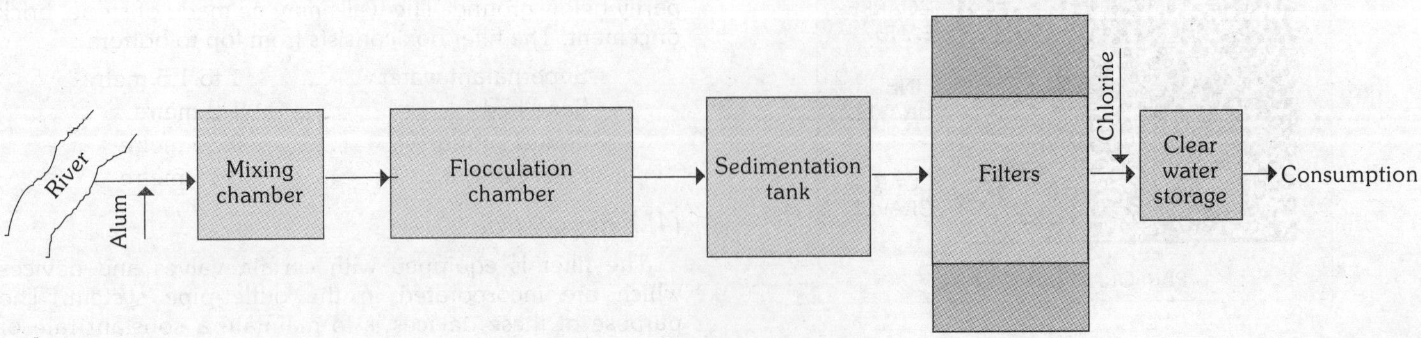

FIG. 6
Flow diagram of a rapid sand filtration plant

Filtration

As filtration proceeds, the "alum-floc" not removed by sedimentation is held back on the sand bed. It forms a slimy layer comparable to the zoogleal layer in the slow sand filters. It adsorbs bacteria from the water and effects purification. Oxidation of ammonia also takes place during the passage of water through the filters. As filtration proceeds, the suspended impurities and bacteria clog the filters. The filters soon become dirty and begin to lose their efficiency. When the "loss of head" approaches 7–8 feet, filtration is stopped and the filters are subjected to a washing process known as "backwashing".

Backwashing

Rapid sand filters need frequent washing daily or weekly, depending upon the loss of head. Washing is accomplished by reversing the flow of water through the sand bed, which is called "backwashing". Backwashing dislodges the impurities and cleans up the sand bed. The washing is stopped when clear sand is visible and the wash water is sufficiently clear. The whole process of washing takes about 15 minutes. In some rapid sand filters, compressed air is used as part of the backwashing processes.

Advantages

The advantages of a rapid sand filter over the slow sand filter are : (1) rapid sand filter can deal with raw water directly. No preliminary storage is needed (2) the filter beds occupy less space (3) filtration is rapid, 40–50 times that of a slow sand filter (4) the washing of the filter is easy (5) there is more flexibility in operation.

Comparison of rapid and slow sand filters

The main features of rapid and slow sand filters are as given in Table 3.

(III) Disinfection

For a chemical or an agent to be potentially useful as a disinfectant in water supplies, it has to satisfy the following criteria :

(a) it should be capable of destroying the pathogenic organisms present, within the contact time available and not unduly influenced by the range of physical and chemical properties of water encountered particularly temperature, pH and mineral constituents;

(b) should not leave products of reaction which render the water toxic or impart colour or otherwise make it unpotable;

(c) have ready and dependable availability at reasonable cost permitting convenient, safe and accurate application to water;

(d) possess the property of leaving residual concentration to deal with small possible recontamination; and

(e) be amenable to detection by practical, rapid and simple analytical techniques in the small concentration ranges to permit the control of the efficiency of the disinfection process.

In water works practice, the term disinfection is synonymous with chlorination.

CHLORINATION

Chlorination is one of the greatest advances in water purification. It is supplement, not a substitute to sand filtration. Chlorine kills pathogenic bacteria, but is has no effect on spores and certain viruses (e.g., polio, viral hepatitis) except in high doses. Apart from its germicidal effect, chlorine has several important secondary properties of value in water treatment : it oxidizes iron, manganese and hydrogen sulphide; it destroys some taste and odour-producing constituents; it controls algae and slime organisms; and aids coagulation.

Action of chlorine : When chlorine is added to water, there is formation of hydrochloric and hypochlorous acids. The hydrochloric acid is neutralized by the alkalinity of the water. The hypochlorous acid ionizes to form hydrogen ions and hypochlorite ions, as follows :–

$$H_2O + Cl_2 \rightarrow HCl + HOCl$$
$$HOCl \rightarrow H + OCl$$

The disinfecting action of chlorine is mainly due to the hypochlorous acid, and to a small extent due to the hypochlorite ions. The hypochlorous acid is the most effective form of chlorine for water disinfection. It is more effective (70–80 times) than the hypochlorite ion. Chlorine acts best as a disinfectant when the pH of water is around 7 because of the predominance of hypochlorous acid. When the pH value exceeds 8.5 it is unreliable as a disinfectant because about 90 per cent of the hypochlorous acid gets ionized to hypochlorite ions. It is fortunate that most waters have a pH value between 6–7.5.

Principles of chlorination : The mere addition of chlorine to water is not chlorination. There are certain rules which should be obeyed in order to ensure proper chlorination : (1) First of all, the water to be chlorinated should be clear and free from turbidity. Turbidity impedes efficient chlorination (2) Secondly, the "chlorine demand" of the

TABLE 3
Comparison of rapid and slow sand filters

		Rapid sand filter	Slow sand filter
1.	Space	Occupies very little space	Occupies large area
2.	Rate of filtration	200 m.g.a.d	2–3 m.g.a.d.
3.	Effective size of sand	0.4–0.7 mm	0.2–0.3 mm
4.	Preliminary treatment	Chemical coagulation and sedimentation	Plain sedimentation
5.	Washing	By back-washing	By scraping the sand bed
6.	Operation	Highly skilled	Less skilled
7.	Loss of head allowed	6–8 feet (2–2.5 m)	4 feet (1.5 m)
8.	Removal of turbidity	Good	Good
9.	Removal of colour	Good	Fair
10.	Removal of bacteria	98–99 per cent	99.9–99.99 per cent

water should be estimated. "The chlorine demand of water is the difference between the amount of chlorine added to the water, and the amount of residual chlorine remaining at the end of a specific period of contact (usually 60 minutes), at a given temperature and pH of the water". In other words, it is the amount of chlorine that is needed to destroy bacteria, and to oxidize all the organic matter and ammonical substances present in the water. The point at which the chlorine demand of the water is met is called the "break-point". If further chlorine is added beyond the break point, free *chlorine* (HOCl and OCl) begins to appear in the water (3) Thirdly the contact period. The presence of free residual chlorine for a contact period of at least one hour is essential to kill bacteria and viruses *(20)*. It should be noted however, that chlorine has no effect on spores, protozoal cysts and helminthic ova, except in higher doses. (4) The minimum recommended concentration of free chlorine is 0.5 mg/L for one hour *(12)*. The free residual chlorine provides a margin of safety against subsequent microbial contamination such as may occur during storage and distribution. (5) The sum of the chlorine demand of the specific water plus the free residual chlorine of 0.5 mg/L constitutes the correct dose of chlorine to be applied.

METHOD OF CHLORINATION

For disinfecting large bodies of water, chlorine is applied either as (1) chlorine gas (2) chloramine or (3) perchloron. Chlorine gas is the first choice, because it is cheap, quick in action, efficient and easy to apply. Since chlorine gas is an irritant to the eyes and poisonous, a special equipment known as "chlorinating equipment" is required to apply chlorine gas to water supplies. Paterson's chloronome is one such device for measuring, regulating and administering gaseous chlorine to water supplies. In some water treatment plants, they use *chloramine* instead of chlorine gas. Chloramines are loose compounds of chlorine and ammonia. They have a less tendency to produce chlorinous tastes and give a more persistent type of residual chlorine. The greatest drawback of chloramines is that they have a slower action than chlorine and therefore they are not being used to any great extent in water treatment. Perchloron or high test hypochlorite (H.T.H.) is a calcium compound which carries 60–70 per cent of available chlorine. Solutions prepared from H.T.H. are also used for water disinfection. As mentioned already, chlorine gas has replaced all the other chlorine derivatives in the disinfection of urban water supplies.

BREAK POINT CHLORINATION

The addition of chlorine to ammonia in water produces chloramines which do not have the same efficiency as free chlorine. If the chlorine dose in the water is increased, a reduction in the residual chlorine occurs, due to the destruction of chloramine by the added chlorine. The end products do not represent any residual chlorine. This fall in residual chlorine will continue with further increase in chlorine dose and after a stage, the residual chlorine begins to increase in proportion to the added dose of chlorine. This point at which the residual chlorine appears and when all combined chlorines have been completely destroyed is the breakpoint and corresponding dosage is the breakpoint dosage. Breakpoint chlorination achieves the same results as superchlorination in a rational manner and can therefore be construed as controlled superchlorination *(4)*.

SUPERCHLORINATION

Superchlorination followed by dechlorination comprises the addition of large doses of chlorine to the water, and removal of excess of chlorine after disinfection, this method is applicable to heavily polluted waters whose quality fluctuates greatly.

ORTHOTOLIDINE (OT) TEST

Orthotolidine test enables both free and combined chlorine in water to be determined with speed and accuracy. The test was developed in 1918. The reagent consists of analytical grade Orthotolidine, dissolved in 10 per cent solution of hydrochloric acid. When this reagent is added to water containing chlorine, it turns yellow and the intensity of the colour varies with the concentration of the gas. The yellow colour is produced by both free and combined chlorine residuals. OT reacts with *free chlorine* instantaneously but reacts more slowly with *combined* chlorine *(12)*.

The test is carried out by adding 0.1 ml of the reagent to 1 ml of water. The yellow colour produced is matched against suitable standards or colour discs. Commercial equipment is available for this purpose. It is essential to take the reading within 10 seconds after the addition of the reagent to estimate *free chlorine* in water *(14)*. The colour that is produced after a lapse, say 15–20 minutes, is due to the action of both free and combined chlorine.

ORTHOTOLIDINE-ARSENITE (OTA) TEST

This is a modification of the OT test to determine the free and combined chlorine residuals separately *(13, 14, 15)*. Further, the errors caused by the presence of interfering substances such as nitrites, iron and manganese all of which produce a yellow colour with Orthotolidine, are overcome by the OTA test *(12)*.

Other agents

While chlorine continues to be the most commonly used sterilizing agent because of its germicidal properties and the comparatively low cost and ease of application, its pre-eminence in water disinfection is being seriously challenged because of the discovery that chlorination of water can lead to the formation of many "halogenated compounds" some of which are either known or suspected carcinogens. As a result, many chlorine alternatives are receiving renewed interest. These include bromine, bromine chloride, iodine and chlorine dioxide – but these do not seem to present a viable alternative to chlorine at the present time. Ozone is showing the greatest promise, and ultra-violet irradiation's limited usefulness as complimentary agents for chlorine in water disinfection.

Ozonation *(19)*

Ozone is a powerful oxidant and has many uses in water treatment, including oxidation of organic chemicals. Ozone can be used as a primary disinfectant. Ozone gas (O_3) is formed by passing dry air or oxygen through a high-voltage electric field. The resultant ozone-enriched air is dosed directly into the water by means of porous diffusers at the base of baffled contactor tanks. The contactor tanks, typically about 5 metre deep, provide 10–20 minutes of contact time. Dissolution of atleast 80% of the applied ozone should be possible, with the remainder contained in the off-gas, which is passed through an ozone destructor and vented to the atmosphere.

The performance of ozonation relies on achieving the desired concentration after a given contact period. For oxidation of organic chemicals, such as some oxidizable pesticides, a residual of about 0.5 mg/l after a contact time of upto 20 minutes is typically used. The doses required to achieve this vary with the type of water, but are typically in the range 2–5 mg/l. Higher doses are needed for untreated waters, because of the ozone demand of the natural background organics.

Ozone reacts with natural organics to increase their biodegradability, measured as assimilable organic carbon. To avoid undesirable bacterial growth in distribution, ozonation is normally used with subsequent treatment, such as biological filtration or granular activated carbon (GAC), to remove biodegradable organics, followed by a chlorine residual, as ozone does not provide a disinfectant residual. Ozone is effective for the degradation of a wide range of pesticides and other organic chemicals.

Membrane processes *(19)*

The membrane processes of most significance in water treatment are reverse osmosis, ultrafiltration, microfiltration and nanofiltration. These processes have traditionally been applied to the production of water for industrial or pharmaceutical applications, but are now being applied to the treatment of drinking-water.

High-pressure processes

If two solutions are separated by a semipermeable membrane (i.e. a membrane that allows the passage of the solvent but not of the solute), the solvent will naturally pass from the lower-concentration solution to the higher-concentration solution. This process is known as osmosis. It is possible however, to force the flow of solvent in the opposite direction, from the higher to the lower concentration, by increasing the pressure on the higher-concentration solution. The required pressure differential is known as the osmotic pressure, and the process is known as reverse osmosis.

Reverse osmosis results in the production of a treated water stream and a relatively concentrated waste stream. Typical operating pressures are in the range 15–50 bar, depending on the application. Reverse osmosis rejects monovalent ions and organics of molecular weight greater than about 50 daltons (membrane pore sizes are less than 0.002 µm). The most common application of reverse osmosis is desalination of brackish water and seawater.

Nanofiltration uses a membrane with properties between those of reverse osmosis and ultrafiltration membranes; pore sizes are typically 0.001–0.01 µm. Nanofiltration membranes allow monovalent ions such as sodium or potassium to pass but reject a high proportion of divalent ions such as calcium and magnesium and some higher molecular weight organics. Operating pressures are typically about 5 bar. Nanofiltration may be effective for the removal of colour-forming organic compounds also.

Lower-pressure processes

Ultrafiltration is similar in principle to reverse osmosis, but the membranes have much larger pore sizes (typically 0.002–0.03 µm) and operate at lower pressures. Ultrafiltration membranes reject organic molecules of molecular weight above about 800 daltons and usually operate at pressure less than 5 bar.

Microfiltration is a direct extension of conventional filtration into the sub-micrometre range. Microfiltration membranes have pore sizes typically in the range 0.01–12 µm and do not separate molecules but reject colloidal and suspended material at operating pressures of 1–2 bar. Microfiltration is capable of sieving out particles greater than 0.05 µm. It has been used for water treatment in combination with coagulation or PAC to remove particulates and some dissolved organic carbon prior to reverse osmosis membranes and to improve permeate flux.

2. PURIFICATION OF WATER ON A SMALL SCALE

(1) Household purification of water

Three methods are generally available for purifying water on an individual or domestic scale. These methods can be used singly or in combination.

(a) BOILING

Boiling is a satisfactory method of purifying water for household purposes. To be effective, the water must be brought to a "rolling boil" for 10 to 20 minutes. It kills all bacteria, spores, cysts and ova and yields sterilized water. Boiling also removes temporary hardness by driving off carbon dioxide and precipitating the calcium carbonate. The taste of water is altered, but this is harmless. While boiling is an excellent method of purifying water, it offers no "residual protection" against subsequent microbial contamination. Water should be boiled preferably in the same container in which it is to be stored to avoid contamination during storage.

(b) CHEMICAL DISINFECTION

(1) *Bleaching powder :* Bleaching powder or chlorinated lime ($CaOCl_2$) is a white amorphous powder with a pungent smell of chlorine. When freshly made, it contains about 33 per cent of "available chlorine". It is, however, an unstable compound. On exposure to air, light and moisture, it rapidly loses its chlorine content. But when mixed with excess of lime, it retains its strength; this is called "stabilized bleach." Bleaching powder should be stored in a dark, cool, dry place in a closed container that is resistant to corrosion. The chlorine content of bleaching powder stocks should be frequently checked.

Appendix III gives in a tabular form the amount of bleaching powder required to disinfect certain quantities of water. The principle in chlorination is to ensure a "free" residual chlorine of 0.5 mg/litre at the end of one hour contact. Highly polluted and turbid waters are not suited for direct chlorination.

(2) *Chlorine solution :* Chlorine solution may be prepared from bleaching powder. If 4 kg of bleaching powder with 25 per cent available chlorine is mixed with 20 litres of water, it will give a 5 per cent solution of chlorine *(13)*. Ready-made chlorine solutions in different strengths are also available in the market. Like bleaching powder, the chlorine solution is subject to losses on exposure to light or on prolonged storage. The solution should be kept in a dark, cool and dry place in a closed container.

(3) *High test hypochlorite :* High test hypochlorite (HTH) or perchloron is a calcium compound which contains 60 to 70 per cent available chlorine. It is more stable than bleaching powder and deteriorates much less on storage. Solutions prepared from HTH are also used for water disinfection. Appendix III (page 824) shows the amount of HTH needed to disinfect certain quantities of water.

(4) *Chlorine tablets :* Under various trade names (viz., halazone tablets) are available in the market. They are quite good for disinfecting small quantities of water, but they are costly. The National Environmental Engineering Research Institute, Nagpur formulated a new type of chlorine tablet which is 15 times better than ordinary halogen tablets. These tablets are manufactured in various strengths and are now available in plenty, in the Indian market at a cheap rate. A single tablet of 0.5 g is sufficient to disinfect 20 litres of water.

(5) *Iodine :* Iodine may be used for emergency disinfection of water. Two drops of 2 per cent ethanol solution of iodine will suffice for one litre of clear water. A contact time of 20 to 30 minutes is needed for effective disinfection. Iodine does not react with ammonia or organic compounds to any great extent; hence it remains in its active molecular form, over a wide range of pH values and water conditions and persists longer than either chlorine or bromine. Iodine is unlikely to become a municipal water supply disinfectant in a broad sense. High costs and the fact that the element is physiologically active (thyroid activity) are its major disadvantages *(17)*.

(6) *Potassium permanganate :* Once widely used it is no longer recommended for water disinfection. Although a powerful oxidizing agent, it is not a satisfactory agent for disinfecting water. It may kill cholera vibrios, but is of little use against other disease organisms*(15)*. It has other drawbacks, too, such as altering the colour, smell and taste of water.

(c) FILTRATION

Water can be purified on a small scale by filtering through ceramic filters such as Pasteur Chamberland filter, Berkefeld filter and "Katadyn" filter. The essential part of a filter is the "candle" which is made of porcelain in the Chamberland type, and of kieselgurh or infusorial earth in the Berkefeld filter (Fig. 8). In the Katadyn filter, the surface of the filter is coated with a silver catalyst so that bacteria coming in contact with the surface are killed by the "oligodynamic" action of the silver ions, which are liberated into the water. Filter candles of the fine type usually remove bacteriae found in drinking water, but not the filter-passing viruses. Filter candles are liable to be logged with impurities and bacteriae. They should be cleaned by scrubbing with a hard brush under running water and boiled at least once a week. Only clean water should be used with ceramic filters. Although ceramic filters are effective in purifying water, they are not quite suitable for widespread use under Indian conditions.

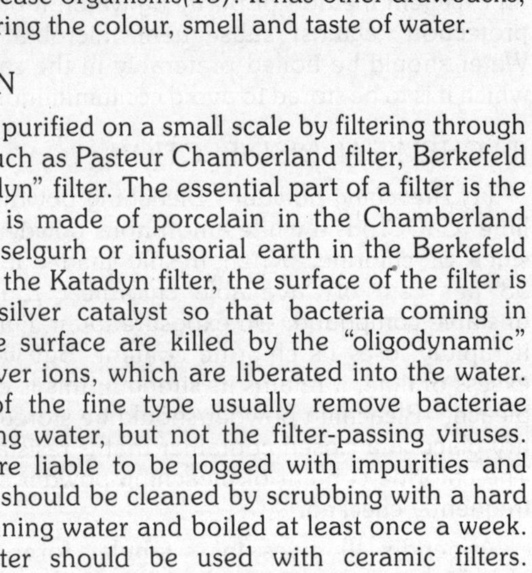

FIG. 8
Berkefeld filter

(d) ULTRAVIOLET IRRADIATION

Germicidal property of UV rays have been recognized for many years. UV irradiation is effective against most microorganisms known to contaminate water supplies like bacteria, yeast, viruses, fungi, algae, protozoa etc.

This method of disinfection involves the exposure of a film of water, upto about 120 mm thick, to one or several quartz mercury vapour arc lamps emitting ultraviolet radiation at a wavelength of 254 (Nano-metre). Applications are limited to individual or institutional systems. The water should be free from turbidity and suspended or colloidal constituents for efficient disinfection.

The advantages are that the exposure is for short period, no foreign matter introduced and no taste and odour produced. Overexposure does not result in any harmful effects. The disadvantages are that no residual effect is available and there is a lack of a rapid field test for assessing the treatment efficiency; moreover, the apparatus needed is expensive.

(e) MULTI-STAGE REVERSE OSMOSIS PURIFICATION OF WATER

Multistage reverse osmosis purification process is used to make water both chemically and microbiologically potable by reducing the total dissolved solids, hardness, heavy metals and disease causing bacteria, virus, protozoa and cysts.

The Fig. 9 shows the diagrammatic form and the various elements of a typical multistage reverse osmosis process.

The clarity cartridge removes the suspended particles such as dust, mud and sand from the water. The Reverse osmosis cartridge reduces the total dissolved solids, hardness, heavy metals (like arsenic, lead, mercury) and eliminates micro-organisms.

(2) Disinfection of wells

Wells are the main source of water supply in the rural areas. The need often arises to disinfect them, sometimes on a mass scale, during epidemics of cholera and gastroenteritis. The most effective and cheapest method of disinfecting wells is by bleaching powder. *Potassium permanganate* should not be used, as it is not a satisfactory disinfecting agent.

STEPS IN WELL DISINFECTION

(1) Find the volume of water in a well

(a) Measure the depth of water column ... (h) metre

(b) Measure the diameter of well ... (d) metre

Take the average of several readings of the above measurements.

(c) Substitute h and d in :

$$\text{Volume (litres)} = \frac{3.14 \times d^2 \times h}{4} \times 1000$$

(d) One cubic metre = 1,000 litres of water

(2) Find the amount of bleaching powder required for disinfection

Estimate the chlorine demand of the well water by *"Horrock's Apparatus* (vide Annex I) and calculate the amount of bleaching powder required to disinfect the well. Annex–III gives the amount of chemicals needed to disinfect water for drinking. Roughly, 2.5 grams of good quality

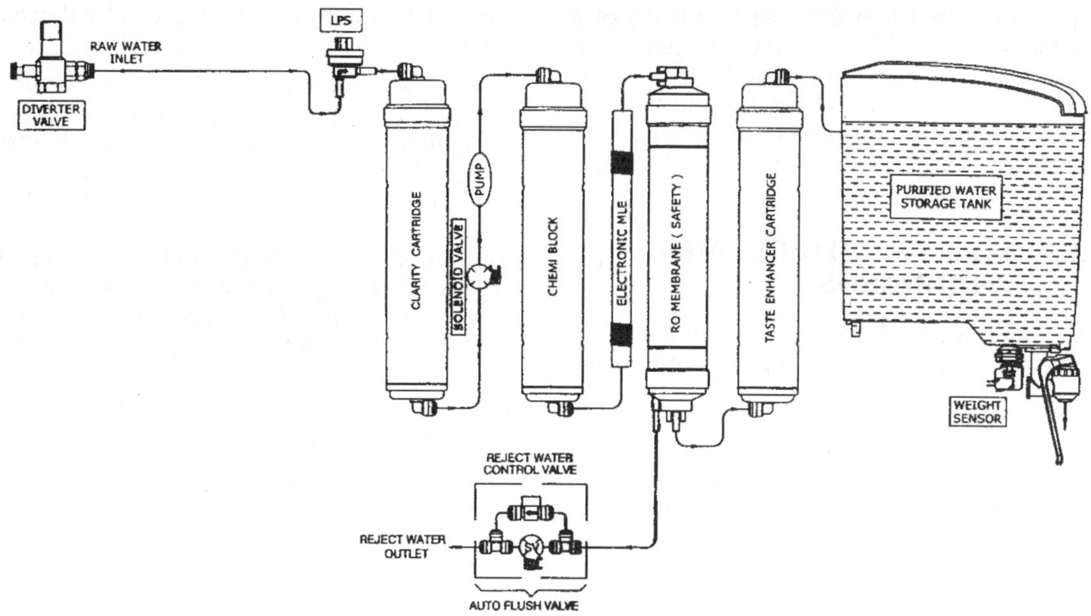

FIG. 9
Multistage reverse osmosis purification of water

bleaching powder would be required to disinfect 1,000 litres of water. This will give an approximate dose of 0.7 mg of applied chlorine per litre of water.

(3) Dissolve bleaching powder in water

The bleaching powder required for disinfecting the well is placed in a bucket (not more than 100 g in one bucket of water) and made into a thin paste. More water is added till the bucket is nearly three-fourths full. The contents are stirred well, and allowed to sediment for 5 to 10 minutes when lime settles down. The supernatant solution which is chlorine solution, is transferred to another bucket, and the chalk or lime is discarded. (Note : the lime sediment should not be poured into the well, as it increases the hardness of well water).

(4) Delivery of chlorine solution into the well

The bucket containing the chlorine solution is lowered some distance below the water surface, and the well water is agitated by moving the bucket violently both vertically and laterally. This should be done several times so that the chlorine solution mixes intimately with the water inside the well.

(5) Contact period

A contact period of one hour is allowed before the water is drawn for use.

(6) Orthotolidine arsenite test

It is good practice to test for residual chlorine at the end of one hour contact. If the "free" residual chlorine level is less than 0.5 mg/litre, the chlorination procedure should be repeated before any water is drawn. Wells are best disinfected at night after the day's draw off. During epidemics of cholera, wells should be disinfected every day.

THE DOUBLE POT METHOD *(13, 18)*

During an emergency, it is desirable to ensure a constant dosage of chlorine to well water. Several simple and effective methods have been devised for this purpose, of which the pot method of chlorination is one which has been used with success in various countries. The double pot method is an improvement devised by the National Environmental Engineering Research Institute, Nagpur, India. This method uses two cylindrical pots, one placed inside the other. The inside height and diameter are 30 cm and 25 cm respectively, for the outer pot. A hole 1 cm in diameter is made in each pot; in the inner pot the hole is in the upper portion, near the rim and in the outer pot it is 4 cm above the bottom.

A mixture of 1 kg of bleaching powder and 2 kg of coarse sand (approx. 2 mm in diameter) is prepared and slightly moistened with water. The inner pot is filled with this mixture up to 3 cm below the level of the hole. The inner pot is introduced into the outer one, and the mouth of the latter closed with polyethylene foil. The use of two pots makes it possible to have larger holes without the risk of over chlorination.

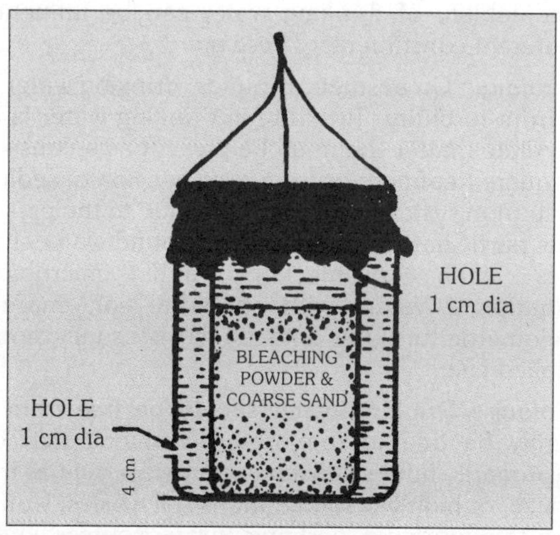

FIG. 10
Double pot

The double pot is lowered into the well by means of a rope attached to the well kerb. The pot should be immersed at least 1 m below the water level to prevent damage by the buckets used for drawing water. It has been found that this device works satisfactorily for 2–3 weeks in small household wells containing about 4,500 litres of water and having a draw-off rate of 360–450 litres per day.

WATER QUALITY – CRITERIA AND STANDARDS

The quest for pure water dates back to antiquity. In modern times, it has led to the formulation of specific standards to provide a basis for judging the quality of water. These standards are exposure limits for bacteriological, viral, chemical and physical agents that have been adopted by governments or appropriate authorities and therefore have legal force. The purpose of standards is to minimise all the known health hazards, since it is obviously impossible to prevent all pollution.

The WHO has published in 1993 vol.1 and in 1996 vol. 2 of second edition, and more recently vol. I and II in 2011 of *guidelines for drinking water quality* intended for use by countries as a basis for the development of standards, which, if properly implemented, will ensure the safety of drinking water supplies. In order to define standards, it is necessary to consider these recommendations in the context of prevailing environmental, social, economic and cultural conditions. These guidelines are intended to supersede the guidelines for drinking water published in 1984 *(19)*.

The guidelines for drinking water quality recommended by WHO (2011) relate to following variables :

- I Acceptability aspects;
- II Microbiological aspects;
- III Chemical aspects; and
- IV Radiological aspects.

I. ACCEPTABILITY ASPECTS

A. Physical parameters

The ordinary consumer judges the water quality by its physical characteristics. The provision of drinking water that is not only safe but also pleasing in appearance, taste and odour is a matter of high priority. The supply of water that is unsatisfactory in this respect will undermine the confidence of consumers, leading to use of water from less safe source. The acceptability of drinking water can be influenced by many different constituents. These are :

1. *Turbidity :* On aesthetic grounds, drinking water should be free from turbidity. Turbidity in drinking water is caused by particulate matter that may be present as a consequence of inadequate treatment or from resuspension of sediment in the distribution system. It may also be due to the presence of inorganic particulate matter in some ground water. Turbidity interferes with disinfection and microbiological determination. Water with turbidity of more than 4 nephelometric turbidity units (NTU) is usually noticeable to the naked eye.

2. *Colour :* Drinking water should be free from colour which may be due to the presence of coloured organic matter (primarily humic substances), metals such as iron and manganese, or highly coloured industrial wastes. Consumers may turn to alternative, perhaps unsafe, sources when their water is coloured to an aesthetically displeasing degree. The guideline value is upto 15 true colour units (TCU) although levels of colour above 15 TCU can be detected in a glass of water.

3. *Taste and odour :* Taste and odour originate from natural and biological sources or processes, from contamination by chemicals, or as a by-product of water treatment (e.g., chlorination). Taste and odour may develop during storage and distribution. It is indicative of some form of pollution or malfunction during water treatment or distribution. The cause should be investigated, particularly if there is substantial change. An unusual taste or odour might be an indication of the presence of potentially harmful substances. No health based guideline value is proposed for taste and odour.

4. *Temperature :* Cool water is generally more palatable. Low water temperature tends to decrease the efficiency of treatment process, including disinfection, and may thus have a deleterious effect on drinking water quality. However, high water temperature enhances the growth of microorganisms and taste, odour, colour and corrosion problem may increase. No guideline value is recommended since its control is usually impracticable.

To sum up, we cannot judge the quality of drinking water by physical characteristics alone. A detailed chemical and microbiological examination is also needed for complete assessment.

B. Inorganic constituents

1. *Chlorides :* All waters including rain water contain chlorides. In the neighbourhood of the sea, the salinity of water tends to be high. Since the chloride content of water varies from place to place, it is necessary, first of all, to determine the normal range of chlorides of the unpolluted surface and ground water in the given locality. Any excess over the normal range should arouse suspicion of water contamination. The standard prescribed for chloride is 200 mg/litre. The maximum permissible level is 600 mg/litre.

2. *Hardness :* Public acceptability of the degree of hardness may vary considerably from one community to another, depending on local conditions. The taste threshold for the calcium ion is in the range of 100–300 mg/litre, depending on the associated anion, and the taste threshold of magnesium is probably less than that for calcium. In some instances water hardness in excess of 500 mg/litre is tolerated by consumers.

Depending on the interaction of other factors, such as pH and alkalinity, water with a hardness of approximately 200 mg/litre may cause scale deposition in the distribution system and will result in excessive soap consumption and subsequent scum formation. On heating, hard water forms deposits of calcium carbonate scale. Soft water, with a hardness of less than 100 mg/litre, may, on the other hand, have a low buffer capacity and so be more corrosive for water pipes *(19)*.

3. *Ammonia :* The term ammonia includes the non-ionized (NH_3) and ionized (NH_4+). Ammonia in the environment originates from metabolic, agricultural and industrial processes and from disinfection with chloramine. Natural levels in ground and surface waters are usually below 0.2 mg/litre. Anaerobic ground waters may contain upto 3mg/litre. Intensive rearing of farm animals can give rise to much higher levels in surface water. Ammonia contamination can also arise from cement mortar pipe linings. Ammonia in water is an indicator of possible bacterial, sewage and animal waste pollution. Ammonia can

compromise disinfection efficiency, result in nitrite formation in distribution systems, can cause the failure of filters for the removal of manganese, and cause taste and odour problems.

4. *pH :* One of the main objectives in controlling the pH is to minimize corrosion and incrustation in the distribution system. pH levels of less than 7 may cause severe corrosion of metals in the distribution pipes and elevated levels of certain chemical substances, such as lead, may result. At pH levels above 8, there is a progressive decrease in the efficiency of the chlorine disinfection process. An acceptable pH drinking water is between 6.5 and 8.5. In the absence of a distribution system, the acceptable range of pH may be broader.

5. *Hydrogen sulphide :* The taste and odour threshold of hydrogen sulphide in water are estimated to be between 0.05 and 0.1 mg/litre. The "rotten eggs" odour of hydrogen sulphide is particularly noticeable in some ground waters and in stagnant drinking water in the distribution system, as a result of oxygen depletion and the subsequent reduction of sulphate by bacterial activity. Sulphide is oxidized rapidly to sulphate in well-aerated water, and hydrogen sulphide level in oxygenated water supplies are normally very low. The presence of hydrogen sulphide in drinking water can be easily detected by the consumer and requires immediate corrective action.

6. *Iron :* Anaerobic ground water may contain ferrous iron at concentrations of upto several mg/litre without discoloration or turbidity in water when directly pumped from the well. On exposure to the atmosphere, however, the ferrous iron oxidizes to ferric iron, giving an objectionable reddish – brown colour to the water. Iron also promotes the growth of "iron bacteria", which derive their energy from the oxidation of ferrous iron to ferric iron, and in the process deposit a slimy coating on the pipe. At level above 0.3 mg/litre, iron stains laundry and plumbing fixtures.

7. *Sodium :* The taste threshold concentration of sodium in water depends on the associated anion and the temperature of the solution. At room temperature, the average taste threshold for sodium is about 200 mg/litre.

8. *Sulphate :* The presence of sulphate in drinking water can cause noticeable taste. Taste impairment varies with the nature of the associated cation. It is generally considered that taste impairment is minimal at levels below 250 mg/litre. It has been found that addition of calcium and magnesium sulphate (but not sodium sulphate) to distilled water improves the taste; optimal taste was recorded at 270 and 90 mg/litre for the two compounds respectively.

9. *Total dissolved solids :* Total dissolved solids (TDS) can have an important effect on the taste of drinking water. The palatability of water with a TDS level of less than 600 mg/litre is generally considered to be good. Drinking water becomes increasingly unpalatable at TDS levels greater than 1,200 mg/litre. Water with extremely low concentrations of TDS may be unacceptable because of its flat, insipid taste. The presence of high level of TDS may also be objectionable to consumers owing to excessive scaling in water pipes, heaters, boilers and household appliances. Water with concentrations of TDS below 1000 mg/litre is usually acceptable to the consumers.

10. *Zinc :* Zinc imparts an undesirable astringent taste to water. Tests indicate a taste threshold concentration of 4 mg/litre (as zinc sulphate). Water containing zinc at concentrations in excess of 5 mg/litre may appear opalescent and develop a greasy film on boiling, although these effects may also be noticeable at concentrations as low as 3 mg/litre. Drinking water seldom contains zinc at concentrations above 0.1 mg/litre, levels in tapwater can be considerably higher because of the zinc used in plumbing material.

11. *Manganese :* Manganese concentrations below 0.1 mg/litre are usually acceptable to consumers, this may vary with local circumstances. At levels above 0.1 mg/litre, manganese in water supplies stains sanitary ware and laundry, and causes an undesirable taste in beverages. It may lead to accumulation of deposits in the distribution system. Even at concentration of 0.2 mg/litre, manganese will often form a coating on pipes, which may slough off as a black precipitate.

12. *Dissolved oxygen :* The dissolved oxygen content of water is influenced by the raw water temperature, composition, treatment and any chemical or biological processes taking place in the distribution system. Depletion of dissolved oxygen in water supplies can encourage microbial reduction of nitrate to nitrite and sulphate to sulphide, giving rise to odour problem. It can also cause an increase in the concentration of ferrous iron in solution. No health-based guideline value has been recommended.

13. *Copper :* The presence of copper in a water supply may interfere with the intended domestic uses of water. It increases the corrosion of galvanized iron and steel fittings. Staining of laundry and sanitary ware occurs at copper concentrations above 1 mg/litre.

14. *Aluminium :* The presence of aluminium at concentrations in excess of 0.2 mg/litre often leads to deposition of aluminium hydroxide floc in distribution system and the exacerbation of discoloration of water by iron.

Substances and parameters in drinking water and the reasons for consumer complaints are listed in Table 4.

II. MICROBIOLOGICAL ASPECTS

(a) **Bacteriological indicators :** Natural and treated waters vary in microbiological quality. Ideally, drinking water should not contain any microorganisms known to be pathogenic. It should also be free from bacteria indicative of pollution with excreta. Failure to provide adequate protection, effective treatment and disinfection of drinking water will expose the community to the risk of outbreaks of intestinal and other infectious diseases. Those at greatest risk of water-borne diseases are infants and young children, people who are debilitated or living under insanitary conditions, the sick and the elderly. For them the infective dose is significantly lower than for the healthy population. The potential consequences of microbial contamination are such that its control must always be of paramount importance and must never be compromised.

The primary bacterial indicator recommended for this purpose is the coliform group of organisms as a whole. Supplementary indicator organisms, such as faecal streptococci and sulphite-reducing clostridia, may sometimes be useful in determining the origin of faecal pollution as well as in assessing the efficiency of water treatment processes.

(1) *Coliform organisms :* The "coliform" organisms include all aerobic and facultative anaerobic, gram-negative, non–sporing, motile and non-motile rods capable of fermenting lactose at 35 to 37 deg. C in less than 48 hours. The coliform group includes both faecal and non-faecal organisms. Typical example of the faecal group is *E. coli* and

TABLE 4
Substances and parameters in drinking-water that may give rise to complaints from consumers

Constituents or characteristics	Levels likely to give rise to consumer complaints	Reasons for consumer complaints
Physical parameters		
Colour	15 TCU	appearance
Taste and odour	–	should be acceptable
Temperature	–	should be acceptable
Turbidity	1 NTU	appearance; for effective terminal disinfection, median turbidity ≤1 NTU,
Inorganic constituents		
Aluminium	0.2 mg/L	depositions, discolouration
Ammonia	1.5 mg/L	odour and taste
Chloride	250 mg/L	taste, corrosion
Copper	1 mg/L	staining of laundry and sanitary ware (health based provisional guideline value 2 mg/L)
Hardness	–	high hardness : scale deposition, scum formation; low hardness; possible corrosion
Hydrogen sulfide	0.05 mg/L	odour and taste
Iron	0.3 mg/L	staining of laundry and sanitary ware
Manganese	0.1 mg/L	staining of laundry and sanitary ware (health-based provisional guideline value 0.4 mg/L)
Dissolved oxygen	–	indirect effects
pH	–	low pH : corrosion; high pH : taste, soapy feel preferably < 8.0 for effective disinfection with chlorine
Sodium	200 mg/L	taste
Sulphate	250 mg/L	taste, corrosion
Total dissolved solids	1000 mg/L	taste
Zinc	4 mg/L	appearance, taste

Source : *(19)*

of the non-faecal group, *Klebsiella aerogens.* From a practical point of view it is assumed that all coliforms are of faecal origin unless a non-faecal origin can be proved.

There are several reasons why coliform organisms are chosen as indicators of faecal pollution rather than the water-borne pathogens directly : (1) the coliform organisms are constantly present in great abundance in the human intestine. It is estimated that an average person excretes 200–400 billion of these organisms per day. These organisms are foreign to potable waters, and hence their presence in water is looked upon as evidence of faecal contamination; (2) they are easily detected by culture methods – as small as one bacteria in 100 ml of water, whereas the methods for detecting the pathogenic organisms are complicated and time-consuming; (3) they survive longer than the pathogens, which tend to die out more rapidly than coliform bacili; and (4) the colifform bacilli have greater resistance to the forces of natural purification than the water borne pathogens. If the coliform organisms are present in a water sample, the assumption is the probable presence of intestinal pathogens.

(2) *Faecal streptococci :* Faecal streptococci regularly occur in faeces, but in much smaller numbers than *E.coli;* in doubtful cases, the finding of faecal streptococci in water is regarded as important confirmatory evidence of recent faecal pollution of water. Streptococci are highly resistant to drying and may be valuable for routine control testing after laying new mains or repairs in distribution systems or for detecting pollution by surface run-off to ground or surface waters.

(3) *C. perfringens :* They also occur regularly in faeces, though generally in much smaller numbers than *E.coli.* The spores are capable of surviving in water for a longer time than organisms of the coliform group, and usually resist chlorination at the doses normally used in waterworks practice. The presence of spores of *C. perfringens* in a natural water suggests that faecal contamination has occurred, and their presence, in the absence of the coliform group, suggests that faecal contamination occurred at some remote time. Its presence in filtered supplies may indicate deficiency in filtration practice.

The guideline values for bacteriological quality are given in Table 5. It is only a guidance required to ensure bacteriologically safe supplies of drinking water whether piped, unpiped or bottled.

(b) **Virological aspects :** It is recommended that, to be acceptable, drinking water should be free from any viruses infections for man. Disinfection with 0.5 mg/L of free chlorine residual after contact period of at least 30 minutes at a pH of 8.0 is sufficient to inactivate virus. This free chlorine residual is to be insisted in all disinfected supplies in areas suspected of endemicity of hepatitis A to take care of the safety of the supply from the virus point of view, which incidently takes care of safety from the bacteriologic point of view as well. For other areas 0.2 mg/L of free residual chlorine for half an hour should be insisted. The turbidity condition of 1 NTU or less, must be fulfilled prior to disinfection of water if adequate treatment is to be achieved. Ozone has been shown to be effective viral disinfectant, preferably for clean water, if residuals of 0.2–0.4 mg/L are maintained for 4 minutes, but it is not possible to maintain an ozone residual in distribution system.

(c) **Biological aspects :** (i) *Protozoa* – Species of protozoa known to have been transmitted by the ingestion of contaminated drinking water include *Entamoeba histolytica, Giardia spp.* and *rarely, Balantidium coli.* These organisms can be introduced into water supply through human or, in some instances, animal faecal contamination. Drinking water should not contain any pathogenic intestinal

TABLE 5

Bacteriological quality of drinking water[a]

Organisms	Guideline value
All water intended for drinking	
E.coli or thermotolerant coliform bacteria[b,c]	Must not be detectable in any 100 ml sample
Treated water entering the distribution system	
E.coli or thermotolerant coliform bacteria[b]	Must not be detectable in any 100 ml sample
Total coliform bacteria	Must not be detectable in any 100 ml sample
Treated water in the distribution system	
E.coli or thermotolerant coliform bacteria[b]	Must not be detectable in any 100 ml sample
Total coliform bacteria	Must not be detectable in any 100 ml sample. In the case of large supplies, where sufficient samples are examined, must not be present in 95% of samples taken throughout any 12 month period.

a. Immediate investigative action must be taken if either *E.coli* or total coliform bacteria are detected. The minimum action in the case of total coliform bacteria is repeat sampling; if these bacteria are detected in the repeat sample, the cause must be determined by immediate further investigation.

b. Although *E.coli* is the more precise indicator of faecal pollution, the count of thermotolerant coliform bacteria is an acceptable alternative. If necessary, proper confirmatory tests must be carried out. Total coliform bacteria are not acceptable indicators of the sanitary quality of rural water supplies, particularly in tropical areas where many bacteria of no sanitary significance occur in almost all untreated supplies.

c. It is recognized that, in the great majority of rural water supplies in developing countries, faecal contamination is widespread. Under these conditions, the national surveillance agency should set medium-term targets for progressive improvement of water supplies.

protozoa. Rapid or slow sand filtration have been shown to be effective in removing a high proportion of pathogenic protozoa. Standard methods are not currently available for the detection of pathogenic protozoa in water supplies in the context of a routine monitoring programme; (ii) *Helminths* : The infective stages of many parasitic roundworms and flatworms can be transmitted to man through drinking water. A single mature larva or fertilized egg can cause infection and such infective stages should be absent from drinking water. However, the water route is relatively unimportant except in the case of *Dracunculus medinensis* (guinea worm) and the human schistosomes, which are primarily hazards of unpiped water supplies. Source protection is the best approach to prevention. The methods for detection of these parasites are unsuited for routine monitoring; (iii) *Free-living organisms* : Free living organisms that may occur in water supplies include fungi, algae etc. The most common problem with these are their interference in the operation of water treatment process, colour, turbidity, taste and odour of finished water.

III. CHEMICAL ASPECTS

The health risk due to toxic chemicals in drinking water differs from that caused by microbiological contaminants. There are few chemical constituents of water that can lead to acute health problems except through massive accidental contamination of a supply. Moreover, experience shows that, in such incidents the water usually becomes undrinkable owing to unacceptable taste, odour and appearance.

The chemicals selected for the development of guideline value include those considered potentially hazardous to human health, those detected relatively frequently in drinking water and those detected in relatively high concentrations. The problem associated with chemical constituents of drinking water arise primarily from their ability to cause adverse health effects after prolonged periods of exposure; of particular concern are contaminants that have cumulative toxic properties, such as heavy metals and substances that are carcinogenic.

Health-related chemical constituents

The presence of certain chemicals in excess of prescribed limits may constitute ground for rejection of the water as a source of public water supply. These substances may be inorganic or organic *(9)*.

a. Inorganic constituents : These substances include arsenic, cadmium, chromium, cyanide, fluoride, lead, mercury, nickel, nitrate, selenium etc. The guide line value of these constituents are as shown in Table 6.

1. *Arsenic :* Arsenic is introduced into water through the dissolution of minerals and ores, from industrial effluents, and from atmospheric deposition; concentrations in ground water in some areas are sometimes elevated as a result of erosion from natural sources. The average daily intake of inorganic arsenic in water is estimated to be similar to that from food. Intake from air is negligible. A provisional guideline value for arsenic in drinking water of 0.01 mg/litre is established.

TABLE 6

Inorganic chemicals of health significance in drinking water

Constituents	Recommended maximum limit of concentration (mg/litre)	(µg/litre)
Antimony	0.02 (P)	20
Arsenic	0.01 (P)	10
Barium	0.7	700
Boron	2.4	2,400
Cadmium	0.003	0.3
Chromium	0.05 (P)	50
Copper	2	2,000
Fluoride	1.5	1,500
Lead	0.01	10
Manganese	0.4 (P)	400
Mercury (total)	0.006	6
Molybdenum	0.07	70
Nickel	0.07	70
Nitrate (as NO_3)	50	50,000
Nitrite (as NO_2)	3 (P)	3,000
Selenium	0.04	40

Source : *(19)* P – Provisional guideline value

2. *Cadmium* : Cadmium metal is used in the steel industry and in plastics. Cadmium compounds are widely used in batteries. It is released to the environment in waste-water and diffuse pollution is caused by contamination from fertilizers and local air pollution. Contamination in drinking water may also be caused by impurities in the zinc of galvanized pipes and some metal fittings, although levels in drinking water are usually less than 1µg/litre. Absorption of cadmium compound is dependent on the solubility of the compound. Cadmium accumulates primarily in the kidneys and has a long biological half-life in humans of 10–35 years. A guideline value for cadmium is established at 0.3 µg/litre *(19)*.

3. *Chromium* : Chromium is widely distributed in the earth's crust. In general, food appears to be the major source of intake. The absorption of chromium after oral exposure is relatively low and depends on the oxidation state. The guideline value for chromium is 0.05 mg/litre, which is considered to be unlikely to give rise to significant health risks.

4. *Cyanide* : The acute toxicity of cyanide is high. Cyanides can be found in some foods, particularly in some developing countries, and they are usually found in drinking water, primarily as a consequence of industrial contamination. Effects on thyroid and particularly the nervous system were observed in some populations as a consequence of the long-term consumption of inadequately processed cassava containing high levels of cyanide.

5. *Fluoride* : Fluoride accounts for about 0.3 g/kg of the earth's crust. Inorganic fluorine compounds are used in the production of aluminium, and fluoride is released during the manufacture and use of phosphate fertilizers which contain upto 4 per cent fluorine. Levels of daily exposure of fluoride depends on the geographical area. If diets contain fish and tea, exposure *via* food may be particularly high. In specific areas, other foods and indoor air pollution may contribute considerably to total exposure. Additional intake may result from the use of fluoride toothpastes.

Exposure to fluoride from drinking water depends greatly on natural circumstances. Levels in raw water are normally below 1.5 mg/litre, but ground water may contain about 10 mg/litre in areas rich in fluoride – containing minerals. High fluoride levels, above 5 mg/litre, have been found in several countries (e.g., China, India and Thailand). Such high levels have at times led to dental or skeletal fluorosis. Fluoride is sometimes added to drinking water to prevent dental caries. Soluble fluorides are readily absorbed in the gastrointestinal tract after intake in drinking water. The guideline value suggested is 1.5 mg/litre. In setting national standards for fluoride, it is particularly important to consider climatic conditions, volume of water intake and intake of fluoride from other sources (e.g., food and air).

6. *Lead* : Lead is present in tapwater to some extent as a result of its dissolution from natural sources, but primarily from household plumbing systems containing lead in pipes, solder, fittings or the service connections to homes. The amount of lead dissolved from the plumbing system depends on several factors, including pH, temperature, water hardness and standing time of the water, with soft, acidic water being the most plumbosolvent.

Placental transfer of lead occurs in humans as early as twelfth week of gestation and continues throughout development. Young children absorb 4–5 times as much lead as adults, and the biological half-life may be considerably longer in children than in adults. Lead is a general toxicant that accumulates in the skeleton. Infants, children upto six years of age, and pregnant women are most susceptible to its adverse health effects. Lead also interferes with calcium metabolism, both directly and by interfering with vitamin D metabolism. Lead is toxic to both central and peripheral nervous system, inducing sub-encephalopathic neurological and behavioural effects. Renal tumours have been induced in experimental animals exposed to high concentrations of lead compounds in the diet and it is grouped in Group B (possible human carcinogen). The health-based guideline value of lead is 0.01 mg/litre.

Lead is exceptional in that most lead in drinking water arises from plumbing in buildings and the remedy consists principally of removing plumbing and fittings containing lead. This requires much time and money, and it is recognized that not all water will meet the guideline immediately. Measures to control corrosion should also be implemented.

7. *Mercury* : Mercury is present in inorganic form in surface and ground water at concentrations usually less than 0.5 µg/litre. The kidney is the main target organ for inorganic mercury, whereas methyl mercury affects mainly the central nervous system. The guideline value for total mercury is 0.006 mg/litre.

8. *Nitrate and nitrite* : Nitrate and nitrite are naturally occurring ions that are part of the nitrogen cycle. Naturally occurring nitrate level in surface and ground water are generally a few milligrams per litre. In many ground waters, an increase of nitrate level has been observed owing to the intensification of farming practice. In some countries, upto 10 per cent of the population may be exposed to nitrate levels in drinking water of above 50 mg/litre.

In general, vegetables are the main source of nitrate intake when levels in drinking water is below 10 mg/litre. When nitrate level in drinking water exceeds 50 mg/litre, drinking water will become the main source of total nitrate intake. The guideline value for nitrate in drinking water is solely to prevent methaemoglobinaemia, which depends upon the conversion of nitrate into nitrite. Bottle-fed infants of less than 3 months of age are most susceptible.

The guideline value should not be expressed on the basis of nitrate-nitrogen but on the basis of nitrate itself, which is the chemical entity of concern to health and the guideline value for nitrate is 50 mg/litre.

As a result of recent evidence of the presence of nitrite in some water supplies, it was concluded that a guideline value of 3 mg/litre for nitrite should be proposed. Because of the possibility of simultaneous occurrence of nitrite and nitrate in drinking water, the sum of the ratios of the concentration of each to its guideline value should not exceed 1, i.e.

$$\frac{\text{Concentration of nitrate}}{\text{Guideline value of nitrate}} + \frac{\text{Concentration of nitrite}}{\text{Guideline value of nitrite}} = \leq 1$$

9. *Selenium* : Selenium levels in drinking water vary greatly in different geographical areas, and are usually much less than the guideline value of 0.01 mg/litre. Food stuffs are the principal source, and the level depends according to geographical area of production. Selenium is an essential element for humans and forms an integral part of the enzyme glutathione peroxidase. Most selenium compounds are water soluble. In humans, the toxicity of long-term exposure are manifested in nails, hair and liver.

b. Organic constituents : The guideline values of some of the organic chemical constituents in water are as shown in Table 7.

TABLE 7

Guideline values for health related organic constituents

Organic constituents	Upper limit of concentration (μg/litre)
Chlorinated alkanes	
Carbon tetrachloride	2
Dichloromethane	20
Chlorinated ethenes	
Vinyl chloride	55
1,1 – dichloroethene	30
1,2 – dichloroethene	50
Aromatic hydrocarbons	
Benzene	10
Toluene	700
Xylenes	500
Ethylbenzene	300
Styrene	20
Benzolalpyrene	0.7

Source : *(19)*

Polynuclear aromatic hydrocarbons : A large number of polynuclear aromatic hydrocarbons (PAHs) from a variety of combustion and pyrolysis sources have been identified in the environment. The main source of human exposure to PAHs is food, with drinking water contributing only minor amounts.

Little information is available on the oral toxicity of PAHs, especially after long-term exposure. Benzo [a] pyrene, which constitutes a minor fraction of total PAHs have been found to be carcinogenic in mice by the oral route of administration. Some PAH compounds have been found to be carcinogenic by non-oral routes, Benzo [a] pyrene has been found to be mutagenic in a number of *in vitro* and *in vivo* assays.

The following recommendations are made for the PAH group :

- Because of the close association of PAH with suspended solids, the application of treatment, when necessary to achieve the recommended level of turbidity will ensure that PAH levels are reduced to a minimum.
- Contamination of water with PAH should not occur during water treatment or distribution. Therefore, the use of coal-tar-based and similar materials for pipe lining and coatings on storage tanks should be discontinued.
- In situation where contamination of drinking water by PAH has occurred, the specific compounds present and the source of the contamination should be identified, as the carcinogenic potential of PAH compounds varies.

Pesticides : The pesticides that are of importance in connection with water quality include chlorinated hydrocarbons and their derivatives, persistent herbicides, soil insecticides, pesticides that are easily leached out from the soil, and pesticides that are systematically added to water supplies for disease vector control. The recommended guideline value (Table 8) are set at a level to protect human health.

TABLE 8

Guideline values of certain pesticides

Pesticides	Upper limit of concentration (μg/litre)
Aldrin/dieldrin	0.03
Chlordane	0.2
DDT	2
2,4–D	30
Heptachlor and heptachlor epoxide	0.03
Hexachlorobenzene	1
Lindane	2
Methoxychlor	20
Pentachlorophenol	9 (P)

Source : *(19)* P – Provisional value

Drinking water consumption and body weight : The average *daily per capita* consumption of drinking water is usually found to be around 2 litres, but there are considerable variations between individuals as water intake is likely to vary with climate, physical activity and culture, e.g., at temperature above 25°C, there is a sharp rise in fluid intake, largely to meet the demands of an increased sweat rate. In developing the guideline values for potentially hazardous chemicals, a daily *per capita* consumption of 2 litres by a person weighing 60 kg was generally assumed. However, such an assumption may underestimate the consumption of water per unit weight, and this exposure, for those living in hot climates as well as for infants and children, who consume more fluid per unit weight than adults. Where it was judged that this segment of the population was at a particularly high risk from exposure to certain chemicals, the guideline value was derived on the basis of a 10 kg child consuming 1 litre water per day or a 5 kg infant consuming 0.75 litre water per day.

Health-risk assessment : For most kinds of toxicity, it is generally believed that there is a dose below which no adverse effects will occur. For chemicals that give rise to such toxic effects, a tolerable daily intake (TDI) can be derived.

Tolerable daily intake (TDI) *:* The TDI is an estimate of the amount of a substance in food or drinking water, expressed on a body weight basis (mg/kg or μg/kg of body weight), that can be ingested daily over a lifetime without appreciable health risk *(19)*.

Acceptable daily intake (ADI) are established for food additives and pesticide residues that occur in food for necessary technological purposes or plant protection reasons. For chemical contaminants, which usually have no intended function in drinking water the term TDI is seen as more appropriate than ADI, as it signifies permissibility rather than acceptability.

No–observed–adverse–effect level (NOAEL) : The NOAEL is defined as the highest dose or concentration of a chemical in a single study, found by experiment or observation, that causes no detectable adverse health effect *(19)*. Whenever possible, the NOAEL is based on long-term studies, preferably of ingestion in drinking water.

Lowest–observed–adverse–effect level (LOAEL) : LOAEL

is the lowest observed dose or concentration of a substance at which there is a detectable adverse health effect *(19)*. When LOAEL is used instead of NOAEL, an additional uncertainty factor (UF) is normally used.

Uncertainty factors (UF) : The application of uncertainty factors has been widely used in the derivation of ADI for food additives, pesticides and environmental contaminants. The derivation of these factors requires expert judgement and a careful sifting of the available scientific evidence.

In the derivation of the WHO drinking water quality guideline values, uncertainty factors were applied to the lowest NOAEL or LOAEL for the response considered to be most biologically significant and were determined by consensus among a group of experts using the approach outlined below :

Source of uncertainty	Factor
Interspecies variation (animal to humans)	1 – 10
Intraspecies variation (individual variation)	1 – 10
Adequacy of studies or database	1 – 10
Nature and severity of effect	1 – 10

The total uncertainty factor should not exceed 10,000. If the risk assessment would lead to a higher uncertainty factor, then the resulting TDI would be so imprecise as to lack meaning. For substances for which uncertainty factors were greater than 1000, guideline values are designated as provisional in order to emphasize the high level of uncertainty inherent in these values *(19)*.

Derivation of guideline value using a TDI approach : TDI can be calculated by following formula.

$$TDI = \frac{NOAEL\ OR\ LOAEL}{UF}$$

The guideline value (GV) is then derived from the TDI as follows :

$$GV = \frac{TDI \times bw \times P}{C}$$

Where bw = body weight (60 kg for adult, 10 kg for children, 5 kg for infants)

P = fraction of the TDI allocated to drinking water

C = daily drinking water consumption (2 litres for adults, 1 litre for children and 0.75 litre for infants)

IV. RADIOLOGICAL ASPECTS

The effects of radiation exposure are called "somatic" if they become manifest in the exposed individual, and "hereditary" if they affect the descendants. Malignant disease is the most important delayed somatic effect *(30)*. For some somatic effects such as carcinogenesis, the probability of an effect occurring, rather than its severity, is regarded as a function of dose without a threshold (stochastic effect). Whereas for other somatic effects the severity of the effect varies with the dose (non-stochastic effects); a threshold may therefore exist for such effects. The aim of radiation protection is to prevent harmful non-stochastic effects and to reduce the probability of stochastic effects to a level deemed acceptable.

Radioactivity in drinking water should not only be kept within safe limits; it should also, within those limits, be kept as low as is reasonably possible. The guideline values recommended take account of both naturally occurring radioactivity and any radioactivity that may reach the water source as a result of man's activities. From a radiological point of view, they represent a value below which water can be considered potable without any further radiological examination.

The activity of a radioactive material is the number of nuclear disintegration per unit of time. The unit of activity is a becquerel (Bq); 1 Bq = 1 disintegration per second. Formerly, the unit of activity was curie (Ci).

The proposed guideline values are :

gross alpha activity 0.5 Bq / L
gross beta activity 1.0 Bq / L

SURVEILLANCE OF DRINKING WATER QUALITY *(20)*

The activities that ideally should be included in the surveillance function are :

a. approval of new sources (including private-owned supplies);
b. watershed protection;
c. approval of the construction and operating procedures of waterworks, including :
   (i) disinfection of the plant and of the distribution system after repair or interruption of supply,
   (ii) periodic flushing programmes and cleaning of water storage facilities,
   (iii) certification of operators,
   (iv) regulation of chemical substances used in water treatment,
   (v) cross-connection control, back-flow prevention and leak detection control ;
d. sanitary surveys;
e. monitoring programmes, including provision for central and regional analytical laboratory services;
f. development of codes of practice for well construction, pump installation and plumbing;
g. inspection quality control in bottled-water and ice manufacturing operations.

Surveillance of drinking water is essentially a health measure. It is intended to protect the public from water-borne diseases. The elements of a surveillance programme are :

1. Sanitary survey

Sanitary survey is an on-the-spot inspection and evaluation by a qualified person of the entire water supply system. The purpose of the survey is detection and correction of faults and deficiencies. A sanitary survey is essential for adequate interpretation of laboratory results.

2. Sampling

Sampling of water should be done with the thoroughness of a surgical operation, with the observation of similar aseptic precautions, for upon it depends the results of analysis. It should be carried out by competent and trained personnel in strict accordance with the methods and frequency of sampling prescribed in the WHO guidelines for drinking-water quality or the ICMR 'Manual of Standards of

Quality for Drinking Water Supplies' *(21)*. The methods of sampling are set out briefly in Appendix II.

3. Bacteriological surveillance

The tests usually employed in water bacteriology are presumptive coliform test, tests for the detection of faecal streptococci and *C. perfringens* and colony count. A complete bacteriological examination consists of all these tests.

(1) PRESUMPTIVE COLIFORM TEST

(i) *Multiple tube method* : This test is based on estimating the most probable number (MPN) of coliform organisms in 100 ml of water. The test is carried out by inoculating measured quantities of the sample water (0.1, 1.0, 10, 50 ml) into tubes of McConkey's Lactose Bile Salt Broth with bromcresol purple as an indicator. The tubes are incubated for 48 hours. From the number of tubes showing acid and gas, an estimate of the MPN of coliform organisms in 100 ml of the sample water can be obtained from statistical tables. This result is known as "presumptive coliform count", the presumption being each tube showing fermentation, contains coliform organisms. The reaction may occasionally be due to the presence of some other organisms or combination of organisms.

Confirmatory tests : The next step is to confirm the presence of coliform organisms in each tube showing a presumptive positive reaction. Such confirmation is not generally required in case of unchlorinated water, but is required in case of chlorinated water. Confirmation is done by subculturing each presumptive positive tube in 2 tubes of brilliant green bile broth, one of which is incubated at 37 deg C for up to 48 hours for confirmation of the presence of coliform organisms, and the other incubated at 44°C and inspected after 6 and 24 hours to decide whether or not *E. coli* is present. *E. coli* is almost the only coliform organism which is capable of producing gas from lactose at 44 deg C. Further confirmation of the presence of *E. coli*, if desired, can be obtained by testing for indol production at 44°C.

(ii) *Membrane filtration technique* : In some countries membrane filter technique is used as a standard procedure to test for the presence of coliform organisms. A measured volume of the sample is filtered through a membrane specially made of cellulose ester. All the bacteria present in water are retained on the surface of the membrane and by inoculating the membrane face upwards on suitable media and at appropriate temperature, it is possible to count the colonies and obtain results within 20 hours as compared to 72–96 hours required for the usual multiple tube technique.

(2) THE DETECTION OF FAECAL STREPTOCOCCI AND *C. PERFRINGENS*

The presence of faecal streptococci and *C. perfringens* provides useful confirmatory evidence of the faecal pollution of water in doubtful cases.

(3) COLONY COUNT

Colony counts on nutrient agar at 37 deg C and 22 deg C are frequently used in the bacteriological examination of water. Colony counts provide an estimate of the general bacterial purity of water. A single count is of little value, but counts from the same source at frequent intervals may be of considerable value. A sudden increase in the colony count may give the earliest indication of contamination. The recommended plate counts are:

Water at the point of consumption	*Plate count after 2 days at 37 deg C*	*Plate count after 3 days at 22 deg C.*
(i) Disinfected	0	20
(ii) Not-disinfected	10	100

Recent studies indicate that a bacterial plate count on yeast extract agar after incubation at 22 deg C for 7 days might serve as the best general purpose indicator of microbiological quality because in the absence of chlorine residual, the number of bacteria growing at 22 deg C after 7 days incubation can increase enormously *(22)*.

4. Biological examination

Water may contain microscopic organisms such as algae, fungi, yeast, protozoa, rotifers, crustaceans, minute worms, etc. These organisms are collectively called 'plankton'. The plankton organisms produce objectionable tastes and odours in water. They are an index of pollution. The degree of pollution is assessed qualitatively and quantitatively by noting the type and number of organisms prevailing in water.

5. Chemical surveillance

Chemical surveillance of drinking water is assuming greater importance in view of industrial and agricultural pollutants finding their way into raw water sources. Tests for pH, colour, turbidity, chlorides, ammonia, chlorine demand and residual chlorine are the basic tests. Regular measurement of chlorine residuals in supply may in part replace bacteriological surveillance. Tests for iron and manganese are required when these substances are present in the raw water in sufficient amount to influence water treatment. Complete chemical analysis would also include analysis for toxic metals, pesticides, persistent organic chemicals and radioactivity.

HARDNESS OF WATER

Hardness may be defined as the soap destroying power of water. The consumer considers water hard if large amounts of soap are required to produce lather. The hardness in water is caused mainly by four dissolved compounds. These are (1) Calcium bicarbonate (2) Magnesium bicarbonate (3) Calcium sulphate, and (4) Magnesium sulphate. The presence of any one of these compounds produces hardness. There are others which are of less importance. Chlorides and nitrates of calcium and magnesium can also cause hardness but they occur generally in small amounts. Iron, manganese and aluminium compounds also cause hardness, but as they generally are present in such small amounts, it is customary not to consider them in connection with hardness.

Hardness is classified as carbonate and non-carbonate. The carbonate hardness which was formerly designated as "temporary" hardness is due to the presence of calcium and magnesium bicarbonates. The non-carbonate hardness, formerly designated as "permanent" hardness, is due to calcium and magnesium sulphates, chlorides and nitrates.

Hardness in water is expressed in terms of "milli-equivalents per litre (mEq/L)". One mEq/L of hardness-producing ion is equal to 50 mg $CaCO_3$ (50ppm) in one litre of water *(23)*. The terms soft and hard water are used when the levels of hardness are as given in Table 9.

TABLE 9

Classification of hardness in water

Classification	Level of hardness (mEq./litre)
(a) Soft water	Less than 1 (<50 mg/L)
(b) Moderately hard	1–3 (50–150 mg/L)
(c) Hard water	3–6 (150–300 mg/L)
(d) Very hard water	over 6 (> 300 mg/L)

Drinking water should be moderately hardy. Softening of water is recommended when the hardness exceeds 3 mEq/l (150 mg per litre).

DISADVANTAGES OF HARDNESS

Hardness in water presents several disadvantages both to the domestic and industrial consumer. These may be stated as follows: (1) hardness in water consumes more soap and detergents (2) when hard water is heated, the carbonates are precipitated and bring about furring or scaling of boilers. This leads to great fuel consumption, loss of efficiency and may sometimes cause boiler explosions (3) hard water adversely affects cooking; food cooked in soft water retains its natural colour and appearance (4) fabrics washed with soap in hard water do not have a long life (5) there are many industrial processes in which hard water is unsuited and gives rise to economic losses (6) hardness shortens the life of pipes and fixtures.

SPECIAL TREATMENT

(a) Removal of hardness

The methods of removal of hardness are briefly stated as below:

Temporary hardness

(a) Boiling
(b) Addition of lime
(c) Addition of sodium carbonate
(d) Permutit process.

Permanent hardness

(a) Addition of sodium carbonate
(b) Base exchange process.

1. BOILING

Boiling removes the temporary hardness by expelling carbon dioxide, and precipitating the insoluble calcium carbonate. It is an expensive method to soften water on a large scale.

$$Ca(HCO_3)_2 \longrightarrow CaCO_3 + H_2O + CO_2$$

2. ADDITION OF LIME

Lime softening not only reduces total hardness but also accomplishes magnesium reduction. Lime absorbs the carbon dioxide, and precipitates the insoluble calcium carbonate. In the Clark's method of softening water, one ounce of quick lime is added to every 700 gallons of water for each degree (14.25 ppm.) of hardness.

$$Ca(OH)_2 + Ca(HCO_3)_2 \longrightarrow 2CaCO_3 + 2H_2O$$

3. ADDITION OF SODIUM CARBONATE

Sodium carbonate (soda ash) removes both temporary and permanent hardness, as shown below :

(i) $Na_2CO_3 + Ca(HCO_3)_2 \longrightarrow 2NaHCO_3 + CaCO_3$
(ii) $CaSO_4 + Na_2CO_3 \longrightarrow CaCO_3 + Na_2SO_4$

4. BASE EXCHANGE PROCESS

In the treatment of large water supplies, the permutit process is used. Sodium permutit is a complex compound of sodium, aluminium and silica ($Na_2\ Al_2\ Si_2O\ H_2O$). It has the property of exchanging the sodium cation for the calcium and magnesium ions in the water. When hard water is passed through the permutit the calcium and magnesium ions are entirely removed by base exchange and the sodium permutit is finally converted into calcium and magnesium permutit. By this process, water can be softened to zero hardness. Since water of zero hardness is corrosive, a part of the raw water is mixed with the softened water to secure the desired hardness. After permutit has been used for sometime, it loses its effectiveness but it may be regenerated by treating with concentrated solution of sodium chloride or brine and washing away the soluble calcium and magnesium chloride formed. Permutit process removes both temporary and permanent hardness.

Water hardness and cardiovascular diseases

Reports from several countries have shown an inverse statistical association between the hardness of drinking water and the death rate from cardiovascular diseases. Areas supplied with soft drinking water showed a significantly higher prevalence of either arteriosclerotic heart disease, or degenerative heart disease, hypertension, sudden deaths of cardiovascular origin, or a combination of these. The evidence is based solely on circumstantial evidence and statistical association. Further studies are in progress to establish a possible connection between certain water characteristics and the development of cardiovascular diseases *(24)*.

(b) Fluoridation of water

Fluorine is one of the constituents naturally present in water supplies. In fact, the main source of fluorine is drinking water. Deficiency of fluorine in drinking water is associated with dental caries, and excess with dental and skeletal fluorosis. Leading workers in India regard fluorine in concentration of 0.5 to 0.8 ppm in drinking water as optimum (a concentration of 1 ppm is regarded as optimum in temperate climates because the consumption of water is low). The term "fluoridation" has been given to the process of supplementing the natural fluoride content of potable waters to the point of optimum concentration. The WHO in 1969 recommended fluoridation of community water supplies in areas where the total intake of fluorides by the population is below the optimal levels for protection against dental caries. Fluoridation is now an accepted public health procedure in many developed countries *(25)*.

(c) Defluoridation

In some geographic areas, water may contain a high level of fluorides. In such communities, water is defluoridated by phosphate to reduce fluorides to optimum levels.

SELECTION OF SOURCE OF WATER

In selecting a source, attention must be given to possible future developments that may influence the continued suitability of the source. Other considerations include (a) *Quantity (source capacity)* : The quantity of water should be sufficient to meet continuing water demands, taking into account daily and seasonal variations and projected growth in the size of the community being served. (b) *Quality* : The quality of raw water should be such that, with appropriate treatment, it meets the drinking water standards. (c) *Protection* : The watershed must be protected from pollution with human excreta, industrial discharge and agricultural run-off. (d) *Feasibility* : The source should be available at reasonable cost. (e) *Treatability* : The raw water should be treated adequately under locally prevailing conditions.

Potential new sources should be examined in the field by qualified and experienced sanitary surveyors and physical, bacteriological and chemical analysis should be carried out for a period covering seasonal variations prior to final selection of the source. Such information is essential in order to define appropriate water treatment requirements and necessary pollution control measures to protect raw water resources. It is preferable to choose the source that requires the least treatment. The source should be protected from contaminants emanating from septic tanks, sewers, cesspools, sullage water and flooding and from contamination by users. Maintaining adequate residual chlorine levels in the distribution system is the most reliable indicator of protection against contamination resulting from cross-connection, back siphonage, leaks etc.

DISTRIBUTION OF WATER

There are two main systems of water distribution, the intermittent supply and the continuous supply. In the intermittent system, water is delivered only during fixed hours. The disadvantages of the intermittent system are : (1) the pipes may be empty during times of emergency (2) people need to store water in containers which may not be clean always. The safe water is likely to be rendered unsafe through improper storage (3) when the pipes are empty, there is negative pressure and by what is known as back-siphoning, bacteria and foul gases may be sucked in through leaky joints. A number of recorded outbreaks of typhoid and of relapsing fever, among other diseases, have been traced back to the contamination of water in the intermittent piped water supplies. Flowing water available 24 hours is therefore desirable, although it may entail some wastage of water through misuse. The supply of water in most cities in India is intermittent. A WHO Expert Committee (1965) strongly recommended that intermittent and low pressure service should be avoided *(26)*. DUAL WATER SUPPLY: In Kolkata, there was a dual water supply system, i.e., one set of pipes supplying filtered water for personal use and the other set supplying unfiltered water for flushing toilets, washing roads and other civic purposes. The greatest drawback of the dual system is that people may mistake one for the other through ignorance. The WHO Expert Committee (1965) strongly disapproved of the practice of supplying two kinds of water *(26)*. The possibility of cross-connection constitutes a serious health hazard.

SWIMMING POOL SANITATION

Swimming pool water is exposed to (1) faecal contamination and (2) organisms from skin and nasopharynx. The health hazards associated with swimming pools are:

(1) fungal and viral infections of the skin. This includes **Epidermophyton** and **Trichophyton** species which produce "athlete's foot." The papilloma virus is the inciting agent of "plantar warts"
(2) infections of the eye, ear, nose and throat
(3) infections of the upper respiratory tract,
(4) intestinal infections, and
(5) accidents.

SANITATION MEASURES

(1) *Recommended area:* The recommended area is 2.2 sq.m. (24 sq.ft.) per swimmer *(27)*. (2) *Surveillance:* Rules and regulations governing the use of the pool should be posted in a conspicuous place for the information of the users. These are: (a) Persons suffering from skin diseases, sore eyes, cold, nasal or ear discharge or any other communicable disease should not be allowed into the swimming pool. (b) All bathers are strictly instructed to empty the bladder, and if necessary use the toilet. (c) A cleansing shower bath in the nude with soap and water is required before entering the pool. (d) spitting, spouting of water, blowing the nose, etc. are prohibited. (e) The environment of the swimming pool including the shower rooms, walk ways and pool decks should receive proper disinfection to destroy bacterial, viral and fungal agents. (2) *Filtration of water* : Swimming pools are equipped with rapid sand filters. The filtering is continuous such that all the water is refiltered in less than 6 hours. Part of the water, up to 15 per cent, should be replaced by fresh water every day. The function of water replacement is to remove solutes consisting of ammonia, albuminoid, organic and nitrate nitrogen derived from the bathers. These solutes have the capacity to reduce the bactericidal activity of chlorine. (3) *Chlorination* : Chlorination is the most widely used method of pool disinfection. Various workers have stated that a continuous maintenance of 1.0 mg/litre (1 ppm) of free chlorine residual provides adequate protection against bacterial and viral agents *(28)*. The pH of water is kept between 7.4–7.8. (4) *Bacteriological quality* : The bacteriological quality of water should reach, as nearly as possible, the standards prescribed for drinking water.

National Water Supply and Sanitation Programme

The National Water Supply and Sanitation Programme was launched in 1954 by the Govt. of India as part of the Health Plan to assist the States to provide adequate water supply and sanitation facilities in the entire country. Provision has been made in the successive 5-year Plans to improve the water supply *(29)*.

For further details see chapter 7.

Health education

The provision of merely good water supply does not in itself secure freedom from water-borne diseases. People must recognize safe water as a "felt" health need and give up their old, unhygienic habits of polluting water supplies. In these circumstances, health education emerges as an important weapon in creating among people a desire for higher standards of life.

APPENDIX I

HORROCK'S APPARATUS

Horrock's water testing apparatus is designed to find out the dose of bleaching powder required for disinfection of water.

CONTENTS

1. 6 white cups (200 ml capacity each)
2. One black cup with a circular mark on the inside
3. 2 metal spoons (each holds 2g of bleaching powder when filled level with the brim)
4. 7 glass stirring rods
5. One special pipette
6. Two droppers
7. Starch-iodide indicator solution
8. Instruction folder.

PROCEDURE

1. Take one level spoonful (2 g) of bleaching powder in the black cup and make it into a thin paste with a little water. Add more water to the paste and make up the volume upto the circular mark with vigorous stirring. Allow to settle. This is the stock solution.

2. Fill the 6 white cups with water to be tested, upto about a cm below the brim.

3. With the special pipette provided add one drop of the stock solution to the 1st cup, 2 drops to the 2nd cup, 3 drops to the 3rd cup, and so on.

4. Stir the water in each cup using a separate rod.

5. Wait for half an hour for the action of chlorine.

6. Add 3 drops of starch-iodide indicator to each of the white cups and stir again. Development of blue colour indicates the presence of free residual chlorine.

7. Note the first cup which shows distinct blue colour. Supposing the 3rd cup shows blue colour, then 3 level spoonfuls or 6 grams of bleaching powder would be required to disinfect 455 litres of water.

APPENDIX II

SAMPLING

1. Samples for physical and chemical examination

Samples for physical and chemical examination should be collected in clean glass stoppered bottles made of neutral glass, of capacity not less than 2 litres. Stoppered glass bottles technically known as "Winchester Quart bottles" are suitable. Before collecting the sample rinse the bottle well three times with the water, filling it each time about 1/3 full. Then fill it with the water, tie the stopper tightly down, with a piece of cloth over it and seal the string.

2. Samples for bacteriological examination

Samples for bacteriological examination should be collected in clean sterilized bottles made of neutral glass, of capacity 200–250 ml and provided with a ground glass stopper having an overlapping rim. The stopper must be relaxed by an intervening strip of paper to prevent breakage of the bottle during sterilization or jamming of the stopper. The stopper and the neck of the bottle should be protected by a paper or parchment cover. If the water to be sampled contains, or is likely to contain chlorine, a small quantity of sodium thiosulphate (0.1 ml of 3.0 per cent solution or a small crystal of the salt) should be added to the bottle before sterilization. Sterile sampling bottles should be obtained from the laboratory which is to carry out the analysis. The sampling bottle should not be opened until the moment at which it is required for filling.

(1) COLLECTION OF THE SAMPLE FROM A TAP

When the sample is to be taken from a tap in regular use, the tap should be opened fully, and the water run to waste at least for 2 minutes in order to flush the interior of the nozzle and to discharge the stagnant water in the service pipe. In the case of samples to be collected from taps which are not in regular use, the tap should be sterilized by heating it either with a blow lamp or with an ignited piece of cotton soaked in methylated spirit, until it is unbearably hot to the touch. Then the tap should be cooled by allowing the water to run to waste before the sample is collected.

The bottle should be held near the base with one hand and the stopper and paper cover over it removed together and held in the fingers. The sample bottle should be filled from a gentle stream of water from the tap, avoiding splashing. The collection of samples from taps which are leaky, should be avoided because the water might run down the outside of the tap and enter the bottle causing contamination. If this cannot be avoided, special precautions should be taken to clean the outside of the tap and to flame it sufficiently to ensure sterility.

(2) COLLECTION OF SAMPLES FROM RIVERS, LAKES, RESERVOIRS, WELLS, ETC

Samples from rivers and streams should not be taken too near the bank or too far away from the point of draw off. For collecting samples directly from rivers, lakes, tanks, wells etc., a bottle with a string attached to the neck which is fully wrapped in paper and sterilized should be used. Before taking the sample, the paper cover should be removed, taking care not to allow the sides of the bottle to come in contact with anything. Another long clean string should be tied to the end of the sterilized string, and the bottle lowered into the water and allowed to fill up. The bottle should be then raised and the stopper with cover replaced.

Another method of collecting samples from rivers or reservoirs is to hold the bottle by the bottom and plunge its neck down-wards below the surface of the water. The bottle is then turned until the neck points slightly up-wards, the mouth being directed towards the current. If no current exists, as in a reservoir, a current should be artificially created by pushing the bottle horizontally forward in a direction away from the hand. When full, the bottle is raised rapidly above the surface and the stopper replaced.

If a sample is to be taken from a well fitted with a pump, the water should be pumped to waste for about 2 minutes and the sample collected from the pump delivery or from a tap on the discharge.

(3) TRANSPORT AND STORAGE OF SAMPLES

The bacteriological examination of the sample should be commenced as soon as possible after collection. Where this is not feasible, the sample should be kept in ice until it is taken for analysis. All such iced samples should be taken for analysis within 48 hours after collection. Samples not preserved in this manner should not be accepted for bacteriological examination. Certain particulars regarding the date and time of collection and despatch, source of water, particulars of recent rainfall and findings of the sanitary survey should also be supplied with the sample.

APPENDIX III

*QUANTITY OF CHEMICALS NEEDED TO DISINFECT WATER FOR DRINKING**

Water (m^3)	Bleaching powder (25–35%) (g)	High strength calcium hypochlorite (70%) (g)	Liquid bleach (5% sodium hypochlorite) (ml)
1	2.3	1	14
1.2	3	1.2	17
1.5	3.5	1.5	21
2	5	2	28
2.5	6	2.5	35
3	7	3	42
4	9	4	56
5	12	5	70
6	14	6	84
7	16	7	98
8	19	8	110
10	23	10	140
12	28	12	170
15	35	15	210
20	50	20	280
30	70	30	420
40	90	40	560
50	120	50	700
60	140	60	840
70	160	70	980
80	190	80	1,100
100	230	100	1,400
120	280	120	1,700
150	350	150	2,100
200	470	200	2,800
250	580	250	3,500
300	700	300	4,200
400	940	400	5,600
500	1,170	500	7,000

* Approximate dose – 0.7 mg of applied chlorine per litre of water.

Source : *(13)*

APPENDIX IV

WATER CONSERVATION

Declining trend of rainfall and rapid urbanization with industrialization has created increasing demand for water. Growing water shortage is already causing problems in several areas and available resources like rivers, ponds, lakes are shrinking, causing more & more pressure on sub-soil water resources. Already, the rate of water extraction is exceeding the replenishment that takes place by natural processes – mainly recharge due to rainfall. This is causing alarming fall in sub-soil water levels which is going down in and around several cities. Development of agriculture dependent on tube wells has further worsened the situation. The underground water resources, therefore, urgently need conservation. The term conservation implies both, protection of water resources, and further building up the precious water reserves.

Conservation of water resources requires :

(a) PREVENTION OF WASTAGE : Wide-spread awareness needs to be developed among people about economical use of water. It has to be propagated that people should make an effort not to waste water, and help in reducing consumption of the invaluable water reserves. Efficient water management can substantially reduce total water requirement of communities. Domestic consumption of water can be reduced by individuals, by cultivating better habits in kitchen and bathroom use, to avoid free running of water.

(b) WATER HARVESTING : Simple innovative ideas like water harvesting are extremely important to preserve and buildup underground water reserves in urban and semi-urban areas, where considerable water is drawn out by tube wells for domestic consumption. Vast quantity of rainwater is normally discharged in to drains. This rainwater can be easily added to the underground reserves by diversion of rainwater from rooftops and courtyards into soaking pits or trenches, instead of drains. It is also viable to clean and filter this water and divert it into existing tube wells or wells. Various economic designs are suggested by agencies like Central Ground Water Board (CGWB), UNICEF etc. Suitably large pit is filled in layers with big stones, followed by gravel and sand. Collected rainwater from rooftops is brought into the pit by PVC pipes. The rainwater filtered through these layers, then travels by a PVC pipe connecting bottom of the pit into the nearby well or tube well.

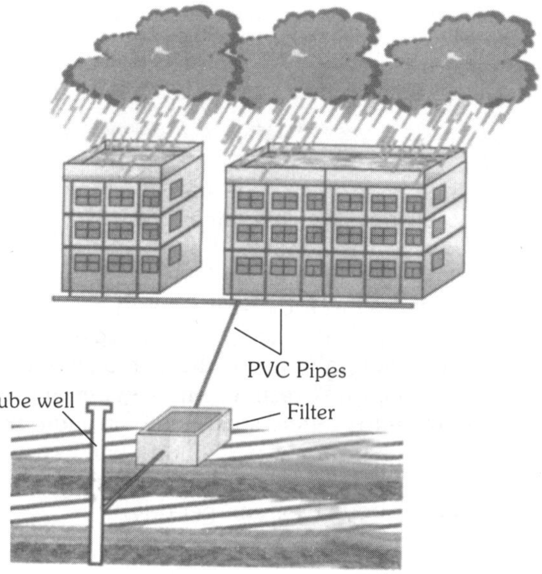

FIG. 11
Water harvesting a tube well

References

1. WHO (1972). *Health Hazards of the Human Environment,* WHO, Geneva.
2. WHO (2022). *World Health Statistics,* 2022.
3. WHO (2021). *State of World's Children, 2021.*
4. Govt. of India (1977). *Manual on Water Supply and Treatment,* Second Edition, Central Public Health and Environmental Engineering Organization, Ministry of Works and Housing, New Delhi.
5. Subrahmanyan, K. and Bhaskaran, T.R. (1948). *Indian J . Med. Res.,* 36, 211.
6. WHO (1969). *The Village Tank as a Source of Drinking Water* WHO/CWS/RD/69–1.
7. Wagner, E.G. and Lanoix, J.N. (1959). *Water Supply for Rural Areas and Small Communities,* WHO.
8. Bhaskaran, T.R. et al (1973). *Indian J.Med.Res.,* 61, 304.
9. WHO (1968). *Techn. Rep. Ser.,* No.406.
10. WHO, *Appropriate Technology for Health,* Water, Newsletter 14–15. (1984), Division of Strengthening of Health Services.
11. Huisman, L. and Wood, W.E. (1974). *Slow Sand Filtration,* WHO, Geneva.
12. WHO (1977). *WHO Chronicle,* 31, 318.
13. Rajagopalan, S. and Shiffman, M.A. (1974). *Guide to Simple Sanitary Measures for the Control of Enteric Diseases, WHO,* Geneva.
14. American Public Health Association, American Water Works Association and Water pollution Control Federation (1971). Standard *Methods for the Examination of Water and Waste Water,* 13th ed., New York.
15. Cox, C.R. (1964). *Operation and Control of Water Treatment Processes, WHO,* Geneva.
16. Bollyky, J. (1976), *Water and Sewage Works,* 123, 66–67.

17. Hoehn, R.C. (1976), *JAWWA*, 68, 302–308.
18. WHO (1970). *Public Health Papers* 40.
19. WHO (2011), *Guidelines For Drinking Water Quality* Vol. 1 & Vol. II Recommendations, 4th Edition.
20. WHO (1976). *Surveillance of Drinking Water Quality*, Geneva
21. Indian Council of Medical Research (1975). *Manual of Standards of Quality for Drinking Water*, Spl, Rpt, Ser, 44.
22. Water Research Centre (1976). *Notes on Water Research*, No. 6, 1–4.
23. WHO (1971). *International Standards for Drinking Water*, Geneva.
24. WHO (1972). *Hazards of the Human Environment*, Geneva.
25. WHO (1970). *Fluorides and Human Health*, Geneva.
26. WHO (1965). *Techn. Rep. Ser.*, No.297.
27. Salvato, J.A. (1976). *Guide to Sanitation in Tourist Establishments*, WHO Geneva.
28. Fish. N.A. (1969). *Canad J. Public Health*, 60, 279.
29. Govt. of India (1981). *India*, A Reference Annual 1981 Publication Division, Ministry of Information and Broadcasting.
30. WHO (1984), *Guidelines For Drinking Water Quality*, Vol. Recommendations.

AIR

The immediate environment of man comprises of air on which depends all forms of life. Apart from supplying the life-giving oxygen, air and atmospheric conditions serve several functions. The human body is cooled by the air contact; the special senses of hearing and smell function through air-transmitted stimuli ; disease agents may be conveyed by air. Pollution of air by dust, smoke, toxic gases and chemical vapours has resulted in sickness and death. Man's adventure into outer space has broadened our concept of air environment. Human beings need a continuous supply of air to exist. The requirement for air is relatively constant (about 10–20m^3 per day)

Composition

Air is a mechanical mixture of gases. The normal composition of external air by volume is approximately as follows: Nitrogen – 78.1 per cent; Oxygen – 20.93 per cent; Carbon dioxide – 0.03 per cent. The balance is made up of other gases which occur in traces, e.g., argon, neon, krypton, xenon and helium. In addition to these gases, air also contains water vapour, traces of ammonia and suspended matter such as dust, bacteria, spores and vegetable debris.

Air is rendered impure by (1) Respiration of men and animals (2) Combustion of coal, gas, oil, etc. (3) Decomposition of organic matter and (4) Trade, traffic and manufacturing processes which give off dust, fumes, vapours and gases. Under ordinary conditions, the composition of outdoor air is remarkably constant. This is brought about by certain self-cleansing mechanisms which operate in nature (1) *Wind :* Wind dilutes and sweeps away the impurities by its movement. Because of wind movement, impurities do not accumulate in any one place; (2) *Sunlight :* The atmospheric temperature and sunlight play their own part by oxidizing impurities, and killing bacteria; (3) *Rain :* It cleanses the atmosphere by removing the suspended and gaseous impurities; (4) *Plant life :* The green plants utilize the carbon dioxide and generate oxygen; this process is reversed during the night time. When the rate of pollution becomes too high or when the cleansing process becomes ineffective, it constitutes a health hazard.

The air of occupied room

Human occupancy and activity vitiate air in occupied rooms and give a sense of discomfort to the occupants. The changes in air that take place in confined places are both chemical and physical. (a) *CHEMICAL CHANGES :* The air becomes progressively contaminated by carbon dioxide and the oxygen content decreases due to metabolic processes. An average person at rest gives off 0.7 c.ft. of carbon dioxide per hour; this may increase up to 2 c.ft. during physical activity. In a mixed gathering comprising all age groups, the per capita output of carbon dioxide is taken as 0.6 c.ft. per hour, (b) *PHYSICAL CHANGES :* The most important changes that occur due to human occupancy are the physical changes. These are (i) *Rise in temperature :* The indoor temperature tends to rise as a result of the emanation of body heat. A man at rest gives off approximately 400 Btu per hour. One Btu (British Thermal Unit) is the quantity of heat required to raise the temperature of one pound of water by 1 deg. F. Under conditions of physical exertion, the heat output may go up to 4,000 Btu. (ii) *Increase of humidity :* There is an increase in the relative humidity due to moisture evaporated from the skin and lungs. The expired air contains about 6 per cent of water vapour. An adult person at rest releases an average 700 gms. of water vapour per 24 hours in the form of perspiration. It has been calculated that a human being releases 18.4 gms of water vapour per hour when sleeping and upto 175 gms of water vapour when engaged in really vigorous exercise *(1)*. (iii) *Decrease in air movement :* In crowded places, the natural movement of air is impeded. (iv) *Body odours :* Unpleasant odours arise from foul breath, perspiration, bad oral hygiene, dirty clothes and other sources. The production of body odours depends upon the social status, age and personal hygiene of the people. (v) *Bacterial pollution :* The exhaled air contains microorganisms in suspension. These are principally saprophytic bacteria and may include pathogenic bacteria. These organisms are discharged into the air during conversation, coughing, sneezing and loud talking.

Unless the vitiated air is replaced by fresh air, it may adversely affect the comfort, health and efficiency of the occupants. It is known that a feeling of suffocation or discomfort is experienced by the occupants in insufficiently ventilated rooms and also complaints of headache, drowsiness and inability to concentrate. There is also the risk of droplet infection and lowered resistance to disease (on prolonged exposure).

Discomfort

Discomfort is a subjective sensation which people experience in ill-ventilated and crowded rooms. For a long time it was believed to be due to increased carbon dioxide and decreased oxygen, resulting from respiration. This theory has since been refuted. Studies have shown that the oxygen content may be reduced to 18 per cent and the carbon dioxide content may be raised to over 5 per cent, without adverse effects, provided the temperature and humidity are kept satisfactory. In the 'Black Hole of Kolkata', 146 prisoners were imprisoned in a room, 18 × 14 × 10 out of whom only 23 survived. There were two small windows which were adequate to supply all the oxygen needs – even then only 23 survived. It was concluded that the deaths were due to changes in the physical condition of the air, leading to 'heat retention'. It is now established that the causes of discomfort are not due to chemical changes but physical changes. These are temperature, humidity, air movement and heat radiation. These factors determine the "cooling power" of the air with respect to the human body. It has been so well said by Professor Lee that "The problems of ventilation are physical, not chemical; cutaneous not respiratory".

Indices of thermal comfort

Thermal comfort is a complex entity. Much work was done in the past to determine what constitutes "thermal comfort". Several indices have been put forward from time to time to express thermal comfort and heat stress. These are as follows : (1) AIR TEMPERATURE : For a long time, air temperature was used as an index of thermal comfort, but it was realised that air temperature alone was not an adequate index of thermal comfort. (2) AIR TEMPERATURE AND HUMIDITY : Later, air temperature and humidity were considered together to express thermal comfort: even this was found to be unsatisfactory. (3) COOLING POWER : Still later, air temperature, humidity and air movement were considered together and expressed as "cooling power" of the air. An instrument was devised by Hill called the Kata Thermometer to measure the cooling power. A dry Kata reading of 6 and above, and a wet Kata reading of 20 and above, were regarded as indices of thermal comfort. Further researches have shown that the Kata cooling powers are also not reliable indices of comfort conditions. (4) EFFECTIVE TEMPERATURE : Effective temperature is an arbitrary index which combines into a single value the effect of temperature, humidity and movement of the internal air on the sensation of warmth or cold felt by the human body. The numerical value of effective temperature is that of the temperature of still, saturated air which would induce the same sensation of warmth or cold as that experienced in the given conditions. For example, if the environment has an ET value of 30 deg.C (86 deg.F), it implies that the subjective sensation of it will be same as in a saturated atmosphere of 30 deg.C (86 deg.F) with no air movement. This scale was evolved in 1923 after a long series of experiments carried out in the Pittsburgh Laboratory of the American Society of Heating and Ventilation Engineers by Houghton and Yaglou. Two scales are available one of which refers to men who are stripped to the waist and the other to men who are fully clad in indoor clothing. Effective temperature may be obtained from special charts by reference to the three variables (Fig. 1). A criticism of the effective temperature scale is that it ignores the effects of a radiation from the surrounding structures. (5) CORRECTED EFFECTIVE TEMPERATURE : This Index is an improvement over the Effective Temperature Index. Instead of the dry bulb temperature, the reading of the Globe Thermometer is used to allow for radiant heat. That is, the C.E.T. scales deal with all the four factors namely, air temperature, velocity, humidity and mean radiant heat. Whenever a source of radiation is present, it is preferable to take C.E.T., the C.E.T. may be readily obtained from prepared nomograms by reference to the globe thermometer temperature, the wet bulb temperature and air speed. At present, effective temperature and C.E.T. scales are widely used as indices of thermal comfort *(1)*. McARDLE'S MAXIMUM ALLOWABLE SWEAT RATE : McArdle and associates took 4.5 litres of sweat excreted in four hours as the maximum allowable sweat rate compatible with physiological normal reaction of acclimatized, healthy young men for repeated exposures to heat. They prepared a chart from which the "predicted four-hour sweat rate" (P_4SR) can be obtained from any combination of dry and wet bulb temperature of the air, mean radiant air temperature and air velocity, under different work intensity. McArdle has put P_4SR value of 3 as upper limit of comfort zone *(3)*.

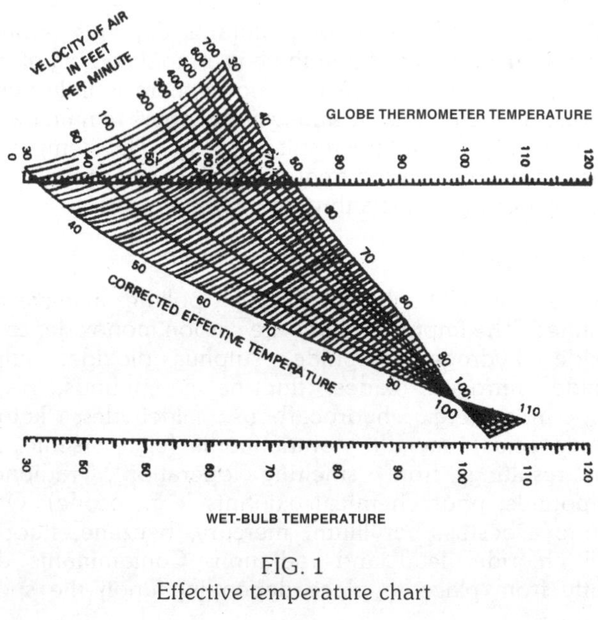

FIG. 1
Effective temperature chart

Comfort zones

Comfort zones may be defined as the range of ETs over which the majority of adults feel comfortable. There is no unanimous decision on a single zone of comfort for all people because comfort is quite a complex subjective experience which depends not only on physical, physiological factors, but also on psychological factors which are difficult to determine. Considering only the environmental factors, 'comfortable thermal conditions are those under which a person can maintain normal balance between production and loss of heat, at normal body temperature and without sweating'. Comfort zones evaluated in India are as below :

		Corrected effective temperature deg C
1. Pleasant and cool	.....	20
2. Comfortable and cool	.....	20–25
3. Comfortable	.....	25–27
4. Hot and uncomfortable	.....	27–28
5. Extremely hot	.....	28 +
6. Intolerably hot	.....	30 +
		Predicted four-hour sweat rate (P_4SR)
1. Comfort zone	.....	1–3 litres
2. Just tolerable	.....	3–4.5 litres
3. Intolerable	.....	4.5 + litres

AIR POLLUTION

The phenomenon called "pollution" is an inescapable consequence of the presence of man and his activities. The term "air pollution" signifies the presence in the ambient (surrounding) atmosphere of substances (e.g., gases, mixtures of gases and particulated matter) generated by the activities of man in concentrations that interfere with human health, safety or comfort, or injurious to vegetation and animals and other environmental media resulting in chemicals entering the food chain or being present in drinking-water and thereby constituting additional source of human exposure. The direct effect of air pollutants on plants, animals and soil can influence the structure and function of ecosystems, including self regulation ability, thereby affecting the quality of life *(2)*. In the past, air pollution meant smoke pollution. Today, air pollution has become more subtle and recognizes no geographical or political boundaries. Air pollution is one of the present-day health problems throughout the world.

Basic definitions *(4)*

Before discussing in detail the sources of air pollutants it is necessary to establish a few basic principles that will place the information on sources in context. Air pollutants may be either emitted into the atmosphere or formed within the atmosphere itself.

Primary air pollutants : Primary air pollutants are those that are emitted into the atmosphere from a source such as a factory chimney or exhaust pipe, or through suspension of contaminated dusts by the wind. In principle, therefore, it is possible to measure the amounts emitted at the source itself.

Secondary air pollutants : Secondary air pollutants are those formed within the atmosphere itself. They arise from chemical reactions of primary pollutants, possibly involving the natural components of the atmosphere, especially oxygen and water. The most familiar example is ozone, which arises almost entirely from chemical reactions that differ with altitude within the atmosphere. Because of this mode of formation, secondary pollutants cannot readily be included in emissions inventories, although it is possible to estimate formation rates per unit volume of atmosphere per unit time.

Another important distinction must be made in relation to the physical state of a pollutant.

Gaseous air pollutants : Gaseous air pollutants are those present as gases or vapours, i.e. as individual small molecules capable of passing through filters, provided they do not adsorb to or chemically react with the filter medium. Gaseous air pollutants are readily taken into the human respiratory system, although if water-soluble, they may very quickly be deposited in the upper respiratory tract and not penetrate to the deep lung.

Particulate air pollutants : Particulate air pollutants comprise material in solid or liquid phase suspended in the atmosphere. Such particles can be either primary or secondary and cover a wide range of sizes. Newly formed secondary particles can be as small as 1–2 μm in diameter, while coarse dust and sea salt particles can be as large as 100 μm in diameter. (Please note :– 1 μm is one millionth of a metre = 1 micron = 0.001 mm)

Local scale : Some pollutants, by virtue of their source or of having a very short atmospheric lifetime, are only encountered in appreciable concentrations close to where they are emitted. For example in less developed countries, poorly controlled household and neighbourhood sources, often involving the burning of biomass fuels, cause serious local pollution.

Urban scale : Pollutants from urban sources, such as nitrogen oxides and carbon monoxide generated by road traffic, tend to be present at high concentrations throughout the city and at significantly reduced concentrations in adjacent rural areas. Their atmospheric lifetimes are not long (typically hours) and therefore concentrations in the remote background atmosphere tend to be very low (except in the case of carbon monoxide, which is more persistent).

Regional scale : Pollutants in the form of fine particles (<2.5 μm diameter, but not ultrafine particles) and some gas-phase pollutants such as ozone have atmospheric lifetimes of days or even weeks, which permit them to be transported on a regional scale. Pollutants such as sulphate particles and ozone readily travel thousands of kilometres in a process known as long-range transport, crossing national boundaries in doing so.

Hemispheric and global scales : Some pollutants, and especially those associated with greenhouse warming effects (carbon dioxide, nitrous oxide and methane) have atmospheric lifetimes of years and are therefore capable of distribution throughout a hemisphere and ultimately globally.

Sources of air pollution

The main sources of air pollution are : (a) AUTOMOBILES : Motor vehicles are a major source of air pollution throughout the urban areas. They emit hydrocarbons, carbon monoxide, lead, nitrogen oxides and particulate matter. In strong sunlight, certain of these hydrocarbons and oxides of nitrogen may be converted in the atmosphere into "photochemical" pollutants of oxidizing nature. In addition, diesel engines, when misused or badly adjusted are capable of emitting black smoke and malodorous fumes. (b) INDUSTRIES : Industries emit large amounts of pollutants into the atmosphere. Combustion of fuel to generate heat and power produces smoke, sulphur dioxide, nitrogen oxides and fly ash. Petrochemical industries generate hydrogen fluoride, hydrochloric acid and organic halides. Many industries discharge carbon monoxide, carbon dioxide, ozone, hydrogen sulphide and sulphur dioxide. Industries discharge their wastes from high chimneys at high temperature and high speed. (c) DOMESTIC SOURCES : Domestic combustion of coal, wood or oil is a major source of smoke, dust, sulphur dioxide and nitrogen oxides. The London disaster of air pollution in 1952 in which thousands had died was due to domestic coal burning. (d) The most direct and important source of air pollution affecting the health of many people is tobacco smoke. Even those who do not smoke may inhale the smoke produced by others ("passive smoking"). (e) MISCELLANEOUS : These comprise burning refuse, incinerators, pesticide spraying, natural sources (e.g., wind borne dust, fungi, molds, bacteria) and nuclear energy programmes. All these contribute to air pollution.

Meteorological factors

Although the Earth's atmosphere extends to several layers above the surface, it is only the first 30 km that hold the major portion of the atmospheric gases. Man is most directly concerned with only the 8–10 km of the atmosphere *(3)*.

The level of atmospheric pollution at any one time depends upon meteorological factors, e.g., topography, air movement and climate. Winds help in the dispersal and dilution of pollutants. If the topography is dominated by mountains (or tall buildings) the winds become weak and calm, and pollutants tend to concentrate in the breathing zone.

The vertical diffusion of pollutants depends upon the temperature gradient. When there is a rapid cooling of lower layers of air (temperature inversion), there is little vertical motion and the pollutants and water vapours remain trapped at the lower levels and the result is "smog". The "temperature inversion" which is more frequent in the winter months than in spring or summer, is a threat to human health.

Air pollutants

More than 100 substances which pollute air have been identified. The important ones are carbon monoxide, carbon dioxide, hydrogen sulphide, sulphur dioxide, sulphur trioxide, nitrogen oxides, fluorine compounds, organic compounds (e.g., hydrocarbons, aldehydes, ketones, organic acids), metallic contaminants (e.g., arsenic, zinc, iron resulting from smelting operation), radioactive compounds, photochemical oxidants (e.g., ozone). Others include asbestos, beryllium, mercury, benzene, fluorides, vinyl chloride, lead and radiation. Contaminants differ greatly from place to place depending upon the specific complex of contaminant source. Pollutants may be in the form of solids, liquids (vapours) or gases. The combination of smoke and fog is called "smog".

(1) **Carbon monoxide :** Carbon monoxide is one of the most common and widely distributed air pollutants. It is a product of incomplete combustion of carbon containing materials, such as in automobiles, industrial process, heating facilities and incinerators. Estimates of man-made carbon monoxide emission vary from 350 to 600 million tonnes per annum *(2)*. Some widespread natural non-biological and biological sources have also been identified. Concentrations in urban areas depend on weather and traffic density. It varies with the density of petrol-powered vehicles and most cities have carbon monoxide peak levels that coincide with the morning and evening rush-hours. Variations in these levels are also influenced by topography. The fluctuation in ambient concentrations is only slowly reflected in the carboxyhaemoglobin levels in humans, as it takes 4–12 hours for approximate equilibrium between air levels and blood levels to occur. Thus environmental concentrations tend to be expressed in terms of 8 hour average concentrations.

(2) **Sulphur dioxide :** It is one of the several forms in which sulphur exists in air. The others include H_2S, H_2SO_4 and sulphate salts. Sulphur dioxide (SO_2) is a colourless gas with a sharp odour, results from the combustion of sulphur containing fossil fuel, the smelting of sulphur-containing ores, and other industrial processes. Domestic fires, power generation and motor vehicles can also produce emissions containing sulphur dioxide.

SO_2 can affect the respiratory system and the function of lungs, and causes irritation of eyes. Inflammation of the respiratory tract causes coughing, mucus secretion, aggravation of asthma and chronic bronchitis, and makes people more prone to infections of the respiratory tract. Hospital admissions for cardiac disease and mortality increase on days with higher SO_2 levels. When SO_2 combines with water, it forms sulphuric acid; this is the main component of acid rain which is a cause of deforestation. A SO_2 concentration of 500 $\mu g/m^3$ should not be exceeded over average periods of 10 minutes duration. Studies indicate that a proportion of people with asthma experience changes in pulmonary function and respiratory symptoms after periods of exposure to SO_2 as short as 10 minutes. The revision of 24-hour guideline for SO_2 from 125 to 20 $\mu g/m^3$ is based on the health effects known to be associated with much lower levels of SO_2 than previously believed *(5)*.

(3) **Lead :** People can become exposed to lead through occupational and environmental sources. This mainly results from : (a) inhalation of lead particles generated by burning materials containing lead, for example, during smelting, recycling, stripping leaded paint and using leaded gasoline or leaded aviation fuel; (b) ingestion of lead-contaminated dust, water (from leaded pipes), food (from lead-glazed or lead soldered containers); and (c) The use of some traditional cosmetics and medicines can also result in lead exposure *(14)*.

Once lead enters the body, it is distributed to organs such as the brain, kidneys, liver and bones. The body stores lead in the teeth and bones where it accumulates over time. Lead stored in bone may be remobilized into the blood during pregnancy, thus exposing the fetus. Undernourished children are more susceptible to lead because their bodies absorb more lead if other nutrients, such as calcium, are lacking. Children at highest risk are the very young (including the developing fetus) and the impoverished.

Lead has serious consequences for the health of children. At high levels of exposure, lead attacks the brain and central nervous system to cause coma, convulsions and even death. Children who survive severe lead poisoning may be left with mental retardation and behavioural disorders. At lower levels of exposure that cause no obvious symptoms, and that previously were considered safe, lead is now known to produce a spectrum of injury across multiple body systems. In particular, lead affects children's brain development resulting in reduced intelligence quotient (IQ), behavioural changes such as reduced attention span and increased antisocial behaviour, and reduced educational attainment. Lead exposure also causes anaemia, hypertension, renal impairment, immunotoxicity and toxicity to the reproductive organs. The neurological and behavioural effects of lead are believed to be irreversible *(14)*.

Lead also causes long-term harm to adults, including risk of hypertension and kidney damage. Exposure of pregnant women to high levels of lead can cause miscarriage, stillbirth, premature birth and low birth weight, as well as minor malformations *(14)*.

(4) **Carbon dioxide :** This is not commonly regarded as an air pollutant, although man generates enormous amount of it in combustion process using coal, oil and gas. Carbon dioxide is a natural constituent of the air. It does not take part in any significant chemical reactions with other substances in the air. However, its global concentration is rising above the natural level by an amount that could increase global temperature enough to affect climate markedly *(6)*.

(5) **Hydrocarbons :** Man-made sources of hydrocarbons include incineration, combustion of coal, wood, processing and use of petroleum. Hydrocarbons exert their pollutant action by taking part in the chemical reactions that cause photochemical smog.

(6) **Cadmium :** The steel industry, waste incineration, volcanic action and zinc production seem to account for the largest emissions. Incineration is increasingly chosen as a method of refuse disposal in European countries. This source of atmospheric cadmium pollution is of growing concern. Tobacco contains cadmium, and smoking may contribute significantly to the uptake of cadmium. Cigarettes may contain from 0.5 to 3 μg cadmium per gram of tobacco, depending on the country of origin.

(7) **Hydrogen sulphide :** Human activities can release naturally occurring hydrogen sulphide into ambient air. In Industry, hydrogen sulphide can be formed whenever elemental sulphur or sulphur containing compounds come in contact with organic material at high temperatures. Hydrogen sulphide is formed during coke production, in viscose rayon production, waste-water treatment plants, wood pulp production using the sulphate method, sulphur extraction process, oil refining and in tanning industry. Hydrogen sulphide is the main toxic substance involved in livestock rearing systems with liquid manure storage *(7)*. The first noticeable effect of hydrogen sulphide at low concentration is its unpleasant odour. Conjunctival irritation is the next subjective symptom. Workers exposed to hydrogen sulphide concentrations of less than 30 $\mu g/m^3$ are reported to have rather diffuse neurological and mental symptoms *(2)*.

(8) **Ozone :** Ozone at ground level – not to be confused with the ozone layer in the upper atmosphere – is one of the major constituents of photochemical smog. It is formed by the photochemical reaction of sunlight with pollutants such as nitrogen oxides from vehicle, industry emissions and volatile organic compounds (VOCs) emitted by vehicles, solvents and industry. The highest levels of ozone pollution

occurs during periods of sunny weather. Excessive ozone in the air can have a marked effect on human health. It can cause breathing problems, trigger asthma, reduce lung function and cause lung diseases. In Europe it is currently one of the air pollutants of most concern. Several European studies have reported that the daily mortality rises by 0.3% and that for heart diseases by 0.4%, per 10 μg/m^3 increase in ozone exposure. The previously recommended limit, which was fixed at 120 μg/m^3 of 8-hour mean, has been reduced to 100 μg/m^3 based on recent conclusive associations between daily mortality and ozone levels occurring at ozone concentrations below 120 μg/m^3 *(5)*.

(9) **Oxides of nitrogen :** Emission of oxides of nitrogen occur predominantly in the form of nitric oxide, which comprises around 95 per cent of nitrogen oxides from a combustion source. Coal is the most important fuel in this context, other sources are road traffic and electricity generation. The pollutant of far greater concern in relation to human health is nitrogen dioxide. Epidemiological studies have shown that symptoms of bronchitis in asthmatic children increase in association with long-term exposure to nitrogen dioxide. Reduced lung function growth is also linked to nitrogen dioxide at concentrations currently measured (or observed) in the cities of Europe and North America. The current WHO guideline value of 40 μg/m^3 (annual mean) set to protect the public from the health effects of gaseous nitrogen dioxide remains unchanged from the level recommended in the previous AQGs.

(10) **Polycyclic aromatic hydrocarbons (PAH) :** Polycyclic aromatic hydrocarbons (PAHs) (also known as polynuclear aromatic hydrocarbons) are a group of approximately 10,000 compounds. The examples are Benzo (a) pyrene (BaP), Benzanthracene, Benzo (b) fluoranthene, fluoranthene, Nephthalene etc. BaP is commonly used as an indicator species for PAH contamination and most available data refer to this compound. Most PAHs in the environment are produced by incomplete burning of carbon containing material like wood, garbage, coal and oil. Automobile exhaust, industrial emission and smoke from burning wood, charcoal and tobacco contain high levels of PAHs. In general, more PAHs form when materials burn at low temperatures, such as in wood fires and cigarettes. The fine PAH particles can bind with ash particles and can move long distances. PAHs can also be toxic when ingested or when they come in contact with skin (they are used in some skin creams and anti-dandruff shampoos). When inhaled some PAHs are carcinogenic, mutagen and reproductive toxin (BaP is one of the most potent carcinogens among the known PAHs). A person who smokes one pack of unfiltered cigarettes per day is exposed daily to 2 to 5 μg of carcinogenic PAHs. Occupational exposure can occur through inhalation and dermal contact. People with highest exposure are smokers, people who live with or work with smokers, roofers, road builders and people who live near major highways or industrial sources.

Based on epidemiological data from studies on coke-oven workers, a unit risk for lung cancer for PAH mixture is estimated to be 8.7×10^{-5} ng/m^3 BaP. This is the guideline for PAH in indoor air. The corresponding concentration of lifetime exposure to BaP producing excess lifetime cancer risk of 1/10,000, 1/100,000 and 1/1,000,000 are approximately 1.2, 0.12 and 0.012 ng/m^3 respectively *(8)*.

(11) **Particulate matter :** Airborne particulate matter represents a complex mixture of organic and inorganic substance. Particles are generally classified by their size measured in μm (micro metre, i.e. one millionth of a metre). Initially guidelines were directed at very general measure of PM concentration including total suspended particulate (TSP) matter in US, and black smoke (BS) in Europe. In 1987, USEPA promulgated a standard for PM – less than 10 μm in aerodynamic diameter (PM_{10}). In 1997, a standard for PM less than 2.5 μm in aerodynamic diameter ($PM_{2.5}$) was added. By definition PM_{10} includes $PM_{2.5}$ and thoracic coarse mass PM (the difference between PM_{10} and $PM_{2.5}$ is referred to as coarse mass PM). PM_{10} includes those inhalable particles that are sufficiently small to penetrate to the thoracic region; the fine fraction of PM_{10} is cut-off from coarse fraction at 2.5 μm, a size fraction with a high probability of deposition in the smaller conducting airways and alveoli.

The major components of PM are sulfate, nitrates, ammonia, sodium chloride, black carbon, mineral dust and water. It consists of a complex mixture of solid and liquid particles of organic and inorganic substances.

The large particles usually contain earth's crustal material and fugitive dust from roads and industries. Particulate matter of respirable size may be emitted from a number of sources, some of them natural (e.g. dust storms) and many others that are more widespread and more important (e.g., power plants and industrial processes, vehicular traffic, domestic coal burning, industrial incinerators). The particulate matter of diameter smaller than 2.5 μm are more dangerous since, when inhaled, they may reach the peripheral regions of the bronchioles, and interfere with gas exchange inside the lungs. The effects of PM on health occur at levels of exposure currently being experienced by most urban and rural populations in both developed and developing countries. Chronic exposure to particles contributes to the risk of developing cardiovascular and respiratory diseases, as well as of lung cancer. In developing countries, exposure to pollutants from indoor combustion of solid fuels on open fires or traditional stoves increases the risk of acute lower respiratory infections and associated mortatlity among young children; indoor air pollution from solid fuel use is also a major risk factor for chronic obstructive pulmonary disease and lung cancer among adults. The mortality in cities with high levels of pollution exceeds that observed in relatively cleaner cities by 15–20 per cent. The 2005 AQG set for the first time a guideline value for particular matter (PM) as 10 μg/m^3 annual mean and 25 μg/m^3 24-hour mean for $PM_{2.5}$, and 20 μg/m^3 annual mean and 50 μg/m^3 24-hour mean for PM_{10} *(5)*. The aim is to achieve the lowest concentrations possible. As no threshold for PM has been identified below which no damage to health is observed, the recommended value should represent an acceptable and achievable objective to minimize health effects in the context of local constraints, capabilities and public health priorities.

Indoor air pollution *(4)*

The indoor environment represents an important microenvironment in which people spend a large part of their time each day. As a result, indoor air pollution, originating from both outdoor and indoor sources, is likely to contribute more to population exposure than the outdoor environment. The extent and magnitude of consequent health risks, however, remain poorly understood. The large number of indoor air pollutants, including chemical and biological contaminants, and the influence of a variety of factors such as the nature and location of sources, air exchange between indoor and outdoor environments, and individual behaviour make accurate estimations of health effects very difficult.

The major sources of indoor air pollution worldwide include combustion of solid fuels indoors, tobacco smoking, outdoor air pollutants, emissions from construction materials and furnishings, and improper maintenance of ventilation and air conditioning systems (Table 1). There are, however, marked variations in the importance of these different sources in different areas of the world, closely related to the level of socio-economic development.

Although relatively clean sources of household energy predominate in developed countries, improvements in energy efficiency have led to homes being relatively airtight, reducing ventilation and raising indoor pollutant levels.

4.3 million people die every year prematurely from illness attributable to the household air pollution caused by inefficient use of solid fuels. Among these deaths 12 per cent are due to pneumonia, 34 per cent from stroke, 26 per cent from ischaemic heart disease, 22 per cent from COPD and 6 per cent from lung cancer.

Exposure to household air pollution almost doubles the risk for childhood pneumonia. Over half of deaths among children less than 5 years old from acute lower respiratory infections (ALRI) are due to particulate matter inhaled from indoor air pollution from household solid fuels.

Nearly one quarter of all premature deaths due to stroke (i.e. about 1.4 million deaths of which half are in women) can be attributed to the chronic exposure to household air pollution caused by cooking with solid fuels. Approximately 15% of all deaths due to ischaemic heart disease, accounting for over a million premature deaths annually, can be attributed to exposure to household air pollution. Over one-third of premature deaths from chronic obstructive pulmonary disease (COPD) in adults in low and middle-income countries are due to exposure to household air pollution. Women exposed to high levels of indoor smoke are 2.3 times as likely to suffer from COPD than women who use cleaner fuels. Among men (who already have a heightened risk of COPD due to their higher rates of smoking), exposure to indoor smoke nearly doubles that risk. Approximately 17% of annual premature lung cancer deaths in adults are attributable to exposure to carcinogens from household air pollution caused by cooking with solid fuels like wood, charcoal or coal. The risk for women is higher, due to their role in food preparation. More generally, small particulate matter and other pollutants in indoor smoke inflame the airways and lungs, impairing immune response and reducing the oxygen-carrying capacity of the blood. There is also evidence of links between household air pollution and low birth weight, tuberculosis, cataract, nasopharyngeal and laryngeal cancers *(4A)*.

TABLE 1

Major health-damaging pollutants generated from indoor sources

Pollutant	Major indoor sources
Fine particles	Fuel/tobacco combustion, cleaning operations, cooking
Carbon monoxide	Fuel/tobacco combustion
Polycyclic aromatic hydrocarbons	Fuel/tobacco combustion, cooking
Nitrogen oxides	Fuel combustion
Sulphur oxides	Coal combustion
Arsenic and fluorine	Coal combustion
Volatile and semi-volatile organic compounds	Fuel/tobacco combustion, consumer products, furnishings, construction materials, cooking
Aldehydes	Furnishings, construction materials, cooking
Pesticides	Consumer products, dust from outside
Asbestos	Remodelling/demolition of construction materials
Lead	Remodelling/demolition of painted surfaces
Biological pollutants	Damp materials/furnishings, components of climate control systems, occupants, outdoor air, pets
Radon	Soil under buildings, construction materials
Free radicals and other short-lived, highly reactive compounds	Indoor chemistry

Source : *(4)*

Monitoring of air pollution

The best indicators of air pollution are sulphur dioxide, smoke and suspended particles. These are monitored on a daily basis over several sites. The results are then collected by a central agency. (a) *Sulphur dioxide :* This gas is a major contaminant in many urban and industrial areas. Its concentration is estimated in all air pollution surveys. (b) *Smoke or soiling index :* A known volume of air is filtered through a white filter paper under specified conditions and the stain is measured by photoelectric meter. Smoke concentration is estimated and expressed as micrograms/ cubic metre of air as an average level over a period of time. (c) *Grit and dust measurement :* Deposit gauges collect grit, dust and other solids. These are analyzed monthly. (d) *Coefficient of haze :* A factor used, particularly in the USA in assessing the amount of smoke or other aerosol in air. (e) *Air pollution index :* It is an arbitrary index which takes into account one or more pollutants as a measure of the severity of pollution. For example, the following index has been used in USA : 10 times the sulphur dioxide concentration plus twice the carbon monoxide concentration (both in ppm by volume) plus twice the coefficient of haze. It was considered to be a cause for alarm when the value of this index rose from its value of about 12–50 or more.

The WHO (1987) in its publication "Air quality guidelines for Europe" and more recently 2020 ed. has described approved methods of determining the concentration of common air pollutants and their health hazards. The emphasis in the guideline is placed on exposure, since this is the element that can be controlled to lessen the dose and hence lessen response. The starting point for the derivation of guideline value was to define the lowest concentration at which adverse effects are observed. On the basis of the body of scientific evidence and judgements of protection (safety) factors, the guideline values were established. The regulatory approach to controlling air pollution differs from country to country as several sources of air pollutants having unique national components are best subject to national control procedures. The approach taken in the preparation of the air quality guidelines was to evaluate data on health effects of individual compounds. As part of this approach, each chemical is considered in isolation. Inevitably, there is little emphasis on such factors as interaction between pollutants that might lead to synergistic effects and on the environmental fate of the pollutants. For some of the substances, a direct relationship between concentrations in air and possible toxic effects is very difficult to establish. This is especially true of those metals for which a greater body-burden results from ingestion than from inhalation. For example, available data show that the food chain is, for most people, the critical route of non-occupational exposure to lead and cadmium.

On the basis of the evidence concerning adverse effects, judgements about the protection factors needed to minimize health risks were made. Averaging times were included, since the time of exposure is critical in determining the toxicity.

Table 2 shows the maximum upper limit with averaging time.

TABLE 2

Guideline values for individual substances based on effects other than cancer or odour/annoyance

Substance	Time-weighted average	Averaging time
Cadmium	1–5 ng/m³ 10–20 ng/m³	1 year (rural areas) 1 year (urban areas)
Carbon disulphide	100 µg/m³	24 hours
Carbon monoxide	100 mg/m³ 60 mg/m³ 30 mg/m³ 10 mg/m³	15 minutes 30 minutes 1 hour 8 hours
1,2-Dichloroethane	0.7 mg/m³	24 hours
Dichloromethane (Methylene chloride)	3 mg/m³	24 hours
Formaldehyde	100 µg/m³	30 minutes
Hydrogen sulphide	150 µg/m³	24 hours
Lead	0.5–1.0 µg/m³	1 year
Manganese	1 µg/m³	1 year
Mercury	1 µg/m³ (indoor air)	1 year
Nitrogen dioxide	400 µg/m³ 150 µg/m³	1 hour 24 hours
Ozone	150–200 µg/m³ 100–120 µg/m³	1 hour 8 hours
Styrene	800 µg/m³	24 hours
Sulphur dioxide	500 µg/m³ 350 µg/m³	10 minutes 1 hour
Tetrachloroethylene	5 mg/m³	24 hours
Toluene	8 mg/m³	24 hours
Trichloroethylene	1 mg/m³	24 hours
Vanadium	1 µg/m³	24 hours

Source : *(2)*

Air pollution monitoring in India

The National Air Quality Monitoring Programme, sponsored by the Central Pollution Control Board (CPCB) since 1990, has generated database over last 14 years in 10 major Indian cities, viz. Ahmedabad, Mumbai, Kolkata, Delhi, Hyderabad, Jaipur, Kanpur, Kochi, Chennai and Nagpur. The programme facilitates evaluation of long-term air quality trends for health-related criteria pollutants such as inhalable dust, sulphur dioxide, nitrogen dioxide, lead, hydrogen sulphide, ammonia and PAH. The trend analysis showed that Suspended Particulate Matter (SPM) exceeds the CPCB standards in all cities most of the time throughout the year. The concentration ratio of < P10 fraction (human respirable particles) to the total SPM varies between 30 to 60 per cent, with coastal cities showing higher percentages. The concentration of respirable suspended particulate matter is invariably higher at the industrial sites. The PAH in suspended particles at various cities did not show specific trend. The BaP concentration was higher than the CPCB standard at Ahmedabad, Mumbai, Kolkata, Delhi and Nagpur in winter months. Chromium, copper, nickel, arsenic, lead, iron, zinc, sulphate, nitrate, chloride, fluoride, ammonia, sodium and potassium are secondary pollutants analyzed for the assessment of dry deposition of air pollutants. Wet deposition of air pollution has also been evaluated by analyzing rain water samples at all monitoring stations. The successive three years data indicates that the first rain event has the maximum concentration of pollutants with low pH values and higher sulphate and nitrate contents. The acid rain phenomenon thus prevails, albeit for a limited period, in the urban atmosphere of Indian cities *(9)*.

Effects of air pollution

About 1.3 billion urban residents worldwide are exposed to air pollution level above recommended limits. Air quality in the developed countries has generally improved in the past two decades, but in many developing countries air quality has deteriorated because of rising industrial activity, increasing power generation and the congestion of streets with poorly maintained motor vehicles that use leaded fuel. Air pollution can affect by two ways :

(a) **Health aspects** : The health effects of air pollution are both immediate and delayed. The immediate effects are borne by the respiratory system, the resulting state is acute bronchitis. If the air pollution is intense, it may result even in immediate death by suffocation. This has taken place in the air pollution epidemic which occurred in London in 1952. The delayed effects most commonly linked with air pollution are chronic bronchitis, lung cancer, bronchial asthma, emphysema, and respiratory allergies.

Lead poisons many systems in the body and is particularly dangerous to children developing brain and nervous system. Elevated lead levels in children have been associated with impaired neuropsychologic development as measured by loss of IQ, poor school performance and behavioural difficulties *(10)*. Table 3 shows the major air pollutants, their source and adverse effects on health.

TABLE 3

Major air pollutants, their sources and adverse effects

Noxious agent	Sources	Adverse effects
Oxides of nitrogen	Automobile exhaust, gas stoves and heaters, wood-burning stoves, kerosene space heaters	Respiratory tract irritation, bronchial hyperactivity, impaired lung defences, bronchiolitis obliterans
Hydrocarbons	Automobile exhaust, cigarette smoke	Lung cancer
Ozone	Automobile exhaust, high altitude aircraft cabins	Cough, substernal discomfort, bronchoconstriction, decreased exercise performance, respiratory tract irritation
Sulphur dioxide	Power plants, Smelters, oil refineries, kerosene space heaters	Exacerbation of asthma and COPD, respiratory tract irritation, hospitalization may be necessary, and death may occur in severe exposure
Lead	Automobile exhaust using leaded gasoline	Impaired neuropsychological development in children

COPD – Chronic obstructive pulmonary disease

Source : *(11, 12)*

Precise estimates of the risk of air pollution to health are difficult to quantify because of problems in estimating the degree of exposure of individuals and the influence of possible confounding variables such as smoking, nutrition, occupation and climate. Air pollution damages the human respiratory and cardio respiratory system in various ways. The elderly, children, smokers and those with chronic respiratory difficulties are most vulnerable. Under the assumption that achievable reduction in urban air pollution can prevent 5 per cent of all infections and chronic respiratory diseases, these reductions could avert 0.6 per cent of the global burden of disease. Epidemiological studies have shown that a sudden increase in the air pollution has often been associated with immediate increase in morbidity and mortality.

(b) **Social and economic aspects :** These comprise destruction of plant and animal life; corrosion of metals; damage to buildings; cost of cleaning and maintenance and repairs and aesthetic nuisance. Air pollution also reduces visibility in towns. It can soil and damage clothings.

Prevention and control of air pollution

The control of air pollution is ultimately an engineering problem. The WHO has recommended the following procedures for the prevention and control of air pollution : (a) *Containment :* That is, prevention of escape of toxic substances into the ambient air. Containment can be achieved by a variety of engineering methods such as enclosure, ventilation and air cleaning. A major contribution in this field is the development of "arresters" for the removal of contaminants. (b) *Replacement :* That is, replacing a technological process causing air pollution, by a new process that does not. Increased use of electricity, solar power generation, natural gas, and central heating in place of coal have greatly helped in smoke reduction. There is a move now to reduce lead in petrol which is a cumulative poison. In India also deleaded petrol is being used. (c) *Dilution :* Dilution is valid so long as it is within the self-cleaning capacity of the environment. For example, some air pollutants are readily removed by vegetation. The establishment of "green belts" between industrial and residential areas is an attempt at dilution. The capacity for dilution is, however, limited and trouble occurs when the atmosphere is overburdened with pollutants. (d) *Legislation :* Air pollution is controlled in many countries by suitable legislation, e.g., Clean Air Acts. Legislation covers such matters as height of chimneys, powers to local authorities to carry out investigations, research and education concerning air pollution, creation of smokeless zones and enforcement of standard for ambient air quality. To decrease the nuisance of air pollution, the Government of India have enacted "The Air (Prevention and Control of Pollution) Act" in 1981. (e) *International action :* To deal with air pollution on a world-wide scale, the WHO has established an international network of laboratories for the monitoring and study of air pollution. The network consists of two international centres at London and Washington, three centres at Moscow, Nagpur and Tokyo and 20 laboratories in various parts of the world *(13)*. These centres will issue warnings of air pollution where and when necessary.

Disinfection of air

In recent years, disinfection of air has received much attention. The methods employed are : (1) MECHANICAL VENTILATION : This reduces vitiated air and bacterial density. (2) ULTRAVIOLET RADIATION : This has been found to be effective in special situations such as operation theatres and infectious disease wards. Since direct exposure to ultraviolet rays is a danger to the eyes and skin, the ultraviolet lamps are shaded and located in the upper portion of the rooms near the inlet of air. Ultraviolet rays have proved effective for general use in public assembly and school rooms. (3) CHEMICAL MISTS : Triethylene glucol vapours have been found to be effective air bactericides, particularly against droplet nuclei and dust. (4) DUST CONTROL : Application of oil to floors of hospital wards reduces the bacterial content of the air. Air disinfection is still in the experimental stage.

References

1. Diamant, R.M.E. (1971), *"The International Environment of dwellings"*, Hutchinson Educational, London.
2. WHO (1987) *Air Quality Guidelines for Europe,* WHO Regional Publication, European Series No.23, Copenhagen.
3. Zutsi, P.K. (1970) *Science Today,* Oct 70.
4. WHO (2006), *Air Quality Guidelines, Global Update 2005,* Vol I, Europe Region.

4A. WHO (2016), *Household air pollution and Health,* Fact Sheet No. 292, Feb. 2016.

5. WHO (2016), *Ambient Air Quality and Health,* Fact sheet, Sept. 2016.
6. American Chemical Society (1969), *Cleaning Our Environment, The Chemical Basis for Action,* Washington, D.C.
7. Donham, K.J. et al., Acute Toxic exposure to gases from liquid manure, *Journal of Occupational Medicine,* 24 : 142–145, 1982.
8. WHO (2010), *Selected Pollutant, WHO Guidelines for indoor Air Quality.*
9. NEERI (1994) National Environmental Engineering Research Institute, *Directors Report.*
10. Maxcy – Rosenau – Last, *Public Health and Preventive Medicine,* 13th Edition, 1992.
11. World Development Report (1993), *Investing in Health* Published for the World Bank, Oxford University Press.
12. *Current Medical Diagnosis and Treatment,* 34th Ed (1995), Edited by Lawrence M Tierney, Stephen J. Mcphee and Maxine A Papadakis, LANGE.
13. WHO (1971), *WHO Chronicles* 25, 91.
14. WHO (2016), *Lead Poisoning and Health,* Fact Sheet, Aug. 2016.

VENTILATION

The modern concept of ventilation implies not only the replacement of vitiated air by a supply of fresh outdoor air, but also control of the quality of incoming air with regard to its temperature, humidity and purity with a view to provide a thermal environment that is comfortable and free from risk of infection.

Standards of ventilation

The fixing of standards of ventilation is a matter of much difficulty. Most of the standards of ventilation have been based on the efficiency of ventilation in removing body odour. (1) *Cubic space :* Different workers have advocated standards for the minimal fresh air supply ranging from 300 to 3,000 c.ft. per hour per person *(1)*. The widely quoted standard is that of De Chaumont who advocated a fresh air supply of 3,000 c.ft. per person per hour on the following grounds: It was observed that so long as the amount of carbon dioxide due to respiration was not more than 2 parts in 10,000 parts of air, the air of the rooms seemed fresh and did not sensibly differ from outdoor air. Assuming that an average person expires 0.6 c.ft. of carbon dioxide per hour, and that 0.0002 c.ft. of CO_2 in one c.ft. of air as the "permissible impurity", it was calculated that 0.6/0.0002 or

3,000 c.ft. of air would be required by a man at rest per hour. This standard of ventilation is no longer followed. (2) *Air change :* It is now established that the carbon dioxide theory is not quite correct because even if the CO_2 content of air is raised to over 5 per cent and the O_2 content reduced to 18 per cent, there were no deleterious effects so long as the "cooling power" of the air was satisfactory. Air change is more important than the cubic space requirement. It is recommended that in the living rooms, there should be 2 or 3 air changes in one hour; in work rooms and assemblies 4 to 6 air changes. If the air is changed more frequently, i.e., more than 6 times in one hour, it is likely to produce a draught which should be avoided. Based on this concept, it is now considered that a space of 1,000 to 1,200 c.ft. per person is quite sufficient. The number of air changes per hour is calculated by dividing the total hourly air supply to the room by the cubic capacity of the room *(1)*. (3) *Floor space :* Floor space per person is even more important than cubic space. Heights in excess of 10 to 12 feet are ineffective from the point of view of ventilation, as the products of respiration tend to accumulate in the lower levels. Therefore, in calculating cubic space requirements, heights over 10 to 12 feet are not taken into account. The optimum floor space requirements per person vary from 50 to 100 sq.ft.

Types of ventilation

1. *NATURAL VENTILATION*

Natural ventilation is the simplest system of ventilating small dwellings, schools and offices. In this method, reliance is placed on certain forces which operate in nature. These are: (1) THE WIND : The wind is an active force in ventilation. When it blows through a room, it is called *perflation.* When there is an obstruction, it bypasses and exerts a suction action at its tail end – this is called aspiration. Doors and windows facing each other provide "cross-ventilation". Back to back houses do not permit cross ventilation and therefore, their construction is not allowed. (2) DIFFUSION : Air passes through the smallest openings or spaces by diffusion. This is a slow process and therefore, is not relied upon as the sole means of ventilation. (3) INEQUALITY OF TEMPERATURE : Air flows from high density to low density; it rises when slightly heated and escapes from openings provided high up in the room. The outside air which is cooler and more dense will enter the room through inlets placed low. The greater the temperature difference between outside and inside air, the greater the velocity of the incoming air. In the tropics the outside air may be hotter than the inside and the reverse may take place *(2)*. These properties of air are utilized to best advantage by the proper location of windows, doors, ventilators and skylights. The chief drawback of natural ventilation is that it is not possible to regulate the velocity of the incoming air nor to adjust its temperature or humidity.

2. *MECHANICAL VENTILATION*

Mechanical or artificial ventilation may be of the following types :

(1) Exhaust ventilation. (2) Plenum ventilation. (3) Balanced ventilation. (4) Air conditioning.

(1) EXHAUST VENTILATION : In this system, air is extracted or exhausted to the outside by exhaust fans usually driven by electricity. As air is exhausted, a vacuum is created which induces fresh air to enter the room through windows, doors and other inlets. Exhaust ventilation is generally provided in large halls and auditoria for removal of vitiated air. The exhaust fans are housed in apertures in the external walls, high up near the roof which facilitate removal of the upper layers of the heated light air. The ventilation may be regulated by adjusting the speed of the fans. Local exhaust ventilation is widely used in industries to remove dusts, fumes and other concentrated contaminants at their source. (2) PLENUM VENTILATION : In this system, fresh air is blown into the room by centrifugal fans so as to create a positive pressure, and displace the vitiated air. Plenum or propulsion system is used for supplying air to air-conditioned buildings and factories. Air is delivered through ducts at desired points. This system is of limited utility. (3) BALANCED VENTILATION: This is a combination of the exhaust and plenum systems of ventilation. The blowing fan must balance the exhaust fan. When this system is employed, the natural system of ventilation is entirely dispensed with. (4) AIR CONDITIONING : Air conditioning is defined as "the simultaneous control of all, or at least the first three of those factors affecting both the physical and chemical conditions of the atmosphere within any confined space or room. These factors include temperature, humidity, air movement, distribution, dust, bacteria, odours and toxic gases, most of which affect in greater or lesser degree the human health and comfort". Air conditioning is popular in large institutions, hospitals, industries and dwellings. Its use in operation theatres is of particular value in control of pathogenic organisms in the air. The air is filtered when drawn into an airconditioner system from the room. Excess humidity is removed and the air is circulated back into the room after heating or cooling it, to bring room temperature to required comfort zone. Mixing some percentage of fresh air with recirculated air is regulated. Large institutions or hospitals often install central airconditioning system for entire building, instead of installing equipments for individual rooms. Better controls and economy is achieved in central airconditioning.

Where the temperature difference is large between outside atmosphere and airconditioned room, "transition room" is sometimes provided, which maintains temperature in between the two, so as to prevent sudden exposure to high or low temperature.

References

1. Bedford, T (1964). *Basic Principles of Ventilation and Heating.* Lewis, London.
2. Wilkie, W. (1965), *Jordan's Tropical Hygiene and Sanitation*, Bailliere Tindall & Co.

LIGHT

The requirements of good lighting

Good lighting is essential for efficient vision. If the lighting conditions are not ideal, the visual apparatus is put to strain which may lead to general fatigue and loss of efficiency. For efficient vision, the following light factors are essential : (1) SUFFICIENCY: The lighting should be sufficient to enable the eye to discern the details of the object as well as the surroundings without eye strain. An illumination of 15 to 20 foot candles (1 foot candle = 10.76 Lux) is accepted as a basic minimum for satisfactory vision. The illumination requirements vary from as little as 5 foot candles in stairways and corridors to 100 foot candles in some industries. (2) DISTRIBUTION : The distribution of light should be uniform, having the same intensity, over the whole field of work. If there are contrast differences in light, it will strain the eyes and affect adversely the visual acuity. Proper dispersal of light, without the production of shadows is therefore necessary for efficient vision. (3) ABSENCE OF GLARE : Glare is excessive contrast. The best example of glare is the automobile headlights at night, the same lights during daylight would not cause glare owing to the absence of excessive contrast. Glare may be a direct glare from a light source or reflected glare from sources such as table tops and polished furniture. Glare causes annoyance. The eye cannot tolerate glare because it causes acute discomfort and reduces critical vision. (4) ABSENCE OF SHARP SHADOWS : Slight shadows are inevitable, but sharp and contrasting shadows are disturbing. Like glare, shadows cause confusion to the eye and therefore should not be present in the field of vision. (5) STEADINESS : The source of light should be constant. It should not flicker because flickering causes eye strain and may lead to accidents. (6) COLOUR OF LIGHT : The colour of light is not very important so long as the intensity is adequate. Since natural light has a soothing effect on the eye, the artificial light should as far as possible approximate the daylight colour. (7) SURROUNDINGS : When a black object is viewed against a dark background, recognition is difficult. High levels of illumination will be required where there is little colour contrast. For efficient vision, colour schemes in rooms are important. Ceilings and roofs should have a reflection factor of 80 per cent; walls 50 to 60 per cent; furniture 30 to 40 per cent. There should not be much reflection from the floor, not more than 15 to 20 per cent. Contrasting colours are often used to prevent accidents, e.g., culverts, bridges, etc.

Measurement of light

What we perceive as light is a narrow wavelength band of electromagnetic radiation from about 380 to 780 nm (nano metre). Light containing all visible waves is perceived as white. There is considerable confusion about units of light measurement. There are four measures of importance. For each of these four measures again, there are a number of terms and also a great variety of names. These are given in Table 1. The four measures are : (1) *Luminous intensity,* which is the "power" of a light source considered as a point radiating in all directions; this is measured as candela or candle power. (2) *Luminous flux,* which is the flow of light related to a unit of solid angle measured in lumen. (3) *Illumination or illuminance,* which is the amount of light reaching a surface measured in lux per unit area; and (4) *Brightness* or *luminance* which is the amount of light reflected from a surface measured in *lamberts.*

TABLE 1
Light measurement units

Description	Quantity measured Name	Recommended Unit*	Other Units
1. Brightness of point source	Luminous intensity	Candela	Candle power
2. Flow of light	Luminous flux	Lumen	
3. Amount of light reaching surface	Illumination Illuminance	Lux (Phot)	Foot candle Lumen/cm^2
4. Amount of light re-emitted by surface	Brightness Luminance	Lambert	Foot lambert Candles/cm^2

* Recommended by the International Organization for Standardization

Natural lighting

Natural lighting is derived partly from the visible sky and partly from reflection. In fact, much light comes to the rooms by reflection from light coloured objects. Efficient utilization of natural light calls for careful design, location and orientation of buildings and relationship between buildings (town planning). Natural lighting also depends upon the time of the day, season, weather and atmospheric pollution. Since natural light is accompanied by radiant heat, all attempts should be made to exclude radiant heat while admitting daylight.

Suggestions for improving daylight illumination : The following general principles are taken into consideration in planning for the best utilization of daylight. (1) ORIENTATION : The brightness of the sky is not constant on the east and west and therefore the illumination is subject to variation in buildings facing east or west. Further, the direct penetration of sunlight from the east or west may heat up the rooms unduly in the tropics, especially during summer. Buildings are therefore oriented, wherever possible, towards north or south for uniform illumination. This is particularly important in respect of schools, factories and laboratories where uniform lighting is required in all the rooms. This rule may not be strictly observed with regard to dwelling houses, as uniform lighting is not required in all the rooms. When a building faces east and west, window shades are provided to protect against the direct penetration of sunlight. (2) REMOVAL OF OBSTRUCTIONS : Removal of obstructive items either wholly or partially is likely to give the most effective single improvement in lighting. (3) WINDOWS : Windows should be properly planned, as the natural lighting within any room is influenced by the amount of visible sky, the size, shape and arrangement of the window openings. A tall window gives greater penetration of light; a broad window gives greater diffusion of light. The rule that window area should not be less than 10 per cent of the floor area is now outdated. In modern practice, window area is correlated to the purpose the room is intended to serve. The usefulness of the windows is reduced by covering them unnecessarily with curtains and screens. (4) INTERIOR OF THE ROOMS : In order to obtain the full benefit of the natural illumination, the ceiling should be white; the upper portions of the walls light-tinted; and lower portions somewhat darker so as to give comfortable contrast to the eyes. The desirable reflection factors of the walls, roof and furniture have already been discussed.

Measurement of daylight

Since the intensity of daylight illumination is liable to change from moment to moment, it is not measured in terms of foot candles. Reliance is placed on a factor called the DAYLIGHT FACTOR (D.F.). It is the ratio of illumination at a given point to illumination at a point exposed simultaneously to the whole hemisphere of the sky (taken as 500 foot candles) excluding direct sunlight. The daylight factor may be summarized as follows :

$$\text{D.F.} = \frac{\text{Instantaneous illumination INDOORS}}{\text{Simultaneously occurring illumination OUTDOORS}} \times 100$$

The daylight factor in a building may be rapidly determined by a modified photo-electric meter known as a Daylight Factor Meter. It is recommended that in living rooms, the daylight factor should be at least 8 per cent and in kitchens about 10 per cent *(4)*.

Artificial lighting

Daylight may not meet the requirements of illumination during all hours, and especially during cloudy days. It should be supplemented by artificial illumination for adequate illumination. Artificial lighting should be as close as possible to daylight in composition. There are five systems of artificial lighting : direct, semi-direct, indirect, semi-indirect and direct-indirect. (1) DIRECT LIGHTING : In direct lighting, 99 to 100 per cent of the light is projected directly towards the working area. Direct lighting is efficient, economical, but tends to cast sharp shadows. It should not fall into the eyes. (2) SEMI-DIRECT : Here 10 to 40 per cent of the light is projected upwards so that it is reflected back on the object by the ceiling. (3) INDIRECT : light does not strike a surface directly, because 90 to 100 per cent of the light is projected towards the ceiling and walls. This gives a general illumination of the whole room but not of any object. (4) SEMI-INDIRECT : Here, 60 to 90 per cent of the light is directed upwards, and the rest downwards. (5) DIRECT-INDIRECT : Here, light is distributed equally, No one system can be recommended to the exclusion of others.

Methods of artificial illumination

(1) FILAMENT LAMPS : These are widely used. The electric current heats up the tungsten filament and the light emitted depends upon the temperature. The hotter filaments produce the bluer light. Accumulation of dust on the bulbs reduces illumination by 30 to 40 per cent. The bulbs and shades therefore should be cleaned frequently. (2) FLUORESCENT LAMPS : Fluorescent lamps are economical in the use of electric current; they are cool and efficient; the light emitted simulates natural light. The lamps consist of a glass tube filled with mercury vapour and an electrode fitted at each end. The inside of the tube is coated with fluorescent chemicals, which absorb practically all the ultraviolet radiation and remit the radiation in the visible range.

The total emission of energy from the 2 lamps is as follows *(1)*.

		Light	*Heat*
Filament	.....	5%	95%
Fluorescent	.....	21%	79%

Lighting standards

The eye responds to a range of illumination ranging from 0.1 lux (full moonlight night) to 100,000 lux (bright sunshine). There is considerable confusion about standards because of the adaptability of the eye. Many standards have been published but these standards are arbitrary. The visual efficiency increases with the increase of illumination, but the curve flattens out at higher levels. The law of diminishing return applies. A useful rule of thumb is that the illumination level should be 30 times higher than the level at which the task can just be done. It is worth repeating there are no exact lighting standards and it is usually better to err on the side of too much light, provided glare can be avoided. For practical situations and various activities, the following values (in lux) have been suggested by the Illuminating Engineer Society *(1)*.

TABLE 2
Recommended illumination (the IES Code)

Visual task	Illumination (lux)
Casual reading	100
General office work	400
Fine assembly	900
Very severe tasks	1,300–2,000
Watch making	2,000–3,000

Biological effects of light *(2, 3)*

Considerable attention has been focused on the biological effects of light. The observation that daylight could cause the *in vitro* degradation of bilirubin is now being used as a therapeutic measure in premature infants with hyperbilirubinaemia. Other biological effects of light include effect on biological rhythms of body temperature, physical activity, the stimulation of melanin synthesis, the activation of precursors of vitamin D, adrenocortical secretion and food consumption.

References

1. Koenigsberger, O.H. et al (1973). *Manual of Tropical Housing and Building,* Part I Climatic Design, Orient Longman, Bombay.
2. Gorodischer, R. (1970), *The New Eng. Jr. of Medicine,* 282, 375.
3. Wurtman, R.J. (1970). *Ibid,* 282, 394.
4. *Newford Standards* Architects Data, Page 26.

NOISE

Noise is often defined as "unwanted sound", but this definition is subjective because of the fact that one man's sound may be another man's noise. Perhaps a better definition of noise is : "wrong sound, in the wrong place, at the wrong time". Man is living in an increasingly noisy environment. The 20th Century has been described as the "Century of Noise". Noise has become a very important "stress factor" in the environment of man. The term "Noise Pollution" has been recently coined to signify the vast cacophony of sounds that are being produced in the modern life, leading to health hazards.

Sources : The sources of noise are many and varied. These are automobiles, factories, industries, air-crafts etc. Noise levels are particularly acute near railway junctions, traffic round-abouts, bus terminuses and airports. Use of pressure horns, recreational noise of loudspeakers with full volume during festivities particularly at night are other sources of noise production. The domestic noises from the radios, transistors, T.V sets – all add to the quantum of noise in daily life.

Properties : Noise has two important properties : loudness or intensity; and frequency.

(1) LOUDNESS : Loudness or intensity depends upon the amplitude of the vibrations which initiated the noise. The loudness of noise is measured in decibels (dB). When we say that sound is 60 dB, it means that it is 60 dB more intense than the smallest distinguishable noise or the "reference" sound pressure, which is understood to be 0.0002 microbar or dynes/cm^2. A dyne is 1/1000,000th of atmospheric pressure. Normal conversation produces a noise of 60–65 dB; whispering, 20–30 dB; heavy street traffic, 60–80 dB; and boiler factories, about 120 dB. A daily exposure upto 85 dB is about the limit people can tolerate without substantial damage to their hearing. The community noise levels are given in Fig.1.

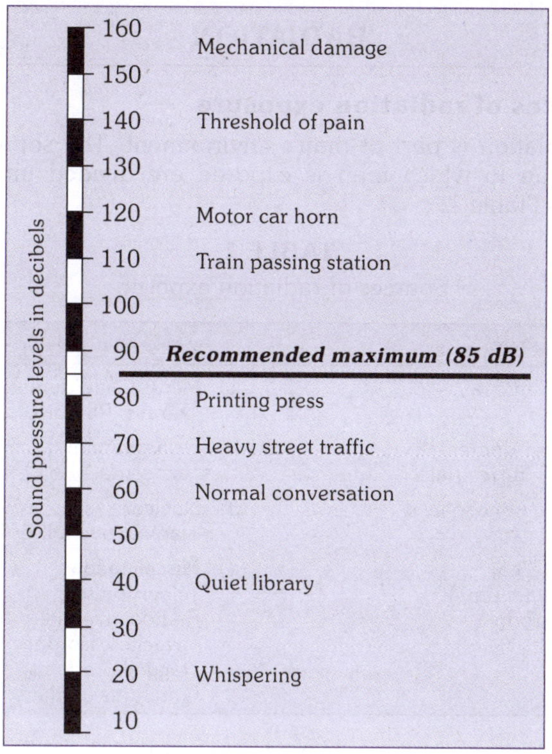

FIG.1
Community noise levels

It has been observed that the human ear responds in a non-uniform way to different sound-pressure levels, that is, it responds not to the real loudness of a sound, but to the perceived intensity. A weighting curve, called curve A has been constructed which takes into account the subjective effects of that sound. Sound-pressure levels are therefore expressed in dB (A), that is in decibels conforming to the weighting curve A, because this reflects the perception of that sound emission by the normal human ear. Acceptable noise levels are as given in Table 1.

TABLE 1

Acceptable noise levels (dBA)

Residential	Bed room	25
	Living room	40
Commercial	Office	35–45
	Conference	40–45
	Restaurants	40–60
Industrial	Workshop	40–60
	Laboratory	40–50
Educational	Class room	30–40
	Library	35–40
Hospitals	Wards	20–35

Source : *(1)*

(2) FREQUENCY : The frequency is denoted as Hertz (Hz.) One Hz is equal to one wave per second. The human ear can hear frequencies from about 20 to 20,000 Hz, but this range is reduced with age and other subjective factors. The range of vibrations below 20 Hz are infra-audible; and those above 20,000 Hz ultrasonic. Many animals (e.g., dogs) can hear sounds inaudible to the human ear. Sometimes noise is expressed in psycho-acoustic terms – the phon. The *phon* is a psycho-acoustic index of loudness. It takes into consideration intensity and frequency.

The sound level of some of the noises are as given in Table 2.

TABLE 2

Sound levels of some noises

Source of noise	Sound level (dB)
Whisper	20
Speech, 2–3 people	73
Speech on radio	80
Music on radio	85
Children shouting	79
Children crying	80
Vacuum cleaner	76
Piano	86
Jet take-off	150

The basic instruments used in studies on noise are : (1) the "Sound Level Meter" which measures the intensity of sound in dB or dB (A); (2) the "Octave Band Frequency Analyzer," which measures the noise in octave bands. The resulting plot shows the "sound spectrum" and indicates the characteristics of the noise, whether it is mainly high-pitched, low-pitched or of variable pitch, and; (3) the "Audiometer" which measures the hearing ability. The zero line at the top in the audiogram represents normal hearing. Noise-induced hearing loss shows a characteristic dip in the curve at the 4000 Hz frequency.

Effects of noise exposure *(2,3)*

The effects of noise exposure are of two types : auditory and non-auditory. (1) AUDITORY EFFECTS. (a) *Auditory fatigue :* It appears in the 90 dB region and greatest at 4000 Hz. It may be associated with side effects such as whistling and buzzing in the ears. (b) *Deafness :* The most serious pathological effect is deafness or hearing loss. The victim is generally unaware of it in early stages. The hearing loss may be temporary or permanent. Temporary hearing loss results from a specific exposure to noise; the disability disappears after a period of time up to 24 hours following the noise exposure. Most temporary hearing loss occurs in frequency range between 4,000 to 6,000 Hz. Repeated or continuous exposure to noise around 100 decibels may result in a permanent hearing loss; in this, the inner ear damage may vary from minor changes in the hair cell endings to complete destruction of the organs of Corti. When this occurs as a result of occupation in industries, it is called 'occupational hearing loss'. Exposure to noise above 160 dB may rupture the tympanic membrane and cause permanent loss of hearing. (2) NON-AUDITORY EFFECTS : These are : (a) *Interference with speech :* Noise interferes with speech communication. In everyday life, the frequencies causing most disturbance to speech communication lie in the 300–500 Hz range. Such frequencies are commonly present in noise produced by road and air traffic. For good speech intelligibility, it is considered that the speech sound level must exceed the SIL (Speech Interference Level) by approximately 12 dB. (b) *Annoyance :* This is primarily a psychological response. Neurotic people are more sensitive to noise than balanced people. Workmen exposed to higher intensity of noise in occupational capacities, were often irritated, short tempered and impatient and more likely to resort to agitation and disrupt production. (c) *Efficiency :* Where mental concentration is to be undertaken, a low level of noise is always desired. Reduction in noise has been found to increase work output. (d) *Physiological changes :* A number of temporary physiological changes occur in the human body as a direct result of noise exposure. These are : a rise in blood pressure, a rise in intracranial pressure, an increase in heart rate and breathing and an increase in sweating. General symptoms such as giddiness, nausea and fatigue may also occur. Noise interferes with sleep. Noise is also said to cause visual disturbance. It is said to cause a narrowing of pupil, affect colour perception and reduce night vision. (e) Besides affecting health, noise is also a significant factor in economic losses. The potential cost of noise induced hearing loss to industry is quite great.

Control of noise

A variety of approaches may be needed to control noise. These include : (1) CAREFUL PLANNING OF CITIES : In planning cities, the following measures should be taken to reduce noise; (a) division of the city into zones with separation of areas concerned with industry and transport; (b) the separation of residential areas from the main streets by means of wide green belts. House fronts should lie not less than 15 metres from the road and the intervening space should be thickly planted with trees and bushes; (c) widening of main streets to reduce the level of noise penetration into dwellings. (2) CONTROL OF VEHICLES : Heavy vehicles should not be routed into narrow streets. Vehicular traffic on residential streets should be reduced. Indiscriminate blowing of the horn and use of pressure horn should be prohibited. (3) TO IMPROVE ACOUSTIC INSULATION OF BUILDING : From the acoustic standpoint, the best arrangement is construction of detached buildings rather than a single large building or one that is continuous. Installations that produce noise or disturb the occupants within dwellings should be prohibited. Buildings should be sound-proof where necessary. (4) INDUSTRIES AND RAILWAYS : Control of noise at source is possible in industries. Special areas must be earmarked, outside residential areas, for industries, for railways, marshalling yards and similar installations. When these demands cannot be met, protective green belts must be laid down between the installations and residential areas. (5) PROTECTION OF EXPOSED PERSONS : Hearing protection is recommended for all workers who are consistently exposed to noise louder than 85 decibels in the frequency bands above 150 Hz. Workers must be regularly rotated from noisy areas to comparatively quiet posts in factories. Periodical audiogram check-ups and use of ear plugs, ear muffs are also essential as the situation demands. (6) LEGISLATION: Many states have adopted legislation providing for controls which are applicable to a wide variety of sources *(4)*. Workers have the right to claim compensation if they have suffered a loss of ability to understand speech. (7) EDUCATION : No noise abatement programme can succeed without people's participation. Therefore, their education through all available media is needed to highlight the importance of noise as a community hazard.

References

1. Koenigsberger, O.H. et al (1973). *Manual of Tropical Housing and Building,* Part I, Climatic Design, Orient Longman Bombay.
2. WHO (1966). *Noise,* An Occupational Hazard and Public Nuisance. Public Health Papers 30.
3. Dougherty, J.D. (1966). *N. Eng. J. Med.,* 275, 759.
4. The Noise Advisory Council (1971). *Neighbourhood Noise,* Report of the Working Group on the Noise Abatement Act, HMSO, London.

RADIATION

Sources of radiation exposure

Radiation is part of man's environment. The sources of radiation to which man is exposed are divided into two groups (Table 1) :

TABLE 1

Sources of radiation exposure

Natural	Man-made
(1) Cosmic rays	(1) Medical and dental: X-rays, Radioisotopes
(2) Environmental: (a) Terrestrial	(2) Occupational exposure
(b) Atmospheric	(3) Nuclear: radioactive fall-out
(3) Internal: Potassium-40 Carbon-14	(4) Miscellaneous: Television sets, Radioactive dial watches, Isotope tagged products, Luminous markers.

(1) *Natural sources :* Man is exposed to natural radiation from time immemorial. Natural background radiation arises from three sources : (a) *Cosmic rays :* The cosmic rays which originate in outer space are weakened as they pass through the atmosphere. At ordinary living altitudes, their impact is about 35 mrad a year. At altitudes above 20 km cosmic radiation becomes important. It has been calculated that a commercial jet pilot receives about 300 mrad per year from cosmic radiation *(1)*. (b) *Environmental :* (i) *Terrestrial radiation :* Radioactive elements such as thorium, uranium, radium and an isotope of potassium (K_{40}) are present in man's environment, e.g., soil, rocks, buildings. It is estimated that man derives about 50 mrad per year from terrestrial radiation. Areas exist (e.g., Kerala in India) where there are rock formations containing uranium, it can be as high as 2,000 mrad a year, (ii) *Atmospheric radiation :* The external radiation dose from the radioactive gases radon and thoron in the atmosphere is rather small : about 2 mrad per year. (c) *Internal radiation :* Man is also subjected to internal radiation, i.e., from radioactive matter stored in the body tissues. These radioactive materials include minute quantities of uranium, thorium, and related substances, and isotopes of potassium (K_{40}), strontium (Sr_{90}), and carbon (C_{14}). Internal radiation is thought to inflict about 25 mrad a year on the body as a whole, but may be as high as 70 or 80. All in all, it is estimated that the total natural radiation to which the average person is subjected comes to approximately 0.1 rad a year.

(2) *Man-made sources :* In addition to natural radiation, man is exposed to artificial or man-made sources. These are : (a) *X-rays :* The greatest man-made source of radiation exposure to the general population at the present time is medical and dental X-rays. Two distinct groups are involved : (i) patients and (ii) radiologists and medical technicians. When optimum radiographic techniques are employed, the skin dose to the patient from a single X-ray film varies roughly from 0.02 to 3.0 rad. (b) *Radioactive fallout :* Nuclear explosions release a tremendous amount of energy in the form of heat, light, ionizing radiation and many radioactive substances, the important being the isotopes of carbon (C_{14}), iodine (I_{131}), cesium (Cs_{137}) and

strontium (Sr_{90}). Cs_{137} and Sr_{90} are considered most important because they are liberated in large amounts and remain radioactive for many years. The "half-life" of Sr_{90} is about 28 years and that of Cs_{137} is 30 years. These radioactive particles released into the atmosphere float down to earth for some years afterwards. Because of air currents, the particles are distributed fairly evenly over the whole human race. Measurements made in 1963 in Germany (F.R.), a country where there had been no explosions, showed that a dose of 33 mrems per person was received from this source. (c) *Miscellaneous* : Some everyday appliances (e.g., TV sets, luminous wrist watches) are radioactive. But radiation from these sources at present is too small to be important.

Types of radiation

The term "ionizing radiation" is applied to radiation which has the ability to penetrate tissues and deposit its energy within them. Ionizing radiation may be divided into two main groups : (1) *electromagnetic radiations* – X-rays and gamma rays, and (2) *corpuscular radiations* – alpha particles, beta particles (electrons) and protons. Some common types of environmental radiations are as given in Table 2.

TABLE 2

Some common environmental radiations

Type of radiation	Approximate penetrating ability		
	Air	Tissue	Lead
Alpha particles	4 cm	0.05 mm	0
Beta particles	6–300 cm	0.06–4.0 mm	0.005–0.3 mm
Gamma rays	400 metres	50 cm	40 mm
X-rays	120–240 metres	15–30 cm	0.3 mm
Cosmic rays		some components very high	

Source : *(1)*

Alpha particles are 10 times as harmful as X-rays, beta particles or gamma rays. Alpha particles, luckily, have little penetrating force. On the other hand, they are quite dangerous if radioactive substance has entered the body (by inhalation or through a wound). Gamma rays and X-rays have short wave lengths; they are deep penetrating radiations. X-rays are manmade, while gamma rays are emitted spontaneously by radioactive elements during their disintegration. Otherwise there is no material difference between gamma rays and X-rays. Cosmic rays also contain ionizing radiations.

The term "non-ionizing radiation" refers to several forms of electromagnetic radiation of wavelengths longer than those of ionizing radiation. As wavelength elongates, the energy value of electromagnetic radiation decreases. So all non-ionizing forms of radiation have less energy than cosmic, gamma, and X-radiation have. In order of increasing wavelength, non-ionizing radiation includes ultraviolet (UV) radiation, visible light, infrared radiation, microwave radiation and radio frequency radiation.

Radiation units

The activity of a radioactive material is the number of nuclear disintegration per unit of time. The unit of activity is a becquerel (Bq); 1 Bq is equal to 1 disintegration per second. Formerly, the unit of activity was curie (Ci) and 1 Bq corresponds approximately to 27 picocuries.

The potency of radiation is measured in three ways : (1) *Roentgen:* Roentgen is the unit of exposure. It is the amount of radiation absorbed in air at a given point, i.e., number of ions produced in 1 ml of air. (2) *Rad* : Rad is the unit of absorbed dose. It is the amount of radioactive energy absorbed per gram of tissue or any material. 1mrad = 0.001 rad (3) *Rem* : Rem is the product of the absorbed dose and the modifying factors. The rem indicates the degree of potential danger to health. The radiation to which the average citizen is exposed is made up almost of the fast moving, highly penetrating X-rays and gamma rays, where rem and rad are equal *(2)*.

The radiation units (viz roentgen, rad, rem) are being replaced by the new SI Units (International System of Units) which are : (a) *Coulomb per kilogram* (C/Kg) replacing the roentgen. 1 roentgen is equal to 2.58×10^{-4} C kg^{-1}. It is the unit for exposure. There is no special name for this. (b) Gray (Gy) replacing the rad. It is the unit of absorbed dose, defined as the dose of ionizing radiation that impart 1 joule of energy to 1 kg of absorbing material. 1 rad is equal to 0.01 Gy. *(1)*, and (c) Sievert (Sv) replacing the rem. It is the SI unit of dose equivalent. The dose equivalent of 1 sievert is equal to 100 rems.

Dose equivalent (H) : As all types of radiation do not produce the same biological effect per unit of energy absorbed, the concept of dose equivalent has been introduced. The dose equivalent, M (Sieverts) is equal to the absorbed dose, D (grays), multiplied by a quality factor Q which depends upon the density of ionization produced in the tissue by the radiation.

$$H = DQ$$

The factor Q for X-rays and Y-rays and electrons is equal to 1, whereas for α particle it is 20 *(3)*.

Biological effects of radiation

Biological effects of radiation are divided into two categories. The first category consists of exposure to high doses of radiation over a short period of time producing acute or short term effects. The second category represents exposure to low doses of radiation over an extended period of time producing chronic or long-term effect. High doses tend to kill cells, causing organ damage. This inturn may cause whole body response often called "Acute Radiation Syndrome". The effects of ionizing radiation can be somatic or genetic as shown below :

SOMATIC
- *Immediate*
  - (1) Radiation sickness
  - (2) Acute radiation syndrome
- *Delayed* :
  - (1) Leukaemia
  - (2) Carcinogenesis
  - (3) Foetal developmental abnormalities
  - (4) Shortening of life

GENETIC
- (1) Chromosome mutations
- (2) Point mutations

The biological response of high dose of radiation is as follows *(4)* :

< 5 rad : No immediate observable effects

~ 5 rad to 50 rad : Slight blood changes may be detected by medical evaluations

~ 50 rad to 150 rad : Slight blood changes will be noted and symptoms of nausea, fatigue, vomiting etc. likely.

~ 150 rad to 1,100 rad : Severe blood changes will be noted and symptoms appear immediately. Approximately 2 weeks later, some of those exposed may die. At about 300–500 rad, upto one half of the people exposed will die within 60 days without intensive medical attention. Death is due to destruction of the blood forming organs. Without white blood cells, infection is likely. At the lower end of the dose range, isolation, antibiotics, and transfusions may provide the bone marrow time to generate new blood cells and full recovery is possible. At the upper end of the dose range, a bone marrow transplant may be required to produce new blood cells.

~ 1,100 rad to 2,000 rad : The probability of death increases to 100% within one to two weeks. The initial symptoms appear immediately. A few days later, things get very bad, very quickly since the gastrointestinal system is destroyed. Once the GI system ceases to function, nothing can be done, and medical care is for comfort only.

>2,000 rad : Death is a certainity. At doses above 5,000 rad, the central nervous system (brain and muscles) can no longer control the body functions, including breathing and blood circulation. Everything happens very quickly. Nothing can be done, and medical care is for comfort only.

As noted, there is nothing that can be done if the dose is high enough to destroy the gastrointestinal or central nervous system. That is why bone marrow transplants don't always work.

GENETIC EFFECTS : While somatic effects are recognizable within the life span of the irradiated person, genetic effects would be manifest in the more or less remote offspring. Genetic effects result from injury to chromosomes – chromosome mutations and point mutations. Chromosome mutation is associated with sterility. Point mutation affects the genes.

Radiation protection

The amount of radiation received from outer space and background radiation has been estimated to be 0.1 rad a year. Apparently, this does not at present constitute a hazard. The additional permissible dose from man-made sources should not exceed 5 rad a year. Of the man-made sources, the X-rays constitute the greatest hazard. In routine fluoroscopy, a dose of 4 rad is delivered to a part of the body in about one minute. This implies that unnecessary X-ray examinations should be avoided, especially in the case of children and pregnant women *(5)*. It also implies adequate control and surveillance of X-ray installations, protection of workers, improvement in techniques and improvements leading to dose reduction *(6)*. Effective protective measures include proper use of lead shields and lead rubber aprons. Lead aprons (0.5 mm of lead) will reduce the intensity of scattered X-rays over 90 per cent and should be worn by all workers regularly associated with X-ray procedures *(1)*. Workers must wear a film badge or dosimeter which shows accumulated exposure to radiation since last time the instrument was charged. Besides, periodic medical examinations, regular working hours, recreation, and holidays must be ensured to workers to maintain their state of health.

Radiation protection is the youngest branch of hygiene, and is called radiation hygiene. The International Commission on Radiological Protection (ICRP), the International Atomic Energy Agency (IAEA) and the World Health Organization (WHO) have been active in this field. The ICRP's recommendations on radiation dose levels *(7)* for occupational workers and for the general population have been adopted by many countries. It has been recommended that the genetic dose to the whole population from all sources additional to the natural background radiation, should not exceed 5 rems over a period of 30 years. The WHO has published permissible radiation levels in drinking water. The IAEA has sponsored many symposia on radioactive waste disposal and associated subjects *(8)*. Its main concern has been to promote peaceful uses of atomic energy and to assure that these uses do not imperil peace or health. In short, there has been a worldwide interest in preparing safety standards, codes of practice for the safe operation of nuclear power plants and enunciating the basic principles of radiation protection.

References

1. Little, J.B. (1966). *N. Eng. J. of Med.*, 275929.
2. Plant, R. (1969). *World Health*, Jan. 1969.
3. WHO (1993). *Guidelines for drinking water quality*, Recommendations vol.1, second ed.
4. United States Nuclear Regulatory Commission, *Biological effects of Radiation*, Reactor Concept Manual.
5. WHO (1963). *Techn. Rep. Ser.*, No.254.
6. WHO (1965). *Techn. Rep. Ser.*, No.306.
7. International Commission on Radiological Protection (1959, 1964). *ICRP Publications*, 2, 6. New York, Pergamon.
8. Straub, C.P. (1970). *Public Health Implications of Radioactive Waste Releases, Geneva.*

METEOROLOGICAL ENVIRONMENT

The elements which comprise the meteorological environment are: (1) atmospheric pressure (2) air temperature (3) humidity (4) rainfall (5) direction and speed of wind and (6) movement of clouds and character of weather *(1)*. The term "climate" is a geographical concept representing a summation of the whole range of meteorological phenomena.

Atmospheric pressure

The atmospheric pressure at earth's surface close to the sea level averages 760 mm of Hg. This is called "one atmosphere of pressure". Man is physiologically adapted to live at 760 mm of Hg pressure or close to it. The atmospheric pressure falls as altitude increases, and rises as altitude decreases. Thus, at an altitude of 100,000 feet above mean sea level, the atmospheric pressure is less than 10 mm. of Hg. The pressure increases at the rate of "one atmosphere" for each 33 feet depth below sea level.

Measurement

The instruments used for measuring atmospheric pressure are known as barometers of which there are three well-known kinds : Fortin's Barometer; the Kew Pattern Station Barometer and the Barograph. The 'Kew Pattern' Station Barometer is widely used by the Indian Meteorological Department for measuring the atmospheric pressure. Barograph is an instrument for obtaining a continuous record of atmospheric pressure. It is a circular box, the walls of which collapse or distend when the atmospheric pressure rises or falls.

Effects of atmospheric pressure on health

HIGH ALTITUDES

The air is less dense at higher altitudes, and consequently the partial pressure of oxygen is also less. Man cannot survive at an altitude of 25,000 feet without breathing equipment. When man is exposed to low pressures, the physiological effects are : (1) increase in respiration (2) increase in the concentration of haemoglobin (3) increase in cardiac output.

Two conditions have been described as a result of sudden exposure to high altitude : (1) *Acute Mountain Sickness :* This is a relatively common, harmless, and transient condition characterised by headache, insomnia, breathlessness, nausea, vomiting and impaired vision. It has not been conclusively proved whether all these symptoms are due to the effect of hypoxia or due to the various intricate biochemical and hormonal disturbances in the body. (2) *High Altitude Pulmonary Oedema :* The symptoms generally appear on about the third day at high altitude and are indistinguishable from those of ordinary mountain sickness. But as pulmonary oedema develops, the patient develops a cough, and may experience irregular or Cheyne-Stokes breathing, oligurea, mental confusion and hallucinations, stupor, seizures and coma. The condition is rare below 12,000 ft. (3,600 m.). The condition does not respond to antibiotics. The patient should be carried to lower altitudes as soon as possible. At present, the causes and mechanism of high altitude pulmonary oedema are not well understood. The main knowledge of this condition has been gained by medical officers in the Indian Army, who have seen many cases among troops transported from the lowlands to Himalayan stations *(2,3)*.

LOW ALTITUDES

The atmospheric pressure increases by one atmosphere for every 33 feet depth below sea level. The greatest depth so far reached are the equivalent of 10 atmospheres. When man is exposed to high pressure, the gases in the air namely oxygen, carbon dioxide and nitrogen are dissolved in the blood and tissues proportionately to the partial pressure of these gases. Excess concentration of nitrogen excerts a narcotic action leading to loss of mental functions and consciousness; excess of carbon dioxide increases the narcotic action of nitrogen; excess of oxygen can lead to convulsions and death. When the person comes up to the surface, the gases which are dissolved in the blood under pressure are released and cause air embolism, the effects of which are fatal. The effects of increased pressure are best observed in persons working in diving bells and compressed air chambers (Caisson disease).

AIR TEMPERATURE

The temperature of air varies in different parts of the day and also in the different seasons. The factors which influence the temperature are latitude of the place, altitude, direction of wind and proximity to sea. The temperature of the ground surface is always higher than that of the air.

MEASUREMENT

Thermometers are instruments used for measuring temperature. Mercury thermometers are widely used, as mercury boils at a high temperature, has a regular expansion and its level can be easily seen. Alcohol thermometers are also used. Alcohol has the advantage of not solidifying even at the lowest known temperature. The essential conditions for the use of the thermometers are that:- (1) the air should have free access to the bulbs of the thermometers and (2) the thermometer should be protected against radiant heat. These conditions are fulfilled by mounting the thermometers on a special approved screen called the "Stevenson Screen" which is used in all the meteorological observatories in India.

Dry bulb thermometer

This is an ordinary thermometer which measures the air temperature. For accurate readings, it is mounted on the 'Stevenson Screen', at a height of 1.20 to 1.80 m above the ground level. The screen protects against radiant heat, direct sun and rain.

Wet bulb thermometer

The wet bulb thermometer is precisely the same as the dry bulb thermometer excepting that the bulb is kept wet by a *muslin* cloth fed by water from a bottle through a wick. The evaporation of water from the muslin cloth lowers the temperature of the mercury. The wet bulb thermometer therefore shows a lower temperature reading than the dry bulb thermometer. The drier the air, the lower the wet bulb reading. If the wet and dry bulb thermometers record the same temperature, it means that the air is completely saturated with moisture, which is rare.

Maximum thermometer

This is a mercury thermometer so designed that there is a very fine constriction near the neck of the bulb. When the temperature rises, mercury expands; when the temperature falls, mercury cannot get back into the bulb. The end of the mercury thread at the distal end gives the maximum temperature reached. The thermometer is set each time by swinging briskly when the mercury retreats into the bulb.

Minimum thermometer

The liquid inside the minimum thermometer is spirit, in which is immersed a dumb-bell shaped index. When the temperature falls, the spirit drags the index towards the bulb end; when the temperature rises, the spirit expands and runs past the index.

Six's maximum and minimum thermometer

This is combination of the maximum and minimum thermometers. This instrument is not used in the Indian Meteorological Observatories.

Globe thermometer

The globe thermometer is used for the direct measurement of the mean radiant temperature of the surroundings. The instrument consists of a hollow copper bulb 6 inches (15 cm) in diameter and is coated on the outside with mattblack paint which absorbs the radiant heat from the surrounding objects. A specially calibrated mercury thermometer is inserted, with its bulb at the centre of the globe (Fig. 1). The globe thermometer registers a higher temperature than the ordinary air temperature thermometer because it is affected both by the air temperature and *radiant heat.* The difference between the globe thermometer temperature and that of the ordinary dry bulb is a measure of the radiant heat. The globe thermometer is also influenced by the velocity of air movement. The standard globe instrument reaches equilibrium with its environment in 15 to 20 minutes. A modified form of globe thermometer has been developed by Hellon and Crockford, which reaches equilibrium in about half this time, i.e., 8 to 10 minutes. The modified globe is made up from lighter gauge metal than the standard type, i.e., half the gauge and it is also provided with an internal air stirring mechanism consisting of a small fan driven by a miniature 6 volt motor *(4)*.

Wet globe thermometer *(5)*

This instrument is designed for environmental heat measurement. It consists of a dial thermometer with the heat sensing portion enclosed by a blackened copper sphere that is completely covered with wet black cloth. The Wet Globe exchanges heat with the surroundings by conduction, convection, evaporation and radiation similar to the way a perspiring man does, so the equilibrium temperature of the globe provides a comprehensive measure of the cooling capacity of the work environment *(5)*.

Silvered thermometer

The bright metallic surface reflects as much of the incident radiant heat as possible. This gives a more accurate reading of the air temperature.

Kata thermometer

The word "kata" is a Greek word meaning "down". The Kata thermometer (Fig. 2) is an alcohol thermometer with a glass bulb 4 cm long and 1.8 cm in diameter. The readings on the stem are marked from 100 deg. to 95 deg.F. Two instruments are used, the bulb of one is covered with a wet muslin cloth, the *wet kata* and the other *dry kata*. Before taking the readings, the bulbs are immersed in hot water to warm them slightly above 130 deg.F, when the alcohol rises into a small reservoir at the top of the instrument. The bulb of the dry Kata is wiped dry. Then both the instruments are suspended in air at the point of observation. The time in seconds required for the spirit to fall from 100 deg. to 95 deg.F is noted with a stop watch. This is repeated at least 4 times. The first reading is discarded and the average of the last three is taken. The length of time depends upon the "cooling power" of the air. Each Kata has a "factor" called the Kata Factor marked on the stem. This factor is determined for each instrument by the manufacturers. This factor, divided by the average cooling time gives the rate of cooling in millicalories per sq. centimetre per second. The Kata thermometer was originally devised for measuring the "cooling power" of the air. A dry Kata reading of 6 and above, and a wet Kata reading of 20 and above were regarded as indices of thermal comfort. The Kata thermometer is now largely used as an anemometer for recording low air velocities rather than the cooling power of the air.

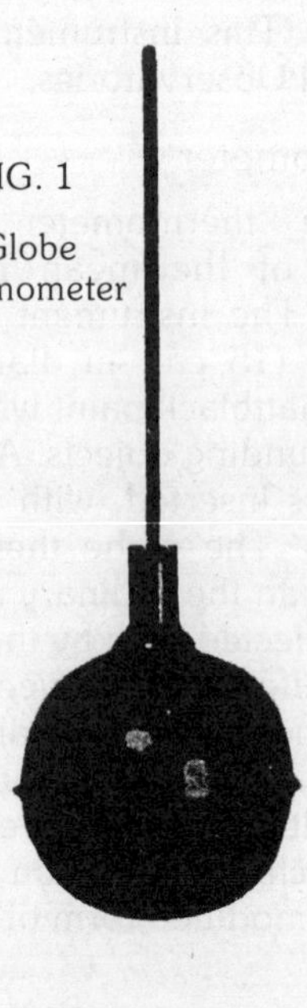

FIG. 1 Globe thermometer

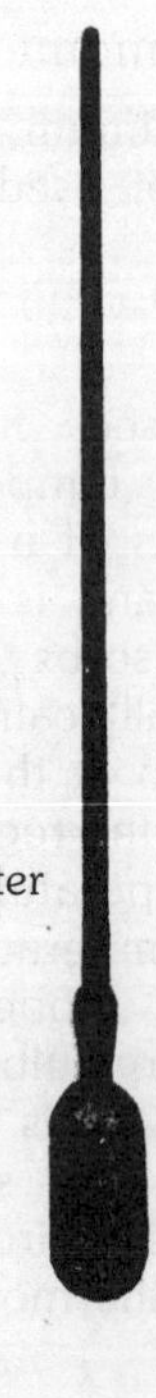

FIG. 2 Kata thermometer

Kata thermometers are available to cover the following 5 deg.F cooling ranges : (1) The standard Kata – cooling range between 100 deg. – 95 deg.F. (2) the High Temperature Kata – cooling range between 130 deg. – 125 deg.F. and (3) the Extra High Temperature Kata – cooling range between 150 deg. – 145 deg.F. In tropical countries, the atmospheric temperature may be well above 100 deg.F when the standard Kata cannot be used, but the other instruments can be used. The three types of Kata are readily distinguished by the colour of the alcohol. The standard Kata is coloured red; the high temperature instrument dark blue; and the extra high instrument magenta. Kata thermometers have silvered bulbs to reduce the errors due to radiation.

Heat stress indices *(6,7)*

Heat stress is the burden or load of heat that must be dissipated if the body is to remain in thermal equilibrium. The factors which influence heat stress are metabolic rate, air temperature, humidity, air movement and radiant temperature. The amount of heat gained by the body must be equalled by the amount of heat lost from it.

Many heat stress indices have been devised, but none is adequate to be valid in all possible complexities of work rate, air temperature, air movement, etc. These include : Equatorial Comfort Index, Heat Stress Index, and Predicted Four Hour Sweat Rate (P_4SR). (a) *Equatorial comfort index :* This denotes the temperature of still and saturated air which is equivalent physiologically to the climate under consideration. (b) *Heat stress index :* This takes into consideration the metabolic rate and the principal channels of heat exchange between the human body and the environment. The heat stress index represents the percentage of the heat storage capacity of an average man. Nomograms have been provided from which the value of the heat stress index could be easily calculated. An interpretation of the HSI values are as given below :

0	.....	No thermal stress
10–30	.....	Moderate to mild heat strain
40–60	.....	Severe heat strain
70–90	.....	Very severe heat strain
100	.....	Upper limit of heat tolerance

(c) *Predicted four hour sweat rate :* The rate at which a man sweats is a good index of the heat stress to which he is subjected. A sweat rate of 4.5 litres in 4 hours is the upper limit of tolerance in health for work in hot environment. A sweat rate of 2.5 litres in 4 hours is considered optimal for a working man. P_4SR is applicable only in the situation where sweating occurs.

Effects of heat stress

As many as 14 disorders resulting from exposure to heat have been recognized and documented *(8)*. The important ones are : (1) HEAT STROKE : This is attributed to failure of the heat regulating mechanism. It is characterized by very high body temperature which may rise to 110°F (43.3°C) and profound disturbances including delirium, convulsions and partial or complete loss of consciousness. The skin is dry and hot. Classically, sweating is absent or diminished, but many victims of clear-cut heat stroke perspire profusely. The outcome is often fatal, even when patients are brought quickly to medical attention; death/case ratios of 40 per cent or more have been reported. The treatment consists of rapidly cooling the body in ice water bath till the rectal temperature falls below 102°F (38.9°C). The rectal temperature should be monitored continuously, both to monitor the efficacy of hypothermia treatment and to guard against the development of clinically significant hypothermia, which can occur if cooling is continued too long. Further treatment is supportive and directed towards the many potential complications of hyperthermia. Hypovolaemia, hyperkalaemia, rhabdomyolysis, hypocalcaemia and bleeding diathesis may require intensive supportive treatment. The patient should be kept in bed for several days until the temperature control becomes stable. (2) HEAT HYPERPYREXIA : This is attributed to impaired functioning of the heat-regulating mechanism but without characteristic features of heat stroke. It is arbitrarily defined as a temperature above 106°F *(8)*. It may proceed to heat stroke. (3) HEAT EXHAUSTION : Unlike heat stroke, heat exhaustion is not because of failure of thermo-regulation. It is a milder illness than heat stroke and is caused primarily by the imbalance or inadequate replacement of water and salts lost in perspiration due to thermal stress. Heat exhaustion typically occurs after several days of high temperature. Body temperature may be normal or moderately elevated, but it is uncommon to exceed 102°F (38.9°C). The symptoms, primarily dizziness, weakness and fatigue, are those of circulatory distress. It may be severe enough to require hospitalization, especially in elderly patients. Treatment is directed towards normalizing fluid and electrolyte balance. (4) HEAT CRAMPS : Heat cramps occur in persons who are doing heavy muscular work in high temperature and humidity. There are painful and spasmodic contractions of the skeletal muscles. The cause of heat cramps is loss of sodium and chlorides in the blood. (5) HEAT SYNCOPE : This is a common ill-effect of heat. In its milder form, the person standing in the sun becomes pale, his blood pressure falls and he collapses suddenly. There is practically no rise in body temperature. The condition results from pooling of blood in lower limbs due to dilatation of blood vessels, with the result that the amount of blood returning to the heart is reduced, which in turn is responsible for lowering of blood pressure and lack of blood supply to the brain. This condition is quite common among soldiers when they are standing for parades in the sun *(10)*. Treatment is quite simple. The patient should be made to lie in the shade with the head slightly down; recovery usually comes within 5 to 10 minutes.

PREVENTIVE MEASURES

The ill effects of high temperature may be prevented by observing the following precautions : (1) REPLACEMENT OF WATER : Persons working under conditions of high temperature and humidity should be encouraged to drink cool water. It has been found in India that a man doing hard work in the sun requires about one litre of water per hour. For a sedentary worker, the requirement is nearly half this quantity. There is a widespread belief that extra salt intake during the summer helps prevent the ill-effects of heat. Studies have shown that the normal intake of salt in the Indian diet is far more than is actually needed. Further, salt losses through sweat are small since the concentration of salt in sweat is considerably low. Therefore, there is no need to add salt to water. However, extra salt is needed by unacclimatized persons during the first ten days of their exposure to heat *(10)*. (2) REGULATION OF WORK : The duration of exposure to a hot environment should be cut down. There should be periods of rest in between intense work. If signs, such as headache and dizziness appear, the person should be removed to a cooler environment, and the necessary treatment given. (3) CLOTHING : The clothing worn should be light, loose and of light colours. (4) PROTECTIVE DEVICES : Protective goggles, shields and helmets are helpful. (5) WORK ENVIRONMENT : The temperature and humidity in the work environment may be controlled by proper ventilation and air-conditioning.

Effects of cold stress

Injury due to cold may be general or local. In general cold injury (hypothermia), the individual is said to be suffering from exposure to cold. This is characterised by numbness, loss of sensation, muscular weakness, desire for sleep, coma and death. Local cold injury may occur at temperatures above freezing (wet-cold conditions) as in *immersion* or *trench foot.* At temperatures below freezing (dry-cold conditions) *frostbite* occurs; the tissues freeze and ice crystals form in between the cells *(11)*. Frostbite is common at high altitudes. It is extremely important to dress for the temperature with which the part will be in contact. The affected part should be warmed using water at 44 deg. C. Warming should last about 20 minutes at a time. Intake of hot fluids promotes general rewarming.

Global warming

Emission of green-house gases into the atmosphere have been increasing ever since the beginning of the industrial revolution. A major component of emission of carbon dioxide is from the combustion of fossil fuels. It is generally conceded that the main effects of this include an increase of about 3°C in the average global surface temperature by the year 2030, a rise in the sea level of 0.1–0.3 metres by 2050, and an increase in the occurrence of extreme climatic events such as cyclones, heatwaves and draughts *(12)*. The temperature rise could overwhelm the capacity of many species to adapt. A change of this magnitude would affect local, regional and global ecosystem, sea levels and ocean currents, prevailing winds, fresh water supplies, agriculture, forests, fisheries, industry, transport, urban planning, demographics and human health. Some effects are mutually reinforcing, so a small additional change in the existing trend could have massive consequences, in accordance with the mathematics of catastrophe theory *(13)*.

Changes in the configuration of jet streams, prevailing winds and ocean currents could alter the distribution of rainfall in many regions, making some wetter, others drier. The summers are becoming hotter. Temperate zone warming induces a decline in soil moisture that impairs grain production. This will also change the distribution of vegetation. The distribution of insect vectors of disease will change. The "heat island" phenomenon that makes cities warmer than surrounding rural areas will lead to longer and more severe heat waves than we are accustomed to now *(13)*.

HUMIDITY

Humidity or moisture is always present in the atmosphere. The amount of moisture which air can hold depends upon its temperature. If the air is cooled, the excessive moisture precipitates for the particular temperature. This is called *Dew Point.* Humidity may be expressed *as absolute humidity* or *relative humidity.*

(a) ABSOLUTE HUMIDITY is the weight of water vapour in a unit volume of air. It is expressed as grammes per kilogram or grammes per cubic metre of air.

(b) RELATIVE HUMIDITY: Relative humidity is the most common way of describing atmospheric moisture. It does not indicate the actual amount of water vapor in the air, instead, it tells us how close the air is to being saturated. The relative humidity (RH) is the ratio of the amount of water vapor actually in the air to the maximum amount of water vapor required for saturation at that particular temperature (and pressure). It is the ratio of the air's water vapour content to its capacity; thus

$$RH = \frac{\text{Water vapour content}}{\text{Water vapour capacity}}$$

It can also be expressed as

$$RH = \frac{\text{Actual vapour pressure}}{\text{Saturation vapour pressure}} \times 100 \text{ per cent}$$

Relative humidity is given as a per cent. Air with a 50 per cent RH actually contains one-half the amount required for saturation. Air with a RH greater than 100 per cent is said to be supersaturated. A change in RH can be brought about in two ways : (a) by changing the air's water vapour content; and (b) by changing the air temperature with a constant amount of water vapour, cooling the air raises the RH and warming the air lowers it *(14)*.

Very low RH in the house can have an adverse effect on things living inside and including house plants. Very low RH causes rapid evaporation of moisture from exposed skin causing crack, dry flake, or itch. It also irritates mucous membranes in the nose and throat, causing an itchy throat. Dry nasal passage permit inhaled bacteria to incubate, causing persistent infection. The remedy for most of these problems is to increase the RH.

(c) DEW POINT : It represents the temperature to which air would have to be cooled (with no change in air pressure or moisture content) for saturation to occur. The dew point is determined with respect to a flat surface of water. When the dew point is determined with respect to a flat surface of ice, it is called frost point. The dew point is an important measurement used to predict the formation of dew, frost, fog and even minimum temperature. High due point indicate high water vapour content; and low dew point indicate low water vapour content.

Measurement

There are several instruments which may be used for measuring humidity. The ones commonly used are described below :

DRY AND WET BULB HYGROMETER

This is the most widely used instrument for measuring humidity. The instrument consists of two similar thermometers – a dry bulb thermometer and a wet bulb thermometer, which are mounted side by side on a stand. The dry bulb measures the air temperature (DBT). The bulb of the second one is covered with a gauze or wick and is kept moist. The wet bulb temperature (WBT) is usually lower than the DBT. If both the readings are the same, it indicates that the atmosphere is 100 per cent saturated with moisture, which never occurs in reality. After obtaining the readings of the dry and wet bulb thermometers, the corresponding RH can be found from specially constructed psychrometric charts or slide rule. Humidity values are high in early morning and are near the minimum value in the afternoon at about 15.00 hours. For accurate readings of the wet bulb thermometer, the air should pass over the bulb with a speed of about 800 ft/min (5 m/sec). The sling psychrometer (described below) achieves this when rotated rapidly.

SLING PSYCHROMETER

The sling or whirling psychrometer (Fig. 3) consists of 2 mercury thermometers (wet and dry) mounted side by side, on a suitable wooden frame, and provided with a handle for rotating the instrument. The underlying principle is that by rotating, the bulbs are exposed to air at a definite velocity. The wet bulb is first moistened with distilled water and the instrument is whirled or rotated standing with the back to the sun, for about 15 seconds at the rate of 4 revolutions per second, so as to obtain the desirable air speed of about 5 metres per second. The reading of the wet bulb is then noted. The instrument is again whirled for about 10 seconds and the wet bulb reading is noted. This is repeated several times till 2 successive readings of the wet bulb are identical. The reading of the dry bulb is then noted. By use of suitable tables or charts, the relative humidity of the air may be obtained from the readings of the psychrometer.

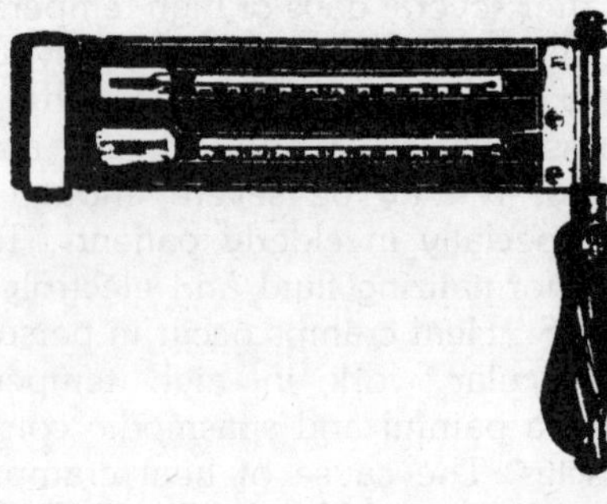

FIG.3
Sling psychrometer

ASSMANN PSYCHROMETER

This is a portable instrument specially designed to give accurate measurement of the wet and dry bulb temperature of the air. In this instrument, air is drawn at a speed higher than 5 metres per second by a clock-work fan. The bulbs of the thermometer are protected from the effects of solar radiation so that the instrument can be used even in strong sunshine.

PRECIPITATION

The term precipitation is the collective term used for rain, snow, hail, dew and frost – that is, all forms of water precipitated from the atmosphere. It is measured by rain-gauges. The rain-gauge prescribed by the Government of India for use at rainfall measuring stations in India is known as the "Symon's Rain-gauge". The funnel for receiving the rainfall has a diameter of 5 inches. Great care is exercised in selecting a suitable site for the erection of rain-gauge. The Rain-gauge should be set on a level ground, away from trees, buildings, or other obstructions. The rule which must be strictly adhered to in the erection of a Rain-gauge is that its rim should be exactly horizontal, and one foot above the ground level, the instrument having been fixed in a masonry or concrete foundation. The rainfall is measured in millimetres per a time unit (mm/day; mm/month).

AIR VELOCITY

Air velocity

The air velocity is measured by an instrument called the *anemometer.* It consists of four hemispherical cups, attached to the ends of 2 crossed metal arms. There is a vertical spindle which is attached to the 'anemometer box'. The velocity of the wind is indicated on a counter called the cyclometer, placed in the anemometer box.

Wind velocities are normally recorded in open flat country at a height of 10 m. Velocities are measured in metres per second (m/s.). When the wind speed is 0.5 m/s, it is described as complete calm with smoke rising vertically; when it is 3.3 m/s, it is described as *slight breeze* with leaves rustling; when it is 10 m/s, it is described as *strong wind* with larger branches of trees moving; when it is 15–20 m/s, it is called *storm;* when it is 25–30 m/s, it is called *gale;* and over 30–50 m/s, it is called *hurricane.*

KATA THERMOMETER : The Kata thermometer is quite sensitive to slight air movements. It can record air velocities as low as 10 feet per minute. This instrument has already been described.

Wind direction

The wind direction is observed by an instrument called the *wind vane.* There is an arrow which turns freely about a vertical axis. The wind vane is erected at a height of 10 m above ground level. If the arrow is motionless for 3 minutes, the wind is described as 'calm'. The wind direction may also be noted by letting off bits of paper in the air, which gives the approximate direction. Directions are grouped into 4 main categories (N,E,S, and W) and 8 or 16 sub-categories.

Clouds and weather observations

In all meteorological stations, clouds are observed for their form, amount, direction and height. Such observations give an insight into the sequence of weather in the particular locality. From the state of the sky and evolution of clouds, weather is described as fine weather, fair weather, unsettled weather, bad weather and thunderous sky. Meteorological satellites are now being used for automatic picture taking to give an idea of the clouds. The satellites can also measure temperature and humidity in the atmosphere.

References

1. Govt. of India (1954). *Instruction to Observers at the Surface Observations,* Part I, India Meteorological Department, Manager of Publications, Delhi.
2. Singh, et al (1969). *N. Eng. J. Med.,*280 175.
3. Editorial (1972). *Brit. Med. J.,* 3, 65.
4. Hellon, R.J. and Crockford, G.W. (1959). *J. Appl. Phys.* 14, 649.
5. Botsford, J.H. (1971). *An Ind.Hyg.Ass.J.,* 32, 1–10.
6. WHO (1969). *Techn. Rep. Ser.,* No.412.
7. Director General Factory Advice Service (1973). *Heat and Ventilation in Factory Building,* Central Labour Institute, Bombay.
8. Medical Research Council (1958). *Brit. Med. J.,* 1, 1533.
9. Goldberger, E (1970). *A Primer of Water, Electrolyte and Acid-Base Syndromes.* 4th Ed., Lea & Febiger, Philadelphia.
10. Malhotra, M.S. (1971). *Science Today,* May 1971, A Times of India Publication.
11. Ward, M. (1974). *Brit. Med. J.,* 1, 67.
12. WHO (1992). *Global Health Situation and Projections* P–24.
13. Maxcy–Rosenau–Last, *Public Health and Preventive Medicine,* 13th Ed., 1992.
14. C. Donald Ahrens, *Meteorology Today,* 8th Ed., 2007.

HOUSING

"Housing", in the modern concept includes not only the 'physical structure' providing shelter, but also the immediate surroundings, and the related community services and facilities. It has become part of the concept of "human settlement", which is defined as "all places in which a group of people reside and pursue their life goals; the size of the settlement may vary from a single family to millions of people".

A WHO Expert Group (1961) on public health aspects of housing prefers to use the term "residential environment" which is defined as the physical structure that man uses and the environs of the structure including all necessary services, facilities, equipment and devices needed or desired for the physical and mental health and the social well-being of the family and the individual *(1).* The immediate surroundings of residential building are often referred to as the neighbourhood or microdistrict.

Social goals of housing

Goals are statements about desirable or projected conditions. The generally accepted goals of housing are : (1) *Shelter :* That the house should provide a sanitary shelter, which is a basic need. (2) *Family life:* That the house should provide adequate space for family life and related activities, viz. preparation and storage of food, meeting, sleeping, individual activities and other basic activities. The adequacy of housing at this level has been found to have a direct impact on such things as worker productivity and family stability. (3) *Access to community facilities :* A third element of housing is accessibility to community services and facilities such as health services, schools, shopping areas, places of worship etc. (4) *Family participation in community life :* Family is part of the wider community. Community is important to family in many ways – it can offer help in times of need; it is an important source of friends. Communities are able to pool their efforts and improve their living conditions. (5) *Economic stability :* Housing is a form of investment of personal savings. It provides for economic stability and well being of the family.

The implementation of social goals in housing requires that government should (1) introduce social housing schemes; (2) establish both minimum and maximum standards; (3) create financial and fiscal institutions geared to helping low income people obtain credit for building or improving their houses.

CRITERIA FOR HEALTHFUL HOUSING

An Expert Committee of the WHO *(3)* recommended the following criteria for healthful housing similar to the Basic Principles of Healthful Housing published by the American Public Health Association *(4)* :

1. Healthful housing provides physical protection and shelter;
2. provides adequately for cooking, eating, washing, and excretory functions;
3. is designed, constructed, maintained and used in a manner such as to prevent the spread of communicable diseases;
4. provides for protection from hazards of exposure to noise and pollution;
5. is free from unsafe physical arrangements due to construction or maintenance, and from toxic or harmful materials; and

6. encourages personal and community development, promotes social relationships, reflects a regard for ecological principles, and by these means promotes mental health.

Housing standards

With the broadening concept of housing, the concept of housing standards has also changed. The standards are no longer confined to narrow health criteria like per capita space and floor space. Social and economic characteristics such as family income, family size and composition, standard of living, life style, stage in life cycle, education and cultural factors must be taken into consideration in determining housing standards. Because of cultural diversity and other factors such as climate and social traditions, standards of housing must vary from country to country and from region to region. In short, there cannot be rigid, uniform standards.

However, minimum standards are still maintained by building regulations, the aim being improvement of housing and environmental conditions for the majority of families within the limits set by available resources and objectives. The standards in India are those recommended by the EHC (1947). These are as below :

SITE : (a) The site should be elevated from its surroundings so that it is not subject to flooding during rains (b) the site should have an independent access to a street of adequate width (c) it should be away from the breeding places of mosquitoes and flies (d) it should be away from nuisances such as dust, smoke, smell, excessive noise and traffic (e) it should be in pleasing surroundings (f) the soil should be dry and safe for founding the structure and should be well drained. "Made-soil", i.e., ground that is levelled by dumping refuse is very unsatisfactory for building purposes for at least 20 to 25 years. The subsoil water should be below 10 feet (3 metres).

SET BACK : For proper lighting and ventilation, there should be an open space all round the house – this is called "set back". In rural areas it is recommended that the built-up area should not exceed one-third of the total area; in urban areas where land is costly, the built-up area may be upto two-thirds. The set back should be such that there is no obstruction to lighting and ventilation.

FLOOR : The floor should be pucca and satisfy the following criteria : (a) it should be impermeable so that it can be easily washed and kept clean and dry. Mud floors tend to break up and cause dust; they are not recommended, (b) the floor must be smooth and free from cracks and crevices to prevent the breeding of insects and harbourage of dust, (c) the floors should be damp proof, (d) the height of the plinth should be 2 to 3 feet (0.6 to 1 metre).

WALLS : The walls should be (a) reasonably strong (b) should have a low heat capacity i.e., should not absorb heat and conduct the same (c) weather resistant (d) unsuitable for harbourage of rats and vermin (e) not easily damaged and (f) smooth. These standards can be attained by 9-inch brick-wall plastered smooth and coloured cream or white.

ROOF : The height of the roof should not be less than 10 feet (3 m) in the absence of air-conditioning for comfort. The roof should have a low heat transmittance coefficient.

ROOMS : The number of living rooms should not be less than two, at least one of which can be closed for security. The other may be open on one side if that side is a private courtyard. The number and area of rooms should be increased according to size of family, so that the recommended floor space per person may be made available.

FLOOR AREA : The floor area of a living room should be at least 120 sq.ft. (12 sq. m.) for occupancy by more than one person and at least 100 sq.ft. (10 sq. m.) for occupancy by a single person. The floor area available in living rooms per person should not be less than 50 sq.ft; the optimum is 100 sq.ft.

CUBIC SPACE : Unless means are provided for mechanical replacement of air the height of rooms should be such as to give an air space of at least 500 c.ft. *per capita, preferably 1,000 c.ft.*

WINDOWS : (a) Unless mechanical ventilation and artificial lighting are provided, every living room should be provided with at least 2 windows, and at least one of them should open directly on to an open space, (b) the windows should be placed at a height of not more than 3 feet (1 m) above the ground in living rooms (c) window area should be 1/5th of the floor area. Doors and windows combined should have 2/5th the floor area.

LIGHTING : The daylight factor should exceed 1 per cent over half the floor area.

KITCHEN : Every dwelling house must have a separate kitchen. The kitchen must be protected against dust and smoke; adequately lighted; provided with arrangements for storing food, fuel and provisions; provided with water supply; provided with a sink for washing utensils and fitted with arrangements for proper drainage. The floor of the kitchen must be impervious.

PRIVY : A sanitary privy is a MUST in every house, belonging exclusively to it and readily accessible. In the more developed areas of the world, the majority of dwelling units are equipped with water carriage systems.

GARBAGE AND REFUSE : These should be removed from the dwelling at least daily and disposed off in a sanitary manner.

BATHING AND WASHING : The house should have facilities for bathing and washing belonging exclusively to it and providing proper privacy.

WATER SUPPLY : The house should have a safe and adequate water supply available at all times.

Rural housing

In rural areas, the "approved" standards may be lower than in towns. The following minimum standards have been suggested : (1) there should be at least two living rooms (2) ample verandah space may be provided (3) the built-up area should not exceed one-third of the total area (4) there should be a separate kitchen with a paved sink or platform for washing utensils (5) the house should be provided with a sanitary latrine (6) the window area should be at least 10 per cent of the floor area (7) there should be a sanitary well or a tube well within a quarter of a mile from the house (8) it is insanitary to keep cattle and livestock in dwelling houses. Cattle sheds should be at least 25 feet away from dwelling houses. A cattle shed should be open on all sides; an area 8 ft.×4 ft. is sufficient for each head of cattle (9) there should be adequate arrangement for the disposal of waste water, refuse and garbage *(5)*.

Housing and health

Housing is part of the total environment of man and

being a part, it is to some extent responsible for the status of man's health and well-being. It is difficult, however, to demonstrate the specific cause and effect relationships because housing embraces so many facets of environment. By deductive reasoning, a strong relationship can be established between poor housing and the following conditions :

(1) RESPIRATORY INFECTIONS : Common cold, tuberculosis, influenza, diphtheria, bronchitis, measles, whooping cough, etc.

(2) SKIN INFECTIONS : Scabies, ringworm, impetigo, leprosy.

(3) RAT INFESTATION : Plague.

(4) ARTHROPODS : Houseflies, mosquitoes, fleas and bugs.

(5) ACCIDENTS : A substantial proportion of house accidents are caused by some defect in the home and its environment.

(6) MORBIDITY AND MORTALITY : High morbidity and mortality rates are observed where housing conditions are sub-standard.

(7) PSYCHOSOCIAL EFFECTS : These effects must not be overlooked. The sense of isolation felt by persons living in the upper floors of high buildings is now well known to have harmful effects. Often, also, people living in densely populated urban areas feel a similar sense of isolation which may lead to neurosis and behaviour disorders.

If the definition of health given by WHO is applied, we have also to take into consideration the broader aspects of mental and social well-being of individuals and families, i.e., factors related to satisfaction of physiological, psychological and social needs.

Overcrowding

Overcrowding refers to the situation in which more people are living within a single dwelling than there is space for, so that movement is restricted, privacy secluded, hygiene impossible, rest and sleep difficult *(8)*. In general the risks as regards *physical health* are clear enough – infectious diseases spread rapidly under conditions of overcrowding. The effects on psychosocial health are not so clear-cut, viz. irritability, frustration, lack of sleep, anxiety, violence and mental disorders. Children are said to be more affected. In short, it is a psychosocial stress, leading to unhappiness and very probably to psychosomatic and mental disorders.

Overcrowding is a health problem in human dwellings. It may promote the spread of respiratory infections such as tuberculosis, influenza and diphtheria. High morbidity and mortality rates are observed where housing conditions are substandard. The accepted standards with respect to overcrowding are as below :

(1) PERSONS PER ROOM : The degree of overcrowding can best be expressed as the number of persons per room, i.e., number of persons in the household divided by the number of rooms in the dwelling. The accepted standards are :

1 room	.....	2 persons
2 rooms	.....	3 persons
3 rooms	.....	5 persons
4 rooms	.....	7 persons
5 or more rooms	.....	10 persons (additional 2 for each further room)

(2) FLOOR SPACE : The accepted standards are :

110 sq.ft. (11 sq. m.) or more	.....	2 persons
90–100 sq.ft. (9–10 sq. m.)	.....	$1\frac{1}{2}$ persons
70–90 sq.ft. (7–9 sq. m.)	.....	1 person
50–70 sq.ft. (5–7 sq. m.)	.....	$\frac{1}{2}$ person
Under 50 sq.ft (5 sq. m.)	.....	nil

(A baby under 12 months is not counted; children between 1 to 10 years counted as half a unit).

SEX SEPARATION : Overcrowding is considered to exist if 2 persons over 9 years of age, not husband and wife, of opposite sexes are obliged to sleep in the same room.

Indicators of housing

In recent years the use of indicators has become widespread for the measurement of quality of life. The indicators for housing may be classified as :

(1) *Physical* : These are based on floor space, cubic space, room height, persons per room, rooms per dwelling, environmental quality (e.g., air, light, water, noise, sewage disposal, etc).

(2) *Economic indicators* : These are cost of the building, rental levels, taxes, expenditure on housing, etc.

(3) *Social indicators* : The following were proposed at an inter-regional seminar on the Social Aspects of Housing, organized by the UN in 1975.

(a) Indicators related to prevention of illness :
- (1) Frequency of illness due to inadequate sewage and garbage collection.
- (2) Frequency of illness associated with contaminated water source.
- (3) Frequency of insect borne diseases
- (4) Frequency of illness due to overcrowding.
- (5) Frequency of illness due to accidents.
- (6) Frequency of illness due to proximity to animals.
- (7) Access to medical facility.

(b) Indicators related to comfort :
- (1) Thermal comfort
- (2) Acoustic comfort
- (3) Visual comfort
- (4) Spatial comfort.

(c) Indicators related to mental health and social well-being
- (1) Frequency of suicides in the neighbourhood
- (2) Neglected and abandoned youth in the neighbourhood
- (3) Drug abuse (including alcohol) in the neighbourhood.

Public policy

In every country where housing conditions in general are unsatisfactory the need for government intervention has been recognized. The approach to public policy on housing in India is indicated in the Five Year Plans. In 1952, a separate Ministry of Works and Housing was created at the Centre. The Government Housing Programmes consists of two categories – public sector housing and social housing schemes. The former provides mainly for government employees, while the latter attempts to provide assistance particularly to low and middle income groups through various housing schemes. For promoting housing activities, statutory Housing Boards have been established at the state level. Four organizations, viz., The National Buildings Organization (NBO), National Buildings Construction Corporation Ltd., Housing and Urban Development Corporation (HUDCO) and the Hindusthan Housing Factory are functioning under the aegis of the Union Ministry of works and Housing to deal with various aspects of housing.

According to an assessment by NBO, the housing stock in 1961 was estimated to be 14.1 million in urban areas and 65.2 million in rural areas (total 79.3 million). This increased to 93 million in 1971, 116.7 million in 1981 and 148.8 million in 1991 *(6)*. In 2001 census, the total number of houses counted were 249 million *(10)* and according to 2011 census, the total number of houses counted were 330.84 million. This includes 220.7 million houses in rural areas and 110.14 million houses in urban areas *(11)*. Urban housing crisis has manifested itself in many ways of which the most significant is the growth of slums and squatter settlement. It was estimated that about 48.8 million persons were living in slums in 1990. About 40 per cent of this population was in million-plus cities. The overall rate of construction of new houses recommended by the expert body of the UN is 10 houses per 1000 persons per year *(7)*.

The Eighth and subsequent Five Year Plans have strategy for the National Housing Policy consisting of creating an enabling environment for housing activity, viewed as an important component of the national economy, by eliminating various constraints and providing direct assistance to the specially disadvantaged groups including rural and urban poor household, SC/ST, physically handicapped, widows and single women *(6)*.

House site and construction assistance : The scheme was included in the State Sector as a part of Minimum Needs Programme and formed the core of the rural housing programme during Seventh and subsequent Five Year Plans. This scheme has two components – provision of free house sites and construction assistance with varying proportion of subsidy and loan in different states. Construction assistance is planned to benefit 3.5 million families directly as part of MNP. This is exclusive of other special rural housing programmes intended for specific beneficiary groups.

Indira Awas Yojana (IAY) : The Indira Awas Yojana was introduced in the Central Sector in 1985–86 as part of the Rural Landless Employment Guarantee Programme. This type of houses have one room, one kitchen attached with latrine, bathroom and a smokeless chullah *(9)*.

References

1. WHO (1961). *Techn. Rep. Ser.*, No.225.
2. WHO (1965). *Techn. Rep. Ser.*, No.297.
3. WHO (1974). *Techn. Rep. Ser.*, No.544.
4. American Public Health Association (1959). *Am. J. Public Health*, 59, 841.
5. Govt. of India (1949). *Report of the Environmental Hygiene Committee,* Ministry of Health, New Delhi.
6. *Bookhive's 8th Five Year Plan (1992-97)* by E. Chandran, Issues of current interest series No.4.
7. UN (1977). *The Social Impact of Housing,* Report of an Inter-regional Seminar, Department of Economic and Social Affairs, ESA/OCT/SEM/77/2, New York.
8. WHO (1975). *Promoting Health in the human Environment* P–26.
9. *Social Welfare,* Housing Feb. 1987.
10. Govt. of India, *Census of India 2001 series 1*, tables on houses, household amenities and assets, Registrar General and Census Commissioner of India.
11. State of Housing in India, A statistical compendium (2013), Govt. of India, NBO.

DISPOSAL OF WASTES

Disposal of wastes is now largely the domain of sanitarians and public health engineers. However, health professionals need to have a basic knowledge of the subject since improper disposal of wastes constitutes a health hazard. Further the health professional may be called upon to give advice in some special situations, such as camp sanitation or coping with waste disposal problems when there is a disruption or breakdown of community health services in natural disasters. These aspects are considered in this section.

SOLID WASTES

The term "solid wastes" includes garbage (food wastes) rubbish (paper, plastics, wood, metal, throw-away containers, glass), demolition products (bricks, masonry, pipes), sewage treatment residue (sludge and solids from the coarse screening of domestic sewage), dead animals, manure and other discarded material. Strictly speaking it should not contain nightsoil. In India and similar other countries, it is not uncommon to find nightsoil in collection of refuse*(3)*. The output of daily waste depends upon the dietary habits, life styles, living standards and the degree of urbanization and industrialization. The per capita daily solid waste produced ranges between 0.25 to 2.5 kg in different countries.

Solid waste, if allowed to accumulate, is a health hazard because:

a. it decomposes and favours fly breeding
b. it attracts rodents and vermin
c. the pathogens which may be present in the solid waste may be conveyed back to man's food through flies and dust.
d. there is a possibility of water and soil pollution, and
e. heaps of refuse present an unsightly appearance and nuisance from bad odours.

There is a correlation between improper disposal of solid wastes and incidence of vector-borne diseases. Therefore, in all civilized countries, there is an efficient system for its periodic collection, removal and final disposal without risk to health.

Sources of refuse

(1) Refuse that is collected by the street cleansing service or scavenging is called *street refuse.* It consists of leaves, straw, paper, animal droppings and litter of all kinds. (2) Refuse that is collected from markets is called *market refuse.* It contains a large proportion of putrid vegetable and animal matter. (3) Refuse that is collected from stables is called *stable litter.* It contains mainly animal droppings and left-over animal feeds. (4) *Industrial refuse* comprises a wide variety of wastes ranging from completely inert materials such as calcium carbonate to highly toxic and explosive compounds. (5) The *domestic refuse* consists of ash, *rubbish* and *garbage.* Ash is the residue from fire used for cooking and heating. Rubbish comprises paper, clothing, bits of wood, metal, glass, dust and dirt. Garbage is waste matter arising from the preparation, cooking and consumption of food. It consists of waste food, vegetable peelings and other organic matter. *Garbage* needs quick removal and disposal because it ferments on storage.

Storage

The first consideration should be given to the proper storage of refuse, while awaiting collection. The galvanized steel dust bin with close fitting cover is a suitable receptacle for storing refuse. The capacity of a bin will depend upon the number of users and frequency of collection. The output of refuse per capita per day in India is estimated to vary from $^1/_{10}$ to $^1/_{20}$ c.ft. For a family of 5 members, a bin having a capacity of 5/10 or 1/2 c.ft. would be needed. If collection is done once in 3 days, a bin having a capacity of $1^1/_2$ or 2 c.ft. would be adequate. A recent innovation in the western countries is the "paper sack." Refuse is stored in the paper sack, and the sack itself is removed with the contents for disposal and a new sack is substituted. *Public bins :* Public bins cater for a larger number of people. They are usually without cover in India because people do not like to touch them. They are kept on a concrete platform raised 2 to 3 inches above ground level to prevent flood water entering the bins. In bigger municipalities, the bins are handled and emptied mechanically by lorries fitted with cranes.

Collection

The method of collection depends upon the funds available. House-to-house collection is by far the best method of collecting refuse. Only at some places in the urban areas this kind of facility is available. In majority of places in India, there is no house-to-house collection system. People are expected to dump the refuse in the nearest public bin, which is usually not done. Refuse is dispersed all along the street, and some is thrown out in front and around the house. As a result, an army of sweepers is required for sweeping the streets in addition to the gang for collecting the refuse from public bins. The refuse is then transported in refuse collection vehicles to the place of ultimate disposal. Dead animals are directly transported to the place of disposal.

The collection methods normally practised in this country need drastic revision and improvement in the interest of better hygiene. The Environmental Hygiene Committee (1949) recommended that municipalities and other local bodies should arrange for collection of refuse not only from the public bins but also from individual houses *(4)*. A house-to-house collection will result in a simultaneous reduction in the number of public bins *(5)*. The open refuse cart should be abandoned and replaced by enclosed vans. Mechanical transport should be used wherever possible as it is more practical and economical than the 19th century methods. There is a wide variety of refuse collection vehicles of all shapes and sizes. The latest arrival in the western countries is the "Dustless Refuse Collector" which has a totally enclosed body.

Methods of disposal

There is no single method of refuse disposal which is equally suitable in all circumstances. The choice of a particular method is governed by local factors such as cost and availability of land and labour. The principal methods of refuse disposal are :–

(a) Dumping
(b) Controlled tipping or sanitary land-fill
(c) Incineration
(d) Composting
(e) Manure pits
(f) Burial.

(a) Dumping

Refuse is dumped in low lying areas partly as a method of reclamation of land but mainly as an easy method of disposal of dry refuse. As a result of bacterial action, refuse decreases considerably in volume and is converted gradually into humus. Kolkata disposes of its refuse by dumping and the reclaimed land is leased out for cultivation. The drawbacks of open dumping are : (1) the refuse is exposed to flies and rodents, (2) it is a source of nuisance from the smell and unsightly appearance, (3) the loose refuse is dispersed by the action of the wind, and (4) drainage from dumps contributes to the pollution of surface and ground water. A WHO Expert Committee (1967) condemned dumping as "a most insanitary method that creates public health hazards, a nuisance, and severe pollution of the environment". Dumping should be outlawed and replaced by sound procedures *(6)*.

(b) Controlled tipping

Controlled tipping or sanitary landfill is the most satisfactory method of refuse disposal where suitable land is available. It differs from ordinary dumping in that the material is placed in a trench or other prepared area, adequately compacted, and covered with earth at the end of the working day. The term "modified sanitary landfill" has been applied to those operations where compaction and covering are accomplished once or twice a week *(7)*.

Three methods are used in this operation : the trench method, the ramp method and the area method *(7, 8)*.

(1) *The trench method :* Where level ground is available, the trench method is usually chosen. A long trench is dug out – 2 to 3 m (6–10 ft.) deep and 4 to 12 m, (12–36 ft.) wide, depending upon local conditions. The refuse is compacted and covered with excavated earth. Where compacted refuse is placed in the fill to a depth of 2 m (6 ft.), it is estimated that one acre of land per year will be required for 10,000 population *(7)*.

(2) *The ramp method :* This method is well suited where the terrain is moderately sloping. Some excavation is done to secure the covering material.

(3) *The area method :* This method is used for filling land depressions, disused quarries and clay pits. The refuse is deposited, packed and consolidated in uniform layers up to 2 to 2.5 m (6–8 ft.) deep. Each layer is sealed on its exposed surface with a mud cover at least 30 cm (12 inches) thick. Such sealing prevents infestation by flies and rodents and suppresses the nuisance of smell and dust. This method often has the disadvantage of requiring supplemental earth from outside sources.

Chemical, bacteriological and physical changes occur in buried refuse. The temperature rises to over 60 deg. C within 7 days and kills all the pathogens and hastens the decomposition process. Then it takes 2 to 3 weeks to cool down. Normally it takes 4 to 6 months for complete decomposition of organic matter into an innocuous mass. The tipping of refuse in water should not be done as it creates a nuisance from odours given off by the decomposition of organic matter. The method of controlled tipping has been revolutionized by mechanization. The bulldozer achieves the tasks of spreading trimming and spreading top soil.

(c) Incineration

Refuse can be disposed of hygienically by burning or

incineration. It is the method of choice where suitable land is not available. Hospital refuse which is particularly dangerous is best disposed of by incineration. Incineration is practised in several of the industrialized countries, particularly in large cities due to lack of suitable land. Incineration is not a popular method in India because the refuse contains a fair proportion of fine ash which makes the burning difficult. A preliminary separation of dust or ash is needed. All this involves heavy outlay and expenditure, besides manipulative difficulties in the incinerator. Further, disposal of refuse by burning is a loss to the community in terms of the much needed manure. Burning, therefore, has a limited application in refuse disposal in India.

(d) Composting

Composting is a method of combined disposal of refuse and nightsoil or sludge. It is a process of nature whereby organic matter breaks down under bacterial action resulting in the formation of relatively stable humus-like material, called the compost which has considerable manurial value for the soil. The principal by-products are carbon dioxide, water and heat. The heat produced during composting, about 60 deg C or higher, over a period of several days, destroys eggs and larvae of flies, weed seeds and pathogenic agents. The end product, or compost, contains few or no disease producing organisms, and is a good soil builder containing small amounts of the major plant nutrients such as nitrates and phosphates *(9)*. The following methods of composting are now used :

(1) Bangalore method (Anaerobic method)

(2) Mechanical composting (Aerobic method)

(1) BANGALORE METHOD *(Hot fermentation process)*

As a result of investigations carried out under the auspices of the Indian Council of Agricultural Research at the Indian Institute of Science, Bangalore, a system of anaerobic composting, known as *Bangalore method* (hot fermentation process) has been developed. It has been recommended as a satisfactory method of disposal of town wastes and nightsoil *(10)*.

Trenches are dug 90 cm (3 ft.) deep, 1.5 to 2.5 m (5–8 ft.) broad and 4.5 to 10 m (15–30 ft.) long, depending upon the amount of refuse and nightsoil to be disposed of. Depths greater than 90 cm (3 ft.) are not recommended because of slow decomposition. The pits should be located not less than 800 m (1/2 mile) from city limits. The composting procedure is as follows : First a layer of refuse about 15 cm (6 in) thick is spread at the bottom of the trench. Over this, nightsoil is added corresponding to a thickness of 5 cm (2 in). Then alternate layers of refuse and nightsoil are added in the proportion of 15 cm (6 in) and 5 cm (2 in) respectively, till the heap rises to 30 cm (1 ft.) above the ground level. The top layer should be of refuse, at least 25 cm (9 in) thickness. Then the heap is covered with excavated earth. If properly laid, a man's legs will not sink when walking over the compost mass *(10)*.

Within 7 days as a result of bacterial action considerable heat (over 60 deg C) is generated in the compost mass. This intense heat which persists over 2 or 3 weeks, serves to decompose the refuse and nightsoil and to destroy all pathogenic and parasitic organisms. At the end of 4 to 6 months, decomposition is complete and the resulting manure is a well decomposed, odourless, innocuous material of high manurial value ready for application to the land. The Environmental Hygiene Committee (1949) did not recommend composting by municipalities with a population of over 100,000 *(4)*. Bigger municipalities should install underground sewers to transport human excreta.

(2) MECHANICAL COMPOSTING

Another method of composting known as 'Mechanical composting' is becoming popular. In this, compost is literally manufactured on a large scale by processing raw materials and turning out a finished product. The refuse is first cleared of salvageable materials such as rags, bones, metal, glass and items which are likely to interfere with the grinding operation. It is then pulverised in a pulverising equipment in order to reduce the size of articles to less than 2 inches. The pulverised refuse is then mixed with sewage, sludge or nightsoil in a rotating machine and incubated. The factors which are controlled in the operation are a certain carbon-nitrogen ratio, temperature, moisture, pH and aeration. The entire process of composting is complete in 4 to 6 weeks. This method of composting is in vogue in some of the developed countries, e.g., Holland, Germany, Switzerland, Israel. The Government of India is considering the installation of mechanical composting plants in selected cities. Cities such as Delhi, Nagpur, Mumbai, Chennai, Pune, Allahabad, Hyderabad, Lucknow and Kanpur have offered to join the Government for setting up pilot plants for mechanical composting *(3)*.

(e) Manure pits

In rural areas in India, there is no system for collection and disposal of refuse. Refuse is thrown around the houses indiscriminately resulting in gross pollution of the soil. The problem of refuse disposal in rural areas can be solved by digging 'manure pits' by the individual householders. The garbage, cattle dung, straw, and leaves should be dumped into the manure pits and covered with earth after each day's dumping. Two such pits will be needed, when one is closed, the other will be in use. In 5 to 6 month's time, the refuse is converted into manure which can be returned to the field. This method of refuse disposal is effective and relatively simple in rural communities.

(f) Burial

This method is suitable for small camps. A trench 1.5 m wide and 2 m deep is excavated, and at the end of each day the refuse is covered with 20 to 30 cm of earth. When the level in the trench is 40 cm from ground level, the trench is filled with earth and compacted, and a new trench is dug out. The contents may be taken out after 4 to 6 months and used on the fields. If the trench is 1 m in length for every 200 persons, it will be filled in about one week *(8)*.

Public education

Refuse disposal cannot be solved without public education. People have very little interest in cleanliness outside their homes. Many municipalities and corporations usually look for the cheapest solution, especially in regard to refuse disposal. What is needed is public education on these matters, by all known methods of health education, viz., pamphlets, newspapers, broadcasting, films etc. Police enforcement of the laws may also be needed at times.

Economics and finance

If refuse disposal is to be carried out efficiently, hygienically and economically, heavy capital outlay will be needed whatever system of disposal is adopted. In the highly industrialized countries up to 20 per cent of municipal budgets are spent on the collection and disposal of solid wastes, and even more will be required if the job is to be done adequately *(6)*.

International cooperation

An organization was formed – the International Solid Wastes and Public Cleansing Association (ISWA) in 1970, to assist countries in the general endeavour to improve sanitary services. A WHO International Reference Centre has also been set up in Switzerland to collect, evaluate and disseminate information on wastes-disposal practices and to foster research *(9)*.

References

1. WHO (1971). *Techn. Rep. Ser.*, No.484.
2. National Environmental Engineering Research Institute, Nagpur (1971). *Technical Digest* No.15, March 1971.
3. Bopardikar M.V. (1967). *Environmental Health*, 9, 349.
4. Govt. of India (1949). *Report of the Environmental Hygiene Committee,* Ministry of Health, New Delhi.
5. Kawata, K. (1963). *Environmental Sanitation in India,* Christian Medical College, Ludhiana Punjab.
6. WHO (1967). *Techn. Rep. Ser.*, No. 367.
7. Ehlers, V.M. et al (1965). *Municipal and Rural Sanitation* Mc Graw-Hill.
8. Assar, M. (1971). *Guide to Sanitation in Natural Disorders,* WHO, Geneva.
9. WHO (1969). *Problems in Community Wastes Management,* Public Health Papers NO.38.
10. Acharya, C.N. (1950). *Preparation of Compost Manure from Town Wastes* the ICAR Monograph, Delhi.

EXCRETA DISPOSAL

Public health importance

Human excreta is a source of infection. It is an important cause of environmental pollution. Every society has a responsibility for its safe removal and disposal so that it does not constitute a threat to public health. The HEALTH HAZARDS of improper excreta disposal are : (1) soil pollution, (2) water pollution, (3) contamination of foods, and (4) propagation of flies. The resulting diseases are typhoid and paratyphoid fever, dysenteries, diarrhoeas, cholera, hookworm disease, ascariasis, viral hepatitis and similar other intestinal infections and parasitic infestations. These diseases are not only a burden on the community in terms of sickness, mortality and a low expectation of life, but a basic deterrent to social and economic progress. Proper disposal of human excreta, therefore, is a fundamental environmental health service without which there cannot be any improvement in the state of community health.

How disease is carried from excreta

Let us consider how the faecal-borne diseases are transmitted to a new host. The human excreta of a sick person or a carrier of disease is the main focus of infection. It contains the disease agent which is transmitted to a new host through various channels : (1) water, (2) fingers, (3) flies, (4) soil and (5) food. These events are as shown in Fig. 1.

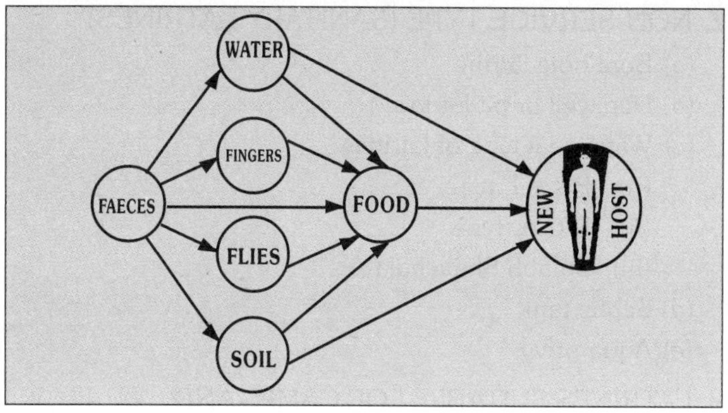

FIG. 1
Transmission of faecal-borne diseases *(1)*

Sanitation barrier

Community medicine aims at breaking the disease cycle at vulnerable points. The disease cycle (Fig. 1) may be broken at various levels : segregation of faeces, protection of water supplies, protection of foods, personal hygiene and control of flies. Of these, the most effective step would be to segregate the faeces and arrange for its proper disposal so that the disease agent cannot reach the new host, directly or indirectly. Fig. 2 shows the segregation of the excreta by imposing a barrier called the "sanitation barrier". In simple terms, this barrier can be provided by a 'sanitary latrine' and a disposal pit. The more elaborate schemes envisage installation of a sewerage system and sewage treatment plants.

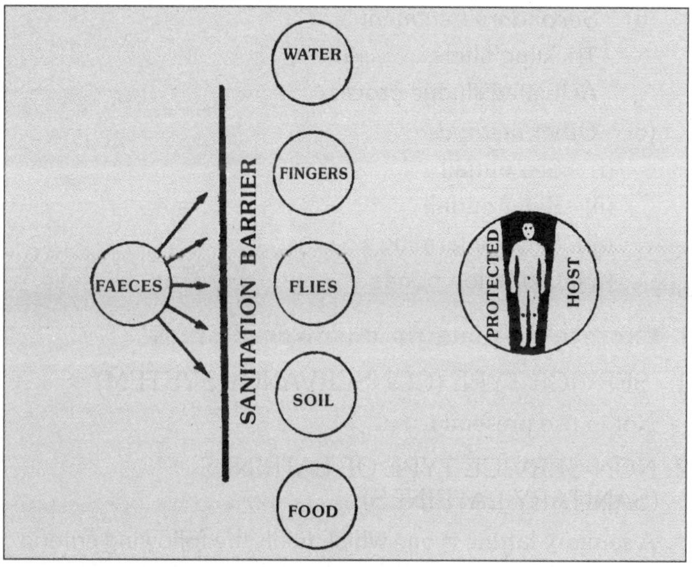

FIG. 2
Sanitation barrier to transmission of faecal-borne diseases *(1)*

Methods of excreta disposal

There are a number of methods of excreta disposal. Some are applicable to unsewered areas, and some to sewered areas. A classification and description of the various methods of excreta disposal is given below :

I. Unsewered areas

1. SERVICE TYPE LATRINES (CONSERVANCY SYSTEM)

Nightsoil is collected from pail or bucket type of latrines by human agency, and later disposed off by burying or composting.

2. NON-SERVICE TYPE (SANITARY LATRINES)
   (a) Bore hole latrine
   (b) Dug well or pit latrine
   (c) Water-seal type of latrines
      (i) P.R.A.I. type
      (ii) R.C.A. type
      (iii) Sulabh Shauchalaya.
   (d) Septic tank
   (e) Aqua privy.

3. LATRINES SUITABLE FOR CAMPS AND TEMPORARY USE
   (a) Shallow trench latrine
   (b) Deep trench latrine
   (c) Pit latrine
   (d) Bore hole latrine

II. Sewered areas

1. WATER-CARRIAGE SYSTEM AND SEWAGE TREATMENT
   (a) *Primary treatment*
      Screening
      Removal of grit
      Plain sedimentation
   (b) *Secondary treatment*
      Trickling filters
      Activated sludge process
   (c) *Other methods*
      (i) Sea outfall
      (ii) River outfall
      (iii) Sewage farming
      (iv) Oxidation ponds

I. Excreta disposal in unsewered areas

1. SERVICE TYPE (CONSERVANCY SYSTEM)

Not in use presently.

2. NON-SERVICE TYPE OF LATRINES (SANITARY LATRINES)

A sanitary latrine is one which fulfils the following criteria :

(1) Excreta should not contaminate the ground or surface water
(2) Excreta should not pollute the soil
(3) Excreta should not be accessible to flies, rodents, animals (pigs, dogs, cattle, etc.) and other vehicles of transmission.
(4) Excreta should not create a nuisance due to odour or unsightly appearance.

A brief description of some of the well-known types of sanitary latrines is given below :

WATER SEAL LATRINE

A further improvement in the designing of sanitary latrines for rural families is the hand-flushed "water seal" type of latrine (Fig. 3). Here, the squatting plate is fitted with a *water seal.* The water seal performs two important functions : (1) it prevents access by flies. That is, the nightsoil is sealed off from flies, by a small depth of water contained in a bent pipe called the trap, (2) it prevents escape of odours and foul gases and thereby eliminates the nuisance from smell. Once the latrine is flushed, nightsoil is no longer visible. These merits have rendered the water seal type of latrine more acceptable to rural people than the bore hole or pit privy without water seal. Several designs of water seal latrines have been tested in the field, and two types have gained recognition for wide use. These are : (1) the P.R.A.I. type, evolved by the Planning, Research and Action Institute, Lucknow (Uttar Pradesh) and (2) the RCA type, designed by the Research cum Action Projects in Environmental Sanitation of the Ministry of Health, Government of India. Of these two types, the RCA latrine has been accepted as a suitable design for wide adoption in different parts of the country *(2).* A brief description of the RCA latrine is given below :

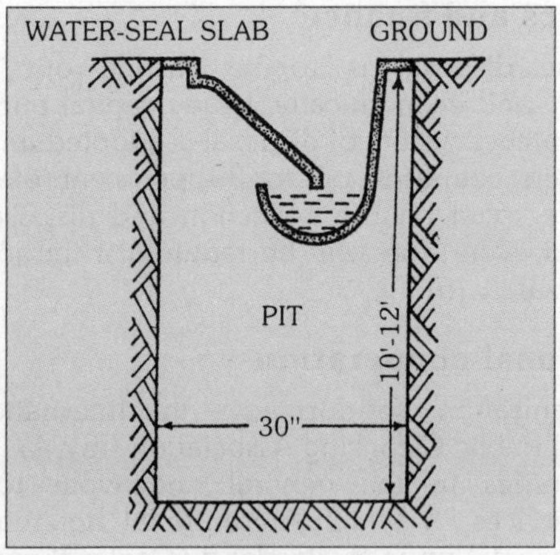

FIG. 3
Water seal latrine (direct type)

The parts of a water-seal latrine, whether RCA type or PRAI type, are essentially the same (Fig. 3 & 7). The differences are in matters of minor engineering detail. The *essential features* of a RCA latrine and its installation are described below :

RCA LATRINE

(1) LOCATION

The safe distance between the latrine and a source of water supply will depend upon the porosity of the soil, level of ground water, its slope and direction of flow. In general, it may be stated, that latrines of any kind should not be located within 15 m (50 ft) from a source of water supply, and should be at a lower elevation to prevent the possibility of bacterial contamination of the water supply. Where possible, latrines should not be located in areas usually subject to flooding.

(2) SQUATTING PLATE

The squatting plate or slab (Fig. 4) is an important part of a latrine. It should be made of an impervious material so that it can be washed and kept clean and dry. If kept dry, it will not facilitate the survival of hookworm larvae. In recommending squatting plates, due consideration should be paid to the habits of Indian people who defecate in the squatting position and use water for anal washing. The slab of the RCA latrine has been designed to meet the above needs. It is made of cement concrete with minimum dimensions of 90 cm (3 ft) square and 5 cm (2 in.) thickness at the outer edge. There is a slope 1/2 inch towards the pan. This allows drainage into the latrine of the water used for ablution or cleansing purposes. A circular squatting plate of 90 cm (3 ft.) diameter and of 5 cm (2 in.) uniform thickness, has also been found satisfactory. For the convenience of the users, raised footrests are included in the squatting plate.

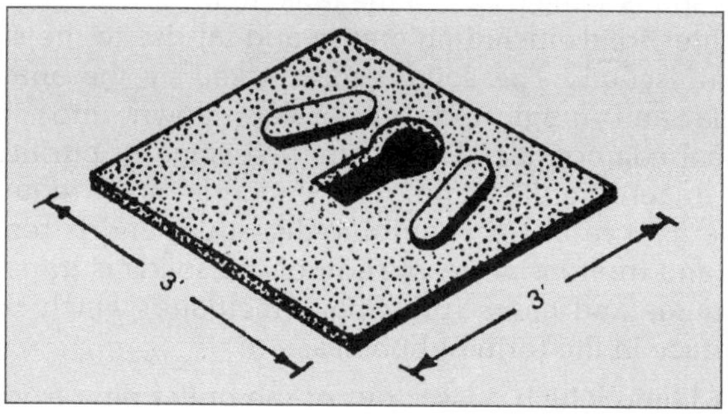

FIG. 4

Squatting plate

(3) PAN

The pan (Fig. 5) receives the nightsoil, urine and wash water. The length of the pan is 42.5 cm (17 in.). The width of the front portion of the pan has a minimum of 12.5 cm (5 in.) and the width at its widest portion is 20 cm (8 in.). There is a uniform slope from front to back of the pan. The pan is given a smooth finish.

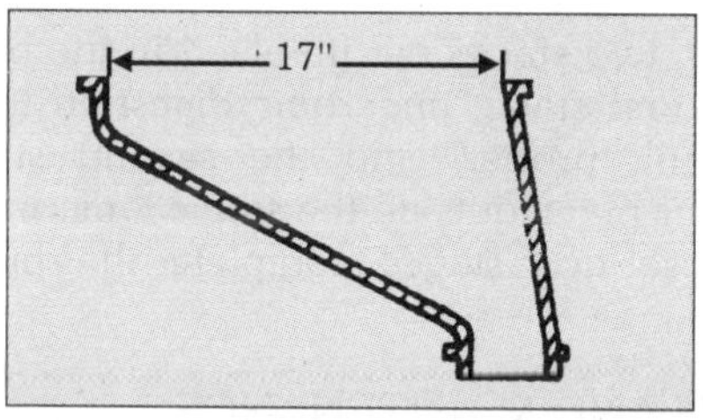

FIG.5

Latrine pan

(4) TRAP

The trap (Fig. 6) is a bent pipe, about 7.5 cm (3 in.) in diameter and is connected with the pan. It holds water and provides the necessary 'water seal'. The water seal is the distance between the level of water in the trap and the lowest point in the concave upper surface of the trap. The depth of the water seal (AB) in the RCA latrine is 2 cm (3/4 in.) (Fig. 6). The water seal prevents the access by flies and suppresses the nuisance from smell.

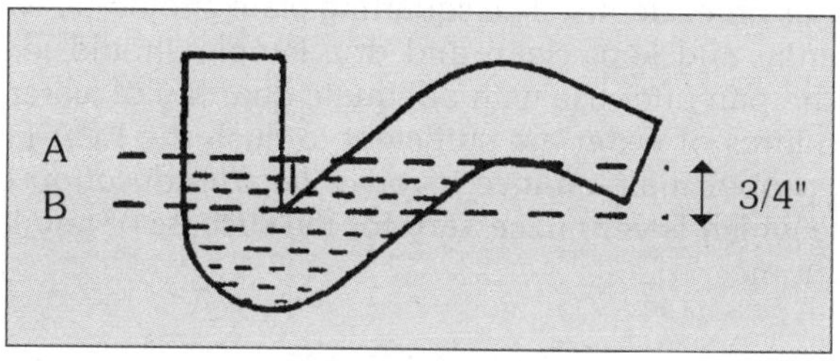

FIG. 6

Trap

(5) CONNECTING PIPE

When the pit is dug, away from the squat plate, the trap is connected to the pit by a short length of connecting pipe 7.5 cm (3 in.) in diameter and at least 1 m (3 ft.) in length with a bend at the end (Fig. 7).

A latrine of this type is called the Indirect type because the pit is sited away from the squatting plate. In the direct type there is no need for a connecting pipe (Fig. 3). The direct type is best suited for areas where the ground is hard and does not easily cave in. The direct type is cheaper and easier to construct and occupies less space *(2)*. An advantage with the indirect type is that when the pit fills up, a second pit can be put into operation by merely changing the direction of the connecting pipe. Therefore, the indirect type is usually preferred.

(6) DUG WELL

The dug well or pit is usually 75 cm (30 in.) in diameter, and 3 to 3.5 m (10–12 ft.) deep and is covered. In loose soil and where the water table is high a lining of earthenware rings or bamboo matting can be used to prevent caving in of the pit *(2)*. When the pit fills up, a second pit is dug nearby and the direction of the connecting pipe is changed into the second pit. When the second pit fills up, the first one may be emptied and reused.

(7) SUPERSTRUCTURE

The desired type of superstructure may be provided for privacy and shelter. An attractive superstructure with a neat finish is desirable as this will be generally well maintained.

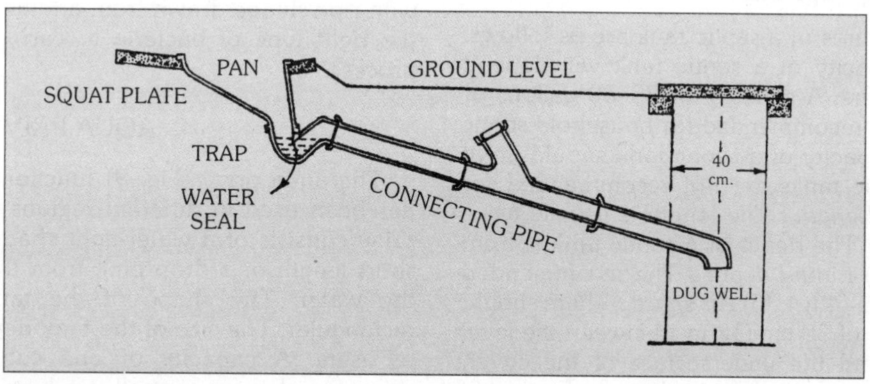

FIG. 7

RCA Latrine (Indirect type)

(8) MAINTENANCE

The life of a latrine will depend upon several factors such as care in usage and maintenance. The latrine should be used only for the purpose intended and not for disposal of refuse or other debris. The squatting plate should be washed frequently and kept clean and dry. People should learn to flush the pan after use with adequate quantity of water. One to two litres of water are sufficient to flush the RCA latrine. Thus, proper maintenance involves *health education* of the people which is very necessary for the success of any latrine programme.

SEPTIC TANK

The septic tank (Fig. 8) is water-tight masonry tank into which household sewage is admitted for treatment. It is a satisfactory means of disposing excreta and liquid wastes from individual dwellings, small groups of houses and institutions which have adequate water supplies but do not have access to a public sewerage system.

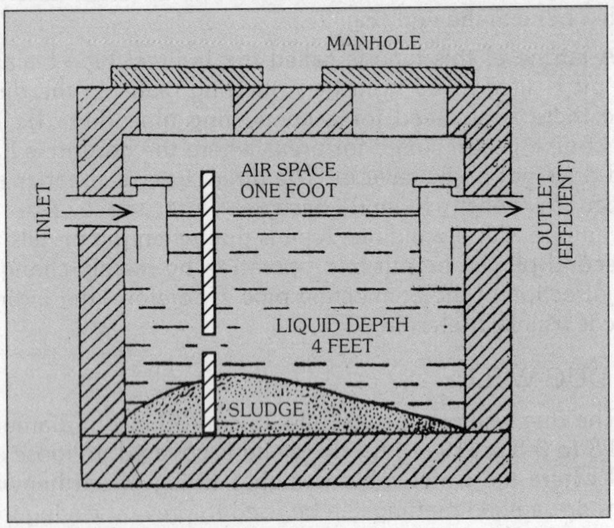

FIG. 8
Septic tank

DESIGN FEATURES

There are various designs in septic tanks. Some are double chambered and some single chambered. A single chambered septic tank has been found satisfactory for small installations. Tanks with more than two compartments are expensive and have shown little advantage over the two or multiple chambered septic tank *(3)*.

The main design features of a septic tank are as follows. (1) *Capacity* : The capacity of a septic tank will depend upon the number of users. A capacity of 20–30 gallons or $2^1/_2$–5 c.ft. per person is recommended for household septic tanks. The minimum capacity of a septic tank should be at least 500 gallons. Septic tanks are not recommended for large communities. (2) *Length* : The length is usually twice the breadth. (3) *Depth* : The depth of a septic tank is from 1.5 to 2 m (5–7 ft.). (4) *Liquid depth* : The recommended liquid depth is only 1.2 m (4 ft.). (5) *Air space* : There should be a minimum air space of 30 cm (12 in.) between the level of liquid in the tank and the undersurface of the cover. (6) *Bottom* : In some septic tanks, the bottom is sloping towards the inlet end. This facilitates retention of solids. (7) *Inlet and outlet* : There is an inlet and outlet pipe, which are submerged. (8) *Cover* : The septic tank is covered by a concrete slab of suitable thickness and provided with a manhole. (9) *Retention Period* : Septic tanks are designed in this country to allow a retention period of 24 hours. Too long a retention period will result in undue septicity of the effluent whereas too short a period gives insufficient treatment.

WORKING OF A SEPTIC TANK

The solids settle down in the tank, to form "sludge", while the lighter solids including grease and fat rise to the surface to form "scum". The solids are attacked by the anaerobic bacteria and fungi and are broken down into simpler chemical compounds. This is the first stage of purification, called anaerobic digestion. The sludge is much reduced in volume as a result of anaerobic digestion, and is rendered stable and inoffensive. A portion of the solids is transferred into liquids and gases (principally methane) which rises to the surface in the form of bubbles.

The liquid which passes out of the outlet pipe from time to time is called the "effluent". It contains numerous bacteriae, cysts, helminthic ova and organic matter in solution or fine suspension. The effluent is allowed to percolate into the sub-soil. It is dispersed by means of perforated or open-jointed pipes laid in trenches 90 cm (3 ft.) deep and the trenches are then covered with soil. The effluent percolates into the surrounding soil. There are millions of aerobic bacteria in the upper layers of the soil, which attack the organic matter present in the effluent. As a result, the organic matter is oxidized into stable end-products, i.e., nitrates, carbon dioxide and water. This stage of purification is called *aerobic oxidation*.

To sum up, two stages are involved in the purification of sewage. The first stage, *anaerobic digestion* takes place in the septic tank proper, and the second stage, aerobic oxidation takes place outside the septic tank, in the sub-soil. Together, these two stages complete the purification of sewage.

OPERATION AND MAINTENANCE

(1) The use of soap water and disinfectants such as phenol should be avoided as they are injurious to the bacterial flora in the septic tank. (2) Undue accumulation of sludge reduces the capacity of the septic tank and interferes with proper working. Therefore, the contents of the septic tank should be bailed out at least once a year. This operation is called "desludging". The bailed out sludge is disposed of by trenching. (3) Newly built septic tanks are first filled with water up to the outlet level and then seeded with ripe sludge drawn from another septic tank, to provide the right type of bacteria to carry out the decomposition process.

AQUA PRIVY

The aqua privy (Fig. 9) functions like a septic tank and has been used in different regions in the country *(2)*. The privy consists of a water-tight chamber filled with water. A short length of a drop pipe from the latrine floor dips into the water. The shape of the tank may be circular or rectangular. The size of the tank depends upon the number of users. A capacity of one cubic metre (35 cu.ft.) is recommended for a small family, allowing 6 years or more for cleansing purposes. Aqua privies are designed for public use also.

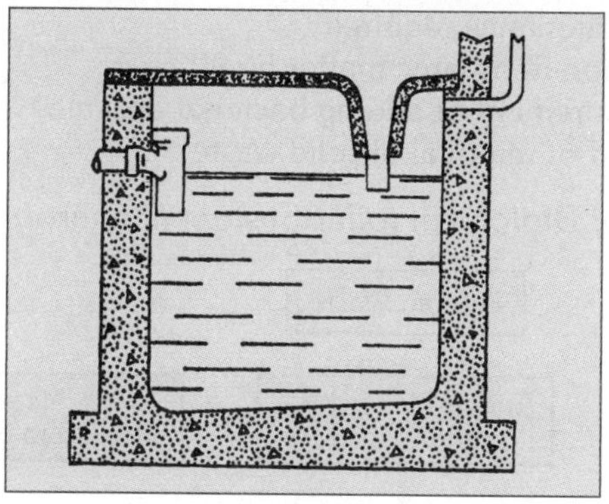

FIG. 9
Aqua privy

Night soil undergoes purification by anaerobic digestion. Since there is evolution of gases, a vent should be provided for the escape of gases into the atmosphere, the vent should be open above the roof of dwellings. The effluent is far from innocuous. It contains finely divided faecal matter in suspension and may carry parasitic and infective agents. It should be treated in the same manner as the effluent from a septic tank by sub-soil irrigation or absorption. The digested sludge which accumulates in the tank should be removed at intervals.

SULABH SHAUCHALAYA

The "Sulabh Shauchalaya" model, the invention of a Patna-based firm, is a low cost pour-flush, water-seal type of latrine, which is now being used in many parts of India. Basically it is an improved version of the standard handflush latrine (e.g., RCA type). It consists of a specially designed pan and a water-seal trap. It is connected to a pit 3 feet square and as deep. Excreta undergoes bacterial decomposition and is converted to manure (compost). The method requires very little water.

Sulabh International, the investors, not only build but also maintain the system of Sulabh **Community Latrines**. Their usual structure is a lavatory block of several dozen seats, with a bathing block adjoining. The system is to charge Rs. 5 per user. Delhi has opted for this system in all its slums. This system has drawn praise from ecologists and planners.

CHEMICAL CLOSET

It has very limited use under Indian conditions. The closet consists of a metal tank containing a disinfectant fluid. The active ingredients of the fluid are formaldehyde and quaternary ammonium compounds. In addition, a harmless water dye and a deodorizing substance are usually incorporated *(4)*. A seat with a cover is placed directly over the tank. Nothing except the toilet paper should be thrown into the chemical closet.

WATER CARRIAGE SYSTEM

The water carriage system or sewerage system implies collecting and transporting of human excreta and waste water from residential, commercial and industrial areas, by a network of underground pipes, called *sewers* to the place of ultimate disposal. It is the method of choice for collecting and transporting sewage from cities and towns where population density is high. There are two types in water carriage system – the combined sewer system and the separate sewer system. In the *combined* system, the sewers carry both the sewage and surface water. In the separate system, surface water is not admitted into sewers. The *separate system* is considered the system of choice today. Although the first sewers were laid in 1867 in Calcutta, the Mudaliar Committee (1962) reported that not more than 15 per cent of the urban population in India had the amenity of a sewerage system. The problem is one of economics – a heavy outlay of capital is needed to install a water-carriage system. Since water is needed for flushing the toilets and for conveying the human wastes, there can be no sewerage system without a piped water supply.

A water carriage system consists of the following elements.

1. Household sanitary fittings (plumbing system of buildings)
2. House sewers
3. Street sewers or trunk sewers
4. Sewer appurtenances : manholes, traps, etc.

1. Household sanitary fittings

Where sewers exist, every house is expected to be connected to the nearest sewer. The usual household sanitary fittings are : (i) water closet, (ii) urinal and (iii) wash basin.

WATER CLOSETS may be broadly divided into two types : Indian squatting type (Fig. 4) and the Western commode type. An ideal water closet bowl (western type) is shown in Fig. 10. It is recommended that for efficient performance : (a) the water seal area should not be more than 7.5 cm *(5)*. (b) there should not be any sharp corners in the trap design. (c) the volume of water in trap should be as little as possible, preferably not exceeding 1.75 litres to maintain a minimum of 50 mm deep water seal, and (d) the interior of the bowl should be vertical at least 50 to 75 mm just above the surface of water seal *(6)*. The water closets are provided with a 'flushing rim'. Human excreta is directly received into the water in the closet without soiling the sides. The flushing removes all traces of excreta from the sides and keeps the closet clean. The closet is connected to a small cistern by a pipe 2.5 to 3.75 cm (1–1.5 in.) in diameter. The flushing cistern normally holds 15 litres (3 gallons) of water and works by syphonic action. The flushing cisterns can be classified as high level, low level and integrated depending upon the height of location above the water closet bowl or pan. The Indian squatting type W.C. pans are used with a high level flushing cisterns.

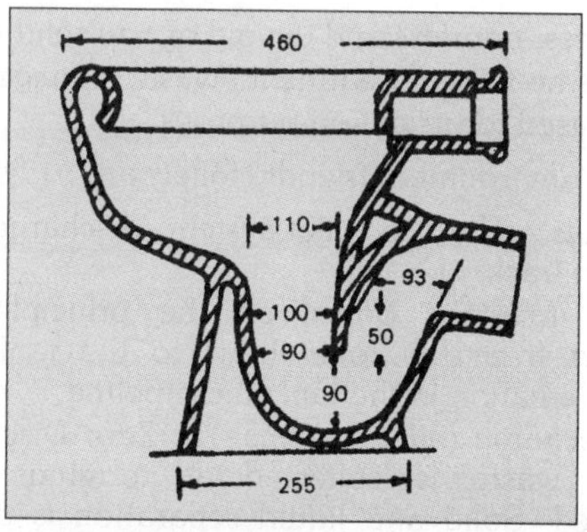

FIG. 10
An ideal water closet (western type)

2. House drain

The house drain is usually 10 cm (4 in.) in diameter and is laid in the courtyard about 15 cm (6 in.) below the ground level on a bed of cement concrete with sufficient gradient towards the main drain. The house drain empties the sewage into the main sewer or public drain.

3. Public sewer

The trunk sewers are not less than 22.5 cm (9 in.) in diameter; bigger ones may be 2 to 3 m (8–10 ft.) in diameter. They are laid on a bed of cement concrete, about 3 m (10 ft.) below the ground level, with sufficient gradient to ensure what is known as "self-cleansing" velocity; this varies from 2 to 3 feet per second. The trunk sewers collect sewage from several houses and transport to the main outfall or place of final disposal.

4. Sewer appurtenances

These are (a) manholes and (b) traps which are installed in the sewerage system. MANHOLES are openings built into the sewerage system. They are placed (a) whenever there is a change in the direction of sewers, (b) at the meeting point of two or more sewers, and (c) at distances of 100 metres in long straight runs. These openings permit a man to enter the sewer for inspection, repairs and cleaning. Workers entering the manholes are liable to gas poisoning and asphyxiation. Due precautions should be taken to ensure their safety. TRAPS are of various kinds, these are devices designed to prevent foul gases entering the houses and to remove sand, grit and grease from sewage. Traps are placed in three situations : (a) under the basin of water closets, (b) where the house drain joins the public drain (intercepting trap), and (c) where surface waste water enters the drains.

The installation of a sewerage system is a huge engineering problem. It involves considerable planning, designing, construction, operation, maintenance and administration – each calling for specialized skills. Sewer systems are designed, like water supplies, for service for one generation (30 years).

Environment Friendly Bio-Toilet *(7)*

A Bio-Toilet is a complete waste management solution which reduces solid human waste to Bio-gas and water, with the help of a bacterial Inoculum. Biological decomposition of Human waste is done in bio-digester tanks with the help of anaerobic bacteria which is developed at bacteria generation plant at Motibagh Workshop SECRLy, Nagpur & DRDE/Gwalior. Bio-Toilet is an innovative technology for disposal of solid human waste in an eco-friendly, economical and hygienic manner.

The residual water from Bio-Toilet

- Is colorless, odorless and devoid of any solid particles.
- Requires no further treatment / waste management.
- Can be used for irrigation purposes.

Types of Environment friendly toilets are :

- *Bio toilets* - The Bio toilet system, discharge processed waste on track
- *Vacuum toilets* - Based on the principle of direct transport from the toilet bowl to the tank aided by vacuum creation in the tank and pipeline.
- *Zero discharge toilet systems* - In Zero Discharge toilet system, waste is collected at terminus and then processed. Solid and liquid separation is done in the tank itself and liquid is recycled as flush water.

Advantage of IR-DRDO Bio-Digester over Conventional Toilet system:-

- No bad smell in toilets from the tanks
- No infestation of Cockroaches & flies
- Fecal matter in the tank not visible
- No clogging of digester
- Effluent is free from off odour and solid waste
- No maintenance required
- Reduction in organic matter by 90%
- No requirement of adding bacteria/ enzyme
- No need of removal of solid waste

Working of Biological toilet System (Anaerobic)

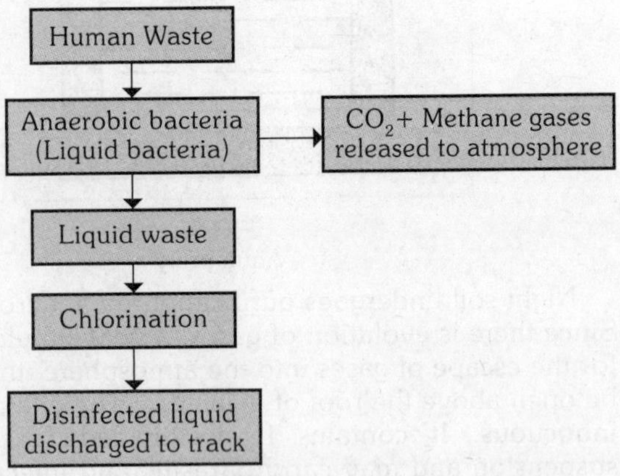

Note: System does not require oxygen and also does not require regular cleaning

Source : *(7)*

Sewage

What is sewage ?

Sewage is waste water from a community, containing solid and liquid excreta, derived from houses, street and yard washings, factories and industries. It resembles dirty water with an unpleasant smell. The term "sullage" is applied to waste water which does not contain human excreta, e.g., waste water from kitchens and bathrooms. The amount of sewage that flows in the sewers depends upon : (a) *Habits of the people :* If people use more water, there will be more sewage. (b) *Time of day :* Sewage does not flow uniformly throughout the day. It is subject to variations depending upon the time of day and during different seasons. In the morning, when people tend to use more water there is greater quantity and flow; in mid-day the flow is less, and again there is a slight increase in the evening. The average amount of sewage which flows through the sewerage system in 24 hours is called the "dry weather flow."

Health aspects

Unless prompt measures are taken to provide proper means of sewage disposal, the following environmental problems may be created :

a. creation of nuisance, unsightliness and unpleasant odours.
b. breeding of flies and mosquitoes
c. pollution of soil and water supplies
d. contamination of food, and
e. increase in the incidence of disease, especially enteric and helminthic diseases.

Composition of sewage

Sewage contains 99.9 per cent of water. The solids which comprise barely 0.1 per cent are partly organic and partly inorganic; they are partly in suspension and partly in solution. The offensive nature of the sewage is mainly due to the organic matter which it contains. The organic matter decomposes according to the laws of nature during which process it gives off offensive odours. In addition, sewage is charged with numerous living organisms derived from faeces, some of which may be agents to disease. It is estimated that one gram of faeces may contain about 1,000 million of *E. coli,* 10 to 100 million of faecal streptococci, and 1 to 10 million spores of *C. perfringens* besides several others. The average adult person excretes daily some 100 grams of faeces.

Aim of sewage purification

Raw sewage or inadequately treated sewage should not be discharged into rivers, sea or other sources of water supply. This is because, the oxygen in the water supply is used up by the numerous aerobic bacteria found in the sewage. Depletion of oxygen may lead to the death of the plant and animal life in water. Furthermore, the water may yield an offensive smell because of the release of hydrogen sulphide.

The aim of sewage treatment is to "stabilize" the organic matter so that it can be disposed off safely; and, to convert the sewage water into an effluent of an acceptable standard of purity which can be disposed off in to land, rivers or sea. A standard test which is an indicator of the organic content of the sewage is biochemical oxygen demand (BOD).

The "strength" of the sewage is expressed in terms of (a) BIOCHEMICAL OXYGEN DEMAND (BOD) : It is the most important test done on sewage. It is defined as the amount of oxygen absorbed by a sample of sewage during a specified period, generally 5 days, at a specified temperature, generally 20 deg.C for the aerobic destruction or use of organic matter by living organisms *(8)*. BOD values range from about 1 mg per litre for natural waters to about 300 mg per litre for untreated domestic sewage. If the BOD is 300 mg/L and above, sewage is said to be "strong"; if it is 100 mg/L, it is said to be "weak" (b) CHEMICAL OXYGEN DEMAND (COD) : The COD test measures the oxygen equivalent of that portion of the organic matter in a sample which is susceptible to oxidation by a strong chemical oxidiser. If wastes contain toxic substances, this test may be the only practical method for determining the organic load. (c) SUSPENDED SOLIDS : The suspended solids are yet another indicator of the "strength" of sewage. The amount of suspended solids in domestic sewage may vary from 100 to 500 ppm (mg/L). If the amount of suspended solids is 100 mg/L, the sewage is said to be weak : if the amount is 500 mg/L the sewage is said to be strong.

Decomposition of organic matter

The decomposition of organic matter in sewage takes place by two processes : aerobic and anaerobic processes.

(1) *Aerobic process* : It is the most efficient method of reducing the organic matter in sewage. The process requires a continuous supply of free dissolved oxygen. The organic matter is broken down into simpler compounds namely CO_2, water, ammonia, nitrites, nitrates and sulphates by the action of bacterial organisms including fungi and protozoa.

(2) *Anaerobic process* : Where the sewage is highly concentrated and contains plenty of solids, the anaerobic process is highly effective. The end-products of decomposition are methane, ammonia, CO_2 and H_2. In anaerobic decomposition, the reactions are slower and the mechanism of decomposition extremely complex.

MODERN SEWAGE TREATMENT

Modern sewage treatment plants are based on biological principles of sewage purification, where the purification is brought about by the action of *anaerobic* and *aerobic* bacteria. Fig. 11 shows the flow diagram of a modern sewage treatment plant. The treatment of sewage may be divided into two stages, primary treatment and secondary treatment. In primary treatment, the solids are separated from the sewage partly by screening and partly by sedimentation and subjected to anaerobic digestion which is the first stage in purification; in secondary treatment, the effluent is subjected to aerobic oxidation, which is the second stage in purification.

a. PRIMARY TREATMENT

1. Screening

Sewage arriving at a disposal work is first passed through a metal screen which intercepts large floating objects such as pieces of wood, rags, masses of garbage and dead animals. Their removal is necessary to prevent clogging of the treatment plant. The screen consists of vertical or inclined steel bars usually set 5 cm (2 in) apart. In some plants, the screens are of the fixed type while in others, the screens are of the moving type. The screenings are removed from time to time either manually or mechanically, and disposed off by trenching or burial.

2. Grit chamber

Sewage is then passed through a long narrow chamber called the *grit chamber* or detritus chamber. This chamber is approximately 10 to 20 metres in length; it is so designed as to maintain a constant velocity of about 1 foot per second, with

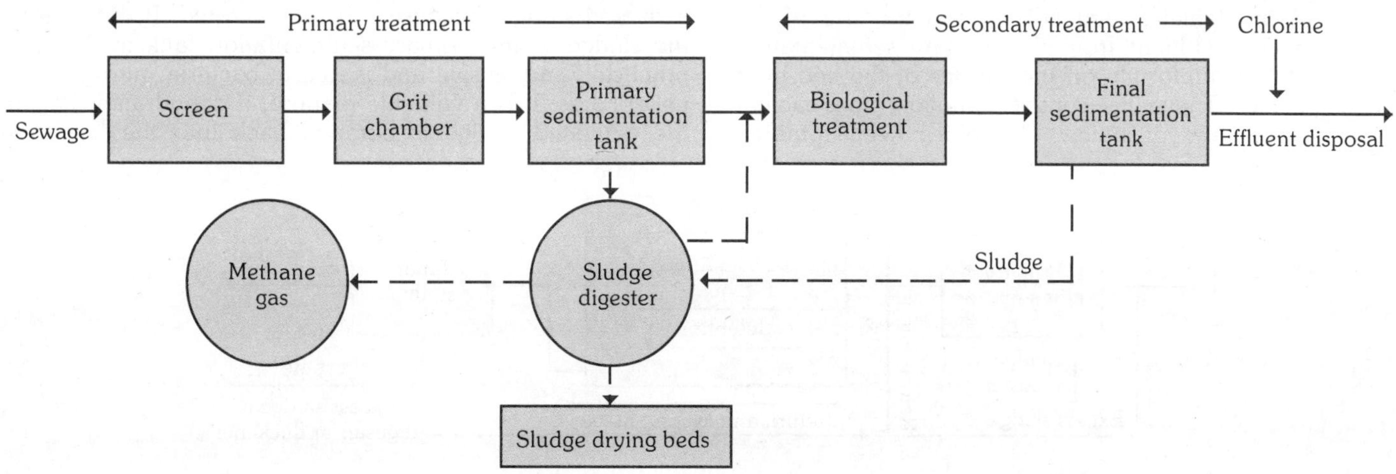

FIG. 11
Flow diagram of a modern sewage treatment plant

a detention period of 30 seconds to 1 minute *(8)*. The function of the grit chamber is to allow the settlement of heavier solids such as sand and gravel, while permitting the organic matter to pass through. The grit which collects at the bottom of the chamber is removed periodically or continuously, and disposed off by plain dumping or trenching.

3. Primary sedimentation

Sewage is now admitted into a huge tank called the *primary sedimentation tank*. It is a very large tank, holding from $^1/_4$ to $^1/_3$ the dry weather flow. There are various designs in primary sedimentation tank. By far the commonest is the rectangular tank. Sewage is made to flow very slowly across the tank at a velocity of 1–2 feet per minute. The sewage spends about 6–8 hours in the tank. During this long period of relatively still conditions in the tank, a very considerable amount of purification takes place mainly through sedimentation of suspended matter. Nearly 50–70 per cent of the solids settle down under the influence of gravity. A reduction of between 30 to 40 per cent in the number of coliform organisms is obtained *(9)*. The organic matter which settles down is called *sludge* and is removed by mechanically operated devices, without disturbing the operation in the tank. While this is going on, a small amount of biological action also takes place in which the microorganisms present in the sewage attack complex organic solids and break them down into simpler soluble substances and ammonia. A certain amount of fat and grease rise to the surface to form *scum* which is removed from time to time and disposed off. When the sewage contains organic trade wastes, it is treated with chemicals such as lime, aluminium sulphate and ferrous sulphate. Addition of one of these chemicals precipitates the animal protein material quickly.

b. SECONDARY TREATMENT

The effluent from the primary sedimentation tank still contains a proportion of organic matter in solution or colloidal state, and numerous living organisms. It has a high demand for oxygen and can cause pollution of soil or water. It is subjected to further treatment, aerobic oxidation, by one of the following methods :

(a) Trickling filter method

(b) Activated sludge process

(a) TRICKLING FILTER METHOD

The trickling filter or percolating filter is a bed of crushed stones or cinker, 1 to 2 m (4–8 ft.) deep and 2 to 30 m (6–100 ft.) in diameter, depending upon the size of the population. The effluent from the primary sedimentation tank is sprinkled uniformly on the surface of the bed by a revolving device. The device consists of hollow pipes each of which have a row of holes. The pipes keep rotating, sprinkling the effluent in a thin film on the surface of the filter. Over the surface and down through the filter, a very complex biological growth consisting of algae, fungi, protozoa and bacteria of many kinds occurs. This is known as the "zoogleal layer". As the effluent percolates through the filter bed, it gets oxidized by the bacterial flora in the zoogleal layer. The action of the filter is thus purely a biological one, and not one of filtration as the name suggests. The term "filter" is a misnomer. The trickling filters are very efficient in purifying sewage. They do not need rest pauses, because wind blows freely through the beds supplying the oxygen needed by the zoogleal flora. The biological growth or zoogleal layer lives, grows and dies. The dead matter sloughs off, breaks away and is washed down the filter. It is a light green, flocculent material and is called "humus". The oxidized sewage is now led into the secondary sedimentation tanks or humus tanks.

(b) ACTIVATED SLUDGE PROCESS

Activated sludge process (Fig. 12) is the modern method of purifying sewage, in place of the trickling filter. The "heart" of the activated sludge process is the aeration tank. The effluent from the primary sedimentation tank is mixed with sludge drawn from the final settling tank (also known as activated sludge or return sludge; this sludge is a rich culture of aerobic bacteria). The proportion of activated sludge to the incoming effluent is of the order of 20 to 30 per cent. The mixture is subjected to aeration in the aeration chamber for about 6 to 8 hours *(8)*. The aeration is accomplished either by mechanical agitation or by forcing compressed air continuously from the bottom of the aeration tank. This latter method, also known as 'diffuse aeration' is considered a better method of aeration. During the process of aeration, the organic matter of the sewage gets oxidized into carbon dioxide, nitrates and water with the help of the aerobic bacteria in the activated sludge. The typhoid and cholera organisms are definitely destroyed, and the coliforms greatly reduced. Activated sludge plants occupy less space, require skilled operations. One acre of activated sludge plant does the work of 10 acres of percolating filter. Activated sludge process is therefore, best suited for larger cities and the percolating filter for smaller towns because they are cheaper to install and easier to operate.

Secondary sedimentation

The oxidized sewage from the trickling filter or aeration chamber is led into the secondary sedimentation tank where it is detained for 2–3 hours. The sludge that collects in the secondary sedimentation tank is called 'aerated sludge' or activated sludge, because it is fully aerated. It differs from the sludge in the primary sedimentation tank in that it is practically inoffensive and is rich in bacteria, nitrogen and phosphates. It is a valuable manure, if dehydrated. Part of the activated sludge is pumped back into the "aeration

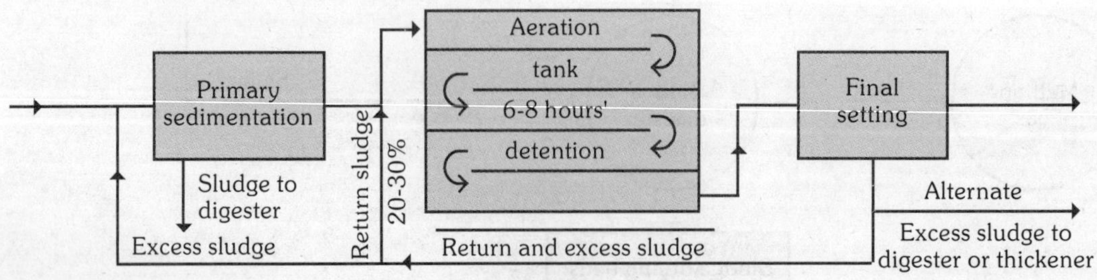

FIG. 12
Activated sludge process

tanks" in the activated sludge process and the rest pumped into the sludge digestion tanks for treatment and disposal.

Sludge digestion

One of greatest problems associated with sewage treatment is the treatment and disposal of the resulting sludge. One million gallons of sewage produces 15–20 tons of sludge. The sludge is a thick, black mass containing 95 per cent of water, and it has a revolting odour. There are a number of methods of sludge disposal : (a) *Digestion :* Modern sewage treatment plants employ digestion of sludge as the method of treatment. If sludge is incubated under favourable conditions of temperature and pH, it undergoes anaerobic auto-digestion in which complex solids are broken down into water, carbon dioxide, methane and ammonia. The volume of sludge is also considerably reduced. It takes 3–4 weeks or longer for complete sludge digestion. The residue is in-offensive, sticky and tarry mud which will dry readily and form an excellent manure. Sludge digestion is carried out in special tanks known as "sludge digestion tanks". Methane gas, which is a by-product of sludge digestion, can be used for heating and lighting purposes. (b) *Sea disposal:* Sea coast towns and cities can dispose of sludge by pumping it into the sea (c) *Land :* Sludge can be disposed off by composting with town refuse.

Disposal of effluent

(a) *Disposal by dilution :* Disposal into water courses such as rivers and streams is called 'disposal by dilution'. The effluent is diluted in the body of water and the impurities are oxidized by the dissolved oxygen in water. The diluting capacity of the river or the receiving body of water and its dissolved oxygen contents, are important considerations before discharging the effluent into a river or any body of water. Since people use river water for drinking purpose, the effluent must be rendered free from pathogenic organisms by adequate chlorination. The Royal Commission in England in its Fifth Report (1908) recommended that an effluent from a sewage treatment plant should not have more than 30 mg/litre of suspended solids and the 5 day B.O.D. of the effluent including the suspended matter, should not exceed 20 mg/litre. These standards assumed that the river or body of water into which the effluent passed would provide an 8 :1 dilution. These standards have been the backbone of subsequent work on the purity of sewage effluent. During the past few years, industry has developed hundreds of new chemicals which are released into the sewerage system. Some of these chemicals are not removed by biological treatment. Consequently, the effluent may contain substances toxic to man, or substances that can kill fish, damage agriculture or interfere with the normal functioning of a stream. In many places in the UK, effluent standards have been raised from the original Royal Commission values of 30 mg per litre of suspended solids and 20 mg per litre of B.O.D. to 10 mg per litre of each *(9)*. The World Health Organization is seized with this problem, and is fostering research in "tertiary" methods of treatment or "polishing" the effluent further. (b) *Disposal on land :* If suitable land is available the effluent can be used for irrigation purposes (e.g., the Okhla Sewage Treatment Plant in Delhi).

OTHER METHODS OF SEWAGE DISPOSAL

(a) Sea outfall
(b) River outfall
(c) Land treatment
(d) Oxidation ponds
(e) Oxidation ditches

(a) Sea outfall

Sea coast towns and cities may dispose off their sewage by discharging it into the sea. For instance, nearly two-thirds of untreated sewage of Greater Mumbai is discharged every day into the Arabian Sea. Purification takes place by dilution in the large body of sea water, and the solids get slowly oxidized. The drawback of this method is that the offensive solid matter may be washed back to the shore and create public nuisance. In order to prevent this, the sewage outfall is designed to discharge the sewage into deep water at many points.

(b) River outfall

Raw sewage should never be discharged into rivers. The present day practice is to purify the sewage before it is discharged into rivers. How far the sewage should be purified depends upon the dilution the river provides to carry on aeration and self-purification.

(c) Land treatment (sewage farming)

If sufficient and suitable land (porous soil) is available, sewage may be applied to the land after grit removal, screening and a short period of settlement. This type of treatment is practised in some Indian towns and cities and is known as *Sewage Farming* or *Broad Irrigation.* An acre of land would be required to treat the sewage of 100–300 persons. The land is first laid into ridges and furrows. Sewage is fed into the furrows *intermittently* and crops are grown on the ridges. The crops that are found suitable to grow are those which do not come in contact with sewage and likely to be eaten raw. Fodder grass and potatoes seem to be the most paying crops. Fruit trees whose fruits are high above the ground (e.g., plantain) can be grown. But sugar cane, coriander, cucumber, tomato, onion, etc. should not be grown. The farm should be under the direction of a competent agricultural expert. During the rainy season, it may not be possible to operate the sewage farms. Badly managed farms stink, a condition described as "sewage sickness" because of lack of sufficient aeration and rest pauses to the land. Alternate methods of disposal may have to be provided during the rainy season.

(d) Oxidation pond *(10)*

A cheap method of sewage treatment is the *oxidation pond* which has been referred to by many different names – waste stabilization pond, redox pond, sewage lagoons, etc. The term "waste stabilization pond" is more appropriate. The term 'waste' includes both sewage and industrial wastes. Although an old method of purifying sewage, oxidation pond has attracted the attention of public health engineers only recently. Over 50 ponds are working at present in India. The first large-scale installation was the one at Bhilai where it serves a population of 100,000.

The oxidation pond is an open, shallow pool 1 to 1.5 m (3–5 ft.) deep with an inlet and outlet (Fig. 13). To qualify as an oxidation pond, there must be the presence of (1) algae (2) certain types of bacteria which feed on decaying organic matter, and (3) sunlight. The organic matter contained in the sewage is oxidized by bacteria (hence oxidation pond) to simple chemical compounds such as carbon dioxide, ammonia and water. The algae, with the help of sunlight,

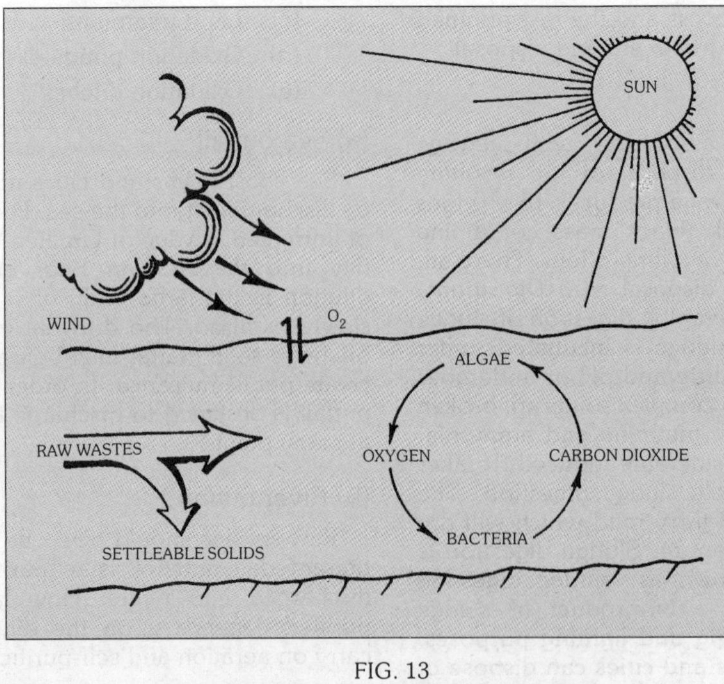

FIG. 13
Oxidation pond

utilize the carbon dioxide, water and inorganic minerals for their growth, Thus there is a mutually beneficial biological balance between the algae and bacteria in oxidation ponds. Oxygen that is needed for oxidation is derived to a small extent from the atmosphere but mostly from the algae which liberates oxygen under the influence of sunlight. Consequently, sunlight is an important factor in the proper functioning of oxidation ponds. Cloudy weather definitely lowers the efficiency of the process.

The oxidation ponds are predominantly aerobic during sunshine hours as well as some hours of the night. In the remaining hours of the night, the bottom layers are generally *anaerobic*. Thus the sewage purification in oxidation ponds is brought about by a combination of aerobic and anaerobic types of bacteria. The effluent may be used for growing vegetable crops (land irrigation) or may be discharged into a river or other water courses after appropriate treatment. Mosquito nuisance is avoided by keeping weed growth in the neighbourhood of oxidation ponds to a minimum and the water line free from marginal vegetation. There is no odour nuisance associated with these ponds when they are properly maintained. Oxidation ponds have become an established method of purifying sewage for small communities.

(e) Oxidation ditches

Other methods recommended are (1) oxidation ditches and (2) aerated lagoons. These methods make use of mechanical rotors for extended aeration. For treatment of the wastes of a population between 5,000 to 20,000 an oxidation ditch requires an area of one acre as compared to 22 acres for an oxidation pond and 2.5 acres for an aerated lagoon. These are low cost treatment methods for the purification of sewage.

SOCIAL ASPECTS OF EXCRETA DISPOSAL IN INDIA

India is a land of villages and about 70 per cent of its population lives in villages. The problem of sanitation therefore is one of "Rural sanitation". Surveys have shown that substantial per cent of the population "go to the open fields" for defecation. This habit of indiscriminate fouling of the surroundings with human excrement is generations-old, and rooted firmly in the cultural behaviour of the village people.

In urban areas, the latrine is considered a necessary part of a house. In rural areas, by and large, people have not accepted latrines with any enthusiasm, and even when installed only a few used them regularly. The problem in rural sanitation is how to overcome the resistance of the village people, and induce them to use sanitary latrines. Research studies have indicated that there is only one way to solve the problem, i.e., through *health education*. Social scientists have listed the reasons why villagers do not accept latrines. Some of the reasons found in the surveys are : (1) latrines are associated with bad smell (2) they are the breeding places of flies (3) they are something foul and dirty so that one should not have them close to houses (4) latrines are costly and beyond their means to install, and (5) they do not know how faecal-borne diseases are spread. Secondly, using a latrine goes against a DAILY habit pattern of going to the fields. The use of latrines involves a drastic change in the day to day behaviour of a large number of people.

The solution to the problem lies in teaching the people first the reasons why latrines are important. The teaching should be undertaken by all known methods of health education – direct discussion, group discussion, latrine demonstration, and use of visual aids and above all service facilities. The ultimate goal of health education will be to *motivate* the rural people towards acceptance and use of sanitary latrines.

Surface water drainage in urban areas

Many low income communities in developing countries consider stormwater drainage to be their most urgent need as far as urban infrastructure is concerned. It is the coastal regions of the world that have the highest average rainfall, but the flat estuarine terrain and often impermeable alluvial soil make drainage difficult. Even in the arid areas where average rainfall is low, tropical rainfall – when it comes – is more intense than in temperate climates, and the lack of vegetation and of adequate drainage means that torrents of water can form in minutes, causing damage to homes and property, which will take years to repair. The lack of drainage is especially serious where the ground is either steeply sloping, as in Hongkong or very flat as in Kolkata, Bangkok and Manila.

Deaths due to drowning in floods or burial beneath landslides or collapsing homes are perhaps the most dramatic signs of the suffering that drainage can help to alleviate. Less noticeable to an outsider, but of greater impact on the residents living in a poor community, is the steady toll of disease, disability and death by standing water.

First in public health importance are the many "faecal-oral" infections acquired by consumption of contaminated food and drink. Children are particularly exposed to infection when playing or bathing in surface water. Surface water becomes contaminated with pathogens from blocked sewers and overflowing septic tanks. This contaminated surface water can infect people in many ways.

Another important group of diseases related to poor drainage is transmitted by mosquitoes, and malaria is the best example. Transmission can be particularly intense in urban areas where there are relatively few animals to divert the vector species of mosquito from human blood meals. Drainage construction is an effective mosquito control measure. It is cheaper than application of insecticides and does not have to be repeated regularly. Unlike insecticides, it can have no detrimental effect on the environment; on the contrary, it constitutes an environmental improvement.

Urban poor may often build on land with drainage problems, but good urban planning can help to avoid making these problems worse. One of the simplest planning measure is to set out regular plots before house building starts in an area, leaving space for well aligned roads. Adequate road width and alignment will make it much easier to build drains when they are needed later.

References

1. Wager and Lanoix, *Excreta Disposal for Rural Areas and Small Communities,* WHO Monograph Series No.38, 1958.
2. Indian Council of Medical Research (1966). *Review of Work done on Rural Latrines in India,* Spl. Rep. Ser., No. 54.
3. Kawata, K. (1963). *Environmental Sanitation in India,* Christian Medical College, Ludhiana, Punjab.
4. News & Queries (1974) *The Practitioner,* 212, 169.
5. Directorate General of Health Services, Ministry of Health, New Delhi (1962). *Rural Latrine Programmes,* 2nd Ed., 1962.
6. Balakrishana Rao, P. et al (1970) *Environmental Health* 12.39.
7. Govt. of India (2015). *Compendium on IR-DRDO Bio-Toilets for Indian Railways,* Ministry of Railways, New Delhi.
8. Okun. D.A. and Ponghis, G (1975). *Community Waste-water collection and Disposal,* WHO Geneva.
9. WHO (1969). *Problems in Community Wastes Management,* Public Health Papers No. 38.
10. Arceivala, S.J. et al (1970) *Waste Stabilization Ponds, Design, Construction and Operation in India.* National Environmental Engineering Research Institute, Nagpur, India.

MEDICAL ENTOMOLOGY

Arthropods comprise the most numerous and varied of the living things in the environment of man. Some of them are man's allies helping in the fertilization of flowers, but the majority of arthropods, in general, are either of no use to man or are his most dangerous enemies. They destroy man's crops and his food reserves; and some which live close to man act as *vectors* or carriers of disease. A study of the arthropods of medical importance is known as medical entomology which is an important branch of preventive medicine.

Arthropods of medical importance

The arthropods of medical importance are as given in Table 1.

TABLE 1

Arthropods of medical importance

Class : Insecta	Class : Arachnida	Class : Crustacea
1. *Mosquitoes :* *Anophelines* *Culicines*	1. *Ticks :* Hard ticks Soft ticks	1. *Cyclops*
2. *Flies :* Houseflies Sandflies Tsetse flies Blackflies	2. *Mites (Chiggers) :* Leptotrombidium and trombiculid mites; Itch mite	
3. *Human Lice :* Head and body lice; Crab lice		
4. *Fleas :* Rat fleas Sand fleas		
5. *Reduviid bugs*		

Distinctive characters

The distinctive characters of the above arthropods are as given in Table 2.

TABLE 2

Distinctive characters of arthropods of medical importance

	Insecta	Arachnida	Crustacea
1. Body divisions	Head. thorax abdomen	Cephalothorax and abdomen (no division) in some cases	Cephalothorax and abdomen
2. Legs	3 pairs	4 pairs	5 pairs
3. Antennae	1 pair	None	2 pairs
4. Wings	One or two pairs; some are wingless	None	None
5. Where found	On land	On land	In water

Arthropod-borne diseases

Arthropod-borne diseases constitute a major health problem in India. Malaria continues to be an important vector-borne disease with an annual morbidity of 4 to 5 million cases. Filaria is another important arthropod-borne disease with an estimated 236 million people living in filaria-endemic areas. Scabies is a widespread disease, especially in rural areas. Dengue, haemorrhagic fever, Japanese encephalitis and KFD are also among the important arthropod-borne virus diseases in India. The prevalence rates for trachoma which is a major cause of blindness in India vary from 0.5 per cent in West Bengal to 79 per cent in Punjab and

Haryana. Thus, arthropods are responsible for much ill-health and deaths (Table 3).

TABLE 3

Arthropod-borne diseases

Arthropod	Diseases transmitted
1. Mosquito	Malaria, filaria, viral encephalitis (e.g., Japanese encephalitis), viral fevers (e.g., dengue, West Nile, viral haemorrhagic fevers (e.g., yellow fever, dengue haemorrhagic fever)
2. Housefly	Typhoid and paratyphoid fever, diarrhoea, dysentery, cholera, gastro-enteritis, amoebiasis, helminthic infestations, poliomyelitis, conjunctivitis, trachoma, anthrax, yaws, etc.
3. Sandfly	Kala-azar, oriental sore, sandfly fever, oraya fever.
4. Tsetse fly	Sleeping sickness
5. Louse	Epidemic typhus, relapsing fever, trench fever, pediculosis
6. Rat flea	Bubonic plague, endemic typhus, chiggerosis, hymenolepis diminuta.
7. Blackfly	Onchocerciasis.
8. Reduviid bug	Chagas disease.
9. Hard tick	Tick typhus, viral encephalitis, viral fevers, viral haemorrhagic fever, (e.g., Kyasanur forest disease), tularemia, tick paralysis, human babesiosis.
10. Soft tick	Q fever, relapsing fever.
11. Trombiculid mite	Scrub typhus, Rickettsial-pox.
12. Itch-mite	Scabies.
13. Cyclops	Guinea-worm disease, fish tapeworm (D. latus).
14. Cockroaches	Enteric pathogens.

Transmission of arthropod-borne diseases

Three types of transmission cycles are involved in the spread of arthropod-borne disease : (1) DIRECT CONTACT : In this method of spread, the arthropods are directly transferred from man to man through close contact, e.g., scabies and pediculosis, (2) MECHANICAL TRANSMISSION : The disease agent is transmitted mechanically by the arthropod. The transmission of diarrhoea, dysentery, typhoid, food poisoning and trachoma by the housefly – are examples of mechanical transmission of the disease agent by the vector. (3) BIOLOGICAL TRANSMISSION : When the disease agent multiplies or undergoes some developmental change with or without multiplication in the arthropod host, it is called biological transmission. This may be of three types : (a) *Propagative :* When the disease agent undergoes no cyclical change, but multiplies in the body of the vector, transmission is said to be propagative, e.g., plague bacilli in rat fleas (b) *Cyclo-propagative :* The disease agent undergoes cyclical change, and multiplies in the body of the arthropod, e.g., malaria parasite in anopheline mosquito (c) *Cyclo-developmental :* When the disease agent undergoes cyclical change but does not multiply in the body of the arthropod, e.g., filarial parasite in culex mosquito and guineaworm embryo in cyclops.

In communicable disease terminology, the word vector means an "arthropod or other invertebrate which transmits infection by inoculation into or through the skin or mucous membrane by biting, or by deposit of infective materials on the skin or on food or other objects". The period of time necessary for the development of the disease agent in the arthropod host is called *extrinsic incubation period.* For example, the extrinsic incubation periods in malaria and filaria are from 10 to 14 days or longer depending upon the environmental temperature. The host in which the sexual cycle of the agent occurs is called the *definitive host,* e.g., mosquito is the definitive host in malaria. The host in which the asexual cycle of the agent occurs is called the *intermediate host* e.g., mosquito in filaria and cyclops in guinea-worm disease. By *infestation* is meant the lodgement, development and reproduction of arthropods on the surface of the body or in the clothing e.g., louse infestation.

Principles of arthropod control

The general principles of arthropod control are :

1. Environmental control
2. Chemical control
3. Biological control
4. Genetic control

(1) *Environmental control :* This offers the best approach to the control of arthropods, because the results are likely to be permanent. Examples of environmental manipulation are : elimination of breeding places (source reduction); filling and drainage operation; carefully planned water management; provision of piped water supply; proper disposal of refuse and other wastes; cleanliness in and around houses, etc. Intensive health education of the public as well as political support are essential prerequisites. (2) *Chemical control :* A wide range of insecticides belonging to the organochlorine, organo-phosphorus and carbamate groups of compounds (Fig. 17, page 909) are available for vector control. It must be mentioned that vector control by insecticides alone is no longer fully effective because resistance has appeared in over 100 species of arthropods of public health importance. This coupled with the danger of environmental contamination has led to restricted use of many insecticides in some countries. To avoid undue environmental pollution, it is now considered essential to replace gradually the highly persistent compounds such as DDT with compounds which are readily "biodegradable" and less toxic to man and animals such as methoxychlor, abate and dursban *(1)*. As there is no alternate control method which is as efficient and economical as the insecticides, it is postulated that most of the developing countries will have to depend, for sometime to come, on the organochlorine compounds for the control of vectors. (3) *Biological control :* To minimize environmental pollution with toxic chemicals, great emphasis is now being placed on biological control. The use of larvivorous fish especially Gambusia is well known in mosquito control. Fungi of the genus Coelomomyces are also known to be pathogenic to mosquitoes. A variety of other biological agents (e.g., bacteria, fungi, nematodes, protozoa and viruses) are under study for the control of insects. But the fear exists that the introduction of biological agents for the control of arthropods may pose a direct hazard to the health of man himself *(2)*. (4) *Genetic control :* Much progress has taken place in recent years in the theoretical and applied

aspects of genetic control of arthropods. The WHO/ICMR Research Unit at New Delhi has contributed massively to the techniques of genetic control of mosquitoes *(3)*. Techniques such as sterile male technique, cytoplasmic incompatibility and chromosomal translocations have been found to be effective in small field trials. In conclusion, it may be stated that these methods are nowhere near the stage where they can be used large-scale in an effective way. (5) *Newer methods :* New and innovative methods are being sought for pest control. These are (a) insect growth regulators (b) chemosterilants, and (c) sex attractants or pheromones *(4)*.

Integrated approach

Since no single method of control is likely to provide a solution in all situations, the present trend is to adopt an "integrated approach" for vector control combining two or more methods with a view to obtain maximum results with the minimum effort and to avoid the excessive use of any one method *(5)*.

MOSQUITO

General description

Mosquitoes constitute the most important single family of insects from the standpoint of human health. They are found all over the world. The four important groups of mosquitoes in India which are related to disease transmission are the *Anopheles, Culex, Aedes* and *Mansonia*.

The body of a mosquito consists of three parts : head, thorax and abdomen, (a) HEAD : The head is semi-globular in outline, and bears the following structures :– (i) a pair of large compound eyes (ii) a long needle-like structure, called the *proboscis* with which the mosquito bites (iii) a pair of *palpi,* each a four jointed structure, situated on either side of the proboscis and (iv) a pair of *antennae* or feelers. The antennae are bushy in the male, and not quite so in the female. They provide an easy means of distinguishing the male from the female (b) THORAX : The thorax is large and rounded in appearance and bears :– (i) a pair of wings dorsally (ii) three pairs of legs ventrally. The wings of the mosquito are characterised by a fringe of scales on the posterior border and the first, third and sixth veins on the wings are not branched. When the mosquito is at rest, the wings are folded. The buzzing noise which the mosquitoes produce is due to the beating of their wings, and not to "singing". (c) ABDOMEN : The abdomen is long and narrow and is composed of 10 segments, the last two of which are modified to form the external genitalia.

Life history

There are four stages in the life history of mosquitoes (Fig. 1): egg, larva, pupa and adult. Metamorphosis is complete.

(1) EGG : Eggs are laid on the surface of water, 100–250 at a time. The *Anopheles* lays her eggs singly; the eggs are boat-shaped and possess lateral floats. The *Culex* lays her eggs in small clusters or rafts; the eggs do not possess lateral floats. The *Aedes* lays her eggs singly; the eggs are cigar-shaped and do not possess lateral floats. The *Mansonia* lays her eggs in star-shaped clusters attached to the under-surface of the leaves of certain aquatic plants, notably the pisita plant. Under favourable conditions, the egg stage of mosquitoes lasts for 1–2 days. The period that elapses from the moment a blood meal is taken until the eggs are laid is called the "gonotrophic cycle", it is about 48 hours in hot and humid tropical areas.

(2) LARVA : The larva is a free swimming creature with an elongated body divisible into head, thorax and abdomen. It feeds on algae, bacteria and vegetable matter and passes through four stages of growth called "instars" with moulting between each stage. The larva of the *Anopheles* floats horizontally in the water, and has no siphon tube at the tip of its abdomen. The *Culicine* (e.g., Culex, Aedes, and Mansonia) larvae, in contrast, are suspended in water with their heads downwards; they all possess a siphon tube, which is situated on the 8th abdominal segment. The larvae of the *Mansonia* are peculiar in the respect that they are attached to the rootlets of certain aquatic plants by their siphon tubes; they obtain air from the plant rootlets. The larval stage occupies 5–7 days.

(3) PUPA : The pupa is comma shaped in appearance, with a large rounded cephalothorax and a narrow abdomen. Two small respiratory tubes or trumpets project from the upper surface of the thorax. The pupa represents the resting stage in the life history of the mosquito; it does not feed but prefers to stay quiet at the water surface. But when disturbed it swims rapidly downwards into the water. The pupal stage lasts for 1–2 days.

(4) ADULT : When the development is complete, the

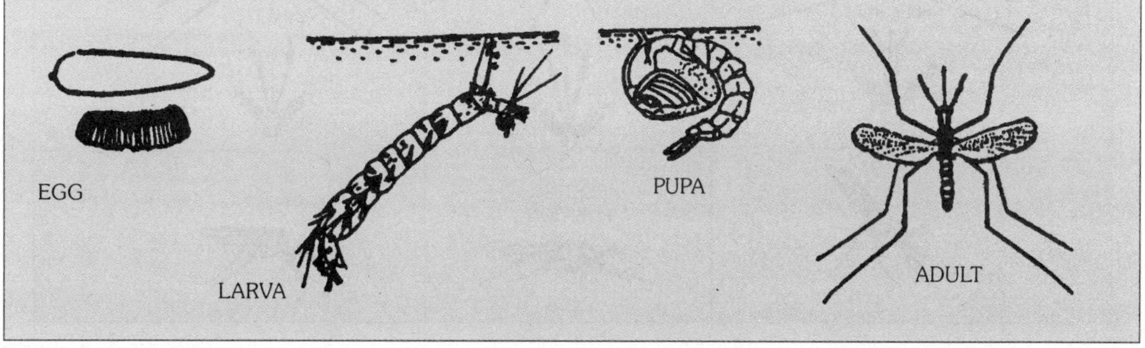

FIG. 1
Life cycle of a mosquito

pupal skin splits along the back and the adult mosquito or imago emerges. It rests for a while on the pupal skin to allow its wings to expand and harden and then flies away. Under favourable conditions of temperature and food supply the life cycle from the egg to adult is complete in 7–10 days. Normally the adult mosquito lives for about 2 weeks. The males are generally short lived.

Differentiation between anophelines and culicines

There are two main *tribes* of mosquitoes – Tribe *Anophelini* and Tribe *Culicini*. The tribe anophelini contains only one genus, *Anopheles*. The tribe *Culicini* is represented in India by 15 genera of which the important ones are *Culex, Aedes* and *Mansonia*. The main points of difference between the two tribes, *Anophelini* and *Culicini* are as given in Table 4 (See Fig. 2).

(1) Anopheles

Some 45 species of anopheles mosquitoes have been found in India but only a few of them have been incriminated as vectors or carriers of malaria. They are (1) *An. culicifacies* (2) *An. fluviatilis* (3) *An. minimus* (4) *An. philippinensis* (5) *An. stephensi* (6) *An. sundaicus* and (7) *An. leucosphyrus*. The areas of distribution of these mosquitoes are different : *An. fluviatilis* and *An. minimus* are found in the foot-hill regions; *An. sundaicus* and *An.stephensi* are found in the coastal regions; and *An. culicifacies* and *An. philippinensis* are found in the plains. An accurate guide to the identification of the known species of anopheles mosquitoes in India may be found in Health Bulletin No.10 entitled : "Synoptic Table for the Identification of the Anopheles Mosquitoes in India *(6)*."

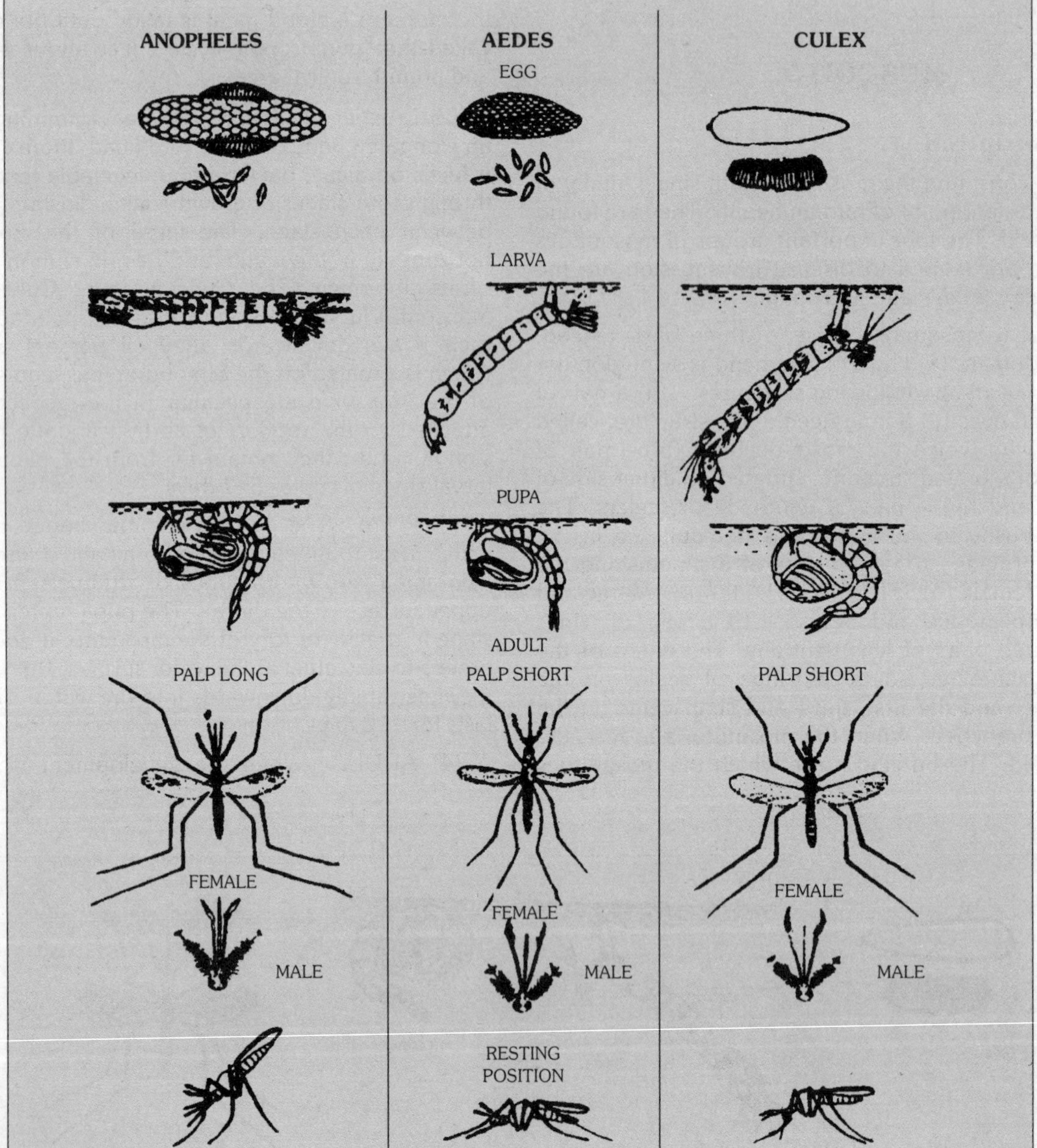

FIG. 2
Characteristics of anopheles, aedes and culex

TABLE 4

Differentiation between anophelini and culicini

Tribe Genus	Anophelini anopheles	Culicini Culex, Aedes, Mansonia
EGGS	(1) Laid singly. (2) Eggs are boat-shaped, and provided with lateral floats.	(1) Laid in clusters or rafts, each raft containing 100–250 eggs (except-Aedes). (2) Eggs are oval-shaped, and not provided with lateral floats.
LARVAE	(1) Rest parallel to water surface. (2) No siphon tube. (3) Palmate hairs present on abdominal segments.	(1) Suspended with head downwards at an angle to water surface. (2) Siphon tube present. (3) No palmate hairs.
PUPAE	Siphon tube is broad and short.	Siphon tube is long and narrow.
ADULTS	(1) When at rest, inclined at an angle to surface. (2) Wings spotted. (3) Palpi long in both sexes.	(1) When at rest, the body exhibits a hunch back. (2) Wings unspotted. (3) Palpi short in female.

(2) Culex

Mosquitoes of the genus *Culex* are the common "nuisance mosquitoes" which are terrible pests of man. An important member of this group is *Culex fatigans,* the vector of Bancroftian filariasis in India. *Culex fatigans* is essentially a domestic species and is found everywhere in India in and around dwellings. Rapid urbanization and industrialization without adequate drainage facilities are responsible for its increased spread. It breeds profusely in dirty water collections, viz. stagnant drains, cesspools, septic tanks, burrow pits, and in fact, in all types of water collection. *Culex fatigans* is a strong-winged mosquito; its dispersal has been found to be 11 km in the rural areas of Delhi *(7)*. The species is highly anthrophilic. It enters the houses at dusk and reaches maximum density by midnight. The peak biting time is about midnight. Legs, particularly below the knee are the preferred biting sites. During day, it may be seen resting indoors on walls, underneath furniture, inside empty pots and in dark corners.

(3) Aedes (Stegomyia)

Aedes mosquitoes are easily distinguished by white stripes on a black body. Because of the striped or banded character of their legs they are sometimes referred to as "tiger mosquitoes". Important members of this group of mosquitoes are : *Aedes aegypti, Aedes vittatus* and *Aedes albopictus.* Aedes mosquitoes are most abundant during rainy season.

Aedes aegypti occupies a very special position in preventive medicine. It is the first proved vector of a virus disease – yellow fever. Aedes aegypti is widely distributed in India. It breeds in artificial accumulations of water in and around human dwellings, such as water found in discarded tins, broken bottles, fire buckets, flower pots, coconut shells, earthen pots, tree holes and the like. It lays eggs singly, and the eggs are cigar-shaped. The females are fearless biters, and they bite chiefly during the day. They do not fly over long distances – usually less than 100 metres (110 yards). This factor facilitates its eradication. Under the WHO International Health Regulations (IHR), all international airports and seaports are kept free from all types of mosquitoes for a distance of 400 metres around the perimeter of the ports. Under the International Health Regulations, *Aedes aegypti index* is defined as "the ratio, expressed as percentage, between the number of houses in a limited well-defined area on the premises of which actual breeding of *Aedes aegypti* are found, and the total number of houses examined in that area" *(8)*. This index is kept at zero at all ports.

(4) Mansonia

The mosquitoes of this genus are big, black or brown mosquitoes with speckling on their wings and legs. The common Indian species are : *M.annulifera, M.uniformis, M. indiana* and *M. longipalpis.* The *mansonoides mosquitoes* are peculiar in their breeding habits. They breed in ponds and lakes containing certain aquatic plants, especially the floating types like *Pistia stratiotes* and water hyacinth. The eggs are laid in star-shaped clusters on the under surface of the leaves of these aquatic plants. The larvae and pupae are found attached to the rootlets of these plants by their siphon tubes; they obtain their air supply from these rootlets. When about to become adults, the pupae come to the surface of water and the fully formed adults emerge and escape. The control of mansonoides mosquitoes is easy by the removal or destruction of the aquatic host plants by herbicides.

Habits of mosquitoes

The habits of mosquitoes have been extensively studied by entomologists. A knowledge of these habits is essential from the point of view of controlling the mosquitoes as well as for a proper understanding of the part they play in disease transmission. The following are some of their important habits : (1) FEEDING HABITS : The males never bite : they subsist on plant juices. The females on the contrary are haematophagous. They require a blood meal, once in 2–3 days for the development of eggs. The females differ in their feeding habits. Some species (anthrophilic) prefer human blood, some (zoophillic) prefer animal blood, and some indifferent in their choice and feed on both man and animals. (2) TIME OF BITING : In general mosquitoes bite in the evening or in the early part of the night, but there are great variations among the species. (3) RESTING HABITS : Mosquitoes obscure themselves during the day in dark and cool corners. Some rest indoors (endophilia), and some outdoors (exophilia). The indoor resting places are usually the dark corners of houses, upper part of walls, behind pictures and under furniture. The outdoor resting places are usually the vegetation, shrubs, tree holes, cattle sheds and wells. (4) BREEDING HABITS : In general, the *anophelines* prefer clean water for breeding; the *culicines* prefer dirty and polluted water; the *aedes* prefer artificial collections of water. The *mansonia* breed in water containing certain types of aquatic vegetation. (5) HIBERNATION : Mosquitoes are known to hibernate in the adult stage when the environmental conditions are not favourable. Severe winters are tided over by hibernation. (6) DISPERSAL : Mosquitoes do not generally fly far from the place where they breed unless swept by currents of wind. The range of flight varies with the species, and may range upto 11 kms. Aircrafts and ships have increased the possibility of the dispersal of mosquitoes from country to country, and have created fresh problems of public health. The danger of introduction of mosquitoes infected with yellow fever into

India where the population have no past experience of the disease is well recognised. (7) LIFE SPAN : The life of a mosquito is influenced by temperature and humidity. Both high and low temperatures are fatal. The normal life span of mosquitoes varies from 8 to 34 days. The males, as a rule, are short lived.

Mosquito-borne diseases

Apart from their pestiferous nature, mosquitoes play an important role in the transmission of human disease. They act as vectors of many diseases in India : (Table 5).

TABLE 5

Mosquito-borne diseases in India

Type of mosquito	Disease
1. Anopheles	Malaria Filaria (not in India)
2. Culex	Bancroftian filariasis Japanese encephalitis West Nile fever Viral arthritis (epidemic/polyarthritis)
3. Aedes	Yellow fever (not in India) Dengue Dengue haemorrhagic fever Chikungunya fever Chikungunya haemorrhagic fever Rift valley fever Filaria (not in India)
4. Mansonoides	Malayan (Brugian) filariasis Chikungunya fever

MOSQUITO CONTROL MEASURES

While there are many methods of mosquito control, experts now recommend an "integrated approach", that is, an approach which avoids the excessive use of any one method (e.g., insecticides) but tries to combine one or more methods with a view to obtain maximum results with minimum inputs and also to prevent environmental pollution with toxic chemicals and development of insecticide resistance. The various methods of mosquito control may be classified as below :

1 ANTI-LARVAL MEASURES
- (a) Environmental control
- (b) Chemical control
- (c) Biological control

2 ANTI-ADULT MEASURES
- (a) Residual sprays
- (b) Space sprays
- (c) Genetic control

3 PROTECTION AGAINST MOSQUITO BITES
- (a) Mosquito net
- (b) Screening
- (c) Repellents

1. ANTI-LARVAL MEASURES

(a) Environmental control

The most important step in reducing the numbers of mosquitoes is to eliminate their breeding places. This is known as "source reduction", and comprises minor engineering methods such as filling, levelling and drainage of breeding places; and water management (such as intermittent irrigation). These are proven methods of larval control. Source reduction also implies rendering the water unsuitable for mosquito breeding, as for example, changing the salinity of water. Source reduction requires an accurate knowledge of the breeding habits of mosquitoes. If *Culex* mosquitoes are a problem, there should be a programme for the abolition of domestic and peridomestic sources of breeding such as cesspools and open ditches; and arrangements should be made for adequate collection, removal and disposal of sewage and waste water. If *Aedes* mosquitoes are a problem, the environment should be cleaned up and got rid of water holding containers such as discarded tins, empty pots, broken bottles, coconut shells and similar other artificial collections of water. If *Anopheles* mosquitoes are a problem, their breeding places should be looked for and abolished by appropriate engineering measures such as filling and drainage. If *Mansonia* mosquitoes are a problem, the aquatic plants to which the larvae attach themselves should be removed or destroyed by herbicides. Source reduction methods generally produce results that are permanent.

(b) Chemical control

The commonly used larvicides are :

(i) Mineral oils
(ii) Paris green
(iii) Synthetic insecticides

(i) *Mineral oils :* The application of oil to water is one of the oldest known mosquito control measure. The oils most widely used are the diesel oil, fuel oil, kerosene and various fractions of crude oils. Special oils (e.g., Mosquito Larvicidal Oil) are also available. Oil kills larvae and pupae within a short time after application. When applied on water, oil spreads and forms a thin film, which cuts off the air supply to the mosquito larvae and pupae. Oil probably has also a specific toxic action on these insect stages. The usual application rate for oils is 40 to 90 litres per hectare *(9)*. Since the life cycle of a mosquito occupies about 8 days, it is customary to apply oil once a week on all breeding places. Oil has also certain disadvantages, it renders water unfit for drinking; it kills fish. Nevertheless, oil is eminently suited for the control of mosquito larvae.

(ii) *Paris green :* Paris green or copper acetoarsenite is an emerald green, microcrystalline powder practically insoluble in water. A good sample of paris green must contain 50 per cent arsenious oxide. Paris green is a stomach poison and to be effective it must be ingested by the larvae. Paris green kills mainly the *Anopheles* larvae because they are surface-feeders. Bottom-feeding larvae are also killed when paris green is applied as a special granular formulation *(9)*. Paris green is applied as 2 per cent dust which is prepared by mixing 2 kg of paris green and 98 kg of a diluent such as soapstone powder or slaked lime in a "rotary mixer". The resulting mixture must be fine with the size of the particles ranging from 20–25 microns. The dusting is accomplished by hand blowers or rotary blowers. The recommended dose is 1 kg of actual paris green per hectare of water surface *(9)*. In the dosage applied, paris green does not harm fish, man or domestic animals.

(iii) *Synthetic insecticides* : Fenthion, Chlorpyrifos, and Abate are the most effective larvicides *(10)*. These organophosphorous compounds hydrolyze quickly in water. Abate at a concentration of 1.0 ppm has been found to be a very effective larvicide, and also the least toxic. Dosage of these toxicants are given in Table 6. The organochlorine compounds (e.g., DDT, HCH) are not recommended for larviciding operations because of their long residual effect, water contamination and increased risk of developing resistance in the vector mosquitoes.

TABLE 6

Toxicants employed as larvicides in mosquito control

Toxicant	Dosage (g/ha)
Abate	56–112
Malathion	224–672
Fenthion	22–112
Chloropyrifos	11–16

Biological control

A wide range of small fish feed readily on mosquito larvae. The best known are the *Gambusia affinis* and *Lebister reticulatus* (sometimes known as Barbados Millions). These fish can be used in burrow pits, sewage oxidation ponds, ornamental ponds, cisterns and farm ponds. In recent years, there has been a revival of interest in the biological control of mosquitoes through the use of fish *(11)*. It is however recognized that biological control can be effective only when used in conjunction with other methods.

2. ANTI-ADULT MEASURES

(a) Residual sprays

Adult mosquitoes are most commonly controlled by spraying houses with residual insecticides. DDT is the insecticide of choice and dosages of 1–2 grams of pure DDT per sq. metre are applied 1–3 times a year to walls and other surfaces where mosquitoes rest. In areas where DDT resistance is encountered, malathion and propoxur (OMS-33), and to a lesser extent gamma-HCH (lindane) are recommended *(12)*. Dosages and average duration of effectiveness are as given in Table 7.

TABLE 7

Toxicants suitable against malaria vectors as residual spray applications

Toxicant	Dosage in g/m^2	Average duration of effectiveness (months)
DDT	1 to 2	6 to 12
Lindane	0.5	3
Malathion	2	3
OMS-33	2	3

Resistance to insecticides has become common among mosquitoes, especially after several years of exposure. Resistance to organophosphorus insecticides is also becoming widespread. It is essential that periodic tests should be made to determine the susceptibility of different species of mosquitoes to the various insecticides so that only potent insecticides can be applied.

(b) Space sprays

Space sprays are those where the insecticidal formulation is sprayed into the atmosphere in the form of a mist or fog to kill insects. The common space sprays are : (i) *Pyrethrum extract* : An extract of pyrethrum flowers is an excellent space spray. The active principle (pyrethrin) is a nerve poison and kills insects instantly on mere contact. Pyrethrum is sprayed at a dosage of 1 oz of the spray solution (containing 0.1 per cent of the active principle, pyrethrin) per 1,000 C. ft. of space. The doors and windows are kept closed for half an hour. For domestic purposes, the hand gun with a fine nozzle is all that is necessary, but for application on a large scale, power sprayers or "aerosol" dispensers may be needed. Pyrethrum sprays are effective in reducing the number of mosquitoes but the reduction is only temporary since it has no residual action. Reinfestation from outside sources generally occurs within a short time. (ii) *Residual Insecticides* : New equipment has been developed for ULV (ultra low volume) space spraying. The most extensively used insecticides are malathion and fenitrothion for ULV fogging *(13)*.

(c) Genetic control *(14, 15)*

In recent years, control of mosquitoes by genetic methods such as sterile male technique, cytoplasmic incompatibility, chromosomal translocations, sex distortion, and gene replacement have been explored. Their use is still in the "Research Phase". These techniques have great potential in mosquito control *(3)*. They also have certain advantages over chemical methods, being cheaper and potentially more efficient and above all not subject to vector resistance.

3. PROTECTION AGAINST MOSQUITO BITES

(a) Mosquito net

The mosquito net offers protection against mosquito bites during sleep. The material of the net should be white, to allow easy detection of mosquitoes. The top as well as the sides of the net should be of netting. The best pattern is the rectangular net. There should not be a single hole or rent in the net. The size of the openings in the net is of utmost importance – the size should not exceed 0.0475 inch in any diameter. The number of holes in one square inch is usually 150.

(b) Screening

Screening of buildings with copper or bronze gauze having 16 meshes to the inch is recommended. The aperture should not be larger than 0.0475 inch. Screening of buildings is costly, but gives excellent results.

(c) Repellents

Diethyltoluamide (deet) has been found to be an outstanding all purpose repellent *(10)*. It has been found to remain active against *C. fatigans* for 18–20 hours. There are others also which are effective: indalone, dimethyl phthalate, dimethyl carbate, ethyl hexanediol, etc. Repellents or *culicifuges* are used mainly for application on the skin, and their chief advantage is the short duration of protection.

HOUSEFLIES

Houseflies are the commonest and most familiar of all insects which live close to man. They occur in abundance all the year round in India. The majority of house-frequenting flies in India are non-biting. The most important of these are : *Musca domestica, M. vicinia, M. nebulo* and *M. sorbens (16)*. Houseflies should be regarded as a sign of insanitation, and their number as an index of that insanitation.

General characters

The common housefly (*M. domestica*) is mouse-grey in colour. The body is divided into head, thorax and abdomen. (1) HEAD : The head bears a pair of antennae, a pair of large compound eyes and a retractile proboscis, which is adapted for sucking liquid foods. The eyes of the male are close together; those of the female are set apart widely. (2) THORAX : The thorax is marked with 2 to 4 dark longitudinal stripes, which is characteristic of the genus, *musca*. The thorax bears a pair of wings and three pairs of legs. Each leg is provided with a pair of pads which enables the fly to walk on highly polished surfaces. The legs and the body are covered with numerous short and stiff hairs, called the *tenent hairs* which secrete a sticky substance. (3) ABDOMEN : The abdomen is segmented and shows light and dark markings.

Life history

The housefly undergoes a complete metamorphosis with four stages in its life cycle : egg, larva (maggot), pupa and adult (Fig. 3).

(1) EGG : The female lays from about 120 to 150 eggs at one sitting in moist decaying organic matter such as human and animal excreta, manure heaps, garbage and vegetable refuse. The Indian *M. domestica* and *M. vicinia* breed profusely in human excreta. The eggs are pearly-white in colour and about 1 mm long. They can be readily seen by the naked eye. The fly lays from 600 to 900 eggs during her life time. The eggs hatch in 8 to 24 hours; during summer, in India, they may hatch within 3 hours. (2) LARVA : The larvae or maggots measure 1 to 2 mm in length at birth. They are white, segmented and footless with a narrow anterior end, and a broad posterior end. They eat voraciously and moult twice in the course of development. The full grown larva may measure up to 12 mm in length. The larvae resent light; they bury themselves under manure heaps. When about to pupate, they migrate to dry outer regions. The larval period lasts from 2 to 7 days, but this stage may be prolonged in cold weather. (3) PUPA : The pupa are dark-brown and barrel shaped and measure about quarter of an inch. The pupal stage in the tropics occupies 3 to 6 days. In winter months, the pupal stage may be considerably prolonged. (4) ADULT : The complete life cycle from egg to adult may take 5 to 6 days during summer in India, but at other times it may take 8 to 20 days. Flies do not generally live longer than 15 days in summer and 25 days during winter.

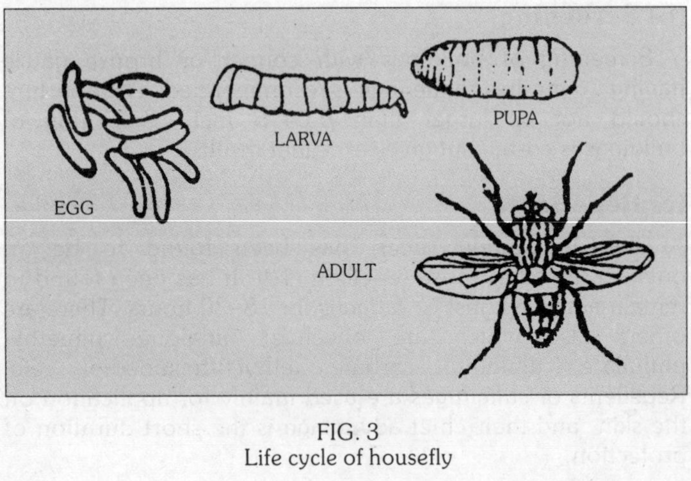

FIG. 3
Life cycle of housefly

Habits

The habits of housefly make it eminently suited for the spread of disease. (1) BREEDING HABITS : The most important breeding places of flies in order of importance are (a) fresh horse manure (b) human excreta (c) manure of other animals (d) garbage (e) decaying fruits and vegetables (f) rubbish dumps containing organic matter and (g) ground where liquid wastes are spilled. (2) FEEDING HABITS : The housefly does not bite. It is attracted to food by its sense of smell. It cannot eat solid foods; it vomits on solid food to make a solution of it and sucks in a liquid state. Adult flies delight in sputum, faeces, discharges from wounds and open sores. (3) RESTLESSNESS : The fly is a restless insect and moves back and forth between food and filth. This helps in the spread of infection mechanically. (4) VOMIT DROP : The fly vomits frequently. The "vomit drop" is often a culture of disease agents. (5) DEFECATION : The housefly has the habit of defecating constantly all the day. Thus it deposits countless bacteria on exposed food. (6) RESTING HABITS : Flies have a tendency to rest on vertical surfaces and hanging objects. They have a tendency to fly towards light. (7) DISPERSAL : Normally houseflies remain close to their breeding places, but they disperse frequently up to 4 miles, and sometimes even more from the point of their origin.

Transmission of disease

Flies are potential vectors of many diseases : typhoid and paratyphoid fevers, diarrhoeas and dysenteries, cholera, and gastroenteritis, amoebiasis, helminthic infestations, poliomyelitis, conjunctivitis, trachoma, anthrax, yaws, in fact, most diseases that can be spread by mechanical transmission.

Flies transmit disease in the following ways : (1) MECHANICAL TRANSMISSION : Houseflies are exceptionally efficient mechanical spreaders of disease. They transport microorganisms on their feet and hairy legs. Pathogenic organisms, ova and cysts have been recovered from the bodies of the common housefly. Houseflies are therefore called "porters of infection". (2) VOMIT DROP : The regurgitated stomach contents or "vomit drop" is a rich bacterial culture. By its habit of frequent vomiting, the housefly infects food and thereby transmits disease. (3) DEFECATION : The excrement of housefly has been found to contain numerous microorganisms as well as cysts and ova of intestinal parasites. By its habit of constant defecation, the housefly spreads these diseases.

FLY CONTROL MEASURES

1. Environmental control

The best way to control houseflies is to eliminate their breeding places and to bring about an overall improvement in the environmental sanitation on a community-wide basis. This, in effect, implies the following : (1) storing garbage, kitchen wastes and other refuse in bins with tight lids, pending disposal. (2) efficient collection, removal and disposal of refuse by incineration, composting or sanitary landfill. (3) provision of sanitary latrines, e.g., pit privies, septic tanks, water-seal latrines and sanitary system. (4) stopping open air defecation. (5) sanitary disposal of animal excreta, and (6) stepping up general sanitation. A clean house with clean surroundings is the best answer to the fly problem.

2. Insecticidal control *(17,18)*

(1) RESIDUAL SPRAYS : Since it first showed resistance to DDT in 1948, *M. domestica* has developed resistance to the other organo-chlorine compounds as well as to organophosphorus and carbamate pesticides. Susceptible flies may be killed by DDT (5%), methoxychlor (5%), lindane (0.5%), or chlordane (2.5%) sprayed at about 5 litres per 100 square metres of surface; for flies resistant to these, diazinon (2%) dimethoate (2.5%), fenthion (2.5%), malathion (5%), or ronnel (5%) may be used. The addition of sugar to insecticidal formulations enhances their effectiveness. Special care should be taken to prevent contamination of food or water during spraying operations. (2) BAITS : Baits may be solid or liquid. Poisoned baits containing 1 or 2 per cent diazinon, malathion, dichlorvos, ronnel and dimethoate have been tried with success. Liquid baits containing 0.1 to 0.2 per cent of the same insecticides and 10 per cent sugar water have given good results. The cheapest bait is one that is made by mixing 3 teaspoons of commercial formalin with one pint of water or milk to which is added a little sugar, (3) CORDS AND RIBBONS : Cords and strips impregnated with diazinon, fenthion, or dimethoate have been tried with success. These are hung like festoons from ceilings. The period of effectiveness ranges from 1 to 6 months. (4) SPACE SPRAYS : Space sprays containing pyrethrin and DDT or HCH are available commercially. These may be applied indoors or outdoors using hand or power sprayers. Space sprays in general have little or no residual action. They produce only a temporary effect on adult fly populations; consequently, repeated applications are necessary. (5) LARVICIDES: Insecticides such as 0.5% diazinon, 2% dichlorovos, 2% dimethoate or 1% ronnel applied at the rate of 28–56 litres per 100 sq. metres have been used for the treatment of fly breeding places, but it is found that they cause or accelerate the development of resistance. In summary, it may be stated that insecticides, at best, are only a supplement, but not a substitute for sanitation.

3. Fly papers

Sticky fly papers are useful adjuncts to other methods of control. These papers can be easily made by mixing 2 lbs of resin and one pint of castor oil which should be heated together until the mixture resembles molasses. This should, while hot, be smeared on paper by using an ordinary paint brush. The adhesive mixture can also be applied to strips of wire and hung up in places where flies abound. Although a slight reduction of flies may occur, no lasting benefits will result from the use of fly papers.

4. Protection against flies

Screening of houses, hospitals, food markets, restaurants and all other similar establishments will give considerable relief from houseflies. Screens with 14 meshes to the inch will keep out houseflies but finer screens will also keep out the other insects. Screening is expensive for general use.

5. Health education

It is difficult to achieve fly control without the willing co-operation of the people. A "fly consciousness" should be created among the people, through health education. Fly control campaigns require *organized individual* and *community effort* which is the basis of a successful public health programme. It is only through health education that people can be motivated with a desire to get rid of flies permanently.

SANDFLIES

Sandflies are small insects, light or dark-brown in colour. They are smaller than mosquitoes, measuring 1.5 to 2.5 mm in length with their bodies and wings densely clothed with hair. Some 30 species of sandflies have been recorded in India. The important ones are : *Phlebotomus argentipes, P. papatasii, P. sergenti,* and *Sergentomyia punjabensis.* Our knowledge of the Indian sandflies is meagre, and needs more studies *(19)*.

General characters

The body of a sandfly is divided into head, thorax and abdomen, (1) HEAD : The head bears a pair of long, slender and hairy antennae; palpi and a proboscis. Only the females bite, the males live on vegetable juices. (2) THORAX : The thorax bears a pair of wings and three pairs of legs. The wings are upright, lanceolate in shape and densely hairy. The second longitudinal vein on the wings branches twice, the first branching takes place in the middle of the wing. This is a characteristic feature of the genus, Phlebotomus. The legs are long and slender and out of proportion to the size of the body. (3) ABDOMEN : The abdomen has 10 segments and is covered with hair. In the female, the tip of the abdomen is rounded; in the male, there are claspers, which are conspicuous and attached to the last abdominal segment.

Sandflies may be distinguished from mosquitoes by the following characteristics : (1) *Size :* Sandflies are smaller than mosquitoes. (2) *Wings :* The wings of the sandfly are up-right and lanceolate in shape; the second longitudinal vein branches twice, the first branching taking place in the middle of the wing. (3) *Legs :* The legs of the sandfly are longer compared with the size of the body. (4) *Hairs :* Sandfly is a hairy insect. (5) *Hopping:* Sandflies hop about, and do not fly by choice.

Life history

The life history of the sandfly is characterised by complete metamorphosis, having four stages : egg, larva, pupa and adult (Fig. 4).

(1) EGG : The eggs are laid in damp dark places in the vicinity of cattle sheds and poultry. The eggs are comparatively large, and torpedo-shaped with longitudinal wavy lines on the outside. The eggs hatch within 7 days. (2) LARVA : The larvae are hairy maggots with a distinct head, thorax and abdomen. The last abdominal segment carries two pairs of long stout hairs; one pair is remarkably long. The larva feeds on decaying organic matter and becomes a pupa in about 2 weeks. (3) PUPA : The pupal stage lasts for about 1 week. (4) ADULT : The average life of a sandfly is about 2 weeks.

Habits

Sandflies are troublesome nocturnal pests. Their bite is irritating and painful, while their presence is scarcely observed. They infest dwellings during night, and take shelter during day in holes and crevices in walls, holes in trees, dark rooms, stables and store rooms. The females

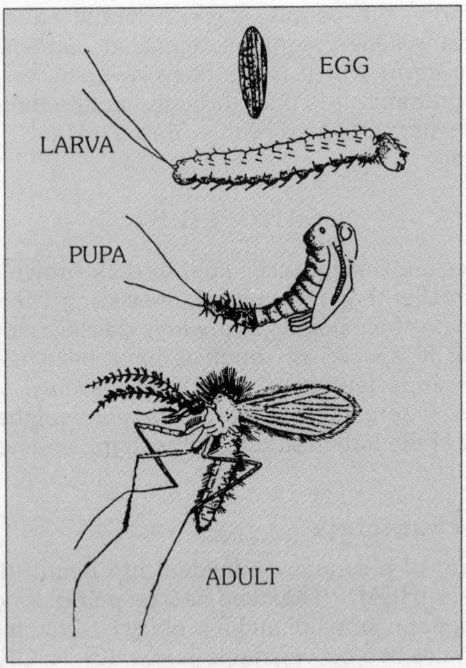

FIG. 4
Life cycle of a sandfly

alone bite, as they require a blood meal every third or fourth day for oviposition. Sandflies are incapable of flying over long distances; they merely hop about from one place to another. Sandflies are generally confined to within 50 yards of their breeding places.

Diseases transmitted

SPECIES	DISEASES CARRIED
Phlebotomus argentipes	Kala-azar
Phlebotomus papatasii	Sandfly fever
	Oriental sore
Phlebotomus sergenti	Oriental sore
S. punjabensis	Sandfly fever

Control of sandflies

Sandflies are easily controlled because they do not move long distances from the place of their breeding. (1) INSECTICIDES : Resistance to DDT has not been demonstrated. A single application of 1 to 2 g/m^2 of DDT or 0.25 g/m^2 of lindane has been found effective in reducing sandflies. DDT residue may remain effective for a period of 1 to 2 years, and lindane only for a period of 3 months *(17)*. Spraying should be done in the human dwellings, cattle sheds and other places. (2) SANITATION : Sanitation measures such as removal of shrubs and vegetation within 50 yards of human dwellings, filling up cracks and crevices in walls and floors, and location of cattle sheds and poultry houses at a fair distance from human habitations should receive attention.

TSETSE FLIES

Tsetse flies or the Glossina are bloodsucking flies, which present a general resemblance to the common housefly. They are yellow or dark-brown in colour, and measure about half an inch long. Their wings, when folded, overlap each other like the blades of a scissors. They have a proboscis which is rigid and non-retractile and adapted for piercing the skin and sucking blood. Tsetse flies are only found in African continent. Regions infested with tsetse flies are called "fly belts". For centuries, the tsetse fly has ravaged vast areas of tropical Africa, and hampered economic and social progress; it continues to be a menace even today.

Life history

The life history of the tsetse fly is somewhat abnormal. The female does not lay eggs, but gives birth to a living larva, one at a time, at 10–day intervals. The female produces only a few offspring in its life time. Soon after birth the larva crawls away to a suitable place and buries itself in the earth, usually at a depth of an inch or so beneath the surface. Pupation then takes place, within a few hours. The pupal stage lasts for 20–40 days. At the end of the pupal stage, the adult fly emerges. The tsetse lives less than 100 days.

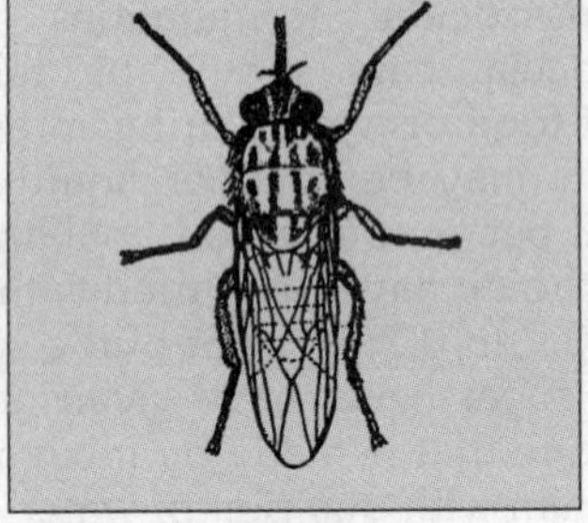

FIG. 5
Tsetse fly

Species and habits

More than 30 species of the *Glossina* have been recognised, but only four species are dangerous to man. They are : *G.palpalis, G.tachinoides, G.morsitans,* and *G.pallidepes.* The first two species are sometimes called "riverine species" because they inhabit the woodland vegetation near water courses; the latter two are called "savannah species" because they prefer to live and breed in woodland vegetation in savannah country.

Tsetse flies attack man, animals, wild game of all kinds, birds, lizards and snakes. Both the sexes bite, mainly during day. The riverine species (e.g., *G. palpalis* and *G. tachinoides*) have a distinct attraction to man; the savannah species prefer to feed on game rather than man. Tsetse flies rarely enter houses, but they are known to follow travellers both by road and rail for considerable distance in order to obtain a blood meal. Tsetse flies are vectors of trypanosomiasis or "sleeping sickness". The disease affects man, domestic animals and wildgame – being particularly lethal to man, and his domestic stock.

Control of tsetse flies

There are four main techniques in the control of tsetse flies : (1) INSECTICIDES : Resistance to insecticides has not been reported in *Glossina*. At present, DDT (25%) and dieldrin (18–20%) are the most commonly used pesticides for tsetse fly control *(17)*. The insecticide is applied from aircraft when large areas are to be covered quickly. (2) CLEARING OF VEGETATION : Clearing of vegetation where tsetse flies live and breed is now the technique most widely adopted for controlling tsetse flies. Used alone, this method gives slow results, but in conjunction with the application of residual insecticides, it has given a speedy reduction of flies. (3) GAME DESTRUCTION : Large tracts of Africa have been cleared of the tsetse flies by the destruction of wild game. This method is now given up. (4) GENETIC CONTROL : Currently, research is centred round genetic control of tsetse flies using the "sterile male release" technique *(20)*.

BLACKFLIES

Blackflies or *Simuliidae* are small robust flies with short stout legs, large broad wings and a short proboscis (Fig. 6). They are very often all black. *Simulum indicum* is the Indian species *(21)*. Blackflies attack domestic animals and man and suck blood. They are vectors of onchocerciasis in Africa, Mexico, and Central and South America. The eggs are laid on submerged stones and water weeds. The larvae are aquatic; they fix themselves to stones or plants, usually at a depth of 1 foot. The larval stage occupies 3 to 4 weeks. They pupate in water; the pupal stage occupies 1 to 3 weeks. In India, *Simuliidae* breed in hill streams. Control of the adult fly is difficult, because the range of the fly is about 100 miles. Therefore, the attack is levelled at the larvae. Abate is used which kills the blackfly larvae without causing harmful effects to mammals or other aquatic fauna. It is added to river water in weekly doses of 0.05 to 0.1 mg/litre over a period of 10 minutes *(22)*.

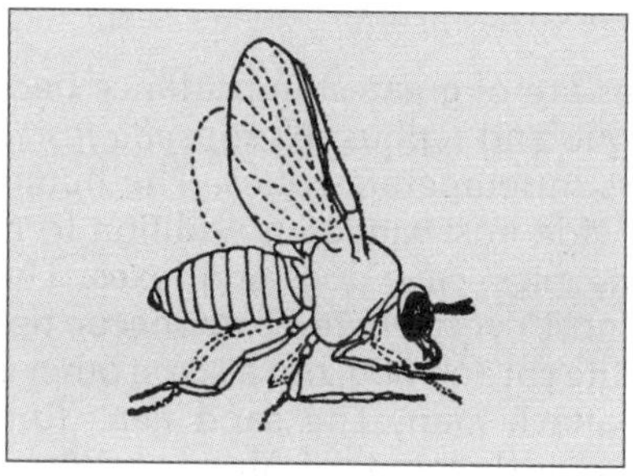

FIG. 6
Simulum

LICE

Lice are small wingless ectoparasites of mammals and birds. They bite severely and are annoying pests. The lice that infest man are of three kinds : head louse (*Pediculus capitis*), body louse (*Pediculus corporis*), and pubic or crab louse (*Phthirus pubis*). Human lice occur in all parts of the world wherever standards of hygiene are low, but people in colder climates are affected more frequently than those in warmer regions. Infestation by lice is called *pediculosis.*

Head and body lice

The head and body lice differ very little in structure except in their habitat. The head lice inhabit the hairs of the scalp, and the body lice occur mainly in the seams of clothing and on the bodies of the hosts. The body of a louse is flattened dorso-ventrally, and is divided into head, thorax and abdomen. (1) HEAD : The head is pointed in front and bears a pair of 5-jointed antennae. The mouth parts are adapted for sucking blood. (2) THORAX : The thorax is a fused mass and is shaped somewhat like a square. Three pairs of legs are attached ventrally to the thorax. The legs are strongly developed and are provided with claws which help the insect to cling to the hair and clothing. (3) ABDOMEN : The abdomen is elongated and consists of 9 segments. The last abdominal segment is pointed in the case of males, and bilobed in the case of females.

Life history

There are three stages in the life history of lice : egg, larva and adult. Metamorphosis is gradual (Fig. 7).

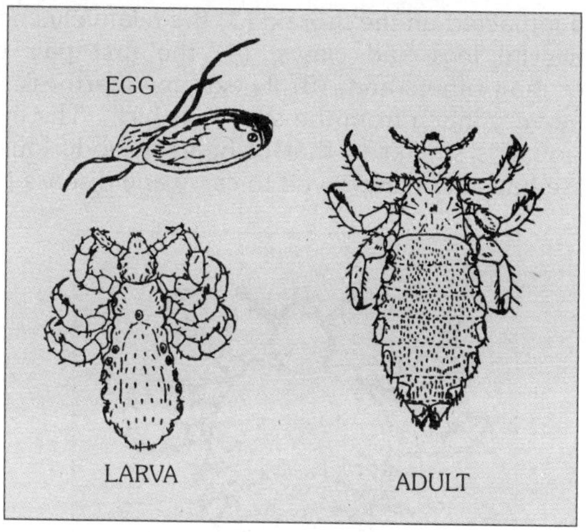

FIG. 7
Life cycle of a louse

(1) EGG : The eggs, called "nits" are laid singly or in groups, firmly attached to the hair or seams of clothing by a cementing substance. The eggs are small, white ovoid bodies, pointed at one end and truncated and pitted at the other end. A female lays up to 300 eggs, at the rate of 4 to 9 eggs a day. Under favourable conditions of temperature, the eggs will hatch in 6 to 9 days. The eggs will not hatch if the temperature is below 22 deg. C (71.6 deg.F). (2) LARVA OR NYMPH : The larva looks very much like an adult, except for its smaller size. It feeds on the host and develops into an adult after passing through 3 moults. The larval stage may take 10 to 15 days. (3) ADULT : The entire life cycle from the laying of an egg to the appearance of the adult louse takes about 15 to 17 days under favourable conditions. Adult lice lives from 30 to 50 days.

Dissemination

(1) DIRECT CONTACT : Lice are disseminated by close contact with lousy or infested persons. Overcrowding provides an excellent opportunity for the direct transference of lice from one person to another. Children get easily infested at school when their heads come together at work or play. (2) INDIRECT CONTACT : Lice may also be acquired from clothing, bedding, combs or brushes used by lousy persons. Lice have been seen to be blown by puffs of wind from heavily infested persons. Lice tends to leave the host whose temperature rises above or falls below the normal.

Lice and disease

Lice are vectors of the following diseases :

DISEASE		CAUSATIVE AGENT
1. Epidemic typhus	.....	Rickettssia prowazeki
2. Relapsing fever	.....	Borrelia recurrentis
3. Trench fever	.....	Rickettssia quintana
4. Dermatitis	.....	Due to scratching and secondary infection

Crab louse

The crab louse or pubic louse (*Phthirus pubis*) is generally found in the pubic and perineal region, but at times it may occur in the other parts of the body as well. It adheres close to the skin, and its removal is a matter of difficulty. The crab louse has a characteristic body form, and is readily recognized by (1) its small size and square body,

(2) head impacted on the thorax, (3) the relatively enormous and powerful legs and claws, (4) the first pair of legs slenderer than others and, (5) its extreme inertness. It does not move very much from the site of its birth. The life cycle of crab louse is similar to that of head or body louse. The crab louse has not been proved to carry any disease (Fig. 8).

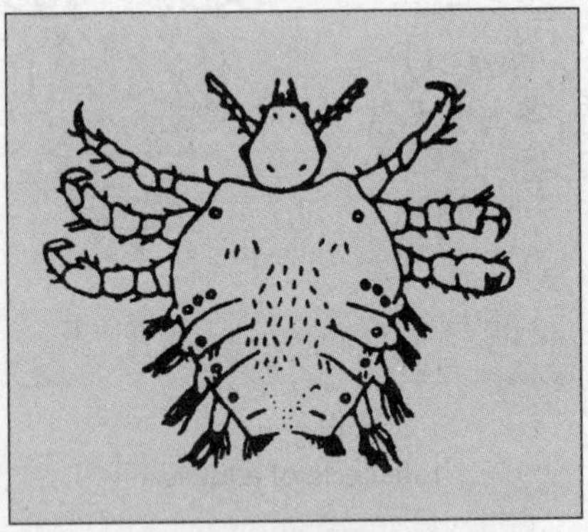

FIG. 8
Phthirus pubis

Control of lice *(17,18)*

(1) INSECTICIDAL CONTROL : Insecticides appear to be the only means at present for the control of lice. There are reports that lice have become resistant in many areas to DDT and HCH, and there are some reports of resistance to malathion. It is of utmost importance to monitor periodically louse susceptibility to insecticides to assess which insecticide should be used *(13)*. (a) *Head and crab lice :* The present recommended treatment is a lotion containing 0.5 per cent malathion. The lotion should be left on for 12 to 24 hours when the hair can be washed. Malathion, if correctly used, will kill lice and nits. Dust containing carbaryl is also effective as louse powder. (b) *Body Lice :* Since lice have become resistant to DDT and HCH, a powder containing 1 per cent malathion will obviously be the treatment of choice. Dust containing carbaryl may also be used. The powder is applied to the inner surface of the clothing as well as socks and the body of the persons. "Mass delousing" of large numbers of people is carried out with hand operated dusters. The powder is blown down the neck of the shirt, up the sleeves, and into the loosened trousers from several angles at the front and back. With this type of treatment, the clothing is not removed and about 50 g. (2 ozs.) of the insecticidal powder are required for one person. Normally a single application will eradicate an infestation, but a second application may be made in 7 days to kill late-hatching lice.

(2) PERSONAL HYGIENE : Delousing procedures should be accompanied by improvements in personal hygiene. Lice require very close contact with humans, frequent blood meals and a relatively constant temperature. They cannot survive in communities where people regularly bathe, change and launder their clothes. A daily bath with soap and water is essential in a country like India to prevent lice infestation. Women with long hair should wash and clean their hair frequently. Clothing, towels and sheets should be washed in hot water and soap and pressed with hot iron. Autoclaving of clothes and bedding in steam sterilizers may be required for body louse control. The long-term control policy should be based on improvement of personal hygiene, partly by simple health education and also by improving living standards.

FLEAS

Fleas are small, bilaterally compressed, wingless insects with a hard chitinous exoskeleton and covered with backwardly directed strong bristles. They are blood sucking ecto-parasites of mammals and birds. The fleas found on one particular kind of animal host will not usually seek the blood of another species of animal, unless compelled by necessity.

Types of fleas

More than a thousand different species of fleas have been described; some 37 species are known to occur in India. The fleas of importance in public health are :

1.	Rat fleas *(Oriental)*	–	*Xenopsylla cheopis*
		–	*Xenopsylla astia*
		–	*Xenopsylla braziliensis*
2.	Rat fleas *(Temperate zone)*	–	*Nosopsylla fasciatus*
3.	Human fleas	–	*Pulex irritans*
4.	Dog and cat fleas	–	*Ctenocephalus canis*
		–	*Ctenocephalus felis*
5.	Sand fleas *(Jigger or chigoe fleas)*	–	*Tunga penetrans*

The rat fleas are of greatest importance because they are vectors of plague and typhus. *Nosopsylla fasciatus* is rare in India; it occurs in temperate zones. The human flea, *Pulex irritans* has a wide host range; in addition to man, it infests commensal rats, pigs, cats, dogs and foxes. The *cat* and *dog fleas* occur almost everywhere. They occur not only on the specific hosts, the cat and dog, but also on other animals. They are prone to attack man. The sand flea, *Tunga penetrans* occurs in the tropical regions of Africa and America.

Rat fleas

The body of a flea is divided into head, thorax and abdomen. (1) HEAD : The head is conical in shape and is attached to the thorax without a neck. The head bears short, piercing mouth parts which are conspicuous and project downwards from the head. The mouth parts are adapted for piercing and sucking blood. (2) THORAX : The thorax is composed of three segments – the prothorax, mesothorax and metathorax. There are three pairs of strong legs attached to the thorax. The flea has no wings. (3) ABDOMEN : The abdomen consists of 10 segments. The sexes are easily distinguished. In the male, there is a coiled structure, the penis, in the abdomen. In the female, there is a short, stumpy structure, the *spermatheca*, in the posterior part of the abdomen. The shape of the *spermatheca* helps in the identification of the species.

Life history

There are four stages in the life history of fleas : egg, larva, pupa and adult. Metamorphosis is complete (Fig. 9).

(1) EGG : The eggs are small (0.5mm), ovoid and white in colour. They are deposited among the hairs of the animal host or in and near the nest or haunts of its host. A female may lay 300–400 eggs in its life time – 2 to 6 or even more at a time. The eggs hatch in 2 to 7 days, depending upon temperature. (2) LARVA : The larvae are small, legless caterpillars, whitish in colour, and bear sparse long hair on their bodies. They are found in the dust and debris, in on near the nests or lairs of the host. They feed on organic matter and the blood in the faeces of the adult flea. There are three larval stages; the last stage spins a cocoon, to which dust particles adhere. The duration of the larval stage is about 2 weeks. (3) PUPA : The

pupa develops inside the cocoon. The pupal stage lasts for 1 to 2 weeks, depending upon temperature and other environmental influences. (4) ADULT : The life cycle of a flea may be completed within 3 weeks, under favourable conditions. The fleas live normally for a month or so under tropical conditions. Infected fleas may live for one year, and certain species may survive in the burrow microclimate for as long as 4 years *(17)*.

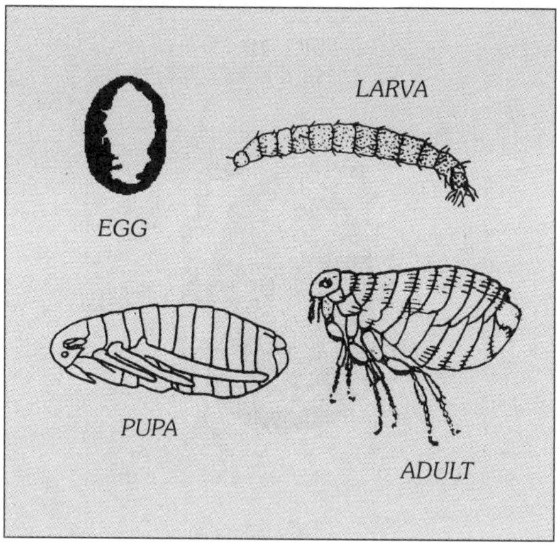

FIG. 9
Life cycle of rat flea

Habits

Fleas are found on their normal hosts and in the nests, burrows and lairs of their hosts. They are also found in the dwellings, on the ground, in cracks and crevices, and under carpets. Both the sexes bite and suck blood. They feed at frequent intervals, usually once a day and sometimes more often. Fleas cannot fly, but they are capable of making vertical jumps of about 4 inches when starved, and about 3 inches when gorged. The distance they can cover by horizontal jumps is less than 6 inches. Fleas are passively transported by (a) their hosts (b) transport vehicles (c) humans – on the person or in the luggage, and (d) the movement of goods like grain, raw cotton, gunny bags, rags and hides.

Flea indices

The following indices are used in flea surveys : (1) GENERAL FLEA INDEX : It is the average number of fleas of all species per rodent. (2) SPECIFIC FLEA INDEX : (*X.cheopis index; X.astia index, etc.*) It is the average number of fleas of each species, found per rodent. (3) PERCENTAGE INCIDENCE OF FLEA SPECIES : It is the percentage of fleas of each species, found per rodent. (4) RODENT INFESTATION RATE : It is the percentage of rodents infested with the various flea species.

Flea indices do not in themselves indicate an imminent plague epidemic. But flea indices serve as useful indicators of the potential explosiveness of the situation, should a plague outbreak occur in an endemic area *(23)*. Specific flea indices are more significant than are overall flea indices.

Fleas and human disease

Fleas are known to transmit the following diseases : (1) Plague (bubonic), (2) Endemic or murine typhus, (3) Chiggerosis, and (4) Hymenolepis diminuta.

MODE OF TRANSMISSION : Fleas convey disease by (1) *Biting* : The chief method of transmission, in the case of plague, is by the bite of hungry 'blocked' fleas. Some fleas which ingest plague bacilli become blocked due to the multiplication of plague bacilli in their proventriculus or stomach. Fleas affected in this way are called 'blocked' fleas. The blockage of the food passage renders the flea unable to obtain further blood feeds. Because of hunger, the flea begins to bite more ferociously and makes frantic efforts to suck blood. Each time it bites, instead of sucking blood, it injects plague bacilli into the wound. Such 'blocked' fleas play a great role in the spread of plague. (2) *Mechanical transmission* : Mechanical transmission takes place from the proboscis of the fleas, which had recently fed on an infected rodent. (3) *Faeces* : The fleas are apt to defecate while feeding. The faecal drop of infected fleas may contain numerous bacilli. When the host scratches over the flea-bitten area, there is direct inoculation of the infective agent into the angry spot.

Control of fleas *(17, 18)*

(1) INSECTICIDAL CONTROL : The cheapest and most widely used formulation has been 10 per cent DDT dust. As the rodents pass over the dust, they pick it up on their fur where it kills the fleas. In a number of plague areas, the rat fleas have developed resistance to DDT and/or to gamma-HCH and dieldrin. In such areas, carbaryl or diazinon (2%) or malathion (5%) should prove effective *(9)*. The sprays should be applied to floors and walls up to a height of about 1 ft. *Patch dusting* with insecticides has also been found to be an effective method of controlling fleas. The insecticidal powder is dusted over rat runs, under gunny bags, and other harbourage areas. The insecticidal dust should also be blown into the rodents' burrows with the help of dust-blowers at about 30 g. per burrow. Animal hosts like cats and dogs and their quarters and premises should also be treated with insecticidal dusts, sprays or dips. (2) REPELLENTS : Diethyltoluamide is an efficient flea repellent. Clothing impregnated with diethyltoluamide repels fleas for more than a week. Benzyl benzoate is also a good flea repellent. (3) RODENT CONTROL : Flea control should be followed by rodent control. This subject is treated elsewhere in this chapter.

SAND FLEA

Sand fleas occur in the tropical regions of Africa and America. They are also known as Jigger or Chigoe fleas. Of particular importance is the sand flea, *Tunga penetrans*. The fertilized female burrows into the skin of the feet, often beneath the nail and causes ulcers. Tetanus and gas gangrene frequently occur because of secondary infection. *T. penetrans* has been recorded in the western parts of India; it has not yet been able to gain foothold in India. It flourishes best in sandy soil. Its hosts are usually domestic animals (Fig. 10).

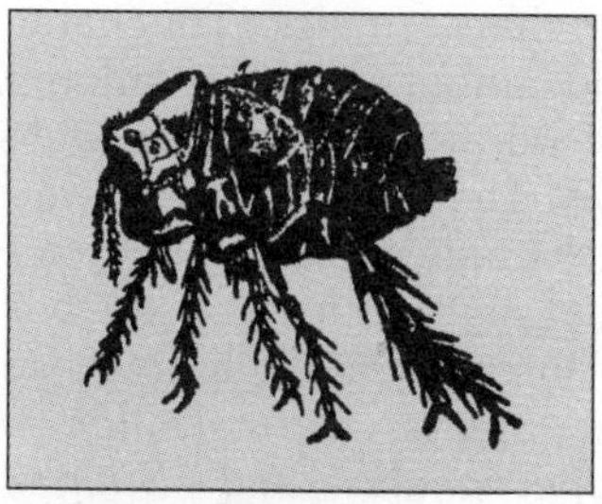

FIG. 10
Sand flea

REDUVIID BUGS

Reduviid bugs, also known as cone-nose bugs, are vectors of Chagas' disease in Mexico and Central and South America. All are of large size, about an inch or more in length. Adults have wings. These bugs live exclusively on the blood of animals including man and transmit *Trypanosoma cruzi,* the causative agent of Chagas' disease. These bugs occur in India *(21),* but are not incriminated in the transmission of any disease. These bugs frequently attack man and their bites may cause intense itching, nausea, flushed face, palpitation of the heart, etc. (Fig. 11).

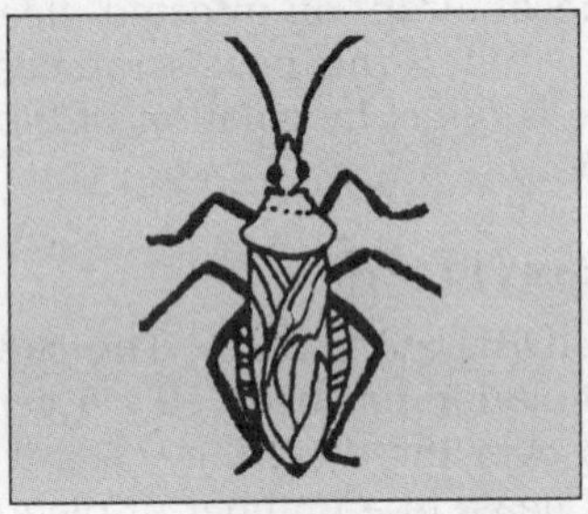

FIG. 11
Reduviid bug

Reduviid bugs live in cracks, fissures and other hiding places in walls and ceilings of human dwellings and in animal habitations and nests. They emerge only to feed and then retreat into their hiding places. Where housing is primitive, conditions may be ideal for these bugs. Residual spraying with HCH (0.5 g/m^2 or dieldrin (1 g/m^2) is commonly used for control of these bugs *(17).*

TICKS AND MITES

Ticks and mites comprise one of the largest and most important orders (acarina) of the phylum Arthropod. They are ectoparasites of vertebrate animals, and they all suck blood.

Ticks

Ticks are of two kinds : hard ticks (*ixodidae*) and soft ticks *(argasidae)*

The body of a tick is oval in shape and is not distinctly separated into head, thorax and abdomen. They have four pairs of legs, and no antennae. The hard ticks are covered on their dorsal surface by a chitinous shield, called scutum , this in the male covers the entire back, and in the female only a small part in front. The scutum or dorsal shield is absent in soft ticks. Hard ticks have a "head" or capitulum at anterior end; soft ticks have a head on underside, which is entirely invisible from above (Fig. 12 & 13). The males are generally smaller than females. The hard ticks feed both night and day and cannot stand starvation; the soft ticks, on the other hand, feed at night and can withstand starvation for several months. The hard ticks are always found on their hosts; the soft ticks hide in cracks and crevices during the day and emerge at night to feed on the host. The common hard ticks which infest domestic animals such as dogs and cattle in India are : *Dermacentor, Haemophysalis, Hyalomma, Rhipecephalus* and *Boophilus.* From the medical standpoint, the soft tick of importance is *Ornithodorus moubata,* which transmits relapsing fever.

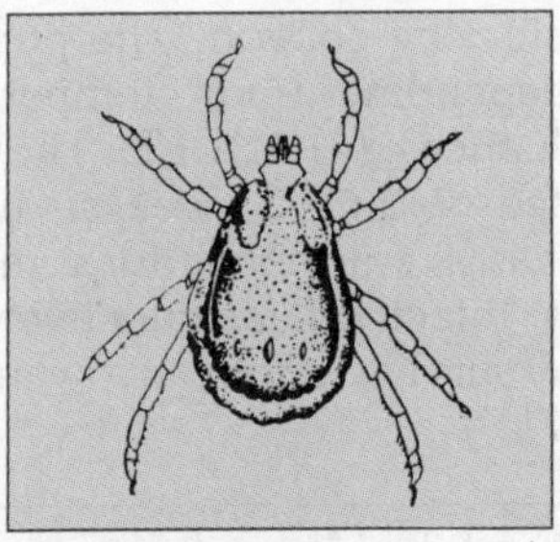

FIG. 12
Hard tick

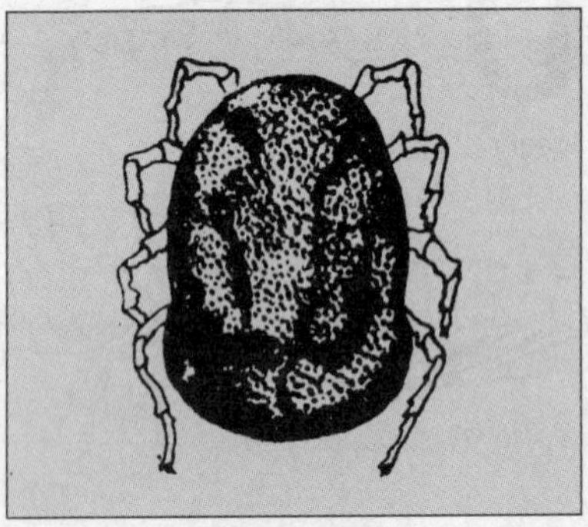

FIG. 13
Soft tick

Life history

There are four stages in the life history of ticks; egg, larva, nymph and adult. (1) EGG : Hard ticks lay eggs in a few hundreds or even thousands, all at one time, after which the female is exhausted and dies. The soft ticks lay eggs in batches of 20 to 100 over a long period. The eggs are deposited on the ground and hatch in 1 to 3 weeks. (2) LARVA : The larva of the tick possesses 3 pairs of legs. It lies in wait among grass and herbiage till a suitable host appears to which it attaches itself. After a blood meal, it drops off, and in course of time it moults to become a nymph. The duration of the larval stage may vary from 3 to 13 days. (3) NYMPH : The nymph resembles the adult in having 4 pairs of legs, but it has no genital pore. The nymphs are all blood suckers, and they attach themselves to suitable hosts for a blood meal. There are 5 nymphal stages in the life history of soft ticks. (4) ADULT : The duration of the life cycle from egg to adult is about 2 months in the case of hard ticks, and from 9 to 10 months in the case of soft ticks. Adult ticks may live for a year or more. Soft ticks live longer than hard ticks.

Public health importance

Hard ticks transmit the following diseases :

(a) Tick typhus (Rocky mountain spotted fever)
(b) Viral encephalitis (e.g., Russian spring-summer encephalitis)
(c) Viral fevers (e.g., Colorado tick fever)
(d) Viral haemorrhagic fevers (e.g. KFD in India)
(e) Tularaemia
(f) Tick paralysis, and
(g) Human babesiosis

Soft ticks transmit :

(a) Q fever
(b) Relapsing fever, and
(c) KFD

The tick attaches itself to its host by means of its mouth parts. The rostrum is burrowed into skin to enable it to suck blood. At the same time saliva is secreted, which contains a neurotoxin. Mature ticks, especially gravid female ticks, may remain attached for a comparatively long time but the male usually drops off the body after a few days. As the tick feeds, it gradually becomes engorged with blood.

Ticks transmit disease by biting; The larva and nymph are also capable of transmitting disease by biting (i.e., infection is maintained transstadially). Experiments have also shown transovarian transmission of infection through successive generations.

Hard and soft ticks compared

Hard and soft ticks are compared as shown in Table 8.

TABLE 8
Comparison of hard and soft ticks

	Hard ticks (Ixodidae)	Soft ticks (Argasidae)
1. Scutum	Covers the entire back in males; only a small portion in front in females	Absent
2. Head	Situated at anterior end	Lies ventrally; not seen from above
3. Spiracles	Situated behind IV coxa	Situated between III and IV coxa
4. Eggs	Several hundreds or thousands laid at one sitting	Laid in batches of 20–100 over a long period
5. Nymphal stages	One	Five
6. Habits	Cannot stand starvation; feed night and day	Can stand starvation for a year or more
7. Diseases transmitted	Tick typhus Viral encephalitis Haemorrhagic fever Tularaemia Tick paralysis Human babesiosis	Relapsing fever
8. Important species	*Dermacentor andersoni* *Haemophysalis spinigera*	*Ornithodorus moubata*

Mites (Chiggers)

Mites (chiggers) resemble ticks in their general appearance, having 4 pairs of legs and a body not well demarcated into head, thorax and abdomen. From the public health standpoint, two mites are important; (1) the trombiculid mite, and (2) the itch mite (*Acarus scabiei*).

TROMBICULID MITES

These are spider-like arthropods. The important species are *Leptotrombidium deliense* and *L. akamushi* which are vectors of scrub typhus in Asia and South Pacific.

Life History

The *life history* of a mite consists of 4 stages (Fig. 14) : egg, larva nymph and adult. (1) EGG : Eggs are laid singly; they hatch in about a week. (2) LARVA : The larva is very small, pale orange in colour, and has 3 pairs of legs. It attacks vertebrate hosts (rodents or man). When gorged with blood, it drops down to the ground for moulting. The larval stage lasts for 1 to 2 weeks. (3) NYMPH : The nymph is brick-red in colour and has 4 pairs of legs. It lives on vegetable juices. The nymphal stage lasts for 1 to 3 weeks. (4) ADULT : The adult male lives in soil. It has 4 pairs of legs, the first pair being the largest. The mite lives for about 6 months.

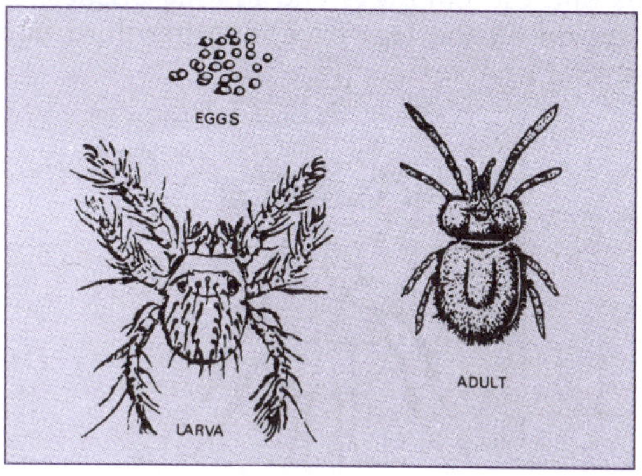

Fig. 14
Life cycle of a mite

Control of ticks and mites

(1) INSECTICIDAL CONTROL : Great success has been obtained in destroying ticks and mites by the use of modern insecticides. DDT, chlordane, dieldrin, lindane, malathion and toxaphane at rates of 1 to 2 lbs per acre give effective control. Either dusting or spray formulations can be employed. A thorough knowledge of the habits of a given species of tick must be obtained before planning a control programme. Animals like dogs may be freed of ticks by treating them with insecticidal sprays or dusts. Not only the animals, but also the premises which they frequent should be treated with insecticides (2) ENVIRONMENTAL CONTROL : Cracks and crevices in ground particularly near buildings and paths should be filled up. Animal hosts such as wild rodents and dogs should be reduced. (3) PROTECTION OF WORKERS : Exposed workers should be encouraged to wear protective clothing impregnated with an insect-repellent. The best repellents against ticks and mites are indalone, diethyltoluamide and benzyl benzoate. Further, persons working in tick-infested areas should be trained to examine themselves for ticks both during the lunch hour and at the end of work and to remove promptly any ticks found on their person. This is achieved by painting the tick with petrol paraffin or a camel-hair brush with which the dead tick can be brushed off the skin *(25)*. It may be necessary to extract the head gently with forceps and in that event care should be taken not to break the mouth parts.

ITCH MITE

The discovery in 1687 of the itch mite marks scabies as the first disease of man with known cause *(26)*. The itch mite (*Sarcoptes scabiei* or *Acarus scabiei*) is an extremely small, globular arthropod just visible to the naked eye. The female parasite burrows into the epidermis where it breeds and causes the condition known as scabies or itch. Species of the genus *sarcoptes* also infest animals such as dog, cattle and horse. The human acarus is morphologically indistinguishable from the animal variety but it is quite distinct physiologically. Therefore, animal scabies cannot flourish on the human skin.

General description

The itch mite is just visible to the naked eye, measuring 0.4 mm in size and has a body shaped like a tortoise, rounded above and flattened below. The body shows no demarcation into cephalothorax or abdomen. The body surface is thrown into folds and is covered with short bristles. The parasite has two pairs of legs in front, and two pairs behind. The front legs end in long tubular processes known as suckers and the hind legs end in long bristles. The male has suckers on all the legs excepting the third pair, which distinguishes it from female (Fig. 15).

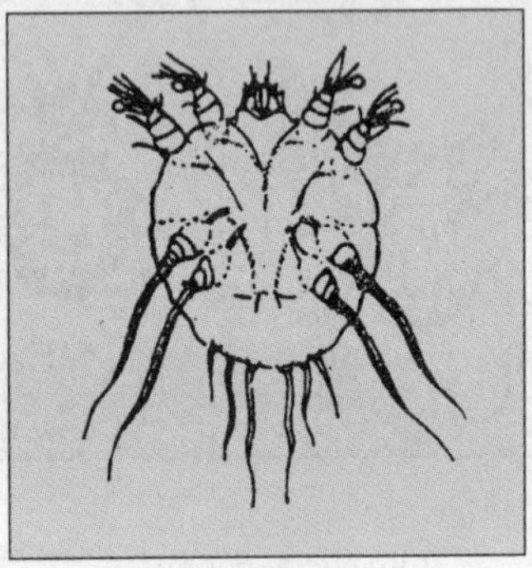

Fig. 15
Itch mite

Life history

There are four stages in the life history of an itch mite : egg, larva, nymph and adult. (1) EGG : The female burrows within the stratum corneum, and lays eggs in the burrow. A single female may lay up to 30 eggs at the rate of 2 to 3 per day, and ultimately dies at the end of the burrow. The eggs hatch into larvae in 3 to 4 days. (2) LARVA : The larvae are three legged. They leave the burrows, come to the surface and bore into the hair follicles where vesicles form. The larvae mature into nymphs in about 3 days. (3) NYMPH : The nymphs develop into adults in 6 to 8 days. (4) ADULT : The life cycle from egg to adult may take 10 to 15 days. The adult mites live for 1 to 2 months.

Mode of spread

(1) CLOSE CONTACT : Scabies is usually transmitted by close contact with an infested person. This is often due to sleeping in the same bed or by children playing with each other or nursing an infested person. Because of close contact, the disease tends to spread through families. Scabies is therefore called a familial or household infection. (2) CONTAMINATED CLOTHES : the disease may be acquired sometimes from contaminated clothes and bed linen.

Site of lesions

The disease classically affects the hands and wrist (63%), The extensor aspect of elbows being next (10.9%). The axillae, buttocks, lower abdomen, feet and ankles, palms in infants are all common sites of infestation. The disease also affects the breasts in women and the genitals in men.

Diagnosis of scabies

The main diagnostic features of scabies are : (1) the patient complains of itching which is worse at night, (2) examination reveals follicular lesions at the affected site, (3) secondary infection leads to crusted papules and pustules, (4) the diagnosis is probable if the other members of the household are affected, (5) confirmation of the diagnosis may be made by searching for the parasite in the skin debris under microscope.

Control of scabies

In the control of scabies, it is essential to treat all members of the affected household simultaneously whether or not they appear to be infested. Before commencing the treatment the patient is given a good scrub with soap and hot water. (1) BENZYL BENZOATE : Benzyl benzoate (25 per cent) is an effective sarcopticide. It should be applied with a paint brush or shaving brush to every inch of the body below the chin including the soles of the feet and allowed to dry. In the case of babies, the head must also be treated, The application should be repeated after 12 hours, and after a further 12 hours a bath given and all underclothes, clothes and sheets changed and washed. Not more than two applications of benzyl benzoate should be given per week as excessive use can cause an irritant dermatitis *(27)*. (2) HCH : 0.5 to 1.0 per cent strength of gamma-HCH (lindane) in coconut oil or any vegetable oil or vanishing cream is an efficient sarcopticide. The preparation should be rubbed on the affected parts of the skin on one or two occasions separated by an interval of 2 to 3 days. (3) TETMOSOL : A 5 per cent solution of tetmosol is also an efficient sarcopticide, three daily applications are recommended (4) SULPHUR OINTMENT : 2.5 to 10 per cent daily for 4 days is a cheap remedy.

CYCLOPS

Cyclops or water flea is a crustacean present in most collections of fresh water. It is a tiny arthropod, not more than 1 mm in length and just visible to the trained eye. It has a pear shaped semi-transparent body, a forked tail, 2 pairs of antennae, 5 pairs of legs and a small pigmented eye (Fig. 16). It swims in water with characteristic jerky movements. The average life of a cyclops is about 3 months.

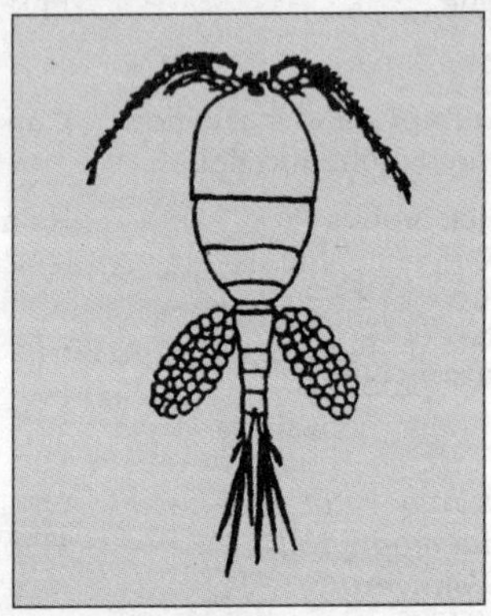

FIG. 16
Cyclops

Public health importance

(1) Cyclops is the intermediate host of Dracunculiasis or guinea-worm disease. Man acquires infestation by drinking water containing infected cyclops.

(2) Cyclops mediates also as one of the intermediate hosts of fish tape worm, *Diphyllobothrium latum* infestation. The disease is rare in India.

Control of cyclops

Cyclops may be controlled by the use of physical, chemical or biological methods *(29)*. (1) PHYSICAL : (a) *Straining :* Straining of water through a piece of fine cloth is sufficient to remove cyclops. (b) *Boiling :* Cyclops is readily killed by heat at 60°C. The physical methods are useful for individual prophylaxis. (2) CHEMICAL : (a) *Chlorine :* Chlorine destroys cyclops and larvae of guinea worm in a strength of 5 ppm. This high concentration of chlorine gives an objectionable smell and taste to drinking water. The excess chlorine needs to be removed by dechlorinating agents *(21)*. (b) *Lime :* Lime at a dosage of 4 gram per gallon of water is found to be very efficient for killing cyclops. (c) *Abate :* The organophosphorus insecticide, *Abate* (OMS – 786) has been found effective in killing cyclops at a concentration of 1 mg/litre *(30)*. This indicates that Abate is potentially useful in the chemical control of the guinea-worm infection. (3) BIOLOGICAL : Certain kinds of small fish, e.g., barbel fish and gambusia fish have been found to feed on cyclops. These fish were used successfully in eradicating guinea-worm in parts of Karnataka State *(31)*. The most satisfactory and permanent method of controlling cyclops in drinking water is to provide piped water supply or tube wells. Abolition of step wells and provision of sanitary wells should receive attention in rural areas.

INSECTICIDES

Insecticides are substances which are used to kill insects. The word pesticide is a general term that includes insecticides, fungicides rodenticides, herbicides, disinfectants, repellents, and other chemicals used for the control of pests. The control of arthropod borne diseases by insecticides is one of the greatest triumphs of public health during the 20th century. Insecticides have not only controlled malaria, plague, typhus and other diseases transmitted by insects, but also brought vast economic and social benefits through better health and increased food production.

Insecticides are classified into three groups : contact poisons, stomach poisons and fumigants. CONTACT POISONS are those which kill insects primarily by contact e.g., pyrethrum, DDT, HCH, dieldrin. STOMACH POISONS are those which when ingested cause the death of the insects, e.g., paris green, sodium fluoride. FUMIGANTS are those which give off vapours which have a lethal effect on the insects, e.g., sulphur dioxide. This classification is by no means a rigid one, because a contact poison can also be a stomach poison.

Most of the present day insecticides available for vector control (excluding inorganic chemicals and larvicidal oils) may be classified conveniently into 3 groups *(10)* :

Group I – *Organochlorine compounds :* DDT, HCH, dieldrin, chlordane, methoxychlor, etc.

Group II – *Organophosphorous compounds :* malathion, fenthion, chlorpyrifos, abate, etc.

Group III – *Carbamates :* Propoxur, carbaryl.

A detailed list of insecticides in public health use is given in Fig. 17. The problem of insecticide resistance and environmental contamination has restricted the use of many insecticides. A brief description of the insecticides in current use is given below :

1. DDT

DDT (Dichloro-diphenyl-trichloroethane) was first synthesized in 1874, by a German chemist, Ziedler. It was in 1939, its insecticidal properties were discovered by the Swiss scientist, Paul Muller. (a) PROPERTIES : DDT is a white

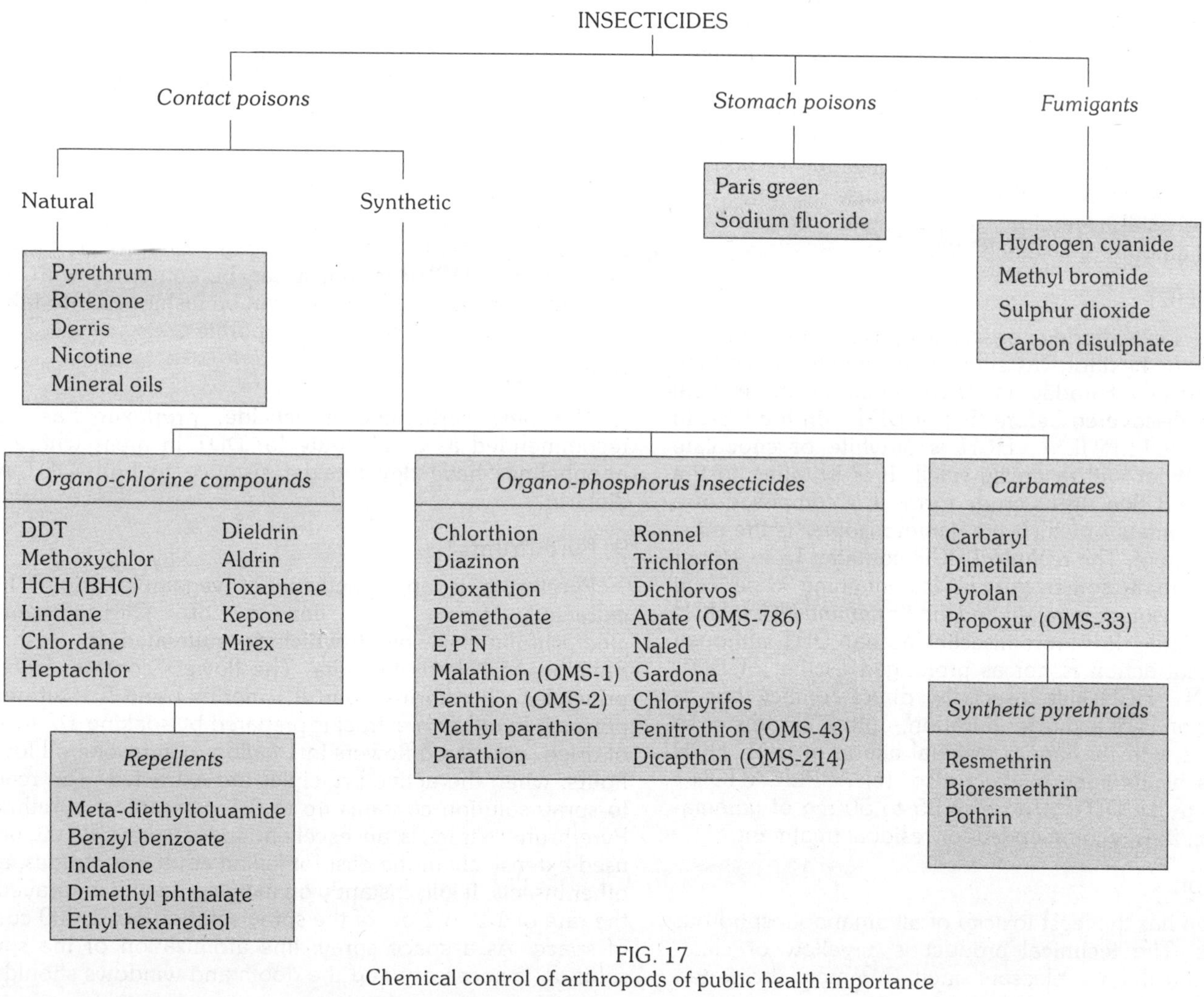

FIG. 17
Chemical control of arthropods of public health importance

amorphous powder with a mild, but not unpleasant smell. It is insoluble in water but dissolves in most organic solvents. The 'technical' DDT contains 70–80 per cent of the *Para, Para isomer,* which is the most active fraction of DDT. (b) ACTION : DDT is primarily a contact poison. It acts on the nervous system of insects. It permeates into the insect body through the cuticle, after dissolving in the waxy covering of the feet, and causes paralysis of legs and wings, convulsions and finally death. DDT does not cause immediate death, but it takes several hours to kill. The residual action of DDT may last as long as 18 months depending upon the treated surface. On mud walls, the prolonged action however, is decreased by absorption. DDT has no repellent action on insects. (c) APPLICATION : As a residual spray, DDT is applied at a dosage of 100–200 mg. per square foot area. The formulation of choice is a 5 per cent suspension of DDT, which when sprayed at a rate of 1 gallon over an area of 1,000 sq. feet, gives a dosage of 200 mg. per sq. ft. As a dust, DDT is used in 5 to 10 per cent strength for the control of lice, fleas, ticks and bugs. In aerosol or space sprays, DDT is one of the main constituents. DDT is still one of the most widely used insecticides.

In recent years DDT has earned the reputation of being an "environmental pollutant". Its persistence in the living organisms and plants and also its adverse effects on certain species of wild animals have led to the controversy on its use. Many developed countries (e.g., U.K., Sweden, Norway) have restricted the use of DDT because of its potential danger to ecosystems of wild life in the environment. But the benefits from the application of DDT in health programmes far outweigh the hazards. It has been responsible for saving millions of lives throughout the world. No toxic effects have been reported in the past 20 years among 200,000 spraymen employed in malaria campaigns nor among the 600 to 1,000 million people living in repeatedly sprayed houses. A WHO Expert Committee pointed out that "there is no valid reason to discontinue the use of DDT, for application in houses, against malaria or other diseases because its safety for human use still remains unchallenged despite the tremendous amount of research" *(32)*.

2. HCH (BHC)

Benzene hexachloride or hexachlorocyclo-hexane or gammexane or hexidol was synthesized much earlier than DDT by Michael Faraday in 1825. Even its insecticidal activity was discovered before that of DDT – in the USA in 1933. (a) PROPERTIES : HCH is a white or chocolate coloured powder with a musty smell. It is irritating to the eyes, nose and skin. In its crude form, it is composed of a number of isomers of which the *gamma isomer* is the most active constituent. The *technical* HCH contains 13 to 16 per cent of the gamma isomer. Pure HCH containing 99 per cent of the gamma isomer is called *lindane* or *gamma HCH*. HCH is slightly volatile. It is more insecticidal than DDT, although its insecticidal action is not as prolonged as that of DDT. (b) ACTION : HCH kills insects by direct contact, but its residual action is of a shorter duration, upto 3 months or so as compared with the longer residual action of DDT. HCH kills insects by its vapour effect also. (c) APPLICATION : HCH is used like DDT. A dose of 25 to 50 mg of gamma-HCH per sq. ft. is recommended for residual treatment.

3. Malathion

Malathion has the least toxicity of all organophosphorous compounds. The technical product is a yellow or clear-brown liquid with an unpleasant smell. Commercially, water-dispersible powders are available. Malathion is used in doses of 100–200 mg. per sq. ft., every 3 months. Because of its low toxicity, malathion has been recommended as an alternative insecticide to DDT. As a low volume (ULV) spray, malathion has been widely used for killing adult mosquitoes to prevent or interrupt dengue-haemorrhagic fever, and mosquito-borne encephalitis epidemics *(9)*.

4. Abate

Abate (Temephos) is an organophosphorus compound. It is a brown viscous liquid, soluble in petroleum solvents. Because of its low toxicity, it has been extensively used in India for the control of *A.stephensi* in wells and in domestic water containers with good results at a dosage not greater than 1.0 ppm. Abate is less effective as adulticide *(9)*.

5. Diazinon

Diazinon is a liquid product. Being volatile, it kills insects not only by direct contact, but also by fumigant action. It has proved effective in the control of DDT– resistant insects. At a dosage of 60 to 100 mg per sq. foot, it has given satisfactory control of flies and mosquitoes. Diazinon is more toxic to man than malathion or fenthion.

6. Fenthion

Fenthion or baytex is a brown liquid smelling slightly of garlic. It is practically insoluble in water. Water dispersible powders are available containing 20 to 40 per cent fenthion. Fenthion is found to be as effective as DDT. The usual dosage for residual sprays is 100 mg./sq ft. As a larvicide, fenthion is reported to be very powerful. Granules containing 2 per cent fenthion have been used in anti-larval work. The WHO Filariasis Research unit in Rangoon found fenthion, applied at the rate of 1 ppm, highly effective in controlling the larvae of *C. fatigans*.

7. Dichlorvos

Dichlorvos or DDVP is highly volatile liquid insecticide, which kills insects by fumigant action. It has been successfully used for disinfecting aircraft. A special advantage of DDVP is that it can be combined with solid substances such as wax, which can be fashioned into tablets or bricks from which it slowly evaporates.

8. Propoxur

The new carbamate insecticide, propoxur has been recommended as a substitute for DDT in areas where the anophelines have developed resistance to both DDT and dieldrin.

9. Pyrethrum

Pyrethrum is an insecticide of vegetable origin. It is extracted from the flowers of *Chrysanthemum cinerariifolium,* a plant which is cultivated in Kashmir, Shimla and Nilgiris in India. The flowers contain 4 active principles : Pyrethrins I and II, cinerins I and II – all nerve poisons. Pyrethrum extract is prepared by soaking 1/2 to 1 lb of dried, powdered flowers in 1 gallon of kerosene oil for 72 hours, when the active principles are extracted. The ready-to-spray solution contains up to 0.1 per cent of pyrethrins. Pyrethrum extract is an excellent space spray. It has been used extensively in the past for killing adult mosquitoes, and other insects. It kills instantly on mere contact. It is sprayed at the rate of 1/2 to 1 oz. of the spray solution per 1,000 cu. ft. of space. As a space spray, fine atomization of the spray solution is necessary and the doors and windows should be kept closed for 1/2 hour after spraying. Pyrethrum suffers from the disadvantage that it does not possess the residual action of DDT and other synthetic insecticides.

10. Pyrethrum and DDT

Most space sprays contain pyrethrum and DDT or other synthetic insecticides, which are added for synergistic action. The standard reference aerosol recommended by the WHO consists of (a) pyrethrum extract (25% pyrethrins) – 1.6 per cent, and (b) DDT technical – 3 per cent to be dispersed at the rate of 10 g. per 1,000 cu. ft. of space in the treatment of aircraft. About one-third of this dosage, 3.3 g. per 1,000 cu. ft. may be used for routine treatment of dwellings.

11. Synthetic pyrethroids

Synthetic pyrethroids are now being developed to replace natural pyrethrins. Some of the newly developed synthetic pyrethroids have been found to be as much as 10 times as effective as naturally occurring pyrethrins. Among the synthetic pyrethroids developed so far, tetramethrin, resethrin, prothrin and proparthin seem to be the most promising ones *(33)*.

12. Rotenone

Rotenone is obtained from the roots of a plant, *Derris elliptica*. The roots are dried and powdered and then are blended to give a rotenone content between 4 to 5 per cent and used as insecticidal dust. An extract of rotenone may be made in organic solvents such as chloroform. Rotenone was once widely used in the control of lice, fleas, mites and ticks.

13. Mineral oils

Oils such as kerosene, crude oil, malariol have been extensively used to kill mosquito larvae and pupae. Oils suffocate and poison the aquatic stages of the mosquito. The killing power of oil is increased greatly by the addition of DDT, HCH and other chemicals. Oils are injurious to vegetation and fish when improperly used.

14. Paris green

Paris green or copper acetoarsenite is an emerald green microcrystalline powder, practically insoluble in water but soluble in ammonia and concentrated acids. A good sample of paris green contains over 50 per cent of arsenious oxide. Paris green is a stomach poison. Till the advent of DDT, paris green was extensively used in the control of anopheline larvae, by spraying as a 2 per cent dust over breeding places once a week. The use of paris green was largely responsible for the eradication of *A. gambiae* from Brazil in 1940, and the near eradication of the same species in Egypt in 1944.

INSECTICIDE RESISTANCE

The widespread use of synthetic insecticides has given rise to the serious problem of insecticide resistance practically all over the world. The magnitude of the problem can be appreciated from the fact that, whereas in 1946 resistance to insecticides was reported in only 2 species of insects of public health importance, in 1962, the number rose to 81 species and in 1980 to 134. Evidence has accumulated to show that resistance in many vectors has been caused as a side effect of agricultural pesticide usage.

Resistance has been defined by WHO (1957) as "the development of an ability in strain of insects to tolerate doses of toxicants which would prove lethal to the majority of individuals in normal population of the same species" *(34)*. Resistance is due to *biochemical* and *genetic* factors. In the former, the toxicant is converted into a non-toxicant form in the body of the insect by various enzymes; in the latter, resistance is transmitted through genes, single or multiple.

A knowledge of insecticide resistance is important from the point of view of proper selection of insecticides. Generally speaking, organo-chlorine insecticide resistance is divided into two groups : resistance to DDT and its analogues; and the other to HCH-dieldrin group of insecticides. Resistance to DDT amounts to resistance to a number of DDT analogues such as methoxychlor, but not to HCH-dieldrin group. Similarly resistance to HCH amounts to resistance to dieldrin but not to DDT. Many insects now have developed "double resistance", that is, resistance to the two groups of organochlorine insecticides. When an insect develops resistance to DDT and HCH, the only effective action that can be taken is to change over to organo-phosphorus and carbamate insecticides. The change to organo-phosphorus and carbamate compounds involves substantial increase in cost, as these are all costly insecticides. Furthermore, cases of resistance towards them have already appeared. There is cross resistance between most carbamates and most organo-phosphorus compounds. To sum up, the problem of insecticide resistance which is growing in magnitude, is no doubt, steadily diminishing the choice of effective insecticides for vector control.

TOXICITY OF INSECTICIDES

1. Organo-chlorine compounds

DDT and its chemical relations are all nerve poisons. They increase the nervous excitability, and cause tremors and convulsions. Of the three commonly used compounds namely DDT, HCH and dieldrin, DDT is the least toxic. The median lethal dose for the humans is about 250 mg per kg. of body weight. Gamma HCH is about twice as toxic as DDT, and dieldrin is about 5 to 8 times as toxic as DDT. Dieldrin poisoning is met with more frequently than DDT or HCH poisoning : the reason is, dieldrin is absorbed through the skin whereas DDT and HCH are not absorbed through the skin in the solid state. TREATMENT : Poisoning with chlorinated hydrocarbons is treated with barbiturates, specially phenobarbitone. Stomach washouts are generally necessary, purgative may be useful but no oils or fats should be given.

2. Organophosphorus compounds and carbamates

These insecticides interfere with the mechanism of transmission of nerve impulses. They act by inhibiting cholinesterase, the enzyme which catalyses the degradation of acetyl choline in the synapse of striated muscle. Consequently there is accumulation of acetyl choline. The effects of poisoning are headache, giddiness, apprehension, restlessness, cold sweating, salivation, uncontrolled urination and defecation, unconsciousness and in extreme cases, ataxia and paralysis of respiratory centre. TREATMENT : Atropine is the specific antidote for poisoning by organo-phosphorus insecticides. It should be injected in doses of 1 to 2 mg intramuscularly and repeated if necessary at 30 minutes interval. Three more specific drugs are available at present – 2 PAM iodine, 2 PAM chloride, and P2S *(35)*. Atropine should be combined with one of these compounds. It is necessary that drugs be supplemented by other measures such as removal of the contaminated clothes, and washing of the exposed skin with soap and water.

Cases of poisoning due to organophosphorus compounds are on the increase in India. Those who are called upon to render First Aid and/or treat cases of pesticide poisoning would do well to refer to "Instructions for Safe use of Pesticides" issued by the Plant Protection Advisor to Government of India, Faridabad, Haryana wherein specific antidotes for groups of pesticides are given. The passing of "Indian Insecticide Act" by Parliament with a view to regulating the manufacture, transport, distribution, sale and use of pesticides is a step in the right direction.

A summary of treatment of poisoning with insecticides may be found in the WHO Publication "Safe Use of Pesticides" Technical Report Series No. 513 on page 52.

RODENTS

Rats and mice are part of man's environment. Often their numbers exceed human population. A female rat can have 100 offsprings each year. By living in close proximity to man, they not only cause substantial economic loss by damaging buildings, consuming and contaminating foodstuffs (36%) and other commodities, but also act as sources or reservoirs of some important communicable diseases such as plague and typhus fever. It implies therefore, that destruction of rats and elimination of their habitat is an important environmental health measure.

Rodents may be classified into two distinct groups : domestic and wild. (1) DOMESTIC RODENTS : The rodents of chief public health concern are those that live in close association with man, namely the black rat (*Rattus rattus*) and the Norway rat (*R. norvegicus*) and the house mouse (*Mus musculus*). Rattus rattus is a domestic animal whose area of movement is usually restricted. It readily infests ships, and therefore its public health importance is considerable. *Rattus rattus* is also a good climber and infestation generally occurs in the roofs of houses, though in some places it does burrow. *R. norvegicus*, on the other hand is a semidomestic animal which frequents sewers, drains as well as houses. Characteristics which are easily ascertainable of *R. rattus* and *R. norvegicus* are illustrated in Fig. 1.

(2) WILD RODENTS : The common wild rodents in India are *Tatera indica, Bandicota bengalensis varius (Gunomys kok), B.indica, Millardia meltada, M. gleadowi* and *Mus booduga.* In India, *Tatera indica* has been found to be the natural reservoir of plague.

Rodents and disease *(36)*

A number of diseases are associated with rodents. Broadly these are : (1) *Bacterial :* plague, tularaemia, salmonellosis; (2) *Viral :* Lassa fever, haemorrhagic fever, encephalitis (3) *Rickettsial :* scrub typhus, murine typhus, rickettsial pox; (4) *Parasitic :* hymenolepis diminuata, leishmaniasis, amoebiasis, trichinosis, Chagas disease; and (5) *Others :* rat bite fever, leptospirosis, histoplasmosis, ring worm etc.

The mode of transmission may be directly through rat bite (e.g., rat bite fever); some through contamination of food or water (e.g., salmonellosis, leptospirosis) and some through rat fleas (e.g., plague and typhus).

Antirodent measures

1. *Sanitation measures :* Sound environmental sanitation is the most effective weapon in deratization campaign. Rats require three things : food, water and shelter. If these are denied, rats will naturally decrease in density. The environmental sanitation measures comprise : (1) proper storage, collection and disposal of garbage, (2) proper storage of food-stuffs, (3) construction of rat-proof buildings, godowns and warehouses, and (4) elimination of rat burrows by blocking them with concrete. Sanitation is therefore essential to the permanent control of rats and mice, and all measures should be regarded as supplementary to sanitation.

2. *Trapping :* Trapping of rats is a simple operation. But it causes temporary reduction in the number of commensal rodents. It is recommended that the number of traps laid should be at least 5 per cent of the human population. The 'wonder trap' developed by the Haffkine Institute, Mumbai is credited to trap as many as 25 rats at a time. The traps are

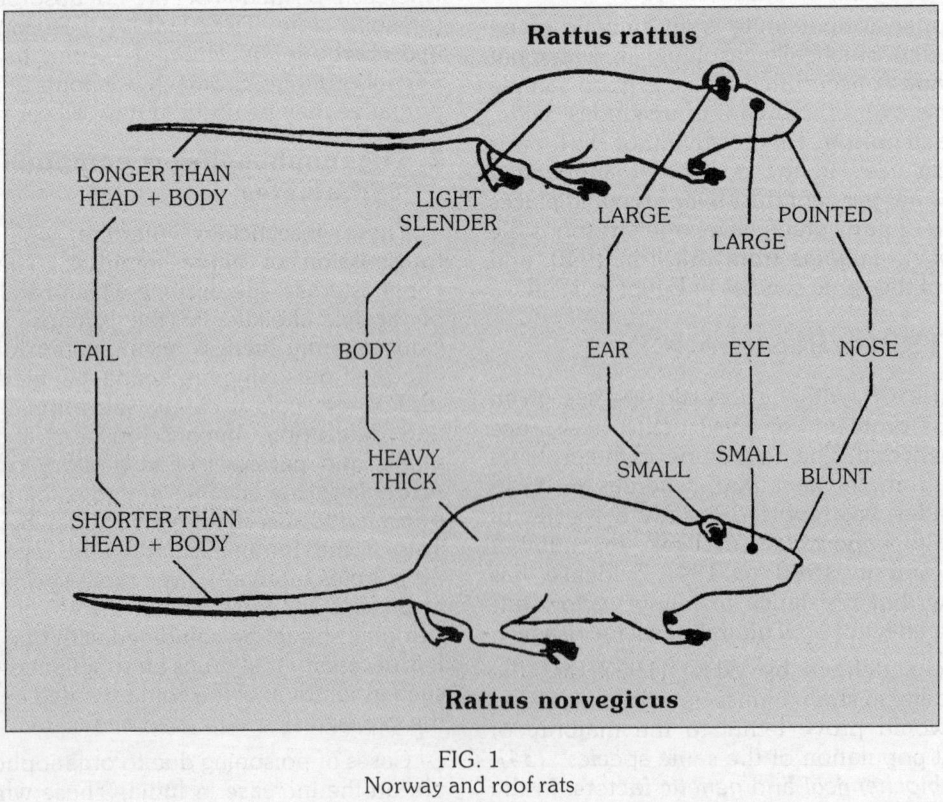

FIG. 1
Norway and roof rats

usually baited with indigenous foods of the locality. The captured rats must be destroyed which may be done by drowning them in water. Rats by nature are suspicious animals, and will soon become "trap-wise" and avoid baited traps. Trapping therefore should be considered supplementary to other methods of rodent control.

3. *Rodenticides* : Rodenticides are of two main types – single-dose (acute) and multiple-dose (cumulative). The former are lethal to the rat after a single feeding, while the latter require repeated feedings over a period of 3 more days *(17)*.

An Expert Committee of the WHO *(37)* grouped the "acute" rodenticides as below :

1. *Those requiring ordinary care*
   - Red squill
   - Norbromide
   - Zinc phosphide
2. *Those requiring maximal precaution*
   - Sodium fluorocetate
   - Fluoroacetamide
   - Strychnine
3. *Too dangerous for use*
   - Arsenic trioxide
   - Phosphorus
   - Thallium sulphate
   - ANTU
   - Gophacide

The commonly used poisons in this country are : (i) *Barium carbonate* : This is a white tasteless powder, and is very cheap. It is mixed with wheat or rice flour in the ratio of 1 part to 4 parts of flour. The mixed material is moistened with water and made into small round marbles. The poisoned baits are placed near the rat burrows and in dark, secluded places. On eating the pills, rats are killed in 2 to 24 hours. Barium carbonate is a weak rodenticide of uneven performance, and probably easily detected by rats in many baits. In the opinion of many workers, in view of the availability of more efficient rodenticides, barium carbonate should not be used any more *(38)*. (ii) *Zinc phosphide* : Zinc phosphide is an efficient rodenticide. When moist, the chemical slowly gives off phosphine whose garlic odour is repellent to man and domestic animals, but seems to have no adverse effect on rats. Zinc phosphide is now extensively used in India. It is used in the ratio of 1 part to 10 parts of wheat or rice flour and mixed with a few drops of edible oil in order to render it more attractive to rats. Rats are killed in about three hours. The use of rubber gloves is recommended in handling zinc phosphide as it is highly poisonous. Special bait boxes have been designed for the administration of very toxic compounds such as zinc phosphide to eliminate the risk to man and domestic animals. Because of its good safety record, low cost and reasonably high effectiveness, Zinc phosphide is recommended for large scale use against rats *(38)*.

The *multiple-dose* (cumulative) poisons are : warfarin, diphacinone, coumafuryl and pindone *(17)*. As anticoagulants, they cause internal haemorrhage and slow death in 4 to 10 days. The continued use of anticoagulant rodenticides has led to the appearance of resistant Norway rat populations in several European countries. In some countries, the use of chronic rodenticides has been given up. All rodent poisons are toxic to mammals including man and call for the utmost care in their use.

(4) *Fumigation* : Fumigation is an effective method of destroying, both rats and rat fleas. The fumigants used in anti-rat campaigns are calcium cyanide (often called cyanogas or cymag), carbon disulphide, methyl bromide, sulphur dioxide, etc. Cyanogas has been extensively used in India for the fumigation of rat burrows. This chemical is prepared in powder form and is pumped into rat burrows by a special foot pump called the "Cyanogas pump" (Fig. 2). About 2 ounces of the poison are pumped into each rat burrow after closing the exit openings and the burrow is then promptly sealed with wet mud. On contact with moisture, the cynogas powder gives off hydrogen cyanide gas which is lethal to both rats and their fleas. Trained personnel are required to carry out fumigation because of its extreme danger to man and livestock. For the eradication of rats from ships, either cyanogas or sulphur dioxide is used.

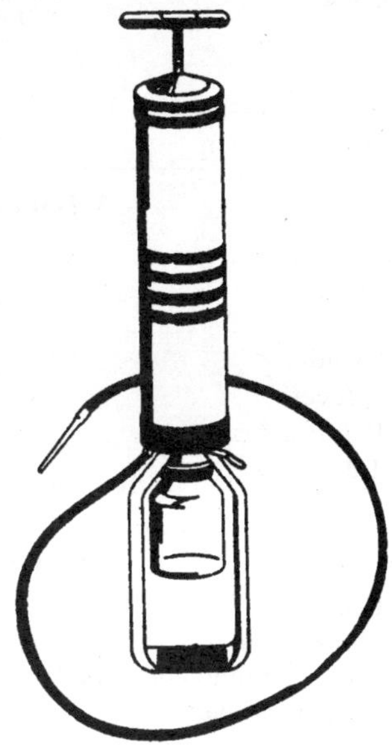

FIG. 2
Cyanogas foot pump

(5) *Chemosterilants* : A chemosterilant is a chemical that can cause temporary or permanent sterility in either sex or both sexes. Rodent chemosterilants are still in the experimental stage *(39)*.

ZOONOSES

Animals are part of man's biological environment. Some of them act as reservoir hosts of a number of diseases. The WHO records more than 150 diseases and infections of animals communicable to man *(40)* – these are termed "zoonoses". The Joint FAO/WHO Expert Committee (1967) defined zoonoses as "those diseases and infections which are naturally transmitted between vertebrate animals and man".

Zoonotic diseases may be due to viruses, bacteriae, rickettisiae, fungi, helminths, protozoa, arthropods or insects. The WHO (1967) classified zoonoses into different groups *(40)*. Some of the important zoonoses are as given in Table 1.

India has the largest animal population in the world which is nearly 11 per cent of the total world animal population. Being an agricultural country the relationship between man and animals is the closest in this country. It is not uncommon to see animals and human beings living under the same roof. The available information indicates that a large number of zoonotic infections (e.g., brucellosis, rabies, tuberculosis, leptospirosis, hydatid disease) occur in different parts of the country. Except for rabies, the prevalence of other diseases in human being is not well mapped out. The National Centre for Disease Control, Delhi is making efforts to organize systematic and collaborative studies with other Institutions on different zoonotic infections. The WHO has a section of Veterinary Public Health in its Division of Communicable Diseases. The control of zoonoses is a challenge facing the veterinary public health today.

TABLE 1
Partial list of zoonoses

Disease in man	Animal principally involved
	A. Bacterial infections
Anthrax	Herbivores, pigs
Brucellosis	Cattle, sheep, goats, camels, pigs, dogs, horses, buffaloes
Ornithosis	Wild and domestic birds
Q fever	Cattle, sheep, goats, wild animals
Leptospirosis	Rodents, mammals
Tuberculosis	Cattle, sheep, goats, pigs, cats, dogs
Plague	Rodents
	B. Viral infections
Cowpox	Cattle
Monkeypox	Monkeys, rodents
Easternequine encephalitis	Horses, rodents
Ross river fever	Horses, cattle, goats, sheep, dogs, rats, bats, pigs
Yellow fever	Monkeys
Japanese encephalitis	Wild birds
Lassa fever	Multi-mammate rat
Rabies	Dog, fox, shunk, mongoose, bat and jackal
	C. Protozoan infections
Leishmaniasis	Dogs, cats, swine
Toxoplasmosis	Cats, mammals, birds
Trypanosomiasis	Game animals, cattle
Babesiosis	Cattle
	D. Helminthic infections
Clonorchiasis	Dogs, cats, swine, wild mammals, fish
Fasciolopsis	Swine, dogs
Schistosomiasis	Rodents
Echinococcosis	Dogs, wild carnivores, domestic and wild ungulates
Taeniasis	Cattle
Trichinellosis	Swine, rodents, wild carnivores, marine mammals

Source : *(41, 42)*

Control of zoonoses

The principal components of control are : (a) *Control in animals :* The measure comprise diagnosis of the zoonotic condition, treatment, destruction, quarantine and immunization. (b) *Control of vehicles of transmission :* These include establishment of food hygiene practices, ensuring safety of animal products such as wool, hides, horn, bones, fat, etc.; proper disposal of animal carcasses and wastes, and disinfection procedures. (c) *Prevention and treatment in man :* This involves protection of high risk groups, by immunization, chemoprophylaxis, monitoring of health status including occupational health programmes, prevention of spread by man, early diagnosis and treatment of the condition in man, health education, prevention of environmental contamination, prevention of food contamination, and improvement of diagnostic facilities *(42)*.

During the past 50 years, the concept of environment has become broad-based. Modern ecologists use the term in its widest sense. The concept of environment covers first the general environment, for instance water and air pollution, to which an individual is exposed. Secondly, it refers to the personal environment created by the individual himself – including such cultural habits as cigarette smoking, alcohol, drug addiction. This has been described as "chemical environment". The concept that the general everyday chemical environment could also be dangerous to human health developed slowly. Evidence is accumulating that environmental factors, especially factors in the chemical environment, play a major role in carcinogenesis, and that many cancers may be theoretically preventable *(43)*.

It is now current jargon to advocate an "integrated" approach to the environmental problems where all aspects of a given problem are looked at from all angles. It implies an unprecedented cooperation between different services and disciplines. The United Nations Environmental Programme (UNEP), UNESCO's Man and Biosphere (MAB) Programme, WHO's Environmental Health Criteria Programme, and the UN's International Drinking Water Supply and Sanitation Decade, 1981–1990 are efforts in the direction to promote health in the human environment.

References

1. Singh, K.R.P. (1976). *J. Com. Dis.*, 8,147–153.
2. Smith, R.F. (1973). *Bull. Wld. Hlth. Org.*, 48.686.
3. Rao, T.R. (1974). *J. Com. Dis.*, 6.57.
4. WHO (1974). *Techn. Rep. Ser.*, No. 586.
5. Sharma, M.I.D. (1974) *J. Com. Dis.*, 6.136.
6. Puri, I.M. (1955). *Synoptic Table for the identification of the Anopheline Mosquitoes in India,* Health Bulletin No. 10, Manager of Publications, Govt. of India Press, Delhi.
7. Sharma, V.P. (1974). *J. Com. Dis.*, 6, 127–135.
8. WHO (1971). *International Health Regulations, (Wld, Hlth, Org. Tech. Ser.,*
9. WHO (1973). *Manual on Larval Control Operations in Malaria,* Geneva.
10. WHO (1975). *Techn. Rep. Ser.*, No. 561.
11. Bay Ernest. C. (1967). *WHO Chronicle,* 21, 415.
12. WHO (1972). *Vector Control in International Health,* Geneva.
13. WHO (1976). *Techn. Rep. Ser.*, No. 585.
14. Pal, R. (1967). *WHO chronicle,* 21, 348.
15. WHO (1968). *Techn. Rep.*, No. 398.
16. Puri, I.M. (1948). *The House–Frequenting Flies, their relation to Disease and their control.* Health Bulletin No. 31, Manager of Publications, Govt. of India Press, Delhi.
17. WHO (1970). *Techn. Rep. Ser.*, No. 443.
18. WHO (1966). *Control of Arthropods of Public Health Importance.* WHO Training Leaflet, No. 1 Vector Control Series Geneva.
19. Kaul, H.N. et al (1973). *Indian J. Med. Res.*, 61, 528.
20. WHO (1967). *WHO Chronicle.* 21, 523.
21. Roy, D.N. and Brown, A.W.A. (1954), *Entomology, Medical and Veterinary,* Excelssior Press, Calcutta.
22. WHO (1976). *World Health,* April, 1976 p. 9.
23. WHO (1976). *Techn. Rep. Ser.*, No. 553.
24. Garnham. P.C.C. et al (1969). *Brit. Med. J.*, 4, 768.
25. Drew, R. (1970). *The Medical Annual,* p. 446.
26. Orkin, M. (1971). *JAMA,* 217, 593.
27. Morley, N. (1970). *The Practitioner,* 204, 107.
28. Chatterji, K.D. (1952). *Human Parasites and Parasitic Diseases,* Calcutta.
29. Maplestone, P.A. and Sunder Rao, S. (1939). *Dracontiasis,* Health Bulletin No. 7, Manager of Publications, Govt. of India, New Delhi.
30. Lyons, G.R.L. (1973). *Bull. Wld. Hlth. Org.*, 49, 215.
31. Singh J. and Raghavan, N.G.S. (1965). *Bull. Nat. Soc. Ind. Mal. Mosq. Diseases,* 5, 143.
32. Dhir, S.L. (1970). *Swasth Hind,* 14, 269.
33. Nishizawa, Y. (1971). *Bull. Wld. Hlth. Org.*, 44, 325–336.
34. WHO (1957). *Techn. Rep. Ser.*, No. 125.
35. WHO (1963). *Techn. Rep. Ser.*, No. 265.
36. WHO (1974). *Techn. Rep. Ser.*, No. 553.
37. WHO (1973). *Techn. Rep. Ser.*, No. 513.
38. Gratz, N.G. (1973). *Bull. Wld. Hlth. Org.*, 48, 469.
39. Marsh, R.E. et al (1973). *Bull. Wld. Hlth. Org.*, 48, 309.
40. WHO (1967). *Techn. Rep. Ser.*, No. 378.
41. WHO (1979). *Tech. Rep. Ser.* No.637
42. WHO (1982). *Tech. Rep. Ser.* No.682
43. WHO (1978). *World Health,* June

16 Hospital Waste Management

Let the wastes of "the sick" not contaminate the lives of "the healthy"

The waste produced in the course of healthcare activities carries a higher potential for infection and injury than any other type of waste. Therefore, it is essential to have safe and reliable method for its handling. Inadequate and inappropriate handling of healthcare waste may have serious public health consequences and a significant impact on the environment. Appropriate management of healthcare waste is thus a crucial component of environmental health protection, and it should become an integral feature of healthcare services.

Definition

According to Bio-Medical Waste (Management and Handling) Rules, 1998 of India, "Bio-medical waste" means any waste, which is generated during the diagnosis, treatment or immunization of human beings or animals, or in research activities pertaining thereto or in the production or testing of biologicals.

Between 75 to 90 per cent of the waste produced by the healthcare providers is non-risk or "general" healthcare waste, comparable to domestic waste. It comes mostly from administrative and house keeping functions of the healthcare establishments, and may also include waste generated during maintenance of healthcare premises. The remaining 10–25 per cent healthcare waste is regarded as hazardous and may create a variety of health risk *(2)*.

Sources of healthcare waste

The institutions involved in generation of bio-medical waste are :

- Government hospitals;
- Private hospitals;
- Nursing homes;
- Physician's office/clinics;
- Dentist's office/clinics;
- Dispensaries;
- Primary health centres;
- Medical research and training establishments;
- Mortuaries;
- Blood banks and collection centres;
- Animal houses;
- Slaughter houses;
- Laboratories;
- Research organizations;
- Vaccinating centres; and
- Biotechnology institutions/production units.

All these healthcare establishments generate waste and are therefore, covered under Bio-Medical Waste (BMW) Rules *(1)*.

Healthcare waste generation

Several surveys have provided an indication of typical healthcare waste generation, and it shows that this differs not only from country to country but also within the country. Waste generation depends on numerous factors such as established waste management methods, type of healthcare establishment, hospital specializations, proportion of reusable items employed in healthcare, and proportion of patients treated on a day-care basis.

In middle and low income countries, healthcare waste generated is lower than in high-income countries. Developing countries that have not performed their own surveys of healthcare waste, find the following estimates for an average distribution of healthcare wastes useful for preliminary planning of waste management *(2)* :

- 80 per cent general healthcare waste, which may be dealt with by the normal domestic, and urban waste management system;
- 15 per cent pathological and infectious waste;
- 1 per cent sharps waste;
- 3 per cent chemical and pharmacological waste;
- Less than 1 per cent special waste, such as radioactive or cytotoxic waste, pressurized containers, or broken thermometers and used batteries.

Table 1 shows average composition of waste obtained from 10 large hospitals in Mumbai, Kolkata, Delhi, and Nagpur during the period 1993–1996.

TABLE 1

Average composition of hospital waste in India

Material	Percentage (wet-weight basis)
Paper	15
Plastics	10
Rags	15
Metal (sharps etc.)	1
Infectious waste	1.5
Glass	4.0
General waste (food waste, sweepings from hospital premises etc.)	53.5

Source : (National Environmental Engineering Research Institute 1997)

A survey done in Bangalore revealed that the quantity of solid wastes generated in hospitals and nursing homes generally varies from 1/2 to 4 kg per bed per day in Govt. hospitals, 1/2 to 2 kg per bed per day in private hospitals, and 1/2 to 1 kg per bed per day in nursing homes. The total quantity of hospital wastes generated in Bangalore is about 40 tonnes per day. Out of this nearly 45 to 50 per cent is infectious. Segregation of infectious wastes from non-infectious wastes is done only in about 30 per cent of hospitals *(3)*.

Health hazards of healthcare waste

Exposure to hazardous health-care waste can result in disease or injury due to one or more of the following characteristics :

(a) it contains infectious agents; (b) it contains toxic or hazardous chemicals, pathological waste or pharmaceuticals; (c) it contains sharps; (d) it is genotoxic; (e) it is radioactive; and (f) non-hazardous or general waste.

All individuals exposed to such hazardous healthcare waste are potentially at risk, including those who generate the waste or those who either handle such waste or are exposed to it as a consequence of careless management. The main groups at risk are :

- medical doctors, nurses, healthcare auxilliaries, and hospital maintenance personnel;
- patients in healthcare establishments;
- visitors to healthcare establishments;
- workers in support service allied to healthcare establishments such as laundries, waste handling and transportation; and
- workers in waste disposal facilities such as land-fills or incinerators including scavengers.

1. Hazards from infectious waste and sharps

Pathogens in infectious waste may enter the human body through a puncture, abrasion or cut in the skin, through mucous membranes by inhalation or by ingestion. There is particular concern about infection with HIV and hepatitis virus B and C, for which there is a strong evidence of transmission *via* healthcare waste. Bacteria resistant to antibiotics and chemical disinfectants, may also contribute to the hazards created by poorly managed waste.

2. Hazards from chemical and pharmaceutical waste

Many of the chemicals and pharmaceuticals used in healthcare establishments are toxic, genotoxic, corrosive, flammable, reactive, explosive or shock-sensitive. Although present in small quantity they may cause intoxication, either by acute or chronic exposure, and injuries, including burns. Disinfectants are particularly important members of this group. They are used in large quantities and are often corrosive, reactive chemicals may form highly toxic secondary compounds.

3. Hazards from genotoxic waste

The severity of the hazards for healthcare worker responsible for handling or disposal of genotoxic waste is governed by a combination of the substance toxicity itself and the extent and duration of exposure. Exposure may also occur during the preparation of or treatment with particular drug or chemical. The main pathway of exposure is inhalation of dust or aerosols, absorption through the skin, ingestion of food accidentally contaminated with cytotoxic drugs, chemicals or wastes etc.

4. Hazards from radioactive waste

The type of disease caused by radioactive waste is determined by the type and extent of exposure. It can range from headache, dizziness and vomiting to much more serious problems. Because it is genotoxic, it may also affect genetic material.

5. Public sensitivity

Apart from health hazards, the general public is very sensitive to visual impact of healthcare waste particularly anatomical waste.

Treatment and disposal technologies for health-care waste *(2)*

Incineration, used to be the method of choice for most hazardous healthcare wastes, and is still widely used. However, recently developed alternative treatment methods are becoming increasingly popular. The final choice of treatment should be made on the basis of factors, many of which depend on local conditions.

I. Incineration

Incineration is a high temperature dry oxidation process, that reduces organic and combustible waste to inorganic incombustible matter and results in a very significant reduction of waste-volume and weight. The process is usually selected to treat wastes that cannot be recycled, reused or disposed off in a land fill site.

The flow diagram of incinerator is as shown in Fig. 1.

Incineration requires no pre-treatment, provided that certain waste types are not included in the matter to be incinerated. Characteristics of the waste suitable for incineration are : (a) low heating volume – above 2,000 kcal/kg for single-chamber incinerators, and above 3,500 kcal/kg for pyrolytic double-chamber incinerators; (b) content of combustible matter above 60 per cent; (c) content of non-combustible solids below 5 per cent; (d) content of non-combustible fines below 20 per cent; and (e) moisture content below 30 per cent *(2)*.

Waste types not to be incinerated are : (a) pressurized gas containers; (b) large amount of reactive chemical wastes; (c) silver salts and photographic or radiographic wastes; (d) Halogenated plastics such as PVC; (e) waste with high mercury or cadmium content, such as broken thermometers, used batteries, and lead-lined wooden panels; and (f) sealed ampules or ampules containing heavy metals *(2)*.

TYPES OF INCINERATORS

Incinerators can range from very basic combustion unit that operates at much lower temperature to extremely sophisticated, high temperature operating plants. It should be carefully chosen on the basis of the available resources, the local situation, and the risk-benefit consideration.

Three basic kinds of incineration technology are of interest for treating healthcare waste :

(a) Double-chamber pyrolytic incinerators which may be especially designed to burn infectious healthcare waste; (b) Single-chamber furnaces with static grate, which should be used only if pyrolytic incinerators are not affordable; and (c) Rotary kilns operating at high temperatures, capable of causing decomposition of genotoxic substances and heat-resistant chemicals.

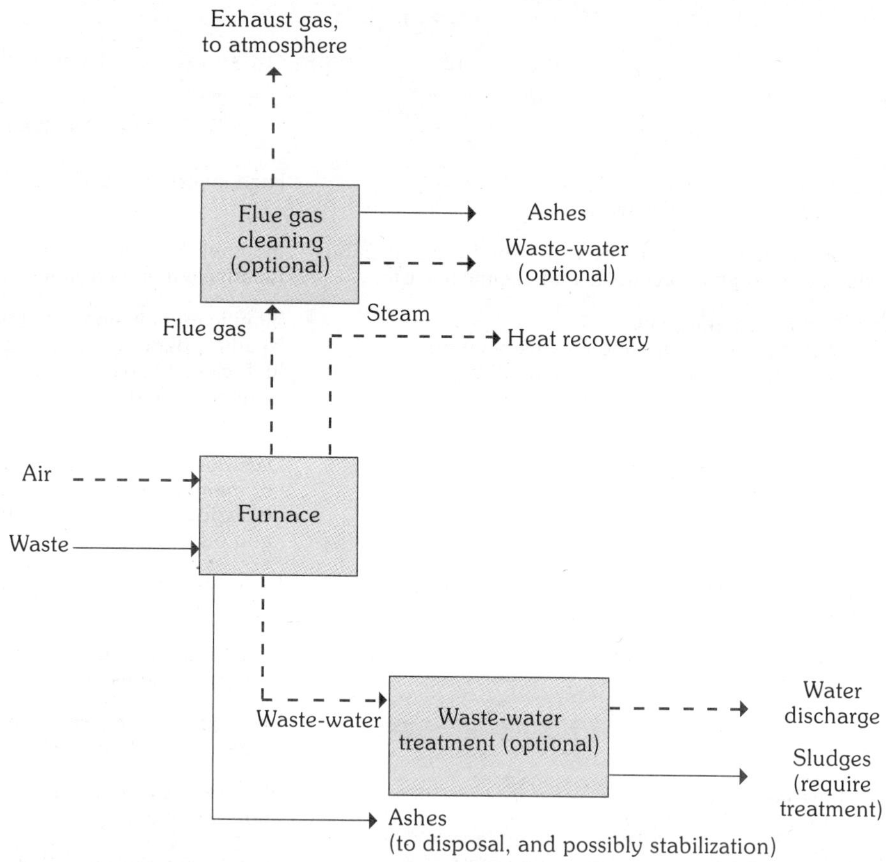

FIG. 1
Simplified flow scheme of incinerator

Source : *(2)*

II. Chemical disinfection

Chemicals are added to waste to kill or inactivate the pathogens it contains, this treatment usually results in disinfection rather than sterilization. Chemical disinfection is most suitable for treating liquid waste such as blood, urine, stools or hospital sewage. However, solid wastes including microbiological cultures, sharps etc. may also be disinfected chemically with certain limitations.

III. Wet and dry thermal treatment

WET THERMAL TREATMENT : Wet thermal treatment or steam disinfection is based on exposure of shredded infectious waste to high temperature, high pressure steam, and is similar to the autoclave sterilization process. The process is inappropriate for the treatment of anatomical waste and animal carcasses, and will not efficiently treat chemical and pharmaceutical waste.

SCREW-FEED TECHNOLOGY : Screw-feed technology is the basis of a non-burn, dry thermal disinfection process in which waste is shredded and heated in a rotating auger. The waste is reduced by 80 per cent in volume and by 20–35 per cent in weight. This process is suitable for treating infectious waste and sharps, but it should not be used to process pathological, cytotoxic or radioactive waste.

IV. Microwave irradiation

Most microorganisms are destroyed by the action of microwave of a frequency of about 2450 MHz and a wave length of 12.24 nm. The water contained within the waste is rapidly heated by the microwaves and the infectious components are destroyed by heat conduction. The efficiency of the microwave disinfection should be checked routinely through bacteriological and virological tests.

V. Land disposal

MUNICIPAL DISPOSAL SITES : If a municipality or medical authority genuinely lacks the means to treat waste before disposal, the use of a landfill has to be regarded as an acceptable disposal route. There are two types of disposal land–open dumps and sanitary landfills. Healthcare waste should not be deposited on or around open dumps. The risk of either people or animals coming into contact with infectious pathogens is obvious.

Sanitary landfills are designed to have at least four advantages over open dumps : geological isolation of waste from the environment, appropriate engineering preparation before the site is ready to accept waste, staff present on site to control operations, and organized deposit and daily coverage of waste.

VI. Inertization

The process of "inertization" involves mixing waste with cement and other substances before disposal, in order to minimize the risk of toxic substances contained in the wastes migrating into the surface water or ground water. A typical proportion of the mixture is: 65 per cent pharmaceutical waste, 15 per cent lime, 15 per cent cement and 5 per cent water. A homogeneous mass is formed and cubes or pellets are produced on site and then transported to suitable storage sites.

The main advantages and disadvantages of various treatment and disposal options are listed in Table 2.

TABLE 2

Main advantages and disadvantages of treatment and disposal options

Treatment / disposal method	Advantages	Disadvantages
Rotary kiln	Adequate for all infectious waste, most chemical waste and pharmaceutical waste.	High investment and operating costs.
Pyrolytic incineration	Very high disinfection efficiency. Adequate for all infectious waste and most pharmaceutical and chemical waste.	Incomplete destruction of cytotoxics. Relatively high investment and operating costs.
Single-chamber incineration	Good disinfection efficiency. Drastic reduction of weight and volume of waste. The residues may be disposed off in landfills. No need for highly trained operators. Relatively low investment and operating costs.	Significant emissions of atmospheric pollutants. Need for periodic removal of slag and soot. Inefficiency in destroying thermally resistant chemicals and drugs such as cytotoxics.
Drum or brick incinerator	Drastic reduction of weight and volume of the waste. Very low investment and operating costs.	Destroys only 99% of microorganisms. No destruction of many chemicals and pharmaceuticals. Massive emission of black smoke, fly ash, toxic flue gas, and odours.
Chemical disinfection	Highly efficient disinfection under good operating conditions.	Requires highly qualified technicians for operation of the process.
	Some chemical disinfectants are relatively inexpensive.	Uses hazardous substances that require comprehensive safety measures.
		Inadequate for pharmaceutical, chemical and some types of infectious waste.
Wet thermal treatment*	Environmentally sound.	Shredders are subject to frequent breakdowns and poor functioning.
	Relatively low investment and operating costs.	Operation requires qualified technicians.
		Inadequate for anatomical, pharmaceutical, chemical waste and waste that is not readily steam-permeable.
Microwave irradiation	Good disinfection efficiency under appropriate operating conditions.	Relatively high investment and operating costs.
	Drastic reduction in waste volume. Environmentally sound.	Potential operation and maintenance problems.
Encapsulation	Simple, low-cost, and safe. May also be applied to pharmaceuticals.	Not recommended for non-sharp infectious waste.
Safe burying	Low costs. Relatively safe if access to site is restricted and where natural infiltration is limited.	Safe only if access to site is limited and certain precautions are taken.
Inertization	Relatively inexpensive.	Not applicable to infectious waste.

* May not apply to more sophisticated, self-contained, commercial methods.

Source : *(2)*

National legislation is the basis for improving healthcare waste disposal practices in any country. It establishes legal control, and permits the national agency responsible for the disposal of healthcare waste, usually the Ministry of Health, to apply pressure for their implementation. The Ministry of Environment may also be involved. There should be a clear designation of responsibilities before the law is enacted.

The United Nations Conference on the Environment and Development (UNCED) in 1992 recommended the following measures :

(a) Prevent and minimize waste production;

(b) Reuse or recycle the waste to the extent possible;

(c) Treat waste by safe and environmentally sound methods; and

(d) Dispose off the final residue by landfill in confined and carefully designed sites.

Bio-Medical Waste Management in India *(1, 4)*

Bio-Medical Waste (Management and Handling) Rule 1998, prescribed by the Ministry of Environment and Forests, Government of India, came into force on 28th July 1998. This rule applies to those who generate, collect, receive, store, dispose, treat or handle bio-medical waste in any manner. The Act is now superceded by Bio-Medical Waste Management Rules, 2016, which came into force from 28th March 2016. Table 3 shows the categories of bio-medical waste, types of waste and treatment and disposal options under Rule 2016.

TABLE 3

Schedule I, Part 1

Biomedical wastes, categories and their segregation, collection, treatment , processing and disposal options

Category	Type of waste	Type of bag or container to be used	Treatment and disposal options
Yellow	**(a) Human anatomical waste:** Human tissues, organs, body parts and foetus below the viability period.	Yellow coloured non-chlorinated plastic bags.	Incineration or plasma pyrolysis or deep burial*
	(b) Animal anatomical waste: Experimental animal carcasses, body parts, organs, tissues, including the waste generated from animals used in experiments or testing in veterinary hospitals or colleges or animal houses.		
	(c) Soiled waste: Items contaminated with blood, body fluids like dressings, plaster casts, cotton swabs and bags containing residual or discarded blood and blood components.		Incineration or plasma pyrolysis or deep burial*. In absence of above facilities, autoclaving or micro-waving/ hydroclaving followed by shredding or mutilation or combination of sterilization and shredding. Treated waste to be sent for energy recovery.
	(d) Expired or discarded medicines: Pharmaceutical waste like antibiotics, cytotoxic drugs including all items contaminated with cytotoxic drugs along with glass or plastic ampoules, vials etc.	Yellow coloured non-chlorinated plastic bags or containers.	Expired cytotoxic drugs and items contaminated with cytotoxic drugs to be returned back to the manufacturer or supplier for incineration at temperature > 1200° C or to a common bio-medical waste treatment facility or hazardous waste treatment, storage and disposal facility for incineration at > 1200° C or Encapsulation or Plasma Pyrolysis at > 1200° C. All other discarded medicines shall be either sent back to manufacturer or disposed by incineration.
	(e) Chemical waste: Chemicals used in production of biological and used or discarded disinfectants.	Yellow coloured containers or non-chlorinated plastic bags.	Disposed of by incineration or Plasma Pyrolysis or Encapsulation in hazardous waste treatment, storage and disposal facility.
	(f) Chemical liquid waste: Liquid waste generated due to use of chemicals in production of biological and used or discarded disinfectants, Silver X-ray film developing liquid, discarded formalin, infected secretions, aspirated body fluids, liquid from laboratories and floor washings, cleaning, house-keeping and disinfecting activities etc.	Separate collection system leading to effluent treatment system.	After resource recovery, the chemical liquid waste shall be pre-treated before mixing with other wastewater. The combined discharge shall conform to the discharge norms given in Schedule-III.
	(g) Discarded linen, mattresses, beddings contaminated with blood or body fluid.	Non-chlorinated yellow plastic bags or suitable packing material.	Non-chlorinated chemical disinfection followed by incineration or Plasma Pyrolysis or for energy recovery. In absence of above facilities, shredding or mutilation or combination of sterilization and shredding. Treated waste to be sent for energy recovery or incineration or Plasma Pyrolysis.
	(h) Microbiology, biotechnology and other clinical laboratory waste: Blood bags, laboratory cultures, stocks or specimens of micro-organisms, live or attenuated vaccines, human and animal cell cultures used in research, industrial laboratories, production of biological, residual toxins, dishes and devices used for cultures.	Autoclave safe plastic bags or containers.	Pre-treat to sterilize with non-chlorinated chemicals on-site as per National AIDS Control Organisation or World Health Organisation guidelines thereafter for Incineration.
Red	**Contaminated waste (Recyclable) :** Wastes generated from disposable items such as tubing, bottles, intravenous tubes and sets, catheters, urine bags, syringes (without needles and fixed needle syringes) and vacutainers with their needles cut) and gloves.	Red coloured non-chlorinated plastic bags or containers.	Autoclaving or micro-waving/hydroclaving followed by shredding or mutilation or combination of sterilization and shredding. Treated waste to be sent to registered or authorized recyclers or for energy recovery or plastics to diesel or fuel oil, or for road making, whichever is possible. Plastic waste should not be sent to landfill sites.
White (Trans-lucent)	**Waste sharps including metals:** Needles, syringes with fixed needles, needles from needle tip cutter or burner, scalpels, blades or any other contaminated sharp object that may cause puncture and cuts. This includes both used, discarded and contaminated metal sharps.	Puncture proof, Leak proof, tamper proof containers.	Autoclaving or Dry Heat Sterilization followed by shredding or mutilation or encapsulation in metal container or cement concrete; combinations of shredding cum autoclaving; and sent for final disposal to iron foundries (having consent to operate from the State Pollution Control Boards or Pollution Control Committees) or sanitary landfill or designated concrete waste sharp pit.
Blue	**(a) Glassware:** Broken or discarded and contaminated glass including medicine vials and ampoules except those contaminated with cytotoxic wastes.	Cardboard boxes with blue coloured marking.	Disinfection (by soaking the washed glass waste after cleaning with detergent and Sodium Hypochlorite treatment) or through autoclaving or microwaving or hydroclaving and then sent for recycling.
	(b) Metallic body implants	Cardboard boxes with blue coloured marking.	

* Disposal by deep burial is permitted only in rural or remote areas where there is no access to common bio-medical waste treatment facility. This will be carried out with prior approval from the prescribed authority and as per the standards specified in Schedule-III. The deep burial facility shall be located as per the provisions and guidelines issued by Central Pollution Control Board from time to time.

Source: *(4)*

Part-2

1. All plastic bags shall be as per BIS standards as and when published, till then the prevailing plastic waste management rules shall be applicable.
2. Chemical Treatment using at least 10% Sodium Hypochlorite having 30% residual chlorine for twenty minutes or any other equivalent chemical reagent that should demonstrate $Log_{10}4$ reduction efficiency for micro-organisms.
3. Mutilation or shredding must be to an extent to prevent unauthorized reuse.
4. There will be no chemical pretreatment before incineration, except for microbiological, lab and highly infectious waste.
5. Incineration ash (ash from incineration of any bio-medical waste) shall be disposed through hazardous waste treatment, storage and disposal facility, if toxic or hazardous constituents are present beyond the prescribed limits as given in the Hazardous Waste (management, handling and transboundary movement) Rules, 2008, or as revised from time to time.
6. Dead foetus below the viability period (as per the Medical Termination of Pregnancy Act 1971, amended from time to time) can be considered as human anatomical waste. Such waste should be handed over to the operator of common bio- medical waste treatment and disposal facility in yellow bag with a copy of the official medical termination of pregnancy certificate from the obstetrician or the medical superintendent of hospital or healthcare establishment.

(7) Cytotoxic drug vials shall not be handed over to unauthorized person under any circumstances. These shall be sent back to the manufacturers for necessary disposal at a single point. As a second option, these may be sent for incineration at common bio-medical waste treatment and disposal facility of TSDFs or plasma pyrolysis at temperature > 1200° C.

8. Residual or discarded chemical wastes, used or discarded disinfectants and chemical sludge can be disposed at hazardous waste treatment, storage and disposal facility. In such case, the waste should be sent to hazardous waste treatment, storage and disposal facility through operator of common bio-medical waste treatment and disposal facility only.
9. On-site pre-treatment of laboratory waste, microbiological waste, blood samples, blood bags should be disinfected or sterilized as per the guidelines of World Health Organisation or National AIDS Control Organisation and then given to the common bio-medical waste treatment and disposal facility.
10. Installation of in-house incinerator is allowed. However in case there is no common biomedical facility nearby, the same may be installed by the occupier after taking authorization from the State Pollution Control Board.
11. Syringes should be either mutilated or needles should be cut and or stored in tamper proof, leak proof and puncture proof containers for sharp storage. Wherever the occupier is not linked to a disposal facility it shall be the responsibility of the occupier to sterilize and dispose in the manner prescribed.
12. Bio-medical waste generated in households during healthcare activities shall be segregated as per these rules and handed over in separate bags or containers to municipal waste collectors. Urban Local Bodies shall have tie up with the common bio-medical waste treatment and disposal facility to pickup this waste from the Material Recovery Facility (MRF) or from the house hold directly, for final disposal in the manner as prescribed in this schedule.

The bio-medical waste should be segregated into containers/bags at the point of generation of the waste. The colour coding and the type of containers used for disposal of waste are as shown in Fig. 2 shows the label for bio-hazards symbol and cytotoxic hazard symbol which should be prominently visible and non-washable.

Bio-hazard Symbol **Cytotoxic Hazard Symbol**

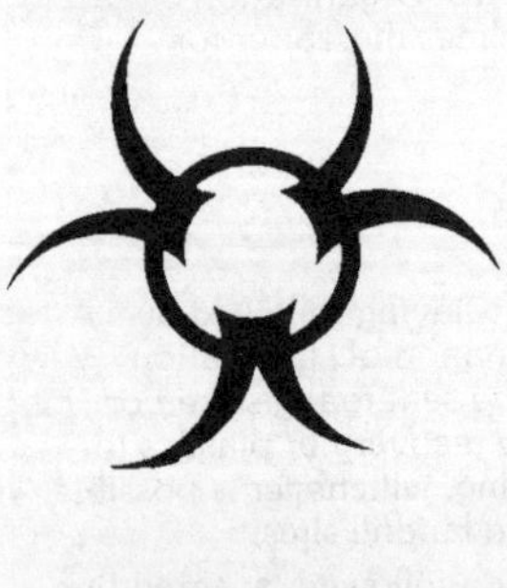

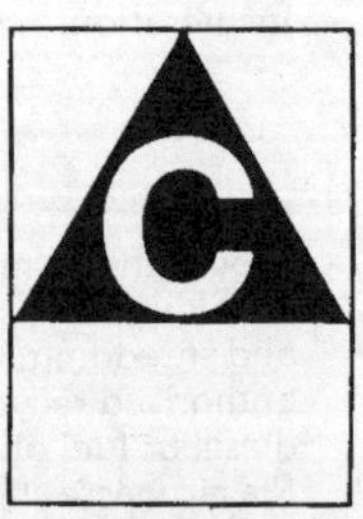

Bio-hazard **Cytotoxic**

HANDLE WITH CARE

FIG. 2

Schedule III

Label for bio-medical waste containers/bags

Note : Label shall be non-washable and prominently visible.

COVID-19 has had a serious impact on all aspects of our society, and waste management is no exception. There have been an increased amount of potentially infected waste which requires additional, careful handling and treatment processes to safeguard the waste handlers and sanitation workers associated with such healthcare facilities. Foot operated lids in colour-coded bins must be introduced to avoid contact. General solid waste should not be contaminated by patient's secretions and body fluids. Wet and dry solid waste bags must be tied securely. As precaution, double layered bags (using 2 bags) should be used for collection of waste from COVID-19 isolation wards so as to ensure adequate strength and no leaks. It should be labelled as "COVID-19 Waste". All the waste handlers must follow the preventive measures like hand washing, using gloves and mask, and other personal protective equipments *(5)*.

References

1. Sharma, A.K. (1998). *Bio-Medical Waste (Management & Handling) Rules, 1998,* Suvidha Law House, Bhopal.
2. Pruss, A., Cirouit, E., and Rushbrook, P. (1999) *Safe Management of Wastes from Healthcare Activities,* WHO, 1999.
3. Rao, H.V.N. (1995). *Disposal of Hospital Wastes in Bangalore and Their Impact on Environment,* Appropriate Waste Management Technologies for Developing Countries, 3rd International Conference 25–26 Feb 1995, Nagpur, Technical Papers Vol. II.
4. Govt. of India (2016). Ministry of Environment, Forest and Climate Change, Notification published in the Gazette of India, *Bio-Medical Waste Management Rule 2016.*
5. Govt. of India (2022). *Revision 5, Guidelines for handling treatment and disposal of waste generated during treatment/ diagnosis/quarantine of COVID-19 patients,* 26th April, 2022.

17 Disaster Management

A stitch in time, saves nine

The United Nations Office for Disaster Risk Reduction (UNISDR) (2009) defines disaster as: "A serious disruption of the functioning of a community or a society involving widespread human, material, economic or environmental losses and impacts, which exceed the ability of the affected community or society to cope using its own resources". UNISDR considers disaster to be a result of the combination of many factors such as the exposure to hazards, the conditions of vulnerability that are present, and insufficient capacity or measures to reduce or cope with the potential negative consequences. Disaster impacts may include loss of life, injuries, disease and other negative effects on human physical, mental and social well-being, together with damage to property, destruction of assets, loss of services, social and economic disruption and environmental degradation *(1)*.

The Disaster Management Act 2005 of India uses the following definition for disaster:

"Disaster means a catastrophe, mishap, calamity or grave occurrence in any area, arising from natural or manmade causes, or by accident or negligence which results in substantial loss of life or human suffering or damage to, and destruction of property, or damage to, or degradation of, environment, and is of such a nature or magnitude as to be beyond the coping capacity of the community of the affected area" *(1)*.

As per the definition adopted by UNISDR, "hazard" is a dangerous, phenomenon, substance, human activity, or condition that may cause loss of life, injury or other health impacts, property damage, loss of livelihoods and services, social and economic disruption, or environmental damage. India, due to its physiographic and climatic conditions is one of the most disaster prone areas in the world *(1)*.

Emergencies and disasters do not only affect health and well-being of people; frequently, large number of people are displaced, killed or injured, or subjected to greater risk of epidemics. Considerable economic harm is also common. Disasters cause great harm to the existing infrastructure and threaten the future of sustainable development.

Disasters are not confined to a particular part of the world; they can occur any where and at any time. Major emergencies and disasters have occurred throughout history and as the world's population grows and resources become more limited, communities are increasingly becoming vulnerable to the hazards that cause disaster. Statistics gathered since 1969 show a rise in the number of people affected by disasters. Since there is little evidence that the actual events causing disasters are increasing in either intensity or frequency, it can only be concluded that vulnerability to disaster is growing. For each disaster listed in officially recognized disaster database, there are some 20 other smaller emergencies with destructive impact on local communities that are unacknowledged.

Types of Disasters

Primarily disasters are triggered by natural hazards or are human-induced, or result from a combination of both. In particular, human-induced factors can greatly aggravate the adverse impacts of a natural disaster. Even at a larger scale, globally, the UN Inter-Governmental Panel on Climate Change (IPCC) has shown that human-induced climate change has significantly increased both the frequency and intensity of extreme weather events. While heavy rains, cyclones, or earthquakes are all natural, the impacts may, and are usually, worsened by many factors related to human activity. The extensive industrialization and urbanization increases both the probability of human-induced disasters, and the extent of potential damage to life and property from both natural and human-induced disasters. The human society is also vulnerable to chemical, biological, radiological and nuclear (CBRN) disasters *(1)*.

A. Natural Hazards

The widely accepted classification system used by the Disaster Information Management System of Deslnventar classifies disasters arising from natural hazards into five major categories (Deslnventar 2016). The classification is not a water tight one. In real life situations, many disasters are a combination of different types of disasters. In addition, secondary disaster may occur after a disaster has occurred *(1)*.

1. Geophysical :

(a) Earthquake/Mass movement of earth material
(b) volcano
(c) Tsunami - A series of waves (with long wavelengths when traveling across the deep ocean) that are generated by a displacement of massive amounts of water through underwater earthquakes, volcanic eruptions or landslides. Tsunami waves travel at very high speed across the ocean but as they begin to reach shallow water, they slow down and the wave grows steeper.

2. Hydrological :

(a) Flood - flash flood
(b) Landslides - Avalanche, debri flow, mud flow, rockfall
(c) Wave action - Wind generated surface waves of water over oceans, rivers or lakes.

3. Meteorological :

(a) Cyclone, storm surge, tornado, convective storm, extratropical storm, high wind

(b) Cold wave, derecho
(c) Extreme temperature, fog, frost, freeze, hail, heat-wave
(d) Lightning, heavy rain
(e) Sand-storm, dust-storm
(f) Snow, ice, winter storm, blizzard

4. *Climatological :*
(a) Drought
(b) Extreme hot/cold conditions
(C) Forest wildfire
(d) Glacial lake outburst
(e) Subsidence

5. *Biological :*
(a) Epidemics: viral, bacterial, parasitic, fungal or prion infections
(b) Insect infestations

B. Human-induced disasters

The rise in population, rapid urbanization and industrialization, development within high-risk zones, environmental degradation, and climate change aggravates the vulnerabilities to various kinds of disasters. Due to inadequate disaster preparedness, communities, and animals are at increased risk from many kinds of human-induced hazards arising from accidents (industrial, road, air, rail, on river or sea, building collapse, fires, mine flooding, oil spills, etc.). Chemical, biological, radiological, and nuclear (CBRN) hazards rank very high among the human-induced risks. Terrorist activities and secondary incidents add to these risks and call for adequate preparedness and planning. Warfare is a special category, because damage is the intended goal of action.

Every catastrophic event has its own special features. Some can be predicted several hours or days before-hand, as in the case of cyclones or floods, others such as earthquakes occur without warning.

The relative number of injuries and deaths differ, depending on a number of factors such as the type of disaster, the density and distribution of the population, condition of the environment, degree of the preparedness and opportunity of the warning. Injuries usually exceed death in explosions, earthquakes, typhoons, hurricanes, fires, tornadoes etc. Death frequently exceeds injuries in landslides, avalanches, volcanic eruptions, tidal waves, floods etc. *(2)*.

The types of emergency vary according to the kind of disaster, and how and when it strikes. In *earthquakes*, there is a high level of mortality, as a result of people being crushed by falling objects. The risk is greater inside or near dwellings but is very small in the open. Consequently earthquakes at night are more deadly. During the night fractures of pelvis, thorax and spine are common, because earthquake strikes while people are lying in bed. In the daytime injuries to the arms and skull are common. In *volcanic eruptions* mortality is high in the case of mudslides (e.g., 23,000 deaths in Colombia in 1985) and glowing clouds (e.g., 30,000 deaths at Saint-pierre in Martinique). There may be injuries, burns and suffocation. In *floods*, mortality is high only in case of sudden flooding e.g., flash floods, collapse of dams or tidal waves. Fractures, injuries and bruises may occur. If weather is cold, cases of accidental hypothermia may occur. In *cyclones* and *hurricanes*, mortality is not high unless tidal waves occur. The combined, effect of wind and rain may cause houses to collapse. A large number of objects may be lifted in the air and carried along by the wind. This may give rise to injuries. In *draughts*, mortality may increase considerably in areas where drought cause famines, in which case there may be protein–calorie malnutrition and vitamin deficiencies particularly vitamin A deficiency, leading to xerophthalmia and blindness. In famine conditions measles, respiratory infections, diarrhoea accompanied by dehydration may bring about a massive increase in infant mortality. When people migrate and settle down on the outskirts of famine hit areas, poor hygiene and overcrowding may facilitate the spread of endemic communicable diseases e.g., tuberculosis, parasitic diseases and malaria *(3)*.

On the whole, morbidity which results from a disaster situation can be classified into four types :

a. Injuries;
b. Emotional stress;
c. Epidemic of disease; and
d. Increase in indigenous diseases.

The short-term effects of major disasters are summarized in Table 1.

TABLE 1
Short-term effects of major disasters

Effect	Earthquakes	High winds (without flooding)	Tidal waves / flash floods	Slow - onset floods	Landslides	Volcanoes / Lahars
Death[a]	Many	Few	Many	Few	Many	Many
Severe injuries requiring extensive treatment	Many	Moderate	Few	Few	Few	Few
Increased risk of communicable diseases	Potential risk following all major disasters (Probability rising with overcrowding and deteriorating sanitation)					
Damage to health facilities	Severe (structure and equipment)	Severe	Severe but localized	Severe (equipment only)	Severe but localized	Severe (structure and equipment)
Damage to water systems	Severe	Light	Severe	Light	Severe but localized	Severe
Food shortage	Rare (may occur due to economic and logistic factors)		Common	Common	Rare	Rare
Major population movements	Rare (may occur in heavily damaged urban areas)		Common (generally limited)			

[a] Potential lethal impact in absence of preventive measures.

Source : *(4)*

DISASTER MANAGEMENT

The UNISDR defines disaster risk management as the systematic process of using administrative decisions, organizations, operational skills and capacities to implement policies, strategies and coping capacities of the society and communities to lessen the impacts of natural hazards and related environmental and technological disasters. This comprises of all forms of activities, including structural and non-structural measures to avoid (prevention) or to limit (mitigation and preparedness) adverse effects of hazards.

There are three fundamental aspects of disaster management :

a. disaster response ;
b. disaster preparedness ; and
c. disaster mitigation.

These three aspects of disaster management correspond to different phases in the so-called *"disaster cycle"* as shown in Fig. 1.

Disaster impact and response

Medical treatment for large number of casualties is likely to be needed only after certain types of disaster. Most injuries are sustained during the impact, and thus, the greatest need for emergency care occurs in the first few hours. The management of mass casualties can be further divided into search and rescue, first aid, triage and stabilization of victims, hospital treatment and redistribution of patients to other hospitals if necessary.

Search, rescue and first-aid

After a major disaster, the need for search, rescue and first aid is likely to be so great that organized relief services will be able to meet only a small fraction of the demand. Most immediate help comes from the uninjured survivors.

Field care

Most injured persons converge spontaneously to health

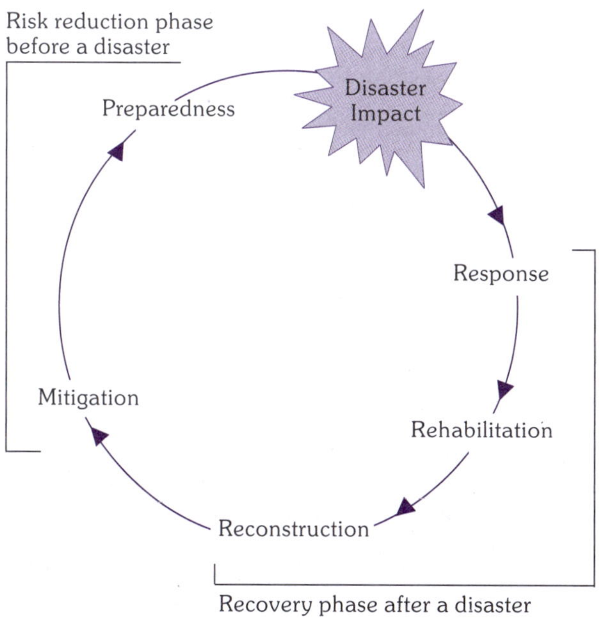

FIG. 1

Management sequence of a sudden-onset disaster

Source : *(4)*

facilities, using whatever transport is available, regardless of the facilities, operating status. Providing proper care to casualties requires that the health service resources be redirected to this new priority. Bed availability and surgical services should be maximized. Provisions should be made for food and shelter. A centre should be established to respond to inquiries from patient's relatives and friends. Priority should be given to victim's identification and adequate mortuary space should be provided.

Triage (4)

When the quantity and severity of injuries overwhelm the operative capacity of health facilities, a different approach to medical treatment must be adopted. The principle of "first come, first treated", is not followed in mass emergencies. Triage consists of rapidly classifying the injured on the basis of the severity of their injuries and the likelihood of their survival with prompt medical intervention. It must be adopted to locally available skills. Higher priority is granted to victims whose immediate or long-term prognosis can be dramatically affected by simple intensive care. Moribund patients who require a great deal of attention, with questionable benefit, have the lowest priority. Triage is the only approach that can provide maximum benefit to the greatest number of injured in a major disaster situation.

Although different triage systems have been adopted and are still in use in some countries, the most common classification uses the internationally accepted four colour code system. Red indicates high priority treatment or transfer, yellow signals medium priority, green indicates ambulatory patients and black for dead or moribund patients.

Triage should be carried out at the site of disaster, in order to determine transportation priority, and admission to the hospital or treatment centre, where the patient's needs and priority of medical care will be reassessed. Ideally, local health workers should be taught the principles of triage as part of disaster training.

Persons with minor or moderate injuries should be treated at their own homes to avoid social dislocation and the added drain on resources of transporting them to central facilities. The seriously injured should be transported to hospitals with specialized treatment facilities.

Tagging

All patients should be identified with tags stating their name, age, place of origin, triage category, diagnosis, and initial treatment.

Identification of dead

Taking care of the dead is an essential part of the disaster management. A large number of dead can also impede the efficiency of the rescue activities at the site of the disaster. Care of the dead includes : (1) removal of the dead from the disaster scene; (2) shifting to the mortuary; (3) identification; (4) reception of bereaved relatives. Proper respect for the dead is of great importance.

The health hazards associated with cadavers are minimal if death results from trauma, and corps are quite unlikely to cause outbreaks of disease such as typhoid fever, cholera or plague. If human bodies contaminate streams, wells, or other water sources as in floods etc., they may transmit gastroenteritis or food poisoning to survivors. The dead bodies represent a delicate social problem.

Relief phase

This phase begins when assistance from outside starts to reach the disaster area. The type and quantity of humanitarian relief supplies are usually determined by two main factors : (1) the type of disaster, since distinct events have different effects on the population, and (2) the type and quantity of supplies available locally.

Immediately following a disaster, the most critical health supplies are those needed for treating casualties, and preventing the spread of communicable diseases. Following the initial emergency phase, needed supplies will include food, blankets, clothings, shelter, sanitary engineering equipment and construction material. A rapid damage assessment must be carried out in order to identify needs and resources. Disaster managers must be prepared to receive large quantities of donations. There are four principal components in managing humanitarian supplies : (a) acquisition of supplies; (b) transportation; (c) storage; and (d) distribution.

Epidemiologic surveillance and disease control

Disasters can increase the transmission of communicable diseases through following mechanisms :

1. Overcrowding and poor sanitation in temporary resettlements. This accounts in part, for the reported increase in acute respiratory infections etc. following the disasters.
2. Population displacement may lead to introduction of communicable diseases to which either the migrant or indigenous populations are susceptible.
3. Disruption and the contamination of water supply, damage to sewerage system and power systems are common in natural disasters.
4. Disruption of routine control programmes as funds and personnel are usually diverted to relief work.
5. Ecological changes may favour breeding of vectors and increase the vector population density.
6. Displacement of domestic and wild animals, who carry with them zoonoses that can be transmitted to humans as well as to other animals. Leptospirosis cases have been reported following large floods (as in Orissa, India, after super cyclone in 1999). Anthrax has been reported occasionally.
7. Provision of emergency food, water and shelter in disaster situation from different or new source may itself be a source of infectious disease.

Outbreak of gastroenteritis, which is the most commonly reported disease in the post-disaster period, is closely related to first three factors mentioned above. Increased incidence of acute respiratory infections is also common in displaced population. Vector-borne diseases will not appear immediately but may take several weeks to reach epidemic levels.

Displacement of domesticated and wild animals increases the risk of transmission of zoonoses. Veterinary services may be needed to evaluate such health risks. Dogs, cats and other domestic animals are taken by their owners to or near temporary shelters. Some of these animals may be reservoirs of infections such as leptospirosis, rickettsiosis etc. Wild animals are reservoirs of infections which can be fatal to man such as equine encephalitis, rabies, and infections still unknown in humans.

The principals of preventing and controlling communicable diseases after a disaster are to – (a) implement as soon as possible all public health measures, to reduce the risk of disease transmission; (b) organize a reliable disease reporting system to identify outbreaks and to promptly initiate control measures; and (c) investigate all reports of disease outbreaks rapidly *(4)*.

Vaccination *(4)*

Health authorities are often under considerable public and political pressure to begin mass vaccination programmes, usually against typhoid, cholera and tetanus. The pressure may be increased by the press media and offer of vaccines from abroad.

The WHO does not recommend typhoid and cholera vaccines in routine use in endemic areas. The newer typhoid and cholera vaccines have increased efficacy, but because they are multidose vaccines, compliance is likely to be poor. They have not yet been proven effective, as a large-scale public health measure. Vaccination programme requires large number of workers who could be better employed elsewhere. Supervision of sterilization and injection techniques may be impossible, resulting in more harm than good. And above all, mass vaccination may lead to false sense of security about the risk of the disease and to the neglect of effective control measures. However, these vaccinations are recommended for health workers. Supplying safe drinking water and proper disposal of excreta continue to be the most practical and effective strategy.

Significant increase in tetanus incidence have not occurred after natural disasters. Mass vaccination of population against tetanus is usually unnecessary. The best protection is maintenance of a high level of immunity in the general population by routine vaccination before the disaster occurs, and adequate wound cleaning and treatment. If tetanus immunization was received more than 5 years ago in a patient who has sustained an open wound, a tetanus toxoid booster is an effective preventive measure. In previously unimmunized injured patients, tetanus toxoid should be given only at the discretion of a physician. If routine vaccination programmes are being conducted in camps with large number of children, it is prudent to include vaccination against tetanus.

Natural disasters may negatively affect the maintenance of on going national or regional eradication programmes against polio and measles. Disruption of these programmes should be monitored closely.

If cold-chain facilities are inadequate, they should be requested at the same time as vaccines. The vaccination policy to be adopted should be decided at senior level only.

Nutrition

A natural disaster may affect the nutritional status of the population by affecting one or more components of food chain depending on the type, duration and extent of the disaster, as well as the food and nutritional conditions existing in the area before the catastrophe. Infants, children, pregnant women, nursing mothers and sick persons are more prone to nutritional problems after prolonged drought or after certain types of disasters like hurricanes, floods, land or mudslides, volcanic eruptions and sea surges involving damage to crops, to stocks or to food distribution systems.

The immediate steps for ensuring that the food relief programme will be effective include : (a) assessing the food supplies after the disaster ; (b) gauging the nutritional needs of the affected population ; (c) calculating daily food rations and need for large population groups ; and (d) monitoring the nutritional status of the affected population.

Rehabilitation

The final phase in a disaster should lead to restoration of the pre-disaster conditions. Rehabilitation starts from the very first moment of a disaster. Too often, measures decided in a hurry, tend to obstruct re-establishment of normal conditions of life. Provisions by external agencies of sophisticated medical care for a temporary period has negative effects. On the withdrawal of such care, the population is left with a new level of expectation which simply cannot be fulfilled.

In first weeks after disaster, the pattern of health needs, will change rapidly, moving from casualty treatment to more routine primary health care. Services should be reorganized and restructured. Priorities also will shift from health care towards environmental health measures. Some of them are as follows :

Water supply

A survey of all public water supplies should be made. This includes distribution system and water source. It is essential to determine physical integrity of system components, the remaining capacities, and bacteriological and chemical quality of water supplied.

The main public safety aspect of water quality is microbial contamination. The first priority of ensuring water quality in emergency situations is chlorination. It is the best way of disinfecting water. It is advisable to increase residual chlorine level to about 0.2–0.5 mg/litre. Low water pressure increases the risk of infiltration of pollutants into water mains. Repaired mains, reservoirs and other units require cleaning and disinfection.

Chemical contamination and toxicity are a second concern in water quality and potential chemical contaminants have to be identified and analyzed.

The existing and new water sources require the following protection measures : (1) restrict access to people and animals, If possible, erect a fence and appoint a guard; (2) ensure adequate excreta disposal at a safe distance from water source; (3) prohibit bathing, washing and animal husbandry, upstream of intake points in rivers and streams; (4) upgrade wells to ensure that they are protected from contamination; and (5) estimate the maximum yield of wells and if necessary, ration the water supply.

In many emergency situations, water has to be trucked to disaster site or camps. All water tankers should be inspected to determine fitness, and should be cleaned and disinfected before transporting water.

Food safety

Poor hygiene is the major cause of food-borne diseases in disaster situations. Where feeding programmes are used (as in shelters or camps) kitchen sanitation is of utmost importance. Personal hygiene should be monitored in individuals involved in food preparation.

Basic sanitation and personal hygiene

Many communicable diseases are spread through faecal contamination of drinking water and food. Hence, every effort should be made to ensure the sanitary disposal of excreta. Emergency latrines should be made available to the displaced, where toilet facilities have been destroyed. Washing, cleaning and bathing facilities should be provided to the displaced persons.

Vector control

Control programme for vector-borne diseases should be intensified in the emergency and rehabilitation period, especially in areas where such diseases are known to be endemic. Of special concern are dengue fever and malaria (mosquitoes), leptospirosis and rat bite fever (rats), typhus (lice, fleas), and plague (fleas). Flood water provides ample breeding opportunities for mosquitoes.

A major disaster with high mortality leaves a substantial displaced population, among whom are those requiring medical treatment and orphaned children. When it is not possible to locate the relatives who can provide care, orphans may become the responsibility of health and social agencies. Efforts should be made to reintegrate disaster survivors into the society, as quickly as possible through institutional programmes coordinated by ministries of health and family welfare, social welfare, education, and NGOs.

Disaster mitigation in health sector

Emergency prevention and mitigation involves measures designed either to prevent hazards from causing emergency or to lessen the likely effects of emergencies. These measures include flood mitigation works, appropriate land-use planning, improved building codes, and reduction or protection of vulnerable population and structures.

In most cases mitigation measures aim to reduce the vulnerability of the system. Medical casualties can be drastically reduced by improving the structural quality of houses, schools and other public and private buildings. Although mitigation in these sectors has clear health implications, the direct responsibility of the health sector is limited to ensuring the safety of health facilities and public health services, including water supply and sewerage systems. When water supplies are contaminated or interrupted, in addition to the social cost of such damage, the cost of rehabilitation and reconstruction severely strains the economy. Mitigation complements the disaster preparedness and disaster response activities.

Disaster preparedness

Emergency preparedness is "a programme of long-term development activities whose goals are to strengthen the overall capacity and capability of a country to manage efficiently all types of emergency. It should bring about an orderly transition from relief through recovery, and back to sustained development" *(5)*.

The objective of disaster preparedness is to ensure that appropriate systems, procedures and resources are in place to provide prompt effective assistance to disaster victims, thus facilitating relief measures and rehabilitation of services.

The individuals are responsible for maintaining their well-being. Community members, resources, organizations, and administration should be the cornerstone of an emergency preparedness programme. The reasons of community preparedness are : (a) Members of the community have the most to lose from being vulnerable to disasters and the most to gain from an effective and appropriate emergency preparedness programme; (b) Those who first respond to an emergency come from within the community. When transport and communications are disrupted, an external emergency response may not arrive for days ; (c) Resources are most easily pooled at the community level and every community possesses capabilities. Failure to exploit these capabilities is poor resource management ; (d) Sustained development is best achieved by allowing emergency-affected communities to design, manage, and implement internal and external assistance programme *(6)*.

Disaster preparedness is an on-going multisectoral activity. It forms an integral part of the national system responsible for developing plans and programmes for disaster management, prevention, mitigation, preparedness, response, rehabilitation and reconstruction. The system, known by a variety of names depending on the country, depends on the coordination of a variety of sectors to carry out the following tasks *(4)* :

1. Evaluate the risk of the country or particular region to disaster ;
2. Adopt standards and regulations ;
3. Organize communication, information and warning systems ;
4. Ensure coordination and response mechanisms ;
5. Adopt measures to ensure that financial and other resources are available for increased readiness and can be mobilized in disaster situation ;
6. Develop public education programmes ;
7. Coordinate information sessions with news media ; and
8. Organize disaster simulation excercises that test response mechanisms.

The emergency preparedness and emergency management do not exist in a vacuum. To succeed, emergency programmes must be appropriate to their context. This context will vary from country to country and from community to community.

Policy development *(6)*

The policy development is "the formal statement of a course of action". Policy is strategic in nature and performs the following functions :

(a) establish long-term goals;
(b) asign responsibilities for achieving goals;
(c) establish recommended work practice; and
(d) determine criteria for decision making.

While policies tend to be "top-down" that is authorized by higher levels, implementation of the strategies that arise from a policy tend to be "bottom-up", with the higher levels assisting lower levels. The form of emergency preparedness policy varies from country to country. Six sectors are required for response and recovery strategies. These sectors are communication, health, social welfare, police and security, search and rescue and transport.

Personal protection in different types of emergencies *(6)*

In addition to considering action by rescuers, thought must be given to personal protection measures in different types of emergencies. Making people aware of what is expected of them in case of an emergency can make large difference to the organized management efforts. By taking precautions, the individual assists the collective effort to reduce the effects of an emergency.

A number of measures must be observed by all persons in all types of emergency:

- Do not use the telephone, except to call for help, so as to leave telephone lines free for the organization of response.
- Listen to the messages broadcast by radio and the various media so as to be informed of development.
- Carry out the official instructions given over the radio or by loudspeaker.
- Keep a family emergency kit ready.

In all the different types of emergency, it is better:

- to be prepared than to get hurt;
- to get information so as to get organized;
- to wait rather than act too hastily.

FLOODS

What to do before-hand

While town planning is a government responsibility, individuals should find out about risks in the area where they live. For example, people who live in areas downstream from a dam should know the special signals (such as foghorns) used when a dam threatens to break. Small floods can be foreseen by watching the water level after heavy rains and regularly listening to the weather forecasts.

Forecasting of floods or tidal waves is very difficult, but hurricanes and cyclones often occur at the same time of year, when particular vigilance must be exercised. They are often announced several hours or days before they arrive.

During a flood

- Turn off the electricity to reduce the risk of electrocution.
- Protect people and property:
  - as soon as the flood begins, take any vulnerable people (children, the old, the sick, and the disabled) to an upper floor;
  - whenever possible, move personal belongings upstairs or go to raised shelters provided for use in floods.
- Beware of water contamination – if the taste, colour, or smell of the water is suspicious, it is vital to use some means of purification.
- Evacuate danger zones as ordered by the local authorities it is essential to comply strictly with the evacuation advice given. Authorities will recommend that families take with them the emergency supplies they have prepared.

After a flood

When a flood is over, it is important that people do not return home until told to do so by the local authorities, who will have ensured that buildings have not been undermined by water. From then on it is essential to:

- wait until the water is declared safe before drinking any that is untreated;
- clean and disinfect any room that has been flooded;
- sterilize or wash with boiling water all dishes and kitchen utensils;
- get rid of any food that has been in or near the water,

including canned foods and any food kept in refrigerators and freezers;
- get rid of all consumables (drinks, medicines, cosmetics, etc.).

STORMS, HURRICANES AND TORNADOES

What to do before-hand

Above all, it is vital that people find out about the kinds of storm liable to strike their region so that they can take optimum preventive measures, and:

- choose a shelter in advance, before the emergency occurs – a cellar, a basement, or an alcove may be perfectly suitable;
- minimize the effects of the storm – fell dead trees, prune tree branches, regularly check the state of roofs, the state of the ground, and the drainage around houses;
- take measures against flooding;
- prepare a family emergency kit.

During an emergency

- Listen to the information and advice provided by the authorities.
- Do not go out in a car or a boat once the storm has been announced.
- Evacuate houses if the authorities request this, taking the family emergency package.
- If possible, tie down any object liable to be blown away by the wind; if there is time, nail planks to the doors and shutters, open the windows and doors slightly on the side opposite to the direction from which the wind is coming so as to reduce wind pressure on the house.
- If caught outside in a storm, take refuge as quickly as possible in a shelter; if there is no shelter, lie down flat in a ditch.
- In a thunderstorm keep away from doors, windows, and electrical conductors, unplug electrical appliances and television aerials. Do not use any electrical appliances or the telephone.
- Anyone who is outside should
  - look for shelter in a building (never under a tree);
  - if out in a boat, get back to the shore;
  - keep away from fences and electric cables;
  - kneel down rather than remain standing.

After an emergency

After the storm has subsided

- follow the instructions given by the authorities;
- stay indoors and do not go to the stricken areas;
- give the alert as quickly as possible;
- give first aid to the injured;
- make sure the water is safe to drink and check the contents of refrigerators and freezers;
- check the exterior of dwellings and call for assistance if there is a risk of falling objects (tiles, guttering, etc.).

EARTHQUAKES

What to do before-hand

The movement of the ground in an earthquake is rarely the direct cause of injuries; most are caused by falling objects or collapsing buildings. Many earthquakes are followed (several hours or even days later) by further tremors, usually of progressively decreasing intensity. To reduce the destructive effects of earthquakes a number of precautions are essential for people living in risk areas:

- Build in accordance with urban planning regulations for risk areas.
- Ensure that all electrical and gas appliances in houses, together with all pipes connected to them, are firmly fixed.
- Avoid storing heavy objects and materials in high positions.
- Hold family evacuation drills and ensure that the whole family knows what to do in case of an earthquake.
- Prepare a family emergency kit.

During an earthquake

- Keep calm, do no panic.
- People who are indoors should stay there but move to the central part of the building.
- Keep away from the stairs, which might collapse suddenly.
- People who are outside should stay there, keeping away from buildings to avoid collapsing walls and away from electric cables.
- Anyone in a vehicle should park it, keeping away from bridges and buildings.

After an earthquake

- Obey the authorities' instructions.
- Do not go back into damaged buildings since tremors may start again at any moment.
- Give first-aid to the injured and alert the emergency services in case of fire, burst pipes, etc.
- Do not go simply to look at the stricken areas: this will hamper rescue work.
- Keep emergency packages and a radio near at hand.
- Make sure that water is safe to drink and food stored at home is fit to eat (in case of electricity cuts affecting refrigerators and freezers).

CLOUDS OF TOXIC FUMES

What to do before-hand

People in a risk area should:

- find out about evacuation plans and facilities;
- familiarize themselves with the alarm signals used in case of emergency;
- equip doors and windows with the tightest possible fastenings;
- prepare family emergency kits.

During an emergency

- Do not use the telephone; leave lines free for rescue services.
- Listen to the messages given by radio and other media.
- Carry out the instructions transmitted by radio or loudspeaker.
- Close doors and windows.
- Stop up air intakes.
- Seal any cracks or gaps around windows and doors with adhesive tape.

- Organize a reserve of water (by filling wash basins, baths, etc.).
- Turn off ventilators and air conditioners.

After an emergency

- Comply with the authorities' instructions and do not go out until there is no longer any risk.
- Carry out necessary decontamination measures.

MAN-MADE DISASTERS

There are many disasters which have large elements of human causation either accidental or intended. These can also be divided into three categories. (a) Sudden disasters such as Bhopal Gas Tragedy in India on 3rd December 1984 in which a leakage in the storage tank of Union Carbide Pesticide Plant released tons of methyl isocyanate into the air. Wind conditions and an atmospheric inversion, along with delayed warning and a population that had not been taught the nature of risks and the appropriate response increased the impact. About 2 million people were exposed to the gas leaving about 3,000 dead. People are still suffering from the adverse effects of the gas. The second example is the accident at reactor 4 of the Chernobyl nuclear power station in the Soviet Union on April 26, 1986, which resulted in the largest reported accidental release of radioactive material in the history of nuclear power. It deposited more than 7 million curies of Iodine 131, Cesium 134 and 137, Strontium 90 and other isotopes throughout the northern hemisphere, *(2)*; (b) Insidious disasters, such as insidious chemical exposure and insidious radiation exposure, as in nuclear weapons production factories, research laboratories resulting in release of radioactive substances into the air, soil and underground water. Chemical plants releasing their toxic by-products into rivers and other water sources is another example. Other form of long term and continuing human-made disaster include global warming (the "green house effect") caused by the heat-trapping gases in the atmosphere released by burning of fossil fuels, and depletion of ozone layer due to the use of the aerosolized chlorofluorohydrocarbons etc.; and (c) Wars and civil conflicts. The latest example is the attack on twin buildings of World Trade Centre in New York in which about 6000 people lost their lives and thousands were injured.

Since World War II, there have been about 127 wars and 21.8 million war-related deaths involving more than 50 per cent of civilians *(2)*. Recently the proportion of civilians among dead has been increasing. Air-borne power and wide–ranging nature of modern war puts an entire population at risk, disrupting food production and supply routes, imperiling fragile ecosystem and forcing refugees by hundred of thousands to flee. More than half of the civilian deaths in current hostilities resulted from war-related famines. As for causes of most wars, most frequent objectives were gain of land assets, and independence. However, civil wars, representing power conflicts within nations, have increased sharply in the twentieth century, and are now, by far the major form of warfare.

The public health response to man-made disaster is the primary prevention, i.e., prevention of occurrence of the disaster. Much can be done to prevent not only the consequences but also the occurrences of fires, explosions, crashes, and sudden chemical and radiation exposures. This includes tighter regulations of chemical plants and other hazardous facilities and insistence that the chemical plants be built away from dense populous areas. Other measures include appropriate engineering and technological measures (like building codes, dam designs, containment of toxic materials), early warning, if possible, and protection against human errors.

During the first half of the twentieth century, two world wars and many regional conflicts provided the experience for governments, to develop civil defence programmes. They were reshaped after the introduction of nuclear weapons and massive air attacks occuring with little warning. Weapons of mass destruction are indiscriminate, killing and injuring civilians as well as military personnel, and destroying and contaminating ecosystem over wide areas. People around the world have turned towards efforts to stop the arms race and prevent nuclear war.

Disasters in India

With a wide range of topographic and climatic conditions, India is the highly disaster-prone country in Asia–Pacific region with an average of 8 major natural calamities a year. While floods, cyclones, draughts, earthquakes and epidemics are frequent from time to time, major accidents happen in railways, mines and factories causing extensive damage to human life and property.

Northern mountain regions, including the foot hills are prone to snow-storms, land-slides and earthquakes. The eastern coastal areas are prone to severe floods and cyclones (Andhra Pradesh, West Bengal, Orissa, etc.). Bihar, Assam and Uttar Pradesh get major floods almost every year. Western desert areas are prone to draughts. There is hardly a year when some or the other part of the country does not face the spectre of drought, floods or cyclone. Orissa had super cyclone on 29th October 1999, when thousands lost their lives and many more became homeless. Gujarat had a severe earthquake in which about 16,480 people died and lacs became homeless. Indian ocean tsunami killed more than 200,000 persons in India in Dec. 2004 and major earthquake in Jammu & Kashmir (7.4 RS) left 2,100 dead and 30,000 injured, more recently, in June 2013 in Uttarakhand, cloudburst causing floods that killed about 5,748 people in Kedarnath, and the floods in Kashmir valley in 2014. India also saw world's worst man-made disaster in 1984, when methyl isocyanate gas leaked at Union Carbide Pesticide Plant in Bhopal killing about 3,000 people. People are still suffering from variety of diseases, as an after effect of this tragedy.

In the federal structure of India, the state governments are responsible for the execution of relief work in wake of natural disasters. Government of India plays a supportive role, in terms of supplementation of final resources to the states. An administrative system has been developed to combat and minimize the adverse impact of the natural disasters. The overall coordination of disaster management vests with the Ministry of Home Affairs (MHA). The Cabinet Committee on Security (CCS) and the National Crisis Management Committee (NCMC) are the key committees involved in the top-level decision-making with regard to disaster management. The National Disaster Management Authority (NDMA) is the lead agency responsible for the preparation of Disaster Management (DM) plans and the execution of DM functions at the national level. The Disaster Management Act of 2005 provides for the setting up of NDMA at national level and the SDMA at the state level *(1)*. Since health is an important part of disaster management, in the DGHS under the ministry of Health and Family Welfare there is a special wing called the Emergency Medical Relief Wing which coordinates all activities related to health *(7)*.

In a vast country like India, it is not practicable for the government machinery alone, to undertake disaster reduction programmes without involvement of NGOs. Public education and community involvement plays a vital role here. As part of the International Decade for Natural Disaster Reduction activities, every year, the second wednesday of October has been designated as *World Disaster Reduction Day*.

Indian Meteorological Department (IMD) plays a key role in forwarning the disaster. It has five centres in Kolkata, Bhubaneswar, Visakhapatnam, Chennai and Mumbai for detection and tracing of cyclone storms. Satellite imagery facilities and cyclone warning radars are provided to various Cyclone Warning Centres. In addition, it has 31 special observation posts set up along east coast of India. For all ships out at sea, warnings are issued six times a day. Insat Disaster Warning System (DWS) receivers have been installed primarily in the coastal areas of Tamil Nadu and Andhra Pradesh. This has proved very reliable form of communication system. The Snow and Avalanche Study Establishment (SASE) in Manali has been issuing warning to people about avalanches 24 to 48 hours in advance.

INTERNATIONAL AGENCIES PROVIDING HEALTH HUMANITARIAN ASSISTANCE

Every country is a potential source of health humanitarian assistance for some other disaster-striken nation. Bilateral assistance, whether personnel, supplies or cash is probably the most important source of external aid. Several international or regional agencies have established special funds, procedures and offices to provide humanitarian assistance. United Nation's Agencies are United Nations Office for the Coordination of Humanitarian Affairs (OCHA), World Health Organization (WHO), UNICEF, World Food Programme (WFP), Food and Agriculture Organization (FAO). Inter-governmental organizations are European Community Humanitarian Office (ECHO), Organization of American States (OAS), Centre of Coordination for Prevention of Natural Disasters in Central America, Caribbean Disaster Emergency Response Agency. Some Non-Governmental Organizations are CARE, International Committee of Red Cross, International Council of Voluntary Agencies (ICVA), International Federation of Red Cross and Red Crescent Societies (IFRC) etc.

References

1. Govt. of India (2016), *National Disaster Management Plan 2016,* A Publication of the National Disaster Management Authority, Govt. of India, May 2016, New Delhi.
2. Maxy – Rosenay – Last (1992), *Public Health and Preventive Medicine*, 13th Edition.
3. WHO (1989). *Coping with Natural Disasters* : The Role of Local Health Personnel and the Community.
4. PAHO (2000). *Natural Disasters, Protecting the Public's Health*, Scientific Publication No. 575.
5. WHO (1995). *Coping with major emergencies* – Strategy and Approaches to Humanitarian Action, Geneva, World Health Organization, 1995.
6. WHO (1999). *Community Emergency Preparedness* : a manual for managers and policy – makers, WHO.
7. Govt. of India (2001). *Annual Report 2000–2001*, Ministry of Health and Family Welfare, New Delhi.

18 Occupational health

"Prevention is better than cure"

Occupational health is essentially preventive medicine. The Joint ILO/WHO Committee on Occupational Health, in the course of its first session, held in 1950, gave the following definition: "Occupational health should aim at the *promotion* and maintenance of the highest degree of physical, mental and social well-being of workers in all occupations; the *prevention* among workers of departures from health caused by their working conditions; the protection of workers in their employment from risks resulting from factors adverse to health; the placing and maintenance of the worker in an occupational environment adapted to his physiological and psychological equipment, and, to summarize, the adaptation of work to man and of each man to his job *(1)*.

Preventive medicine and occupational health have the same aim – the prevention of disease and maintenance of the highest degree of physical, mental and social well-being of workers in all occupations; the levels of application of preventive measures are the same – health promotion, specific protection, early diagnosis and treatment, disability limitation and rehabilitation; the tools are the same – epidemiologic approach, statistics, health screening, health education etc. *(2)*. Occupational health, therefore, is the application of preventive medicine in all places of employment.

In the past, it was customary to think of occupational health entirely in relation to factories and mines; hence the terms "industrial hygiene" or "industrial health" were in vogue. Modern concepts of occupational health now embrace all types of employment including mercantile and commercial enterprises, service trades, forestry and agriculture and includes the subjects of industrial hygiene, industrial diseases, industrial accidents, toxicology in relation to industrial hazards, industrial rehabilitation and occupational psychology. Occupational health in agriculture and ergonomics (human engineering) are relatively new concepts *(3,4)*.

ERGONOMICS is now a well recognized discipline and constitutes an integral part of any advanced occupational health service. The term "ergonomics" is derived from the Greek *ergon,* meaning work and *nomos,* meaning law. It simply means: "fitting the job to the worker". Training in ergonomics involves designing of machines, tools, equipment and manufacturing processes, lay-out of the places of work, methods of work and environment in order to achieve greater efficiency of both man and machine *(5)*. The object of ergonomics is "to achieve the best mutual adjustment of man and his work, for the improvement of human efficiency and well-being". The application of ergonomics has made a significant contribution to reducing industrial accidents and to the overall health and efficiency of the workers *(5)*.

HEALTH OF THE WORKER

Industrial workers constitute only a segment of the general population, and the factors that influence the health of the population also apply equally to industrial workers, i.e., housing, water, sewage and waste disposal, nutrition, and education. A detailed consideration of these factors can be found in Chapter 2. In addition to these factors, the health of the industrial workers, in a large measure, will also be influenced by conditions prevailing in their work place. One of the declared aims of occupational health is to provide a safe 'occupational environment' in order to safeguard the health of the workers and to step up industrial production.

Occupational environment

By "occupational environment" is meant the sum of external conditions and influences which prevail at the place of work and which have a bearing on the health of the working population. The industrial worker today is placed in a highly complicated environment which is getting more complicated as man is becoming more ingenious. Basically, there are three types of interaction in a working environment:

(a) Man and physical, chemical and biological agents

(b) Man and machine

(c) Man and man.

MAN AND PHYSICAL, CHEMICAL AND BIOLOGICAL AGENTS

(1) *Physical agents:* The physical factors in the working environment which may be adverse to health are heat, cold, humidity, air movement, heat radiation, light, noise, vibrations and ionizing radiation. The factors act in different ways on the health and efficiency of the workers, singly or in different combinations. The amount of working and breathing space, toilet, washing and bathing facilities are also important factors in an occupational environment. (2) *Chemical agents:* These comprise a large number of chemicals, toxic dusts and gases which are potential hazards to the health of the workers. Some chemical agents cause disabling respiratory illnesses, some cause injury to skin and some may have a deleterious effect on the blood and other organs of the body. (3) *Biological agents:* The workers may be exposed to viral, rickettsial, bacterial and parasitic agents which may result from close contact with animals or their products, contaminated water, soil or food.

MAN AND MACHINE

An industry or factory implies the use of machines driven by power with emphasis on mass production. The unguarded machines, protruding and moving parts, poor installation of the plant, lack of safety measures are the causes of accidents which is a major problem in industries. Working for long hours in unphysiological postures is the cause of fatigue, backache, diseases of joints and muscles and impairment of the worker's health and efficiency.

MAN AND MAN

There are numerous psychosocial factors which operate at the place of work. These are the human relationships amongst workers themselves on the one hand, and those in authority over them on the other. Examples of psychosocial factors include the type and rhythm of work, work stability, service conditions, job satisfaction, leadership style, security, workers participation, communication, system of payment, welfare conditions, degree of responsibility, trade union activities, incentives and a host of similar other factors, all entering the field of human relationships. In modern occupational health, the emphasis is upon the people, the conditions in which they live and work, their hopes and fears and their attitudes towards their job, their fellow-workers and employers *(2)*.

The occupational environment of the worker cannot be considered apart from his *domestic environment.* Both are complementary to each other. The worker takes his worries home, and brings to his work disturbances which arise in his domestic environment. Stress at work may disturb his sleep, just as stress at home may affect his work. Severe prolonged stress, no matter where it has been aroused, may produce serious physical or mental symptoms which do not allow man to work efficiently. According to ecological approach, occupational health represents a dynamic equilibrium or adjustment between the industrial worker and his occupational environment.

OCCUPATIONAL HAZARDS

An industrial worker may be exposed to five types of hazards, depending upon his occupation:

(a) Physical hazards
(b) Chemical hazards
(c) Biological hazards
(d) Mechanical hazards
(e) Psychosocial hazards.

a. Physical hazards

(1) HEAT AND COLD: The common physical hazard in most industries is heat. The direct effects of heat exposure are burns, heat exhaustion, heat stroke and heat cramps; the indirect effects are decreased efficiency, increased fatigue and enhanced accident rates. Many industries have local "hot spots" – ovens and furnaces, which radiate heat. Radiant heat is the main problem in foundry, glass and steel industries, while *heat stagnation* is the principal problem in jute and cotton textile industry *(7)*. High temperatures are also found in mines for instance in the Kolar Gold Mines of Mysore which is the second deepest mine of the world (11,000 feet), temperatures as high as 65 deg. C are recorded *(8)*. Physical work under such conditions is very stressful and impairs the health and efficiency of the workers. For gainful work involving sustained and repeated effort, a reasonable temperature must be maintained in each work room. The Indian Factories Act has not laid down any specific temperature standard. However, the work of Rao (1952, 1953) and Mookerjee et al. (1953) indicate that a corrected effective temperature of 69 to 80 deg. F (20°C to 27°C) is the comfort zone in this country and temperatures above 80 deg. F (27°C) cause discomfort *(7)*.

Important hazards associated with cold work are chilblains, erythrocyanosis, immersion foot, and frostbite as a result of cutaneous vasoconstriction. General hypothermia is not unusual *(9)*.

(2) LIGHT: The workers may be exposed to the risk of poor illumination or excessive brightness. The *acute* effects of poor illumination are eye strain, headache, eye pain, lachrymation, congestion around the cornea and eye fatigue. The *chronic* effects on health include "miner's nystagmus". Exposure to excessive brightness or "glare" is associated with discomfort, annoyance and visual fatigue. Intense direct glare may also result in blurring of vision and lead to accidents. There should be sufficient and suitable lighting, natural or artificial, wherever persons are working.

(3) NOISE: Noise is a health hazard in many industries. The effects of noise are of two types: (i) *Auditory effects* which consist of temporary or permanent hearing loss. (ii) *Non-auditory effects* which consist of nervousness, fatigue, interference with communication by speech, decreased efficiency and annoyance. The degree of injury from exposure to noise depends upon a number of factors such as intensity and frequency range, duration of exposure and individual susceptibility.

(4) VIBRATION: Vibration, especially in the frequency range 10 to 500 Hz, may be encountered in work with pneumatic tools such as drills and hammers. Vibration usually affects the hands and arms. After some months or years of exposure, the fine blood vessels of the fingers may become increasingly sensitive to spasm (white fingers). Exposure to vibration may also produce injuries of the joints of the hands, elbows and shoulders *(9)*.

(5) ULTRAVIOLET RADIATION : Occupational exposure to ultraviolet radiation occurs mainly in arc welding. Such radiation mainly affects the eyes, causing intense conjunctivitis and keratitis (welder's flash). Symptoms are redness of the eyes and pain, these usually disappear in a few days with no permanent effect on the vision or on the deeper structures of the eye *(9)*.

(6) IONIZING RADIATION : Ionizing radiation is finding increasing application in medicine and industry, e.g., X-rays and radioactive isotopes. Important radioisotopes are cobalt 60 and phosphorus 32. Certain tissues such as bone marrow are more sensitive than others and from a genetic standpoint, there are special hazards when the gonads are exposed. The radiation hazards comprise genetic changes, malformation, cancer, leukaemia, depilation, ulceration, sterility and in extreme cases death. The International Commission of Radiological Protection has set the maximum permissible level of occupational exposure at 5 rem per year to the whole body *(10)*.

b. Chemical hazards

There is hardly any industry which does not make use of chemicals. The chemical hazards are on the increase with the introduction of newer and complex chemicals. Chemical agents act in three ways : local action, inhalation and ingestion. The ill-effects produced depend upon the duration of exposure, the quantum of exposure and individual susceptibility.

(1) LOCAL ACTION : Some chemicals cause dermatitis, eczema, ulcers and even cancer by *primary irritant action;* some cause dermatitis by an allergic action. Some

chemicals, particularly the aromatic nitro and amino compounds such as TNT and aniline are *absorbed* through the skin and cause systemic effects. Occupational dermatitis is a big problem in industry. Rao and Banerji (1952) were the first to draw attention in India to the prevalence of occupational dermatitis due to machine oil, rubber, X-rays, caustic alkalies and lime *(7)*.

(2) INHALATION : (i) *DUSTS* : Dusts are finely divided solid particles with size ranging from 0.1 to 150 microns. They are released into the atmosphere during crushing, grinding, abrading, loading and unloading operations. Dusts are produced in a number of industries – mines, foundry, quarry, pottery, textile, wood or stone working industries. Dust particles larger than 10 microns settle down from the air rapidly, while the smaller ones remain suspended indefinitely. Particles smaller than 5 microns are directly inhaled into the lungs and are retained there. This fraction of the dust is called "respirable dust", and is mainly responsible for pneumoconiosis. Dusts have been classified into *inorganic* and *organic* dusts; *soluble* and *insoluble dusts*. The inorganic dusts are silica, mica, coal, asbestos dust, etc.; the organic dusts are cotton, jute and the like. The soluble dusts dissolve slowly, enter the systemic circulation and are eventually eliminated by body metabolism. The insoluble dusts remain, more or less, permanently in the lungs. They are mainly the cause of pneumoconiosis. The most common dust diseases in this country are silicosis and anthracosis. (ii) *GASES* : Exposure to gases is a common hazard in industries. Gases are sometimes classified as *simple gases* (e.g., oxygen, hydrogen), *asphyxiating gases* (e.g. carbon monoxide, cyanide gas, sulphur dioxide, chlorine) and *anaesthetic gases* (e.g., chloroform, ether, trichlorethylene). Carbon monoxide hazard is frequently reported in coal-gas manufacturing plants and steel industry. (iii) *METALS AND THEIR COMPOUNDS:* A large number of metals, and their compounds are used throughout the industry. The chief mode of entry of some of them is by inhalation as dust or fumes. The industrial physician should be aware of the toxic effects of lead, antimony, arsenic, beryllium, cadmium, cobalt, manganese, mercury, phosphorus, chromium, zinc and others. The ill-effects depend upon the duration of exposure and the dose or concentration of exposure. Unlike the pneumoconiosis, most chemical intoxications respond favourably to cessation, exposure and medical treatment.

(3) INGESTION: Occupational diseases may also result from ingestion of chemical substances such as lead, mercury, arsenic, zinc, chromium, cadmium, phosphorus etc. Usually these substances are swallowed in minute amounts through contaminated hands, food or cigarettes. Much of the ingested material is excreted through faeces and only a small proportion may reach the general blood circulation.

c. Biological hazards

Workers may be exposed to infective and parasitic agents at the place of work. The occupational diseases in this category are brucellosis, leptospirosis, anthrax, hydatidosis, psittacosis, tetanus, encephalitis, fungal infections, schistosomiasis and a host of others. Persons working among animal products (e.g., hair, wool, hides) and agricultural workers are specially exposed to biological hazards.

d. Mechanical hazards

The mechanical hazards in industry centre round machinery, protruding and moving parts and the like. About 10 per cent of accidents in industry are said to be due to mechanical causes.

e. Psychosocial hazards

The psychosocial hazards arise from the workers' failure to adapt to an alien psychosocial environment. Frustration, lack of job satisfaction, insecurity, poor human relationships, emotional tension are some of the psychosocial factors which may undermine both physical and mental health of the workers. The capacity to adapt to different working environments is influenced by many factors such as education, cultural background, family life, social habits, and what the worker expects from employment.

The health effects can be classified in two main categories: (a) Psychological and behavioural changes : including hostility, aggressiveness, anxiety, depression, tardiness, alcoholism, drug abuse, sickness, absenteeism; (b) Psychosomatic illhealth : including fatigue, headache; pain in the shoulders, neck and back; propensity to peptic ulcer, hypertension, heart disease and rapid aging.

Reports from various parts of the world indicate that physical factors (heat, noise, poor lighting) also play a major role in adding to or precipitating mental disorders among workers. The increasing stress on automation, electronic operations and nuclear energy may introduce newer psychosocial health problems in industry. Psychosocial hazards are therefore, assuming more importance than physical or chemical hazards.

OCCUPATIONAL DISEASES

There is no internationally accepted definition for the term "occupational disease" *(3)*. However, occupational diseases are usually defined as diseases arising out of or in the course of employment. For convenience, they may be grouped as under:

I. Diseases due to physical agents

(1) Heat	: Heat hyperpyrexia, heat exhaustion, heat syncope, heat cramps, burns and local effects such as prickly heat.
(2) Cold	: Trench foot, frost bite, chilblains
(3) Light	: Occupational cataract, miner's nystagmus
(4) Pressure	: Caisson disease, air embolism, blast (explosion)
(5) Noise	: Occupational deafness
(6) Radiation	: Cancer, leukaemia, aplastic anaemia, pancytopenia
(7) Mechanical factors	: Injuries, accidents
(8) Electricity	: Burns.

II. Diseases due to chemical agents

(1) Gases: CO_2, CO, HCN, CS_2, NH_3, N_2, H_2S, HCl, SO_2 – these cause gas poisoning.

(2) Dusts (Pneumoconiosis)

(i) Inorganic dusts :

(a) Coal dust	..	Anthracosis
(b) Silica	..	Silicosis
(c) Asbestos	..	Asbestosis, cancer lung
(d) Iron	..	Siderosis

(ii) Organic (vegetable) dusts

(a) Cane fibre	..	Bagassosis

(b) Cotton dust .. Byssinosis

(c) Tobacco .. Tobacossis *(11)*

(d) Hay or grain dust .. Farmers' lung

(3) Metals and their compounds

Toxic hazards from lead, mercury, cadmium, manganese, beryllium, arsenic, chromium etc.

(4) Chemicals : Acids, alkalies, pesticides

(5) Solvents : Carbon bisulphide, benzene, trichloroethylene, chloroform, etc.

III. Diseases due to biological agents

Brucellosis, leptospirosis, anthrax, actinomycosis, hydatidosis, psittacosis, tetanus, encephalitis, fungal infections, etc.

IV. Occupational cancers

Cancer of skin, lungs, bladder.

V. Occupational dermatosis

Dermatitis, eczema.

VI. Diseases of psychological origin

Industrial neurosis, hypertension, peptic ulcer, etc.

PNEUMOCONIOSIS

Dust within the size range of 0.5 to 3 micron, is a health hazard producing, after a variable period of exposure, a lung disease known as pneumoconiosis, which may gradually cripple a man by reducing his working capacity due to lung fibrosis and other complications. The hazardous effects of dusts on the lungs depend upon a number of factors such as (a) chemical composition (b) fineness (c) concentration of dust in the air (d) period of exposure and (e) health status of the person exposed. Therefore, the threshold limit values for different dusts are different. In addition to the toxic effect of the dust on the lung tissues, the super-imposition of infections like tuberculosis may also influence the pattern of pneumoconiosis. The important dust diseases are silicosis, anthracosis, byssinosis, bagassosis, asbestosis and farmer's lung. As no cure for the pneumoconiosis is known, it is essential to prevent these diseases from arising. A brief account of these conditions is given below :

1. Silicosis

Among the occupational diseases, silicosis is the major cause of permanent disability and mortality. It is caused by inhalation of dust containing free silica or silicon dioxide (SiO_2). It was first reported in India from the Kolar Gold Mines (Mysore) in 1947. Ever since, its occurrence has been uncovered in various other industries, e.g., mining industry (coal, mica, gold, silver, lead, zinc, manganese and other metals), pottery and ceramic industry, sand blasting, metal grinding, building and construction work, rock mining, iron and steel industry and several others.

In the mica mines of Bihar, out of 329 miners examined, 34.1 per cent were found suffering from silicosis. In a ceramic and pottery industry, the incidence of silicosis was found to be 15.7 per cent *(12)*. The incidence of silicosis depends upon the chemical composition of the dust, size of the particles, duration of exposure and individual susceptibility. The higher the concentration of free silica in the dust, the greater the hazard. Particles between 0.5 to 3 micron are the most dangerous because they reach the interior of the lungs with ease. The longer the duration of exposure, the greater the risk of developing silicosis. It is found that the incubation period may vary from a few months up to 6 years of exposure, depending upon the above factors.

The particles are ingested by the phagocytes which accumulate and block the lymph channels. Pathologically, silicosis is characterized by a dense "nodular" fibrosis, the nodules ranging from 3 to 4 mm in diameter. Clinically the onset of the disease is insidious. Some of the early manifestations are irritant cough, dyspnea on exertion and pain in the chest. With more advanced disease, impairment of total lung capacity (TLC) is commonly present. An X-ray of the chest shows "snow-storm" appearance in the lung fields. Silicosis is progressive and what is more important is that silicotics are prone to pulmonary tuberculosis, a condition called "silico-tuberculosis." In recent years doubts have been raised, whether silico-tuberculotics are really tubercular or purely silicotics. It is because, sputum in silico-tuberculotics rarely shows tubercle bacilli; children and women of silico-tuberculotics do not develop tuberculosis; post-mortems on silico-tuberculotics failed to prove the existence of tuberculosis disease, but showed them to be cases of pure silicosis. The radiological evidence in the two conditions is so similar that one is apt to mistake a case of silicotic to be a case of tuberculosis of lungs *(13)*. The final answer to this question is still awaited.

There is no effective treatment for silicosis. Fibrotic changes that have already taken place cannot be reversed. The only way that silicosis can be controlled (if not altogether eliminated) is by (a) rigorous dust control measures, e.g., substitution, complete enclosure, isolation, hydroblasting, good house-keeping, personal protective measures and (b) regular physical examination of workers *(14)*.

Silicosis was made a notifiable disease under the Factories Act 1948 and the Mines Act 1952.

2. Anthracosis

Previously it was thought that pulmonary "anthracosis" was inert. Studies *(15)* indicate that there are two general phases in coal miners pneumoconiosis – (1) the first phase is labelled *simple pneumoconiosis* which is associated with little ventilatory impairment. This phase may require about 12 years of work exposure for its development (2) the second phase is characterised by *progressive massive fibrosis* (PMF); this causes severe respiratory disability and frequently results in premature death. Once a background of simple pneumoconiosis has been attained in the coal worker, a progressive massive fibrosis may develop out of it without further exposure to it. From the point of view of epidemiology, the risk of death among coal miners has been nearly twice that of the general population *(15)*. Coal-miners' pneumoconiosis has been declared a notifiable disease in the Indian Mines Act of 1952, and also compensatable in the Workmen's Compensation (Amendment) Act of 1959.

3. Byssinosis

Byssinosis is due to inhalation of cotton fibre dust over long periods of time. The symptoms are chronic cough and progressive dyspnoea, ending in chronic bronchitis and emphysema. India has a large textile industry employing nearly 35 per cent of the factory workers. Incidence of byssinosis is reported to be 7 to 8 per cent in three independent surveys carried out in Mumbai, Ahmedabad and Delhi *(12)*.

4. Bagassosis

Bagassosis is the name given to an occupational disease of the lung caused by inhalation of bagasse or sugarcane dust. It was first reported in India by Ganguli and Pal in 1955 in a cardboard manufacturing firm near Kolkata. India has a large cane-sugar industry. The sugarcane fibre which earlier went to waste, is now utilized in the manufacturing of paper, cardboard and rayon.

Bagassosis has been shown to be due to a thermophilic actinomycete for which the name *Thermoactinomyces sacchari* was suggested *(18)*. The symptoms consist of breathlessness, cough, haemoptysis and slight fever. Initially there is acute diffuse bronchiolitis. Skiagram may show mottling in lungs or shadow. There is impairment of pulmonary function *(17)*. If treated early, there is resolution of the acute inflammatory condition of the lung. If left untreated, there is diffuse fibrosis, emphysema and bronchiectasis.

PREVENTIVE MEASURES : (1) *DUST CONTROL* : Measures for the prevention and suppression of dust such as wet process, enclosed apparatus, exhaust ventilation etc., should be used. (2) PERSONAL *PROTECTION* : Personal protective equipment (masks or respirators with mechanical filters or with oxygen or air supply) may be necessary. (3) *MEDICAL CONTROL* : Initial medical examination and periodical medical check-ups of the workers are indicated. (4) *BAGASSE CONTROL* : By keeping the moisture content above 20 per cent and spraying the bagasse with 2 per cent propionic acid, a widely used fungicide, bagasse can be rendered safe for manufacturing use *(18)*.

5. Asbestosis

Asbestos is the commercial name given to certain types of fibrous materials. They are silicates of varying composition; the silica is combined with such bases as magnesium, iron, calcium, sodium and aluminium. Asbestos is of two types – serpentine or chrysolite variety and the amphibole type. Ninety per cent of the world's production of asbestos is of the serpentine variety, which is hydrated magnesium silicate, the amphibole type contains little magnesium. The amphibole type occurs in different varieties, e.g., crocidolite (blue), amosite (brown), and anthrophyllite (white) *(9)*. Asbestos fibres are usually from 20 to 500 μ in length and 0.5 to 50 μ in diameter. Asbestos is used in the manufacture of asbestos cement, fire-proof textiles, roof tiling, brake lining , gaskets and several other items. Asbestos is mined in Andhra Pradesh (Cuddapah), Bihar, Jharkhand, Karnataka, and Rajasthan – but most of it is imported from USSR, Canada, US and South Africa.

Asbestos enters the body by inhalation, and fine dust may be deposited in the alveoli. The fibres are insoluble. The dust deposited in the lungs causes pulmonary fibrosis leading to respiratory insufficiency and death; carcinoma of the bronchus; mesothelioma of the pleura or peritoneum; and cancer of the gastro-intestinal tract. In Great Britain, an association was reported between mesothelioma and living within 1 km of an asbestos factory *(19)*. The risk of bronchial cancer is reported to be high if occupational exposure to asbestos is combined with cigarette smoking. Mesothelioma, a rare form of cancer of the pleura and peritoneum, has been shown to have a strong association with the crocidolite variety of asbestos *(9)*. The disease does not usually appear until after 5 to 10 years of exposure *(20)*. The fibrosis in asbestosis is due to mechanical irritation, and is peri-bronchial, diffuse in character, and basal in location in contrast to silicosis in which the fibrosis is nodular in character and present in the upper part of the lungs. Clinically the disease is characterized by dyspnoea which is frequently out of proportion to the clinical signs in the lungs. In advanced cases, there may be clubbing of fingers, cardiac distress and cyanosis. The sputum shows "asbestos bodies" which are asbestos fibres coated with fibrin. An X-ray of the chest shows a ground-glass appearance in the lower two-thirds of the lung fields. Once established, the disease is progressive even after removal of the worker from contact *(2)*.

The *preventive measures* consists of : (1) use of safer types of asbestos (chrysolite and amosite); (2) substitution of other insulants: glass fibre, mineral wool, calcium silicate, plastic foams, etc.; (3) rigorous dust control; (4) periodic examination of workers; biological monitoring (clinical, X-ray, lung function), and (5) continuing research.

6. Farmer's lung

Farmer's lung is due to the inhalation of mouldy hay or grain dust *(22)*. In grain dust or hay with a moisture content of over 30 per cent bacteria and fungi grow rapidly, causing a rise of temperature to 40 to 50 deg. C. This heat encourages the growth of thermophilic actinomycetes, of which *Micropolyspora faeni* is the main cause of farmer's lung *(23)*. The acute illness is characterized by general and respiratory symptoms and physical signs. Repeated attacks cause pulmonary fibrosis and inevitable pulmonary damage and cor pulmonale. It is quite possible that this condition might be widespread in India considering the bulk of the population engaged in agricultural work.

LEAD POISONING

More industrial workers are exposed to lead than to any other toxic metal. Lead is used widely in a variety of industries because of its properties : (1) low boiling point (2) mixes with other metals easily to form alloys (3) easily oxidised and (4) anticorrosive. All lead compounds are toxic – lead arsenate, lead oxide and lead carbonate are the most dangerous; lead sulphide is the least toxic.

INDUSTRIAL USES : Over 200 industries are counted where lead is used – manufacture of storage batteries; glass manufacture; ship building; printing and potteries; rubber industry and several others.

NON-OCCUPATIONAL SOURCES : The greatest source of environmental (non-occupational) lead is gasoline. Thousands of tons of lead every year is exhausted from automobiles. Lead is one of the few trace metals that is abundantly present in the environment. Lead exposure may also occur through drinking water from lead pipes; chewing lead paint on window sills or toys in case of children.

MODE OF ABSORPTION : Lead poisoning may occur in three ways : (1) *INHALATION* : Most cases of industrial lead poisoning is due to inhalation of fumes and dust of lead or its compounds. (2) *INGESTION* : Poisoning by ingestion is of less common occurrence. Small quantities of lead trapped in the upper respiratory tract may be ingested. Lead may also be ingested in food or drink through contaminated hands. (3) *SKIN* : Absorption through skin occurs only in respect of the organic compounds of lead, especially tetraethyl lead. Inorganic compounds are not absorbed through the skin.

BODY STORES : The body store of lead in the average adult population is about 150 to 400 mg and blood levels average about 25μg/100 ml. An increase to 70μg/100 ml blood is generally associated with clinical symptoms. Normal adults ingest about 0.2 to 0.3 mg of lead per day largely from food and beverages *(24)*.

DISTRIBUTION IN THE BODY: Ninety per cent of the ingested lead is excreted in the faeces. Lead absorbed from the gut enters the circulation, and 95 per cent enters the erythrocytes. It is then transported to the liver and kidneys and finally transported to the bones where it is laid down with other minerals. Although bone lead is thought to be 'metabolically inactive', it may be released to the soft tissues again under conditions of bone resorption. Lead probably exerts its toxic action by combining with essential SH-groups of certain enzymes, for example some of those involved in prophyrin synthesis and carbohydrate metabolism. Lead has an effect on membrane permeability and potassium leakage has been demonstrated from erythrocytes exposed to lead *(25)*.

CLINICAL PICTURE : The clinical picture of lead poisoning or plumbism is different in the inorganic and organic lead exposures. The toxic effects of *inorganic* lead exposure are abdominal colic, obstinate constipation, loss of appetite, blue-line on the gums, stippling of red cells, anaemia, wrist drop and foot drop. The toxic effects of *organic* lead compounds are mostly on the central nervous system – insomnia, headache, mental confusion, delirium, etc.

DIAGNOSIS *(26, 27)*

Diagnosis of lead poisoning is based on : (1) HISTORY : a history of lead exposure (2) CLINICAL FEATURES : such as loss of appetite, intestinal colic, persistent headache, weakness, abdominal cramps and constipation, joint and muscular pains, blue line on gums, anaemia, etc. (3) LABORATORY TESTS : (a) *Coproporphyrin in urine (CPU)* : Measurement of CPU is a useful screening test. In non-exposed persons, it is less than 150 microgram/litre. (b) *Amino levulinic acid in urine (ALAU)* : If it exceeds 5 mg/litre, it indicates clearly lead absorption. (c) *Lead in blood and urine* : Measurement of lead in blood or urine requires refined laboratory techniques. They provide quantitative indicators of exposure. Lead in urine of over 0.8 mg/litre (normal is 0.2 to 0.8 mg) indicates lead exposure and lead absorption. A blood level of 70μg/100 ml is associated with clinical symptoms. (d) *Basophilic stipling of RBC* : Is a sensitive parameter of the haematological response.

PREVENTIVE MEASURES

(1) *Substitution* : That is, where possible lead compounds should be substituted by less toxic materials. (2) *Isolation* : All processes which give rise to harmful concentration of lead dust or fumes should be enclosed and segregated. (3) *Local exhaust ventilation:* There should be adequate local exhaust ventilation system to remove fumes and dust promptly (4) *Personal protection* : Workers should be protected by approved respirators. (5) *Good house-keeping* : Good house-keeping is essential where lead dust is present. Floors, benches, machines should be kept clean by wet sweeping. (6) *Working atmosphere* : Lead concentration in the working atmosphere should be kept below 2.0 mg per 10 cu. metres of air, which is usually the permissible limit or threshold value. (7) *Periodic examination of workers* : All workers must be given periodical medical examination. Laboratory determination of urinary lead, blood lead, red cell count, haemoglobin estimation and coproporphyrin test of urine should be done periodically. Estimation of basophilic stippling may also be done. An Expert Committee of the WHO states that in the case of exposure to lead, it is not only the average level of lead in the blood that is important, but also the number of subjects whose blood level exceeds a certain value (e.g., 70μg/ml or whose ALA in the urine exceeds 10 mg/litre) (8) *Personal hygiene* : Hand-washing before eating is an important measure of personal hygiene. There should be adequate washing facilities in industry. Prohibition on taking food in work places is essential. (9) *Health education* : Workers should be educated on the risks involved and personal protection measures.

MANAGEMENT : The major objectives in management of lead poisoning are the prevention of further absorption, the removal of lead from soft tissues and prevention of recurrence. Early recognition of cases will help in removing them from further exposure. A saline purge will remove unabsorbed lead from the gut. The use of D-penicillamine has been reported to be effective. Like Ca–EDTA, it is a chelating agent and works by promoting lead excretion in urine. Lead poisoning is a notifiable and compensatable disease in India since 1924.

OCCUPATIONAL CANCER

Occupational cancer is a serious problem in Industry. The sites of the body most commonly affected are skin, lungs, bladder, and blood-forming organs.

1. Skin cancer

Percival Pott was first to draw attention to cancer of scrotum in chimney sweeps in 1775. It was subsequently found that cancer of the scrotum and of the skin in other parts of the body was caused by coal tar, X-rays, certain oils and dyes. Statistics now show that nearly 75 per cent of occupational cancers are skin cancer *(28)*. Skin cancers are an occupational hazard among gas workers, coke oven workers, tar distillers, oil refiners, dye-stuff makers, road makers and in industries associated with the use of mineral oil, pitch, tar and related compounds.

2. Lung cancer

Lung cancer is a hazard in gas industry, asbestos industry, nickel and chromium work, arsenic roasting plants and in the mining of radioactive substances (e.g., uranium). Nickel, chromates, asbestos, coal tar (presumably 3–4 benzpyrene), radioactive substances and cigarette-smoking are proved carcinogens for the lungs. Arsenic, beryllium and isopropyl oil are suspected carcinogens. More than nine-tenths of lung cancer are attributed to tobacco smoking, air pollution and occupational exposure.

3. Bladder cancer

Cancer bladder was first noted in man in aniline industry in 1895. In more recent years, it was noted in the rubber industry. It is now known that bladder cancer is caused by aromatic amines, which are metabolized in the body and excreted in the urine. The industries associated with bladder cancer are the dye-stuffs and dyeing industry, rubber, gas and the electric cable industries. The following have been mentioned as possible bladder carcinogens. : Beta-naphthylamines, benzidine, para-amino-diphenyl, auramine and magenta *(28)*.

4. Leukaemia

Exposure to benzol, roentgen rays and radioactive

substances give rise to leukaemia. Benzol is a dangerous chemical and is used as a solvent in many industries. Leukaemia may appear long after exposure has ceased.

The characteristics of occupational cancer are : (1) they appear after prolonged exposure, (2) the period between exposure and development of the disease may be as long as 10 to 25 years, (3) the disease may develop even after the cessation of exposure, (4) the average age incidence is earlier than that for cancer in general, (5) the localization of the tumours is remarkably constant in any one occupation *(29)*.

Personal hygiene is very important in the prevention of occupational cancer.

Control of industrial cancer

The control measures comprise the following : (1) elimination or control of industrial carcinogens. Technical measures like exclusion of the carcinogen from the industry, well-designed building or machinery, closed system of production, etc., (2) medical examinations, (3) inspection of factories, (4) notification, (5) licensing of establishments, (6) personal hygiene measures, (7) education of workers and management, and (8) research *(30)*.

OCCUPATIONAL DERMATITIS

Occupational dermatitis is a big health problem in many industries. The causes may be; *Physical* – heat, cold, moisture, friction, pressure, X-rays and other rays; *Chemical* – acids, alkalies, dyes, solvents, grease, tar, pitch, chlorinated phenols etc. *Biological* – living agents such as viruses, bacteria, fungi and other parasites; *Plant products* – leaves, vegetables, fruits, flowers, vegetable dust, etc.

The dermatitis-producing agents are further classified into : (1) primary irritants, and (2) sensitizing substances. Primary irritants (e.g. acids, alkalies, dyes, solvents, etc.) cause dermatitis in workers exposed in sufficient concentration and for a long enough period of time. On the other hand, allergic dermatitis occurs only in small percentage of cases, due to sensitization of the skin.

PREVENTION : Occupational dermatitis is largely preventable if proper control measures are adopted : (1) *Pre-selection* : The workers should be medically examined before employment, and those with an established or suspected dermatitis or who have a known pre-disposition to skin disease should be kept away from jobs involving a skin hazard. (2) *Protection* : The worker should be given adequate protection against direct contact by protective clothing, long leather gloves, aprons and boots. The protective clothing should be frequently washed and kept in good order. There are also, what are known as *barrier creams* which must be used regularly and correctly. There is no barrier cream so far invented which will prevent dermatitis in all occupations. (3) *Personal hygiene* : There should be available a plentiful supply of warm water, soap and towels. The worker should be encouraged and educated to make frequent use of these facilities. Adequate washing facilities in industry are a statutory obligation under the Factories Act. (4) *Periodic inspection* : There should be a periodic medical check-up of all workers for early detection and treatment of occupational dermatitis. If necessary, the affected worker may have to be transferred to a job not exposing him to risk. The worker should be educated to report any skin irritation, no matter how mild or insignificant.

RADIATION HAZARDS

A number of industries use radium and other radioactive substances, e.g., painting of luminous dials for watches and other instruments, manufacture of radioactive paints. Exposure to radium also occurs in mining of radioactive ores, monazite sand workers and handling of their products. X-rays are used both in medicine and industry. Exposure to ultraviolet rays occurs in arc and other electric welding processes. Infrared rays are produced in welding, glass blowing, foundry work and other processes where metal and glass are heated to the molten state, and in heating and drying of painted and lacquered objects.

Effects of radiation

Occupational hazards due to ionizing radiation may be acute burns, dermatitis and blood dyscrasias; chronic exposure may cause malignancies and genetic effects. Lung cancer may develop in miners working in uranium mines due to inhalation of radioactive dust.

Preventive measures

(1) Inhalation, swallowing or direct contact with the skin should be avoided. (2) In case of X-rays, shielding should be used of such thickness and of such material as to reduce the exposure below allowable exposures. (3) The employees should be monitored at intervals not exceeding 6 months by use of the film badge or pocket electrometer devices. (4) Suitable protective clothing to prevent contact with harmful material should be used. (5) Adequate ventilation of workplace is necessary to prevent inhalation of harmful gases and dusts. (6) Replacement and periodic examination of workers should be done every 2 months. If harmful effects are found, the employees should be transferred to work not involving exposure to radiation, and (7) Pregnant women should not be allowed to work in places where there is continuous exposure.

OCCUPATIONAL HAZARDS OF AGRICULTURAL WORKERS

Occupational health in agriculture sector is a new concept. From the standpoint of capital investment and number of persons employed, agriculture may be termed as "big industry". Agricultural workers have a multitude of health problems – a fact which is often forgotten because of the widespread misconception that occupational health is mainly concerned with industry and industrialized countries. The health problems of workers in agriculture may be enumerated as below *(3, 31)*.

(1) ZOONOTIC DISEASES : The close contact of the agricultural worker with animals or their products increases the likelihood of contracting certain zoonotic diseases such as brucellosis, anthrax, leptospirosis, tetanus, tuberculosis, bovine and Q fever. The extent of the occupational occurrence of these diseases in most parts of the world is not known.

(2) ACCIDENTS : Agricultural accidents are becoming more frequent, even in developing countries, as a result of the increasing use of agricultural machinery. Insect and snake bites are an additional health problem in India.

(3) TOXIC HAZARDS : Chemicals are being used increasingly in agriculture either as fertilizers, insecticides or pesticides. Agricultural workers are exposed to toxic hazards from these chemicals. Associated factors such as malnutrition and parasitic infestation may increase

susceptibility to poisoning at relatively low levels of exposure.

(4) PHYSICAL HAZARDS : The agricultural worker may be exposed to extremes of climatic conditions such as temperature, humidity, solar radiation, which may impose additional stresses upon him. He may also have to tolerate excessive noise and vibrations, inadequate ventilation and the necessity of working in uncomfortable positions for long periods of time.

(5) RESPIRATORY DISEASES : Exposure to dusts of grains, rice husks, coconut fibres, tea, tobacco, cotton, hay and wood are common where these products are grown. The resulting diseases – e.g., byssinosis, bagassosis, farmer's lung and occupational asthma, appear to be widespread.

ACCIDENTS IN INDUSTRY

Accidents are a common feature in most industries. In fact, some industries are known for accidents, e.g., coal and other mining industries, quarries, construction work. It was estimated that nearly 3 million mandays are lost yearly in India because of accidents. To the worker, the loss is in terms of his wages, apart from human suffering; to the industry, it is in terms of compensation costs, provision of medical care, lowered morale, lowered production and damage to machinery and goods; to the nation in terms of lost production.

CAUSES

The causes of accidents are several and may be grouped under two headings : human and environmental *(33)*.

(a) HUMAN FACTORS : Most authorities consider human factors much more important than environmental factors in accident causation, the former being responsible for 85 per cent of all accidents *(34)*. These factors are : (1) *PHYSICAL :* The physical capabilities of the worker may not meet the job requirements; his visual acuity may be inadequate; his hearing may be inadequate. (2) *PHYSIOLOGICAL FACTORS :* (a) *Sex :* Studies have shown that women are known to have less accidents than men, doing comparative jobs. In a study from the Physiological and Industrial Hygiene Section of the All India Institute of Hygiene and Public Health, Kolkata the ratio was 5:24 reportable accidents in Bengal (b) *Age :* Younger ages are known to be involved more in accidents than older age groups. The very old again are more prone to accidents. (c) *Time :* Accidents are minimum at the beginning of the day and increase gradually as fatigue sets in. (d) *Experience :* Approximately 50 per cent of the employees had accidents in their first 6 months of employment, 23 per cent in the next 6 months and only 3 per cent subsequently in certain industrial undertakings. Thus experience is an important factor in the occurrence of accidents. (e) *Working hours :* An increase in accidents is found whenever the daily or weekly working hours increases. (3) *PSYCHOLOGICAL :* These are mental factors that might involve a person in accidents – carelessness, inattentiveness, overconfidence, slow cerebration, ignorance, inexperience, emotional stress and accident proneness. Psychological factors appear to be more important factors than physiological factors.

(b) ENVIRONMENTAL FACTORS : Amongst the environmental factors known to influence the incidence of accidents are the temperature, poor illumination, humidity, noise and unsafe machines. Causes directly attributable to unsafe machines account for 10–20 per cent of all accidents.

Prevention

Accident prevention is a fascinating problem. Studies have shown that 98 per cent of the accidents are preventable. The principles of accident prevention are : (1) adequate preplacement examination. (2) adequate job training. (3) continuing education. (4) ensuring safe working environment. (5) establishing a safety department in the organization under a competent safety engineer. (6) periodic surveys for finding out hazards. (7) careful reporting, maintenance of records and publicity.

SICKNESS ABSENTEEISM

Sickness absence is an important health problem in industry. It may seriously impede production with serious cost repercussions, both direct as well as indirect. As the production techniques become more sophisticated, absenteeism tends to increase the adverse repercussions. Absenteeism is a useful index in industry to assess the state of health of workers, and their physical, mental and social well-being.

INCIDENCE : India has a working force of about 30 million in registered factories. Research undertaken by the National Productivity Council (N.P.C.) into absenteeism showed a marked increase from around 8 to 13 per cent in the early 1950s to around 15 to 20 per cent or even more in recent years. The rate of absenteeism was reported to be 8 to 10 days per head per year *(36)*.

CAUSES : The causes of sickness-absenteeism may not be entirely due to sickness : (a) *Economic causes :* Studies have shown that if the worker is entitled to sick leave with pay, he tends to avail of this privilege by reporting sick. It is so well remarked that in industry the workers declare themselves fit or unfit for work, at their choice. (b) *Social causes :* Certain social factors appear to influence sickness absenteeism in India. These are the social and family obligations such as weddings, festivals, repair and maintenance of ancestral house and similar other causes. Some of the workers who come from rural areas go back to their villages, for short or long periods, during sowing and harvest seasons. (c) *Medical causes :* About 10 per cent of the days lost were found to be due to occupational accidents. Respiratory and alimentary illnesses have also been found to be important causes. (d) *Non-occupational causes :* Certain non-occupational causes such as nutritional disorders, alcoholism and drug addiction have also been found to be responsible for sickness-absenteeism.

PREVENTION: The prevention/reduction of sickness absenteeism would result in better utilization of resources and maximising the production. The methods for reducing sickness absenteeism include : (1) good factory management and practices (2) adequate preplacement examination (3) good human relations and (4) application of ergonomics.

HEALTH PROBLEMS DUE TO INDUSTRIALIZATION

Industrialization implies the transformation of a peasant society into a community dependent upon the industries. It involves individual and collective technical skills for the manufacture of particular goods through highly specialized processes. There is division of work under the same roof with emphasis on mass production and community profit. In short, industrialization means a social and economic revolution in the culture of a nation. Any such revolution is bound to carry with it some associated hazards.

The community health problems arising out of industrialization may be enumerated as follows. (1) ENVIRONMENTAL SANITATION PROBLEMS (a) HOUSING : A rise in the number of slums and insanitary dwellings is one of the chief problems in all industrial areas due to migration of people from the country-side for employment. The effect of sub-standard housing on the health of the population is discussed elsewhere in detail. (b) WATER POLLUTION : Water pollution is one of the tragic aftermath of rapid industrialization due to discharge of industrial wastes without treatment, into water courses. *Industrial wastes* may contain acids, alkalies, oils and other organic and inorganic chemicals, some of which may be toxic; synthetic detergents and radioactive substances. It requires legal, administrative and technical measures to deal with the situation. Pollution control measures should be instituted in the planning stage itself in the process of industrialization. (c) AIR POLLUTION : This is an important problem in industrial areas which may have an adverse effect on the health of the population. Air pollution is due to the discharge of toxic fumes, gases, smoke and dusts into the atmosphere. It requires proper town planning and zoning to eliminate this hazard. (d) SEWAGE DISPOSAL : There is bound to be pressure on the existing sanitation services if proper planning is not undertaken before locating industries. Lack of facilities for the disposal of sewage leads to pollution of water supply, contamination of soil with parasites and their ova. (2) COMMUNICABLE DISEASES : The main problems in industrial areas are tuberculosis, venereal diseases, and food and water borne infections. These are in addition to the specific diseases associated with specific industries. Industrial areas without proper sewage disposal have become hot-beds for filariasis owing to the breeding of the mosquito vectors in contaminated water. (3) FOOD SANITATION : The standards of food sanitation are bound to be lowered due to industrialization, if proper precautions are not taken. Food-borne infections such as typhoid fever and viral hepatitis are all too common in India. (4) MENTAL HEALTH : Mental health problems are due to altered living conditions. People are removed from the warmth of village community life and are transplanted in an alien environment which calls for certain adjustments. Failure of adjustment leads to mental illness, psychoneurosis, behaviour disorders, delinquency. etc. (5) ACCIDENTS : Accidents are a public health problem in industrial areas due to congestion, vehicular traffic and the increased tempo of life. These accidents are in addition to those that occur in the factories. (6) SOCIAL PROBLEMS : Alcoholism, drug addiction, gambling, prostitution, increased divorces, breaking up of home, juvenile delinquency, higher incidence of crime are some of the social problems due to industrialization. (7) MORBIDITY AND MORTALITY : Vital statistical rates indicate that industrial areas are characterized by high morbidity and mortality from certain diseases. For example the incidence of chronic bronchitis and lung cancer is higher in industrialized areas than in rural areas. The crude death rate and infant mortality rate tend to be high in industrial areas. India has special problems due to industrialization. It is because the level of public health is generally low, the average expectation of life is less than that in industrially advanced countries.

MEASURES FOR HEALTH PROTECTION OF WORKERS

The aim of occupational health is "the promotion and maintenance of the highest degree of physical, mental and social well-being of workers in all occupations". The measures for the general health protection of workers was the subject of discussion by an ILO/WHO Committee on Occupational Health in 1953. The Committee recommended the following *(38)*.

1. Nutrition

In many developing countries, malnutrition is an important factor contributing to poor health among workers and low work output. Malnutrition may also affect the metabolism of toxic agents and also the tolerance mechanisms. Under the Indian Factories Act, it is obligatory on the part of the industrial establishments to provide a canteen when the number of employees exceed 250. The aim is to provide balanced diets or snacks at reasonable cost under sanitary control. It is important to combine this action with the education of the workers on the value of a balanced diet. If the worker carries his own lunch to work, provision should be made for a safe and uncontaminated place to store the food before it is eaten to avoid spoilage or contamination. Likewise, some place separate from the workroom should be provided so that the meal may be eaten in sanitary surroundings.

2. Communicable disease control

The industry provides an excellent opportunity for early diagnosis, treatment, prevention and rehabilitation. It is a general objective everywhere, to detect cases of communicable disease and to render them non-infectious to others by treatment or removal from the working environment, or both. The communicable diseases of special importance in India are tuberculosis, typhoid fever, viral hepatitis, amoebiasis, intestinal parasites, malaria and sexually transmitted diseases. There should be an adequate immunization programme against preventable communicable diseases. Anthrax, undulant fever, and Q fever are examples of communicable diseases which may be of occupational origin. Their control calls for special sanitary measures in the handling of working materials and substances.

3. Environmental sanitation

Within the industrial establishment, the following needs attention for the prevention of the spread of communicable diseases by water, food or other means : (1) WATER SUPPLY : A sufficient supply of wholesome drinking water is one of the basic requirements in all industrial establishments. The common glass tumbler for drinking water should be abandoned as it spreads infection. Installation of drinking water fountains, at convenient points should be encouraged. (2) FOOD : If food is sold, its sanitary preparation, storage and handling are essential. Education of food handlers and other measures may be necessary to prevent outbreaks of gastro-intestinal disease. (3) TOILET : There should be sufficient number of latrines and urinals of the sanitary type, separate for males and females, conveniently situated. It is recommended that there should be at least one sanitary convenience for every 25 employees (males and females separate) for the first 100 employees, and thereafter one for every 50. Garbage and waste disposal should be such as to avoid the breeding of flies and vermin. (4) GENERAL PLANT CLEANLINESS : The walls, ceilings and passages should be painted with water washable paint and repainted at least once in 3 years and washed at least once in every 6 months. The dust which settles down on the floor and machinery should be promptly removed by vacuum cleaners or by wetting agents before it is redistributed into the atmosphere by the vibration of the machinery or buildings. A high standard of general cleanliness is one of the fundamentals of accident prevention. It also contributes to the efficiency and high morale of the workers. (5) SUFFICIENT SPACE : Sufficient floor space and cubic space are essential to prevent not only respiratory infections but also to ensure a comfortable working environment. The recommended standard is a minimum of 500 Cu. ft. of space for every worker; space more than 14 feet above the floor level is not to be taken into consideration. (6) LIGHTING : The results of poor industrial illumination are workers' eye fatigue, increased accidents, decreased production and more rejections of finished products. Furthermore, defective illumination over a long period of time may result in permanent impairment of vision. There should be sufficient and suitable lighting, natural or artificial or both, in every part of a factory where workers are working or passing through. The standards of illumination for different kinds of work have been set out – precision work for a high degree of accuracy may require 50–75 foot candles; where people work regularly, 6 to 12 foot candles may be sufficient. Illumination in corridors and passages should be at least 0.5 foot candles. (7) VENTILATION AND TEMPERATURE: Poor ventilation not only increases the chances of infection from person to person, but also affects the mental and physical efficiency of the workers. Proper ventilation is also needed for the control of noxious vapours, fumes and dusts and prevention of fatigue and industrial accidents. Effective and suitable provision should be made for maintaining adequate ventilation by circulation of fresh air in every work room; and such a temperature which will secure to workers therein, reasonable conditions of comfort and prevent injury to health. (8) PROTECTION AGAINST HAZARDS: There should be adequate environmental controls designed to protect the workers against exposure to dusts, fumes and other toxic hazards. (9) HOUSING: There is usually an acute shortage of housing in industrial areas. Most workers come from rural areas. The housing of workers near a plant must be correlated to essential community amenities and to social and sanitary facilities. Town planning and zoning are highly desirable.

4. Mental health

The objective of an occupational health service is not only to keep the workers physically healthy, but mentally and psychologically stable. Industrial workers are susceptible to the effects of love, recognition, rejection, job satisfaction, rewards and discipline. The master-servant era is now disappearing from industry. The workers, individually and collectively, like to be recognized, like to have a measure of control over their own affairs, like to have the opportunity to develop skills appropriate to their individual capacity.

The goals of mental health in industry are : (1) to promote the health and happiness of the workers, (2) to detect signs of emotional stress and strain and to secure relief of stress and strain where possible, (3) the treatment of employees suffering from mental illness, and (4) the rehabilitation of those who become ill.

5. Measures for women and children

Women workers require special protection because (1) the developing embryo may be more susceptible to noxious agents than the exposed mother (e.g., in the case of methylmercury poisoning, (2) females may be less suited for some work tasks than men; pregnancy may decrease the capacity to cope with many work factors, (3) women tend to feed themselves less substantially than men and also restrict their nourishment in difficult economic circumstances, (4) the infant mortality is higher amongst children of women employed in industrial work. The Government has notified the Maternity Benefit (Amendment) Act, 2017 on 28th March, 2017 and the provisions of the Amendment Act have come into force with effect from 1st April, 2017 *(35)*.

The following types of protection are available for women workers in India : (1) Expectant mothers are given maternity leave for 26 weeks, of which upto 8 weeks precede the expected date of confinement; during this period they are allowed 'maternity benefit', which is a cash payment, under the Employees State Insurance Act, 1948. After 2 children, the duration of paid maternity leave shall be 12 weeks (6 weeks pre and 6 weeks post delivery) (2) Provision of free antenatal, natal and postnatal services. (3) The Factories Act (Section 66) prohibits night work between 7 p.m. and 6 a.m.; Section 34 prohibits carrying of excessive weights beyond a certain schedule which has been laid down. (4) The Indian Mines Act (1923) prohibits work underground. (5) Maternity Benefit Act, 2017 provides for creches in factories where more than 50 women workers are employed *(35)*, and also prohibits the employment of women and children in certain dangerous occupations. Regarding protection of children, the Constitution of India declared: "No child below the age of fourteen shall be employed to work in any factory or mine or engaged in any other hazardous employment" (Chapter III, Fundamental Rights – Article 24). Further, The Child Labour (Prohibition and Regulation) Amendment Rules were notified on 20th April, 2017 giving protection to children *(38)*.

6. Health education

Health education is a basic health need. It is an important health promotional measure. Health education in the industrial setting should be envisaged at all levels – the management, the supervisory staff, the worker, the trade union leaders and the community. The content varies from matters of personal hygiene and protection to participation of the workers in the planning and operation of the total health service programme in industry.

7. Family planning

Family planning is now recognized a decisive factor for the quality of life, and this applies to industrial workers also. The workers must adopt the small family norm.

PREVENTION OF OCCUPATIONAL DISEASES

The various measures for the prevention of occupational diseases may be grouped under three heads: medical, engineering and statutory or legislative.

1. MEDICAL MEASURES

1. Pre-placement examination

Pre-placement examination is the foundation of an efficient occupational health service. It is done at the time of employment and includes the worker's medical, family, occupational and social history; a thorough physical examination and a battery of biological and radiological examinations, e.g., chest X-ray, electro-cardiogram, vision testing, urine and blood examination, special tests for endemic disease. A fresh recruit may either be totally rejected or given a job suited to his physical and mental abilities. The purpose of preplacement examination is to place the right man in the right job, so that the worker can perform his duties efficiently without detriment to his health. This is ergonomics. The following is a list of some occupations in which it is risky to employ men suffering from certain diseases *(39)*.

Hazard	*Undesirable conditions*
(1) Lead	Anaemia, hypertension, nephritis, peptic ulcer
(2) Dyes	Asthma; skin, bladder and kidney diseases; precancerous lesions
(3) Solvents	Liver and kidney disease, dermatitis, alcoholism
(4) Silica	Healed or active tuberculosis of lungs, chronic lung disease
(5) Radium and X-rays	Signs of ill-health, especially any blood disease.

Pre-placement examination will also serve as a useful benchmark for future comparison. It may be mentioned that in most countries, many workers start employment without the benefit of a pre-employment medical examination. This is particularly true of workers in small-scale industries and mines and those engaged in construction and agricultural work in the developing countries.

2. Periodical examination

Many diseases of occupational origin require months or even years for their development. Their slow development, very often, leads to their non-recognition in the early stages and this is harmful to the worker. This is the reason why a periodical medical check-ups of workers is very necessary when they handle toxic or poisonous substances.

The frequency and content of periodical medical examinations will depend upon the type of occupational exposure. Ordinarily workers are examined once a year. But in certain occupational exposures (e.g., lead, toxic dyes, radium) monthly examinations are indicated. Sometimes, even daily examinations may be needed such as when irritant chemicals like dichromates are handled *(39)*. The periodical examinations may be supplemented, where necessary by biological and radiological examinations. Particular care should be given to workers returning from medical leave, to assess the nature and degree of any disability and to assess suitability or otherwise of returning to the same job.

3. Medical and health care services

The medical care of occupational diseases is a basic function of an occupational health service. In India, the Employees State Insurance Scheme provides medical care not only for the worker but also his family. Within the factory, first aid services should be made available. Properly applied first aid can reduce suffering and disability and hasten recovery. Immunization is another accepted function of an occupational health service.

4. Notification

National Laws and Regulations (Factories Act, 1976; Mines Act, 1952; Dock Labourers Act, 1948; etc.) require the notification of cases and suspected cases of occupational disease. In the Factories Act, a list of 22 diseases is included while in the Mines Act 3 diseases and in the Dock Regulations 8 diseases are listed. These diseases are recognized internationally for the purpose of workmen's compensation. The main purpose of notification in industry is to initiate measures for prevention and protection and ensuring their effective application; and to investigate the working conditions and other circumstances which have caused or suspected to have caused occupational diseases *(26)*.

5. Supervision of working environment

Periodic inspection of working environment provides information of primary importance in the prevention of occupational disabilities. The physician should pay frequent visits to the factory in order to acquaint himself with the various aspects of the working environment such as temperature, lighting, ventilation, humidity, noise, cubic space, air pollution and sanitation which have an important bearing on the health and welfare of the workers. He should be acquainted with the raw materials, processes and products manufactured. He should also study the various aspects of occupational physiology such as occurrence of fatigue, night–work, shift-work, weight carried by the workers and render advice to the factory management on all matters connected with the health and welfare of the workers. For studies of this kind the physician should enlist the cooperation of safety engineers, industrial hygienists and psychologists.

6. Maintenance and analysis of records

Proper records are essential for the planning, development and efficient operation of an occupational health service. The worker's health record and occupational disability record must be maintained. Their compilation and review should enable the service to watch over the health of the workers, to assess the hazards inherent in certain types of work and to devise or improve preventive measures.

7. Health education and counselling

Ideally, health education should start before the worker enters the factory. All the risks involved in the industry in which he is employed and the measures to be taken for personal protection should be explained to him. The correct use of protective devices like masks and gloves should also be explained. Simple rules of hygiene – hand-washing, paring the nails, bodily cleanliness and cleanliness of clothes, should be impressed upon him. He should be frequently reminded about the dangers in industry through the media of health education such as charts, posters and hand bills. The purpose of health education is to assist the worker in his process of adjustment to the working, home and community environment.

2. ENGINEERING MEASURES

1. Design of building

Measures for the prevention of occupational diseases should commence in the blue-print stage. The type of floor, walls, height, ceiling, roof, doors and windows, cubic space are all matters which should receive attention in the original plan of the building which is put up by the industrial architect. Once the building is constructed, it would be difficult to introduce alterations without much trouble and expense.

2. Good house-keeping

Good house-keeping is a term often applied to industry,

and means much the same as when used domestically. It covers general cleanliness, ventilation, lighting, washing, food arrangements and general maintenance. Good housekeeping is a fundamental requirement for the control or elimination of occupational hazards. It also contributes to efficiency and morale in industry. The walls, ceilings, and passages should be white-washed at least once a year. The dust which settles down on the floor, ledges, beams, machinery and other stationary objects should be promptly removed by vacuum cleaners or by wetting agents. Masks, gloves, aprons and other protective equipment should be kept clean and in a state of good repair. To prevent accidents, the right thing should be in the right place. Not only the inside, but the outside of the plant should also be kept clean and tidy.

3. General ventilation

There should be good general ventilation in factories. It has been recommended that in every room of a factory, ventilating openings shall be provided in the proportion of 5 sq. feet for each worker employed in such room, and the openings shall be such as to admit a continued supply of fresh air. In rooms where dust is generated there should be an efficient exhaust ventilation system. Good general ventilation decreases the air-borne hazards to the workers, especially hazards from dusts and gases. The Indian Factories Act has prescribed a minimum of 500 cu. ft. of air space for each worker.

4. Mechanization

The plant should be mechanized to the fullest possible extent to reduce the hazard of contact with harmful substances. Dermatitis can be prevented if hand-mixing is replaced by mechanical devices. Acids can be conveyed from one place to another through pipes. There may be other similar situations where mechanisation can be substituted to hand-operation.

5. Substitution

By substitution is meant the replacement of a harmful material by a harmless one, or one of lesser toxicity. A classical example is the substitution of white phosphorus by phosphorus sesquisulphide in the match industry, which resulted in the elimination of necrosis of jaw (Phossy jaw). Zinc or iron paints can be used in place of harmful lead paints; silver salts can be used in place of mercury salts; acetone can be used in place of benzene. But substitution is not always possible in industry. Where possible, it should be used to the fullest possible extent.

6. Dusts

Dusts can be controlled at the point of origin by water sprays, e.g., wet drilling of rock. Inclusion of a little moisture in the materials will make the processes of grinding, sieving and mixing comparatively dust-free. Wet methods should be tried to combat dust before more elaborate and expensive methods are adopted.

7. Enclosure

Enclosing the harmful materials and processes will prevent the escape of dust and fumes into the factory atmosphere. For example, grinding machinery can be completely enclosed. Such enclosed units are generally combined with exhaust ventilation.

8. Isolation

Sometimes it may be necessary to isolate the offensive process in a separate building so that workers not directly connected with the operation are saved from exposure. Isolation may not be only in space, but also in the fourth dimension of time. Certain operations can be done at night in the absence of the usual staff.

9. Local exhaust ventilation

By providing local exhaust ventilation dusts, fumes and other injurious substances can be trapped and extracted "at source" before they escape into the factory atmosphere. The heart of the local exhaust ventilation is the hood which is placed as near as possible to the point of origin of the dust or fume or other impurity. Dusts, gases and fumes are drawn into the hood by suction and are conveyed through ducts into collecting units. In this way, the breathing zone of workers may be kept free of dangerous dust and poisonous fumes.

10. Protective devices

Respirators and gas masks are among the oldest devices used to protect workers against air-borne contaminants and they are still used for that purpose. There are two classes of respirators : (i) those which remove contaminants from air, (ii) those to which fresh air is supplied. The workers should know what kinds to use, and when and how to use. Respiratory devices should not be used as substitute for other control methods. The other protective devices comprise ear plugs, ear muffs, helmets, safety shoes, aprons, gloves, gum boots, barrier creams, screens and goggles. The worker should be instructed in the correct use of protective devices.

11. Environmental monitoring

An important aspect of occupational health programme is environmental monitoring. It is concerned with periodical environmental surveys, especially sampling the factory atmosphere to determine whether the dusts and gases escaping into the atmosphere are within the limits of permissible concentration. The use of "permissible limits" has played an important part in reducing occupational exposure to toxic substances. Thermal environment, ventilation, lighting would also have to be monitored. Such monitoring should be done by joint collaboration of doctors and engineers.

12. Statistical monitoring

Statistical monitoring comprises review at regular intervals of collected data on health and environmental exposure of occupational groups. The main objective of these reviews is to evaluate the adequacy of preventive measures and occupational health criteria, including permissible exposure levels.

13. Research

Research in occupational health offers fertile ground for study which can provide a better understanding of the industrial health problems. There are two kinds of research – pure research and research for the improvement of, or in connection with a manufactured product. Both are important. Study of the permissible limits of exposure to dusts and toxic fumes, occupational cancer, accident prevention, industrial fatigue and vocational psychology are some aspects of research in occupational health.

3. LEGISLATION

Society has an obligation to protect the health of the worker engaged in diverse occupations. It has grown out of the realisation that the worker is more important than the machine which he operates. The worker cannot be permitted to endanger his life and limb in an occupation, while the employer makes a fortune. Factory laws, therefore, have been framed in every country to govern the conditions in industry and to safeguard the health and welfare of the worker. The most important factory laws in India today are:

(1) The Factories Act, 1948
(2) The Employees' State Insurance Act, 1948

There are other specialized Acts adapted to the particular circumstances of the industry, e.g., the Mines Act, the Plantation Act, the Minimum Wages Act, the Maternity Benefit Act, etc. All these Acts lay down certain standards to which the employer must comply to ensure health and safety to workers.

The Factories Act, 1948

The first Indian Factories Act dates as far back as 1881. The Act was revised and amended several times, the latest being the Factories (Amendment) Act, 1987. A brief description of the Act is given below:

(1) SCOPE: The Act defines factory as an establishment employing 10 or more workers where power is used, and 20 or more workers where power is not used. There is no distinction between perennial and seasonal factories. The 1976 amendment modifies the definition of the term 'worker' so as to include within its meaning contract labour employed in the manufacturing process. The Act applies to the whole of India except the State of Jammu and Kashmir. The State Governments are authorized to appoint besides the Chief Inspector of Factories as many Additional Chief Inspectors, Joint Chief Inspectors, Deputy Chief Inspectors and Inspectors as they think fit to enforce the provisions of the law.

(2) HEALTH, SAFETY AND WELFARE : (Chapter III, IV, IVA, & V). Elaborate provisions have been made in the Act with regard to health, safety and welfare of the workers. In addition to such matters as cleanliness, lighting and ventilation, the Act provides for the treatment of wastes and effluents so as to render them innocuous, and for their disposal, the elimination of dusts and fumes, the provision of spittoons, control of temperature, supply of cool drinking water during summer and for the employment of cleaners to keep the water closets clean. A minimum of 500 Cu.ft of space for each worker has been prescribed (not taking into account space more than 14 feet above the ground level). For factories installed before the 1948 Act, a minimum of 350 Cu.ft of space has been prescribed.

The Act also prescribes in detail the precautions which should be taken for ensuring the safety of workers. Some of the safety provisions relate to the casing of new machinery, devices for cutting off the power, hoists and lifts, cranes and other lifting devices, protection of the eyes and precautions against dangerous fumes, explosive and inflammable material. The Act provides that no worker shall be required to lift or carry loads which are likely to cause him injury. The State Governments are empowered to prescribe maximum weights which may be lifted or carried by men, women and children. The 1976 amendment (Section 40 B) provides for the appointment of 'Safety Officers' in every factory wherein 1,000 or more workers are ordinarily employed.

The Act contains a separate Chapter (Chapter V) relating to specific welfare measures, e.g., washing facilities, facilities for storing and drying clothes, facilities for sitting, first-aid appliances, shelters, rest-rooms and lunch rooms, canteens and creches. The Act specifies that wherein more than 250 workers are ordinarily employed, a canteen shall be provided. The 1976 amendment provides for creches in every factory wherein more than 30 women workers are ordinarily employed. In every factory, wherein 500 or more workers are ordinarily employed, there should be a Welfare Officer.

(3) EMPLOYMENT OF YOUNG PERSONS: The Act prohibits employment of children below the age of 14 years and declares persons between the ages 15 and 18 to be adolescents. Adolescents should be duly certified by the "Certifying Surgeons" regarding their fitness for work. Restrictions have been laid down on employment of women and children in certain dangerous occupations. Child who has not completed his fourteenth year of age has been restricted from employment in any factory. Adolescent employee is allowed to work only between 6 A.M. & 7 P.M.

(4) HOURS OF WORK: The Act has prescribed a maximum of 48 working hours per week, not exceeding 9 hours per day with rest for at least $^1/_2$ hour after 5 hours of continuous work. For adolescents, the hours of work have been reduced from 5 to $4^1/_2$ per day. The 1976 amendment makes a provision to increase the spread-over period of work (including rest intervals) of an employee in a factory upto 12 hours from the existing $10^1/_2$ hours. The total number of hours of work in a week including overtime shall not exceed 60.

(5) LEAVE WITH WAGES: The Act lays down that besides weekly holidays, every worker will be entitled to leave with wages after 12 month's continuous service at the following rate; adult – one day for every 20 days of work, children – one day for every 15 days of work. The leave can be accumulated up to 30 days in case of adults and 40 days in case of children.

(6) OCCUPATIONAL DISEASES: It is obligatory on the part of the factory management to give information regarding specified accidents which cause death, serious bodily injury or regarding occupational diseases contracted by employees. The Act gives a schedule of notifiable diseases. The 1976 amendment includes Byssinosis, Asbestosis, occupational dermatitis and noise-induced hearing loss among the list of notifiable diseases and provides for enquiry in every case of a fatal accident. Provision has also been made in the 1976 amendment for safety and occupational health surveys in factories and industries.

(7) EMPLOYMENT IN HAZARDOUS PROCESSES : The Central Govt. has incorporated a new Chapter IV-A by the Factories (Amendment) Act, 1987, relating to hazardous processes. Site Appraisal Committee consisting of Chief Inspector and other members, not more than 14 in number, for examination of service conditions of employees in a factory, involving hazardous processes, is to be constituted for recommendations. Specific responsibility of the occupier in relation to hazardous processes were also made with workers' participation in safety management. List of industries involving hazardous processes is prescribed in 1st schedule of the Act.

The Employees State Insurance Act, 1948 *(40, 42)*

The ESI Act passed in 1948 (amended in 1975, 1984, 1989, 2010, 2019 and 2022) is an important measure of social security and health insurance in this country. It provides for certain *cash* and *medical benefits* to industrial employees in case of sickness, maternity and employment injury.

SCOPE

The Act extends to the whole of India. The ESI Act of 1948 covered all power-using factories other than seasonal factories wherein 10 or more persons were employed (excluding mines, railways and defence establishments). The provisions of the ESI (Amendment) Act of 1975 were extended to the following new classes of establishments :

a) Small factories employing 10 or more persons, whether power is used in the process of manufacturing or not.
b) Shops;
c) Hotels and restaurants;
d) Cinemas and theatres;
e) Road-motor transport establishments;
f) Newspaper establishments; and
g) The scheme has been extended to private medical and educational institutions employing 20 or more persons in some states.

With effect from 1.5.2010 the Act covers all employees – manual, clerical, supervisory and technical getting upto Rs.15,000 per month. This has been further revised to Rs.21,000 per month as per notification of ESIC on 6.9.2016. The provisions of the Act can be extended to any other agricultural or commercial establishment.

ADMINISTRATION

The administration of the ESI Scheme under the Act is entrusted to an autonomous body called the ESI *Corporation.* The Union Minister for Labour is the Chairman and the Secretary to Govt. of India Ministry of Labour is the Vice-Chairman of this corporation. It consists of members representing Central and State Governments, employers and employees' organizations, medical profession and Parliament. There is a Standing Committee, constituted from the members of the Corporation, which acts as an executive body for the administration of the Scheme. The chief executive officer of the Corporation is the Director General who is assisted by four Principal Officers – (1) Insurance Commissioner (2) Medical Commissioner (3) Financial Commissioner (4) Actuary. There is a Medical Benefit Council which is headed by the Director General of Health Services, Government of India who is assisted by the Medical Commissioner in all matters relating to medical relief. Besides the head office in New Delhi, the corporation has 24 regional offices and 39 sub-regional offices at 1 divisional office, 2 camp offices, and 592 branch offices, 800 cash offices and 422 inspection offices all over the country for the administration of the scheme as on 31.03.21.

Given the huge number of beneficiaries – about 13.16 crores by 31.3.2021 – the corporation has set up a wide spread network of service outlets for prompt delivery of benefits in cash and kind that includes full medical care. ESI gives coverage to about 339 lakh family units of about 7.83 lakh factories and establishments, as on 31.3.2021.

Medical facilities are provided through a network of 1520 ESI dispensaries, over 2100 panel clinics, 307 diagnostic centres, besides 143 ESI hospitals and 43 hospital annexes with over 27,000 beds. For providing super-speciality medical care the corporation has tie up arrangements with advanced medical institutions in the country, both in public and private sector. The medical benefit is administered with the active co-operation of state governments.

The payment of cash benefits is made at the grass root level through as many as 592 branch offices, 800 cash offices that function under the direct control of the corporation.

There are 406 inspection offices throughout the country to inspect factories and for checking insurability of employees and correct payment of contributions *(41, 43)*.

FINANCE

The scheme is run by contributions by employees and employers and grants from Central and State Governments. The employer contributes 3.25 per cent of total wage bill; the employee contributes 0.75 per cent of wages (revised rates w.e.f. 1.7.19). Employees getting daily wages of below Rs.176 are exempted from payment of contribution. The State Government's share of expenditure on medical care is 1/8 of total cost of medical care; the ESI Corporation's share of expenditure on medical care is 7/8 of total cost of medical care.

BENEFITS TO EMPLOYEES

The Act has made provision for the following benefits to insured persons or, to other dependants as the case may be:

(1) Medical benefit
(2) Sickness benefit
(3) Maternity benefit
(4) Disablement benefit
(5) Dependant's benefit
(6) Funeral expenses
(7) Rehabilitation allowance.

1. Medical benefit

Medical benefit consists of "full medical care" including hospitalization, free of cost, to the insured persons in case of sickness, employment injury and maternity. The services comprise : (1) out-patient care (2) supply of drugs and dressings (3) specialist services in all branches of medicine (4) pathological and radiological investigations (5) domiciliary services (6) antenatal, natal and postnatal services (7) immunization services (8) family planning services (9) emergency services (10) ambulance services (11) health–education and (12) in-patient treatment. In complicated cases where specialized treatment is necessary, patients are sent for institutional treatment even outside their State at the expense of the ESI Corporation.

Medical care is provided either *directly* through the agency of ESI hospitals and dispensaries, or *indirectly* through a panel of private medical practitioners (panel system) appointed as "insurance medical practitioners". DIRECT PATTERN : (1) In areas having a concentration of 1,000 or more employees' family units, service dispensaries are established with full-time medical and para-medical personnel. On an average, a doctor will attend to about 80 cases in the out-patient department per day, and makes one home visit a day. (2) In areas where the employees are less than 750, part-time ESI dispensaries are established. (3) If the residential concentration of employees is scattered over a long distance, mobile dispensaries are established. INDIRECT PATTERN: This is known as "panel system".

Registered medical practitioners designated as Insurance Medical Practitioners are appointed to provide medical care.

Medical care is also extended to families of workers where requisite arrangements could be made. A start has been made by providing "restricted medical care", i.e., only out-patient care. Where facilities are available "expanded medical care" i.e., full medical care short of hospitalization is given.

OTHER MEDICAL FACILITIES :(1) Dentures, spectacles and hearing aids are provided free to patients who are incapacitated due to employment injury (2) Artificial limbs are provided free to insured persons who lose their limbs in employment injury or otherwise (3) Special appliances such as hernia belts, walking callipers, surgical boots, spinal braces and jackets are provided as prescribed by specialists.

COST OF MEDICAL BENEFIT: The per capita cost of medical benefit under the ESI Scheme has been steadily increasing. It was Rs. 23.79 in 1961–62, Rs. 58.91 in 1969–70, Rs. 67.53 in 1973–74, Rs. 406.78 in 1992–93 and Rs. 905 in 2001–02, and has been rising further since then. Expenditure on medical benefit were Rs. 4058 crores in 2012–13, Rs. 9368 crores in 2020 and Rs. 9530 crores by 2022 *(41)*.

2. Sickness benefit

It consists of periodical cash payment to an insured person in case of sickness, if his sickness is duly certified by an Insurance Medical Officer or Insurance Medical Practitioner. The benefit is payable for a maximum period of 91 days, in any continuous period of 365 days, the daily rate being about 70% of the average daily wages. A person receiving the sickness benefit is required to remain under medical treatment provided under the Act i.e., in order to qualify for sickness benefit the insured person is required to contribute for 78 days in a contribution period of 6 months *(40)*.

EXTENDED SICKNESS BENEFIT: In addition to 91 days of sickness benefit, insured persons suffering from certain long-term diseases are entitled to Extended Sickness Benefit as shown below, for a maximum period of two years.

34 diseases for which Extended Sickness Benefit with effect from 1.1.2000 is payable, in case where the insured person has been in continuous employment for 2 years :

I. Infectious Diseases

1. Tuberculosis.
2. Leprosy.
3. Chronic empyema.
4. AIDS.

II. Neoplasms

5. Malignant diseases.

III. Endocrine, Nutritional and Metabolic Disorders

6. Diabetes mellitus with proliferative retinopathy/ Diabetic foot/Nephropathy.

IV. Disorders of Nervous Systems

7. Monoplegia.
8. Hemiplegia.
9. Paraplegia.
10. Hemiparesis.
11. Intracranial space occupying lesion.
12. Spinal Cord compression.
13. Parkinson's disease.
14. Myasthenia Gravis/Neuromuscular dystrophy.
15. Immature cataract with vision 6/60 or less.
16. Detachment of retina.
17. Glaucoma.

V. Diseases of Cardiovascular System

18. Coronary Artery Disease
    a. Unstable angina.
    b. Myocardial infarction with ejection less than 45%.
19. Congestive Heart Failure – Left, Right.
20. Cardiac valvular diseases with failure/complications.
21. Cardiomyopathies.
22. Heart disease with surgical intervention alongwith complications.

VI. Chest Diseases

23. Bronchiectasis.
24. Interstitial Lung Disease.
25. Chronic Obstructive Lung Diseases (COPD) with congestive heart failure (Cor Pulmonale).

VII. Diseases of the Digestive System

26. Cirrhosis of liver with ascities/chronic active hepatitis.

VIII. Orthopaedic Diseases

27. Dislocation of vertebra/prolapse of intervertebral disc.
28. Non union or delayed union of fracture.
29. Post Traumatic Surgical amputation of lower extremity.
30. Compound fracture with chronic osteomyelitis.

IX. Psychosis

31. Sub-group under this head are listed for clarification
    a. Schizophrenia.
    b. Endogenous depression.
    c. Manic Depressive Psychosis (MDP).
    d. Dementia.

X. COVID-19

32. The insured person and/or his family members in case of being infected with COVID-19 can avail free of cost medical care in any of the ESIC/ESIS hospital which has been declared as COVID-19 dedicated hospital. Presently 21 ESIC hospitals run directly by ESIC with 3676 COVID isolation beds, 229 ICU beds and 163 ventilator beds and 26 ESI scheme hospitals run by State Govts. having 2023 beds are functioning as COVID-19 dedicated hospitals *(44)*.

XI. Others

33. More than 20% burns with infection/complication
34. Chronic renal failure.
35. Reynaud's disease/Burger's disease.

The insured person is protected from dismissal or discharge from service by the employer during the period of sickness.

Cash benefit is also payable to insured persons in the productive age group for undergoing sterilisation operation, viz. vasectomy/ tubectomy.

- Enhanced sickness benefit is payable to insured women for 14 days for tubectomy and for 7 days in case of vasectomy in respect of male IPs.
- The amount payable is double the standard sickness benefit rate, that is, equal to full wages.

3. Maternity benefit

The benefit is payable in cash to an insured woman for confinement/miscarriage or sickness arising out of pregnancy/confinement or premature birth of child or miscarriage. For confinement, the duration of benefit is 26 weeks, for miscarriage 6 weeks and for sickness arising out of confinement etc. 30 days. The benefit is allowed at about full wages. The rate of confinement expenses has been increased from Rs. 5,000 to Rs. 7,500 per confinement.

4. Disablement benefit

The Act provides for cash payment, besides free medical treatment, in the event of temporary or permanent disablement as a result of employment injury as well as occupational diseases. The rate of temporary disablement benefit is about 90 per cent of the wages as long as the temporary disablement lasts. In case of total permanent disablement, the insured person is given life pension worked out on the basis of loss of earning capacity determined by a medical board, while in cases of partial permanent disablement a portion of it is granted as life pension.

5. Dependant's benefit

In case of death, as a result of employment injury, the dependants of an insured person are eligible for periodical payments. Pension at the rate of 90 per cent of the wages is payable, shared by dependants in a fixed ratio, on monthly basis in accordance with the prescribed share. An eligible son or daughter is entitled to dependant's benefit up to the age of 18; the benefit is withdrawn if the daughter marries earlier.

6. Funeral expenses

Funeral benefit is a cash payment payable on the death of an insured person towards the expenses on his funeral, the amount not exceeding Rs. 15,000/-.

7. Rehabilitation

On monthly payment of Rs 10, the insured person and his family members continue to get medical treatment after permanent disablement, or retirement.

The ESI Scheme has been implemented in 35 States/Union territories. The Scheme, by 31.03.2021, covered 2.46 crores employees; including 61.63 lakhs women, and the total number of beneficiaries were around 13.16 crores *(40, 41)*.

Benefits to employers

(1) Exemption from the applicability of Workmen's Compensation Act 1923
(2) Exemption from Maternity Benefit Act 1961
(3) Exemption from payment of Medical allowance to employees and their dependants or arranging for their medical care
(4) Rebate under the Income Tax Act on contribution deposited in the ESI Account
(5) Healthy work-force.

RAJIV GANDHI SHRAMIK KALYAN YOJNA *(40, 41)*

The ESI Corporation has launched a new Yojna for the employees covered under the ESI scheme. This scheme provides an unemployment allowance for the employees covered under ESI scheme who are rendered unemployed involuntarily due to retrenchment/closure of factory etc. after fulfilling certain eligibility conditions. The scheme came into effect from 1st April, 2005.

As per this scheme, an insured person going out of insurable employment involuntarily, on account of closure of a factory or establishment, retrenchment, or permanent invalidity arising out of non-employment injury, after rendering insurable employment and having contributed under the scheme for two or more years, is entitled to claim unemployment allowance equal to 50% of wage for a maximum period of upto two years during the life time.

The allowance can be availed in one spell or in different spells of not less than one month.

The daily rate of unemployment allowance is the "standard benefit rate" as specified in the table on standard benefit rates under rule-54 of ESI (Central) Rules, 1950 corresponding to the average daily wage drawn by the insured person.

During the period for which a person is entitled for unemployment allowance, he is also eligible for medical care for himself and his/her family from ESI dispensaries, ESI panel clinics and ESI hospitals to which he/she was attached prior to the date of loss of employment.

OCCUPATIONAL HEALTH IN INDIA

The trend in India is towards industrialization. As industries develop, both in size and complexity, occupational health will pose new and more difficult problems. The National Government have recognised the need for protecting the health of the workers. The Directive Principles of State Policy, in the Indian Constitution are important in this context. The relevant portions are :

(a) "The State shall, in particular, direct its policy towards securing that the health and strength of the workers, man, woman, and the tender age of the children are not abused, and that citizens are not forced by economic necessity to enter avocations unsuited to their strength.
(b) The State shall make provisions for securing just and humane conditions of work",

To assess the health conditions of the workers, a number of inquiries have been conducted and were submitted to the Government of India by many experts. The important reports in this connection are: Adarkar's Report of Health Insurance for Industrial Workers (1945); Report of the Health Survey and Development Committee (1946); Report of the Health of the Industrial Workers (Thomas Bedford, 1946) and Report on the Health of Workers in Plantation (Jones, 1947). The Government of India have given practical shape to some of the recommendations contained in these reports and have introduced certain legislative measures pertaining to both the curative and preventive aspects of occupational health. Most important among these measures are the Indian Factories Act 1948, the Coal Mines Labour Welfare Act (1947) and the Employees State Insurance Act (1948).

At present, there is no comprehensive occupational health service in India. However, there are various organizations active in the field of occupational health. The Organization of the Chief Adviser of Factories – now Directorate General, Factory Inspection and Advisory Service – was set up in 1945, to function as an integrated service to advise the Government, industries, and other interests concerned in matters relating to health, welfare and safety of industrial workers. The Organization deals with questions relating to the administration of the Factories Act and other Acts and the rules framed thereunder and the training of Factory Inspectors.

For scientific study of the various aspects of occupational health, particularly the "human factor" in industry, the Central Labour Institute was set up in Mumbai in 1960. Three Regional Labour Institutes at Kanpur, Kolkata and Chennai have also been set up. These institutes are dealing with a variety of activities important in the field of safety and health. They have (a) a Museum of Industrial Health, Safety and Welfare (b) Industrial Hygiene Laboratory (c) Training section (d) Library cum Information Centre (e) Industrial psychology and (f) Occupational Physiology sections.

At the State level, the Departments of Health and Labour, through the Chief Inspector of Factories and Industrial Health Inspection Service are rendering assistance by making studies and undertaking surveys at the plant level and enforcing the legal standards laid down in the various Acts.

In addition to the above, the following Research Institutes are active in the field of occupational health : (1) The Central Mining and Research Station, Dhanbad under the Council of Scientific and Industrial Research (CSIR). (2) Industrial Toxicology Research Centre, Lucknow under the CSIR. (3) Occupational Health Research Institute, Ahmedabad under the Indian Council of Medical Research (4) National Environmental Engineering Research Institute at Nagpur (5) The All India Institute of Hygiene and Public Health, Kolkata. (6) Indian Institute of Technology, Kanpur. Besides these, the Indian Council of Medical Research has an occupational health division. The Indian Association of Occupational Health is playing an important role in the promotion of occupational health.

References

1. WHO (1950). *Unpublished Working Document*, WHO/Occ. Health/2, Geneva, 1950.
2. Dastur, H.P. (1960). *A Doctor's Approach to Industrial Medicine*, Tata Institute of Social Sciences, Bombay.
3. WHO (1962). *Techn. Rep. Ser.*,No. 246.
4. WHO (1969). *World Health*, March 1969.
5. Chanda, S.L. (1971). In: *Report on the Symposium on Academic, Education and Training in Occupational Health and Hygiene*, WHO/SEA/Occ/Hlth.6.
6. WHO (1960). *WHO Chronicle*, 7, 279.
7. Rao, M.N. and Lundgren. N.P.V. (1955). *A Review of Occupational Health Research in India*, ICMR, New Delhi.
8. Chakraborty, M.K. (1967). *Ind. J. Indust. Med.*, 13, 121.
9. WHO (1962). *Health Hazards of the Human Environment*, Geneva.
10. Nagaratnam, A. (1968). *Ind. J. Industr. Med.*, 14, 212.
11. Shivram, C. et al (1970). *Ind. J. Industr. Med.*, 16, 20-24.
12. Thacker, P.V. (1967). *Souvenir, Indian Public Health Association*, 12th Annual conference, Poona, p. 65.
13. Ghosh, P.K. (1969). *Ind. J. Industr. Med.*, 15, 1.
14. Sen, J.R. (1968). *Ind. J. Industr. Med.*, 14, 186.
15. Wyatt, J.P. (1971). *Amer. J. Pathology*, 64, 197.
16. Gupta, M.N. (1969). *Indian J. Med. Res.*,57, 1776-1789.
17. Gupta, M.N. (1970). *Technical Review on Pneumoconiosis in India*, ICMR, Spl.Rep.Ser.,No.4 New Delhi.
18. Editorial (1970). *Brit. Med. J.*, 2 : 496.
19. Editorial (1973). *Brit. Med. J.*, 4, 312.
20. Banerji, D.P. (1968). *Ind. J. Industr. Med.*, 14, 157.
21. Gilson, J.C. (1973). *Proceedings of the Royal Society of Medicine*, 66, 395.
22. Quinlan, J.J. et al (1969). *Canad.J.Public Health*, 60, 15.
23. Editorial (1970). *Brit. Med. J.*, 2, 496.
24. Coyer, R.A. (1971). *Amer. J.of Pathology*, 64, 167.
25. Barltrop, D. (1968). *Post Graduate Med.,J.* 44, 537.
26. Govt. of India (1965). *Occupational Diseases, A Guide to Recognition and Notification*, Chief Adviser Factories, Ministry of Labour and Employment, New Delhi.
27. WHO (1975). *Techn.Rep.Ser.*, No.571.
28. Bhansali, K.N. (1967).*Ind. J. Industr. Med.*, 13, 45.
29. Donald Hunter (1959). *Health in Industry*, Pelican Book.
30. Mendonca, Lobo (1970). *The Antiseptic*,67, 455.
31. WHO (1976). *WHO Chronicle*,30, 318.
32. Gupta, M.N. (1961). *Swasth Hind*, 5, 74.
33. Sabnis, C.V. and Rao, M.N. (1961). *Swasth Hind*, 5, 81.
34. ILO (1967). *Accident Prevention*, A Worker's Education Manual, Geneva.
35. Govt. of India (2017). *Press note*, Maternal benefit (Amendment Act) May, 2017.
36. Govt. of India (1969). *Swasth Hind*, 13, 109.
37. Banerji, B. and Chakraborty, S. (1969). *Ind. J. Industr. Med.*,15, 85.
38. Govt. of India (2017). *Ministry of Labour and Employment*, Notification 20th April, 2017.
39. Lobo-Mendonca, R. (1965). *Protecting the Indian Worker*, Society for the Study of Industrial Medicine, Bombay.
40. ESI Corporation (2021). website www.esic.nic.in
41. ESI Corporation (2021), *Annual Report 2020–21*.
42. The Gazette of India, Employees State Insurance (Central) Amendment Rules, 2022.
43. ESIC, Corporation (2022), Citizen's charter, website www.esic.in/web/esic/citizen-s-charter.
44. ESIC, Press Release, Dated 29.04.2021 website : www.esic.nic.in/www.esic.in.

19 Genetics and health

"Human genetics is much more than the study of mere inborn abnormalities"

The basic principles of genetics were laid down by Mendel and Galton towards the close of the 19th century. But it is only during the past few years the science of genetics including human genetics has made rapid progress. The discovery of the biological role of nucleic acids, the uncovering of the structure of genetic information and its role in regulating life processes are discoveries, the importance of which can hardly be over estimated.

With increasing control of communicable diseases and infant mortality, inherited abnormalities are assuming a proportionately greater importance in medical practice. Over 2,300 hereditary diseases have been identified and more are added to the list every year. According to many authors, genetically conditioned diseases or diseases with a clear genetic component account for 25–40 per cent of all cases treated by the health services *(1)*.

Human genetics is much more than the study of mere hereditary diseases. It has emerged as a basic biological science for understanding the endogenous factors in health and disease and the complex interaction between nature and nurture. Owing to rapid specialization, several branches in genetics have come into being, e.g., cytogenetics, biochemical genetics, clinical genetics, pharmacogenetics, immunogenetics, microbial genetics, population genetics and so on. Achievements in these fields have created a basis for effective medical and preventive intervention in many diseases, and also possibly of "genetic engineering", i.e., of controlling the traits of an individual.

Cytologic facts

In 1956, Tjio and Levan surprised the scientific world by reporting that they could find only 46 chromosomes in the normal human karyotype. This was immediately confirmed by other workers. There is now universal agreement that the normal human body cell (except the sex cells) contains 46 chromosomes, i.e., 22 pairs of autosomes and a pair of sex chromosomes, XX in the female and XY in the male. The chromosomes vary in length, the longest being about 5 times as long as the smallest. Each pair of chromosomes is homologous. The autosomes are numbered according to their length, the first pair being the longest and the last pair the shortest. The sex chromosomes are not included in the numbering, but are merely termed X and Y. Barr and his group discovered that the normal female cell nucleus contains in addition a dark-staining area at the periphery of cell nucleus, called a Barr body or "sex chromatin" body which is not present in normal males.

The autosomes have been classified and divided on the basis of length and certain morphological similarities into 7 groups as follows :

Group A	.....	1 to 3	pairs
Group B	.....	4 and 5	pairs
Group C	.....	6 to 12	pairs
Group D	.....	13 to 15	pairs
Group E	.....	16 to 18	pairs
Group F	.....	19 and 20	pairs
Group G	.....	21 and 22	pairs

The X-chromosome is included in Group 'C' with chromosomes 6–12, and the Y-chromosome is included in Group G with chromosomes 21 and 22.

Mitosis

During ordinary cell division, each chromosome divides lengthwise into two sister chromosomes called *chromatids*. The chromatids are joined together for a short time at a point called *centromere*. Then the chromatids separate, one goes to one daughter cell, and one to the other daughter cell. In this manner, each daughter cell inherits the same number and kind of sister chromosomes. This process of nuclear division is called *mitosis*.

Meiosis

The reproductive cells (sperms and ova) are produced in a different manner. There are two nuclear divisions and only one chromosome division. This form of division is called 'reduction division' or *meiosis*. A detailed description of meiosis is unnecessary here. Broadly, the main events in meiosis are : (1) The homologous chromosomes first come together. This is called "pairing". (2) The chromosomes then replicate – each doubling into two chromatids which are held together at centromere. (3) At this stage there is "crossing over" and a redistribution of genetic material. (4) Then the homologous chromosomes separate – one goes to one pole of the nucleus and the other to the other pole. The chromosome number is thus reduced to half, i.e., 23. (5) The cell divides and the nucleus of each daughter cell contains 23 chromosomes. (6) The second meiotic division follows : the centromeres divide and the chromatids move apart. (7) The cell divides again so that the daughter cells each contain 23 chromosomes. During fertilization, the two half-sets come together and restore the full complement of 46. The full complement of 46 chromosomes is called the *diploid* number, and the half set of 23 is called the *haploid* number.

Chromosomes

Chromosomes are rod-like condensations of chromatin. They become visible in the nucleus only during cell division. They occur in pairs – one member of each pair comes from the father, and other from the mother. The largest chromosome measures about 7 μ and is about five times the length of the shortest. Biochemically, the chromosomes are made up of deoxyribonucleic acid (DNA). Genetically, they consists of genes arranged like the beads of a necklace. The number of chromosomes in each species is fixed. All individuals of the same species have the same number of chromosomes (with exceptions). Thus the total number for man is 46, the fruit fly 8, garden peas 14 and potato 48.

Methods of Chromosomal Study : Buccal smears, peripheral blood, bone marrow, skin and in some instances testis tissue are used to study chromosomes. More information can be obtained by using cell cultures. Cells, which are usually peripheral white blood cells, are cultured in the proper medium and incubated for 3 days. Colchicine is then added to arrest cells in metaphase. After further incubation for 3 to 5 hours, the cells are placed in a hypotonic solution which causes them to swell and the chromosomes to disperse within the cell. The cells are fixed, stained and examined for chromosomes. A more recent discovery in cytogenetics is the fluorescent staining of chromosomes. It has been shown that human chromosomes treated with quinacrine hydrochloride (Atabrine) or quinacrine mustard exhibit distinct fluorescence *(2)*.

Genes

Genes are the units of heredity. They contain the hereditary information encoded in their chemical structure for transmission from generation to generation. They affect development and function, both normal and abnormal. Though genes are not seen with a microscope, much is known about them by indirect methods. It is said we inherit about 50,000 genes from the father and 50,000 from the mother. The genes occupy a specific position or *locus* on the chromosomes. For example, the locus for the ABO blood groups is in chromosome 9 and the *locus* for the major histocompatibility complex is in chromosome 6. The Y-chromosome contains genes that determine the normal development of testis. It is known that the human X-chromosome carries the genes governing a blood group haemophilia, red-green colour-blindness, glucose-6-phosphate dehydrogenase, muscular dystrophy, height and gonadal development *(3)*. Presumably, some thousands of loci are contained in chromosomes. More than 20 loci have been assigned to chromosome '1' including the Rh locus. More than 100 loci have been assigned to X-chromosome *(4)*.

Since genes are contained in the chromosomes, genes also occur in pairs. If the genes comprising a pair are alike (AA), the individual is described as *homozygous* for that gene, and if it is different (Aa) the individual is described as heterozygous.

A gene is said to be *dominant* when it manifests its effect both in the heterozygous and the homozygous state. A gene is said to be *recessive* when it manifests its effect only in the homozygous state. Genes whose combined action affects one particular character are known as *polygenes* or "multiple genes". In man three genes have been identified as being responsible for muscular dystrophy – one is a sex-linked recessive gene, the second is an autosomal recessive, and the third is an autosomal dominant gene. Many instances are known in which the same character is controlled by several genes – the colour of our skin, height and weight, life span, degree of resistance to disease, rate of heart beat, arterial blood pressure and many other inherited traits. These genes may occupy separate positions in the chromosomes; some may be widely distributed on several non-homologous chromosomes *(3)*. The extent to which a genetically determined condition is expressed in an individual is called *penetrance.* Lack of penetrance is one reason for skipped generations and unexpected pedigree patterns *(4)*.

Genes are usually stable, but sometimes normal genes may be converted into abnormal ones – this change is called mutation. Mutation is a regular phenomenon in nature. The natural mutation rate is increased by exposure to mutagens such as ultraviolet rays, radiation or chemical carcinogens *(5)*.

Genotype and phenotype

The term *genotype* refers to the total genetic constitution of an individual and the term *phenotype* to the outward expression of the genetic constitution. Taking the ABO blood group system, the possible genotypes are AA, AB, BB, AO, BO and OO but the phenotypes are A, B and O. The colour, form, size and stature of individuals are all phenotypical expression of a particular genetic constitution. Certain phenotype characteristics of an individual may change from infancy to adulthood such as height, weight, muscularity, body shape, but the genotype is relatively stable throughout the life of an individual. Thus there are two aspects of the genetic material – one fixed and the other plastic. The fixed characters are the genotype, and the plastic ones are the phenotype. These two types may best be compared to a given pellet of clay which may be moulded into any desired shape by an artist but the weight, volume, density and chemical constitution of the pellet will remain the same *(6)*. *Therefore,* it is said that medicine is the science of management of the human phenotype *(7)*.

Chromosomal abnormalities

Chromosomal abnormalities (numerical or structural alterations) occur from time to time in human beings. They arise in various ways : (1) *Non-disjunction :* By an error in nuclear division called "non-disjunction" a pair of chromosomes may fail to separate and both are carried to one pole. The resulting daughter cells contain an unequal number of chromosomes, 45 or 47. This numerical abnormality in which the chromosome number is not an exact multiple of the haploid number is called aneuploidy. If a particular pair of chromosomes has three chromosomes instead of two, it is called "trisomy"; if there is only one chromosome instead of two in any given pair of chromosomes, it is called "monosomy". Non-disjunction may occur during gametogenesis or during mitosis. (2) *Translocation :* Sometimes during nuclear division, a portion of one chromosome breaks away and becomes attached to another which is not homologous to the first. This is called translocation. (3) *Deletion :* A piece of a chromosome may become detached and lost from the karyotype resulting in the loss of one or more genes. If the loss is severe, it may be incompatible with live birth. (4) *Duplication :* Some genes may appear twice in the same chromosome. This is called duplication. (5) *Inversion :* Sometimes a chromosomal segment becomes inverted and then the order of sequence of genes is altered. (6) *Isochromosomes :* These are a special class of structurally abnormal chromosomes, arising because of misdivision, i.e., transverse division instead of the normal longitudinal division. (7) *Mosaicism :* The cells of the body are compounded of cells of two or more genetically different chromosomal types. This can result by mutation or non-disjunction either during embryo or later life.

Laws of inheritance

Mendel crossed two races of the common pea (Pisum sativum) a tall and a short. The first generation (F_1 generation) consisted entirely of tall offspring. But when the F_1 generation was inbred, they gave rise to a mixed generation of tall and short in the ratio of 3:1, i.e., three-fourths tall and one-fourth short. This generation is known as the F_2 generation or the second filial generation. All the short plants of the F_2 generation bred true, producing short plants only. But the tall plants of the F_2 generation gave rise to a mixture of tall and short offspring in the same ratio of 3:1. The F_2 generation is therefore 1:2:1, i.e., one-fourth pure talls, half mixed talls and one-fourth pure shorts. From the result of his experiments, Mendel formulated certain laws to explain the inheritance of characters : (1) *Law of unit characters :* All characters are units by themselves, and certain factors (now called genes) control the expression of these characters during the development of the organism. (2) *Law of dominance :* The factors or genes occur in pairs. One factor may mask the expression of the other. The character that expresses itself in the F_1 generation is said to be dominant, and the character that does not appear in the F_1 generation is said to be recessive. (3) *Law of segregation :* When germ cells are formed, Mendel supposed, that the opposed factors are separated or segregated so that each germ cell carries one or other of the two factors and not both. Mendel's work provided the basis of the study of inheritance.

Classification of genetic disorders

These may be classified as :

a. Chromosomal abnormalities
b. Unifactorial (single gene or Mendelian) diseases
c. Multifactorial disorders

CHROMOSOMAL DISORDERS

More than 300 numerical and structural types of chromosome aberrations have been described *(8)*. A significant portion of embryonic and foetal wastage is due to chromosomal anomalies. The incidence of chromosomal abnormalities is 5.6 per 1000 live births. Of these, 2 per 1000 live births represent sex aneuploidies, 1.7 per 1000 live births autosomal aneuploidies, and 1.9 per 1000 live births chromosomal translocations. For the most part, these disorders are not inherited *(4)*.

1. Relating to sex chromosomes

The following are some of the well-known syndromes associated with abnormalities of sex chromosomes :

(a) Klinefelter's syndrome : This is a common sex - chromosome aneuploidy. Persons suffering from this syndrome are abnormal males having two or more X-chromosomes in addition to one Y-chromosome (XXY, XXXY). They have a normal autosomal set of 22. The main features of this syndrome are that the affected persons are eunuchoid males with non-functional testis. Spermatozoa are absent in their ejaculations. The growth of hair on face, axillae and pubes is scanty. The condition is associated with gynaecomastia and mental retardation. The incidence of this syndrome is about 1 in 1000 among males at birth *(9)*.

(b) XYY syndrome : The male with an extra Y-chromosome has attracted much attention because of his reported tendency to anti-social, aggressive and often criminal behaviour. However, the relationship is not yet clear. The principal features of this syndrome appear to be exceptional height (usually six feet and over) and a serious personality disorder leading to behavioural disturbances *(10)*. The incidence of this syndrome is about '1' in 1000 males at birth *(9)*.

(c) Turner's syndrome : This anomaly is probably the most common chromosome disorder in humans, but about 98 per cent of the conceptuses abort spontaneously. The remaining 2 per cent that reach term, account for an incidence of 1 in 7,500 live born girls *(9)*. They have an increased risk of dying in the neonatal period. Persons suffering from this syndrome are apparent females with underdeveloped sex glands. They have 45 chromosomes instead of the normal complement of 46. Their sex chromosome constitution is XO instead of XX ('O' represents the missing chromosome). This abnormal condition is due to non-disjunction of the sex chromosomes. Clinically the patients are of short stature, infertile and have primary amenorrhoea. They often show other congenital defects such as coarctation of the aorta, pulmonary stenosis, renal malformations and mental retardation.

(d) "Super females" : Females with 3 to 5 X-chromosomes (XXX, XXXX, XXXXX) have been found. In general, the higher the number of X-chromosomes, the greater the degree of mental retardation and congenital abnormalities, e.g., underdeveloped external genitalia, uterus and vagina.

2. Relating to autosomes

There are many syndromes associated with abnormalities of autosomes. A full description of these conditions is beyond the scope of this book. A brief account of *mongolism* which is a public health problem in some countries is given here. *Mongolism* or Down's Syndrome was described by Langdon Down in 1866. Most cases of mongolism are caused by an extra chromosome which occurs on the 21st pair. The anomaly is therefore sometimes described as "Trisomy 21". The syndrome is easily recognized in the older child and adult by the short stature and small round head, narrow, tilted eye-slits, mal-formed ears, short broad hands, lax limbs, mental retardation and quite a few other abnormalities especially internal congenital defects such as cardiac defects and atresia of the alimentary tract. In communities of European origin the incidence of mongolism at birth is reported to be one in 900 births *(9)*.

One observation which is important is that the frequency of mongolism increases with rising maternal age but is unaffected by the age of the father. The risk for a woman of 20 is estimated at about 1 in 3,000 and that for a woman of 45, 1 in 50 *(11)*.

Autosomal monosomies are rare. Loss of an entire chromosome is very serious genetic defect; the fertilised ovum may not survive.

MENDELIAN DISEASES

Mendelian diseases are inherited according to the Mendelian Laws. These are the dominant, recessive and sex-linked diseases. (a) An individual with an autosomal dominant trait will produce two kinds of gametes with respect to the mutant gene – half with the mutant gene and half with the normal allele. The offspring of such an individual has a 50:50 chance of being affected, provided the other parent is normal. The sexes are equally affected. (b) Abnormalities caused by recessive genes occur when both the parents are heterozygous. Each off-spring of such parents has a chance of 1:4 being affected. Autosomal recessive diseases occur sporadically in the children of outwardly normal parents. (c) In sex linked inheritance, a mutant gene on X-chromosome in males will express itself readily as there is no normal allele, while a mutant gene on X-chromosome in females will not express itself in the presence of the normal allele. This is the basis of sex-linked inheritance of which haemophilia is an outstanding example. If an affected male marries a normal female, the gene is transmitted to all the daughters, but the sons escape. But if a carrier female marries a normal male, 50 per cent of her daughters will be carriers and 50 per cent normal; 50 per cent of her sons will be affected and 50 per cent normal. Fig.1 shows the patterns of inheritance.

Mendelian diseases are individually rare since there is strong selection against them and gene mutations are rare events. Mutation usually occurs at random. If mutation is confined to a single gene it is called "point" mutation, which is responsible for many human diseases and defects.

It is estimated that the combined incidence in man of diseases and disabilities in this category is about 1 per cent of all live-born individuals *(12)*. Rare as these diseases are, as many as 793 autosomal dominant phenotypes, 629 autosomal recessive traits and 123 sex-linked diseases have been catalogued to date *(10)*. A short list of these abnormalities is given in Table 1.

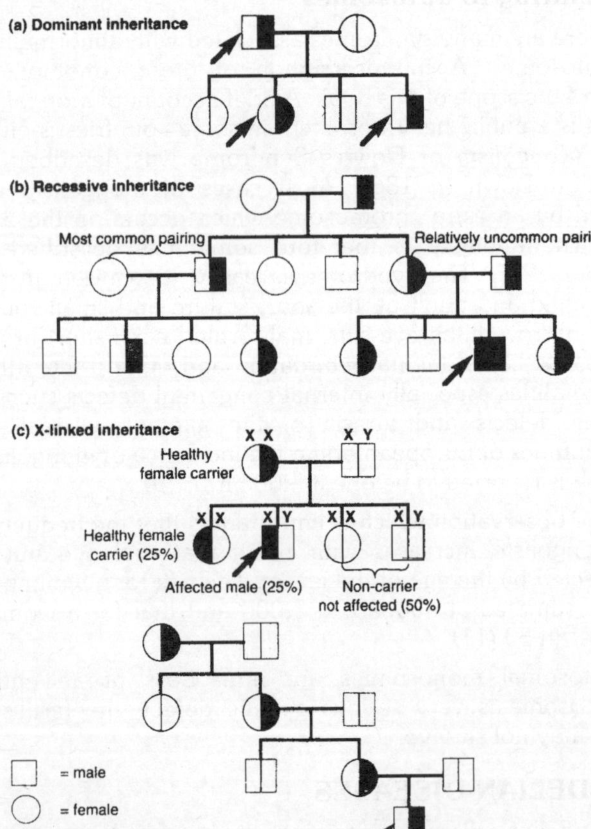

FIG. 1
Classical mendelian patterns of inheritance

Source : *(5)*

TABLE 1

Some dominant, recessive and sex-linked diseases

Autosomal dominant traits	Achondroplasia Huntington's chorea Neurofibromatosis Polyposis coli, familial Brachydactylia Marfan's syndrome Retinoblastoma ABO blood group system Hyperlipoproteinaemia I, II, III, IV Polycystic, kidney Polydactyly Spherocytosis, hereditary
Autosomal recessive traits	Fibrocystic disease of the pancreas Phenylketonuria Albinism Tay-Sachs disease Agammaglobulinaemia, Swiss type Alkaptonuria Cystic fibrosis Galactosaemia Haemoglobinopathies Maple syrup urine disease Megacolon (Hirschsprung's disease)
Recessive sex-linked traits	Haemophilia type A and B Duchenne type of muscular dystrophy Colour blindness G6PD Deficiency Hydrocephalus Retinitis pigmentosa Agammaglobulinaemia, Bruton type.
Dominant X-linked traits	Vit. D resistant rickets Familial hypophosphataemia Blood group Xg

Source : *(4)*

Blood groups

Early genetic studies centred round blood groups in man. Blood groups are determined by genes. At present 14 blood group systems have been discovered in man; the well-known ones are the ABO and Rh blood groups.

ABO SYSTEM

The genotypes and phenotypes in the ABO system are shown in Table 2 :

TABLE 2

Genotypes and phenotypes in ABO system

Genotype	Phenotype (Blood Group)	Approximate frequency in Indian population
OO	O	40 per cent
AA AO	A A	22 per cent "
BB BO	B B	33 per cent "
AB	AB	5 per cent

Source : *(13)*

Gene O is recessive; the red blood cells of a person whose blood group is O have no antigens. Genes A and B are co-dominant; when both are present, the red blood cells carry antigen-A and antigen-B. Blood groups provide valuable evidence in cases where there is a question of true parentage; they are also extensively used to determine whether the twins are identical or not.

RHESUS SYSTEM

The Rhesus system depends upon three genes which are designated by the letter C, D and E and their alleles by the small letters c, d and e. The Rh-antigens develop very early and have been demonstrated in a 38-day old foetus. It had been established that the Rh-antigens are present only on the surface of red cells *(14)*.

The possible genotypes in the rhesus system will be CDE, CDe, cDE, cdE, cDe and cde. The diploid individual inherits any two of these units, e.g., CDe/cde. Of the rhesus antigens, the most potent is the antigen D; so much so, the term "Rhesus-positive" has come to mean possessing this antigen and "Rhesus-negative" lacking it. In India, it is found that about 93 per cent of the population are Rhesus-positive as compared to 85 per cent in countries of Northern Europe and North America *(11)*. The importance of the rhesus system in preventive medicine is exemplified in the fatal disease in the newborn, Erythroblastosis foetalis.

Erythroblastosis foetalis

If the foetus is Rh-positive and the mother Rh-negative, certain consequences are likely. Some of the foetal red cells cross the placenta and enter the maternal circulation where they act as foreign antigen and the production of Rh antibodies.

The Rh antibodies are of two main types : (a) the "strong" or saline antibodies and (b) the "weak" or albumin antibodies. The latter are small 7S gammaglobulins which cross the placental barrier and pass back into the blood circulation of the foetus. When this happens, the RBC of the foetus are destroyed. If the damage is severe, the foetus is killed *in utero* and results in miscarriage; if the damage is less severe, the infant may be born with jaundice, anaemia and oedema. This symptom complex is known as Rh-haemolytic disease or erythroblastosis foetalis.

Blood groups and disease

During the past 10 years researchers have been trying to find out the association of certain diseases with particular blood groups. However, only two disease conditions have shown such association with the ABO groups. Duodenal ulcer and gastric ulcer are common in 'O' group and stomach cancer in 'A' group individuals. A number of other diseases appear to be associated with particular blood groups, especially carcinoma of the uterine cervix and pernicious anaemia with group 'A', and rheumatic heart disease with a lack of group 'O'. Haemolytic tendencies appear to be associated with group 'O', and thrombosis with group 'A'. An 'A' group woman taking an oral contraceptive is at greater risk of thrombotic episodes than an 'O' group woman *(15)*. The demonstration of associations between blood groups and certain diseases is an important contribution of human genetics.

Sickle cell anaemia

Sickle cell anaemia is an autosomal recessive disorder in which an abnormal haemoglobin leads to chronic haemolytic anaemia with a variety of severe clinical consequences. The disorder is a classic example of disease caused by a point mutation in DNA. Individuals with one gene of this disease are clinically healthy, but their RBC look abnormal under the microscope. Persons with 2 genes (homozygous) of this disease suffer from acute anaemia and in most cases die before puberty. The rate of sickling is influenced by a number of factors, most importantly by concentration of haemoglobin S in the individual red blood cell.

The disease is prevalent among blacks, specially in certain parts of Africa. It has been found that the areas where the disease is most prevalent also showed the higher frequencies of malaria. The haemoglobin S gene is carried in 8 per cent of American blacks, and one birth out of 400 in American blacks will produce a child with sickle cell anaemia. In India, it is an important disorder on account of its high incidence in certain regions.

The disorder has its onset during the first year of life, when haemoglobin F level falls. These patients are prone to delayed puberty. On examination, patients are often chronically ill and jaundiced. There is hepatomegaly, but the spleen is not palpable in adult life. The heart is enlarged, with hyperdynamic precardium and systolic murmurs. Non-healing ulcers may be present. Sickle cell anaemia becomes a chronic multisystem disease, with death from organ failure commonly occurring between ages 20 and 40 years.

No specific treatment is available for the primary disease. However, both longevity and quality of life may be improved by comprehensive medical management. Prenatal diagnosis is now available for couples at risk of producing a child with sickle cell anaemia. DNA from foetal cells can be directly examined, and the presence of the sickle cell mutation can be accurately diagnosed. Genetic counselling should be made available to such couples *(9)*.

Thalassaemias

The thalassaemias are hereditary disorders characterized by reduction in the synthesis of globin chain (alpha or beta). Reduced globin chain synthesis causes reduced haemoglobin synthesis and eventually produces a hypochromic microcytic anaemia because of defective haemoglobinization of red cells. Thalassaemias can be considered among hypo-proliferative anaemias, the haemolytic anaemias, and the anaemias related to abnormal haemoglobin, since all of these factors may play a role.

Alpha thalassaemia is primarily due to gene deletion directly causing reduced a – globin chain synthesis. Beta thalassaemia are usually caused by point mutations rather than large deletions. Signs of thalassaemia develop after 6 months of age, because this is the time when haemoglobin synthesis switches from haemoglobin F to haemoglobin A. Prenatal diagnosis is available for couples at risk of producing a child with one of the severe thalassaemia syndromes. Asian couples whose parents on both sides have alpha thalassaemia trait are at risk of producing an infant with hydrops foetalis. Mediterranean people with both parents heterozygous for beta thalassaemia, are at risk of producing homozygous child *(9)*.

Haemophilia *(16)*

Haemophilia is a hereditary bleeding disorder affecting 15-20 of every 100,000 males born, with equal incidence in all ethnic groups and geographical areas that have been surveyed. Prevalence, which depends on survival, varies according to available medical care. There are an estimated 420,000 people with haemophilia worldwide.

There are different forms of haemophilia. While the disorder affects males, it is carried by females, who are only occasionally affected, usually mildly. The disorder concerns the absence, decrease or deficient function of blood coagulating factor, leading to excessive, prolonged or delayed bleeding. In severe cases it most commonly occurs in the large joints of the limbs. Unless such bleeding is controlled promptly by infusion of the deficient factor, there is progressive joint disease and muscle atrophy, leading to serious physical, psychological and social handicaps. Until recently, the foremost cause of death was haemorrhage, especially in the skull.

In countries with highly developed haemophilia care programmes, therapy with plasma derivatives has reduced mortality. In the past decade, the main causes of death have stemmed from infections as the side-effects of treatment, including AIDS and liver disease secondary to hepatitis. Survival in patients without these infections is almost the same as that of the general population.

Cystic fibrosis *(16)*

Cystic fibrosis is a genetic disease occurring worldwide, which affects the respiratory and gastrointestinal tracts and the sweat glands. Incidence ranges from 2.5 to 5 per 10,000 live births in most European populations. The condition is less common in blacks, and rare in orientals.

Until a few years ago, life expectancy of children with the disease was below 5 years of age. Now that it is recognized and treated earlier and more effectively, life expectancy in developed countries is about 30 years, and projections for young children alive with cystic fibrosis now suggest that they may live for 40 years or more, even without the development of new treatments. However, upto 95% of cases in Latin America are never diagnosed, and the life expectancy of those that are diagnosed is only about 10 years.

The gene defect in cystic fibrosis was identified in 1989, since then there has been unprecedented progress in understanding the disease, leading to new approaches to drug treatment and hopes for gene therapy. Such treatments are expected to be available within the lifetime of most current patients, with a corresponding anticipated improvement in outlook.

Phenylketonuria (PKU)

Phenylketonuria is an autosomal recessive disorder resulting in a deficiency of the liver enzyme phenylalanine hydroxylase which converts phenylalanine to tyrosine. The name PKU is derived from the build-up of phenylpyruvic acid in the urine, a characteristic of the disease. The frequency of the disease is about 1 in 10,000 births *(5)*.

Phenylalanine accumulates in the blood and tissues and has a toxic effect on the brain leading to mental retardation. Tests for elevated blood levels of phenylalanine are much more desirable than tests for urine phenylketone, since blood levels must be elevated before urine detection is possible. Testing of bottle-fed infants should be done no sooner than 48 hours after the first successful formula feeding. Breast-fed babies, however, are tested at 7 days, since breast milk often has little protein content before the 5th day *(17)*.

MULTIFACTORIAL DISORDERS

The frequency of multifactorial disorders is high compared with that of Mendelian and chromosomal disorders. There are indications that most of the common disorders of adult life such as essential hypertension, schizophrenia, mental retardation, duodenal ulcer, ischaemic heart disease of early onset, diabetes, congenital heart malformations are conditions with a multifactorial aetiology. A small minority of cancers (family cancer syndromes) are clearly inherited; these include familial polyposis coli, familial non-polyposis colon cancer and some thyroid cancers. Also known is a major genetic component in cancer of the colon and breast, although in these relatively common conditions it can be difficult to distinguish familial from non-familial cases.

In a disorder such as cancer or coronary heart disease, features that should arouse suspicion of an inherited predisposition include : early onset; similarly affected parents and/or siblings; when there is a difference in frequency between the sexes, occurrence in the less commonly affected sex (e.g., coronary heart disease in women); in ethnic groups in which there is a high incidence of a particular condition (e.g., spina bifida is 40 times more common in Caucasians – and even more frequent among the Irish – than in Asians.

The mode of inheritance of multifactorial disorders is complex because environmental factors are also involved, as for instance, the influence of smoking, diet, obesity and lack of exercise on ischaemic heart disease. Campbell (1965) stressed that environmental agents and genetic constitutions usually interact closely in producing abnormalities. He summarizes his conclusions in saying that some genetic factors are effective only under certain environmental conditions *(17)*. The relative contributions of genetic predisposition and environmental factors to the aetiology will vary greatly from patient to patient.

Role of genetic predisposition in common disorders *(16)*

Although the limits of intelligence, physical ability and longevity are genetically determined, external and environmental influences such as infections, malnutrition and war have long been the main determinants of health and survival. Now, with increased control of the environment, genetic make-up is becoming an ever-more important determinant of individual health. Genetic predisposition may lead to the premature onset of common diseases of adult life such as cancer, coronary heart disease, diabetes, hypertension and mental disorders.

Cancer : It is not yet certain whether most cancers are hereditary. But a genetic predisposition may be involved in as many as 10–25% of cases of cancer of the breast or colon. Numerous genes are being identified that may affect susceptibility to tumour development. This may lead to a general improvement in the diagnosis and treatment of cancer. For example, a DNA screening test for breast cancer could soon be available. Advice could be offered on the chemoprevention of cancers, tailored for families with different types of cancer risk.

Coronary heart disease : Until recently, it was generally believed that environmental factors alone cause coronary heart disease. But investigating family histories often uncover genetic risks. Mapping the human genome will make the genetic predisposition to CHD much easier. High blood pressure and high blood cholesterol levels, major risk factors in CHD, are also genetically influenced. A combination of risk detection and lifestyle counselling, with drug treatment, might cut the incidence of heart attacks to the low levels as two or three generations ago.

Diabetes : Evidence for a genetic element in insulin-dependent diabetes mellitus has emerged from studies showing a higher concordance in identical twins (25–30%) than in non-identical twins (5–10%). About 85% of cases of diabetes in developed countries are of the non-insulin-dependent form of the disease, which has a particularly strong familial tendency. Diabetes of all types is an important candidate for future treatments such as gene therapy of pancreatic tissue transplantation.

Mental disorders : Evidence from family and twin studies demonstrate the existence of genetic predisposition to some common mental diseases. Alzheimer's disease, the most common form of senile dementia, has a strong familial tendency and is known to be caused by at least four different genes. Research may lead to the development of drugs useful in preventing or delaying the onset of the disease.

Enough is already known about the genetics of common diseases to introduce a family-oriented approach into basic as well as specialist medical practice. A major effort is being made to study the genetic factors involved, develop appropriate therapies, and determine how these approaches can best be applied in practice.

Application and uses of genomics *(18)*

DNA technology depends on a number of basic tools that have been gradually developed over the past 30 years or so. A wide range of enzymes involved in DNA and RNA synthesis and repair have been identified and become available for laboratory use, nucleotide bases are available as laboratory reagents, and specific DNA sequences can be synthesized at will. DNA diagnostic methods have been greatly simplified over the past 20 years. DNA has many advantages for genetic diagnosis. It is easy to obtain, since every cell of an individual or foetus contains the full DNA complement of that individual. Genes can be studied whether they are actively producing their product or not. A definitive diagnosis can usually be made in all genetic conditions. A short list of application and uses of genomics are as follows :

Gene therapy (5)

Gene therapy is the introduction of a gene sequence into a cell with the aim of modifying the cell's behaviour in a clinically relevant fashion. It may be used in several ways, e.g., to correct a genetic mutation (as for cystic fibrosis), to kill a cell (as for cancer) or to modify susceptibility (as for coronary artery disease).

The gene may be introduced using a virus (usually a retrovirus or adenovirus) or by means of lipid or receptor targeting. There is now almost universal agreement that gene delivery to somatic cell to treat disease is ethical, and that gene therapy should take its place alongside other forms of medical treatment.

The human genome project (5)

The human genome project is an attempt to systematize the research on mapping and isolating human genes that is already in progress in many countries, in order to create a single linear map of the human genome, with each coding gene defined and sequenced.

Agencies with a role in coordinating human genome data include UNESCO, the Genome Data Base, HUGO, the National Institute of Health/Department of Energy (USA), the Medical Research Council (UK), Genethon (France) and the European Union.

The human genome diversity project (5)

As part of the work of HUGO, the Human Genome Diversity Project is aimed at increasing understanding of human evolution. The major objective is to define the genetic relationships between human populations and interpret them in terms of natural selection, genetic drift, migration, etc. For example, the frequency and distribution of rare single-gene disorders are related to the history of human migration. Differences in distribution between populations may often be accounted for by "founder

Application	Use
Human genomics for medical purposes	• Risk assessment (carrier screening, prenatal screening tests, newborn, child, and adult screening) • Diagnosis of disease, both single gene and common disorders • Treatment selection, including pharmacogenomics to target therapies and reduce adverse events, gene editing, and gene therapy • Disease prognosis and monitoring
Microbial genomics for medical purposes	• Identification of infectious agents and development of diagnostic tests for the disease • Contact tracing of infectious agents • Investigation of cluster outbreaks to identify potential sources of the infectious agent • Mapping chains of transmission of infectious agents within a community • Assessment of characteristics such as infectivity and severity of associated disease • Design of vaccines and prediction of responses to vaccines and medications
Agriculture and aquaculture genomics	• Catalogue of genetic diversity in the wild and in founder stocks • Identification of new traits and disease susceptibility • Selection of traits in genetic programmes
Biological and medical research	• Discovery of genes influencing disease • Rational drug development • Identification of genetic signatures in combination with other biomarkers
Other	• Assessment of ancestry and parentage • Environmental and ecological sciences • Forensic science

Source : *(18)*

effects". When a population expands from a relatively few founding members, some contribute more, and some less, to the genetic make-up of subsequent generations. If one prolific founder carries a genetic abnormality, this can lead to a localized cluster of affected individuals. Studies of isolated and aboriginal populations can be particularly informative.

Factors which influence the gene frequencies

The Hardy-Weinberg law assumes that human population is static. But in reality, human population and consequently human gene pool is never static. There are several factors which influence the human gene pool. The following are some : *(a) Mutation :* Mutation implies a change in the genetic material of an organism which results in a new inherited variation. Mutation is a rather regular phenomenon in nature. It is now recognized that mutant genes are so wide-spread in their occurrence that every one of us might be harbouring a few or many of them. According to modern geneticists, the entire body structure of man and every other animal and plant cell have been built through hundreds of millions of years by means of a long succession of mutation *(7)*. The cause of spontaneous mutation is not yet known. But we know that certain external influences such as ionizing radiation and certain chemicals are capable of producing mutations experimentally and there is no reason to believe that man is an exception. Most mutant genes are believed to be harmful. But there are instances where a mutant gene could be beneficial, e.g., sickle cell anaemia. The heterozygotes of sickle cell trait were found to be resistant to falciparum malaria. Some mutant genes remain "neutral" in that they do not harm or impair the survival ability of the carriers. Such genes may persist indefinitely in the population for many generations. Specialists in population genetics are interested in mutation rates. It is said that each gene has its own characteristic mutation rate which is estimated anywhere from 10^4 to 10^6 per generation. During the past 30 years, mutation rates have probably risen owing to increased use of X-rays and chemical mutagens. *(b) Natural selection :* Darwin proposed the theory of natural selection or survival of the fittest to explain evolution. Natural selection is the process whereby harmful genes are eliminated from the gene pool and genes favourable to an individual tend to be preserved and passed on to the offspring. When DDT was first used, it was lethal to houseflies. Today, not many houseflies are killed by DDT. This is an example of natural selection in response of DDT; the resistant variety of houseflies has become the usual form. The forces which operate in the animal kingdom do not apply in human populations because man by his superior intelligence has interfered with natural selection in every conceivable way by changing the environmental conditions under which people live and by advances in technology, public health and medical care services. *(c) Population movements :* Because of industrialization, increased facilities for earning, ways of living and education, people are moving – sometimes on a large scale – from rural to urban areas. There is also a migration of people between countries. Such population movements will lead to changes in the distribution of genes, affecting both the areas of immigration and emigration. The intermixing of people makes new genetic combinations possible. *(d) Breeding structure :* If all marriages were to occur in a random fashion, the effect would be the attainment of a genetic equilibrium. In practice, however, matings tend to occur selectively within various subgroups based on religion, economic and educational status and family relationships. In open societies, there is more freedom in mating. For instance doctors tend to marry doctors or nurses; musicians tend to marry musicians. This type of mating is called "assortative mating", or birds of the same feather flocking together. The genetic consequences of assortative mating have not been adequately studied. *(e) Public health measures :* Advances in public health and medical care services do affect the genetic endowment of people as a whole. More lives are now being saved by advances in medical sciences than ever before. For instance, Ramstedt's operation which was introduced in 1912 has saved many children suffering from congenital pyloric stenosis. Individuals with genetically conditioned retinoblastoma may be saved by timely surgery. The provision of insulin has saved the lives of diabetics. The carriers of hereditary diseases, malformations and constitutional weaknesses are able to survive and pass their genes to their progeny. Public health measures are thus decreasing the selection rates and increasing the genetic burden. This has led some scientists to prophesy that "medicine will harm people in the long run by helping them in the short run" *(12)*.

PREVENTIVE AND SOCIAL MEASURES

1. Health promotional measures

(a) EUGENICS : Galton proposed the term eugenics for the science which aims to improve the genetic endowment of human population. Eugenics has both negative and positive aspects.

(i) Negative eugenics : Hitler sought to improve the German race by killing the weak and defective; this was negative eugenics. But nobody in the civilized world would approve of such a measure to improve the human race.

On the other hand, if people who are suffering from serious hereditary diseases are sterilized or otherwise debarred from producing children, there should be no serious objection to marriage. The aim of negative eugenics is to reduce the frequency of hereditary disease and disability in the community to as low as possible. However, the question one would ask is how far negative eugenic measures would be helpful in eliminating genetic defects? The simple answer is that in spite of eugenic sterilization, new cases of hereditary diseases will continue to arise in the population partly because of fresh mutations, and partly because of marital alliances between hidden carriers (heterozygotes) of recessive defects. Nevertheless, it may be hoped that should eugenic measures be applied, hereditary diseases would become less frequent *(12)*.

(ii) Positive eugenics : This is a more ambitious programme than negative eugenics. It seeks to improve the genetic composition of the population by encouraging the carriers of desirable genotypes to assume the burden of parenthood. At present, positive eugenics has very little application. Its realization is difficult for 2 reasons (i) The majority of socially valuable traits – let us say – intelligence and positive character features, though partially determined biologically are not inherited in such a simple way as, say blood groups. These traits have a complex, multifactorial determination, both genetical and environmental. It would be difficult to expect, therefore, that positive eugenic measures will yield direct results (ii) Secondly, we cannot determine which gene we transmit to our children *(7)*.

(b) EUTHENICS : Mere improvement of the genotype is of no use unless the improved genotype is given access to a suitable environment, an environment which will enable the genes to express themselves readily. Throughout the course of history, man has been adapting environment to his genes more than adapting his genes to the environment. Studies with mentally retarded (mild) children indicated that exposure to environmental stimulation improved their IQ. Thus the solution of improving the human race does not lie in contrasting heredity and environment, but rather in the mutual interaction of heredity and environmental factors. This environmental manipulation is called euthenics and has considerable broader prospects for success.

(c) GENETIC COUNSELLING *(19)* : The most immediate and practical service that genetics can render in medicine and surgery is genetic counselling *(12)*. Genetic counselling may be prospective or retrospective *(8)*.

(i) Prospective genetic counselling : This allows for the true prevention of disease. This approach requires identifying heterozygous individuals for any particular defect by screening procedures and explaining to them the risk of their having affected children if they marry another heterozygote for the same gene. In other words, if heterozygous marriage can be prevented or reduced, the prospects of giving birth to affected children will diminish. The application in this field, for example, are sickle cell anaemia and thalassemia. It is possible that this kind of prevention may find wider application to cover a number of other recessive defects *(12)*.

(ii) Retrospective genetic counselling : Most genetic counselling is at present retrospective, i.e., the hereditary disorder has already occurred within the family. A survey carried out by the WHO showed that genetic advice was chiefly sought in connection with congenital abnormalities, mental retardation, psychiatric illness and inborn errors of metabolism and only a few sought premarital advice. The WHO recommends the establishment of genetic counselling centres in sufficient numbers in regions where infectious disease and nutritional disorders have been brought under control and in areas where genetic disorders have always constituted a serious public health problem (e.g., sickle cell anaemia and thalassaemia) *(12)*.

The methods which could be suggested under retrospective genetic counselling are : (i) contraception (ii) pregnancy termination and (iii) sterilization depending upon the attitudes and cultural environment of the couples involved *(8)*.

(d) OTHER GENETIC PREVENTIVE MEASURES : *(i) Consanguineous marriages* : When blood relatives marry each other there is an increased risk in the offspring of traits controlled by recessive genes, and those determined by polygenes. Examples are albinism, alkaptonuria, phenylketonuria and several others. An increased risk of premature death is also noted in such offspring. For instance, in a certain Japanese city, a death rate of 116 per 1,000 was found during the first 8 years of life amongst the offspring of first cousins, against 55 amongst the controls *(12)*. Therefore, a lowering of consanguineous marriages would be advantageous to the health of the community.

(ii) Late marriages : The pendulum is swinging in favour of early marriages. The discovery of "Trisomy 21" in mongols coupled with the knowledge that mongolism is more frequent in children born of elderly mothers, lends support to the view that early marriage of females is better than late marriage from the point of view of preventing mongolism. Its incidence in a mother at age 20 is only 1 : 3000; by the age 40, it is 1:40.

2. Specific protection

Increasing attention is now being paid to the protection of individuals and whole communities against mutagens such as X-rays and other ionizing radiations and also chemical mutagens. Patients undergoing X-ray examination should be protected against unnecessary exposure of the gonads to radiation. X-ray examination of the pregnant uterus to determine the presence of twins or the lie of the foetus is to be strongly deprecated. Rh haemolytic disease of the newborn which is a genetically determined immunological disorder is now preventable by immunization by anti-D globulin.

3. Early diagnosis and treatment

(a) Detection of genetic carriers : It is now possible to identify the healthy carriers of a number of genetic disorders, especially the inborn errors of metabolism. The female carriers of Duchenne type of muscular dystrophy, an X-linked disorder, can now be detected by elevated levels of serum creatine kinase in 80 per cent of carriers. In some conditions, carriers can be recognized with a high degree of certainty (e.g., acatalasia); in some only a proportion of carriers can be detected (e.g., haemophilia, PKU, galactosaemia); in other conditions, no method has yet been found which will distinguish carriers (e.g., alkaptonuria) *(20)*.

(b) Prenatal diagnosis : Amniocentesis in early pregnancy (about 14–16 weeks) has now made it possible for prenatal diagnosis of conditions associated with chromosomal anomalies (e.g., Down's Syndrome); many inborn errors of metabolism (e.g., Tay-Sach's disease, galactosaemia, Maple syrup urine disease, Alpha-thalassaemia and neural tube defects). The indications for prenatal diagnosis are listed in Table 3.

TABLE 3

Indications for prenatal diagnosis

Indications	Methods
a. Advanced maternal age, previous child with chromosome aberration, intrauterine growth delay	Cytogenetics (amniocentesis, chorionic villus sampling)
b. Biochemical disorders	Protein assay, DNA diagnosis
c. Congenital anomaly	Sonography, fetoscopy
d. Screening for neural tube defects and trisomy	Maternal serum alpha-fetoprotein and chorionic gonadotropin

Source : *(9)*

Amniocentesis : Examination of a sample of amniotic fluid makes possible the prenatal diagnosis of chromosomal anomalies and certain metabolic defects. The procedure can be used as early as 14th week of pregnancy when abortion of the affected fetus is still feasible. The diagnosis of chromosomal anomalies is made by culture and Karyotyping of fetal cells from the amniotic fluid, and of metabolic defects by biochemical analysis of the fluid.

Amniocentesis is called for in the following circumstances if the parents are prepared to consider abortion.

1. A mother aged 35 years or more (because of high risk of Down's syndrome with advanced maternal age).
2. Patients who have had a child with Down's syndrome or other chromosomal anomalies.
3. Parents who are known to have chromosomal translocation.

4. Parents who have had a child with a metabolic defect – detectable by amniocentesis. The most common are defects of the neural tube, anencephaly and spina bifida which can be detected by an elevation of alpha fetoprotein in the amniotic fluid.
5. When determination of the sex is warranted, given a family history of a sex-linked genetic disease e.g., certain muscular dystrophies.

For the detection of neural tube defects there is now the possibility of widespread screening by the determination of alpha-fetoprotein levels in the maternal serum. If the test is positive it can be confirmed by amniocentesis.

(c) Screening of newborn infants : We have today a long list of screening tests for the early diagnosis of genetic abnormalities – sex chromosome abnormalities, congenital dislocation of hip, PKU, congenital hypothyroidism, sickle cell disease, cystic fibrosis, Duchenne muscular dystrophy, congenital adrenal hyperplasia, G6PD deficiency etc.

Neonates should be routinely examined for congenital abnormalities, particularly dislocation of the hip, which can be simply corrected at this stage. Biochemical screening of newborn infants was first used for PKU in 1966. Heel-prick blood samples are usually collected at 5–10 days after birth. Several drops of blood are collected on filter paper (the Guthrie card), which is sent to screening laboratory. Screening of newborns for congenital hypothyroidism is carried out in most developed countries. Sickle-cell disease can be detected cheaply and reliably by haemoglobin electrophoresis using Guthrie blood spots. Neonatal screening for cystic fibrosis is based on the measurement of immunoreactive trypsin in Guthrie blood spots.

(d) Recognizing pre-clinical cases : We have today a pretty long list of screening tests for the early diagnosis of hereditary diseases. For example, heterozygotes for phenylketonuria can be detected by a phenylalanine tolerance test. A simple urine examination for sugar after morning breakfast is good enough to detect diabetics. Examination of sibs and close relatives of diabetics by a glucose tolerance test will often reveal preclinical cases of acholuric jaundice. A raised serum uric acid should arouse suspicion of gout. Sickle cell trait can be uncovered by subjecting the red cells to reduced oxygen tension. Thalassaemia minor can be detected by studying the blood picture.

Genetic counselling can have the greatest impact when individuals or couples at genetic risk are identified prospectively, i.e., before they have developed symptoms themselves or produced their first affected child. Prospective counselling is technically possible only when carriers can be accurately identified. To some extent, the established genetic population-screening services listed in Table 4 may serve as models for the development of future genetic screening programmes *(5)*.

Once diagnosed, some of the genetic conditions can be treated with complete or partial success by medical and surgical measures. For example, diets low in phenylalanine are now prescribed as treatment for PKU children. Persons suffering from haemophilia can be greatly helped by administering antihaemolytic globulin, which promotes the clotting of blood. Modern surgical techniques have brought great improvements in dealing with cases of spina bifida.

Rehabilitation

Finally, rehabilitation. With many genetic or partially genetic conditions causing physical or mental disability, much can be done for the patient and for his family in helping him to lead a better and more useful life.

TABLE 4

Established genetic population-screening services

Type of service	Conditions	Preventive or screening action
Primary prevention	Rhesus haemolytic disease	Postpartum use of Anti-D globulin
	Congenital rubella	Immunization of girls
	Congenital malformations	Addition of folic acid to the maternal diet (may prevent neural tube defects) Control of maternal diabetes; Avoidance of mutagens and teratogens such as alcohol, certain drugs and possibly tobacco
Antenatal screening	Congenital malformations	Ultrasound foetal anomaly scan, maternal serum alpha-fetoprotein estimation
	Chromosomal abnormalities	Noting maternal age and maternal serum factor levels Checking family history
	Inherited disease	Carrier screening for haemoglobinopathies, Tay-Sach's disease
Neonatal screening	Congenital malformations	Examination of the newborn for early treatment (e.g., of congenital dislocation of the hip)
	Phenylketonuria, congenital hypothyroidism, sickle-cell disease	Biochemical tests for early treatment

Source : *(5)*

References

1. Wald, I. (1976) in *"Health, Medicine and Society"* - Proceedings of the International conference on the Sociology of Medicine, D. Reidel Publ. Co., Boston.
2. Editorial (1971). *N. Eng. J. Med.*, 284, 788.
3. Koller, P.C. (1968). *Chromosomes and Genes,* Oliver and Boyd, Edinburgh.
4. Porter, I.H. (1980). in Maxy-Rosenau : *Public Health and Preventive Medicine,* 11th Ed., John M last (ed), Appleton - Century - Crofts, New York.
5. WHO (1996). *Tech. Rep. Ser.* No.865.
6. May, J.M. (1958). *The Ecology of Human Disease,* MD Publications, Inc., New York.
7. Corwin, E.H.L. (1949). *Ecology of Health,* The Commonwealth Fund, New York.
8. WHO (1972). *Techn. Rep. Ser.,* No.49.
9. Lawrence M tierney, Jr., Stephen J. McPhee, and Maxine A. Papadakis (Edt.), 34th Ed. (1995). *Current Medical Diagnosis and Treatment,* A LANGE Medical Book.
10. Indian Council of Medical Research (1972). *Genetics and Our Health* Techn. Rep. Ser., No.20.
11. Crew, F.A.E. (1965). *Health, Its Nature and Conservation,* Pergamon P.
12. WHO (1964). *Techn. Rep. Ser.,* No.282.
13. Ranganathan, K.S. (1967). *Essentials of Blood Grouping and Clinical Applications,* Varadachary, Madras.
14. Finn. R. (1970). *British Medical Journal,* 2, 219.
15. Mourant, A.E. (1973). *Bull, Wld. Hlth. Org.,* 49, 93.
16. WHO (1997). *The World Health Report* 1997, Conquering Suffering, Enriching Humanity, Report of the Director - General WHO.
17. Rakel, R.E. (1977). *Principles of Family Medicine,* Saunders.
18. WHO (2022). *Accelerating access to genomics for global health; promotion implementation, collaboration, and ethical, legal and social issues,* A report of the WHO science council.
19. Hecht F. (1970). *Paediat. Chn. N. Amer.,* 17, 1039.
20. Emery, A.E.H. (1974). *Elements of Medical Genetics,* 3rd Ed. Livingstone, London.

20 Mental Health

"A mentally healthy person feels right towards others"

Health is defined as a state of complete physical, mental and social well-being and not merely the absence of disease or infirmity. A sound mind in a sound body has been recognised as a social ideal for many centuries. The Indian sages and seers had paid particular attention to the unconscious, wherein lay the suppressed unfulfilled desires and compulsions of several kinds which led the individual astray; by mastering their minds, they attained the highest level of emotional equilibrium. Mental health is thus the balanced development of the individual's personality and emotional attitudes which enable him to live harmoniously with his fellow-men. Mental health is not exclusively a matter of relation between persons; it is also a matter of relation of the individual towards the community he lives in, towards the society of which the community is a part, and towards the social institutions which for a large part guide his life, determine his way of living, working, leisure, and the way he earns and spends his money, the way he sees happiness, stability and security.

By definition, "mental health is a state of well-being in which an individual realizes his or her own abilities, can cope with the normal stress of life, can work productively and is able to make a contribution to his or her community" *(1)*. Mental health is fundamental to our collective and individual ability as humans to think, emote, interact with each other, earn a living and enjoy life. On this basis, the promotion, protection and restoration of mental health can be regarded as a vital concern of individuals, communities and societies throughout the world.

Problem statement

WORLD: Mental disorders are not the exclusive preserve of any special group; they are truly universal. Mental and behavioural disorders are found in people of all regions, all countries and all societies. There are many different mental disorders, with different presentations. They are generally characterized by a combination of abnormal thoughts, perceptions, emotions, behaviour and relationship with others. The burden of mental disorders continue to grow with significant impact on health and major social, human rights and economic consequences in all countries of the world. The tentative global estimates of the major mental disorders are depression 300 million, bipolar affective disorders 60 million, schizophrenia and other psychosis 23 million and dementia 50 million *(2)*.

INDIA : National Mental Health Survey (NMHS) was carried out in the country to identify the prevalence, pattern, outcome, treatment gap, disabilities along with the current status of medical health services and facilities. The survey was done in the year 2015, in 12 states. i.e. Kerala, Tamil Nadu, Gujarat, Rajasthan, West Bengal, Jharkhand, Chhattisgarh, Madhya Pradesh, Assam and Manipur. The key findings of the survey are as follows *(3)*:

1. NMHS indicates that nearly 150 million Indians aged 13 and above are likely to be suffering from one or more mental health problems and are in need of services.
2. Mental health problems are comparatively more prevalent in urban areas.
3. The proportion of those with a mental health disorder in young adolescents was 7.3%
4. Neurosis and stress related disorders (phobias and anxiety disorders) affected twice as many women compared to man.
5. Alcohol use disorder in men was 4.6% amongst the 18+ population while, illicit substance use disorders (dependence +abuse) was 0.6%
6. Less than 2% had a severe mental illness like psychosis or bipolar disorder. Amongst those with the disorder, nearly 50% had moderate to severe disability.
7. A growing concern has also been the risk of suicide in India and data indicates that 0.9% are at a high risk of suicide.
8. The economic impact of mental disorder is huge as the median monthly expenditure ranged between INR 1000 to 2500 and varied across conditions.

Based on uniform and standardized data collection procedures from a nationally representative population, it is estimated that, excluding tobacco use disorders, mental morbidity of individuals above the age of 18 years currently was 10.6 per cent. The life time prevalence in the surveyed population was 13.7 per cent. This estimate includes a range of mental disorder categories and are summarized in Fig. 1 *(4)*.

Characteristics of a mentally healthy person

Mental Health is not mere absence of mental illness. A mentally healthy person has three main characteristics: (1) He feels comfortable about himself, that is, he feels reasonably secure and adequate. He neither underestimates nor overestimates his own ability. He accepts his shortcomings. He has self-respect. (2) The mentally healthy person feels right towards others. This means that he is able to be interested in others and to love them. He has friendships that are satisfying and lasting. He is able to feel a part of a group without being submerged by it. He is able to like and trust others. He takes responsibility for his neighbours and his fellow-men. (3) The mentally healthy

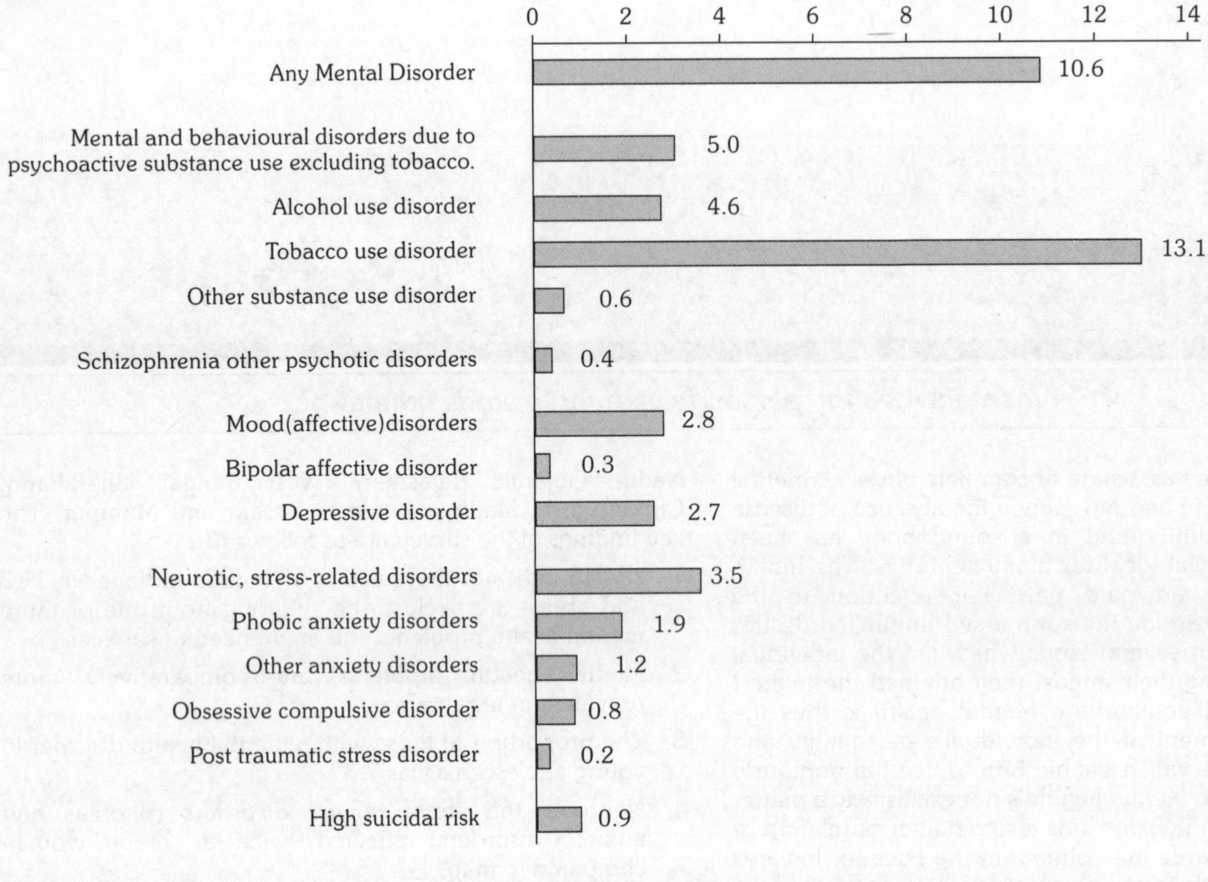

FIG. 1
Prevalence of mental disorders (weighted per cent)

person is able to meet the demands of life. He does something about the problems as they arise. He is able to think for himself and to take his own decisions. He sets reasonable goals for himself. He shoulders his daily responsibilities. He is not bowled over by his own emotions of fear, anger, love or guilt.

Warning signals of poor mental health

William C. Menninger, President of the Menninger Foundation, Topeka, Kansas, United States of America drew up the following questions to aid in taking one's own mental health pulse:

1. Are you *always* worrying ?
2. Are you *unable* to concentrate because of unrecognized reasons?
3. Are you *continually* unhappy without justified cause?
4. Do you lose your *temper easily* and *often*?
5. Are you troubled by *regular* insomnia?
6. Do you have wide fluctuations in your moods from depression to elation, back to depression, which *incapacitate* you?
7. Do you *continually* dislike to be with people?
8. Are you *upset* if the routine of your life is disturbed?
9. Do your children *consistently* get on your nerves ?
10. Are you "browned off" and *constantly* bitter?
11. Are you afraid *without* real cause?
12. Are you *always* right and the other person *always* wrong?
13. Do you have numerous aches and pains for which no doctor can find a physical cause?

The conditions chartered in these questions are the major warning signals of poor mental health in one degree or another. According to Dr. Menninger, help is necessary if the answer to any of these questions is definitely "yes".

Types of mental illness

Mental and behavioural disorders are understood as clinically significant conditions characterized by alteration in thinking, mood (emotions) or behaviour associated with personal distress and/or impaired functioning. Any classification of mental disorder classifies syndromes and conditions. Individuals may suffer from one or more disorders during one or more periods of their life. One incidence of abnormal behaviour or a short period of abnormal mood does not of itself, signify the presence of a mental or behavioural disorder.

The International Classification of Diseases (ICD–10) classifies the mental and behavioural disorders as *(5)*:

- *Organic, including symptomatic, mental disorders* – e.g., dementia in Alzheimer's disease, delirium.
- *Mental and behavioural disorders due to psychoactive substance use* – e.g., harmful use of alcohol, opioid dependence syndrome.
- *Schizophrenia, schizotypal and delusional disorders* – e.g., paranoid schizophrenia, delusional disorders, acute and transient psychotic disorders.
- *Mood (affective) disorders* – e.g., bipolar affective disorder, depressive episode.
- *Neurotic, stress-related and somatoform disorders* – e.g., generalized anxiety disorders, obsessive-compulsive disorders.

- *Behavioural syndromes associated with physiological disturbances and physical factors* – e.g., eating disorders, non-organic sleep disorders.
- *Disorders of adult personality and behaviour* – e.g., paranoid personality disorder, trans-sexualism.
- *Mental retardation.*
- *Disorders of psychological development* – e.g., specific reading disorders, childhood autism.
- *Behavioural and emotional disorders with onset usually occurring in childhood and adolescence* – e.g., hyperkinetic disorders, conduct disorders, tic disorders.
- *Unspecified mental disorder.*

Mental illness is a vast subject, broad in its limits and difficult to define precisely. There are major and minor illnesses. The major illnesses are called *psychoses*. Here, the person is "insane" and out of touch with reality. There are three major illnesses: (1) SCHIZOPHRENIA (split personality) in which the patient lives in a dream world of his own. (2) MANIC DEPRESSIVE PSYCHOSIS in which the symptoms vary from heights of excitement to depths of depression, and (3) PARANOIA which is associated with undue and extreme suspicion and a progressive tendency to regard the whole world in a framework of delusions. The minor illnesses are of two groups: (a) NEUROSIS OR PSYCHONEUROSIS: In this the patient is unable to react normally to life situations. He is not considered "insane" by his associates, but nevertheless exhibits certain peculiar symptoms such as morbid fears, compulsions and obsessions, (b) PERSONALITY AND CHARACTER DISORDERS: This group of disorders are the legacy of unfortunate childhood experiences and perceptions.

Causes of mental ill-health

Mental illness like physical illness is due to multiple causes. There are many known factors of agent, host and environment in the natural histories of mental disorders. Among the known factors are the following: (1) ORGANIC CONDITIONS: Mental illnesses may have their origin in organic conditions such as cerebral arteriosclerosis, neoplasms, metabolic diseases, neurological diseases, endocrine diseases and chronic diseases such as tuberculosis, leprosy, epilepsy, etc. (2) HEREDITY: Heredity may be an important factor in some cases. For example, the child of two schizophrenic parents is 40 times more likely to develop schizophrenia than is the child of healthy parents. (3) SOCIAL PATHOLOGICAL CAUSES: To produce any disease, there must be a combination of genetic and environmental factors. The social and environmental factors associated with mental illhealth comprise : worries, anxieties, emotional stress, tension, frustration, unhappy marriages, broken homes, poverty, industrialization, urbanization, changing family structure, population mobility, economic insecurity, cruelty, rejection, neglect and the like. The social environment not only determines the individual's attitudes but also provides the "framework" within which mental health is formulated.

Environmental factors other than psychosocial ones capable of producing abnormal human behaviour are: (1) *Toxic substances* – carbon disulfide, mercury, manganese, tin, lead compounds, etc. (2) *Psychotropic drugs* – barbiturates, alcohol, griseofulvin. (3) *Nutritional factors* – deficiency of thiamine, pyridoxine. (4) *Minerals* – deficiency of iodine. (5) *Infective agents* – infectious disease (e.g., measles, rubella) during the prenatal, perinatal and post-natal periods of life may have adverse effects on the brain's development and the integration of mental functions. (6) *Traumatic factors* – road and occupational accidents and (7) *Radiation* – nervous system is most sensitive to radiation during the period of neural development.

Crucial points in the lifecycle of human beings

There are certain key points in the development of the human being which are important from the point of view of mental health. These are : (1) *Prenatal period :* Pregnancy is a stressful period for some women. They need help not only for their physical but also emotional needs. (2) *First 5 years of life*: The roots of mental health are in early childhood. The infant and young child should experience a warm, intimate and continuous relationship with his mother and father. It is in this relationship where underlies the development of mental health. It follows that broken homes are likely to produce behaviour disorders in children and this has been confirmed by several studies. (3) *School child :* Everything that happens in the school affects the mental health of the child. The programmes and practices of the school may satisfy or frustrate the emotional needs of the child. Children who have emotional problems may need child guidance clinic or psychiatric services. From the standpoint of the child's mental health and his effectiveness in learning, proper teacher-pupil relationship and climate of the class room are very important. (4) *Adolescence :* The transition from adolescence to manhood is often a stormy one and fraught with dangers to mental health, manifested in the form of mental illhealth among the young, and juvenile delinquents in particular. The basic needs of the adolescents are: (a) the need to be needed by others, (b) the need for increasing independence, (c) the need to achieve adequate adjustment to the opposite sex and (d) the need to rethink the cherished beliefs of one's elders. The failure to recognize and understand these basic needs may prevent sound mental development. (5) *Old age :* The mental health problems of the aged have received considerable attention in recent times in the developed countries. The causes of mental illness in the aged are organic conditions of the brain, economic insecurity, lack of a home, poor status and insecurity.

Thus throughout his life, the needs of man remain the same (1) the need for affection, (2) the need for belonging, (3) the need for independence, (4) the need for achievement, (5) the need for recognition or approval, (6) the need for a sense of personal worth and (7) the need for self-actualization. These needs only differ in degree and qualitative importance at various ages.

Mental disorders often affect, and are affected by, other diseases such as cancer, cardiovascular disease and HIV infection/AIDS, and as such require common services and resource mobilization efforts. For example, there is evidence that depression predisposes people to myocardial infarction and diabetes, both of which conversely increase the likelihood of depression. Many risk factors such as low socioeconomic status, alcohol use and stress are common to both mental disorders and other non-communicable diseases. There is also substantial concurrence of mental disorders and substance use disorders. Taken together, mental, neurological and substance use disorders exact a high toll, accounting for 13% of the total global burden of disease. Depression alone accounts for 4.3% of the global burden of disease and is among the largest single causes of disability worldwide (11% of all years lived with disability globally), particularly for women. The economic consequences of these health losses are equally large: a recent study estimated that the cumulative global impact of mental disorders in terms of lost economic output will amount to US$ 16.3 trillion between 2011 and 2030.

Mental disorders frequently lead individuals and families into poverty. Homelessness and inappropriate incarceration are far more common for people with mental disorders than for the general population, and exacerbate their marginalization and vulnerability. Because of stigmatization and discrimination, persons with mental disorders often have their human rights violated and many are denied economic, social and cultural rights, with restriction on the right to work and education, as well as reproductive rights and the right to the highest attainable standard of health. They may also be subject to unhygienic and inhuman living conditions, physical and sexual abuse, neglect, and harmful and degrading treatment practices in health facilities. They are often denied civil and political rights such as right to marry and found a family, personal liberty, the right to vote and to participate effectively and fully in public life, and the right to exercise their legal capacity on other issue affecting them, including their treatment and care. As such persons with mental disorders often live in vulnerable situations and may be excluded and marginalized from society, which constitutes a significant impediment to the achievement of national and international development goals. The convention on the rights of persons with disabilities, which is binding on States Parties that have ratified or acceded to it, protects and promotes the rights of all persons with disabilities, including persons with mental and intellectual impairments, and also promotes their full inclusion in international cooperation including international development programmes.

Mental health services

Mental health services in a community are concerned not only with early diagnosis and treatment, but also with the preservation and promotion of good mental health and prevention of mental illness. The mental health services comprise:

(1) Early diagnosis and treatment;
(2) Rehabilitation;
(3) Group and individual psychotherapy;
(4) Mental health education;
(5) Use of modern psychoactive drugs; and
(6) After-care services.

Comprehensive mental health programme

Since 95 per cent of psychiatric cases can be treated with or without hospitalization close to their homes, the current trend is full integration of psychiatric services with other health services. The Community Mental Health Programme includes all community facilities pertinent in any way to prevention, treatment and rehabilitation. The philosophy of Community Mental Health Programme consists of the following essential elements : (1) In-patient services (2) Out-patient services (3) Partial hospitalization (4) Emergency services (5) Diagnostic services (6) Pre-care and aftercare services including foster home placement and home visiting (7) Education services (8) Training, and (9) Research and evaluation.

ALCOHOLISM AND DRUG DEPENDENCE

Definition

The word "drug" is defined as "any substance that, when taken into the living organism, may modify one or more of its functions" (WHO). "Drug abuse" is defined as self-administration of a drug for non-medical reasons, in quantities and frequencies which may impair an individual's ability to function effectively, and which may result in social, physical, or emotional harm. "Drug dependence" is described as "a state, psychic and sometimes also physical, resulting from the interaction between a living organism and a drug, characterized by behavioural and other responses that always include a compulsion to take the drug on a continuous or periodic basis in order to experience its psychic effects, and sometimes to avoid the discomfort of its absence. A person may be dependent upon more than one drug *(6)*.

Agent factors

Dependence-producing drug

A dependence-producing drug is one that has the capacity to produce dependence, as described above. The specific characteristics of dependence varies with the type of drug involved. ICD–10 recognizes the following psychoactive drugs, or drug classes, the self administration of which may produce mental and behavioural disorders, including dependence :

1. Alcohol
2. Opioids
3. Cannabinoids
4. Sedatives or hypnotics
5. Cocain
6. Other stimulants including caffeine
7. Hallucinogens
8. Tobacco
9. Volatile solvents
10. Other psychoactive substances, and drugs from different classes used in combination.

Although the dependence-producing properties and public health problems caused by tobacco were recognized since long, its acute effects on behaviour were minimal. The WHO Expert Committee on drug dependence at its meeting in Sept. 1992 felt that tobacco and other forms of nicotine use warranted their inclusion in the report. Furthermore, it recommended that WHO should consider expanding the Committee's term of reference to include substances such as anabolic steroids, which are used because of their performance-enhancing effects. Anabolic steroids are being abused by people who wish to increase muscle mass for cosmetic reasons or for greater strength. In addition to the medical problems, the practice is associated with significant mood swings, aggressiveness, and paranoid delusions. Alcohol and stimulant use is higher in these individuals. Withdrawal symptoms of steroid dependency include fatigue, depressed mood, restlessness, and insomnia *(7)*. This form of use is described in ICD–10 under the category F-55, "Abuse of non-dependence-producing substances". The development of other performance enhancing drugs may present new types of drug use problems in the future.

The drugs which are in common use today are *(8,9)* :

(1) AMPHETAMINES AND COCAINE : Amphetamines are synthetic drugs, structurally similar to adrenaline. In

medical practice, they are used to treat obesity, mild depression, narcolepsy and certain behaviour disorders in children. The ordinary therapeutic dose is 10–30 mg a day. There are various brands of amphetamines: the common names are Benzedrine, Dexedrine, Methedrine, etc. These drugs act on the central nervous system. They produce mood elevation, elation, a feeling of well-being and increased alertness and a sense of heightened awareness. Because they give a tremendous boost to self-confidence and energy, while increasing endurance, they are called "superman" drugs. The use of these drugs results in psychic dependence. With large doses, such dependence, is often rapid and strong.

Cocaine is derived from the leaves of the coca plant. It was formerly used in medical practice as a potent local anaesthetic. Cocaine is a central nervous stimulant. It produces a sense of excitement, heightened and distorted awareness and hallucinations. Unlike amphetamines, it produces no tolerance. There is a 'no physical dependence; no withdrawal symptoms', *per se*. The chewing of coca leaves is a very common practice in Bolivia and Peru in South America.

(2) BARBITURATES: If amphetamines stimulate, barbiturates sedate. They are a major ingradient in sleeping pills. The drug-users generally prefer short-acting barbiturates such as pentobarbital and secobarbital to long acting ones. The addiction to barbiturates is one of the worst forms of suffering. It leads to craving, or both physical and psychic dependence.

(3) CANNABIS: Perhaps, the most widely used drug today is *Cannabis*, which is a very ancient drug obtained from the hemp plants – *Cannabis sativa, C.indica and C. americana.* The resinous exudate from the flowering tops of the female plant contains most of the active ingradients – called *hashish or charas.* The dried leaves and flowering shoots are called *bhang;* the resinous mass from the small leaves and brackets of inflorescence is called *ganja*. In USA, the term *marijuana* is used to refer to any part of the plant which induces somatic and psychic changes in man.

Most commonly the plant is cut, dried, chopped and incorporated into cigarettes. It is also taken with drinks or incorporated in foods like sweets and cakes. A marijuana cigarette will produce intoxication within minutes and lasts from 1 to 4 hours. The oral consumption results in a delayed onset of action and a prolonged effect lasting many hours.

The most common reaction is the development of a dreamy state of altered consciousness. Relaxation, euphoria, and an increased tendency to laugh, greater awareness of colours and sounds, interference with perception of both time and space, and paranoia are among the psychological effects reported by marijuana users. Human death appears to be a rare phenomenon. There is a psychic dependence.

(4) HEROIN: Heroin, morphine, codein, methadone, pethidine are narcotic analgesics. Addiction to heroin is perhaps the worst type of addiction because it produces craving. With narcotics generally psychic dependence is strong and tends to develop early. Tolerance to narcotics also occurs rapidly, making it necessary to take increasing doses of the drug to achieve the same effect.

(5) LSD: Lysergic acid diethylamide (LSD) was synthesized in 1938 by Hoffmann in the Sandoz Laboratories in Switzerland. Its psychic properties were noticed much later in 1943, when he accidentally sniffed a few micrograms of it.

LSD is a potent psychotogenic agent. Although amounts as low as 20–25 µg may produce subjective disturbances, oral doses in the range of 100–250 µg are usually required to effect intense depersonalization. The lethal dose in man is not known.

LSD alters the normal structuring of perception. The individual perceives the world in a different manner. There is intensification of colour perception and auditory acuity; body image distortions, visual illusions, fantasies pseudohallucinations are common. Colours are heard and music becomes palpable. Subjective time is deranged so that seconds seem to be minutes and minutes pass as slowly as hours.

Physical dependence does not develop with LSD; hence there is no addiction liability. No characteristic abstinence syndrome is manifest upon abrupt discontinuation of chronic use of the drug.

(6) ALCOHOL: By pharmacological definition, alcohol is a drug and may be classified as a sedative, tranquillizer, hypnotic or anaesthetic, depending upon the quantity consumed. Of all the drugs, alcohol is the only drug whose self-induced intoxication is socially acceptable.

Alcohol is rapidly absorbed from the stomach and small intestine. Within 2–3 minutes of consumption, it can be detected in the blood – the maximum concentration is usually reached about one hour after consumption. The presence of food in the stomach inhibits the absorption of alcohol because of dilution.

Over the past 30–40 years, increasing percentages of young people have started to drink alcoholic beverages, their alcohol consumption has increased in quantity and frequency, and the age at which drinking starts has declined *(8)*. This situation is disturbing because the young people concerned may run a greater risk of alcoholic problems in later life and also, in the short term, because of increased rates of drunkenness and involvement in road accidents.

In 2016, the harmful use of alcohol resulted in some 3 million deaths worldwide and 132.6 million DALYs - i.e. 5.1 % of all DALYs in that year. Mortality resulting from alcohol consumption is higher than that caused by diseases such as TB, HIV/AIDS and diabetes. Among men, in 2016, an estimated 2.3 million deaths and 106.5 million DALYs were attributable to the consumption of alcohol. Women experienced 0.7 million deaths and 26.1 million DALYs attributable to alcohol. In 2016, of all deaths attributable to alcohol consumption worldwide, 28.7 per cent were due to injuries, 21.3 per cent due to digestive disease, 19 per cent due to cardiovascular diseases, 12.9 per cent due to infectious diseases and 12.6 per cent due to cancers. About 49 per cent of alcohol attributable DALYs are due to non-communicable diseases and mental health conditions, and about 40 per cent due to injuries *(10)*. Numerically, harmful use of alcohol caused 1.7 million deaths from non-communicable diseases in 2016, including some 1.2 million deaths from digestive and cardiovascular diseases and 0.4 million deaths from cancers. Globally, an estimated 0.9 million injury deaths were attributable to alcohol, including around 370,000 deaths due to road injuries, 150,000 due to self-harm and around 90,000 due to interpersonal violence *(10)*.

Globally in 2016, there were about 2.3 billion current drinkers. Alcohol is consumed by more than half of the population in only three WHO regions - The Americas, Europe and Western Pacific. Total alcohol per capita consumption in the world's population over 15 years of age rose from 5.5 liters of pure alcohol in 2005 to 6.4 liters in

2016. The highest levels of per capita alcohol consumption are observed in countries of European region. Globally, 44.8 per cent of total alcohol is consumed in the form of spirits. The second most consumed type of beverage is beer (34.3 per cent) followed by wine (11.7 per cent). Worldwide there have been only minor changes in beverage preferences since 2010 *(10)*. Prevalence of heavy episodic drinking, defined as 60 or more grams of pure alcohol on at least one occasion at least once per month, has decreased globally from 22.6 per cent in 2000 to 18.2 per cent in 2016 *(10)*. Prevalence of heavy episodic drinkers is lower among adolescents (15–19 years) than in the total population but it increases and peaks at 20–24 years when it becomes higher than total population.

Alcohol policy development and implementation have improved globally but are still far from accomplishing effective protection of populations from alcohol-related harm.

The mortality data is as follows:

Cause	ASDR*		AAF %		AAD **
	Male	Female	Male	Female	(number)
Liver cirrhosis	45.8	14.7	60.0	33.3	140632
Road traffic injuries	5.3	10.3	33.7	18.3	92878
Cancer	107.2	95.3	6.5	0.8	30958

* ASDR : Age standardized death rate per 100,000 population (15+)
** AAD : Alcohol-attributable deaths, both sexes
AAF : Alcohol-attributable fractions

While alcohol is used traditionally by men, its use by women is now on the increase. The proportion of dependent users is large. Issues of concern include pay-day drinking, violence including domestic violence, alcohol's contribution to poverty, illicit and home-brewed alcohol, and reduction in average age of initiation. Alcohol use is considered a risk factor for high risk sexual behaviour leading to sexually transmitted diseases including HIV/AIDS.

Alcohol has a marked effect on the central nervous system. It is not a "stimulant" as long believed, but a primary and continuous depressant. Alcohol produces psychic dependence of varying degrees from mild to strong. Physical dependence develops slowly.

According to current concepts, alcoholism is considered a disease and alcohol a "disease agent" which causes acute and chronic intoxication, cirrhosis of the liver, toxic psychosis, gastritis, pancreatitis, cardiomyopathy and peripheral neuropathy. Also, evidence is mounting that it is related to cancer of the mouth, pharynx, larynx and oesophagus. Further, alcohol is an important aetiologic factor in suicide, automobile and other accidents, and injuries and deaths due to violence. The health problems for which alcohol is responsible are only part of the total social damage which includes family disorganization, crime and loss of productivity.

The health, safety and socio-economic problems attributable to alcohol can be effectively reduced and requires actions on the levels, patterns and contexts of alcohol consumption and the wider social determinants of health.

Countries have a responsibility for formulating, implementing, monitoring and evaluating public policies to reduce the harmful use of alcohol. Substantial scientific knowledge exists for policy-makers on the effectiveness and cost-effectiveness of the following strategies *(11)*:

- Regulating the marketing of alcoholic beverages (in particular to younger people);
- Regulating and restricting the availability of alcohol;
- Enacting appropriate drink-driving policies;
- Reducing demand through taxation and pricing mechanisms;
- Raising awareness of public health problems caused by harmful use of alcohol and ensuring support for effective alcohol policies;
- Providing accessible and affordable treatment for people with alcohol-use disorders; and
- Implementing screening and brief intervention programmes for hazardous and harmful drinking in health services.

(7) TOBACCO : Tobacco is in legal use everywhere in the world. Yet it causes far more deaths than all other psychoactive sustances combined. About 7 million premature deaths a year are already attributed to tobacco smoking. More than 6 million of those deaths are the result of direct tobacco use while around 890,000 are the result of non-smokers being exposed to second-hand smoke. Around 80 per cent of the world's 1.1 billion smokers live in low-middle-income countries where burden of tobacco-related illness and death is heaviest. Tobacco epidemic is one of the biggest public health threats the world has ever faced *(12)*.

More people die from tobacco related diseases other than cancer such as stroke, myocardial infarction, aortic aneurysm and peptic ulcer. Young people who take up smoking have been shown to experience an early onset of cough, phlegm production, and shortness of breath on exertion. There is evidence that the earlier a person begins to smoke, the greater is the risk of life-threatening diseases such as chronic bronchitis, emphysema, cardiovascular disease, and lung cancer. Experimentation with smoking as a symbol of "adult" behaviour is common in adolescence. It is suggested that three factors are associated with young people smoking : peer pressure, following the example of siblings and parents, and employment outside the home. If a child's older sibling and both parents smoke, the child is four times as likely to smoke as one with no smoking model in the family *(8)*.

Women who smoke run even more risks than men. For example, the adverse effects of oral contraceptive use are markedly increased in women smokers. Osteoporosis is accelerated with tobacco use. Some evidence indicates that fertility is impaired with smoking. Tobacco use is also associated with a higher rate of spontaneous miscarriages. In pregnancy, smoking contributes to perinatal complications such as bleeding, which is dangerous for both mother and fetus, especially in low income countries where health facilities are inadequate. Intrauterine growth retardation and low-birth-weight babies are known outcomes of smoking during pregnancy *(13)*. The babies of mothers who smoke may weigh, on an average, 200 grams less at birth than those of non-smokers *(9)*. The harm from maternal smoking can extend beyond pregnancy, affecting the child's growth and development. This is often compounded by the child's exposure to second-hand smoke from parents and other adults.

Passive smoking

Second-hand tobacco smoke is the combination of smoke emitted from the burning end of a cigarette or other tobacco products and smoke exhaled by the smoker.

Smoking harms non-smokers too. The first conclusive evidence of the danger of passive smoking came from a study carried out by Takeshi Hirayama, in 1981, on lung cancer in non-smoking Japanese wives married to men who smoked. Surprising at the time, those women showed a significantly increased risk of dying from lung cancer, despite never having smoked a cigarette. Hirayama believed that passive smoking (i.e. breathing in the smoke from their husbands) caused these women's excess cancer risk. About 40 further studies have confirmed this link.

Today, research indicates that passive smoking can also give rise to other potentially fatal diseases such as heart disease and stroke, and new scientific evidence on the adverse effects of second-hand smoke continues to accumulate *(13)*.

Per capita consumption of tobacco is decreasing slowly in developed countries. By contrast, per capita tobacco consumption is rising in many developing countries among both men and women. Because of the long delay between the cause and full effect, people tend to misjudge the hazards of tobacco. When a generation of young adults begin to smoke, they do not witness the high morbidity and mortality associated with their behaviour until they reach middle age. The best documented example of this delay is that of men in the USA, among whom the main increase in smoking took place before 1945. In 1945 smoking was common but lung cancer was rare as in developing countries today. Over the next forty years (1945–1985) the smoking habit did not change greatly, but lung cancer in this population rose sharply – about twenty fold, whereas non-smokers lung cancer remained approximately constant at a low level during 1945–1985. About half of those killed by tobacco were still in middle age (35–69) and thereby lost almost twenty-five years of non-smoker life expectancy *(9)*.

The age standardized prevalence of tobacco smoking has decreased steadily since the beginning of the twenty-first century. WHO estimates that 20.2 per cent of the world's population aged ≥ 15 years were currently smoking in 2015, indicating that smoking rates have decreased by 6.7 per cent globally since year 2000 and by 4.1 per cent since the WHO frame work Convention on Tobacco Control (FCTC) came into force in the year 2005 *(14)*.

WHO estimates that worldwide, there are at least 367 million smokeless tobacco users aged ≥ 15 years. More males used smokeless tobacco products (237 million) than females (129 million). Although smokeless tobacco is used in all regions, the SEAR has by far the largest number of users (301 million) representing 82 per cent of all users globally. Every WHO region has atleast 8 million smokeless users, although 86 per cent live in lower middle-income countries *(15)*.

INDIA : The Global Adult Tobacco Survey GATS-2 was done in the year 2016–17. The key findings of the survey are : Prevalence of tobacco use has decreased by six percentage points from 34.6 per cent in GATS-1 in 2009–10, to 28.6 per cent in 2016–17; 19.0 per cent of men, 2.0 per cent of women and 10.7 per cent of all adults currently smoke tobacco; 42.4 per cent of men, 14.2 per cent of women and 28.6 per cent of all adults currently either smoke tobacco and/or use smokeless tobacco; khaini and bidi are the most commonly used tobacco products; 49 per cent of smokers and 32 per cent of smokeless tobacco users were advised by health care providers to quit tobacco; three in every 10 adults who work indoors were exposed to second-hand smoke at their work-place; 62 per cent of cigarette smokers and 54 per cent of bidi smokers thought of quitting smoking because of warning lable on the packets; and 92 per cent of adults believe that smoking causes serious illness and 96 per cent of adults believe that use of smokeless tobacco causes serious illness *(16)*.

A variety of smokeless tobacco products are consumed in South East Asia Region. Pan masala, gutkha (industrially manufactured chewing tobacco product), khaini (chewing of dry tobacco leaves and lime), and chewing tobacco with areca nuts are common in India, Bangladesh, Bhutan, Nepal and Myanmar. Smokeless tobacco use is more prevalent among men than among women in these countries excepting in Bangladesh, where smokeless tobacco use is more prevalent among women *(15)*.

The adverse health effects of smoking are as shown in Table 1.

The withdrawal symptoms include irritability, anxiety, craving, sleep problems, headache, tremors, and lethargy. Withdrawal symptoms may continue for 4–6 weeks, and craving may continue for many months.

(8) VOLATILE SOLVENTS : In a number of countries, the sniffing of substances such as glue, petrol, diethyl ether, chloroform, nitrous oxide, paint thinner, cleaning fluids, typewriter correction fluid etc., is causing increasing concern, as it can result in death, even on the first occasion. These substances are central nervous system depressants and produce effects comparable to those produced by alcohol. There may be initial euphoria and exhilaration, followed by confusion, disorientation and ataxia. Some of the substances like petrol and toluene may also produce marked euphoria, grandiosity, recklessness, delusions and hallucinations and a substantial loss of self-control. With increasing doses, there may be convulsions, coma and death. In chronic abusers damage to the brain, peripheral nervous system, kidney, liver, heart or bone marrow may occur *(8)*. Lead encephalopathy can be associated with sniffing lead gasoline.

(9) CAFFEINE : Caffeine is one of the most commonly used drug worldwide. About 10 billion pounds of coffee are consumed yearly throughout the world. Tea, cocoa, and cola drinks also contribute to an intake of caffeine that is often very high in a large number of people. The approximate content of caffeine in a cup (180 ml) of beverage is as follows : brewed coffee 80–140 mg; instant coffee 60–100 mg; decaffeinated coffee 1–6 mg; black leaf tea 30–80 mg; tea bags 25–75 mg; instant tea 30–60 mg; cocoa 10–50 mg; and 12 oz cola drinks 30–65 mg. Symptoms of caffeinism (usually associated with ingestion of over 500 mg/day) include anxiety, agitation, restlessness, insomnia and somatic symptoms referable to the heart and gastrointestinal tract. Withdrawal from caffeine can produce headache, irritability, lethargy, and occasional nausea *(7)*.

Host factors

Many attempts have been made to define the host factors. Studies employing questionnaires or structured interviews report motives for drug dependence with descriptive words such as pleasure, desire to experiment, sense of adventure, wish for self-knowledge, and desire to escape. Increasingly, people are unwilling to accept even minor discomforts and are looking to drugs for solutions. Many of them have shown symptoms of social and psychological maladjustment resulting from personal handicaps of all sorts.

TABLE 1

Adverse health effects of smoking

Body system or organ	Established or suspected adverse health effect of cigarette smoking	Body system or organ	Established or suspected adverse health effect of cigarette smoking
Lungs	– Lung cancer – Chronic obstructive pulmonary disease – Increased severity of asthma – Increased risk of developing various respiratory infections	*Bones*	– Disc degeneration – Osteoporosis – Osteoarthritis – Less successful back surgery – Delayed fracture healing – Musculoskeletal injury
Heart	– Coronary heart disease – Angina pectoris – Heart attack – Increased risk of repeat heart attack – Arrhythmia – Aortic aneurysm – Cardiomyopathy	*Reproduction*	– Infertility – Impotence – Decreased sperm motility and density – Miscarriage – Earlier menopause
Blood vessels	– Peripheral vascular disease – Thromboangiitis obliterans (Buerger's disease)	*The unborn child*	– Fetal growth retardation – Prematurity – Stillbirth – Enhanced transmission of HIV to fetus – Birth defects – Intellectual impairment – Sudden infant death syndrome
Skin	– Earlier wrinkling – Fingernail discoloration – Psoriasis – Palmoplantar pustulosis	*Brain*	– Transient ischaemic attack – Stroke – Worsened multiple sclerosis
Cancer	– Lung cancer – Esophageal cancer – Laryngeal cancer – Oral cancer – Bladder cancer – Kidney cancer – Stomach cancer – Pancreatic cancer – Vulvular cancer – Cervical cancer – Colorectal cancer	*Others*	– Cataract – Macular degeneration – Snoring – Periodontal disease – Stomach and duodenal ulcers – Crohn's disease – Impaired immunity

Source : *(13)*

The average age of drug users has decreased considerably in recent years. Multiple drug-use has also become more common. Concern over drug-use by teenagers increased in the late 1960s, particularly in the developed countries. In countries with long experience of heavy drug use, there is a tendency to prefer a single drug, perhaps because a continuous supply is less problematic. Multiple drug use may be more common where drug abuse is a relatively recent occurrence.

Symptoms of drug addiction

1. Loss of interest in sports and daily routine ;
2. Loss of appetite and body weight ;
3. Unsteady gait, clumpsy movements, tremors ;
4. Reddening and puffiness of eyes, unclear vision ;
5. Slurring of speech ;
6. Fresh, numerous injection marks on body and blood stains on clothes ;
7. Nausea, vomiting and body pain ;
8. Drowsiness or sleeplessness, lethargy and passivity ;
9. Acute anxiety, depression, profuse sweating ;
10. Changing mood, temper, tantrums ;
11. Depersonalization and emotional detachment ;
12. Impaired memory and concentration; and
13. Presence of needles, syringes and strange packets at home.

Environmental factors

Among the environmental factors attributed to drug dependence are rapid technological developments with associated need for extended periods of education, along with the in-applicability of old solutions to novel problems. Television, world travel, affluence, freedom to speculate and experiment have encouraged youngsters to question and often reject the values and goals of their parents. Established social values are perceived as irrelevant, all to be stripped away, partly through the use of drugs in order to reveal the real person, the real humanity, and the real goals of mankind. Studies confirm that those who take drugs usually form part of a small antisocial and often criminal subculture.

The problem exists in virtually all societies and socio-economic groups. Some of the social and environmental factors associated with a high risk for drug abuse are listed in Table 2.

TABLE 2
Factors associated with a high risk for drug abuse

– unemployment	– certain occupations (tourism, drug production or sale)
– living away from home	– areas with high rates of crime or vice
– migration to cities	– areas where there are drug - using gangs
– relaxed parental control	– areas where delinquency is common
– alienation from family	
– early exposure to drugs	
– leaving school early	
– broken homes; one parent families	
– large urban environments	
– areas where drugs are sold, traded, or produced	

Source : *(8)*

Magnitude of substance abuse in India *(18)*

A National Survey was conducted between December 2017 and October 2018. The primary objective of the survey was to assess the extent and pattern of substance use in each state/UT. The key findings of the use of psychoactive substances in India is as follows *(18)*.

1. *Alcohol* : Alcohol is the most common psychoactive substance used by Indians. Nationally, about 14.6 per cent of the population between 10 and 75 years of age uses alcohol. In terms of absolute numbers, about 16 crore persons consume alcohol in India. It is considerably higher in men (27.3 per cent) than women (1.6 per cent). Among alcohol users, country liquor or desi sharab (about 30 per cent) and spirit or Indian made foreign liquor (about 30 per cent) are predominantly consumed beverages. Of the 14.6 per cent (16 crore) users, 5.7 crore (5.2 per cent) are problem users and 2.9 crore (2.7 per cent) are dependent users.
2. *Cannabis* : Cannabis are the next commonly used substance. About 2.8 per cent of the population (3.1 crore individuals) report having used any cannabis product within the previous year. The legal form (bhang) was used by 2.2 crore (2 per cent) and 1.3 crore (1.2 per cent) persons used illegal form (ganja and charas). Out of 3.1 crore cannabis users, about 72 lakhs are problem users and 25 lakhs are dependent users. The highest use of cannabis was recorded in Uttar Pradesh, Punjab, Sikkim, Chhattisgarh and Delhi.
3. *Opioid* : About 2.1 per cent (2.3 crore) population in India use opioids which includes opium or its variants like poppy husk known as doda/phukki, heroin or its impure form – smack or brown sugar and a variety of pharmaceutical opioids. Out of 2.3 crore users, about 77 lakh are problem users (opium 11 lakhs, heroin 63 lakhs and pharma opioid 25 lakhs), and 28 lakhs are dependent users.
4. A sizeable number of people use other drugs like sedatives and inhalants. In the general population, about 0.2 per cent of Indians need help for their sedative use problems. At the national level, an estimated 4.6 lakhs children and 18 lakhs adults need help for their inhalant use (harmful use/dependence). In terms of absolute numbers, states with high population of children needing help for inhalant use are : Uttar Pradesh, Madhya Pradesh, Maharashtra, Delhi and Haryana. The number of people dependent on cocaine, ATS and Hallucinogens is extremely small in comparison to the size of country's population.
5. Nationally, it is estimated that there are about 8.5 lakh people who inject drugs (PWID). Opioid group of drugs are predominantly injected by PWID (heroin – 46 per cent and pharmaceutical opioids – 46 per cent). A substantial proportion of PWID report risky injecting practices. High numbers of PWID are estimated in Uttar Pradesh, Punjab, Delhi, Andhra Pradesh, Telangana, Haryana, Karnataka, Maharashtra, Manipur and Nagaland.

Prevention

Approaches to prevention of drug dependence should have realistic aims. Over-ambitious hopes of *eradicating* a drug problem in a short time are likely to lead to policies that are unrealistic and self-discrediting. Changes in culture attitudes and alteration in relevant aspects of the environment can be brought about only slowly.

Legal approach : The legal control on the distribution of drugs, when effectively applied has been and remains an important approach in the prevention of drug abuse. Controls may be designed to impose partial restriction or to make a drug completely unavailable. Legislation may be directed at controlling the manufacture, distribution, prescription, price, time of sale, or consumption of a substance.

Legislation restricting or prohibiting advertisements that directly or indirectly promote use of tobacco and alcohol has been increasingly common in recent years. The anti-smoking measures suggested are : (a) prohibition of the sale of tobacco products to minors; (b) restriction on the sale of cigarettes from automatic vending machines; (c) prohibition of smoking in schools and other places frequented by young people; (d) prohibition of smoking in public; (e) prohibition of cigarette advertising at times, and in places and ways, calculated to ensure its maximum impact on adolescents; (f) establishment of mandatory public health education on health consequences of smoking; (g) insisting on the placing of mandatory health warning on cigarette packets.

The minimum age at which minors may legally have access to alcoholic beverages, has been raised in some countries. There is also legislation controlling the distribution of alcohol in some countries. Mandatory jail sentences for drunken driving have not been very effective.

Educational approach : Educational approaches to the prevention of drug use and drug-related problems have been used in many countries. Common approaches have included educational programmes for school children and public information campaigns on electronic media. General principles of communication can be applied to increase the effectiveness of educational approach. The message should be clear and unambiguous to the intended audience, and come from credible source of information. The message should also provide specific advice, rather than general, and as far as possible the information should be new to the audience and should be capable of provoking discussion or action. Educational approach should not be planned and carried out as isolated activity. To be effective, such approaches should be regarded as a part of integrated plan of action involving other strategies.

Community approach : The non-medical use of the drugs individually as well as in its mass appearance involves a complex interaction of drug, man, and his environment, including social, economic, cultural, political and other elements of varying character and strength. The rapid changes taking place at the present time in relations between individuals, groups and nations are also reflected in a rapidly changing pattern of drug abuse in many parts of the world. There should be a strong emphasis on action at the community level to prevent drug abuse. Initiating preventive interventions in the community brings preventive action to the level of people's every day lives and actions, and contributes to emphasis on strengthening primary health care. Action at the community level is also important since communities often bear the main burden of dealing with the harmful use of drugs and drug related problems.

A popular approach to the prevention of drug abuse is provision of alternative activities which may help to prevent drug abuse – e.g., *teen centres* providing activities attractive to the adolescents who might otherwise drift in to drug taking subculture. Such activities include the establishment of groups or organizations interested in athletics, sports, music, public policy, religion, artistic activities of various kinds, and improvement of the environment through the prevention of pollution. Non-governmental organizations play a crucial role in the development of such activities and are likely to become important.

Treatment

Treatment cannot take place unless the individual attends for treatment. He must come to terms with the possibility of a life without drug taking. Unfortunately, drug takers, as a rule, have little or no motivation to undergo treatment. Alcoholics tend to deny that their consumption is abnormal; others openly defend their habits. Long term treatment is not only a medical problem, but needs the cooperation of psychologists and sociologists. There is a high relapse rate with all treatment methods *(9)*.

Though drug addiction may be considered as a social problem, the first step in its management is medical care, which includes :

- identification of drug addicts and their motivation for detoxication
- detoxication (requires hospitalization)
- post-detoxication counselling and follow-up (based on clinic and home visits), and
- rehabilitation.

Simultaneously with medical treatment, changes in environment (home, school, college, social circles) are important. The patient must effect a complete break with his group, otherwise the chances of relapse are 100 per cent. Psychotherapy has a valuable place in the management of the addict.

Rehabilitation *(6)*

The rehabilitation of former drug user, regardless of age, is in most cases a long and difficult process. Relapses are very frequent. Success of the treatment necessitates the adoption of mature and realistic attitude by the local community and the avoidance of panic, moral condemnation and discrimination. Facilities for vocational training and sometimes the provision of sheltered work opportunities are useful in rehabilitation and help to prevent relapse. Generally speaking, facilities for the registration, diagnosis, treatment, after-care, etc., of drug-dependent individuals and groups should be regarded as indispensable integrated parts of the health and social services structure of any community in which drug-dependence exists.

Comprehensive mental health action plan 2013–2020 *(17)*

The vision of the action plan is a world in which mental health is valued, promoted and protected, mental disorder are prevented and persons affected by these disorders are able to exercise the full range of human rights and to access high quality, culturally-appropriate health and social care in a timely way to promote recovery, all in order to attain the highest possible level of health and participate fully in society and at work free from stigmatization and discrimination.

Its overall goal is to promote mental well-being , prevent mental disorders, provide care, enhance recovery, promote human rights and reduce the mortality, morbidity and disability for persons with mental disorders.

The action plan has the following objectives:

(1) To strengthen effective leadership and governance for mental health;

(2) To provide comprehensive integrated and responsive mental health and social care services in community-based settings;

(3) To implement strategies for promotion and prevention in mental health;

(4) To strengthen information systems, evidence and research for mental health.

The global targets established for each objective provide the basis for measurable collective action and achievement by Member States towards global goals.

It is suggested that when there is evidence of significant "alienation" among a group, especially of younger persons, it should be regarded as indication of possible presence of actual or potential drug-takers, and should lead to an analysis of the situation and to such preventive or remedial action as may be indicated.

References

1. WHO (2014), *Mental Health : A State of well-being updated,* Aug. 2014.
2. WHO (2018), *Fact sheet on Mental disorder,* 9 April, 2018.
3. Govt. of India (2018), *Annual Report 2017–18,* Ministry of Health and Family welfare, New Delhi.
4. Govt. of India (2016), *National Mental Health Survey of India, 2015–16,* Prevalence, Pattern and outcomes, supported by Ministry of Health and Family Welfare, New Delhi.
5. WHO (2001), *World Health Report 2001,* Mental Health : New Understanding, New Hope.
6. WHO (1993). *Expert Committee on Drug Dependence.,* Twenty-eighth Report, No.836.
7. Current *Medical Diagnosis and Treatment,* 34th Edition (1995), Edited by Lawrence M. Tierney, Jr., stephen J. Mcphee, and Maxine A. Papadakis, A Lange Medical book.
8. WHO (1986). *Tech. Rep. Ser.,* No. 731.
9. World Development Report 1993, *Investing in Health,* Published for the World Bank, Oxford University Press.
10. WHO (2018), *Global Status Report on alcohol and health.*
11. WHO (2018), *Fact sheet on Alcohol,* Sept. 2018.
12. WHO (2018), *Fact Sheet on Tobacco,* March 2018.
13. WHO (2004), *Building Blocks for Tobacco Control : A Hand Book.*
14. WHO (2017), *Global Report on Trends in Prevalence of Tobacco Smoking 2000–2025,* 2nd Ed.
15. WHO (2008), *Health Situation in the South-East Asia Region, 2001-2007.*
16. Govt. of India (2017), *Global Adult Tobacco Survey Fact Sheet,* India 2016–17 GATS-2.
17. WHO (2013), *Comprehensive mental health action plan 2013–2020.*
18. Govt. of India (2019), *Magnitude of substance use in India,* 2019, Ministry of Social Justice and Empowerment, New Delhi.

21 Health Information and Basic Medical Statistics

"As a general rule, the most successful man in life is the man who has the best information"

Health information is an integral part of the national health system. It is a basic tool of management and a key input for the progress of any society. A health information system is defined as :

> *"a mechanism for the collection, processing, analysis and transmission of information required for organizing and operating health services, and also for research and training" (1, 2).*

The primary objective of a health information system is to provide reliable, relevant, up-to-date, adequate, timely and reasonably complete information for health managers at all levels (i.e., central, intermediate and local), and at the sharing of technical and scientific (including bibliographical) information by all health personnel participating in the health services of a country; and also to provide at periodic intervals, data that will show the general performance of the health services and to assist planners in studying their current functioning and trends in demand and work load.

Unfortunately, it is still very difficult to get the information where it matters most – i.e., at the community level. It is conceded that no country at the present time has such a thoughtfully constructed system of health information in operation, but the concept is receiving much attention. The whole science of health statistics has undergone considerable changes in the past two decades *(3)*. In 1973, the World Health Assembly stressed the need for complete reconstruction of the health information system.

Distinction between data and information

There is more than a subtle semantic difference between "data", "information" and "intelligence". **Data** consists of discrete observations of attributes or events that carry little meaning when considered alone; data as collected from operating health care systems or institutions are inadequate for planning. Data need to be transformed into **information** by reducing them, summarizing them and adjusting them for variations, such as the age and sex composition of the population so that comparisons over time and place are possible. It is the transformation of information through integration and processing with experience and perceptions based on social and political values that produces **intelligence** *(4)*.

Data that are not transformed into *information,* and information that is not transformed into *intelligence* to guide decision-makers, policy-makers, planners, administrators and health care personnel themselves, are of little value.

Requirements to be satisfied by health information systems

A WHO Expert Committee *(5)* identified the following requirements to be satisfied by the health information systems :

(1) The system should be population-based;
(2) The system should avoid the unnecessary agglomeration of data;
(3) The system should be problem-oriented;
(4) The system should employ functional and operational terms (e.g., episodes of illness, treatment regimens, laboratory tests);
(5) The system should express information briefly and imaginatively (e.g., tables, charts, percentages); and
(6) The system should make provision for the feed-back of data.

Components of a health information system

The health information system is composed of several related subsystems. A comprehensive health information system requires **information** and **indicators** on the following subjects *(6)* :

(1) demography and vital events;
(2) environmental health statistics;
(3) health status : mortality, morbidity, disability, and quality of life;
(4) health resources : facilities, beds, manpower;
(5) Utilization and non-utilization of health services : attendance, admissions, waiting lists;
(6) indices of outcome of medical care; and
(7) financial statistics (cost, expenditure) related to the particular objective.

Uses of health information

The important uses to which health information may be applied are :

(1) to measure the health status of the people and to quantify their health problems and medical and health care needs;
(2) for local, national and international comparisons of health status. For such comparisons the data need to be subjected to rigorous standardization and quality control;
(3) for planning, administration and effective management of health services and programmes;

(4) for assessing whether health services are accomplishing their objectives in terms of their effectiveness and efficiency;

(5) for assessing the attitudes and degree of satisfaction of the beneficiaries with the health system; and

(6) for research into particular problems of health and disease.

Sources of health information

The lifeblood of a health information system is the routine health statistics. Information requirements will vary according to the administrative level at which planning is envisaged. For example, the information requirements of a public health administrator will be different from the information requirements of a hospital administrator. These different contexts require different sources of information. These are discussed in this section.

1. Census

The census is an important source of health information. It is taken in most countries of the world at regular intervals, usually of 10 years. A census is defined by the United Nations as "the total process of collecting, compiling and publishing demographic, economic and social data pertaining at a specified time or times, to *all* persons in a country or delimited territory" *(7)*. Census is a massive undertaking to contact every member of the population in a given time and collect a variety of information. It needs considerable organization, a vast preparation and several years to analyse the results. This is the main drawback of census as a data source – i.e., the full results are usually not available quickly.

The first regular census in India was taken in 1881, and others took place at 10-year intervals. The last census was held in March 2011. The census is usually conducted at the end of the first quarter of the first year in each decade, the reason being, most people are usually resident in their own homes during that period. The legal basis of the census is provided by the Census Act of 1948. The supreme officer who directs, guides and operates the census is the Census Commissioner for India.

Although the primary function of census is to provide demographic information such as total count of population and its breakdown into groups and subgroups such as age and sex distribution, it represents only a small part of the total information collected. The census contains a mine of information on subjects not only demographic, but also social and economic characteristics of the people, the conditions under which they live, how they work, their income and other basic information. These data provide a frame of reference and base line for planning, action and research not only in the field of medicine, human ecology and social sciences but in the entire governmental system. Population census provides basic data (such as population by age and sex) needed to compute vital statistical rates, and other health, demographic and socio-economic indicators. Without census data, it is not possible to obtain quantified health, demographic and socio-economic indicators.

2. Registration of vital events

Whereas census is an intermittent counting of population, registration of vital events (e.g., births, deaths) keeps a continuous check on demographic changes. If registration of vital events is complete and accurate, it can serve as a reliable source of health information. Much importance is therefore given to the registration of vital events in all countries. It is the precursor of health statistics. Over the years, it has dominated the health information system.

The United Nations defines a vital events registration system as including "legal registration, statistical recording and reporting of the occurrence of, and the collection, compilation, presentation, analysis and distribution of statistics pertaining to **vital events**, i.e., live births, deaths, foetal deaths, marriages, divorces, adoptions, legitimations, recognitions, annulments and legal separations" *(7)*. Registration of vital events has been the foundation of vital statistics.

India has a long tradition of registration of births and deaths. In 1873, the Govt. of India had passed the Births, Deaths and Marriages Registration Act, but the Act provided only for voluntary registration. Subsequently, individual States like Tamil Nadu, Karnataka and Assam passed their own Acts. However, the Registration system in India tended to be very unreliable, the data being grossly deficient in regard to accuracy, timeliness, completeness and coverage. This is because of illiteracy, ignorance, lack of concern and motivation. There are also other reasons such as lack of uniformity in the collection, compilation and transmission of data which is different for rural and urban areas, and multiple registration agencies (e.g., health agency, panchayat agency, police agency and revenue agency).

The Central Births and Deaths Registration Act, 1969

In an effort to improve the civil registration system, the Govt. of India promulgated the Central Births and Deaths Registration Act in 1969. The Act came into force on 1st April 1970. The Act provides for compulsory registration of births and deaths throughout the country, and compilation of vital statistics in the States so as to ensure uniformity and comparability of data. The implementation of the Act required adoption of rules for which also, model guidelines have been provided. The Act also fixes the responsibility for reporting births and deaths. While the public (e.g., parents, relatives) are to report events occurring in their households, the heads of hospitals, nursing homes, hotels, jails or dharmashalas are to report events occurring in such institutions to the concerning Registrar. The time limit for registering the event of births and that of deaths is 21 days uniformly all over India. In case of default a late fee can be imposed. The Act makes the beginning of a new era in the history of vital statistics registration in India. More recently, from October 2018, Aadhaar number is a must for registration of death.

Lay reporting

Because of slow progress in the development of a comprehensive vital registration system, some countries have attempted to employ first-line health workers (e.g., village health guides) to record births and deaths in the community. Indeed, one of the important functions of a primary health worker is to collect and record data on vital events and other health information in his or her community.

In order to obtain this information, a new approach has been developed in several countries. This approach is known as "lay reporting of health information" *(8)*. Lay reporting is defined as the collection of information, its use, and its transmission to other levels of the health system by non-professional health workers *(9)*.

In large majority of countries properly functioning vital events registers do not exist and it is necessary to resort to demographic surveys, etc. as an alternative source. The demographic survey, however, can never lead to the desired goal of complete recording of all vital events in a country. Thus, where a vital events registration system is not functioning, the demographic survey should be regarded as a temporary substitute rather than a replacement *(7)*.

3. Sample Registration System (SRS)

Since civil registration is deficient in India, a Sample Registration System (SRS) was initiated in the mid-1960s to provide reliable estimates of birth and death rates at the National and State levels. The SRS is a dual-record system, consisting of continuous enumeration of births and deaths by an enumerator and an independent survey every 6 months by an investigator-supervisor. The half-yearly survey, in addition to serving as an independent check on the events recorded by the enumerator, produces the denominator required for computing rates.

The SRS now covers the entire country. It is a major source of health information. Since the introduction of this system, more reliable information on birth and death rates, age-specific fertility and mortality rates, infant, under-five and adult mortality, etc. have become available.

4. Notification of diseases

Historically notification of infectious diseases was the first health, information sub-system to be established. The primary purpose of notification is to effect prevention and/or control of the disease. Notification is also a valuable source of morbidity data i.e., the incidence and distribution of certain specified diseases which are notifiable.

Lists of notifiable diseases vary from country to country, and also within the same country between the States and between urban and rural areas. Usually diseases which are considered to be serious menaces to public health are included in the list of notifiable diseases. Notification system is usually operative through certain legal Acts (e.g., Madras Public Health Act, 1930). Some State Governments in India do not have any specific Act, except invoking the Epidemic Diseases Act of 1897, and extending the same from year to year. The notification system is linked up with the vital statistics machinery and the reporter is often the village chowkidar or headman. With the introduction of village Health Guides and multipurpose workers, the reporting responsibility is now shifted from the village chowkidar to the health workers. Since the legal provision is an essential pre-requisite for any notification system, the enactment of a uniform Act similar to the Registration of Births and Deaths Act, 1969 is deemed necessary for any improvement in the notification system in India.

At the international level, the following diseases are notifiable to WHO in Geneva under the International Health Regulations (IHR), viz. cholera, plague and yellow fever. A few others – louseborne typhus, relapsing fever, polio, influenza, malaria, rabies and salmonellosis are subject to international surveillance. This information is published by WHO on a worldwide basis. The Expert Committee on Health Statistics in its third Report *(10)* recommended that yearly data of notification should be detailed by age and sex.

Although notification is an important source of health information, it is common knowledge that it suffers from serious limitations : (a) notification covers only a small part of the total sickness in the community (b) the system suffers from a good deal of under-reporting (c) many cases especially atypical and subclinical cases escape notification due to non-recognition, e.g., rubella, non-paralytic polio, etc. The accuracy of diagnosis and thereby of notification depends upon the availability of facilities for bacteriological, virological and serological examination. The lack of such facilities in the rural areas of India also works against the correct reporting of the causes of sickness.

In spite of the above limitations, notification provides valuable information about fluctuations in disease frequency. It also provides early warning about new occurrences or outbreaks of disease. The concept of notification has been extended to many non-communicable diseases and conditions notably cancer, congenital malformations, mental illness, stroke and handicapped persons.

5. Hospital records

In a country like India, where registration of vital events is defective and notification of infectious diseases extremely inadequate, hospital data constitute a basic and primary source of information about diseases prevalent in the community. The eighth report of the WHO Expert Committee on Statistics *(11)* recommended that hospital statistics be regarded in all countries as an integral and basic part of the National Statistical Programme.

The main drawbacks of hospital data are : (a) they constitute only the "tip of the iceberg" – i.e., they provide information on only those patients who seek medical care, but not on a representative sample of the population. Mild cases may not attend hospitals; subclinical cases are always missed (b) the admission policy may vary from hospital to hospital; therefore hospital statistics tend to be highly selective (c) population served by a hospital (population at risk) cannot be defined. There are no precise boundaries to the catchment area of a hospital. In effect, hospital statistics provide only the **numerator** (i.e., the cases), not the denominator. Extrapolation of hospital data to an entire community is highly conjectural in estimating frequency rates of disease. Therefore, hospital statistics are considered a poor guide to the estimation of disease frequency in a community.

In spite of the above limitations, a lot of useful information about health care activities and utilization can be derived from hospital records. For example, hospital discharge sheets contain much useful information on diagnosis, medical and surgical procedures, complications, length of stay, laboratory data, etc. A study of hospital data provides information on the following aspects: (a) geographic sources of patients (b) age and sex distribution of different diseases and duration of hospital stay (c) distribution of diagnosis (d) association between different diseases (e) the period between disease and hospital admission (f) the distribution of patients according to different social and biological characteristics, and (g) the cost of hospital care. Such information may be of great value in the planning of health care services *(3, 12)*. Indices such as bed-occupancy rates, duration of stay, cost-effectiveness of treatment policies are useful in monitoring the use of hospital facilities. For the development of hospital statistics, the importance of establishing a medical record department in each hospital cannot be overemphasized. It is now felt that computerization of medical records will enable medical care to be more effectively rendered, better planned, and better evaluated.

6. Disease registers

The term "registration" implies something more than "notification". A register requires that a permanent record be established, that the cases be followed up, and that basic statistical tabulations be prepared both on frequency and on survival. In addition, the patients on a register should frequently be the subjects of special studies *(13)*.

Morbidity registers exist only for certain diseases and conditions such as stroke, myocardial infarction, cancer, blindness, congenital defects and congenital rubella. Tuberculosis and leprosy are also registered in many countries where they are common.

Morbidity registers are a valuable source of information as to the duration of illness, case fatality and survival. These registers allow follow-up of patients and provide a continuous account of the frequency of disease in the community. Even in the absence of a defined population base, useful information may be obtained from registers on the natural course of disease, especially chronic diseases in different parts of the world *(13)*. If the reporting system is effective and the coverage is on a national or representative basis, the register can provide useful data on morbidity from the particular diseases, treatment given and disease-specific mortality.

7. Record linkage

The term **record linkage** is used to describe the process of bringing together records relating to one individual (or to one family), the records originating in different times or places *(14)*. The term **medical record linkage** implies the assembly and maintenance for each individual in a population, of a file of the more important records relating to his health *(14)*. The events commonly recorded are birth, marriage, death, hospital admission and discharge. Other useful data might also be included such as sickness absence from work, prophylactic procedures, use of social services, etc. Record linkage is a particularly suitable method of studying associations between diseases; these associations may have aetiological significance *(13)*.

The main problem with record linkage is the volume of data that can accumulate. Therefore in practice record linkage has been applied only on a limited scale e.g., twin studies, measurement of morbidity, chronic disease epidemiology and family and genetic studies. At the moment, record linkage is beyond the reach of many developing countries.

8. Epidemiological surveillance

In many countries, where particular diseases are endemic, special control/eradication programmes have been instituted, as for example national disease control programmes against malaria, tuberculosis, leprosy, filariasis, etc. As part of these programmes, surveillance systems are often set up (e.g., malaria) to report on the occurrence of new cases and on efforts to control the diseases (e.g., immunizations performed). These programmes have yielded considerable morbidity and mortality data for the specific diseases.

9. Other health service records

A lot of information is also found in the records of hospital out-patient departments, primary health centres and subcentres, polyclinics, private practitioners, mother and child health centres, school health records, diabetic and hypertensive clinics, etc. For example, records in MCH centres provide information about birth weight, weight, height, arm-circumference, immunization, disease specific mortality and morbidity. However, the drawback with this kind of data is that it relates only to a certain segment of the general population. Further the data generated by these records are mostly kept for administrative purposes rather than for monitoring.

10. Environmental health data

Another area in which information is generally lacking is that relating to the environment. Health statistics are now sought to provide data on various aspects of air, water and noise pollution; harmful food additives; industrial toxicants, inadequate waste disposal and other aspects of the combination of population explosion with increased production and consumption of material goods. Environmental data can be helpful in the identification and quantification of factors causative of disease. Collection of environmental data remains a major problem for the future *(3)*.

11. Health manpower statistics

Information on health manpower is by no means least in importance. Such information relates to the number of physicians (by age, sex, speciality and place of work), dentists (classified in the same way), pharmacists, veterenarians, hospital nurses, medical technicians, etc. Their records are maintained by the State medical/dental/ nursing councils and the Directorates of Medical Education. The census also provides information about occupation. The Institute of Applied Manpower Research attempts estimates of manpower, taking into account different sources of data, mortality and out-turn of qualified persons from the different institutions. The Planning Commission also gives estimates of active doctors for different States. Regarding medical education, statistics of numbers admitted, numbers qualified, are given every year in "Health Information of India", published by the Government of India, in the Ministry of Health & Family Welfare.

12. Population surveys

A health information system should be population-based. The routine statistics collected from the above sources do not provide all the information about health and disease in the community. This calls for population surveys to supplement the routinely collected statistics. The statistics available for cholera, malaria, plague, respiratory diseases, fevers and diarrhoea are of use for public health administration.

The term "health surveys" is used for surveys relating to any aspect of health – morbidity, mortality, nutritional status, etc. When the main variable to be studied is disease suffered by the people, the survey is referred to as "morbidity survey". Broadly, the following types of surveys would be covered under health survey *(15)* :

a. surveys for evaluating the health status of a population, that is community diagnosis of problems of health and disease. It is information about the distribution of these problems over time and space that provides the fundamental basis for planning and developing needed services *(16)*.

b. surveys for investigation of factors affecting health and disease, e.g., environment, occupation, income, circumstances associated with the onset of illness, etc. These surveys are helpful for studying the natural history of disease, and obtaining more information about disease aetiology and risk factors; and

c. surveys relating to administration of health services, e.g., use of health services, expenditure on health, evaluation of population health needs and unmet needs, evaluation of medical care, etc.

Population surveys can be conducted in almost any setting; sampling techniques have been developed so that estimates at any level of precision desired within the constraints of available resources can be achieved *(17)*. Health surveys may be cross-sectional or longitudinal; descriptive or analytic or both *(18)*. Health surveys on a permanent basis are in operation in only a few countries, viz. in Japan since 1953, USA since 1957 and UK since 1971. The first methodological general health survey was carried out in Singur Health Centre by Lal and Seal in 1944–46.

Survey methods

From the point of view of the method employed for data collection, health surveys can be broadly classified into 4 types :

a. Health interview (face-to-face) survey
b. Health examination survey
c. Health records survey
d. Mailed questionnaire survey

Each method has its advantages and disadvantages. When information about morbidity is needed, **Health examination surveys** generally provide more valid information than health interview surveys. The survey is carried out by teams consisting of doctors, technicians and interviewers. The main disadvantage of a health examination survey is that it is expensive and cannot be carried out on an extensive scale. The method also requires consideration of providing treatment to people found suffering from certain diseases. **The health interview (face-to-face) survey** is an invaluable method of measuring subjective phenomena such as perceived morbidity, disability and impairment; economic loss due to illness, expenditure incurred on medical care; opinions, beliefs and attitudes; and some behavioural characteristics. It has also the advantage of giving population-based data. **The National Sample Survey Organization** in India has been active in conducting interview surveys; these surveys have provided some country-wide data on general morbidity, family planning and vital events, but the morbidity data is not reliable because of the limitation of the interview method. This is why interviews are often combined with health examination surveys and/or laboratory measurements. An alternative method of measuring subjective phenomena is the self-administered **Questionnaire,** i.e., a questionnaire without an interviewer. The use of questionnaires is simpler and cheaper, and they may be sent, for example, by mail to persons sampled from a given target population. A certain level of education, and skill is expected from the respondents when a questionnaire is administered. There is usually a high rate of non-response. **Health records survey** involves collection of data from health service records. This is obviously the cheapest method of collecting data. This method has several disadvantages : (a) the estimates obtained from the records are not population based (b) reliability of data is open to question, and (c) lack of uniform procedures and standardization in the recording of data.

Unless the aim of survey is to derive information from a special group (e.g., school children or a particular occupational group), the **household** is the most common sampling unit. It is one that allows for the collection of most social, economic and health information in a convenient way. National Family Health Survey and District Level Health Survey are some of the examples.

The size of the sample, necessary for a household survey, depends upon the measurement being taken and the degree of precision needed. Many national samples typically cover between 5,000 to 10,000 households. This is usually considered adequate for providing national estimates on such variables as health care status, anthropometric measurements, food consumption, income, expenditure, housing, literacy, etc. *(7)*.

Surveys carried out by either single or repeat visits provide direct estimates of vital events. A single survey obtains the necessary information retrospectively and is subject to problems of recall and omission. Follow-up surveys on the same households within short intervals (e.g., 6 months) appear to provide more accurate estimates of vital events, but may be too expensive for monitoring purposes *(7)*.

Data must be gathered under standardized conditions with quality control. The collection of data should be limited to those items for which there is a clearly defined use or need; the fact that data might be of interest or use to someone, someday, somewhere is not a valid reason for collecting them *(16)*. The data that is collected should be transformed into information by reducing them, summarizing them and adjusting them for variations in the age and sex composition of the population so that comparisons over time and place are possible.

13. Other routine statistics related to health

The following list, which is not comprehensive, merely serves to give examples of sources of data that have already been put to good use by epidemiologists :

(1) *Demographic :* In addition to routine census data, statistics on such other demographic phenomena as population density, movement and educational level.

(2) *Economic :* consumption of such consumer goods as tobacco, dietary fats and domestic coal; sales of drugs and remedies; information concerning per capita income; employment and unemployment data.

(3) *Social security schemes :* medical insurance schemes make it possible to study the occurrence of illnesses in the insured population. Other useful data comprise sickness absence, sickness and disability benefit rates.

14. Non-quantifiable information

Hitherto, the health information system concentrated mainly on quantifiable (statistical) data. Health planners and decision makers require a lot of non-quantifiable information, for instance, information on health policies, health legislation, public attitudes, programme costs, procedures and technology. In other words, a health information system has multi-disciplinary inputs. There should be proper **storage, processing** and **dissemination** of information.

ELEMENTARY STATISTICAL METHODS

In any field of inquiry or investigation, data is first obtained which is subsequently classified, analysed and tested for accuracy by statistical methods. Data that is obtained directly from an individual is called *primary data.* The census of 1991 is an example of collecting primary data relating to the population. The collection of data about the health and sickness of a population is primary data. Data that is obtained from outside source is called *secondary data.* If we are studying the hospital records and want to use the census data, the census data becomes secondary data. Primary data gives the precise information wanted which the secondary data may not give.

Presentation of Statistical Data

Statistical data, once collected, must be arranged purposively, in order to bring out the important points clearly and strikingly. Therefore the manner in which statistical data is presented is of utmost importance. There are several methods of presenting data – tables, charts, diagrams, graphs, pictures and special curves. A brief description of these methods is given below :

TABULATION

Tables are devices for presenting data simply from masses of statistical data. Tabulation is the first step before the data is used for analysis or interpretation. A table can be simple or complex, depending upon the number or measurement of a single set or multiple sets of items. Whether simple or complex, there are certain general principles which should be borne in mind in designing tables : (a) The tables should be numbered e.g., Table 1, Table 2, etc. (b) A title must be given to each table. The title must be brief and self-explanatory, (c) The headings of columns or rows should be clear and concise, (d) The data must be presented according to size or importance; chronologically, alphabetically or geographically, (e) If percentages or averages are to be compared, they should be placed as close as possible, (f) No table should be too large, (g) Most people find a vertical arrangement better than a horizontal one because, it is easier to scan the data from top to bottom than from left to right, (h) Foot notes may be given, where necessary, providing explanatory notes or additional information. Some examples of tabulation are given below :

1. Simple tables

(a) **TABLE 1**

Population of some states in India*

States	Population 1st March 2011
Andhra Pradesh	8,46,65,533
Bihar	10,38,04,637
Madhya Pradesh	7,25,97,565
Uttar Pradesh	19,95,81,477

*Source : Census of India, 2011

(b) **TABLE 2**

Population of India*

Year	Population
1901	238,396,000
1921	251,321,000
1981	685,185,000
1991	843,930,000
2001	1027,015,247
2011	1210,193,422

* Source : Census of India, 2011

2. Frequency distribution table

In a frequency distribution table, the data is first split up into convenient groups (class intervals) and the number of items (frequency) which occur in each group is shown in the adjacent column.

Example : The following figures are the ages of patients admitted to a hospital with poliomyelitis. Construct a frequency distribution table.

8, 24, 18, 5, 6, 12, 4, 3, 3, 2, 3, 23, 9, 18, 16, 1, 2, 3, 5, 11, 13, 15, 9, 11, 11, 7, 10 6, 9, 5, 16, 20, 4, 3, 3, 3, 10, 3, 2, 1, 6, 9, 3, 7, 14, 8, 1, 4, 6, 4, 15, 22, 2, 1, 4, 7, 1, 12,3, 23, 4, 19, 6, 2, 2, 4, 14, 2, 2, 21, 3, 2, 9, 3, 2, 1, 7, 19

The data given above may be conveniently analyzed as shown below :

Age group		Frequency
0–4	𝍸 𝍸 𝍸 𝍸 𝍸 𝍸 𝍸	35
5–9	𝍸 𝍸 𝍸 ///	18
10–14	𝍸 𝍸 /	11
15–19	𝍸 ///	8
20–24	𝍸 /	6

The data, analysed above, is prepared in the form of a frequency table as shown below :

TABLE 3

Age distribution of polio patients

Age	Number of Patients
0–4	35
5–9	18
10–14	11
15–19	8
20–24	6

In the above example, the age is split into groups of five. These are known as *class intervals.* The number of observations in each group is called *frequency.* In constructing frequency distribution tables, the questions that arise are : Into how many groups the data should be split ? And what class intervals should be chosen ? As a practical rule, it might be stated that when there is large data, a maximum of 20 groups, and when there is not much data, a minimum of 5 groups, could be conveniently taken. As far as possible, the class intervals should be equal, so that observations could be compared. The merits of a frequency distribution table are, that it shows at a glance how many individual observations are in a group, and where the main concentration lies. It also shows the range, and the shape of distribution.

CHARTS AND DIAGRAMS

Charts and diagrams are useful methods of presenting simple statistical data. They have a powerful impact on the imagination of people. Therefore, they are a popular media of expressing statistical data, especially in newspapers and magazines. The impact of the picture depends on the way it is drawn. A few general remarks need be mentioned about charts and diagrams. Diagrams are better retained in the memory than statistical tables. The data that is to be presented by diagrams ought to be simple. Then there is no risk that the reader will misunderstand. However, simplicity may be obtained only at the expense of details and accuracy. That is, lot of details of the original data may be lost in the charts and diagrams. If we want the real study, we have to go back to the original data.

1. Bar charts

Bar charts are merely a way of presenting a set of numbers by the length of a bar – the length of the bar is proportional to the magnitude to be represented. Bar charts are a popular media of presenting statistical data because they are easy to prepare, and enable values to be compared visually. The following are some examples of bar charts.

(a) SIMPLE BAR CHART

Bars may be vertical or horizontal (Fig. 1 and Fig. 2). The bars are usually separated by appropriate spaces with an eye to neatness and clear presentation. A suitable scale must be chosen to present the length of the bars.

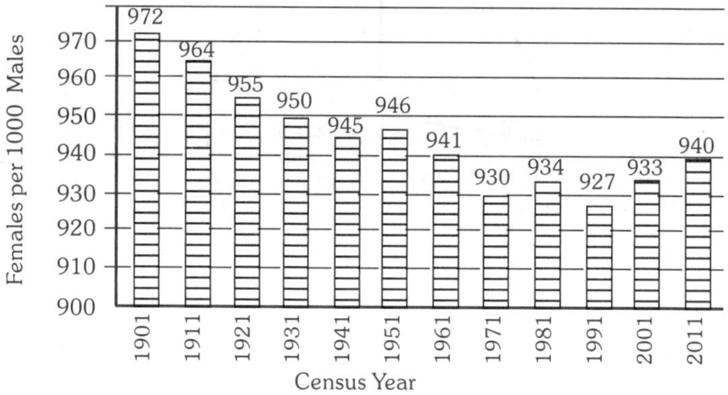

FIG. 1
India; Sex Ratio 1901-2001

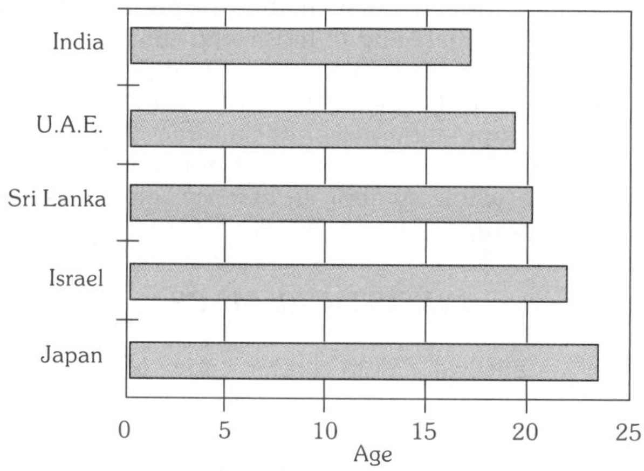

FIG. 2
Mean age at marriage (Females) in some countries

(b) MULTIPLE BAR CHART

Fig. 3 gives an example of a multiple bar chart or a compound bar chart. Two or more bars can be grouped together. In Fig. 3, population and land area by region are compared.

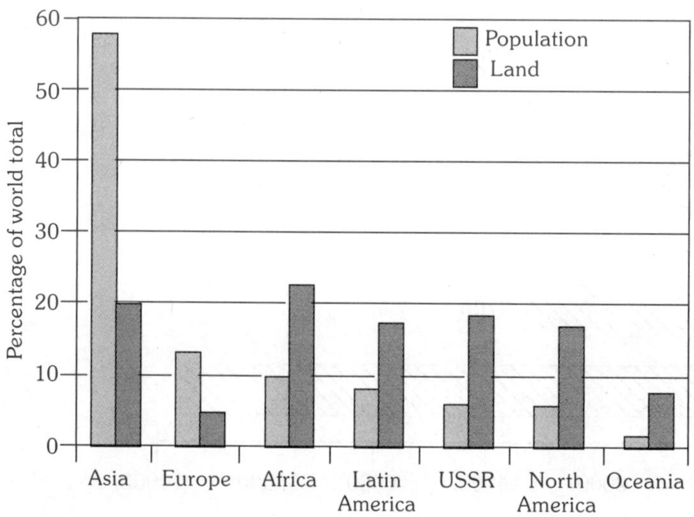

FIG. 3
Population and land area by Region,

(c) COMPONENT BAR CHART

The bars may be divided into two or more parts ... each part representing a certain item and proportional to the magnitude of that particular item (Fig. 4).

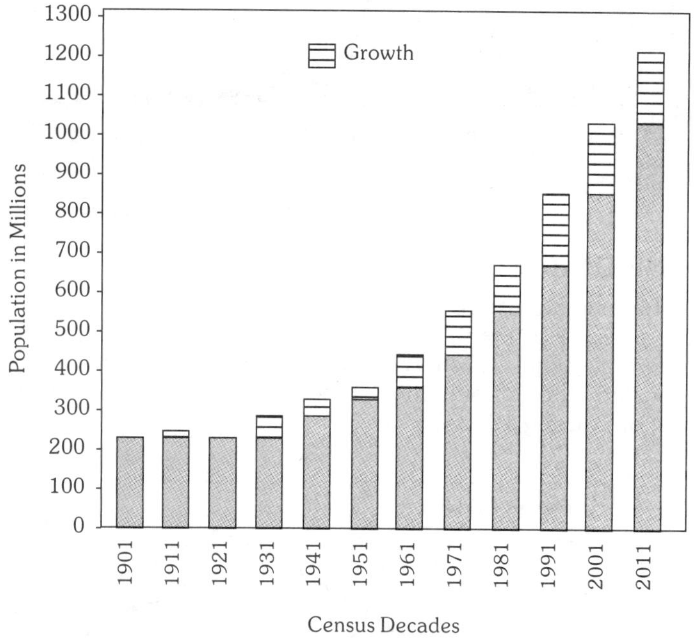

FIG. 4
India : Growth of population 1901 to 2011

2. Histogram

It is a pictorial diagram of frequency distribution. It consists of a series of blocks (Fig. 5). The class intervals are given along the horizontal axis and the frequencies along the vertical axis. The area of each block or rectangle is proportional to the frequency. Fig. 5 is the histogram of the frequency distribution of blood pressure in females 45–64 years.

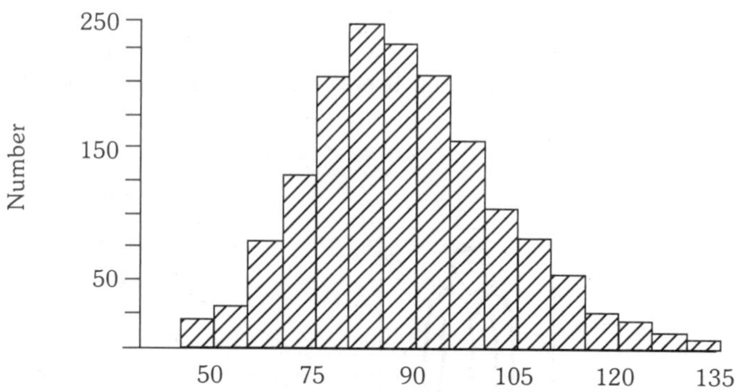

FIG. 5
Frequency distribution of diastolic blood pressure in females aged 45–64 years

FREQUENCY POLYGON

A frequency distribution may also be represented diagrammatically by the frequency polygon. It is obtained by joining the mid-points of the histogram blocks. Fig. 6 is the frequency polygon of the distribution of readings of systolic blood pressure in a community.

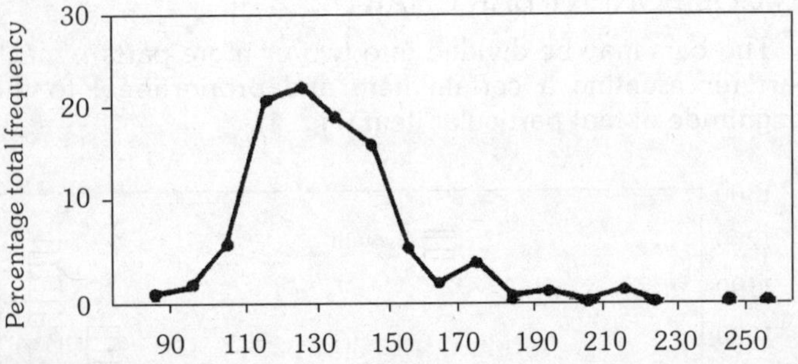

FIG.6
Frequency distribution of readings of systolic blood pressure

LINE DIAGRAM

Line diagrams are used to show the trend of events with the passage of time. The following is an example of a line diagram, (Fig. 7) showing the trend of malaria cases reported throughout the world (excluding the African Region) during 1972–78.

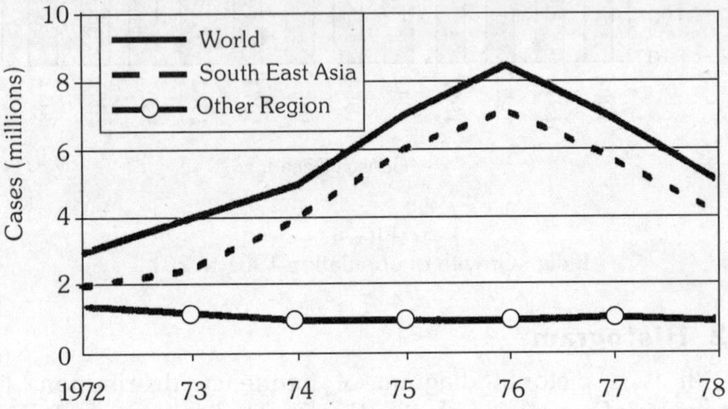

FIG. 7
Malaria cases reported, 1971-1978 (excluding African Region)

3. Pie charts

Instead of comparing the length of a bar, the areas of segments of a circle are compared. The area of each segment depends upon the angle. Pie charts are extremely popular with the laity, but not with statisticians who consider them inferior to bar charts. It is often necessary to indicate the percentages in the segments (Fig. 8) as it may not be sometimes very easy, virtually, to compare the areas of segments.

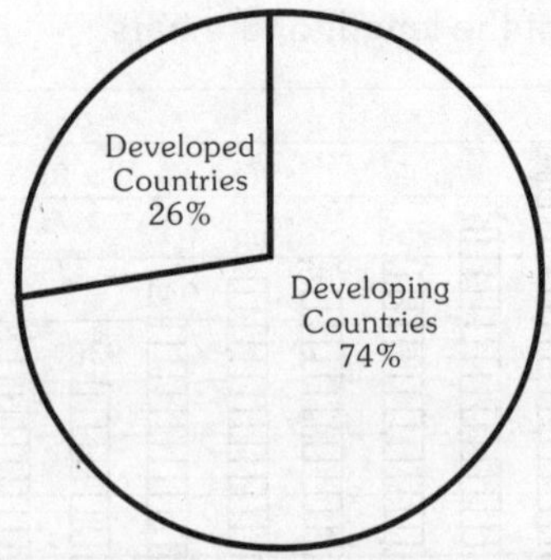

FIG. 8
World population

4. Pictogram

Pictograms are a popular method of presenting data to the "man in the street" and to those who cannot understand orthodox charts. Small pictures or symbols are used to present the data. For example, a picture of doctor to represent the population per physician (Fig. 9). Fractions of the picture can be used to represent numbers smaller than the value of a whole symbol. In essence, pictograms are a form of bar charts.

STATISTICAL MAPS

When statistical data refer to geographic or administrative areas, it is presented either as "Shaded Maps" or "Dot maps" according to suitability. The shaded maps are used to present data of varying size. The areas are shaded with different colours, or different intensities of the same colour, which is indicated in the key.

Scatter diagram shows the relationship between two variables, e.g., Fig. 10 shows a positive correlation between the intakes of fat and sugar in the average diets of 41 countries. Populations with more income are known to consume more protein, fat and also sugar (Source : Yudkin, J. (1964) : *Lancet,* 2, 5)

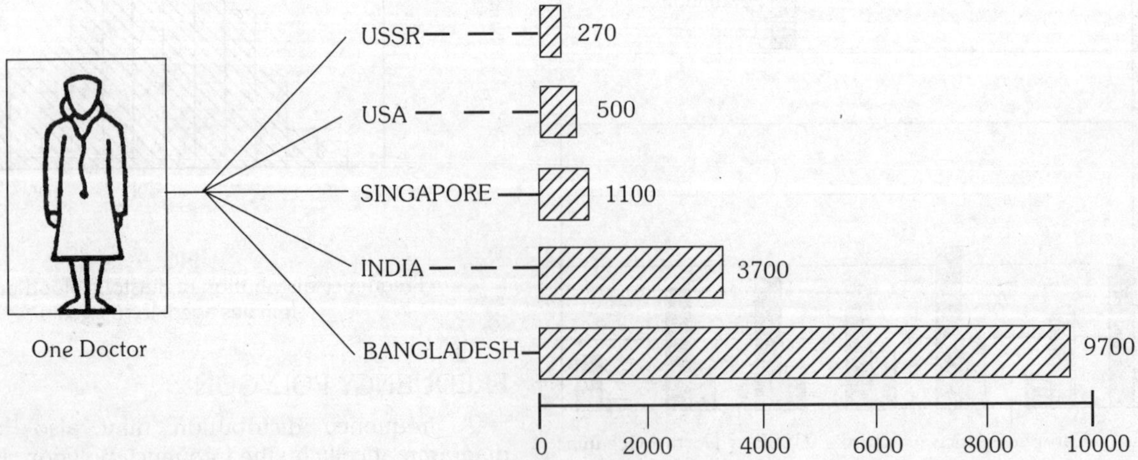

FIG. 9
Population per physician

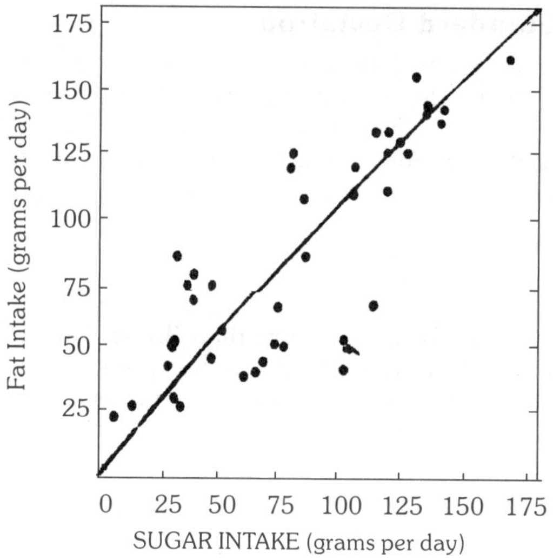

FIG. 10
Relation between average fat intake and sugar intake in 41 countries

If the dots cluster round a straight line, it shows evidence of a relationship of a linear nature. If there is no such cluster, it is probable that there is no relationship between the variables.

STATISTICAL AVERAGES

The word "average" implies a value in the distribution, around which the other values are distributed. It gives a mental picture of the central value. There are several kinds of averages, of which the commonly used are : – (1) The Arithmetic Mean, (2) Median, and (3) The Mode.

The Mean

The arithmetic mean is widely used in statistical calculation. It is sometimes simply called *Mean.* To obtain the mean, the individual observations are first added together, and then divided by the number of observations. The operation of adding together is called 'summation' and is denoted by the sign Σ or S. The individual observation is denoted by the sign η and the mean is denoted by the sign $\bar{x}$ (called "X bar").

The mean ($\bar{x}$) is calculated thus : the diastolic blood pressure of 10 individuals was 83, 75, 81, 79, 71, 95, 75, 77, 84, 90. The total was 810. The *mean* is 810 divided by 10 which is 81.0.

The advantages of the *mean* are that it is easy to calculate and understand. The disadvantages are that sometimes it may be unduly influenced by abnormal values in the distribution. Sometimes it may even look ridiculous; for instance, the average number of children born to a woman in a certain place was found to be 4.76, which never occurs in reality. Nevertheless, the arithmetic mean is by far the most useful of the statistical averages.

The Median

The *median* is an average of a different kind, which does not depend upon the total and number of items. To obtain the median, the data is first arranged in an ascending or descending order of magnitude, and then the value of the middle observation is located, which is called the *median.* For example, the diastolic blood pressure of 9 individuals was as follows : (Fig. 11).

The *median* is 79, which is the value of the middle observation (Fig. 12).

Diastolic Blood Pressure
83
75
81
79
71
95
75
77
84

FIG. 11
Data unarranged

Diastolic Blood Pressure	
71	
75	
75	
77	
79	Median
81	
83	
84	
95	

FIG. 12
Data arranged in order of magnitude

If there are 10 values instead of 9, the median is worked out by taking the average of the two middle values. That is, if the number of items or values is even, the practice is to take the average of the two middle values. For example, the diastolic blood pressure of 10 individuals was : Fig. 13.

In the *example* given, the median will be 79+81 divided by 2 which is 80 (Fig. 14).

Diastolic Blood Pressure
83
75
81
79
71
95
75
77
84
90

FIG. 13
Data unarranged

Diastolic Blood Pressure	
71	
75	
75	
77	
79	$\frac{79 + 81}{2}$
81	
83	
84	= 80
90	
95	

FIG. 14
Data arranged in order of magnitude

The relative merits of median and mean may be examined from the following example : The income of 7 people per day in Rupees was as follows :

5, 5, 5, 7, 10, 20, 102 = (Total 154)

The mean is 154 divided by 7 which is 22; the median is 7 which is the value of the middle observation. In this example, the income of the seventh individual (102) has seriously affected the mean, whereas it has not affected the median. In an example of this kind median is more nearer the truth, and therefore more representative than the mean.

The Mode

The *mode* is the commonly occurring value in a distribution of data. It is the most frequent item or the most "fashionable" value in a series of observations. For example, the diastolic blood pressure of 20 individuals was :

85, 75, 81, 79, 71, 95, 75, 77, 75, 90,
71, 75, 79, 95, 75, 77, 84, 75, 81, 75

The mode or the most frequently occurring value is 75. The advantages of mode are that it is easy to understand, and is not affected by the extreme items. The disadvantages are that the exact location is often uncertain and is often not clearly defined. Therefore, mode is not often used in biological or medical statistics.

MEASURES OF DISPERSION

The daily calorie requirement of a normal adult doing sedentary work is laid down as 2,400 calories. This clearly is not universally true.

There must be individual variations. If we examine the data of blood pressure or heights or weights of a large group of individuals, we will find that the values vary from person to person. Even within the same subject, there may be variation from time. The questions that arise are : What is normal variation ? And how to measure the variation ?

There are several measures of variation (or "dispersion" as it is technically called) of which the following are widely known :

(a) The Range
(b) The Mean or Average Deviation
(c) The Standard Deviation

(a) The Range

The range is by far the simplest measure of dispersion. It is defined as the difference between the highest and lowest figures in a given sample. For example, from the following record of diastolic blood pressure of 10 individuals –

83, 75, 81, 79, 71, 90, 75, 95, 77, 94.

It can be seen that the highest value was 95 and the lowest 71. The range is expressed as 71 to 95 or by the actual difference *(24)*. If we have grouped data, the range is taken as the difference between the *mid-points* of the extreme categories. The range is not of much practical importance, because it indicates only the extreme values between the two values and nothing about the dispersion of values between the two extreme values.

(b) The Mean Deviation

It is the average of the deviations from the arithmetic mean. It is given by the formula :

$$\text{M.D.} = \frac{\Sigma(x - \bar{x})}{\eta}$$

Example : The diastolic blood pressure of 10 individuals was as follows : 83, 75, 81, 79, 71, 95, 75, 77, 84 and 90. Find the mean deviation.

Answer (Mean deviation)

Diastolic B.P. x	Arithmetic Mean $\bar{x}$	Deviation from the Mean $(x - \bar{x})$
83	81	2
75	81	−6
81	81	0
79	81	−2
71	81	−10
95	81	14
75	81	−6
77	81	−4
84	81	3
90	81	9
Total = 810		Total = 56(ignoring ± sign)

$\text{Mean} = \frac{810}{10} = 81$ The Mean Deviation $= \frac{56}{10} = 5.6$

(c) The Standard Deviation

The standard deviation is the most frequently used measure of deviation. In simple terms, it is defined as "Root – Means – Square – Deviation." It is denoted by the Greek letter sigma σ or by the initials S.D. The standard deviation is calculated from the basic formula :

$$\text{S.D.} = \sqrt{\frac{\Sigma(x - \bar{x})^2}{\eta}}$$

When the sample size is more than 30, the above basic formula may be used without modification. For smaller samples, the above formula tends to underestimate the standard deviation, and therefore needs correction, which is done by substituting the denominator (η−1) for η. The modified formula is as follows :

$$\text{S.D.} = \sqrt{\frac{\Sigma(x - \bar{x})^2}{\eta - 1}}$$

The steps involved in calculating the standard deviation are as follows :

(a) First of all, take the deviation of each value from the arithmetic mean,
$(x - \bar{x})$

(b) Then, square each deviation -
$(x - \bar{x})^2$

(c) Add up the squared deviations -
$\Sigma(x - \bar{x})^2$

(d) Divide the result by the number of observations η :
[or (η – 1) in case the sample size is less than 30]

(e) Then take the square root, which gives the standard deviation.

Example : The diastolic blood pressure of 10 individuals was as follows : 83, 75, 81, 79, 71, 95, 75, 77, 84, 90. Calculate the standard deviation.

Answer

x	$(x - \bar{x})$	$(x - \bar{x})^2$
83	2	4
75	−6	36
81	0	–
79	−2	4
71	−10	100
95	14	196
75	−6	36
77	−4	16
84	3	9
90	9	81
$\bar{x} = 81$ η = 10		Total = 482

$$\text{S.D.} = \sqrt{\frac{\Sigma(x - \bar{x})^2}{\eta - 1}} = \sqrt{\frac{482}{10 - 1}} = \sqrt{\frac{482}{9}}$$

$$= \sqrt{53.55} = 7.31$$

The meaning of standard deviation can only be appreciated fully when we study it with reference to what is described as *normal curve.* For the present, we may contend with the basic significance of standard deviation – that it is an abstract number; that it gives us an idea of the 'spread' of the dispersion; that the larger the standard deviation, the greater the dispersion of values about the mean.

NORMAL DISTRIBUTION

The normal distribution or 'normal curve' is an important concept in statistical theory. Let us suppose, we collect the haemoglobin values of a very large number of people and make a frequency distribution with narrow class intervals, we are likely to get a smooth, symmetrical curve. Such a curve is called a normal distribution or normal curve. The shape of the curve will depend upon the mean and standard deviation which in turn will depend upon the number and nature of observations. It follows, therefore, there will be an infinite number of normal curves.

It is useful to note at this stage that in a normal curve (Fig. 15) : (a) the area between one standard deviation on either side of the mean ($\bar{x} \pm 1\sigma$) will include approximately 68 per cent of the values in the distribution, (b) the area between two standard deviations on either side of the mean ($\bar{x} \pm 2\sigma$) will cover most of the values, i.e., approximately 95 per cent of the values, and (c) the area between ($\bar{x} \pm 3\sigma$) will include 99.7 per cent of the values. These limits on either side of the mean are called "confidence limits" and are as shown in Fig. 15.

Supposing we are considering the 95 per cent confidence limits ($\bar{x} \pm 2\sigma$). When we say this, we mean that 95 per cent of the *area* of the normal curve, and hence 95 per cent of the values in the distribution will be included between the limits $\bar{x} \pm 2\sigma$. Therefore, the probability of a reading falling outside the 95 per cent confidence limits is 1 in 20 (P = 0.05).

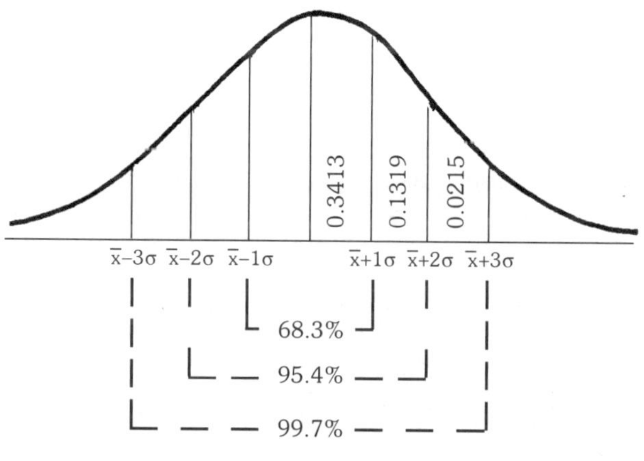

FIG. 15
Normal curve

Standard normal curve

Although there is an infinite number of normal curves depending upon the mean and standard deviation, there is only one **standardized** normal curve, which has been devised by statisticians to estimate easily the area under the normal curve, between any two ordinates. The standard normal curve is a smooth, bell-shaped, perfectly symmetrical curve, based on an infinitely large number of observations. The total area of the curve is 1; its mean is zero; and its standard deviation is 1. The mean, median and mode all coincide. The distance of a value (x) from the mean ($\bar{x}$) of the curve in units of standard deviation is called "relative deviate or standard normal variate" and is usually denoted by Z. The standard normal deviate or Z is given by the formula :

$$Z = \frac{(x - \bar{x})}{\sigma}$$

A random variable (x) is said to have been standardized when it has been adjusted so that its mean is zero and its standard deviation is 1. Standardization can be effected by subtracting the mean of x, from x and dividing the resulting difference by σ, the standard deviation of x. Thus $\frac{(x - \bar{x})}{\sigma}$ is a standardized variable. An important concept of mathematical statistics is that the new variate "Z" like the variate "x" also follows a normal distribution. The mean of the transformed distribution is zero (0), and the standard deviation (σ) is 1.

Areas under the standard normal curve are frequently needed. They have been computed for values of different relative deviate $\frac{(x - \bar{x})}{\sigma}$.

An extract of these values is given in Table 4.

TABLE 4

Areas of the standard normal curve with mean 0 and standard deviation 1

Relative deviate (z) $\frac{(x - \bar{x})}{\sigma}$	Proportion of area from middle of the curve of designated deviation
0.00	.0000
0.50	.1915
1.00	.3413
1.50	.4332
2.00	.4772
3.00	.4987
4.00	.49997
5.00	.4999998

Source : *(20)*

Estimation of probability (Example)

Let us suppose, the pulse of a group of normal healthy males was 72, with a standard deviation of 2. What is the probability that a male chosen at random would be found to have a pulse of 80 or more ?

$$\text{The relative deviate (z)} = \frac{(x - \bar{x})}{\sigma} = \frac{80 - 72}{2} = 4$$

The area of the normal curve corresponding to a deviate 4=0.49997 (Table 4). Since we are dealing with only half the total area (i.e., 0.5) the area beyond 0.49997 is equal to 0.5 – 0.49997 or 0.00003. Therefore, the probability is that only 3 out of 100,000 individuals would likely have a pulse rate of 80 or higher.

SAMPLING

When a large proportion of individuals or items or units have to be studied, we take a *sample*. It is easier and more economical to study the sample than the whole population or universe. Great care therefore is taken in obtaining a sample. It is important to ensure that the group of people or items included in the sample are representative of the whole population to be studied.

The Sampling frame

Once the *universe* has been defined, a sampling frame must be prepared. A sampling frame is a listing of the members of the universe from which the sample is to be drawn. The accuracy and completeness of the sampling frame influences the quality of the sample drawn from it.

Sampling Methods

The following three methods are most commonly used :

(1) *Simple random sample :* This is done by assigning a number to each of the units (the individuals or households) in the sampling frame. A table of random numbers is then used (see page 853) to determine which units are to be included in the sample. Random numbers are a haphazard collection of certain numbers, arranged in a cunning manner to eliminate personal selection of unconscious bias in taking out the sample. With this procedure, the sample is drawn in such a way that each unit has an equal chance of being drawn in the sample. This technique provides the greatest number of possible samples.

(2) *Systematic random sample :* This is done by picking every 5th or 10th unit at regular intervals. For example, to carry out a filaria survey in a town, we take 10 per cent sample. The houses are numbered first. Then a number is selected at random between 1 and 10 (say four). Then every 10th number is selected from that point on 4, 14, 24, 34, etc. By this method, each unit in the sampling frame would have the same chance of being selected, but the number of possible samples is greatly reduced.

(3) *Stratified random sample :* The sample is deliberately drawn in a systematic way so that each portion of the sample represents a corresponding strata of the universe. This method is particularly useful where one is interested in analysing the data by a certain characteristic of the population, viz. Hindus, Christians, Muslims, age-groups etc. – as we know these groups are not equally distributed in the population.

It is useful to note at this stage that Greek letters are usually used to refer to population characteristics : mean (μ), standard deviation (σ), and Roman letters to indicate sample characteristics : mean ($\bar{x}$), standard deviation (s).

Sampling Errors

If we take repeated samples from the same population or universe, the results obtained from one sample will differ to some extent from the results of another sample. This type of variation from one sample to another is called *sampling error.* It occurs because data were gathered from a sample rather than from the entire population of concern. Presuming that the sampling procedure is such that all the individuals in the population are favoured equally to come to the sample, the factors that influence the sampling error are : (a) the size of the sample and (b) the natural *variability* of the individual readings. As the size of the sample increases, sampling error will decrease. As the individual readings vary widely from one another, we get more variability from one sample to another.

Non-Sampling Errors

The sampling error is not the only error which arises in a sample survey. Errors may occur due to inadequately calibrated instruments, due to observer variation, as well as due to incomplete coverage achieved in examining the subjects selected and conceptual errors. These are often more important than the sampling errors.

Standard Error

If we take a random sample (η) from the population, and similar samples over and over again we will find that every sample will have a different mean ($\bar{x}$). If we make a frequency distribution of all the sample means drawn from the same population, we will find that the distribution of the mean is nearly a *normal* distribution and the mean of the sample means practically the same as the population mean (μ). This is a very important observation that the sample means are distributed *normally* about the population mean (μ). The standard deviation of the means is a measure of the sample error and is given by the formula $\sigma/\sqrt{\eta}$ which is called the standard error or the *standard error of the mean.* Since the distribution of the means follows the pattern of a normal distribution, it is not difficult to visualize that 95 per cent of the sample means will lie within limits of two standard error [$\mu \pm 2\ (\sigma/\sqrt{\eta})$] on either side of the true or population mean. Therefore standard error (S.E.) is a measure which enables us to judge whether the mean of a given sample is within the set confidence limits or not.

TESTS OF SIGNIFICANCE

We have observed till now that *standard error* indicates how reliable an estimate of the mean is likely to be. The concept of standard error is applied with appropriate formulae to all statistics, i.e., mean, standard deviation, etc. It is proposed to consider briefly the following :-

(a) Standard Error of the Mean
(b) Standard Error of Proportion
(c) Standard Error of Difference
(d) Standard Error of Difference between two Proportions.

(a) Standard Error of the Mean

We have already considered in some detail the meaning of the "standard *error* of the mean" which is also called simply the *standard error,* and the distribution of the sample means about the true mean of the universe. In actual practice, we don't take repeated samples usually from a population. We take only one sample from the universe and calculate the mean and standard deviation. The questions that arise are : How accurate is the mean of our sample ? What can be said about the true mean of the universe ? In order to answer these questions, we calculate the standard error of the mean and set up 'confidence limits' within which the mean (μ), of the population (of which we have only one sample) is likely to lie.

Example : Let us suppose, we obtained a random sample of 25 males, age 20–24 years whose mean temperature was 98.14 deg. F with a standard deviation of 0.6. What can we say of the true mean of the universe from which the sample was drawn ?

We use the *standard error* as the yard stick :

$$\text{S.E. } \bar{x} = S/\sqrt{(\eta)} = 0.6/\sqrt{(25)} = 0.12$$

We now set up confidence limits on the basis of the normal curve distribution. If the limits are set out at twice the standard error from the mean (95 per cent confidence limits) the range of the population mean would be 98.14 ± (2 × 0.12) = 97.90 deg. F. to 98.38 deg. F. The chances will be only 1 in 20 (P = 0.05) that the population mean would be outside these limits.

Very often we come across in scientific terminology the word 'significant'. When we say that "this difference is significant", we mean that it is unlikely to be merely due to chance. It has become customary to regard as significant, when P<0.05 (1 in 20) and more significant, when P < 0.01 (1 in 100).

(b) Standard Error of Proportion

Let us suppose, the proportion of males in a certain village was 52 per cent. A random sample of 100 people was taken, and the proportion of males was found to be only 40 per cent. What conclusions could be drawn from the sample ? What possible range of males could we expect in a sample of 100, within 95 per cent confidence limits ?

In an example of this kind, we are not dealing with means but with proportions in a sample and its universe. We may designate these proportions as *p* and *q* and proceed to calculate the standard deviation round that expected 52 per cent. This is called the *standard error of proportion* and is given by the formula :

$$\text{Standard Error of Proportion} = \sqrt{\frac{pq}{n}}$$

where p = proportion of males; q = proportion of females and n = size of the sample. Substituting the values, we get :

$$\text{S.E. (Proportion)} = \sqrt{\frac{52 \times 48}{100}} = 5.0$$

We take two standard errors on either side of 52 as our criterion. That is, If the sample is a truly representative one, we might get by chance a value in the range 52+2 (5) = 62 and 52 – 2 (5) = 42. In other words, the proportion of males in our sample could vary from 42 to 62. Since the observed proportion of males was only 40 per cent and well outside the confidence limits, we consider the difference between the observed and expected values "significant" and is not likely to have arisen by chance. The *relative deviate* in this particular case, in units of a standard error of 5, will be :-

$$\text{Relative deviate} = \frac{52 - 40}{5} = 2.4$$

Since the relative deviate exceeded 2, it is obvious in the present example, that the deviation was 'significant'. This significance test is applicable in situations where the population consists of only 2 classes or proportions, e.g., males and females, sick and healthy, successes and failures, etc.

(c) Standard Error of Difference Between two Means

Very often, in biological work the investigator is faced with the problem of comparing results between two groups. One may be the control group and the other experimental group. The question arises, whether the difference between the means of the two groups is significant to indicate that the samples represent two different universes. We proceed to tackle this problem by calculating the *standard error of difference* between the two means.

Let us suppose, we are testing the effect of a drug on mice. 24 mice, comparable in all respects, were randomly divided into 2 groups. Group A was the control group, i.e., no treatment. The other group, the experimental group was given a drug for a certain period of time. At the end of the experiment, the mice were sacrificed and the kidney of each animal was weighed in milligrams. The effects of the treatment on the kidney weights was as follows :

	Number	Mean	Standard Deviation
Control group	12	318	10.2
Experimental group	12	370	24.1

Let us determine whether the difference between the kidney weights of the two groups is significant.

We apply the formula for the *standard error of difference between the two means :*

$$\text{S.E. (d) between the means} = \sqrt{\frac{\sigma^2_1}{n_1} + \frac{\sigma^2_2}{n_2}}$$

$$= \sqrt{\frac{(10.2)^2}{12} + \frac{(24.1)^2}{12}}$$

$$= \sqrt{8.67 + 48.4}$$

$$= \sqrt{57.07}$$

$$= 7.5$$

The standard error of difference between the two means is 7.5. The actual difference between the two means is (370 – 318) = 52, which is more than twice the standard error of difference between the two means, and therefore "significant". We conclude that the treatment affected the kidney weights.

(d) Standard Error of Difference Between Proportions

Instead of means, sometimes we may have to test the significance of difference between two proportions or ratios to find out if the difference between the two proportions or ratios have occurred by chance. In this case, we calculate the *standard error of difference between two proportions.*

Confidence limits	Normal deviate (N.D.) $= \frac{x - \mu}{\sigma / \sqrt{\eta}}$	Significance
μ is outside the 95 per cent confidence limits	N.D. > 2	P < 0.05 Significant at 5 per cent level
μ is just within 95 per cent confidence limits	N.D. = 2	P = 0.05 Just significant at 5 per cent level
μ is within the 95 per cent confidence limits	N.D. < 2	P > 0.05 Not significant at 5 per cent level

Let us suppose, we are making a trial of 2 whooping cough vaccines. The results of the field trial were as follows :

Vaccine	No. Vaccinated	No. of Exposures	No. of cases	Attack Rate
A	2,400	90	22	24.4%
B	2,300	86	14	16.2%

From the above it appears that vaccine B is superior to vaccine A. Is there any significance ?

We calculate the standard error of difference between the two proportions :

$$\text{S.E. of Difference between two proportions} = \sqrt{\frac{p_1 q_1}{n_1} + \frac{p_2 q_2}{n_2}}$$

$$= \sqrt{\frac{24.4 \times 75.6}{90} + \frac{16.2 \times 83.8}{86}}$$

$$= \sqrt{20.49 + 15.78} = \sqrt{36.27} = 6.02$$

The standard error of difference is 6 whereas the observed difference (24.4 – 16.2) was 8.2. In other words, the observed difference between the two groups is less than twice the S.E. of difference, i.e., 2 × 6. We infer that there was no strong evidence of any difference between the efficacy of the two vaccines. Therefore, the observed difference might be easily due to chance.

Alternatively, we can use the CHI-SQUARE (χ^2) Test in an example of this kind.

CHI-SQUARE TEST

Chi-square (χ^2) Test offers an alternate method of testing the significance of difference between two proportions. It has the advantage that it can also be used when more than two groups are to be compared.

Let us consider the previous example : we were making a trial of 2 whooping cough vaccines. The results of the field trial were as below:

Vaccine	Attacked	Not Attacked	Total	Attack Rate
A	22	68	90	24.4%
B	14	72	86	16.2%
Total	36	140	176	–

Apparently, vaccine B was superior to vaccine A. The question that arises is whether the vaccine B was really superior to vaccine A, or whether the difference was merely due to chance.

(1) TEST THE 'NULL HYPOTHESIS'

First, we set up a hypothesis, called the *Null Hypothesis* that there was no difference between the effect of the two vaccines, and then proceed to test the hypothesis in quantitative terms. It is done in the following manner :

We first pool the results from the two vaccines. The proportion of people attacked will be 36/176 = 0.204. The proportion of people not attacked will be 140/176 = 0.795. From these proportions, we now calculate the *expected* number of attacks or cases, and those not attacked. The expected number of attacks by vaccine A will be 90 × 0.204 = 18.36; the expected number not attacked will be 90 × 0.795 = 71.55. Similarly, the expected number of attacks by vaccine B will be 86 × 0.204 = 17.544; the expected number not attacked will be 86 × 0.795 = 68.37. We shall now rewrite the previous table, showing the *observed* (O) and *expected* (E) values in each cell :

Vaccine	Attacked	Not Attacked
A	O = 22 E = 18.36 + 3.64	O = 68 E = 71.55 3.55
B	O = 14 E = 17.54 – 3.54	O = 72 E = 68.37 + 3.63

(2) APPLYING THE χ^2 TEST

$$\chi^2 = \frac{\Sigma\,(O-E)^2}{E}$$

$$\chi^2 = \frac{(3.64)^2}{18.36} + \frac{(3.55)^2}{71.55} + \frac{(3.54)^2}{17.54} + \frac{(3.63)^2}{68.37}$$

$$= 0.72 + 0.17 + 0.71 + 0.19 = 1.79$$

(3) FINDING THE DEGREE OF FREEDOM

The next step in the calculation is to find out what is known as the *degree of freedom* (d.f.). This depends upon the number of columns and rows in the original table, and given by the formula :

d.f. = (c – 1) (r – 1)
c = Number of columns
r = Number of rows

In our table (cited above), there are two rows (attacked and not attacked) and two columns (vaccine A and vaccine B). It is a 2 × 2 contingency table. The degree of freedom will be :

d.f. = (c – 1) (r – 1)
= (2 – 1) (2 – 1) = 1

(4) PROBABILITY TABLES

We next turn to the published probability tables given below. On referring to χ^2 Table, with 1 *degree of freedom*, the value of χ^2 for a probability of 0.05 is 3.84. Since the observed value (1.79) is much lower we conclude that the *null hypothesis* is true and that vaccine B is not superior to vaccine A. The test is valid only if the expected number in each cell is not less than two.

CORRELATION AND REGRESSION

Meaning of Correlation

Often we wish to know whether there is linear relation between two variables, e.g., height and weight, temperature and pulse, age and vital capacity, etc. In order to find out whether there is significant association or not between two variables (we may call them x and y), we calculate what is known as *Co-efficient of Correlation*, which is represented by the symbol "r".

Suppose, we have 2 variables x and y and we have n individuals who have each one reading of x and one reading of y. The correlation coefficient is given by the formula :

$$r = \frac{\Sigma\,(x-\bar{x})\,(y-\bar{y})}{\sqrt{\Sigma\,(x-\bar{x})^2\ \Sigma\,(y-\bar{y})^2}}$$

TABLE OF χ^2

Probability (P)

D.F.	.50	.10	.05	.02	.01	.005	.001
1.	0.45	2.71	3.84	5.41	6.64	7.88	10.83
2.	1.39	4.61	5.99	7.82	9.21	10.60	13.82
3.	2.37	6.25	7.82	9.84	11.34	12.64	16.27
4.	3.36	7.78	9.49	11.67	13.28	14.86	18.47
5.	4.35	9.24	11.07	13.39	15.09	16.75	20.51
6.	5.35	10.65	12.59	15.03	16.81	18.55	22.46
7.	6.35	12.02	14.07	16.62	18.48	20.28	24.32
8.	7.34	13.36	15.51	18.17	20.09	21.96	26.13
9.	8.34	14.68	16.92	19.68	21.67	23.59	27.88
10.	9.34	15.99	18.31	21.16	23.21	25.19	29.59

TABLE OF RANDOM NUMBERS*

76	58	30	83	64	87	29	25	58	84	86	50	60	00	25
47	56	91	29	34	05	87	31	06	95	12	45	57	09	09
10	80	21	38	84	90	56	35	03	09	43	12	74	49	14
00	95	01	31	76	17	16	29	56	63	38	78	94	49	81
07	28	37	07	61	11	16	36	27	03	78	86	72	04	95
20	26	36	31	62	68	69	86	95	44	84	95	48	46	45
31	56	34	19	09	79	57	92	36	59	14	93	87	81	40
98	40	07	17	81	22	45	44	84	11	24	62	20	42	31
24	33	45	77	58	80	45	67	93	82	75	70	16	08	24
01	31	60	10	39	53	58	47	70	93	85	81	56	39	38
50	78	13	69	36	37	68	53	37	31	71	26	35	03	71
90	78	50	05	62	77	79	13	57	44	59	60	10	39	66
46	72	60	18	77	55	66	12	62	11	08	99	55	64	57
47	21	61	88	32	27	80	30	21	60	10	92	35	36	12
12	73	73	99	12	49	99	57	94	82	96	88	57	17	91
23	54	20	83	85	23	86	66	99	07	36	37	34	92	09
65	76	36	95	90	18	48	27	45	68	27	23	65	30	72
37	55	85	78	78	01	48	41	19	10	35	19	54	07	73

*Taken from Table XXXIII of : Fisher, R.A. & Yates, F. *Statistical tables for biological, agricultural and medical research*, 6th ed., Longman Group Ltd., London, 1974.

The correlation coefficient r tends to lie between – 1.0 and + 1.0. If r is near + 1, it indicates a strong positive association between x and y i.e., when one variable increases the other variable also increases. A value near – 1 indicates a strong negative association i.e. when one variable increases the other decreases. If r = 0, it indicates there is no association between x and y. There are also tests to show whether or not the correlation could be due to chance. However, it needs to be noted that correlation does not necessarily prove *causation.*

Meaning of Regression

If we wish to know in an individual case the value of one variable, knowing the value of the other, we calculate what is known as the *regression coefficient* of one measurement to the other. It is customary to denote the independent variate by x and the dependent variate by y. The formula for obtaining the regression coefficient is as follows :

$$y = \bar{y} + b\,(x - \bar{x})$$

where $\bar{y}$ = mean of $y_1, y_2, y_3 \ldots\ldots\ldots\ldots y_n$

$\bar{x}$ = mean of $x_1, x_2, x_3 \ldots\ldots\ldots\ldots x_n$

$$b = \frac{\Sigma\,(x - \bar{x})\,(y - \bar{y})}{\Sigma\,(x - \bar{x})^2}$$

The value of b is called the *regression coefficient* of y upon x. Similarly, we can obtain the regression of x upon y.

$$x = \bar{x} + b^1\,(y - \bar{y})$$

$$b^1 = \frac{\Sigma\,(x - \bar{x})\,(y - \bar{y})}{\Sigma\,(y - \bar{y})^2}$$

Where b^1 is the regression coefficient of x upon y. The function of regression is to provide a means of estimating the value of one variable from the value of another.

References

1. Alderson, M.R. (1974). *WHO Chronicle,* 28 : 52.
2. WHO/EURO (1973). *Conference on Health Information System.*
3. WHO (1976). *WHO Chronicle,* 30 (2) 58.
4. WHO (1977). *Public Health Paper* No.67.
5. WHO (1971). *Techn. Rep. Ser.,* No.472.
6. WHO (1979). *WHO Chronicle,* 33 (5) 177-179.
7. WHO (1981). *Health for All,* Sr.No.4.
8. WHO (1978). *Lay Reporting of Health Information.*
9. WHO (1981). *Health for All,* Sr.No.9.
10. WHO (1952). *Techn. Rep. Ser.,* No.53.
11. WHO (1963). *Techn. Rep. Ser.,* No.261.
12. WHO (1968). *Techn. Rep. Ser.,* No.389.
13. WHO (1967). *Techn. Rep. Ser.,* No.365.
14. Hogarh, J. (1978). *Glossary of Health Care Terminology, WHO* Reg. Office, Europe.
15. WHO (1966). *Techn. Rep. Ser.,* No.336.
16. White, K.L. (1978). *In : Basic Health Care* in Developing Countries, B.S. Hetzel (ed), Oxford.
17. White, K.L. et al (1977). *Public Health Paper* No. 67.
18. Abramson, J.H. (1974). *Survey Methods in Community Medicine,* Edinburgh, Churchill Livingstone.
19. Bancroft, H. (1957). *Introduction to Biostatistics,* Hoeber-Harper, N.Y.

22 Communication for Health Education

"The only thing more expensive than education is ignorance"

Communication can be regarded as a two-way process of exchanging or shaping ideas, feelings and information. Broadly it refers "to the countless ways that humans have of keeping in touch with one another" *(1)*.

Communication is more than mere exchange of information. It is a process necessary to pave way for desired changes in human behaviour, and informed individual and community participation to achieve predetermined goals. Communication has, in recent years, developed into an interdisciplinary science drawing richly from social sciences. With the development of newer methods of communication and information explosion, the mental development of the humans has expanded considerably for clearer thinking, better social inter-sectoral coordination.

Communication and education are interwoven. Communication strategies can enhance learning. The ultimate goal of all communication is to bring about a change in the desired direction of the person who receives the communication. This may be at the **cognitive** level in terms of increase in knowledge; it may be **affective** in terms of changing existing patterns of behaviour and attitudes; and it may be **psychomotor** in terms of acquiring new skills. These are referred to as learning objectives *(2)*.

Communication is part of our normal relationship with other people. Our ability to influence others depends on our **communication skills**, e.g., speaking, writing, listening, reading and reasoning. These skills are much needed in health education. The developing countries are now beginning to exploit the current "communication revolution" to put today's health information at the disposal of families, to help people to achieve health by their own actions and efforts. It is said that without communication an individual could never become a human being, without mass communication, he could never become a part of modern society *(3)*.

THE COMMUNICATION PROCESS

Communication which is the basis of human interaction is a complex process. It has the following main components (Fig. 1) :

1. sender (source)
2. receiver (audience)
3. message (content)
4. channel(s) (medium)
5. feedback (effect)

1. Sender

The sender (communicator) is the originator of the message. To be an effective communicator, he must know:

- his objectives, clearly defined
- his audience : it's interests and needs
- his message
- channels of communication
- his professional abilities and limitations

The impact of the message will depend on his own social status (authority), knowledge and prestige in the community.

2. Receiver

All communications must have an audience, this may be a single person or a group of people. Without the audience, communication is nothing more than mere noise. It is this element of audience and their frame of mind (e.g., opinions, attitudes, prejudices) which lends meaning to all the different types of communication.

The audience may be of two types : the controlled and the uncontrolled. A controlled audience is one which is held together by a common interest. It is a homogeneous group. An uncontrolled or "free" audience is one which has

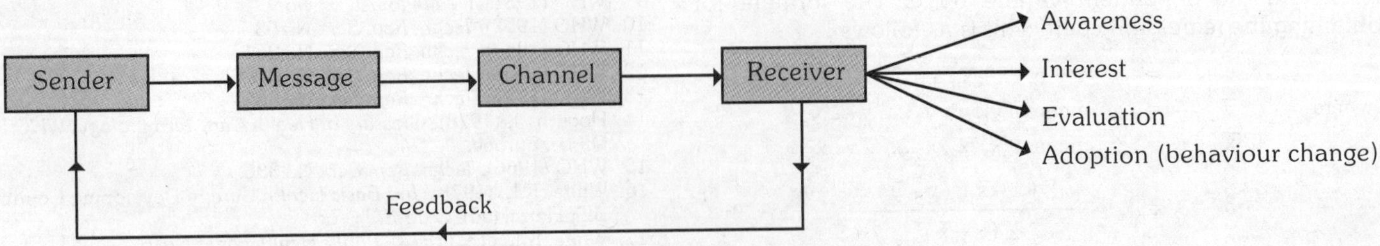

FIG. 1
Communication process

gathered together from motives of curiosity. This type of audience poses a challenge to the ability of the educator. The more homogeneous the audience is, the greater are the chances of an effective communication.

3. Message

A message is the information (or "technical know-how") which the communicator transmits to his audience to receive, understand, accept and act upon. It may be in the form of words, pictures or signs. Health communication may fail in many cases, if its message is not adequate.

A good message must be :

- in line with the objective (s)
- meaningful
- based on felt needs
- clear and understandable
- specific and accurate
- timely and adequate
- fitting the audience
- interesting
- culturally and socially appropriate

Transmitting the right message to the right people at the right time is a crucial factor in successful communication.

4. Channels of communication

By channel is implied the "physical bridges" or the media of communication between the sender and the receiver.

Media systems

The total communication effort is based on three media systems :

a. Interpersonal communication
b. Mass media
c. Traditional or folk media

a. Interpersonal communication

The most common channel of communication is the interpersonal or face-to-face communication. Being personal and direct it is more persuasive and effective than any other form of communication. Interpersonal communication is particularly important in influencing the decisions of the undecided persons. The superiority of interpersonal communication over mass media for creation of motivational effect has been well documented *(4)*.

When the message relayed *via* mass media gets diffused in the community, it is picked up by the interpersonal and informal networks. The message is then subject to debate and discussion by interpersonal communications. On the basis of this scrutiny a consensus is gradually built up in the community whether to accept or reject the message *(5)*.

b. *Mass media*

In mass communication, the channel is one or more of the following "mass media", viz., TV, radio, printed media, etc. Mass media have the advantage of reaching a relatively larger population in a shorter time than is possible with other means. Being one-way channels of communication, mass media carry messages only from the centre to the periphery ; feedback mechanisms are poorly organized. Being impersonal media, they are usually not effective in changing established modes of behaviour.

c. *Folk media*

Every community has its own network of traditional or folk media such as folk dances, singing, dramas, *Nautanki* in Uttar Pradesh, *Burrakatha* in Andhra Pradesh and *Harikatha* in Western India besides informal group gatherings, caste or religious meetings. These are important channels of communication close to the cultural values of the rural population. They have been the principal instruments of preserving the cultural heritage. Health messages may be communicated through these traditional media.

Every channel of communication has its advantages and limitations. For instance, knowledge of surgery cannot be effectively transmitted by verbal communication, demonstrations are needed. The proper selection and use of channels results in successful communication. Since effective communication is seldom achieved through the use of one method alone, an attempt should be made to combine a variety of methods to accomplish the educational purpose. Health education uses a variety of methods to help people understand their own situations and choose actions that will improve their health.

5. Feedback

It is the flow of information from the audience to the sender. It is the reaction of the audience to the message. If the message is not clear or otherwise not acceptable the audience may reject it outright. The feedback thus provides an opportunity to the sender to modify his message and render it acceptable. In interpersonal communication the feedback is immediate. In mass communication it takes some time to get feedback. Feedback is generally obtained through opinion polls, attitude surveys and interviews. It can rectify transmission errors.

TYPES OF COMMUNICATION

1. One-way communication (Didactic Method)

The flow of communication is "one-way" from the communicator to the audience. The familiar example is the lecture method in class rooms. The drawbacks of the didactic method are :

- knowledge is imposed
- learning is authoritative
- little audience participation
- no feedback
- does not influence human behaviour

2. Two-way communication (Socratic method)

The Socratic method is a two-way method of communication in which both the communicator and the audience take part. The audience may raise questions, and add their own information, ideas and opinions to the subject. The process of learning is active and "democratic". It is more likely to influence behaviour than one-way communication.

3. Verbal communication

The traditional way of communication has been by word of mouth. The advent of written and printed matter are of comparatively recent origin. Direct verbal communication by word of mouth may be loaded with hidden meanings. It is persuasive. Non-direct or written communication may not be as persuasive as the spoken word.

4. Non-verbal communication

Communication can occur even without words. It includes a whole range of bodily movements, postures, gestures, facial expressions (e.g., smile, raised eye brows, frown, staring, gazing etc.). Silence is non-verbal communication. It can speak louder than words.

5. Formal and informal communication

Communication has been classified into formal (follows lines of authority) and informal (grape-vine) communication. Informal network (e.g., gossip circles) exists in all organizations. The informal channels may be more active, if the formal channels do not cater to the information needs.

6. Visual communication

The visual forms of communication comprise : charts and graphs, pictograms, tables, maps, posters etc.

7. Telecommunication and internet

Telecommunication is the process of communicating over distance using electromagnetic instruments designed for the purpose. Radio, TV and internet etc. are mass communication media, while telephone is known as point-to-point telecommunication systems. The point-to-point systems are closer to interpersonal communication. With the launching of satellites, a big explosion of electronic communication has taken place all over the world.

BARRIERS OF COMMUNICATION

Health education may often fail due to communication barriers between the educator and the community – these may be:

1. Physiological – difficulties in hearing, expression.
2. Psychological – emotional disturbances, neurosis, levels of intelligence, language or comprehension difficulties.
3. Environmental – noise, invisibility, congestion.
4. Cultural – illiteracy, levels of knowledge and understanding, customs, beliefs, religion, attitudes, economic and social class differences, language variations, cultural difficulties between foreigners and nationals, between urban education and the rural population.

Even when health services are readily available, the social and cultural barriers can present serious problems to the achievement of health behaviour change. These barriers should be identified and removed.

HEALTH COMMUNICATION

Health is the concern of everyone for everyone. Health communication is therefore an important area of communication. The term "health communication" is often used synonymously with health education, which itself suggests "outward and downward" communication of knowledge *(6)*. Health education is the foundation of a preventive health care system.

Functions of health communication

Health communication has to cater to the following needs:

1. Information
2. Education
3. Motivation
4. Persuasion
5. Counselling
6. Raising morals
7. Health development
8. Organization

1. Information

The primary function of health communication is to provide scientific knowledge or information to people about health problems and how to maintain and promote health. People rarely seek such information although they have a right to know the facts about health and disease.

Information should be easily accessible to the people. Exposure to the right kind of health information can

- eliminate social and psychological barriers of ignorance, prejudice and misconceptions people may have about health matters;
- increase awareness of the people to the point that they are able to perceive their health needs ; and
- influence people to the extent that unfelt needs become felt needs, and felt needs become demands.

The government, the media and health providers have an important social responsibility to provide factual and balanced health and health related information to the people and awaken their interest on the basis of which they can make informed decisions. But, the assumption that the acquisition of information will mean a change in an individual's behaviour and attitudes is fallacious. Most people make important decisions regarding their health only after much thought, perhaps over a period of time and after serval educational contacts. The cultural values, beliefs and norms of the people influence their acceptance of health information. Correct information is a basic part of health education.

2. Education

Education of the general public is an integral part of a prevention oriented approach to health and disease problems; and, the basis of all education is communication. Education can help to increase knowledge. It is often assumed that knowledge determines attitudes and attitudes determine behaviour *(7)*.

Health education can bring about changes in life styles and risk factors of disease. Most of the world's major health problems and premature deaths are preventable through changes in human behaviour at low cost *(8)*. But education *alone* is insufficient to achieve optimum health. The target population must have access to proven preventive measures or procedures.

3. Motivation

It is the power that drives a person from within to act. One of the goals of health communication is to motivate individuals to translate health information into personal behaviour and lifestyle for their own health. Motivation includes the stages of interest, evaluation and decision making. Health communication assists the individual in passing from the state of awareness and interest to the final stage of decision making and adoption of the new idea or programme. Motivation may not be long-lasting; it may diminish with lapse of time. The best channels of success involve programmes directed at individuals who already have some strong motivation, in patients with chronic illness or a disability, those facing acute crisis such as surgery or childbirth. This suggests that probably the quickest pay off will come in the area of patient education.

4. Persuasion

Persuasion is the art of winning friends and influencing people. It is an art that does not employ force or deliberate manipulation. The sole purpose of communication is to influence. Persuasion is "a conscious attempt by one individual to change or influence the general beliefs, understanding, values and behaviour of another individual or group of individuals in some desired way". Persuasive communication is more effective than coercion or authoritative communication. Persuasion can change life style and modify the risk factors of disease.

When persuasive communication is deliberately employed to manipulate feelings, attitudes and beliefs, it becomes "propaganda" or "brain washing" *(1)*.

5. Counselling

Counselling is a process that can help people understand better and deal with their problems and communicate better with those with whom they are emotionally involved. It can improve and reinforce motivation to change behaviour. It can provide support at times of crisis. It helps them face up to their problems and to reduce or solve them.

Counselling is different from advising. It implies choice, not force. Advising amounts to directing people and cautioning them to some do's and dont's.

In different circumstances different people can undertake counselling. A counsellor should be able:

- to communicate information
- to gain the trust of the people
- to listen sympathetically to people who are anxious, distressed and possibly hostile.
- to understand other person's feelings and to respond to them in such a way that the other person can feel free to express his feelings
- to help people reduce or resolve their problems.

Thus counselling relies heavily on communication and relationship skills. Counselling is an important part of treatment, disease prevention and health promotion. It helps people to avoid illness and to improve their lives through their own efforts *(9)*. Counselling develops positive attitudes. It is an integral part of all health care programmes.

6. Raising morale

Morale is "the capacity of a group of people (or team) to pull together persistently or consistently. Communication – vertical and horizontal, internal and external is the first step in any attempt to raise morale of the health team or a group of people.

7. Health development

Communication can play a powerful role in health development by helping to diffuse knowledge in respect of the goals of development and preparing the people for the roles expected of them. But its own role is essentially, supportive *(5)*. Judicial use of communication media can contribute to health development *(10)*.

8. Health organization

Communication is the life and blood of an organization. There are two major directions in which communications within an organization flow. These are vertical and horizontal communications. Vertical communication can be downward or upward. Horizontal or cross communication takes place usually between equals at any level. The downward communication extends from top administrator down through the hierarchy of professionals and non-professionals to the beneficiaries or employees. The direction in which communication flows in an organization suggests the degree of freedom in the internal communication network *(1)*.

Communication is an important dimension of health organization. It is an important means of intra – and inter–sectoral coordination.

HEALTH EDUCATION

Health education is a term commonly used and referred to by health professionals.

Definitions

Health education is indispensable in achieving individual and community health. It can help to increase knowledge and to reinforce desired behaviour patterns. But there is no single acceptable definition of health education. A variety of definitions exist. Concepts of health education as a process or an activity for inducing behavioural changes are emphasized in the following definitions :

1. Health education is the translation of what is known about health, into desirable individual and community behaviour patterns by means of an educational process *(11)*.
2. The definition adopted by John M Last is "The process by which individuals and groups of people learn to behave in a manner conducive to the promotion, maintenance or restoration of health" *(12)*.
3. Any combination of learning opportunities and teaching activities designed to facilitate voluntary adaptations of behaviour that are conducive to health *(13)*.
4. The definition adopted by the National Conference on Preventive Medicine in USA is "Health education is a process that informs, motivates and helps people to adopt and maintain healthy practices and lifestyles, advocates environmental changes as needed to facilitate this goal and conducts professional training and research to the same end" *(14)*.
5. Health education is the part of health care that is concerned with promoting healthy behaviour *(9)*.

Alma-Ata Declaration

The Declaration of Alma-Ata (1978) by emphasizing the need for "individual and community participation" gave a new meaning and direction to the practice of health education. The dynamic definition of health education is now as follows :

- "a process aimed at encouraging people to want to be healthy, to know how to stay healthy, to do what they can individually and collectively to maintain health, and to seek help when needed" *(6)*.

The Alma-Ata Declaration has revolutionized the *concepts* and *aims* of health education :

The modern concept of health education emphasizes on health behaviour and related actions of people.

Health education and behaviour

The behaviours to be adopted or modified may be that of individuals, groups (such as families, health professionals, organizations or institutions) or entire community.

Strategies designed to influence the behaviour of individuals or groups will vary greatly depending upon the specific disease (or health problem) concerned and its distribution in the population as well as upon the characteristics and acceptability of available methods preventing or controlling that disease (or health problem).

Health education can help to increase knowledge and to reinforce desired behaviour patterns.

It is clear that education is necessary, but education *alone* is insufficient to achieve optimum health. The target population must have access to proven preventive measures or procedures.

Changing concepts

Historically health education has been committed to disseminating information and changing human behaviour. Following the Alma-Ata Declaration adopted in 1978, the emphasis has shifted from *(6)* :

- Prevention of disease to promotion of healthy lifestyles;
- the modification of individual behaviour to modification of "social environment" in which the individual lives ;
- community participation to community involvement; and
- promotion of individual and community "self-reliance"

Aims and objectives

The definition adopted by WHO in 1969 *(15)* and the Alma-Ata Declaration adopted in 1978 provide a useful basis for formulating the aims and objectives of health education, which may be stated as below :

1. to encourage people to adopt and sustain health promoting lifestyle and practices;
2. to promote the proper use of health services available to them;
3. to arouse interest, provide new knowledge, improve skills and change attitudes in making rational decisions to solve their own problems; and
4. to stimulate individual and community self-reliance and participation to achieve health development through individual and community involvement at every step from identifying problems to solving them.

The educational objectives are aimed at the group to be taught in the educational programme. The objectives flow from the health needs which have been discovered. They should be carefully unambiguously defined in terms of knowledge to be acquired, behaviour to be acquired or actions to be mastered. They must be pertinent if the programme is to be appropriate and successful.

The focus of health education is on people and on action *(15)*. Its goal is to make realistic improvements in the basic quality of life. Many health education programmes hope, in some way, to influence behaviour or attitudes. The implication of these new concepts is that health education is an integral part of the national health goals. The fact remains that effective health education has the potential for saving many more lives than has any one research discovery in the foreseeable future.

Role of health care providers

It is clear that education is necessary, but education alone is not sufficient to achieve optimum health. The role of health care providers in this regard comprise to *(6)*:

a. provide opportunities for people to learn how to identify and analyze health and health related problems, and how to set their own targets and priorities ;
b. make health and health related information easily accessible to the community;
c. indicate to the people alternative solutions for solving the health and health-related problems they have identified; and
d. people must have access to proven preventive measures.

APPROACH TO HEALTH EDUCATION

There are 4 well-known approaches to health education :

1. Regulatory approach (Managed prevention)

Regulation in the context of health education may be defined as any governmental intervention, direct or indirect, designed to alter human behaviour. Regulations may be promulgated by the State by a variety of administrative agencies. Regulations may take many forms ranging from prohibition to imprisonment.

The coercive or regulatory approach seeks change in health behaviour and improvement in health through a variety of external control or laws placed on people, as for example, The Child Marriage Restraint Act in India and the use of compulsory seat belts in the western countries. The legislative approach may seem to be simplest and quickest way to improve health or bring about desired changes in society, but there are also important failures of laws, e.g., prohibition of alcohol.

The reasons for the failure of the coercive approach are not far to seek; in the first place, the cause of disease (medical or social) cannot be eradicated by legislation, at the most the government can make laws to prevent a person spreading disease in his community, as for example vaccination in an emergency. Secondly in areas involving personal choice (e.g., diet, exercise, smoking) no government can pass legislation to force people to eat a balanced diet or not to smoke. It amounts to taking away some of the rights of the individual. The disastrous sterilization campaign of 1976 in India which led to the Congress defeat in the 1977 elections is a case in point. The lesson learnt is that it is difficult to enforce a law unless the majority of people are in favour of it and if it does not interfere with the rights of the individual.

However, laws may be useful in times of emergency or in limited situations such as control of an epidemic disease or management of fairs and festivals. Even in cases where it is the duty of the government to make laws to prevent the spread of disease (e.g., AIDS) it is difficult to enforce laws without a vast administrative infrastructure and considerable expenditure. To a degree, the people must be ready to accept a law. In short, the coercive approach runs counter to the basic tenet of health education, that is, in health education, we do not force people to change. In specific situations, legislation can be used to reinforce the pressure to change collective behaviour.

2. Service approach

This approach was tried by the Basic Health Services in 1960's. It aimed at providing all the health services needed by the people at their door steps on the assumption that people would use them to improve their own health. This approach proved a failure because it was not based on the felt-needs of the people. For example, when water-seal latrines were provided by the government, free of cost, many people in the rural areas did not make use of them because it was not their habit to use latrines. The lesson is simple – the people will not accept a programme or service, even if it is offered free of cost, unless it is based on their felt-needs.

3. Health education approach

There are many problems (e.g., cessation of smoking, use of safe water supply, fertility control) which can be solved only through health education. It is a general belief in western democracies that people will be better off if they have autonomy over their own lives, including health affairs on which an informed person should be able to make decisions to protect his own health. These are the higher goals of health education. However, if the necessary behaviour changes are to take place, people must be educated through planned learning experiences what to do, and be informed, educated and encouraged to make their own choice for a healthy life. This approach is consistent with democratic philosophy which does not "order" the individual. The results are slow, but enduring. The mass media and social organizations must be mobilized to help introduce new attitudes and new habits without conflicting with the masses and the collective reaction to particular change.

Since attitudes and behavioural patterns are formed early in life. We must move back in time and start health education with young population. The assumption is that behaviour is more easily controlled or developed in young population than adults *(16)*.

4. Primary health care approach

This is a radically new approach starting from the people with their full participation and active involvement in the planning and delivery of health services based on principals of primary health care, viz. community involvement and intersectoral coordination. The underlying objective is to help individuals to become self-reliant in matters of health. This, in turn, can be done if the people receive the necessary guidance from health care providers in identifying their health problems and finding workable solutions. This approach is a fundamental shift from the earlier approaches.

Health education versus propaganda

Health education is not health propaganda; it is more than mere information or propaganda. To *educate* means to cause or facilitate learning; propaganda means to spread particular systemized doctrine. The differences between health education and propaganda drawn up by the Central Health Education Bureau, Government of India are given in Table 1.

MODELS OF HEALTH EDUCATION

During the past few decades, a number of health education models have been developed *(6)*. They include the following :

1. Medical model

Most health education in the past has relied on knowledge transfer to achieve behaviour changes. The medical model is primarily interested in the recognition and treatment of disease (curing) and technological advances to facilitate the process. It is concerned with disease (as defined by the doctor) or opposed to illness (as defined by the client).

Originally health education developed along the lines of the bio-medical views of health and disease. The emphasis was on dissemination of health information based on scientific facts. The assumption was that people would act on the information supplied by health professionals to improve their health. In this model social, cultural and psychological factors were thought to be of little or no importance. The medical model did not bridge the gap between knowledge and behaviour.

2. Motivation model

When people did not act upon the information they received, health education started emphasizing "motivation" as the main force to translate health information into the desired health action. But the adoption of a new behaviour or idea is not a simple act, it is a process consisting of several stages through which an individual is likely to pass

TABLE 1

Health education and propaganda

	Education	*Propaganda or publicity*
1.	Knowledge and skills actively acquired.	Knowledge instilled in the minds of people.
2.	Makes people think for themselves.	Prevents or discourages thinking by ready-made slogans.
3.	Disciplines primitive desires.	Arouses and stimulates primitive desires.
4.	Develops reflective behaviour. Trains people to use judgement before acting.	Develops reflexive behaviour; aims at impulsive actions.
5.	Appeals to reason.	Appeals to emotion.
6.	Develops individuality, personality and self-expression.	Develops a standard pattern of attitudes and behaviours according to the mould used.
7.	Knowledge acquired through self-reliant activity.	Knowledge is spoon-fed and passively received.
8.	The process is behaviour centred – aims at developing favourable attitudes, habits and skills.	The process is information centred – no change of attitude or behaviour designed.

before adoption. In this regard, sociologists have described 3 stages in the process of change in behaviour (Fig. 2).

1. Awareness	Interest
2. Motivation	Evaluation
	Decision-making
3. Action	Adoption or acceptance

FIG. 2
Adoption model

The individual first goes through AWARENESS or getting general information about the subject. In health education, we must first create awareness of health needs and problems through a programme of public information. Mere awareness is not of much value unless it leads to motivation. Motivation includes the stages of interest, evaluation and decision-making. The individual evinces interest in the subject; he may seek more detailed information about the usefulness, limitations or applicability of the new idea or practice. He then evaluates the various aspects (social, psychological, economic) of the information received, if necessary by consulting others. Such an evaluation is a mental exercise and results in decision-making. He finally decides whether to accept or reject the new idea, programme or proposal. At this stage, interpersonal communication (friends, kinship groups, technical persons) is vital to lend support to his decision. Conviction leads to action, adoption or acceptance of the new idea. The new idea or acquired behaviour becomes part of his own existing values. This is called **Internalization**. Effective communication strategy should be evolved to help the individual in passing from one stage to another.

The above stages are not necessarily rigid; there may be skipping of stages. It is also found that in the same community, people may be in different stages of the adoption process. Adoptions are slow at first and increase as more and more people accept the practice.

3. Social intervention model

Soon, however, it was realized that the public health problems facing us today are so complex that the traditional motivation approach is insufficient to achieve behavioural change, as for example, reducing smoking, adoption of small family norm, raising the age of marriage, elimination of dowry, etc.

The motivation model ignored the fact that in a number of situations, it is not the individual who needs to be changed but the **social environment** which shapes the behaviour of individual and the community. It is often found that people will not readily accept and try something new or novel until it has been "legitimated" (or approved) by the group to which they belong. Most of us prefer to do only the things commonly done by our group. This highlights the importance of group support in helping reaching the decisions and taking action. Adoption of a new idea such as vasectomy or loop insertion is facilitated if there is a group support. This gave birth to the development of social intervention model of health education. An effective health education model is based on precise knowledge of human ecology and understanding of the interaction between the cultural, biological, physical and social environmental factors.

In sum, a coherent strategy needs to be developed involving *all the ways* to change behaviour and to recognize that the approach will differ for different behaviour one wants to change. The need is for a programme of pacts. Reliance on only one method is likely to lead to failures. A combination of approaches using all methods to change life-style and appropriate use of medical care will be necessary.

CONTENTS OF HEALTH EDUCATION

The scope of health education extends beyond the conventional health sector. It covers every aspect of family and community health. While no definite training curricula can be proposed, the content of health education may be divided into the following divisions for the sake of simplicity. Since health education has a limited impact when directed from general education, most of the needed information must be integrated into the educational system (by way of books, classroom material, etc.) and must have the young population as the principal target.

1. *Human biology*

Understanding health, demands an understanding of the human biology, i.e., the structure and functions of the body; how to keep physically fit – the need for exercise, rest and sleep; the effects of alcohol, smoking and drugs on the body; cultivation of healthy lifestyles, etc. Reproductive biology is another area of current interest. UNICEF's "State of the World's Children report 1989" has drawn up a basic list of health information which it believes, every family has a right to know. The list comprises of child spacing, breast-feeding, safe motherhood, immunization, weaning and child growth, diarrhoeal disease, respiratory infections, house hygiene – which could enable families to bring about significant improvements in their own and their children's health *(8)*.

The best place to teach human biology is the school. It is only the school, through its sequential health curriculum, which can provide continuous in-depth learning experiences for millions of students. The provision of information and advice on human biology and hygiene is vital for each new generation.

2. *Nutrition*

The aim of nutrition education is to guide people to choose optimum and balanced diets, remove prejudices and promote good dietary habits – not to teach the familiar jargon of calories and the biochemistry of nutrients. Nutritional problems such as ignorance about the value of breast feeding beyond the first year of life, misconceptions about proper weaning, ignorance of the appropriateness of certain diets for infants and pregnant women, traditional food allocation pattern within the families, etc. can be best solved by nutrition education. In recent years, the link between dietary habits and certain chronic diseases of middle age such as obesity, diabetes and cardio-vascular diseases has been established. Nutrition education is a major intervention for the prevention of malnutrition, promotion of health and improving the quality of life.

3. *Hygiene*

This has two aspects – personal and environmental. The aim of personal hygiene is to promote standards of personal cleanliness within the setting of the condition where people live. *Personal hygiene* includes bathing, clothing, washing hands after toilet; care of nails, feet and teeth; spitting, coughing, sneezing, personal appearance and inculcation of clean habits in the young. Training in personal hygiene should begin at a very early age and must be carried through school age. ENVIRONMENTAL HYGIENE has two aspects – domestic and community. Domestic hygiene comprises that of the home, use of soap, need for fresh air, light and ventilation; hygienic storage of foods; hygienic disposal of wastes, need to avoid pests, rats, mice and insects. Improvement of environmental health is a major concern of many governments and related agencies throughout the world. In the developing countries, the emphasis is on the improvement of basic sanitary services consisting of water supply, disposal of human excreta, other solid and liquid wastes, vector control, food sanitation and housing which are fundamental to health. In many areas, poor sanitary practices among the people have their roots in centuries – old customs, styles of living and habits. These are not easily altered *(17)*.

An environmental sanitation programme should include health education. It is not enough to provide sanitary wells, latrines and waste collecting facilities. People will continue to suffer from the diseases caused by poor sanitation if they do not use the facilities. If a health education approach is taken the people will participate from the beginning in identifying their sanitation problems and will choose the solutions and facilities they want. They will then be more likely to use these facilities and improve their health.

4. *Family health*

The family is the first defence, as well as the chief reliance for the well-being of its members. Health largely depends on the family's social and physical environment and its lifestyle and behaviour. The role of the family in health promotion and in prevention of disease, early diagnosis and care of the sick is of crucial importance. One of the main tasks of health education is to promote the family's self-reliance, especially regarding the family's responsibilities in childbearing, child rearing, self-care and in influencing their children adopt a healthy lifestyle.

5. *Disease prevention and control*

Drugs alone will not solve health problems without health education, a person may fall sick again and again from the same disease. The experiences of western countries have shown the role of education in the eradication of cholera, typhoid, malaria and tuberculosis etc. Education of the people about the prevention and control of locally endemic diseases is the first of eight essential activities in primary health care. Several public health programmes are in operation on a national scale to eradicate diseases such as malaria, tuberculosis, leprosy, filaria, goitre, etc. The recent experience of malaria eradication has indicated that anti-malarial spray with insecticides cannot solve the problem without health education.

6. *Mental health*

Mental health problems occur everywhere. They become more prominent when major killer diseases are brought under control. There is a tendency to an increase in the prevalence of mental diseases when there is a change in the society from an agricultural to an industrial economy, and when people move from the warm intimacy of a village community to the isolation found in big cities. The aim of education in mental health is to help people to keep mentally healthy and to prevent a mental breakdown. People should enjoy their relationships with others and learn to live and work without mental breakdown. There are certain special situations when mental health is of great importance – mother after child birth; child at entry into school for the first time, school child entering the secondary school, decision about a future career, starting a new family and at the time of widowhood. These are critical periods of life when external pressure tends to breakdown mental health. Health workers should help people achieve mental health by showing sympathy, understanding and by social contact.

7. *Prevention of accidents*

Accidents are a feature of the complexity of modern life. In the developed countries, they are taking an increasing toll of life and limb. Accidents occur in three main areas : the home, road and the place of work. Safety education should be directed to these areas. It should be the concern of the engineering department and also the responsibility of the police department to enforce rules of road safety. Accidents occur in workshops, factories, railways and mines. Management must provide a safe environment and promote general order and cleanliness. There should be a place for everything, and everything should be in its place in the factory, in the home, and in the office. The predominant factor in accidents is carelessness and the problem can be tackled through health education.

8. *Use of health services*

Many people particularly in rural areas do not know what health services are available in their community, and many more do not know what signs to look for that indicate a visit to the doctor is necessary. Studies indicate that the public attitude towards health services is still apprehensive. There is a communication gap between the public and the state health administration in the form of "feedback" for further improvement of health services.

One of the declared aims of health education is to inform the people about the health services that are available in the community and how they can utilize them (e.g., screening programmes, immunization, family planning services etc.) and use the health care resources.

PRINCIPLES OF HEALTH EDUCATION

Before we come to the practice of health education, we must know the principles involved. Health education brings together the art and science of medicine, and the principles and practice of general education. The link is to be found in the social and behavioural sciences – sociology, psychology and social anthropology.

Health education cannot be "given" to one person by another. It involves, among other things, the teaching, learning and inculcation of habits concerned with the objective of healthful living. Psychologists have given a great deal of attention to the learning process. Every individual learns and through learning develops the modes of behaviour by which he lives. Learning and teaching is a two-way process of transactions in human relations, between the teacher and taught. The teacher cannot teach unless the pupil wants to learn. Learning takes place not only in the class room, but also outside in the wider world. There is internal learning by which a man grows into an adult individual. It is possible to abstract certain principles of learning and use them in health education. These include :

(1) *Credibility :* It is the degree to which the message to be communicated is perceived as trustworthy by the receiver. Good health education is based on facts – that means it must be consistent and compatible with scientific knowledge and also with the local culture, educational system and social goals. Unless the people have trust and confidence in the communicator, no desired action will ensue after receiving the message.

(2) *Interest :* It is a psychological principle that people are unlikely to listen to those things which are not to their interest. It is salutary to remind ourselves that health teaching should relate to the interests of the people. The public is not interested in health slogans such as "Take care of your health" or "be healthy". A health education programme of this kind would be as useless as asking people to "be healthy", as a nutrition programme asking people to "eat good food". Health educators must find out the real health needs of the people. Psychologists call them "felt-needs", that is needs the people feel about themselves. If a health programme is based on "felt needs" people will gladly participate in the programme; and only then it will be a people's programme. Very often, there are groups who may have health needs of which they are not aware. This is especially true in India where about 25 per cent of the people are illiterate. The health educator will have to bring about a recognition of the needs before he proceeds to tackle them.

(3) *Participation :* Participation is a key word in health education. It is based on the psychological principle of active learning. Health education should aim at encouraging people to work actively with health workers and others in identifying their own health problems and also in developing solutions and plans to work them out. Participation of family members in patient care will create opportunity for more effective, practically based health education. A high degree of participation tends to create a sense of involvement, personal acceptance and decision-making. It provides maximum feedback. The Alma-Ata Declaration states : "The people have a right and duty to participate individually and collectively in the planning and implementation of their health care" *(18)*. If community participation is not an integral part, health programmes are unlikely to succeed *(19)*.

(4) *Motivation :* In every person, there is a fundamental desire to learn. Awakening this desire is called motivation. There are two types of motives – primary and secondary. Primary motives (e.g. sex, hunger, survival) are driving forces initiating people into action; these motives are inborn desires. Secondary motives are based on desires created by outside forces or incentives. Some of the secondary motives are praise, love, rivalry, rewards and punishment, and recognition. In health education, motivation is an important factor; that is, the need for incentives is a first step in learning to change. The incentives may be positive (the carrot) or negative (the stick). To tell a lady, faced with the problem of overweight, to reduce her weight because she might develop cardiovascular disease or it might reduce her life span, may have little effect; but to tell her that by reducing her weight she might look more charming and beautiful, she might accept health advice. When a father promises his child a reward for getting up early everyday, he is motivating the child to inculcate a good habit. In health education, we make use of motivation to change behaviour. Motivation is contagious; one motivated person may spread motivation throughout a group. For example, men who have already had vasectomies are among the best advertisements for male sterilization.

(5) *Comprehension :* In health education we must know the level of understanding, education and literacy of people to whom the teaching is directed. One barrier to communication is using words which cannot be understood. A doctor asked the diabetic to cut down starchy foods; the patient had no idea of starchy foods. A doctor prescribed medicine in the familiar jargon "one teaspoonful three times a day"; the patient, a village woman, had never seen a teaspoon, and could not follow the doctor's directions. In health education, we should always communicate in the language people understand, and never use words which are strange and new to the people. Teaching should be within the mental capacity of the audience.

(6) *Reinforcement :* Few people can learn all that is new in a single period. Repetition at intervals is necessary. If there is no reinforcement, there is every possibility of the individual going back to the pre-awareness stage. If the message is repeated in different ways, people are more likely to remember it.

(7) *Learning by doing :* Learning is an action – process; not a "memorizing" one in the narrow sense. The Chinese proverb : "If I hear, I forget; if I see, I remember; if I do, I know" illustrates the importance of learning by doing.

(8) *Known to unknown :* In health education work, we must proceed "from the concrete to the abstract"; "from the particular to the general"; "from the simple to the more complicated;" "from the easy to more difficult"; and "from the known to the unknown". These are the rules in teaching. We start where the people are and with what they understand and then proceed to new knowledge. We use the existing knowledge of the people as pegs on which to hang new knowledge. In this way systematic knowledge is built up. New knowledge will bring about a new, enlarged understanding which can give rise to an insight into the problem. The way in which medicine has developed from religion to modern medicine serves us as an illustration, the growth of knowledge from the unknown to the known. It is a long process full of obstacles and resistance, and we must not expect quick results.

(9) *Setting an example :* The health educator should set a good example in the things he is teaching. If he is explaining the hazards of smoking, he will not be very successful if he himself smokes. If he is talking about the "small family norm", he will not get very far if his own family size is big.

(10) *Good human relations :* Sharing of information, ideas and feelings happen most easily between people who have a good relationship. Building good relationship with people goes hand in hand with developing communication skills.

(11) *Feedback :* Feedback is one of the key concepts of the systems approach. The health educator can modify the elements of the system (e.g., message, channels) in the light of feedback from his audience. For effective communication, feedback is of paramount importance.

(12) *Leaders :* Psychologists have shown and established that we learn best from people whom we respect and regard. In the work of health education, we try to penetrate the community through the local leaders – the village headman, the school teacher or the political worker. Leaders are agents of change and they can be made use of in health education work. If the leaders are convinced first about a given programme, the rest of the task of implementing the programme will be easy. The attributes of a leader are : he understands the needs and demands of the community; provides proper guidance, takes the initiative, is receptive to the views and suggestions of the people; identifies himself with the community; self-less, honest, impartial, considerate and sincere; easily accessible to the people; able to control and compromise the various factions in the community; possesses the requisite skill and knowledge of eliciting cooperation and achieving coordination of the various official and non-official organizations.

PRACTICE OF HEALTH EDUCATION

Educational material should be designed to focus attention to provide new knowledge, to facilitate interpersonal and group discussion and to reinforce or clarify prior knowledge and behaviour.

1. Audio-visual aids

No health education can be effective without audio-visual aids. They help to simplify unfamiliar concepts; bring about understanding where words fail; reinforce learning by appealing to more than one sense, and provide a dynamic way of avoiding monotony. Modern science has made available an endless array of audio-visual aids which can be classified into three groups *(20)*:

(1) AUDITORY AIDS

Radio, tape-recorder, microphones, amplifiers, earphones.

(2) VISUAL AIDS

(a) *Not requiring projection* : Chalk-board, leaflets, posters, charts, flannelgraph, exhibits, models, specimens, etc.

(b) *Requiring projection* : Slides, film strips.

(3) COMBINED A-V AIDS

Television, sound films (Cinema), slide-tape combination.

A knowledge of the advantages, disadvantages and limitations of each audio-visual aid is necessary in order to make proper use of them. Audio-visual aids are means to an end, not an end in themselves.

2. Methods in health communication

The methods in health communication may be grouped as in Fig. 3.

A rundown of the assets of mass media and personal communication methods is as shown in Table 2.

Any one or a combination of these methods can be used selectively at different times, depending upon the objectives to be achieved, the behaviour to be influenced and available funds.

1. Individual approach

There are plenty of opportunities for individual health education. It may be given in personal *interviews* in the consultation room of the doctor or in the health centre or in the homes of the people. The individual comes to the doctor or health centre because of illness. Opportunity is taken in educating him on matters of interest – diet, causation and nature of illness and its prevention, personal hygiene, environmental hygiene, etc. Topics for health counselling may be selected according to the relevance of the situation. By such individual health teaching, we will be equipping the individual and the family to deal more effectively with the health problems. The responsibility of the attending physician in this regard, is very great because he has the confidence of the patient. The patient will listen more readily to the physician's health counselling. A hint from the doctor may have a more lasting effect than volumes of printed word. The nursing staff have also ample opportunities for undertaking health education. Florence Nightingale said that the nurse can do more good in the home than in the hospital. Public health nurses, health visitors and health inspectors are visiting hundreds of homes, they have plenty of opportunities for individual health teaching. In working with individuals, the health educator must first create an atmosphere of friendship and allow the individual to talk as much as possible. The biggest advantage of individual health teaching is that we can discuss, argue and persuade the individual to change his behaviour. It provides opportunities to ask questions in terms of specific interests. The limitation of individual health teaching is that the numbers we reach are small, and health education is given only to those who come in contact with us.

2. Group approach

Our society contains groups of many kinds – school children, mothers, industrial workers, patients, etc. Group teaching is an effective way of educating the community. The choice of subject in group health teaching is very important; it must relate directly to the interest of the group. For example, we should not broach the subject of tuberculosis control to a mother who has come for delivery; we should talk to her about child-birth and baby care.

Health Communication

Individual approach
1. Personal contact
2. Home visits
3. Personal Letters

Group approach
1. Lectures
2. Demonstrations
3. Discussion methods
   - Group discussion
   - Panel discussion
   - Symposium
   - Workshop
   - Conferences
   - Seminars
   - Role play

Mass approach
1. Television
2. Radio
3. News paper
4. Printed material
5. Direct mailing
6. Posters
7. Health museums and exhibitions
8. Folk methods
9. Internet

FIG. 3
Methods in health communication

TABLE 2

A rundown of assets of mass media and personal communication

Mass Media (TV, radio, newspaper)	Personal communication (Interpersonal and group methods)
1. Reaches the widest population	1. Capitalizes on warmth and understanding and knowledge of communication
2. Gets public attention	2. Provides the opportunity for involvement, for asking questions, expressing fears, and learning more
3. Gives greater support for concentrated programmes such as those for a week or month	3. Can get people to make changes in personal habits more readily, when discussion presents reasonable explanations for these changes.
4. More effective among those with above average educational level	4. More influential with average and below average educational level.

Similarly, school children may be taught about oral hygiene; tuberculosis patients about tuberculosis; and industrial workers about accidents. We have to select also the suitable method of health education including audio-visual aids for successful group health education. A brief account of the methods of group teaching is given below :

(1) Chalk and talk (Lecture)

A lecture may be defined as carefully prepared oral presentation of facts, organized thoughts and ideas by a qualified person. The "chalk" lends the visual component. The chalk and talk communication has still a very important place in small group education. Its effectiveness depends to a large extent on the speaker's ability to write legibly and to draw with chalk on a black board. The talk should be based on a topic of current interest or health needs of the group. The group should not be more than 30 and the talk should not exceed 15 to 20 minutes. If the talk is too long people may become bored and restless.

The lecture method can be made more effective by combining with suitable audio-visual aids such as : (a) *Flipcharts* : They consist of a series of charts (or posters), about 25 by 30 cms or more, each with an illustration pertaining to the talk to be given. They are meant to be shown one after another. Each chart is "flashed" or displayed before a group as the talk is being given. The message on the charts must be brief and to the point. These charts are primarily designed to hold attention of the group and help the lecture to proceed. (b) *Flannelgraph* : A piece of rough flannel or khadi fixed over a wooden board provides an excellent background for displaying cut-out pictures, graphs, drawings and other illustrations. The cut-out pictures and other illustrations are provided with a rough surface at the back by pasting pieces of sand paper, felt or rough cloth and they adhere at once when put on the flannel. Flannelgraph offers the advantage that pre-arranged sequence of pictures displayed one after another helps maintain continuity and adds much to the presentation. The other advantages are that the flannelgraph is a very cheap medium, easy to transport and promotes thought and criticism (c) *Exhibits :* Objects, models, specimens, etc. convey a specific message to the viewer. They are essentially mass media of communication, which can also be used in group teaching. (d) *Films and charts :* These are mass media of communication. If used with discrimination, they can be of value in educating small groups.

Lectures can be faulted on a number of grounds. Their disadvantages include the following : students are involved to a minimum extent; learning is passive; do not stimulate thinking or problem-solving capacity; the comprehension of a lecture varies with the student; and the health behaviour of the listeners is not necessarily affected.

(2) Demonstrations

A demonstration is a carefully prepared presentation to show how to perform a skill or procedure. Here a procedure (e.g. lumber puncture, disinfection of a well) is carried out step by step before an audience or the target group, the demonstrator ascertaining that the audience understands how to perform it. The demonstrator involves the audience in discussion.

Demonstration (a) dramatizes by arousing interest (b) persuades the onlookers to adopt recommended practices (c) upholds the principles of "seeing is believing" and "learning by doing", and (d) can bring desirable changes in the behaviour pertaining to the use of new practice.

Demonstration as a means of communication has been found to have a high educational value in programmes like environmental sanitation (e.g., installation of a hand-pump, construction of a sanitary latrine); mother and child health (e.g. demonstration of oral rehydration technique) and control of diseases (e.g., scabies). The clinical teaching in hospitals is based on demonstrations. This method has a high motivational value.

(3) Group discussion

A "group" is an "aggregation of people interacting in a face-to-face situation". This contrasts sharply to the group of students in a class room situation. Group discussion is considered a very effective method of health communication. It permits the individuals to learn by freely exchanging their knowledge, ideas and opinions. Group discussion provides a wider interaction among members than is possible with other methods. Where long term compliance is involved (e.g., cessation of smoking, obesity reduction) group discussion is considered valuable.

For effective group discussion, the group should comprise not less than 6 and not more than 12 members. The participants are all seated in a circle, so that each is fully visible to all the others (Fig. 4). There should be a group leader who initiates the subject, helps the discussion in the proper manner, prevents side-conversations, encourages everyone to participate and sums up the discussion in the end. If the discussion goes well, the group may arrive at decisions which no individual member would have been able to make alone. It is also desirable to have a person to record whatever is discussed. The "recorder" prepares a report on the issues discussed and agreements reached. In a group discussion, the members should observe the following rules : (a) express ideas clearly and concisely (b) listen to what others say (c) do not interrupt when others are speaking (d) make only relevant remarks (e) accept criticism gracefully and (f) help to reach conclusions *(9)*. Group discussion is successful if the members know each other beforehand, when they can discuss freely.

A well conducted group discussion with adequate resources (Fig. 4) is very effective in reaching decisions, based on the ideas of ALL people. The decision taken by the group tends to be adopted more readily than in situations where the decision is a solitary one. Thus the group acceptance has a binding effect on the individual member to translate their acceptance into action. A well-conducted group discussion is effective for changing attitudes and the health behaviour of people.

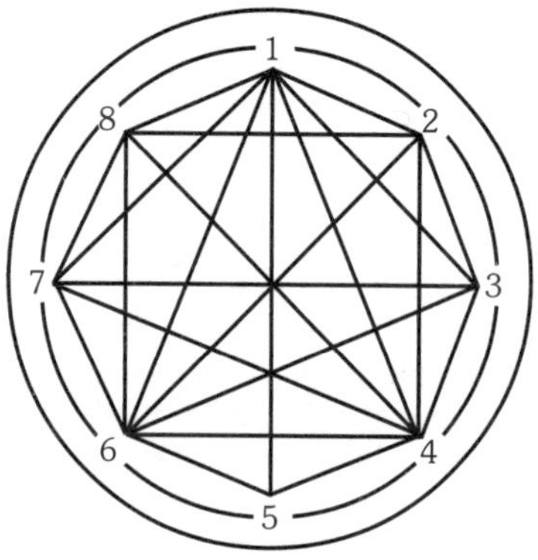

FIG. 4
A good group discussion

Limitations : Group discussion is not without limitations. Those who are shy may not take part in the discussions. Some may dominate the discussion (Fig. 5). Thus there may be unequal participation of members in a group discussion, unless properly guided. Some members may deviate from the subject and make the discussion irrelevant or unprofitable.

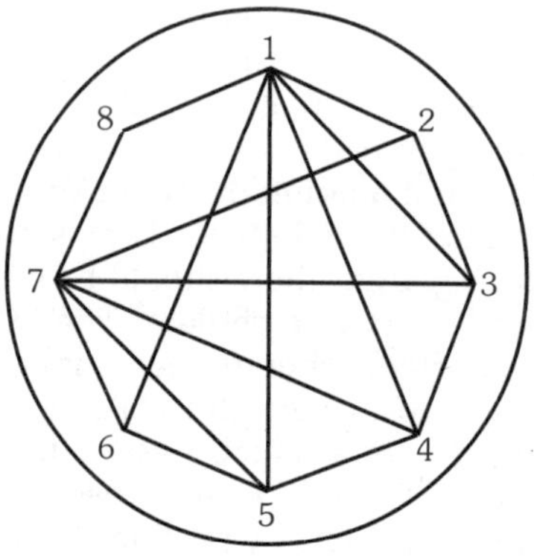

FIG. 5
A dominated group. No.1 and No.7 dominate the discussion

(4) Panel discussion

In a panel discussion, 4 to 8 persons who are qualified to talk about the topic sit and discuss a given problem, or the topic, in front of a large group or audience. The panel comprises, a chairman or moderator and from 4 to 8 speakers. The chairman opens the meeting, welcomes the group and introduces the panel speakers. He introduces the topic briefly and invites the panel speakers to present their points of view. There is no specific agenda, no order of speaking and no set speeches *(21)*. The success of the panel depends upon the chairman; he has to keep the discussion going and develop the train of thought. After the main aspects of the subject are explored by the panel speakers, the audience is invited to take part. The discussion should be spontaneous and natural. If members of the panel are unacquainted with this method, they may have a preliminary meeting, prepare the material on the subject and decide upon the method and plan of presentation. Panel discussion can be an extremely effective method of education, provided it is properly planned and guided.

(5) Symposium *(21,22)*

A symposium is a series of speeches on a selected subject. Each person or expert presents an aspect of the subject briefly. There is no discussion among the symposium members like in panel discussion. In the end, the audience may raise questions. The chairman makes a comprehensive summary at the end of the entire session.

(6) Workshop *(21, 22, 23)*

The workshop is the name given to a novel experiment in education. It consists of a series of meetings, usually four or more, with emphasis on individual work, within the group, with the help of consultants and resource personnel. The total workshop may be divided into small groups and each group will choose a chairman and a recorder. The individuals work, solve a part of the problem through their personal effort with the help of consultants, contribute to group work and group discussion and leave the workshop with a plan of action on the problem. Learning takes place in a friendly, happy and democratic atmosphere, under expert guidance. The workshop provides each participant opportunities to improve his effectiveness as a professional worker.

(7) Role playing *(21, 22)*

Role playing or socio-drama is based on the assumption that many values in a situation cannot be expressed in words, and the communication can be more effective if the situation is dramatised by the group. The group members who take part in the socio-drama enact their roles as they have observed or experienced them. The audience is not passive but actively concerned with the drama. They are supposed to pay sympathetic attention to what is going on, suggest alternative solutions at the request of the leader and if requested, come up and take an active part by demonstrating how they feel a particular role should be handled, or the like. The size of the group is thought to be best at about 25. Role playing is a useful technique to use in providing discussion of problems of human relationship. It is a particularly useful educational device for school children. Role playing is followed by a discussion of the problem.

(8) Conferences and seminars

This category contains a large component of commercialized continuing education. The programmes are usually held on a regional, state or national level. They range from once half-day to one week in length and may cover a single topic in depth or be broadly comprehensive. They usually use a variety of formats to aid the learning process from self instruction to multimedia.

3. Mass approach – Education of the general public

No health worker or health team can mount an effective health education programme for the whole community, except through **mass media** of communication. The evolution of the media has been rapid. Uptill the early 1920s, mass communication depended largely on what was printed – posters, pamphlets, books, periodicals and newspapers. Then came the radio and with it a new dimension of experience. TV went a gigantic step further and has become a very powerful weapon. The press caters primarily to the eye, the radio appeals to the ear, and TV to both eye and ear. A final word about radio and TV – they come close to the warmth and motivational effect of a person-to-person communication. They have become part of the fabric of modern civilization.

Mass media are a "one-way" communication. They are useful in transmitting messages to people even in the remotest places. The number of people who are reached usually count in millions. Their effectiveness can give high returns for the time and money involved.

Mass media alone are generally inadequate in changing human behaviour. For effective health communication, they should be used in combination with other methods. The power of mass media in creating a political will in favour of health, raising the health consciousness of the people, setting norms, delivering technical messages, popularising health knowledge and fostering community involvement are well recognized *(6)*. Public health methodologies should be culturally appropriate; they should be carefully thought-out before use. A brief account of the mass media is given below :

1. Television

Television has become the most popular of all media. It is effective in not only creating awareness, but also to an extent influencing public opinion and introducing new ways of life. It is raising levels of understanding and helping people familiarise with things they have not seen before, including crime and violence which are shown as part of feature programmes. TV is a one-way channel. It can only be an aid to teaching. It cannot cover all areas of learning. It has much potential for health communication.

2. Radio

Radio is found nearly in every home. In many developing countries the radio has a broader audience than TV. Both radio and TV can reach illiterate population not accessible through printed word. It is a purely didactic medium. It can be valuable aid in "putting across" useful health information, in the form of straight talks, plays, questions and answers and quiz programmes. Radio is much cheaper than TV. Doctors and health workers may speak out on radio. Local health issues may be identified and discussed leading to increased general awareness.

3. Internet

This new means of computer based communication system has opened vast capability of transfer of knowledge, and has made it possible to get into direct and instant communication across the world by means of e-mail and even a online chat. This is a fast growing communication media and holds very large potential to become a major health education tool. Already a fairly large number of persons in India are using this media, and the numbers are growing everyday. Vast amount of health related literature from WHO and other health agencies is available on line. The Health related information from the ministry of health and family welfare Govt. of India, is also available on their website.

4. Newspapers

Newspapers are the most widely disseminated of all forms of literature. News must be newsworthy before it is printed. Whereas many people turn to radio or TV for entertainment, newspaper readers are often seeking newspapers. Newspapers should, therefore provide more factual, detailed and even statistical material *(7)*. Unfortunately, health problems have little of value to newspapers. Newspapers have limitation of having low readership in rural areas because of illiteracy. They reach only a limited group, i.e. the literates in the community.

5. Printed material

Magazines, pamphlets, booklets and hand-outs have long been in use for health communication. They are aimed at those who can read. Their usefulness lies in the fact that they can convey detailed information. They can be produced in bulk for very little cost, and can be shared by others in the family and community.

6. Direct mailing

This is a new innovation in health communication in India. The intention is to reach the remote areas of the country with printed word (e.g., folders and newsletters and booklets on family planning, immunization and nutrition etc.). These are sent directly to village leaders, literate persons, panchayats and local bodies and others who are considered as opinion leaders. Direct mailing has been a successful mass media in creating public awareness. It is possibly the most personal of mass communication.

7. Posters, billboards and signs

These are intended to catch the eye and create awareness. Therefore, the message to be communicated must be simple, and artistic. Posters are not expensive when one considers they are seen by a large number of people. Motives such as humour and fear are introduced into posters in order to hold the attention of the public. In places where the exposure time is short (e.g., streets), the message of the poster should be short, simple, direct and one that can be taken at a glance and easy to understand immediately. In places where people have some time to spend (e.g., bus stops, railway stations, hospitals, health centres) the poster can present more information. The right amount of matter should be put up in the right place and at the right time. That is, when there is an epidemic of viral hepatitis, there should be posters displayed on viral jaundice, but not on cholera. The life of a poster is usually short; posters should be changed frequently, otherwise they will lose their effect. As a media of health education, posters have much less effect in changing behaviour than its enthusiastic users would hope. Indiscriminate use of posters by pasting them on walls serves no other useful purpose than covering the wall.

8. Health museums and exhibitions

If properly organized, health museums and exhibitions can attract large numbers of people. By presenting a variety of ideas, they do increase knowledge and awareness. Photographic panels attract more persons than graphic panels. This is because photos give a humanized touch to the communication. The three dimensional models with lighted visuals are even more effective than photos.

In exhibitions, there is a big element of personal communication through workers who explain each item on the exhibit. Printed literature explaining the exhibits is often freely distributed. Health exhibitions and museums thus offer a package of both personal and impersonal methods of communication.

9. Folk media

The term "mass communication" ought to refer to the totality of communication which takes within its compass not only the electronic media, but also folk (or indigenous) media such as keerthan, katha, folk songs, dances and dramas and puppet shows which have roots in our culture. The muslims have their own traditional folk forum like the ghazals, the kawali.

The mass media are only "instruments". As such they are neither good nor bad; what matters is the message they carry and the way the message is delivered *(6)*. There is no single way to do public education. Health education is still art rather than a science. Each community and country should develop techniques that meet its own needs.

PLANNING AND MANAGEMENT

Health education cannot be planned in a vacuum. It is planned in connection with a specific health programme or health service. Therefore, the specifics of a health education strategy in a local community have to be formulated in accordance with its socio-cultural, psycho-social, political, economic and situational characteristics. The planners should be fully conversant with the health education needs of the particular programme for which health education is to be planned.

Health education planning follows the main steps in scientific planning, which are :

1. Collecting information on specific problems as seen by the community
2. Identification of the problem
3. Deciding on priorities
4. Setting goals and measurable objectives
5. Assessment of resources
6. Consideration of possible solutions
7. Preparation of a plan of action :
   (i) What will be done ?
   (ii) When ?
   (iii) By whom ?
8. Implementing the plan
9. Monitoring and evaluating the degree to which stated objectives have been achieved
10. Reassessment of the process of planning. Planning and evaluation are essential for effective health education. The subject of planning is discussed more fully in chapter 23.

All health education work requires continuous evaluation to measure the effectiveness of health education activities in achieving stated objectives and to assess the importance on programme performance of such variables as knowledge, attitudes, behaviour change and consumer satisfaction.

ADMINISTRATION AND ORGANIZATION

Governments have a responsibility for assisting and guiding the health education of the general public. At the national level, the Government of India in 1956 established a Central Health Education Bureau in the Ministry of Health, New Delhi to promote and coordinate health education work in the country. Many state governments in India have now Health Education Bureaux in their Health Directorate.

There are also other official agencies in the country such as the Directorate of Advertising and Visual Publicity (DAVP), Press Information Bureau, Doordarshan and All India Radio which are active in health education work. Several voluntary agencies such as Indian Red Cross are also engaged in the health education work. At the international level, there is an International Union for Health Education with headquarters in Paris, whose main task is to promote the creation of national societies for health education. The South East Asia Regional Bureau (SEARB) of the International Union for Health Education was established in 1983 with headquarters at Bangalore.

A new division of Health Education and Health Promotion has been established by the WHO. The division will support regional offices of WHO in strengthening national capabilities in health education and promotion, and develop and test new ideas and tools. (The former Division of Public Information and Education for Health is now called Division of Public Information and Public Relations).

Health education is a complex activity in which different individuals and organizations play a part. Among them are parents, teachers, friends, physicians, nurses, health workers and various organizations, governmental and non-governmental. No country in the world, least of all a country with a large population and small resources such as India, can afford to employ institutionally trained health workers. Therefore, health education should be the concern of everybody engaged in any form of community welfare work.

References

1. Kumar, K.J. (1982). *Business Communication,* A Modern Approach, Jaico Publication House Mumbai.
2. Lilbert, J.J., (1977). *Educational Hand Book for Health Personnel,* WHO (offset publication No. 35).
3. Kumar, K.J. (1987). *Mass Communication in India,* Jaico Publication House Mumbai.
4. Dr. Dubey and A.K. Devgan (1969). *Family Planning Communication Studies in India,* NIHAE New Delhi.
5. O.P. Dahama and O.P. Bhatnagar (1987). *Education and Communication for Development 2nd Ed.,* Oxford and IBH New Delhi.
6. *T R S* 690 P 8 1983.
7. *T R S* 695 1983.
8. UNICEF *State of World's Children* 1989.
9. WHO (1988), *Education for Health :* A manual on health education in primary health care.
10. *T R S* 766 1988.
11. NIHAE : *A Guide to Communication System in Hospitals* Tech. Rept 16 Glossary P 33.
12. Last J M Dictionary.
13. Green L W (1979). *Int. J. of Health Education* 22: 161 - 168.
14. Somers, Anne R. (1977). *Prev. Medicine,* 6 (3) 406.
15. *T R S* 409 (1969). P 8.
16. Haggerty R.J. (1977). *Preventive Medicine* 6 : 282.
17. WHO (1974). *WHO Offset Publication* No. 7.
18. Health For All Sr. No. 1.
19. *T R S* 782 (1982) 41 - 42.
20. WHO (1972). *Public Health Papers* No.47, p. 53.
21. Subramanian, R. (1966). *Health Education.* A Practical Guide for Health Personnel, The State Health Education Bureau, Directorate of Health Services Trivandrum.
22. Garland, J.V. (1951). *Discussion Methods,* M.H. Wilson, New York.
23. Kelley E.C. (1950). *The Workshop Way of Learning,* Harper & Row, N.Y.

23 Health Planning and Management

"Plan ahead - it was not raining when Noah built the ark"

Planning and management are relatively new subjects. Planning is for tomorrow, and management is for today. These subjects have acquired great importance during the past two decades. The purpose of planning is (1) to match the limited resources with many problems; (2) to eliminate wasteful expenditure or duplication of expenditure; and (3) to develop the best course of action to accomplish a defined objective. The increasing demand for medical and health care services, in the face of limited resources, has brought out the need for careful planning and management of health services. Planning and management are considered essential if higher standards of health and health care are to be achieved *(1)*.

Planning in its broadest sense includes three steps:

(a) Plan formulation;
(b) Execution; and
(c) Evaluation

Planning is a matter of team work and consultation. The planning team consists of not only specialists within the field, but also specialized in other fields, viz. economics, statistics, sociology, management, etc.

DEVELOPMENT PLANNING

Every country has its own plan for national development. The purpose of national planning is to achieve a rapid, balanced, economic and social development of the country as a whole. The National Development Plan of a country is a combination of sectoral plans which comprise the following sectors, viz. food and agriculture, education, health and family planning, industry, transport and communications, housing, power, social welfare, etc. All these sectors compete for national resources *(2)*.

In this context, National Development Planning has been defined as "continuous, systematic, coordinated, planning for the investment of the resources of a country (men, money and materials) in programmes aimed at achieving the most rapid economic and social development possible *(3)*.

HEALTH PLANNING

Health planning is a concept of recent origin. It is part of national development planning. Health planning is necessary for the economic utilisation of material, man-power and financial resources. The purpose of health planning is to improve the health services.

In this context, National Health Planning has been defined as "the orderly process of defining community health problems, identifying unmet needs and surveying the resources to meet them, establishing priority goals that are realistic and feasible and projecting administrative action to accomplish the purpose of the proposed programme" *(3)*.

Health needs and demands

The purpose of health planning is to meet the health needs and demands of the people. Health needs have been defined as "deficiencies in health that call for preventive, curative, control or eradication measures" *(3)*; The need for medical care, safe water supply, adequate nutrition, immunization, family planning are all community health needs. It may be mentioned that the health needs as seen by the people are not exactly the same as seen by experts. Some needs may not be perceived at all; others vaguely perceived, and still others awaken only on contact with new ways of life. People's needs are conditioned by their aspirations. In a democratic society, people's needs may be presented as demands.

Resources

The term "resources" is widely used in health planning. It implies the manpower, money, materials, skills, knowledge, techniques and time needed or available for the performance or support of action directed towards specified objectives. The resources can be readily wasted if there is no proper planning and management.

Objectives, targets and goals

A number of words are used to describe the end results of planning – objective, target, goal. These words are drawn from military and sports terminology. An important element of planning is the setting of clear-cut objectives, targets and goals. Let us consider the meaning of these words:

An OBJECTIVE (point) is precise – it is either achieved or not achieved. It is a planned end-point of all activities. A TARGET often refers to a discrete activity such as the number of blood films collected or vasectomies done; it permits the concept of degree of achievement. Targets are thus concerned with the factors involved in a problem, whereas objectives are concerned directly with the problem itself.

GOAL is defined as the ultimate desired state towards which objectives and resources are directed. Unlike objectives and targets, goals are not constrained by time or existing resources, nor are they necessarily attainable. Goals formulated at the highest level are generally broad. A goal is usually described in terms of (1) what is to be attained; (2) the extent to which it is to be attained; (3) the population or section of the environment involved; (4) the geographic area in which the proposed programme will operate; and (5) the length of time required for attaining the goal *(3)*.

Plan

Planning results in the formulation of a Plan. A "Plan" is a blue print for taking action. It consists of five major elements; objectives, policies, programmes, schedules and budget.

A "programme" is a sequence of activities designed to implement policies and accomplish objectives. A programme gives a step-by-step approach to guide the action necessary to reach a predetermined goal. Programmes must be closely integrated with objectives.

A "schedule" is a time sequence for the work to be done. "Procedures" are a set of rules for carrying out work which, when observed by all, help to ensure the maximum use of the resources and efforts. "Policies" are the guiding principles stated as an expectation, not as a commandment.

Pre-planning

Pre-planning is preparation for planning. The important preconditions are : *(a) Government interest :* Any plan for the health and welfare of a country must be based on a strong 'political will' as manifested by clear directives or policies given by the political authority. *(b) Legislation :* The social and health policies formulated may have to be translated into legislation. As an example may be cited the enactment of the Medical Termination of Pregnancy Act, 1971, by the Indian Parliament to protect the health of mothers. *(c) Organization for planning :* There should be an organizational structure for the preparation of the various parts of the plan. The Planning Commission in India serves this function. It is composed of fulltime planners who are advised by representatives and technical experts in the field of social and economic development as well as political leaders. *(d) Administrative capacity :* One of the essential pre-conditions of planning is administrative capacity for proper coordination of activities and implementation of the plan at all levels. For the health plan, administrative capacity is vested in the Central and State Ministries of Health.

PLANNING CYCLE

Planning is the broad foundation on which much of the management is based. Planning may be defined as a process of analysing a system, or defining a problem, assessing the extent to which the problem exists as a need, formulating goals and objectives to alleviate or ameliorate those identified needs, examining and choosing from among alternative intervention strategies, initiating the necessary action for its implementation and monitoring the system to ensure proper implementation of the plan and evaluating the results of intervention in the light of stated objectives. Planning thus involves a succession of steps *(3, 4, 5)*. These are as shown in Fig. 1.

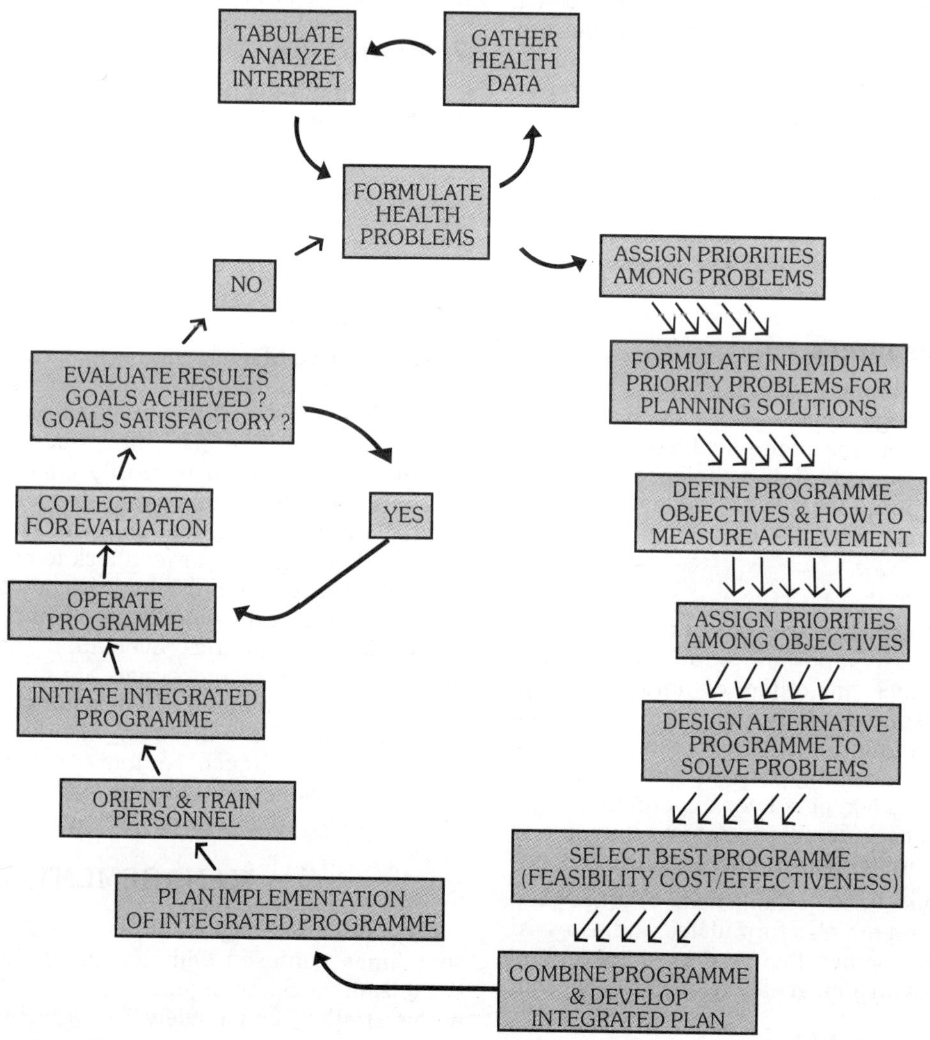

FIG. 1
The planning cycle

1. Analysis of the health situation

The first step in health planning is analysis of the health situation. It involves the collection, assessment and interpretation of information in such a way as to provide a clear picture of the health situation. The following items of data are the minimum essential requirements for health planning:

(a) The population, its age and sex structure;
(b) Statistics of morbidity and mortality;
(c) The epidemiology and geographical distribution of different diseases;
(d) Medical care facilities such as hospitals, health centres, and other health agencies – both public and private;
(e) The technical manpower of various categories;
(f) Training facilities available; and
(g) Attitudes and beliefs of the population towards disease, its cure and prevention.

The analysis and interpretation of the above data brings out the health problems, the health needs and health demands of the population.

2. Establishment of objectives and goals

Objectives and goals are needed to guide efforts. Unless objectives are established, there is likely to be haphazard activity, uneconomical use of funds and poor performance. Objectives must be established at all levels, down to the smallest organizational unit. At upper levels, objectives are general; at successively lower levels, they become more specified and detailed. The objectives may be short-term or long-term. In setting these objectives, time and resources are important factors. Objectives are not only a guide to action, but also a yard-stick to measure work after it is done. Modern management techniques such as "cost-benefit" analysis, and "input-output" study of health services are being used for defining goals, objectives and targets in more definite terms than hitherto.

3. Assessment of resources

The term resources implies the manpower, money, materials, skills, knowledge and techniques needed or available for the implementation of the health programmes. These resources are assessed and a balance is struck between what is required and what is available, or likely to be available in terms of resources.

4. Fixing priorities

Once the problems, resources and objectives have been determined, the next most important step in planning is establishment of priorities in order of importance or magnitude, since the resources always fall short of the total requirement. In fixing priorities, attention is paid to financial constraints, mortality and morbidity data, diseases which can be prevented at low cost, saving the lives of younger people in whom there has been considerable social investment; and also political and community interests and pressures.

Once priorities have been established, ALTERNATE PLANS for achieving them are also formulated and assessed in order to determine whether they are practicable and feasible. Alternate plans with greater effectiveness are chosen.

5. Write-up of formulated plan

The next major step in the planning process is the preparation of the detailed plan or plans. The plan must be complete in all respects for the execution of a project. For each proposed health programme, the resources (inputs) required are related to the results (outputs) expected. Each stage of the plan is defined and costed and the time needed to implement is specified. The plan must contain working guidance to all those responsible for execution. It must also contain a "built-in" system of evaluation. It will be left to the central planning authority and the government to consider modifications of the plan relating to allocation of resources.

6. Programming and implementation

Once the health plan has been selected and approved by the policy making authorities, programming and implementation are begun. Plan execution depends upon the existence of effective organization. The organizational structure must incorporate well-defined procedures to be followed and sufficient delegation of authority to and fixation of responsibility of different workers for achieving the predetermined objectives during the period prescribed. It is at the implementation stage that shortcomings often appear in practice. Many well considered plans have fallen down because of delays in critical supplies, inappropriate use of staff, and similar factors. The main considerations at the implementation stage include: (a) definition of roles and tasks (b) the selection, training, motivation and supervision of the manpower involved (c) organization and communication, and (d) the efficiency of individual institutions such as hospitals or health centres.

7. Monitoring

Monitoring is the day-to-day follow-up of activities during their implementation to ensure that they are proceeding as planned and are on schedule. It is a continuous process of observing, recording, and reporting on the activities of the organization or project. Monitoring, thus, consists of keeping track of the course of activities and identifying deviations and taking corrective action if excessive deviations occur.

8. Evaluation

The purpose of evaluation is to assess the achievement of the stated objectives of a programme, its adequacy, its efficiency and its acceptance by all parties involved. While monitoring is confined to day-to-day or ongoing operations, evaluation is mostly concerned with the final outcome and with factors associated with it. Good planning will have a built-in evaluation to measure the performance and effectiveness and for feedback to correct deficiencies or fill up gaps discovered during implementation. In the words of the WHO Expert Committee on National Health Planning in Developing Countries, evaluation "measures the degree to which objectives and targets are fulfilled and the quality of the results obtained. It measures the productivity of available resources in achieving clearly defined objectives. It measures how much output or cost-effectiveness is achieved. It makes possible the reallocation of priorities and of resources on the basis of changing health needs" *(6)*.

MANAGEMENT *(7)*

The term "management" is used in many senses. It is sometimes confused with administration; sometimes with organization. Some equate the terms, management and administration. Others view it as a technique of leadership. The widely prevalent view is that administration broadly means "getting things done" and management as "the purposeful and effective use of resources – manpower, materials and finances – for fulfilling a pre-determined objective". In theory, management consists of four basic activities :

(i) *planning*: determining what is to be done.
(ii) *organizing:* setting up the framework or apparatus and making it possible for groups to do the work.
(iii) *communicating*: motivating people to do the work.
(iv) *monitoring (controlling):* checking to make sure the work is progressing satisfactorily.

Management techniques are familiar in business, industry, defence and other fields. The current emphasis by WHO and many governments is on improving the efficiency of the health care delivery systems through the application of modern management methods and techniques.

MANAGEMENT METHODS AND TECHNIQUES *(1, 8, 9)*

Management techniques are many. They are based on principles of behavioural sciences as well as *quantitative* methods. These techniques have been developed by experts of management science to help the managers of any organization to achieve the stated goals more efficiently. Efforts are being made by the WHO for making these techniques more popular for application in the health field. A brief account of these techniques is given below :

Methods based on behavioural sciences

1. ORGANIZATIONAL DESIGN

Poor organization results in waste of resources. It is a theory of management that organization must be suited to its current situation and the needs to be serviced. The organization of health services should, therefore, be designed so as to meet the health needs and demands of the people. Further, the organizational design should be reviewed every few years because of changing concepts or purpose, changing problems and changing technology. Efficient delivery of health services depends upon the existence of an effective organization.

2. PERSONNEL MANAGEMENT

This is skilful use of human resources. Proper methods of selection, training and motivation; division of responsibility; distribution of roles; elimination of "square pegs in round holes" (i.e., professional staff not suited to administration, either through training, selection or natural inclination, should not be entrusted with administrative and management burdens); incentive for better work; opportunities for promotion and professional advancement; effective design of "health teams" are all fundamental techniques of personnel management which could contribute to the efficiency of health service delivery.

3. COMMUNICATION

Better communication contributes to effective functioning of an organization. Communication roadblocks exist at various levels: between the doctor and the patient; doctor and nurse; between the senior officials and juniors; between the directorate and the health ministry; between the health ministry and other ministries and rest of the government. Communication barriers are responsible for delays in regular reporting and notification; delays in the compilation of statistics; delays in the release of supplies and salaries; delays in the institution of prompt remedial measures. In fact, these are some of the major weaknesses in health ministries. One of the tasks of health management is to solve the communication problems by establishing suitable vertical and horizontal communication channels.

4. INFORMATION SYSTEMS

Information is needed for day-to-day management of the health system. Information comes from many sources – both formal and informal. The information system should be tailored according to the management needs of the individual health services. The functions of an information system consist of collection, classification, transmission, storage, retrieval, transformation and display of information. A good information system provides data for monitoring and evaluation of health programmes and gives the requisite feedback to health administrators and planners at all levels. Computers can play a great role in improving the health information system.

5. MANAGEMENT BY OBJECTIVES (MBO)

Objectives are set forth for different units and subunits, each of which prepares its own plan of action – usually on a short-term basis. This helps in achieving the results more effectively and smoothly.

Quantitative methods

Quantitative methods are derived from the field of economics, operation research and budgeting. Some of these techniques have a great role in the management of health services :

1. COST-BENEFIT ANALYSIS

This is a management technique which has attracted the widest attention for application in the health field. The economic benefits of any programme are compared with the cost of that programme. The benefits are expressed in monetary terms to determine whether a given programme is economically sound, and to select the best out of several alternate programmes. The main drawback with this technique is that the benefits in the health field, as a result of a particular programme, cannot always be expressed in monetary terms. We generally express the benefit in terms of births or deaths prevented, or illness avoided or overcome. Hence the scope of applying this method is rather vague.

2. COST-EFFECTIVE ANALYSIS

This is a more promising tool for application in the health field than cost-benefit analysis. It is similar to cost-benefit analysis except that benefit, instead of being expressed in monetary terms is expressed in terms of results achieved, e.g., number of lives saved or the number of days free from disease. However, even cost-effective analysis is not possible in many cases.

3. COST-ACCOUNTING *(10)*

It provides basic data on cost structure of any programme. Financial records are kept in a manner permitting costs to be associated with the purpose for which they are incurred. Cost-accounting has three important purposes in health services : (a) cost control; (b) planning and allocation of people and financial resources; and (c) pricing of cost reimbursement.

4. INPUT-OUTPUT ANALYSIS

Input-output analysis is an economic technique. In the

health field, "input" refers to all health service activities which consume resources (manpower, money, materials and time); and "output" refers to such useful outcomes as cases treated, lives saved or inoculations performed. An input-output table shows how much of each "input" is needed to produce a unit amount of each "output". It enables calculations to be made of the effects of changing the inputs.

5. MODEL

The model is a basic concept of management science. It is an aid to understand how the factors in a situation affect one another. It is an abstraction of the reality, not the reality itself. The decision process includes the use of a model.

6. SYSTEMS ANALYSIS

The purpose of systems analysis is to help the decision maker to choose an appropriate course of action by investigating his problem, searching out objectives, finding out alternative solutions, evaluation of the alternatives in terms of cost-effectiveness, re-examination of the objectives if necessary and finding the most cost-effective alternative. Systems analysis is essentially finding the cost-effectiveness of the available alternatives. The system can be a hospital supply system, an information system, a total community health service system, an outpatient clinic or any other system with problems of management. A system may be made of independent subsystems.

7. NETWORK ANALYSIS

A network is a graphic plan of all events and activities to be completed in order to reach an end objective (Fig. 2). It brings greater discipline in planning. The two common types of network technique are (a) PERT and (b) CPM.

(a) PERT (Programme Evaluation and Review Technique) is a management technique which makes possible more detailed planning and more comprehensive supervision. Every housewife who plans a meal so that each part of the menu is completed at the same time is using the basic technique of PERT.

The essence of PERT is to construct an Arrow Diagram (Fig. 2). The diagram represents the logical sequence in which events must take place. It is possible with such a diagram to calculate the time by which each activity must be completed, and to identify those activities that are critical. This simple technique provides a basic discipline by which all concerned in a project can know what is expected of them and to minimise any delays or crises in the implementation of the plan.

PERT is a useful management technique which can be applied to a great variety of projects. It aids in planning, scheduling and monitoring the project; it allows better communication between the various levels of management; it identifies potential problems; it furnishes continuous, timely progress reports; it forms a solid foundation upon which to build an evaluation and checking system.

(b) CRITICAL PATH METHOD (CPM) : The longest path of the network (Fig. 2) is called "critical path". If any activity along the critical path is delayed, the entire project will be delayed *(11)*.

8. PLANNING–PROGRAMMING–BUDGETING SYSTEM (PPBS)

The Planning–Programming–Budgeting System (PPBS) is primarily a system to help decision makers to allocate resources so that the available resources of an organization are used in the most effective way in achieving its objectives. The PPBS does not call for changes in the existing organization. It calls for grouping of *activities* into *programmes* related to each *objective.* Another approach is known as the 'Zero Budget Approach", i.e., all budgets start at zero and no one gets any budget that he cannot specifically justify on a year-to-year basis.

9. WORK SAMPLING

It is systematic observation and recording of activities of one or more individuals, carried out at predetermined or random intervals. It provides quantitative measurement of the various activities. The major parameters that are analysed are the type of activities performed and the time needed to do specified jobs. Work sampling studies have been done on doctors, nurses, pharmacists and laboratory technicians. Work sampling permits judgments to the appropriateness of current staff, job description and training. It helps in standardising the methods of performing jobs and determining the manpower needs in any organization.

10. DECISION MAKING

Decision making is just like the basic discipline of differential diagnosis in medical practice. It is an adage that decisions should be made at the level where the best decisions can be made; it does not follow that the best decision is always made at the top of an organization. Decisions should not be made with incomplete data. In the health sector, decisions have to be made about development of resources, optimum work load for medical and paramedical workers, strategies for providing health care, etc.

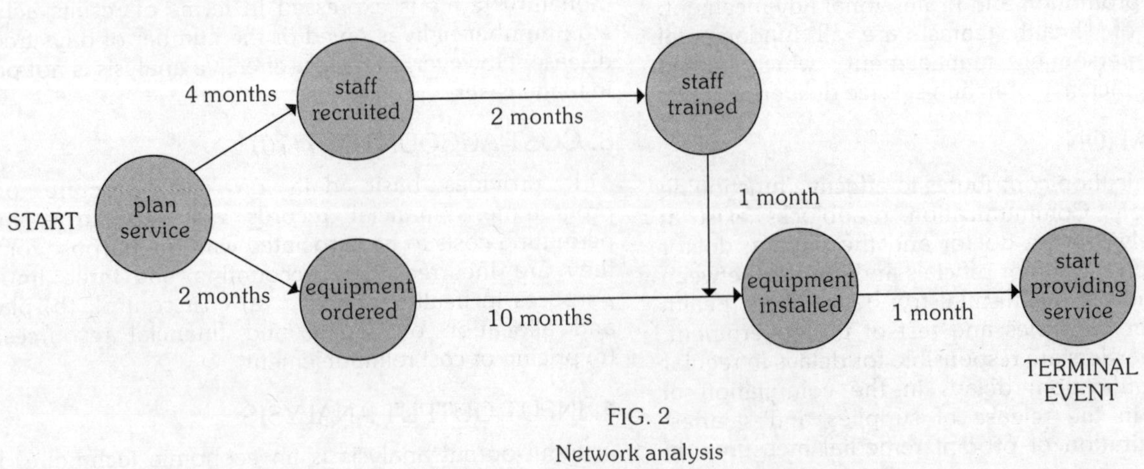

FIG. 2
Network analysis

NATIONAL HEALTH POLICY–2017 *(12)*

The National Health Policy of 1983 and the National Health Policy of 2002 have served well in guiding the approach for the health sector in the Five-year plans. Now 14 years after the last health policy, the context has changed in four major ways. First, the health priorities are changing. Although maternal and child mortality have rapidly declined, there is growing burden on account of non-communicable diseases and some infectious diseases. The second important change is the emergence of a robust health care industry estimated to be growing at double digit. The third change is the growing incidences of catastrophic expenditure due to health care costs, which are presently estimated to be one of the major contributors to poverty. Fourth, a rising economic growth enables enhanced fiscal capacity. Therefore, a new health policy responsive to these contextual changes was required.

The primary aim of the National Health Policy, 2017, is to inform, clarify, strengthen and prioritize the role of the Government in shaping health systems in all its dimensions - investments in health, organization of healthcare services, prevention of diseases and promotion of good health through cross sectoral actions, access to technologies, developing human resources, encouraging medical pluralism, building knowledge base, developing better financial protection strategies, strengthening regulation and health assurance.

Specific Quantitative Goals and Objectives: The indicative, quantitative goals and objectives are outlined under three broad components viz. (a) health status and programme impact (b) health systems performance and (c) health system strengthening. These goals and objectives are aligned to achieve sustainable development in health sector in keeping with the policy thrust.

A. Health status and programme impact

1. Life expectancy and healthy life

a. Increase life expectancy at birth from 67.5 to 70 by 2025.
b. Establish regular tracking of Disability Adjusted Life Years (DALY) index as a measure of burden of disease and its trends by major categories by 2022.
c. Reduction of TFR to 2.1 at national and sub-national level by 2025.

2. Mortality by age and/or cause

a. Reduce under five mortality to 23 by 2025 and MMR from current levels to 100 by 2020.
b. Reduce infant mortality rate to 28 by 2019.
c. Reduce neo-natal mortality to 16 and still birth rate to "single digit" by 2025.

3. Reduction of disease prevalence/ incidence

a. Achieve global target of 2020 which is also termed as target of 90:90:90, for HIV/AIDS i.e. – 90% of all people living with HIV know their HIV status, – 90% of all people diagnosed with HIV infection receive sustained antiretroviral therapy and 90% of all people receiving antiretroviral therapy will have viral suppression.
b. Achieve and maintain elimination status of leprosy by 2018, Kala-azar by 2017 and lymphatic filariasis in endemic pockets by 2017.
c. To achieve and maintain a cure rate of >85% in new sputum positive patients for TB and reduce incidence of new cases, to reach elimination status by 2025.
d. To reduce the prevalence of blindness to 0.25/1000 by 2025 and disease burden by one third from current levels.
e. To reduce premature mortality from cardiovascular diseases, cancer, diabetes or chronic respiratory diseases by 25% by 2025.

B. Health systems performance

1. Coverage of health services

a. Increase utilization of public health facilities by 50% from current levels by 2025.
b. Antenatal care coverage to be sustained above 90% and skilled attendance at birth above 90% by 2025.
c. More than 90% of the newborn are fully immunized by one year of age by 2025.
d. Meet need of family planning above 90% at national and sub-national level by 2025.
e. 80% of known hypertensive and diabetic individuals at household level maintain 'controlled disease status' by 2025.

2. Cross sectoral goals related to health

a. Relative reduction in prevalence of current tobacco use by 15% by 2020 and 30% by 2025.
b. Reduction of 40% in prevalence of stunting of under-five children by 2025.
c. Access to safe water and sanitation to all by 2020 (Swachh Bharat Mission).
d. Reduction of occupational injury by half from current levels of 334 per lakh agricultural workers by 2020.
e. National/state level tracking of selected health behaviour.

C. Health systems strengthening

1. Health finance

a. Increase health expenditure by Government as a percentage of GDP from the existing 1.15% to 2.5% by 2025.
b. Increase state sector health spending to > 8% of their budget by 2020.
c. Decrease in proportion of households facing catastrophic health expenditure from the current levels by 25% by 2025.

2. Health infrastructure and human resource

a. Ensure availability of paramedics and doctors as per Indian Public Health Standard (IPHS) norm in high priority districts by 2020.
b. Increase community health volunteers to population ratio as per IPHS norm, in high priority districts by 2025.
c. Establish primary and secondary care facility as per norms in high priority districts (population as well as time to reach norms) by 2025.

3. Health management information

a. Ensure district-level electronic database of information on health system components by 2020.
b. Strengthen the health surveillance system and

establish registries for diseases of public health importance by 2020.

c. Establish federated integrated health information architecture, health information exchanges and national health information network by 2025.

HEALTH PLANNING IN INDIA

Health planning in India is an integral part of national socio-economic planning *(2, 13)*. The guidelines for national health planning were provided by a number of committees dating back to the Bhore committee in 1946. These committees were appointed by the Government of India from time to time to review the existing health situation and recommend measures for further action.

The Alma-Ata Declaration on primary health care and the National Health Policy of the Government gave a new direction to health planning in India, making primary health care the central function and main focus of its national health system. The goal of national health planning in India was to attain Health for All by the year 2000.

PLANNING COMMISSION

The Government of India set up a Planning Commission in 1950 to make an assessment of the material, capital and human resources of the country, and to draft developmental plans for the most effective utilization of these resources. In 1957, the Planning Commission was provided with a Perspective Planning Division which makes projections into the future over a period of 20 to 25 years. The Planning Commission consists of a Chairman, Deputy Chairman and 5 members. The Planning Commission works through 3 major divisions – Programme Advisers, General Secretariat and Technical Divisions which are responsible for scrutinizing and analyzing various schemes and projects to be incorporated in the Five Year Plans. Over the years, the Planning Commission has been formulating successive Five Year Plans. By its terms of reference, the Planning Commission also reviews from time to time the progress made in various directions and to make recommendations to Government on problems and policies relevant to the pursuit of rapid and balanced economic development. The planning process was decentralised towards Decentralised District Planning by the year 2000.

NITI AAYOG

Government of India has established NITI Aayog (National Institution for Transforming India) to replace Planning Commission on 1st January 2015. It will seek to provide a critical directional and strategic input into the development process. NITI Aayog will emerge as a "think-tank" that will provide Governments at the central and state levels with relevant strategic and technical advice across the spectrum of key elements of policy. In addition, the NITI Aayog will monitor and evaluate the implementation of programmes, and focus on technology upgradation and capacity building.

HEALTH SECTOR PLANNING

Since "health" is an important contributory factor in the utilization of manpower, the Planning Commission gave considerable importance to health programmes in the Five Year Plans. For purposes of planning, the health sector has been divided into the following sub-sectors *(25)*.

(1) Water supply and sanitation;

(2) Control of communicable diseases;

(3) Medical education, training and research;

(4) Medical care including hospitals, dispensaries and primary health centres;

(5) Public health services;

(6) Family planning; and

(7) Indigenous systems of medicine.

All the above sub-sectors have received due consideration in the Five Year Plans. However, the emphasis has changed from Plan to Plan depending upon the felt-needs of the people and technical considerations. To give effect to a better coordination between the Centre and State Governments, a Bureau of Planning was constituted in 1965 in the Ministry of Health, Govt. of India. The main function of this Bureau is compilation of National Health Five Year Plans. The Health Plan is implemented at various levels, e.g., Centre, State, District, Block and Village.

FIVE YEAR PLANS *(26, 27, 28)*

The five year plans were conceived to re-build rural India, to lay the foundations of industrial progress and to secure the balanced development of all parts of the country. Recognising "health" as an important contributory factor in the utilisation of manpower and the uplifting of the economic condition of the country, the Planning Commission gave considerable importance to health programmes in the five year plans. The broad objectives of the health programmes during the five year plans have been :

(1) Control or eradication of major communicable diseases;

(2) Strengthening of the basic health services through the establishment of primary health centres and subcentres;

(3) population control; and

(4) development of health manpower resources.

Twelfth Five Year Plan (2012–2017)

The health of a nation is an essential component of development, vital to the nation's economic growth and internal stability. Assuring a minimal level of health care to the population is a critical constitutent of the development process.

Since independence, India has built up a vast health infrastructure and health personnel at primary, secondary and tertiary care in public, voluntary, and private sectors. For producing skilled human resources, a number of medical and paramedical institutions including Ayurveda, Yoga and Naturopathy, Unani, Siddha and Homeopathy (AYUSH) institutions have been set up.

Considerable achievements have been made over the last six decades in the efforts to improve health standards, such as life expectancy, child mortality, infant mortality, and maternal mortality. Smallpox, guineaworm, poliomyelitis have been eradicated. Nevertheless, problems abound. Malnutrition affects a large proportion of children. An unacceptably high proportion of the population continues to suffer and die from new diseases that are emerging; apart from continuing and new threats posed by the existing ones. Pregnancy and childbirth related complications also contribute to the suffering and mortality.

The strong link between poverty and ill-health needs to be recognized. The onset of a long and expensive illness can drive the non-poor into poverty. Ill health creates immense stress even among those who are financially secure. The country has to deal with rising costs of health care and growing expectations of the people. The challenge of quality health services in remote rural regions has to be urgently met. Given the magnitude of the problem, there is a need to transform public health care into an accountable, accessible, and affordable system of quality services during the Twelfth Five Year Plan.

One of the 12th Plan long-term objective was to establish a system of Universal Health Coverage in the country. This means that each individual would have assured access to a defined essential range of medicines and treatment at an affordable price, which should be entirely free for a large percentage of the population. The High Level Expert Group (HLEG) has defined the Universal Health Coverage as "Ensuring equitable access for all Indian citizens in any part of the country, regardless of income level, social status, gender, caste or religion, to affordable, accountable and appropriate, assured quality health services (promotive, preventive, curative and rehabilitative) as well as services addressing wider determinants of health delivered to individuals and populations, with the government being the guarantor and enabler, although not necessarily the only provider of health and related services" *(29)*. This definition affirms that the system must be available for all who want it, though some, typically the upper income groups, may opt out.

In order to achieve health goals, the universal health coverage (UHC) must build on universal access to services that are determinants of health, such as safe drinking water and sanitation, wholesome nutrition, basic education, safe housing and hygienic environment. Therefore, it may be necessary to realise the goal of UHC in two parallel steps : (1) clinical services at different levels, defined in an Essential Health Package, which the government would finance and ensure provision through the public health system, supplemented by contracted-in private providers; (2) the universal provision of high impact, preventive and public health interventions which the government would universally provide within the 12th Five Year Period (as shown in Table 2).

TABLE 3

12th Five year health goals for communicable diseases

Disease	Twelfth plan goal
Tuberculosis	Reduce annual incidence and mortality by half
Leprosy	Reduce prevalence to <1/10,000 population and incidence to zero in all districts
Malaria	Annual malaria incidence of <1/1,000
Filariasis	<1 per cent microfilaria prevalence in all districts
Dengue	Sustaining case fatality rate of <1 per cent
Chikungunya	Containment of outbreaks
Japanese Encephalitis	Reduction in mortality by 30 per cent
Kala-azar	Elimination by 2015, that is, <1 case per 10,000 population in all blocks
HIV/AIDS	Reduce new infections to zero and provide comprehensive care and support to all persons living with HIV/AIDS and treatment services for all those who require it.

TABLE 2

List of preventive and public health interventions funded and provided by government

1. Full immunization among children under three years of age, and pregnant women.
2. Full antenatal, natal and postnatal care.
3. Skilled birth attendance with a facility for meeting need for emergency obstetric care.
4. Iron and Folic acid supplementation for children, adolescent girls and pregnant women.
5. Regular treatment of intestinal worms, especially in children and reproductive age women.
6. Universal use of iodine and iron fortified salt.
7. Vitamin A supplementation for children aged 9 to 59 months.
8. Access to a basket of contraceptives, and safe abortion services.
9. Preventive and promotive health educational services, including information on hygiene, hand-washing, dental hygiene, use of potable drinking water, avoidance of tobacco, alcohol, high calorie diet and obesity, need for regular physical exercise, use of helmets on two-wheelers and seat belts; advice on initiation of breast-feeding within one hour of birth and exclusively upto six months of age, and complimentary feeding thereafter, adolescent sexual health, awareness about RTI/STI; need for screening for NCDs and common cancers for those at risk.
10. Home based newborn care, and encouragement for exclusive breast-feeding till six months of age.
11. Community based care for sick children, with referral of cases requiring higher levels of care.
12. HIV testing and counselling during antenatal care.
13. Free drugs to pregnant HIV positive mothers to prevent mother to child transmission of HIV.
14. Malaria prophylaxis, using Long Lasting Insecticide Treated Nets (LLIN), diagnosis using Rapid Diagnostic Kits (RDK), and appropriate treatment.
15. School check-up of health and wellness, followed by advice, and treatment if necessary.
16. Management of diarrhoea, especially in children, using Oral Rehydration Solution (ORS).
17. Diagnosis and treatment of Tuberculosis, Leprosy including Drug and Multi-Drug Resistant cases.
18. Vaccines for hepatitis B for high risk groups.
19. Patient transport systems including emergency response ambulance services of the 'dial 108' model.

Three Year Action Agenda of Niti Aayog (2017–18 to 2019–2020)

On 1st January 2015, The National Institution for Transforming India (NITI Aayog) came into existence as the Government's premier think tank. It was told to prepare a 15 year vision, Seven Year Strategy and Three Year Action Agenda documents. Accordingly, the Vision Strategy and Action Agenda is a departure from the Five Year Plan process. The 12th Five Year Plan was the last of these plans. The Three Year Action Agenda offers ambitious proposals for policy changes within a relatively short period. The proposed Agenda is wide-ranging and the specific health goals to be achieved by the year 2020 are as follows *(29)*:

1. Reduce maternal mortality ratio to 120/100,000 live births (2013 estimate: 167/100,000 live births).
2. Reduce infant mortality rate to 30/1,000 live births (2013 estimate: 40/1,000 live births).
3. Reduce under 5 mortality rate to 38/1,000 live births (2015 estimate: 48/1,000 live births).
4. Reduce Total Fertility Rate to 2.1 (2013 estimate: 2.3).
5. Reduce incidence of TB to 130/100,000 (2015 estimate: 217/100,000).
6. Reduce incidence of malaria (annual parasite incidence) to less than1/1,000 in 90% of districts (2016 estimate: 74% of districts have achieved an API of less than 1).
7. Eliminate Kala-azar (2015 estimate: 80% of endemic blocks have eliminated) and Lymphatic Filariasis (2015 estimate: 87% of endemic districts have eliminated).
8. Reduce premature mortality from cardiovascular diseases, cancer, diabetes or chronic respiratory diseases by 1/4th of National Family Health Survey-4 (NFHS-4) levels.
9. Reduce out-of-pocket spending to 50% of the total health expenditure (2014 estimate: 62.4%).

HEALTH SYSTEM IN INDIA

India is a Union of 29 States and 7 Union territories. Under the Constitution of India, the States are largely independent in matters relating to the delivery of health care to the people. Each State, therefore, has developed its own system of health care delivery, independent of the Central Government. The Central responsibility consists mainly of policy making, planning, guiding, assisting, evaluating, and coordinating the work of the State Health Ministries, so that health services cover every part of the country, and no State lags behind for want of these services. The health system in India has 3 main links, i.e., Central, State and Local or peripheral.

I – AT THE CENTRE

The official "organs" of the health system at the national level consist of : (1) The Ministry of Health and Family Welfare; (2) The Directorate General of Health Services; and (3) The Central Council of Health and Family Welfare.

1. Union Ministry of Health and Family Welfare

(1) ORGANIZATION

The Union Ministry of Health and Family Welfare is headed by a Cabinet Minister, a Minister of State and a Deputy Health Minister. These are political appointments. Currently, the Union Health Ministry has the following departments: (1) Department of Health and (2) Department of Family Welfare. The Health Department is headed by a Secretary to the Government of India as its executive head, assisted by joint secretaries, deputy secretaries and a large administrative staff. The Department of Family Welfare was created in 1966 within the Ministry of Health and Family Welfare. The Secretary to the Govt. of India in the Ministry of Health and Family Welfare is in overall charge of the Department of Family Welfare. He is assisted by an Additional Secretary & Commissioner (Family Welfare), and one Joint Secretary.

(2) FUNCTIONS

The functions of the Union Health Ministry are set out in the seventh schedule of Article 246 of the Constitution of India under (a) the Union list and (b) the Concurrent list.

(a) Union list: The functions given in the Union list are: (1) International health relations and administration of port quarantine (2) Administration of central institutes such as the All India Institute of Hygiene and Public Health, Kolkata; National Centre for Disease Control, Delhi, etc. (3) Promotion of research through research centres and other bodies (4) Regulation and development of medical, pharmaceutical, dental and nursing professions (5) Establishment and maintenance of drug standards (6) Census, and collection and publication of other statistical data (7) Immigration and emigration (8) Regulation of labour in the working of mines and oil fields and (9) Coordination with States and with other ministries for promotion of health.

(b) Concurrent list: The functions listed under the concurrent list are the responsibility of both the Union and State governments. The Centre and the States have simultaneous powers of legislation; the powers of the latter are restricted to the framework of such legislation as may be undertaken by the Centre. The concurrent list includes: (1) Prevention of extension of communicable diseases from one unit to another (2) Prevention of adulteration of foodstuffs (3) Control of drugs and poisons (4) Vital statistics (5) Labour welfare (6) Ports other than major (7) Economic and social planning, and (8) Population control and Family Planning.

2. Directorate General of Health Services

(a) ORGANIZATION : The Director General of Health Services is the principal adviser to the Union Government in both medical and public health matters. He is assisted by an additional Director General of Health Services, a team of deputies and a large administrative staff. The Directorate comprises of three main units, e.g., medical care and hospitals, public health and general administration.

(b) FUNCTIONS: The GENERAL functions are surveys, planning, coordination, programming and appraisal of all health matters in the country. The SPECIFIC functions are (1) International health relations and quarantine: All the major ports in the country (Kolkata, Visakhapatnam, Chennai, Cochin, Mumbai, Kandla) and international air ports (Mumbai-Santa Cruz, Kolkata-Dum Dum, Chennai-Meenambakkam, Tiruchirapalli, Delhi-Palam) are directly controlled by the Directorate General of Health Services. All matters relating to the obtaining of assistance from International agencies and the coordination of their activities in the country are undertaken by the Directorate General of Health Services. (2) Control of drug standards: The Drugs Control Organization is part of the Directorate General of Health Services, and is headed by the Drugs Controller. Its primary function is to lay down and enforce standards and control the manufacture and distribution of drugs through both Central and State Government Officers.

The Drugs Act (1940) vests the Central Government with the powers to test the quality of imported drugs (3) Medical store depots: The Union Government runs medical store depots at Mumbai, Chennai, Kolkata, Karnal, Guwahati and Hyderabad. These depots supply the civil medical requirements of the Central Government and of the various State Governments. These depots also handle supplies from foreign agencies. The Medical Stores Organization endeavours to ensure the highest quality, cheaper bargain and prompt supplies. (4) Post graduate training: The Directorate General of Health Services is responsible for the administration of national institutes, which also provide postgraduate training to different categories of health personnel. Some of these institutes are :– the All India Institute of Hygiene and Public Health at Kolkata, All India Institute of Mental Health at Bangalore, College of Nursing at Delhi, National Tuberculosis Institute at Bangalore, National Institute of Communicable Diseases at Delhi, Central Research Institute at Kasauli, National Institute of Health and Family Welfare at Delhi, etc. (5) Medical education: The Central Directorate is directly in charge of the following medical colleges in India: the Lady Hardinge, the Maulana Azad and the medical colleges at Puducherry, and Goa. Besides these, there are many medical colleges in the country which are guided and supported by the Centre. (6) Medical Research : Medical Research in the country is organised largely through the Indian Council of Medical Research, founded in 1911 in New Delhi. The Council plays a significant role in aiding, promoting and coordinating scientific research on human diseases, their causation, prevention and cure. The research work is done through the Council's several permanent research institutes, research units, field surveys and a large number of ad-hoc research enquiries financed by the Council. It maintains Cancer Research Centre, Tuberculosis Chemotherapy Centre at Chennai, Virus Research Centre at Poona, National Institute of Nutrition at Hyderabad and Blood Group Reference Centre at Mumbai. The funds of the Council are wholly derived from the budget of the Union Ministry of Health. (7) Central Govt. Health Scheme. (8) National Health Programmes : The various national health programmes for the eradication of malaria and for the control of tuberculosis, filaria, leprosy, AIDS and other communicable diseases involve expenditure of crores of rupees. Health programmes of this kind can hardly succeed without the help of the Central Government. The Central Directorate plays a very important part in planning, guiding and coordinating all the national health programmes in the country. (9) Central Health Education Bureau: An outstanding activity of this Bureau is the preparation of education material for creating health awareness among the people. The Bureau offers training courses in health education to different categories of health workers. (10) Health Intelligence: The Central Bureau of Health Intelligence was established in 1961 to centralise collection, compilation, analysis, evaluation and dissemination of all information on health statistics for the nation as a whole. It disseminates epidemic intelligence to States and international bodies. The Bureau has an Epidemiological Unit, a Health Economics Unit, a National Morbidity Survey Unit and a Manpower Cell. (11) National Medical Library: The Central Medical Library of the Directorate General Health Services was declared the National Medical Library in 1966. The aim is to help in the advancement of medical, health and related sciences by collection, dissemination and exchange of information.

3. Central Council of Health

A large number of health subjects fall in the Concurrent list which calls for continuous consultation, mutual understanding and cooperation between the Centre and the States. The Central Council of Health was set up by a Presidential Order on 9th August, 1952 under Article 263 of the Constitution of India for promoting coordinated and concerted action between the Centre and the States in the implementation of all the programmes and measures pertaining to the health of the nation. The Union Health Minister is the Chairman and the State Health Ministers are the members.

FUNCTIONS : The functions of the Central Council of Health are: (1) To consider and recommend broad outlines of policy in regard to matters concerning health in all its aspects such as the provision of remedial and preventive care, environmental hygiene, nutrition, health education and the promotion of facilities for training and research. (2) To make proposals for legislation in fields of activity relating to medical and public health matters and to lay down the pattern of development for the country as a whole. (3) To make recommendations to the Central Government regarding distribution of available grants-in-aid for health purposes to the States and to review periodically the work accomplished in different areas through the utilisation of these grants-in-aid. (4) To establish any organisation or organisations invested with appropriate functions for promoting and maintaining cooperation between the Central and State Health administrations.

II – AT THE STATE LEVEL

Historically, the first milestone in State health administration was the year 1919, when the States (then known as provinces) obtained autonomy, under the Montague-Chelmsford reforms, from the Central Government, in matters of public health. By 1921–22, all the States had created some form of public health organization. The Government of India Act, 1935 gave further autonomy to the States. The health subjects were divided into three groups: federal, concurrent and state. The "state" list which became the responsibility of the State included provision of medical care, preventive health services and pilgrimages within the State. The position has largely remained the same, even after the new Constitution of India came into force in 1950. The State is the ultimate authority responsible for all the health services operating within its jurisdiction.

State health administration

At present there are 28 States and 9 UTs in India, with each one having its own health administration. In all the States, the management sector comprises the State Ministry of Health and a Directorate of Health.

1. State Ministry of Health

The State Ministry of Health is headed by a Minister of Health and Family Welfare and a Deputy Minister of Health and Family Welfare. In some States, the Health Minister is also in charge of other portfolios. The Health Secretariat is the official organ of the State Ministry of Health and is headed by a Secretary who is assisted by Deputy Secretaries, Under Secretaries and a large administrative staff. The Secretary is a senior officer of the Indian Administrative Service. The Bhore Committee (1946) recommended that the Director of Health Services should also be Secretary to the State Government to facilitate administration, but this recommendation has not been implemented.

2. State Health Directorate

For a long time, two separate departments, medical and public health, were functioning in the States; the heads of these departments were known as Surgeon General and Inspector General of Civil Hospitals and Director of Public Health respectively. The Bhore Committee (1946) recommended that the medical and public health organizations should be integrated at all levels and therefore, should have a single administrative officer for the curative and preventive departments of health. West Bengal led the process of integrating health services at the State level by creating a post of the Director of Health Services in August 1947; the process was completed by Maharashtra in May 1970.

The Director of Health Services (known in some States as Director of Medical and Health Services) is the chief technical adviser to the State Government on all matters relating to medicine and public health. He is also responsible for the organization and direction of all health activities. With the advent of family planning as an important programme, the designation of Director of Health Services has been changed in some States and is now known as Director of Health and Family Welfare. A recent development in some States is the appointment of a *Director of Medical Education* in view of the increasing number of medical colleges. Some experts feel that there is no justification for the removal of medical education from general health services under the Director of Health Services. The health services and training institutions should develop into one logical whole designed to an end – the protection of the health of the people.

The Director of Health and Family Welfare is assisted by a suitable number of deputies and assistants. The Deputy and Assistant Directors of Health may be of two types – regional and functional. The Regional Directors inspect all the branches of public health within their jurisdiction, irrespective of their speciality. The Functional Directors are usually specialists in a particular branch of public health such as mother and child health, family planning, nutrition, tuberculosis, leprosy, health education etc. The Public Health Engineering Organization in most States is part of the Public Works Department of the State Government. It has been recommended by experts in the public health that the public health engineering organization in every State should be part of the State Health Department, and that the Chief Engineer of Public Health should have the status of an Additional Director of Health Services.

III – AT THE DISTRICT LEVEL

The District

The principal unit of administration in India is the district under a Collector. There are 718 (year 2020) districts in India. There is no "average" district, that is the districts vary widely in area and population. Within each district again, there are 6 types of administrative areas :

1. Sub-divisions;
2. Tahsils (Talukas);
3. Community Development Blocks;
4. Municipalities and Corporations;
5. Villages; and
6. Panchayats.

Most districts in India are divided into two or more sub-divisions, each in charge of an Assistant Collector or sub-Collector. Each division is again divided into tahsils (taluks), in charge of a Tahsildar. A tahsil usually comprises between 200 to 600 villages. Since the launching of the Community Development Programme in India in 1952, the rural areas of the district have been organized into Blocks, known as Community development blocks, the area of which may or may not coincide with a tahsil. The block is a unit of rural planning and development, and comprises approximately 100 villages and about 80,000 to 1,20,000 population, in charge of a Block Development Officer. Finally there are the village panchayats, which are institutions of rural local self-government.

The urban areas of the district are organized into the following institutions of local self-government :

1. Town area committees – (in areas with population ranging between 5,000 and 10,000).
2. Municipal Boards – (in areas with population ranging between 10,000 and 2 lakhs).
3. Corporations – (with population above 2 lakhs).

The Town area committees are like panchayats. They provide sanitary services. The Municipal Boards are headed by a Chairman/President, elected usually by the members. The term of a Municipal Board ranges between 3–5 years. The functions of a municipal board are: construction and maintenance of roads, sanitation and drainage, street lighting, water supply, maintenance of hospitals and dispensaries, education, registration of births and deaths, etc. Corporations are headed by Mayors. The councillors are elected from different wards of the city. The executive agency includes the Commissioner, the Secretary, the Engineer and the Health Officer. The activities are similar to those of the municipalities, but on a much wider scale.

Health organization

The Bhore Committee (1946) recommended integrated preventive and curative services at all levels and the setting up of a unified health authority in each district. Subsequent expert committees, appointed by the Government of India have also recommended the same. Since "health" is a state subject, there is no uniform "model" of a district health organization in India, each State developed its own pattern to suit its policy and convenience.

Under the Multi-Purpose Workers Scheme, it has been suggested to the States to have an integrated set-up at the district level by having a Chief Medical Officer with three Deputy CMOs (existing Civil Surgeons, District Health Officers and District Family Welfare Officers) with each of the Dy. CMOs being incharge of one-third of the district for all the Health, Family Welfare and MCH programmes. The recent Working Group on Health for All by 2000 AD, appointed by the Planning Commission, recommended that the District Hospitals should be converted into District Health Centres, each centre monitoring all preventive, promotive and curative services of one million population. It has been recommended that the district set-up should be reorganized on the basis of the number of primary health centres it comprises *(23)*.

PANCHAYATI RAJ *(32, 33)*

The Panchayati Raj is a 3-tier structure of rural local self-government in India, linking the village to the district. The three institutions are:

(1) *Panchayat* – at the village level;

(2) *Panchayat Samiti* – at the block level; and

(3) *Zilla Parishad* – at the district level.

The Panchayati Raj institutions are accepted as agencies of public welfare. All development programmes are channelled through these bodies. The Panchayati Raj institutions strengthen democracy at its root, and ensure more effective and better participation of the people in the government.

1. At the Village level

The Panchayati Raj at the village level consists of:

(i) the Gram Sabha;

(ii) the Gram Panchayat; and

(iii) the Nyaya Panchayat.

Gram Sabha : It is the assembly of all the adults of the village, which meets at least twice a year. The gram sabha considers proposals for taxation, discusses the annual programme and elects members of the gram panchayat.

Gram Panchayat : It is the executive organ of the gram sabha, and an agency for planning and development at the village level. Its strength varies from 15 to 30, and the population covered also varies widely from 5,000 to 15,000 or more. The members of the panchayat hold office for a period of 3 to 4 years. Every panchayat has an elected President (Sarpanch or Sabhapati or Mukhiya), a Vice-President and a Panchayat Secretary. The powers and functions of the Panchayat Secretary are very wide – they cover the entire field of civic administration, including sanitation and public health; and of social and economic development of the village.

2. At the Block level

The block consists of about 100 villages and a population of about 80,000 to 1,20,000. The Panchayati Raj agency at the block level is the Panchayat Samiti / Janpada Panchayat. The Panchayat Samiti consists of all Sarpanchas (heads) of the village panchayats in the Block; MLAs, MPs residing in the block area; representatives of women, scheduled castes, scheduled tribes and cooperative societies. The Block Development Officer (BDO) is the ex-officio secretary of the Panchayat Samiti. The prime function of the Panchayat Samiti is the execution of the community development programme in the block, The funds provided by the Government for Stage I and Stage II development are channelled through the Panchayat Samiti. The Block Development Officer and his staff give technical assistance and guidance to the village panchayats engaged in development work.

3. At the District level

The Zilla Parishad / Zilla Panchayat is the agency of rural local self-government at the district level. The members of the Zila Parishad include all heads of the Panchayat Samitis in the district; MPs, MLAs of the district; representatives of scheduled castes, scheduled tribes and women; and 2 persons of experience in administration, public life or rural development. The Collector of the district is a non-voting member. Thus, the membership of the Zilla Parishad is fairly large varying from 40 to 70.

The Zilla Parishad is primarily supervisory and coordinating body. Its functions and powers vary from state to state. In some states, the Zilla Parishads are vested with administrative functions. In Gujarat, the District Health Officer and the District Family Planning and MCH Officers are under the control of the Zilla Parishad.

RURAL DEVELOPMENT

Terms such as village improvement, rural upliftment, rural reconstruction and community development have been in vogue for many years to denote certain aspects of rural development. It is only during the last four decades that they have become comprehensive in content.

Community Development Programme

Community development was defined as "a process designed to create conditions of economic and social progress for the whole community with its active participation and the fullest possible reliance upon the community's initiative" *(34)*. The United Nations defined community development as "the process by which the efforts of the people themselves are united with those of governmental authorities to improve the economic, social and cultural conditions of communities, to integrate those communities with the life of the nation and to enable them to contribute fully to national progress" *(33)*.

A beginning was made in India in 1952 during the First Five Year Plan to involve the rural population in the process of planning their own welfare measures. A Programme known as the Community Development Programme was launched on 2nd October 1952 for the all-round development of the rural areas, where nearly 72 per cent of India's population live. The programme was hailed as a programme "of the people, for the people, by the people" to exterminate the three ills of poverty, disease and illiteracy.

Under the Community Development Programme, the rural areas of the country have been organized into Community Development Blocks – each Block comprising approximately 100 villages and a population of one lakh. There are about 6,000 Community Development Blocks in the country, each Block is headed by a Block Development Officer. Over the years, the CD Block has emerged as a permanent unit of rural planning and development.

The Community Development Programme was envisaged as a multipurpose programme covering the following main activities – improvement of agriculture, improvement of communications, education, health and sanitation (through the establishment of primary health centres and sub-centres), improvement of housing through self-help, social welfare and training in rural arts, crafts and industries to local people.

Each Block passed through two stages of development – Stage I of 5 years intensive development followed by Stage II of another 5 years. The Central Government supported the programme substantially by providing funds to the tune of Rs.12 lakhs during Stage I and Rs.5 lakhs during Stage II phases of development. At the end of 10 years, the Blocks entered post-stage II phase and their financial arrangements became the responsibility of the State Governments. The Block continues to be the permanent infrastructure for rural planning and development.

Although the Community Development Programme has made its own contribution to rural development, it has not succeeded in bringing about an all-round improvement in rural areas and in eliminating rural poverty and unemployment. The hope that people would unite their efforts with those of the Government to build the village community on a pattern in which disparities in income and wealth would disappear was not realised. In fact, the benefits of the programme did not reach the weaker sections of the community.

Integrated Rural Development Programme (IRDP)

Another innovation in the continuous search for appropriate strategies to attack poverty is the IRDP. It was launched in April 1978 to eliminate rural poverty and improve the quality of life of the rural poor. The target families are generally agricultural labourers, small cultivators, village artisans and craftsmen. They are provided with resources and skills, bank loans and subsidies by the government. The IRDP is being implemented through District Rural Development Agency (DRDA).

During Ninth Five Year Plan it was implemented through an integrated approach under which the existing schemes of Training of Rural Youth for Self Employment (TRYSEM) and Supply of Improved Toolkits to Rural Artisans (SITRA), Development of Women and Children in Rural Areas (DWCRA) and Ganga Kalyan Yojana (GKY) were merged in to IRDP. There will be a strategic shift from an individual beneficiary approach to formation of Self-Help Groups. This approach will focus on the identification of few specified viable activities based on the local resources and occupational skills of the people of that area.

The Village Level Worker

The village level worker (gram sevak) is the key person responsible for transforming the economic and social life of the people. Each gram sevak is in charge of 10 villages and attends to 5 or 6 thousand people. He lives with the people and keeps in close touch with them and their families. He probes into their "felt-needs" and seeks to arouse in them interest in all-round family and village development. In short, he functions as a multi-purpose worker and a link between the people and governmental agencies.

EVALUATION OF HEALTH SERVICES

Health services have become complex. There has been a growing concern about their functioning both in the developed and developing countries. Questions are raised about the quality of medical care *(35)*, utilization and coverage of health services *(36)*, benefits to community health in terms of morbidity and mortality reduction *(37)* and improvement in the health status of the recipients of care. An evaluation study addresses itself to these issues.

General steps of evaluation

The basic steps involved are as follows :

1. Determine what is to be evaluated;
2. Establish standards and criteria;
3. Plan the methodology to be applied;
4. Gather information;
5. Analyze the results;
6. Take action; and
7. Re-evaluate.

1. Determine what is to be evaluated

Generally speaking, there are three types of evaluation : **(a) Evaluation of "structure":** This is evaluation of whether facilities, equipment, manpower and organization meet a standard accepted by experts as good. **(b) Evaluation of "process":** The process of medical care includes the problems of recognition, diagnostic procedures, treatment and clinical management, care and prevention. The way in which the various activities of the programme is carried out is evaluated by comparing with a predetermined standard. An objective and systematic way of evaluating the physician (or nurse) performance is known as "Medical (or nursing) Audit" *(38)*. **(c) Evaluation of "outcome":** This is concerned with the end results, that is, whether persons using health services experience measurable benefits such as improved survival or reduced disability. The traditional outcome components are the "5 Ds" of ill-health, viz. disease, discomfort, dissatisfaction, disability and death.

2. Establishment of standards and criteria

Standards and criteria must be established to determine how well the desired objectives have been attained. Naturally such standards are a prerequisite for evaluation. Standards and criteria must be developed in accordance with the focus of *evaluation – structural criteria :* e.g., physical facilities and equipment; process criteria: e.g., every prenatal mother must receive 6 check-ups; every laboratory technician must examine 100 blood smears, etc; outcome criteria: e.g., alterations in patient health status (cured, death, disability); or behaviour resulting from health care (satisfaction, dissatisfaction); or the educational process (e.g., cessation of smoking, acceptance of a small family norm), etc.

3. Planning the methodology

A format in keeping with the purpose of evaluation must be prepared for gathering information desired. Standards and criteria must be included at the planning stage.

4. Gathering information

Evaluation requires collection of data or information. The type of information required may include political, cultural, economic, environmental and administrative factors influencing the health situation as well as mortality and morbidity statistics. It may also concern health and related socio-economic policies, plans and programmes as well as the extent, scope and use of health systems, services and institutions *(39)*. The amount of data required will depend on the purpose and use of the evaluation.

5. Analysis of results

The analysis and interpretation of data and feedback to all individuals concerned should take place within the shortest time feasible, once information has been gathered. In addition, opportunities should be provided for discussing the evaluation results.

6. Taking action

For evaluation to be truly productive, emphasis should be placed on actions – actions designed to support, strengthen or otherwise modify the services involved. This may also call for shifting priorities, revising objectives, or development of new programmes or services to meet previously unidentified needs.

7. Re-evaluation

Evaluation is an on-going process aimed mainly at rendering health activities more relevant, more efficient and more effective.

Elements of evaluation

Evaluation is perhaps the most difficult task in the whole area of health services. The components of the evaluation process are:

(a) Relevance: Relevance or requisiteness relates to the appropriateness of the service, whether it is needed at all *(40)*. If there is no need, the service can hardly be of any value. For example, vaccination against smallpox is now irrelevant because the disease no longer exists.

(b) Adequacy: It implies that sufficient attention has been paid to certain previously determined courses of action. For example, the staff allocated to a certain programme may be described as inadequate if sufficient attention was not paid to the quantum of work-load and targets to be achieved.

(c) Accessibility: It is the proportion of the given population that can be expected to use a specified facility, service, etc. The barriers to accessibility may be physical (e.g., distance, travel, time); economic (e.g., travel cost, fee charged); or social and cultural (e.g., caste or language barrier) *(41)*.

(d) Acceptability: The service provided may be accessible, but not acceptable to all, e.g., male sterilization, screening for rectal cancer *(42)*.

(e) Effectiveness: It is the extent to which the underlying problem is prevented or alleviated. Thus it measures the degree of attainment of the predetermined objectives and targets of the programme, service or institution – expressed, if possible, in terms of health benefits, problem reduction or an improvement of an unsatisfactory health situation. The ultimate measures of effectiveness will be the reduction in morbidity and mortality rates. *(45)*.

(f) Efficiency: It is a measure of how well resources (money, men, material and time) are utilized to achieve a given effectiveness. The following examples will illustrate: the number of immunizations provided in an year as compared with an accepted norm; the percentage of bed occupancy, cost per day in hospital, cost per patient treated, etc *(43, 44, 45)*.

(g) Impact: It is an expression of the overall effect of a programme, services or institution on health status and socio-economic development. For example, as a result of malaria control in India, not only the incidence of malaria dropped down, but all aspects of life – agricultural, industrial and social-showed an improvement. If the target of 100 per cent immunization has been reached, it must also lead to reduction in the incidence or elimination of vaccine-preventable diseases. If the target of village water supply has been reached, it must also lead to a reduction in the incidence of diarrhoeal diseases.

Planning and evaluating must be viewed as a continuous interactive process, leading to continual modification both of objectives and plans. Successful evaluation may also depend upon whether the means of evaluation were built into the design of the programme before it was implemented *(46)*.

HISTORY OF PUBLIC HEALTH IN INDIA

1. Early History

India has one of the most ancient civilizations in recorded history. Thousands of years before the Christian era, there existed a civilization in the Indus Valley, known as the Indus Valley Civilization. Excavations in the Indus Valley (e.g., Mohenjodaro and Harappa), showed relics of planned cities with drainage, houses and public baths built of baked bricks suggesting the practices of environmental sanitation, by ancient people as far back as 3,000 B.C. India was invaded by the Aryans around 1,400 B.C. It was probably during this period, the Ayurveda and the Siddha systems of medicine came into existence. Ayurveda or the Science of Life developed a comprehensive concept of health. The Manu Samhita prescribed rules and regulations for personal health, dietetics and hygienic ritual at the time of birth and death, and also emphasised the unity of the physical, mental and spiritual aspects of life *(47)*. Sarve Jana Sukhino Bhavatu (May all men be free from disease and may all be healthy) was an ancient saying of the Indian sages. This concept of happiness has its roots in the ancient Indian philosophy of life, which conceived the oneness and unity of all people, wherever they lived.

The Post-Vedic period (600 B.C.–600 A.D.) was dominated by the religious teachings of Buddhism and Jainism. Medical education was introduced in the ancient universities of Taxila and Nalanda, leading to the titles of Pranacharya and Pranavishara *(47)*. A hospital system was developed during the reign of Rahula Sankirtyana (son of the Buddha) for men, women and animals and the system was continued and expanded by King Ashoka.

The next phase in Indian history (650–1850 A.D.) witnessed the rise and fall of the Moghul empire The Muslim rulers introduced into India around 1,000 A.D. the Arabic system of medicine, popularly known as the Unani system, the origin of which is traced to Greek medicine. The Unani system since then became part of Indian medicine. With changes in the political conditions in India, the torch which was lighted thousands of years ago by the ancient sages grew dim, medical education and medical services became static, and the ancient universities and hospitals disappeared.

2. Public Health in British India

Please refer to 24th Ed. of this book for details.

3. Public Health in the Post-independence era

India became independent in 1947. For the first time in India's long history, a democratic regime was set up with its economy geared to a new concept, the establishment of a "Welfare State". The burden of improving the health of the people, and widening the scope of health measures fell upon the national government. The Bhore Committee's report and recommendations became the basis for most of the planning and measures adopted by the national government. The significant events in the history of public health since 1980 are as follows:

1980 : (1) On May 8th, 1980, smallpox was officially declared eradicated from the entire world by World Health Assembly (2) Sixth Five Year Plan (1980-1985) was launched.

1981 : (1) The 1981 census was taken (2) WHO and Member Countries adopted the Global strategy for Health for All (3) Report of the Working Group on Health for All, set up by the Planning Commission, was published (4) India is committed to the goal of providing safe drinking water and adequate sanitation for all by 1990, under the International Drinking water Supply and Sanitation Decade 1981-1990. (5) The Air (Prevention and Control of Pollution) Act of 1981 was enacted.

1982 : (1) The New 20 Point Programme was announced. (2) The Govt. of India announced its National Health Policy.

1983 :(1) India launched a National Plan of Action against avoidable disablement, known as "IMPACT India". (2) National Leprosy Control Programme to be called National Leprosy Eradication Programme. (3) Medical Education Review Committee submitted its report. (4) National Health Policy was approved by the Parliament (5) Guineaworm eradication Programme was launched.

1984 :(1) Bhopal gas tragedy, the worst ever industrial accident in history occurred on the night of Dec. 2/3 taking a toll of at least 3000 people and no fewer than 50,000 affected (2) The ESI (Amendment) Bill, 1984 was approved by Parliament (3) The Workmen's Compensation (Amendment) Act, 1984 came into force from July 1st. (4) Juvenile Justice Act 1986 came into force.

1985 :(1) Seventh Five Year Plan (1985-1990) was launched (2) Universal Immunization Programme was launched (3) The Lepers Act, 1898 was repealed by Parliament (4) A separate Department of Women and Child Development was set up under the newly created Ministry of Human Resource Development.

1986 :(1) The Environment (Protection) Act 1986 promulgated (2) 20-point plan restructured (3) Parliament voted Mental Health Bill (4) Juvenile Justice Act 1986 came into force.

1987 :(1) New 20 - point programme was launched (2) Indian Standards institution (ISI) renamed: Bureau of Indian Standards (3) A worldwide "safe motherhood" campaign was launched by World Bank. (4) National Diabetes Control Programme and National AIDS Control Programme initiated.

The Factories (Amendment) Act 1987 operated - with provisions to protect employees exposed to hazardous processes.

1989 : Blood Safety Programme was launched. The ESI (Amendment) Act 1989 operated - Modifications in dependent, employee, family, factory and seasonal factory definitions and provisions in original Act.

1990 : Control of Acute Respiratory Infection (ARI) Programme initiated as a pilot project in 14 districts.

1991 : India stages the last decadal Census of the Century.

1992 : (1) Eighth Five Year Plan (1992–97) was launched (2) Child Survival and Safe Motherhood Programme (CSSM) was launched on 20th August (3) The Infant Milk substitute, Feeding Bottles and Infant Foods (Regulation of Production, Supply and Distribution) Act 1992 came into force.

1993 : (1) Revised National Tuberculosis Programme with DOTS introduced as Pilot Project in the country (2) National Nutrition Policy 1993 formulated.

1994 : (1) Return of plague after 28 years of silence (2) The Panchayati Raj Act came into force with all States completing the process of legislation.

1995 : (1) ICDS renamed as Integrated Mother and child Development Services (IMCD) (2) The legislation on Transplantation of Human Organs was enacted to regulate the removal, storage and transplantation of human organs for therapeutic purposes and for prevention of commercial dealings in human organs (3) Expert committee on Malaria submitted its report and recommended guidelines for Malaria Action Plan

1996 : (1) Pulse Polio Immunization, the largest single day public health event took place on 9th December 1995 and 20th January 1996. The second phase of PPI was conducted on 7th December 1996 and 18th January 1997. (2) Family planning programme made target-free from 1st April 1996 (3) Prenatal Diagnostic Technique (Regulation and Prevention of Misuse) Act 1994 came into force from January 1996 (4) Yaws eradication programme launched.

1997 : (1) Reproductive and Child Health Programme launched. (2) Ninth five Year Plan Launched

1998–99 : (1) National Family Health Survey-II undertaken covering 90,000 women aged 15-49 years. (2) National Malaria Eradication Programme renamed as National Anti-Malaria Programme. (3) Phase II of National AIDS Control Programme became effective. (4) National Policy for older persons announced.

2000 : (1) Government of India announced National Population Policy-2000. (2) Declared guineaworm free country (3) Signatory to UN Millennium Declaration. (4) National Commission on Population constituted.

2001 : (1) India stages first census of the century (2) National Policy for empowerment of women launched on 20th March 2001.

2002 : (1) National Health Policy 2002 announced. (2) Government announces National AIDS Prevention and Control Policy 2002. (3) Tenth Five Year Plan launched 2003. Emergence of SARS.

2003 : (1) Parliament approves the Cigarettes and other Tobacco Products (Prohibition, Regulation of Trade and Commerce, Production, Supply and Distribution) Act (2) National Vector Borne Disease Control Programme approved as umbrella programme for prevention of vector borne diseases viz. malaria, filaria, Kala-azar, dengue/DHF, and Japanese encephalitis.

2004 : (1) Vandemataram Scheme launched (2) Revised Programme of Nutritional Support to Primary Education (Mid-day meal scheme) launched (3) Low osmolarity oral rehydration salt replaces the existing formula (4) Integrated Disease Surveillance Project launched (5) National Guidelines on Infant and Young Child Feeding formulated in Aug. 2004.

2005 : (1) RCH II launched (2) Janani Suraksha Yojana launched (3) National Rural Health Mission launched (4) Indian Public Health Standards for Community health centres formulated (5) India achieved leprosy elimination target by end of 2005 (6) National Plan of Action for Children 2005 formulated.

2006 : (1) WHO releases new paediatric growth chart based on breast-fed children (2) Ban on child labour as domestic servant (3) RNTCP covers whole country since March 2006 (4) National Family Health Survey-3 conducted (5) Ministry of Women and Child Development carved out of the Ministry of Human Resources and Development (6) IMNCI was launched in 16 states.

2007 : (1) 11th Five Year Plan launched (2) NACP III launched (3) Indian Public Health Standards for PHC and sub-centres formulated (4) Maintenance and Welfare of Parents and Senior Citizens Bill 2007 passed.

2008 : (1) Non-communicable Disease Programme as pilot project launched on 4th Jan.

2009 : Pandemic Influenza A (H_1N_1) 2009 outbreak, New ICDS Mother and Child Protection Card came into use.

2010 : ICMR announces nutrients requirements and recommended dietary allowances for Indians.

2011 : India stages second census of the century.

2013 : National Health Mission launched, RMNCH+A strategy launched.

2014 : (1) India Newborn Action Plan launched on 27th March. (2) India declared polio free country. (3) Mission Indradhanush launched on 25th December.

2015 : (1) NITI Aayog replaces Yojana Aayog on 1st January 2015; (2) Use of IPV in immunization schedule from Nov. 2015; (3) Juvenile Justice Act 2015; and (4) Swachh Bharat Abhiyan launched.

2016 : (1) Sustainable Development Goals officially came in to force on 1st Jan. 2016; (2) Anganwadi workers are now government employees; (3) Malaria eradication plan (2016–2030) launched; and (4) Switch from tOPV to bOPV in April 2016.

2017 : (1) Aadhaar number must for death certificate from Oct. 2017; (2) National Health Policy 2017.

2018 : (1) National Health Protection Scheme; (2) Ayushman Bharat launched.

2019 : RNTCP renamed National Tuberculosis Elimination Programme (NTEP).

2020 : (1) New commission replaces MCI "National Medical Commission" on 25.9.20; (2) COVID-19 Pandemic played havoc in the world.

2021 : Digital health ID project.

References

1. WHO (1974). *Modern Management Methods and the Organization of Health Services,* Public Health papers 55.
2. WHO (1972). *Approaches to National Health Planning,* Public Health Papers 46.
3. WHO (1971). *Planning and Programming for Nursing Services,* Public Health Papers 44.
4. Sharma, H.R. (1968). *NIHAE Bulletin* 1, No.2, pp. 24–33.
5. Gupta, J.R. et al (1972). *NIHAE Bulletin, 5,* 261–290.
6. WHO (1967). *Techn. Rep. Ser.,* No.350.
7. Koontz, H. et al (1959). *Principles of Management,* McGraw-Hill.
8. WHO (1973). *Health Practice Research,* Public Health Papers 51.
9. WHO (1973). *Application of Modern Management Methods and Techniques for the improved delivery of Health Services,* SEA/PHA/ 120, WHO, New Delhi.
10. Srivastava, A.B.L. et al (1974). *NIHAE Bulletin, 7,* 29–55.
11. Sharma, H.R. (1969). *NIHAE Bulletin,* 2 No.1, pp. 29–39.
12. Govt. of India (2017). *National Health Policy–2017,* Department of Health, Ministry of Health and Family Welfare, New Delhi.
13. Rao, S.K. (1969). *NIHAE Bulletin,* 2, No.3, pp. 5–19.
14. Govt. of India (1946). *Report of the Health Survey and Development Committee,* Govt. of India Press, Shimla.
15. Govt. of India (1962). *Report of the Health Survey and Planning Committee,* Ministry of Health, New Delhi.
16. Chadha, M.S. (1963). *Report of the Special Committee on the preparation for entry of the NMEP into the Maintenance Phase,* Ministry of Health, Govt. of India.
17. Mukherjee, B. (1966). *Report on Reorganization of Family Planning Services, Administration and Basic Health Services.* Ministry of Health. Govt. of India.
18. Govt. of India (1967). *Report of the Committee on Integration of Health Services,* Directorate General of Health Services, Ministry of Health, New Delhi.
19. Govt. of India (1973). *Report of the Committee on Multipurpose Workers under Health and Family Planning Programme,* Department of Family Planning, Ministry of Health and Family Planning, New Delhi.
20. Govt. of India (1975). Ministry of Health and Family Planning (1975). *Report of Group on Medical Education and Support Manpower,* New Delhi.
21. Govt. of India (1976). *Swasth Hind,* 20, 233.
22. Sharad Kumar (1976). *NIHAE Bulletin,* IX, 105–109.
23. Govt. of India (1981). *Report of the Working Group on Health for All by 2000 AD,* Ministry of Health and Family Welfare.
24. ICSSR and ICMR (1980). *Health for All – An Alternative Strategy,* Indian Institute of Education, Pune.
25. Shrivastav, J.B. (1972). *Indian J.Med.Edu.,* XI,99.
26. Dhir, S.L. et al (1972). *NIHAE Bulletin,* 5, 179–186.
27. Govt. of India, Planning Commission (1974). *Draft Fifth Five Year Plan,* 1974–79, vol.I & II, Controller of Publications, Delhi.
28. Govt. of India (1987). *India A Reference Annual,* 1986 Director, Publications Division, Ministry of Information and Broadcasting.
29. Govt. of India (2014), *Twelfth Five Year plan (2012-2017),* Social Sector, Vol. II, Planning Commission, Govt. of India.
30. Niti Aayog (2017), *Three Year Action Agenda 2017–18 to 2019–2020,* Govt. of India, New Delhi.
31. Govt. of India (2019). *Bulletin on Rural Health Statistics in India,* 2018–19, Infrastructure Division, Ministry of Health and Family Welfare, New Delhi.
32. Govt. of India (1964). *Panchayati Raj,* Ministry of Community Development, New Delhi.
33. Govt. of Madhya Pradesh, Bhopal (1962). *Guide Notes,* Training of Officials and Non–officials in Panchayati Raj, Govt. Central Press, Bhopal.
34. Barkat Narain (1961). *Swasth Hind,* Souvenir, Feb. 1961, p. 189.
35. Deniston, O.L. et al (1968). *Public Health Reports,* 83: 323.
36. Tanahasi, T. (1978). Bull WHO, 56: 295.
37. Dept. of Health and Social Security, Scottish Office (1969). *The Fluoridation Studies in the UK and results achieved after 11 years.* Report on Public Health and Medical Subjects No.22, HMSO, London.
38. Sanazaro, P.J. (1974). *Brit.Med.J.,* 1: 271.
39. WHO (1981). *Health for All* Sr.No.6, WHO Geneva.
40. Abramson, J.H. (1979). *Survey Methods in Community Medicine,* 2nd ed. Churchill Livingstone.
41. WHO, SEARO (1984). *Health Planning and Management Glossary,* SEARO Reg. Health Papers No.2, New Delhi.
42. Alderson, M.R. and Robin D. (1979). *Health Surveys and Related Studies,* Pergamon Press.
43. Cochrane, A.L. (1972). *Effectiveness and Efficiency,* Nuffield Provincial Hospital Trust, London.
44. Deniston, O.L. et al (1968). *Public Health Reports,* 83: 603.
45. WHO (1971). Techn. Rep. Ser., No.472.
46. Knox, E.G. (1979). *Epidemiology in Health Care Planning.* Oxford University Press.
47. Rao, K.N. (1966). *The Nation's Health,* The Publications Division, Delhi–6.

24 Essential Medicines and Counterfeit Medicines

"Counterfeit medicines are a crime against humanity"

The concept of essential medicines *(1)*

Essential medicines are those that satisfy the priority health care needs of the population. Essential medicines are intended to be available within the context of functioning health systems at all times in adequate amounts, in the appropriate dosage forms, with assured quality and adequate information, and at a price the individual and the community can afford. The implementation of the concept of essential medicines is intended to be flexible and adaptable to many different situations; exactly which medicines are regarded as essential remains a national responsibility. Experience has shown that careful selection of a limited range of essential medicines results in a higher quality of care, better management of medicines (including improved quality of prescribed medicines), and a more cost-effective use of available health resources.

National list of essential medicines of India–2022 *(2)*

The first National List of Essential Medicines in India was prepared in the year 1996, this list was subsequently revised in the year 2003, 2011, 2015 and 2022.

The medicines have been categorized according to therapeutic use, hence, it is possible that a medicine with more than one indication appears in more than one category.

India has adopted the concept of Essential Medicines as pronounced by the WHO. However, India's list of essential medicines is different from the list issued by WHO due to differences in national circumstances. The list of essential medicines contains such medicines that satisfy the priority health needs of the country's population, addressing its own disease burden. The medicines used in various national health programmes, emerging and re-emerging infections are included in this list of essential medicines. The criteria used for inclusion of a medicine in national list is as follows *(3)* :

1. The medicine should be approved/licensed in India;
2. The medicine should be useful in disease which is a public health problem in India;
3. It should have proven efficacy and safety profile based on valid scientific evidence;
4. It should be cost effective;
5. It should be aligned with the current treatment guidelines for the disease;
6. It should be stable under the storage conditions in India;
7. Price of the total treatment to be considered and not the unit price of a medicine;
8. Fixed dose combination are generally not included unless the combination has unequivocally proven advantage over individual ingredients administered separately in terms of increasing efficacy, reducing side effects and/or improving compliance;
9. The list of essential medicines is based according to the level of health care i.e. Primary (P), Secondary (S) and tertiary (T) because the treatment facility, training, experience and availability of health care personnel differ at these levels.

Dosage forms/formulations of a medicine

Formulation of a medicine may be available in different dosage forms. Oral solid dosage form includes tablet, capsule, sachet etc. Tablets include immediate-release tablets like film coated, uncoated, sugar coated, crushable, chewable and dispersible etc. Enteric coated on the other hand, modified drug release. Crushable, chewable and dispersible tablets may be easier to administer to paediatric and elderly cases. Capsules include hard gelatin capsule, soft gelatin capsule etc. (unless specified, capsules mentioned in the list are considered as hard gelatin capsules).

Oral liquid dosage forms include syrup, suspension, elixirs etc. Injectable dosage forms include conventional liquid injection or powder for injection, as well as delivery system like depot, liposomal/ lipid complex etc. Topical dosage forms include ointment, cream, lotion, drops etc.

Monitoring of medicine safety and pharmacovigilance

Safety monitoring is an important part of the overall surveillance of medicine use. The aims of the various forms of pharmacovigilance are to identify new, previously unrecognized adverse effects of medicines, to quantify their risks, and to communicate these to drug regulatory authorities, health professionals, and when relevant, the public. Voluntary reporting of adverse effects of medicines, on which the International WHO Programme for Drug Monitoring is based, has been effective in identifying a number of previously undescribed effects. The magnitude of the risk of adverse effects is generally evaluated using observational epidemiological methods, such as case-control, cohort and case-population studies.

The Government of India approved list of essential medicines is as follows. Medicines are listed in alphabetical order within sections *(2)*.

National List of Essential Medicines – 2022

	Medicines	Level of Healthcare	Dosage form and strength
	Section 1 : Anaesthetic agents		
	1.1 : General Anaesthetics and oxygen		
1.1.1	Halothane	S,T	Inhalation
1.1.1	Halothane	S,T	Liquid for inhalation
1.1.2	Isoflurane	S,T	Liquid for inhalation
1.1.3	Ketamine	P,S,T	Injection 10 mg/ml Injection 50 mg/ml
1.1.4	Nitrous oxide	P,S,T	As licensed for medical purpose
1.1.5	Oxygen	P,S,T	As licensed for medical purpose
1.1.6	Propofol	P,S,T	Injection 10 mg/ml
1.1.7	Sevoflurane	S,T	Liquid for inhalation
1.1.8	Thiopentone	P,S,T	Powder for injection 0.5 g Powder for injection 1 g
	1.2 : Local anaesthetics		
1.2.1	Bupivacaine	S,T	Injection 0.25% Injection 0.5% Injection 0.5% with 7.5 % glucose
1.2.2	Lignocaine	P,S,T	Topical forms 2-5 % Injection 1% Injection 2% Injection 5% with 7.5% glucose
1.2.3	Lignocaine (A) + Adrenaline (B)	P,S,T	Injection 1% (A) + 1:200000 (5 mcg/ml) (B) Injection 2% (A) + 1:200000 (5 mcg/ml) (B)
	1.3 : Preoperative medication and sedation for short term procedures		
1.3.1	Atropine	P,S,T	Injection 0.6 mg/ml
1.3.2	Glycopyrrolate	S,T	Injection 0.2 mg/ml
1.3.3	Midazolam	P,S,T	Tablet 7.5 mg Nasal Spray 0.5mg Nasal Spray 1.25 mg Injection 1 mg/ml Injection 5 mg/ml
1.3.4	Morphine	P,S,T	Injection 10 mg/ml Injection 15 mg/ml
	1.4 : Muscle relaxants and cholinesterase inhibitors		
1.4.1	Atracurium	S,T	Injection 10 mg/ml
1.4.2	Baclofen	S,T	Tablet 5 mg Tablet 10 mg Tablet 20 mg
1.4.3	Neostigmine	S,T	Tablet 15 mg Injection 0.5 mg/ml
1.4.4	Succinylcholine	S,T	Injection 50 mg/ml
1.4.5	Vecuronium	S,T	Powder for injection 4 mg Powder for injection 10 mg
	Section 2 : Analgesics, antipyretics, non steroidal anti- inflammatory medicines, medicines used to treat gout and disease modifying agents used in rheumatoid disorders		
	2.1 : Non-opioid analgesics, antipyretics and non-steroidal anti-inflammatory drugs		
2.1.1	Acetylsalicylic acid	P,S,T	Tablet 300 mg to 500 mg Effervescent/ Dispersible/ Enteric coated Tablet 300 mg to 500 mg
2.1.2	Diclofenac	P,S,T	Tablet 50 mg Injection 25 mg/ml
2.1.3	Ibuprofen	P,S,T	Tablet 200 mg Tablet 400 mg Oral liquid 100 mg/5 ml (p)
2.1.4	Mefenamic acid	P,S,T	Tablet 250 mg Oral liquid 100 mg/5 ml (p)
2.1.5	Paracetamol	P,S,T	Tablet 500 mg Tablet 650 mg Oral liquid 120 mg/5 ml (p) Oral liquid 125 mg/5 ml (p) Oral liquid 250 mg/5 ml (p) Injection 150 mg/ ml Suppository 80 mg Suppository 170 mg
	2.2 : Opioid analgesics		
2.2.1	Fentanyl	S,T	Injection 50 mcg/ml
2.2.2	Morphine	P,S,T	Tablet 10 mg Injection 10 mg/ml Injection 15 mg/ml
2.2.3	Tramadol	S,T	Capsule 50 mg Capsule 100 mg Injection 50 mg/ml
	2.3 : Medicines used to treat gout		
2.3.1	Allopurinol	P,S,T	Tablet 100 mg Tablet 300 mg
2.3.2	Colchicine	P,S,T	Tablet 0.5 mg
	2.4 : Disease modifying agents used in rheumatoid disorders		
2.4.1	Azathioprine	S,T	Tablet 25 mg (p) Tablet 50 mg
2.4.2	Hydroxy-chloroquine	P,S,T	Tablet 200 mg Tablet 400 mg
2.4.3	Methotrexate	P,S,T	Tablet 2.5 mg Tablet 5 mg Tablet 10 mg
2.4.4	Sulfasalazine	S,T	Tablet 500 mg
	Section 3 : Antiallergics and medicines used in anaphylaxis		
3.1	Adrenaline	P,S,T	Injection 1 mg/ml
3.2	Cetirizine	P,S,T	Tablet 10 mg Oral liquid 5 mg/5 ml (p)
3.3	Dexamethasone	P,S,T	Tablet 0.5 mg Tablet 2 mg Tablet 4 mg Oral liquid 0.5 mg/5 ml (p) Injection 4 mg/ml
3.4	Hydrocortisone	P,S,T	Tablet 5 mg Tablet 10 mg Powder for Injection 100mg Powder for Injection 200mg
3.5	Pheniramine	P,S,T	Injection 22.75 mg/ml
3.6	Prednisolone	P,S,T	Tablet 5 mg Tablet 10 mg Tablet 20 mg Oral liquid 5 mg/5 ml (p) Oral liquid 15 mg/5 ml (p)
	Section 4 : Antidotes and other substances used in management of poisonings/envenomation		
	4.1 : Nonspecific		
4.1.1	Activated charcoal	P,S,T	Powder (as licensed)
	4.2 : Specific		
4.2.1	Atropine	P,S,T	Injection 0.6 mg/ml
4.2.2	Calcium gluconate	P,S,T	Injection 100 mg/ml

	Medicines	Level of Healthcare	Dosage form and strength
4.2.3	D-Penicillamine	P,S,T	Capsule 150 mg (p) Capsule 250 mg
4.2.4	Desferrioxamine	S,T	Powder for Injection 500 mg
4.2.5	Methylthioninium chloride (Methylene blue)	S,T	Injection 10 mg/ml
4.2.6	N-acetylcysteine	P,S,T	Sachet 200 mg Injection 200 mg/ml
4.2.7	Naloxone	P,S,T	Injection 0.4 mg/ml
4.2.8	Neostigmine	P,S,T	Injection 0.5 mg/ml
4.2.9	Pralidoxime chloride (2-PAM)	P,S,T	Injection 25 mg/ml
4.2.10	Snake venom antiserum	P,S,T	Soluble/ liquid polyvalent - As licensed Lyophilized polyvalent - As licensed
4.2.11	Sodium nitrite	S,T	Injection 30 mg/ml
4.2.12	Sodium thiosulphate	S,T	Injection 250 mg/ml

Section 5 : Medicines used in neurological disorders

5.1 : Anticonvulsants/Antiepileptics

	Medicines	Level of Healthcare	Dosage form and strength
5.1.1	Carbamazepine	P,S,T	Tablet 100 mg Tablet 200 mg Tablet 400 mg Modified Release Tablet 200 mg Tablet 400 mg Oral liquid 100 mg/5 ml (p)
5.1.2	Clobazam	S,T	Tablet 5 mg Tablet 10 mg
5.1.3	Diazepam	P,S,T	Oral liquid 2 mg/5 ml (p) Injection 5 mg/ml Suppository 5 mg
5.1.4	Levetiracetam	S,T	Tablet 250 mg Tablet 500 mg Tablet 750 mg Modified Release Tablet 750 mg Oral liquid 100 mg/ml (p) Injection 100 mg/ml
5.1.5	Lorazepam	P,S,T	Tablet 1 mg Tablet 2 mg Injection 2 mg/ml Injection 4 mg/ml
5.1.6	Magnesium sulphate	S,T	Injection 500 mg/ml
5.1.7	Midazolam	P,S,T	Tablet 7.5 mg Tablet 15 mg Nasal Spray 0.5mg/actuation Nasal Spray 1.25 mg/actuation Injection 1 mg/ml Injection 5 mg/ml
5.1.8	Phenobarbitone	P,S,T	Tablet 30 mg Tablet 60 mg Oral liquid 20 mg/5 ml (p)
		S,T	Injection 200 mg/ml
5.1.9	Phenytoin	P,S,T	Tablet 50 mg Tablet 100 mg Tablet 300 mg Modified Release Tablet 300 mg Oral liquid 30 mg/5 ml (p) Oral liquid 125 mg/5 ml (p) Injection 25 mg/ml Injection 50 mg/ml
5.1.10	Sodium Valproate	P,S,T	Tablet 200 mg Tablet 300 mg Tablet 500 mg Modified Release - Tablet 300 mg Tablet 500 mg Oral liquid 200 mg/5 ml (p)
		S,T	Injection 100 mg/ml

5.2 : Antimigraine medicines

	Medicines	Level of Healthcare	Dosage form and strength
5.2.1	Acetylsalicylic acid	P,S,T	Tablet 300 mg to 500 mg Effervescent/ Dispersible/ Enteric coated Tablet 300 mg to 500 mg
5.2.2	Ibuprofen	P,S,T	Tablet 200 mg Tablet 400 mg Oral liquid 100 mg/5 ml (p)
5.2.3	Paracetamol	P,S,T	Tablet 500 mg Tablet 650 mg Oral liquid 120 mg/5ml (p) Oral Liquid 125 mg/5ml (p) Oral Liquid 250 mg/5ml (p)
5.2.4	Sumatriptan	P,S,T	Tablet 25 mg Tablet 50 mg

5.2.1 : For prophylaxis

	Medicines	Level of Healthcare	Dosage form and strength
5.2.1.1	Amitriptyline	P,S,T	Tablet 10 mg Tablet 25 mg Tablet 75 mg
5.2.1.2	Flunarizine	P,S,T	Tablet 5 mg Tablet 10 mg
5.2.1.3	Propranolol	P,S,T	Tablet 10 mg Tablet 20 mg Tablet 40 mg

5.3 : Antiparkinsonism medicines

	Medicines	Level of Healthcare	Dosage form and strength
5.3.1	Levodopa (A) + Carbidopa (B)	P,S,T	Tablet 100 mg (A) + 10 mg (B) Tablet 100 mg (A) + 25 mg (B) Tablet 250 mg (A) + 25 mg (B) Modified Release - Tablet 100 mg (A) + 25 mg (B) Tablet 200 mg (A) + 50 mg (B)
5.3.2	Trihexyphenidyl	P,S,T	Tablet 2 mg

5.4 : Medicines used in dementia

	Medicines	Level of Healthcare	Dosage form and strength
5.4.1	Donepezil	S,T	Tablet 5 mg Tablet 10 mg

Section 6 : Anti infective medicines

6.1 : Anthelminthics

6.1.1 : Intestinal anthelminthics

	Medicines	Level of Healthcare	Dosage form and strength
6.1.1.1	Albendazole	P,S,T	Tablet 400 mg Chewable Tablet 400 mg Oral liquid 200 mg/5 ml (p)
6.1.1.2	Mebendazole	P,S,T	Tablet 100 mg Oral liquid 100 mg/5 ml (p)

6.1.2 : Antifilarial

	Medicines	Level of Healthcare	Dosage form and strength
6.1.2.1	Albendazole	P,S,T	Tablet 400 mg Chewable Tablet 400 mg Oral liquid 200 mg/5 ml (p)
6.1.2.2	Diethylcarbamazine (DEC)	P,S,T	Tablet 50 mg Tablet 100 mg Oral liquid 120 mg/5 ml (p)
6.1.2.3	Ivermectin	P,S,T	Tablet 6 mg Tablet 12 mg

	Medicines	Level of Healthcare	Dosage form and strength
6.1.3 : Anti-schistosomal & anti-trematodal medicine			
6.1.3.1	Praziquantel	S,T	Tablet 600 mg
6.2 : Antibacterials			
6.2.1 : Beta-lactam medicines			
6.2.1.1	Amoxicillin	P,S,T	Capsule 250 mg Capsule 500 mg Oral liquid 125 mg/5 ml (p) Oral liquid 250 mg/5 ml (p) Powder for Injection 250mg Powder for Injection 500mg Powder for Injection 1000 mg
6.2.1.2	Amoxicillin (A) + Clavulanic acid (B)	P,S,T	Tablet 500 mg (A) + 125 mg (B) Oral liquid 200 mg (A) + 28.5 mg (B)/5 ml (p) Dry Syrup 125 mg (A) + 31.25(B)/ 5 ml (p)
		S,T	Powder for Injection 500 mg (A)+ 100 mg (B) Powder for Injection 1 g (A) + 200 mg (B)
6.2.1.3	Ampicillin	P,S,T	Powder for Injection 500mg Powder for Injection 1000 mg
6.2.1.4	Benzathine benzylpenicillin	P,S,T	Powder for Injection 6 lac units Powder for Injection 12 lac units Powder for injection 24 lac units
6.2.1.5	Benzylpenicillin	P,S,T	Powder for injection 5 lac units Powder for injection 10 lac units
6.2.1.6	Cefadroxil	P,S,T	Tablet 500 mg Tablet 100 mg Oral liquid 125 mg/5 ml (p)
6.2.1.7	Cefazolin	P,S,T	Powder for Injection 500mg Powder for Injection 1000 mg
6.2.1.8	Cefixime	S,T	Tablet 200 mg Tablet 400 mg Oral liquid 50 mg/5 ml (p) Oral liquid 100 mg/5 ml (p)
6.2.1.9	Cefotaxime	S,T	Powder for Injection 250mg Powder for Injection 500mg Powder for Injection 1000 mg
6.2.1.10	Ceftazidime	S,T	Powder for Injection 250mg Powder for Injection 1000 mg
6.2.1.11	Ceftriaxone	S,T	Powder for Injection 250mg Powder for Injection 500mg Powder for Injection 1000 mg Powder for Injection 2000 mg
6.2.1.12	Cloxacillin	P,S,T	Capsule 250 mg Capsule 500 mg Oral liquid 125 mg/5 ml (p) Powder for Injection 250mg
6.2.1.13	Piperacillin (A) + Tazobactam (B)	T	Powder for Injection 1000 mg(A) + 125 mg (B) Powder for Injection 2000 mg(A) + 250 mg (B) Powder for Injection 4000 mg(A) + 500 mg (B)

	Medicines	Level of Healthcare	Dosage form and strength
6.2.1.14	Meropenem	T	Powder for Injection 500 mg (as trihydrate) Powder for Injection 1000 mg (as trihydrate)
6.2.2 : Other antibacterials			
6.2.2.1	Azithromycin	P,S,T	Tablet 250 mg Tablet 500 mg Oral liquid 200 mg/5ml (p) Powder for Injection 500mg
6.2.2.2	Cefuroxime	P,S,T	Tablet 500 mg Oral liquid 125 mg/ 5 ml (p) Injection 1500 mg
6.2.2.3	Ciprofloxacin	P,S,T	Tablet 250 mg Tablet 500 mg Oral liquid 250 mg/ 5 ml (p) Injection 200 mg/ 100 ml
6.2.2.4	Clarithromycin	S,T	Tablet 250 mg Tablet 500 mg Oral liquid 125 mg/5 ml (p)
6.2.2.5	Clindamycin	P,S,T	Capsule 150 mg Capsule 300 mg Injection 150 mg /ml
6.2.2.6	Co-trimoxazole [Sulphamethoxazole(A) + Trimethoprim (B)]	P,S,T	Tablet 400 mg (A) + 80 mg (B) Tablet 800 mg (A) + 160 mg (B) Oral liquid 200 mg (A) + 40 mg (B)/5 ml (p)
6.2.2.7	Doxycycline	P,S,T	Capsule 100 mg Dry Syrup 50 mg/5 ml (p) Powder for Injection 100mg
6.2.2.8	Gentamicin	P,S,T	Injection 10 mg/ml Injection 40 mg/ml
6.2.2.9	Metronidazole	P,S,T	Tablet 200 mg Tablet 400 mg Oral liquid 200 mg/5 ml (p) Injection 500 mg/100 ml
6.2.2.10	Nitrofurantoin	P,S,T	Tablet 100 mg Oral liquid 25 mg/5 ml (p)
6.2.2.11	Phenoxymethyl penicillin	P,S,T	Tablet 250 mg
6.2.2.12	Procaine Benzylpenicillin	P,S,T	Powder for Injection 1000 mg (=1 million IU)
6.2.2.13	Vancomycin	S,T	Capsule 125 mg Capsule 250 mg Powder for Injection 250mg Powder for Injection 500mg Powder for Injection 1000 mg
6.3 : Antileprosy medicines			
6.3.1	Clofazimine	P,S,T	Capsule 50 mg Capsule 100 mg
6.3.2	Dapsone	P,S,T	Tablet 50 mg Tablet 100 mg
6.3.3	Rifampicin	P,S,T	Capsule 150 mg Capsule 300 mg
6.4 : Antituberculosis medicines			
6.4.1	Amikacin	S,T	Injection 100 mg/ml Injection 250 mg/ml Injection 500 mg/ml
6.4.2	Bedaquiline	T	Tablet 100 mg
6.4.3	Clarithromycin	S,T	Tablet 250 mg Tablet 500 mg Tablet 750 mg
6.4.4	Clofazimine	S,T	Capsule 50 mg Capsule 100 mg

	Medicines	Level of Healthcare	Dosage form and strength
6.4.5	Cycloserine	S,T	Capsule 125 mg Capsule 250 mg
6.4.6	Delamanid	T	Tablet 50 mg
6.4.7	Ethambutol	P,S,T	Tablet 200 mg Tablet 400 mg Tablet 600 mg Tablet 800 mg
6.4.8	Ethionamide	S,T	Tablet 125 mg Tablet 250 mg
6.4.9	Isoniazid	P,S,T	Tablet 100 mg Tablet 300 mg Oral Liquid 50 mg/5 ml (p)
6.4.10	Levofloxacin	P,S,T	Tablet 250 mg Tablet 500 mg Tablet 750 mg
6.4.11	Linezolid	P,S,T	Tablet 300 mg Tablet 600 mg
6.4.12	Moxifloxacin	P,S,T	Tablet 400 mg
6.4.13	Para-aminosalicylic acid	S,T	Granules (As licensed)
6.4.14	Pyrazinamide	P,S,T	Tablet 500 mg Tablet 750 mg Tablet 1000 mg Tablet 1500 mg Oral liquid 250 mg/5 ml (p)
6.4.15	Rifampicin	P,S,T	Capsule 150 mg Capsule 300 mg Capsule 450 mg Capsule 600 mg Oral liquid 100 mg/ 5 ml (p)
6.4.16	Streptomycin	P,S,T	Powder for Injection 750mg Powder for Injection 1000 mg
	6.5 : Antifungal medicines		
6.5.1	Amphotericin B	S,T	a) Amphotericin B (conventional) - Injection 50 mg/vial b) Lipid Amphotericin B Injection 50 mg/vial c) Liposomal Amphotericin B - Injection 50 mg/vial
6.5.2	Clotrimazole	P,S,T	Pessary 100 mg
6.5.3	Fluconazole	P,S,T	Tablet 50 mg Tablet 100 mg Tablet 150 mg Tablet 200 mg Tablet 400 mg Oral liquid 50 mg/ 5 ml (p)
		S,T	Injection 200 mg / 100 ml
6.5.4	Griseofulvin	P,S,T	Tablet 125 mg Tablet 250 mg Tablet 375 mg
6.5.5	Itraconazole	S,T	Capsule 100 mg Capsule 200 mg Oral liquid 10 mg/ml
6.5.6	Mupirocin	P,S,T	Ointment 2%
6.5.7	Nystatin	S,T	Pessary 1 Lac IU Oral Liquid 1 Lac IU/ml (p)
6.5.8	Terbinafine	P,S,T	Cream 1%
	6.6 : Antiviral medicines		
	6.6.1 : Antiherpes medicines		
6.6.1.1	Acyclovir	P,S,T	Tablet 200 mg Tablet 400 mg Powder for Injection 250mg Powder for Injection 500mg Oral liquid 400 mg/5 ml

	Medicines	Level of Healthcare	Dosage form and strength
	6.6.2 : Anti cytomegalovirus (CMV) medicines		
6.6.2.1	Valganciclovir	S, T	Tablet 450 mg Powder for oral solution 50 mg/ml
	6.7 : Medicines used in the management of HIV		
	6.7.1 : Nucleoside reverse transcriptase inhibitors		
6.7.1.1	Abacavir	S,T	Tablet 60 mg (p) Tablet 300 mg
6.7.1.2	Abacavir (A) + Lamivudine (B)	S,T	Tablet 60 mg (A) + 30 mg (B) (p) Tablet 600 mg (A) + 300 mg (B)
6.7.1.3	Lamivudine	S,T	Tablet 100 mg Tablet 150 mg
6.7.1.4	Tenofovir Disproxil Fumarate (TDF)	S,T	Tablet 300 mg
6.7.1.5	Tenofovir Disproxil Fumarate (A) + Lamivudine (B)	S,T	Tablet 300 mg (A) + 300 mg (B)
6.7.1.6	Tenofovir Disproxil Fumarate (A) + Lamivudine (B) + Dolutegravir (C)	P,S,T	Tablet 300 mg (A) + 300 mg (B)+ 50 mg (C)
6.7.1.7	Tenofovir Disproxil Fumarate (A) + Lamivudine (B) + Efavirenz (C)	S,T	Tablet 300 mg (A) + 300 mg (B)+ 600 mg (C)
6.7.1.8	Zidovudine	S,T	Tablet 300 mg Oral liquid 50 mg/5 ml (p)
6.7.1.9	Zidovudine (A) + Lamivudine (B)	S,T	Tablet 60 mg (A) + 30 mg (B) (p) Tablet 300 mg (A) + 150 mg (B)
6.7.1.10	Zidovudine (A) + Lamivudine (B) + Nevirapine (C)	S,T	Tablet 60 mg (A) + 30 mg (B) + 50 mg (C) (p) Tablet 300 mg (A) + 150 mg (B)+ 200 mg (C)
	6.7.2 : Non-nucleoside reverse transcriptase inhibitors		
6.7.2.1	Efavirenz	S,T	Tablet 200 mg (p) Tablet 600 mg
6.7.2.2	Nevirapine	P,S,T	Tablet 200 mg Dispersible Tablet 50mg (p) Oral liquid 50 mg/ 5 ml (p)
	6.7.3 : Integrase inhibitors		
6.7.3.1	Dolutegravir	S,T	Tablet 50 mg
6.7.3.2	Raltegravir	S,T	Tablet 400 mg
	6.7.4 : Protease inhibitors		
6.7.4.1	Atazanavir (A) + Ritonavir (B)	S,T	Tablet 300 mg (A) + Tablet 100 mg (B)
6.7.4.2	Darunavir	S,T	Tablet 600 mg
6.7.4.3	Darunavir (A) + Ritonavir (B)	S,T	Tablet 600 mg (A) + Tablet 100 mg (B)
6.7.4.4	Lopinavir (A) + Ritonavir (B)	S,T	Tablet 100 mg (A) + 25 mg (B) Tablet 200 mg (A) + 50 mg (B) Oral liquid 80 mg (A) + 20 mg (B) /ml (p) Capsule/ Sachet (containing pellets granules) 40 mg (A) + 10 mg (B) (p)
6.7.4.5	Ritonavir	S,T	Tablet 100 mg

	Medicines	Level of Healthcare	Dosage form and strength
	6.7.5 : Medicines for treating opportunistic infections in people living with HIV		
6.7.5.1	Acyclovir	P,S,T	Injection 250 mg
6.7.5.2	Cefotaxime	P,S,T	Injection 1000 mg
6.7.5.3	Clindamycin	P,S,T	Tablet 300 mg
6.7.5.4	Clotrimazole	P,S,T	Ointment 1 %
6.7.5.5	Valganciclovir	S,T	Tablet/Capsule 450 mg
	6.7.6 : Additional medicines for syndromic management of sexually transmitted infections		
6.7.6.1	Azithromycin	P,S,T	Tablet 1000 mg
	6.8 : Medicines used in Hepatitis B and Hepatitis C		
6.8.1	Daclatasvir	S,T	Tablet 30 mg Tablet 60 mg
6.8.2	Entecavir	S,T	Tablet 0.5 mg Tablet 1 mg Oral liquid 0.05 mg/ml (p)
6.8.3	Ribavirin	S,T	Capsule 200 mg
6.8.4	Sofosbuvir	S,T	Tablet 400 mg
6.8.5	Tenofovir Alafenamide Fumarate (TAF)	S,T	Tablet 25 mg
6.8.6	Tenofovir Disproxil Fumarate (TDF)	S,T	Tablet 300 mg
	6.9 : Antiprotozoal Medicines		
	6.9.1 : Medicines for amoebiasis and other parasitic infections		
6.9.1.1	Metronidazole	P,S,T	Tablet 200 mg Tablet 400 mg Injection 500 mg/100 ml Oral liquid 200 mg/5 ml (p)
	6.9.2 : Antileishmaniasis medicines		
6.9.2.1	Amphotericin B	S,T	a) Amphotericin B (conventional) - Injection 50 mg b) Lipid Amphotericin B Injection 50 mg c) Liposomal Amphotericin B - Injection 50 mg
6.9.2.2	Miltefosine	P,S,T	Capsule 50 mg
6.9.2.3	Paromomycin	P,S,T	Injection 375 mg/ml
	6.9.3 : Antipneumocystosis and antitoxoplasmosis medicines		
6.9.3.1	Clindamycin	P,S,T	Capsule 150 mg Capsule 300 mg
6.9.3.2	Co-trimoxazole [Sulphamethoxazole(A) + Trimethoprim (B)]	P,S,T	Tablet 400 mg (A) + 80 mg (B) Tablet 800 mg (A) + 160 mg (B) Oral liquid 200 mg (A) + 40 mg (B)/5 ml (p)
	6.10 : Antimalarial medicines		
	6.10.1 : For curative treatment		
6.10.1.1	Artemether (A) + Lumefantrine (B)	P,S,T	Tablet 20 mg (A) + 120 mg (B) Tablet 40 mg (A) + 240 mg (B) Tablet 80 mg (A) + 480 mg (B)
6.10.1.2	Artesunate	P,S,T	Powder for Injection 60 mg Powder for Injection 120 mg
6.10.1.3	Artesunate (A) + Sulphadoxine - Pyrimethamine (B)	P,S,T	Combi pack (A+B) 1 Tablet 25 mg (A) + 1 Tablet (250 mg + 12.5 mg) (B) 1 Tablet 50 mg (A) + 1 Tablet (500 mg +25 mg) (B) 1 Tablet 100 mg (A) + 1 Tablet (750 mg + 37.5 mg) (B) 1 Tablet 150 mg (A) + 2 Tablet (500 mg + 25 mg) (B) 1 Tablet 200 mg (A) + 2 Tablet (750 mg + 37.5 mg) (B)
6.10.1.4	Chloroquine	P,S,T	Tablet 150 mg Oral liquid 50 mg/5 ml
6.10.1.5	Clindamycin	P,S,T	Capsule 150 mg Capsule 300 mg
6.10.1.6	Primaquine	P,S,T	Tablet 2.5 mg Tablet 7.5 mg Tablet 15 mg
6.10.1.7	Quinine	P,S,T	Tablet 300 mg Injection 300 mg/ml
	6.10.2 : For prophylaxis		
6.10.2.1	Doxycycline#	P,S,T	Capsule 100 mg Oral liquid 50 mg/ 5ml #for prophylaxis of *P. vivax*
6.10.2.2	Mefloquine#	T	Tablet 250 mg #Only for use as chemoprophylaxis for long term travellers like military and travel troops, travelling from low endemic to high endemic area.
	Section 7 : Anti-cancer agents including immunosuppressives and medicines used in palliative care		
	7.1 : Antineoplastic medicines		
7.1.1	5-Fluorouracil	T	Injection 250 mg/ 5 ml
7.1.2	6-Mercaptopurine	T	Tablet 50 mg
7.1.3	Actinomycin D	T	Powder for Injection 0.5 mg
7.1.4	All-trans retinoic acid	T	Capsule 10 mg
7.1.5	Arsenic trioxide	T	Injection 1mg/ ml
7.1.6	Bendamustine hydrochloride	T	Injection 25 mg/ vial Injection 100 mg/vial
7.1.7	Bleomycin	T	Powder for Injection 15 units
7.1.8	Bortezomib	T	Powder for Injection 2 mg
7.1.9	Calcium folinate	T	Tablet 15 mg Injection 3 mg/ml
7.1.10	Capecitabine	T	Tablet 500 mg
7.1.11	Carboplatin	T	Injection 10 mg/ml
7.1.12	Chlorambucil	T	Tablet 2 mg Tablet 5 mg
7.1.13	Cisplatin	T	Injection 1mg/ml
7.1.14	Cyclophosphamide	T	Tablet 50 mg Powder for Injection 500mg
7.1.15	Cytosine-arabinoside	T	Injection 100 mg/vial Injection 500 mg/vial Injection 1000 mg/vial
7.1.16	Dacarbazine	T	Powder for Injection 200mg Powder for Injection 500mg

	Medicines	Level of Healthcare	Dosage form and strength
7.1.17	Daunorubicin	T	Injection 5 mg/ml
7.1.18	Docetaxel	T	Powder for Injection 20 mg Powder for Injection 80 mg
7.1.19	Doxorubicin	T	Injection 2 mg/ml
7.1.20	Etoposide	T	Capsule 50 mg Injection 20 mg/ml
7.1.21	Gefitinib	T	Tablet 250 mg
7.1.22	Gemcitabine	T	Powder for Injection 200mg Powder for Injection 1000 mg
7.1.23	Hydroxyurea	T	Capsule 500 mg
7.1.24	Ifosfamide	T	Powder for Injection 1000 mg Powder for Injection 2000 mg
7.1.25	Imatinib	T	Tablet 100 mg Tablet 400 mg
7.1.26	Irinotecan HCl trihydrate	T	Solution for injection 20 mg/ ml
7.1.27	L-Asparaginase	T	Powder for Injection 5000 KU Powder for Injection 10000 KU
7.1.28	Lenalidomide	T	Capsule 5 mg Capsule 25 mg
7.1.29	Melphalan	T	Tablet 2 mg Tablet 5 mg
7.1.30	Methotrexate	S,T	Tablet 2.5 mg Tablet 5 mg Tablet 10 mg Injection 50 mg/ml
7.1.31	Oxaliplatin	T	Injection 5 mg/ml in 10 ml vial Injection 5 mg/ml in 20 ml vial
7.1.32	Paclitaxel	T	Injection 30 mg/5 ml Injection 100 mg/16.7 ml
7.1.33	Rituximab	T	Injection 10 mg/ml
7.1.34	Temozolomide	T	Capsule 20 mg Capsule 100 mg Capsule 250 mg
7.1.35	Thalidomide	T	Capsule 50 mg Capsule 100 mg
7.1.36	Trastuzumab	T	Injection 440 mg/50 ml
7.1.37	Vinblastine	T	Injection 1 mg/ml
7.1.38	Vincristine	T	Injection 1 mg/ml
	7.2 : Hormones and anti-hormones used in cancer therapy		
7.2.1	Bicalutamide	T	Tablet 50 mg
7.2.2	Letrozole	T	Tablet 2.5 mg
7.2.3	Leuprolide acetate	T	Powder for injection 3.75 mg Powder for injection 11.25 mg Powder for injection 22.5 mg
7.2.4	Prednisolone	S,T	Tablet 10 mg Tablet 20 mg Tablet 40 mg Oral liquid 5 mg/5 ml (p) Oral liquid 15 mg/5 ml (p) Injection 20 mg/2 ml
7.2.5	Tamoxifen	T	Tablet 10 mg Tablet 20 mg

	Medicines	Level of Healthcare	Dosage form and strength
	7.3 : Immunosuppressive Medicines		
7.3.1	Azathioprine	T	Tablet 50 mg
7.3.2	Cyclosporine	T	Capsule 25 mg Capsule 50 mg Capsule 100 mg Oral liquid 100 mg/ml (p) Injection 50 mg/ml
7.3.3	Mycophenolate mofetil	T	Tablet 250 mg Tablet 500 mg
7.3.4	Tacrolimus	T	Capsule 0.5 mg Capsule 1 mg Capsule 2 mg
	7.4 : Medicines used in Palliative Care		
7.4.1	Allopurinol	S,T	Tablet 100 mg
7.4.2	Amitriptyline	S,T	Tablet 10 mg Tablet 25 mg
7.4.3	Dexamethasone	S,T	Tablet 0.5 mg Tablet 4 mg Injection 4 mg/ml
7.4.4	Diazepam	S,T	Tablet 2 mg Tablet 5 mg Injection 5 mg/ml
7.4.5	Filgrastim	T	Injection 300 mcg
7.4.6	Fluoxetine	S,T	Capsule 20 mg
7.4.7	Haloperidol	S,T	Tablet 1.5 mg Tablet 5 mg Injection 5 mg/ml
7.4.8	Lactulose	S,T	Oral liquid 10 g/15 ml
7.4.9	Loperamide	S,T	Tablet 2 mg
7.4.10	Metoclopramide	S,T	Tablet 10 mg Oral liquid 5 mg/5 ml (p) Injection 5 mg/ml
7.4.11	Mesna	T	Injection 100 mg/ml
7.4.12	Midazolam	S,T	Injection 1 mg/ml
7.4.13	Morphine	S,T	Tablet 10 mg Modified Release Tablet 30 mg
7.4.14	Ondansetron	S,T	Tablet 4 mg Tablet 8 mg Oral liquid 2 mg/5 ml (p) Injection 2 mg/ml
7.4.15	Tramadol	S,T	Capsule 50 mg Capsule 100 mg Injection 50 mg/ml
7.4.16	Zoledronic acid	T	Powder for Injection 4 mg
	Section 8 : Medicines affecting blood		
	8.1 : Antianaemia medicines		
8.1.1	Erythropoietin	S,T	Injection 2000 IU/ml Injection 10000 IU/ml
8.1.2	Ferrous salts (a) Iron Dextran (b) Iron sorbitol citrate complex	P,S,T	Tablet equivalent to 60 mg of elemental iron Injection 50 mg/ml Injection 50 mg/ml
8.1.3	Ferrous Salt (A) + Folic acid (B)	P,S,T	Tablet 45 mg elemental iron (A)+ 400 mcg (B) Tablet 100 mg elemental iron(A) + 500 mcg (B) Oral liquid 20 mg elemental iron(A)+100 mcg/ml(B) (p)
8.1.4	Folic Acid	P,S,T	Tablet 1 mg Tablet 5 mg
8.1.5	Hydroxocobalamin	P,S,T	Injection 1 mg/ml
8.1.6	Hydroxyurea	S,T	Capsule 500 mg
8.1.7	Iron sucrose	S,T	Injection 20 mg/ml

	Medicines	Level of Healthcare	Dosage form and strength
	8.2 : Medicines affecting coagulation		
8.2.1	Enoxaparin	S,T	Injection 40 mg/ 0.4 ml Injection 60 mg/ 0.6 ml
8.2.2	Heparin	S,T	Injection 1000 IU/ml Injection 5000 IU/ml
8.2.3	Phytomenadione (Vitamin K_1)	P,S,T	Tablet 10 mg Injection 10 mg/ml
8.2.4	Protamine Sulphate	S,T	Injection 10 mg/ml
8.2.5	Tranexamic acid	P,S,T	Tablet 500 mg Injection 100 mg/ml
8.2.6	Warfarin	S,T	Tablet 1 mg Tablet 2 mg Tablet 3 mg Tablet 5 mg
	Section 9 : Blood products and plasma substitutes		
	9.1 : Blood and blood components		
9.1.1	Fresh frozen plasma	S,T	As licensed
9.1.2	Platelet rich plasma/ Platelet concentrates	S,T	As licensed
9.1.3	Red blood cells/ Packed RBCs	S,T	As licensed
9.1.4	Whole blood	S,T	As licensed
	9.2 : Plasma substitutes		
9.2.1	Dextran-40	S,T	Injection 10%
	9.3 : Plasma fractions for specific use		
9.3.1	Coagulation factor IX	S,T	Powder for Injection 600 IU
9.3.2	Coagulation factor VIII	S,T	Powder for Injection 250 IU Powder for Injection 500 IU
9.3.3	Cryoprecipitate	S,T	As licensed
	Section 10 : Cardiovascular medicines		
	10.1 : Medicines used in angina		
10.1.1	Diltiazem	P,S,T	Tablet 30 mg Tablet 60 mg Modified Release Tablet 180 mg
		S, T	Injection 5 mg/ml
10.1.2	Glyceryl trinitrate	P,S,T	Sublingual Tablet 0.5 mg
		S,T	Injection 5 mg/ml
10.1.3	Isosorbide dinitrate	P,S,T	Tablet 5 mg Tablet 10 mg
10.1.4	Metoprolol	P,S,T	Tablet 25 mg Tablet 50 mg Tablet 100 mg Modified Release Tablet 100 mg
		S,T	Injection 1 mg/ml
	10.2 : Antiarrhythmic medicines		
10.2.1	Adenosine	S,T	Injection 3 mg/ml
10.2.2	Amiodarone	S,T	Tablet 100 mg Tablet 200 mg Injection 50 mg/ml
10.2.3	Digoxin	S,T	Tablet 0.25 mg Oral liquid 0.05 mg/ml Injection 0.25 mg/ml
10.2.4	Esmolol	S,T	Injection 10 mg/ml
10.2.5	Lignocaine	S,T	Injection 2%
10.2.6	Verapamil	S,T	Tablet 40 mg Tablet 80 mg Injection 2.5 mg/ ml

	Medicines	Level of Healthcare	Dosage form and strength
	10.3 : Antihypertensive medicines		
10.3.1	Amlodipine	P,S,T	Tablet 2.5 mg Tablet 5 mg Tablet 10 mg
10.3.2	Enalapril	P,S,T	Tablet 2.5 mg Tablet 5 mg
10.3.3	Hydrochloro-thiazide	P,S,T	Tablet 12.5 mg Tablet 25 mg
10.3.4	Labetalol	P,S,T	Tablet 50 mg Tablet 100 mg
		P,S,T	Injection 5 mg/ml
10.3.5	Ramipril	P,S,T	Tablet 2.5 mg Tablet 5 mg
10.3.6	Sodium nitroprusside	S, T	Injection 10 mg/ml
10.3.7	Telmisartan	P,S,T	Tablet 20 mg Tablet 40 mg Tablet 80 mg
	10.4 : Medicines used in shock and heart failure		
10.4.1	Digoxin	S,T	Tablet 0.25 mg Oral liquid 0.05 mg/ml Injection 0.25 mg/ml
10.4.2	Dobutamine	S,T	Injection 50 mg/ml
10.4.3	Dopamine	S,T	Injection 40 mg/ml
10.4.4	Noradrenaline	S,T	Injection 2 mg/ml
10.4.5	Spironolactone	P,S,T	Tablet 25 mg Tablet 50 mg
	10.5 : Antiplatelet and antithrombotic medicines		
10.5.1	Acetylsalicylic acid	P,S,T	Conventional/Effervescent/ Dispersible/ Enteric coated Tablets 150 mg Conventional/Effervescent/ Dispersible/ Enteric coated Tablets 325 mg Enteric coated Tablet 75 mg Enteric coated Tablet 100 mg
10.5.2	Clopidogrel	P,S,T	Tablet 75 mg Tablet 150 mg
10.5.3	Dabigatran	S, T	Tablet 110 mg Tablet 150 mg
10.5.4	Enoxaparin	S,T	Injection 40 mg/ 0.4 ml Injection 60 mg/ 0.6 ml
10.5.5	Heparin	S,T	Injection 1000 IU/ml Injection 5000 IU/ml
10.5.6	Streptokinase	S,T	Injection 750,000 IU Injection 15,00,000 IU
10.5.7	Tenecteplase	S,T	Injection 30 mg/vial Injection 40 mg/vial
	10.6 : Hypolipidemic medicines		
10.6.1	Atorvastatin	P,S,T	Tablet 10 mg Tablet 20 mg Tablet 40 mg Tablet 80 mg
	Section 11 : Dermatological medicines (Topical)		
	11.1 : Antifungal medicines		
11.1.1	Clotrimazole	P,S,T	Cream 1%, Lotion 1%
	11.2 : Antibacterial medicines		
11.2.1	Framycetin	P,S,T	Cream 1%
11.2.2	Fusidic acid	P,S,T	Cream 2%
11.2.3	Silver sulphadiazine	P,S,T	Cream 1%

	Medicines	Level of Healthcare	Dosage form and strength
	11.3 : Antiinflammatory and Antipruritic Medicines		
11.3.1	Betamethasone valerate	P,S,T	Cream 0.05% Cream 0.1%
11.3.2	Calamine	P,S,T	Lotion (As per IP)
	11.4 : Keratolytic agents		
11.4.1	Benzoyl peroxide	P,S,T	Gel 2.5% - 5%
11.4.2	Coal tar (A) + Salicylic Acid (B)	P,S,T	Solution 1% (A) + 3% (B)
11.4.3	Podophyllin resin	S,T	Solution 20%
11.4.4	Salicylic acid	P,S,T	Ointment 3-6%
	11.5 : Scabicides and pediculicides		
11.5.1	Permethrin	P,S,T	Lotion 1%, Cream 5%
	11.6 : Miscellaneous		
11.6.1	Glycerin/glycerol (as mentioned in IP)	P,S,T	Topical
	Section 12 : Diagnostic agents		
	12.1 : Ophthalmic medicines		
12.1.1	Fluorescein	S,T	Ophthalmic Strips
12.1.2	Proparacaine	S,T	Eye Drops 0.5%
12.1.3	Tropicamide	S,T	Eye drop 1%
	12.2 : Radiocontrast media		
12.2.1	Barium sulphate	S,T	Oral Liquid 95% w/v
12.2.2	Gadobenate dimeglumine	T	Injection 529 mg/ml
12.2.3	Iohexol	S,T	Injection 140 to 350 mg iodine/ml
12.2.4	Meglumine diatrizoate	S,T	Injection 60% w/v Injection 76% w/v
	Section 13 : Dialysis components (Haemodialysis and Peritoneal Dialysis)		
13.1	Haemodialysis fluid	S,T	As licensed
13.2	Peritoneal dialysis solution	S,T	As licensed
	Section 14 : Antiseptics and disinfectants		
	14.1 : Antiseptics		
14.1.1	Chlorhexidine	P,S,T	Solution 5% (Concentrate)
14.1.2	Ethyl alcohol (Denatured)	P,S,T	Solution 70%
14.1.3	Hydrogen peroxide	P,S,T	Solution 6%
14.1.4	Methylrosanilinium chloride (Gentian Violet)	P,S,T	Topical preparation 0.25% to 2%
14.1.5	Povidone iodine	P,S,T	Solution 4% to 10%
	14.2 : Disinfectants		
14.2.1	Glutaraldehyde	S,T	As Licensed
14.2.2	Potassium permanganate	P,S,T	Crystals for topical solution
	Section 15 : Diuretics		
15.1	Furosemide	P,S,T	Tablet 40 mg Oral liquid 10 mg/ml Injection 10 mg/ ml
15.2	Hydrochlorothiazide	P,S,T	Tablet 25 mg Tablet 50 mg
15.3	Mannitol	P,S,T	Injection 10% Injection 20%
15.4	Spironolactone	P,S,T	Tablet 25 mg Tablet 50 mg

	Medicines	Level of Healthcare	Dosage form and strength
	Section 16 : Ear, nose and throat medicines		
16.1	Budesonide	P,S,T	Nasal Spray 50 mcg/dose Nasal Spray 100 mcg/dose
16.2	Ciprofloxacin	P,S,T	Drops 0.3%
16.3	Clotrimazole	P,S,T	Drops 1%
16.4	Xylometazoline	P,S,T	Nasal drops 0.05% Nasal drops 0.1%
	Section 17 : Gastrointestinal medicines		
	17.1 : Antiulcer medicines		
17.1.1	Omeprazole	P,S,T	Capsule 10 mg Capsule 20 mg Capsule 40 mg Powder for oral liquid 20 mg
17.1.2	Pantoprazole	S,T	Injection 40 mg
	17.2 : Antiemetics		
17.2.1	Domperidone	P,S,T	Tablet 10 mg Oral Liquid 1 mg/ml
17.2.2	Metoclopramide	P,S,T	Tablet 10 mg Injection 5 mg/ml
17.2.3	Ondansetron	S,T	Tablet 4 mg Oral Liquid 2 mg/5 ml (p) Injection 2 mg/ ml
	17.3 : Anti-inflammatory medicines		
17.3.1	5-aminosalicylic acid (Mesalazine/ Mesalaine)	S, T	Tablet 400 mg Suppository 500 mg Retention Enema
	17.4 : Antispasmodic medicines		
17.4.1	Dicyclomine	P,S,T	Tablet 10 mg Oral Solution 10 mg/5ml Injection 10 mg/ ml
17.4.2	Hyoscine butyl bromide	P,S,T	Tablet 100 mg Injection 20 mg/ ml
	17.5 : Laxatives		
17.5.1	Bisacodyl	P,S,T	Tablet 5 mg Suppository 5 mg
17.5.2	Ispaghula	P,S,T	Granules/ Husk/ Powder
17.5.3	Lactulose	S,T	Oral Liquid 10 g/15 ml
	17.6 Medicines used in diarrhea		
17.6.1	Oral rehydration salts	P,S,T	As licensed
17.6.2	Zinc Sulphate	P,S,T	Dispersible Tablet 20 mg
	17.7 : Other medicines		
17.7.1	Somatostatin	T	Powder for Injection 3 mg
	Section 18 : Hormones, other endocrine medicines and contraceptives		
	18.1 : Adrenal hormones and synthetic substitutes		
18.1.1	Dexamethasone	S,T	Tablet 0.5 mg Injection 4 mg/ml
18.1.2	Fludrocortisone	S,T	Tablet 0.1 mg
18.1.3	Hydrocortisone	P,S,T	Tablet 5 mg Tablet 10 mg Tablet 20 mg Powder for Injection 100mg
18.1.4	Methylprednisolone	S,T	Injection 40mg/ml
18.1.5	Prednisolone	P,S,T	Tablet 5 mg Tablet 10 mg Tablet 20 mg Oral liquid 5 mg/5 ml (p) Oral liquid 15 mg/5 ml (p)

	Medicines	Level of Healthcare	Dosage form and strength
	18.2 : Contraceptives		
	18.2.1 : Hormonal contraceptives		
18.2.1.1	Ethinylestradiol (A) + Levonorgestrel (B)	P,S,T	Tablet 0.03 mg (A) + Tablet 0.15 mg (B)
18.2.1.2	Levonorgestrel	P,S,T	Tablet 0.75 mg Tablet 1.5 mg
18.2.1.3	Ormeloxifene (Centchroman)	P,S,T	Tablet 30 mg
	18.2.2 : Intrauterine devices		
18.2.2.1	Hormone releasing IUD	T	Contains 52 mg of Levonorgestrel
18.2.2.2	IUD containing Copper	P,S,T	As licensed
	18.2.3 : Barrier methods		
18.2.3.1	Condom	P,S,T	As Licensed as per the standards of Drugs Rules, 1945
	18.3 : Medicines used in diabetes mellitus		
	18.3.1 : Insulins and other antidiabetic agents		
18.3.1.1	Glimepiride	P,S,T	Tablet 1 mg Tablet 2 mg
18.3.1.2	Insulin (Soluble)	P,S,T	Injection 40 IU/ml
18.3.1.3	Insulin Intermediate Acting (NPH)	P,S,T	Injection 40 IU/ml
18.3.1.4	Insulin Glargine	P,S,T	Injection 100 IU/ml
18.3.1.5	Insulin Premix Injection 30:70 (Regular : NPH)	P,S,T	Injection 40 IU/ml
18.3.1.6	Metformin	P,S,T	Tablet 500 mg Tablet 1000 mg Modified release Tablet 1000 mg
18.3.1.7	Teneligliptin	P,S,T	Tablet 20 mg
	18.3.2 : Medicines used to treat Hypoglycaemia		
18.3.2.1	Glucose	P,S,T	Injection 25%
	18.4 : Ovulation inducers		
18.4.1	Clomiphene citrate	T	Tablet 50 mg Tablet 100 mg
18.4.2	Human chorionic gonadotropin	S,T	Injection 2000 IU Injection 5000 IU Injection 10000 IU
	18.5 : Progestogens		
18.5.1	Medroxyprogesterone acetate	P,S,T	Tablet 5 mg Tablet 10 mg Injection 150 mg/ ml
18.5.2	Norethisterone	P,S,T	Tablet 5 mg
	18.6 : Thyroid and antithyroid medicines		
18.6.1	Carbimazole	P,S,T	Tablet 5 mg Tablet 10 mg Tablet 20 mg
18.6.2	Levothyroxine	P,S,T	Tablet 12.5 mcg to 150 mcg* (*Several strengths are available in market such as 12.5, 25, 50, 62.5, 75, 88, 100, 112mcg. Therefore, it was considered to give a range of available strengths)

	Medicines	Level of Healthcare	Dosage form and strength
	Section 19 : Immunologicals		
	19.1 : Diagnostic agents		
19.1.1	Tuberculin, Purified Protein derivative	P,S,T	As Licensed
	19.2 : Sera and immunoglobulins (Liquid/ Lyophilized)		
19.2.1	Anti-rabies immunoglobulin	P,S,T	As Licensed
19.2.2	Anti-tetanus immunoglobulin	P,S,T	As Licensed
19.2.3	Anti-D immunoglobulin	S,T	As Licensed
19.2.4	Diphtheria antitoxin	P,S,T	As Licensed
19.2.5	Hepatitis B immunoglobulin	S,T	As Licensed
19.2.6	Human normal immunoglobulin	T	As Licensed
19.2.7	Snake Venom Antiserum	P,S,T	a) Soluble/ liquid polyvalent - As Licensed b) Lyophilized polyvalent - As Licensed
	19.3 : Vaccines **For universal immunization**		
19.3.1	BCG vaccine	P,S,T	As licensed
19.3.2	DPT+ Hib+ Hep B vaccine	P,S,T	As licensed
19.3.3	DPT vaccine	P,S,T	As licensed
19.3.4	Hepatitis B vaccine	P,S,T	As licensed
19.3.5	Japanese encephalitis vaccine	P,S,T	As licensed
19.3.6	Measles vaccine	P,S,T	As licensed
19.3.7	Oral poliomyelitis vaccine	P,S,T	As licensed
19.3.8	Rotavirus vaccine	P,S,T	As licensed
19.3.9	Tetanus toxoid	P,S,T	As licensed
	19.4 : For specific group of individuals		
19.4.1	Rabies vaccine	P,S,T	As licensed
	Section 20 : Medicines for neonatal care		
20.1	Alprostadil	S,T	Injection 0.5 mg/ml
20.2	Caffeine	S,T	Oral liquid 20 mg/ml Injection 20 mg/ml
20.3	Surfactant	S,T	Suspension for intratracheal instillation (As licensed)
	Section 21 : Ophthalmological medicines		
	21.1 : Anti-infective medicines		
21.1.1	Acyclovir	P,S,T	Ointment 3%
21.1.2	Ciprofloxacin	P,S,T	Drops 0.3% Ointment 0.3%
21.1.3	Natamycin	P,S,T	Drops 5%
21.1.4	Povidone iodine	P,S,T	Drops 5%
	21.2 : Antiinflammatory medicine		
21.2.1	Prednisolone	P,S,T	Drops 1%
	21.3 : Local anaesthetic		
21.3.1	Proparacaine	P,S,T	Drops 0.5%
	21.4 : Miotics and antiglaucoma medicines		
21.4.1	Acetazolamide	P,S,T	Tablet 250 mg
21.4.2	Latanoprost	P,S,T	Drops 0.005%

	Medicines	Level of Healthcare	Dosage form and strength
21.4.3	Pilocarpine	P,S,T	Drops 2% Drops 4%
21.4.4	Timolol	P,S,T	Drops 0.25% Drops 0.5%
	21.5 : Mydriatics		
21.5.1	Atropine	P,S,T	Drops 1% Ointment 1%
21.5.2	Homatropine	P,S,T	Drops 2%
21.5.3	Phenylephrine	P,S,T	Drops 5% Drops 10%
21.5.4	Tropicamide	P,S,T	Drops 1%
	21.6 : Miscellaneous		
21.6.1	Carboxymethyl cellulose	P,S,T	Drops 0.5% Drops 1%
21.6.2	Hydroxypropyl methylcellulose	T	Injection 2%
	Section 22 : Oxytocics and antioxytocics		
	22.1 : Oxytocics and abortifacient		
22.1.1	Dinoprostone	S,T	Tablet 0.5 mg Gel 0.5 mg
22.1.2	Methylergo-metrine	P,S,T	Tablet 0.125 mg Injection 0.2 mg/ml
22.1.3	Mifepristone	P,S,T	Tablet 200 mg
22.1.4	Misoprostol	P,S,T	Tablet 100 mcg Tablet 200 mcg
22.1.5	Oxytocin	P,S,T	Injection 5 IU/ml Injection 10 IU/ml
	22.2 : Medicines used in preterm labour		
22.2.1	Betamethasone	P,S,T	Injection 4 mg/ml
22.2.2	Nifedipine	S,T	Tablet 10 mg
	Section 23 : Medicines used in treatment of psychiatric disorders		
	23.1 : Medicines used in psychotic disorders		
23.1.1	Clozapine	T	Tablet 25 mg Tablet 50 mg Tablet 100 mg
23.1.2	Fluphenazine	P,S,T	Injection 25 mg/ml
23.1.3	Haloperidol	S,T	Tablet 2 mg Tablet 5 mg Tablet 10 mg Tablet 20 mg Oral liquid 2 mg/5 ml Injection 5 mg/ml
23.1.4	Risperidone	P,S,T	Tablet 1 mg Tablet 2 mg Tablet 4 mg Oral liquid 1 mg/ml Injection (Long acting) 25 mg Injection (Long acting) 37.5 mg
	23.2 : Medicines used in mood disorders		
	23.2.1 : Medicines used in depressive disorders		
23.2.1.1	Amitriptyline	P,S,T	Tablet 10 mg Tablet 25 mg Tablet 50 mg Tablet 75 mg
23.2.1.2	Escitalopram	P,S,T	Tablet 5 mg Tablet 10 mg Tablet 20 mg
23.2.1.3	Fluoxetine	P,S,T	Capsule 10 mg Capsule 20 mg Capsule 40 mg Capsule 60 mg

	Medicines	Level of Healthcare	Dosage form and strength
	23.2.2 : Medicines used in bipolar disorders		
23.2.2.1	Lithium	S,T	Tablet 300 mg
23.2.2.2	Sodium valproate	P,S,T	Tablet 200 mg Tablet 300 mg Tablet 500 mg Modified Release - Tablet 300 mg Tablet 500 mg
23.2.2.3	Carbamazepine	P,S,T	Tablet 100 mg Tablet 200 mg Tablet 400 mg Modified Release - Tablet 200 mg Tablet 400 mg Oral liquid 100 mg/5 ml (p)
	23.3 : Medicines used in generalized anxiety and sleep disorders		
23.3.1	Clonazepam	P,S,T	Tablet 0.25 mg Tablet 0.5 mg Tablet 1 mg
23.3.2	Zolpidem	P,S,T	Tablet 5 mg Tablet 10 mg
	23.4 : Medicines used in obsessive compulsive disorders and panic attacks		
23.4.1	Clomipramine	P,S,T	Capsule 10 mg Capsule 25 mg Capsule 75 mg
23.4.2	Fluoxetine	S,T	Capsule 10 mg Capsule 20 mg Capsule 40 mg Capsule 60 mg
	23.5 : Medicines used in disorders due to psychoactive substance abuse		
23.5.1	Buprenorphine	P,S,T	Tablet (Sub-lingual) 0.4 mg
23.5.2	Buprenorphine (A) + Naloxone (B)	P,S,T	Tablet (Sub-lingual) 0.4 mg (A)+ 0.1 mg (B) Tablet (Sub-lingual) 2 mg (A) +0.5 mg (B)
23.5.3	Nicotine (for nicotine replacement therapy)	P,S,T	Oral Dosage forms 2 mg Oral Dosage forms 4 mg
	Section 24 : Medicines acting on the respiratory tract		
	24.1 : Antiasthmatic medicines		
24.1.1	Budesonide	P,S,T	Inhalation (MDI/DPI) 100 mcg/dose Inhalation (MDI/DPI) 200 mcg/dose Respirator solution for use in nebulizer 0.5 mg/ml Respirator solution for use in nebulizer 1 mg/ml
24.1.2	Budesonide (A) + Formoterol (B)	P,S,T	Inhalation (MDI/DPI) 100 mcg (A)+ 6 mcg (B) Inhalation (MDI/DPI) 200 mcg (A)+ 6 mcg (B) Inhalation (MDI/DPI) 400 mcg (A)+ 6 mcg (B)
24.1.3	Hydrocortisone	P,S,T	Powder for Injection 100mg Powder for Injection 200mg
24.1.4	Ipratropium	P,S,T	Inhalation (MDI/DPI) 20 mcg/dose Respirator solution for use in nebulizer 250 mcg/ml
24.1.5	Montelukast	S,T	Tablet 4 mg Tablet 5 mg (including chewable tablets) Tablet 10 mg

	Medicines	Level of Healthcare	Dosage form and strength
24.1.6	Salbutamol	P,S,T	Tablet 2 mg Tablet 4 mg Oral liquid 2 mg/5 ml Inhalation (MDI/DPI*) 100 mcg/dose Respirator Solution (Solution for Nebulizer 5 mg/ml)
24.1.7	Tiotropium	P,S,T	Inhalation (MDI) 9 mcg/dose Inhalation (DPI) 18 mcg/dose MDI- Metered Dose Inhaler DPI- Dry Powder Inhaler
	Section 25 : Solutions correcting water, electrolyte disturbances and acid-base disturbances		
25.1.1	Glucose	P,S,T	Injection 5% Injection 10% Injection 25% Injection 50%
25.1.2	Glucose(A) + Sodium chloride (B)	P,S,T	Injection 5% (A) + 0.9% (B)
25.1.3	Oral rehydration salts	P,S,T	As licensed
25.1.4	Potassium chloride	P,S,T	Oral liquid 500 mg/5 ml
		S,T	Injection 150 mg/ml
25.1.5	Ringer lactate	P,S,T	Injection (as per IP)
25.1.6	Sodium bicarbonate	P,S,T	Injection (as per IP)
25.1.7	Sodium chloride	P,S,T	Injection 0.9%
		S,T	Injection 3%
	25.2 : Miscellaneous		
25.2.1	Water for Injection	P,S,T	Injection
	Section 26 : Vitamins and minerals		
26.1	Ascorbic acid (Vitamin C)	P,S,T	Tablet 100 mg Tablet 500 mg
26.2	Calcium carbonate	P,S,T	Tablet 625 mg (equivalent to elemental calcium 250 mg) Tablet 1250 mg (equivalent to elemental calcium 500 mg)
26.3	Calcium gluconate	P,S,T	Injection 100 mg/ml
26.4	Cholecalciferol	P,S,T	Solid oral dosage form 1000 IU Solid oral dosage form 60000 IU Oral liquid 400 IU/ml
26.5	Pyridoxine	P,S,T	Tablet 10 mg Tablet 50 mg Tablet 100 mg
26.6	Riboflavin	P,S,T	Tablet 10 mg
26.7	Thiamine	P,S,T	Tablet 100 mg Injection 100 mg/ml
26.8	Vitamin A	P,S,T	Capsule/Tablet 50000 IU (including Chewable Tablet) Oral liquid 100000 IU/ml Injection 50000 IU/ml
	Section 27 : Medicines for COVID 19 management		
27.1	Dexamethasone	P,S,T	Tablet 0.5 mg Tablet 2 mg Tablet 4 mg Oral liquid 0.5 mg/5 ml (p) Injection 4 mg/ml
27.2	Enoxaparin	S,T	Injection 40 mg/ 0.4 ml Injection 60 mg/ 0.6 ml
27.3	Methylpred-nisolone	S,T	Injection 40 mg/ml
27.4	Paracetamol	P,S,T	Tablet 500 mg Tablet 650 mg Oral liquid 120 mg/5 ml (p) Oral liquid 125 mg/5 ml (p) Oral liquid 250 mg/5 ml (p)
27.5	Oxygen	P,S,T	As licensed for medical purpose

COUNTERFEIT MEDICINES

According to WHO's definition, a drug/medicine is counterfeit if it is produced with an intention to cheat. This can include mis-labelling (including fudging expiry date), or no active ingredients, a wrong ingredient, or the correct ingredient in an insufficient quantity. Both branded and generic products can be counterfeited *(3)*.

Sub-standard medicines, also called "out of specification" medicines are authorized medical products that fail to meet either their quality standards or specifications, or both *(4)*.

Falsified medical products that deliberately/fraudulently misrepresent their identity, composition or source *(4)*.

Unregistered/unlicensed medical products that have not undergone evaluation and/or approval by the National or Regional Regulation Authority for the market in which they are marketed/distributed or used, subject to permitted conditions under national or regional regulation and legislation *(4)*.

Falsified medical products may contain no active ingredient, the wrong active ingredient or the wrong amount of correct active ingredient. They are also commonly found to contain corn starch, potato starch or chalk. Some sub-standard and falsified medical products have been toxic in nature with either fatal levels of the wrong active ingredient or other toxic chemicals. Anti-malarials and antibiotics are amongst the most commonly reported sub-standard and falsified medical products. Both generic and innovator medicines can be falsified. An estimated 10 per cent medical products in low and middle-income countries is sub-standard or falsified. These products contribute to antimicrobial resistance and drug-resistant infections *(4)*.

Unregulated websites, social media platforms and smartphone applications can also be direct conduits of sub-standard and falsified medical products. Risks to consumers are increased when they obtain medicines from unlicensed and unregulated sources. Consumers should be cautious of the following *(4)*;

1. spam email advertising medicines;
2. lack of authenticity or no verification logo or certificate;
3. spelling mistakes and poor grammar on packaging;
4. websites that do not display a physical address or landline; and
5. websites offering prescription only medicines without a

prescription.

Identifying a sub-standard or falsified medical product

Some falsified medical products are almost visually identical to the genuine product and very difficult to detect. However, many can be identified by *(4)*:

- examining the packaging for condition, spelling mistakes or grammatical errors;
- checking the manufacture and expiry dates and ensuring any details on the outer packaging match the dates shown on the inner packaging;
- ensuring the medicine looks correct, is not discoloured, degraded or has an unusual smell;
- discussing with your pharmacist, doctor or other healthcare professional as soon as possible if you suspect the product is not working properly or you have suffered an adverse reaction; and
- reporting suspicious medical products to your National Medicines Regulatory Authority.

In 2006, WHO launched the international medical products Anti-Counterfeiting Task Force (IMPACT) and in 2013, WHO launched the Global Surveillance and Monitoring System to encourage countries to report incidence of sub-standard and falsified medical products in a structured and systematic format, to help develop a more accurate and validated assessment of the problem.

Measures for combating counterfeit medicines so far have included: actions taken by drug regulatory authorities and co-operation initiatives between different law enforcement agencies; providing simple, easily interpretable and cheap markers of authenticity; coordinating international surveillance for fake and sub-standard drugs; and educating patients and healthcare workers.

Legislation forms the basis for drug regulation. Medicines need to be safe, effective and of good quality in order to produce the expected therapeutic effect. Ensuring these properties requires the creation of competent national drug regulatory authorities with the necessary human and other resources to control the manufacture, importation, distribution and sale of medicines.

Legislation must be complemented with effective law enforcement. Governments need to develop strategies to reduce corruption and criminal activity and promote intersectoral co-operation between regulatory authorities, police, customs services and the judiciary to effectively control the drug market and enforce drug regulation.

QUALITY CONTROL IN DRUG SECTOR IN INDIA

Central Drug Standard Control Organization *(5)*

The quality control of the drugs marketed in the country is regulated under the Drugs and Cosmetics Act, 1940 and Drugs & Cosmetics Rules, 1945. The Central Drugs Standard Control Organization (CDSCO), in the Directorate of Director General of Health Services, along with Drug Control Organization in the States are responsible for safety, efficacy and quality of drugs, their import, manufacture, distribution, sale and standards.

The CDSCO at the Centre is headed by the Drugs Controller General (India), in the Directorate of Director General of Health Services, under the Ministry of Health and Family Welfare. The Drug Control Organization in the States is generally headed by the State Drug Controllers appointed by the State Governments.

The main functions of the CDSCO include control of the quality of drugs imported into the country, coordination of the activities of the States/UTs Drug Control Authorities, approval of new drugs proposed to be imported or manufactured in the country, laying down standards and regulatory measures and acting as the Central License Approving Authority in respect of whole human blood and its products, large volume parenterals (IV fluids), sera and vaccines and rDNA products. Quality of cosmetics manufactured and marketed in the country are also regulated under the Drugs and Cosmetics Act.

The CDSCO has a network of six Zonal Offices located at Mumbai, Ghaziabad, Kolkata, Hyderabad, Ahmedabad and Chennai, six sub-zonal offices and 16 port offices responsible for ensuring quality of imports and 7 laboratories. The Zonal Officers inspect the drug manufacturing units, blood banks and approved drug testing laboratories, either jointly with State Drug Control Authorities or independently, and deficiencies observed during these inspections are invariably brought to the notice of State Drug Control Authorities. The port offices monitor import and export of drugs.

References

1. WHO (2005), *Tech. Rep. Ser. No. 933*, The Selection and Use of Essential Medicines.
2. Govt. of India (2022), *National List of Essential Medicines*, 2022.
3. WHO (2006), Fact Sheet M. 275, *Counterfeit Medicines.*
4. WHO (2018), Fact Sheet, *Sub-standard and falsified Medical Products*, 31st Jan. 2018.
5. Govt. of India (2019), *Annual Report 2018–19*, Ministry of Health and Family Welfare, New Delhi.

25 International Health

"Medicine is one of the pillars of peace"

"Nothing on earth is more international than disease", said Paul Russel. Health and disease have no political or geographical boundaries. Disease in any part of the world is a constant threat to other parts. History is replete with examples of the spread of pestilences – particularly of plague and cholera, along trade routes. In order to protect against the spread of disease from one country to another, many attempts were made in the past by individual rulers and States to place barriers against infection by detection and isolation of incoming travellers. In the 14th century, a procedure known as "quarantine" was introduced in Europe to protect against the importation of plague. Ships, crews, travellers and cargoes, suspected of harbouring infection, were detained for a 40-day period. The underlying idea was that the passage of time would give dormant disease to manifest itself or die out. Quarantine soon became an established practice in many countries, and different countries adopted different quarantine procedures. This was the origin of international health work.

Quarantine failed in its objective because of the lack of scientific knowledge regarding the causation and mode of spread of disease. Opposition to quarantine came from several quarters because the 40-day detention obstructed and caused serious inconveniences to international trade and travel. It became necessary for international agreement and cooperation on quarantine matters to control communicable diseases. International conferences were held and organizations set up for discussion, agreement and cooperation on matters of international health. A brief account of these endeavours and of the early health organizations which preceded the World Health Organization is given below.

First International Sanitary Conference (1851)

The origin of international health cooperation dates back to 1851, when an international sanitary conference – the first of its kind – was convened in Paris. The Conference was attended mainly by European countries – Austria, France, Great Britain, Greece, Portugal, Russia, Spain and four Sovereign States (Sardinia, the two Sicilies, the Papal States, Tuscany) that were later to form a united Italy *(1)*. Turkey also participated in this Conference. The objective of this Conference was very limited i.e., to introduce some order and uniformity into quarantine measures which varied from country to country. The conference lasted six months with no lasting results. Some members opposed quarantine, and some took an intermediate position. Despite the many difficulties involved, an international sanitary code was prepared, comprising 137 articles dealing with cholera, plague and yellow fever *(2)*. But, the sanitary code never came into force as it was ratified by only three countries – France, Portugal and Sardinia of which Portugal and Sardinia withdrew in 1865. Thus the conference was generally regarded as having ended in failure. The 1851 conference was followed in rapid succession by further conferences – no less than 10 conferences took place between 1851 and 1902, but they were equally unable to reach an agreement on quarantine measures *(2)*.

Pan American Sanitary Bureau (1902)

The next important milestone in international health work was the establishment of Pan American Sanitary Bureau (PASB) in 1902 in the Americas. It was primarily intended to coordinate quarantine procedures in the American States. In 1924 an important document was signed by the American Republic namely "The Pan American Sanitary Code" which is still in force between the States. In 1947, the Bureau was reorganized and the organization was called the Pan American Sanitary Organization (PASO). In 1949, an agreement was reached whereby the PASO would serve as the WHO Regional Office for the Americas. In 1958, the name was changed to Pan American Health Organization (PAHO) *(3)*. Over the years, PAHO has grown from a small information centre to a major health agency with its headquarters in Washington, D.C. The Pan American Sanitary Bureau was the World's first international health agency *(4)*.

Office International D'Hygiene Publique (1907)

At the 1903 International Sanitary Conference, a step of fundamental importance was taken, that is, to establish a permanent International Health Bureau *(1)*. This decision was probably influenced by the fact that the American republics had already established a similar bureau, the Pan American Sanitary Bureau in 1902. Accordingly in 1907, the "Office International d'Hygiene Publique" (OIHP), generally known as the "Paris Office" was created to disseminate information on communicable diseases and to supervise international quarantine measures. At its inception, the OIHP was predominantly European, but later on a considerable degree of cooperation grew up between OIHP and PASB. Sixty other countries, including British India, joined the OIHP, giving the Office an international character *(5)*.

Although the OIHP had no field staff to undertake investigation of epidemics it did remarkable work in disseminating knowledge of communicable diseases and their control, and also information on a variety of health problems of worldwide interest. The OIHP continued to exist until 1950, by which time its responsibilities had been taken over by the WHO.

The Health Organization of the League of Nations (1923)

After the first World War (1914–18), the League of Nations was established to build a better world. It included a 'Health Organization' to "take steps in matters of international concern for the prevention and control of disease". Although the League of Nations was a failure on the political side, its Health Organization, which was established in 1923, did creditable work. Not confining itself to quarantine regulations and epidemiological information or even larger problems of epidemic diseases, the Health Organization of the League branched out into such matters as nutrition, housing and rural hygiene, the training of public health workers and the standardization of certain biological preparations. The League analysed epidemiological information received, and started the series of periodical epidemiological reports now issued by the WHO. It also established the Far Eastern Bureau at Singapore. It laid down lines for technical studies (including the use of expert committees) which are substantially followed by the WHO. The WHO owes much to the work done and methods devised by the Health Organization of the League. It may be mentioned that efforts to amalgamate the OIHP, PASB and the Health Organization of the League of Nations proved a failure, and all the three organizations were co-existing during the years between the two World Wars. In 1939, the League of Nations was dissolved but its Health Organization in Geneva continued to deal as best it could with requests for information and the publication of the Weekly Epidemiological Records was never suspended.

The United Nations Relief and Rehabilitation Administration (1943)

The United Nations Relief and Rehabilitation Administration (UNRRA) was set up in 1943 with the general purpose of organizing recovery from the effects of the Second World War. The UNRRA had a health division to care for the health of the millions of displaced persons, to restore and help services and to revive the machinery for international interchange of information on epidemic diseases.

UNRRA did outstanding work of preventing the spread of typhus and other diseases, so that they never reached serious epidemic levels anywhere. Similarly, UNRRA'S assistance to malaria control in such countries as Greece and Italy, where war had disrupted peace–time anti-malaria services, was on an immense scale. The world renowned campaign for the eradication of malaria from Sardinia was begun as a joint effort of UNRRA, the Rockefeller Foundation and the Italian Government *(5)*.

At the end of 1946, UNRRA terminated its official existence and its health activities and financial assets were taken over by the Interim Commission on the WHO.

Birth of the WHO

The WHO has its origin in April 1945, during the conference held at San Francisco to set up the United Nations. The representatives of Brazil and China proposed that an international health organization should be established and that a conference to frame its constitution should be convened. The constitution was drawn up at an international health conference in New York in 1946. The same conference set up an "Interim Commission" to prepare the ground for the new organization and to carry out urgent tasks until the WHO constitution had been accepted by the required number of UN Member States. The ratifications were secured by 7th April 1948; the formal existence of the WHO as a specialised agency began on that date. The formation of WHO represents the culmination of efforts to establish a single worldwide intergovernmental health agency.

WORLD HEALTH ORGANIZATION

The World Health Organization is a specialized, non-political, health agency of the United Nations, with headquarters at Geneva. In 1946, the Constitution was drafted by the "Technical Preparatory Committee" under the chairmanship of Rene Sand, and was approved in the same year by an International Health Conference of 51 nations in New York. The constitution came into force on 7th April, 1948 which is celebrated every year as "World Health Day". A World Health day theme is chosen each year to focus attention on a specific aspect of public health.

Objective

The objective of the WHO is "the attainment by all people's of the highest level of health" which is set out in the preamble of the Constitution. The current objective of WHO is the attainment by all people of the world a level of health that will permit them to lead a socially and economically productive life. The preamble of the Constitution states :

> "Health is a state of complete physical, mental and social well-being and not merely the absence of disease or infirmity.
>
> The enjoyment of the highest attainable standard of health is one of the fundamental rights of every human being without distinction of race, religion, political belief, economic and social condition.
>
> The health of all people is fundamental to the attainment of peace and security and is dependent upon the fullest cooperation of individuals and States.
>
> The achievement of any State in the promotion and protection of health is of value to all.
>
> Unequal development in different countries in the promotion of health and control of disease, especially communicable disease, is a common danger.
>
> Healthy development of the child is of basic importance; the ability to live harmoniously in a changing total environment is essential to such development.
>
> The extension to all people of the benefits of medical, psychological and related knowledge is essential to the fullest attainment of health.
>
> Informed opinion and active cooperation on the part of the public are of the utmost importance in the improvement of the health of the people.
>
> Governments have a responsibility for the health of their peoples which can be fulfilled only by the provision of adequate health and social measures".

The WHO is unique among the UN Specialized Agencies in that it has its own constitution, own governing bodies, own membership and own budget. It is part of, but not subordinate to, the United Nations.

Two major policy developments have influenced the WHO. First, the Alma-Ata Conference in 1978 on primary health care which provided both WHO and UNICEF with a common charter for health, and secondly, the Global Strategy for Health for All by 2000, and more recently Millennium Development Goals.

Membership

Membership in WHO is open to all countries. While most countries are members of both the UN and of WHO, there are some differences. For example, Switzerland is a member of WHO, but not of the United Nations. Territories which are not responsible for the conduct of their international relations may be admitted as associate members. Associate members participate without vote in the deliberations of the WHO. Each member state contributes yearly to the budget and each is entitled to the services and aid the organization can provide. In 1948, the WHO had 56 Members. WHO now has 194 member states and two associate members.

Work of WHO

WHO's first Constitutional function is to act as the directing and coordinating authority on all international health work. This function permits WHO's Member States to identify collectively priority health problems throughout the world, to define collectively health policies and targets to cope with them, to devise collectively strategies, principles and programmes to give effect to these policies and to attain the targets. The WHO also has specific responsibilities for establishing and promoting international standards in the field of health, which comprise the following broad areas :

1. PREVENTION AND CONTROL OF SPECIFIC DISEASES

Almost all communicable diseases are or have been at sometime the subject of WHO activities. The global eradication of smallpox is an outstanding example of international health cooperation. With the same energy and commitment with which WHO eradicated smallpox, it is now directing the global battle against poliomyelitis.

An important activity of WHO is epidemiological surveillance of communicable diseases. The WHO collects and disseminates epidemiological information on diseases subject to International Health Regulations and occasionally other communicable diseases of international importance through an Automatic Telex Reply Service (ATRS) and the "Weekly Epidemiological Record" (WER). The latter contains more complete details and brief reviews of communicable diseases of international importance *(7)*. Member States can also make use of the "WHO Emergency Scheme for Epidemics" whenever necessary *(8)*. The aim of International Health Regulations is to ensure maximum security against international spread of diseases with the minimum interference with world traffic.

The WHO has also paid attention in its programme of work to non-communicable disease problems such as cancer, cardiovascular diseases, genetic disorders, diabetes, blindness, mental disorders, drug addiction and dental diseases.

The activities of WHO have also branched out into the fields of vector biology and control, immunology, quality control of drugs and biological products, drug evaluation and monitoring and health laboratory technology as these activities are relevant to the control of both communicable and non-communicable diseases. Immunization against common diseases of childhood (Expanded Programme on Immunization) is now a priority programme of the WHO.

2. DEVELOPMENT OF COMPREHENSIVE HEALTH SERVICES

WHO's most important single function is to promote and support national health policy development and the development of comprehensive national health programmes. This broad field of endeavour encompasses a wide variety of activities such as organizing health systems based on primary health care, the development of health manpower and utilization, building of long-term national capability, particularly in the areas of health infrastructure development, and managerial capabilities (including monitoring and evaluation) and health services research. Appropriate Technology for Health (ATH) is another new programme launched by the WHO to encourage self-sufficiency in solving health problems. The new programme is part of WHO's efforts to build up primary health care.

3. FAMILY HEALTH

Family health is one of the major programme activities of WHO since 1970, and is broadly subdivided into maternal and child health care, human reproduction, nutrition and health education. The chief concern is improvement of the quality of life of the family as a unit.

4. ENVIRONMENTAL HEALTH

Promotion of environmental health has always been an important activity of WHO. WHO advises governments on national programmes for the provision of basic sanitary services. The activities are directed to protection of the quality of air, water and food; health conditions of work, radiation protection and early identification of new hazards originating from new technological developments. A number of programmes have been developed such as the 'WHO Environmental Health Criteria Programme' and 'WHO Environmental Health Monitoring Programme' towards improving environmental health.

5. HEALTH STATISTICS

From its earliest days in 1947, WHO has been concerned with the dissemination of a wide variety of morbidity and mortality statistics relating to health problems. The data is published in the (a) Weekly Epidemiological Record (b) World Health Statistics Quarterly and (c) World Health Statistics Annual. Readers interested in current data may obtain it from the Chief Statistician, Dissemination of Statistical Information, WHO, Geneva. In order that statistics from different countries may be comparable, WHO publishes 'International Classification of Diseases' which is updated every 10th year. The Tenth Revision of ICD came into effect from 1st January 1993. Assistance is also given to countries in the improvement of their medical records, and in the planning and operating national health information systems.

6. BIOMEDICAL RESEARCH

The WHO does not itself do research, but stimulates and coordinates research work. It has established a worldwide network of WHO collaborating centres, besides awarding grants to research workers and research institutions for promoting research. There are Regional Advisory Committees on health research which define regional health research priorities and a Global Advisory Committee, which in close collaboration with the regional committee deals with policy issues of global import. Six tropical diseases (malaria, schistosomiasis, trypanosomiasis, filariasis, leishmaniasis and leprosy) are the target of the WHO Special Programme for Research and Training in Tropical Diseases to develop new tools, strengthen research institutions and training workers in the countries affected.

7. HEALTH LITERATURE AND INFORMATION

WHO acts as a clearing house for information on health problems. Its publications comprise hundreds of titles on a wide variety of health subjects. The WHO library is one of the satellite centres of the Medical Literature Analysis and Retrieval System (MEDLARS) of the U.S. National Library of Medicine. MEDLARS is fully computerised indexing system covering the whole of medicine on an international basis. The WHO has also a public information service both at headquarters and each of the six regional offices.

8. COOPERATION WITH OTHER ORGANIZATIONS

WHO collaborates with the UN and with the other specialized agencies, and maintains various degrees of working relationships. Besides, WHO has also established relations with a number of international governmental organizations.

Structure

The WHO consists of three principal organs : the World Health Assembly, the Executive Board and the Secretariat.

(a) THE WORLD HEALTH ASSEMBLY : This is the "Health Parliament" of Nations and the supreme governing body of the organization. It meets annually, usually in May, and generally at the headquarters in Geneva, but from time to time in other countries. The Assembly is composed of delegates representing Member States, each of which has one vote. The main functions of the Health Assembly are : (i) to determine international health policy and programmes (ii) to review the work of the past year (iii) to approve the budget needed for the following year and (iv) to elect Member States to designate a person to serve for three years on the Executive Board, and to replace the retiring members. The Health Assembly also appoints the Director General on the nomination of the Executive Board. It is now the practice to organize on the occasion of each Health Assembly, "technical discussions" on some subjects of world interest.

(b) THE EXECUTIVE BOARD : The Board had originally 18 members, each designated by a Member State. Subsequently, the number was raised to 24 and 30. The Health Assembly (1976) increased the membership from 30 to 31, providing that no fewer than three are to be elected from each of the WHO regions *(11)*. The board now has 34 members. The members of the Board are to be "technically qualified in the field of health"; they are designated by, but do not represent their governments. One-third of the membership is renewed every year. The Executive Board meets at least twice a year, generally in January and shortly after the meeting of the World Health Assembly in May. The main work of the Board is to give effect to the decisions and policies of the Assembly. The Board also has power to take action itself in an emergency, such as epidemics, earthquakes and floods where immediate action is needed.

(c) THE SECRETARIAT : The secretariat is headed by the Director General who is the chief technical and administrative officer of the Organization. The primary function of the WHO secretariat is to provide Member States with technical and managerial support for their national health development programmes. While in 1948, WHO staff counted 250 persons, the Organization in 1985 counted 4475 international public servants. The secretariat, by 2010, is staffed by about 8000 health and other experts and support staff. At WHO headquarters in Geneva, there are 5 Assistant Director Generals each of whom is responsible for the work of such divisions as may from time to time be assigned to him by the Director General. On 31st December, 1985, the WHO Secretariat comprised of the following divisions.

1. Division of epidemiological surveillance and health situation and trend assessment.
2. Division of communicable diseases.
3. Division of vector biology and control.
4. Division of environmental health.
5. Division of public information and education for health.
6. Division of mental health.
7. Division of diagnostic, therapeutic and rehabilitative technology.
8. Division of strengthening of health services.
9. Division of family health.
10. Division of non-communicable diseases.
11. Division of health manpower development.
12. Division of information systems support.
13. Division of personnel and general services.
14. Division of budget and finance.

Regions

In order to meet the special health needs of different areas, WHO has established six regional organizations. (Table 1).

TABLE 1

WHO Regional Organizations

Region	Headquarters
1. South East Asia	New Delhi (India)
2. Africa	Brazzaville (Congo)
3. The Americas	Washington D.C. (U.S.A.)
4. Europe	Copenhagen (Denmark)
5. Eastern Mediterranean	Alexandria (Egypt)
6. Western Pacific	Manila (Philippines)

The regional organizations are an integral part of the WHO and have under the constitution an important part in implementing the policies and programmes of the WHO. The regional office is headed by the Regional Director, who is assisted by technical and administrative officers, and members of the secretariat. There is a regional committee composed of representatives of the Member States in the region. Regional Committees meet once a year to review health work in the region and plan its continuation and development. Regional plans are amalgamated into overall plans for the Organization by the Director General at WHO's headquarters in Geneva.

The South East Asia Region

The headquarters of the South East Asia Regional Office (SEARO) is in New Delhi, the official address being World Health House, Indraprastha Estate, New Delhi. The Region has now 11 members (Table 2).

TABLE 2

WHO: SEARO Member countries

Year of joining	Member country SEARO	Population (mid 2018) (million)
1972	Bangladesh	166.4
1982	Bhutan	0.8
1948	India	1371.3
1950	Indonesia	265.2
1973	Korea (Dem.People's Rep.)	25.6
1965	Maldives Islands	0.4
1948	Myanmar	53.9
1953	Nepal	29.7
1948	Sri Lanka	21.7
1947	Thailand	66.2
2002	Timor-Leste	1.2

The WHO activities in South East Asia Region cover a wide range of subjects such as malaria eradication, tuberculosis control, control of other communicable diseases, health laboratory services and production of vaccines, health statistics, public health administration and rural health services, maternal and child health, nursing, environmental health and water supply, health education, nutrition, mental health, dental health, medical rehabilitation, quality control of drugs and medical education.

OTHER UNITED NATIONS AGENCIES

UNICEF

UNICEF (United Nations International Children's Emergency Fund) is one of the specialized agencies of the United Nations. It was established in 1946 by the United Nations General Assembly to deal with rehabilitation of children in war ravaged countries. In 1953, when the emergency functions were over, the General Assembly gave it a new name "U.N. Children's Fund" but retained the initials, UNICEF. UNICEF's regional office is in Kathmandu, Nepal; the region is known as the South Central Asian Region which covers Afghanistan, Sri Lanka, India, the Maldives, Pakistan, Bhutan, Bangladesh and Nepal. UNICEF is governed by a thirty six nation Executive Board as in 2010. The headquarters of the UNICEF is at United Nations, New York.

UNICEF works in close collaboration with WHO, and the other specialized agencies of the United Nations like UNDP, FAO and UNESCO. In the early years, UNICEF and WHO worked together on urgent problems such as malaria, tuberculosis and venereal diseases. Later, its assistance to countries covered such fields as maternal and child health, nutrition, environmental sanitation (especially the provision of water supplies to rural communities), health centres and health education and programmes which would directly or indirectly, benefit child health.

More recently, the tendency has been for UNICEF to turn away from campaigns for the eradication of specific diseases unless they are of direct benefit to mothers and children. Greater attention is being given to the concept of the "whole child" meaning that assistance should hence forward be geared not only to health and nutrition, as before, which are of immediate benefit to children, but also to their long-term personnel development and to the development of the countries in which they live. This approach is also known as 'country health programming' in which UNICEF is currently interested so as to meet the needs of children as an integral part of the country's development effort.

Content of services *(12)*

(a) Child health : UNICEF has provided substantial aid for the production of vaccines and sera in many countries. UNICEF has supported India's BCG vaccination programme from its inception. It has also assisted in the erection of a penicillin plant, near Pune; donated a DDT plant; two plants for the manufacture of triple vaccine and iodized salt. UNICEF has also assisted environmental sanitation programmes emphasizing safe and sufficient water for drinking and household use in rural areas. The purpose is not only to reduce child illness and death, but to improve the quality of life in the villages. Currently, UNICEF is focusing attention on providing primary health care to mothers and children. Emphasis is placed on immunization; infant and young child care; family planning aspects of family health; safe water and adequate sanitation. The services contemplated are intended to be so organized that the local community can participate in planning personnel and material support. The services will be delivered economically at the village level through resident volunteers or part time primary health workers selected for the purpose with the agreement of the local community.

(b) Child nutrition : UNICEF gives high priority to improving child nutrition. Its aid for child nutrition, which first took the form of supplementing child feeding began to expand in mid–1950s with the development of low-cost protein-rich food mixtures. In collaboration with FAO, UNICEF also began aiding "applied nutrition" programmes through such channels as community development, agricultural extension, schools and health services so as to stimulate and help the rural population to grow and eat the foods it required for better child nutrition. The UNICEF has supplied equipment for modern dairy plants in various parts of India, viz. Maharashtra, Gujarat, Karnataka, Uttar Pradesh, West Bengal, Andhra Pradesh. Specific aid is also given for intervention against nutritional deficiency diseases, viz. provision of large doses of vitamin A in areas where xerophthalmia is prevalent; enrichment of salt with iodine in areas of endemic goitre; provision of iron and folate supplements to combat anaemias and enrichment of foods. More recently, FAO, UNICEF and WHO have been encouraging the development of national food and nutrition policies that make provision for child nutrition.

(c) Family and child welfare : The purpose is to improve the care of children, both within and outside their homes through such means as parent education, day-care centres, child welfare and youth agencies and women's clubs. These services are carried out not as separate projects but as part of health, nutrition and education or home economics extension programmes.

(d) Education – formal and non-formal : In collaboration with UNESCO, UNICEF is assisting India in the expansion and improvement of teaching science in India. Science laboratories' equipment, workshop tools, library books, audiovisual aids are being made available to educational institutions. Emphasis is placed on the kind of schooling relevant to the environment and future life of the children.

The UNICEF is promoting a campaign known as GOBI campaign to encourage 4 strategies for a "child health revolution" :

- G for growth charts to better monitor child development;
- O for oral rehydration to treat all mild and moderate dehydration;

- B for breast feeding; and
- I for immunization against measles, diphtheria, polio, pertussis, tetanus and tuberculosis.

Since 1976, UNICEF has been participating in Urban Basic Services (UBS). The aim of the UBS projects is to upgrade basic services (e.g., health, nutrition, water supply, sanitation and education) – especially for children and women – in selected cities and towns. The overall objective is to improve the degree and quality of survival and development of the children of urban low-income families.

In short, UNICEF activities cover programmes assisting in child survival, protection and development; interventions like immunization, improved infant feeding practices; child growth monitoring, homebased diarrhoea management, drinking water, environmental sanitation, birth spacing, education of girls and income-generating activities for women.

As full partners in primary health care, UNICEF and WHO have been developing joint strategies in support of its implementation at country level.

UNDP

The United Nations Development Programme (UNDP) was established in 1966. It is the main source of funds for technical assistance. The member countries – rich and poor – of the United Nations meet annually and pledge contributions to the UNDP.

The basic objective of the UNDP is to help poorer nations develop their human and natural resources more fully. The UNDP projects cover virtually every economic and social sector – agriculture, industry, education and science, health, social welfare, etc.

UN Fund for Population Activities

The United Nations Fund for Population Activities (UNFPA) has been providing assistance to India since 1974. In addition to funding national level schemes, Area Projects for intensive development of health and family welfare infrastructure and improvement in the availability of services in the rural areas have been under implementation in eleven districts of Bihar and 4 districts of Rajasthan.

The UNFPA inputs are designed to develop national capability for the manufacture of contraceptives, to develop population education programmes, to undertake organized sector projects, to strengthen programme management as well as to improve output of grass-root level health workers and introduction of innovative approaches to family planning and MCH care *(16)*.

FAO

The Food and Agriculture Organization (FAO) was formed in 1945 with headquarters in Rome. It was the first United Nations Organization specialized agency created to look after several areas of world cooperation. The chief aims of FAO are : (1) to help nations raise living standards (2) to improve nutrition of the people of all countries (3) to increase the efficiency of farming, forestry and fisheries (4) to better the condition of rural people and, through all these means, to widen the opportunity of all people for productive work. FAO's prime concern is the increased production of food to keep pace with the ever-growing world population. The most important aspect of FAO's work is towards ensuring that the food is consumed by the people who need it, in sufficient quantities and in right proportions, to develop and maintain a better state of nutrition throughout the world *(13)*. In this context, the FAO has organized a world Freedom from Hunger Campaign (FFHC) in 1960. The main object of the Campaign is to combat malnutrition and to disseminate information and education. The FAO is also collaborating with other international agencies in the Applied Nutrition Programmes. The joint WHO/FAO expert committees have provided the basis for many cooperative activities – nutritional surveys, training courses, seminars and the coordination of research programmes on brucellosis and other zoonoses *(4)*.

ILO

Soon after the First World War, it was recognized that problems of industry, like disease, know no frontiers. In 1919, the International Labour Organization (I.L.O.) was established as an affiliate of the League of Nations to improve the working and living conditions of the working population all over the world. The purposes of ILO are : (1) to contribute to the establishment of lasting peace by promoting social justice (2) to improve, through international action, labour conditions, and living standards and (3) to promote economic and social stability. The International Labour Code is a collection of international minimum standards related to health, welfare, living and working conditions of workers all over the world. The ILO also provides assistance to organizations interested in the betterment of living and employment standards. There is a close collaboration between ILO and WHO in the field of health and labour. The headquarters of ILO is in Geneva, Switzerland.

WORLD BANK

World Bank is a specialized agency of the United Nations. It was established with the purpose of helping less developed countries raise their living standards. The powers of the Bank are vested in a Board of Governors. The Bank gives loans for projects that will lead to economic growth (e.g., India's Population Projects). The projects are usually concerned with electric power, roads, railways, agriculture, water supply, education, family planning, etc. Health and environmental components have been added to many projects. Cooperative programmes exist between WHO and the Bank, e.g., projects for water supply, World Food Programme, Population Control, and the control of onchocerciasis programme in West Africa *(14)*.

HEALTH WORK OF BILATERAL AGENCIES

USAID

The US Government presently extends aid to India through three agencies : (1) United States Agency for International Development (USAID); (2) The Public Law 480 (Food for Peace) Programme; and (3) The US Export–Import Bank. The USAID was created in 1961; it is in charge of activities previously administered by the Technical Cooperation Mission (TCM). A USAID mission functions in New Delhi. Both grants and loans are extended by the Agency.

The US has been assisting in a number of projects designed to improve the health of India's people. These are : (1) malaria eradication; (2) medical education; (3) nursing education; (4) health education; (5) water supply and sanitation; (6) control of communicable diseases; (7) nutrition; and (8) family planning *(15)*. The recent trend in assistance from the USA is increasingly in the support of agricultural and family planning programmes, with some reduction in aid in the general public health field *(5)*.

THE COLOMBO PLAN

At a meeting of the commonwealth Foreign Ministers at Colombo in January 1950, a programme was drawn up for cooperative economic development in South and South East Asia. Membership comprises 20 developing countries within the region and 6 non-regional members – Australia, Canada, Japan, New Zealand, UK and USA. The bulk of Colombo Plan assistance goes into industrial and agricultural development, but some support has also been given to health promotion, mostly through fellowships. The All India Institute of Medical Sciences at New Delhi was established with financial assistance from New Zealand. The Plan provides for visits to countries by experts who can offer advice on local problems and train the local people. The contribution of Canada in supplying Cobalt Therapy Units to medical institutions in India was an important item of aid under the Colombo plan *(5)*. Colombo plan seeks to improve living standards of the people of the area by reviewing developmental plans and coordinating development assistance.

SIDA

The Swedish International Development Agency is assisting the National Tuberculosis Control Programme since 1979. The SIDA assistance is usually spent on procurement of supplies like X-ray unit, microscopes and anti-tuberculosis drugs.

DANIDA

The Government of Denmark is providing assistance for the development of services under National Blindness Control Programme since 1978.

NON-GOVERNMENTAL AND OTHER AGENCIES

Rockefeller Foundation

The Rockefeller Foundation is a philanthropic organization chartered in 1913 and endowed by Mr. John D. Rockefeller. Its purpose is to promote the well-being of mankind throughout the world. In its early years, the Foundation was active chiefly in public health and medical education. Subsequently, its interest was expanded to include the advancement of life sciences, the social sciences, the humanities and the agricultural sciences *(13)*.

The work of the Rockefeller Foundation in India began in 1920 with a scheme for the control of hookworm disease in the then Madras Presidency. Since then, the Foundation has been associated with several medical and public health programmes in India. The establishment of the All India Institute of Hygiene and Public Health at Kolkata was in a large measure due to the cooperation of the Rockefeller Foundation. The Foundation's programme included the training of competent teachers and research workers; training abroad of candidates from India through fellowships and travel grants; the sponsoring of visits of a large number of medical specialists from the USA; providing grants-in-aid to selected institutions: development of medical college libraries; population studies; assistance to research projects and institutions (e.g., National Institute of Virology at Pune and more recently the setting up of a field demonstration area (Ballabhgarh) in connection with a department of preventive and social medicine, as well as to the All India Institute of Medical Sciences. At present the Foundation is directing its support to the improvement of agriculture, family planning and rural training centres as well as to medical education *(5)*.

Ford Foundation

Whereas the Rockefeller Foundation earlier concentrated most of its assistance on universities and post-graduate institutions, on professional education and on research, the Ford Foundation has been active in the development of rural health services and family planning *(5)*. The Ford Foundation has helped India in the following projects : (1) Orientation training centres : The orientation training centres at Singur, Poonamalle and Najafgarh were set up with help from the Ford Foundation. The centres provide training courses in public health for medical and paramedical personnel from all over India. (2) Research–cum–action projects : These projects were aimed at solving some of the basic problems in environmental sanitation, e.g., designing and construction of hand-flushed acceptable sanitary latrines in rural areas (3) Pilot project in rural health services, Gandhigram (Tamil Nadu) : Among a rural population of 100,000 people, an attempt was made to develop and operate a coordinated type of health service which will provide a useful model for health administrators in the country. (4) Establishment of NIHAE: In the last few years, the Ford Foundation has supported the establishment of the National Institute of Health Administration and Education at Delhi. The Institute provides a senior staff-college type training for health administrators. (5) Calcutta water supply and drainage scheme : The Foundation has helped in the preparation of a master plan for water supply, sewerage and drainage for the city of Calcutta in collaboration with other international agencies. (6) Family planning programme : The Foundation is supporting research in reproductive biology and in the family planning fellowship programmes.

CARE

CARE (Cooperative for Assistance and Relief Everywhere) was founded in North America in the wake of the Second World War in the year 1945. It is one of the world's largest independent, non-profit, non-sectarian international relief and development organization. CARE provides emergency aid and long term development assistance.

CARE began its operation in India in 1950. Till the end of 1980s, the primary objective of CARE – India was to provide food for children in the age group of 6–11 years. From mid 1980s, CARE–India focused its food support in the ICDS programme and in development of programmes in the areas of health and income supplementation. It is helping in the following projects : Integrated Nutrition and Health Project; Better Health and Nutrition Project; Anaemia Control Project; Improving Women's Health Project; Improved Health Care for Adolescent Girl's Project; Child Survival Project; Improving Women's Reproductive Health and Family Spacing Project; Konkan Integrated Development Project etc.

CARE–India works in partnership with the Government of India, State Governments, NGOs etc. Currently it has projects in Andhra Pradesh, Bihar, Madhya Pradesh, Maharashtra, Orissa, Rajasthan, Uttar Pradesh and West Bengal.

International Red Cross

The Red Cross is a non-political non-official international humanitarian organization devoted to the service of mankind in peace and war. It was founded by Henry Dunant, a young Swiss businessman, who when travelling through North Italy in 1859 happened to be on the scene of one of the most savage battles of history, the battle of Solferino. Appalled by the neglect of thousands of the wounded and dying soldiers, Dunant recruited volunteers from nearby villages to help relieve their suffering. Later, in his book "Un Souvenir de Solferine" and in countless interviews with eminent persons, throughout Europe, Dunant urged that voluntary national societies be founded "which in time of war would render aid to the wounded without distinction of nationality". He proposed further that these societies should have a protective emblem and trained workers and their services to the wounded should be protected by international treaty.

Dunant's plea met with success. The First Geneva Convention took place in 1864 and a treaty was signed for the relief of the wounded and the sick of the armies in the field. Thus came into being the International Committee of the Red Cross (ICRC), an independent, neutral institution, the founder organization of the Red Cross. It has since grown into a mighty mission with branches all over the world symbolising the spirit of compassion and universal brotherhood. In 1919, the League of the Red Cross Society was created with headquarters in Geneva to coordinate the work of the national societies, which now number more than 90.

Role of Red Cross

In the beginning, the role of the Red Cross, as conceived by Dunant, was largely confined to humanitarian service on behalf of the victims of war. Soon thereafter, it was realised that natural disasters too bring in their wake great human suffering and that on such occasions there is equally great need for help among nations "as good neighbours". Later on the work of the Red Cross was extended to other programmes which would prevent human suffering. These comprise service to armed forces, service to war veterans, disaster service, first aid and nursing, health education and maternity and child welfare services.

Indian Red Cross

The Red Cross Society of India was established by an Act of the Indian Legislature in 1920 with the three objectives of the improvement of health, prevention of disease and mitigation of suffering. In peacetime, the Society provides military hospitals with such amenities as newspapers, periodicals, musical instruments and other comfort goods. The Red Cross Home at Bangalore for disabled ex-servicemen is one of the pioneer institutions of its kind in Asia. Disaster services comprise distribution of milk, medicines, Vitamin tablets, codliver oil and hundred other items to the famine stricken people and to those who have been hit by the floods. In the development of maternity and child welfare services, the Society has done pioneering work and has functioned as an auxiliary of the country's health services.

The JUNIOR RED CROSS is one of the most active sections of the Society. It gives an opportunity to lakhs of boys and girls all over India to be associated with activities like the village uplift, first aid, antiepidemic work and building up of an international fraternity of youth, thus promoting international friendliness, understanding and cooperation.

There are numerous other non-governmental organizations (NGO's). Some of these are: Oxfam, Save-the-Children Fund, International Planned Parenthood Federation, The Population Council, Voluntary Health Association of India, All India Women's Conference, India Medical Association, Trained Nurses Association of India, International Agency for the Prevention of Blindness, World Federation of the Deaf, International Leprosy Association, World Federation of Medical Education, International Union against Cancer, and so on. Non-governmental organizations constitute a valuable resource in promoting health care.

References

1. WHO (1976). *Introducing WHO.*
2. WHO (1963). *World Health,* March, 1963.
3. WHO (1977). *WHO Chronicle,* 31, 479.
4. WHO (1969). *WHO Chronicle,* 23, 16.
5. WHO (1967). *Twenty Years in South East Asia,* 1948–1967, Regional Office for South East Asia, New Delhi.
6. UNICEF–WHO (1987). *Joint Committee on Health Policy,* 1987.
7. WHO (1979). *WHO Chronicle,* 33 : 233.
8. WHO (1979). *WHO Chronicle,* 33 : 263.
9. WHO (1986). *The Work of WHO 1984–85,* Biennial Report of the D. G.
10. WHO (1977). *WHO Chronicle,* 31 : 492.
11. WHO (1976). *WHO Chronicle,* 30 : 304.
12. UNICEF (1975). *UNICEF – A GUIDE.* Current Policies and Working Methods, E/ICEF/Misc.258.
13. Central Health Education Bureau (1965). *Swasth Hind,* 9, 196
14. WHO (1977). *WHO Chronicle,* 31 : 94.
15. US Information Services (1971). *Fact Sheet–US Economic Assistance to India. 1951–71. New Delhi.*
16. Govt. of India (1987). *Annual Report 1986–87,* Ministry of Health and Family Welfare, New Delhi.

ABBREVIATIONS

ABER	Annual blood examination rate
ACD	Active case detection
ACT	Artemisinin-based combined therapy
ADB	Asian Development Bank
ADLA	Acute dermatolymphangioadenitis
AEFI	Adverse events following immunization
AES	Acute encephalitis syndrome
AFB	Acid fast bacillus
AFP	Acute flaccid paralysis
AIDS	Acquired immuno deficiency syndrome
AIIMS	All India Institute of Medical Sciences
ALRI	Acute lower respiratory tract infections
ANC	Antenatal care
ANCDR	Annual new case detection rate
ANM	Auxiliary Nurse Midwife
API	Annual parasite incidence
AR	Attributable risk
ARC	AIDS-related complex
ARI	Acute respiratory infections
ART	Anti-retroviral therapy
ASFR	Age-specific fertility rate
ASHA	Accredited social health activist
ASMFR	Age-specific marital fertility rate
AURI	Acute upper respiratory tract infection
AUWSP	Accelerated Urban Water Supply Programme
AWC	Anganwadi centre
AWW	Anganwadi worker
AYUSH	Ayurvedic, Yoga, Unani, Siddha & Homeopathy, system of medicine
BCC	Behaviour change communication
β-cells	Bone-marrow derived lymphocytes
BCG	Bacillus calmette-guarin
BDO	Block development officer
BEO	Block extension officer
BEE	Block extension educator
BFHI	Baby friendly hospital initiatives
BLAC	Block level awareness campaign
BMI	Body mass index
BPL	Below poverty line
CABG	Coronary artery bypass grafting
CARE	Cooperative assistance and relief everywhere
CBR	Crude birth rate
CDPO	Child development project officer
CDSCO	Central Drug Standard Control Organization
CGHS	Central Government Health Scheme
CHC	Community health centre
CHW	Community health worker
CMO	Chief Medical Officer
CNS	Central nervous system
COPD	Chronic obstructive pulmonary disease
CPCB	Central Pollution Control Board
CPM	Critical path method
CPR	Couple protection rate
CRY	Child Relief and You
CSF	Cerebrospinal fluid
CSSM	Child survival and safe motherhood
CVD	Cardiovascular diseases
DALY	Disability adjusted life year
DANIDA	Danish International Development Agency
DBCS	District blindness control society
DDC	Drug distribution centre in malaria control
DEC	Diethylcarbamazine
DES	Diethylstilbestrol
DFWO	District family welfare officer
DGHS	Director General of Health Services
DHF	Dengue haemorrhagic fever
DHO/DMO	District health/medical officer
DHS	Directorate of health services
DM	Diabetes mellitus
DMC	Designated microscopy centre
DOTS	Directly observed therapy, short-course
DPT	Diphtheria, pertussis, and tetanus vaccine
DSS	Dengue shock syndrome
DT	Diphtheria-Tetanus toxoid
dta	Diphtheria-tetanus adult type
DTC	District tuberculosis centre
DTP	District tuberculosis programme
dTpa	Diphtheria, tetanus, acellular pertussis
DTPw	Diphtheria, tetanus, whole-cell-pertussis
% E	Percentage of total energy
EAA	Essential amino acids
EAG	Empowered action group
EFA	Essential fatty acids
ELF	Elimination of lymphatic filariasis
EPI	Expanded programme on immunization
EQA	External quality assessment
ESI	Employees state insurance scheme
ETEC	Enterotoxin Escherichia coli
FAO	Food and Agriculture Organization
F-IMNCI	Facility based IMNCI
FLEP	Focused leprosy elimination plan
FRUs	First referral units
FSW	Female sex worker
FTD	Fever treatment depot
GDP	Gross domestic product
GFR	General fertility rate
GMFR	General marital fertility rate
GNI	Gross national income
GNP	Gross net product
HAV	Hepatitis A virus
HBIG	Hepatitis B immunoglobulin
HBNC	Home based newborn care

HBV	Hepatitis B virus
HCV	Hepatitis C virus
HDL	High density lipoproteins
HDV	Hepatitis D virus
HEV	Hepatitis E virus
HFA	Health for all
Hib Vaccine	Haemophilus influenzae type B vaccine
HIV	Human immunodeficiency virus
HPS	High performing states
HPV	Human papilloma virus
HRD	Human resource development
HW (F)	Health worker female
HW (M)	Health worker male
ICDS	Integrated child development service
ICMR	Indian Council of Medical Research
ICTC	Integrated counselling and testing centre
IDD	Iodine deficiency disorder
IDDM	Insulin dependent diabetes mellitus
IDSP	Integrated disease surveillance project
IVDU	Intravenous drug users
IEC	Information, education & communication
IEC	Information Education Commission
IFA	Iron & folic acid
IFC	International Classification of Functioning, Disability and Health
IHD	Ischaemic heart disease
IHR	International Health Regulations
ILO	International labour organization
IMCI	Integrated management of childhood illness
IMR	Infant mortality rate
INH	Isoniazid
IMNCI	Integrated management of neonatal & childhood illness
IOL	Intraocular lens
IPHS	Indian public health standards
IPPI	Intensified pulse polio immunization
IPV	Inactivated polio vaccine
IRC	International red cross
IRLs	Intermediate Reference Laboratories
IRS	Indoor residual spray
ISM	Indian system of medicine
ITN	Insecticide treated bed nets
IUCD	Intrauterine contraceptive device
IUD	Intrauterine device
JE	Japanese encephalitis
JSSK	Janani shishu suraksha karyakram
JSY	Janani suraksha yojana
KFD	Kyasanur forest disease
LBW	Low birth weight
LDL	Low density lipoproteins
LECs	Leprosy elimination campaigns
LEM	Leprosy elimination monitoring
LHV	Lady health visitor
LLIN	Long lasting insecticide nets
LPS	Low performing states
LSD	Lysergic acid diethylamide
MAP	Malaria Action Plan
MB	Multibacillary
MCH	Maternal & child health
MDA	Mass drug administration
MDGs	Millennium Development Goals
MDMP	Mid-day meal programme
MDR-TB	Multi-drug resistant tuberculosis
MDT	Multi-drugs therapy
MDT	Multi-drugs therapy of tuberculosis
Mf	Microfilaria
MLEC	Modified leprosy elimination campaign
MMR	Maternal mortality ratio
MNP	Minimum needs programme
MO	Medical Officer
MOPHC	Medical Officer at primary health centre
MOU	Memorandum of understanding
MPO	Modified Plan of Operation
MPW	Multipurpose worker
MRFIT	Multiple risk factor intervention trial
MSM	Men having sex with men
MTCT	Mother to child transmission
MTP	Medical termination of pregnancy
MUFA	Monounsaturated fatty acids
MVA	Manual vaccum aspiration
NACO	National AIDS control organization
NAMP	National antimalaria programme
NBCC	Newborn care corner
NBSU	Newborn stabilization unit
NCCP	National cancer control programme
NCD	Non-communicable disease
NCDC	National centre for disease control
NCDs	Non-communicable diseases
NFCP	National Filaria Control Programme
NFHS	National family health survey
NGO	Non-government organization
NHP	National health policy
NID	National immunization day
NIMH	National Institute for Mentally Handicapped
NIMR	National Institute of Malaria Research
NLCP	National leprosy control programme
NLEP	National leprosy eradication programme
NMCP	National malaria control programme
NMEP	National malaria eradication programme
NMHP	National mental health programme
NNMR	Neonatal mortaliy rate
NNR	Net reproduction rate
NORAD	Norwegian agency for development cooperation
NPAC	National plan of action for children
NPSU	National polio surveillance unit
NPU	Net protein utilization

NRCS	Nutritional rehabilitation centres
NRHM	National rural health mission
NSI	The nutrition society of India
NTCP	National tuberculosis control programme
NTP	National tuberculosis programme
NVBDCP	National vector borne disease control programme
OPV	Oral polio vaccine
ORS	Oral rehydration salts
ORT	Oral rehydration therapy
PB	Paucibacillary
PCD	Passive case detection
PCV-7	Pneumococcal conjugate vaccine
PEM	Protein energy malnutrition
PERT	Programme evaluation and review technique
PFA	Prevention of food adulteration act
PHA	Polynuclear aromatic hydrocarbons
PHC	Primary health care/centre
PHFI	Public health foundation of India
PHI	Peripheral health institutions
PLHA	People living with HIV/AIDS
PMDT	Programmatic management of drug resistant-TB
PNDT	Prenatal diagnostic technique act
POCSO	Protection of children from sexual offence
PPBS	Planning-programming-budgeting system
PPD	Purified protein derivative
PPP	Purchasing power parity
PPTCT	Prevention of parent to child transmission
PPV23	Pneumococcal polysaccharide-non-conjugate vaccine containing 23 serotypes
PRAI	Planning, Research and Action Institute, Lucknow
PTB	Pulmonary tuberculosis
PTCA	Percutaneous transluminal coronary angiography
PTCT	Parent-to-child transmission
PUFA	Polyunsaturated fatty acids
PWB	Patient-wise boxes
RBM	Roll back malaria
RCA	Research-cum-Action projects
RCH	Reproductive and child health
RCT	Randomized controlled trials
RDT	Rapid diagnostic test
RF	Rheumatic fever
RHME	Representative, re-sampled, routine household interveiw of mortality with medical evaluation
RLF	Retrolental fibroplasia
RMP	Rifampicin
RNTCP	Revised national tuberculosis control programme
RR	Relative risk
RTI	Reproductive Tract Infection
SAARC	South asian association for regional cooperation
SACS	State AIDS control society
SAPEL	Special action project for elimination of leprosy
SAR	Secondary attack rate
SARS	Severe acute respiratory syndrome
SC	Sub-centre
SDGs	Sustainable Development Goals
SEAR	South-East Asia Region
SEARO	South-East Asian Regional Office
SFD	Small for date baby
SIA	Supplemental immunization activities
SIDA	Swedish international development agency
SMR	Standard mortality ratio
SNCU	Special newborn care unit
SNID	Sub-national immunization day
SRS	Sample registration system
STDs	Sexually transmitted diseases
STI	Sexually transmitted infections
TB	Tuberculosis
TBA	Trained birth attendant
TFR	Total fertility rate
TG	Triglycerides
T-lymphocytes	Thymus-derived lymphocytes
TMFR	Total marital fertility rate
Torch agents	Toxoplasma gondii, rubella virus, cytomegalo virus and herpes virus
TT	Tetanus toxoid
TU	Tuberculosis Unit
UCI	Universal child immunization
UHC	Urban health center
UIP	Universal immunization program
UN	United Nations
UNDP	United Nations Development Programme
UNESCO	United Nations Educational, Scientific and Cultural Organization
UNFPA	United Nations Fund for population activities
UNICEF	United Nations International Children's Emergency Fund
USAID	The United States Agency for International Development
UT	Union territory
VBDs	Vector borne diseases
VCTC	Voluntary Counselling and Testing Centre
VDPV	Vaccine derived poliovirus
VHAI	Voluntary health association of India
VLDL	Very low density lipoproteins
VPD	Vaccine preventable disease
VVM	Vaccine vial monitor
WB	World Bank
WHO	World Health Organization
WIC	Walk-in-cooler
WPV1	Wild poliovirus type 1
WPV2	Wild poliovirus type 2
WPV3	Wild poliovirus type 3
WTO	World Trade Organization
XDR-TB	Extensively drug resistant tuberculosis
ZDV	Zudovudine

INDEX

E